FOOD ALLERGY AND INTOLERANCE

2nd Edition

Edited by

Jonathan Brostoff

MA, DM, DSc(Med), FRCP, FRCPath
Professor Emeritus of Allergy and Environmental Health
King's College London,
London, UK

Stephen J Challacombe

PhD, BDS, FRCPath, FDSRCSE, FMedSci
Head, Division of Oral Medicine and
Pathology, Microbiology and Immunology
Guy's Hospital, London, UK

SAUNDERS

London Edinburgh New York Philadelphia St Louis Sydney Toronto 2002

To DB and CBC

SAUNDERS
An imprint of Elsevier Science

First edition published 1987
Reprinted 1989
Second edition published 2002

ISBN 0702020389

British Library Cataloguing in Publication Data
A catalogue record for this book is available from the British Library

Library of Congress Cataloging in Publication Data
A catalog record for this book is available from the Library of Congress

Note
Medical knowledge is constantly changing. As new information becomes
available, changes in treatment, procedures, equipment and the use of drugs
become necessary. The editors, contributors and the publishers have taken
care to ensure that the information given in this text is accurate and up to
date. However, readers are strongly advised to confirm that the information, especially with regard to drug usage, complies with the latest legislation and standards of practice.

Commissioning Editor: Cathy Carroll
Project Development Manager: Tim Kimber
Project Manager: Shuet-Kei Cheung
Design Manager: Jayne Jones

The
publisher's
policy is to use
**paper manufactured
from sustainable forests**

Printed in Spain

Contents

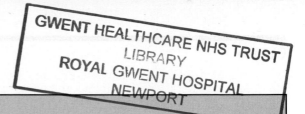

Contents

List of Contributors

HM Anthony MB, ChB
Specialist in Allergy and Environmental Medicine, Leeds, UK

Jon Ayres BSc, MD, FRCP
Professor of Respiratory Medicine, Birmingham Heartlands Hospital, Birmingham, UK

Michael Bailey BVSc, PhD
Lecturer in Immunology, University of Bristol, Bristol, UK

Christine Baker SRD
Birmingham Heartlands Hospital, Birmingham, UK

Dean Befus PhD
Professor of Medicine and Astra Chair in Asthma Research, University of Alberta, Canada

Iris Bell MD, PhD
Associate Professor of Psychiatry, Psychology and Family and Community Medicine, The University of Arizone College of Medicine, Tucson, USA

John Bienenstock PhD, MD
Professor, Medicine and Pathology, McMaster University, Hamilton, Canada

Ian Bier ND, PhD
Medical Director, Dietary Research Foundation, Durham, USA

Graham Bird MD, FRCP, FRCPath
Consultant Clinical Immunologist, Churchill Hospital, Oxford, UK

Stephan Bischoff MD
Specialist in Gastroenterology and Allergy, Medical School of Hannover, Hannover, Germany

Ingvar Bjarnason MSc, MD, DSc, FRCP, FRCPath
Professor of Digestive Diseases, Guy's, King's and St Thomas', Medical School, London, UK

Bengt Björkstén MD, PhD
Executive Director and Professor of Allergy Prevention, Centre for Allergy Research, Karolinska Institutet, Stockholm, Sweden

Paul Bland BSc, BAgr PhD
Senior Lecturer in Immunology, University of Bristol, Bristol UK

Dale Bockman PhD
Professor and Chairman, Medical College of Georgia, Augusta, USA

Per Brandtzaeg DDS, MS, PhD, Professor, Institute of Pathology, University of Oslo Rikshospitalet, Norway

Jonathan Brostoff MA, DM, DSc(Med), FRCP, FRCPath
Professor Emeritus of Allergy and Environmental Health, King's College, London, UK

Stephen Challacombe PhD, BDS, FDSRCSE, FRCPath, FMedSci
Professor of Oral Medicine and Pathology, Guy's Hospital, London, UK

Paul Ciclitira MD, PhD, FRCP
Professor of Gastroenterology, St Thomas' Hospital, London, England

Anthony Corfield BSc, PhD, CChem, FRSC
Senior Research Fellow, Mucin Research Group, Division of Medicine, Bristol Royal Infirmary, Bristol, UK

Timothy Cox MD, FRCP, FMedSci
Professor of Medicine, University of Cambridge, and, Honorary Consultant Physician, Addenbrooke's Hospital, Cambridge, UK

John Cummings MBChB, MRCP, MSc, MD, FRCP(Lon), FRCP(Edin)
Honorary Consultant and Clinical Professor of Gastroenterology Ninewells Hospital and University of Dundee Medical School, Dundee, UK

Charlotte Cunningham-Rundles MD, PhD
Professor of Medicine, Pediatrics and Immunobiology, Mount Sinai Medical Center, New York, USA

Cecil Czerkinsky DMD, PhD, Dr Sci
Director INSERM Laboratory of Mucosal Immunity and Vaccinology, Faculté de Médecine-Pasteur, Nice, France

Gail Darlington MD, FRCP
Consultant in General Internal Medicine and Rheumatology, Epsom General Hospital, Epsom, UK

Keith Dear MD, MRCP
Consultant Gastroenterologist, Chesterfield & North Derbyshire NHS Trust, Chesterfield, UK

Keith Eaton LRCPS(Ed), LRFPS(Glas)
Consultant Physician, Biolab Medical Unit, London, UK

Alan Ebringer BSc, MD, FRCP, FRACP, FRCPath
Professor of Immunology, King's College London, London, UK

Joseph Egger MD
Neurology Department, Royal Aberdeen Children's Hospital, Aberdeen, UK

H J Ellis BSc, PhD
Senior Research Fellow, Gastroenterology Unit, St Thomas' Hospital, London, England

Said Elsayed PhD
Professor of Clinical Biochemistry, University Hospital Bergen, Bergen, Norway

William Fickling MB BChir, MRCP
Research Registrar, Royal United Hosiptal, Bath, UK

RPK Ford MD, FRACP
Community Paediatrician, Primary Health Division, Christchurch, New Zealand

AW Frankland MA, DM, FRCP
Consulting Allergist, London Allergy Clinic, London, UK

David Freed MB, ChB, MD, CBiol, MIBiol
Consulting Allergist, Salford Allergy Clinic, Salford, UK

Lionel Fry BSc, MD, FRCP
Professor of Dermatology, Imperial College of Science, Technology and Medicine, London, UK

Michael Gardner BSc, PhD, DSc, FIBiol
Professor of Physiological Biochemistry, University of Bradford, Bradford, UK

John Gerrard DM (Oxon), FRCP
Professor Emeritus of Paediatrics, Saskatoon, Canada

Armond Goldman MD
Professor Emeritus, Department of Pediatrics, University of Texas Medical Branch, Galveston, USA

Ellen Goudsmit PhD
Chartered Health Psychologist and Medical Archivist, Teddington, UK

Malcolm Greaves MD, PhD, FRCP
Professor of Dermatology, St Thomas's Hospital, London, UK

Anthony Ham Pong MBBS
Consultant in Allergy and Clinical Immunology, Smyth Medical Centre, Ottawa, Canada

Susan Hefle PhD
Assistant Professor, Food Allergy Research and Resource Program, Department of Food Science and Technology, University of Nebraska, Lincoln, USA

David J Hendrick MD, FRCP
Professor of Occupational Respiratory Medicine and Consultant Physician, Royal Victoria Infirmary, Newcastle upon Tyne, UK

Sally Hicks PhD
Senior Research Fellow, School of Applied Sciences, University of Wales Institute Cardiff, Cardiff, UK

David Hughes BSc, PhD
Head of Immunology, Institute of Food Research, Norwich, UK

John Hunter MA, MD, FRCP
Consultant Physician and Director of Gastroenterology, Addenbrooke's Hospital, Cambridge, UK

Lasse Kanerva MD, PhD
Chief, Finish Institute of Occupational Health, Helsinki, Finland

Gisele Kanny PhD
Centre Hospitalier Universitaire de Nancy, Nancy, France

Anand Kantak MB BS, FAAAI
Assistant Professor of Pediatrics, University of North Dakota, Fargo, USA

Natasha Kapur BSc, MBBS, MRCP
Specialist Registrar in Dermatology, The Royal Free Hospital, London, UK

David King PhD
Chief Neuropsychologist, Kaiser Permanente, Sacramento, USA

Jonathan Leonard BSc, MD, FRCP
Consultant Dermatologist, St Mary's Hospital, London, UK

Colin Little MB BS, MRCP, FRACP, FACA
Allergist and Physician, Mt Waverley, Australia

Robert Longman BSc, MBChB, FRCS, PhD
Specialist Registrar in Surgery, Bristol Royal Infirmary, Bristol, UK

Jonathan Maberly FRCP, FRACP
Consultant Physician, Airedale Allergy Clinic, Keighley, UK

Thomas MacDonald PhD, FRCPath
Professor of Immunology and Director of the Division of Infection, Allergy, Inflammation and Repair, University of Southampton School of Medicine, Southampton, UK

GT Macfarlane BSc, PhD
Professor of Bacteriology, Ninewells Hospital Medical School, University of Dundee, Dundee, UK

Timothy Maher PhD
Sawyer Professor of Pharmaceutical Sciences and Dean, Research and Graduate Studies, Massachusetts College of Pharmacy and Health Sciences, Boston, USA

Christopher Mallinson FRCP
Consultant Gastroenterologist, Harley Street, London, UK

Michael Marsh DSc, DM, FRCP
Reader (Emeritus), Department of Medicine, University of Manchester, Salford, UK

Julika Mayer MD
Medical School of Hannover, Hannover, Germany

Len McEwen MA, BM BCh
McEwen Laboratories Ltd, Pangbourne, UK

Ian Menzies FRCPath, DPath, MBBS(Lon)
Formerly Senior Lecturer/Consultant (Retired), Chemical Pathology Department, St Thomas's Hospital, London
Correspondence: Villiers Lodge, 1 Cranes Park, Surbiton, Surrey, UK

Jiri Mestecky MD, PhD
Professor of Microbiology and Medicine, University of Alabama at Birmingham, Birmingham, USA

Rita Mirakian MD
St Bartholomew's and Royal London School of Medicine and Dentistry, London

D A Moneret-Vautrin MD
Professor of Internal Medicine Centre Hospitalier Universitaire de Nancy, Nancy, France

MMC Mullan SRD
Research Dietician, Addenbrooke's Hospital, Cambridge, UK

Neil Myerscough BSc, MSc
Research Associate, Division of Medicine, Bristol Royal Infirmary, Bristol, UK

Zdenek Pelikan MD, PhD
Director of the Department of Allergology and Immunology, Institute of Medical Sciences "De Klokkenberg", Breda, The Netherlands

Mary Perdue MD
Professor of Pathology and Director, Intestinal Disease Research Program, McMaster University, Hamilton, Canada

Julia Phillips-Quagliata PhD
Professor of Pathology, New York University School of Medicine, New York, USA

Gail Pollard MSc, SRD
Specialist Dietician, The Royal Free Hampstead NHS Trust , London, UK

Christopher Probert MD, MRCP (UK)
Consultant Senior Lecturer, University of Bristol, and Bristol Royal Infirmary, Bristol, UK

Richard S H Pumphrey MD, FRCPath
Regional Immunology Service, St Mary's Hospital, Manchester, UK

Michael Radcliffe MB, ChB, MRCGP, FAAEM
Clinical Allergist, The Royal National Throat Nose and Ear Hospital, London, UK

William Rea MD, FACS, FAAEM, FACN, FRSM, FACAI, FACPM
Director and Founder, and Cardiovascular General Surgeon, The Enviromental Health Center-Dallas, Dallas, USA

Duncan Robertson BSc, MD, FRCP
Consultant Physician and Gastroenterologist, Royal United Hospital, Bath, UK

Gerald Ross MD, CCFP, FAAEM, DABEM, FRSM
Private Practice of Environmental Medicine, Bountiful, UT, USA

MW Russell PhD
Professor of Microbiology, University of Buffalo, Buffalo, USA

Malcolm Rustin BSc, MD, FRCP
Consultant Dermatologist, Department of Dermatology, The Royal Free Hospital, London, UK

Douglas Sandberg MD
Nephrologist, Miami, USA

Jeremy Sanderson MD, FRCP
Consultant Gastroenterologist, St Thomas' Hospital, London, UK

Ian Sanderson MD, FRCP, FRCPCH
Professor of Paediatric Gastroenterology, St Bartholomew's and Royal London School of Medicine and Dentistry, London, UK

Javier Santos MD
McMaster University, Hamilton, Canada

Stephen Schoenthaler PhD
Professor, Department of Sociology and Criminal Justice, California State University, Stanislaus, Turlock, USA

Tarek Shirazi MB BS, MRCP
Specialist Registrar in Gastroenterology, Royal Devon and Exeter Hospital, Exeter, UK

Grant Stenton PhD
Research Scientist, Inflazyme Pharmaceuticals Ltd, Richmond, Canada

Christopher Stokes BSc, PhD
Professor of Mucosal Immunology, University of Bristol, Bristol, UK

Jessica Strid MSc
Institute of Child Health and Great Ormond Street Hospital for Children, London, UK

Stephan Strobel MD, PhD, FRCP, FRCPCH
Professor of Clinical Immunology and Paediatrics, Institute of Child Health and Great Ormond Street Hospital for Children, London, UK

Steve Taylor PhD
Professor, Food Allergy Research and Resource Program, Department of Food Science and Technology, University of Nebraska, Lincoln, USA

Francis Waickman MD
Allergist, Akron, USA

Allan Walker MD
Professor of Pediatrics, Massachusetts General Hospital, Boston, USA

John Walker-Smith MD, FRCP(Lon), FRCP(Ed), FRACP, FRCPCH
Emeritus Professor of Paediatric Gastroenterology, The Wellcome Trust for the History of Medicine at UCL, London, UK

Rosemary Waring DSc, FRCPath
Reader in Human Toxicology, University of Birmingham, Birmingham, UK

Suzanna Widmer MA
Research Psychologist, Institute of Psychiatry, London, UK

Clyde Wilson PhD
Senior Research Fellow, Division of Life Sciences, King's College London, London, UK

David Wray MD, FDSRCPS, FDSRCS(Edin), FMedSci
Dean of the Dental School and Professor of Oral Medicine, University of Glasgow Dental School, Glasgow, UK

Lawrence Youlten FRCP(Edin)
Consultant in Allergy, London Allergy Clinic, London, UK

Preface to the Second Edition

This second edition of *Food Allergy and Intolerance* identifies the ways in which the subject has changed and advanced over the last few years. More is known about the biochemical and immunological idiosyncracies of patients with food intolerance, and how biochemical interventions might help the patient. More is also known about the elements of foods that impact on the immunological system and how IgE is induced. This knowledge is leading not only to the identification of those food peptides causing disease but also to those that can tolerise 'allergic' T cells and allow the patient to become tolerant of their culprit food following immunotherapy.

As before, we feel that it is crucial to understand the 'nuts and bolts' of the gut and its relationship to the immune system. The first section of the book has been brought completely up to date with added sections describing gut epithelial cells, neurological interations with immunity, mast cells and mucins as well as individual chapters on T cells, B cells, and anatomy and physiology of the gut. We encourage clinicians to read this part of the book, as an understanding of structure and function of the gut will give them further insights and understanding of the symptoms relating to food allergy or intolerance in their patients.

The clinical chapters are aimed at illuminating both the diagnosis and treatment of patients with food allergy and intolerance in relation to systems in the body. New chapters relate to 'Hyperventilation' which can mimic many of the indeterminate symptoms sometimes found in patients who are food sensitive. Other new chapters include 'Nutritional effects on immune function', 'Exorphins', 'Food induced asthma', 'Skin contact reactions to foods', 'Addiction and criminal behaviour' and 'Psychological aspects of food intolerance'.

The lining of the gut is the first port of call for food entering the body, and the health of this huge surface area is crucial for the health of the whole patient. The public are perhaps more aware than the medical profession that a healthy gut is a necessity for a healthy body - no longer only 'in mens sana, in corpore sano'!

The awareness of the public has been a great stimulus to trying to identify ways of treating the patient with more consideration and understanding – especially in the area of food intolerance. 'Systemic Candidiasis' is a controversial diagnosis sometimes used when a patient feels systemically ill with Irritable Bowel Syndrome. But is there any truth in it? The concept may be wrong but empirical dietary management can be successful. Patients can be sensitive to yeasts and a change in diet can be dramatic – whether or not it is Candida that is the cause and whether or not 'whatever it is' is systemic. This subject is critically reviewed in Chapter 23.

The vast increase in the sales of minerals, vitamins, prebiotics and probiotics attests to the value that the public place on the concept of a 'healthy gut'.

As always, the patient poses the clinical question that we as clinical scientists have to answer. The more we understand about mechanisms, the more we can refine our diagnostic tests and the better we can treat patients – that must be our goal.

We hope that our new edition will at least fulfill part of these aims.

Jonathan Brostoff
Stephen Challacombe
2002

Preface to the First Edition

As all who deal in the field will know, food allergy is an exciting, challenging, exasperating and sometimes controversial subject. Its study should be a clinical science with diagnosis based on a combination of clinical observations and scientific investigations.

The study of food allergy is incomplete without a fundamental knowledge of how food is processed by the body, in both normal and abnormal conditions, and of how the majority of us are tolerant from an immunological point of view of large quantities of foreign protein to which the body is exposed each day. This is a triumph of the body's adaptation to man's eating habits. It is when this tolerance is broken that maladaptation and disease occur.

The field of food allergy has generally been considered to be a clinical art rather than a laboratory science. There is more than an element of truth in this since clinical observations have often not been supported by reliable diagnostic tests or even laboratory data. This has led to scepticism of some of the clinical associations, especially when the mechanisms of any proposed food allergies are not understood.

Clinical pragmatism is accepted as fundamental in most of the major specialties, but food allergy seems to be an exception. Here there has been a strong tendency for the conventional physician to say that if the mechanism is not understood then food allergy does not exist, especially if the symptoms of the patient do not fit into a conventional diagnostic pigeonhole. This is of course unacceptable.

Clinical medicine is the practice of an art which combines clinical ability with sound judgement based on experience and an understanding of the scientific basis of the specialty. To make a diagnosis certainly requires clinical skill but does not necessarily need a complete understanding of the mechanisms underlying the disease process or an exact understanding of the aetiology. Clinical observation comes before scientific understanding and this is highlighted by many of the names that we give diseases such as Intrinsic Asthma, Essential Hypertension, Minimal Change Nephropathy, Nummular Eczema, and Irritable Bowel Syndrome. These are labels of ignorance and are hardly enlightening as to mechanism or cause.

In this book we have attempted to provide a scientific basis for the clinical observations of food allergy and intolerance. The importance attached to understanding the basic mechanisms underlying food allergy is, we hope, emphasized by a comprehensive review of the structure and function of the gut, its immune cells and secretions, the mechanisms of normal antigen handling, and the contribution that animal models can make to our understanding. This section also emphasizes the fact that, under normal conditions, processing of antigens in the gut may lead to protective effects at distant sites, especially with regard to secretory immunity and oral tolerance.

Certain food allergens have now been chemically characterized, and in the second section of the book the relevance of these in food allergic disease and as models for yet uncharacterized antigens or allergies is discussed.

A major part of the book is devoted to end-organ effects of food allergy or intolerance. Our objective has been to review the evidence for the involvement of reactions to foods in the manifestation of disease at different sites and in different organs. We have brought together a group of scientists and clinicians whose main aim is to help us understand the immunopathological and other processes in our patients. Their points of view are diverse and some are considered unorthodox. There is no suggestion that, because we have invited particular authors to contribute to our book, we necessarily agree with their view. Occasionally the reverse is true! Differing views in clinical medicine are more the rule than the exception, but we hope that these chapters provide the link between clinical art and laboratory science.

A thread running through all these chapters and those in Parts IV and V is that the cornerstone of diagnosis of food intolerance is the removal of that food from the patient's diet with concomitant improvement (or not) of the patient's symptoms and their reappearance on adding that food back—preferably in a double-blind manner. At the clinical level, the effect of the manoeuvre is all that matters to the patient—the mechanism is irrelevant. However, the more that is understood about mechanisms the closer we come to diagnostic tests, and the value of in vivo or in vitro tests in diagnosis has been critically reviewed.

The objective of increased understanding of food allergic disease must be the application of this knowledge to the treatment and prevention of disease in the patient. Antigen avoidance, hyposensitization, the usefulness of drugs and immunological intervention are all discussed in the final section. The prevalence of food allergy in the population is unknown, but it is possible that it may be as high as that of classical atopy (about 15%). It should be one of the easiest diseases to treat (by avoidance), which should therefore obviate the need for treatment with drugs.

We hope that the emphasis placed in this book on the correct methods for the diagnosis of food allergy may result in fewer patients being classified as food allergic without good evidence; but in contrast we hope too that increased understanding of food allergy will make physicians more aware that at least some of their polysymptomatic patients may have an organic basis for their complaints.

For many of the reasons outlined above, we feel that this is an exciting book which we hope will be found useful, stimulating and challenging. Increased understanding of the mechanisms of antigen handling, more accurate clinical diagnosis and the rapid development of laboratory tests all suggest that the extent of the role of food allergy or intolerance in disease will become even clearer in the near future.

As a postscript we would like to refer our readers to the words of Sir Peter Medawar which encapsulate what we must all be striving for.

Jonathan Brostoff
Stephen Challacombe
1987

xi

Why do we eat?

Although physiologists have described a number of possible mechanisms that can operate to drive an individual to seek food, it is doubtful if any of these are of much importance in the life of those living in affluent Western societies. Here, with a wide variety of attractive foods freely available, eating would seem to be governed by social custom rather than necessity. The characteristic pattern of three meals a day, interspersed with mid-morning and afternoon coffee or tea (or 'coke') breaks, and possibly even a last nibble before bed, scarcely leaves any time for classical hunger to develop. Indeed, the fact that most individuals maintain a reasonably constant, albeit often excessive, weight despite the frequency of presentation of ample portions of attractive foods, directs attention to the reasons for a person desisting from eating further at a particular meal, i.e. the attainment of satiety.

Although the three meal pattern, as mentioned, would obviously preclude many of the classical hunger drive mechanisms, the matter may not be so simple. Many people working in the business and professional sectors adopt a rather different meal habit. Breakfast for them may consist merely of a cup of coffee, and so they go from their evening meal to the midday meal, a matter of some 17–18 hours, without significant food or concern about its absence. Such a prolonged abstinence should call into play classical hunger mechanisms, particularly as normal carbohydrate reserves should be exhausted. Clearly the particular eating habit and a metabolic adjustment can override the effect of the physiological stimuli to the hypothalamic hunger centres that would be expected in a person not accustomed to such an eating pattern.

In considering such mechanisms and their overriding, it is salutary to consider what drastic changes have taken place in the eating habits of the affluent in a relatively short time compared to the tens of thousands of years of existence wherein the dominant pattern of eating was firstly governed by the limits of hunter-gatherer societies and then by the greatly improved food situation provided by the larger agrarian societies. However, for the vast majority of mankind, even at best, food was usually in short supply, ranging from subsistence to the occasional modest surplus. This remains true today probably for the majority of the peoples of the earth. But for some hundreds of millions of people who now make up the burgeoning affluent society the situation is quite different. For them ample supplies of a wide variety of attractive foods are freely available. It needs to be appreciated that this situation is in reality a dramatically new development in human affairs. In fact its full flowering has only occurred during the past few decades, although the seeds were planted in the latter part of the eighteenth century, when the Industrial Revolution began. The first century of this was primarily concerned with the development of large-scale industries and thus the development of great wealth for relatively few. The welfare of the many was not considered a matter of importance by governments. In matters of nutrition, the factory workers, formerly farm workers, were in many areas markedly worse off. The twentieth century saw the shift in Western societies from a dominance of heavy industries to light industries and, of particular importance, an enormous expansion of the so-called service industries. This has produced an unprecedented growth of the middle classes. Their relative wealth, wider spread within society and their wider aspirations have led to their designation as the affluent society, an important new subclassification of populations. Little noticed during these developments was another revolution, at first apparently wholly beneficial, but now in question, namely intensive animal husbandry or factory farming.

The Second World War necessitated moving millions of soldiers great distances, particularly the deployment of United States forces to Europe and the Pacific fighting areas. The supply of food to these soldiers was a major and critical problem. This was largely solved by scientists who, by applying genetic and physiological knowledge with the financial resources available due to the exigencies of war, managed to transform and amplify the production of eggs and poultry meat. Thus modern intensive farming came into being, the greatest transformation in farming practice since the introduction of the sowing and harvesting of crops. In the postwar years intensive farming techniques were rapidly developed and soon eggs from 'battery hens' dominated the marketplace and the luxury roast chicken was transformed into the ubiquitous and cheap 'broiler' chicken. Labour-intensive factory farming methods now dominate the production of animal protein. Turkeys, ducks, pigs, calves, beef and even fish can now be raised on a vast scale. Not only has production been intensified but also marketing, and not only of meat and poultry. The supermarket chains with their huge turnovers of all kinds of foods depend themselves upon the mass production of food products, many in the form of so-called 'convenience' foods. The mass production of foodstuffs depends upon a complex technology which necessitates the use of a wide range of chemicals such as preservatives, emulsifiers, stabilizers, antioxidants, flavourings and colourings. In all it has been estimated that over 2000 such nonnutritive food additives are used in the manufacture and marketing of foodstuffs. The supermarket is not the only source of 'convenience' foods. The complex social changes that have accompanied the growth of the service industries has produced a situation where, in order to afford the consumer products manufactured by the consumer society, it is now common for both husband and wife to be wage earners. Hence the role of the wife as a preparer of meals from carefully selected raw materials has diminished as the availability of tasty takeaway meals from a wide variety of small restaurants has increased. Thus the latter part of the twentieth century has seen fundamental changes in nutrition and life styles. These have come about mainly because of economic factors, i.e. the wider disposition of wealth in societies and the consequential forces of the marketplace, with little consideration for actual human needs.

It comes as no surprise, therefore, that affluent societies can be characterized by an apparent increase in susceptibility to certain diseases, particularly chronic diseases such as atherosclerosis, cardiovascular diseases, diabetes and some forms of cancer, and there is growing awareness of the possibility that underlying some of these manifestations of disease is an increase in autoimmune dysfunction. Thus, just as there are the diseases of destitution, so there are the diseases of affluence. Nutritional and environmental factors, particularly overnutrition and stress, are increasingly implicated; but which stress factors are important, and which particular nutrients are in excess remain matters of considerable controversy. Apart from the above considerations the affluent society is also exposed, possibly even more so in some cases, to the increasing pervasiveness of toxic chemicals in the domestic and general environments. Thus although the reasons for the ill-health characteristic of an affluent society are undoubtedly multifactorial there remains the concern that the basis of good health and the resistance to disease factors resides in proper nutrition and that, in the midst of apparent plenty, this is just what many people do not achieve. Thus the question—Why do we eat?—asked in the context of an affluent society needs serious consideration because it seems that, in a situation of free choice, many people are not selecting the correct mix of foods needed to supply all the molecules in the right balance necessary to maintain adequately a healthy body.

The human metabolic machinery is highly evolved and dependent upon a constant supply of molecules, some of them extremely complex. These in turn are synthesized from simple organic and mineral substances by less evolved organisms. Recent advances in molecular biology have provided new insights into not only the incredible complexity of these metabolic processes but, perhaps of greater practical significance, the extraordinary rapidity of turnover of the constituents of many important systems. Some idea of this can be gained from the magnitude of overall protein turnover, which is some 200 g per day in an adult weighing 65 kg. This is over five times the daily protein requirement. This is, however, only a crude estimate of activity. A more meaningful idea of the intensity of synthetic activity is given by the turnover of tissues. For example, the entire mucosa of the gastrointestinal tract is renewed in one to two days, and it has been estimated that some one million B lymphocytes are produced each second. This represents, among other molecules such as DNA and RNA, the daily synthesis of about 25 g of highly specialized proteins, particularly enzymes, to which can be added about 10 g of serum albumin and 2 g of fibrinogen with probably at least this amount of immunoglobulins. These few examples show that, quite apart from the activity of the liver and secretory glands, there is an enormous turnover of complex molecules each second needed for the maintenance of basic metabolic and protective functions.

Thus one essential aspect of eating can be easily identified. This is the supply of the raw materials needed to maintain the highly specialized metabolic activity of the vital tissues. The quantities needed are not large; for example, some 30 g of protein should suffice to supply the amino acid requirement—that is about one medium steak. However, at the level of the vital 'core' tissues it is the quality of the input that matters not the quantity. In particular it is the crucial supply of micronutrients that must be maintained, because many of them, for example vitamin C, cannot be stored in the body. Although knowledge of the importance of many micronutrients, such as the vitamins and trace elements, has been known for decades, their mode of action at the molecular level remains in many cases obscure, as does their requirement particularly when the dynamics of supply are considered in a situation of metabolic stress. Another aspect of eating that has been well publicized in a calorie-conscious age is the need for energy to drive the biological machine. This is the function of the fats and carbohydrates of the diet. However, this simple statement is proving extemely difficult to translate into quantitative practical terms such as what kind, how much and in what ratios. One of the problems of the affluent society is the question of so-called empty calories that come from excess consumption of energy-rich foods, especially alcoholic beverages. It is held by some that prolonged excess consumption results in endocrine and metabolic changes that underlie the diseases of affluence.

It is now appreciated that food contains, in addition to its useful constituents, useless and even potentially dangerous substances and, even though these latter may be in minute quantities, their low-level prolonged intake can result in serious diseases such as cancer. Such toxic molecules are widespread in natural products, for example the aflatoxins, and some may be produced by the process of cooking itself, particularly grilling and toasting. Human metabolic processes have evolved to detoxify many of these substances. Such detoxifications do, however, depend upon a supply of specialized intracellular molecules, such as glutathione, and these in turn depend upon a suitable supply of substrate molecules from the diet. In addition it is now known that certain micronutrients such as vitamin C, vitamin E and b-carotene play a crucial role as anti-carcinogens. A further problem in this context arises from the ubiquity of the products of the chemical industry in the domestic and general environments, a phenomenon of the mid-twentieth century. Toxicologists have discovered that a few widely used chemicals were, rather surprisingly, carcinogens. The identification of vinyl chloride monomer, the basis of the plastic polythene, as a carcinogen was the first intimation of the possible dangers of new classes of man-made molecules. Since that discovery many potentially dangerous chemicals have been identified and eliminated. However there are thousands of chemicals in common use about which little is known toxicologically. There is concern that some of these may produce health effects as yet unidentified because the possibility is not considered, despite the growing evidence from animal studies.

The intracellular detoxification of molecules is one aspect of the defence system of the body against foreign material. Molecules too large to enter cells, macromolecules or microorganisms that gain entrance to the body are dealt with, not always effectively, by the incredibly complex and dynamic immune system. The turnover of its constituents is enormous and is obviously dependent for full efficiency on an adequate and continuing supply of substrate molecules. Thus it can be seen that the diet must provide in addition to the molecules needed for vital functions, maintenance and energy, a further and variable supply of key molecules for the 'nonnutritive' functioning of the defence systems of the body.

Why do we eat?

The importance of nutritional factors in the disease of affluence seems obvious. Thus the question—Why do we eat?—is not trivial. It is necessary to understand why people choose to eat what they eat, and in so doing fail to obtain what they need. It is also obvious that nutritional science has at present no satisfactory understanding of what should constitute an adequate diet. It is to be hoped that the wider perspectives that have come about because of the great advances in molecular biology will stimulate scientists and clinicians to pay greater attention to human nutrition, particularly as what seems apparent in the adult must also have implications for infants, children, the pregnant and the aged.

Morrell Draper

PART I Basic mechanisms

Chapter 1

The structure and organization of lymphoid tissue in the gut

Thomas T. MacDonald

INTRODUCTION

Within the intestinal wall there exist coordinated and specialized lymphoid tissues which protect the most vulnerable and largest surface of the body, the gut mucosa. The gut-associated tissues (Peyer's patches, appendix, colonic and caecal follicles, and isolated lymphoid aggregates), together with mesenteric lymph nodes and the lymphoid elements of the gut epithelium and lamina propria, account for the bulk of the body's lymphoid mass. This mass is largely due to the continuous stimulation of the gut-associated lymphoid tissue (GALT) by food antigens and bacteria and, as will be discussed later in the chapter, one of the most important distinguishing features between the mucosal and systemic lymphoid system is that the former exists in a state of chronic reactivity. It is important to emphasize from the outset that the gut immune system must have a means to sense the antigens in the gut lumen so that recognition and effective anti-pathogen immunity can be generated. Moreover, the gut immune system does not have the option to be unresponsive to enteric antigens, but it responds to all antigens in the gut in a positive fashion (immunity) or in a negative fashion (active downregulation and tolerance). Thus it can be seen that, because of its location, the gut immune system requires unique features not necessary elsewhere. Some of these features have been recognized for many years, such as the dissemination of activated T and B cells from Peyer's patches to the distant lamina propria via the blood, but others are more recent, such as the description of a new primary lymphoid organ in the gut of mice – the cryptopatch.

The lymphoid structures of the gastrointestinal tract have anatomical features in common which distinguish them from other secondary lymphoid tissues. The most obvious of these common features is the lack of a defined capsule or afferent lymphatics and the presence of a specialized covering epithelium, the follicle-associated epithelium (FAE), which facilitates the transmission of antigen from the gut lumen. In this chapter the term GALT is used to describe any organized aggregate of lymphoid tissue with a specialized FAE. Large numbers of lymphoid/myeloid cells are also present in the mucosa between the follicular structures in the epithelium and lamina propria, and these will be considered independently. All evidence suggests that the lymphoid structures in the intestine are the site of induction of mucosal immunity and that the epithelium and lamina propria are the effector sites of mucosal immunity.

STRUCTURE AND CELLULAR COMPOSITION OF ORGANIZED GUT-ASSOCIATED LYMPHOID TISSUE IN MAN

The stomach

The normal human stomach is devoid of organized lymphoid tissue, and lymphoid/myeloid cells are sparse in the lamina propria. There is a scattering of T cells in the lamina propria and a few in the epithelium. In the lamina propria, immunoglobulin (Ig) A plasma cells predominate over IgM and IgG cells. In chronic gastritis, there is an increase in plasma cells of all isotypes, but the increase in IgG cells is especially profound.[12] There is also an increase in epithelial

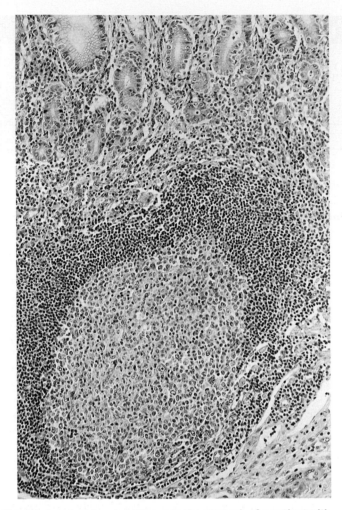

Fig. 1.1 Acquired lymphoid tissue in the stomach of a patient with *Helicobacter pylori* gastritis. Note the large reactive follicle centre (haematoxylin and eosin, original magnification ×100).

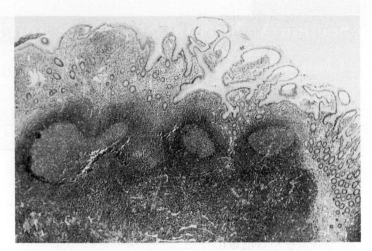

Fig. 1.2 Histological appearance of Peyer's patch in human terminal ileum (haematoxylin and eosin, original magnification ×40).

the same number of Peyer's patches as at birth.[23] The assumption by Cornes that five or more follicles are necessary before a lymphoepithelial structure can be called a Peyer's patch is arbitrary and it is reasonable to categorize even a single nodule as a Peyer's patch providing there is a FAE present. In normal intestine, all organized mucosal follicles can be shown to have a FAE if the tissue is properly orientated for sectioning. There are many Peyer's patches with 1–4 follicles, evident in small intestine both macroscopically and microscopically, and Cornes' estimates, although useful for comparative studies, seriously underestimate the amount of organized lymphoid tissue in the human gut.

Peyer's patch follicle-associated epithelium
The epithelial cells overlying the follicle are derived from crypts of Lieberkuhn adjacent to the follicles. FAE is different from columnar villus epithelium in that it is cuboidal, contains few goblet cells and does not contain secretory component.[7] In addition, there are specialized M cells, also derived from adjacent crypts,[17] so-called because they have microfolds rather than microvilli on their surface.[75] M cells have a number of morphological and functional specializations. They have attenuated processes to adjacent cells and are very closely associated with lymphocytes. Clusters of T and B cells lie next to M cells in the epithelium, which can be identified by their lack of brush border alkaline phosphatase.[8] There are significantly raised CD4+ T cells in follicle epithelium compared to villus epithelium. M cells are deficient in cytoplasmic acid phosphatase and microvillus-associated alkaline phosphatase.[77] They are also probably[7] HLADR-. It is unlikely, therefore, that they play a role in antigen presentation but are more likely to be a portal for antigen entry into the dome area of the follicle. This has been clearly shown for reovirus in mice (which only adheres to and penetrates the M cells of the FAE[121]) poliovirus[99] and horseradish peroxidase, which is also preferentially taken up by M cells.[76] Pathogenic intestinal microbes such as virulent *Salmonella* spp, *Yersinia enterocolitica Yersinia pseudotuberculosis* and *Shigella* all take advantage of the phagocytic capacity of M cells to invade the gut mucosa.[2,45,66,115]

For many years attempts have been made to identify specialized features of M cells over and beyond their phagocytic capacity and their characteristic morphology. However, apart from lectin binding characteristics, this has not been productive. A

T cells.[50] A striking feature of the stomach, however, is the acquisition of organized lymphoid aggregates in association with *Helicobacter pylori* infection (Fig. 1.1). It is from this ectopic lymphoid tissue that gastric B cell lymphomas are thought to arise.[122] In children this is especially striking and leads to antral nodularity which is visible at gastroscopy.[39,123] Whether this acquired lymphoid tissue functionally resembles Peyer's patches, has a FAE-containing M cells and is capable of generating a secretory IgA response to gastric antigens remains to be established.

Peyer's patches of the small intestine
The organized lymphoid tissue of the small intestine was first described by de Peyer in 1667. Structurally, Peyer's patches are organized areas of lymphoid tissue in the mucosa of the small bowel. They usually contain follicle centres and have well defined cellular zonation (Fig. 1.2). They are overlaid by a specialized lymphoepithelium without crypts or villi.

At birth there are approximately 100 Peyer's patches with five or more follicles in human small intestine and the majority of these patches are in the distal small intestine.[22] The number of Peyer's patches increases to 225–300 in the whole small intestine by late adolescence and then decreases with increasing age so that the small intestine from 90-year-old individuals has roughly major advance in this area is the observation that differentiated epithelial cells can transform into M cells when cocultured with B cells, thus explaining the close relationship between these two cell types *in vivo*.[51] There is now the potential to identify M cell-specific gene products using this *in vitro* model. There is clearly a close interaction between B cells and M cells in vivo. B cell deficient mice have very small PP, FAE and few M cells.[33b] RAG1 deficient mice have no T or B cells and have small PP anlagen and a smal FAE, but there are still a few M cells.[25a] Thus the number of M cells in the FAE does largely depend on PP B cells. M cell numbers in the FAE seem to be quite plastic. Infusion of *Streptoccus pneumoniae* into loops of rabbit gut leads to a large increase in M cells at the periphery of the PP within hours.[11a] Whether this is a direct effect on M cell differentiation or is via B cells activated by *S.pneumoniae* is nor known. The B cells which are adjacent to M cells in the FAE have a memory phenotype and are more like germinal centre B cells, and indeed it has been suggested that the B cells in M cell pockets are extensions of germinal centers.[124a]

Morphological and immunohistochemical characteristics of human Peyer's patches

The most prominent feature of Peyer's patches is the follicle centre, which contains centrocytes and centroblasts. The follicle centre is surrounded by a mantle of small lymphocytes which merge into the mixed cell zone of the dome. The dome area also contains plasma cells, dendritic cells macrophages and small B cells with cleaved nuclei (ccntrocyte-like cells) which infiltrate the overlying epithelium.[103] B cells are not seen in villus or crypt epithelium.

T cell populations in Peyer's patches

Immunohistochemical staining of Peyer's patches with anti-CD3 monoclonal antibodies shows T cells to be present in the greatest density in the areas surrounding the high endothelial venulcs (Fig. 1.3). IL2-receptor positive T cells are present in this area. T cells are also present surrounding the follicle, in the mixed cell zone in the dome and in the lymphoepithelium.[103] In man, in contrast to the mouse, the T cell zone extends between the follicle centre and the muscularis mucosa. Occasional T cells are seen in the follicle centre. The majority of the T cells are CD4[+]. It has been established for many years that Peyer's patches are on the major route of lymphocyte recirculation. Small naïve T cells (CD45RA[+], L-selectin[hi]) can enter Peyer's patches because glycosylation of the mucin-like domains of the gut-specific addressin MAdCAM 1 binds L-selectin.[16] If these small naïve T cells become activated in Peyer's patches they lose L-selectin and the presence of CD45RO[+] cells coexpressing high levels of the $\alpha4\beta7$ integrin and L-selectin[lo] near microlymphatics in Peyer's patches suggests that these cells are leaving the patches and are on their way to the lamina propria via the blood.[33] The other site at which activated T cells are seen in Peyer's patches is next to M cells. These cells are also CD45RO[+], L-selectin[lo], CD69[+] and are dividing.[31] It is not known if these are the same cells as are seen near the lymphatics. Although there have been many studies on T cells in mouse Peyer's patches, the literature on human PP is small. Recently, it has been shown that human PP T cells show antigen-specific recall responses to milk protein antigens and the response is predominantly of the Th1 type.[71a]

B cell and plasma cells in Peyer's patches

Human Peyer's patches contain large numbers of B cells (Fig. 1.4). The narrow mantle zone surrounding the follicle centre is composed of cells expressing surface IgM or IgD. The B cells which surround the mantle zone, are present in the mixed cell zone of the dome and infiltrate the epithelium, do not express IgD but do express surface IgM (sIgM) or sIgA.[103] Germinal centre formation is not seen in Peyer's patches in the fetus and develops after antigenic exposure at birth.[15] The adaptive sIgA response is almost certainly generated in the Peyer's patches, the progeny migrating to the lamina propria. In mice, about half of the IgA plasma cells do not follow this route and are instead the progeny of CD5[+] peritoneal B cells, mostly containing germline V region sequences.[57] Recently it has been suggested that about 25% of the mouse secretory IgA response is T-independent and largely of the B1 lineage.[64a] Indeed in mice it has been shown that a secretory IgA response can occur in the absence of PP,[123a] but to deny a role for PP in secretory IgA responses would fly in the face of overwhelming evidence. In man, however, this pathway is less important and IgA plasma cells in the gut are highly mutated, implying selection and affinity maturation in the Peyer's patches germinal centre.[30]

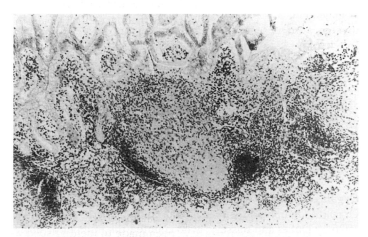

Fig. 1.3 Immunohistochemical localization of CD3[+] cells in human Peyer's patch. Most T cells are in the interfollicular zones (immunoperoxidase, original magnification ×40).

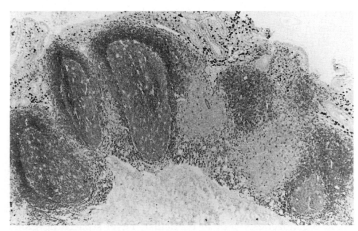

Fig .1.4 Immunohistochemical localization of B cells (CD20[+]) in human Peyer's patch (immunoperoxidase, original magnification ×40).

IL4 appears to be important in the Peyer's patches germinal centre response. IL4 knock-out mice do not have Peyer's patches germinal centres and are defective in sIgA responses to protein antigens.[112] It was originally reported that IL-6 was also crucial secretory IgA responses,[85a] however subsequent studies have not confirmed this observation.[15a, 112a]

Most of the cells with abundant cytoplasmic immunoglobulin (cIg) are in the dome area in human Peyer's patches. Most contain IgA with fewer cIgM cells.[103] Some workers have reported that cIgG plasma cells are as abundant as cIgA(cytoplasmic IgA) cells in the dome.[5] There are also cells with cIgA in the T cell zone surrounding the high endothelial venules (HEV), but the dense accumulation of IgA-containing immunoblasts around the HEV in rodents is not seen in man.[104]

Macrophages and accessory cells in Peyer's patches

In man, B cells, activated T cells, dendritic cells, follicular dendritic cells, and macrophages express Class II molecules necessary for antigen presentation to CD4+ T cells. All of these cell types are present in normal Peyer's patches. Numerous non-lymphoid HLADR+ cells with cytoplasmic processes are present in the dome area of human Peyer's patches and in the T cell zones. The HLADR+ cells in the dome do not stain with antimacrophage markers such as RFD7 or lysozyme (although these cells are abundant in adjacent lamina propria), but do stain with S-100[103] and cystatin A.[91] These cells are probably dendritic cells but the HLADR+ cells between the follicles in the T cell zones are probably interdigitating cells. The dome epithelium[102] itself is also HLADR+ and may also be capable of presenting antigen to the numerous lymphoid cells in the epithelium. The presence of dendritic cells in the mixed cell zone of the dome immediately underlying the M cells (which are Class II−) suggests that, in Peyer's patches, most antigen presentation takes place in the dome region. Functional studies on PP dendritic cells have all been carried out in the mouse. In this species, 2 lineages of dendritic cells have been identified, a population expressing high levels of CD11b of a myeloid lineage and those expressing CD8αα, of a lymphoid lineage. In mouse PP myeloid DC's are present in the subepithelial zone and lymphoid DC's in the interfollicular T cell zone.[43a] There is also a population of double negative dendritic cells within the FAE.[43b] These subpopulations appear to have different functions. Myeloid DC's produce IL-10, whereas lymphoid and double negative DC's produce IL-12.[43b] Functional studies in man are still largely lacking. There is a population of IL-12 p40 containing cells below the FAE in human ileal PP[71a] and it has been proposed that bacterial products crossing the FAE from the gut lumen active IL-12 production in these cells via toll-like receptors.[63a]

Cytokines and their receptors control Peyer's patch organogenesis

One of most exciting features of gene knock-out experiments is the discovery of a totally unexpected phenotype. Immunologists interested in the functions of tumour necrosis factor α (TNFα), lymphotoxin α (LTα), lymphotoxin β(LTβ) and their receptors (TNF-RI, TNF-RII and the lymphotoxin β receptor) have discovered that these molecules play a crucial role in lymphoid tissue organogenesis and, in particular, Peyer's patch development.[67]

It was first observed that mice deficient in TNF-RI had apparently normal systemic lymphoid tissues, but had absent Peyer's patches.[72] This view was, however, revised in later studies in which it was clear that absence of TNF or TNF-RI did have Peyer's patch-specific effects. The phenotype was not absence of Peyer's patches, but rather that they were small and inconspicuous, with disrupted cellular zonation.[79] This was secondary to a defect of follicular organization in all lymphoid tissues, but phenotypically maximal in the Peyer's patch. Thus, TNF and TNF-RI are not important in Peyer's patch morphogenesis, but are important in the zonation and differentiation of the follicles.

Deletion of TNF-RI abolishes signalling through this receptor of soluble TNFα, soluble LTα (which exists as a trimer, LTα3) and membrane-bound LTα2β1 (a cell surface trimer of LTα and membrane bound LTβ). However it will not alter the interaction of membrane bound LTα1β2 with its receptor LTβR. When mice are made homozygous for a null mutation in the LTα gene, however, a dramatic effect is seen. These mice have a normal thymus, an abnormal spleen and no lymph nodes or Peyer's patches.[53] Clearly, therefore, membrane LTαβ complexes are crucial in secondary lymphoid tissue morphogenesis. It would be expected that mice deficient in LTβ would have the same phenotype, but this is not the case, since these mice have mesenteric lymph nodes, although they lack Peyer's patches.[53]

The most interesting recent development in this field is the phenotype of mice heterozygous for null mutations in the LTα and LTβ genes (LTα+/−, LTβ+/−). Such mice are completely normal but lack Peyer's patches,[54] although histology did not show whether a Peyer's patch rudiment remains. There is, therefore, some crucial gene dosage effect which is not yet understood. None the less, mice deficient in Peyer's patches will be a tremendous model in which to study mucosal immunity, hypersensitivity and tolerance.

Cryptopatches

It is unusual for a new primary lymphoid organ to be discovered in the mouse, the most intensely investigated of all species. Yet in 1996, Kanamori and colleagues[49] reported that the intestinal mucosa of mice contained 1500 small clusters of lymphocytes (around 1000 cells per cluster) which had all the features of such a tissue. The phenotype of these cells was consistent with their lymphopoietic role, in that they are dividing, c-kit,+ IL7-R+, with some that are CD25+. Importantly, these cells are CD3−, T cell receptor-negative and RAG 1−, showing that T cell receptor arrangement is not occurring *in situ*. In addition, these cryptopatches are present in germfree and athymic mice, SCID mice and TcR knock-out mice, but are absent in IL7 knock-out mice, as is the thymus. When cells from cryptopatches are grafted into SCID mice, there is preferential repopulation of αβ and γδ T cells in the gut epithelium, but not other tissues.[90]

It is extremely difficult to reconcile these observations with the notion that αβ T cells in the gut derive from Peyer's patches and that γδ T cells, at least in mice, come from the marrow and differentiate in the gut epithelium. It is also not known whether cryptopatches are present in human intestine.

Organized lymphoid tissue of the colon

Organized lymphoid tissue in human colon was first described in 1926 by Dukes and Bussey,[29] who counted the number of single lymphoid follicles in human colon of different ages. They showed that, in children, there were eight follicles per square centimetre of colonic mucosa, which decreased to three follicles per square

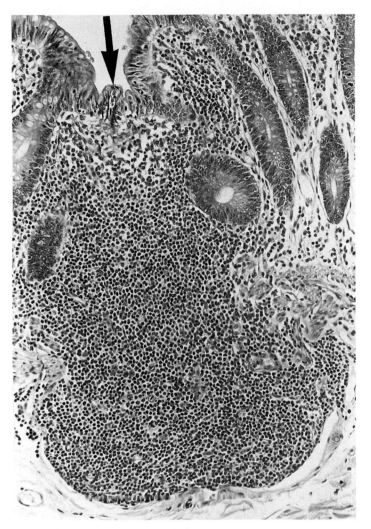

Fig. 1.5 Colonic lymphoid follicle. The small follicle-associated epithelium is arrowed. (haematoxylin and eosin, original magnification ×100).

centimetre in old age. The density of follicles is highest in the rectum. Aggregates of follicles akin to that seen in the multifollicular Peyer's patches in the small bowel are not seen in human colon. The bulk of the lymphoid tissue in colonic lymphoid follicles lies below the muscularis mucosa, the follicles producing points of discontinuity in the latter.[74] Unless colonic lymphoid tissue is properly orientated it may appear as though it has no FAE (Fig. 1.5). Colonic lymphoid follicles also have a dome epithelium with M cells, similar in many regards to the specialized lymphoepithelium overlying Peyer's patches, although in proportion to the mass of lymphoid tissue colonic FAE is less than in Peyer's patches.[44] There have been no functional studies on colonic follicles in man.

Appendix

The human appendix is a blind sac, 5–8 cm long, extending from the caecum near the ileocaecal junction. The most striking feature of the appendix is the presence of numerous lymphoid nodules separated by regions of lamina propria, into which the glandular crypts penetrate. The types of cells and their zonal arrangement is very similar to that of human Peyer's patches. The most prominent feature of the lymphoid nodules is the reactive follicle

centre, surrounded by a narrow mantle of cells which merge with the mixed cell zone below the epithelium. The mantle and mixed cell zone contain CD4+ T cells but are mostly IgM+ IgD− B cells.[102] The FAE, which contains T and B cells, is often HLADR+. The T cell zone lies mostly between the follicle centre and the muscularis mucosa (Fig. 1.6). Lysozyme-containing macrophages are uncommon in the dome region, and most of the HLADR+ cells with cytoplasmic processes stain with S-100 and are probably dendritic cells.[101] S-100+ cells can occasionally be seen in the epithelium.

IgG-producing plasma cells predominate in the region immediately adjacent to the follicles and in the dome, but the majority of plasma cells in the lamina propria between the follicles produce IgA.[6]

The exact role of the appendix is still to be determined. It is somewhat of an orphan organ and is poorly investigated. There is the intriguing observation that appendectomy protects against the development of ulcerative colitis.[89] Somewhat analogous results are seen in T cell receptor α knock-out mice, where removal of the caecal Peyer's patches (mice do not have an appendix) delays the onset of their inflammatory bowel disease.[70]

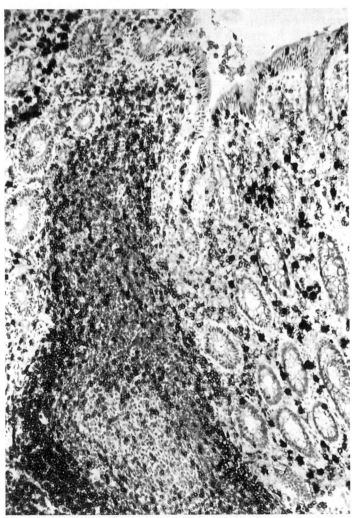

Fig. 1.6 T cells in human appendix (immunoperoxidase with anti-CD3, original magnification ×100).

INTESTINAL MUCOSA

Gut epithelium as a lymphoid tissue

The mucosa between the follicles makes up most of the mass of the intestine. There are extensive lymphoid/myeloid elements in the connective tissue of the lamina propria, and numerous lymphocytes (mostly T cells, but never B cells, macrophages or plasma cells) in the gut epithelium. Small bowel villus enterocytes also express HLADR.[93] Thus it may be considered that both the gut epithelium and lamina propria may be sites at which mucosal immune responses may be initiated. A recent concept is that the gut epithelium can play an immunomodulatory role. Gut epithelial cells secrete IL7, which is a growth factor for lamina propria T cells.[116] In addition, when epithelial cells are invaded by pathogenic microorganisms they rapidly secrete a large number of cytokines and chemokines to draw inflammatory cells to the site of infection.[48] The epithelium may therefore be the most important primary sensor of infections in the gut.

Major histocompatibility complex and related gene expression in the epithelium

All gut epithelial cells are strongly MHC Class I[+]. Gut epithelial cells also express the Class I-related, non-polymorphic, CD1d molecule.[9] There is limited evidence that CD1d on epithelial cells can be a ligand for intraepithelial lymphocytes (IEL). An $\alpha\beta$ T cell line from human IEL lysed CD1d-transfected target cells[3] and there is some evidence that, in a mixed lymphocyte reaction where the stimulator cells are epithelial cells, that CD8 T cells respond to CD1d on the enterocytes.[78] CD1d may also play a role in signalling to the epithelial cell. Cross-linking CD1d on epithelial cell lines rapidly increases production of IL-10 and this may serve as a mechanism to down-regulate mucosal T cell responses.[21a] For many years, Mayer and colleagues have been investigating the activation of non-specific CD8[+] suppressor cells by epithelial cells. They have recently demonstrated that an important CD8 ligand on epithelial cells is a 180 kD heavily glycosylated protein related to carcinoembryonic antigen.[60] The most exciting recent development in this area, however, is the demonstration that stressed epithelial cells rapidly upregulate the MHC-like genes, MIC-A and MIC-B. These molecules are expressed without $\beta2$-microglobulin and peptide.[35] Importantly, epithelial cells expressing MIC-A or MIC-B are lysed by $\gamma\delta$ T cells in man,[36] showing for the first time that $\gamma\delta$ T cells can eliminate damaged enterocytes.

The expression of Class II MHC products on gut epithelium was first seen in the guinea pig[120] and later in human small intestine[93] (Fig. 1.7). In man, normal large intestine and stomach epithelium are HLADR[-],[96,105] as are crypt epithelial cells. Peyer's patch epithelium[102] is also HLADR[+]. In man, normal small intestinal epithelial cells are HLADP and DQ[-].[94] It is now clear that human epithelial cells can present antigen to CD4 cells via class II MHC, after internalisation at the apical surface.[40a] It is quite controversial as to whether other accessory molecules are expressed on epithelial cells. CD58 is expressed constitutively and blocking CD58 inhibits CD4 proliferation to antigen presented by epithelial cells.[33a] The same study failed to detect CD80 or CD86 on epithelial cells. However other investigators have clearly shown CD86 transcripts and protein in normal and inflamed colonic epithelial cells.[71b] The reasons for these different results are unclear.

Epithelial HLADR expression in man is increased in chronic inflammatory bowel disease,[96] coeliac disease,[1] gastritis[105] and

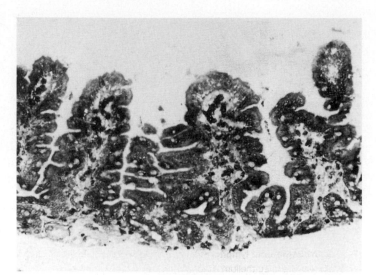

Fig. 1.7 HLADR expression in normal human small intestine. The epithelium is strongly positive, as are many cells in the lamina propria (immunoperoxidase, original magnification ×100).

autoimmune enteropathy.[69] In untreated coeliac disease there is also expression of HLADP and DQ on the surface epithelial cells in some patients.[94] In patients with ulcerative colitis in whom intestinal inflammation has been reduced by steroids the epithelium[84] becomes HLADR[-].

Gamma interferon (IFNγ) can increase DR expression on human transformed intestinal epithelial cell lines and rat epithelial cell lines.[20,100] Activation of lamina propria T cells in explants of human small intestine with mitogens *in vitro* results in IFNγ production and an increase in HLADR expression by crypt epithelial cells.[64] Thus there is good, but circumstantial, evidence that increased epithelial HLADR expression during inflammation is caused by local production of IFNγ by activated mucosal T cells. Whether the increased HLADR expression is of any pathogenic significance or is merely an epiphenomenon is unknown.

Phenotype of intraepithelial lymphocytes

If epithelial cells can present enteric antigens, the cells most likely to be stimulated will be IEL, situated basally above the basement membrane (Fig. 1.8). However, although this hypothesis has been mooted for many years, actual demonstration of this phenomenon using IEL and epithelial cells is still lacking. IEL are a highly unusual population of T cells with many features distinct from cells of the lamina propria and systemic lymphoid tissues. There has been a great deal of work on mouse IEL in the last 10 years, mainly directed at which populations ($\alpha\beta$ or $\gamma\delta$ T cells) are thymus-independent. Much of this work is contradictory, but is well summarized elsewhere.[59] However, it appears that the majority of $\gamma\delta$ T cells in IEL differentiate locally in the epithelium, whereas the majority of the $\alpha\beta$ T cells are thymus-derived. Here, discussion will be restricted to studies in man.

It is well established that the majority of IEL in the small bowel are CD8,[+] with fewer CD4[+] cells, even fewer CD3[+] 4[-] 8[-] cells, and a small number of CD3[-] 7[+] non-T cells concentrated at the villus tips.[46,97,107] There are no B cells or macrophages in mucosal epithelium but it has been reported that dendritic cells are present in the rat gut epithelium.[65] The majority of IEL in man use the $\alpha\beta$ TcR.[13] Only about 10% of IEL in healthy indi-

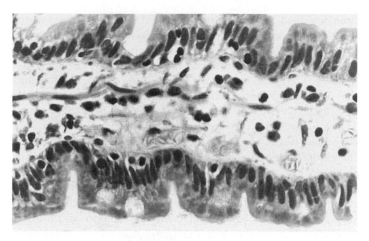

Fig. 1.8 Intraepithelial lymphocytes in human small intestine. Most lie basally within the epithelium (haematoxylin and eosin, original magnification ×100).

viduals use the γδ TcR.[34,47,106] An important difference between blood γδ TcR+ T cells and those in the gut epithelium is that, whereas most in the blood use the Vδ2 gene product, those in the gut use the Vδ1 gene product.[38,106] IEL also bear markers of chronically activated T cells.[14] They are L-selectin[lo] and CD45RO+. Virtually all express the gut-specific integrin αEβ7, whose ligand is epithelial E-cadherin.[19] Interactions between αEβ7 and E-cadherin may help anchor IEL in the epithelium and may also play a functional role. Although E-cadherin is the only ligand for αEβ7 so far defined, there is now some evidence for alternative ligands. In TNSB colitis, treatment of mice with antibodies to αEβ7 ameliorates disease.[0?a] This is a surprise given that TNSB colitis is mediated by CD4 T cells which normally do not express αEβ7. However it has recently been shown that antibodies to αEβ7 partially block binding of cells to gut microvascular endothelial cells, which lack detectable E-cadherin.[107a] Antibodies to αEβ7 therefore might block lymphocyte extravasation into the gut. All evidence in mice suggests that there is virtually no traffic of lymphocytes out of the IEL compartment and that they are longlived and renewed slowly.[81,85] Although it is outwith the remit of this chapter, virtually all of the evidence in mouse and man suggests that CD8+ IEL of both αβ and γδ lineages are cytotoxic cells and that they predominantly secrete IFNγ.[62,114,124]

The observation that some mouse IEL are thymus-independent has led a number of investigators to determine whether this is also the case in man. On balance, however, if IEL arise locally it is to a very minor extent. It was reported that IEL in man expressed transcripts for RAG 1 and RAG 2,[63] but the methodology used was RT-PCR which is liable to contamination and is not quantitative. A compelling negative study[109] is the report that IEL do not contain transcripts for the enzyme terminal deoxytransferase (TdT). During T cell receptor gene recombination, TdT adds nucleotides to the broken strands of the 3′ end of the gene segment encoding the D and J regions (N region insertion), thereby increasing T cell receptor diversity. All studies of T cell receptors used by IEL have shown that there are extensive N region insertions; therefore the lack of TdT clearly shows that the T cell receptor diversity was generated outwith the epithelium.

T cell receptor usage of intraepithelial lymphocytes

It has traditionally been considered that, because the gut is exposed to myriad antigens, the T cell receptors would be very diverse; that is, capable of recognizing many different peptides. However, this is not the case. Both αβ and γδ IEL in normal individuals are markedly oligoclonal and this clonality is stable with time.

Fetal intestinal lamina propria lymphocyte (LPL) and IEL populations contain detectable mRNA for rearranged TCR β loci as early as 13 weeks, but the number of TCR Vβ family members which are detectable is limited at this time.[55] This number increases with gestation such that at birth all 24 Vβ families are detectable as rearranged mRNA transcripts. Analysis of the CDR3 regions of these Vβ transcripts by CDR3 spectratyping and DNA sequencing reveals that they are diverse, with numerous non-templated N region additions. IEL Vβ CDR3s are more restricted in repertoire up to around 19 weeks of gestation, when they become more diverse.

There is a marked disparity between expression of TCR β chains and TCR α in the fetal intestine. Rearranged TCR α chains are undetectable until around 16 weeks of gestation when the repertoire of expressed TCR Vα chains is very limited. Expression of TCR β in the absence of TCR α is strong evidence that TCR locus recombination may be occurring *in situ* in the intestine before birth. Random anchored PCR (polymerase chain reaction) and RACE (Rapid Amplification of CDNA Ends) analysis of TCR α transcripts in the human fetal intestine reveals that a large majority of rearranged TCR α transcripts before 16 weeks of gestation are recombined to an immature precursor segment which replaces Vα. This segment is termed T early alpha (TEA). The TEA locus is located 3′ of Cδ and 5′ of the most upstream Jα.[119]

T early alpha (TEA)

TEA has been postulated to play a role in opening the TCR locus for subsequent rearrangement,[27,28,98] and has been reported to be expressed on thymocytes before the onset of TCR Vα recombination with rearranged TCR J–C segments.[28] In addition, many of the rearranged TCR α transcripts detectable around 16 weeks of gestation are joining segments correctly spliced to constant regions but not recombined with TCR Vα. These transcripts initiate upstream of the Jα loci and may be the result of initiation of transcription of the partially rearranged TCR α genes prior to full recombination of J–C joins with the Vα loci.[86,88,125] TEA becomes less predominant with increasing gestational age and more fully rearranged TCR α transcripts can be detected. This process starts later with IEL than LPL; however, by 23 weeks′ gestation TCR α transcripts with productively rearranged TCR V–J–C segments are detectable in both compartments. TEA is also detected in adult LPL and IEL. In addition to TEA expression as the sole TCR α transcript in IEL and as the predominant TCR α transcript in the gut up to 16 weeks′ gestation, a new T early β transcript (TEB) has been identified as a major TCR β transcript in the fetal intestine from 14 weeks of gestation onwards. Expression of this immature transcript in the gut is evidence that, for many αβ T cells, TCR β recombination has not yet occurred and, like the TCR α locus, may be doing so in the intestine. TEB, like TEA, is also expressed in fetal blood and adult IEL and LPL in addition to the thymus.

Repertoire of intestinal αβ TCR

The repertoire of adult intestinal αβ TCR is remarkably different to that seen in the fetus. Adult IEL express an oligoclonal repertoire of αβ TCR,[3,9,113] and the adult intestinal epithelium contains dominant αβ TCR expressing IEL which are present expressing the same TCR at distal points throughout the intestine.[37] These are thought to be derived from an expansion of a limited number of T cell clones in the Peyer's patches before dissemination throughout the intestine. The ligands which drive this oligoclonal expansion have yet to be elucidated, but it has been shown that CD8[+] IELs can recognize and respond to a cytotoxic response to antigen presented on the MHC I-like non-polymorphic CD1 molecules CD1a, CD1b, CD1c and CD1d.[3] It is very likely that the oligoclonal expansion of IEL bearing αβ TCR is antigen-driven, as the fetal intestinal lumen is effectively sterile until birth, and both fetal LPL and IEL populations utilize a diverse and polyclonal array of αβ TCR.[55]

γ/δ T cells

γ/δ cells arise in the fetal liver and thymus at 6–8 weeks' gestation[56,68,83] and are detectable in the gut at 14 weeks' gestation,[106] where they are located predominantly in the epithelium and comprise 10–30% of the IEL of the fetus. By adulthood, the proportion of γ/δ IEL remains around 10–15% in the small intestine[106] and is up to 40% in the colon.[26,47] However, important changes in the complexity and clonality of the TCR δ repertoire occur in this period. Complexity and specificity of the TCR γ/δ heterodimer is largely contributed by the CDR3 region of the delta chain, which is produced by random joining of the variable, diversity and joining segments in addition to random N region non-templated nucleotide deletion and addition at the coding joints of nucleotides palindromic to the coding ends of the V, D and J segments (P additions[58]). The CDR3 region of the TCR δ chain is generally longer and more variable in length than the α or β chains, and it has been suggested that the ligands for the γ/δ TCR are soluble non-MHC-bound antigens, with the γ/δ TCR recognizing these in a similar fashion to antibody.[87] The TCR δ repertoire of fetal intestinal T cells in the second trimester of gestation is polyclonal, with numerous different CDR3 lengths being observed; however, sequence analysis reveals that the junctional regions of the CDR3 region at this time are limited by a lack of N region addition at the joining ends of the V, D and J segments.[42] In addition, numerous template-encoded P additions are seen at the junctions between the V, D and J regions. Also, numerous identical TCR DV2 transcripts resembling the canonical sequences described in mice can be observed in multiple fetuses.[42] In the early period after birth (from 1 day to 4 weeks), the repertoire of expressed TCR δ transcripts remains polyclonal but, at this time, the junctional regions become more complicated with numerous N region nucleotide insertions in addition to P additions. After birth the TCR δ repertoire becomes increasingly restricted such that at mid-adolescence the diversity of TCR δ usage is comparable with adults in their sixtieth year of life. It is possible that the increasing restriction of the TCR δ repertoire in the gut with increasing age is caused by a change in the diversity of the cognate ligands, currently unidentified in the gut microenvironment with time.

TCR δ usage in adult intestine

The traditional view of TCR δ usage in the adult intestine and peripheral immune compartments has been that Vδ1 is the predominantly used TCR Vδ chain in the gut and that Vδ2 is predominant in the periphery, where the TCR Vδ repertoire has been described as highly diverse.[61,73,108,111] Recent studies describing adult gut and peripheral blood TCR Vδ clonality and diversity have revealed that both the colon and peripheral blood Vδ repertoires are oligoclonal irrespective of whether Vδ1, 2 or 3 is utilized.[21,41] Moreover, in contrast to previous reports, it was found that Vδ1, 2 and 3 are utilized by γ/δ T cells in the colon and, despite the potential of TCR Vδ loci for great junctional diversity, TCR Vδ diversity in the blood and colon is highly restricted. This oligoclonal restriction of TCR δ is unique to each individual and the clones in blood and intestine are separate. The dominant clones are also stable over time in each individual being detected consistently over a 16-month period. This phenotype of stable clones scattered throughout long distances of the colon has been suggested to occur because of positive selection of a limited number of TCR δ-expressing T cells on gut-specific ligands before dissemination throughout the body and homing back to the gut via the α4β7/MAdCAM interaction, and not because of continuous *in situ* V(D)J recombination which would be expected to produce a more polyclonal distribution of TCR δ usage.[21] T cell receptor diversity of IEL at different ages is shown in Table 1.1.

The role of the epithelium in retaining mucosal lymphocytes

Homing of lympoctes to different tissues is now known to involve vascular adressins and chemokines. Cells derived from PP express the α4β7 integrin which binds to MAdCAM on mucosal endothelia and allows cells to extravasate into the lamina propria. Nieve T cells also use MAdCAM to enter PP. The chemokine secondary lymphoid tissue chemokine (SLC) expressed in PP also plays a role in migration to PP at least and is crucial for α4β7/MAdCAM1 ineractions.[77a] Analysis of chemokine receptors on IEL and LPL shows that they predominantly express CXCR3 and CCR2.[1a] The chemokine IP-10 is present in normal colon endothelium and may therefore also play a role in recruiting cells to this site. In addition, in inflammation, epithelial cells make chemokines such as MIP-1α which are ligands for CCR5 and may help draw cells into the gut. More importantly however, colon and small bowel epithelium secrete distinctive chemokines which may attract and retain different lymphocyte subsets. Mucosae associated epithelial chemokine (MEC) is expressed in the colonic epithelium but not small bowel epithelium.[77b] MEC supports migration of memory lymphocytes which express CCR3. However CCR3 is not expressed on human gut lymphocytes,[1a] which might explain the relative paucity of T cells in normal colon. In contrast small bowel epithelium expresses thymus-expressed chemokine(TECK) which is a ligand for CCR9, a chemoreceptor present on all IEL and LPL in the small bowel in man.[57c] Colon T cells however rarely express CCR9. This would help explain the abundance of T cells in normal human small bowel compared to colon.

Intestinal lamina propria

The lamina propria is the layer of connective tissue between the epithelium and muscularis mucosa. It is made of smooth muscle cells, fibroblasts, lymphatics and blood vessels, and makes up the villus core over which the absorptive epithelial cells migrate from the crypts to the villus tips. The most striking feature of adult human large and small intestinal lamina propria is the infiltrate of lymphoid/myeloid cells. The large numbers of macrophages, dendritic cells and T cells in the lamina propria make it likely that antigen crossing the epithelium may be processed and presented to lamina propria CD4[+] T cells. These

Table 1.1 Changes in intestinal α/β and $\gamma\delta$ TCR diversity during development in man.

Changes in intestinal α/β and $\gamma\delta$ TCR diversity during development in man		
Age of development	T cell receptor expression	
	α/β	$\gamma\delta$
5–16 weeks' gestation	Rearranged TCR β mRNA detectable at 13 weeks Polyclonal TCR β usage Extensive N region addition No TCR α rearrangement IEL Vβ expression more restricted than LPL TEA and TEB expression abundant Incomplete TCR α J–C rearrangements transcribed	10–30% IEL express $\gamma\delta$ TCR at 14 weeks Polyclonal $\gamma\delta$ expression Simple V(D)J junctions without N region additions
16 weeks' gestation–term	TEA less common TEB less common Rearranged V–J–C α transcripts detectable TCR α transcripts restricted in diversity before 23 weeks	Polyclonal δ repertoire expressed No N region additions Template encoded P additions at V(D)J joins Canonical Vδ2 transcripts detectable
Birth–teens	TEA and TEB less abundant though still detectable All TCR Vβ and Vα segments utilized Polyclonal TCR Vα/β usage at birth, IEL becoming oligoclonal with age	(1 day–4 weeks) N region additions detectable at V(D)J junctions Polyclonal TCR Vδ usage at birth becoming oligoclonal with time TCR δ expression oligoclonal by mid-teens
Adulthood	TEA and TEB rare but detectable α/β TCR IEL oligoclonal with identical dominant clones throughout the gut LPLs polyclonal	$\gamma\delta$ T cells 5–10% IELs Highly restricted TCR δ expression Identical dominant clones throughout the gut Clonality stable over time (>1 year)

IEL, intraepithelial lymphocytes; LPL, lamina propria lymphocytes; TEA, T early alpha; TEB, T early beta.

cells could then provide B cell help as well as functioning in mucosal cell-mediated immunity.

Plasma cells in the lamina propria

As was first observed almost 35 years ago, the major plasma cell isotype and hence the major immunoglobulin isotype in the intestinal secretions is IgA.[24,110] IgA plasma cells make up 30–40% of the mononuclear cells in human intestinal lamina propria. In the jejunum around 80% of the total plasma cells secrete IgA, around 18% secrete IgM and only 3% secrete IgG.[12,25] These same relative proportions are also seen in the ileum and the colon, although there are fewer IgM plasma cells than in the proximal small intestine. In addition, immediately adjacent to lymphoid follicles throughout the gut there is an increase in IgG plasma cells.[5] IgD or IgE plasma cells are very uncommon. Most of the plasma cells, regardless of isotype, are found in the region around the crypts. Slightly more than half of the IgA plasma cells in the gut secrete IgA2,[25] in contrast to tonsils and lymph nodes where most of the IgA is IgA1. The majority of IgA secreted by the plasma cells is dimeric IgA; 100% of IgA2 immunocytes are J chain-positive and 88% of IgA1 immunocytes are J chain-positive.[52] Dimeric IgA binds specifically via a J chain-secretory component interaction to the basolateral aspect of crypt epithelial cells and is actively transported into the lumen.

There are no plasma cells in the lamina propria at birth,[82] although there is a rapid expansion thereafter. There is also a dramatic reduction in IgA plasma cells in the lamina propria of children with defunctioned colostomies.[118]

T cells in the lamina propria

Scattered throughout the lamina propria of the small bowel and colon are large numbers of T cells. These are mostly CD4+, $\alpha\beta$TcR+. A minority are CD8+ and express the αEβ7 integrin, suggesting that they may be in transit to the epithelium.[32] All the evidence available points strongly to the fact that lamina propria CD4+ T cells in postnatal intestine are derived from Peyer's patch T blasts which have extravasated from the blood using α4β7 integrin binding to MAdCAM 1. Functionally, unstimulated, freshly isolated lamina propria T cells contain a very high frequency of cells which secrete IFNγ, with tenfold less secreting IL4.[18,40] Phenotypically, lamina propria T cells also have all the characteristics of antigen-activated cells. They are L-selectin,[lo] α4β7+, CD25[lo], some are DR+.[4,14,92] They are not dividing. Virtually all express *Fas* and some are *FasL*+.[11] Both unstimulated

A

11

and anti-CD2-activated lamina propria lymphocytes undergo apoptosis *in vitro*, which can be partially reversed with IL2.[11] It is well known that activated T cells are destined to die by apoptosis unless rescued by antigen or common γ chain cytokines such as IL2, IL7 or IL15. The expression of *Fas* and the increased apoptosis of lamina propria T cells is therefore consistent with the idea that, although these cells were generated in the Peyer's patches in response to antigen, in the normal situation, when they extravasate into the lamina propria, the lack of antigen and stimulatory cytokines leads them to enter a default apoptotic pathway. Although data in post-natal intestine is clear that lamina propria T cells are memory/activated type cells, the situation does appear to be different in the fetus. Human small bowel contains extremely large numbers of T cells from about 17 weeks gestion. These cells are dividing, and also have an activated phenoptype, but do not express α4β7. There is circumstantial evedence that mucosal T cells in the fetus are generated from CD3-, 7+ precursor abendant in fetal gut lamina propria.[42a] This process however seems to shut down at birth.

Macrophages and dendritic cells in the lamina propria

The majority of the HLADR[+] cells in the lamina propria of the large and small intestine are macrophages and dendritic cells.[95] It should be emphasized, however, that the distinction between these two cell types in the lamina propria is vague and controversial. It is difficult to isolate these cells in any great number and so most studies have used immunohistological and/or immunochemical techniques to characterize these cells.

The relative proportions of dendritic-type cells to phagocytic-type cells in human gut is unclear. It appears that below the epithelium there is a population of cells with features of classical phagocytic macrophages. Wilders *et al.*[117] first showed that, at the tops of the villi in normal intestine, there is a population of DR[+], strongly acid phosphatase[+] cells. These are probably phagocytic macrophages identical to the population of 25F9[+] cells (a marker of mature macrophages) also identified by others.[43] More recently it has been shown that subepithelial macrophages contain debris of epithelial cells.[71] Thus, although it has traditionally been thought that shed epithelial cells are sloughed into the lumen, it may be that they are ingested by macrophages through processes which extend from the macrophage through the basement membrane and into the epithelium. In contrast, Selby *et al.*[95] reported that, in the normal human small intestine, 80–90% of the DR[+] histiocytes were weakly acid phosphatase[+], weakly non-specific esterase[+], and strongly membrane ATPase[+], suggesting that they are dendritic cells. In normal colon, Selby also reported that most of the DR[+] cells were strongly acid phosphatase and esterase[+] and were weakly ATPase[+].

In the absence of good markers it is difficult to give definitive answers about the distribution of dendritic cells in the mucosa. There is a population of strongly class II[+] cells with long processes around the crypts, and Pavli and colleagues[80] reported that these cells expressed S-100 protein, suggestive that they were more dendritic-like. These results have been extended by Sarsfield and colleagues,[91] who have shown that a similar population of cells expresses CD68 (a classical macrophage marker), but also express factor XIIIa, a marker of dermal dendritic cells in man. However, since it is now known that dendritic cells can be derived from a large number of different cell lineages *in vitro*, it is clear that dendritic cell morphology and function are probably more important than surface markers. The challenge remains to isolate these cells from the gut for functional studies.

REFERENCES

1 Arato A, Savilahti E, Taenio V-M, Verkasalo M, Klemola T. HLA-DR expression, natural killer cells and IgE containing cells in the jejunal mucosa of coeliac children. *Gut* 1987; 28: 988–94.

1a Agace WW, Roberts AI, Wu Lijun, Greineder C, Ebert EC, Parker CM. Human intestinal lamina propria and intraepithelial lymphocytes express receptors specific for chemokines induced by inflammation. *Eur J Immunol* 2000; 30: 819–826

1b Arstila T, Arstila TP, Calbo S, Selz f, Malassis-Seris M, Vassalli P, Kourilsky P, Guy-Grand D. Identical T cell clones are located within the mouse gut epithelium and lamina propria and circulate in the thoracic duct lymph. *J Exp Med* 2000; 191: 823–34

2 Autenrieth IB, Firsching R. Penetration of M cells and destruction of Peyer's patches by *Yersinia enterocolitica*: an ultrastructural and histologic study. *J Med Micro* 1996; 44: 285–94.

3 Balk SP, Ebert EC, Blumenthal RL *et al.* Oligoclonal expansion and CD1 recognition by human intestinal intraepithelial lymphocytes. *Science* 1991; 253: 1411–15.

4 Berg M, Murakawa Y, Camerini D, James SP. Lamina propria lymphocytes are derived from circulating cells that lack the Leu-8 lymph node homing receptor. *Gastroenterology* 1991; 101: 90–99.

5 Bjerke K, Brandtzaeg P. Immunoglobulin- and J chain-producing cells associated with lymphoid follicles in the human appendix, colon and ileum, including Peyer's patches. *Clin Exp Immunol* 1986; 64: 432–41.

6 Bjerke K, Brandtzaeg P, Rognum TO. Distribution of immunoglobulin producing cells is different in normal human appendix and colon mucosa. *Gut* 1986; 27: 667–74.

7 Bjerke K, Brandtzaeg P. Lack of relation between expression of HLA-DR and secretory component (SC) in follicle-associated epithelium of human Peyer's patches. *Clin Exp Immunol* 1988; 71: 502–07.

8 Bjerke K, Brandtzaeg P, Fausa O. T cell distribution is different in follicle-associated epithelium of human Peyer's patches and villous epithelium. *Clin Exp Immunol* 1988; 74: 270–75.

9 Blumberg RS, Terhorst C, Bleicher P *et al.* Expression of a nonpolymorphic MHC Class 1-like molecule, CD1D, by human intestinal epithelial cells. *J Immunol* 1991; 147: 2518–24.

10 Blumberg RS, Yockey CE, Gross GG, Ebert EC, Balk SP. Human intestinal intraepithelial lymphocytes are derived from a limited number of T cell clones that utilize multiple V beta T cell receptor genes. *J Immunol* 1993; 150: 5144–53.

11 Boirivant M, Pica R, DeMaria R, Testi R, Pallone F, Strober W. Stimulated human lamina propria T cells manifest enhanced Fas-mediated apoptosis. *J Clin Invest* 1996; 98: 2616–22.

11a Borghesi C, Taussig MJ, Nicoletti C. Rapid appearance of M cells after microbial challenge is restricted at the periphery of the follicle-associated epithelium of Peyer's patch. *Lab Invest* 1999; 79: 1393–401

12 Brandtzaeg P. The B cell system. In: *Food Allergy and Intolerance*, (J. Brostoff and S. J. Challacombe, eds) Bailliére Tindall, London: 1987, 118–55.

13 Brandtzaeg P, Bosnes V, Halstensen TS, Scott H, Sollid LM, Valnes KN. T lymphocytes in human gut epithelium express preferentially the αβ antigen receptor and are often CD45/UCHL 1-positive. *Scand J Immunol* 1989; 30: 123–28.

14 Brandtzaeg P, Farstad IN, Helgeland L. Phenotypes of T cells in the gut. In: *Chemical Immunology – Mucosal T Cells* (T.T. MacDonald, ed.) Karger, Basel, 1998; 1–26.

15 Bridges RA, Condie RM, Zak SJ, Good RA. The morphologic basis of antibody formation development during the neonatal period. *J Lab Clin Med* 1959; 53: 331–59.

15a Bromander AK, Ekman L, Kopj M, Nedrud JG, Lycke NY. IL-6-deficient mice exhibit normal mucosal IgA responses to local immunizations and Helicobacter felis infection. *J Immunol* 1996; 156: 4290–7.

16 Butcher EJ, Picker LJ. Lymphocyte homing and homeostasis. *Science* 1996; 272: 60–66.

17 Bye WA, Allan CH, Trier JS. Structure, distribution, and origin of M cells in Peyer's patches of mouse ileum. *Gastroenterology* 1984; 86: 789–801.

18 Carol M, Lambrechts A, Van Gossum A, Libin M, Goldman M, Mascart-Lemone F. Spontaneous secretion of interferon-gamma and interleukin-4 by human intraepithelial and lamina propria gut lymphocytes. *Gut* 1998; 32: 643–9.

19 Cepek KL, Shaw SK, Parker CM et al. Adhesion between epithelial cells and T lymphocytes mediated by E-cadherin and αEβ7 integrin. *Nature* 1994; 372: 190–93.

20 Cerf-Bensussan N, Quaroni A, Kurnick JT, Bhan AK. Intraepithelial lymphocytes modulate Ia expression by intestinal epithelial cells. *J Immunol* 1984; 132: 2244–52.

21 Chowers Y, Holtmeier W, Harwood J, Morzycka-Wroblewska E, Kagnoff MF. The Vδ 1 T cell receptor repertoire in human small intestine and colon. *J Exp Med* 1994; 180: 183–90.

21a Colgan SP, Hershberg RM, Furtura GT, Blumberg RS. Ligation of intestinal epithelial CD1d induces bioactive IL-1: critical role of the cytoplasmic tail in autocrine signalling. *Proc Natl Acad Sci USA* 1999; 96: 13938–43.

22 Cornes JS. Number, size, and distribution of Peyer's patches in the human small intestine. The development of Peyer's patches. *Gut* 1965; 6: 225–29.

23 Cornes JS. Number, size and distribution of Peyer's patches in the human small intestine. The effect of age on Peyer's patches. *Gut* 1965; 6: 230–33.

24 Crabbe PA, Heremans JF. The distribution of immunoglobulin containing cells along the human gastrointestinal tract. *Gastroenterology* 1966; 51: 305–16.

25 Crago SS, Kutteh WH, Moro I et al. Distribution of IgA1-, IgA2-, and J chain-containing cells in human tissues. *J Immunol* 1984; 132: 16–18.

25a Debard N, Sierro F, Browning J, Kraehenbuhl JP. Effect of mature lymphocytes and lymphotoxin on the development of the follicle-associated epithelium and M cells in mouse Peyer's patch. *Gastroenterology* 2001; 120: 1173–82.

26 Deusch K, Luling F, Reich K, Classen M, Wagner H, Pfeffer K. A major fraction of human intraepithelial lymphocytes simultaneously express the γδ T cell receptor, the CD8 accessory molecule and preferentially uses the Vδ1 gene segment. *Eur J Immunol* 1990; 21: 1053–59.

27 de Villartay J, Lewis D, Hockett RD, Waldmann TA, Korsmeyer SJ, Cohen DI. Deletional rearrangement in the human T cell receptor α chain locus. *Proc Natl Acad Sci USA* 1987; 84: 8608–12.

28 de Villartay J, Cohen DI. Gene regulation within the TCR α/δ locus by specific deletion of the TCR δ cluster. *Res Immunol* 1990; 141: 618–23.

29 Dukes C, Bussey HJR. The number of lymphoid follicles of the human large intestine. *J Pathol Bact* 1926; 29: 111–16.

30 Dunn-Walters DK, Boursier L, Spencer J. Hypermutation, diversity and dissemination of human intestinal lamina propria plasma cells. *Eur J Immunol* 1997; 27: 2959–64.

31 Farstad I, Halstensen TS, Fausa O, Brandtzaeg P. Heterogeneity of M-cell associated B and T cells in human Peyer's patches. *Immunology* 1994; 83: 457–64.

32 Farstad IN, Halstensen TS, Lien B, Kilshaw PJ, Lazarovitz AI, Brandtzaeg P. Distribution of β7 integrins in human intestinal mucosa and organised gut-associated lymphoid tissue. *Immunology* 1996; 89: 227–37.

33 Farstad IN, Norstein J, Brandtzaeg P. Phenotypes of B and T cells in human intestinal and mesenteric lymph. *Gastroenterology* 1997; 112: 163–73.

33a Framson PE, Cho DH, Lee LY, Hershberg RM. Polarized expression aand function of the costimulator molecule CD58 on human intestinal epithelial cells. *Gastroenterology* 1999; 116: 1054–62.

33b Golovkina TV, Shlomchik M, Hannum L, Chervonsy A. Organogenic role of B lymphocytes in mucosal immunity. *Science* 1999; 286: 1965–8.

34 Groh V, Porcelli S, Fabbi M et al. Human lymphocytes bearing the T cell receptor γ/δ are phenotypically diverse and evenly distributed throughout the lymphoid system. *J Exp Med* 1989; 169: 1277–94.

35 Groh V, Bahram S, Bauer S, Herman A, Beauchamp M, Spies T. Cell stress-regulated human major histocompatability complex class I gene expressed in gastrointestinal epithelium. *Proc Natl Acad Sci USA* 1996; 93: 12445–50.

36 Groh V, Steinle A, Bauer S, Spies T. Recognition of stress-induced MHC molecules by intestinal epithelial γδ T cells. *Science* 1998; 279: 1737–40.

37 Gross GG, Schwartz VL, Stevens C, Ebert EC, Blumberg RS, Balk SP. Distribution of dominant T cell receptor beta chains in human intestinal mucosa. *J Exp Med* 1994; 180: 1337–44.

38 Halstensen TS, Scott H, Brandtzaeg P. Intraepithelial T cells of the TcRγ/δ + CD8- and Vδ 1/Jδ 1+ phenotypes are increased in coeliac disease. *Scand J Gastroenterol* 1989; 30: 665–72.

39 Hassal E, Dimmick JE. Unique features of *Helicobacter pylori* disease in children. *Dig Dis Sciences* 1991; 36: 417–23.

40 Hauer AC, Breese EJ, Walker-Smith JA, MacDonald TT. The frequency of cells secreting interferon-γ, IL-4, IL-5 and IL-10 in the blood and duodenal mucosa of children with cows' milk hypersensitivity. *Ped Res* 1997; 42: 629–38.

40a Ershberg RM, Cho DH, Youakin A, Bradley MB, Lee JS, Framson, H Nepom GT. Highly polarized HLA class II antigen processing and presentation by human intestinal epithelial cells. *J Clin Invest* 1998; 102: 792–803.

41 Holtmeier W, Yehuda C, Lumeny A, Morzycka-Wroblewska E, Kagnoff MF. The δ T cell receptor repertoire in human colon and peripheral blood is oligoclonal irrespective of V region usage. *J Clin Invest* 1995; 96: 1108–17.

42 Holtmeier W, Witthöft T, Hennemann A, Winter HS, Kagnoff MF. The TCR-δ repertoire in human intestine undergoes characteristic changes during fetal to adult development. *J Immunol* 1997; 158: 5632–41.

42a Howie D, Spencer J, DeLord D, Pitzalis C, Wathen NC, Dogan A, Akbar A, MacDonald TT. Extrathymic T cell differentiation in the human intestine early in life. *J Immunol* 1998; 161: 5862–72.

43 Hume DA, Allan W, Hogan PG, Doe WF. Immunohistochemical characterisation of macrophages in human liver and gastrointestinal tract, expression of CD4, HLA-DR, OKM1, and the mature macrophage marker 25F9 in normal and diseased tissue. *J Leukocyte Biol* 1987; 42: 474–84.

43a Iwasaki A, Kelsall BL. Localization of distinct Peyer's patch dendritic cell subsets and their recruitment by chemokines macrophage inflammatory protein (MIP)-3 alpha, MIP-3 beta and secondary lymphoid organ chemokine. *J Exp Med* 2000; 191: 1381–94.

43b Iwasaki A, Kelsall BL. Unique functions of CD11b(+), CD8α+, and double-negative Peyer's patch dendritic cells. *J Immunol* 2001; 166: 4884–90.

44 Jacob E, Baker SJ, Swaminathan SP 'M' cells in the follicle-associated epithelium of the human colon. *Histopathology* 1987; 11: 941–52.

45 Jones BD, Ghori N, Falkow S. *Salmonella typhimurium* initiates murine infection by penetrating and destroying the specialised M cells of the Peyer's patches. *J Exp Med* 1994; 180: 15–23.

46 Janossy G, Tidman N, Selby WS et al. Human T lymphocytes of inducer and suppressor type occupy different microenvironments. *Nature* 1980; 288: 81–84.

47 Jarry A, Cerf-Bensussan N, Brousse N, Selz F, Guy-Grand D. Subsets of CD3+ (T cell receptor α/β or γ/δ) and CD3-lymphocytes isolated from normal human gut epithelium display phenotypical features different from their counterparts in peripheral blood. *Eur J Immunol* 1990; 20: 1097–1104.

48 Jung HC, Eckmann L, Yang S-K et al. A distinct array of pro-inflammatory cytokines is expressed in human colon epithelial cells in response to bacterial invasion. *J Clin Invest* 1995; 95: 55–65.

49 Kanamori Y, Ishimaru K, Nanno M et al. Identification of novel lymphoid tissues in murine intestinal mucosa where clusters of c-kit+ IL-7R+Thy1+ lympho-hemopoetic progenitors develop. *J Exp Med* 1996; 184: 1449–59.

50 Kazi JI, Sinniah R, Jaffrey NA *et al.* Cellular and humoral immune responses in *Campylobacter pylori*-associated chronic gastritis. *J Pathol* 1989; 159: 231–37.

51 Kereneis S, Bogdanova A, Kraehenbuhl J-P, Pringault E. Conversion by Peyer's patch lymphocytes of human enterocytes into M cells that transport bacteria. *Science* 1997; 277: 949–52.

52 Kett K, Brandtzaeg P, Fausa O. J-chain expression is more prominent in immunoglobulin A2 than in immunoglobulin A1 colonic immunocytes and is decreased in both subclasses associated with inflammatory bowel disease. *Gastroenterol* 1988; 94: 1419–25.

53 Koni PA, Sacca R, Lawton P, Browning JL, Ruddle NH, Flavell RA. Distinct roles in lymphoid organogenesis for lymphotoxins α and β revealed in lymphotoxin β-deficient mice. *Immunity* 1997; 6: 491–500.

54 Koni PA, Flavell RA. A role for tumor necrosis factor receptor type 1 in gut-associated lymphoid tissue development: genetic evidence of synergism with lymphotoxin β. *J Exp Med* 1998; 187: 1977–83.

55 Koningsberger JC, Chott A, Logtenberg T *et al.* TCR expression in human fetal intestine and identification of an early T cell receptor β-chain transcript. *J Immunol* 1997; 159: 1775–82.

56 Krangel MS, Yssel H, Brocklehurst C, Spits H. A distinct wave of human T cell receptor γδ lymphocytes in the early fetal thymus: evidence for controlled gene rearrangement and cytokine production. *J Exp Med* 1990; 172: 847–59.

57 Kroese FG, Butcher EC, Stall AM, Lalor PA, Adams S, Herzenberg LA. Many of the IgA producing plasma cells in murine gut are derived from self-replenishing precursors in the peritoneal cavity. *Int Immunol* 1989; 1: 75–84.

57a Kunkel EJ, Campbell JJ, Haraldsen G, Pan J, Boisvert J, Robert AI, Ebert EC, Vierra MA, Goodman SB, Genovese MC, Wardlwa AJ, Greenberg HB, Parker CM, Butcher EC, Andrew DP, Agace WW. Lymphocyte CC Chemokine Receptor 9 and Epithelial Thymus-expressed Chemokine (TECK) Expression Distinguish the Small Intestinal immune Compartment: Epithelial expression of Tissue-specific Chemokines as an organizing Principles in Regional immunity. *J Exp.* 2001; 192: 761–7.

58 Lafaille JJ, Decloux A, Bonneville M, Takagaki Y, Tonegawa S. Junctional sequences of T cell receptor γδ genes: implications for γδ T cell lineages and for a novel intermediate of V(D)J joining. *Cell* 1989; 59: 859–70.

59 Lefrancois L, Puddington L. Extrathymic T-cell development: virtual reality? *Immunology Today* 1995; 16: 16–21.

60 Li Y, Yio XY, Mayer L. Human intestinal epithelial cell-induced CD8+ T cell activation is mediated through CD8 and the activation of CD8-associated p56lck. *J Exp Med* 1995; 182: 1079–88.

61 Loh EY, Elliott JF, Cwirla S, Lanier LL, Davis MM. Polymerase chain reaction with single sided specificity: analysis of the T cell receptor delta chain. *Science* 1989; 243: 217–20.

62 Lundqvist C, Melgar S, Yeung MM-W, Hammarstrom S, Hammarstrom M-L. Intraepithelial lymphocytes in human gut have lytic potential and a cytokine profile that suggests T helper 1 and cytotoxic functions. *J Immunol* 1996; 157: 1926–34.

62a Ludviksson BR, Strober W, Nishikomori R, Hasan SK, Ehrhardt RO. Administration of mAb against alpha E beta 7 prevents and ameliorates immunization-induced colitis in IL-2-/-mice. *J Immunol* 1999; 162: 4975–82

63 Lynch S, Kelleher D, McManus R, O'Farrelly C. RAG1 and RAG2 expression in human intestinal epithelium: evidence of extrathymic T cell differentiation. *Eur J Immunol* 1995; 25: 1143–47.

63a MacDonald TT, Monteleone G. Interleukin-12 and Th1 immune responses in human Peyer's patches. *Trends in Immunology* 2001; 22: 244–247.

64 MacDonald TT, Weinel A, Spencer JM. HLA-DR expression in human fetal intestinal epithelium. *Gut* 1988; 29: 1342–48.

64a Macpherson AJ, Gatto D, Sainsbury E, Harriman GR, Hengartner H, Zinkkernagel RM. A prinitive T cell-independant mechanism of intestinal mucosal IgA responses to commensal bacteria. *Science* 2000; 288: 2222–6.

65 Maric I, Holt PG, Perdue MH, Bienenstock J. Class II MHC antigen (Ia)-bearing cells in the epithelium of the rat intestine. *J Immunol* 1996; 156: 1408–14.

66 Marra A, Isberg RR. Invasin-dependent and invasin-independent pathways for translocation of *Yersinia pseudotuberculosis* across the Peyer's patch intestinal epithelium. *Infect Immun* 1997; 65: 3412–21.

67 Mayrhofer G. Peyer's patch organogenesis-cytokines rule, OK? *Gut* 1997; 47: 707–09.

68 McVay LD, Carding SR. Extrathymic origin of human γδ T cells during fetal development. *J Immunol* 1996; 157: 2873–82.

69 Mirakian R, Richardson A, Milla PJ *et al.* Protracted diarrhoea of infancy, evidence in support of an autoimmune variant. *BMJ* 1986; 293: 1132–36.

70 Mizoguchi A, Mizoguchi E, Chiba C, Bhan AK. Role of appendix in the development of inflammatory bowel disease in TCR-alpha mutant mice. *J Exp Med* 1996; 184: 707–15.

71 Nagashima R, Maeda K, Imai Y, Takahashi T. Lamina propria macrophages in the human gastrointestinal mucosa: their distribution, immunohistological phenotype, and function. *J Histochem Cytochem* 1996; 44: 721–31.

71a Nagata S, McKenzie C, Pender SLF, Bajaj-Eliott M, Fairclough PD. Walker-Smith JA. Monteleone G, MacDonald TT. Human Peyer's patch T cells are sensitised to dietary antigen and display a Th cell type I cytokine profile. *J Immunol* 1999; 117: 536–45.

71b Nakazawa A, Watanabe M, Kanai T, Yajima T, Yamakazi M, Ogata H, Ishil H, Zauma M, Hibi T. Functional expression of costimulatory molecule CD86 on epithelial cells in the inflamed colonic mucosa. *American gastroenterological Association* 1999; 0016–5085/99.

72 Neumann B, Luz A, Pfeffer K, Holzmann B. Defective Peyer's patch organogenesis in mice lacking the 55-Kd receptor for tumor necrosis factor. *J Exp Med* 1996; 184: 259–64.

73 Ohmen JD, Barnes PF, Uyemura K, Lu S, Grisso CC, Modlin RL. The T cell receptor of human gamma/delta T cells reactive to *Mycobacterium tuberculosis* are encoded by specific V genes but diverse V-J junctions. *J Immunol* 1991; 147: 3353–59.

74 O'Leary AD, Sweeney EC. Lymphoglandular complexes of the colon, structure and distribution. *Histopathology* 1986; 10: 267–83.

75 Owen RL, Jones AL. Epithelial cell specialization within human Peyer's patches, an ultrastructural study of intestinal lymphoid follicles. *Gastroenterol* 1974; 66: 189–203.

76 Owen RL. Sequential uptake of horseradish peroxidase by lymphoid follicle epithelium of Peyer's patches in normal unobstructed mouse intestine, An ultrastructural study. *Gastroenterol* 1977; 72: 440–51.

77 Owen RL, Apple RT, Bhalla DK. Morphometric and cytochemical analysis of lysosomes in rat Peyer's patch follicle epithelium, their reduction in volume fraction and acid phosphatase content in M cells compared to adjacent enterocytes. *Anatomical Record* 1986; 216: 521–27.

77a Pachynski RK, Wu SW, Gunn MD, Erle DJ. Secondary lymphoid-tissue chemokine(SLC) stimulates integrin alpha 4 beta 7-mediated adhesion of lymphocytes to mucosal addressin cell adhesion molecule-1 (MAdCAM-1) under flow. *J Immunol* 1998; 161: 952–6.

77b Pan J, Kunkel EJ, Gosslar U, Lazarus N, Langdon P, Broadwell K, Vierra MA, Genovese MC, Butcher EC, Soler D. A novel chemokine ligand for CCR10 and CCR3 expressed by epithelial cells in mucosal tissues. *J Immunol* 2000; 165: 2493–9.

78 Panja A, Blumberg RS, Balk SP, Mayer L. CD1d is involved in T cell–intestinal epithelial cell interactions. *J Exp Med* 1993; 178: 1115–19.

79 Pasparakis M, Alexopoulou L, Grell M, Pfizenmaier K, Bluethmann H, Kolias G. Peyer's patch organogenesis is intact yet formation of B lymphocyte follicles is defective in peripheral lymphoid organs of mice deficient for tumor necrosis factor and 55 kDa receptor. *Proc Natl Acad Sci USA* 1997; 94: 6319–23.

80 Pavli P, Maxwell L, Van de Pol E, Doe W. Distribution of human colonic dendritic cells and macrophages. *Clin Exp Immunol* 1996; 104: 124–32.

81 Penney LM, Kilshaw PJ, MacDonald TT. Regional variation in the proliferative rate and lifespan of alpha beta TCR+ and gamma delta TCR+ intraepithelial lymphocytes in the murine small intestine. *Immunology* 1995; 86: 212–18.

82 Perkkio M, Savilahti E. Time of appearance of immunoglobulin-containing cells in the mucosa of the neonatal intestine. *Pediatric Res* 1980; 14: 953–55.

83 Poggi A, Sargiacomo M, Biassoni R et al. Extrathymic differentiation of T lymphocytes and natural killer cells from human embryonic liver precursors. Proc Natl Acad Sci USA 1993; 90: 4465–69.

84 Poulsen LO, Elling P, Sorensen FB, Hoedt-Rasmussen K. HLA-DR expression and disease activity in ulcerative colitis. Scand J Gastroenterol 1986; 21: 364–68.

85 Poussier P, Edouard P, Lee C, Binnie M, Julius M. Thymus-independent development and negative selection of T cells expressing T cell receptor alpha/beta in the intestinal epithelium; evidence for distinct circulation patterns of gut - and thymus-derived T lymphocytes. J Exp Med 1992; 176: 187–99.

85a Ramsay AJ, Husband AJ, Ramshaw IA, Bao S, Matthaei KI, Koehl G, Kopj M. The role of interleukin-6 in mucosal IgA antibody responses vivo. Science 1994; 264: 561–3.

86 Ricken G, Pluschke G, Krawinkel U. T cell receptor alpha chain germ line transcripts from activated lymphocytes. Immunol Lett 1992; 32: 97–98.

87 Rock EP, Sibbald PR, Davis MM, Chien YH. CDR3 length in antigen specific immune receptors. J Exp Med 1994; 179: 323–28.

88 Roman-Roman S, Ferradini L, Azocar J, Genevee C, Hercend T, Triebel F. Studies on the human T cell receptor alpha/beta variable region genes. I. Identification of 7 additional V alpha subfamilies and 14 J alpha gene segments. Eur J Immunol 1991; 21: 927–33.

89 Russel MG, Dorant E, Brummer RJ et al. Appendectomy and the risk of developing ulcerative colitis or Crohn's disease: results of a large case-control study. Gastroenterol 1997; 113: 377–82.

90 Saito H, Kanamori Y, Takemori T et al. Generation of intestinal T cells from progenitors residing in gut cryptopatches. Science 1998; 280: 275–78.

91 Sarsfield P, Rinne A, Jones DB, Johnson P, Wright DH. Accessory cells in physiological lymphoid tissue from the intestine: an immunohistochemical study. Histopathology 1996; 28: 205–11.

92 Schieferdecker HL, Ullrich R, Hirseland H, Zeitz M. T cell differentiation antigens on lymphocytes in the human intestinal lamina propria. J Immunol 1992; 149: 2816–22.

93 Scott H, Solheim BG, Brandtzaeg P, Thorsby E. HLA-DR-like antigens in the epithelium of the human small intestine. Scand J Immunol 1980; 12: 77–82.

94 Scott H, Sollid LM, Fausa O et al. Expression of major histocompatibility Class II subregion products by jejunal epithelium in patients with coeliac disease. Scand J Immunol 1987; 26: 563–71.

95 Selby WS, Poulter LW, Hobbs S, Jewell DP, Janossy G. Heterogeneity of HLA-DR-positive histiocytes in human intestinal lamina propria, a combined histochemical and immunohistological analysis. J Clin Path 1983; 36: 379–84.

96 Selby WS, Janossy G, Mason DY, Jewell DP. Expression of HLA-DR antigens by colonic epithelium in inflammatory bowel disease. Clin Exp Immunol 1983; 53: 614–18.

97 Selby WS, Janossy G, Bofill M, Jewell DP. Intestinal lymphocyte subpopulations in inflammatory bowel disease, an analysis by immunohistological and cell isolation techniques. Gut 1984; 25: 32–40.

98 Shimizu T, Takeshita S, Muto M, Kibo E, Sado T, Yamagishi H. Mouse germline transcript of TCRα joining region and temporal expression in ontogeny. Int Immunol 1993; 5: 155–60.

99 Sicinski P, Rowinski J, Warchol JB et al. Poliovirus type 1 enters the human host through intestinal M cells. Gastroenterol 1990; 98: 56–58.

100 Sollid LM, Kvale D, Brandzaeg P, Markussen G, Thorsby E. Interferon-γ enhances expression of secretory component, the epithelial receptor for polymeric immunoglobulins. J Immunol 1987; 138: 4303–06.

101 Spencer J, Finn T, Isaacson PG. Gut associated lymphoid tissue, a morphological and immunocytochemical study of the human appendix. Gut 1985; 26: 672–79.

102 Spencer J, Finn T, Isaacson PG. Expression of HLA-DR antigens on epithelium associated with lymphoid tissue in the human gastrointestinal tract. Gut 1986; 27: 153–57.

103 Spencer J, Finn T, Isaacson PG. Human Peyer's patches, an immunohistochemical study. Gut 1986; 27: 405–10.

104 Spencer J, Finn T, Isaacson PG. A comparative study of the gut-associated lymphoid tissue of primates and rodents. Virchows Arch [Cell Pathol] 1986; 51: 509–19.

105 Spencer J, Pugh S, Isaacson PG. HLA-D region antigen expression on stomach epithelium in absence of autoantibodies. Lancet 1986; II: 983.

106 Spencer J, Isaacson PG, Diss TC, MacDonald TT. Expression of disulphide linked and non-disulphide linked forms of the T cell receptor gamma/delta heterodimer in human intestinal intraepithelial lymphocytes. Eur J Immunol 1989; 19: 1335–39.

107 Spencer JO, MacDonald TT, Diss TC, Walker-Smith JA, Ciclitira PJ, Isaacson PG. Changes in intraepithelial lymphocyte subpopulations in coeliac disease and enteropathy associated T cell lymphoma (malignant histiocytosis of the intestine). Gut 1989; 30: 339–46.

107a Strauch UG, Mueller RC, Li XY, Cernadas M, Higgins JM, Binion DG, Parker CM. Integrin alpha(E)(CD103)beta(7) mediates adhesion to intestinal microvascular endothelal cell lines via an e-cadherin independent interaction. J Immunol 2001; 166: 3506–14.

108 Tamura N, Holroyd KJ, Banks T, Kirby M, Okayama H, Crystal RG. Diversity in junctional sequences associated with the common V gamma 9 and V delta 2 gene segments in normal blood and lung compared with the limited diversity in a granulomatous disease. J Exp Med 1990; 172: 169–81.

109 Taplin ME, Franz ME, Canning C, Ritz J, Blumberg RS, Balk SP. Evidence against T-cell development in the adult human intestinal mucosa based upon lack of terminal deoxynucleotidyl transferase expression. Immunology 1996; 87: 402–07.

110 Tomasi TB, Tan EM, Soloman EA, Prendergast RA. Characterisation of an immune system common to certain external secretions. J Exp Med 1965; 121: 101–24.

111 Uyemura K, Deans RJ, Band H, Ohmen J, Panchamoorthy G. Evidence for clonal selection of gamma/delta T cells in response to a human pathogen. J Exp Med 1991; 174: 683–92.

112 Vadjy M, Kosco-Vilbois MH, Kopf M, Kohler G, Lycke N. Impaired mucosal immune responses in interleukin-4 targeted mice. J Exp Med 1995; 181: 41–53.

112a VanCott JL, Franco MA, Greenberg HB, Sabbaj S, Tang B, Murray R, McGhee JR. Protective immunity to rotavirus shedding in the absence of interleukin-6: Th 1 cells and immunoglobulin A develop normally. J Virol 2000;74: 5250–6.

113 Van Kerckhove C, Russell GJ, Deusch K et al. Oligoclonality of human intestinal intraepithelial cells. J Exp Med 1992; 175: 57–63.

114 Viney JL, Kilshaw PK, MacDonald TT. Cytotoxic αβ and γδ T cells in murine intestinal epithelium. Eur J Immunol 1990; 20: 1623–26.

115 Wasef JS, Keren DF, Mailloux JL. Role of M cells in initial antigen uptake and ulcer formation in the rabbit intestinal loop model of shigellosis. Infect Immun 1989; 57: 858–63.

116 Watanabe M, Ueno Y, Yajima T et al. Interleukin 7 is produced by human intestinal epithelial cells and regulates the proliferation of intestinal mucosal lymphocytes. J Clin Invest 1995; 95: 2945–53.

117 Wilders MM, Drexhage HA, Kokje M, Verspaget H, Meuwissen GM. Veiled cells in chronic idiopathic inflammatory bowel disease. Clin Exp Immunol 1984; 55: 377–87.

118 Wijesinha SS, Steer HW. Studies of the immunoglobulin-producing cells of the human intestine, the defunctioned bowel. Gut 1982; 23: 211–14.

119 Wilson A, de Villartay J, Robson MacDonald H. T cell receptor δ gene rearrangement and T early α (TEA) expression in immature αβ lineage thymocytes: implications for αβ/γδ lineage commitment. Immunity 1996; 4: 37–45.

120 Wiman K, Curman B, Forsum U et al. Occurrence of Ia antigens on tissues of non-lymphoid origin. Nature 1978; 276: 711–13.

121 Wolf JL, Rubin DH, Finberg R et al. Intestinal M cells, a pathway for entry of reovirus into host. Science 1981; 212: 471–72.

122 Wotherspoon AC, Ortiz-Hitalgo C, Falzon MR, Isaacson PG. Helicobacter pylori-associated gastritis and primary B cell lymphoma. Lancet 1991; 338: 1175–76.

123 Wyatt JI, Rathbone BJ. Immune response of the gastric mucosa to Campylobacter pylori. Scand J Gastroenterol 1988; 23 (Suppl. 142): 44–49.

123a Yamamoto M, Rennert P, McGhee JR, Kweon MN, Yamamoto S, Dohi T, Otake S, Bluethmann H, Fujihashi K, Kiyono H. Alternate mucosal immune system:organized Peyer's patches are not required for IgA responses in the gastrointestinal tract. *J Immunol* 2000; 164: 5184–91.

124 Yamamoto S, Russ F, Teixeira HC, Conradt P, Kaufmann SH. *Listeria monocytogenes*-induced γ-interferon secretion by intestinal intraepithelial lymphocytes. *Infect Immun* 1993; 61: 2154–61.

124a Yamanaka T, Straumfors A, Morton H, Fausa O, Brandtzaeg P, Farstad I. M cell pockets of human Peyer's patches are specialized extensions of germinal centres. *Eur J Immunol* 2001; 107–17.

125 Yoshikai Y, Kimura N, Toyonaga B, Mak TW. Sequences and repertoire of human T cell receptor alpha chain variable region genes in mature T lymphocytes. *J Exp Med* 1986; 164: 90–103.

Chapter 2

Basic functions of the gut

Jeremy D. Sanderson and Chris Mallinson

INTRODUCTION

This chapter is intended to provide a summary of current understanding of human gastrointestinal physiology. The contents should give the reader an insight into the basic function of the gut and provide a platform from which one can interpret the significance of abnormalities of gut function relating to food intolerance and allergy.

The primary function of the gut is to absorb nutrients. This is achieved by the coordinated activity of motility, secretion and absorption. The introduction of food into the stomach and the expulsion of waste from the colon are purely motor activities. Hence, the oesophagus and anorectal apparatus have no secretory or absorptive functions. The stomach, pancreas, biliary system and the proximal small intestine are the main secretory organs of the gut, rendering a randomly mixed diet absorbable. Motility is coordinated with secretion to facilitate digestion. The first 100 cm of the small intestine are highly adapted to the absorption of nutrients, while the terminal part of the small intestine and the entire colon are involved in reclaiming the large amount of fluid and electrolytes secreted into the proximal gut during the digestive period in response to a meal.

Inevitably, the processes of motility, secretion and absorption are highly integrated in the normal gastrointestinal tract. However, for the purposes of this chapter, the processes will be considered separately.

MOTILITY

The motor activity of the gut is, self-evidently, responsible for the passage of luminal contents through the gut. This is rapid in the oesophagus, whereafter contents are held up in the reservoir of the body of the stomach and are progressively liquidized by the gastric antrum. The antrum also sieves liquid through the remaining solid matter and is responsible for a continuous slow rate of emptying of gastric contents into the duodenum. From here, the food passes down the small intestine to the ileocaecal valve more or less steadily over the succeeding 2–6 hours (Table 2.1). There is evidence that the ileocaecal valve acts as a brake, holding up ileal contents temporarily as well as acting as an antireflux valve. From the caecum onwards, colonic contents move irregularly and more slowly towards the rectum over the next 12 or more hours, undergoing prolonged periods of mixing between brief periods of movement.

Patterns of gastrointestinal motility

Motility in the stomach and small intestine can be divided into two basic types – a *fasting* (or *interdigestive*) pattern and a *fed* pattern.

A

Transit of contents through different parts of the gastrointestinal tract	
Segment	Range of transit time
Oesophagus	4–8 seconds
Stomach	1–2 hours
Small intestine	2–6 hours
Colon	12–24 hours

Table 2.1 Transit of contents through different parts of the gastrointestinal tract.

The fasting pattern

In the fasting state, the smooth muscle of the distal stomach and small intestine exhibits constant, regular, non-contractile electrical activity called *slow-wave activity* resulting from rhythmic changes in membrane potential. In the antrum, these occur at 3 cycles/min, in the duodenum at 12 cycles/min and this rate steadily falls along the small intestine to approximately 8 cycles/min in the distal ileum (Fig. 2.1). Muscular contractions only occur when action potentials (also called spike potentials) occur on the crest of slow waves. In the fasting state, about 10–30% of slow waves lead to spike potentials and contractions (Fig. 2.2). Contractions are therefore phase-locked to slow waves such that the frequency of slow-wave activity in a particular part of the gut imposes a limit on the frequency of contraction at that site. This is important in the small intestine where true peristalsis does not occur but the greater frequency of contraction in the proximal versus distal small intestine results in caudal movement of gut contents even in the absence of peristalsis.[57]

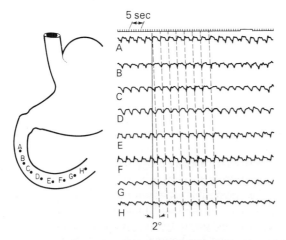

Fig. 2.1 Slow waves recorded simultaneously from closely spaced electrodes in the unanaesthetized cat. Eight monopolar AC-amplified records are shown as recorded from eight chronically implanted needle electrodes spaced uniformly 1 cm apart along the duodenum. Slow-wave configuration is between that of the actual signal and its second derivative. The last few slow waves, at the right, carry spike bursts. Dashed lines are drawn through corresponding slow-wave cycles from each record. The angle, 2°, between these lines and the solid line, the common time-base, is a function of the apparent velocity of spread of slow waves and of the paper speed of the recording polygraph. From Christensen,[9] with permission.

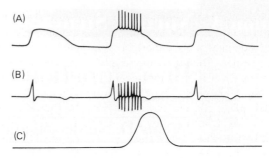

Fig. 2.2 Diagram of time relations between slow waves, spike bursts and contractions. Curve A represents the electromyogram of a single smooth muscle cell, recorded with an intracellular microelectrode. Curve B represents the electromyogram recorded from several cells by a large extracellular volume-recording electrode. Curve C shows tension in the muscle mass. All three traces are drawn to a common time-base. In A, three slow waves appear as a monophasic depolarization from a stable maximal value, the resting membrane potential. Observe that the rate of depolarization is faster than the rate of repolarization. In B, the slow waves appear with two components: an initial biphasic spike, which represents depolarization; and a secondary slower biphasic signal, representing repolarization. The trace shown in B approximates the second derivative of the trace shown in A. The second of the three slow waves bears a burst of spikes, appearing on the plateau of the slow wave. The tension record, in C, shows a contraction beginning during the spike burst, and apparently initiated by it. (From Christensen,[9] with permission.)

The underlying slow-wave activity is added to by a regular sequence of highly organised contractile activity called the *migrating motor complex*.[67]

Migrating motor complexes

The migrating motor complex (MMC) comprises three distinct phases of motor activity occurring in sequence and migrating slowly along the length of the small intestine (Fig. 2.3). A 40-min period of quiescence (phase I) is followed by a period of irregular random contractions (phase II) for a similar time period, which culminates in a short period of intense contractile activity (phase III). Each

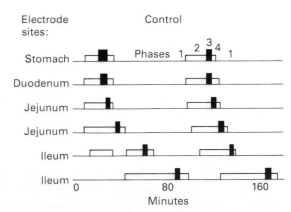

Fig. 2.3 Phases of the interdigestive myoelectric complex at multiple recording sites in the dog. Phase I has slow waves with no action potentials. In Phase II there are an increasing number of slow waves with action potentials. In Phase III each slow wave has action potentials. Phase IV shows a steady diminution in the number of slow waves with action potentials. (From Ref 19, with permission.)

cycle originates in the gastric antrum and proximal duodenum and passes steadily along the intestine at a decreasing velocity, related to the frequency of the underlying slow-wave activity in each part of the intestine. The MMC appears to have a housekeeper function, preventing stasis in the intestine and, hence, preventing bacterial overgrowth. However, Phase III is also accompanied by secretion of gastric juice, bile and pancreatic juice.[36,75] (See also Fig. 2.11.)

The MMC is initiated by a sequence of neural events accompanied by the secretion of the peptide motilin. The propagation of MMC, however, does not depend on motilin but is under intrinsic neural control.[76]

The fed pattern

Feeding almost immediately abolishes the MMC and replaces it with a period of irregular phasic contractile activity mediated by extrinsic autonomic nervous activity, particularly vagal. The intensity of these contractions relates to the nature of the ingested food. Solid food induces much greater activity than a pure liquid meal, and meals high in glucose will induce greater activity than ones high in fat. In the gastric antrum, spike potentials rapidly increase in frequency and soon coincide with every slow wave, to a maximum of 3 cycles/min. Meanwhile, activity is also increased in the duodenum and small intestine, resulting in a more rapid transfer of contents down the small intestine.

The colon

The contractile activity of the colon appears fundamentally different to that of the stomach and small intestine. There are two main types on contraction – haustral contractions and mass contractions – which are superimposed on an underlying pattern of tonic slow pressure variations. Haustral contractions are non-propagating and comprise rapid low-amplitude contractions, resulting in ring-like constrictions along the colon. Mass contractions comprise slow high-amplitude contractions which, in most cases, are propagated aborally towards the rectum at a speed of approximately 1 cm/s.

OESOPHAGEAL FUNCTION

The adult oesophagus is a 24–27 cm muscular tube with tonically contracted sphincters at each end. The oesophagus functions to propel food from mouth to stomach and, importantly, to prevent reflux of gastric contents. The proximal 5% of the oesophagus comprises pure striated muscle, the middle 35–40% mixed striated and smooth muscle and the distal 50–60% pure smooth muscle. The upper oesophageal sphincter (UOS) lies in the region of the cricopharyngeus muscle. The lower oesophageal sphincter (LOS) defines a high-pressure zone at the lower end of the oesophagus, usually just below the diaphragmatic hiatus.

The act of swallowing[49]

Swallowing consists of an *oral phase*, where food is taken into the mouth, chewed to a variable extent and then forced down into the hypopharynx under conscious control. Arrival of food in the hypopharynx triggers the *pharyngeal phase*, in which the food bolus passes through the pharynx by strong peristalsis while simultaneous movements of the soft palate, epiglottis and larynx prevent loss of pressure through the nose and aspiration into the trachea. The UOS then relaxes, allowing passage of the bolus into the upper oesophagus to initiate the *oesophageal phase* of swallowing.

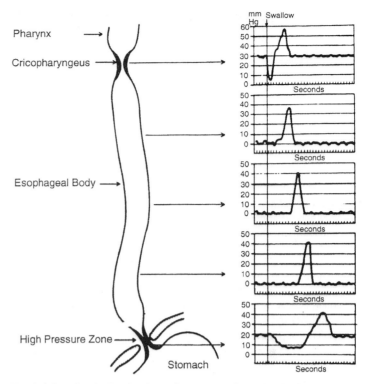

Fig. 2.4 Intraluminal oesophageal pressures in response to swallowing. (From Waters.[77])

In this phase, a true peristaltic contraction moves from the proximal striated muscle to the distal smooth muscle at a rate of 2–4 cm/s, propelling the food bolus down the oesophagus. The LOS relaxes as the peristaltic wave approaches, to allow the bolus to be propelled into the stomach (Fig. 2.4). This is done against a pressure gradient of approximately 12 mmHg from the negative pressure of the thorax to the positive pressure in the abdomen.

Lower oesophageal sphincter

The LOS comprises a zone of high pressure but without any definable conventional muscular sphincter.[21] Instead, the LOS is made up of a specific arrangement of muscle fibres running both as short clasps around the oesophagus and longer gastric sling fibres hooking around the gastric fundus. These two may function as distinct muscle units at the junction of the oesophagus and the stomach.

The LOS is dynamic, asymmetrical and exerts a variable pressure between swallows. The LOS is tonically closed at rest at an average pressure of approximately 20 mmHg. On swallowing, the pressure falls to a level which is still higher than that in the oesophagus or stomach, and oesophageal contents require active peristalsis to pass into the stomach (Fig. 2.5). The resting tone in the LOS is due to a combination of myogenic, neural and hormonal factors.[27] The myogenic component is calcium-dependent; hence, the use of calcium-channel blocking agents in various lower oesophageal motility disorders. The neural component appears predominantly vagal, via release of acetylcholine. Many factors influence LOS pressure (Table 2.2) with many clinical and therapeutic implications.

Relaxation of the lower oesophageal sphincter is triggered by swallowing, belching or vomiting, and by distension of the oesophageal body. This is probably innervated sympathetically.

(a)

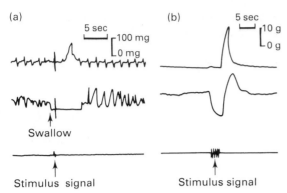

(b)

Swallow

Stimulus signal

Stimulus signal

Fig. 2.5 Normal peristalsis in the body of the oesophagus (upper tracing) and lower oesophageal sphincter relaxation (lower tracing) in the opossum are shown in the left (a). The response of strips of opossum oesophageal circular smooth muscle from the body of the oesophagus (upper tracing) and the lower oesophageal sphincter (lower tracing) to electrical field stimulation are shown on the right (b). It can be seen that the patterns in vivo and in vitro are similar. The fluctuations in resting pressure measured manometrically in the lower oesophageal sphincter are due to movement of the sensing orifice with the sphincter. They are invariably seen if a high-fidelity recording system is used. (From Ref. 19, with permission.)

Tension in lower oesophageal sphincter	
Decreased by:	**Increased by:**
Calcium antagonists	Raised intraabdominal pressure
Glucagon	Acid infusion
Secretin	Gastrin
GIP	
VIP	**No effect:**
	Atropine (in man)

Table 2.2 Tension in lower oesophageal sphincter.

Transient relaxations of the LOS occur independent of swallowing and, whilst these have a physiological role in releasing gastric pressure, they are of considerable importance in the pathophysiology of gastro-oesophageal reflux disease.[16]

THE STOMACH

The stomach stores a meal, liquefies it and empties it into the small intestine in a controlled fashion. At the same time gastric secretion acidifies the meal and adds pepsins and gastric intrinsic factor to the luminal contents. The surface secretion of mucus and bicarbonate protects the gastric mucosa from the effects of acid and peptic digestion, as well as corrosive or abrasive ingested matter.

Motor function

The fasting stomach

The proximal two-thirds of the stomach by volume exhibits no peristaltic activity and remains tonically contracted in the fasting state. The distal stomach exhibits cyclical slow-wave electrical depolarizations as described above; 10–30% of these depolarizations initiate contractions organized as peristaltic waves, which gather speed as they move distally towards the pylorus. A pacemaker for slow-wave activity appears to be located in the mid part of the greater curve of the stomach.

The effects of eating and storage

Cannon observed that the proximal stomach acts as a reservoir and storage area by relaxing in direct relation to the volume of the meal consumed without any increase in intragastric pressure. Isotopic studies confirm that the major part of the meal is stored in the proximal part of the stomach while only small amounts in the antrum. The volume of the body of the stomach diminishes exponentially as emptying proceeds, while the antral portion remains constant in volume until the stomach is nearly empty (Fig. 2.6).

The liquidizer

During the postprandial period, the cone-shaped distal stomach exhibits vigorous peristalsis at 3 cycles/min, which continues for 1.5–2 hours after a standard meal. Gastric peristalsis results in material passing through the pylorus only when it coincides with duodenal peristalsis; thus, the majority of peristaltic waves occur against a closed pylorus. The cone shape and the peristaltic activity of the antrum serve to produce a shearing and streaming effect on the contents, with the result that solid particles are reduced to a diameter of 1 mm or less and not until then do solid particles usually pass the pylorus under normal circumstances (Fig. 2.6).

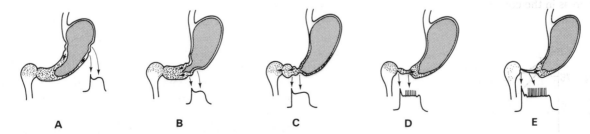

Fig. 2.6 Gastric processing and emptying of solid food. Intracellular electrical potentials, gastric contractions and the effects of contraction on gastric contents are shown. In A, solid food fills the proximal stomach and corpus. Gastric peristalsis begins with gentle contractions of the corpus. Paced by the electrical slow wave, the wave of contraction travels distally, compressing and kneading the solid food and breaking off small pieces (B). These pieces are propelled into the antrum by progressively stronger waves, and small particles of food are accelerated through the still open pylorus by the force of contraction (C). Antral contraction proceeds, and food is squirted through the narrowing pylorus and through the central orifice of the contraction wave (D). The pylorus closes during the terminal antral contraction (E), and all material is forced back to the corpus. Another wave then starts in the corpus, and the cycle is repeated. This pattern of activity results in the mixing and grinding of solid food and in the selective passage of small food particles into the duodenum. (From Ref. 70, with permission.)

Receptive relaxation of the body of the stomach is under vagal control, with vagovagal reflexes also involved. Truncal vagotomy largely abolishes this function and partly explains the sense of fullness commonly experienced after this operation. The regulation of mixing and grinding in the distal stomach is poorly understood but truncal vagotomy reduces this activity, greatly permitting larger particles to pass into the small intestine. In addition, it also reduces the basal MMC activity and, in consequence, the stomach often retains moderate volumes of food residue long after eating.

Gastric emptying

The emptying of the stomach has been studied in detail, in particular using isotopic methods to observe the differential emptying of the liquid and solid components of a meal.[52] In any phase, gastric emptying occurs exponentially in relation to the volume introduced into the stomach. The rate of emptying is inversely related to the nutritional density of the gastric contents, their osmolarity, acidity and the particle size of any solids present (Fig. 2.7). Thus fats will, molecule for molecule, slow gastric emptying more than protein or carbohydrate. The emptying of mixed meals of solids and liquids is complex. Liquids appear to empty before solids, which depend upon the rate at which they can be reduced to 1 mm diameter particles.

The regulation of gastric emptying

This appears to be under neural control and is rapidly adjusted to the nature of the contents entering the upper few centimetres of the small intestine. The observations on gastric emptying can best be explained by postulating the presence of postpyloric receptors in the mucosa of the duodenum and jejunum deep to the brush border enzyme, although such receptors have never been isolated anatomically. One example of their activity is in the slowing of emptying by glucose and starch. Sequential meals of isocaloric content empty at the same rate in the normal individual, although starch has negligible osmolarity and glucose a high osmolarity. The suggestion is that the starch stimulates the slowing of emptying after it has been digested, and absorbed as glucose. In support of this suggestion is the observation that, in patients with severe pancreatic insufficiency where starch is not digested, the slowing of emptying by starch is lost while that by glucose is preserved.[45]

Central nervous system effects

Apart from the influence of the gastric and small intestinal contents, central areas in the cortex, brain stem and, possibly, spinal cord can influence gastric motility. Gastric emptying is slowed in patients in extreme pain or distress. Subclinical nausea induced pharmacologically slows gastric emptying, even when the patient does not appreciate the nausea; this is restored to normal by centrally acting antiemetic drugs.

Gastric secretion

Gastric juice is a mixture of hydrochloric acid, pepsin, bicarbonate, intrinsic factor and mucus. While this combination has some initial digestive function, particularly proteolytic, the main function of the gastric juice is to act as a barrier to ingested micro-organisms.

Gastric acid secretion

Gastric acid secretion is carried out exclusively by the parietal cell of the gastric glands. These are most numerous in the oxyntic mucosa of the gastric body. Hydrogen ions are secreted actively by the H^+/K^+ ATPase pump on the canalicular membrane of the parietal cell.[63] This process involves a one-to-one exchange of hydrogen for potassium ions, a process accompanied by striking morphological alterations of the secretory surface membrane. Tubulovesicles present in the resting parietal cell are transformed into a six- to ten-fold increase in the apical plasma membrane and the appearance of long apical microvilli,[1] referred to as the secretory canaliculus, containing the H^+/K^+ ATPase pump and K^+ and Cl^- conductances.

Stimuli for acid secretion

Histamine, acetylcholine and gastrin are the main stimulants of gastric acid secretion. Histamine acts at specific H_2 receptors and is produced by enterochromaffin-like cells (ECL cells), mast cells and from histaminergic neurones. Binding of histamine to the H_2 receptor leads, via binding of cytosolic guanosine triphosphate (GTP)[71] to activation of adenylate cyclase and production of cyclic AMP. Accumulation of cyclic AMP activates the H^+/K^+ ATPase pump (the proton pump). Acetylcholine is released from parasympathetic neurones in response to vagal stimulation. This stimulates acid production via a muscarinic receptor on the parietal cell, resulting in influx of calcium into the cell and mobilization of intracellular calcium.[53]

Gastrin is produced by the G cells of the gastric antrum (and duodenum) and travels to the parietal cell via the bloodstream. Gastrin release is predominantly under vagal stimulation, via gastrin releasing peptide (GRP), but also occurs in response to gastric distension and the presence of amino acids and peptides in the gastric lumen. Gastrin mediates its effect on acid secretion either directly on the parietal cell or by increasing histamine release.

Phases of acid secretion

The stomach secretes at an extremely low rate in the fasting state even in phase III of the interdigestive cycle. Basal acid output is almost undetectable in the majority of normal subjects. The anticipation of a meal and the postprandial phase is marked by an intense period of acid secretory activity (as well as secretion of electrolytes and macromolecules). Gastric secretion comprises three distinct but overlapping phases. In the *cephalic phase*, the thought, sight, smell or chewing of appetizing food results in vagal stimulation of acid secretion mediated via cholinergic and opioid pathways. In the *gastric phase*, distension of the fundus stimulates acid secretion via vagal pathways. Conversely, antral distension diminishes acid secretion. Food, particularly protein, also stimulates acid secretion

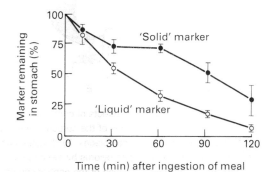

Fig. 2.7 Gastric emptying of solid and liquid phase meal markers. Liquids empty more rapidly than simultaneously ingested solids. (From Heading et al.,[30] with permission. (C) Williams & Wilkins, 1976.)

independent of gastric distension, probably via gastrin release. In the *intestinal phase*, absorbed fat and carbohydrate inhibit acid secretion while absorbed amino acids stimulate secretion further by direct and indirect pathways. As a meal diminishes in volume in the stomach, acid secretion diminishes in absolute amount but is enough to keep the pH of the reducing volume of the contents low (Fig 2.8). In the normal subject, secretion and acidity of gastric contents fall to basal levels within approximately 2 hours of eating (Fig 2.9).

Inhibition of acid secretion

Luminal gastric acid is the main inhibitor of gastric acid secretion, predominantly via a negative feedback on gastrin release once the pH in the stomach falls below 3. A number of gastrointestinal peptide hormones will also inhibit acid secretion, in particular secretin and somatostatin. Many drugs will inhibit acid secretion, the best known being the H_2-receptor antagonists (e.g. ranitidine) and the proton pump inhibitors (e.g. omeprazole, lansoprazole).

Bicarbonate secretion

Bicarbonate is secreted by surface epithelial cells throughout the stomach. These cells contain considerable amounts of carbonic anhydrase. The role of bicarbonate is thought to be to enhance the pH gradient across the surface mucus layer, enhancing the cellu-

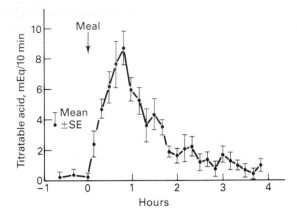

Fig. 2.9 Postprandial gastric acid output in man, showing the cephalic phase, the peak secretion and the lesser phase of secretion after 2 hours. (From Malagelada *et al.*,[46] with permission.)

lar protection from gastric luminal acid and pepsin. This amounts to 10% of gastric ion secretion and would thus provide a high concentration of sodium bicarbonate to neutralize acid impinging on the gastric surface.[56,60]

Gastric mucus secretion

The surface cells and the neck cells of the gastric mucosa secrete mucopolysaccharide and, for the most part, mucus glycoproteins. The latter contain antigens in common with the red blood cell surface antigens belonging to the ABO Lewis blood group system. The mucus layer in conjunction with secreted bicarbonate is speculated to protect the gastric mucosa from acid peptic digestion and from the effects of local trauma to the mucosa (Fig. 2.10) (see Chapter 10). Mucus secretion also provides the mechanism for trapping an unstirred layer over the surface of the stomach, which may in turn hold sodium bicarbonate secreted by the surface cells.[2]

Intrinsic factor

Intrinsic factor (IF) is required for the absorption of vitamin B_{12} (see below) and is secreted by parietal cells. All stimulants of gastric acid secretion also stimulate the secretion of IF.[17] Vitamin B_{12} binds initially to another binding protein, haptocorrin, which is more widely produced in saliva, gastric juice and bile. IF binds to vitamin B_{12} after proteolytic cleavage of the vitamin B_{12} – haptocorrin

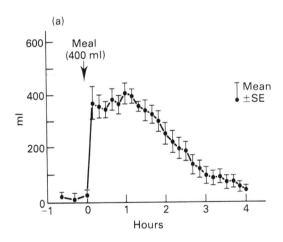

(a)

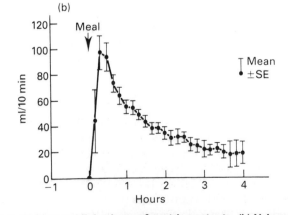

(b)

Fig. 2.8 (a) Postprandial volume of gastric contents. (b) Volume of gastric contents emptied into the duodenum after a meal. The intragastric volume is constant during the first hour after a meal, during which period gastric secretion and emptying rates are at a peak but offset each other. As secretion declines, intragastric volume also falls and pH, not shown, stays steady. (From Malagelada *et al.*,[46] with permission.)

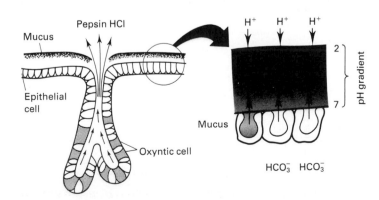

Fig. 2.10 The gastric epithelium, showing the relationship between mucus and bicarbonate secretion by the surface cells, which are probably protected against pepsin and hydrochloric acid secreted by glands. (From Rees and Turnberg,[60] with permission.)

complex. The IF–vitamin B$_{12}$ complex resists proteolysis and carries vitamin B$_{12}$ to the distal small intestine for absorption.[54]

Pepsinogens

Pepsinogens are secreted by the chief cells of the gastric glands. Six or eight pepsinogens are recognized; these are converted, at various pHs, to active pepsin. Pepsinogens are polypeptides with high molecular weight of 42 000 or so and are activated usually at a pH of less than 5. Active pepsins have several functions, the principal one being to initiate the hydrolysis of proteins in the gastric contents both at the terminal bonds and at bonds within the molecule, thus creating large numbers of medium-sized polypeptide fragments. Loss of pepsin secretion, such as occurs in pernicious anaemia or after gastrectomy, does not result in clinically ineffective protein digestion given the large reserves of the pancreas and small intestinal mucosa for proteolysis. The regulation of pepsin secretion is closely connected to that of acid, being predominantly under the influence of vagal stimulation and gastrin.

THE SMALL INTESTINAL LUMEN

The absorption of nutrients by the small intestine is the principal role of the gastrointestinal tract. The ingestion of a meal provokes intense activity in pancreatic secretion, bile flow and intraluminal digestion of complex nutrients during the first hour (Fig. 2.11). Over the next 2–6 hours the contents pass down the small intestine, and by the first 100 cm the major nutritional part of the meal is absorbed. The remainder of the small intestine serves to reclaim the large volume of secreted fluid and electrolyte. The terminal ileum is more highly specialized because of the role of the ileocaecal valve and also being the specific site for absorption of vitamin B$_{12}$ and bile salts.

Pancreatic secretion following a meal[24]

The exocrine functions of the pancreas are carried out by the functional unit of the acinus and its associated ductule, which drains the pancreatic secretions into the main pancreatic duct via an interlobular duct. The acinar cells of the pancreas synthesize and secrete pancreatic enzyme largely under the stimulation

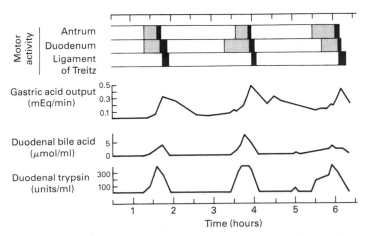

Fig. 2.11 Phases of interdigestive motor activity in association with gastric acid output and duodenal secretion of trypsin and bile acids. Regular recurring interdigestive motor activity: phase I, white portion; phase II, stippled portion; phase III, solid black portion. (From Keane et al.[35], with permission.)

of vagal cholinergic fibres and of the peptide hormone cholecystokinin (CCK), which is secreted by the mucosa of the duodenum and jejunum. In addition, approximately 1 litre/day of water containing isosmotic sodium bicarbonate is secreted mainly by the ductular cells under the influence of secretin in conjunction with CCK. This is largely independent of vagal fibres but is probably influenced by enteropancreatic neural reflexes.

In the fasting state, the pancreas secretes very little. A small amount of water, bicarbonate and enzyme is secreted in phase II and phase III of the interdigestive cycle.

As with gastric acid secretion, in response to a meal there is a cephalic phase of pancreatic secretion. This is vagally mediated and abolished by vagotomy, and may amount to 25% of the total output.[66] This is further augmented by the arrival of food in the stomach, probably mediated through vagovagal reflexes. The greater part of pancreatic enzyme secretion, however, is stimulated by the arrival of nutrients in the duodenum and upper jejunum, which is rapidly followed by the release of CCK. While this hormone is secreted more abundantly in response to hypercalcaemia and the ingestion of solubilized fat, mixed meals even in the absence of fat provide a near-maximal stimulation of pancreatic enzyme secretion. Moreover, this secretion is greatly in excess of any possible requirements provoked by the ingestion of a single meal.[25]

Nature of enzymes

The 8 g or so of enzyme protein secreted each day is composed of a mixture of hydrolases, which are responsible for proteolysis, lipolysis and starch hydrolysis. Bond-splitting of numerous fat-soluble vitamin esters and other lipid esters also possibly occurs without specific hydrolases. The proteolytic enzyme trypsin and the phospholipases are secreted in an inactive form and are only activated within the gastrointestinal lumen under normal circumstances. The remainder are secreted in their active forms.

Pancreatic secretion of bicarbonate and water is stimulated predominantly by the release of secretin, caused by the arrival of acid in the duodenum. However, an additive effect of CCK and enteropancreatic reflexes is also likely to be involved in this process.[78]

Rates of secretion

Following a meal, there is a peak of secretion within the first 45 min, followed by a plateau of high secretion until the duodenum is empty of nutritional contents. Thereafter, secretion dwindles, more by diminishing stimulation than by any specific inhibitory action, although pancreatic polypeptide does inhibit enzyme secretion and may do so physiologically (Fig. 2.12).

Biliary secretion

Bile is a complex solution of water and electrolytes, bilirubin, cholesterol and phospholipid in micellar solution with a critical concentration of bile salts. In the fasting state there is a steady secretion of bile, which is largely diverted to the gall bladder. During interdigestive phases II and III, up to 10 ml of bile are secreted into the gut by the gall bladder accompanied by a brief burst of motor activity in the gall bladder and bile duct.

There is little or no cephalic phase of gall bladder emptying which, nevertheless, begins rapidly after the ingestion of a meal under the influence of cholinergic nerve fibres and CCK, a potent stimulator of gall bladder emptying. At the same time the sphincter of Oddi at the lower end of the common bile duct opens and remains so until the end of the postprandial period, approximately

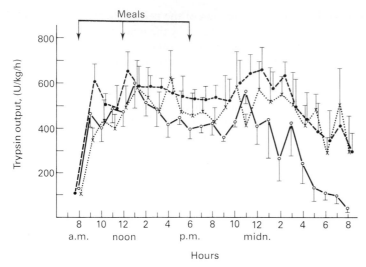

Fig. 2.12 Trypsin secretion into the duodenum (mean ± s.e.) in 18 healthy people ingesting three equicaloric liquid meals: (○), 20 cal/kg; (●), 30 cal/kg; (×), 40 cal/kg. (From Brunner *et al.*,[8] with permission.)

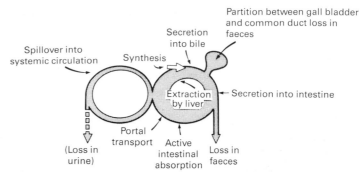

Fig. 2.13 The enterohepatic circulation of bile acids in man. Gall bladder filling is determined by contraction of the sphincter of Oddi (not shown). The movement of the enterohepatic circulation is largely mediated by intestinal motility. The serum level of bile acids is determined by the fraction of bile acids returning from the intestine that are removed by the liver. In a healthy man, individual bile acids are eliminated from the body only in faeces. The composition of the circulatory bile acids reflects hepatic synthesis from cholesterol and bacterial formation of secondary bile acids that are absorbed from the distal intestine (not shown). (From Sleisinger & Fordtran[70], with permission.)

2 hours later. Hepatic bile subsequently bypasses the gall bladder during the postprandial period and passes directly into the duodenum.

Bile acids[38]

Three bile acids are synthesized by the liver and secreted into the bile; they are responsible for the solubilization of cholesterol and phospholipids in bile and are essential to their excretion. Bile acids also play an intrinsic part in the secretion of bile by the hepatocytes. In the gut, bile acids are responsible for the solubilization of lipids and, hence, the absorption of dietary lipid and fat-soluble vitamins. They also have an effect in stimulating pancreatic secretion. Conjugated bile acids remain in the small intestinal lumen until they reach the terminal ileum, where there is a specific receptor for their absorption. Recirculation occurs through the portal blood to the liver and re-secretion by the hepatocytes (*enterohepatic circulation*) (Fig. 2.13). In experimental studies in man the total bile acid pool circulates at least twice per meal. Bile acid synthesis is limited compared with, for example, the exuberant overproduction of pancreatic enzymes. Nevertheless, with modern food and cooking, removal of the gall bladder does not have any obvious adverse effects on the digestion or absorption of fats.

Intraluminal digestion

Very little of the nutrient content of a normal diet is in the form of material that can be absorbed unchanged by the small intestine. High-energy foods such as protein, starches, fat and even vitamins require to be broken down into simpler molecules before absorption can occur. Hence, intraluminal digestion is a vital process taking place in the upper small intestine which results in the enterocyte being presented with nutrients in an absorbable form (Fig. 2.14).

Proteins arriving in the upper small intestine have already been partially fragmented by the activity of gastric pepsin; lipids may be partly digested within the gastric lumen under the influence of lingual lipase, while starch may have been partly digested by salivary amylase in the mouth during chewing. Nevertheless, the burden of hydrolysis falls upon pancreatic enzymes.

Nature of protein digestion

Intraluminal protein digestion is performed by trypsin, chymotrypsin, elastase and carboxypepsidases. Proteolysis occurs both at the terminal linkages of the protein molecules and at the internal bonds, breaking the proteins into oligopeptides. Trypsinogen is converted to active trypsin by the action of intestinal enterokinase, derived from the intestinal brush border. Trypsin then, in turn, activates more trypsinogen. The final products of intraluminal protein digestion are a range of oligopeptides, 2–6 amino acids in length and a number of neutral and basic amino acids.[55]

Fat digestion

Intraluminal fat digestion is more complex.[32] Pancreatic lipase requires the presence of a colipase to function at the neutral pH of the duodenal contents. Moreover, the presence of a critical concentration of bile salt is important to ensure the solubilization of the digestion products into micelles. Pancreatic lipase hydrolyses the bond between fatty acid and glycerol in the 1-position on the glycerol molecule, but internal rearrangement of the residual diglyceride permits hydrolysis to continue, resulting in monoglyceride and fatty acid, both of which are incorporated into the micelle. The fat-soluble vitamins are similarly incorporated (after de-esterification by pancreatic enzyme) in the centre of micelles and are presented in this way to the surface of the enterocyte.

Intraluminal carbohydrate digestion

Pancreatic amylase is the main enzyme for the digestion of starches, which takes place at the α-linkages, producing short oligosaccharides, maltose, maltotriose and α-limit dextrins.

Rates of intraluminal digestion

The process of intraluminal digestion is complex but it is nevertheless extremely rapid, and the rate of absorption and the appearance of the products of absorption in the circulation are just as rapid if the native dietary elements are presented to the intestine as when the primitive amino acids, peptides or monosaccharides are administered. Thus, intraluminal digestion presents no limiting factor in absorption provided the enzymes, bile salt

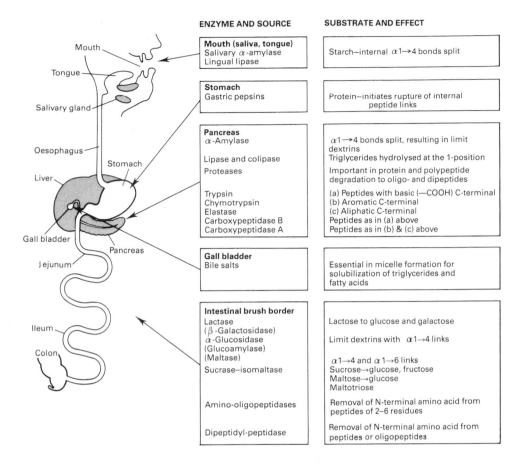

Fig. 2.14 Main sites of enzyme activity.

ENZYME AND SOURCE	SUBSTRATE AND EFFECT
Mouth (saliva, tongue) Salivary α-amylase Lingual lipase	Starch—internal $\alpha1\rightarrow4$ bonds split
Stomach Gastric pepsins	Protein—initiates rupture of internal peptide links
Pancreas α-Amylase	$\alpha1\rightarrow4$ bonds split, resulting in limit dextrins
Lipase and colipase	Triglycerides hydrolysed at the 1-position
Proteases	Important in protein and polypeptide degradation to oligo- and dipeptides
Trypsin Chymotrypsin Elastase Carboxypeptidase B Carboxypeptidase A	(a) Peptides with basic (—COOH) C-terminal (b) Aromatic C-terminal (c) Aliphatic C-terminal Peptides as in (a) above Peptides as in (b) & (c) above
Gall bladder Bile salts	Essential in micelle formation for solubilization of triglycerides and fatty acids
Intestinal brush border Lactase (β-Galactosidase) α-Glucosidase (Glucoamylase) (Maltase)	Lactose to glucose and galactose Limit dextrins with $\alpha1\rightarrow4$ links $\alpha1\rightarrow4$ and $\alpha1\rightarrow6$ links
Sucrase–isomaltase	Sucrose$\rightarrow$glucose, fructose Maltose$\rightarrow$glucose Maltotriose
Amino-oligopeptidases	Removal of N-terminal amino acid from peptides of 2–6 residues
Dipeptidyl-peptidase	Removal of N-terminal amino acid from peptides or oligopeptides

concentration and the luminal milieu are all functioning at a minimum critical requirement.

The role of the small intestinal epithelial cell – the enterocyte
The epithelium covering the villi of the small intestine contains absorptive cells (enterocytes), goblet cells and scattered endocrine cells. The surface of the enterocytes is amplified about 30-fold by the formation of microvilli which are made lined by a highly specialized bimolecular lipid membrane, rich in protein, and containing numerous mucosal enzymes – the brush border enzymes. These enzymes are principally peptidases and carbohydrases. So-called tight junctions exist between the apical borders of the enterocyte, while the basal portions of the enterocytes are separated to form the lateral intercellular spaces (Fig. 2.15). The base of the cell is contiguous with capillary endothelium, while the intercellular spaces communicate more generally with lymphatic channels.

Digestion at the brush border membrane
Disaccharides and small oligosaccharides resulting from intraluminal digestion of starch are presented to the brush border surface by the movements of the bulk phase in the lumen.[69] The enterocytes can only absorb monosaccharides, and the brush border carbohydrases (Fig. 2.16) are responsible for completing the digestion of oligosaccharides.

The sucrase–isomaltase complex is responsible for splitting sucrose into glucose and fructose and for producing glucose from α-limit dextrins. In comparison, lactase is responsible for splitting lactose into glucose and galactose and is important principally in neonatal life during milk-feeding.

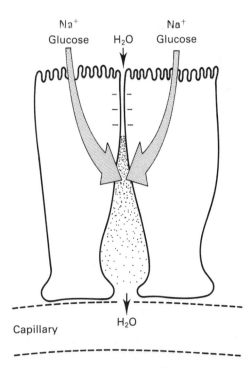

Fig. 2.15 Hypothesis of fluid absorption involving the transport of sodium and glucose into the cell and the subsequent pumping of sodium into the intercellular space. Water is shown to pass through the tight junction between the cells into the lateral space. The increase in hydrostatic pressure in the lateral space so created encourages fluid to move in the direction of least resistance into the capillary. (From Bouchier et al.,[7] with permission.)

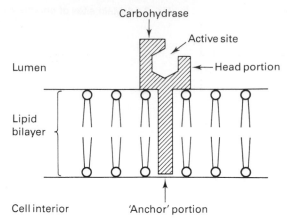

Fig. 2.16 The integration of brush border carbohydrases into lipid cell membrane. The tail within the membrane anchors the head portion, which 'projects' into the lumen. (From Bouchier *et al.*,[7] with permission.)

Peptidases are present in the brush border but are also present in the cytoplasm of the enterocyte and function in a more obscure fashion – see below.[14] Enterokinase is also found in the brush border membrane, but the principal site of trypsinogen activation is nevertheless probably luminal.

INTESTINAL CELLULAR ABSORPTION

A number of mechanisms are involved in the cellular absorption of digested nutrients from the intestinal lumen, including cytosis, diffusion, active transfer and carrier-mediated transfer. Many of these mechanisms are also a means of effecting secretion of various molecules from cell to lumen.

Cytosis

Cytosis is the transfer of discernible particulate matter or solutions within vesicles produced by cell membranes. Secretion in this manner is typified by the secretion of pancreatic enzymes. The transfer of long-chain lipid from the enterocyte into the lateral intercellular space in the form of chylomicrons is another example, and vitamin B_{12}–IF complexes are absorbed by micropinocytosis.

Passive diffusion

Diffusion is the random movement of a substance due to thermal agitation. In solution, substances disperse by diffusion until an even distribution is achieved. The nature of diffusion implies that back-diffusion is bound to occur, although, in many natural systems in which diffusion is responsible for the transfer of material across a membrane, back-diffusion is often reduced by some form of trapping mechanism on one side of the membrane. If this results in a reduced concentration of the original substance, then diffusion will proceed in a directional manner and may mimic an actively assisted process. This is particularly the case in the instance of non-ionic diffusions. A number of lipid-soluble substances are weak acids or bases, as are most pharmacological preparations. Thus a weak acid in solution and largely dissociated on one side of a membrane will diffuse steadily and continuously across that membrane if the physicochemical environment on the far side removes undissociated acid by trapping it or rendering the milieu on the far side more alkaline.

Active transfer

A substance may be moved by active transfer against an electrical or chemical gradient (electrochemical). The implication is that the cell participates in active transfer by devoting metabolic energy to regulate and influence the rate and direction of transfer. The resulting transfer is greater than could be expected from the existence of the known chemical potential, osmotic, hydrostatic and electrical forces. In practice it is often difficult to distinguish between passive transfer, assisted by a trapping mechanism, and an active transfer system.

Carrier-mediated transfer

Hexoses, amino acids and certain ions appear to be transferred by specific carriers, which act as a ferry shuttling across the lipid cell membrane. Carrier-mediated transfer exhibits several characteristics: the rate of transfer exhibits saturation with increasing concentration of substrate; competitive inhibition occurs when substances of similar structure are present; and the transfer is highly specific (for example, transporting D-glucose but not its stereoisomer).

The unstirred layer

Even when the bulk phase luminal contents are energetically stirred at the interface with the cell membrane, a still, unstirred layer of fluid exists which plays an important role in the kinetics of molecular absorption. In particular, the thickness of the unstirred layer has a considerable effect on the absorption of large lipid-soluble molecules such as long-chain fatty acids and on solutes rapidly transported across the apical plasma membrane.[74]

The absorption of sugars

Glucose and galactose are absorbed via an active carrier system coupled to sodium transport (see below) in the brush border membrane. Fructose enters the enterocyte by a process of facilitated diffusion via a specific carrier protein but independent of sodium transport.[22,69]

The cellular absorption of lipid[23]

Lipid in micellar solution impinges on the lipid membrane of the cell and, after disruption of the micelle, most lipid is absorbed by a process of passive diffusion. 'Empty' micelles return through the unstirred layer to the lumen to take up more lipid. A fatty-acid-binding protein facilitates passage of absorbed lipid to the endoplasmic reticulum where the absorbed fat is re-esterified to triglyceride, which appears first in the smooth endoplasmic reticulum near the apex of the enterocyte. This provides a further mechanism for maintaining the concentration gradient of fatty acid across the luminal membrane.

The triglyceride passes slowly through the endoplasmic reticulum to become associated with the Golgi apparatus. Here the triglyceride is enveloped in lipoprotein, the envelope of the lipoprotein being synthesized in the rough endoplasmic reticulum (Fig. 2.17). This forms chylomicrons, which pass through a microtubular system to the lateral basal part of the cell membrane where the chylomicron membrane fuses with the cell membrane and the whole microvesicle passes by exocytosis into the lateral space and thence to the lymphatics.

Medium-chain triglyceride provides a small percentage of dietary fat in humans and is of interest because it can be absorbed without first being solubilized into micelles. It appears to diffuse through the cytosol without metabolic conversion and passes

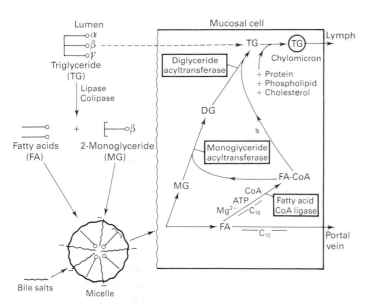

Fig. 2.17 Fat digestion and absorption. Abbreviated structures and names are given. DG indicates diglyceride; C_{10} and C_{15} denote carbon chain length of amino acids. (From Silk & Dawson,[69] with permission.)

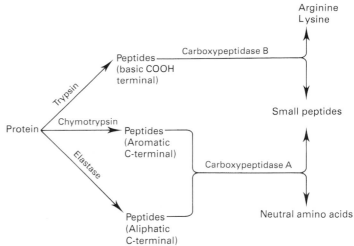

Fig. 2.18 Sequence of events leading to hydrolysis of dietary protein by intraluminal proteases. The fate of the final oligopeptide and amino acid products depends on the intestinal epithelial cell. (From Sleisinger & Fordtran,[70] with permission.)

without chylomicron formation through the basal membrane into the portal circulation. This may be clinically useful in patients with malabsorption of long-chain triglyceride who might be successfully nourished with medium-chain triglyceride.

Absorption of peptides and amino acids[28]

In contrast to carbohydrate, which is absorbed entirely as monosaccharide, the majority of the products of protein digestion are probably absorbed as peptides. The original work suggesting this showed that an oral load of glycine delivered as dipeptide or tripeptide was absorbed more rapidly than glycine itself. More striking evidence came from studies of patients with Hartnup disease, in which there is an intestinal transport defect for neutral amino acids,[48] and in cystinuria, in which there is a transport defect for dibasic amino acids.[50] In these patients the absorption of the affected amino acids was rendered normal if they were presented to the gut as dipeptides.

Following these observations a consistent line of work using intestinal perfusion in man has supported the belief that protein is predominantly absorbed in peptide form by mechanisms independent of those resulting in single amino acid transport (Fig. 2.18).[31] The intestinal brush border is rich in peptidases; however, these have a greater affinity for certain dipeptides than others, and it appears that dipeptides with high affinity for peptidases are likely to undergo mucosal hydrolysis followed by absorption as individual amino acids. Dipeptides with a low affinity for such peptidases are absorbed intact. Existing evidence, while not comprehensive, suggests that unhydrolysed dipeptides and tripeptides are absorbed by an energy- and sodium-dependent carrier mechanism which is saturable. There is conflicting evidence as to whether there is a single peptide carrier or multiple specific carriers.

As with glucose, amino acid absorption is mediated by a sodium-dependent carrier-mediated mechanism. Three major groups of amino acids appear to have group-specific active transport systems: the neutral amino acids, the dibasic amino acids and the dicarboxylic amino acids.

Vitamin absorption

Fat-soluble vitamins

Fat-soluble vitamins, A, D, K and E, are all absorbed from micellar solution in the proximal small intestine. Like a long-chain triglyceride they are extruded into the lymphatic channels in chylomicrons. They are present in small amounts in the diet, and, although they are only required in very small amounts to maintain adequate supplies, any prolongation of absolute bile salt deficiency such as occurs in biliary obstruction results in almost complete absorptive failure. The appearance of deficiency then depends upon body stores, which are small for vitamin K, highly variable for vitamin D and only rarely exhaustible for vitamin A.

Water-soluble vitamins

The water-soluble vitamins are absorbed by a variety of mechanisms. Ascorbic acid and pyridoxine are both absorbed by passive diffusion. Niacin and thiamine are absorbed by a sodium-dependent active-transport system, while the absorption mechanisms for biotin, riboflavin and pantothenic acid are unknown. Nevertheless, even severe small-intestinal disease does not lead to significant deficiency, which is almost invariably due to dietary deficiency.

Vitamin B_{12}

Cooking and gastric digestion release vitamin B_{12} from the animal foodstuffs in which it is largely found, particularly liver, kidney and red meat. In the stomach, vitamin B_{12} is predominantly bound to the R protein, which is derived partly from saliva and which has a higher affinity for vitamin B_{12} than intrinsic factor(IF). However, at neutral pH in the duodenum, the R protein–vitamin B_{12} complex is degraded by pancreatic protease and released vitamin B_{12} binds to IF, which is secreted by the gastric parietal cell. The vitamin B_{12}–IF complex is resistant to trypsin digestion in the intestinal lumen and is absorbed at highly specific receptor sites in the terminal ileum (Fig. 2.19). The complex is extremely large and is thought to be absorbed by endocytosis. The number of receptors is limited such that only a limited amount of vitamin B_{12} can be absorbed from each meal. Furthermore, following exposure to vitamin B_{12} the ileum is refractory to further absorption for up

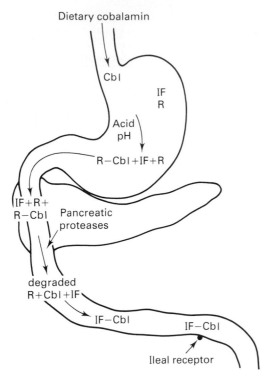

Fig. 2.19 Absorption of cobalamin (Cbl) requires proteolysis and intrinsic factor (IF). The mass of IF secreted is far in excess of that needed for binding the available cobalamin. R protein derived from saliva is also present in great abundance. More R protein and cobalamin are added from biliary secretions into the duodenum. Note that Cbl binds initially to R protein in the stomach at acid pH. Only after R protein is degraded by proteases does Cbl bind IF. After Cbl is absorbed in the ileum, it is bound to transcobalamin II and perhaps TC I and III. (From Sleisinger & Fordtran,[70] with permission.)

to 4 hours. During this time IF is digested from vitamin B_{12} by lysosomal enzymes in the cytosol, and vitamin B_{12} reappears in portal blood after several hours bound to a different carrier protein, transcobalamin II, which is probably synthesized within the ileal enterocyte. Vitamin B_{12} deficiency does not enhance vitamin B_{12} absorption in the ileum and ileal resection is followed by permanent failure of vitamin B_{12} absorption, which is not corrected by the adaptation of more proximal gut. Other causes of deficiency are outlined in Table 2.3.

Folic acid (folate)

Folate occurs naturally in a wide variety of food, particularly offal, nuts and greens. While the average Western diet contains six times the requirement, folate is easily denatured by cooking, storing or leaching out by large volumes of water during food preparation. Absorption takes place predominantly in the duodenum and jejunum with conversion of the various dietary folates to a single, fully reduced monoglutamate derivative, 5-methyl-tetrahydrofolate. Carrier-mediated uptake systems may be present in both brush border and basolateral membranes.

The absorption of minerals

Iron absorption[33]

Iron is present in excess in the Western diet, but as a rule only 5–10% of the dietary intake is absorbed. Worldwide, the combination of dietary deficiency, multiple child-bearing and chronic intestinal parasitic infestations make iron deficiency one of the commonest diseases of the world. Body iron content is controlled by regulating iron absorption.

Peptic digestion releases inorganic ferric iron (Fe^{3+}) from food; this is reduced to ferrous iron (Fe^{2+}) by gastric acid and then bound to mucoproteins in the gastric juice. Reducing substances and low pH favour conversion to ferrous iron, which is absorbable, while the higher pH prevailing in the stomach immediately after food or in pancreatic juice favours the ferric state, which forms insoluble hydroxides (Fig. 2.20). Absorption is more complete from animal food than from vegetable food, which contains more binding material. Haem iron is more readily absorbed than inorganic iron.

Most iron is absorbed in the duodenum and proximal jejunum. Absorption is by an active transport system in the brush border membrane, whence it is transferred slowly across the enterocyte attached to a carrier protein. Ferrous iron is oxidized to the ferric form at the brush border before it can interact with its carrier. The extreme slowness of absorption may result in a substantial proportion of absorbed iron being lost into the gut by desquamation of the mature enterocyte from the villus tips. This increased rate of desquamation can be in part responsible for iron deficiency, e.g. in coeliac disease. This also represents one mechanism whereby excessive iron absorption may be blocked. Nevertheless, it does not explain the comparatively exact control whereby the amount of iron entering the portal blood is approximately relevant to the body's requirements, and is increased in deficiency states.

Abnormalities in cobalamin absorption producing deficiency	
Physiological step	**Disorder**
Impaired food digestion	Gastrectomy, achlorhydria
Decreased intrinsic factor secretion	Pernicious anaemia, gastrectomy
Impaired transfer to intrinsic factor	Pancreatic insufficiency, Zollinger–Ellison syndrome
Abnormal intrinsic factor	Decreased ileal binding
Competition for uptake	Bacterial overgrowth
Impaired attachment to ileal receptor	Ileal disease or resection
Impaired passage through the ileal cell	Familial cobalamin malabsorption
Impaired uptake into blood	Transcobalamin II deficiency

Table 2.3 Abnormalities in cobalamin absorption producing deficiency. (From Sleisinger & Fordtran,[70] with permission.)

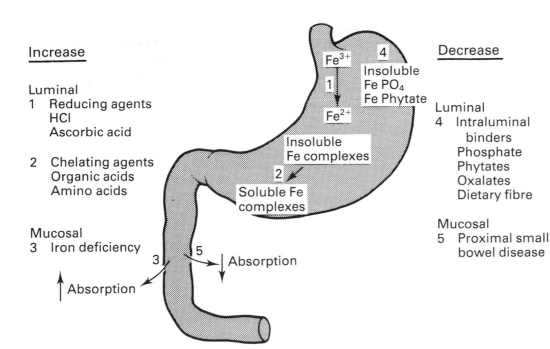

Increase

Luminal
1. Reducing agents
   HCl
   Ascorbic acid

2. Chelating agents
   Organic acids
   Amino acids

Mucosal
3. Iron deficiency

↑ Absorption

Fe^{3+}

1

Fe^{2+}

4

Insoluble
Fe PO_4
Fe Phytate

Insoluble
Fe complexes

2

Soluble Fe
complexes

3 | 5 → Absorption

↓ Absorption

Decrease

Luminal
4. Intraluminal
   binders
   Phosphate
   Phytates
   Oxalates
   Dietary fibre

Mucosal
5. Proximal small
   bowel disease

Fig. 2.20 Factors that affect iron absorption. Non-haem iron absorption is affected both by intraluminal factors (1, 2 and 4) and by the total iron body content (3) as well as by small bowel disease (5). Haem iron absorption is altered only by those factors that affect the mucosa itself (3 and 5). (From Sleisinger & Fordtran,[70] with permission.)

The absorption of calcium and magnesium

To remain in calcium balance and compensate for losses from the skin and urine, approximately 150 mg of calcium must be absorbed from the intestine each day. Calcium is absorbed by both active and passive means. Only the active transport mechanism is vitamin D-dependent and is limited to the small intestine. Passive absorption occurs via tight junctions in both the small and large intestine. Entry of calcium into the enterocyte occurs down a significant concentration gradient. No carrier protein or channel has been identified. However, calmodulin may bind calcium in the brush border membrane. In the cytoplasm, calbindins chelate calcium, which is then extruded at the basolateral membrane via an ATPase-dependent pump.

Various luminal factors will affect calcium absorption. Absorption may be reduced to some extent by binding to phytates, oxalate and dietary fibre. Lactose enhances absorption.

Binding of calcium to calbindin in the enterocyte is the rate-limiting step in calcium absorption. Regulation of calbindin levels by vitamin D is therefore likely to be the main mechanism by which calcium absorption is controlled.

Magnesium differs from calcium in that absorption in the basal state is greater in the ileum than in the jejunum. Vitamin D increases absorption in the jejunum but not in the ileum.[3,26,39]

Absorption of water and electrolytes
Water absorption[39]

Approximately 1.5 litres of water are ingested daily; a further 8–10 litres of fluid enter the gut via secretion daily and a mere 0.1 litre leaves in the stool, the remainder being absorbed largely by the small intestine. The reserve for the absorption of water is large, in that under steady-state conditions the limit appears to be 20 litres, while the colon alone can absorb 6 litres of isotonic normal saline.

The orthodox view of water absorption is that it is inextricably linked to absorption of solutes, particularly sodium and glucose, across the epithelium. These solutes are absorbed across the cell membrane and are then concentrated in the lateral intercellular space. This process, known as 'solvent drag', establishes a hypertonic zone in the intercellular space and water moves into this directly through pores in the tight junctions between the cells (see Fig. 2.15). The flow of water into the hypertonic zone increases the hydrostatic pressure in the space, and capillary or lymphatic flow at the base of the space provides the route of least resistance through which water, sodium and glucose pass. One objection to this hypothesis is that in the jejunum, at least, the tight junctions are calculated to be large and permeable, and would permit more back-flow than is actually observed.

Countercurrent hypothesis

An alternative hypothesis proposes a countercurrent mechanism in the cells at the tip of the villus, similar to that operating in the loop of Henle[29] (Fig. 2.21). This theory has the advantage of explaining why 50% of net water absorption occurs via the lymph, while blood flow in the villus is 500 times greater than lymph flow. It is possible that a combination of these mechanisms occurs in the jejunum.

The presence of pores in the tight junctions is postulated as a result of observed data concerning absorption in the jejunum, ileum and colon. In the proximal small intestine the pores are apparently larger than in the ileum, and in the colon they are smaller than in either proximal or distal small intestine.[15] Water absorption is extremely rapid in the jejunum and slower in the ileum, but active cellular intervention appears to account for the observation that fluid can be absorbed from a more dilute intraluminal solution, thus against a higher concentration gradient. In the colon the channels are apparently tightest, and transit is slow, with the result that water is extracted from progressively drier material against an ever-steeper concentration gradient.

Electrolyte absorption

Sodium enters the enterocyte from the lumen by three key mechanisms. Firstly, sodium can enter the cell linked to the transport of glucose or amino acids via specific transmembrane carrier proteins. Secondly, sodium can enter the cell coupled to the entry of

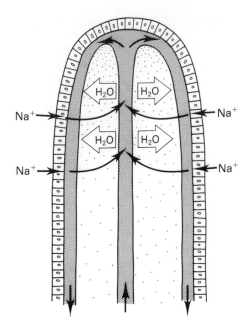

Fig. 2.21 The countercurrent hypothesis for fluid absorption from the small intestine. Active transepithelial absorption of sodium establishes a sodium gradient between the peripheral capillary and the central artery. This results in a cross-diffusion of sodium from capillary to artery, while water travels in the opposite direction from artery to capillary. This effect is multiplied towards the villus tip until very large osmotic gradients are built up. (From Hallback et al.,[29] with permission. © 1978 by The American Gastroenterological Association.)

chloride via a co-transport system in the brush border membrane. In this system, sodium enters the cell via a sodium– hydrogen exchange pump (NHE) driven by the downhill gradient across the apical membrane. The passage of hydrogen out of the cell creates a gradient favouring bicarbonate exit, which in turn promotes entry of chloride into the cell. Finally, sodium will also enter the cell via a specific membrane channel as a result of the downhill electrochemical gradient. This is likely to be the major route of sodium absorption in the colon (Fig 2.22). Once sodium has entered the cell, a sodium–potassium ATPase pump in the basolateral membrane of the enterocyte exchanges intracellular

sodium for extracellular potassium, concentrating sodium in the intercellular space and maintaining the gradient across the cell.

The colon absorbs sodium and water in a different fashion, whereby it is entirely dependent on an intracellular pump mechanism and is adapted to the extraction of sodium from very low concentrations (15 mmol/l) into a cell cytosol of greatly higher concentration.

Transport of potassium across the small intestinal epithelium behaves throughout as though it were a passive process accompanying the diffusion of water into the intercellular space by solvent drag. In the colon, however, there is net secretion of potassium, which is present at highest concentration in the stool.

Active secretion of water and electrolytes
While the enterocytes of the villus are primarily absorptive in function, those of the crypts are involved in the process of secretion of water and electrolytes. Secretion of water and electrolytes is fundamentally linked to changes in permeability to chloride in the apical membrane. Chloride passes into the lumen along its electrochemical gradient setting up an electronegative gradient, which in turn promotes passage of sodium and water into the lumen. Importantly, this is facilitated by an alteration in the permeability of the tight junctions as well as other cellular events. The process of chloride 'secretion' is highly dependent on intracellular mediators, particularly calcium, cyclic AMP, cyclic GMP and GTP-dependent regulatory proteins (G proteins). In turn, various substances, or *secretagogues*, will activate the process, increasing secretion of water and electrolyes into the intestinal lumen.

Secretagogues
There are several agents which act as intestinal secretagogues, all of them by apparently increasing intracellular levels of calcium. Cholera toxin and VIP activate via a surface receptor, adenylate cyclase, thus leading to the formation of cyclic AMP. Other secretagogues, including serotonin, act differently by inducing hydrolysis of phospholipid in the cell membrane, forming channels that enable calcium to enter the cell.

Numerous factors promote secretion or, conversely, promote absorption in the intestine and are summarised in Table 2.4.

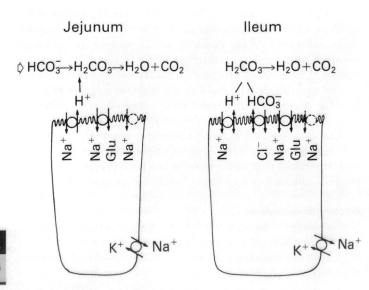

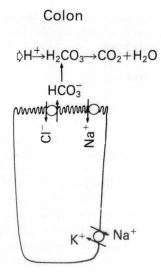

Fig. 2.22 The carrier-mediated mechanisms thought to exist for the absorption of sodium, potassium and chloride across the mucosal and basolateral membranes in the human jejunum, ileum and colon. (From Bouchier et al.,[7] with permission.)

Factors influencing sodium and water absorption and secretion in the intestine	
Factors that increase absorption and/or increase secretion	**Factors that decrease absorption and/or inhibit secretion**
Nutrients	Bacterial toxins
Glucose	Cholera toxin
Amino acids	*E. coli* toxins
Peptides	
Volatile fatty acids (colon)	Luminal contents
	Bile acids
Neurotransmitters/neuromodulators	Long-chain fatty acids (colon)
Neuropeptide Y	
Noradrenaline	Neurotransmitters/neuromodulators
Dopamine	Acetylcholine
Somatostatin	Prostaglandins
Enkephalins	Leukotrienes
Angiotensin	Serotonin
Glucocorticoids	Histamine
	Vasoactive intestinal peptide
	Neurotensin
	Cholecystokinin (CCK)
	Secretin
	Glucagon
	Bradykinin
	Substance P
	Free oxygen radicals
	Platelet activating factor
	Bombesin
	ATP

Table 2.4 Factors influencing sodium and water absorption and secretion in the intestine. (From Read,[59] with permission.)

Role of the enteric nervous system

Most substances that act on secretion do so via the cells of the enteric nervous system (ENS). This is a highly developed system which plays a key role, not only in gut motility (e.g. slow-wave activity and migrating motor complexes) but also the secretory and immunological function of the intestine.[12] The ENS comprises primary afferent neurones, sensitive to chemical and mechanical stimuli, and interneurones and motor neurones, acting upon various effector cells, including smooth muscle, pacemaker cells, blood vessels, glandular cells and enterocytes.

Neural input to the muscular components of the intestine is regulated by a network of pacemaker cells (the interstitial cells of Cajal)[64] and modified by input from other neural, endocrine and paracrine substances. Calcium influx is critical to the action of excitatory transmitters, whereas inhibitory transmitters may work via potassium channels.[65] The enteroendocrine cells (e.g. enterochromaffin cells) act as sensors of the intestinal lumen, initiating neural activity in response to changes in concentration of various substances. For example, the secretion of CCK in response to changes in luminal fat and protein is probably mediated in this way.[20] 5-Hydroxytryptamine (5HT) is the principal mediator released by enteroendocrine cells; it is released across the basolateral membrane and acts on neural cells locally to enhance secretion. This is classically seen in the response to cholera toxin.[43]

COLONIC FUNCTION

The colon is unique in absorbing water and sodium against high concentration gradients and doing so from increasingly drier luminal contents. The colon also has the capacity to absorb short-chain fatty acids derived from bacterial fermentation of carbohydrate in colonic lumen. The motor function of the colon is specifically adapted to slowing the progress of its contents, mixing them thoroughly and pushing the semisolid contents of the left colon towards the rectum and eventual defecation.[58]

Absorption and secretion

The ileum discharges approximately 1500 ml of liquid into the colon every 24 hours, containing approximately 200 mmol of chloride and 50 mmol of bicarbonate.[34] The faeces contain a mere 100 ml of water and as little as 4 mmol of sodium and perhaps 24 mmol of chloride and 20 mmol of potassium. The active absorption against unprecedentedly high concentration gradients occurs mainly in the right colon.

The mechanism of sodium and water absorption in the colon is different from that in the small intestine (see Fig 2.22). Sodium is absorbed actively by a sodium-activated membrane-bound ATPase. This is independent of hydrogen ion exchange, and it is also independent of non-ionic absorption, e.g. by glucose or amino acid, neither of which enhance sodium and water absorption by the colon. Chloride is more readily absorbed than bicarbonate by passive diffusion at high luminal concentration and by active exchange of bicarbonate below 24 mmol/l. Short-chain fatty acids (acetate, propionate, butyrate) are absorbed particularly in the right colon, perhaps via a specific anion exchange mechanism with bicarbonate.[47]

Potassium may be actively secreted into the colon to a concentration of 100 mmol/l, although usually a much lower concentration is found.

Effect of mineralocorticoids

The colonic is unusual in the gut in responding to the influence of mineralocorticoids and antidiuretic hormone in increasing sodium and hence water absorption in conditions of hypovolaemia or mineralocorticoid administration as, for example, in corticosteroid treatment. Conversely, the diarrhoea seen in Addison's disease may represent a failure of mineralocorticoid influence on the colon.

Bidirectional fluxes

The colonic mucosa like the rest of the gut exhibits bidirectional fluxes of all these substances and under normal conditions is strongly in favour of absorption overall. However, there are strict limitations on the capacity of the colon for absorption of water, and an ileal input of greater than 3 litres/day usually results in liquid stool. Likewise, no more than approximately 450 mmol of sodium or chloride can be absorbed per day. The small intestine has a far greater capacity for adaptation to a high fluid input than the colon, and the capacity of the ileum for taking over almost the entire colonic function in the case of ileostomy is well established.[34] This is not so in the case of resection of both ileum and colon when adequate absorption of nutrients is seen, but no adaptation of excessive water and electrolyte is possible. Colonic absorptive function is summarized in Fig 2.23.

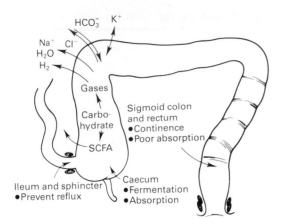

Fig. 2.23 Function of the large bowel (SCFA = short-chain fatty acids). (From Kerlin & Phillips,[37] with permission.)

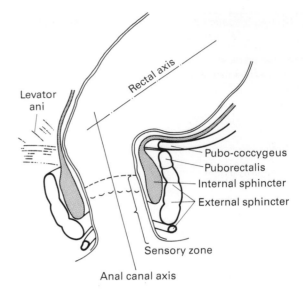

Fig. 2.24 A longitudinal section of the anorectum showing the angulation at the pelvic floor between rectum and anal canal and the disposition of the muscles. The zone of somatic sensation in the anal canal is also indicated (From Duthie & Wormsley,[19] with permission.)

Motor function

The overall transit rate for colonic contents averages 12 hours for caecum to rectum but is highly variable and much modified by activity, discomfort and regular feeding. Progress is intermittent and achieved by two or three mass movements each day, imperceptible to the subject but striking on radiological visualization when a transfer of a large bulk of colonic contents through 30 cm can happen in a few seconds. This progression is much influenced by the combination of eating and exercise.

Segmental movement

The principal movement of the colon is, however, segmentation, which appears to have the function of holding up the passage of contents and mixing them thoroughly.[51,62] This is largely achieved by a series of circular muscular contractions, creating the familiar haustrations seen on imaging of the colon. This is apparently an effective method for mixing the thickening contents of the colon and it is particularly prominent in the right and transverse colon. Segmentation is associated with the generation of high intraluminal pressure, and the slowing of transit encourages greater contact of the bulk phase with the mucosa. Transit is slow in the right colon, tends to be faster in the transverse and in the left colon, which is the site of mass movement, and is then slow again in the sigmoid.

ANORECTAL FUNCTION[19]

The rectum and anal canal work in conjunction with the muscles of the pelvic floor in a highly coordinated manner to retain and expel faeces. The rectum exhibits greater sensitivity to distension than the colon proper. It ends at the proximal part of the anal canal to which it is held at an angle of 80 degrees (Fig. 2.24), largely as a result of the sling action of the puborectalis portion of the levator ani. The anal canal is held gently shut by the internal and external sphincters (Fig. 2.24). There is a low resting pressure within the canal (10–20 mmHg), which is unaffected by ablation of local nerves or cord section, and a ring of high pressure (50–100 mmHg) within the anal canal at the point where the internal and external sphincters overlap (Fig. 2.24). This high pressure is abolished by ablation of local parasympathetic autonomic nerves and is largely the result of internal sphincter activity.

Sensation

The rectum is usually empty and out of mind; it imparts a transient sense of distension at volumes of 80–120 cm³, very much smaller volumes than are sensed by the remainder of the colon. The sensation of distension is continuous but resistible between 200 and 300 cm³, and irresistible above 400 cm³, at which volume explosive defecation occurs. Anal sensation, on the other hand, is that of normal skin, with the capacity to discriminate effectively between contact with gas, fluid or solid.

Anorectal reflexes

Three reflexes combine to maintain anal continence interrupted by flatus and by controlled defecation. The accommodation reflex of the rectum permits increasing volumes of contents to be tolerated unconsciously until a critical volume is reached of approximately 200–300 ml, which varies between individuals and tends to decline with age and most mucosal, muscular or neurological diseases affecting the rectum.

The sampling reflex of the anus, which is illustrated in the tracing in Fig. 2.25, occurs when any transient increase in rectal contents occurs *de novo*. The upper anal sphincter relaxes, the rectal contents descend into the canal and are sampled by the sensitive mucosa. Gas alone is usually permitted to escape by further relaxation of the anus; liquid imparts a burning desire to defecate, which may have to be consciously countered by an extra voluntary squeeze of the anal sphincter; and solid may be expelled or pushed back into the rectum by a sudden squeeze of the sphincter. This sampling reflex, all important to continence, is preserved even with sleeve resection of the anorectal mucosa, and is probably conveyed from sensory nerve endings in the levator ani and the myenteric nerve plexus in the rectal wall. It is not abolished by cord section or pudendal nerve block.

Defecation

The defecation reflex is induced by increasing the volume of rectal contents whereby accommodation is overcome and a

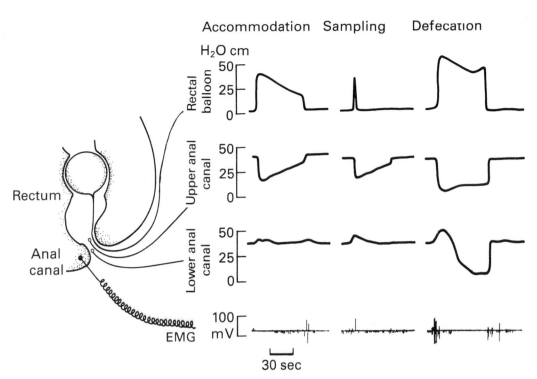

Accommodation Sampling Defecation

rapid sequence of anal relaxation, increased abdominal pressure and relaxation of the puborectalis results in the expulsion of rectal contents. Controlled defecation is the result of released cortical inhibition and a voluntary increase in the intra-abdominal pressure. The assumption of the sitting, and even more so, the squatting position, helps to straighten out the anorectal angle, also facilitating the passage of the rectal bolus through the anus.

GASTROINTESTINAL BACTERIA

Bacteria colonize the human intestine shortly after birth. Within hours of birth, maternal coliforms and streptococci begin to populate the intestine, followed shortly by enterococci and lactobacilli. Within 3 weeks, the number of coliforms decreases and *Bacteroides* organisms begin to establish themselves as the predominant bacterial species in the colon.[6,68] Overall, the gastrointestinal tract contains 10 times as many microbial organisms as there are cells in the human body.[5]

The flora of the gastrointestinal contents are derived from ingested food.[44] Food is seldom completely sterile and is incompletely sterilized by gastric secretion. Thus, after eating, the upper small intestinal contents are transiently colonized by over 100 bacterial species. However, with increasing gastric secretion, the gastric and jejunal contents rapidly become sterile in the hour following a meal. In the distal small intestine, however, ingested bacteria begin to proliferate and even more so in the colon with its slow-moving contents. In the jejunum, lactobacilli, enterococci, Gram-positive aerobes or facultative anaerobes predominate in concentrations of 10^4 organisms/ml. In the terminal ileum, concentrations reach 10^9 organisms/ml. This concentration may reach as high as 10^{12} organisms/ml in the colon, the concentration where *Bacteroides* and other anaerobes are the predominant organisms.

The importance of gastrointestinal bacteria

It is not clear whether the presence of this mass of bacteria represents a well-adjusted symbiosis in the face of inevitable contamination or whether some biological advantage is conferred. There is some evidence to suggest that a stable mixed flora in the lumen, and subsequently attached to the mucus of the gastrointestinal tract, confers additional protection against infection by more pathogenic organisms such as *Salmonella*, *Clostridia*, *Cholera* and *Candida albicans*. Enteric bacteria also perform a variety of metabolic functions which may be of benefit to the host. This includes the fermentation of unabsorbed dietary sugars to short-chain fatty acids, which can be absorbed by the colon, and the production of vitamin K and folate. Conversely, some metabolic bacterial properties may be detrimental, e.g. the production of deoxycholic acid from primary bile acids by bacterial 7-dehydroxylase, which may promote carcinogenesis in the colon.

Several measures exist to prevent the harmful effects of excessive colonization of the gut by bacteria. These are the 'acid trap' of the stomach; antegrade peristalsis, which minimizes bacterial attachment; proteolytic enzyme digestion; the ileo-caecal valve; the intestinal mucus layer; and, finally, the suppressive effects of the gut immune system.

GASTROINTESTINAL GAS[41,42]

The gastrointestinal tract contains, fasting or fed, approximately 200 ml of gas even in subjects complaining of excessive wind. There is, however, a wide difference between normal subjects in the rate of transfer of gas through the gut from 200 to 2000 ml/day, with a mean of 600 ml/day. The mean number of passages of flatus is 15 per day with an extrapolated mean volume of 40 ml per emission. Many foods have been blamed for increasing the volume of intestinal gas but alone amongst them the bean has been carefully studied, with the conclusion that a diet containing 50% of its calories as pork and beans results in an increase of hourly basal flatus volume from 15 to 150 ml. The composition of intestinal gas is a highly variable mixture of nitrogen, carbon dioxide, hydrogen, oxygen and methane.

Origins of gas

Swallowed air is the major contributor to gas in the upper gut, but the composition is modified partly by the eructation of the major part of the swallowed air and then by diffusion of gas into and out of the gut through the intestinal mucosa and, finally, by the products of bacterial decomposition of food residues in the colon.

Nitrogen varies from 90% to 10% of the intestinal gas but is usually the predominant component. Oxygen may vary from 5% to 50% but is usually in very low concentration. Carbon dioxide, resulting from the reaction of gastric acid and pancreatic bicarbonate, is high in the duodenum but is rapidly absorbed unless rates of transit are high. The major component of hydrogen and methane is from bacterial activity in the colon.

The importance of intestinal gas in symptomatology is great but very few scientific studies have been made in this enigmatic field.

REFERENCES

1   Aese S, Dahl E, Roland M, Hars R. Morphometric studies of parietal cells during basal conditions and during stimulation with pentagastrin in healthy subjects. *Gastroenterology* 1983; 18: 913.

2   Allen A, Garner A. Mucus and bicarbonate secretion in the stomach and their possible role in mucosal protection. *Gut* 1980; 21: 249–62.

3   Alcock N, MacIntyre I. Interrelation of calcium and magnesium absorption. *Clin Sci* 1962; 22: 185–93.

4   Baron JH. Studies of basal and peak acid output with an augmented histamine test. *Gut* 1963; 4: 136–44.

5   Bengmark S. Econutrition and health maintenance – a new concept to prevent GI inflammation, ulceration and sepsis. *Clin Nutr* 1996; 15: 1.

6   Bishop RF, Anderson CM. Bacterial flora of the stomach and small intestine in children with intestinal obstruction. *Arch Dis Child* 1960; 35: 487.

7   Bouchier IAD, Allan RN, Hodgson HJF, Keighley MRB (eds). *Textbook of Gastroenterology*. Baillière Tindall, London, 1984.

8   Brunner H, Northfield TC, Hofmann AF *et al*. Gastric emptying and secretion of bile acids, cholesterol, and pancreatic enzymes during digestion. Duodenal perfusion studies in healthy subjects. *Mayo Clin Proc* 1974; 49: 851–60.

9   Christensen J. The controls of oesophageal movement. *Clin Gastroenterol* 1976; 5(1): 15–28.

10 Code CF, Schlegel JR. The gastrointestinal interdigestive housekeeper: motor correlates of the interdigestive myoelectric complex of the dog. In: *Proceedings of the Fourth International Symposium on Gastrointestinal Motility* (Daniel EE *et al*. eds). Mitchell Press, Vancouver, 1973: 631–4.

11 Christensen J. The controls of gastrointestinal movements: some old and new views. *N Engl J Med* 1971; 285: 85.

12 Costa M, Brookes SJH. The enteric nervous system. *Am J Gastroenterol* 1994; 89: 129–37.

13 Craft IL, Geddes D, Hyde CW *et al*. Absorption and malabsorption of glycine and glycine peptides in man. *Gut* 1968; 9: 425–37.

14 Crane CW. Some aspects of protein absorption and malabsorption. In: *Malabsorption* (Girdwood RH, Smith AN, eds). Edinburgh University Press, Edinburgh; 1969: 33.

15 Davis GR, Santa Ana CA, Morawski SG, Fordtran JS. Permeability characteristics of human jejunum, ileum, proximal colon and distal colon. Results of potential difference measurements and unidirectional fluxes. *Gastroenterology* 1982; 83: 844–50.

16 Dodds WJ, Dent J, Hogan WJ. Mechanisms of gastroesophageal reflux in patients with reflux oesophagitis. *N Engl J Med* 1982; 307: 1547–52.

17 Donaldson RM. Intrinsic factor and the transport of cobalamin. In: (Johnson LR ed). *Physiology of the Gastrointestinal Tract*, 2nd edn. Raven Press, New York, 1987: 959.

18 Drasan BS, Shiner M, McLeod GM. Studies on the intestinal flora. I. The bacterial flora of the gastrointestinal tract in healthy and achlorhydric persons. *Gastroenterology* 1969; 56: 71–9.

19 Duthie ML, Wormsley KG (eds). *Scientific Basis of Gastroenterology*. Churchill Livingstone, Edinburgh, 1979.

20 Eastwood C, Maubach K, Kirkup AJ *et al*. The role of endogenous cholecystokinin in the sensory transduction of luminal nutrient signals in the rat jejunum. *Neurosci Lett* 1998; 254: 145–8.

21 Edwards DAW. The anti-reflux mechanism, its disorders and their consequences. *Clin Gastroenterol* 1982; 11(3): 479–96.

22 Fordtran JS. Stimulation of active and passive absorption by sugars in the human jejunum. *J Clin Invest* 1975; 55: 728–37.

23 Gangl A, Ockner RK. Intestinal metabolism of lipids and lipoproteins. *Gastroenterology* 1975; 68: 167–86.

24 Go VLW, DiMagno EP. Assessment of exocrine pancreatic function by duodenal intubation. *Clin Gastroenterol* 1984; 13: 701–15.

25 Go VLW, Hofmann AF, Summerskill WHJ. Simultaneous measurements of total pancreatic, biliary, and gastric outputs in man using a perfusion technique. *Gastroenterology* 1970; 58: 321–8.

26 Golden MH, Golden BE. Trace elements. Potential importance in human nutrition with particular reference to zinc and vanadium. *Br Med Bull* 1981; 37: 31–6.

27 Goyal RK, Rattan S. Genesis of basal sphincter pressure: effect of tetrodotoxin on lower oesophageal sphincter pressure in opossum *in vivo*. *Gastroenterology* 1976; 71: 62–7.

28 Gray GM, Cooper HL. Protein digestion and absorption. *Gastroenterology* 1971; 61: 535–44.

29 Hallback DA, Hulten L, Jodal M *et al*. Evidence for the existence of a countercurrent exchanger in the small intestine of man. *Gastroenterology* 1978; 74: 683–90.

30 Heading RC, Tothill P, McLoughlin GP, Shearman DJC. Gastric emptying rate measurement in man. A double isotope scanning technique for simultaneous study of liquid and solid components of a meal. *Gastroenterology* 1976; 71: 45–50.

31 Hellier MD, Holdsworth CD, Perrett D. Dibasic amino acid absorption in man. *Gastroenterology* 1973; 65: 613–18.

32 Hofmann AF, Borgstrom B. The intraluminal phase of fat digestion in man: the lipid content of the micellar and oil phase of intestinal content obtained during fat digestion and absorption. *J Clin Invest* 1964; 43: 247–57.

33 Jacobs A, Worwood M. Iron metabolism, iron deficiency and overload. In: *Blood and Its Disorders*, 2nd edn. (Hardisty RM, Weatherall DJ, eds). Blackwell Scientific Publications, Oxford, 1982: 149–97.

34 Kanaghinus T, Lubran M, Coghill NF. The composition of ileostomy fluid. *Gut* 1963; 4: 322–38.

35 Keane FD, Dozois RR, Go VLW, DiMagno EP. Interdigestive canine pancreatic juice composition and pancreatic reflux and pancreatic sphincter anatomy. *Dig Dis Sci* 1981; 26: 577–84.

36 Kellow JE, Borody TJ, Phillips SF, Tucker RL, Haddad AC. Human interdigestive motility: variations in patterns from oesophagus to colon. *Gastroenterology* 1986; 91: 386–95.

37 Kerlin P, Phillips SF. Absorption of fluids and electrolytes from the colon with reference to inflammatory bowel disease. In: *Inflammatory Bowel Diseases* (Allen R, Keighley M, Hawkins C, Alexander-Williams J, eds). Churchill Livingstone, Edinburgh.

38 Krag E, Phillips SF. Active and passive bile acid absorption in man. Perfusion studies of the ileum and jejunum. *J Clin Invest* 1974; 53: 1686–94.

39 Sellin JH. Intestinal electrolyle absorption and excretion. In: *Gastrointestinal Disease* (Sleisenger MH, Fordtran JS, eds). WB Saunders, Philadelphia, 1993: 954–76.

40 Krejs GJ, Nicar MJ, Zerwekh JE, Norman DA, Kane MG, Pak CYC. Effect of 1,25-dihydroxyvitamin D_3 on calcium and magnesium absorption in the healthy human jejunum and ileum. *Am J Med* 1983; 75: 973.

41 Lasser RB, Bond JH, Levitt MD. The role of intestinal gas in functional abdominal pain. *N Engl J Med* 1975; 293: 524.

42 Levitt MD. Volume and compositions of human intestinal gas determined by means of an intestinal wash out technique. *N Engl J Med* 1971; 284: 1394.

43 Lundgren O. 5-hydroxytryptamine, enterotoxins and intestinal fluid secretion. *Gastroenterology* 1998; 115: 1009–11.

44 Mackowiak PA. The normal bacterial flora. *N Engl J Med* 1982; 307: 83–93.

45 Mallinson CN. The gastric emptying of starch and glucose in patients with pancreatic insufficiency. *Gut* 1968; 9: 737.

46 Malagelada JR, Longstreth GF, Summerskill WHJ, Go VLW: Measurement of gastric functions during digestion of ordinary solid meals in man. *Gastroenterology* 1976; 70: 203–10.

47 Mascolo N, Rajendran VM, Binder HJ. Mechanism of short-chain fatty acid uptake by apical membrane vesicles of the rat distal colon. *Gastroenterology* 1991; 101: 331–8.

48 Matthews DM, Adibi SA. Peptide absorption. *Gastroenterology* 1976; 71: 151–61.

49 Meyer GW, Castell DO. Physiology of the oesophagus. *Clin Gastroenterol* 1982; 11(3): 439–51.

50 Milne MD, Asatoor AM, Edwards KDG, Loughridge LW. The intestinal absorption defect in cystinuria. *Gut* 1961; 2: 323–37.

51 Misiewicz JJ. Colonic motility. *Gut* 1975; 16: 311–14.

52 Moromtz M, Cook DJ, Collins PJ *et al*. The application of techniques using radionuclides to the study of gastric emptying. *Surg Gynecol Obstet* 1982; 155: 737–44.

53 Negelescu PA, Reenstra WW, Machen TE. Intracellular Ca requirement for stimulus-secretion coupling in parietal cells. *Am J Physiol* 1989; 256: C241.

54 Nicolas J-P, Jimenez M, Marcoullis G, Parmentier Y. *In vivo* evidence that intrinsic factor–cobalamin complex traverses the human intestinal tract. *Biochim Biophys Acta* 1981; 675: 328.

55 Nixon SE, Mawer GE. The digestion and absorption of proteins in man. II. The form in which digested protein is absorbed. *Br J Nutr* 1970; 24: 241.

56 O'Brien P, Rosen S, Trencis-Buck L, Silen W. Distribution of carbonic anhydrase within the gastric mucosa. *Gastroenterology* 1979; 72: 870.

57 Quigley EMM. Small intestinal motor activity: its role in gut homeostasis in health and disease. *Q J Med* 1987; 65: 799–810.

58 Read NW. The relationship between intestinal motility and intestinal transport. *Clin Res Rev* 1981; 1 (suppl 1): 73–81.

59 Read NW. Intestinal transport of fluid and electrolytes (Physiology and Pathophysiology). In: Gastroenterology: Clinical Science and Practice. Bonchics, Allan, Hodgson, Keighley (eds). W.B. Saunders, Philadelphia; 1993; 447–59.

60 Rees WDW, Turnberg LA. Mechanisms of gastric mucosal protection: a role for the mucus–bicarbonate barrier. *Clin Sci* 1982; 62: 343–8.

61 Richardson CT, Walsh JH, Cooper KA *et al*. Studies on the role of cephalic-vagal stimulation in the acid secretory response to eating in normal human subjects. *J Clin Invest* 1977; 60: 345–441.

62 Ritchie JA. Colonic motor activity and bowel function. 1. Normal movement of contents. *Gut* 1968; 9: 442–56.

63 Saccomani G, Helander HF, Mihas AA, Crago S, Sachs G. An acid transporting enzyme in human gastric mucosa. *J Clin Invest* 1979; 64: 627–35.

64 Sanders KM. A case for the interstitial cells of Cajal as pacemakers and mediators of neurotransmission in the gastrointestinal tract. *Gastroenterology* 1996; 11: 492–515.

65 Sanders KM. Post-junctional electrical mechanisms of enteric neurotransmission. *Gut* 2000; 47 (Suppl IV): 23–5.

66 Sarles H, Dani R, Preselin G, Souville C, Figarella C. Cephalic phase of pancreatic secretion in man. *Gut* 1968; 9: 214–21.

67 Sarna SK. Cyclic motor activity; migrating motor complex. *Gastroenterology* 1985; 89: 894–913.

68 Sherman P, Lichtman S. Small bowel bacterial overgrowth syndrome. *Dig Dis Sci* 1987; 5: 157.

69 Silk DBA, Dawson AM. Intestinal absorption of carbohydrate and protein in man. *Int Rev Physiol* 1979; 19: 151–204.

70 Sleisinger MH, Fordtran JS (eds): *Gastrointestinal Disease*. WB Saunders, Philadelphia, 1983.

71 Soll AH, Wollin A. Histamine and cyclic AMP in isolated canine parietal cells. *Am J Physiol* 1979; 237: E444.

72 Stein HJ, Liebermann-Meffert D, DeMeester TR. Three-dimensional pressure image and muscular structure of the human lower oesophageal sphincter. *Surgery* 1995; 117(6): 692–8

73 Sternlieb I. Gastrointestinal copper absorption in man. *Gastroenterology* 1967; 52: 1038–41.

74 Strocchi A, Levitt MD. A reappraisal of the magnitude and implications of the unstirred layer. *Gastroenterology* 1991; 101: 893.

75 Vantrappen GR, Peeters TK, Janssens J. The secretory component of the interdigestive migrating motor complex in man. *Scand J Gastroenterol* 1979; 14: 663–7.

76 Vantrappen GR, Janssens J, Peeters TL, Bloom SR, Cristofides ND, Hellemans J. Motilin in the interdigestive migrating motor complex in man. *Dig Dis Sci* 1979; 24: 497.

77 Waters PF, DeMeester TR. Foregut motor disorders and their surgical management. *Med Clin North Am* 1981; 65: 1237–72.

78 Wormsley KG. Pancreatic function tests. *Clin Gastroenterol* 1972; 1: 27–42.

Chapter 3

Adhesion molecules and circulation and differentiation of lymphocytes in gut-associated lymphoid tissue and mammary glands

Julia M. Phillips-Quagliata

INTRODUCTION

Mammals have evolved a complex immune system capable of generating adaptive immune responses against a variety of infectious agents entering the body through different routes. Protection of mucosae presents a special problem because their surfaces are large and moist, and their secretions provide a milieu in which many microorganisms could potentially thrive. Natural selection has resulted in development of a mucosal immune system that permits uptake of antigens and potential pathogens in a controlled way so that immune responses can be induced against them. Protective immune responses are mounted against pathogens to prevent them, at subsequent exposures, from entering the body. At the same time, digestion of potentially antigenic foods and the survival of harmless commensals on mucosal surfaces is supported.

The external surface of the mucosa-associated lymphoid tissue (MALT) and especially of the gut-associated lymphoid tissue (GALT) is so constructed that microorganisms and macromolecules can be taken up from the mucosal fluid, passed through the epithelium to antigen-presenting cells, and then processed for presentation as antigens to interacting T and B cells capable of recognizing them. Immune effector cells and antibodies can then be delivered via the bloodstream to local and distant mucosae where they can help to ward off potentially invasive organisms.

In the GALT, induction of local protective responses to a given antigen is often coupled with systemic immune suppression to the same antigen (see Chapter 15). This may reflect the necessity of preventing, as far as possible, systemic immunization against any intact food antigens that reach the blood circulation. Much of the early literature on the subject of lymphocyte migration and the mucosal immune response was previously covered in a review article[94] published in 1994. In the interests of space, only recent references and older references that are especially pertinent will be cited here.

One useful way of thinking about MALT is to divide it into two components – one, highly structured and essential for antigen uptake and immunization; the other, more loosely organized, containing the protective mucosal effector cells and antibody-producing cells that are delivered to the mucosae in the blood. Only the GALT, the bronchus-associated lymphoid tissue (BALT) and the nose-associated lymphoid tissue (NALT) have the first component, consisting of a modifed epithelium, crucial for antigen uptake, covering organized lymphoid nodules containing the elements necessary for local immunization. This nodular lymphoid tissue is drained via lymphatics to a second, back-up, regional lymph node in which much of the proliferation and differentiation of cells originally stimulated in the nodular tissue may occur. All MALTs, including GALT, BALT and NALT, as well as MALT in the lactating mammary and lacrimal glands and in the urogenital system have the second, effector cell-containing component. This consists of loosely arranged lymphoid tissue within the lamina propria having the capacity to attract and retain effector T cells and plasma cell precursors entering from blood. The secretory epithelium covering it transmits antibodies to the secretions and is infiltrated with intraepithelial T lymphocytes. This lamina propria lymphoid tissue is drained by lymphatics directly to a regional lymph node, usually bypassing any local nodular lymphoid tissue.

Features of the mucosal immune system

Six key features of the mucosal immune system distinguish it from the peripheral immune system (Table 3.1).

1. It surveys antigens in the fluids outside the body; for example, in the intestinal, bronchial and nasal secretions. Microorganisms and macromolecules capable of penetrating the protective layer of mucus (see Chapters 12 and 13) and adhering to epithelia, thus displaying properties necessary to invasive organisms, can be efficiently taken up into the lymphoid nodules of the mucosal immune system. By contrast, in the systemic immune system, all foreign macromolecules reaching the body fluids are likely to be filtered out either in the spleen or regional lymph nodes, where they can stimulate a systemic immune response.

2. The two components of the mucosal immune system mentioned above are integrated in such a way that the effector cells are distributed throughout the lamina propria at sites quite distant from the organized lymphoid tissue in which their precursors proliferated and differentiated. This situation seems to differ from that in the peripheral immune system, where the bulk of antibody-producing B cells and effector T cells are generally found within the organized lymphoid tissue of the lymph nodes and spleen. The distinction may, however, be somewhat artificial since antibody-producing plasma cells are quite prominent in distant sites such as bone marrow and T cells are known to traverse tissues such as skin. Chronic antigenic stimulation in the mucosae may greatly increase the amount of the effector/delivery component relative to the nodular lymphoid component in MALT. The ability of nodular mucosal lymphoid tissue to generate immune responses against local infectious agents and then distribute effector T and B cells to distant mucosal sites offers antigen-specific protection to hitherto uninfected and even distant mucosae. It

has profound implications for the design and effective use of vaccines against mucosal pathogens.

3. In most mucosae, especially those of the gastrointestinal, respiratory and urinary tracts, the major immunoglobulin (Ig) isotype produced by local plasma cells is IgA, in contrast to the systemic immune system in which IgG predominates.

4. MALT effector cells and epithelia cooperate in producing effector molecules that can be delivered to mucosal secretions rather than to blood. The best example of this is the cooperation between IgA-secreting plasma cells and epithelial cells in producing secretory IgA (SIgA). Transportation of IgA that has been secreted into the interstitial fluid by IgA plasma cells across the secretory epithelium into mucosal secretions is made possible by the poly Ig receptor (pIgR) on the epithelial cells. During its transportation, IgA becomes covalently bound to the pIgR, a portion of which, the so-called secretory component, remains attached to the IgA after its release into the fluids as SIgA. SIgA is especially well adapted to functioning as an antibody in fluids such as those in the intestine because it is to some extent protected from proteolytic digestion by covalently bound secretory component (see Chapters 8 and 11). Another example of effector cell–epithelial cell interaction is manifest when activated mucosal T cells responding to worm infestation produce cytokines that stimulate an increase in mucus secretion by goblet cells (see Chapters 7 and 13).

5. Although the mucosal and peripheral immune systems apparently draw most of their lymphoid cell populations from the same pools in terms, for example, of $\alpha\beta$ T cell receptor and IgV_H and V_κ gene usage, there are unique populations of mucosal intraepithelial T cells distinguished by use of a limited set of $\gamma\delta$ T cell receptor genes, which differs from that used by T cells in skin. About 70% of $\gamma\delta$ and 20% of $\alpha\beta$ mouse intraepithelial T cells lack Thy 1. In addition, a unique set of T cells in mucosae express their CD8 coreceptor as an $\alpha\alpha$ homodimer rather than as the more ubiquitous $\alpha\beta$ heterodimer (see Chapter 7).

6. Mucosal and peripheral lymphoid tissues in adult mammals express different addressins which permit segregation of circulating lymphocytes into MALT *versus* peripheral lymphoid tissue.

ANATOMY OF THE MUCOSAL IMMUNE SYSTEM

As outlined above, the major elements of the mucosal immune system are: (a) the lymphoid nodules of GALT, BALT and NALT in which immunization against local immunogens and commitment to IgA production takes place;[94] (b) the afferent lymphatics connecting the nodules and the lamina propria to the regional lymph nodes and the regional lymph nodes themselves. In these regional lymph nodes, the immunized T and B cells coming from the lymphoid nodules proliferate and mature to an activated blast stage at which they are capable of migrating into lamina propria;[94] in addition, immunization by antigens arriving via lymphatics from the lamina propria may occur; (c) the efferent lymphatics, thoracic duct and blood circulation by which the activated blasts are delivered to the lamina propria; and (d) the lamina propria itself.[94]

The mucosal lymphoid follicles are scattered singly or in clusters in the lamina propria of the intestine and bronchial tree.

Features of mucosal immune system
Survey of external antigens
Generation of effector cells at distant sites
IgA as predominant isotype
Delivery of effector molecules to secretions
Use of limited set of $\gamma\delta$ T cell receptor genes
Distinct addressins for mucosal tissue

Table 3.1 Features of mucosal immune system.

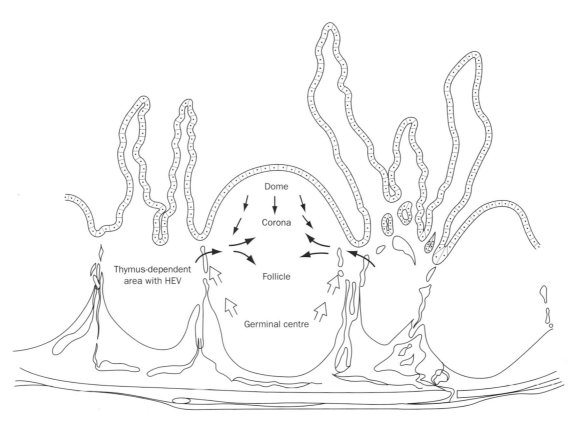

Fig. 3.1 Section of a Peyer's patch drawn from a photomicrograph. The large black arrows indicate the supposed pathways of migration of lymphocytes from the high endothelial venules (HEV) in the thymus-dependent areas through the corona and dome of the nodule; the small black arrows indicate the probable direction of flow of fluid containing antigen that has entered through the M cells in the dome epithelium towards the plexus of lymphatics surrounding the nodule; the open arrows indicate the likely direction of movement of postmitotic cells away from the germinal centre towards the lymphatic plexus.

Large clusters of such follicles constitute the Peyer's patches (Fig. 3.1) and appendix of GALT, and the tonsils and adenoids that make up Waldeyer's ring in human NALT. The epithelium covering the follicles differs from the regional glandular epithelium in that it lacks a glycocalyx, has fewer goblet cells, and has numerous specialized epithelial cells, the so-called M cells, with short, irregular microvilli (see Chapter 1). These M cells transport macromolecules from the lumen of the mucosal organ and release them into the interstitial fluids in the dome of lymphoid tissue lying directly beneath the epithelium. Here they can be taken up by local macrophages and dendritic cells. MHC Class II-bearing dendritic cells[16] are present immediately below the follicle-associated epithelium in humans. The follicles generally contain a large germinal centre (GC), made up of proliferating B cells presumably responding to the many antigens that enter through the follicle-associated epithelium. In germfree mice, the Peyer's patches are very small and underdeveloped. Thymus-dependent (TD) areas containing high endothelial venules (HEV), through which lymphocytes arriving with the blood supply can pass into the nodule, surround each follicle. In Peyer's patches, the TD areas have overlying villi with villous epithelium unlike the modified epithelium containing M cells that overlies the follicle.

Antigen access and the lymphatic system

Lymphoid follicles of the mucosae and lymph nodes differ in that the former lack an organized afferent lymphatic system. Presumably the fluid percolating down through the domes func-tions like afferent lymph, transporting free antigen or antigen associated with macrophages and dendritic cells towards the follicles. Antigen-presenting cells are available in mouse Peyer's patches but precisely where the antigen that has passed through the M cells is presented has not been demonstrated. It is possible, as discussed later, that it differs for primary and secondary exposures to antigen. The follicular fluid eventually collects in a plexus of lymphatics surrounding each follicle and passes from there into the lymphatic network lying in the wall of the mucosal organ. Here it is mixed with lymph from the mucosa surrounding the follicle or group of follicles and the mixed lymph passes into the afferent lymphatics of a regional lymph node: in the case of the NALT, the superficial and deep cervical lymph nodes; in the case of the lungs and bronchi, the mediastinal (bronchial) lymph nodes; in the case of the small intestine, the mesenteric lymph nodes.

A consequence of the lack of afferent lymphatics in MALT nodules is that antigen that enters the mucosa via villous epithelia rather than via the follicle-associated epithelium will probably pass by way of lymphatics directly to the draining lymph nodes instead of to a nearby MALT nodule. In the case of GALT, for example, antigen that enters the intestinal lamina propria by penetrating the villous epithelium is likely to pass directly to the mesenteric lymph nodes. Only the small fraction of antigen that enters through the epithelium of the villi above the TD areas of Peyer's patches may pass into the nodule. In the mesenteric lymph nodes, the antigen may induce not only a mucosal immune response, but also a systemic immune response since the mesenteric lymph node permits entry of T and B cells capable of migrating through peripheral as well as mucosal lymphoid tissue (see later discussion on addressins). Alternatively, antigen may travel via the portal system to the liver, which might render it tolerogenic (see Chapters 13–15). Lymphocytes that leave the blood circulation in the lamina propria will also travel to the draining lymph node rather than to the nearest MALT nodule.

IMMUNIZATION AND THE MUCOSAL IMMUNE SYSTEM

Role of the lymphoid nodule

The role of the lymphoid nodule in the economy of the mucosal immune response has been most intensively studied with respect to Peyer's patches. Efficient immunization of B cells so as to yield antibody-forming cells that can populate the lamina propria requires that, at some stage, antigen be presented via the mucosal lymphoid follicles. Experiments involving instillation of antigen into isolated lengths of rabbit small intestine with or without Peyer's patches (Thiry–Vella loops) have shown that these GALT nodules are essential for specific antibody-forming cells to appear at both local and distant mucosal sites.[94] One possible explanation for this finding is that the antigens used in these experiments can only penetrate the body from the lumen of the small intestine via M cells in the epithelium of the Peyer's patch. An alternative hypothesis is that the follicle in the Peyer's patch is the optimal site for priming and/or selectively boosting B cells capable of eventual mucosal migration. Probably both the antigen-sampling ability of the M cells and the selective expansion of B cell populations capable of mucosal migration play a role.

Germinal centres

The GC of lymph nodes are well known to be sites at which intense proliferation of antigen-specific B and T cells,[71,99] somatic mutation of IgV-region genes, selection for high affinity antibody-forming B cells and deletion of low-affinity or self-reactive B cells take place. Follicular dendritic cells (FDC) are important in GC formation because they bind and retain antigen–antibody complexes and present them on iccosomes to antigen-specific B cells.[125,126] The B cells can then process and present the antigen to T cells which provide the signals necessary for B cell proliferation and differentiation. It is a reasonable supposition that MALT GC fulfil the same function; i.e. that the prominent GC in MALT follicles of conventional animals are maintained by constant antigenic stimulation from enteric antigens in GALT or inhaled antigens in NALT and BALT. The relationship between the B cells in the domes and coronas of the nodules and the proliferating B cells in the GC is not, however, at all clear. It is possible that primary antigen presentation can occur in the domes, where macrophages and dendritic cells as well as both T cells[11] and medium to large IgM+IgD+ B cells are plentiful,[128] or in the follicle. An alternative possibility is that most priming for IgA responses actually takes place in the regional lymph nodes and that the MALT nodule is a site of secondary expansion of antigen-specific mucosa-committed B lymphocytes and of their exposure to TGFβ,[26,121] which induces transcription of the germline Cα gene.[63,68]

About 60% of GALT GC cells express surface IgA,[21,62] which implies that they have already been exposed to T cell help and

inductive influences necessary for switching. The TGFβ needed for switching may be produced by local T cells interacting with the B cells: TGFβ expression is upregulated in the interfollicular (T-dependent) areas of Peyer's patches within 6 h of feeding the cognate antigen in T cell receptor (TCR) transgenic mice.[40] TGFβ is, however, constitutively produced in the intestinal lamina propria of conventional mice[6] and might even be transported in lymph to the mesenteric lymph nodes. Whatever its source, if it becomes activated locally, TGFβ is available to promote switching in GALT. B cell proliferation and commitment to IgA production also appears to take place in the lymphoid nodules of BALT and NALT, though there are many fewer cells expressing surface IgA in rat NALT than in Peyer's patches or BALT.[60]

Site of priming

Both primary and secondary responses to enteric antigen leading to IgA responses may take place in the Peyer's patch. As discussed previously,[94] antigen-specific B and T cells usually disappear from Peyer's patches rapidly after enteric priming, and their numbers then increase in the mesenteric lymph node. This suggests that they actively emigrate, conceivably in association with antigen-bearing dendritic cells. It is usually difficult to induce a mucosal immune response by administering antigen solely by the mucosal route except when viruses, invasive microorganisms or multiple doses of particulate antigens are used,[94] but addition of cholera toxin, a powerful mucosal adjuvant, often dramatically improves priming.[32] It may act by promoting antigen uptake, potentiating antigen processing and presentation, stimulating Th2-type cytokine production, inducing expression of costimulatory molecules and/or enhancing any of a variety of other necessary components to a mucosal immune response (see Chapters 7, 12 and 17).

It is moderately easy to induce a mucosal immune response by priming first via the intraperitoneal route and then boosting via the enteric route.[98] This supports the idea that Peyer's patch follicles may function best as sites of secondary expansion of B cells primed elsewhere than as sites at which priming occurs.[94] Some of the antigen injected via the intraperitoneal route might enter Peyer's patches from its serosal surface,[31] but most probably passes into the mediastinal[23] and mesenteric lymph nodes. If B memory cells responding to enteric antigen were primed in mesenteric lymph nodes by antigen carried there by macrophages and/or dendritic cells in lymph coming from the Peyer's patches, those that expressed mucosal recognition markers could subsequently migrate to Peyer's patches and mount secondary responses to antigen retained there.

MIGRATION OF MUCOSAL B AND T CELLS

Many types of transfer experiments, extensively reviewed in reference 94, have been used to delineate, in broad general terms, the pattern of immunization, isotype switching, maturation and migration of the B2 B cells in the mucosal immune system. At a certain point, cells stimulated in MALT nodules leave and pass into the regional lymph nodes; i.e. the mediastinal in the case of BALT, the mesenteric in the case of GALT, and the cervical in the case of NALT.[60] In the regional lymph nodes, IgA- and mucosa-committed B cells continue to proliferate and mature into activated blast cells capable of migration. They then leave the lymph node in its efferent lymph and pass into the thoracic duct through which they reach the blood circulation that carries them to the lamina propria of various mucosal organs. By the time mesenteric node-derived cells are ready to migrate, they are actively synthesizing DNA, bear surface IgA and lack complement receptors known to be present on their IgM[+]IgD[+] precursors in the Peyer's patch. Populations of GALT-derived T lymphoblasts and of IgG-committed B lymphoblasts also follow the same route. By contrast, B and T lymphoblasts from peripheral lymph nodes tend not to enter either mucosal lymphoid nodules or lamina propria at anything like the same frequency as GALT- and BALT-derived lymphoblasts.

MALT migrants

T and B cells within mucosal nodules are preselected in the sense that, to enter the nodule, their naïve precursors must have expressed a surface molecule necessary for binding to a receptor on the mucosal HEV. Several years ago, evidence that populations of IgA-committed B lymphoblasts activated by antigen in GALT or BALT could traffic to and settle not only in the intestinal[42,72–74,111] and bronchial[72] lamina propria, but also at sites such as the lactating mammary glands,[72,112] uterine cervix,[72] salivary and lacrimal glands,[82] gave rise to the idea that there is a common mucosal immune system. In this system, it was hypothesized that identification markers on the surface of the endothelial cells and receptors for them on the immigrant lymphoid cells might be shared. This idea formed the basis of hope that enteric vaccination with a variety of pathogens would yield populations of immune effector cells that would traffic to and provide protection at distant and unrelated mucosal sites.

It rapidly became clear, however, that regional preferences exist and that there might be several overlapping MALT circuits. For example, lymphocytes from the mediastinal lymph node localize better in the lungs than in the small intestine and the reverse is true of cells from the mesenteric lymph nodes;[72] lymphocyte populations expanded by encounter with antigen in the colon prefer the colon over the jejunum and vice versa;[97] protective immunization of macaques against simian immunodeficiency virus infection in the rectum is most effectively achieved with recombinant gp120 and p27 antigens by immunizing in the internal iliac lymph nodes rather than via the nasal, rectal and intramuscular routes and female genital tract;[66] this route of immunization does not, however, protect against vaginal infection.[69] Immunization of mice against streptococcal surface antigen via the nasal route results in the appearance of IgA antibody-secreting cells not only in the saliva and intestine, but also in the vagina.[134] The last few years have provided a wealth of information on some of the ligand–receptor interactions that govern migration of lymphocytes into MALT and peripheral lymphoid tissues. The endothelial molecules that control the tissue specificity of extravasating lymphocytes are known as vascular **addressins**. A scheme for the migration of mucosally committed lymphocytes is depicted in Fig. 3.2.

MUCOSAL ADDRESSINS

Addressins govern the migration of bloodborne lymphocytes into mucosal and peripheral lymphoid tissues.[20] Traffic into both peripheral and mucosal lymph nodes and MALT nodules of naïve T and B lymphocytes depends upon their ability to pass through HEV located in the paracortical areas of lymph nodes and in the T-dependent areas of MALT nodules. Extravasation of lymphocytes by crossing the endothelium (diapedesis) results from a multistep process[5,19,117,123] that depends first on interaction between L-selectin, present on the lymphocyte surface, and an addressin on the endothelial cells. This initiates rolling of the lymphocyte on the endothelium. Subsequently, integrins on the lymphocyte surface engage receptors on the endothelium, the lymphocyte stops rolling and diapedesis begins (Fig. 3.3).

L-selectin is a glycoprotein with a terminal Ca[++] lectin-like domain that binds to sulfated and sialylated O-linked oligosaccharides on several mucin-like glycoproteins expressed on HEV. Depending on their location primarily in peripheral lymph nodes *versus* Peyer's patches, these glycoproteins are collectively known as the peripheral node addressin (PNAd) or the mucosal addressin (MAdCAM-1), and are held responsible for peripheral node *versus* MALT discrimination by lymphocytes. In mice, both PNAds[49,53,100,109,110,116,135] expressed on peripheral lymph node HEV, and a subset of MAdCAM-1 molecules[84,115,119,124] expressed on MALT HEV bear the carbohydrate epitope recognized by the monoclonal antibody, MECA-79,[5,7] and by L-selectin.[49] Except for a few MAdCAM-1-positive cells in HEV of occasional individual peripheral lymph nodes, the majority of peripheral lymph nodes are MAdCAM-1-negative, expressing only the PNAds.[124] In principle, L-selectin-bearing lymphocytes can interact with the carbohydrate wherever it is present, but MAdCAM-1 is essentially expressed only in MALT, and mucosa-seeking lymphocytes bear a unique integrin, α4β7, that reacts with the protein core of MAdCAM-1.[10,34] Entry of lymphocytes into peripheral lymph nodes depends almost completely on L-selectin interaction with PNAds, but entry into Peyer's patch HEV depends on both L-selectin and α4β7 integrin interacting with MAdCAM-1 and is much less affected by the inhibitory effect of either MECA-79 or antibody to L-selectin.[14,37,124] Interestingly, given their central position in the body, mesenteric lymph nodes appear to have HEV expressing both PNAds and MAdCAM-1. Presumably these permit entry both of GALT-committed α4β7-bearing lymphocytes and of α4β7-negative lymphocytes committed to peripheral migration.

Adhesion mechanisms

Contact between L-selectin at the tips of the microvilli of a lymphocyte circulating in blood and MECA-79-positive molecules on the HEV leads to a rapid change in the behaviour of the lymphocyte: it becomes transiently tethered and then starts to roll on the surface of the endothelium.[5,61] Pertussis toxin-sensitive Gα$_i$-protein coupled receptors of the chemoattractant receptor family on the lymphocytes[122] then become activated. The undefined ligands for these receptors may or may not be chemoattractants.[20,123] Stimulation of the Gα$_i$ protein is thought to trigger rapid allosteric change in the integrins that mediate vascular adhesion.[22] If an endothelial ligand for the activated integrin is encountered in sufficient density, the lymphocyte stops and begins to migrate through the endothelium. If an appropriate ligand is not available, the integrin rapidly reverts to its former state and the lymphocyte goes back to rolling.

In peripheral lymph node HEV, the MECA-79 epitope is plentifully expressed on one or more of the PNAds. Peripheral lymphocytes have no known integrin capable of binding to PNAd that could be considered the equivalent of α4β7 binding to MAdCAM-1. In Peyer's patch HEV, the MECA-79 epitope is expressed on MAdCAM-1 in smaller amounts than on PNAd,[95,109]

A

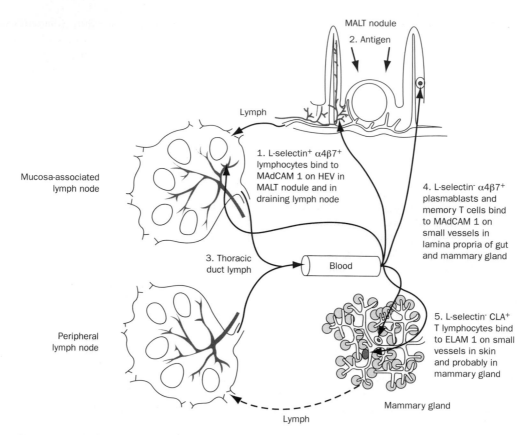

Fig. 3.2 Migration of lymphoctes in the mucosal immune system. Solid vessels in the lymph nodes and MALT nodule represent the venous system; open vessels in the MALT nodule and adjacent villi represent lymphatics. (1) L-selectin⁺ α4β7⁺ naïve T and B lymphocytes and B memory cells extravasate from blood through MAdCAM-1⁺ HEV in both mucosa-associated lymph nodes and MALT nodules. In these lymphoid tissues they encounter antigen (2) that has entered through M cells in the epithelium covering the MALT nodule. (3) After undergoing antigenic stimulation in the presence of costimulators and cytokines that promote switching of the B cells to IgA, activated lymphocytes leave the MALT nodule in the lymph, flowing into afferent lymphatics of the mucosa-associated lymph node. Here they undergo further stimulation and the stimulated B cells mature into plasmablasts. The mature cells, including the lymphocytes initially stimulated in the lymph node itself, leave in the efferent lymph. They enter the thoracic duct and are transported into the bloodstream which carries them to the same or distant lymphoid tissues as well as to lamina propria of MALT and exocrine glands, such as the mammary gland. Plasmablasts derived from the B cells extravasate through MAdCAM-1⁺ vessels in the lamina propria and settle down to become IgA-secreting plasma cells in the lamina propria. Memory B cells that re-express L-selectin recirculate through MAdCAM-1⁺ HEV. Each time these B cells re-encounter their specific antigen, their numbers are expanded such that MALT comes to contain a preponderance of IgA-committed B cells capable of migrating through MALT. Memory T cells lose L-selectin and do not regain it so cannot extravasate through HEV. They can, however, migrate through tissues and arrive in lymph nodes via afferent lymphatics. In the peripheral lymph nodes there may not be much antigenic stimulation, so populations of T and B cells that arrive in peripheral lymph nodes after traversing the lamina propria of the mammary glands may not be greatly expanded. Moreover, even if local antigenic stimulation is provided, the milieu in peripheral lymph nodes is not particularly conducive to IgA switching, so the antibody produced is more usually IgG.

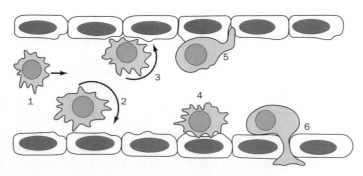

Fig. 3.3 Extravasation of lymphocytes through HEV at mucosal sites. (1) Lymphocytes bearing L-selectin and α4β7 integrin at the tips of microvilli encounter MAdCAM-1 on the HEV, leave the central freeflowing stream and (2 and 3) begin to roll along the surface of the HEV. Upon receipt of an activation signal through a G protein-linked receptor, the lymphocyte stops rolling (4) and binds more strongly to the HEV, using a cooperative interaction between LFA-1, which binds to ICAM-1 and ICAM-2, together with α4β7 binding to MAdCAM-1. Adhesion of the lymphocyte to the HEV is then followed by diapedesis (5 and 6). LFA-1 is expressed on the lymphocyte surface only between the microvilli and does not participate in the rolling interactions.

and effective initial rolling interaction of the mucosa-seeking lymphocyte microvilli with the endothelial cell surface requires cooperative interaction between L-selectin binding to the carbohydrate and $\alpha 4\beta 7$ binding to the core of MAdCAM-1.[5,9] Binding of the lymphocyte to MAdCAM-1 and lymphocyte arrest is then mediated by $\alpha 4\beta 7$ integrin. Subsequently, for adhesion and diapedesis, both peripheral node-seeking and mucosa-seeking lymphocytes utilize the $\alpha 1\beta 2$ integrin,[5] LFA-1, which binds to ICAMs 1 and 2 on the endothelial cell.

Expression of L-selectin and $\alpha 4\beta 7$

The amounts of L-selectin and $\alpha 4\beta 7$ integrin vary on lymphocytes of different lineages at different stages in their careers and significantly affect the way they migrate through HEV in lymphoid tissues *versus* vessels in lamina propria, skin and other tissues. For example, although naïve T and B cells bear L-selectin which enables them to extravasate via HEV, L-selectin disappears from, or is drastically reduced on, the surface of both T and B cells upon antigen-driven activation.[25,57,101] Subsequently, both activated T effector cells and T memory cells tend to be L-selectin-deficient,[1,70] whereas memory B cells re-express L-selectin[57] (Table 3.2). Thus, for memory T lymphocytes to circulate through lymphoid tissue, many or all of them have to extravasate in the tissues and then enter lymphoid tissue by way of afferent lymphatics.[24,70] Memory B cells, on the other hand, can enter lymph nodes by way either of afferent lymphatics or HEV. Given the paucity of afferent lymphatics to lymphoid nodules such as Peyer's patches, it is intriguing that, while the B cells entering Peyer's patches can be either naïve or memory cells, a preponderance of the T_H cells available to interact with them is probably naïve.

Skin T cells[8] and L-selectin-negative memory T lymphocytes thought to be destined to extravasate in skin[96,118] bear a surface carbohydrate named CLA that binds E-selectin, induced on dermal endothelial cells in delayed hypersensitivity reactions[27] and inflamed skin.[96] This mediates rolling of the lymphocytes just like L-selectin binding to PNAd, even though the locations of the lectin (on the endothelium) and carbohydrate (on the lymphocyte) are reversed.

In contrast to MAdCAM-1 expressed on Peyer's patch and mesenteric lymph node HEV, MAdCAM-1 expressed in lamina propria at various mucosal sites lacks the MECA-79 epitope that defines the L-selectin ligand. Activated mucosal B and T effector lymphoblasts have high levels[20] of $\alpha 4\beta 7$, which enable them to extravasate through the endothelium of intestinal lamina propria or any other lamina propria bearing MAdCAM-1 without the need for L-selectin interaction. In contrast, naïve $\alpha 4\beta 7$-bearing cells generally do not have sufficient $\alpha 4\beta 7$ to bind to lamina propria MAdCAM-1 without the cooperation of L-selectin and can only extravasate in HEV. This effectively keeps naïve B cells in the circulation and lymphoid nodules and out of the lamina propria. MAdCAM-1 is expressed in the lamina propria not only of the large intestine but also of the lactating mammary gland.[95,124] The presence of MAdCAM-1 on lactating mammary gland endothelium of course provides a ready explanation for why mesenteric node IgA-committed B lymphoblasts migrate there.[112] Evidence that they only do so if the gland is lactating suggests that expression of MAdCAM-1 at this site is under hormonal control.

It is quite possible that other mucosal addressins, perhaps with their own integrin ligands, have yet to be discovered in BALT and NALT. As discussed earlier, BALT-derived lymphoblasts from mice show some preference for BALT over GALT.[72] Expression of MAdCAM-1 in the lung and associated lymph nodes has been shown to be minimal,[17] and only very low expression of $\alpha 4\beta 7$ integrin is detected on lymphocytes circulating through the lungs of sheep.[1] It may be that lymphocytes in BALT use a different addressin–ligand system from that in GALT. The small amount of data available on the way in which immunization in NALT affects the female urogenital tract suggests that the population of lymphocytes that migrates through MALT at these locations may also use a different addressin–ligand system from that used in GALT.

Types of B cell precursors

Transfer experiments have shown that the B cell pool that contributes to mucosal IgA plasma cells contains a mixture of two types of B cell precursors. One population, often termed 'conventional' B2 cells,[51,57] consists of fetal liver and/or bone marrow-derived cells that mature through stages at which they express high levels of surface IgD.[128] The other population[58] consists of coelomic or B1[51,52] B cells that predominate in the peritoneal and pleural cavities,[46–48] and are also found in the 13-day fetal omentum and liver.[120] B1 B cells express only low levels of IgD and may or may not bear CD5.[46,50] It is difficult to determine the proportions of intestinal IgA plasma cells actually derived from B1 *versus* B2 cell populations in conventional animals because, in transfer experiments using mixed populations, the B1 cells seem to suppress the immunoglobulin secretory activity of B2 cells.[107] Despite several problems in interpreting these experiments, discussed in reference 94, the contribution of B1 cells to lamina propria IgA plasma cells is of tremendous interest and potential importance. Many B1 cells produce germline unmutated antibodies that react both with autoantigens and with common microbial epitopes.[45,91,92,102] Such antibodies could form a highly efficient first line of defence against infection and contribute to local immunity in the lamina propria. In the context of the present discussion, there are several unanswered questions. B1 B cells have germline, unmutated Ig V-region genes and are thought not to enter GC (where antigenic stimulation could lead to mutation and selection). They are virtually absent from Peyer's patches or lymph nodes[59] and presumably reach the lamina propria in the bloodstream. How do they exit the peritoneal and pleural cavities and enter the blood? Do they go through the afferent lymphatics of the mediastinal lymph nodes and then pass rapidly through the subcapsular, cortical and medullary sinuses to the efferent lymph without ever migrating into the B cell areas of the nodes? Do they migrate to lamina

Expression of L-selectin and $\alpha 4\beta 7$ on mucosal cells		
	L-selectin	$\alpha 4\beta 7$
Naïve T and B cells	+++	+
Antigen-activated mucosal T and B cells	+/–	+++
T effector cells	+/–	++
T memory cells	+/–	
B memory cells	++	

Table 3.2 Expression of L-selectin and $\alpha 4\beta 7$ on mucosal cells.

propria in mucosal sites other than the small intestine? Do they bear α4β7? Answers to some of these questions could lead to new ways of thinking about mucosal migration and immune responses as well as about morphogenesis of the mucosal lymphoid tissues.

MORPHOGENESIS OF THE PERIPHERAL AND MUCOSAL LYMPHOID SYSTEMS

Work by early anatomists indicates that the lymphoid system arises first as fluid-filled clefts in the mesenchyme usually at or near vascular junctions.[12] The mesenchymal cells surrounding the clefts acquire endothelial characteristics and the spaces gradually fuse to form lymphatic sacs interconnected by more or less cylindrical lymphatic vessels. More lymphatics are formed by budding out from the existing vessels. Lymph nodes do not appear until after the formation of the primary lymphatic system. The primary nodes, including the deep jugular (deep cervical) and retroperitoneal nodes, then develop from the lymphatic sacs in their region. Secondary nodes, such as the inguinal node, appear later along the course of the lymphatic vessels.

Role of the IL7 receptor

Recent work[2] targeting either IL7 receptor α (IL7Rα) or JAK3, an essential transducer of the IL7Rα signal, indicates that Peyer's patch anlagen develop early in embryogenesis under the control of the IL7Rα. They first appear as VCAM-1-positive spots on the small intestine whether or not lymphocytes are available to populate them, developing in rag 2$^{-/-}$, nu/nu and SCID mice. Nothing is yet known about the inductive signals that make Peyer's patches and lymph nodes form just where they do during normal embryogenesis. Studies using transgenic and gene-targeted 'knock-out' mice have, however, shown that development of both mucosal and peripheral lymphoid tissues is influenced by a variety of cytokines, integrins, chemokines and their receptors, whose effects are presumably mediated by the different transcription factors they activate. It has not been unambiguously demonstrated that any one of the known ligand–receptor pairs is responsible for the initial formation of the lymphoid anlagen itself. Each pair may have several effects on the entry of immigrant lymphoid cells and/or the internal architecture of the organ.[79]

Role of lymphotoxins

Three TNF-related cytokines play major roles in the development of lymphoid tissue: TNFα, LTα and LTβ.[3,56,76,114,130] TNFα, a type II membrane protein, is proteolytically cleaved from the surface of macrophages and T cells as a soluble homotrimer. LTα, secreted as a homotrimer primarily by activated T and B lymphocytes and natural killer (NK) cells, also associates with its homologue LTβ, a type II membrane protein, to form a cell surface heterotrimer, LTα1β2, or a minor form, LTα2β1, on these cells. Both TNFα and secreted LTα bind to a pair of TNF receptors (TNF-R), TNF-RI (p55) and TNF-RII (p78), expressed in different regions of lymphoid tissue. TNF-RI expression is limited to the FDC in the follicles and GC, while TNF-RII is located in the interfollicular areas.[113] TNF-RII does not appear to play a major role in the development of lymphoid tissue[33,76,90,93] and will not be further discussed. The LTα1β2 heterotrimer binds to the LTβ receptor (LTβ-R),[28] which, in vitro, is expressed on most of the same cell lines that express TNF-RI. The minor heterotrimer, LTα2β1, binds to TNF-RI[130] (Table 3.3).

TNF-related cytokines and development of lymphoid tissue			
	Type	**Origin**	**Binds to**
TNFα	Type II membrane protein: soluble homotrimer	Macrophages, T cells	TNF-RI (p55) TNF-RII (p78)
LTα	Type II membrane protein: soluble homotrimer	Activated T, B cells, NK cells	TNF-RI (p55) TNF-RII (p78)
LTβ	Homologue of LTα	Activated T, B cells, NK cells	—
LTα1β2	Surface heterotrimer	Major form	LTβ-R
LTα2β1	Surface heterotrimer	Minor form	TNF-RI

Table 3.3 TNF-related cytokines and development of lymphoid tissue.

Sorting out the roles in lymphoid development of the soluble homotrimers, TNFα and LTα, that bind to and activate TNF-RI *versus* the cell surface heterotrimer LTα1β2 that binds to LTβ-R, has proven to be very difficult. Lately, the work of several groups of researchers using mice with targeted TNFα, LTα, LTβ, TNF-RI and LTβ-R genes and/or exposed to genetically engineered soluble receptors and monoclonal antibodies, is finally yielding fruit. As would be expected, LTα is revealed as a key player since it participates in activating both TNF-RI and LTβ-R.

Effects of gene targeting on splenic architecture

In both LTα$^{-/-}$ (references 4, 30, 76–78, 127) and TNF-RI$^{-/-}$ (reference 65) mice, splenic architecture is disorganized, with defective formation of GC and FDC networks and of B and T cell compartments. The effects of targeting the LTα and TNF-RI genes seem to reflect their normal expression in different cell types: when irradiated LTα$^{-/-}$ mice are given wild type (wt) T-depleted bone marrow (BM) cells, GC and FDC clusters are formed in their spleens, indicating that the defects in splenic architecture caused by LTα deficiency can be at least partially ameliorated by providing a BM-derived cellular component from adult mice, most likely B cells.[127] By contrast, giving wild type (wt) BM cells to TNF-RI-targeted mice does not repair their splenic defects, suggesting that the cells affected by TNF-RI deficiency, most likely the FDC on which TNF-RI are normally expressed, are not BM-derived, at least in adult mice.[77,127]

Effects of gene targeting on development of lymph nodes and Peyer's patches

The effects of targeting LTα, TNFα, TNF-RI and LTβ on lymphoid tissue development indicate that synergistic interactions between different ligand and receptor pairs are responsible for development of individual lymph nodes and Peyer's patches. The intricacy of the interactions is illustrated by the following observations. LTα$^{-/-}$ mice lack virtually all lymph nodes and Peyer's patches at birth,[4,30,56,76] as do wt mice treated *in utero* with both LTβ-R-Ig and TNF-R55-Ig to block signalling by either receptor[105] and mice lacking both TNF-RI and LTβ.[55] By contrast, LTα$^{-/-}$ mice lacking LTα1β2 but expressing soluble LTα from a transgene[114] have cervical, axillary, brachial, mesenteric and para-aortic lymph nodes but still lack Peyer's patches, inguinal and popliteal lymph nodes. LTα[-/-] mice exposed *in utero* to agonist anti-LTβ-R monoclonal antibody develop lymph nodes if exposure begins early in gestation, but not if initial exposure is left too late.[105] TNFα[-/-] mice have normal numbers of lymph nodes of normal size,[56,90] but have reduced numbers of abnormally small, ill-defined Peyer's patches[90] and TNF-RI[-/-] mice resemble them in having normal numbers of normally sized lymph nodes but no true Peyer's patches, only small, undifferentiated lymphoid aggregates in the gut wall.[65,85] LTβ[-/-] mice lack Peyer's patches and most lymph nodes, but usually have mesenteric and cervical lymph nodes.[3,54] Wt mice in which membrane LTα1β2 is blocked *in utero* by LTβ-R-Ig so that it cannot interact with the LTβ-R *in situ* have mesenteric, sacral, lumbar and cervical lymph nodes but lack sciatic, parathymic, iliac and mandibular lymph nodes or Peyer's patches.[104] In contrast to mice heterozygous for deficiency in either LTα or LTβ, which have both lymph nodes and Peyer's patches, mice heterozygous for deficiency in *both* LTα and LTβ[55] lack Peyer's patches, suggesting that quantitative differences in the relative amounts of LTα3 *versus* LTα1β2 that can be formed disrupt the synergy between the TNF-RI and the LTβ-R with deleterious effects on Peyer's patch formation. In LTβ-R[-/-] mice, there are no detectable Peyer's patches and no mesenteric, cervical axillary, inguinal, para-aortic sacral or popliteal lymph nodes.[36]

Need for LTβ-R and TNF-RI

Taken together, the results cited above suggest strongly that signalling via both LTβ-R and the TNF-RI are essential for proper development of Peyer's patches. Signalling via LTβ-R is required for development of most, if not all, lymph nodes but signalling via TNF-RI is not, though it may be required for proper development of the lymphoid architecture. The complete lack of anything more than endothelium-lined spaces where lymph nodes should be in LTβ-R[-/-] mice suggests that signalling via the LTβ-R may be required for formation of the lymphoid anlagen themselves.[36] There is an apparent discrepancy between the total lack of lymph nodes in LTβ-R[-/-] mice[36] and the presence of mucosal lymph nodes in wt mice exposed *in utero* to LTβ-R-Ig.[104] A possible explanation could be that *in utero* exposure to LTβ-R-Ig may have begun too late to prevent the formation of the anlagen. Since, as mentioned above, RAG 2[-/-], nu/nu and SCID mice have Peyer's patches, it seems likely that the ligand responsible for activating LTβ-R in the lymphoid anlagen of fetal mice is not carried to the site on the surface of a T or B lymphocyte.

Once lymphoid anlagen have formed, interaction between LTβ-R and a ligand continues to be necessary for their further development. When it is blocked,[104] both MAdCAM-1 and PNAd are downregulated on the HEV of those lymph nodes that do form, and the B cells that arrive in the nodes are mainly found in the subcapsular region. Presumably these B cells enter the lymph nodes via afferent lymphatics rather than through HEV. Development of Peyer's patches may be more affected than that of mucosal lymph nodes when interaction between LTβ-R and its ligand is blocked because the Peyer's patches lack afferent lymphatics and are more dependent on entry of lymphocytes via HEV. Mucosal lymph nodes act as funnels that collect all the lymph and cells arriving from the considerable amount of lamina propria draining into them. Since the major source of antigenic stimulation in these very clean mice is via mucosa, the mucosal

lymph nodes are likely to contain more lymphocytes arriving via afferent lymphatics than peripheral lymph nodes and many more than Peyer's patches. What is still missing to clinch this argument is any information on the expression of MAdCAM-1 on lamina propria vessels in LTβ-R-Ig-treated mice.

Role of chemokines

In normal mice, mature B cells and a subset of T cells express a G protein-coupled chemokine receptor called BLR1, whose ligand is a CXC chemokine, variously known as B cell-attracting chemokine 1 (BCA-1)[64] or B lymphocyte chemoattractant BLC.[41] BLC is expressed in splenic B cell-rich zones and follicles and in the GC of Peyer's patches, but only sporadically in lymph node follicles. Although they have all other lymph nodes, BLR1[-/-] mice[35] completely lack inguinal lymph nodes and lack or have few, very impaired Peyer's patches. In those Peyer's patches that do develop, the follicles are replaced by multiple B and T cell-rich zones. Despite the defects in the number and structure of the Peyer's patches, the lamina propria of the small intestine appears to be normal with respect to IgA plasma cell content. In the spleen, there are defects in the formation of primary and secondary follicles and GC, but the peripheral and mesenteric lymph nodes appear to be normal. In both the spleen and peripheral blood B cells predominate over T cells.

Transfer experiments indicate that BLR1[-/-] B cells can enter the T cell areas of Peyer's patches and spleen but then fail to migrate into the follicles. In the lymph nodes, by contrast, they distribute themselves normally. These data suggest that B cell follicle formation in Peyer's patches, inguinal lymph nodes and spleen is fundamentally different from that in peripheral and mesenteric lymph nodes. It has been suggested[41] that an additional, thus far unknown, B cell chemoattractant may be of importance in certain lymph nodes, and this raises the possibility that there may also be an additional receptor. It could be that Peyer's patches, spleen and inguinal nodes are highly dependent on BLR1–BLC/BCA1 interaction while most lymph nodes depend on a different chemotactic ligand–receptor combination that allows them to develop normally in BLR1[-/-] mice.

Role of addressins and their ligands

As discussed earlier, entry of small lymphocytes into adult mouse mucosal lymphoid tissue through HEV depends upon the lymphocytes expressing both L-selectin and the α4β7 integrin as well as on the HEV expressing the mucosal addressin MAdCAM-1. By contrast, lymphocytes entering peripheral lymph nodes via HEV use only L-selectin binding to the PNAds. Recent work has revealed a developmental switch in the expression of endothelial vascular addressin and lymphocyte homing receptors.[80] Neonatal lymphocyte entry into lymph nodes before and up to 24 h after birth depends on expression of MAdCAM-1 on the HEV of *both* mucosal and peripheral lymph nodes. The PNAd recognized by MECA-79 appears on HEV no earlier than 24 h after birth and is then expressed together with MAdCAM-1 on both peripheral and mesenteric lymph nodes for about 2 weeks. Thereafter there is a gradual decline in expression of MAdCAM-1 on the HEV of peripheral lymph nodes until it disappears by the fourth week after birth while high levels of MAdCAM-1 continue to be expressed by mesenteric lymph nodes. The first cells to enter peripheral lymph nodes are α4β7-positive and are apparently derived from a minor population of the leukocytes in peripheral blood (2–4%), while the bulk of the peripheral blood leukocytes are L-selectin-positive. Entry of α4β7-positive cells into lymph nodes can be blocked with antibody to MAdCAM-1 but not by antibody to L-selectin.

On the day of birth, the majority of the small numbers of cells entering the lymph nodes using α4β7 and MAdCAM-1 are CD3+CD4+ or CD3+C60+ T cells; there are very few B cells. There is also an extremely interesting population of α4β7-bearing CD4+CD3- cells that enters lymph nodes of fetal mice.[81] Cells of this population, first found in early fetal spleen, bear both LTβ and IL2-Rγ chains and contain message for BLR1, LTβ and Rel B. Upon culture with appropriate cytokines, they can develop into antigen-presenting cells and NK cells but not T or B cells. Upon transfer, they migrate into B cell areas and it has been suggested that they might be FDC precursors. The findings discussed above suggest that expression of the integrin β7 molecule would be likely to be critical for the proper development of all lymphoid tissue, both mucosal and peripheral. It has, however, been reported that in integrin β7−/− mice, while there is overall GALT hypoplasia, with no Peyer's patches visible at the age of 6 weeks, there is no reduction in cellularity of spleen, peripheral and mesenteric lymph nodes.[129] This suggests that L-selectin/PNAd-mediated entry of lymphocytes into the peripheral and mesenteric nodes can take place once these markers appear. What has not yet been established at time of writing is whether the follicular structure and architecture of the lymph nodes are normal.

THE MAMMARY GLAND IN THE CONTEXT OF MUCOSAL IMMUNITY

As the name implies, the key evolutionary feature of mammals, distinguishing them from all other vertebrates, is the presence of mammary glands enabling them to suckle their young. Mammary glands are not only anatomically and physiologically adapted to providing sustenance to the offspring in the form of colostrum and milk, they also transmit antibodies evoked in the mother against microorganisms with which she has been infected via mucosal routes. Suckling therefore provides the immature offspring not only with food, but also with antibody-mediated protection against the microorganisms most likely to be transmitted from the mother during or after birth. Before birth, human fetuses receive, via the placenta, maternal IgG, whose many specificities reflect the systemic antigenic stimulation to which the mother has been exposed. This IgG protects the fetus *in utero* and persists in the infant's circulation for several months after birth while the infant's own immune system is immature. But IgG does not pass from the infant's circulation into mucosal secretions and so does not protect the infant's mucosae from infection. In some mammals, IgG is present in milk early in lactation.[103] In these, the intestinal tract of the immature offspring permits ingested IgG to be absorbed into the circulation for species-defined short periods of time before 'closure'. This IgG, however, comes from the mother's serum pool and does not reflect her mucosal immunity.

Human milk

There is little IgG in human milk at any time. IgA with specificity for microorganisms present in the mother's intestinal and, to a lesser extent, respiratory tract, is the principal antibody isotype transmitted in milk throughout lactation. After it is ingested, IgA antibody is not absorbed by the infant's gastrointestinal tract.

Instead, it passes down the intestine, providing local protection against endemic microorganisms, including potential pathogens. Apart from its specificity for enteric microorganisms, a major reason that IgA is the preferred immunoglobulin for milk is that covalent bonding of secretory component to dimeric IgA during its passage through the mammary gland epithelium renders the SIgA so formed resistant to proteolysis.[18] In areas of the world where sanitation is deficient, the importance of breast feeding in providing passive protection to the developing infants was rightly stressed by healthcare workers until recently, when the risk of transmission of HIV in milk became of serious concern.[13,67]

Milk immunoglobulin A

Most human serum IgA is monomeric so cannot be transcytosed across the mammary epithelium by pIgR, which interacts only with dimeric, J chain-containing IgA. Mice and rats, on the other hand, have appreciable quantities of dimeric IgA in their serum. Early in lactation this can be transported into milk in mice,[44] but not in rats.[29] In human milk, the many plasma cells in the lactating mammary gland are the major source of IgA.[15,38] Their precursors were evidently exposed to intestinal antigens in GALT since specific IgA antibodies to intestinal microorganisms appear in milk in the absence of serum antibodies of any isotype, thus precluding any idea that they could have arisen by systemic immunization.[39,83] There are few plasma cells in the mammary glands of non-pregnant humans or mice, but they increase dramatically during pregnancy and lactation in both humans[15] and mice,[131] and the great majority express IgA. In mice, their increase has been shown to be under hormonal control: in virgin females, injections of oestrogen, progesterone and prolactin enhance the number of IgA plasma cells in mammary gland whereas, in naturally lactating females, injections of testosterone depress it.[132]

Milk lymphocytes

Direct evidence has been obtained using radiolabelled cells that GALT-derived lymphoblasts from mouse mesenteric lymph nodes migrate to mammary glands of lactating, but not virgin, mice much more efficiently than do lymphoblasts from peripheral lymph nodes.[72,112] Moreover, in mice that have been fed ferritin throughout pregnancy, numerous ferritin-specific IgA plasma cells appear in the mammary glands during lactation.[133] At the time of their entry into mammary glands, the plasma cell precursors already bear surface IgA and lack CR2 found on most mature B cells.[112] The addressin by which they recognize mammary gland endothelium is thought to be MAdCAM-1 expressed on small vessels in the lactating gland.[124] That IgA-committed B lymphoblasts migrate from GALT to lactating mammary glands in humans has not been formally demonstrated for obvious reasons, but the evidence acquired in the mouse model suggests very strongly that they do and that this migration accounts for the presence in mother's milk of IgA antibodies against her intestinal microorganisms (Fig. 3.4).

Mammary gland T cells

T cells isolated from human mammary gland and colostrum may represent selected subsets since they do not mirror T cells in the blood circulation with respect to responsiveness to antigens and mitogens or suppressor:helper ratios.[87,88,106] They do not necessarily, however, have a special connection with GALT. There

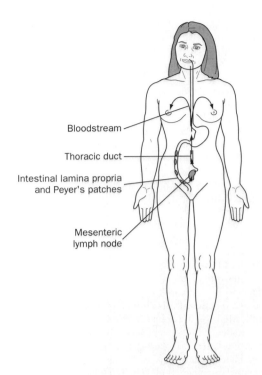

Fig. 3.4 Enteromammary circulation of lymphocytes. IgA-committed B cells that have responded to antigen in the intestine leave the Peyer's patches in the lymph and migrate into the mesenteric lymph nodes. From here, they pass via the thoracic duct into the bloodstream which carries them to the lactating mammary glands where they extravasate and become dimeric IgA-secreting plasma cells.

Bloodstream

Thoracic duct

Intestinal lamina propria
and Peyer's patches

Mesenteric
lymph node

KEY FACTS

1. The mucosal immune system consists of two components: (a) nodular lymphoid tissue, usually containing germinal centres, covered by a modified epithelium that participates in uptake of antigen from mucosal surface, and (b) lymphoid tissue distributed throughout the lamina propria.

2. Lymphocyte migration in the mucosal immune system depends on interaction between sets of ligands and receptors expressed on naïve and memory B and T cells, and on the endothelia through which they extravasate.

3. Both mucosal and peripheral lymphoid tissues express the L-selectin-binding epitope of the peripheral node addressin (PNAd) on high endothelial venules in organized lymphoid tissue, but the mucosal lymphoid tissue expresses much less than the peripheral and does not express it in lamina propria.

4. Mucosa-associated lymphoid tissue is distinguished from peripheral lymphoid tissue by its expression of the mucosal addressin MAdCAM-1 on its endothelium both in the HEV of lymphoid nodues and in the lamina propria vessels.

5. Mucosa-seeking lymphocytes bear a unique integrin, the $\alpha4\beta7$ integrin, which mediates binding to MAdCAM-1.

6. Migration of activated B lymphoblasts from the nodular components of gut-associated lymphoid tissue and bronchus-associated lymphoid tissue to other mucosal sites such as the salivary, lacrimal glands and lactating mammary gland appears to involve interaction between integrin $\alpha4\beta7$ and MAdCAM-1. It is possible that additional ligand receptor pairs may be involved in migration within the nose-associated lymphoid tissue and BALT, and between NALT and the urogenital tract.

7. Migration of antigen-activated IgA-committed B lymphoblasts from GALT and BALT to the lactating mammary gland results in transmission of maternal IgA antibodies against enteric and respiratory microorganisms to the infant's intestine where they can exert a protective effect.

8. The development of mucosal and peripheral lymphoid tissue is controlled by complex interactions between the soluble lymphotoxin α and tumour necrosis factor α homotrimers and one of their receptors, TNF receptor (TNF-R) I, as well as by the cell surface heterotrimer $LT\alpha1\beta2$ and its receptor, the $LT\beta$ receptor.

9. These interactions may be involved in development of certain lymphoid tissue anlagen as well as in the development of the architecture of the lymphoid tissue.

10. Interaction between $LT\alpha1\beta2$ and the $LT\beta$-R is necessary for expression of addressins on HEV in lymphoid tissue.

are, in GALT, populations of T cells that seem to have a similar life cycle to that of GALT B cells participating in mucosal immune responses.[43] When, however, the abilities of populations of rat T lymphoblasts from mesenteric *versus* peripheral lymph node to migrate to the mammary gland were compared, there was no difference between them.[75] The suggestion was made 20 years ago that T cells from GALT may migrate to mammary gland as part of a generalized mucosal immune system, whereas those from peripheral lymph nodes may do so as a manifestation of the tendency of some T cells to go to skin, the tissue of origin of the mammary gland.[89,108] In the light of more recent studies on the loss of L-selectin from activated T cells and T memory cells, and the acquisition by some peripheral node T memory cells of cutaneous lymphocyte antigen (CLA),[8,96,118] this suggestion seems quite prescient. The function of the T cells in the mammary gland and in milk is unknown.

REFERENCES

1 Abitorabi AA, Mackay CR, Jerome EH *et al*. Differential expression of homing molecules on recirculating lymphocytes from sheep gut, peripheral and lung lymph. *J Immunol* 1996; 156: 3111–17.

2 Adachi S, Yoshida H, Honda K *et al*. Essential role of IL-7 receptor α in the formation of Peyer's patch anlage. *Int Immunol* 1998; 10: 1–6.

3 Alimzhanov MB, Kuprash DV, Kosco-Viboius MH *et al*. Abnormal development of secondary lymphoid tissues in lymphotoxin beta-deficient mice. *Proc Natl Acad Sci USA* 1997; 94: 9302–7.

4 Banks T, Rouse BT, Kerley MK *et al*. Lymphotoxin alpha-deficient mice: effects on secondary lymphoid organ development and humoral responsiveness. *J Immunol* 1995; 155: 1685–93.

5 Bargatze RF, Jutila MA, Butcher EC. Distinct roles of L-selectin and integrins $\alpha4\beta7$ and LFA1 in lymphocyte homing to Peyer's patch-HEV *in situ*: the multistep model confirmed and refined. *Immunity* 1995; 3: 99–108.

6 Barnard JA, Warwick GJ, Gold LI. Localization of transforming growth factor beta isoforms in the normal murine small intestine and colon. *Gastroenterology* 1993; 105: 67–73.

7 Berg EL, McEvoy LM, Berlin C *et al.* L-selectin-mediated lymphocyte rolling on MAdCAM-1. *Nature* 1993; 366: 695–8.

8 Berg EL, Yoshino T, Rott L *et al.* The cutaneous lymphocyte antigen is a skin lymphocyte homing receptor for the vascular lectin endothelial cell leukocyte adhesion molecule 1. *J Exp Med* 1991; 174: 1461–1466.

9 Berlin C, Bargatze RF, Campbell JJ *et al.* α4 integrins mediate lymphocyte attachment and rolling under physiologic flow. *Cell* 1995; 80: 413–22.

10 Berlin C, Berg EL, Briskin MJ *et al.* α4β7 integrin mediates lymphocyte binding to the mucosal vascular addressin MAdCAM-1. *Cell* 1993; 74: 185–95.

11 Bjerke K, Brandtzaeg P, Fausa O. T cell distribution is different in follicle-associated epithelium of human Peyer's patches and villous epithelium. *Clin Exp Immunol* 1988; 74: 270–5.

12 Bloom W, Fawcett DW. In: *A Textbook of Histology*, 8th edn. WB Saunders, Philadelphia, 1962; 300–1.

13 Bobat R, Moodley D, Coutsoudis A, Coovadia H. Breastfeeding by HIV-1-infected women and outcome in their infants: a cohort study from Durban, South Africa. *AIDS* 1997; 11: 1627–33.

14 Bradley LM, Watson SR, Swain SL. Entry of naive CD4 T cells into peripheral lymph nodes requires L-selectin. *J Exp Med* 1994; 180: 2401–6.

15 Brandtzaeg P. The secretory immune system of lactating human mammary glands compared with other exocrine organs. *Ann NY Acad Sci* 1983; 409: 353–81.

16 Brandtzaeg P. Research in gastrointestinal immunology – state of the art. *Scand J Gastroenterol* 1985; 20 (Suppl. 114): 137–56.

17 Briskin MJ, McEvoy LM, Butcher EC. MadCAM-1 has homology to immunoglobulin and mucin-like adhesion receptors and to IgA1. *Nature* 1993; 363: 461–4.

18 Brown WR, Newcombe RW, Ishizaka K. Proteolytic degradation of exocrine and serum immunoglobulins. *J Clin Invest* 1970; 49: 1374–80.

19 Butcher EC. Leukocyte-endothelial cell recognition: three (or more) steps to specificity and diversity. *Cell* 1991; 67: 1033–6.

20 Butcher EC, Picker LJ. Lymphocyte homing and homeostasis. *Science* 1996; 272: 60–6.

21 Butcher EC, Rouse RV, Coffman RL *et al.* Surface phenotype of Peyer's patch germinal center cells: implications for the role of germinal centers in B cell differentiation. *J Immunol* 1982; 129: 2698–707.

22 Carr MW, Alon R, Springer TA. The C-C chemokine MCP-1 differentially modulates the avidity of beta 1 and beta 2 integrins on T lymphocytes. *Immunity* 1996; 4: 179–87.

23 Carter PB, Collins FM. The route of enteric infection in normal mice. *J Exp Med* 1974; 139: 1189–203.

24 Catalina MD, Carroll MC, Arizpe H *et al.* The route of antigen entry determines the requirement for L-selectin during immune responses. *J Exp Med* 1996; 184: 2341–51.

25 Chao C-C, Jensen R, Dailey MO. Mechanisms of L-selectin regulation by activated T cells. *J Immunol* 1997; 159: 1686–94.

26 Coffman RL, Lebman DA, Schrader B. Transforming growth factor-β specifically enhances IgA production by lipopolysaccharide-stimulated murine B lymphocytes. *J Exp Med* 1989; 170: 1039–44.

27 Cotran RS, Gimbrone MA Jr, Bevilacqua MP *et al.* Induction and detection of a human endothelial activation antigen *in vivo*. *J Exp Med* 1986; 164: 661–6.

28 Crowe P, VanArsdale TL, Walter BN *et al.* A lymphotoxin-β-specific receptor. *Science* 1994; 264: 707–10.

29 Dahlgren U, Ahlstedt S, Hedman L *et al.* Dimeric IgA in the rat is transferred from serum into bile but not into milk. *Scand J Immunol* 1981; 14: 95–8.

30 DeTogni PD, Goeliner J, Ruddle NH *et al.* Abnormal development of peripheral lymphoid organs in mice deficient in lymphotoxin. *Science* 1994; 264: 703–7.

31 Dunkley ML, Husband AJ. The induction and migration of antigen-specific helper cells for IgA responses in the intestine. *Reg Immunol* 1986; 3: 336–40.

32 Elson CO, Dertzbaugh MT. Mucosal adjuvants. In: *Handbook of Mucosal Immunology*, 1st edn. (Ogra PL, Mestecky J, Lamm ME, Strober W, McGhee JR, Bienenstock J, eds), Academic Press, San Diego, 1994; 391–402.

33 Erickson SL, de Sauvage FJ, Kikly K *et al.* Decreased sensitivity to tumour-necrosis factor but normal T-cell development in TNF receptor-2-deficient mice. *Nature* 1994; 372: 560–3.

34 Erle DJ, Briskin MJ, Butcher EC *et al.* Expression and function of the MAdCAM-1 receptor, integrin α4β7 on human leukocytes. *J Immunol* 1994; 153: 517–28.

35 Förster R, Mattis AE, Kremmer E *et al.* A putative chemokine receptor, BLR1, directs B cell migration to defined lymphoid organs and specific anatomic compartments of the spleen. *Cell* 1996; 87: 1037–47.

36 Fütterer A, Mink K, Luz A *et al.* The lymphotoxin β receptor controls organogenesis and affinity maturation in peripheral lymphoid tissues. *Immunity* 1998; 9: 59–70.

37 Gallatin WM, Weissman IL, Butcher EC. A cell-surface molecule involved in organ-specific homing of lymphocytes. *Nature* 1983; 304: 30–4.

38 Goldblum RM, Ahlstedt S, Carlsson B *et al.* Antibody-forming cells in human colostrum after oral immunization. *Nature* 1975; 257: 797–8.

39 Goldblum RM, Goldman AS. Immunological components of milk: formation and function. In: *Handbook of Mucosal Immunology* 1st edn. (Ogra PL, Mestecky J, Lamm ME, Strober W, McGhee JR, Bienenstock J, eds), Academic Press, San Diego, 1994; 643–52.

40 Gonnella PA, Chen Y, Inobe J-I *et al.* In situ immune response in gut-associated lymphoid tissue (GALT) following oral antigen in TCR-transgenic mice. *J Immunol* 1998; 160: 4708–18.

41 Gunn MD, Ngo VN, Ansel KM. A B-cell-homing chemokine made in lymphoid follicles activates Burkitt's lymphoma receptor 1. *Nature* 1988; 391: 799–803.

42 Guy-Grand D, Griscelli C, Vassalli P. The mouse gut-associated lymphoid system: nature and properties of the large dividing cells. *Eur J Immunol* 1974; 4: 435–43.

43 Guy-Grand D, Griscelli C, Vassalli P. The mouse gut T lymphocyte, a novel type of T cell. Nature, origin and traffic in mice in normal and graft-versus-host conditions. *J Exp Med* 1978; 148: 1661–77.

44 Halsey JF, Mitchell C, Meyer R, Cebra JA. Metabolism of immunoglobulin A in lactating mice: origins of immunoglobulin A in milk. *Eur J Immunol* 1982; 12: 107–12.

45 Hardy RR, Carmack CE, Shinton SA *et al.* A single V$_H$ gene is utilized predominantly in anti-BrMRBC hybridomas derived from purified Ly-1 B cells. *J Immunol* 1989; 142: 3643–51.

46 Hardy RR, Hayakawa K. Development and physiology of Ly-1 B and its human homolog, Leu-1 B. *Immunol Revs* 1986; 93: 53–79.

47 Hayakawa K, Hardy RR, Herzenberg LA. Peritoneal Ly-1 B cells: genetic control, autoantibody production, increased lambda light chain expression. *Eur J Immunol* 1986; 16: 450–6.

48 Hayakawa K, Hardy RR, Honda M *et al.* The 'Ly 1 B' cell subpopulations in normal, immunodefective and autoimmune mice. *J Exp Med* 1983; 157: 202–18.

49 Hemmerich S, Butcher EC, Rosen SD. Sulfation-dependent recognition of high-endothelial venules (HEV)-ligands by L-selectin and MECA-79, an adhesion-blocking monoclonal antibody. *J Exp Med* 1994; 180: 2219–26.

50 Herzenberg LA, Stall AM, Lalor PA *et al.* The Ly-1 B cell lineage. *Immunol Revs* 1986; 93: 81–102.

51 Kantor A. A new nomenclature for B cells. *Immunol Today* 1991; 12: 388.

52 Kantor A. The development and repertoire of B-1 cells (CD5 B cells). *Immunol Today* 1991; 12: 389–91.

53 Kikuta A, Rosen SD. Localization of ligands for L-selectin in mouse peripheral lymph node high endothelial cells by colloidal gold conjugates. *Blood* 1994; 84: 3766–75.

54 Koni PA, Sacca R, Lawton P *et al.* Distinct roles in lymphoid organogenesis for lymphotoxins alpha and beta revealed in lymphotoxin beta-deficient mice. *Immunity* 1997; 6: 491–500.

55 Koni PA, Flavell RA. A role for tumor receptor type 1 in gut-associated lymphoid tissue development: genetic evidence of synergism with lymphotoxin β. *J Exp Med* 1998; 187: 1977–83.

56 Korner H, Cook M, Riminton DS et al. Distinct roles for lymphotoxin-alpha and tumor necrosis factor in organogenesis and spatial organization of lymphoid tissue. Eur J Immunol 1997; 27: 2600–9.

57 Kraal G, Weissman IL, Butcher EC. Memory B cells express a phenotype consistent with migratory competence after secondary but not short-term primary immunization. Cell Immunol 1988; 115: 78–87.

58 Kroese HGM, Butcher EC, Stall AM et al. Many of the IgA producing plasma cells in murine gut are derived from self-replenishing precursors in the peritoneal cavity. Internat Immunol 1989; 1: 75–84.

59 Kroese GM, Kantor AB, Herzenberg LA. The role of B1 cells in mucosal immune responses. In: Handbook of Mucosal Immunology 1st edn. (Ogra PL, Mestecky J, Lamm ME, Strober W, McGhee JR, Bienenstock J, eds), Academic Press, San Diego, 1994; 217–24.

60 Kuper CF, Koornstra PJ, Hameleers DMH et al. The role of nasopharyngeal lymphoid tissue. Immunol Today 1992; 13: 219–24.

61 Lawrence MB, Berg EL, Butcher EC, Springer TA. Rolling of lymphocytes and neutrophils on peripheral node addressin and subsequent arrest on ICAM-1 in shear flow. Eur J Immunol 1995; 25: 1025–31.

62 Lebman DA, Griffin PM, Cebra JJ. Relationship between expression of IgA by Peyer's patch cells and functional IgA memory cells. J Exp Med 1987; 166: 1405–18.

63 Lebman DA, Nomura DY, Coffman RL, Lee FD. Molecular characterization of germ-line immunoglobulin α transcripts produced during transforming growth factor type β-induced isotype switching. Proc Natl Acad Sci USA 1990; 87: 3962–6.

64 Legler DF, Loetscher M, Stuber Roos R et al. B cell-attracting chemokine 1, a human CXC chemokine expressed in lymphoid tissues, selectively attracts B lymphocytes via BLR1/CXCR5. J Exp Med 1998; 187: 655–60.

65 Le Hir M, Bluethmann H, Kosko-Vilbois MH et al. Differentiation of follicular dendritic cells and full antibody responses requires tumor necrosis factor receptor-1 signalling. J Exp Med 1996; 183: 2367–72.

66 Lehner T, Wang Y, Cranage M. Protective mucosal immunity elicited by targeted lymph node immunization with a subunit SIV envelope and core vaccine in macaques. Dev Biol Stand 1998; 92: 225–35.

67 Lewis P, Nduati R, Kreiss JK et al. Cell-free human immunodeficiency virus type 1 in breast milk. J Infect Dis 1998; 177: 34–9.

68 Lin Y-CA, Shockett P, Stavnezer J. Regulation of the antibody class switch to IgA. Immunol Res 1991; 10: 376–80.

69 Lu X, Kiyono H, Lu D et al. Targeted lymph node immunization with whole inactivated simian immunodeficiency virus (SIV) or envelope and core subunit antigen vaccines does not reliably protect rhesus macaques from vaginal challenge with SIVmav251. AIDS 1998; 12: 1–10.

70 Mackay CR. Migration pathways and immunologic memory among T lymphocytes. Semin Immunol 1992; 4: 51–8.

71 MacLennan ICM. Germinal centers. Annu Rev Immunol 1994; 12: 117–39.

72 McDermott MR, Bienenstock J. Evidence for a common mucosal immunologic system. I. Migration of B immunoblasts into intestinal, respiratory and genital tissues. J Immunol 1979; 122: 1892–8.

73 McWilliams M, Phillips-Quagliata JM, Lamm ME. Characteristics of mesenteric lymph node cells homing to gut-associated lymphoid tissue in syngeneic mice. J Immunol 1975; 115: 54–8.

74 McWilliams M, Phillips-Quagliata JM, Lamm ME. Mesenteric lymph node B lymphoblasts which home to the small intestine are precommitted to IgA synthesis. J Exp Med 1977; 145: 866–75.

75 Manning LS, Parmely MJ. Cellular determinants of mammary cell-mediated immunity in the rat I. The migration of radioisotopically labelled T lymphocytes. J Immunol 1980; 125: 2508–14.

76 Matsumoto M, Lo SF, Carruthers JL et al. Affinity maturation without germinal centers in lymphotoxin α-deficient mice. Nature 1996; 382: 462–6.

77 Matsumoto M, Fu YX, Molina H et al. Distinct roles of lymphotoxin alpha and the type I tumor necrosis factor (TNF) receptor in the establishment of follicular dendritic cells from non-bone marrow-derived cells. J Exp Med 1997; 186: 1997–2004.

78 Matsumoto M, Mariathasan S, Nahm MH et al. Role of lymphotoxin and the type I TNF receptor in the formation of germinal centers. Science 1996; 271: 1289–91.

79 Mayrhofer G. Peyer's patch organogenesis. Gut 1997; 41: 707–9.

80 Mebius RE, Streeter PR, Michie S et al. A developmental switch in lymphocyte homing receptor and endothelial vascular addressin expression regulates lymphocyte homing and permits CD4+CD3− cells to colonize lymph nodes. Proc Natl Acad Sci USA 1996; 93: 11019–24.

81 Mebius RE, Rennert P, Weissman IL. Developing lymph nodes collect CD4+CD3-LTβ+ cells that can differentiate to APC, NK cells, and follicular cells but not T or B cells. Immunity 1997; 7: 493–504.

82 Montgomery PC, Ayyildiz A, Lemaître-Coelho IM et al. Induction and expression of antibodies in secretions: the ocular immune system. Ann NY Acad Sci 1983; 409: 428–39.

83 Montgomery PC, Rosner BR, Cohn J. The secretory antibody response. Anti-DNP antibodies induced by dinitrophenylated type III pneumococcus. Immunol Commun 1974; 3: 143–56.

84 Nakache M, Lakey-Berg BT, Streeter PR, Butcher EC. The mucosal vascular addressin is a tissue-specific endothelial adhesion molecule for circulating lymph nodes. Nature 1989; 377: 179–81.

85 Neumann B, Luz A, Pfeffer K, Holzmann B. Defective Peyer's patch organogenesis in mice lacking the 55-kD receptor for tumor necrosis factor. J Exp Med 1996; 184: 259–64.

86 Nieuwenhuis P, van Nouhuijs CE, Eggens JH, Keuning FJ. Germinal centers and the origin of the B cell system. I. Germinal centers in the rabbit appendix. Immunology 1974; 26: 497–507.

87 Ogra SS, Ogra PL. Immunologic aspects of human colostrum and milk. II. Characteristics of lymphocyte reactivity and distribution of E-rosette forming cells at different times after the onset of lactation. J Pediatr 1978; 92: 550–5.

88 Parmely MJ, Beer AE, Billingham RE. In vitro studies on the T-lymphocyte population of human milk. J Exp Med 1976; 144: 358–70.

89 Parrott DMV. Source, identity and locomotor characteristics of lymphocyte populations migrating to mammary glands: problems and predictions. In: Immunology of Breast Milk. (Ogra PL, Dayton DH, eds), Raven Press, New York; 1979; 131–41.

90 Pasparakis M, Alexopoulou L, Episkopou V, Kolias G. Immune and inflammatory responses in TNFα-deficient mice: a critical requirement for TNFα in the formation of primary B follicles, follicular dendritic cell networks and germinal centers, and in the maturation of the humoral immune response. J Exp Med 1996; 184: 1397–411.

91 Pennell CA, Mercolino TJ, Grdina TA et al. Biased immunoglobulin variable region gene expression by Ly-1 B cells due to clonal selection. Eur J Immunol 1989; 19: 1289–95.

92 Pennell CA, Sheehan KM, Brodeur PH, Clarke SH. Organization and expression of VH gene families preferentially expressed by Ly-1+ (CD5) B cells. Eur J Immunol 1989; 19: 2115–21.

93 Peschon JJ, Torrance DS, Stocking KL et al. TNF receptor-deficient mice reveal divergent roles for p55 and p75 in several models of inflammation. J Immunol 1998; 160: 943–52.

94 Phillips-Quagliata JM, Lamm ME. Lymphocyte homing to mucosal effector sites. In: Handbook of Mucosal Immunology 1st edn. (Ogra PL, Mestecky J, Lamm ME, Strober W, McGhee JR, Bienenstock J, eds), Academic Press, San Diego, 1994; 225–39.

95 Picker LJ, Butcher EC. Physiological and molecular mechanisms of lymphocyte homing. Annu Rev Immunol 1992; 10: 561–91.

96 Picker LJ, Kishimoto TK, Smith CW et al. ELAM-1 is an adhesion molecule for skin-homing T cells. Nature 1991; 349: 796–8.

97 Pierce NF, Cray WC Jr. Determinants of the localization and duration of a specific mucosal IgA plasma cell response in enterically immunized animals. J Immunol 1982; 128: 1311–15.

98 Pierce NF, Gowans JL. Cellular kinetics of the intestinal immune response to cholera toxoid in rats. J Exp Med 1975; 142: 1550–63.

99 Przlepa J, Himes C, Kelso G. Lymphocyte development and selection in germinal centers. Curr Topic Microbiol Immunol 1998; 229: 85–104.

100 Puri KD, Finger EB, Gaudernack G, Springer TA. Sialomucin CD34 is the major L-selectin ligand in human tonsil high endothelial venules. J Cell Biol 1995; 131: 261–70.

101 Reichert RA, Gallatin WM, Weissman IL, Butcher EC. Germinal center B cells lack homing receptors necessary for normal lymphocyte recirculation. J Exp Med 1983; 157: 813–27.

102 Reininger L, Ollier P, Poncet P et al. Novel V genes encode virtually identical variable regions of six murine monoclonal anti-bromelain-treated red blood cell autoantibodies. *J Immunol* 1987; 138: 316–23.

103 Renegar KB, Small PA. Passive immunization: systemic and mucosal. In: *Handbook of Mucosal Immunology* 1st edn. (Ogra PL, Mestecky J, Lamm ME, Strober W, McGhee JR, Bienenstock J, eds), Academic Press, San Diego, 1994; 347–56.

104 Rennert PD, Browning JL, Hochman PS. Selective disruption of lymphotoxin ligands reveals a novel set of mucosal lymph nodes and unique effects on lymph node cellular organization. *Int Immunol* 1997; 9: 1627–39.

105 Rennert PD, James D, Mackay F et al. Lymph node genesis is induced by signalling through the lymphotoxin β receptor. *Immunity* 1998; 9: 71–9.

106 Richie ER, Bass R, Meistrich ML, Dennison DK. Distribution of T lymphocyte subsets in human colostrum. *J Immunol* 1982; 129: 1116–19.

107 Riggs JE, Stowers RS, Mosier DE. The immunoglobulin allotype contributed by peritoneal cavity B cells dominates in SCID mice reconstituted with allotype-disparate mixtures of splenic and peritoneal cavity B cells. *J Exp Med* 1990; 172: 475–84.

108 Rose ML, Parrott DMV, Bruce RG. The accumulation of immunoblasts in extravascular tissues including mammary gland, peritoneal cavity, gut and skin. *Immunology* 1978; 35: 415–23.

109 Rosen SD. Cell surface lectins in the immune system. *Semin Immunol* 1993; 5: 237–47.

110 Rosen SD, Bertozzi CR. The selectins and their ligands. *Curr Biol* 1994; 6: 663–73.

111 Roux ME, McWilliams M, Phillips-Quagliata JM, Lamm ME. Differentiation pathway of Peyer's patch precursors of IgA plasma cells in the secretory immune system. *Cell Immunol* 1981; 61: 141–53.

112 Roux ME, McWilliams M, Phillips-Quagliata JM, Lamm ME. Origin of IgA-secreting cells in the mammary gland. *J Exp Med* 1981; 146: 1311–22.

113 Ryffel B, Brockhaus M, Durmuller U, Gudat F. Tumor necrosis factor receptors in lymphoid tissues and lymphomas. *Am J Pathol* 1991; 139: 7–15.

114 Sacca R, Turley S, Soong L et al. Transgenic expression of lymphotoxin restores lymph nodes to lymphotoxin-alpha-deficient mice. *J Immunol* 1997; 159: 4252–60.

115 Sampaio SO, Li X, Takeuchi M et al. Organization, regulatory sequences, and alternatively spliced transcripts of the mucosal addressin cell adhesion molecule-1 (MAdCAM-1) gene. *J Immunol* 1995; 155: 2477–86.

116 Sassetti C, Tangemann K, Singer MS et al. Identification of podocalyxin-like protein as a high endothelial venule ligand for L-selectin: parallels to CD34. *J Exp Med* 1998; 187: 1965–75.

117 Shimizu Y, Newman W, Tanaka Y, Shaw S. Lymphocyte interactions with endothelial cells. *Immunol Today* 1992; 13: 106–10.

118 Shimizu Y, Shaw S, Graber N et al. Activation-independent binding of human memory T cells to adhesion molecule ELAM-1. *Nature* 1991; 349: 799–802.

119 Shyjan AM, Bertagnolli M, Kenney CJ, Briskin MJ. Human mucosal addressin cell adhesion molecule-1 (MAdCAM-1) demonstrates structural and functional similarities to the α4β7-integrin binding domains of murine MAdCAM-1, but extreme divergence of mucin-like sequences. *J Immunol* 1996; 156: 2851–7.

120 Solvason N, Lehuen A, Kearney JF. An embryonic source of Ly 1 but not conventional B cells. *Int Immunol* 1991; 3: 543–50.

121 Sonoda E, Matsumoto R, Hitoshi Y et al. Transforming growth factor-β induces IgA production and acts additively with interleukin 5 for IgA production. *J Exp Med* 1989; 170: 1415–20.

122 Spangrude GJ, Braaten BA, Daynes RA. Molecular mechanisms of lymphocyte extravasation. I. Studies of two selective inhibitors of lymphocyte recirculation. *J Immunol* 1984; 132: 354–62.

123 Springer T. Traffic signals for lymphocyte recirculation and leukocyte emigration: the multistep paradigm. *Cell* 1994; 76: 301–14.

124 Streeter PR, Lakey-Berg E, Rouse BTN et al. A tissue-specific endothelial cell molecule involved in lymphocyte homing. *Nature* 1988; 331: 41–6.

125 Szakal AK, Homes KL, Tew JG. Transport of immune complexes from the subcapsular sinus to lymph node follicles on the surface of non-phagocytic cells, including cells with dendritic morphology. *J Immunol* 1983; 131: 1714–27.

126 Szakal AK, Kosco-Vilbois MH, Tew JG. A novel in vivo follicular dendritic cell-dependent iccosome-mediated mechanism for delivery of antigen to antigen-processing cells. *J Immunol* 1988; 140: 354–60.

127 Tkachuk M, Bolliger S, Ryffel B et al. Crucial role for tumor necrosis receptor 1 expression on non-hematopoietic cells for B cell localization within the splenic white pulp. *J Exp Med* 1998; 187: 469–77.

128 Tseng J. Migration and differentiation of IgA precursor cells in the gut-associated lymphoid tissue. In: *Migration and Homing of Lymphoid Cells Vol. II.* (Husband AJ, ed.) CRC Press, Boca Raton FL; 1988; 77–98.

129 Wagner N, Löhler J, Kunkel EJ et al. Critical role for β7 integrins in formation of the gut-associated lymphoid tissue. *Nature* 1996; 382: 366–70.

130 Ware CF, VanArsdale TL, Crowe PD, Browning JL. The ligands and receptors of the lymphotoxin system. *Curr Top Microbiol Immunol* 1995; 198: 175–218.

131 Weisz-Carrington P, Roux ME, Lamm ME. Plasma cells and epithelial immunoglobulins in the mouse mammary gland during pregnancy and lactation. *J Immunol* 1977; 119: 1306–9.

132 Weisz-Carrington P, Roux ME, McWilliams M et al. Hormonal induction of the secretory immune system in the mammary gland. *Proc Natl Acad Sci USA* 1978; 75: 2928–32.

133 Weisz-Carrington P, Roux ME, McWilliams M et al. Organ and isotype distribution of plasma cells producing specific antibody after oral immunization: evidence for a generalized secretory immune system. *J Immunol* 1979; 123: 1705–8.

134 Wu H-Y, Russell MW. Induction of mucosal immunity by intranasal application of a streptococcal surface protein antigen with the cholera toxin B subunit. *Infect Immun* 1993; 61: 314–22.

135 Young PE, Baumhueter S, Lasky LA. The sialomucin CD34 is expressed on hematopoietic cells and blood vessels during murine development. *Blood* 1995; 85: 96–105.

Chapter 4

Innervation of lymphoid tissue and functional consequences of neurotransmitter and neuropeptide release

Javier Santos, John Bienenstock and Mary Perdue

INTRODUCTION

The mucosal surfaces of the body are the first and critical location where immunogenic particles and molecules (food and microorganism-derived antigens) gain access to the immune system. Antigen processing in this region will determine, when a second contact with the antigen takes place, whether an immunological balanced (mild-to-moderate hypersensitivity reaction) or unbalanced response (anaphylactic reaction) or a permissive one (tolerance) is mounted. Mucosal membranes are covered by epithelial layers, i.e. single-cell-thick in the gastrointestinal tract. In the gastrointestinal and respiratory systems, classical effector cells of immune reactions (lymphocytes, eosinophils, mast cells, neutrophils, macrophages and dendritic cells) are normally present or lie in close proximity to the epithelial layer.

One key concept emerging in the last few years is that non-traditional immune cells that also populate the mucosal membranes, classically viewed as innocent bystanders, may display potentially relevant effector and modulatory functions in antigen processing and immunologic responses. Besides epithelial cells, this structural group includes mesenchymal (fibroblasts, myofibroblasts, muscle cells), endothelial and nerve cells and also acellular components such as the extracellular matrix. In the context of food-allergic hypersensitivity reactions, one also must take into account that, in addition to cellular elements, food itself may be immunomodulatory. In this sense, it has been recently shown that feeding, in contrast to fasting, has important consequences in the redistribution of immune cells in the blood compartment; moreover, food intake itself can also induce changes in the production of several immunoregulatory cytokines.[83]

In the last 10 years our knowledge of the immunoregulatory effects of nerves and neuropeptides has grown tremendously. Considerable and converging evidence coming from anatomical, pharmacological, biochemical, genetic and clinical studies from different research areas (immunology, psychology, neurobiology, gastrointestinal and airways physiology) has firmly established the existence of bidirectional communication between the neural and immune systems (Fig. 4.1). This interaction involves most, if not all, of the immune cells present in mucosal surfaces, and both the central and peripheral nervous systems, including efferent and afferent subdivisions of the autonomic nervous system, sympathetic and parasympathetic, as well as the enteric nervous system. Moreover, those studies have shown the functional relevance of neuroimmune interactions in regulating immunological and inflammatory events in mucosal surfaces, by influencing the transport of macromolecules across the epithelial surface, the expression of adhesion molecules, the release of cytokines, chemokines, neurotransmitters, neuropeptides and other regulatory molecules that participate in the trafficking and homing of immune cells in the mucosal layers, the growth and remodelling of nerves, and even the apoptotic cascade.

A

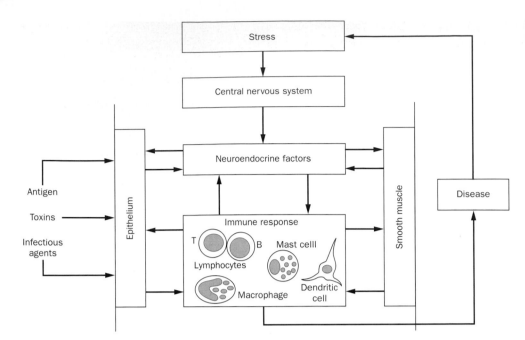

Fig. 4.1 The factors and system interactions that are involved in the regulation of food-allergic reactions.

Although food-allergic reactions may display a broad spectrum of clinical manifestations involving most tissues in the body, it is accepted that primary events predominantly occur at the level of the gastrointestinal mucosa. Thus, for improving the understanding of this chapter, a superficial reference to the organization and composition of the gut-associated lymphoid tissue will be presented to provide a context in which neuro–lymphoid interactions will be discussed.

A distinct characteristic of the complex neuroendocrine and immune systems is the high level of integration of both systems, which together provide the organism with an ultra-fine homeostatic balance (Fig. 4.2). The neuroendocrine system modulates the function of the immune system through the release of neuropeptides, neurohormones and neurotransmitters. In addition, a primary or counteracting immunoregulatory role for immune cells has also been reported which comprises the effects of mediators

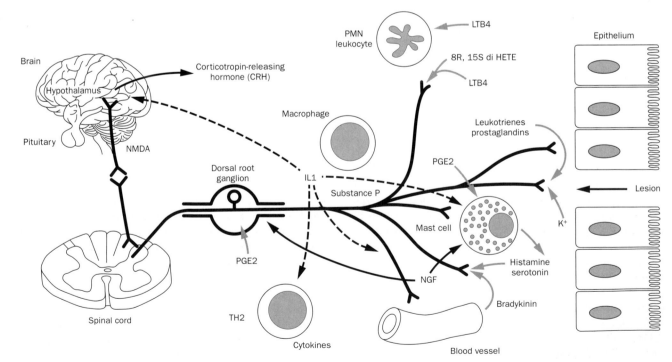

Fig. 4.2 Cells and mediators that participate in the generation of allergic inflammation in the gastrointestinal tract. The neuroendocrine and immune systems share common messengers (neurotransmitters, cytokines, peptides and lipid mediators) that may influence both systems through the activation of specific receptors in paracrine, autocrine and neurocrine pathways. The surrounding epithelium is also able to regulate and effect to some extent, the signals coming from both neuroendocrine and immune systems. After an antigenic exposure, the integration of those signals may dictate the final physiopathological events taking place. *Note*: TH2, lymphocytes T helper type 2; NGF, nerve growth factor; PGE, prostaglandin E; IL, interleukin; NMDA, N-methyl D-aspartate; HETE, hydroxyeicosatetraenoic acid; LTB, leukotriene B; PMN, polymorphonuclear.

released by immunocompetent cells on neuroendocrine function. It is now clear that immune cells are able to synthesize and release neuropeptides and even classical hormones such as growth hormone or prolactin, and that endocrine and neural cells can produce a broad array of cytokines, originally described as being part of the repertoire of immune cells.

This chapter will focus mainly on the efferent limb of the neuro–immune interactions, i.e. the effect of neural mediators on immune cells, particularly lymphocytes. For this purpose, anatomical and functional evidence for the presence and relevance of neural and neuropeptide-containing fibres in lymphoid tissues and immunocompetent cells will be reviewed in detail. However, scattered reference to the effects of mediators released from lymphoid and other immune cells on nerve function will be gathered through this chapter, specifically mast cell–nerve interactions will be briefly overviewed in a separate section, since the authors believe that understanding of physiological responses can be better achieved in the context of bidirectional interactions (for detailed review on those topics readers are directed to recent reviews[15,122,127,138,231] . Finally, experimental and clinical data supporting the potential relevance of this interplay and its significance in the management of food allergy and other allergic and inflammatory disorders will be briefly discussed at the end of the chapter.

GUT-ASSOCIATED LYMPHOID TISSUE ORGANIZATION AND MUCOSAL INNERVATION

Although thoroughly reviewed in other chapters in this book, a short discussion of the composition and organization of mucosa-associated lymphoid tissues (MALT) is suitable here for better understanding of the scope of neuroimmune interactions. MALT comprise a great part of the immune cells in the body. The gut-associated lymphoid tissue (GALT) alone contains almost 90% of immunoglobulin (Ig)-producing cells in the body and as many lymphocytes as the spleen.[18] At the mucosal level the immune system is compartmentalized and includes lymphoid aggregates (Peyer's patches and follicles) that contain mainly B cells bearing surface immunoglobulin A (IgA), and a diffuse population of B and T cells in the lamina propria. Most of the T cells in the lamina propria are CD4+, and there is also a population of intraepithelial lymphocytes, mainly CD8+ cells. On the other hand, the gastrointestinal mucosa is highly innervated, the density of nerves being reported to be up to one per $200 \, \mu m^2$ in rat jejunal mucosa.[212] Apart from the enteric nervous system, the vast majority of extrinsic nerve fibres do not reach the epithelium but terminate at the submucosal or myenteric plexus. From the plexus regions, nerve varicosities extend to surrounding areas, from where neurotransmitters and neuropeptides may be expected to diffuse and reach mucosal targets.

NEURO–LYMPHOID INTERACTIONS: NEUROTRANSMITTERS AND NEUROPEPTIDES AS REGULATORY MOLECULES THAT ARE PRESENT THROUGHOUT THE LYMPHOID SYSTEM

The effect of neural activation is the release of agonist substances (neurotransmitters, neuropeptides and neurohormones) that act through neurocrine, paracrine or endocrine pathways to activate specific receptors on immune cells. For a molecule to be accepted

Characteristics of neurotransmitters
Present in and synthesized by the cell populations
Released upon appropriate stimulation
Exogenous application or endogenous release of the molecule induce similar effects

Table 4.1 Characteristics of neurotransmitters.

as a neurotransmitter it should meet at least three requirements:[46] (a) it is present and synthesized in the cell population studied; (b) it is released upon appropriate stimulation; and (c) exogenous application and endogenous release of the molecule induce similar effects (Table 4.1). Similar criteria, with some restrictions, may apply for neuropeptides and neurohormones. For neurotransmission to be complete, receptors should be present on target cells, where binding of the corresponding ligand molecule exerts its physiological effects.

Requirements for neural-mediated activation of lymphocytes

For endocrine and paracrine communication between the effector and the commander cell physical contact is not required, but for neural-mediated activation close proximity between cells is a requisite. Within the lymphoid system, the classical paradigm of neuroimmune communication is represented by norepinephrine (NE), or noradrenaline, the neurotransmitter of most postganglionic sympathetic fibres, and lymphocytes in the spleen:(1) presence of noradrenergic nerves establishing synapse-like contacts between lymphocytes and NE varicosities;[65] (2) release of NE upon splenic nerve stimulation;[51] and (3) action on NE receptors on lymphocytes resulting in altered lymphocyte function.[71,192] In addition, NE can also act in a paracrine manner, diffusing away from parenchymal nerve ends to be available in the vicinity of immune cells. This is the case in the thymus where, although the criteria for neurotransmission have been fulfilled to a considerable extent, the lack of synaptic-like contacts between thymocytes and noradrenergic nerves[228] has led to the suggestion that paracrine diffusion of NE could explain the effects of sympathetic activity on thymocytes.[228]

Non-splenic neuropeptides and neurotransmitters

The picture for other neurotransmitters and neuropeptides and for NE outside the spleen is not so clear, since fulfilment of the highly demanding criteria for neurotransmission in lymphoid organs has not been strictly demonstrated for these substances. However, despite that lack of fulfilment, the evidence presented in this chapter indicates that these molecules regulate immuno–inflammatory processes. Thus, neuropeptides released from central and peripheral nerve varicosities and by cells of the immune system act as conventional neurotransmitters, transducing environmental signals into specific chemical messages.

Extensive evidence from functional studies indicates that almost all the steps of lymphocyte activation are affected by neuropeptide release.[14,59,228] Moreover, those and other functional studies have been substantiated by anatomical reports showing neuropeptide-like immunoreactivity for numerous peptides including neuropeptide Y (NPY), cholecystokinin, metenkephalin, substance P (SP), calcitonin gene-related peptide (CGRP),

A

neurotensin, somatostatin (SS) and vasoactive intestinal peptide (VIP) in neural profiles in lymphoid tissues.[14,15,122] In addition, the existence of neuropeptide receptors on lymphoid cells in the gastrointestinal mucosa for endorphins, enkephalins, SP, SS and VIP,[14,27] among others, supports the physiological role of neuropeptides as endogenous regulators of the immune response. Commonly, the effects of neuropeptides on immune function are tissue-specific and probably dependent on the resident cell populations within the lymphoid tissue and the surrounding microenvironment. Besides direct effects on immune cells, these peptides may alter the immunological response indirectly by acting on neighbouring cells, such as smooth muscle cells, endothelial cells, nerve and endocrine cells and even epithelial cells. In other cases, the effects of neuropeptides may require the presence of necessary co-signal molecules to exert maximal effects through synergistic action.

INNERVATION OF MUCOSA-ASSOCIATED LYMPHOID TISSUE

Anatomical evidence: neural networks innervating lymphoid tissues

Noradrenergic innervation

Numerous neuroanatomical reports have rendered conclusive evidence for the presence of nerve terminals, mostly noradrenergic in nature, in primary and secondary lymphoid organs.[22,23,61–64,78,162,232] Noradrenergic nerve fibres can be identified by fluorescence histochemistry for catecholamines and by immunocytochemistry, where specific antibodies for tyrosine hydroxylase, the rate-limiting enzyme for NE synthesis, bind to noradrenergic terminals.[22,126] Although, each organ has its own pattern of innervation that varies among species, between different compartments of the same organ and, even during ontogeny, a general model has been described:[2,64] noradrenergic nerves enter the organs near or with the blood vessels and distribute in areas where T cells predominate. Although noradrenergic terminals skipped follicular zones, rich in B cells in most lymphoid territories,[62,64] studies using double-label immunocytohistochemistry for T and B subsets have shown that single fine fibres enter the B cell follicles in the spleen.[61] All primary (bone marrow[23,63] and thymus[22,62,64]), and secondary lymphoid organs (spleen,[2,62,64,113] lymph nodes[62,78,164] and MALT[22,63,64,78,98,239]) have been shown to possess varying degrees and patterns of noradrenergic innervation in several species of mammals, including among many others, rat,[2,27,62,64,78,164] mice,[22,62,64,78] cat,[62,64] rabbit,[62,63,98] guinea-pig,[62,64] dog[64] and humans.[2,62,64,113,164,239]

GALT innervation

GALT innervation has been described in detail in the rabbit appendix, sacculus rotundus and Peyer's patches. In this case, preganglionic sympathetic fibres, whose cell bodies reside in the intermediolateral column of the spinal cord, synapse with neurons in the mesenteric ganglia from where postganglionic fibres arise to enter the gut at the serosal surface in association with large arterial vessels.[63,98] Then these fibres follow smooth muscle and blood vessels inside the muscularis interna until they reach septa between lymphoid nodules, where they turn from a longitudinal to a radial direction towards the apical surface, reaching the lamina propria. At this level, a dense subepithelial network is formed without penetrating the epithelium.[64,212]

Human studies have revealed that palatine tonsils also bear sympathetic fibres that follow a similar pattern of distribution as in the rabbit appendix.[225,239] Using the incomplete polyneuronal marker PGP (protein gene product) 9.5, it has been shown that the human appendix also bears a dense innervation at the submucosal level that extends to the lamina propria, where several fibres reach the outer zone of lymph follicles avoiding the germinal centres.[43] However, the use of PGP 9.5 did not allow the nature of the different types of fibres to be distinguished.

In the bronchus-associated lymphoid tissue (BALT) of cat and rat, tyrosine hydroxylase- and dopamine β-hydroxylase-positive nerves have been reported in association with blood vessels, but only few fibres were seen between lymphocytes in the parenchyma.[162]

Origin of noradrenaline

Studies carried out in mice and rats have suggested that most NE present in lymphoid tissues is of neuronal origin. Thus, by using a selective neurotoxin, 6-hydroxydopamine (6-OHDA), that depletes noradrenergic sympathetic terminals, it has been reported that NE is almost totally depleted in the spleen[236] and lymph nodes.[123] Although, 6-OHDA might have induced loss of spleen NE contents by decreasing catecholamine blood levels, the depletion of NE in the spleen that followed ganglionectomy[12] or surgical transection of the splenic nerve[229] supported the neural origin of NE.

Indirect indication of NE release from spleen sympathetic terminals comes from studies where inhibition of tyrosine hydroxylase with α-methyl-p-tyrosine was paralleled by NE decreases, suggesting the existence of an NE turnover.[2] Direct measurement of basal and stimulated release of NE in the rat, mouse and cat spleen using electrophysiological and in vivo microdialysis techniques[51,214] have confirmed that NE is released at postganglionic sympathetic terminals. Since, the concentrations of NE were higher in the spleen than in the peripheral circulation, these studies also strongly argue in favour of local neural release of NE. Similar electrophysiological approaches have shown that, upon electrical stimulation, NE is released from nerve endings in the rat thymus.[15,22] This NE current was able to inhibit potassium flux across the thymocyte membrane, possibly acting at the level of voltage-dependent potassium channels. These channels, previously described in murine[36,117] as well as human peripheral T lymphocytes,[136] have been shown to be involved in the signalling cascade that ultimately leads to the activation, differentiation and proliferation of T cells.[74]

Since synaptic-like contacts between thymocytes and noradrenergic terminals are absent in the thymus,[228] these studies collectively indicate that NE transmission is an important modulator of lymphocyte physiology, supporting the hypothesis that at this level NE exerts its function through paracrine routes.[228] However, some of the observed release of NE could have been of intracellular origin, since recent reports have demonstrated that catecholamine synthesis is possible in human and murine lymphocytes.[100,155] These reports add a new possibility to the already complex theatre of neuroimmune interactions: lymphocyte generation of neurotransmitters could be involved in autocrine and paracrine regulation of immune responses.

Cholinergic innervation

Conflicting results have been provided by several groups using immunostaining techniques for specific acetylcholinesterase

(AChE), the degrading enzyme for acetylcholine. These reports described the presence of AChE-positive fibres in the bone marrow,[40] thymus,[57] spleen,[113] lymph nodes,[164] appendix[63] and palatine tonsils.[239] The distribution of AChE-positive nerve terminals in the mammalian GALT has been reported to be similar to that of noradrenergic terminals in the rabbit appendix and human palatine tonsils.[63,239] In addition, a dense network of strong AChE-positive areas was found in association with B lymphocytes in appendix nodules and germinal centres in human tonsils. However, in view of light and electron microscopic studies,[64] this staining, far from being specific for cholinergic neurons is also present in other neural (in particular noradrenergic) and non-neural elements,[64] possibly serving different roles from that of acetylcholine degradation.[13,31] Moreover, denervation studies have shown that after vagotomy, the AChE staining did not disappear, suggesting that the affected structures were not neural or at least, if neural, non-cholinergic.[13,158]

Other evidence of cholinergic nerves in lymphoid tissue

Other approaches to determine the presence of cholinergic nerves in lymphoid tissues have included the investigation of the activity and immunoreactivity of choline acetyltransferase (ChAT), the enzyme responsible for acetylcholine synthesis. In rodent lymph tissues ChAT staining is modest or absent,[57,222] whereas ChAT activity seems to vary from organ to organ, during developmental stages, being high in the early postnatal period and declining thereafter, in several different species of mammals.[13,64,222] Consistent with previous reports, retrograde tracing studies have rendered questionable evidence of the presence of cholinergic terminals in the thymus.[158]

The data so far presented suggest that cholinergic innervation of lymphoid tissues is sparse in some organs and absent in others. Since the *in vivo* origin of acetylcholine in lymphoid organs remains disputed, acetylcholine synthesis has been looked for in lymphocytes themselves. AChE has been detected on the surface of human and rodent lymphocytes.[79,216] Moreover, using a radio-enzymatic technique, significant ChAT activity has been reported to be present in isolated thymus lymphocytes as well as in mature B and T cells in different organs.[187] However, the conditions under which lymphocytes may synthesize and secrete acetylcholine remain obscure.

Peptidergic innervation

In the gastrointestinal system neuropeptides are expressed and released from neurons in the enteric nervous system and also from extrinsic afferent varicosities. Both systems share a growing number of neuropeptides but they can be differentiated according to their chemical code and origin (Table 4.2). Thus, while enteric neurons contain only the β-form of CGRP and it is not coexpressed with SP, extrinsic afferent nerves typically contain a variety of bioactive peptides, such as CGRP (mostly α-form), SP and neurokinin A (NKA) and also excitatory amino acids and nitric oxide, that can be coreleased upon appropriate stimulation.[90,127] However, corelease is a common phenomenon for other peptides, such as NPY and VIP in enteric neurons.

Enteric neurons lie in the myenteric and submucosal plexuses, while most gastrointestinal peptidergic afferents emanate from dorsal root ganglia. Furthermore, capsaicin sensitivity of unmyelinated (type C) and thinly myelinated (type Aδ) afferent peptidergic nerves, as opposed to insensitivity of enteric peptidergic

Neuropeptides implicated in peptidergic innervation in lymphoid tissue
Substance P (SP)
Somatostatin (SS)
Vasoactive intestinal peptide (VIP)
Neuropeptide Y (NPY)
Calcitonin gene-related peptide (CGRP (α, β))
Corticotropin-releasing hormone (CRH)
Neurokinin A (NKA)

Table 4.2 Neuropeptides implicated in peptidergic innervation in lymphoid tissue.

neurons, has furnished proof for the role of extrinsic afferent innervation in the modulation of various immune functions. Thus, extrinsic afferent fibres are conveyed through sympathetic and parasympathetic nerves to the gut wall. Then, spinal projections mainly distribute nearby blood vessels, forming a dense para- and perivascular network with some axons, also reaching the lamina propria, enteric plexuses and muscle layers. Moreover, compelling evidence indicates the existence of reciprocal short- and long-term interactions between the afferent innervation and noradrenergic nerves that involve nerve growth factor, which might be involved in the modulation of acute and chronic inflammatory conditions.[127]

Relationship between peptidergic nerves and immune cells

Mounting evidence indicates the presence of close spatial relationships between mast cells, lymphocytes, eosinophils, plasma cells and macrophages and capsaicin-sensitive, peptidergic nerves in various lymphoid organs such as spleen, lymph nodes, thymus, tonsils and lymphoid aggregates in the nasal, lung and gastrointestinal mucosa.[8,11,160,213] This close association has been described for immunoreactive peptidergic fibres containing SP, NKA, VIP, CGRP, NPY, enkephalins and galanin. In lymph nodes capsaicin-sensitive fibres follow a perivascular pattern whereby they reach B and T cell areas,[160,180] while in the thymus and bone marrow these fibres travel in both vascular and paravascular areas.[92,233] Whatever the distribution, it is clear that neuropeptide-containing nerves are strategically located to provide direct or indirect signalling to lymphoid and other immune elements.

Specific patterns of neuropeptide-containing fibres in lymphoid tissues

Substance P

SP is a natural undecapeptide distributed extensively in the central, peripheral and enteric nervous systems and also in primary and secondary lymphoid tissues including spleen, lymph nodes and thymus.[62,174] The pattern of innervation varies among different lymphoid tissues and even throughout the same organ. Thus, in the mesenteric lymph nodes, SP innervation is sparse and mainly related to blood vessels near T cell regions,[180] whereas in Peyer's patches, SP-containing fibres infiltrate T cell zones yet also associate with macrophages.[213] In contrast, in the lamina propria of Peyer's patches, IgA-bearing plasma cells are more likely to be influenced by SP, since they reside in highly innervated areas.[213] SP-containing fibres have also been described in subepithelial areas in rat BALT and in human palatine tonsils.[93]

A

Somatostatin

This 14 amino acid peptide is widely present in the central and peripheral nervous system, in lymphoid tissues including spleen, thymus, Peyer's patches and bursa of Fabricius and throughout the gastrointestinal tract in nerve cells in the myenteric and submucous plexuses as well as in endocrine cells.[4,58,64,183] SS immunoreactive nerve fibres are in some cases in close proximity to lymphocytes and plasma cells.[58]

Vasoactive intestinal peptide

This 28 amino acid peptide is found in the central, enteric and peripheral nervous system, particularly in the peptidergic nerves in mucosal tissues, including the gastrointestinal, upper respiratory and genital tracts, where sometimes it colocalizes with SP.[50] In the gastrointestinal tract, VIP is expressed in all layers of both the small and large intestine.[49,50] VIP-containing nerves have also been found in human and murine lymphoid tissues, including the thymus, spleen, Peyer's patches and in the bursa Fabricii of the chicken.[62,165,169]

Neuropeptide Y

NPY, a 36 amino acid peptide, is the main effector of a group of peptides that also includes peptide YY and pancreatic polypeptide. In the periphery, NPY is often colocalized with NE and dopamine-β-hydroxylase in postganglionic sympathetic nerve fibres in the rat thymus, spleen and lymph nodes.[51,190] It is also extensively expressed in enteric neurons throughout the small and large intestine. Commonly, NPY-containing fibres follow a similar pattern of distribution to that of NE in lymphoid organs. In the gastrointestinal tract, NPY is found in the myenteric plexus in association with SS and cholecystokinin and in mesenteric lymph nodes in the vicinity of lymphocytes.[199] Functional studies have shown that NPY is released from sympathetic splenic nerve terminals upon stimulation of the splenic nerve.[42]

Calcitonin gene-related peptide

CGRP is a 37 amino acid peptide derived from the CGRP/calcitonin gene, which also encodes for amylin and adrenomedullin, other members of this neuropeptide family. CGRP-containing fibres are widely present in central and peripheral nervous systems and in the cardiovascular system.[237] Two differents forms of CGRP (α and β) exist. While CGRPα is the main form expressed in extrinsic gastrointestinal afferents, CGRPβ is the only form present in enteric neurons.[90] CGRP-containing nerves have also been described along the blood vessels in the thymus, spleen, lymph nodes and in the lamina propria of the gut, sometimes in close association with mast cells, where they may be colocalized with SP and other tachykinins.[64,90,180]

Corticotropin-releasing hormone (CRH)

CRH, a 41 amino acid single-chain polypeptide, is the predominant regulator of the neuroendocrine and behavioural responses to stress by inducing the secretion of pituitary pro-opiomelanocortin (POMC)-derived peptides, such as adrenocorticotropic hormone (ACTH) and β-endorphin, and by activation of the sympathetic nervous system and the subsequent release of catecholamines. It is largely present in the central nervous system – in sympathetic and sensory fibres – where sometimes it is colocalized with SP. It is also present in peripheral organs, including the immune, gastrointestinal, cardiorespiratory and endocrine systems.[102] CRH mRNA and immunoreactivity has been demonstrated in several lymphoid tissues, such as the thymus, spleen and mesenteric lymph nodes.[20]

Opioids

The opioid family includes the endorphins, the enkephalins and the dynorphins. Opioids are found mainly in the adrenal medulla and brain. However, immunohistochemical studies have revealed the presence of endorphin, metenkephalin and dynorphin A nerve fibres in lymphoid organs, such as spleen and lymph nodes.[27,78]

Receptors for neurotransmitters on lymphoid tissues and immune cells (Table 4.3)

Adrenergic receptors

In vitro pharmacological studies in the early 1970s showed that human peripheral lymphocyte proliferation enhancement was mediated by α-adrenoceptors, whereas inhibition was mediated by activation of β-receptors.[81] That study, taken together with previous reports showing that reserpine, which depletes NE stores, caused involution in the thymus gland and decreased both cellular and immune responses,[47] and phenoxybenzamine, an α-adrenergic blocker, reduced humoral response to pertussis vaccine,[176] led to the suggestion that sympathetic modulation of the immune response could be mediated by the presence of specific receptors for NE on immune cells.[82]

The presence of receptors for NE on lymphocytes was initially indicated by studies showing attachment of these cells to columns containing adrenergic agonists and antagonists. Later studies using radiolabelled ligands disclosed the presence of β_2-adrenoceptors on murine and human B and T lymphocytes.[19,114,154,179] B cells expressed higher number of β_2-adrenoceptors than T cells and, among T cells, the CD8$^+$ phenotype expressed more than the CD4$^+$.[46,176] Among the CD8$^+$, those with suppressor functions showed higher numbers than those with cytotoxic phenotype.[114] Similar studies have identified α_2-adrenoceptors in human and

Receptors for neurotransmitters in immune cells		
Receptor	**Concentration per cell**	**Cell type**
Adrenergic	?	Lymphocytes
Acetylcholine Nicotinic Muscarinic	2000–50 000	Lymphocytes
Neuropeptides SP SS VIP (2 types) NPY (6 types) CGRZ	190–23 000 ? 490–41 000 ? ?	T, B lymphocytes T, B lymphocytes, esp. Peyer's patch T, B lymphocytes Splenic lymphocytes T, B lymphocytes, macrophages, Langerhans' cells
CRH (3 types)		Mononuclear cells, lymphocytes
Opioids		Lymphocytes

Table 4.3 Receptors for neurotransmitters in immune cells.

guinea-pig lymphocytes,[145,221] whereas rodent lymphocytes seemed to lack them.[19] However, *in vitro* studies have shown that pharmacological modulation of B (antibody generation) and T (proliferation) cell functions was possible in rodents by using α-agonists.[60] In addition, α_2-adrenoceptors have been localized in the spleen and lymph nodes in the rat by autoradiographic techniques.[66] These studies, taken together, suggest that at least some subset(s) of murine lymphocytes express α-adrenoceptors.

Acetylcholine receptors

Radioligand studies have established the presence of both nicotinic and muscarinic receptors on lymphocytes.[15,135,184] The number of muscarinic binding sites varied from 2000 to 50 000 per cell, depending, among others factors, on the stage of maturation, the subpopulation studied and the phase of the immune process.[79,135] Again, controversy exists, since some authors have raised doubts about the expression of specific cholinergic receptors on murine lymphocytes.[181]

Neuropeptide receptors
Substance P
SP receptors (NK1 receptor) have been identified in germinal centres of mesenteric, gastrointestinal and colonic lymph nodes in dogs[8,131] and also in colonic tissues from patients with inflammatory bowel disease.[130] Moreover, receptors for SP are present on human and murine splenic and GALT T and B lymphocytes, with receptor sites varying from 190 to 23 000 per cell.[27,211] Other immune cells, such as macrophages and possibly mast cells, also bear specific tachykinin receptors.[111,199]

Somatostatin
SS receptors have been described in both human B and T and murine lymphocytes.[17,204] Lymphocytes from Peyer's patches disclosed higher binding frequency than those from the spleen and, among B cells, binding affinity varies according to the surface immunoglobulin expressed.[24] In addition, strong evidence that SS is synthesized in cells and organs in the immune system has been recently reported.[4]

Vasoactive intestinal peptide
High affinity and specific VIP receptors have been shown on human and murine B and T cells, with sites per cell ranging between 490 and 41 200.[24,65,167] Both CD4+ and CD8+ T cells express VIP receptors where type I VIP receptors are constitutively present and type II are induced upon T cell activation. Furthermore, VIP receptors are also present on mast cells and macrophages.

Neuropeptide Y
At least six Y receptor types have been described in mammalian tissues.[148] NPY receptors have been identified on splenic lymphocytes[175] and synthesis capacity for NPY has been demonstrated in human lymphocytes.[201]

Calcitonin gene-related peptide
CGRP receptors are expressed mainly in central and peripheral nervous systems and in the cardiovascular system.[237] In addition, receptors for CGRP have been demonstrated on immune cells such as T and B lymphocytes, macrophages and Langerhans' cells.[91,140]

Corticotropin-releasing hormone
CRH mRNA has been detected in the vicinity of the base of the crypts, probably being produced by enterochromaffin cells, while CRH-like immunoreactivity has been described on mononuclear cells, myofibroblasts, myenteric plexi and in sympathetic and sensory ganglia.[223] Furthermore, CRH is synthesized by a wide range of immune cells, including lymphocytes and probably macrophages and fibroblasts.[20]

At least, three different receptor subtypes for CRH have been described: R_1, R_{2a} and R_{2b}. CRH R_1 and R_{2b} subtypes are distributed in both the brain and periphery, including the intestine, while the R_{2a} subtype is mainly restricted to the brain.[119,223] Radioligand studies have disclosed the presence of CRH receptors on monocytes, macrophages and lymphocytes,[110,197] and pharmacological modulation has also rendered convincing evidence for the presence of CRH R_1 receptors on mast cells.[218] Moreover, CRH receptors have been described in gastrointestinal sympathetic ganglia,[224] and their presence on myenteric neurons is supported by direct CRH excitatory effects.[89]

Opioids and other pro-opiomelanocortin-derived peptides
Functional and radioligand studies have identified opioid and antiopioid bindings sites on cells of the immune system, including human and murine lymphocytes.[62,150,206] Besides β-endorphin, other products encoded by the POMC gene include ACTH, α-melanocyte-stimulating hormone and β-lipotropin. These peptides are produced by numerous cell types, including immune cells such as lymphocytes and macrophages.[120] Furthermore, the presence of melanocortin receptors has been reported in several tissues and cells, including the gastrointestinal mucosa and immune cells.[120]

Other neuropeptides
Numerous other neuropeptides and neurohormones have been described to have receptors on immune cells. The list includes prolactin, luteinizing hormone-releasing hormone (LH-RH), thyrotropin, thyrotropin-releasing hormone (TRH), arginine vasopressin, growth hormone, growth hormone-releasing hormone (GH-RH), nerve growth factor and other neurotrophins, pituitary adenylate cyclase-activating polypeptide, neurotensin, glucocorticoids and galanin.[27,54,199,217] The evidence now is that many of these peptides can interact directly with lymphocytes, resulting, in most cases, in a subsequent cascade of intracellular changes that alter effector cell function. In addition, many of these peptides may act in an auto/paracrine manner, since immune cells have been shown to produce many of them under widely different circumstances.[27,231]

Physiological relevance of neural and neuropeptide innervation of lymphoid tissues
Adrenergic effects
The functional role of autonomic innervation of lymphoid tissues is only partially understood. Several *in vitro* observations have shown that β_2- and α_1-adrenergic influence on antibody production and B cell proliferation was stimulatory, but α_2-influence was inhibitory.[192,193] Sympathetic activation has also been shown to increase the cytotoxic activity of CD8+ cells, to inhibit T cell proliferation, natural killer and cytolitic activity through β-receptors[124,136] and to selectively redistribute natural killer and CD8+ cells through β_2-adrenergic activation,[114] while the effects of α-receptor

activation on some of those lymphocyte functions have been controversial.[124]

In vivo experiments

The physiological relevance of sympathetic modulation of immune response has been further investigated using *in vivo* approaches. Although it is very difficult to generalize since the responses are dynamic and affected by an undetermined number of factors, it has been shown that adrenergic activation (Table 4.4) leads to (1) an increased number of circulating B and T cells and lymph flow, with redistribution of natural killer and T helper populations;[52,53,168] (2) a decreased proliferative response to T-dependent mitogens[59] and; (3) enhanced and decreased antibody response, depending on the time of administration and possibly the intracellular signalling pathway required for activation.[41,126] Denervation studies with 6-OHDA have shown a great variability of effects in the modulation of immune responses, depending on the organ, the age, the species and the strain studied, although it has been generally shown that sympathetic denervation in adult rodents increased humoral and reduced cell-mediated responses.[126,206]

Somewhat opposite effects have been rendered in chemically sympathectomized neonates, as well as in adult rodents after surgical sympathectomy.[125,236] Some of those studies support the contention that NE exerts a restraining influence on some lymphocyte functions, such as proliferation and migration, suggesting that for optimal immune responses transient decrease of NE is required.[123,206] NE may also induce changes in the lymph microenvironment itself that could explain some of the differential *in vivo* effects of catecholamines in different lymphocytic populations.[126]

Although the clinical relevance of sympathetic innervation of lymphoid organs is not clear, several studies have documented an important role of NE in modulating inflammatory reactions in animal models of autoimmune disorders, including experimental arthritis, allergic encephalomyelitis, lupus-like syndrome and myasthenia gravis. In the gastrointestinal tract, it has been suggested that sympathetic innervation might play a role in the development of experimental colitis and in the modulation of focal infections in human palatine tonsils.[137,238]

Cholinergic effects

Electrophysiological studies have shown that millimolar concentrations of acetylcholine were able to activate K^+ channels on peripheral human lymphocytes with subsequent inhibition of the proliferative response to phytohaemagglutinin.[77] Acetylcholine or cholinergic agonists have also been shown to stimulate T cell secretion of interleukin 2 (IL2), interleukin 4 (IL4) and interferon γ (IFNγ)[241] and to inhibit that of interleukin 6 (IL6),[186] to increase

Immunological effects of adrenergic activation
Increase in circulating B and T cells
Increased lymph flow
Redistribution of natural killer and T helper cells
Decreased proliferative response for T-dependent mitogens
Modulated antibody response

Table 4.4 Immunological effects of adrenergic activation.

Immunological consequences of acetylcholine and cholinergic agonists
Stimulation of T cell secretion of IL2, IL4, IFNγ
Inhibition of IL6 production by T cells
Increased T cell proliferation
Enhanced cytotoxic activity of T cells
Increased T or B cell mobility
Modulation of antibody secretion
Protection of mature T cells from apoptotic signals

Table 4.5 Immunological consequences of acetylcholine and cholinergic agonists.

T cell proliferation,[121] lytic function of cytotoxic T cells,[215] T and B cell motility,[200] to modulate antibody generation by B cells[188] and suppressor activity of T cells,[185] and to protect mature T cells from apoptotic signals,[7] through differential activation of muscarinic or nicotinic cholinergic receptors (Table 4.5).

Additional support for cholinergic-mediated influence on lymphocyte functions has been provided by *in vivo* studies. For instance, it has been reported that stimulation of the vagus nerve increased the release of lymphocytes from the rat thymus to the blood through nicotinic pathways.[7] In contrast, in the guinea pig spleen, cholinergic agonist stimulation increased lymphocyte mobilization through muscarinic receptors.[191] Moreover, indirect involvement of cholinergic mechanisms in the modulation of lymphocyte functions comes from studies where electrolytic lesions in specific hypothalamic areas resulted in altered muscarinic receptor-binding capacity on thymocytes, while no apparent changes in binding capacity were observed in spleen or peripheral lymphocytes.[80] On the other hand, spleen lymphocytes' binding capacity was increased by both T cell-dependent and independent antigens.[80] Thus, despite controversy regarding cholinergic innervation of lymphoid tissues, substantial evidence points toward cholinergic-mediated receptor modulation of lymphocyte functions as a functionally relevant branch of neuroimmune interactions.

Effects of neuropeptides
Substance P

In vitro studies have shown that SP is able to directly enhance murine B cell production of IgA and IgM at different levels, including gastrointestinal mucosal lymphoid tissues[84,172] and also IgG_3 and IgG_2 in other locations.[107] *In vivo* studies have corroborated that SP acts as a potentiating factor on the secretion of immunoglobulins by B cells.[84,171] Different effects on lymphocyte proliferation has been reported *in vitro* for SP, depending on concentration and time of exposure, with both stimulatory and inhibitory effects,[203] whereas *in vivo* SP definitely increases lymphocyte proliferation.[202] SP has also been shown to increase natural killer and cytotoxic activity of intestinal intraepithelial lymphocytes and human peripheral blood leukocytes,[32,67] to enhance lymphocyte traffic and lymph flow,[153] to decrease T cell adhesion to blood vessels,[116] and to enhance the release of several cytokines, including interleukins IL1, IL2 and IL6, tumour necrosis factor α (TNFα) and granulocyte–macrophage colony-stimulating factor.[210] Similar immunomodulatory effects to SP have been shown for NKA, the co-product of SP encoding gene.[28] In addition, SP in high concentrations was able to degranulate

Observed effects on mucosal immunity by neuropeptides	
Neuropeptide	Effect
Cholecystokinin Thyrotropin-releasing hormone	Increased IgA or IgG in intestinal fluid Normal development of gut intraepithelial lymphocytes Mucosal mast cell activation in ileum
Bombesin	Modulates GALT dysfunction after lack of parenteral nutrition
VIP	Decrease in IgE; increase in IgA in Peyer's patch B cells. Alters migration of T cells to Peyer's patch
SP	Enhances IgA production in mucosal lymphoid tissues. Increases NK and cytotoxic activity of intraepithelial lymphocytes
SS	Inhibits IgA production for Peyer's patches Decreases IL2 expression in LPL

Table 4.6 Observed effects of mucosal immunity by neuropeptides.

mast cells whereas, most importantly, in low concentrations it could prime mast cells to respond to subsequent stimulus without necessarily inducing degranulation (Table 4.6).[97]

Somatostatin

SS inhibited IgA and IgM production *in vitro* by murine mononuclear cells from the Peyer's patches,[209] while at lower concentrations SS increased IgA production.[205] In accordance with previous results, SS also inhibited the rat primary antibody response *in vivo*.[48] In human B cells, SS inhibited IgE production,[107] while it increased that of IgG_2.[106] SS also decreased IgA synthesis and IL2 expression in human intestinal lamina propria lymphocytes.[55] *In vitro* and *in vivo* studies have shown that SS can either inhibit or stimulate murine mitogen-induced T cell proliferation in mucosal lymph tissues[3] while in human lymphocytes its effects are mainly suppressive.[128,173] SS also enhanced T cell adhesion to fibronectin[116] and cytotoxic and natural killer activity,[3] whereas it inhibited colony-stimulating factor release from activated lymphocytes.[88]

Vasoactive intestinal peptide and related peptides

The effects of VIP on immunoglobulin secretion seem to depend on the population of lymphocytes tested.[166] Thus, in the Peyer's patches when T cells receive the first signal, VIP has been shown to increase IgM while diminishing IgA production.[209] In contrast, when human B cells are directly activated by VIP, a rise in IgA, IgM and IgG and a decrease in IgE secretion were obtained.[105,107] In both cases, VIP required costimulatory signals for maximal stimulation. VIP also inhibited mitogen-induced T cell proliferation, probably by reducing IL2 and IL4 synthesis,[167,209] although increased IL2 and IL5 synthesis have also been reported.[161] Moreover, VIP affected the expression of natural killer cell function[189] and altered the migration of T cells into the Peyer's patches and mesenteric lymph nodes.[152,167] Both VIP and the structurally related peptide PACAP (pituitary adenylate cyclase-activating polypeptide) stimulated the adherence and decreased the mobility of peritoneal lymphocytes probably by activating a common

VIP/PACAP receptor[37,65] and protected thymocytes from glucocorticoid-induced apoptosis,[39] while PACAP also regulated the production of certain cytokines by lymphocytes.[133] Therefore, depending on interactions with the local cytokine network, VIP and related peptides may contribute significantly to controlling the amplitude and timing of the inflammatory response to foreign antigens (Table 4.6).

Neuropeptide Y

The effects of NPY on the proliferative activity of lymphocytes may depend on the physiological status of the cell donor, with both stimulatory and inhibitory effects being reported. In addition, NPY inhibited natural killer responses and abolished the primary antibody response.[157] Moreover, NPY has been shown to increase T cell adhesion to the extracellular matrix.[116]

Calcitonin gene-related peptide

Besides being a potent endogenous vasodilator neuropeptide and having a primary role in modulating sensory perception, CGRP has been proved to be a potent immunomodulatory agent. Thus, depending upon experimental conditions, CGRP either inhibited mitogen-induced T cell proliferation[226] or enhanced it,[28] inhibited surface immunoglobulin expression and IL2 production,[139,230] increased T cell adhesion to fibronectin[116] and augmented chemotactic activity of lymphocytes and eosinophils,[68] modulated the effects of SP on inflammation,[237] inhibited cell antigen-presenting activity of both macrophages and Langerhans' cells,[91,163] induced mast cell degranulation,[177] and decreased delayed- and contact-type hypersensitivity *in vivo*.[6]

Corticotropin-releasing hormone

CRH has been shown to inhibit antibody responses,[95] to either stimulate or reduce T cell proliferation,[95,141,196] to stimulate B cell proliferation,[95,141] to suppress *in vivo*[96] or stimulate *in vitro* natural killer activity and chemotaxis,[102,115] and to increase expression of IL2 receptors and IL1, IL2 and IL6 secretion in leukocytes.[102,196,198] CRH seems to play a dual immunomodulatory role: proinflammatory when actions are mediated by CRH receptor activation and anti-inflammatory when effects are mediated through the release of steroids and catecholamines, as has been shown in CRH-deficient mice.[102]

Opioids and other pro-opiomelanocortin-derived peptides

Both, endorphins and enkephalins have been shown to dampen immunoglobulin production in different locations, including the GALT.[26] Opioids also showed opposite dose-dependent effects on mitogen-induced T cell proliferation[178] and enhanced generation of cytotoxic lymphocytes and natural killer activity.[56] Opioids also modulated the expression of surface antigens on lymphocytes,[227] motility of T and B cells,[240] IL2 production[227] and lymphocyte release from peripheral lymph nodes.[168]

ACTH and other POMC-related peptides are potent modulators of immunoglobulin synthesis and B cell proliferation and lymphocytic motility.[6,122] Melanocyte-stimulating hormone α has major anti-inflammatory properties partly mediated by the modulation of the production of cytokines and chemokines in immune cells.[171]

Other neuropeptides and neurohormones

Cholecystokinin has been shown to increase the production of IgA and IgG in intestinal fluid[70] and to modulate T cell proliferation in response to mitogens.[144] Cholecystokinin also exhibited inhibitory effects on lymphocyte chemotaxis.[38]

Neurotensin showed no effect on lymphocyte proliferation but stimulated lymphocyte chemotaxis.[76] Neurotensin has been suggested to be involved in the regulation of microvasculature, specifically during inflammatory conditions, probably due to its striking ability to induce mast cell secretion.[30]

Some of the observed effects of *nerve growth factor* on lymphocyte functions include the stimulation of T and B cell proliferation,[170,219] the increased expression of surface IL2,[220] and either increased or decreased immunoglobulin synthesis.[108,109] In accordance with the well-known trophic effects of nerve growth factor on central and peripheral nerves, it has also been shown that nerve growth factor was able to modulate sympathetic innervation in lymphoid tissues.[25]

Glucocorticoids exerted both enhancing and inhibitory effects on lymphocytic function by modulating B and T cell proliferation, interfering with antigen presentation, altering cytokine production and natural killer and cytotoxic activity and lymphocyte traffic.[122,138,235] Macrophage migration inhibitory factor, the physiological counter-regulator of glucocorticoid actions, has also been shown to exert a key role in the development of delayed-type hypersensitivity reactions and in the induction of antigen-specific T and B cell responses.[21]

TRH increased T cell proliferation and IL2 production, has been shown to be necessary for fetal development of gut-associated intraepithelial lymphocytes, modulated the antibody production of B cells, probably by inducing thyrotropin-stimulating hormone release at several levels including lymphocytes,[112] and induced mucosal mast cell activation in the rat ileum.[194] Growth hormone and prolactin disclosed important immunomodulatory actions, such as increased antibody production and proliferation and natural and cytolytic activity of T cells.[103,156] In addition, several studies have shown that growth hormone might be relevant for the development and maturation of the immune system.[122,138,235] Bombesin has been shown to have no effect or to be antiproliferative on lymphocytes, to increase intestinal release of IgA and IgM and to prevent the decrease and dysfunction of GALT associated with parenteral nutrition.[99,118]

IMMUNOMODULATORY ROLE OF NERVE–MAST CELL INTERACTIONS

Neuroanatomical studies have provided strong evidence for the direct innervation of gastrointestinal mucosal mast cells.[160,213] In addition to specific immune activation, the secretion of mast cell mediators may also be triggered by non-specific stimuli, including neurotransmitters, neuropeptides and nerve stimulation.[51] Numerous neuropeptides such as ACTH, SP, CGRP, SS, VIP, TRH, CRH, nerve growth factor, neurotensin, bradykinin and opiates have been reported to induce mast cells to secrete histamine and other mediators. However, only some of them, including SP, CRH, TRH, nerve growth factor, stem-cell factor and neurotensin, have been shown to activate mucosal mast cells in the gastrointestinal tract.[14,29,147,194,207,218] Mast cell responses to neural stimulation are heterogeneous. Thus, depending upon experimental conditions, NE and sympathetic stimulation may either enhance or inhibit histamine secretion.[5,129] Parasympathetic activation and acetylcholine are also potent secretagogues for mast cells, although this response is, to some extent, dependent

on the presence of IgE.[134] Moreover, Pavlovian-conditioned activation of mast cell secretion indicates that mast cell activity is subject to CNS modulation.[146]

Pharmacological and electrophysiological studies have suggested that the interaction between mast cells and neuropeptide-containing nerves is functionally relevant. For instance, in the gastrointestinal tract, activation of intestinal mast cells is responsible for many of the functional events that take place after an antigenic challenge. In this sense, mast cell activation leads to the release of mediators, many of which markedly alter epithelial ion transport and motility patterns in both animals[34] and humans.[33] But, mast cell products may also promote hypersensitivity reactions in many other ways, either by direct activation of epithelial cells or by indirect stimulation of other neuroimmune cells. Numerous studies support the modulatory role of mast cell mediators in hypersensitivity reactions taking place at mucosal levels such as in the airways, gut, eye and urogenital tracts by altering the antigen presentation, the cytokine production or the proliferation and adhesion to extracellular matrix of T cells.[69,73,85]

CLINICAL IMPLICATIONS ON FOOD ALLERGY

All described (and other potential) interactions occurring among immune–endocrine cells and neural endings in GALT and BALT may be relevant for the regulation and coordination of the *in vivo* inflammatory response against food-derived antigens. However, those interactions must be viewed as a dynamic interplay involving the classical immune and non-immune cellular network that eventually resides in the mucosal tissues and the central, peripheral and enteric neuroendocrine systems. These dynamic interactions are further represented (1) by the migratory capacity of activated immunocytes and (2) by the functional state of effector cells. Thus, for instance, activated lymphocytes are able to cross the blood–brain barrier,[86] allowing direct local cross-talk between different microenvironments. The effectiveness of neuroimmune interplay in the control of immune reactions may largely depend on the functional state of immune cells, since it has been shown that primed cells are more prepared to sense and react against antihomeostatic messages than resting cells. It is also important to remember that both afferent and efferent neuroimmune–endocrine interactions are involved in that interplay. In this circuitry, neural and immune byproducts, including cytokines, chemokines, neurotransmitters, growth factors, antibodies, neurohormones and neuropeptides, act as the chemical messengers.

Food-induced nerve–lymphocyte interactions

Food-allergic hypersensitivity reactions are mounted when the offending antigen is able to crosslink with surface IgE present on mast cells and basophils. This interaction causes release of a broad array of bioactive molecules that alter epithelial and smooth muscle physiology by inducing water and ionic secretion, increased vascular and epithelial permeability to small and large molecules and gross abnormalities in gastrointestinal motility patterns.[34,207] During the course of these events some of the bioactive molecules released by immunocompetent cells activate other immune and non-immune cells, including nerve terminals, which in turn liberate pro- and counter-regulatory substances that purposely help to maintain the homeostatic balance. In this sense, cytokines, antibodies and neuropeptides released by immune cells have been shown to alter electrical activity and neuropeptide secretion by peripheral, enteric and central neurons,[16,87] to modulate neuritogenesis in lymphoid tissues[101] and to regulate neurogenic inflammation in the gastrointestinal tract.[149] The opposite is also true, since nerve stimulation has been shown to inhibit the effects of antigen challenge.[151] The complexity of the response is ultimately represented by the fact that food antigens themselves may induce a variety of effects on the nervous system, leading to lower threshold of discharge to normal stimuli (hyperexcitability or visceral hyperalgesia), which could be responsible for some of the clinical manifestations of food allergy.[234]

Modulation of food-induced immunological reactions by neuropeptides

Numerous experimental studies have confirmed that food-induced immunological reactions are influenced by neural and neuropeptide innervation and cytokine release. Thus, for instance, it has been shown that intestinal secretory responses and permeability, in some cases, to egg ovalbumin luminal challenge were inhibited by systemic capsaicin, tetrodotoxinin and NPY, reduced by interferon α/β but potentiated by SP and opioid antagonists.[34,45,142,143] Additional evidence supports the involvement of capsaicin-sensitive fibres as well as VIP, SP, opioids, CGRP, CRH and many other peptides in the pathogenesis of several immune-mediated inflammatory disorders such as asthma, nasal allergy, contact- and delayed-type hypersensitivity reactions, rheumatoid arthritis, systemic lupus, autoimmune thyroiditis, urticaria, chronic arachnoiditis, inflammatory bowel disease, enteric parasitic infestation and coeliac disease.[1,21,90,132,142,159,208]

Emotion and food-induced immunological reactions

Given the complexity of neuroimmune interactions, it is understandable that an endless list of factors may influence the immune response. In the clinical setting one of the most striking factors that could be involved in the development and reactivation of hypersensitivity reactions is the emotional state of the individual. Clinical and experimental studies have shown that stress, inherited and acquired mental disorders and brain-induced lesions have important consequences on immune functions.[104,138,182,208] Although this aspect is beyond the scope of this chapter, some examples can illustrate this point. Thus, acute exposure to stress induces a predominant suppressive effect on immune parameters *in vitro*; in contrast, chronic stress can enhance immune reactions.[138,182] Conversely, studies *in vivo* have shown that acute stressors induced both immunostimulatory and immunoinhibitory effects. For instance, cold pain induced intestinal mast cell activation in control individuals and food-allergic patients,[195] while wrap-restraint stress activated colonic mast cells in rats.[29] Moreover, gastrointestinal functional changes and clinical symptoms paralleled that activation.[29,195] Likewise, it has also been shown that Pavlovian conditioning was associated with supramaximal secretory responses to antigen and taste aversion was able to modulate the anaphylactic reaction in rats.[44]

AGE EFFECTS

Another important factor that may be involved in the regulation of immune response is age. It is well known that the prevalency of food-allergic reactions is higher during the first years of life and decreases thereafter. Several age-related changes in immune functions have been described, such as decreased natural killer activity, increased vulnerability to the immunosuppressive effects of stress,[95] increased blood levels of catecholamines and NPY[94,110] and increased expression of β-adrenoceptors on lymphocytes.[2] the way that these factors may influence the *in vivo* responses to food-derived antigens remains presently unknown.

CONCLUDING OBSERVATIONS

The therapeutic implications of the growing knowledge of neuroimmune interactions are enormous but remain mostly theoretical and speculative at present. Central and peripheral nervous system manipulation by psychological (hypnosis, behavioural conditioning), pharmacological and other modalities of intervention could turn out to be very valuable weapons against the deleterious effects of stress on the immune system and on the induction of tolerance to food-derived antigens. By modulating the activity of the autonomic nervous system it may be feasible to regulate many immune functions along with some protective factors that contribute to diminish the antigenic load to the intestine, such as acid and pepsin secretion, small intestinal motility, mucus and IgA secretion. Finally, since gastrointestinal inflammation is a major component of allergic reactions to food, progressing in the knowledge of anti/pro-inflammatory properties of certain neuropeptides and cytokines and developing more specific and potent receptor agonists/antagonists of some of these molecules could lead to the opening of new avenues in the treatment and prevention of food-allergic related disorders.

SUMMARY

- Food allergy is an immunologically mediated adverse reaction against antigenic epitopes contained in food that may affect most organs in the body.
- Hypersensitivity reactions to food are regulated by the nervous system and the mucosa-associated immune system.
- Immune and nervous systems display a dynamic and interactive communication based upon the presence of common messengers and receptors.
- This interaction is functionally relevant and may have important clinical implications.
- Modulation of nerve–immune interactions in the gastrointestinal and respiratory tracts may influence the course of hypersensitivity reactions.
- Development of new drugs with blocking or enhancing activity against nerve–immune mediators and receptors may contribute to the prevention and treatment of food-allergic diseases.

Acknowledgement

This work was supported in part by the Grant 1996–97 per estudis a l'estranger from the Acadèmia de Cièncias Mèdiques de Catalunya i Balears i la Societat Catalana de Digestologia (Barcelona, Spain), from whom Javier Santos is a recipient.

REFERENCES

1 Abe Y, Takeda N, Irifune M et al. Effects of capsaicin desensitization on nasal allergy-like symptoms and histamine release in the nose induced by toluene diisocyanate in guinea pigs. Acta Oto Laryngol 1992; 112: 703–9.

2 Ackerman KD, Bellinger DL, Felten SY, Felten DL. Ontogeny and senescence of noradrenergic innervation of the rodent thymus and spleen. In: Psychoneuroimmunology, 2nd edn (Ader R, Felten DL, Cohen N, eds). Academic Press, San Diego, 1991: 71–126.

3 Agro A, Padol I, Stanisz AM. Immunomodulatory activities of the somatostatin analogue BIM 23014c: effects on murine lymphocyte proliferation and natural killer activity. Regul Pept 1991; 32: 129–39.

4 Aguila MC, Dees WL, Haensly WE, McCann SM. Evidence that somatostatin is localized and synthesized in lymphoid organs. Proc Natl Acad Sci USA 1991; 88: 11485–9.

5 Alm PE, Bloom GD. What – if any– is the role of adrenergic mechanisms in histamine release from mast cells. Agents Actions 1981; 11: 60–6.

6 Alvarez Mon M, Kehrl JH, Fauci AS. A potential role for adrenocorticotropin in regulating human B lymphocyte functions. J Immunol 1985; 135: 3823–6.

7 Antonica A, Magni F, Mearini L, Paolocci N. Vagal control of lymphocyte release from rat thymus. J Auton Nerv Syst 1994; 48: 187–97.

8 Arizono N, Matsuda S, Hattori T, Kojima Y, Maeda T, Galli SJ. Anatomical variation in mast cell nerve association in the rat small intestine, heart, lung and skin: similarities of distance between neural processes and mast cells, eosinophils, or plasma cells in the jejunal lamina propria. Lab Invest 1990; 62: 626–34.

9 Asahina A, Hosoi J, Beissert S, Stratigos A, Granstein RD. Inhibition of the induction of delayed-type and contact hypersensitivity by calcitonin gene-related peptide. J Immunol 1995; 154: 3056–61.

10 Audhya T, Jain R, Hollander CS. Receptor-mediated immunomodulation by corticotropin-releasing factor. Cell Immunol 1991; 134: 77–84.

11 Baron R, Janig W. Sympathetic and afferent neurons projecting in the splenic nerve in the cat. Neurosci Lett 1988; 94: 109–13.

12 Bellinger DL, Felten SY, Lorton D, Felten DL. Origin of noradrenergic innervation on the spleen in rats. Brain Behav Immun 1989; 3: 291–311.

13 Bellinger DL, Lorton D, Hamill RW, Felten SY, Felten DL. Acetylcholinesterase staining and choline acetyltransferase activity in the young adult rat spleen: lack of evidence for cholinergic innervation. Brain Behav Immun 1993; 7: 91–204.

14 Bellinger DL, Lorton DN, Romano TA, Olschowska JA, Felten SY, Felten DL. Neuropeptide innervation of lymphoid organs. Ann NY Acad Sci 1990; 594: 17–33.

15 Besedowsky HO, del Rey A. Immune-neuro-endocrine interactions: facts and hypothesis. Endoc Rev 1996; 17. 64–102.

16 Besedowsky HO, Sorkin E, Felix E, Haas H. Hypothalamic changes during the immune response. Eur J Immunol 1977; 7: 323–5.

17 Bhathena SJ, Louie J, Schechter GP, Redman RS, Wahl L, Recant L. Identification of human mononuclear leukocytes bearing receptors for somatostatin and glucagon. Diabetes 1980; 30: 127–31.

18 Brandtzaeg P, Halstensen TS, Kett K et al. Immunobiology and immunopathology of human gut mucosa: humoral immunity and intraepithelial lymphocytes. Gastroenterology 1989; 97: 1562–84.

19 Brodde OE, Engel G, Hoyer D, Block KD, Weber F. The β-adrenergic receptor in human lymphocytes: subclassification by the use of a new radioligand [125 Iodo] cyanopindolol. Life Sci 1981; 29: 2189–98.

20 Brouxhon SM, Prasad AV, Joseph SA, Felten DL, Bellinger DL. Localization of corticotropin-releasing factor in primary and secondary lymphoid organs in the rat. Brain Behav Immun 1998; 12: 107–22.

21 Bucala R. Neuroimmunomodulation by macrophage migration inhibitory factor (MIF). Ann NY Acad Sci 1998; 840: 74–82.

22 Bulloch K, Pomerantz W. Autonomic nervous system innervation of thymic-related lymphoid tissue in wild-type and nude mice. J Comp Neurol 1984; 228: 57–68.

23 Calvo W. The innervation of bone marrow in laboratory animals. Am J Anat 1968; 123: 315–28.

24 Calvo JR, Pozo D, Guerrero JM. Functional and molecular characterization of VIP receptors and signal transduction mechanisms in human and rodent immune systems. Adv Neuroimmunol 1996; 6: 39–47.

25 Carlson SL, Albers KM, Beiting DJ, Parish M, Conner JM, Davis BM. NGF modulates sympathetic innervation in lymphoid tissues. J Neurosci 1995; 15: 5892–9.

26 Carr DJJ, Radulescu RT, de Costa BR, Rice KC, Blalock JE. Differential effects of opioids on immunoglobulin production by lymphocytes isolated from Peyer's patches and spleen. Life Sci 1990; 47: 1059–69.

27 Carr DJJ. Neuroendocrine peptide receptors on cells of the immune system. Chem Immunol 1997; 69: 132–54.

28 Casini A, Geppetti P, Maggi CA, Surrenti C. Effects of calcitonin generelated peptide (CGRP), neurokinin A and neurokinin A (4–10) on the mitogenic response of human peripheral blood mononuclear cells. Naunyn's-Schmiedeberg's Arch Pharmacol 1989; 339: 354–8.

29 Castagliuolo I, LaMont JT, Qui B et al. Acute stress causes mucin release from rat colon. role of corticotropin releasing factor and mast cells. Am J Physiol 1996; 271: G884–92.

30 Castagliuolo I, Leeman SE, Bartolak-Suki E et al. A neurotensin antagonist, SR 48692, inhibits colonic responses to immobilization stress in rats. Proc Natl Acad Sci USA 1996; 93: 12611–15.

31 Chubb IW, Ranieri R, White GH, Hogdson AJ. The enkephalins are amongst the peptides hydrolyzed by purified acetylcholinesterase. Neuroscience 1983; 10: 1369–77.

32 Croitoru K, Ernst PB, Bienenstock J, Padol I, Stanisz AM. Selective modulation of the natural killer activity of murine intestinal intraepithelial leucocytes by the neuropeptide substance P. Immunology 1990; 71: 196–201.

33 Crowe SE, Perdue MH. Anti-immunoglobulin E-stimulated ion transport in human large and small intestine. Gastroenterology 1993; 105: 764–72.

34 Crowe SE, Perdue MH. Gastrointestinal food hypersensitivity: basic mechanisms of pathophysiology. Gastroenterology 1992; 103: 1075–95.

35 Crowe SE, Sestini P, Perdue MH. Allergic reactions of rat jejunal mucosa, ion transport responses to luminal antigen and inflammatory mediators. Gastroenterology 1990; 99: 74–82.

36 DeCoursey TE, Chandy KG, Gupta S, Cahalan MD. Voltage-gated K⁺ channels in human T lymphocytes: a role in mitogenesis. Nature 1984; 307: 465–8.

37 De la Fuente M, Delgado M, Del Rio M et al. VIP modulation of adherence and mobility in rat peritoneal lymphocytes and macrophages. Peptides 1994; 15: 1157–63.

38 De la Fuente M, Campos M, del Rio M, Hernanz A. Inhibition of murine peritoneal macrophage functions by sulfated cholecystokinin octapeptide. Regul Pept 1995; 55: 47–56.

39 Delgado M, Garrido E, Martinez C, Leceta J, Gomariz RP. Vasoactive intestinal peptide and pituitary adenylate cyclase-activating polypeptide (PACAP 27 and PACAP 38) protect CD4⁺ CD8⁺ thymocytes from glucocorticoid-induced apoptosis. Blood 1996; 87: 5152–61.

40 DePace DM, Webber RH. Electrostimulation and morphologic study of the nerves to the bone marrow of the albino rat. Acta Anatomica 1975; 93: 1–18.

41 Depelchin A, Letteson JJ. Adrenalin influence on the immune response. I. Accelerating or suppressor effects according to the time of application. Immunol Lett 1981; 3: 199–205.

42 De Potter WD, Kurzawa R, Miserez B, Coen EP. Evidence against differential release of noradrenaline, neuropeptide Y, and dopamine-β-hydroxylase from adrenergic nerves in the isolated perfused sheep spleen. Synapse 1995; 19: 67–76.

43 Di Sebastiano P, Fink T, Weihe E, Friess H, Beger HG, Bechler M. Changes of protein gene product 9.5 (PGP 9.5) immunoreactive nerves in inflamed appendix. Dig Dis Sci 1995; 40: 366–72.

44 Djuric VJ, Markovic BM, Lazarevic M, Jankovic BD. Conditioned taste aversion in rats subjected to anaphylactic shock. Ann NY Acad Sci 1987; 496: 561–8.

45 Djuric VJ, Wang L, Bienenstock J, Perdue MH. Naloxone exacerbates intestinal and systemic anaphylaxis in the rat. *Brain Behav Immun* 1995; 9: 87–100.

46 Dockray GJ. Physiology of enteric neuropeptides. In: *Physiology of the Gastrointestinal Tract* (Johnson LR, Alpers DH, Christensen J, Jacobson DE, Walsh JH, eds). Raven Press, New York, 1994: 169–209.

47 Draskoci M, Jankovic BD. Involution of thymus and suppression of immune responses in rats treated with reserpine. *Nature* 1964; 202: 408–11.

48 Eglezos A, Andrews PV, Helme RD. *In vivo* inhibition of the rat primary antibody response to antigenic stimulation by somatostatin. *Immunol Cell Biol* 1993; 71: 125–9.

49 Ekblad E, Ekman R, Hakanson R, Sundler F. Projections of peptide-containing neurons in rat colon. *Neuroscience* 1988; 27: 655–74.

50 Ekblad E, Winther C, Ekman R, Hakanson R, Sundler F. Projections of peptide-containing neurons on rat small intestine. *Neuroscience* 1987; 20: 169–88.

51 Elenkov IJ, Vizi ES. Presynaptic modulation of release of noradrenaline from the sympathetic nerve terminals in the rat spleen. *Neuropharmacology* 1991; 30: 1319–24.

52 Ernström U, Sandberg G. Effects of α- and β-receptor stimulation on the release of lymphocytes and granulocytes from the spleen. *Scand J Haematol* 1973; 11: 275–86.

53 Ernström U, Soder O. Influence of adrenaline on the dissemination of antibody-producing cells from the spleen. *Clin Exp Immunol* 1975; 21: 131–40.

54 Evers BM, Bold RJ, Erenfried JA, Li J, Townsend M, Klimpel GR. Characterization of functional neurotensin receptors on human lymphocytes. *Surgery* 1994; 116: 134–9.

55 Fais S, Annibale B, Boirivant M, Santoro F, Pallone F, Delle Fave G. Effect of somatostatin on human intestinal lamina propria lymphocytes. *J Neuroimmunol* 1991; 31: 211–19.

56 Faith RE, Liang HJ, Plotnikoff NP, Murgo AL, Nimeh NF. Neuroimmunomodulation with enkephalins: *in vitro* enhancement of natural killer cell activity in peripheral blood lymphocytes from cancer patients. *Natl Immun Cell Growth Regul* 1987; 6: 88–98.

57 Fatani JA, Qayyum MA, Mehta L, Singh U. Parasympathetic innervation of the thymus: a histochemical and immunocytochemical study. *J Anat* 1986; 147: 115–19.

58 Feher E, Fodor M, Burnstock G. Distribution of somatostatin-immunoreactive nerve fibres in Peyer's patches. *Gut* 1992; 33: 1195–8.

59 Felsner P, Hofer D, Rinner I *et al.* Continuous *in vivo* treatment with catecholamines suppresses *in vitro* reactivity of rat peripheral blood T-lymphocytes via α-mediated mechanisms. *J Neuroimmunol* 1992; 37: 47–57.

60 Felsner P, Hofer D, Rinner I, Porta S, Korsatko W, Schauenstein K. Adrenergic suppression of peripheral blood T cell reactivity in the rat is due to activation of peripheral α_2 receptors. *J Neuroimmunol* 1995; 57: 27–34.

61 Felten DL, Ackerman KD, Wiegand SJ, Felten SY. Noradrenergic sympathetic innervation of the spleen. I. Nerve fibers associated with lymphocytes and macrophages in specific compartments of the splenic white pulp. *J Neurosci Res* 1987; 18: 28–36.

62 Felten DL, Felten SY, Carlson SL, Olschowska JA, Livnat S. Innervation of lymphoid tissue. *J Immunol* 1985; 135: 755–65s.

63 Felten DL, Overhage JM, Felten SY, Schmedtje JF. Noradrenergic sympathetic innervation of lymphoid tissue in the rabbit appendix: further evidence for a link between the nervous and immune systems. *Brain Res Bull* 1981; 7: 595–612.

64 Felten SY, Felten DL. Innervation of lymphoid tissue. In: *Psychoneuroimmunology*, 2nd edn (Ader R, Felten DL, Cohen N, eds). Academic Press, San Diego, 1991: 27–69.

65 Felten SY, Olschowka JA. Noradrenergic sympathetic innervation of the spleen. II. Tyrosine hydroxylase (TH)-positive terminals from synaptic-like contacts on lymphocytes in the splenic white pulp. *J Neurosci Res* 1987; 18: 37–48.

66 Fernandez-Lopez A, Pazos A. Identification of α_2-adrenoceptors in rat lymph nodes and spleen: an autoradiographic study. *Eur J Pharmacol* 1994; 252: 333–6.

67 Flageole H, Senterman M, Trudel JL. Substance P increases *in vitro* lymphokine-activated killer cell activity against fresh colorectal cancer cells. *J Surg Res* 1992; 53: 445–9.

68 Foster CA, Mandak B, Kromer E, Rot A. CGRP is chemotactic for human T lymphocytes. *Ann NY Acad Sci* 1992; 657: 397–404.

69 Fox CC, Jewll SD, Whitacre CC. Rat peritoneal mast cells present antigen to a PPD specific T cell line. *Cell Immunol* 1994; 158: 253–64.

70 Freier S, Eran M, Faber J. Effect of cholecystokinin and of its antagonist, of atropine, and of food on the release of immunoglobulin A and immunoglobulin G specific antibodies in the rat intestine. *Gastroenterology* 1987; 93: 1242–6.

71 Friedman EM, Irwin MR. Modulation of immune cell function by the autonomic nervous system. *Pharmacol Ther* 1997; 74: 27–38.

72 Friedman EM, Irwin MR, Nonogaki K. Neuropeptide Y inhibits *in vivo* specific antibody production in rats. *Brain Behav Immun* 1995; 9: 182–9.

73 Frieri M, Metcalfe DD. Analysis of the effect of mast cell granules on lymphocyte blastogenesis in the absence and presence of mitogen. *J Immunol* 1983; 131: 1942–8.

74 Gallin EK. Ion channels in leukocytes. *Pharmacol Rev* 1991; 71: 775–811.

75 Garrido E, Delgado M, Martinez C, Gomariz RP, De la Fuente M. Pituitary adenylate cyclase-activating polypeptide (PACAP 38) modulates lymphocyte and macrophage functions: stimulation of adherence and opposite effects on mobility. *Neuropeptides* 1996; 30: 583–95.

76 Garrido JJ, Arahuetes RM, Hernanz A, de la Fuente M. Modulation of neurotensin and neuromedin N of adherence and chemotaxis capacity of murine lymphocytes. *Regul Pept* 1992; 41: 27–37.

77 Gaspar R, Varga Z, Bene L, Marcheselli F, Pieri C, Damjanovich S. Effect of acetylcholine on the electrophysiology and proliferative response of human lymphocytes. *Biochem Biophys Res Commun* 1996; 226: 303–8.

78 Giron LT, Crutcher KA, Davis JN. Lymph nodes — a possible site for sympathetic neuronal regulation of immune responses. *Ann Neurol* 1980; 8: 520–2.

79 Gordon MA, Cohen JJ, Wilson B. Muscarinic cholinergic receptors in murine lymphocytes. Demonstration by direct binding. *Proc Natl Acad Sci USA* 1978; 75: 2902–4.

80 Guschin GV, Jakovleva EE, Kataeva GV *et al.* Muscarinic cholinergic receptors of rat lymphocytes: effect of antigen stimulation and local brain lesion. *Neuroimmunomodulation* 1994; 1: 259–64.

81 Hadden JW, Hadden EM, Middleton E. Lymphocyte blast transformation. I. Demonstration of adrenergic receptors in human peripheral lymphocytes. *Cell Immunol* 1970; 1: 583–95.

82 Hadden JW. Sympathetic modulation of immune response. *N Engl J Med* 1971; 285: 178.

83 Hansen K, Sickelmann F, Pietrowsky R, Fehm HL, Born J. Systemic immune challenges following meal intake in humans. *Am J Physiol* 1997; 273: R548–53.

84 Helme RD, Eglezos A, Dandie GW, Andrews PV, Boyd RL. The effect of substance P on the regional lymph node antibody response to antigenic stimulation in capsaicin-pretreated rats. *J Immunol* 1987; 139: 3470–3.

85 Hershkoviz R, Lider O, Baram D, Reshef T, Miron S, Mekori YA. Inhibition of T cell adhesion of extracellular matrix glycoproteins by histamine: a role for mast cell degranulation products. *J Leukocyte Biol* 1994; 56: 495–501.

86 Hickey WF, Hsu BL, Kimura H. T lymphocyte entry into the central nervous system. *J Neurosci Res* 1991; 28: 254–60.

87 Hikawa N, Takenaka T. Sensory neurons regulate immunoglobulin secretion of spleen cells: cellular analysis of bidirectional communications between neurons and immune cells. *J Neuroimmunol* 1996; 70: 191–8.

88 Hinterberger W, Cerny C, Kinast H, Pointner H, Tragl KH. Somatostatin reduces the release of colony-stimulating activity (CSA) from PHA-activated mouse spleen lymphocytes. *Experientia* 1978; 34: 860–2.

89 Höllt V, Garzon J, Schulz R, Herz A. Corticotropin-releasing factor is excitatory in the guinea-pig ileum and activates an opioid mechanism in this tissue. *Eur J Pharmacol* 1984; 101: 165–6.

90 Holzer P. Implications of tachykinins and calcitonin gene-related peptide in inflammatory bowel disease. *Digestion* 1988; 59: 269–83.

A

91 Hosoi J, Murphy GF, Egan CL, Grabbe S, Asahina A, Granstein RD. Regulation of Langerhans cells function by nerves containing calcitonin gene-related peptide. *Nature* 1993; 363: 159–63.

92 Hukannen M, Konttinen YT, Rees RG, Gibson SJ, Santavirta S, Polak JM. Innervation of bone from healthy and arthritic rats by SP and CGRP containing sensory fibers. *J Rheumat* 1992; 19: 1252–9.

93 Inoue N, Magari S, Sakanaka M. Distribution of peptidergic nerve fibers in rat bronchus-associated lymphoid tissue: light microscopy observations. *Lymphology* 1990; 23: 155–60.

94 Irwin MR, Brown M, Patterson T, Hauger R, Mascovich A, Grant I. Neuropeptide Y and natural killer cell activity: findings in depression and Alzheimer caregiver stress. *FASEB J* 1991; 5: 3100–7.

95 Irwin MR, Hauger R, Brown M. Central corticotropin releasing hormone activates the sympathetic nervous system and reduces immune function: increased responsivity in the aged rat. *Endocrinology* 1992; 131: 1047–53.

96 Irwin MR, Hauger RL, Jones L, Provencio M, Britton KT. Sympathetic nervous system mediates central corticotropin-releasing factor induced suppression of natural killer cytotoxicity. *J Pharmacol Exp Ther* 1990; 255: 101–7.

97 Janiszewski J, Bienenstock J, Blennerhassett MG. Picomolar doses of substance P trigger electrical responses in mast cells without degranulation. *Am J Physiol* 1994; C138–45.

98 Jesseph JM, Felten DL. Noradrenergic innervation of the gut-associated lymphoid tissues (GALT) in the rabbit. *Anat Rec* 1984 (Abstract); 208: A81.

99 Jin GF, Guo YS, Houston CW. Bombesin: an activator of specific Aeromonas antibody secretion in rat intestine. *Dig Dis Sci* 1989; 34: 1708–12.

100 Josefsson E, Bergquist J, Erkman R, Tarkowski A. Catecholamines are synthesized by mouse lymphocytes and regulate functions of these cells by induction of apoptosis. *Immunology* 1996; 88: 140–6.

101 Kannan Y, Bienenstock J, Ohta M, Stanisz AM, Stead RH. Nerve growth factor and cytokines mediate lymphoid tissue-induced neurite outgrowth from mouse superior cervical ganglia *in vitro*. *J Immunol* 1996; 156: 313–20.

102 Karalis K, Muglia LJ, Bae D, Hilderbrand H, Majzoub JA. CRH and the immune system. *J Neuroimmunol* 1997; 72: 131–6.

103 Kelley KW. The role of growth hormone in the regulation of the immune response. *Ann NY Acad Sci* 1990; 594: 95–103.

104 Khansari DN, Murgo AJ, Faith RE. Effects of stress on the immune system. *Immunol Today* 1990; 11: 170–5.

105 Kimata H, Fujimoto M. Vasoactive intestinal peptide specifically induces human IgA1 and IgA2 production. *Eur J Immunol* 1994; 24: 2262–5.

106 Kimata H, Yoshida A, Fujimoto M, Mikawa H. Effect of vasoactive intestinal peptide, somatostatin, and substance P on spontaneous IgE and IgG4 production in atopic patients. *J Immunol* 1993; 150: 4630–40.

107 Kimata H, Yoshida A, Ishioka C, Mikawa H. Differential effect of vasoactive intestinal peptide, somatostatin and substance P on human IgE and IgG subclass production. *Cell Immunol* 1992; 144: 429–42.

108 Kimata H, Yoshida A, Ishioka C, Mikawa H. Nerve growth factor inhibits immunoglobulin production but not proliferation of human plasma cell lines. *Clin Immunol Immunopathol* 1991; 69: 145–51.

109 Kimata H, Yoshida A, Kusunoki T, Hosoi S, Mikawa H. Nerve growth factor specifically induces human IgG4 production. *Eur J Immunol* 1991; 21: 137–41.

110 Krall JF, Connelly M, Weisbart R, Tuck ML. Age-related elevation of plasma catecholamine concentration and reduced responsiveness of lymphocyte adenylate cyclase. *J Clin Endocrinol Metab* 1981; 52: 863–7.

111 Krumins SA, Bloomfield CA. Evidence of NK-1 and NK-2 tachykinin receptors and their involvement in histamine release in murine mast cell line. *Neuropeptides* 1992; 21: 65–72.

112 Kruger TE. Immunomodulation of peripheral lymphocytes by hormones of the hypothalamus–pituitary–thyroid axis. *Adv Neuroimmunol* 1996; 6: 387–95.

113 Kudoh G, Hoshi K, Murakami T. Fluorescence microscopic and enzyme histochemical studies of the innervation of the human spleen. *Arch Histol Jap* 1979; 42: 169–80.

114 Landmann R. Beta-adrenergic receptors in human leukocyte subpopulations. *Eur J Clin Invest* 1992; 22 (Suppl 1): 30–6.

115 Leu SJ, Singh VK. Modulation of natural killer cell-mediated lysis by corticotropin-releasing neurohormone. *J Neuroimmunol* 1991; 33: 253–60.

116 Levite M, Cahalon L, Hershkowitz R, Steinman L, Lider O. Neuropeptides, via specific receptors, regulate T cell adhesion to fibronectin. *J Immunol* 1998; 160: 993–1000.

117 Lewis RS, Cahalan MD. Subset-specific expression of potassium channels in developing murine T lymphocytes. *Science* 1988; 239: 771–5.

118 Li J, Kudsk KA, Hamidian M, Gocinski BL. Bombesin affects mucosal immunity and gut-associated lymphoid tissue in intravenously fed mice. *Arch Surg* 1995; 130: 1164–9.

119 Lovenberg TW, Chalmers DT, Liu C, De Souza EB. CRF_{2a} and CRF_{2b} receptor mRNAs are differentially distributed between the rat central nervous system and peripheral tissues. *Endocrinology* 1995; 136: 4139–42.

120 Luger TA, Scholzen T, Brzoska T, Becher E, Slominski A, Paus R. Cutaneous immunomodulation and coordination of skin stress responses by α-melanocyte-stimulating hormone. *Ann NY Acad Sci* 1998; 840: 381–94.

121 MacManus JP, Boyton AL, Whitfield JF, Gillan DJ, Isaacs RJ. Acetylcholine-induced initiation of thymic lymphoblast DNA synthesis and proliferation. *J Cell Physiol* 1975; 85: 321–9.

122 Madden KS, Felten DL. Experimental basis for neural-immune interactions. *Physiol Rev* 1996; 75: 77–106.

123 Madden KS, Felten SY, Felten DL, Hardy CA, Livnat S. Sympathetic nervous system modulation of the immune system. II. Induction of lymphocyte proliferation and migration *in vivo* by chemical sympathectomy. *J Neuroimmunol* 1994; 49: 67–75.

124 Madden KS, Livnat S. Catecholamine action and immunological reactivity. In: *Psychoneuroimmunology*, 2nd edn (Ader R, Felten D, Cohen N, eds). Academic Press, San Diego, 1991: 283–310.

125 Madden KS, Felten SY, Felten DL, Sundaresan PR, Livnat S. Sympathetic neural modulation of the immune system. I. Depression of T cell immunity *in vivo* and *in vitro* following chemical sympathectomy. *Brain Behav Immun* 1989; 3: 72–89.

126 Madden KS, Sanders VM, Felten DL. Cathecholamine influences and sympathetic neural modulation of immune responsiveness. *Annu Rev Pharmacol* 1995; 35: 417–48.

127 Maggi CA. Tachykinins and calcitonin gene-related peptide (CGRP) as co-transmitters released from peripheral endings of sensory nerves. *Prog Neurobiol* 1997; 45: 1–98.

128 Malec P, Zeman K, Markiewicz K, Tchorzewski H, Nowak Z, Baj Z. Short-term somatostatin infusion affects T lymphocyte responsiveness in humans. *Immunopharmacology* 1989; 17: 45–9.

129 Mannaioni PF, Moroni F, Fantozzi R, Masini E. Studies on the ^{14}C-histamine release induced by noradrenaline in mouse neoplastic mast cells. *Agents Actions* 1975; 5: 417–23.

130 Mantyh CR, Gates TS, Zimmerman RP *et al*. Receptor binding sites for SP but not substance K or neuromedin K are expressed in high concentrations by arterioles, venules and lymph nodules in surgical specimens obtained from patients with ulcerative colitis and Crohn disease. *Proc Natl Acad Sci USA* 1988; 85: 3235–9.

131 Mantyh PW, Mantyh CR, Gates T, Vigna SR, Maggio JE. Receptors binding sites for substance P and substance K in the canine gastrointestinal tract and their possible role in inflammatory bowel disease. *Neuroscience* 1988; 25: 817–37.

132 Manzini S, Maggi CA, Geppetti P, Bacciarelli C. Capsaicin desensitization protects from antigen induced bronchospasms in conscious guinea-pigs. *Eur J Pharmacol* 1987; 138: 307–8.

133 Martinez C, Delgado M, Gomariz RP, Ganea D. Vasoactive intestinal peptide and pituitary adenylate cyclase-activating polypeptide-38 inhibit IL-10 production in murine T lymphocytes. *J Immunol* 1996; 156: 4128–36.

134 Masini E, Fantozzi R, Blandina P, Brunelleschi S, Mannaioni PF. The riddle of cholinergic histamine release from mast cells. In: *Progress in Medicinal Chemistry* (Ellis GP, West GB, eds). Elsevier Science Publishers, Amsterdam; 1985; 22. 267–91.

135 Maslinski W, Grabczewska E, Laskowska-Bosek H, Ryzewski J. Expression of muscarinic cholinergic receptors during T cell maturation in the thymus. *Eur J Immunol* 1987; 17: 1059–63.

136 Matteson DR, Deutsch C. K channels in T lymphocytes: a patch-clamp study using monoclonal antibody adhesion. *Nature* 1984; 307: 468–71.

137 McCafferty D-M, Wallace JL, Sharkey KA. Effects of chemical sympathectomy and sensory nerve ablation on experimental colitis in the rat. *Am J Physiol* 1997; 272: G272–80.

138 McEwen BS, Biron CA, Brunson KW et al. The role of adrenocorticoids as modulators of immune function in health and disease: neural, endocrine and immune interactions. *Brain Res Rev* 1997; 23: 79–133.

139 McGillis JP, Humphreys S, Rangnekar V, Ciallella J. Modulation of B lymphocyte differentiation by calcitonin gene-related peptide (CGRP). *Cell Immunol* 1993; 150: 391–416.

140 McGillis JP, Humphreys S, Reid S. Characterization of functional calcitonin gene-related peptide receptors on rat lymphocytes. *J Immunol* 1991; 147: 3482–7.

141 McGillis JP, Park A, Rubin-Fletter P, Turck C, Dallman MF, Payan DG. Stimulation of rat B-lymphocyte proliferation by corticotropin-releasing factor. *J Neurosci Res* 1989; 26: 346–52.

142 McKay DM, Berin MC, Fondacaro JD, Perdue MH. Effects of neuropeptide Y and substance P on antigen-induced ion secretion in rat jejunum. *Am J Physiol* 1996; 271: G987–92.

143 McKay DM, Bienenstock J, Perdue MH. Inhibition of antigen-induced secretion in the rat jejunum by interferon α/β. *Reg Immunol* 1993; 5: 43–59.

144 McMillen MA, Ferrara A, Schaefer HC, Goldenring JR, Zucker KA, Modlin IM. Cholecystokinin mediates a calcium signal in human peripheral blood mononuclear cells and is a co-mitogen. *Ann NY Acad Sci* 1990; 594: 399–402.

145 McPherson GA, Summers RJ. Characteristics and localization of ^{3}H-clonidine binding in membranes prepared from guinea-pig spleen. *Clin Exp Pharmacol Physiol* 1982; 9: 77–87.

146 McQueen G, Marshall J, Perdue M, Siegel S, Bienenstock J. Pavlovian conditioning of rat mucosal mast cells to secrete rat mast cell protease II. *Science* 1989; 243: 83–5.

147 Metcalfe DD, Baram D, Mekori YA. Mast cells. *Physiol Rev* 1997; 77: 1033–81.

148 Michel MC, Beck-Sickinger A, Cox HM et al. XVI. IUPHAR recommendations for the nomenclature of neuropeptide Y, PYY and pancreatic polypeptide receptors. *Pharmacol Rev* 1998; 50: 143–50.

149 Miampamba M, Sharkey KA. Distribution of calcitonin gene-related peptide, somatostatin, substance P and vasoactive intestinal polypeptide in experimental colitis in rats. *Neurogastroenterol Mot* 1988; 10: 315–29.

150 Minault M, Lecron JC, Labrouche S, Simonnet G, Gombert J. Characterization of binding sites for neuropeptide FF on T lymphocytes of the Jurkat cell line. *Peptides* 1995; 16: 105–11.

151 Miura M, Inoue H, Ichinose M, Kimura K, Katsumata U, Takishima T. Nonadrenergic noncholinergic inhibitory nerve stimulation on the allergic reaction in cat airways. *Am Rev Respir Dis* 1990; 141: 29–32.

152 Miura S, Serzawa H, Tsuzuki Y et al. Vasoactive intestinal peptide modulates T lymphocyte migration in Peyer's patches of rat small intestine. *Am J Physiol* 1997; 272: G92–9.

153 Moore TC, Lami JL, Spuck SU. Substance P increases lymphocyte traffic and lymph flow through peripheral lymph nodes of sheep. *Immunology* 1989; 67: 109–114.

154 Motulsky HJ, Insel PA. Adrenergic receptors in man: direct identification, physiologic regulation, and clinical alterations. *N Engl J Med* 1982; 307: 18–29.

155 Musso NR, Brenci S, Setti M, Indiveri F, Lotti G. Catecholamine content and *in vitro* catecholamine synthesis in peripheral human lymphocytes. *J Clin Endocrinol Metabol* 1996; 81: 3553–7.

156 Nagy E, Berczi Y, Friesen HG. Regulation of immunity in rats by lactogenic and growth hormones. *Acta Endocrinol* 1983; 102: 351–7.

157 Nair MPN, Schwartz SA, Wu K, Kronfol Z. Effect of neuropeptide Y on natural killer activity of normal human lymphocytes. *Brain Behav Immun* 1993; 7: 70–8.

158 Nance DM, Hopkins DA, Bieger D. Re-investigation of the innervation of the thymus gland in mice and rats. *Brain Behav Immun* 1987; 1: 134–47.

159 Nilsson G, Ahlstedt S. Increased delayed-type hypersensitivity reaction in rats neuromanipulated with capsaicin. *Int Arch Allergy Appl Immunol* 1989; 90: 256–60.

160 Nilsson G, Alving K, Alstedt S, Hokfelt T, Lundberg JM. Peptidergic innervation of rat lymphoid tissue and lung: relation to mast cells and sensitivity to capsaicin and immunization. *Cell Tissue Res* 1990; 262: 125–33.

161 Nio DA, Moylan RN, Roche JK. Modulation of T lymphocyte function by neuropeptides. *J Immunol* 1993; 150: 5281–8.

162 Nohr D, Weihe E. The neuroimmune link in the bronchus-associated lymphoid tissue (BALT) of cat and rat: peptides and neural markers. *Brain Behav Immun* 1991; 5: 84–101.

163 Nong YH, Titus RG, Ribeiro JM, Remold HG. Peptides encoded by the calcitonin gene inhibit macrophage function. *J Immunol* 1989; 143: 45–9.

164 Novotny GEK. Ultrastructural analysis of lymph node innervation in the rat. *Acta Anat* 1988; 133: 57–61.

165 Ottaway CA. Selective effects of vasoactive intestinal peptide on the mitogenic response of murine T cells. *Immunology* 1987; 62: 291–7.

166 Ottaway CA. Vasoactive intestinal peptide and immune functions. In: *Psychoneuroimmunology*, 2nd edn. (Ader R, Felten D, Cohen N eds). Academic Press, San Diego, 1991: 225–62.

167 Ottaway CA, Greenberg GR. Interaction of vasoactive intestinal peptide with mouse lymphocytes: specific binding and the modulation of mitogenic responses. *J Immunol* 1984; 132: 417–23.

168 Ottaway CA, Husband AJ. Central nervous system influences on lymphocyte migration. *Brain Behav Immun* 1992; 6: 97–116.

169 Ottaway CA, Lewis DL, Asa SL. Vasoactive intestinal peptide-containing nerves in Peyer's patches. *Brain Behav Immun* 1987; 1: 148–58.

170 Otten U, Ehrhard P, Peck R. Nerve growth factor induces growth and differentiation of human B lymphocytes. *Proc Natl Acad Sci USA* 1989; 86: 10059–63.

171 Pascual DW, Beagley KW, Kiyono H, McGhee JR. Substance P promotes Peyer's patch and splenic B cell differentiation. *Adv Exp Med Biol* 1995; 371A: 55–9.

172 Pascual DW, Xu-Amano J, Kiyono H, McGhee JR, Bost KL. Substance P acts directly upon clone B lymphoma cells to enhance IgA and IgM production. *J Immunol* 1991; 146: 2130–6.

173 Payan DG, Hess CA, Goetzl EJ. Inhibition by somatostatin of the proliferation of T lymphocytes and Molt-4 lymphoblasts. *Cell Immunol* 1984; 84: 433–8.

174 Pernow B. Substance P. *Pharmacol Rev* 1983; 35: 85–140.

175 Petitto JM, Huang Z, McCarthy DB. Molecular cloning of NPY-Y1 receptor cDNA from rat splenic lymphocytes: evidence of low levels of mRNA expression and [125]NPY binding sites. *J Neuroimmunol* 1994; 54: 81–6.

176 Pieroni RE, Levine L. Further studies on the adjuvant principle of pertussis vaccine for the mouse. *Nature* 1967; 213: 1015–17.

177 Piotrowski W, Foreman JC. Some effects of CGRP in human skin and on histamine release. *Brit J Dermatol* 1986; 114: 37–46.

178 Plotnikoff NP, Miller GC. Enkephalins as immunomodulators. *Int J Immunopharmacol* 1983; 5: 437–41.

179 Pochet R, Delespesse G, Gausset PW, Collet H. Distribution of β-adrenergic receptors on human lymphocyte subpopulations. *Clin Exp Immunol* 1979; 38: 578–84.

180 Popper P, Mantyh CR, Vigna SR, Maggio JE, Mantyh PW. The localization of sensory nerve fibers and receptor binding sites for sensory neuropeptides in canine mesenteric lymph nodes. *Peptides* 1988; 9: 257–67.

181 Pruett SB, Han Y, Munson AE, Fuchs BA. Assessment of cholinergic influences on a primary humoral immune response. *Immunology* 1992; 77: 428–35.

182 Psychosocial factors, stress, disease and immunity. In: *Psychoneuroimmunology*, 2nd edn. (Ader R, Felten DL, Cohen N eds). Academic Press; San Diego, 1991: 847–1106.

183 Reubi JC, Horisberger U, Waser B, Gebbers JO, Laissue J. Preferential location of somatostatin receptors in germinal centers of human gut lymphoid tissue. *Gastroenterology* 1992; 103: 1207–14.

184 Richmann DP, Antel JP, Burns JB, Arnason BGW. Nicotinic acetylcholine receptor on human lymphocytes. *Ann NY Acad Sci* 1981; 377: 427–35.

185 Richman DP, Arnason BGW. Nicotinic acetylcholine receptor: evidence for a functional distinct receptor on human lymphocytes. *Proc Natl Acad Sci USA* 1979; 76: 4632–5.

186 Rinner I, Felsner P, Falus A *et al*. Cholinergic signals to and from the immune system. *Immunol Lett* 1995; 217–20.

187 Rinner I, Schauenstein K. Detection of choline-acetyltransferase activity in lymphocytes. *J Neurosci Res* 1993; 35: 188–91.

188 Rinner I, Schauenstein K. The parasympathetic nervous system takes part in the immuno-neuroendocrine dialogue. *J Neuroimmunol* 1991; 34: 165–72.

189 Rola-Pleszczynski M, Bolduc D, St-Pierre S. The effects of vasoactive intestinal peptide on human natural killer cells and mast cells. *J Immunol* 1985; 135: 2569–77.

190 Romano TA, Felten SY, Felten DL, Olschowska JA. Neuropeptide-Y innervation of the rat spleen: another potential immunomodulatory neuropeptide. *Brain Behav Immun* 1991; 5: 116–31.

191 Sandberg G. Leukocyte mobilization from the guinea pig spleen by muscarinic cholinergic stimulation. *Experientia* 1994; 15: 40–3.

192 Sanders VM, Munson AE. β-Adrenoceptor mediation of the enhancing effect of norepinephrine on the murine primary antibody response *in vitro*. *J Pharmacol Exp Ther* 1984; 230: 183–92.

193 Sanders VM, Munson AE. Norepinephrine and the antibody response. *Pharmacol Rev* 1985; 37: 229–48.

194 Santos J, Saperas E, Mourelle M, Antolin M, Malagelada JR. Regulation of intestinal mast cells and luminal protein release by cerebral thyrotropin-releasing hormone in rats. *Gastroenterology* 1996; 111: 1465–73.

195 Santos J, Saperas E, Nogueiras C *et al*. Release of mast cell mediators into the jejunum by cold pain stress in humans. *Gastroenterology* 1998; 114: 640–8.

196 Singh VK. Stimulatory effects of corticotropin-releasing neurohormone on human lymphocyte proliferation and interleukin-2 receptor expression. *J Neuroimmunol* 1989; 23: 257–62.

197 Singh VH, Fudenberg HH. Binding of [^{125}I]corticotropin releasing factor to blood immunocytes and its reduction in Alzheimer's disease. *Immunol Lett* 1988; 18: 5–8.

198 Singh VK, Leu SJ. Enhancing effect of corticotropin-releasing neurohormone on the production of interleukin-1 and interleukin-2. *Neurosci Lett* 1990; 120: 151–4.

199 Sirinek LP, O'Dorisio MS. Modulation of immune function by intestinal neuropeptides. *Acta Oncol* 1991; 30: 509–17.

200 Schreiner GF, Unanue ER. The modulation of spontaneous and anti-Ig-stimulated motility of lymphocytes by cyclic nucleotides and adrenergic and cholinergic agents. *J Immunol* 1975; 114: 802–8.

201 Schwartz H, Villiger PM, Von Kempis J, Lotz M. Neuropeptide Y is an inducible gene in the human immune system. *J Neuroimmunol* 1994; 51: 53–61.

202 Scicchitano R, Bienenstock J, Stanisz AM. *In vivo* immunomodulation by the neuropeptide substance P. *Immunology* 1988; 63: 733–5.

203 Scicchitano R, Bienenstock J, Stanisz AM. The differential effect with time of neuropeptides on the proliferative responses of murine Peyer's patch and splenic lymphocytes. *Brain Behav Immun* 1987; 1: 231–7.

204 Scicchitano R, Dazin P, Bienenstock J, Payan DG, Stanisz AM. Distribution of somatostatin receptors on murine spleen and Peyer's patch T and B lymphocytes. *Brain Behav Immun* 1987; 1: 173–84.

205 Scicchitano R, Dazin P, Bienenstock J, Payan DG, Stanisz AM. The murine IgA-secreting plasmacytoma MOPC-315 expresses somatostatin receptors. *J Immunol* 1988; 141: 937–41.

206 Shahahi NA, Linner KM, Sharp BM. Murine splenocytes express a naloxone-insensitive binding site for β-endorphin. *Endocrinology* 1990; 126: 3006–15.

207 Shanahan F, Denburg JA, Fox J, Bienenstock J, Befus AD. Mast cell heterogeneity. Effects of neuroenteric peptides on histamine release. *J Immunol* 1985; 135: 1331–7.

208 Stanisz AM. Neuronal factors modulating immunity. *Neuroimmunomodulation* 1994; 1: 217–30.

209 Stanisz AM, Befus D, Bienenstock J. Differential effects of vasoactive intestinal peptide on proliferation by lymphocytes from Peyer's patches, mesenteric lymph nodes and spleen. *J Immunol* 1986; 136: 152–6.

210 Stanisz AM, Scicchitano R. Neuroimmune interactions in the gastrointestinal mucosa. *Reg Immunol* 1994; 6: 378–81.

211 Stanisz AM, Scicchitano R, Dazin P, Bienenstock J, Payan DG. Distribution of substance P receptors on murine spleen and Peyer's patch T and B cells. *J Immunol* 1987; 139: 749–54.

212 Stead RH, Kosecka-Janiszewska U, Oestreicher AB, Dixon MF, Bienenstock J. Remodeling of B-50 (GAP-43)- and NSE-immunoreactive mucosal nerves in the intestines of rats infected with *Nippostrongylus brasiliensis*. *J Neurosci* 1991; 11: 3809–21.

213 Stead RH, Tomioka M, Quinonez G, Simon GT, Felten SY, Bienenstock J. Intestinal mucosal mast cells in normal and nematode-infected rat intestines are in intimate contact with peptidergic nerves. *Proc Natl Acad Sci USA* 1987; 84: 2975–9.

214 Straub RH, Lang B, Falk W, Schölmerich J, Singer EA. *In vitro* superperfusion method for the investigation of nerve–immune cell interaction in murine spleen. *J Neuroimmunol* 1995; 61: 53–60.

215 Strom TB, Deisseroth A, Morganroth J, Carpenter CB, Merrill JP. Alteration of cytotoxic action of sensitized lymphocytes by cholinergic agents and activators of adenylate cyclase. *Proc Natl Acad Sci USA* 1972; 69: 2995–9.

216 Szelenyi J, Paldi-Haris P, Hollan S. Changes in the cholinergic system of lymphocytes due to mitogenic stimulation. *Immunol Lett* 1987; 16: 49–54.

217 Tatsuno I, Gottschall PE, Arimura A. Inhibition of mitogen-stimulated proliferation of murine splenocytes by a novel neuropeptide, pituitary adenylate cyclase-activating polypeptide: a comparative study with vasoactive intestinal peptide. *Endocrinology* 1991; 128: 728–34.

218 Theoharides TC, Singh LK, Boucher W *et al*. Corticotropin-releasing hormone induces skin mast cell degranulation and increased vascular permeability, a possible explanation for its proinflammatory effects. *Endocrinology* 1998; 139: 403–13.

219 Thorpe LW, Perez Polo JR. The influence of nerve growth factor on the *in vitro* proliferation response of rat spleen lymphocytes. *J Neurosci Res* 1987; 18: 134–9.

220 Thorpe LW, Werbach-Perez K, Perez Polo JR. Effect of nerve growth factor on the expression of interleukin-2 receptors on cultured human lymphocytes. *Ann NY Acad Sci* 1987; 496: 310–11.

221 Titinchi S, Clark B. Alpha$_2$-adrenoceptors in human lymphocytes: direct characterisation by [^{3}H]yohimbine binding. *Biochem Biophys Res Commun* 1984; 121: 1–7.

222 Tria MA, Vantini G, Fiori MG, Rossi A. Choline acetyltransferase activity in murine thymus. *J Neurosci Res* 1992; 31: 380–6.

223 Turnbull AV, Rivier C. Corticotropin-releasing factor (CRF) and endocrine responses to stress: CRF receptors, binding protein, and related peptides. *Proc Soc Exp Biol Med* 1997; 215: 1–10.

224 Udelsman R, Harwood JP, Millan MA *et al*. Functional corticotropin-releasing factor receptors in the primate peripheral nervous system. *Nature (London)* 1986; 319: 146–50.

225 Ueyama T, Kozuki K, Houtani T *et al*. Immunolocalization of tyrosine hydroxylase and vasoactive intestinal polypeptide in nerve fibers innervating human palatine tonsil and paratonsillar glands. *Neurosci Lett* 1990; 116: 70–4.

226 Umeda Y, Takamiya M, Yoshikazi H, Arisawa M. Inhibition of mitogen stimulated T lymphocyte proliferation by calcitonin gene-related peptide. *Biochem Biophys Res Commun* 1988; 154: 227–35.

227 van der Bergh P, Rozing J, Nagelkerken L. Two opposing modes of action of β-endorphin on lymphocyte function. *Immunology* 1991; 72: 537–43.

228 Vizi ES, Orsó E, Osipenko ON, Haskó G, Elenkov IJ. Neurochemical, electrophysiological and immunocytochemical evidence for a noradrenergic link between the sympathetic nervous system and thymocytes. *Neuroscience* 1995; 68: 1263–76.

229 Vriend CY, Wan W, Greenberg AH, Nance DM. Cutting the splenic nerve differentially affects catecholamine and neuropeptide levels in the spleen. *Soc Neurosci* 1993 (Abstract); 388: 5.

230 Wang F, Millet I, Bottomly K, Vignery A. Calcitonin gene-related peptide inhibits interleukin 2 production by murine T lymphocytes. *J Biol Chem* 1992; 267: 21052–7.

231 Weigent DA, Blalock JE. Interactions between the neuroendocrine and immune systems: common hormones and receptors. *Immunol Rev* 1987; 100: 79–108.

232 Weihe E, Krekel J. The neuroimmune connection in human tonsils. *Brain Behav Immun* 1991; 5: 41–54.

233 Weihe E, Muller S, Fink T, Zentel HJ. Tachykinins, calcitonin gene-related peptide and neuropeptide Y in nerves of the mammalian thymus: interactions with mast cells in autonomic and sensory immunomodulation? *Neurosci Lett* 1989; 100: 77–82.

234 Weinreich D, Unolem BJ, Leal-Caroloso JM. Functional effects of mast cell activation in sympathetic ganglia. *Ann NY Acad Sci* 1992; 664: 293–308.

235 Wilder RL. Neuroendocrine–immune system interactions and autoimmunity. *Annu Rev Immunol* 1995; 13: 307–38.

236 Williams JM, Peterson RG, Shea PA, Schmedtje JF, Bauer DC, Felten DL. Sympathetic innervation of murine thymus and spleen: evidence for a functional link between the nervous and the immune systems. *Brain Res Bull* 1981; 6: 83–94.

237 Wimalawansa SJ. Calcitonin gene-related peptide and its receptors: molecular genetics, physiology, pathophysiology, and therapeutic potentials. *Endoc Rev* 1996; 17: 533–85.

238 Yamashita T, Kozuki K, Kubo N, Kumazawa H, Otani K, Kumazawa T. Participation of autonomic nerve in tonsillar focal infection. *Acta OtoLaryngol* 1988; 454 (Suppl): 237–40.

239 Yamashita T, Kumazawa H, Kozuki K, Amano H, Tomoda K, Kumazawa T. Autonomic nervous system in human palatine tonsil. *Acta OtoLaryngol* 1984; Suppl 416: 63–71.

240 Ye S, Applegreen RR, Davis JM, Cheung HJ. Modulation of lymphocyte motility by β-endorphin and met-enkephalin. *Immunopharmacology* 1989; 17: 81–9.

241. Yi Q, Ahlberg R, Pirskanen R, Lefvert AK. Acetylcholine receptor-reactive T cells in myasthenia gravis: evidence for the involvement of different subpopulation of T helper cells. *Neuroimmunol* 1994; 50: 177–86.

Chapter 5

Macrophages

Dale E. Bockman

INTRODUCTION

Macrophages are a dominant cell type in the lamina propria of the gastrointestinal tract. They are present in the submucosa, and in solitary lymphoid follicles, Peyer's patches and the appendix. They are found in smaller numbers within the epithelium, muscle and serosa.

The functions of macrophages in the gastrointestinal tract may be generalized or specific. As examples of general activity, particulate material which has penetrated the epithelial barrier, or effete lymphocytes in the lamina propria and epithelium, are phagocytized. On the other hand, macrophages may be mediators and regulators of quite specific immune reactivity. They do not exist and function alone, but release substances which affect other cells involved in the immune response and react to other cells and their products. These interactions modulate the environment, including the extracellular matrix, and affect circulation and coagulation. Generalized and specific activity usually occur simultaneously *in vivo*.

A complete understanding of normal and pathological responses to antigens, including food antigens, must encompass the functions which are performed by macrophages. This chapter begins with a consideration of some general characteristics of macrophages, and then proceeds to macrophages in the gastrointestinal tract proper, including those in lymphoepithelial tissue, which is important for the handling of gut antigens.

The approach to the functions of macrophages must include consideration of the interaction and functions of other cells, such as dendritic cells, lymphocytes, neutrophils, eosinophils and epithelial cells. Also, macrophages associated with the mammary glands will be discussed because of the association of colostrum and milk with gastrointestinal immune function in infants.

Finally, some discussion of macrophage involvement in selected diseases and disorders of the gastrointestinal tract will be undertaken for the purpose of trying to establish some generalizations which might be helpful when applied to the problems of food intolerance and allergy.

CHARACTERISTICS OF MACROPHAGES

Morphology

Macrophages are large mononuclear cells. In routine histological sections, a large, slightly irregular nucleus is surrounded by abundant, pinkish, granular cytoplasm which may have numerous vacuoles or inclusions. Many dense granules are evident in the cytoplasm upon examination by phase contrast microscopy. Transmission electron microscopy clearly shows a heterogeneous population of granules dispersed among cytoplasmic membranes and mitochondria, and frequently among phagocytic vacuoles and phagolysosomes. These granules are lysosomes, and a lysosomal enzyme marker, acid phosphatase, usually may be detected in macrophages by biochemical or cytochemical techniques. Other common characteristics of macrophages are positive reactions for nonspecific esterase and ATPase.[58,88] Numerous surface antigens, some limited to macrophages and some shared by other cells, are amenable to detection. Active macrophages have a characteristic appearance when viewed by scanning electron microscopy (Fig. 5.1), due to elaborate folding or ruffling of the cell membrane, and sometimes by extension of filamentous protrusions. Isolated macrophages adhere to glass or plastic surfaces, and are capable of considerable phagocytic activity.

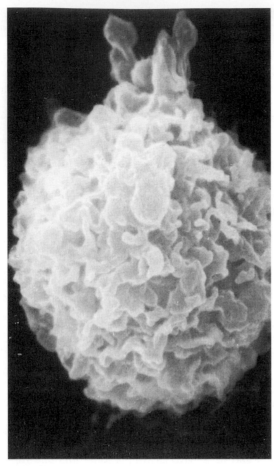

Fig. 5.1 Scanning electron micrograph of a macrophage from the peritoneal cavity of a rat. The surface membrane is highly convoluted or ruffled. × 8000. (Reproduced from Ref. 11, with permission of the *Journal of the Reticuloendothelial Society.*)

Some pertinent factors regulating macrophage activity	
Endotoxin/lipopolysaccharide (LPS)	Interferon γ (IFNγ)
Prostaglandin E$_2$ (PGE$_2$)	Interleukin 2 (IL2)
Macrophage colony-stimulating factor (M-CSF)	Interleukin 4 (IL4)
Granulocyte–macrophage colony-stimulating factor (GM-CSF)	Interleukin 10 (IL10)
Leukotrienes	Tumour necrosis factor (TNF)

Table 5.1 Some pertinent factors regulating macrophage activity.

changes. The resulting activated macrophages express more microbicidal activity than non-stimulated macrophages.

Activation implies that macrophages are responding to stimuli by developing characteristics not necessarily expressed constitutively. It is accomplished through modulation of the pattern of gene expression, and may take a number of pathways.[40] Macrophages are activated efficiently in response to interferon γ (IFNγ) acting in cooperation with lipopolysaccharide (LPS, endotoxin). Stimulation of macrophage activity may be accomplished by cytokines and colony stimulating factors. Other factors, such as prostaglandin E$_2$ (PGE$_2$), suppress the process by which activation is achieved. Some of the substances that are active in regulating macrophage activity are listed in Table 5.1.

Phagocytosis
The process of phagocytosis consists of two separable steps: attachment to the cell membrane and internalization. These processes are illustrated in Fig 5.2 and 5.3. During phagocytosis, potent oxidizing agents such as superoxide, hydrogen peroxide and hydroxyl radical, which may be effective in killing internalized organisms and breaking down ingested and surrounding material, are released.[68]

The end stage of breakdown finds most of the material degraded to nonantigenic fragments through the action of the hydrolytic enzymes of lysosomes, but some antigen remains undegraded. Some of this may be released into the environment and some may be found on the surface membrane of the macrophages. For continued reactivity to the antigen, there is an essential interaction between macrophages and T lymphocytes. In this interaction macrophages are said to be carrying out accessory cell function.

MACROPHAGE ACTIVITY AND REGULATION

Antigen presentation
Some of the peptides in the endosomes within macrophages that have engulfed and processed an antigen bind to Class II major histocompatibility complexes (Class II MHCs) on the endosomal membrane. The complexes of peptide antigens and Class II MHCs are exteriorized when the endosomes fuse with the surface membrane. The antigens are thus 'presented' on the surface of the macrophage. T cell receptors on helper T lymphocytes recognize the antigen when presented with the Class II MHC protein. If the antigen is presented along with another signal from the

Heterogeneity among macrophages is produced because they have a large number of characteristics which are acquired or lost with time, in response to multiple stimuli present in the local microenvironment, during differentiation of their cell line. Macrophages are not normally replenished by cell division *in situ*, but through the differentiation of cells which arise elsewhere and are transported to the site of activity. Monocytes are produced from more primitive cells in the bone marrow, enter the bloodstream for transport and differentiate into macrophages in the connective tissues.[20,22,93] Under appropriate stimulation, macrophages differentiate further into epithelioid cells and giant cells.

Activation
Macrophages acquire heightened activity and distinct morphological and functional characteristics when 'activated'. Macrophages harvested from animals combating infection or stimulated by the proper agents display an increased capacity for phagocytosis, ruffling of the surface membrane, increased adherence and spreading on a glass or plastic surface, increased numbers of phagolysosomes and endocytic vesicles, altered metabolism and increased secretions.[21,49,68,69] Living or dead microbes, endotoxin, foreign serum proteins, immune complexes and lymphokines are among the agents capable of initiating these kinds of

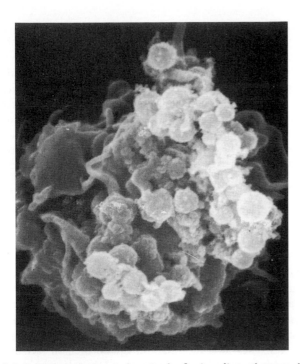

Fig. 5.2 Scanning electron micrograph of rat peritoneal macrophage after ferritin-coated zymogen granules have been added to the culture medium and become attached to the cell membrane. × 7000. (Reproduced from Ref. 11, with permission of the *Journal of the Reticuloendothelial Society*.)

macrophage, either interleukin 1 (IL1) or membrane-bound B7 protein, the helper T cell is stimulated to produce a number of signalling molecules that can activate lymphocytes and macrophages.

Secretion

Many interactions between macrophages and lymphocytes, and between macrophages and other elements in the environment, are mediated through secretory products. There are well over 50 secretory products of mononuclear phagocytes.[68] Some of the pertinent factors secreted by macrophages are listed in Table 5.2. Macrophages secrete both lymphocyte activating factors and factors inhibiting replication of lymphocytes. Products of lymphocytes may stimulate macrophages to secrete such diverse products as lysosomal enzymes, interferon, collagenase and plasminogen activator.[92] Macrophage secretory products may promote

Some pertinent factors secreted by macrophages	
Tumour necrosis factor α (TNFα)	Collagenase
Transforming growth factor β (TGFβ)	Elastase
Interleukin 1 (IL1)	Plasminogen activator
Interleukin 6 (IL6)	Lysozyme
Interleukin 8 (IL8)	Lysosomal enzymes
Interleukin 10 (IL10)	α_2-Macroglobulin
Interleukin 12 (IL12)	α_1-Antitrypsin inhibitor
Prostaglandins	Nitric oxide (NO)
Tissue inhibitors of metalloproteinases (TIMPs)	

Table 5.2 Some pertinent factors secreted by macrophages.

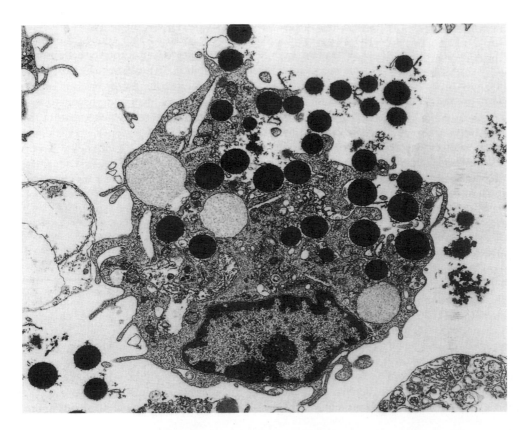

Fig. 5.3 Transmission electron micrograph of a macrophage which has been incubated with ferritin-coated zymogen granules. Both surface adherence and internalization are obvious. ×9000. (Reproduced from Ref. 11, with permission of the *Journal of the Reticuloendothelial Society*.)

replication of myeloid and erythroid precursors, fibroblasts and endothelial cells. Secreted prostaglandins may affect circulation. Macrophages secrete lysozyme, which causes bacterial breakdown; interferon, which inhibits viral replication; many complement factors; and α_1-antitrypsin inhibitor. The endogenous pyrogen which they secrete produces fever and causes granulocytes to release lactoferrin.

Regulation of macrophage activity
Signalling molecules and interaction

Macrophages signal other cells (e.g. lymphocytes and other macrophages) and themselves through the elaboration and release of molecules, many of which react with cell surface receptors on the responding cells.[67] In response to IFNγ from lymphocytes, the macrophage is activated to increase the quantity of nitric oxide synthase so that nitric oxide is produced and released. Interleukin 1 (IL1) from activated macrophages stimulates lymphocytes to release IL2, IL4, macrophage colony-stimulating factor (M-CSF) and granulocyte–macrophage colony-stimulating factor (GM-CSF), which, in turn, stimulate macrophages. Interferon β (IFNβ) from lymphocytes induces increased Class II MHCs in the macrophage membrane, enhancing the potential for immune reactivity. Tumour necrosis factor α (TNFα), released from macrophages in response to lipopolysaccharide (LPS, endotoxin), can lead to septic shock. TNFα also acts in autocrine and paracrine fashion to elicit the synthesis and release of IL1, IL6, IL8, IL10 and IL12 from macrophages.

Some products of macrophages have inhibitory effects on the immune system.[67] Prostaglandin E_2 (PGE$_2$), secreted by macrophages, nevertheless inhibits activation of macrophages. Transforming growth factor β (TGFβ) inhibits T and B cell proliferation and macrophage cytokine synthesis.

Extracellular matrix

TGFβ enhances the proliferation of fibroblasts and deposition of extracellular matrix components, and initiates angiogenesis.[67] On the other hand, macrophages secrete matrix metalloproteinases that break down the extracellular matrix. Collagenase and elastase lyse their connective tissue substrates. Remarkably, macrophages also secrete α_2-macroglobulin, which inhibits collagenase and elastase.

The cell membrane

The surface membranes of macrophages present a heterogeneous array of substances which contribute to their functional characteristics and provide markers for their presence and activity. A large number of membrane components of macrophages may be grouped under the general designation of surface antigens. Class II MHCs have been discussed already. Surface antigens may be identified by the use of specific antibodies, frequently monoclonal antibodies. Macrophages are identified immunohistochemically by the presence of the membrane protein CD68.[64] Subpopulations of mononuclear phagocytes may be identified through the profiles of surface antigens present, sometimes in combination with other characteristics. Some antigens reflect the differentiative steps achieved by mononuclear phagocyte cell lines, and marked heterogeneity among these cells is evident.[4,33] Plasma membrane ectoenzymes, such as 5′-nucleotidase usually decrease markedly with activation.[21] Laminin and fibronectin are detectable on the surface of macrophages, and may be important in cell–cell and cell–matrix adhesive properties.[45,97]

Receptors for the Fc portion of immunoglobulins (Igs), including receptors for IgG, IgE and IgA,[13] the C3b fragment of complement and lactoferrin, are on the macrophage membrane.[68,76,94] The binding of lactoferrin to the membrane may modulate macrophage secretion and thus play a role in immune regulation.[68] Binding of IgG through its Fc receptor is important in phagocytosis of particles coated with IgG (opsonization). Complement binding may augment opsonization is some cases.

Receptors for IgE[16,42] on macrophages may assist adhesion and killing of parasites. IgE–antiIgE complexes stimulate IL1 secretion by monocytes cultured in GM-CSF.[61]

Inflammatory cells

Macrophages attract and interact with inflammatory cells. Eosinophils and neutrophils (polymorphonuclear leukocytes) are normally found in gut mucosa. They are most prominent in the lamina propria, but occasionally may be found within the epithelium under normal conditions.[23,86] The number and apparent activity of these granulocytes increases dramatically with inflammation.

Under the appropriate conditions both types of granulocytes phagocytize material. Eosinophils phagocytize antigen–antibody complexes. They have receptors for IgE on their surface and can phagocytize, for instance, microfilariae of *Dipetalonema*, mediated by IgE antibodies, degranulating on the ingested material.[42] This does not, however, kill the microfilariae, whereas macrophages kill and degrade them after phagocytosis mediated by the same antibody.

The surface receptors for immunoglobulins on neutrophils are somewhat similar to those on macrophages, in that receptors for IgA and IgG, but not IgM, are present.[32,38] IgG may opsonize for phagocytosis by neutrophils from peripheral blood. Coating erythrocytes with IgA causes binding to peripheral blood neutrophils, but not internalization. IgA can augment the phagocytosis mediated by IgG. Furthermore, neutrophils from the oral cavity carry out phagocytosis mediated by IgA alone, indicating the possibility that environmental effects (such as high concentrations of IgA) may increase the number of IgA receptors on the cell surface, thus modulating reactive capability.[32] This raises the possibility that neutrophils in the IgA-rich environment of the gut lamina propria might be able to carry out IgA-mediated phagocytosis.

Drainage from the gastrointestinal tract via blood leads to the liver. Lymph drains to mesenteric lymph nodes. Particulate and soluble material, free in the fluid or associated with cells, may be intercepted in these locations. Kupffer cells dispersed along the sinusoids of the liver are highly phagocytic and form an important part of the system of mononuclear phagocytes. Mesenteric lymph nodes also contain a plethora of phagocytes and, in addition, may serve as a location for a stage in maturation of lymphocytes which have been stimulated in the gastrointestinal tract.

MACROPHAGES IN THE LAMINA PROPRIA

Macrophages are quite conspicuous in the extensive cellular collection in the lamina propria.[29,86] The macrophages collect mainly in the upper 100–150 μm of the mucosa so that they, along with fibroblasts, are prominent in the subepithelial region, and thus are quite evident between crypts and in villi in the small intestine, and immediately beneath the lining epithelium in the colon.[23,29,78] Collan[23] has shown that macrophages immediately beneath the epithelium may insert long pseudopodia through the basal lamina

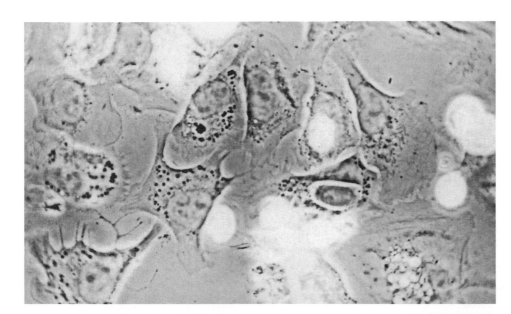

Fig. 5.4 Human intestinal macrophages after 24 hours in culture. The cytoplasm contains many phase-dense granules, and cellular extensions are prominent. × 400. (Reproduced from Ref. 98, with permission of *Gastroenterology*.)

into the epithelial layer proper and there make contact with intraepithelial lymphocytes. Macrophages occasionally are found within the epithelial layer.[86] Other cell types which are common in the lamina propria include plasma cells, lymphocytes, mast cells, neutrophils and eosinophils. Close associations and contacts between macrophages and some of these cells have been demonstrated by electron microscopic study, showing the possibility of interactions which may depend on cell–cell contacts.[23,27]

Macrophages in the lamina propria have a heterogeneous morphology, dependent upon their developmental and functional history. Some may be similar to monocytes, others may display the features of mature phagocytes. Cytoplasmic granules (Fig. 5.4) and vacuoles are prominent when observed by phase microscopy[37,98] and by electron microscopy.[27,91] Dead cells and degenerating cell fragments commonly are seen in phagolysosomes, indicating that *in situ* phagocytosis and breakdown of lymphocytes and other cells is a normal function of gut-associated macrophages.[23,78] It is presumed that most of the cells to be phagocytized undergo apoptosis.

Phagocytosis and pinocytosis of foreign material may be demonstrated as well. Ferritin, a large protein molecule with micelles of iron, administered by either subcutaneous or intraperitoneal injection, is taken up and concentrated within macrophages in intestinal villi and surrounding intestinal crypts (Figs. 5.5 and 5.6). Bovine serum albumin may be demonstrated in lamina propria macrophages after 2 days of feeding this substance.[2]

Lamina propria macrophages have been isolated and characterized. Golder & Doe[37] characterized macrophages from human colon after EDTA (ethylenediaminetetraacetic acid) and enzyme dispersal, collection by Percoll density gradients, then adherence to plastic. Winter *et al.*[98] prepared their cells by adherence to cover slips coated with fibronectin. The cells thus isolated were capable of phagocytosis mediated by Fc receptors, had receptors for complement, were positive for Class II MHC antigens and nonspecific esterase, were negative for peroxidase, synthesized complement and secreted lysozyme. Thus they had many of the basic characteristics described previously for macrophages derived from other sites.

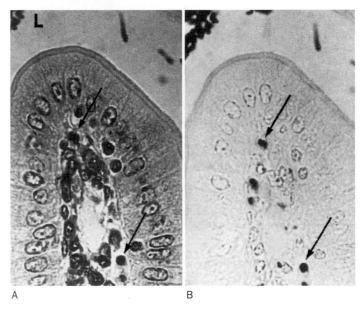

Fig. 5.5 Intestinal villus from hamster after previous intraperitoneal injections of ferritin. Paraffin section is treated with Prussian blue reagents to reveal the iron moiety of ferritin. The arrows point to macrophages containing ferritin. A, photographed with regular light; B, photographed with red filter to emphasize the location of blue reaction product. × 760. (Reproduced from Ref. 10, with permission of the *Anatomical Record*).

Macrophages in the lamina propria are demonstrably responsive to luminal contents. Takeuchi *et al.*[86] studied the response of the intestinal mucosa in guinea pigs made susceptible to infection with *Shigella flexneri* by starvation. Macrophages increased in size and number, became quite active phagocytically and, along with other inflammatory cells, breached the epithelium. Donnellan[29] studied colonic mucosa from patients during chronic colonic obstruction. Although there was absence of apparent bacterial invasion, macrophages were markedly increased. Lamina propria macrophages must be considered as constantly interacting with material from the lumen of the gastrointestinal tract.

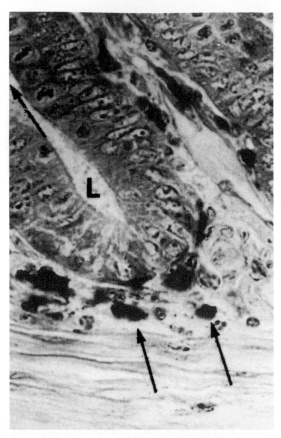

Fig. 5.6 Intestinal crypt region after intraperitoneal injections of ferritin, and localization of ferritin with the Prussian blue reaction. Arrows indicate ferritin-laden macrophages. × 475. (Reproduced from Ref. 10, with permission of the *Anatomical Record*.)

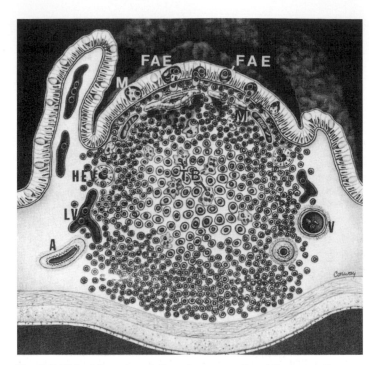

Fig. 5.7 Pictorial representation of some pertinent features of Peyer's patch. Tingible body macrophages (TB) are prominent in the germinal centre. Macrophages (M) are located within and beneath the epithelium; some are associated closely with follicle-associated epithelial (FAE) cells. A, artery; V, vein; LV, lymphatic vessel; HEV, high endothelial venule. (Reproduced from Ref. 6, with permission from Pergamon Press.)

LYMPHOEPITHELIAL TISSUE

The unit of organization of gut-associated lymphoepithelial tissue is the lymphoid follicle. Lymphoid follicles occur singly along the gastrointestinal tract (solitary follicles or nodules) and, in addition, are grouped together in large numbers up to the highly organized arrays present in Peyer's patches and the appendix. Solitary follicles take up and respond to luminal contents, and are similar morphologically to the follicular units in more complex lymphoepithelial tissue.[46,51]

Distribution of macrophages and dendritic cells

Macrophages are prominent in lymphoepithelial tissue.[19,25,31,41,56,57,80,83] They are found throughout each follicle. Within the germinal centre, numerous so-called tingible body macrophages commonly are concentrated (Fig. 5.7). These are macrophages with many engulfed cells, mostly lymphocytes in various stages of breakdown, in their cytoplasm. The disintegrating cellular products stain densely. Other macrophages are found closer to the periphery of the follicle. There is a concentration of macrophages in the subepithelial region of each follicle (Fig. 5.8), and some may be found within the epithelial layer proper.[1,6,8,25,71,95]

Dendritic cells also are prominent in lymphoepithelial tissue. They, like macrophages, are derived from cells that originate in the bone marrow. They, like macrophages, are 'professional' antigen presenters. Dendritic cells are more efficient at antigen

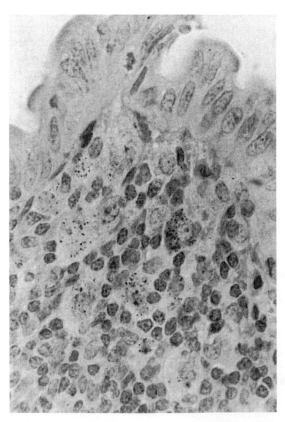

Fig. 5.8 Light micrograph of mouse Peyer's patch after ingestion of Fe$_2$O$_3$. The small dense particles are localized within macrophages in the dome area. (Provided through the courtesy of Drs ME LeFevre and DD Joel.)

presentation than macrophages, and macrophages are more efficient at phagocytosis. Dendritic cells are distributed differently from macrophages in lymphoepithelial collections. Distinct populations of dendritic cells are present in the subepithelial dome and T cell regions of Peyer's patches in mice, indicating a likely role in presenting antigens brought into the lymphoid tissue through overlying M cells.[50]

Uptake of soluble and particulate material

The macrophages in lymphoepithelial tissue obviously are responsive to the contents of the intestinal lumen. There are fewer macrophages in lymphoepithelial tissue of germ-free animals as compared with conventional animals.[89] Particulate material can be transmitted through enterocytes to the lamina propria,[10,60] although M cells accomplish this much more efficiently. When luminal contents are transmitted through the specialized M cells in the dome epithelium over each follicle[9,12,72] or the epithelial barrier is breached, they likely will be processed by macrophages and dendritic cells. Naturally occurring bacteria in the lumen of the rabbit appendix penetrate the epithelium to be taken up by intraepithelial macrophages (Fig. 5.9) or by subepithelial macrophages.[7,12,80]

Macrophage activity in lymphoepithelial tissue has been demonstrated clearly by histological examination at various times after gavage or long-term feeding (in drinking water) of carbon particles.[41,46] The carbon was taken up to a much greater extent in lymphoid follicles (solitary follicles and follicles in Peyer's patches) than in the remaining intestine (Figs 5.10 and 5.11). Subepithelial macrophages with engulfed carbon particles were identified on the second day of gavage. After chronic ingestion for 2 months, concentrations of carbon were heaviest in the sub-epithelial region and toward the periphery of the serosal pole of each follicle, but carbon-containing macrophages were present throughout the follicle. Many tingible body macrophages had

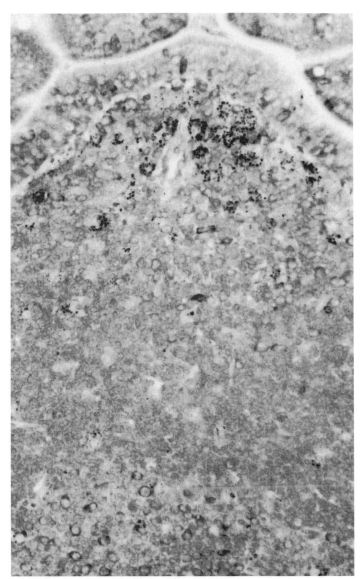

Fig. 5.10 Peyer's patch follicle from mouse after ingestion of carbon particles. The dense particles are concentrated in macrophages in the dome. Compare with particles in Fig. 5.12. (Provided through the courtesy of Drs ME LeFevre and DD Joel.)

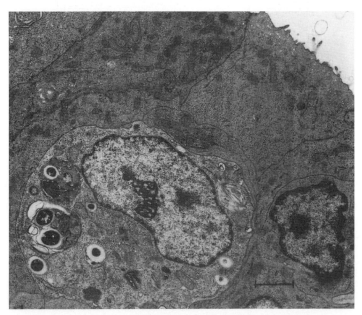

Fig. 5.9 Electron micrograph of an intraepithelial macrophage in rabbit appendix. Phagocytized bacteria are evident in the cytoplasm. × 3700. (Reproduced from Ref. 8, with permission from *Scanning Electron Microscopy*.)

carbon particles in the cytoplasm in addition to the degenerating cells. Carbon particle-laden macrophages were identified in mesenteric lymph nodes (Fig. 5.12). After cessation of carbon feeding, clearance of carbon from the subepithelial zone took over 2 months. Carbon particles could be identified in the dome epithelium 40 days after termination of carbon exposure. It is possible that this carbon was in intraepithelial macrophages, but the histological technique did not allow this to be verified or denied.

Uptake of organisms

Uptake of organic material by Peyer's patch macrophages has been demonstrated in several studies. Kimura[52] studied rabbit Peyer's patches after intravenous immunization with a bacterial antigen and subsequent oral administration of killed bacteria. The number of intraepithelial macrophages increased, and phagocytized bacteria could be found in the intra- and subepithelial

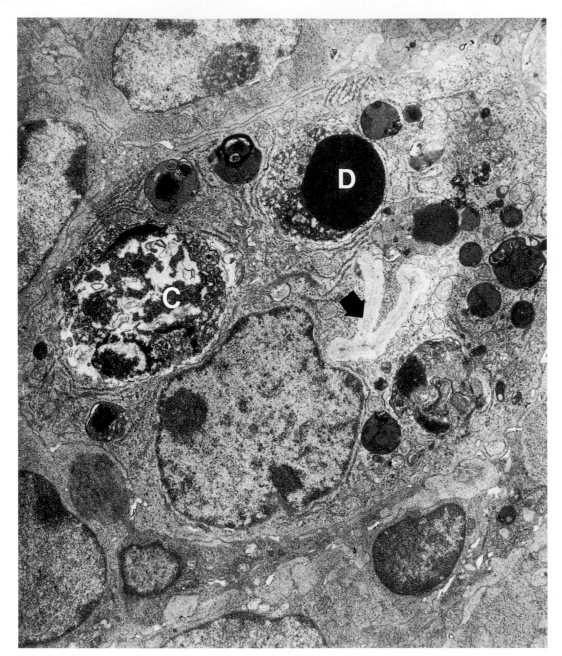

Fig. 5.11 Electron micrograph of macrophage in dome of mouse Peyer's patch follicle. Fluffy masses of carbon (C) and cellular debris (D) are seen in the cytoplasm. The configuration at the arrow indicates vigorous uptake activity. (Provided through the courtesy of Drs R Hammer, ME LeFevre and DD Joel.)

macrophages of immunized animals, but not of controls. Intraepithelial macrophages may phagocytize and degrade cells which they encounter in the epithelial layer, including plasma cells (Fig. 5.13). Ferritin, administered as a tracer in the intestinal lumen, may be transmitted through M cells to the intercellular space, where intraepithelial macrophages may internalize it (Fig. 5.14). Owen *et al.*[73] studied the reaction by Peyer's patches in mice experimentally infected with *Giardia muris*. These organisms inserted themselves between epithelial cells near dying and desquamating columnar cells. Macrophages beneath the basal lamina extended pseudopods into the epithelial layer to engulf the *Giardia*. Some macrophages entered the epithelium for phagocytosis. Macrophages containing remnants of digested organisms could be identified deep in the follicle dome.

Accessory cell function

Peyer's patch macrophages and dendritic cells are capable of accessory cell function. There is ample evidence, however, that differences exist between Peyer's patches and other lymphoid organs with respect to the methods necessary to prepare functional macrophages, the *in vitro* techniques necessary to reveal those functions and, perhaps, in the nature of the accessory cells.

Stimulation

Kagnoff & Campbell[47] prepared cells from spleen and Peyer's patches similarly, by mechanical disruption, to compare the capabilities to produce antibodies to erythrocytes *in vitro*. While spleen cells could perform this function, Peyer's patch cells could not, until adherent peritoneal cells or 2-mercaptoethanol were

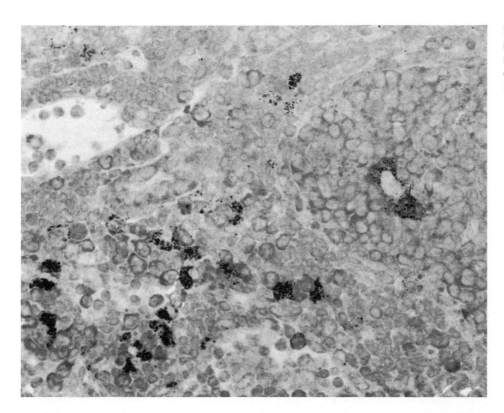

Fig. 5.12 Dense accumulations of carbon porticles are seen in a mesenteric lymph node from a mouse after long-term ingestion of carbon. (Provided through the courtesy of Drs ME LeFevre and DD Joel.)

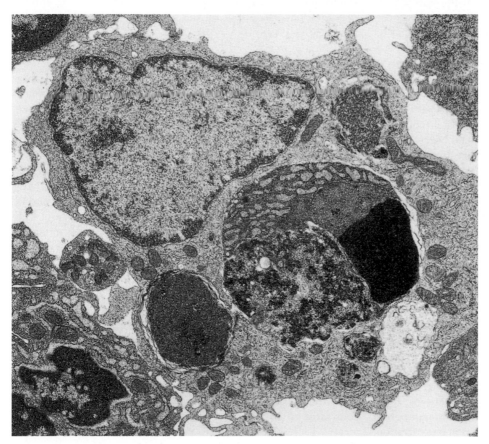

Fig. 5.13 Electron micrograph of macrophage within the epithelium covering a dome in a rat Peyer's patch. Cellular debris, including the remnants of a plasma cell, are seen in the cytoplasm. × 9000. (Reproduced from Ref. 55, with permission from *Cell and Tissue Research.*)

added. Cytotoxic allograft reactions *in vitro* also were deficient. Similarly, spleen cells, but not Peyer's patch cells, could display antibody-dependent cell-mediated cytotoxicity.[48] It was suggested that Peyer's patches were deficient in an accessory cell type or types necessary for the generation of these activities. Tomasi *et al.*[90] found adherent cells from Peyer's patches could not present antigens such as ovalbumin, human gammaglobulin or purified protein derivative to sensitized lymph node cells, whereas

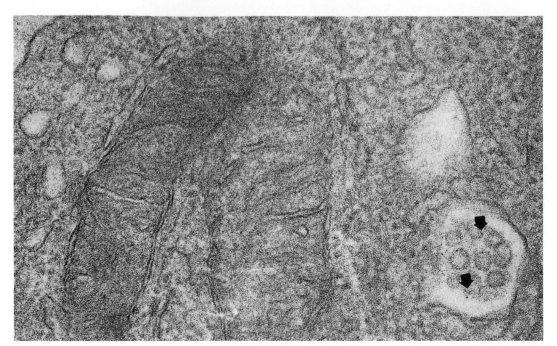

Fig. 5.14 Part of an intraepithelial macrophage from a rat given ferritin in the gut lumen 1 hour prior to sacrifice. Tiny dense dots representing ferritin molecules are seen in the intercellular space (upper left) and in a multivesicular body (arrows). × 57 000. (Reproduced from Ref. 55, with permission from *Cell and Tissue Research*.)

adherent cells from spleen, lymph node and peritoneal exudate induced marked stimulation, indicating antigen presentation. Low-density Peyer's patch cells were capable of presenting poly L-glutamine:L-alanine:L-tyrosine to T cells, although less efficiently than spleen cells. Low-density spleen cells were said to have large numbers of cells (40% or more) with the morphological characteristics of dendritic cells, while Peyer's patch low-density cells had less than 5%.

Evidence for more complete accessory cell function has been presented by other workers. Richman *et al.*[77] compared Peyer's patch macrophages with spleen macrophages in their ability to present ovalbumin to primed lymph node cells. Macrophages prepared from Peyer's patches by collagenase digestion were able to present antigen at least as well as those from spleen. Cells prepared from Peyer's patches not incubated with collagenase frequently were unable to present antigen. Furthermore, these workers demonstrated that Peyer's patch macrophages from animals fed ovalbumin could stimulate primed lymph node cells without the need for antigen to be added *in vitro*.

Other clear evidence that the macrophages of Peyer's patches show accessory cell function has come from study of the cell populations after dispersal of tissue by a neutral protease.[53,63] *In vitro* cultures prepared in this manner demonstrated plaque-forming cell responses similar to those in spleen cell cultures. Priming mice orally with sheep erythrocytes prior to *in vitro* exposure to sheep erythrocytes produced high IgA plaque-forming cell responses. The enzymatic extraction of Peyer's patches produced greater than 10-fold higher numbers of esterase-positive macrophages than conventional methods.

Peyer's patch macrophages are heterogeneous in a number of ways, as judged by characteristics such as adherence, expression of Class II MHC antigens, nonspecific esterase and phagocytosis.[30,54,55,74] Accessory cell function may be carried out by Peyer's patch cells which are low-density, non-adherent and lack Fc receptors.[84,89] It seems quite possible that the antigen-presenting cells in lymphoepithelial tissue may differ from their counterparts in other lymphoid organs because of a heterogeneity generated by

the extent of differentiation of characteristic features, interacting with the local microenvironment. It also should be kept in mind, as elucidated by Challacombe,[18] that the nature of the antigen may well have an effect on the reactivity by lymphoepithelial tissue.

Induction of tolerance

Feeding of certain antigens in the appropriate manner can induce a state of tolerance rather than producing stimulation of an immune response, a condition referred to as oral tolerance. Antigen-presenting cells such as macrophages or dendritic cells participate in the induction of tolerance through their interaction with lymphocytes.[43] If antigen coupled with Class II MHCs is presented to lymphocytes without costimulation, such as that due to the interaction of B7 on the antigen-presenting cell with CD28 on the lymphocyte, tolerance is induced.[36] It may also be possible that interaction of B7 with the cell surface molecule CTLA-4 on lymphocytes will lead to tolerance.[5] For the induction of oral tolerance, antigen in the intestinal lumen transits the M cells overlying lymphoid follicles and is presented by cells in the lymphoid tissue in a manner that usually induces nonresponsiveness by IgG and IgE classes, but not IgA (see Chapter 15).

MACROPHAGES ASSOCIATED WITH MAMMARY GLANDS

Milk and colostrum have remarkably high quantities of IgA and many cells. IgA antibodies and cellular immunity are transferred from the mother through colostrum and milk to the offspring soon after birth.[70]

Cellular components of colostrum and milk

The cells in colostrum and milk include macrophages, neutrophils, lymphocytes and epithelial cells.[24,44,79,81] Total leukocyte counts in early postpartum colostrum range from 500 to 8000 per cubic millimetre. Macrophages and neutrophils are the predominant cell types. Eosinophils are seen occasionally.

Mammary gland macrophages

Colostral and milk macrophages range from 8 to 40 μm in diameter; most are mononuclear, but the larger ones may be multinucleate and have ingested cellular material in their cytoplasm.[44] Leukocytes penetrate the epithelium of the mammary gland to gain access to the lumina of the alveoli and ducts even before lactation begins (Fig. 5.15).[79] The cytoplasm of many of the macrophages becomes filled with numerous, rather uniform, fat droplets (Fig. 5.16). Neutrophils also display lipid-containing vacuoles. Colostral macrophages are positive for nonspecific

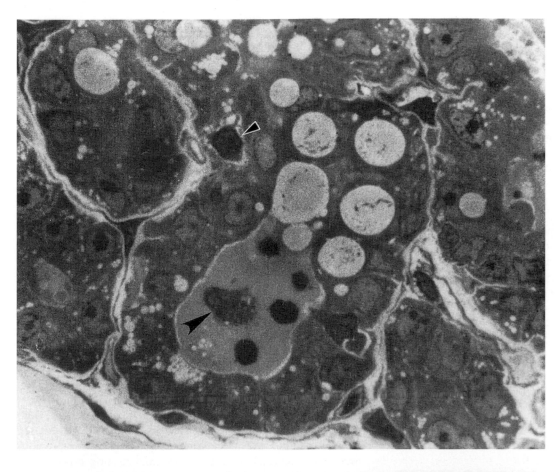

Fig. 5.15 Light micrograph showing a portion of human mammary gland late in pregnancy. A macrophage is present in the alveolar lumen (large arrow). Leukocytes are migrating through the epithelium (small arrow). × 1000. (Reproduced from Ref. 79, with permission from *Biology of Reproduction*.)

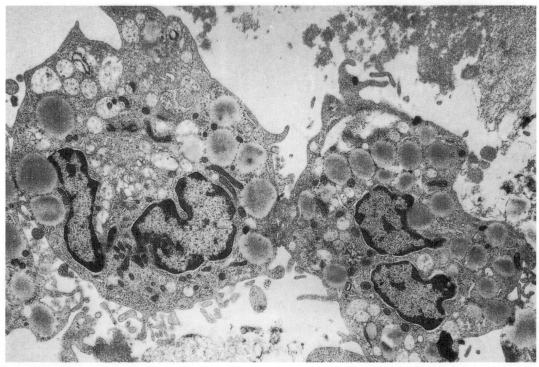

Fig. 5.16 Electron micrograph of macrophages from milk of rat. Fat vacuoles are prominent in the cytoplasm. × 10 500. (Provided through the courtesy of Dr L Seelig.)

esterase and acid phosphatase. Many do not adhere to glass readily.[24] They are phagocytic, capable of including newly presented material in the cytoplasm along with the numerous lipid droplets.[44] Breast milk macrophages have demonstrable Class II MHC antigens on their surfaces.[3] Macrophages and lymphocytes may be shown to interact by cell–cell contact.[24,82] Milk macrophages have been shown to act as accessory cells in T cell proliferative response.[65] While they are deficient in stimulating tumouricidal activity,[3] they may mediate antibody-dependent cytotoxicity.[59]

Transport of IgA

Macrophages from mammary glands contain large quantities of IgA, which is released during phagocytosis.[75,96] It has been suggested, in fact, that macrophages may be important in the mammary glands as transporters of immunoglobulin.[75] This possibility has not been ruled out, but the coincidental appearance of immunoglobulins with secretory component in macrophages has been advanced as an argument that uptake occurred after transport of IgA through epithelial cells.[24] Brandtzaeg[15] found no evidence for a significant role of macrophages for the translocation of IgA into colostrum in the mammary gland tissue from a woman early in her 8th month of pregnancy. Some intraepithelial and intraluminal IgA-positive macrophages were found in ducts adjacent to occasional interlobular accumulations of macrophages in the mammary gland tissue from a woman who had been breast feeding regularly for 8 months.

Although macrophages from the mammary gland obviously have characteristics which allow them to participate in immune reactivity, the full extent of their role in protection of the infant is not yet appreciated. Part of this activity may take place in the gut lumen. Colostrum and milk have non-immunological protective factors as well. The nonspecific defence factors lysozyme and lactoferrin must be derived, at least in part, from the macrophages and neutrophils.

INFECTION AND DISEASES IN THE DIGESTIVE SYSTEM

Macrophages clearly are involved in a number of disease processes associated with the digestive system.[56] Inflammatory bowel diseases involve macrophages in addition to other inflammatory cells. Crohn's disease develops with the accumulation of lymphocytes and plasma cells in small ulcers in the intestine, an influx of macrophages and the formation of granulomata by epithelioid cells.[14] The dense cellular infiltrate in ulcerative colitis includes macrophages, neutrophils and lymphocytes.[14] In these conditions, cytokines such as TNFα and IL1 are released from macrophages to contribute to the inflammatory reaction.

Pathogenic microorganisms and their toxic products are reacted to by macrophages and dendritic cells upon passing the epithelial barrier. Microorganisms breach the epithelial barrier in various ways: some take advantage of minute breaks in the epithelium, while others attack enterocytes directly. However, a common pathway is through the M cells of lymphoepithelial tissue.[26,35,50]

Involvement of lymphoepithelial tissue

Lymphoepithelial tissue is an initial focus for some intestinal diseases.[87] It is likely that the earliest lesion of Crohn's disease is in

solitary lymphoid follicles and Peyer's patches.[39,66] M cells seem to be intimately involved in the establishment of the primary focus of infection by many viruses and bacteria, including human immunodeficiency virus, reoviruses, *Shigella flexneri*, *Salmonella* and *Vibrio cholerae*.[17,26,35,50] Many of these involve uptake by macrophages after transcytosis through the epithelium.

Killing and maintenance

Uptake by macrophages is not sufficient for protection, however, for it does not necessarily signify the killing of all of the organisms.[42] Live tubercle bacilli can be carried by macrophages until cell-mediated immunity is induced.[56] The characteristic bacilli of Whipple's disease[28] can crowd the cytoplasm of gut-associated macrophages and not be killed. Although macrophages may be shown to degrade viruses very rapidly,[34] they also may be the vector for virus replication and spread.[26]

Epithelioid and giant cells

The reaction carried out by macrophages in gastrointestinal diseases frequently involves the formation of epithelioid cells and giant cells.[85] Examination of surgical specimens from patients with ulcerative colitis and Crohn's disease usually will reveal granulomas composed of epithelioid and giant cells.[66] Production of these lesions through recruitment of monocytes is followed by differentiation *in situ* into macrophages which fuse with each other to form multinucleated giant cells.[62] Figure 5.17 shows a granuloma in the small intestine.

CONCLUSION

There can be little doubt that gut-associated macrophages are active participants in gastrointestinal function. Reaction to the contents of the gut lumen begins with macrophages and dendritic cells once the material has traversed the epithelial barrier. Depending upon the nature of the material and the previous experience and capabilities of the responding antigen-presenting cells, the reaction may take many directions. It may be generalized or immunologically specific. It may provide immediate

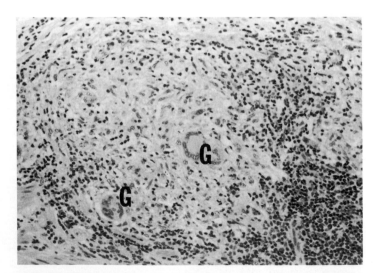

Fig. 5.17 Granuloma from human small intestine. Multinucleated giant cells (G) are surrounded by epithelioid cells. Lymphocyte infiltration is greatest at lower right. (Provided through the courtesy of Dr Luther Mills.)

protection, delayed reactivity, tolerance, or be the focus of continuing difficulty.

Macrophages are important in the well-being of the gastrointestinal tract and the whole organism. While macrophages and dendritic cells in Peyer's patches certainly are important in day-to-day gut immunity, we have more to learn about their characteristics and capabilities, and therefore their full functions. Many of the functions ascribed solely to macrophages in the past are now known to be carried out by dendritic cells. The way these antigen-presenting cells function in parallel to produce stimulation under certain circumstances and tolerance under others remains to be determined in detail. Acquisition of knowledge about the interaction necessary for regulation of gut immune reaction, including tolerance, will provide new ideas about what aberrations lead to food intolerance and allergy.

Acknowledgement

The original chapter was written while the author was supported by Fogarty Senior International Fellowship TW00789, N.I.H., for work in the INSERM Unité de Recherche de Pathologie Digestive, Marseille, France, Professor Henri Sarles, Director.

REFERENCES

1 Abe K, Ito T. Fine structure of the dome in Peyer's patches of mice. *Arch Histol Jpn* 1978; 41: 195–204.

2 Bienenstock J, Dolezel J. Peyer's patches: lack of specific antibody-containing cells after oral and parenteral immunization. *J Immunol* 1971; 106: 938–45.

3 Biondi A, Peri G, Colombo J, Bolis G, Montovani A. Antibody-dependent and independent cytotoxicity of human mononuclear phagocytes: defective stimulation of tumoricidal activity in milk macrophages. *Clin Exp Immunol* 1982; 50: 701.

4 Biondi A, Rossing TH, Bennett J, Todd RF III. Surface membrane heterogeneity among human mononuclear phagocytes. *J Immunol* 1984; 132: 1237–43.

5 Bluestone JA. Is CTLA-4 a master switch for peripheral T cell tolerance? *J Immunol* 1997; 158: 1989–93.

6 Bockman DE. Range of function of gut-associated lymphoepithelial tissue. In: *Aspects of Developmental and Comparative Immunology I* (Solomon JB, ed.) Pergamon Press, Oxford, 1980: 273–7.

7 Bockman DE. Functional histology of appendix. *Arch Histol Jpn* 1983; 46: 271–92.

8 Bockman DE, Boydston WR. Participation of follicle associated epithelium (FAE), macrophages, and plasma cells in the function of appendix. *Scan Electron Microsc* 1982; 3: 1341–50.

9 Bockman DE, Cooper MD. Pinocytosis by epithelium associated with lymphoid follicles in the bursa of Fabricius, appendix, and Peyer's patches. An electron microscopic study. *Am J Anat* 1973; 136: 455–78.

10 Bockman DE, Winborn WB. Light and electron microscopy of intestinal ferritin absorption. Observations in sensitized and non-sensitized hamsters (*Mesocricetus auratus*). *Anat Rec* 1966; 155: 603–22.

11 Bockman DE, Lause DB, Doran JE, Waldrep JC. Preparation of protein-coated zymogen granules for use in studies of phagocytosis, vascular distribution and adherence techniques. *J Reticuloendothel Soc* 1979; 26: 539–48.

12 Bockman DE, Boydston WR, Beezhold DH. The role of epithelial cells in gut-associated immune reactivity. *Ann NY Acad Sci* 1983; 409: 129–43.

13 Boltz-Nitulescu G, Willheim M, Spittler A, Leutmezer F, Tempfer C, Winkler S. Modulation of IgA, IgE, and IgG Fc receptor expression on human mononuclear phagocytes by 1 alpha, 25-dihydroxyvitamin D3 and cytokines. *J Leukocyte Biol* 1995; 58: 256–62.

14 Braegger CP, MacDonald TT. Immune mechanisms in chronic inflammatory bowel disease. *Ann Allergy* 1994; 72: 135–41.

15 Brandtzaeg P. The secretory immune system of lactating human mammary glands compared with other exocrine organs. *Ann NY Acad Sci* 1983; 409: 353–82.

16 Capron A, Dessaint J-P, Capron M. Specific IgE antibodies in immune adherence of normal macrophages to *Schistosoma mansoni* schistosomules. *Nature* 1975; 253: 474–5.

17 Carter PB, Collins FM. The route of enteric infection in normal mice. *J Exp Med* 1974; 139: 1189–1203.

18 Challacombe SJ. Salivary antibodies and systemic tolerance in mice after oral immunization with bacterial antigens. *Ann NY Acad Sci* 1983; 409: 177–92.

19 Chin KN, Hudson G. Ultrastructure of Peyer's patches in the normal mouse. *Acta Anat* 1971; 78: 306–18.

20 Cohn ZA. The structure and function of monocytes and macrophages. *Adv Immunol* 1968; 9: 163–214.

21 Cohn ZA. The activation of mononuclear phagocytes: fact, fancy, and future. *J Immunol* 1978; 121: 813–6.

22 Cohn ZA, Hirsch JG, Fedorko ME. The *in vitro* differentiation of mononuclear phagocytes. IV. *J Exp Med* 1966; 123: 747–57.

23 Collan Y. Characteristics of nonepithelial cells in the epithelium of normal rat ileum. *Scand J Gastroenterol* 1972; 7(Suppl. 18): 1–66.

24 Crago SS, Prince SJ, Pretlow TG, McGhee JR, Mestecky J. Human colostral cells. I. Separation and characterization. *Clin Exp Immunol* 1979; 38: 585–97.

25 Crabb ED, Kelsall MA. Organization of the mucosa and lymphatic structures in the rabbit appendix. *J Morphol* 1940; 67: 351–67.

26 Davis IC, Owen RL. The immunopathology of M cells. *Springer Semin Immunopathol* 1997; 18: 421–48.

27 Deane HW. Some electron microscopic observations of the lamina propria of the gut, with comments on the close association of macrophages, plasma cells and eosinophils. *Anat Rec* 1964; 149: 453–74.

28 Dobbins WO, Kawanishi H. Bacillary characteristics in Whipple's disease: an electron microscopic study. *Gastroenterology* 1981; 80: 1468–75.

29 Donnellan WL. The structure of the colonic mucosa. The epithelium and subepithelial reticulohistiocytic complex. *Gastroenterology* 1965; 49: 496–514.

30 Eldridge JH, Lee Y, Kiyono H *et al*. Peyer's patch accessory cells bear Ia. *Ann NY Acad Sci* 1983; 409: 819–21.

31 Faulk WP, McCormick JN, Goodman JR, Yoffey JM, Fudenberg HH. Peyer's patches: morphologic studies. *Cell Immunol* 1970; 1: 500–20.

32 Fanger MW, Goldstine SN, Shen L. The properties and role of receptors for IgA on human leukocytes. *Ann NY Acad Sci* 1983; 409: 552–62.

33 Flotte TJ, Springer TA, Thorbecke GJ. Dendritic cell and macrophage staining by monoclonal antibodies in tissue sections and epidermal sheets. *Am J Path* 1983; 111: 112–24.

34 Friend DS, Rosenau W, Winfield JS, Moon HD. Uptake and degradation of T2 bacteriophage by rat peritoneal macrophages. I. Electron microscopic and immunologic studies. *Lab Invest* 1969; 20: 275–82.

35 Gebert A, Rothkötter H-J, Pabst R. M cells in Peyer's patches of the intestine. *Int Rev Cytol* 1996; 167: 91–159.

36 Gimmi CD, Freeman GJ, Gribben JG, Gray G, Nadler LM. Human T-cell clonal anergy is induced by antigen presentation in the absence of B7 costimulation. *Proc Natl Acad Sci USA* 1993; 90: 6586–90.

37 Golder JP, Doe WF. Isolation and preliminary characterization of human intestinal macrophages. *Gastroenterology* 1983; 84: 795–802.

38 Goldstine SN, Tsai A, Kemp CJ, Fanger MW. Role of IgA antibody in phagocytosis by human polymorphonuclear leukocytes. *Ann NY Acad Sci* 1983; 409: 824.

39 Hadfield G. The primary histological lesion of regional ileitis. *Lancet* 1939; 2: 773–5.

40 Hamilton TA, Ohmori Y, Narumi S, Tannenbaum CS. Regulation of diversity of macrophage activation. In: *Mononuclear Phagocytes in Cell*

biology. (Lopez-Berestein G, Klostergaard J, eds). CRC Press, Boca Raton, 1993: 47–70.

41 Hammer R, Joel DD, LeFevre ME. Ultrastructure of macrophages of the murine Peyer's patch dome. *Exp Cell Biol* 1983; 51: 61–9.

42 Haque A, Ouaissi A, Joseph M, Capron M, Capron A. IgE antibody in eosinophil- and macrophage-mediated *in vitro* killing of *Dipetalonema viteae* microfilariae. *J Immunol* 1981; 127: 716–25.

43 Harper HM, Cochrane L, Williams NA. The role of small intestinal antigen-presenting cells in the induction of T-cell reactivity to soluble protein antigens: association between aberrant presentation in the lamina propria and oral tolerance. *Immunology* 1996; 89: 449–56.

44 Ho FCS, Wong RLC, Lawton JWM. Human colostral and breast milk cells. A light and electron microscopic study. *Acta Paediatr Scand* 1979; 68: 389–96.

45 Hopper KE, Geczy CL, Davies WA. A mechanism of migration inhibition in delayed-type hypersensitivity reactions. I. Fibrin deposition on the surface of elicited peritoneal macrophages *in vivo*. *J Immunol* 198; 126: 1052–8.

46 Joel DD, Laissue JA, LeFevre ME. Distribution and fate of ingested carbon particles in mice. *J Reticuloendothel Soc* 1978; 24: 477–87.

47 Kagnoff MF, Campbell S. Functional characteristics of Peyer's patch lymphoid cells. I. Induction of humoral antibody and cell-mediated allograft reactions. *J Exp Med* 1974; 139: 398–406.

48 Kagnoff MF, Campbell S. Antibody-dependent cell-mediated cytotoxicity. Comparative ability of murine Peyer's patch and spleen cells to lyse lipopolysaccharide-coated and uncoated erythrocytes. *Gastroenterology* 1976; 70: 341–6.

49 Karnovsky ML, Lazdins JK. Biochemical criteria for activated macrophages. *J Immunol* 1978; 121: 809–13.

50 Kelsall BL, Strober W. Host defenses at mucosal surfaces. In: *Clinical Immunology* (Rich RR, ed.). Mosby, St. Louis, 1996: 299–332.

51 Keren DF, Holt PS, Collins HH, Gemski P, Formal SB. The role of Peyer's patches in the local immune response of rabbit ileum to live bacteria. *J Immunol* 1978; 120: 1892–6.

52 Kimura A. The epithelial–macrophagic relationship in Peyer's patches: an immunopathological study. *Bull Osaka Med School* 1977; 23: 67–91.

53 Kiyono H, McGhee JR, Wannemuehler MJ *et al*. *In vitro* immune responses to a T cell-dependent antigen by cultures of disassociated murine Peyer's patch. *Proc Natl Acad Sci USA* 1982; 79: 596–600.

54 Krco CJ, Challacombe SJ, Lafuse WP, David CS, Tomasi TB Jr. Expression of Ia antigens by mouse Peyer's patch cells. *Cell. Immunol* 1981; 57: 420–6.

55 Lause DB, Bockman DE. Heterogeneity, position, and functional capability of the macrophages in Peyer's patches. *Cell Tiss Res* 1981; 218: 557–66.

56 LeFevre ME, Hammer R, Joel DD. Macrophages of the mammalian small intestine: a review. *J Reticuloendothel Soc* 1979; 26: 553–73.

57 LeFevre ME, Joel DD. The Peyer's patch epithelium: an imperfect barrier. In: *Toxicology of Intestinal Function* (Schiller M, ed.). Raven Press, New York, 1984: 45–56.

58 Li CY, Lam KW, Yam LT. Esterases in human leukocytes. *J Histochem Cytochem* 1973; 21: 1–12.

59 Mandyla H, Xanthou M, Maravelias C, Baum D, Matsaniotis N. Antibody-dependent cytotoxicity of human colostrum phagocytes. *Pediatr Res* 1982; 16: 995.

60 Mathiowitz E, Jacob JS, Jong YS *et al*. Biologically erodable microspheres as potential oral drug delivery systems. *Nature* 1997; 386: 410–14.

61 Matz J, Williams J, Rosenwasser LJ, Borish LC. Granulocyte–macrophage colony-stimulating factor stimulates macrophages to respond to IgE via the low affinity IgE receptor. *J Allergy Clin Immunol* 1994; 93: 650–7.

62 Meunet G, Bitzi A, Hammer G. Macrophage turnover in Crohn's disease and ulcerative colitis. *Gastroenterology* 1978; 74: 501–3.

63 Michalek SM, McGhee JR, Kiyono H *et al*. The IgA response: inductive aspects, regulatory cells, and effector functions. *Ann NY Acad Sci* 1983; 409: 48–71.

64 Mikkelsen HB, Rumessen JJ. Characterization of macrophage-like cells in the external layers of human small and large intestine. *Cell Tiss Res* 1992; 270: 273–9.

65 Mori M, Hayward AR. Phenotype and function of human milk monocytes as antigen presenting cells. *Clin Immunol Immunopathol* 1982; 23: 94.

66 Morson BC. Regional enteritis (Crohn's disease). Part I. Pathology. In: *Gastroenterology Vol. 2*, (Bockus HL, ed.). WB Saunders, Philadelphia, 1976: 550–61.

67 Mosmann T. Cytokines and immune regulation. In: *Clinical Immunology* (Rich RR, ed.). Mosby, St. Louis, 1996: 217–30.

68 Nathan CF, Murray HW, Cohn ZA. The macrophage as an effector cell. *N Engl J Med* 1980; 303: 622–6.

69 North RJ. The concept of the activated macrophage. *J Immunol* 1978; 121: 806–9.

70 Ogra SS, Weintraub D, Ogra PL. Immunologic aspects of human colostrum and milk. III. Fate and absorption of cellular and soluble components in the gastrointestinal tract of the newborn. *J Immunol* 1977; 119: 245–8.

71 Owen RL. Macrophage function in Peyer's patch epithelium. *Adv Exp Med Biol* 1982; 149: 507–13.

72 Owen RL, Jones AL. Epithelial cell specialization within human Peyer's patches: an ultrastructural study of intestinal lymphoid follicles. *Gastroenterology* 1974; 66: 189–203.

73 Owen RL, Allen CL, Stevens DP. Phagocytosis of *Giardia muris* by macrophages in Peyer's patch epithelium in mice. *Infect Immun* 1981; 33: 591–601.

74 Pappo J, Ebersole J, Taubman M, Smith D. Isolation and characterization of M cells and macrophages in rat Peyer's patches. *Fed Proc* 1982; 41: 434.

75 Pittard WB, Polmar SH, Fanaroff AA. The breast milk macrophage: a potential vehicle for immunoglobulin transport. *J Reticuloendothel Soc* 1977; 22: 597–603.

76 Reynolds HY, Atkinson JP, Newball HH, Frank MM. Receptors for immunoglobulin and complement on human alveolar macrophages. *J Immunol* 1975; 114: 1813–20.

77 Richman LK, Graeff AS, Strober W. Antigen presentation by macrophage-enriched cells from the mouse Peyer's patch. *Cell Immunol* 1981; 62: 110–18.

78 Sawicki W, Kucharczyk K, Szamska K, Kujawa M. Lamina propria macrophages of intestine of guinea pig. *Gastroenterol* 1977; 73: 1340–4.

79 Seelig LL Jr, Beer AE. Intraepithelial leukocytes in the human mammary gland. *Biol Rep* 1981; 24: 1157–63.

80 Shimizu Y, Andrew W. Studies on the rabbit appendix. I. Lymphocyte–epithelial relationships and the transport of bacteria from lumen to lymphoid nodule. *J Morphol* 1967; 123: 231–50.

81 Smith CW, Goldman AS. The cells of human colostrum. I. *In vitro* studies of morphology and functions. *Pediatr Res* 1968; 2: 103–9.

82 Smith CW, Goldman AS. Interactions of lymphocytes and macrophages from human colostrum: characteristics of the interacting lymphocyte. *J Reticuloendothel Soc* 1970; 8: 91.

83 Sobhon P. The light and the electron microscopic studies of Peyer's patches in non-germ-free adult mice. *J Morphol* 1971; 135: 457–82.

84 Spalding DM, Koopman WJ, McGhee JR. Identification of a nonadherent accessory cell in murine Peyer's patches. *Ann NY Acad Sci* 1983; 409: 880–1.

85 Spector WG. Epithelioid cells, giant cells, and sarcoidosis. *Ann NY Acad Sci* 1976; 278: 3–6.

86 Takeuchi A, Sprinz H, LaBrec EH, Formal SB. Experimental bacillary dysentery. An electron microscopic study of the response of the intestinal mucosa to bacterial invasion. *Am J Pathol* 1965; 47: 1011–44.

87 Tandon HD, Prakash A. Pathology of intestinal tuberculosis and its distinction from Crohn's disease. *Gut* 1972; 13: 260–9.

88 Tew JG, Thorbecke GJ, Steinman RM. Dendritic cells in the immune response: characteristics of recommended nomenclature. (A report from the Reticuloendothelial Society Committee on Nomenclature.) *J Reticuloendothel Soc* 1982; 31: 371–80.

89 Tlaskalova-Hogenova H, Sterzl J, Stepankova R *et al*. Development of immunological capacity under germfree and conventional conditions. *Ann NY Acad Sci* 1983; 409: 96–113.

90 Tomasi TB, Barr WG, Challacombe SJ, Curran G. Oral tolerance and accessory-cell function of Peyer's patches. *Ann NY Acad Sci* 1983; 409: 145–63.

91 Trier JS, Phelps PC, Rubin CE. Electron microscopy of mucosa of small intestine. *J Am Med Assoc* 1963; 183: 768–74.

92 Unanue ER. The regulatory role of macrophages in antigenic stimulation. Part Two: symbiotic relationship between lymphocytes and macrophages. *Adv Immunol* 1981; 31: 1–136.

93 van Furth R. Origin and kinetics of mononuclear phagocytes. *Ann NY Acad Sci* 1976; 278: 161–75.

94 Vray B. Expression of Fc and C3b receptors and intracellular distribution of bacteria in rat macrophages. *Adv Exp Med Biol* 1982; 141: 567–73.

95 Watanabe Y, Tashiro Y. An electron microscopic observation of the lymphoid tissue from the rabbit appendix. *Recent Adv Respir Res* 1971; 10: 51–80.

96 Weaver EA, Goldblum RM, Davis CP, Goldman AS. Enhanced immunoglobulin A release from human colostral cells during phagocytosis. *Infect Immun* 1981; 34: 498–502.

97 Wicha MS, Huard TK. Macrophages express cell surface laminin. *Exp Cell Res* 1983; 143: 475–90.

98 Winter HS, Cole FS, Huffer LM, Davidson CB, Katz AJ, Edelson PJ. Isolation and characterization of resident macrophages from guinea pig and human intestine. *Gastroenterology* 1983; 85: 358–63.

Chapter 6

Intestinal mast cells

Grant R. Stenton and A. Dean Befus

INTRODUCTION

An understanding of the roles of mast cells (MC) in many inflammatory responses and pathological conditions is evolving rapidly. There are functionally distinct subpopulations of MC that contain a diversity of mediators and respond differently to stimuli and inhibitors of mediator secretion. One of the best known examples of MC heterogeneity is the distinction between intestinal mucosal MC (IMMC) and peritoneal MC (PMC) from rats. Human MC also exhibit heterogeneity, best shown by differences in proteinase content.

MC are widely distributed and are found in association with the external environment, in sites such as respiratory and gastrointestinal tracts, skin and mucosal tissues.[206] Their wide tissue distribution and ability to increase dramatically in number in several pathological conditions led to a diversity of postulates about their functions. MC bear high affinity IgE receptors, Fcε-RI, and release a spectrum of mediators following crosslinking of IgE. These mediators are believed to play pathophysiological roles in allergic and inflammatory conditions such as inflammatory bowel disease (IBD), pulmonary fibrosis, asthma and food allergy, making the MC a target for therapeutic control of such disorders.[16,50,97,220] While MC activation in these conditions is generally viewed as unwanted, MC are also important in host resistance to parasitic infections, regulation of gastric acid secretion, control of the microvasculature, and in tissue repair and remodelling.[14,75,155,156] In this overview of MC, the origin, heterogeneity, and function are considered, as well as some of the more recent and exciting developments in MC biology; namely, an improved understanding of their role in food hypersensitivity and host defence, and of their production of proteinases, cytokines and nitric oxide.

ORIGIN OF MAST CELLS

Mast cell precursors originate in the bone marrow

Human and rodent MC are derived from multipotent stem cells in bone marrow. Following partial differentiation in the bone marrow,[18] MC progenitors leave the bone marrow and are carried in the blood to mucosal and connective tissue sites, where they complete their differentiation[118] (Fig. 6.1).

MC progenitors may differentiate from either erythrocyte/megakaryocyte or monocyte/macrophage lineages.[206] However, because the repertoire of surface markers on MC precursors is not fully understood, the precise differentiation pathway remains unclear. Nevertheless, some factors involved in MC differentiation have been defined. Treatment of human bone marrow mononuclear cells with human recombinant interleukin 3 (hrIL3) gives rise to MC, and stimulation of CD34+ stem cells with various factors produces MC-committed progenitors.[8,118] Elimination of CD34+ cells depletes the potential to produce MC-committed progenitors,[195] while CD34+ cells cultured with the c-*kit* ligand stem cell factor (SCF), hrIL3 or 3T3 fibroblasts were shown to develop into MC.[117,118] Because MC develop from CD34+, CD45+ stem cells upon exposure to SCF and IL3, these progenitors are thought to express the surface markers CD34, CD45, c-*kit* (SCF$_R$) and IL3 receptors (Fig. 6.1).

Mast cell progenitors in the circulation

The earliest detectable progenitors that are committed to a MC lineage have recently been found in murine blood.[193] These progenitors are Thy1[lo] c-*kit*[hi] and contain cytoplasmic granules and MC proteinases, etc. However, these MC-committed progenitors do not express Fcε-RI, the high affinity IgE receptor.[193] Circulating MC progenitors in humans have been identified as c-*kit*+, CD34+, CD14-, CD17- and ly- cells.[3] Recently, Li *et al.*[130] reported higher numbers of cells expressing the surface marker for basophils,

Bsp1, in the blood of allergic patients compared with normal patients. Many of the Bsp1+ cells from allergic patients also expressed the MC surface marker c-*kit*+ and the MC proteinases tryptase, chymase and carboxypeptidase A, whereas Bsp1+ cells from normal patients express very little, if any, of these MC markers. These cells may release mediators into the peripheral blood of allergic individuals.

Maturation of mast cells in peripheral tissues

After the MC progenitors leave the blood, further differentiation occurs in mucosal or connective tissues under the control of growth factors, cytokines and other factors.[18] In rodents, fibroblast-derived SCF and IL3 are important cytokines controlling MC development. SCF alone can promote survival and proliferation of rat connective tissue MC (CTMC) and PMC,[228] but it cannot stimulate proliferation and maturation of rat MC progenitors.[192] IL3 can promote survival of mature murine CTMC, but not their proliferation.[229] However, IL3 can promote the proliferation of less mature mouse MC.[85] In rats, SCF promotes survival and proliferation of both connective tissue MC and bone marrow-derived MC (BMMC), which express a mucosal phenotype,[84] whereas IL3 can stimulate BMMC but not CTMC survival and proliferation.[83] Thus the effects of SCF and IL3 on MC maturity depend on the host (rat *versus* mouse), and MC phenotype (mucosal *versus* connective tissue). In addition, IL4, IL9 and IL10 act synergistically with IL3 to enhance murine MC growth and proliferation,[118,192] while IL4 potentiates SCF-mediated proliferation of immature murine MC.[192] In addition to SCF, fibroblasts can produce nerve growth factor (NGF), which in rats promotes PMC survival but not proliferation.[100] NGF can also increase MC colony production from rat bone marrow cultures when given with suboptimal doses of IL3.[100,148]

In humans, SCF is the predominant cytokine involved in MC maturation. Unlike rodent MC, human lung MC and the human MC line HMC1 do not express IL3 receptors.[118,231] IL4 inhibits the expression of c-*kit* and tryptase by human fetal liver MC progenitors. However, as these MC progenitors mature, they become less affected by IL4.[172] Unlike rodent MC, IL9 and IL10 do not appear to promote human MC development.[106,199]

In addition to cytokines which promote MC maturation, differentiation and survival, some cytokines inhibit these processes. For example, transforming growth factor β1 (TGFβ1) inhibits IL3-dependent proliferation of murine BMMC.[38] Interferon γ (IFNγ) suppresses proliferation of committed MC progenitors from murine bone marrow cells without affecting the growth of mature MC.[168] Granulocyte–macrophage colony stimulating factor (GMCSF) downregulates murine IL3-dependent MC differentiation.[195] However, contrary to previous reports that IL4 has stimulatory effects and IFNγ has inhibitory effects on MC development,[195] it has also been reported that IFNγ increases MC induction from murine splenocytes and promotes survival of human cultured MC, while IL4 was inhibitory if added during the first 4 days of culture.[102] Thus, opposing regulatory effects of cytokines may occur at different phases in MC development.

TECHNIQUES FOR ISOLATION OF MAST CELLS FROM TISSUES

To help understand the pathophysiological roles of MC, procedures have been developed to isolate and purify MC from different

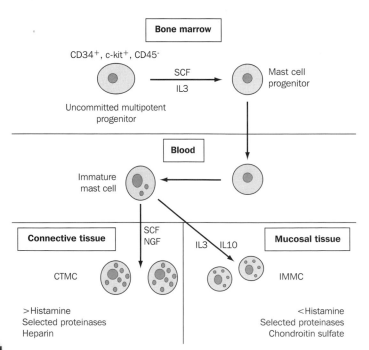

Fig. 6.1 Phases of mast cell development from pluripotent progenitor cells in the bone marrow to differentiation, and the effects of cytokines on this differentiation.

species and anatomical sites, using enzymatic and mechanical means. Perhaps the most thoroughly studied MC is that from the peritoneal cavity of the rat. Isolation and purification of PMC by density gradients of media such as Percoll have been well documented.[216] Modifications of these procedures have been used to isolate and enrich rat[21,33,126,183] and human IMMC.[19,28,72] In addition, antibodies to c-kit (SCF$_R$) have been used to enrich human IMMC[215] and lung MC[177] to a higher purity than can be obtained using Percoll. MC have also been isolated and enriched from human skin,[29] lung[98,178] and uterus.[147]

IN VITRO CULTURE OF MAST CELLS

MC or their progenitors have been isolated and primary cultures or long-term cell lines have been established in order to improve accessibility and reduce variability. The phenotype of these primary cultures or MC lines differs: some are clearly immature, whereas others express markers of more mature CTMC or MMC. RBL-2H3, originally thought to be a basophilic cell line, was later discovered to express an MMC proteinase, RMCP 2, and is the most thoroughly studied rat MC line.[213] Another line, rat cultured MC (RCMC), also expresses RMCP 2.[46] Murine P815, an immature mastocytoma, and MC9 release mediators such as histamine.[165,176] In addition, primary cultures of BMMC have been grown from IL3-treated bone marrow cells isolated from mice and rats.[84,139] Studies of mediator content and responsiveness to secretory stimuli have indicated that rat BMMC are mucosal in phenotype, similar to freshly isolated intestinal mucosal MC.[138]

An immature human MC line (HMC 1) has also been developed from a patient with leukaemia.[40] HMC 1 lacks Fcε-RI (the IgE receptor),[171] but exhibits several MC markers, such as tryptase, and can be activated to release histamine and cytokines.[159,171,196,214] Recently, Bischoff and colleagues established cultures of human IMMC which can last for several months with SCF but for only 2 weeks in its absence.[27] SCF selectively supported MC survival, thus increasing IMMC purity over time in culture.

While there are several advantages to using cultured cells, cell lines are not fully representative of freshly isolated cells. Thus, information obtained from cell lines must be confirmed by using freshly isolated MC, or MC in situ.

HETEROGENEITY OF MAST CELLS

As outlined above, mature MC in rodents are broadly classified as MMC and CTMC. Human MC are described as MC^{TC} (tryptase and chymase positive), MC^T (tryptase positive only) or MC^C (chymase positive only), according to their expression of neutral proteinases.[132] However, the concept of distinct populations and distinct anatomical locations of MC subsets is simplified. MC populations probably exist as a continuum of phenotypes with great potential to alter their gene expression and thus phenotype. While certain MC populations may be phenotypically similar, the extremes of heterogeneity indicate that no MC is exactly like another in its spectrum of gene expression, or even like itself at a different time or location.

Rodent mast cell heterogeneity
Structural and metachromatic heterogeneity
The concept of MC heterogeneity was introduced by Maximow in 1906 when he observed that MC from different tissues vary in their

properties.[152] Enerbäck, in 1966, further clarified this heterogeneity in a series of important studies demonstrating that rat IMMC differ from CTMC.[62-64] CTMC are larger (18 μm mean diameter) than IMMC (12 μm mean diameter) and appear to be more heavily granulated than their IMMC counterparts. CTMC also differ from IMMC in their sensitivity to fixation procedures and metachromatic properties. These differences are due to CTMC predominantly expressing the proteoglycan heparin, while IMMC do not express heparin, but predominantly express chondroitin sulfate.

Heterogeneity in rodent mast cell function
MC from various anatomical sites differ in their content of mediators such as neutral proteinases. Serine proteinases and metalloproteinases are abundant in MC and are excellent markers for different MC phenotypes (Table 6.1). Rat IMMC selectively express the chymase MC proteinase 2 (RMCP 2), while CTMC selectively express RMCP 1.[17,137] Rat CTMC also produce the chymase RMCP 5 and the tryptases RMCP 6 and 7, as well as the metalloproteinase, carboxypeptidase A, all of which are not expressed by IMMC.[17,137] By contrast, IMMC produce a newly described subfamily of chymases RMCP 8, 9 and 10, which are related to T cell granzymes.[138] Similarly, mice express 15 proteinases to date, including the chymases murine MC proteinases (MMCP 1, 2, 3, 4, 5, 8, 9 and 10), the metalloproteinase carboxypeptidase A, cathepsin G and granzyme B, as well as the tryptases MMCP 6, 7 and 11.[104,149] These proteinases appear to be differentially expressed by murine IMMC and CTMC, with mRNA for MMCP 1 and 2 only expressed in IMMC, while mRNA for MMCP 5, 6 and 7 and carboxypeptidase A is only expressed in CTMC.

MC also exhibit heterogeneity in their expression of other mediators. For example, histamine is stored in both rat IMMC and CTMC, but CTMC contain more histamine (10–30 pg/cell) than IMMC (1–3 pg/ml).[21] In addition, CTMC can produce 7.5 ng/10^6 cells of prostaglandin D$_2$ (PGD$_2$), but cannot produce leukotrienes (LT),[163] whereas IMMC produce little PGD$_2$ but significant amounts[91] of LTB$_4$ and LTC$_4$.

Differential expression of proteinases in rodent mast cells		
Rat		
	IMMC	**CTMC**
Chymase	RMCP 2,8,9,10	RMCP 1,5
Tryptase	No	RMCP 6,7
Carboxypeptidase A	No	Yes
Mouse		
	IMMC MMCP 1,2	**CTMC** MMCP 5,6,7
Carboxypeptidase	No	Yes
Cathepsin G	Yes	Yes
Granzyme B	Yes	Yes

Table 6.1 Differential expression of proteinases in rodent mast cells.

Activation of mast cells

In rodents, MC heterogeneity is also characterized by different responsiveness to various secretagogues, antiallergic drugs and cytokines. Although IMMC and CTMC are both activated in response to Fcε-RI stimulation, rat CTMC but not IMMC can be stimulated by compound 48/80, bradykinin, vasoactive intestinal peptide (VIP) and bee venom[30] (Table 6.2). Disodium cromoglycate (DSCG) and nedocromil sodium (NED) and the cytokine interferon gamma (IFNγ) inhibit Fcε-RI-induced histamine release from CTMC but not from IMMC, whereas histamine release from both cell types is inhibited by the antiallergic drug doxantrazole.[183] In addition, while DSCG, NED and IFNγ do not inhibit IgE-dependent histamine release from IMMC, they inhibit the release of TNF from both CTMC and IMMC.[32] These data suggest that the mechanisms of histamine release by IMMC and CTMC are different, while the regulation of TNF release in the two MC phenotypes is similar.

Human mast cell heterogeneity
Structural and biochemical heterogeneity

As with rodents, human MC express multiple proteinases. For example, four different tryptase cDNA (α, βI, βII, βIII) have been identified from human lung[157,158] and skin mRNA.[234] Several tryptase encoding genes have been identified on human chromosome 16p13.3–; however, which genes are expressed by human MC remains to be determined.[181] To date, two distinct populations of human MC, MC^{TC} and MC^T, have been identified *in vivo* by their expression of chymase and/or tryptase.[19] In addition, human MC expressing chymase only (MC^C) have also been identified in cultures and *in situ*.[131] While rodent MMC and CTMC can be found in distinct anatomical sites, human MC^{TC} and MC^T usually coexist, even though one of the phenotypes may be more abundant in a given site. For example, the majority of MC present in human intestinal mucosa are MC^T (81%), with only 19% of the total MC exhibiting the MC^{TC} phenotype.[105] Conversely, the predominant MC phenotype in human intestinal submucosa is MC^{TC} (77%), with only 23% of the total MC exhibiting the MC^T phenotype.[105] MC^T are the predominant MC phenotype found in the lung, with a small population of MC^{TC} in the lung submucosa,[43] while MC^{TC} predominate in the skin[125] (Table 6.3).

Granules

Human MC also exhibit heterogeneity in the ultrastructure of their granules. Although several granule patterns can be observed in all tissue locations, a predominance for one granule type is common. For example, while human uterine MC contain scroll,

Heterogeneity of human mast cells		
	MC^{TC}	**MC^T**
Chymase	Yes	No
Tryptase	Yes	Yes
Intestinal mucosa	19%	81%
Intestinal submucosa	77%	23%
Lung	Few in submucosa	Predominant
Skin	Predominant	Few
Proteoglycan content	Similar	Similar

Table 6.3 Heterogeneity of human mast cells.

crystal and combined granule patterns, human lung and gut MC generally contain scroll patterns, while granules in human skin MC have a predominance of crystalline patterns.[147] Less common than other types of granules, particle pattern granules can be found in human IMMC and lung MC, but not uterine MC. The factors determining the expression of particular granule patterns are not well understood. Different structural patterns may reflect a fundamental developmental property, a pathological condition of the tissue, the preparation procedure, or activation status of the MC.

Similarities between MC^{TC} and MC^T

In addition to proteinase differences between MC^{TC} and MC^T, similarities exist between MC^{TC} and MC^T. For example, unlike rat IMMC and CTMC, which predominantly express chondroitin sulfate or heparin, respectively, human MC^{TC} and MC^T are believed to express similar quantities of the proteoglycans, heparin and chondroitin sulfate, which are responsible for the metachromatic properties of MC. However, since highly pure populations of MC^{TC} or MC^T are difficult to isolate, the precise proteoglycan content of these cell populations cannot be determined accurately. Furthermore, the different proteoglycan content of rodent MC, predominantly heparin in CTMC and chondroitin sulfate in IMMC, accounts for the difference in formalin sensitivity during fixation. However, despite human MC^{TC} and MC^T having similar proteoglycan content, the existence of formalin-sensitive and -insensitive populations within the same tissue has been demonstrated. Therefore, formalin sensitivity of human MC may not depend entirely on proteoglycan content. For example, formalin fixation of human lung MC results in a 90% reduction in histochemically detectable MC.[191,205,217,239] Furthermore, human intestinal mucosa contains similar numbers of formalin-sensitive and -insensitive MC, while MC isolated from the muscle of the human large intestine (submucosa) are almost all formalin-insensitive.[179] It appears, therefore, that human MC populations with higher MC^{TC} content are more resistant to formalin fixation.

Heterogeneity in human mast cell function

Human MC also exhibit differential cytokine expression. In bronchial biopsies, MC^T expressed IL4, IL5, IL6 and TNF, whereas MC^{TC} from the same biopsy specimens exclusively expressed IL4.[37]

Activation of rat mast cells		
	IMMC	**CTMC**
Fcε-RI stimulation	Yes	Yes
Compound 48/80	No	Yes
Bradykinin, VIP, bee venom	No	Yes

VIP, vasoactive intestinal peptide.

Table 6.2 Activation of rat mast cells.

As with rodent MC, human MC phenotypes respond differently to secretagogues and antiallergic drugs.[206,224] MC isolated from human skin, which are predominantly MC^{TC}, can be activated by cationic secretagogues such as substance P, but their histamine secretion is not inhibited by DSCG. Immunological stimulation of human skin MC induces histamine release that is partially inhibited by DSCG.[206] However, human lung MC and IMMC, characterized as <10% MC^{TC} and >60% MC^{TC}, respectively, are unresponsive to substance P, while DSCG can inhibit immunologically induced histamine release from these cells.[206,224]

Thus, while rodent MC can be divided into distinct populations based on their structural and functional properties, human MC populations are not so easily subdivided. MC^{T}, MC^{TC} and even MC^{C} coexist and may respond differently to stimuli or inhibitors in the same location. Further studies of MC characteristics are essential to elucidate the roles of distinct MC populations in various pathophysiological conditions.

MAST CELL ACTIVATION

MC can be activated by an IgE-dependent pathway (Fcε-RI-dependent) or by several IgE-independent stimuli. Despite considerable research, the signal transduction mechanisms are incompletely understood. A better understanding of these activation pathways may lead to the rational design of new and more effective anti-allergic and anti-inflammatory drugs.

IgE-dependent mast cell activation

IgE binds to high affinity IgE receptors (Fcε-RI) on the MC, forming an IgE–Fcε-RI receptor complex that is free to move in the MC membrane. The binding of multivalent antigens to two or more specific IgE antibodies crosslinks IgE receptor complexes and initiates MC degranulation.[69] Fcε-RI aggregation activates several tyrosine kinases including the src family member, Lyn, and the zap-70 member, Syk.[6] Subsequent downstream events involve a pertussis toxin-insensitive G protein,[200] phospholipase C (PLC),[182] and protein kinase C (PKC) activation.[77] Activation of these signalling molecules leads to the production of several second messengers, including inositol 1,4,5-trisphosphate (IP$_3$) and diacylglycerol (DAG). However, the complete sequence of second messenger production leading to MC degranulation is unknown. The phosphatidylinositol system is a widely used signalling pathway activated by neurotransmitters, hormones, growth factors and Fcε-RI-dependent MC activation.[57] Activation of MC leads to the hydrolysis of phosphatidylinositol 4,5-bisphosphate (PIP$_2$) by PLC, yielding IP$_3$ and DAG; the former releases calcium from intracellular stores in the endoplasmic reticulum,[67] while the latter activates another signalling molecule PKC.[246]

Many studies have examined the role of the flux of calcium and chloride ions in MC degranulation. Fcε-RI-dependent mediator secretion requires extracellular calcium.[114] Two phases of change in free intracellular calcium concentration occur:[245] a rapid transient rise in free intracellular calcium caused by IP$_3$-dependent release of calcium from intracellular stores,[204] followed by a lower, but stable elevation of free intracellular calcium, believed to result from an influx of calcium across the plasma membrane.[184] This calcium influx may occur via a calcium-specific channel, identified

as I$_{CRAC}$ (calcium release-activated calcium channel),[101,184] believed to be activated by the release of calcium from intracellular stores, but I$_{CRAC}$ is not the only calcium channel which can allow influx of extracellular calcium in MC. Low conductance (50 pS) and higher (250 pS) conductance non-specific cation channels on MC membranes may also play a role in calcium influx following cell stimulation.[66,101,175,184]

Fcε-RI-dependent MC activation also induces chloride influx, an area which has received relatively little attention.[150] This chloride influx is thought to hyperpolarize the MC, initially depolarized by the release of calcium from intracellular stores, thus providing the driving force for influx of extracellular calcium. Following cellular activation, the free intracellular calcium is believed to interact with calmodulin, causing conformational changes which result in calmodulin-mediated activation of other enzymes, such as calmodulin-dependent protein kinase, and eventually MC degranulation.[45]

The final mechanisms involved in exocytosis are incompletely known, but recently emphasis has been placed on several proteins and pathways, including synaptotagmins, synaptobravins, Rab and Rac. Undoubtedly, in the next few years the detailed mechanisms will be more clearly defined and opportunities for therapeutic advances may be uncovered.

The latter stages of IgE-dependent MC activation involve degranulation and mediator release, followed by mediator-dependent pathophysiological responses. However, in addition to degranulation, Fcε-RI-mediated MC activation induces the synthesis and release of many other mediators, such as cytokines and chemokines. The synthesis of these mediators requires gene transcription, protein synthesis, processing and secretion. The functions of some of these cytokines are discussed below.

IgE-independent mast cell activation

There are several IgE-independent MC secretagogues, but in many cases their biological relevance is not understood. For example, calcium ionophore A23187 and cationic compounds such as compound 48/80, substance P, neutrophil defensins, bee venom peptides and complement-derived anaphylatoxin C3a are non-cytotoxic MC secretagogues. These secretagogues activate MC by mechanisms distinct from Fcε-RI-dependent pathways,[20,69,123,162] although there are some similarities in the pathways such as the dependence on a rise in free intracellular calcium concentration. In addition, the anaphylatoxin C5a, may also activate MC in a cationic-dependent manner. However, the human MC line (HMC 1) and MC populations isolated from human skin, heart and kidney, but not lung, uterine or tonsil MC, have recently been shown to express the receptor for C5a (CD88), suggesting that C5a-mediated activation of MC may occur, at least in part, via this receptor.[74]

Of all non-cytotoxic MC secretagogues, calcium ionophore A23187 arguably has the simplest mechanism of action, because it increases free intracellular calcium concentration by a mechanism which circumvents membrane-associated G proteins from directly transporting calcium ions from the extracellular medium into the cell.[70] Cationic secretagogues activate a pertussis toxin-sensitive G protein which is distinct from the pertussis toxin-insensitive G protein activated by Fcε-RI stimulation (Table 6.4).[169,200] The cationic MC secretagogues appear to act by electrostatic and hydrophobic interactions with the cell membrane and with the anionic C terminus of the G protein α subunit.[161] Following direct

IgE-independent mast cell activation	
Type	**Activation**
Calcium ionophore A23187	G protein independent
Cationic secretagogues	G protein dependent

Table 6.4 IgE-independent mast cell activation.

G protein activation by cationic secretagogues, PLC is activated, resulting in the formation of IP_3 and DAG and, as with Fcε-RI-mediated MC activation, production of IP_3 induces a transient increase in free intracellular calcium[122,226] followed by an influx of extracellular calcium. Despite the similarities, there are differences between calcium influx induced by cationic secretagogues and Fcε-RI-induced activation. The cationic secretagogue compound 48/80 can produce higher concentrations of free intracellular calcium than Fcε-RI-dependent activation, and also releases significant, albeit reduced, levels of histamine in the absence of extracellular calcium,[122,226] whereas Fcε-RI-mediated histamine release is substantially inhibited under conditions of reduced extracellular calcium.

NEUROGENIC INFLAMMATION

Because of their proximity to neurons, it has long been hypothesized that MC and neurons interact. This interaction suggests a role for MC in neurogenic inflammation. It is widely accepted that activation of capsaicin-sensitive primary afferent neurons results in neurogenic inflammation, characterized by induction of vasodilatation, vascular permeability and other inflammatory changes. Capsaicin, a component of chilli peppers, selectively depletes sensory neurons of substance P and other neuropeptides.[23] In addition to their afferent functions, capsaicin-sensitive neurons have efferent functions, including bronchoconstriction, increased peristalsis in the gastrointestinal tract and contraction of the urinary bladder.[23] Because of the diversity of functions exhibited by capsaicin-sensitive neurons and their widespread distribution, it is not surprising that neurogenic inflammation has been identified in many organs.[23,115,120,121]

Role of mast cell

The role played by MC in neurogenic inflammation is controversial. Since human skin MC can be activated by substance P to release mediators,[162] it was suggested that substance P and perhaps other neuropeptides released from capsaicin-sensitive neurons, induce the release of MC mediators which themselves induce vasodilatation and permeability changes observed during neurogenic inflammation.[71,115] In addition, MC appear to be involved in capsaicin-induced increases in gastric mucosal blood flow.[238] However, there is evidence suggesting that MC activation is not essential in cutaneous neurogenic inflammation.[12,121] Perhaps MC are important in some neurogenic inflammatory situations, but not all.

In addition to capsaicin-sensitive neurons, there is evidence that the adrenergic and cholinergic systems have proinflammatory and anti-inflammatory effects. For example, β-agonists suppress IgE-mediated histamine and TNF release from human MC.[29,247]

Furthermore, cholinergic and capsaicin-sensitive nerves, as well as MC mediators, are involved in antigen-induced alteration of intestinal epithelial transport.[51,241] Therefore it may not be appropriate to disregard the interactions of non-capsaicin-sensitive neurons with MC when studying neurogenic inflammation.

Neural regulation

Evidence of neural regulation of MC function was obtained following bilateral decentralization or ganglionectomy of the superior cervical ganglia of rats. This surgery resulted in substantial inhibition of systemic and pulmonary inflammation following systemic antigen challenge.[189] Furthermore, there were reduced histamine levels in the bronchoalveolar lavage fluid of challenged rats, suggesting that the sympathetic nervous system regulates MC function.[189]

Clearly, neurons can activate MC. Likewise, there is evidence that MC regulate the functions of the nervous system. For example, murine sympathetic neurons grow towards MC *in vitro*, suggesting that MC have a neurotropic effect.[35] A series of studies has also shown that MC mediators can modulate neural excitability. Challenge of sensitized guinea pig bronchus with antigen resulted in the release of histamine and PGD_2 from MC, which correlated with increased excitability of bronchial parasympathetic ganglion neurons.[166,167] Furthermore, this antigen-mediated increase in neuronal excitability was mimicked[166,167] with the addition of histamine and PGD_2. Similarly, antigen-induced histamine release from guinea pig superior cervical ganglion (SCG) MC, as well as exogenously added histamine, depolarized neurons in the SCG.[47] Antigen was also observed to mediate long-term potentiation of nicotinic synaptic transmission in the SCG, which was proposed to be MC-dependent.[244]

It is evident that there is a functional interdependence between the nervous system and MC.[15] Neurogenic inflammation suggests a role for MC in relaying messages from the peripheral tissues to the peripheral nervous system, perhaps even to the central nervous system, and likewise from the central or peripheral nervous systems to the peripheral tissues. This potentially important role deserves further study to elucidate the precise involvement of MC.

MAST CELL MEDIATOR RELEASE

MC activation induces pathophysiological changes such as bronchoconstriction and mucous secretion in asthma.[97] Similarly, induction of epithelial secretion and altered smooth muscle activity occurs in the intestine following IMMC activation.[16] Such responses are due to the release of a plethora of MC mediators, including histamine, serotonin (5HT), prostaglandins, leukotrienes, heparin and chondroitin sulfate proteoglycans, proteinases, nitric oxide (NO), platelet activating factor (PAF), and numerous cytokines. MC can also release chemotactic factors for eosinophils, neutrophils and macrophages which contribute to late-phase hypersensitivity reactions by releasing a second pool of mediators that amplify the physiological response (Fig. 6.2). These mediators can be placed in one of three categories, depending on whether they are preformed, newly synthesized or cytokines.

Preformed mediators

Several mediators are synthesized and stored within MC granules before MC activation (Table 6.5). The most thoroughly studied

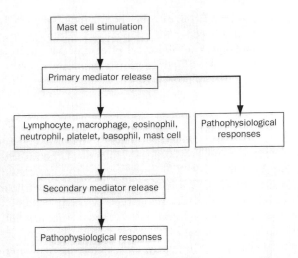

Fig. 6.2 Cascade of allergic inflammation: recruitment and activation of other inflammatory cells following mast cell activation and mediator release, leading to the generation of a second pool of mediators which amplify the allergic response.

Mast cell mediators	
Preformed	**Newly synthesized**
Histamine	Arachidonic acid derivatives
Acid hydrolases	Prostaglandins
Proteinases	Leukotrienes
Some cytokines	PAF
	Chemokines, cytokines

Table 6.5 Mast cell mediators.

of these mediators is histamine. Histamine is produced from L-histidine by histidine decarboxylase, after which it is stored in the cytoplasmic granules at an acidic pH, keeping it in a positively charged state. The positively charged histamine is attracted to the negatively charged proteoglycan–protein matrix of the granule, a mechanism which facilitates storage of other preformed mediators as well.[206] Upon MC stimulation, external sodium ions facilitate a cation exchange at neutral pH, thus allowing the dissociation of histamine from the granules.[206] In addition to the release of histamine and other mediators by this ion exchange mechanism, proteoglycans can dissociate from the granule and produce various biological effects. MC granules also contain acid hydrolases which are released upon MC activation and degranulation. These include arylsulfatase A, β-hexosaminidase, β-glucuronidase and β-D-galactosidase, which act at acidic pH and are believed to degrade proteoglycans and glycoproteins.[206]

The numerous proteinases found in MC are also preformed and stored and released during MC degranulation. They are thought to have many biological actions, including stimulation of fibroblast proliferation and neuropeptide extracellular matrix degradation.[206] Knowledge of MC proteinases has evolved rapidly and a more detailed discussion of their biology is presented below.

Newly synthesized mediators

Fcε-RI-mediated and cationic compound-mediated activation of MC induces synthesis of arachidonic acid derivatives including prostaglandins (PG) and leukotrienes (LT).[48,153] However, the amount and types of PG or LT synthesized depends on the activating stimulus. To date, two phospholipase A_2 (PLA_2) enzymes have been identified: secretory PLA_2 ($sPLA_2$) and constitutive PLA_2 ($cPLA_2$), both of which liberate arachidonic acid from cellular membranes. Both $cPLA_2$ and $sPLA_2$ appear to be involved in the production of arachidonic acid metabolites by MC.[163,223] Arachidonic acid can be metabolized by the cyclo-oxygenase pathway, resulting in the formation of PGD_2,[65,128,219] a potent constrictor of bronchial smooth muscle.[87] When MC are activated there is an initial release of PGD_2 which is complete within 30 min, followed by a second phase of PGD_2 release 4–8 h after activation. In MC there are two cyclo-oxygenase (COX) enzymes responsible for production of PGD_2, constitutive COX (COX 1) and inducible COX (COX 2). Moreover, recent studies using COX inhibitors suggested that COX 1 is responsible for the early PGD_2 release and COX 2 is responsible for the second phase release.[112]

Arachidonic acid can also be metabolized by 5-lipoxygenase to produce LT through the intermediates 5-hydroperoxyeicosatetraeonic acid (5-HPETE) and 5-hydroxyeicosatetraenoic acid (5-HETE). LTA_4 is produced first and then converted to LTB_4 or LTC_4.[219] LTB_4 is a powerful chemotactic agent for neutrophils and eosinophils,[68,79] while LTC_4 causes the contraction of bronchial smooth muscle.[129] Rat IMMC activation can produce LTB_4 and LTC_4,[91] whereas rat PMC cannot produce significant LTB_4 or LTC_4 release.[128] Human lung MC produce LTC_4 in excess of LTB_4.[127]

PAF is another lipid mediator produced by MC. PAF has a wide range of pharmacological actions, such as platelet aggregation, vasodilatation, increased vascular permeability, and the induction of release of chemotactic mediators from neutrophils.[171]

Mast cell-derived chemokines and cytokines

MC also synthesize and release a selection of cytokines and chemokines such as IL3, IL4, IL5, IL6, GM-CSF, RANTES, TNF and IFNγ.[133] This list of MC-derived cytokines is growing rapidly (Table 6.6), but their significance in most settings is unclear. Some reports are restricted to the identification of mRNA in MC lines and few studies have identified cytokine production by MC in human tissue *in situ*. While this review cannot discuss the functions of all the cytokines and chemokines listed in Table 6.6, the pathophysiological effects of several of the better known cytokines found in MC are discussed below.

RECENT DEVELOPMENTS IN MAST CELL BIOLOGY

Recently, significant advances have been made in understanding the roles of MC and some of their mediators in inflammation, host defences and pathophysiology. This chapter will focus on MC-derived proteinases, NO and superoxide, cytokines and the role of stem cell factor (SCF) *in vivo*.

Mast cell proteinases

Proteinases are excellent markers of MC subpopulations in rodents and humans. The presence of RMCP 2 or human MC

Protein and/or mRNA expression of cytokines and chemokines from cultured or freshly isolated rodent and human mast cells				
	Rodent mast cells		Human mast cells	
Cytokines	Cell culture	Freshly isolated	Cell culture	Freshly isolated
TNF	+	+	+	+
Lymphotoxin			+	
NGF			+	
TGFβ1	+	+	+	
GM-CSF	+		+	
IFNγ	+	+		
IFNα/β	+			
RANTES			+	+
MCP1			+	+
I-309	+		+	
MIP1α	+		+	
MIP1β	+		+	
MIP2		+		
FGF	+	+	+	+
Lymphotactin	+		+	
Endothelin	+	+		
PDGFAB			+	
VEGF			+	
LIF	+	+		
BDNF			+	
IL1α	+			
IL1β	+		+	
IL2	+		+	
IL3	+	+	+	
IL4	+	+	+	+
IL5	+	+	+	+
IL6	+	+	+	+
IL8		+	+	+
IL10	+		+	
IL12	+			
IL13	+		+	+
IL16			+	

NGF (nerve growth factor), GM-CSF (granulocyte–macrophage colony stimulating factor), MCP1 (monocyte chemotactic factor 1), I-309 (ligand for chemokine receptor CCR8), MIP (macrophage inflammatory protein), PDGFAB (platelet-derived growth factor AB), VEGF (vascular endothelial growth factor), LIF (leukaemia inhibitory factor), FGF (fibroblast growth factor), BDNF (brain-derived neurotropic factor).

Table 6.6 Protein and/or mRNA expression of cytokines and chemokines from cultured or freshly isolated rodent and human mast cells.

tryptase in the circulation or other body fluids is a good marker of activation of a specific MC population. Although relatively little is know about the biological effects of MC proteinases, recent advances in their identification, cloning and expression, as well as the discovery of proteinase-activated receptors (PAR) and their functions, hold much promise.

A role in gut anaphylaxis
RMCP 2 release from IMMC is thought to mediate components of intestinal anaphylaxis, because challenge of the rat intestine with antigen induced RMCP 2 release, and this correlated with increased mucosal permeability.[211] This may involve in part the degradation by MC proteinases of type IV collagen found in the basal lamina of the epithelium.[198] Although this has not been studied in humans, human MC proteases may play a role in damaging epithelial barrier integrity, thus increasing macromolecule permeability, enhancing antigen uptake, and further facilitating local and systemic inflammatory responses.

A role in host resistance
The chymase MMCP 1, a murine analogue of RMCP 2, is constitutively released into the jejunum and blood of normal mice, suggesting that it has a physiological function.[242] Following infection with *N. brasiliensis*, increased levels of MMCP 1 were found in the jejunum and serum, together with an upregulation of MMCP 1 gene transcription and mucosal MC hyperplasia. Immunohistochemical studies showed MMCP 1 in intraepithelial MC of the jejunum, gastric mucosa and major airways, but not in submucosal and peritoneal MC. Interestingly, only 20% of MMC from the jejunum of normal mice contained MMCP 1, whereas MMC in the stomach were negative for MMCP 1.[210] However, after nematode infection, 100% of jejunal MMC expressed MMCP 1, as did a small number of gastric mucosal MC. MMC in the intestine and gastric mucosa are thus phenotypically distinct and presumably this has some functional significance. The constitutive storage and release of MMCP 1 in normal mice and its upregulation in parasite-infected mice suggest that there are both normal physiological and pathological functions for this MC proteinase.

A role in weaning
In rats, weaning is associated with increased numbers of IMMC, evidence of their activation and increased levels of RMCP 2 in serum. After weaning, serum levels of RMCP 2, IMMC numbers and morphology returned to normal, suggesting a role for IMMC and RMCP 2 during this phase of intestinal development.[56] The immunosuppressant cyclosporin A reduces the numbers of intraepithelial lymphocytes, suppresses RMCP 2 secretion and inhibits maturation of the small intestine, suggesting that the immune system is involved in MC-mediated changes associated with weaning.[54,55] Neurogenic activation of IMMC does not appear to be involved during weaning, because substance P depletion with capsaicin does not prevent weaning-dependent IMMC activation.[53]

Biological activity of human mast cell proteinases
No *in vivo* study of MC proteinase function has been performed in humans, in contrast to rodent MC proteinases. Tryptase has several biological effects, including increased bronchial contractility and the cleavage of a protein closely related to type IV collagenase in the epidermis, suggesting a role in tissue remodelling

or matrix degradation.[1,135,136,212] Human MC tryptase can also stimulate DNA synthesis and proliferation of a human lung epithelial cell line[41] H292, human umbilical vein endothelial cells,[51] and a human lung fibroblast cell line[42] MRC 5, suggesting that tryptase may be involved in epithelial renewal and fibrosis.

In addition, tryptase can potentiate inflammatory responses by inducing neutrophil and eosinophil recruitment. Human MC tryptase stimulates the release of IL8, a potent granulocyte chemoattractant from epithelial[41] and endothelial cells,[42,241] and upregulates the intracellular adhesion molecule ICAM 1 from a human epithelial cell line.[41] Human MC tryptase injected into guinea pig skin or the peritoneum of mice also induces neutrophil and eosinophil recruitment.[50,89] Furthermore, intraperitoneal injection of mice with murine tryptase, MMCP 6, induces a significant and prolonged peritoneal neutrophilia associated with induction by enzymatically active MMCP 6 (but not MMCP 7) of large amounts of IL8 by endothelial cells.[103]

Human MC tryptase may have direct effects on MC as it can induce histamine release from guinea pig skin and lung MC as well as from human tonsil MC, but not from human skin MC.[88,90] Tryptase may also amplify the signal for IgE- and ionophore-induced histamine release, since incubation of human tonsil or skin MC with the tryptase inhibitor APC366 suppressed IgE- and ionophore-induced histamine release.[88] The effects of tryptase on the production of newly generated mediators and on cytokine production from MC must be studied.

Human MC chymase has received less study than tryptase, but some actions have been identified. It can cleave both VIP and substance P,[44] thus attenuating the biological actions of these peptides. Since VIP and substance P can activate some MC, it is possible that, by degrading VIP and substance P, chymase can inhibit MC activation by these peptides.[44,73] Furthermore, chymase mediated cleavage of VIP and substance P can reduce the direct physiological effects of these peptides on smooth muscle.

Proteinase-activated receptors

Recently, a new receptor family known as proteinase-activated receptors (PAR) has been identified which will shed light on biological functions of MC proteinases. Four PAR[59,99,107,235,237] have now been described (PAR$_{1-4}$) and are activated by the serine proteinases thrombin (PAR$_1$, PAR$_3$ and PAR$_4$) and tryptase (PAR$_2$ and PAR$_4$). PAR are activated when thrombin or tryptase cleave an extracellular portion of the PAR, exposing a tethered ligand which binds to an intramolecular site to activate the receptor. Small peptides with sequences similar to the active site on the tethered ligand have been synthesized and used to study the activation of PAR. These PAR-activating peptides (PAR-AP) are designed to activate one PAR selectively.

PAR are widespread and have a multitude of effects. For example, PAR$_2$ and PAR$_3$ are found in the gastrointestinal tract, while PAR$_1$ has yet to be identified in the gut.[59] While little is known of PAR$_3$ in the gut, PAR$_2$ is highly expressed on the apical and basolateral membranes of enterocytes in the gastrointestinal tract and its activation induces PGE synthesis.[119] While the physiological significance of this PAR$_2$ activation is not clear, PGE regulates multiple intestinal functions. Furthermore, tryptase activates PAR$_2$ in the muscularis externa of rat colon,[49] preventing the peristaltic activity of the colon. This suggests that MC tryptase may contribute to MC-dependent motility disturbances of the colon associated with MC degranulation. Recently, trypsin was

shown to regulate intestinal ion transport via a PAR$_2$-dependent increase of short circuit current (Isc).[236]

In addition to PAR-mediated effects on the gastrointestinal tract, activation of PAR$_1$ and PAR$_2$ in human endothelial cells induces vasodilatation and inflammation.[59] Thrombin and MC tryptase can also increase intracellular calcium mobilization in human dermal fibroblasts and keratinocytes respectively, through PAR.[203]

Other effects of thrombin and tryptase may be PAR-mediated. For example, thrombin-mediated activation of mouse cultured BMMC, mobilization of intracellular calcium and mediator release may indeed be PAR-mediated.[11,186,190] Thrombin has also been reported to induce histamine release from rat PMC.[222] Furthermore, PAR-mediated thrombin-induced rat paw oedema is suppressed if MC function is compromised by in vivo administration[236] with compound 48/80. However, the precise mechanism underlying the MC dependency of thrombin (PAR)-mediated inflammation is unknown. Future work using specific PAR-AP and PAR antagonists, thrombin and tryptase will help to determine the cellular distribution and specific functions of PAR, and will likely indicate which MC proteinases and PAR are involved in pathophysiological conditions such as gut anaphylaxis.

Mast cell nitric oxide and superoxide production

In the last decade there has been much research on endothelium-derived relaxing factor, nitric oxide (NO). Rat MMC and CTMC produce low levels of NO[34,60,111,143,201] that appear to be significant in tissue homeostasis and pathophysiological responses.[58,109,110,146,197] In addition, mediator release from MC can be regulated by NO. For example, NO suppresses secretion of histamine, PAF and RMCP 2 from MC.[110,146,202] Conversely, reduction of NO production by NO synthase (NOS) inhibitors increases histamine release from rat PMC.[110,140] The relatively selective inhibitor of constitutive NOS (cNOS), N^G-nitro-L-arginine methyl ester (L-NAME), causes a rapid release of mediators from IMMC thought to be responsible for increased ileal epithelial permeability.[110] A recent report confirmed that NOS inhibitors induced RMCP 2 release, while NO donors decreased RMCP 2 release.[188] Whether NO that suppresses release of MC mediators is derived from MC or from other cell types, e.g. macrophages,[60] is a question that requires additional study (Fig. 6.3). NO is also involved in suppression of cytokine production[13,227] and neutrophil adhesion,[173] suggesting that it has widespread anti-inflammatory activities. For example, L-NAME-mediated inhibition of NO synthesis led to an ICAM 1-dependent neutrophil adhesion to endothelial cells in the presence of MC.[173] In addition, NO donors reversed the L-NAME-mediated increase in neutrophil adhesion. When MC were absent, NO inhibition did not affect neutrophil adhesion, suggesting that in this system MC are the source of NO which regulates neutrophil adhesion.

Proinflammatory action of nitric oxide

In addition to potential anti-inflammatory roles for NO, there is evidence that it may have proinflammatory roles. Inflammatory conditions are often associated with elevated production of NO by the inducible form of NOS (iNOS). Intestinal injury in sepsis correlates with increased NO metabolites and iNOS activity. Some controversy exists about the treatment rationale for this inflammatory condition since one report suggested that iNOS inhibition reduced sepsis-mediated intestinal injury, while another showed that inhibition of iNOS worsened sepsis.[36,86] The sources

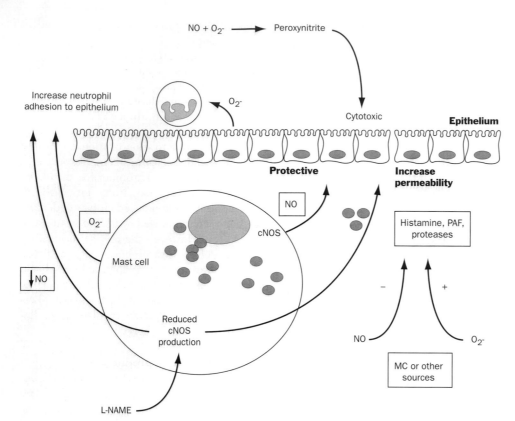

Fig. 6.3 Effects of nitric oxide (NO) and superoxide (O^{2-}) derived from intestinal mast cells (MC) and other cells in the regulation of intestinal epithelial barrier function and a possible protective role for the MC in modulating epithelial barrier integrity. Since constitutive NO production by MC helps to maintain the epithelial barrier integrity, L-NAME-mediated suppression of NO production leads to epithelial damage, perhaps via upregulating the release of preformed mediators which increase epithelial permeability. Preformed mediator release from intestinal MC is suppressed by NO production, but enhanced with superoxide generation by MC or other cells. Reduced NO and increased superoxide production from MC increases neutrophil adhesion to epithelium, as does superoxide release from epithelial cells. Peroxynitrite can be formed from the reaction of NO and superoxide generated by mast cells or other cells. Figure adapted from Alican and Kubes,[5] and Stenton et al.[220]

of iNOS in human intestinal inflammation are unclear. However, iNOS can be upregulated in macrophages and its inhibition can reduce inflammation.[172] Low levels of NO produced by cNOS may be beneficial in many settings, whereas markedly enhanced production of NO by iNOS can be detrimental.[5] Highly specific inhibitors of each form of NOS are becoming available and promise to help clarify the source and significance of NO in host defence and tissue injury.

Superoxide

MC also produce superoxide, a strong oxidizing molecule with many actions, such as neutrophil attraction and adhesion to endothelial cells.[93,94,173] In addition to superoxide production by endothelial cells, superoxide generation by MC may play a role in inflammatory conditions (Fig. 6.3). Furthermore, since NO and superoxide can be converted to the highly cytotoxic product peroxynitrite, it is possible that MC-derived NO and superoxide can be converted to peroxynitrite, resulting in tissue damage.[164] Interestingly, MC also produce the antioxidants superoxide dismutase and peroxidase which can metabolize and inhibit oxidants such as superoxide.[93,94] Clearly, in addition to discovering that MC may produce NO, the recent suggestion that MC can produce oxidizing mediators such as superoxide is important and may be valuable in elucidating the roles of MC in inflammation.

Therefore, MC are a source of NO and can be affected by elevated or decreased NO levels. The release of MC mediators fluctuates accordingly, with subsequent physiological or pathological effects. In addition to NO production, MC activation can release superoxide and generate peroxynitrite, both of which damage tissue and cause inflammation. More work is needed to establish the exact role of MC and their production of, and regulation by, NO, superoxide and peroxynitrite in various inflammatory disorders.

Mast cell cytokines

MC activation releases several chemotactic, growth and regulatory factors believed to be in part responsible for late phase reactions.[16,133] Many cytokines and chemokines are released by MC, including TNF, IFNγ, IL3, IL4, IL6, IL8, IL16 and RANTES (Table 6.1). Moreover, MC of different phenotypes do not store or synthesize the same cytokines. For example, IL4, IL10 and IL13 are constitutively released by mouse BMMC cultured in IL3, but in the absence of exogenous stimulation.[144,218] However, BMMC that develop in the presence of SCF only produced IL10 and IL13 after Fcε-RI-mediated activation or stimulation with exogenous IL3. Despite these interesting and important results, the factors that influence the expression, storage and/or secretion of different cytokines in MC are inadequately understood, especially in the human. Furthermore, cells other than MC can produce the same cytokines and whether MC or other cells are the most important source remains to be determined.

Recent reports suggest that some MC cytokines exhibit anti-inflammatory properties. IL4, IL10 and IL13 can be released by MC and have been shown to reduce the release of TNF by monocytes and macrophages (Fig. 6.4).[7,108,154,248] Furthermore, IL10 may inhibit IFNγ-mediated damage to the epithelial barrier.[2,140] Interestingly, clinical trials have since shown that 50% of patients with Crohn's disease treated with IL10 experienced complete remission within 3 weeks of treatment, compared to 23% of those who received placebo.[232] Whether MC-derived IL10 plays such a regulatory role in vivo remains to be determined.

TNF is produced by both rodent and human MC, and has many actions, such as stimulation of neutrophil degranulation and the production of IL1, IL6 and GM-CSF.[22,80,134,221] Patients with IBD often have elevated levels of TNFα in serum and stool samples[141,170] and a single intravenous infusion of monoclonal anti-

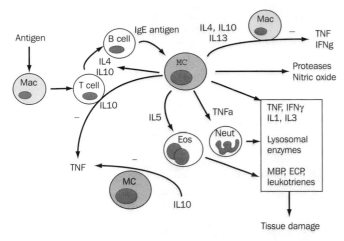

Fig. 6.4 Pathophysiology of allergic inflammation and cytokine-mediated cell–cell interaction. Pathways labelled with (–) represent an inhibitory action of mast cell cytokines on the production of cellular mediators and may represent tissue protective pathways. Abbreviations: MC (mast cell), Mac (macrophage), Eos (eosinophil), Neut (neutrophil). Figure adapted from Stenton et al.[220]

bodies to TNF improved symptoms in patients with Crohn's disease.[225,233] Since IMMC produce TNF, they may play a role in TNF-mediated effects in the intestine. Interestingly, MC-derived IL10 may play an autocrine role in regulating TNF release from MC (Fig. 6.4).[132] When antibodies to IL10 were used to neutralize MC IL10, TNF release from resting and antigen-activated MC was significantly increased.

Stem cell factor and mast cell activation

SCF is an important growth and differentiation factor for MC and has also been shown to induce or modulate mediator secretion. When fibroblasts and bone marrow cells are cocultured in IL3 and SCF, histamine and eotaxin can be released.[96] This suggests that bone marrow cells differentiate into histamine and eotaxin secreting MC. Moreover, eotaxin and histamine release was suppressed by anti-SCF antibody, or following separation of the fibroblasts from the MC,[96] suggesting that fibroblast–mast cell contact and SCF plays an important role in histamine release and eotaxin production. In rats, SCF alone does not induce histamine release, but it can potentiate Fcε-RI-dependent release of histamine, RMCP 2 and β-hexosaminidase, but not Fcε-RI-independent histamine release.[95,111] Interestingly, SCF did not potentiate Fcε-RI-mediated production of TNF or NO from rat PMC, suggesting that SCF differentially regulates mediator release.[132,134]

Human studies

Similar experiments have been performed on MC isolated from resected specimens of non-inflamed human intestine. Stimulation of these MC with SCF or anti-IgE did not release histamine or LT, whereas costimulation with SCF and antigen induced significant histamine and LT release.[28] This SCF potentiation of antigen-induced histamine release was more apparent with MC isolated from intestines of patients with IBD. By contrast, a recent study showed that, while SCF or IgE stimulation of human lung MC induced low levels of mediator release, costimulation with SCF and anti-IgE did not potentiate mediator release compared to additive effects of anti-IgE and SCF alone.[78] Similar data were

obtained using human interlobar bronchi without isolating MC.[230] SCF mimicked the actions of anti-IgE in releasing histamine and arachidonic acid metabolites from the bronchi, while SCF did not potentiate anti-IgE-induced mediator release.[230] Furthermore, treatment with SCF or anti-IgE caused contraction of the bronchi, which could be blocked by pretreatment with LT and histamine receptor antagonists.[230] Hence SCF can induce significant mediator release from human lung MC, but not from human intestinal MC, whereas SCF can potentiate anti-IgE-induced mediator release from both lung and intestinal MC. Clearly, additional study of the effects of SCF on MC activation is needed.

Mast cells and host defence
Mast cells and innate immunity to bacteria

A growing body of evidence suggests that MC are likely to be involved in innate immunity to bacterial infection. For example, MC are activated and release mediators in response to the bacterial product lipopolysaccharide (LPS).[76] Furthermore, bacterial infection can activate complement, which in turn activates MC directly or indirectly.[187] Indeed, while mice deficient in complement C3 exhibit suppressed MC mediator release, reduced neutrophil recruitment and diminished bacterial clearance in a caecal ligation and puncture model of acute peritonitis (CLP), treatment of C3-deficient mice with C3 protein before CLP reduced the mortality rate.[187] TNF is one MC-derived mediator believed to be important in mediating immunity to bacteria. In addition to the observation that MC-derived TNF mediates recruitment of bactericidal neutrophils, MC promote the clearance of *Klebsiella pneumoniae* from the peritoneal cavity and lungs of mice and reduce mortality rates associated with peritoneal infection.[142] Moreover, reconstitution of MC-deficient mice with MC reduced the mortality rate induced by CLP, suggesting that MC have antibacterial properties.[61] This MC-dependent antibacterial effect was at least in part TNF-mediated as shown by TNF neutralizing antibodies. Furthermore, recombinant TNF treatment of MC-deficient mice was also protective.[61]

Finally, since a reduction in MC numbers correlated with reduced immunity to bacterial infections, it was not surprising that an increase in MC numbers mediated by repeat administration of SCF increased immunity to bacterial infection induced by CLP in mice.[151] While MC may play a role in mediating immunity to bacterial infections in mice, less is known of the role of human MC in innate immunity to bacterial infections. However, it may be clinically useful to potentiate MC activity in immunocompromised humans to control or suppress bacterial infections.

Mast cells and acquired immunity to parasites

It is well recognized that there is a marked hyperplasia of IMMC and synthesis of IgE in response to helminth infections.[14,155,156,194] Parasitic infection stimulates IL3 production, which is a multipotent haematopoietic growth factor[133,180] and acts to induce MC differentiation and proliferation. As a result there is an increase in MC progenitors and maturation in the intestinal lamina propria.[82] Furthermore, in IL3-deficient mice, mastocytosis and worm expulsion were impaired following infection with *Strongyloides venezuelensis*.[124] Moreover, MC activation and mediator release correlates with expulsion of *Trichinella spiralis*.[4] In addition to IL3-deficient mice, in MC-deficient mice worm expulsion is either delayed or unaffected by the absence of MC.[155,194] Helminth infection induces intestinal mastocytosis, and elimination of this increase in MC slows down parasite expulsion. Pharmacological studies, which either inhibit MC degranulation or antagonize the released mediators, provide strong evidence that histamine[194] and arachidonic acid metabolites[160] play important roles in parasite expulsion. For example, activation of MC released LTB_4 which killed the protozoan *Toxoplasma gondii*.[92] Incubation with A-63162 and MK-866, two agents that specifically block LT production, prevented killing of this parasite, whereas incubation with the COX inhibitor indomethacin, which prevents PG synthesis, had no effect on MC-mediated killing. Thus there is substantial evidence implicating MC in host defence.

Overview of mast cells and food intolerance

Gastrointestinal food allergy is a significant problem in about 5% of the population, with a higher prevalence in children than in the elderly. Abundant evidence has implicated MC in intestinal hypersensitivity reactions to food since 1940, when food antigen-dependent reactions were observed *in vitro* following passive sensitization of human ileum and colon.[81] While the exact mechanisms of action are not clear, MC mediators such as histamine may be important in intestinal anaphylaxis, since patients with food allergy show elevated histamine release from the duodenum after antigen challenge compared with normal subjects.[10,24]

Animal models

The use of animal models of intestinal anaphylaxis and pharmacological agents designed to block the effects of MC mediators have provided considerable information about the role of MC in intestinal inflammation. MC mediators such as histamine, PG, LT and 5HT increase intestinal motility in a similar manner to challenge with food allergens, and antagonists to many of the MC mediators reduce these symptoms.[39,207,240] For example, in rats sensitive to hen egg ovalbumin (OVA), the $5HT_1$ receptor antagonist methysergide and the cyclo-oxygenase inhibitor, indomethacin, blocked allergen-mediated increase in motility.[208,209] The MC stabilizers DSCG and doxantrazole also inhibited antigen-induced changes in motility of rat jejunal smooth muscle, while compound 48/80 and concanavalin A, MC secretagogues, induced changes in motility, providing strong evidence for MC involvement in these motility changes.[208,209] MC stabilizers, inhibitors of PG and LT synthesis, and LT and PAF antagonists all inhibited antigen-mediated contraction of colonic smooth muscle. However, histamine and 5HT antagonists as well as atropine and tetrodotoxin did not.[179] These studies suggest that antigen-mediated increase in jejunal motility and colonic contraction were MC-dependent, but differentially regulated; serotonin was involved in jejunal motility but not colonic contraction. Moreover, antigen challenge reduced the number of granulated MC in the colon.[179] Pharmacological agents also implied a role for MC in food allergen-induced alteration of intestinal transit of food[185] and ion transport in intestinal epithelium.[52]

Transforming growth factor β and interferon γ

Intestinal MC may also be involved in the normal tolerance to food antigens. For example, TGFβ, a cytokine with anti-inflammatory properties in the intestine, prevents colitis in normal mice.[145,243] It has been suggested that food antigens induce intestinal production of IFNγ by Th1 cells and TGFβ production by antigen non-specific suppressor T cells.[243] Usually, the latter prevails, and oral tolerance for the ingested antigen is established. When IL12 is coadministered with a food antigen, TGFβ production and oral tolerance is enhanced.[145] Furthermore, when anti-TGFβ is coadministered with a food antigen, inflammatory disease occurs, probably because of the removal of the anti-inflammatory properties of TGFβ.[145] Thus, it seems likely that there is a balance in IFNγ and TGFβ production in non-diseased intestine and that an alteration of this balance towards excess IFNγ production leads to intestinal inflammation and colitis. This IFNγ and TGFβ balance may play an important role in human colitis.[9]

Recent studies have shown that TGFβ1 suppresses IgE-mediated histamine and TNF release, but not NO production by rat PMC.[33] Furthermore, treatment of cells with anti-TGFβ1 abrogated the TGFβ1-mediated suppression of mediator release and potentiated the spontaneous release of histamine and TNF from untreated PMC.[96] Therefore, in non-inflamed intestine it is possible that the constitutive production of TGFβ has anti-inflammatory properties by suppressing mediator release from MC. Another possible role for MC in TGFβ-mediated inhibition of intestinal inflammation stems from the observation that human and rodent MC contain TGFβ,[33,114,159] and that this TGFβ is released spontaneously.[33,159] Thus, MC may play a role in maintaining oral tolerance to food antigens by constitutively releasing TGFβ. Further study of MC in food tolerance will provide knowledge that may be useful in treatment of patients with food allergies.

Diagnosis of food intolerance

In addition to existing clinical techniques for identifying intolerance to allergens found in food, a new technique called colonoscopic allergen provocation (COLAP) has recently been reported to be a useful tool for the diagnosis of food allergy in humans.[25,26] During endoscopy, antigen is injected into the intestinal mucosa, and positive or negative reactions are recorded. This test may be more useful than existing tests since some patients exhibit positive colonic responses to certain food antigens in the absence of positive skin or RAST tests.

SUMMARY

MC have a variety of effects in regulating allergic and physiological responses to various stimuli. Intestinal MC clearly have a role in many pathological conditions such as food intolerance. On the other hand, intestinal MC appear to play important physiological roles, such as in weaning and in host resistance to parasitic and microbial infections. They have both beneficial and harmful effects, but the mechanisms that control the balance of these effects are poorly known. Various cytokines are involved and, recently, MC-derived NO and superoxide have been identified as other important factors in regulating pathophysiological responses. In addition, further study of MC proteinases will markedly enhance our understanding of MC functions. The ability of the nervous system to modulate MC function and the effects of MC on the nervous system are areas of enormous potential that may lead to new opportunities for therapeutic and management strategies.

REFERENCES

1 Adams JC, Watt FM. Fibronectin inhibits the terminal differentiation of human keratinocytes. *Nature* 1989; 340: 307–9.

2 Adams RB, Planchon SM, Roche JK. IFN-gamma modulation of epithelial barrier function. Time course, reversibility, and site of cytokine binding. *J Immunol* 1993; 150: 2356–63.

3 Agis H, Willheim M, Sperr WR *et al*. Monocytes do not make mast cells when cultured in the presence of SCF. Characterization of the circulating mast cell progenitor as a c-*kit*+, CD34 +, Ly–, CD14–, CD17–, colony-forming cell. *J Immunol* 1993; 151: 4221–7.

4 Ahmad A, Wang CH, Bell RG. A role for IgE in intestinal immunity. Expression of rapid expulsion of *Trichinella spiralis* in rats transfused with IgE and thoracic duct lymphocytes. *J Immunol* 1991; 146: 3563–70.

5 Alican I, Kubes P. A critical role for nitric oxide in intestinal barrier function and dysfunction. *Am J Physiol* 1996; 270: G225–37.

6 Amoui M, Draberova L, Tolar P, Draber P. Direct interaction of Syk and Lyn protein tyrosine kinases in rat basophilic leukemia cells activated via type 1 Fc epsilon receptors. *Eur J Immunol* 1997; 27: 321–8.

7 Armstrong L, Jordan N, Millar A. Interleukin 10 (IL-10) regulation of tumour necrosis factor alpha (TNF-α) from human alveolar macrophages and peripheral blood monocytes. *Thorax* 1996; 51: 143–9.

8 Ashman RI, Jarboe DJ, Conrad DH, Huff TF. The mast cell-committed progenitor. In vivo generation of committed progenitors from bone marrow. *J Immunol* 1991; 146: 211–16.

9 Babyatsky MW, Rossiter G, Podolsky DK. Expression of transforming growth factor alpha and beta in colonic mucosa in inflammatory bowel disease. *Gastroenterology* 1996; 110: 975–84.

10 Baenkler HW, Lux G. Antigen-induced histamine-release from duodenal biopsy in gastrointestinal food allergy. *Ann Allergy* 1989; 62: 449–52.

11 Baranes D, Liu FT, Razin E. Thrombin and IgE antigen induce formation of inositol phosphates by mouse E-mast cells. *FEBS Lett* 1986; 206: 64–8.

12 Baraniuk JN, Kowalski ML, Kaliner MA. Relationship between permeable vessels, nerves and mast cells in rat cutaneous neurogenic inflammation. *J Appl Physiol* 1990; 68: 2305–11.

13 Bauer H, Jung T, Tsikas D *et al*. Nitric oxide inhibits the secretion of T helper 1- and T-helper 2-associated cytokines in activated human T cells. *Immunology* 1997; 90: 205–11.

14 Befus AD. Mast cells that are polymorphic! *Reg Immunol* 1989; 2: 176–87.

15 Befus AD. Reciprocity of mast cell nervous–system interactions. In: *Innervation of the Gut: Pathophysiological Implications*. (Taché Y, Wingate DL, Burks TF, eds). CRC Press, Boca Raton, 1993: 315–29.

16 Befus AD. The immunophysiology of mast cells in intestinal immunity and symbiosis. In: *Infections of the Gastrointestinal Tract*. (Blaser MJ, Smith PD, Ravdin JI, Greenberg HB, Guerrant RL, eds). Raven Press, New York 1995: 227–36.

17 Befus AD, Chin B, Pick J *et al*. Proteinases of rat mast cells. Peritoneal but not intestinal mucosal mast cells express mast cell proteinase 5 and carboxypeptidase. *J Immunol* 1995; 155: 4406–11.

18 Befus AD, Denburg JA. Basophilic leucocytes: mast cells and basophils. In: *Winthrobe's Clinical Hematology* (Lee GR, Foerster J, Lukens J *et al*., eds). Williams and Wilkins, Baltimore; 1998: 362–76.

19 Befus AD, Dyck N, Goodacre R, Bienenstock J. Mast cells from human intestinal lamina propria. Isolation, histochemical subtypes, and functional characterization. *J Immunol* 1987; 138: 2604–10.

20 Befus AD, Mowat C, Hu J *et al*. Neutrophil defensins induce histamine secretion from mast cells: mechanisms of action. *J Immunol* 1999; 163: 947–53.

21 Befus AD, Pearce FL, Gauldie J *et al*. Mucosal mast cells. I. Isolation and functional characteristics of rat intestinal mast cells. *J Immunol* 1982; 128: 2475–80.

22 Benyon RC, Bissonnette EY, Befus AD. Tumor necrosis factor-alpha dependent cytotoxicity of human skin mast cells is enhanced by anti-IgE antibodies. *J Immunol* 1991; 147: 2253–8.

23 Bevan S, Szolcsanyi J. Sensory neuron-specific actions of capsaicin: mechanisms and applications. *Trends Pharmacol Sci* 1990; 11: 30–3.

24 Bischoff SC, Grabowski J, Manns MP. Quantification of inflammatory mediators in stool samples of patients with inflammatory bowel disorders and controls. *Dig Dis Sci* 1997; 42: 394–403.

25 Bischoff SC, Mayer J, Meier PN *et al*. Clinical significance of the colonoscopic allergen provocation test. *Int Arch Allergy Immunol* 1997; 113: 348–51.

26 Bischoff SC, Mayer J, Wedemeyer J *et al*. Colonoscopic allergen provocation (COLAP): a new diagnostic approach for gastrointestinal food allergy. *Gut* 1997; 40: 745–53.

27 Bischoff SC, Schwenberg S, Raab R, Manns MP. Functional properties of human intestinal mast cells cultured in a new culture system: enhancement of IgE receptor-dependent mediator release and response to stem cell factor. *J Immunol* 1997; 159: 5560–7.

28 Bischoff SC, Schwengberg S, Wordelmann K *et al*. Effect of c-kit ligand, stem cell factor, on mediator release by human intestinal mast cells isolated from patients with inflammatory bowel disease and controls. *Gut* 1996; 38: 104–14.

29 Bissonnette EY, Befus AD. Anti-inflammatory effect of β2-agonists: Inhibition of TNF-α release from human mast cells. *J Allergy Clin Immunol* 1997; 100: 825–31.

30 Bissonnette EY, Befus AD. Modulation of mast cell function in the gastrointestinal tract. In: *Immunopharmacology of the Gastrointestinal System*. (Wallace JL, ed.) London: Academic Press, 1993: 95–103.

31 Bissonnette EY, Chin B, Befus AD. Isolation and characterization of rat intestinal mucosal mast cells. In: *Methods in Gastrointestinal Pharmacology*. (Gaginella TS, ed.) CRC Press, 1995: 401–18.

32 Bissonnette EY, Enciso JA, Befus AD. Interferon and antiallergic drug regulation of histamine and tumour necrosis factor-alpha (TNF-alpha) in rat mast cell subsets. *Intl Arch Allergy Immunol* 1995; 107: 156–7.

33 Bissonnette EY, Enciso JA, Befus AD. TGF-beta 1 inhibits the release of histamine and tumor necrosis factor-alpha from mast cells through an autocrine pathway. *Am J Rep Cell Mol Biol* 1997; 16: 275–82.

34 Bissonnette EY, Hogaboam CM, Wallace JL, Befus AD. Potentiation of tumor necrosis factor-alpha-mediated cytotoxicity of mast cells by their production of nitric oxide. *J Immunol* 1991; 147: 3060–5.

35 Blennerhassett MG, Tomioka M, Bienenstock J. Formation of contacts between mast cells and sympathetic neurons *in vitro*. *Cell Tissue Res* 1991; 265: 121–8.

36 Boughton-Smith NK, Evans SM, Laszlo F *et al*. The induction of nitric oxide synthase and intestinal vascular permeability by endotoxin in the rat. *Br J Pharmacol* 1993; 110: 1189–95.

37 Bradding P, Okayama Y, Howarth PH *et al*. Heterogeneity of human mast cells based on cytokine content. *J Immunol* 1995; 55: 297–307.

38 Broide DH, Wasserman SI, Alvaro-Garcia J *et al*. Transforming growth factor-β1 selectively inhibits IL-3 dependent mast cell proliferation without affecting mast cell function or differentiation. *J Immunol* 1989; 143: 1591–7.

39 Burakoff R, Nastos E, Won S, Percy WH. Comparison of the effects of leukotrienes B4 and D4 on distal colonic motility in the rabbit in vivo. *Am J Physiol* 1989; 257: G860–4.

40 Butterfield JH, Weiler D, Dewald G, Gleich GJ. Establishment of an immature mast cell line from a patient with mast cell leukemia. *Leukemia Res* 1988; 12: 345–55.

41 Cairns JA, Walls AF. Mast cell tryptase is a mitogen for epithelial cells. Stimulation of IL-8 production and intercellular adhesion molecule-1 expression. *J Immunol* 1996; 156: 275–83.

42 Cairns JA, Walls AF. Mast cell tryptase stimulates the synthesis of type I collagen in human lung fibroblasts. *J Clin Invest* 1997; 99: 1313–21.

43 Caughey GH. The structure and airway biology of mast cell proteinases. *Am J Resp Cell Mol Biol* 1991; 4: 387–94.

44 Caughey GH, Leidig F, Viro NF, Nadel JA. Substance P and vasoactive intestinal peptide degradation by mast cell tryptase and chymase. *J Pharmacol Exp Ther* 1988; 244: 133–7.

45 Chakravarty N. The role of protein kinase C in histamine secretion from mast cells. *Acta Physiol Scand* 1990; 139: 319–31.

46 Chan BMC, Neill K, Froese A. Factor-independent tissue cultured mast cells: establishment from rat peritoneal mast cells. *Immunol Lett* 1988; 18: 37–42.

47 Christian EP, Undem BJ, Weinreich D. Endogenous histamine excites neurons in the guinea pig superior cervical ganglion *in vitro*. *J Physiol* 1989; 409: 297–312.

48 Church MK, el-Lati S, Okayama Y. Biological properties of human skin mast cells. *Clin Exp Allergy* 1991; 21 (Suppl 3): 1–9.

49 Corvera CU, Déry O, McConalogue K *et al.* Mast cell tryptase regulates rat colonic myocytes through proteinase-activated receptor 2. *J Clin Invest* 1997; 100: 1383–93.

50 Costa JJ, Weller PF, Galli SJ. The cells of the allergic response: mast cells, basophils, and eosinophils. *JAMA* 1997; 278: 1815–22.

51 Crompton SJ, Cairns JA, Holgate ST, Walls AF. The role of mast cell tryptase in regulating endothelial cell proliferation, cytokine release, and adhesion molecule expression: tryptase induces expression of mRNA for IL-1 beta and IL-8 and stimulates selective release of IL-8 from human umbilical vein endothelial cells. *J Immunol* 1998; 161: 1939–46.

52 Crowe SE, Sestini P, Perdue MH. Allergic reactions of rat jejunal mucosa. Ion transport responses to luminal antigen and inflammatory mediators. *Gastroenterology* 1990; 99: 74–82.

53 Cummins AG, Antoniou D, Thompson FM. Neuropeptide depletion by capsaicin does not prevent mucosal mast cell activation in the rat at weaning. *Immunol Cell Biol* 1994; 72: 230–3.

54 Cummins AG, Labroy JT, Shearman DJ. The effect of cyclosporin A in delaying maturation of the small intestine during weaning in the rat. *Clin Exp Immunol* 1989; 75: 451–6.

55 Cummins AG, Munro GH, Ferguson A. Effect of cyclosporin A on rat mucosal mast cells and the associated proteinase RMCPII. *Clin Exp Immunol* 1988; 72: 136–40.

56 Cummins AG, Munro GH, Miller HR, Ferguson A. Association of maturation of the small intestine at weaning with mucosal mast cell activation in the rat. *Immunol Cell Biol* 1988; 66: 417–22.

57 Dar O, Pecht I. Fcε receptor mediated Ca^{2+} influx into mast cells is modulated by the concentration of cytosolic free Ca^{2+} ions. *FEBS Letters* 1992; 310: 123–8.

58 Davies NM, Jamali F. Pharmacological protection of NSAID-induced intestinal permeability in the rat: effect of tempo and metronidazole as potential free radical scavengers. *Hum Exp Toxicol* 1997; 16: 345–9.

59 Déry O, Corvera CU, Steinhoff M, Bunnet NW. Proteinase-activated receptors: novel mechanisms of signaling by serine proteinases. *Am J Physiol* 1998; 43: C1429–C52.

60 Eastmond NC, Banks EM, Coleman JW. Nitric oxide inhibits IgE-mediated degranulation of mast cells and is the principal intermediate in IFN-gamma-induced suppression of exocytosis. *J Immunol* 1997; 159: 1444–50.

61 Echtenacher B, Männel DN, Hültner L. Critical protective role of mast cells in a model of acute septic peritonitis. *Nature* 1996; 381: 75–7.

62 Enerbäck L. Mast cells in rat gastrointestinal mucosa. I. Effect of fixation. *Acta Path Micro Scand* 1966; 66: 289–302.

63 Enerbäck L. Mast cells in rat gastrointestinal mucosa. II. Dye binding and metachromatic properties. *Acta Path Micro Scand* 1966; 66: 303–12.

64 Enerbäck L. Mast cells in rat gastrointestinal mucosa. III. Reactivity towards compound 48/80. *Acta Path Micro Scand* 1966; 66: 312–22.

65 Ennis M, Barrow SE, Blair IA. Prostaglandin and histamine release from stimulated rat peritoneal mast cells. *Agents Actions* 1984; 14: 397–400.

66 Fasolato C, Hoth M, Matthews G, Penner R. Ca^{2+} and Mn^{2+} influx through receptor-mediated activation of non-specific cation channels in mast cells. *Proc Natl Acad Sci USA* 1993; 90: 3068–72.

67 Ferris CD, Huganir RL, Supattapone S, Snyder SH. Purified inositol 1,4,5-trisphosphate receptor mediates calcium flux in reconstituted lipid vesicles. *Nature* 1989; 342: 87–9.

68 Ford-Huchinson AW, Bray MA, Doig MV *et al.* Leukotriene B, a potent chemokinetic and aggregating substance released from polymorphonuclear leukocytes. *Nature* 1980; 286: 264–5.

69 Foreman JC. Non-immunological stimuli of mast cells and basophil leukocytes. In: *Immunopharmacology of Mast Cells and Basophils.* (Foreman JC, ed.). Academic Press, San Diego, 1993: 57–69.

70 Foreman JC, Mongar JL, Gomperts BD. Calcium ionophores and movement of calcium ions following the physiological stimulus to a secretory process. *Nature* 1973; 245: 249–51.

71 Foreman JC, Piotrowski W. Peptides and histamine release. *J Allergy Clin Immunol* 1984; 74: 127–31.

72 Fox CC, Dvorak AM, Peters SP *et al.* Isolation and characterization of human intestinal mucosal mast cells. *J Immunol* 1985; 135: 483–91.

73 Franconi GM, Graf PD, Lazarus SC *et al.* Mast cell tryptase and chymase reverse airway smooth muscle relaxation induced by vasoactive intestinal peptide in the ferret. *J Pharmacol Exp Ther* 1989; 248: 947–51.

74 Fureder W, Agis H, Willheim M *et al.* Differential expression of complement receptors on human basophils and mast cells. Evidence for mast cell heterogeneity and CD88/C5aR expression on skin mast cells. *J Immunol* 1995; 155: 3152–60.

75 Galli SJ. The mast cell: a versatile effector cell for a challenging world. *Int Arch Allergy Immunol* 1997; 113: 14–22.

76 Galli SJ, Maurer M, Lantz CS. Mast cells as sentinels of innate immunity. *Curr Opin Immunol* 1999; 11: 53–9.

77 Germano P, Gomez J, Kazanietz MG *et al.* Phosphorylation of the gamma chain of the high affinity receptor for immunoglobulin E by receptor-associated protein kinase C-delta. *J Biol Chem* 1994; 269: 23102–7.

78 Gibbs BF, Arm JP, Gibson K *et al.* Human lung mast cells release small amounts of interleukin-4 and tumour necrosis factor-alpha in response to stimulation by anti-IgE and stem cell factor. *Eur J Pharmacol* 1997; 327: 73–8.

79 Goetzl EJ, Picket WC. Novel structural determinants of the human neutrophil chemotactic activity of leukotriene B. *J Exp Med* 1982; 153: 482–7.

80 Gordon JR, Galli SJ. Release of both preformed and newly synthesized tumor necrosis factor alpha (TNF-alpha)/cachectin by mouse mast cells stimulated via the Fc epsilon RI. A mechanism for the sustained action of mast cell-derived TNF-alpha during IgE-dependent biological responses. *J Exp Med* 1991; 174: 103–7.

81 Gray I, Harten M, Walzer M. Studies in mucous membrane hypersensitiveness. IV. The allergic reaction in the passively sensitized mucous membranes of the ileum and colon in humans. *Am J Int Med* 1940; 13: 2050–61.

82 Guy-Grand D, Dy M, Luffau G, Vassalli P. Gut mucosal mast cells: origin, traffic and differentiation. *J Exp Med* 1984; 160: 12–28.

83 Haig DM, Huntley JF, Mackellar A *et al.* Effects of stem cell factor (*kit*-ligand) and interleukin-3 on the growth and serine proteinase expression of rat bone marrow-derived or serosal mast cells. *Blood* 1994; 83: 72–83.

84 Haig DM, Menamin C, Redmond J *et al.* Rat IL-3 stimulates the growth of rat mucosal mast cells in culture. *Immunology* 1988; 65: 205–11.

85 Harada M, Sumichika H, Hamano S *et al.* IL-3 derived from CD4+ T cells is essential for the in vitro expansion of mast cells from the normal adult mouse spleen. *Clin Exp Immunol* 1996; 106: 149–55.

86 Harbrecht BG, Billiar TR, Stadler J *et al.* Inhibition of nitric oxide synthesis during endotoxemia promotes intrahepatic thrombosis and an oxygen radical-mediated hepatic injury. *J Leukoc Biol* 1992; 52: 390–4.

87 Hardy CC, Robinson C, Tattersfield AE, Holgate ST. The bronchoconstrictor effect of inhaled prostaglandin D_2 in normal and asthmatic men. *N Engl J Med* 1984; 311: 209–13.

88 He S, Gaca MD, Walls AF. A role for tryptase in the activation of human mast cell: modulation of histamine release by tryptase and inhibitors of tryptase. *J Pharmacol Exp Ther* 1998; 286: 289–97.

89 He S, Peng Q, Walls AF. Potent induction of a neutrophil and eosinophil-rich infiltrate in vivo by human mast cell tryptase: selective enhancement of eosinophil recruitment by histamine. *J Immunol* 1997; 159: 6216–25.

90 He S, Walls AF. Human mast cell tryptase: a stimulus of microvascular leakage and mast cell activation. *Eur J Pharmacol* 1997; 328: 89–97.

91 Heavey DJ, Ernst P, Stevens RL *et al.* Generation of leukotriene C4, leukotriene B4 and prostaglandin D2 by immunologically activated rat intestinal mucosa mast cells. *J Immunol* 1988; 140: 1953–7.

92 Henderson WR, Chi EY. The importance of leukotrienes in mast cell-mediated *Toxoplasma gondii* cytotoxicity. *J Infect Dis* 1998; 177: 1437–43.

93 Henderson WR, Kaliner M. Immunologic and non-immunologic generation of superoxide from mast cells and basophils. *J Clin Invest* 1978; 61: 187–96.

94 Henderson WR, Kaliner M. Mast cell granule peroxidase: location secretion and SRS-A inactivation. *J Immunol* 1979; 122: 1322–8.

95 Hill PB, MacDonald AJ, Thornton EM *et al*. Stem cell factor enhances immunoglobulin E-dependent mediator release from cultured rat bone marrow-derived mast cells: activation of previously unresponsive cells demonstrated by a novel ELISPOT assay. *Immunology* 1996; 87: 326–33.

96 Hogaboam C, Kunkel SL, Streiter RM *et al*. Novel role of transmembrane SCF for mast cell activation and eotaxin production in mast cell–fibroblast interactions. *J Immunol* 1998; 160: 6166–71.

97 Holgate SJ. The immunopharmacology of mild asthma. *J Allergy Clin Immunol* 1996; 98: S7–S16.

98 Holgate ST, Burns GB, Robinson C, Church MK. Anaphylactic- and calcium-dependent generation of prostaglandin D_2 (PGD_2), thromboxane B2, and other cyclooxygenase products of arachidonic acid by dispersed human lung cells and relationship to histamine release. *J Immunol* 1984; 133: 2138–44.

99 Hollenberg MD. Proteinase-mediated signalling: new paradigms for cell regulation and drug development. *Trends Pharmacol Sci* 1996; 17: 3–6.

100 Horigome K, Bullock ED, Johnson EM Jr. Effects of nerve growth factor on rat peritoneal mast cells. Survival promotion and immediate-early gene induction. *J Biol Chem* 1994; 269: 2695–702.

101 Hoth M, Penner R. Depletion of intracellular calcium stores activates a calcium current in mast cells. *Nature* 1992; 355: 353–5.

102 Hu ZQ, Zenda N, Shimamura T. Down-regulation by IL-4 and up-regulation by IFN-γ of mast cell induction from mouse spleen cells. *J Immunol* 1996; 156: 3925–31.

103 Huang C, Friend DS, Qiu WT *et al*. Induction of a selective and persistent extravasation of neutrophils into the peritoneal cavity by tryptase mouse mast cell proteinase 6. *J Immunol* 1998; 160: 1910–9.

104 Huang C, Šali A, Stevens RL. Regulation and function of mast cell proteases in inflammation. *J Clin Immunol* 1998; 18: 169–83.

105 Irani AM, Bradford TR, Kepley CL *et al*. Detection of MC^T and MC^{TC} types of human mast cells by immunohistochemistry using new monoclonal anti-tryptase and anti-chymase antibodies. *J Histochem Cytochem* 1989; 37: 1509–15.

106 Irani AM, Nilsson G, Miettinen U *et al*. Recombinant human stem cell factor stimulates differentiation of mast cells from dispersed human fetal liver cells. *Blood* 1992; 80: 3009–21.

107 Ishihara H, Connolly AJ, Zeng D *et al*. Proteinase activated receptor 3 is a second thrombin receptor in humans. *Nature* 1997; 386: 502–6.

108 Kambayashi T, Jacob CO, Strassmann G. IL-4 and IL-13 modulate IL-10 release in endotoxin-stimulated murine peritoneal mononuclear phagocytes. *Cell Immunol* 1996; 171: 153–8.

109 Kanwar S, Tepperman BL, Payne D *et al*. Time course of nitric oxide production and epithelial dysfunction during ischemia/reperfusion of the feline small intestine. *Circ Shock* 1994; 42: 135–40.

110 Kanwar S, Wallace JL, Befus D, Kubes P. Nitric oxide synthesis inhibition increases epithelial permeability via mast cells. *Am J Physiol* 1994; 266: G222–9.

111 Kawasaki H, Inagaki N, Kimata M *et al*. Selective potentiation of IgE-dependent histamine release from rat peritoneal mast cells by stem cell factor. *Life Sci* 1995; 57: 2377–83.

112 Kawata R, Reddy ST, Wolner B, Herschman HR. Prostaglandin synthase 1 and prostaglandin synthase 2 both participate in activation-induced prostaglandin D_2 production in mast cells. *J Immunol* 1995; 155: 818–25.

113 Kazimierczak W, Diamant B. Mechanisms of histamine release in anaphylactic and anaphylactoid reactions. *Prog Allergy* 1978; 24: 295–365.

114 Kendall JC, Li XH, Galli SJ, Gordon JR. Promotion of mouse fibroblast proliferation by IgE-dependent activation of mouse mast cells: role for mast cell tumor necrosis factor-alpha and transforming growth factor-beta 1. *J Allergy Clin Immunol* 1997; 99: 113–23.

115 Kiernan JA. A pharmacological and histological investigation of the involvement of mast cells in cutaneous axon reflex vasodilatation. *Q J Exp Physiol* 1975; 60: 123–30.

116 Kirshenbaum AS, Goff JP, Kessler SW, Mican JM, Zsebo KM, Metcalfe DD. Effects of IL-3 and stem cell factor on the appearance of human basophils and mast cells from CD34+ pluripotent progenitors. *J Immunol* 1992; 148: 772–7.

117 Kirshenbaum AS, Kessler SW, Goff JP, Metcalfe DD. Demonstration of the origin of human mast cells from CD34+ bone marrow progenitor cells. *J Immunol* 1991; 146: 1410–5.

118 Kitamura Y, Kasugai T, Nomura S, Matsuda H. Development of mast cells and basophils. In: *Immunopharmacology of Mast Cells and Basophils* (Foreman JC, ed.). Academic Press, London, 1993: 5–27.

119 Kong W, McConalogue K, Khitin LM *et al*. Luminal trypsin may regulate enterocytes through proteinase-activated receptor 2. *Proc Natl Acad Sci USA* 1997; 94: 8884–9.

120 Kowalski ML, Didier A, Kaliner MA. Neurogenic inflammation in the airways. 1. Neurogenic stimulation induces plasma protein extravasation into the rat airway lumen. *Am Rev Resp Dis* 1989; 140: 101–9.

121 Kowalski ML, Kaliner MA. Neurogenic inflammation, vascular permeability, and mast cells. *J Immunol* 1988; 140: 3905–11.

122 Kuno M, Kawaguchi J, Mukai M, Nakamura F. PT pretreatment inhibits 48/80-induced activation of Ca^{2+}-permeable channels in rat peritoneal mast cells. *Am J Physiol* 1990; 259: C715–22.

123 Lagunoff D, Martin TW. Agents that release histamine from mast cells. *Ann Rev Pharmacol Toxicol* 1983; 23: 331–51.

124 Lantz CS, Boesiger J, Song CH *et al*. Role of interleukin-3 in mast cell and basophil development and in immunity to parasites. *Nature* 1998; 392: 90–3.

125 Lazarus GS. Mastocytosis: new understandings in cutaneous pathophysiology. *J Dermatol* 1996; 23: 769–72.

126 Lee TDG, Sterk A, Ishizaka T *et al*. Number and affinity of receptors for IgE on enriched populations of isolated rat intestinal mast cells. *Immunology* 1985; 55: 363–6.

127 Leung KBP, Flint KC, Hudspith BN *et al*. Some further properties of human pulmonary mast cells recovered by bronchoalveolar lavage and enzymic dispersion of lung tissue. *Agents Actions* 1987; 20: 213–5.

128 Lewis R, Soter NA, Diamond PT *et al*. Prostaglandin D_2 generation after activation of rat and human mast cells with anti-IgE. *J Immunol* 1982; 129: 1627–31.

129 Lewis RA, Austen KF, Soberman RJ. Leukotrienes and other products of the 5-lipoxygenase pathway. *N Engl J Med* 1990; 323: 645–55.

130 Li L, Li Y, Reddel SW *et al*. Identification of basophilic cells that express mast cell granule proteases in peripheral blood of asthma, allergy and drug-reactive patients. *J Immunol* 1998; 161: 5079–86.

131 Li L, Meng XW, Krilis SA. Mast cells expressing chymase but not tryptase can be derived by culturing human progenitors in conditioned medium obtained from a human mastocytosis cell strain with c-*kit* ligand. *J Immunol* 1996; 156: 4839–44.

132 Lin TJ, Befus AD. Differential regulation of mast cell function by IL-10 and stem cell factor. *J Immunol* 1997; 159: 4015–23.

133 Lin TJ, Befus AD. Mast cells and eosinophils in mucosal defenses and pathogenesis. In: *Mucosal Immunology*, 2nd edn, (Ogra PL, Mestecky J, Lamm ME *et al*. eds). Academic Press, San Diego, 1998: 469–82.

134 Lin TJ, Bissonnette EY, Hirsh A, Befus AD. Stem cell factor potentiates histamine secretion by multiple mechanisms, but does not affect tumour necrosis factor-alpha release from rat mast cells. *Immunology* 1996; 89: 301–7.

135 Little SS, Johnson DA. Human mast cell tryptase isoforms: separation and examination of substrate-specificity differences. *Biochem J* 1995; 307: 341–6.

136 Lohi J, Harvima I, Keski-Oja J. Pericellular substrates of human mast cell tryptase: 72,000 dalton gelatinase and fibronectin. *J Cell Biochem* 1992; 50: 337–49.

137 Lutzelschwab C, Pejler G, Aveskogh M, Hellman L. Secretory granule proteinases in rat mast cells. Cloning of 10 different serine proteinases and a carboxypeptidase A from various rat mast cell populations. *J Exp Med* 1997; 185: 13–29.

138 MacDonald AJ, Haig DM, Bazin H *et al*. IgE-mediated release of rat mast cell proteinase II, β-hexosaminidase and leukotriene C_4 from bone marrow-derived rat mast cells. *Immunology* 1989; 67: 414–8.

139 MacDonald AJ, Pick J, Bissonnette EY, Befus AD. Rat mucosal mast cells: the cultured bone marrow-derived mast cell is biochemically and

functionally analogous to its counterpart *in vivo*. *Immunology* 1998; 93: 533–9.

140 Madara JL, Stafford J. Interferon-gamma directly affects barrier function of cultured intestinal epithelial monolayers. *J Clin Invest* 1989; 83: 724–7.

141 Mahmud N, O'Connell MA, Stinson J *et al*. Tumour necrosis factor-alpha and microalbuminuria in patients with inflammatory bowel disease. *Eur J Gastroenterol Hepatol* 1995; 7: 215–9.

142 Malaviya R, Ikeda T, Ross E, Abraham N. Mast cell modulation of neutrophil influx and bacterial clearance at sites of infection through TNF-α. *Nature* 1996; 381: 77–80.

143 Mannaioni PF, Bello MG, Di Bello MG *et al*. Interaction between histamine and nitric oxide in rat mast cells and in isolated guinea pig hearts. *Int Arch Allergy Immunol* 1997; 113: 297–9.

144 Marietta EV, Chen Y, Weis JH. Modulation of expression of the anti-inflammatory cytokines interleukin-13 and interleukin-10 by interleukin-3. *Eur J Immunol* 1996; 26: 49–56.

145 Marth T, Strober W, Kelsall BL. High dose oral tolerance in ovalbumin TCR-transgenic mice: systemic neutralization of IL-12 augments TGF-beta secretion and T cell apoptosis. *J Immunol* 1996; 157: 2348–57.

146 Masini E, Salvemini D, Pistelli A *et al*. Rat mast cells synthesize a nitric oxide like-factor which modulates the release of histamine. *Agents Actions* 1991; 33: 61–3.

147 Massey WA, Guo CB, Dvorak AM *et al*. Human uterine mast cells: isolation, purification, characterization, ultrastructure and pharmacology. *J Immunol* 1991; 147: 1621–7.

148 Matsuda H, Yukiko K, Hiroko U *et al*. Nerve growth factor induces development of connective tissue-type mast cells *in vitro* from murine bone marrow cells. *J Exp Med* 1991; 174: 7–14.

149 Matsumoto R, Sali A, Ghildyal N *et al*. Packaging of proteases and proteoglycans in the granules of mast cells and other hematopoietic cells, a cluster of histidines on mouse mast cell protease 7 regulates its binding to heparin serglycin proteoglycans. *J Biol Chem* 1995; 270: 19524–31.

150 Matthews G, Neher E, Penner R. Chloride conductance activated by external agonists and internal messengers in rat peritoneal mast cells. *J Physiol* 1989; 418: 131–44.

151 Maurer M, Echtenacher B, Hültner L *et al*. The c-kit ligand, stem cell factor, can enhance innate immunity through effects on mast cells. *J Exp Med* 1998; 188: 2343–8.

152 Maximow A. Über die zellformen des lockeren bindegewebes. *Arch Mikrosk Anat Entwicklungsmech* 1906; 67: 680–757.

153 Metcalfe DD. Mast cell mediators with emphasis on intestinal mast cells. *Ann Allergy* 1984; 53: 563–75.

154 Mijatovic T, Kruys V, Caput D *et al*. Interleukin-4 and -13 inhibit tumour necrosis factor-alpha mRNA translational activation in lipopolysaccharide-induced mouse macrophages. *J Biol Chem* 1997; 272: 14394–8.

155 Miller HRP: Mast cells: Their function and heterogeneity. In: *Allergy and Immunity to Helminths. Common Mechanisms or Divergent Pathways?* (Moqbel R, ed.). Taylor and Francis, London, 1992; 228–48.

156 Miller HRP. Jarrett WFH. Immune reactions to mucous membranes. 1. Intestinal mast cells response during helminth expulsion in the rat. *Immunology* 1971; 20: 277–8.

157 Miller JS, Moxley G, Schwartz LB. Cloning and characterization of a second complimentary DNA for human tryptase. *J Clin Invest* 1990; 86: 864–70.

158 Miller JS, Westin EH, Schwartz LB. Cloning and characterization of complimentary DNA for human tryptase. *J Clin Invest* 1989; 84: 1188–95.

159 Möller A, Henz BM, Grützhau A *et al*. Comparative cytokine gene expression: regulation and release by human mast cells. *Immunology* 1998; 93: 289–95.

160 Moqbel R, King SJ, MacDonald AJ *et al*. Enteral and systemic release of leukotrienes during anaphylaxis of *Nippostrongylus brasiliensis*-primed rats. *J Immunol* 1986; 146: 3563–70.

161 Mousli M, Bueb JL, Bronner C *et al*. G protein activation: a receptor-independent mode of action for cationic amphiphilic neuropeptides and venom peptides. *Trends Pharmacol Sci* 1990; 11: 358–62.

162 Mousli M, Hugli TE, Landry Y, Bronner C. Peptidergic pathway in human skin and rat peritoneal mast cell activation. *Immunopharmacology* 1994; 27: 1–11.

163 Murakami M, Austen KF, Arm JP. Cytokine regulation of arachidonic acid metabolism in mast cells. In: *Biological and Molecular Aspects of Mast Cells and Basophil Differentiation and Function*. (Kitamura Y, Yamamoto S, Galli SJ, Greaves MW, eds.). Lippincott-Raven, New York, 1995: 25–37.

164 Murphy MP, Packer MA, Scarlett JL, Martin SW. Peroxynitrite: a biologically significant oxidant. *Gen Pharmacol* 1998; 31: 179–86.

165 Musch MW, Siegel MI. Antigenic stimulated release of arachidonic acid, lipoxygenase activity and histamine release in a cloned murine mast cell MC9. *Biochem Biophys Res Commun* 1985; 126: 517–25.

166 Myers AC, Undem BJ, Weinreich D. Influence of antigen on membrane properties of guinea pig bronchial ganglion neurons. *J Appl Physiol* 1991; 71: 970–6.

167 Myers AC, Undem BJ. Antigen depolarizes guinea pig bronchial parasympathetic ganglion neurons by activation of histamine H1 receptors. *Am J Physiol* 1995; 268: L879–L84.

168 Nafziger J, Arock M, Guillosson JJ, Wietzerbin J. Specific high-affinity receptors for interferon-γ on mouse bone marrow-derived mast cells: inhibitory effects of interferon-γ on mast cell precursors. *Eur J Immunol* 1990; 20: 113–7.

169 Nakamura T, Ui M. Islet-activating protein, pertussis toxin, inhibits Ca²⁺-induced and guanine nucleotide-dependent release of histamine and arachidonic acid from rat mast cells. *FEBS Lett* 1984; 261: 171–4.

170 Nicholls S, Stephens S, Braegger CP *et al*. Cytokines in stools of children with inflammatory bowel disease or infective diarrhoea. *J Clin Pathol* 1993; 46: 757–60.

171 Nilsson G, Blom T, Kusche-Gullberg M *et al*. Phenotypic characterization of the human mast-cell line HMC-1. *Scand J Immunol* 1994; 39: 489–98.

172 Nilsson G, Miettinen U, Ishizaka T *et al*. Interleukin-4 inhibits the expression of kit and tryptase during stem cell factor-dependent development of human mast cells from fetal liver cells. *Blood* 1994; 84: 1519–27.

173 Niu XF, Ibbotson G, Kubes P. A balance between nitric oxide and oxidants regulates mast cell-dependent neutrophil–endothelial cell interaction. *Circ Res* 1996; 79: 992–9.

174 Nussler AK, Billiar TR. Inflammation, immunoregulation, and inducible nitric oxide synthase. *J Leukoc Biol* 1993; 54: 171–8.

175 Obukov AG, Jones SVP, Degtiar VE *et al*. Ca²⁺-permeable large-conductance non-selective cation channels in rat basophilic cells. *Am J Physiol* 1995; 269: C119–C25.

176 Ohtsu H, Kuramuasu A, Suzuki S *et al*. Histidine decarboxylase expression in mouse mast cell line P815 is induced by mouse peritoneal cavity incubation. *J Biol Chem* 1996; 271: 28439–44.

177 Okayama Y, Hunt TC, Kassel O *et al*. Assessment of the anti-c-kit monclonal antibody YB5.B8 in affinity magnetic enrichment of human lung mast cells. *J Immunol Methods* 1994; 169: 153–61.

178 Okayama Y, Petit-Frére C, Kassel O *et al*. IgE-dependent expression of mRNA for IL-4 and IL-5 in human lung mast cells. *J Immunol* 1995; 155: 1796–1808.

179 Oliver MR, Tan DT, Scott RB. Intestinal anaphylaxis: mediation of the response of colonic longitudinal muscle in rat. *Am J Physiol* 1995; 268: G764–71.

180 Palacios R, Garland J. Distinct mechanisms may account for the growth-promoting activity of interleukin 3 on cells of lymphoid and myeloid origin. *Proc Natl Acad Sci USA* 1984; 81: 1208–11.

181 Pallaoro M, Fejzo MS, Shayesteh L *et al*. Characterization of genes encoding known and novel human mast cell tryptases on chromosome 16p13.3±. *J Biol Chem* 1999; 274: 3355–62.

182 Park DJ, Min HK, Rhee SG. IgE-induced tyrosine phosphorylation of phospholipase C-gamma 1 in rat basophilic leukemia cells. *J Biol Chem* 1991; 266: 24237–40.

183 Pearce FL, Befus AD, Gauldie J, Bienenstock J. Mucosal mast cells. II. Effects of anti-allergic compounds on histamine secretion by isolated intestinal mast cells. *J Immunol* 1982; 128: 2481–6.

184 Penner R, Matthews G, Neher E. Regulation of calcium influx by second messengers in rat mast cells. *Nature* 1988; 334: 499–504.

185 Perdue MH, Gall DG. Transport abnormalities during intestinal anaphylaxis in the rat: effect of antiallergic agents. *J Allergy Clin Immunol* 1985; 76: 498–503.

186 Pervin R, Kanner BI, Marx G, Razin E. Thrombin-induced degranulation of cultured bone marrow-derived mast cells: effect on calcium uptake. *Immunology* 1985; 56: 667–72.

187 Prodeus AP, Zhou X, Maurer M *et al.* Impaired mast cell-dependent natural immunity in complement C3-deficient mice. *Nature* 1997; 390: 172–5.

188 Qiu B, Pothoulakis C, Castagliuolo I *et al.* Nitric oxide inhibits rat intestinal secretion by *Clostridium difficile* toxin A but not *Vibrio cholerae* enterotoxin. *Gastroenterology* 1996; 111: 409–18.

189 Ramaswamy K, Mathison R, Carter L *et al.* Marked anti-inflammatory effects of decentralization of the superior cervical ganglia. *J Exp Med* 1990; 172: 1819–30.

190 Razin E, Marx G. Thrombin-induced degranulation of cultured bone marrow-drived mast cells. *J Immunol* 1984; 133: 3282–5.

191 Rees PH, Hillier K, Church MK. The secretory characteristics of mast cells isolated from the human large intestinal mucosa and muscle. *Immunology* 1988; 65: 437–42.

192 Rennick D, Hunte B, Holland G, Thompson-Snipes L. Co-factors are essential for stem cell factor-dependent growth and maturation of mast cell progenitors: comparative effects of interleukin-3 (IL-3), IL-4, IL-10 and fibroblasts. *Blood* 1995; 85: 57–65.

193 Rodelwald HR, Dessing M, Dvorak AM, Galli SJ. Identification of a committed precursor for the mast cell lineage. *Science* 1996; 271: 818–22.

194 Rothwell TL. Immune expulsion of parasitic nematodes from the alimentary tract. *Int J Parasitol* 1989; 19: 139–68.

195 Rottem M, Metcalfe DD. Development and maturation of mast cells and basophils. In: *Asthma and Rhinitis*. (Busse WW, Holgate ST, eds). Blackwell Scientific Publications, Boston; 1995: 167–81.

196 Rumsaeng V, Cruikshank WW, Foster B *et al.* Human mast cells produce the CD4+ T lymphocyte chemoattractant factor, IL-16. *J Immunol* 1997; 159: 2904–10.

197 Sababi M, Nylander O. Comparative study of the effects of nitric oxide synthase and cyclo-oxygenase inhibition on duodenal functions in rats anaesthetized with inactin, urethane or alpha-chloralose. *Acta Physiol Scand* 1996; 158: 45–52.

198 Sage H, Woodbury RG, Bornstein P. Structural studies on human type IV collagen. *J Biol Chem* 1979; 254: 9893–900.

199 Saito H, Hatake K, Dvorak AM. Selective differentiation and proliferation of hematopoietic cells induced by recombinant human interleukins. *Proc Natl Acad Sci USA* 1988; 85: 2288–92.

200 Saito H, Okajima F, Molski TF *et al.* Effect of a ADP-ribosylation of GTP-binding protein by pertussis toxin on immunoglobulin E-dependent histamine release from mast cells and basophils. *J Immunol* 1987; 138: 3927–34.

201 Salvemini D, Masini E, Anggard E *et al.* Synthesis of a nitric oxide-like factor from L-arginine by rat serosal mast cells: stimulation of guanylate cyclase and inhibition of platelet aggregation. *Biochem Biophys Res Com* 1990; 169: 596–601.

202 Salvemini D, Masini E, Pistelli A *et al.* Nitric oxide: a regulatory mediator of mast cell reactivity. *J Cardiovasc Pharmacol* 1991; 17: S258–64.

203 Schechter NM, Brass LF, Lavker RM, Jensen PJ. Reaction of mast cell proteinases tryptase and chymase with proteinase activated receptors (PARs) on keratinocytes and fibroblasts. *J Cell Physiol* 1998; 176: 365–73.

204 Schneider H, Cohen-Dayag A, Petch I. Tyrosine phosphorylation of phospholipase C gamma 1 couples the Fc epsilon receptor mediated signal to mast cell secretion. *Int Immunol* 1992; 4: 447–53.

205 Schulman ES, Pollack RB, Post TJ, Peters SP. Histochemical heterogeneity of dispersed human lung mast cells. *J Immunol* 1990; 144: 4195–201.

206 Schwartz LB, Huff T. Biology of mast cells and basophils. In: *Allergy Principles and Practice* (Middleton E, ed.). Mosby, St Louis, 1994: 135–68.

207 Scott RB, Diamant SC, Gall DG. Motility effects of intestinal anaphylaxis in the rat. *Am J Physiol* 1988; 255: G505–11.

208 Scott RB, Gall DG, Maric M. Mediation of food protein-induced jejunal smooth muscle contraction in sensitized rats. *Am J Physiol* 1990; 259: G6–14.

209 Scott RB, Maric M. Mediation of anaphylaxis-induced jejunal circular smooth muscle contraction in rats. *Dig Dis Sci* 1993; 38: 396–402.

210 Scudamore CL, Millan L, Thornton EM *et al.* Mast cell heterogeneity in the gastrointestinal tract: variable expression of mouse mast cell proteinase-1 (MMCP-1) in intraepithelial mucosal mast cells in nematode-infected and normal BALB/c mice. *Am J Pathol* 1997; 150: 1661–72.

211 Scudamore CL, Thornton EM, Millan L *et al.* Release of the mucosal mast cell granule chymase, rat mast cell proteinase-II, during anaphylaxis is associated with the rapid development of paracellular permeability to macromolecules in rat jejunum. *J Exp Med* 1995; 182: 1871–81.

212 Sekizawa K, Caughey GH, Lazarus SC *et al.* Mast cell tryptase causes airway smooth muscle hyperresponsiveness in dogs. *J Clin Invest* 1989; 83: 175–9.

213 Seldin DC, Adelman S, Austen KF *et al.* Homology of the rat basophilic leukemia cell and the rat mucosal mast cells. *Proc Natl Acad Sci USA* 1985; 82: 3871–5.

214 Selvan RS, Butterfield JH, Krangel MS. Expression of multiple chemokine genes by a human mast cell leukemia. *J Biol Chem* 1994; 269: 13893–8.

215 Shah PM, Husby S, Damsgaard TE *et al.* Purification of human colonic and gastric mast cells. *J Immunol Meth* 1998; 214: 141–8.

216 Shanahan F, Denburg JA, Fox J *et al.* Mast cell heterogeneity: effects of neuroenteric peptides on histamine release. *J Immunol* 1985; 135: 1331–7.

217 Shanahan F, MacNiven I, Dyck N *et al.* Human lung mast cells: distribution and abundance of histochemically distinct subpopulations. *Int Arch Allergy Appl Immunol* 1987; 83: 329–31.

218 Smith TJ, Ducharme LA, Weis JH. Preferential expression of interleukin-12 or interleukin-4 by murine bone marrow mast cells derived in mast cell growth factor or interleukin-3. *Eur J Immunol* 1994; 24: 822–6.

219 Smith WL. The eicosanoids and their biochemical mechanism of action. *Biochem J* 1989; 259: 315–24.

220 Stenton GR, Vliagoftis H, Befus AD. Role of intestinal mast cells in modulating gastrointestinal pathophysiology. *Ann Allergy Asthma Immunol* 1998; 81: 1–15.

221 Strieter RM, Kunkel SL, Bone RC. Role of tumor necrosis factor-alpha in disease states and inflammation. *Crit Care Med* 1993; 21: S447–63.

222 Strukova SM, Dugina TN, Khlgatian SV *et al.* Thrombin-mediated events implicated in mast cell activation. *Semin Thromb Hemost* 1996; 22: 145–50.

223 Tada K, Murakami M, Kambe T, Kudo I. Induction of cyclooxygenase-2 by secretory phospholipases A₂ in nerve growth factor-stimulated rat serosal mast cells is facilitated by interaction with fibroblasts and mediated by a mechanism independent of their enzymic functions. *J Immunol* 1998; 161: 5008–15.

224 Tainsh KR, Lau HY, Liu WL, Pearce FL. The human skin mast cell: a comparison with the human lung cell and a novel mast cell type, the uterine mast cell. *Agents Actions* 1991; 33: 16–9.

225 Targan SR, Hanauer SB, van Deventer SJ *et al.* A short-term study of chimeric monoclonal antibody cA2 to tumor necrosis factor alpha for Crohn's disease. Crohn's disease cA2 study group. *New Engl J Med* 1997; 337: 1029–35.

226 Tasaka K, Mio M, Okamoto M. Intracellular calcium release induced by histamine releasers and its inhibition by some anti-allergic drugs. *Ann Allergy* 1986; 56: 464–9.

227 Thomassen MJ, Buhrow LT, Connors MJ *et al.* Nitric oxide inhibits inflammatory cytokine production by human alveolar macrophages. *Am J Respir Cell Mol Biol* 1997; 17: 279–83.

228 Tsai M, Takeishi T, Thompson H *et al.* Induction of mast cell proliferation, maturation and heparin synthesis by the rat c-kit ligand, stem cell factor. *Proc Natl Acad Sci USA* 1991; 88: 6382–6.

229 Tsuji K, Nakahata T, Takagi M *et al.* Effects of interleukin-3 and interleukin-4 on the development of connective tissue-type mast cells: interleukin-3 supports their survival and interleukin-4 triggers and supports their proliferation synergistically with interleukin-3. *Blood* 1990; 75: 421–7.

230 Undem BJ, Lichtenstein LM, Hubbard WC *et al.* Recombinant stem cell factor-induced mast cell activation and smooth muscle contraction in human bronchi. *Am J Respir Cell Mol Biol* 1994; 11: 646–50.

231 Valent P, Besemer J, Sillaber C *et al.* Failure to detect IL-3 binding sites on human mast cells. *J Immunol* 1990; 145: 3432–7.

232 Van Deventer SJ, Elson CO, Fedorak RN. Multiple doses of intravenous interleukin 10 in steroid-refractory Crohn's disease. Crohn's Disease Study Group. *Gastroenterology* 1997; 113: 383–9.

233 Van Dullemen HM, van Deventer SJ, Hommes DW *et al.* Treatment of Crohn's disease with anti-tumor necrosis factor chimeric monoclonal antibody (cA2). *Gastroenterology* 1995; 109: 129–35.

234 Vanderslice P, Ballinger SM, Tam EK *et al.* Human mast cell tryptase: multiple cDNAs and genes reveal a multigene serine protease family. *Proc Natl Acad Sci USA* 1990; 87: 3811–5.

235 Vergnolle N, Hollenberg MD, Wallace JL. Pro- and anti-inflammatory actions of thrombin: a distinct role for proteinase-activated receptor-1 (PAR₁). *Br J Pharmacol* 1998; 126: 1262–8.

236 Vergnolle N, MacNaughton WK, Al-Ani B *et al.* Proteinase-activated receptor 2 (PAR₂)-activating peptides: identification of a receptor distinct from PAR₂ that regulates intestinal transport. *Proc Natl Acad Sci USA* 1998; 95: 7766–71.

237 Vu TK, Hung DT, Wheaton VI, Coughlin SR. Molecular cloning of a functional thrombin receptor reveals a novel proteolytic mechanism of receptor activation. *Cell* 1991; 64: 1057–68.

238 Wallace JL, McKnight GW, Befus AD. Capsaicin-induced hyperemia in the stomach: possible contribution of mast cells. *Am J Physiol* 1992; 263: G209–14.

239 Walls AF, Jones DB, Williams JH *et al.* Immunohistochemical identification of mast cells in formaldehyde-fixed tissue using monoclonal antibodies specific for tryptase. *J Pathol* 1990; 162: 119–26.

240 Wang YZ, Cooke HJ. H2 receptors mediate cyclical chloride secretion in guinea pig distal colon. *Am J Physiol* 1990; 258: G887–93.

241 Wang YZ, Palmer JM, Cooke HJ. Neuroimmune regulation of colonic secretion in guinea pigs. *Am J Physiol* 1991: 260: G307–14.

242 Wastling JM, Scudamore CL, Thornton EM *et al.* Constitutive expression of mouse mast cell proteinase-1 in normal BALB/c mice and its up-regulation during intestinal nematode infection. *Immunology* 1997; 90: 308–13.

243 Weiner HL. Oral tolerance: immune mechanisms and treatment of autoimmune diseases. *Immunol Today* 1997; 18: 335–43.

244 Weinreich D, Undem BJ, Taylor G, Barry MF. Antigen-induced long-term potentiation of nicotinic synaptic transmission in the superior cervical ganglion of the guinea pig. *J Neurophysiol* 1995; 73: 2004–16.

245 White JR, Ishizaka T, Ishizaka K, Sha'afi RI. Direct demonstration of increased intracellular concentration of free calcium as measured by quin-2 in stimulated rat peritoneal mast cells. *Proc Natl Acad Sci USA* 1984; 81: 3978–82.

246 White JR, Zembryki D, Hanna N, Mong S. Differential inhibition of histamine release from mast cells by protein kinase C inhibitors: staurosporine and K-252a. *Biochem Pharmacol* 1990; 40: 447–56.

247 White SR, Stimler-Gerard NP, Munoz NM *et al.* Effect of beta-adrenergic blockade and sympathetic stimulation on canine bronchial mast cell response to immune degranulation *in vivo. Am Rev Respir Dis* 1989; 139: 73–9.

248 Zurawski G, de Vries JE. Interleukin 13, an interleukin 4-like cytokine that acts on monocytes and B cells, but not on T cells. *Immunol Today* 1994; 15: 19–26.

Chapter

7

The mucosal T cell

J. Strid and S. Strobel

INTRODUCTION

The intestinal mucosa is a major barrier limiting and controlling foreign antigen access to the body. As the first line of defence, the intestinal epithelium has been particularly well investigated and it has been known for many years that non-epithelial cells are present in large numbers within the epithelium.[24,37,98] The cellular infiltrate consists of granular and non-granular lymphocytes, dendritic cells, macrophages, eosinophils, mast cells and the occasional neutrophil (Fig. 7.1). These cell types can be demonstrated both in the epithelium and the lamina propria; B cells and plasma cells are normally restricted to the latter.

The gut-associated lymphoid tissue (GALT) has the inherent property of protecting the host from adverse reactions to pathogens and ingested proteins. As a framework for understanding mucosal immune responses, it is helpful to divide GALT into inductive and effector sites. The primary inductive sites are the (organized) lymphoid aggregates present in the wall of the small and large intestine termed Peyer's patches (PP). They are found in all mammals and, although there are some differences in structure and cell populations between species, most features are remarkably conserved. The main effector sites for intestinal immune responses are the lamina propria, which contains mature T and B cells as well as other cells necessary for an adaptive immune response, and the epithelium, which contains a unique population of T cells called intraepithelial lymphocytes (IELs).

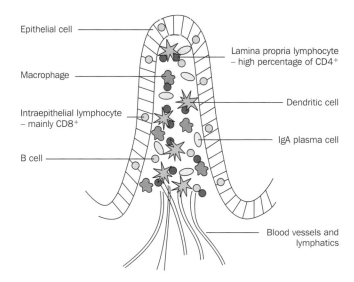

Fig. 7.1 An intestinal villus, showing the general structure of the epithelium and the lamina propria as well as major cell populations present.

T lymphocytes primed in the Peyer's patch may 'home' back to the intestinal mucosa or to other mucosal sites.

The intestinal lamina propria and epithelium represent the largest T cell sites in humans. The relative T cell contribution by organized GALT is estimated to amount to nearly 10% of the total number of lymphocytes.[132] T lymphocytes resident in the GALT either as organized PP or as microfollicles play a pivotal role in host defence and in (immune-) regulation of gastrointestinal function.

This chapter discusses the origins and roles of intraepithelial and lamina propria lymphocytes (LPLs) in humans and selected experimental models, with reference to their heterogeneity and their role in food-related hypersensitivity reactions.

ONTOGENY OF MUCOSAL LYMPHOCYTES

Intraepithelial lymphocytes

The origin and fate of IELs are still a matter of controversy, and lymphoid as well as non-lymphoid origins have been proposed.[39,51–53,77,88] In humans, they appear as early as the 20th gestational week and increase in numbers of up to 6–40 per 100 epithelial cells in the normal human small intestine.[37,98] The small intestine of the mouse has been estimated to contain 50–100 × 10[6] IEL.[38,92] In mice, there is a steady increase after birth from 0.3 to 0.5 per 100 epithelial cells 2 days after birth to about 2 per 100 epithelial cells at 1 week of age, to around 8–11 per 100 epithelial cells in adult mice, dependent on the environmental conditions under which the animals are kept.

IEL development

Most IELs seem to originate from the bone marrow and develop into T cells in the intestinal epithelium. Others develop in the thymus and migrate to the epithelium directly or via the Peyer's patches. Over 30 years ago, Fichtelius proposed that gut IELs, then called theliolymphocytes, were not thymus-derived cells, and suggested that the intestinal epithelium was itself a first-level lymphoid organ.[41] Subsequently, a number of reports have supported that conclusion.[5,39,67] The presence of T cells within the intestinal epithelium but not in the periphery of athymic nude mice is well documented,[5] and suggests that the intestinal epithelium can support some T cell development in the absence of a functional thymus.

Likewise, neonatal thymectomy prevents the production of peripheral T cells, but the number of IELs recovered from the small intestine is only slightly reduced compared with age-matched normal control animals.[39] Experiments performed in athymic and euthymic mice suggest that selection of intestinal T cells occur locally. Unlike thymic selection, however, where potentially autoreactive cells are deleted, the self-reactive cells developing in the intestinal epithelium are functionally inactivated so that they are refractory to signalling through their TCR.[78,104,110] This lack of responsiveness cannot be overcome by the addition of exogenous cytokines.[8] Despite strong evidence that the intestinal epithelium can support extrathymic T cell development, it has been suggested that, although this development occurs extrathymically, it is not entirely thymus-independent.[77,79,81]

IEL 'homing'

Once the IELs are mature they do not seem to recirculate in a manner similar to conventional T cells[103] but rather show a distinct tissue-specific migration behaviour. Adoptively transferred labelled IELs appear to selectively lodge in the intestinal epithelium, whereas adoptively transferred labelled cells from other lymphoid compartments do not.[128]

It has been demonstrated by measurements of DNA synthesis that 70% of IELs are short-lived with a half-life of about 3 weeks. However, a small proportion of long-lived small lymphocytes can also be demonstrated.[111] The IELs are capable of local division within the epithelium and, as an indicator, mitotic figures can be seen both in humans[40,86] and in laboratory rodents.[40,111]

Lamina propria lymphocytes

The lamina propria undergoes a characteristic differentiation during development. The extracellular matrix consists of stromal cells, which are in intimate association with T cells, immunoglobulin A (IgA) plasma cells, dendritic cells and macrophages. The association between immune cells and the lamina propria stromal cells is laid down ontogenetically, independent of antigen. At 11 weeks of gestation, just after the villi have formed and the epithelium becomes columnar, the lamina propria is filled with accessory cells.[123] T cells appear in the lamina propria a few weeks later.[121]

Lamina propria lymphocyte ontogeny involves the thymus followed by induction in the PP and the lymphoid follicles within the mucosa. Naive T cells enter mucosal lymphoid follicles, encounter antigen, enter the peripheral circulation, and 'home' back to the lamina propria.[60,61,141] Unlike IELs and blood lymphocytes (BLs), the nature of the ligand–receptor interactions that direct LPLs to home back to the mucosa is unclear. LPLs and IELs constitutively express chemokine receptors (e.g. CXCR3, CCR5, CCR2) whose expression is upregulated during inflammation, suggesting that they could play a role in lymphocyte localization within the intestinal mucosa.[142] LPLs are likely to express other adhesion molecules that facilitate homing to the lamina propria, some of which may be lost once the lymphocytes have reached the mucosa.[1] (See Chapter 1 for a detailed discussion.)

MORPHOLOGY AND HISTOCHEMISTRY

The major morphological characteristic of IELs noted in early reports is the presence of intracytoplasmic granules. These are easily recognized in Giemsa-stained tissue sections from most species.[88,89,101] They have abundant pale blue cytoplasm and a densely stained nucleus, thus exhibiting staining patterns typical of blood lymphocytes. Perforin and granzymes have been identified in IEL granules: however, these granules do not contain histamine, as observed in intraepithelial cells of mast cell origin, nor do they express Fcε receptors.[51,101] The intracytoplasmic granules are thus similar in many aspects to those of natural killer (NK) cells; however, granules are not essential for cytotoxicity, as lytic activity is also present in non-granule-containing IEL subsets.

In humans, 25–50% of IELs are granulated.[19] In mice, up to 60% are granulated,[100] reaching over 90% in some inbred strains. Over 30% of the IELs in rats and rabbits are granulated.[88,112] Attempts to identify granulated IELs in tissue sections of different species have yielded widely divergent results, most likely due to differences in fixation and staining properties.[33,87,125] The majority of IELs are medium sized.[37,111] With the exception of a small subset (~15%) of larger densely granulated cells, they are often indistinguishable from lymphocytes in other tissues based on cell size.[17,34,52,69] Most protocols for isolation of IELs involve the use of Percoll gradients to separate IELs from contaminating epithelial cells. Using cell density as a criterion, IELs show an inverse relationship to splenic lymphocytes when separated on Percoll gradients.[8,68] The low-density nature of IELs compared with splenic lymphocytes may indicate that IELs are proliferating at a higher rate.

PHENOTYPE OF MUCOSAL T LYMPHOCYTES

IELs and LPLs can be divided into two broad categories based on the surface T cell receptor (TCR) type: those expressing αβ TCRs and those expressing γδ TCRs. Further subsets can be distinguished by expression of the CD8 (αα homodimer or αβ heterodimer) or CD4 coreceptors. Circulating T cells consist predominantly of two populations: TCRαβ CD8αβ⁺ and TCRαβ

CD4⁺ cells. The mucosal T lymphocytes are phenotypically heterogeneous and substantially different from circulating BLS. The phenotypes of mucosal T lymphocytes also differ markedly between the epithelial and lamina propria compartments. Table 7.1 lists the most important phenotypic markers of IELs and LPLs and compares their prevalence to that of circulating lymphocytes.

Intraepithelial lymphocytes
IELs have a number of characteristics that distinguish them from the majority of blood T cells, thymocytes and LPLs.

Phenotypic markers of IELs and LPLs						
Cell surface markers	Cellular expression	Functions	Family relationships	IEL (%)	LPL (%)	BL (%)
CD3	Thymocytes, T cells	Associated with the T cell antigen receptor (TCR). Required for cell surface expression of and signal transduction by the TCR	Immunoglobulin superfamily (γ, δ, ε) ζ/η related to FcRγ chain	>80	40–90	~60
CD4	Thymocyte subsets, helper and inflammatory T cells, monocytes, macrophages	Coreceptor for MHC Class II molecules	Immunoglobulin superfamily	20	65	65
CD8	Thymocyte subsets, cytotoxic T cells	Coreceptor for MHC Class I molecules	Immunoglobulin superfamily	80	35	35
αβ TCR	Thymocytes, T cells	Antigen recognition and MHC restriction	Immunoglobulin superfamily	50	95	95
γδ TCR	Thymocytes, T cells	Unknown, restricted recognition pattern (aberrant Class I and heat shock proteins)	Immunoglobulin superfamily	50	3	3
α_Eβ_7 (CD103, HML 1)	Intraepithelial lymphocytes and lamina propria lymphocytes	Homing and adhesion. Intestinal activation marker. Involved in lymphoepithelial interactions	Integrin superfamily of adhesion molecules	90	30–40	0
CD25 (α-chain IL2R)	Activated T and B cells, macrophages	IL2 receptor	α: CCP and β: cytokine receptor superfamilies	15–30	15–30	<5
CD45RO	T cell subsets, B cell subsets, monocytes, macrophages	CD45 augments signalling through antigen receptor of T and B cells. CD45RO is an isoform of CD45 containing none of the A, B and C exons	Fibronectin type III	85	65–95	30–50
CD45RA	T cell subsets (naive T cells), B cells, monocytes	Isoform of CD45 containing the A exon	Fibronectin type III	15–20	10–22	60–90

Table 7.1 Phenotypic markers of IELs and LPLs.

Immunohistochemical staining *in situ* and extensive analysis of freshly isolated IELs by flow cytometry show that IELs in both the small and large intestine are predominantly T cells. Over 80% of IELs express CD3 and are intracytoplasmic and cell surface immunoglobulin negative (Ig⁻). Immunoglobulin positive (Ig⁺) cells are confined to the lamina propria. On the basis of TCR and coreceptor expression, IELs can be separated into five main subsets: TCRγδ CD8αα, TCRαβ CD8αα, TCRαβ CD8αβ, TCRαβ CD4 and TCRαβ CD4 CD8αα. There are also two small intraepithelial populations of TCR positive, double negative cells (CD8⁻, CD4⁻) and cells without T cell receptors.[76,93] Human[27,84] and mouse[12,50] small and large intestinal IELs contain a much higher percentage of γδ T cells than are found in other lymphoid sites. Analysis of IELs in the small intestine has revealed an approximately equal number of cells using TCRαβ and TCRγδ receptors – however, a considerable variation in the ratio of TCRαβ:TCRγδ is found between studies.

TCRγδ IELs are first to occur in the gut, and the subsequent expansion of TCRαβ IELs is dependent on antigen exposure. The number of TCRαβ IELs is greatly reduced in germ-free mice.[134] Thus, diet, housing conditions and age are all factors that seem to influence the TCRαβ:TCRγδ IEL ratio, although the specific factors which are likely to control the TCR expression ratios on IELs in various species and in different strains of mouse are not known. An interesting characteristic of IELs is their predominant expression of the CD8 molecule. Within the IEL compartment CD8 can be expressed as a CD8αβ heterodimer or a CD8αα homodimer. The CD8αα homodimer is unique to IELs, and evidence is accumulating that this molecule is a phenotypic marker for thymus-independent development of at least one population of IELs.[51,109]

Surface molecule coexpression

Coexpression of accessory (CD2, CD5, Thy 1, CD45RO⁺ or RA⁺), costimulatory (CD28), adhesion and homing (α_Eβ_7, CD62L), activation (CD25, CD69) and NK associated molecules (CD16, NK2.1, Ly49) has allowed further characterization of IELs into distinct subpopulations with different activities (Table 7.1).

The composition of IELs within the mucosa is affected by their location along the small and large intestine. In general, IELs from the large intestine are more similar in phenotype to splenic and lymph node T cells than small intestine IELs.[16,58] The variation in IEL composition as related to anatomical location is probably due to the necessity for differing functional roles in distinct sites.

Lamina propria lymphocytes

The study of both human and murine LPLs has been facilitated by methods of enzymatic digestion of freshly isolated intestinal mucosa.[25,135] Approximately 40–90% of LPLs are T cells expressing the CD3 surface marker. The vast majority of LPLs (~95%) bear an αβ TCR complex.[46,133] Compared with the 50% of IELs that express the γδ TCR, only 3% of CD3⁺ LPLs express this form of TCR[133] – a situation similar to that in blood.

Likewise, the ratio between cells being positive for the coreceptors CD4 or CD8 in the lamina propria is similar to that found in blood, with a high percentage of CD4⁺ cells (35–65%).[62,117] Although BLs and LPLs share several common phenotypic features, LPLs differ in their maturational state. Analysis of cell surface markers and application of functional assays have demon-

strated that CD4⁺ lamina propria cells are predominantly of a memory/activated phenotype.

Naive T cells can be characterized as CD45RA^hi, LFA-3^lo, CD2^lo, LFA-1^lo, CD45RO^lo and CD29^lo and memory T cells represent the reciprocal subset. In contrast to BLs, most LPL TCRαβ (~80%) and TCRγδ (75%) express the memory marker CD45RO.[35,54] Moreover, approximately 15% of LPLs express the putative memory marker CD45RB, whereas only a minority show a truly naive (CD45RA⁺) phenotype.[54] In the BL population the distribution of memory and naive phenotypes is more even. However, expression of another marker of memory T cells, CD29, is not increased in the lamina propria compared with peripheral blood.

Activation markers

Another distinguishing feature of LPLs is their frequent expression of cell surface markers associated with activation. This is probably the result of the continuous antigenic and mitogenic challenge encountered within the gut. T cell activation is followed by an early expression of the interleukin 2 (IL2) receptor. It has been shown by flow cytometry that 15–30% of freshly isolated intestinal LPLs are CD25+ (IL2 receptor α chain), while less than 5% of other lymphoid population are CD25⁺. The increased CD25 expression of LPLs correlates with a high proliferative response to low doses of IL2.[115,140] In addition, a putative marker of recent activation, CD69, is expressed by 80–90% of CD4⁺, 90–100% CD8⁺ and on all TCRγδ LPLs, while it is virtually absent on the circulating counterparts.[26] Other activation markers found on LPLs include major histocompatibility complex (MHC) Class II (HLADR) antigens[140] and a frequent expression of the α_Eβ_7 integrin, which is expressed during activation. Approximately 40% of LPLs show an α_Eβ_7⁺ phenotype, where fewer than 1% of circulating T cells are positive for α_Eβ_7.[20,116]

In summary, the phenotypic studies of LPLs give a clear indication that T cells in the human intestinal lamina propria are a specialized T cell subset with a phenotype consistent with that of memory cells and with a higher percentage expression of activation markers (Table 7.1).

FUNCTIONAL ROLE OF MUCOSAL T LYMPHOCYTES

The precise effector function of mucosal T lymphocytes is controversial and remains essentially unresolved. An increasing list of activities can be attributed to these cells and there is accumulating evidence that a disturbance of the homeostasis of the lymphocyte-mediated immunoregulation in the gut is associated with a variety of intestinal diseases, some of which are discussed elsewhere in this book. T lymphocytes associated with the human gastrointestinal tract have unique characteristics, which reflect their specialized roles in host defence. The presumed and known functional properties of T lymphocytes in the epithelial and lamina propria compartment are summarized in Table 7.2.

Intraepithelial lymphocytes

In accordance with their anatomical location, the following roles have been attributed to IELs:

1. surveillance of the intestinal epithelial layer for detection of microbial pathogens

Comparison of functional features of T lymphocytes in the epithelial and lamina propria compartments		
Function	**IEL**	**LPL**
Cytokine production	CD8$^+$: IFNγ >> IL5, IL6 CD4$^+$: IL4, IL5, IL6 >> IFNγ γδ: IFNγ, TGFβ, TNFα, IL5	IL4, IL5, IL10 >> IFNγ
Cytotoxic T cell activity	+++++	++
B cell help	Yes: CD4$^+$ subset (not CD8$^+$)	Yes: terminal differentiation of sIgA$^+$ B cells
CD8 suppressor activity	+++	+/–
CD4 suppressor activity	+++	+/–
Preferential activation pathways	↓ Proliferation to TCR stimuli; ↑ IL2 secretion with CD2 stimulation	↓ Proliferation and cytokine secretion to TCR stimuli; ↑ Proliferation and cytokine secretion with CD2 (± CD28) stimulation (IFNγ, TNFα, IL2, IL4)

Table 7.2 Comparison of functional features of T lymphocytes in the epithelial and lamina propria compartments.

2. removal of damaged or transformed epithelial cells
3. maintenance of epithelial integrity via secretion of trophic factors important for epithelial cell growth and differentiation
4. regulation of local cell-mediated or humoral immune responses.[3]

Poor proliferation

IELs proliferate only minimally in response to mitogens, such as phytohaemagglutinin (PHA); to superantigens, such as staphylococcal exotoxin B (SEB); and to antibody against CD3. This low proliferative response is not enhanced by addition of IL2 or by autologous irradiated blood monocytes. The proliferation is also unaffected by the addition of IL1β, IL4 or IL6.[29] In contrast, IELs seem to proliferate vigorously to stimulation via the CD2 receptor, with a marked increase in the production of IL2 and interferon γ (IFNγ).[30,97]

Cytotoxic activity

Most IELs are CD8$^+$ and many contain cytoplasmic granules, which contain perforin and serine esterases. A large number of IELs also express asialo GM1 and other NK markers and phenotypically some IELs resemble large granular lymphocytes. Altogether this would suggest that IELs are capable of cytotoxicity. Indeed IELs can mediate various forms of cytotoxicity, including NK activity, antigen-specific-MHC restricted CTL activity, alloreactive CTL activity, antibody-dependent cell-mediated cytotoxicity (ADCC), activity in redirected cytotoxicity assays and spontaneous cytotoxicity.[8] The heterogeneity of the IEL population may explain their multiple activities in cytotoxicity assays.

Cytotoxic activities can be mediated by at least two distinct mechanisms: one involves the release of perforin and granzyme molecules; the other involves the expression of Fas ligand on cytotoxic T cells, which then delivers an apoptotic death signal via the Fas signalling pathway.[48]

Classical cell-mediated immune reactions such as allograft rejections and graft-versus-host disease produce characteristic alterations in gut morphology, such as raised numbers of IELs, increased crypt length and villus atrophy (Fig. 7.2). The extent to which cytotoxic responses contribute to the mucosal damage observed during delayed hypersensitivity reactions is unknown (see below).

Cytokines

IELs have the potential to secrete a wide array of cytokines. The cytokine profile of the IEL seems to be determined by the type of activation signal provided. The cytokines can be divided into Th1 cytokines (IL2, IFNγ, tumour necrosis factor α (TNFα)) and Th2 cytokines (IL4, IL5, IL10), which are commonly associated with cell-mediated immunity and humoral immunity, respectively. Determination of cytokine mRNA levels by semiquantitative reverse transcriptase-polymerase chain reaction (RT-PCR) has revealed expression of mRNA for IL1, IL2, IL4, IL5, IL10, IFNγ TNFα and transforming growth factor β (TGFβ) in freshly isolated, unsorted IELs from the small and large intestine of mice.[7]

IELs do not display the normal polarization toward either a Th1 or Th2 phenotype, despite being morphologically in an activated state.[129] In situ analyses demonstrate that IELs in the resting state produce IFNγ and IL5.[130,131] However, after activation, the majority of IELs adopt a Th1 cytokine profile, expressing cytokines somewhat similar to that of other CD8$^+$ T cells. Although the cytokine profile produced after in vitro activation or in vivo inflammation resembles a Th1 profile and is associated with increased cytotoxic activity,[83,84] there is a subset of IELs that is capable of B cell help.[45] A further subset may provide contrasuppressor activity capable of abrogating oral tolerance.[43] The subset capable of B cell help appears to be TCRαβ$^+$ and produces IL5, whereas the cells associated with a 'contrasuppressor' function seem to be TCRγδ$^+$ and do not produce IL5.[43]

It is probable that cytokines produced by IELs are intimately involved in immune responses within the epithelium and/or can affect responses in the underlying lamina propria.

Role of IELs in immunoregulation and homeostasis

Studies examining the potential immunoregulatory function of IELs have suggested that IELs are capable of supporting the

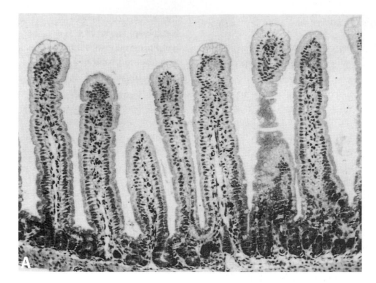

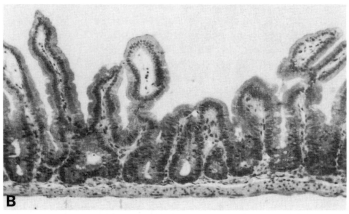

Fig. 7.2 Intestinal damage due to a classical cell-mediated immune response: graft-*versus*-host disease. A Jejunum of a 15-day-old mouse, 14 days after intraperitoneal injection of syngeneic spleen cells (control): Note the long finger-shaped villi and short crypts. The villus/crypt ratio is 5:1 (original magnification × 160). **B** Jejunum of a 15-day-old mouse, 14 days after intraperitoneal injection of parental spleen cells (graft-*versus*-host disease). Note the irregular villus pattern with elongated crypts, shortened villi, mucosal oedema and the only sparsely populated lamina propria. The villus/crypt ratio is reduced to 1.8:1 (original magnification × 160).

differentiation of Peyer's patch B cells into immunoglobulin-producing cells. This helper activity was confined to the CD4+ and CD4+ CD8+ double positive IEL subsets and was not present in the CD8+ subset.[45] B cell help was shown to occur in an antigen-specific and MHC Class II restricted manner. Although the intraepithelial compartment is devoid of B cells, IELs could potentially interact *in vivo* with lamina propria B cells via cytokine secretion and by cell contact through fenestrations in the basement membrane.[82]

More data have suggested an immunoregulatory role for IELs expressing the γδ TCR. It seems that this subset may play an important role in regulating responses to antigen encountered via the oral route in such a way that antigen-specific responses can be mounted in the gut at the same time as systemic responses are suppressed.[43]

The proximity of IELs to the intestinal epithelial cells (IECs) ensures that IEL activities produce effects that modify epithelial function. It has been demonstrated that TCRγδ IELs produce

some trophic factors important for the differentiation and physiology of IECs. It is known that γδ but not αβ IELs are capable of producing keratinocyte growth factor (KGF), which may be important for IEC growth or repair of damaged IECs.[11] IELs may also directly remove damaged or transformed IECs through cytotoxic mechanisms. IELs might also be involved in homeostasis of the intestinal epithelium and of the resident immune system by virtue of their cytokine production.

Delayed-type hypersensitivity reaction

The function of isolated mucosal lymphocytes can be examined *in vivo* upon transfer to naive syngeneic recipients. It has been reported that oral immunization of mice with a protein antigen can induce delayed-type hypersensitivity effector cells in the IEL population capable of transferring a classical delayed-type hypersensitivity reaction to unimmunized recipient mice.[118] Although there is no evidence to suggest that oral immunization *per se* causes a gastrointestinal lesion in these animals, it would be interesting to examine those situations where oral immunization and challenge does lead to small intestinal pathology,[94] to determine whether specific delayed hypersensitivity effector cells can be found in the IEL population. Ferguson and colleagues have studied three animal models: allograft rejection of fetal gut grafts,[85] graft-*versus*-host disease induced in inbred mice by injecting parental spleen cells into F1 offspring[95] and local hypersensitivity reactions produced by oral immunization and challenge using a soluble protein antigen.[94,124] In all three models there were comparable alterations in gut morphology and cell kinetics: increased numbers of IELs (Fig. 7.3), increased crypt cell proliferation rates and increased crypt lengths. Based on these observations, the infiltration of the epithelium by lymphocytes has been examined in a number of clinical situations and their potential relevance to the pathogenesis will be discussed below.

Lamina propria lymphocytes

Lamina propria lymphocytes exist in an increased state of activation, which has been attributed to a continuous exposure to antigens and mitogens in the gut lumen. Although LPLs display an increased expression of activation markers, dividing T lymphocytes within the normal lamina propria are rare.[36] Generally, the pattern of weak proliferative and cytokine responses mirrors that of the IELs, and is probably a manifestation of these cells' maturation/differentiation stage.

Cytotoxic activity

There are several ways in which cytotoxic lymphocytes may play an important role in the function of the intestinal immune system and in the pathogenesis of intestinal disease.[64] Both phenotypic and functional studies are consistent with the conclusion that the effector cells of NK and ADCC activity are infrequent in the intestinal lamina propria,[63,99] and the main cytotoxic activities seem to be confined to the IEL population. It has also been shown that granzyme-containing cells are infrequent in the lamina propria compared with other sites and that they are predominantly of the NK cell phenotype rather than belonging to the CD8+ cytotoxic lymphocyte population.[73]

Cytokines

Many of the functions carried out by T cells in the gastrointestinal immune system are thought to be mediated at least in part by

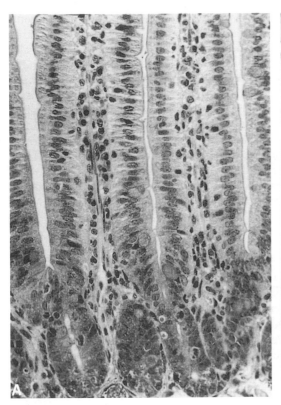 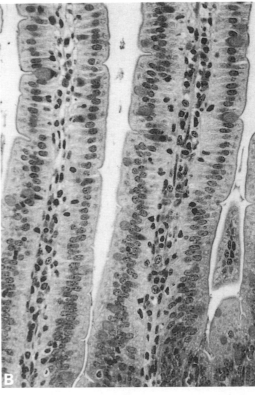

Fig. 7.3 Intraepithelial lymphocyte numbers during a cell-mediated immune response to ovalbumin in the mouse. Original magnification × 320, haematoxylin–eosin stain. **A** Normal morphology and normal crypt cell kinetics in control animals. Intraepithelial lymphocyte count is 11:1 per 100 epithelial cells. **B** Jejunum after induction of a cell-mediated immune reaction to oral ovalbumin administration after injection of the adjuvant N-acetylmuramyl-dipeptide. Increased number of intraepithelial lymphocytes: 18.6 per 100 epithelial cells; otherwise, normal morphology.

their secreted cytokines. In humans, freshly isolated LPLs contain a high frequency of cytokine-secreting cells compared with blood T cells from the same individual.[18,57] Intestinal LPLs have been shown to have the capacity to express IL2, IFNγ, IL4 and IL5 mRNA. Human LPLs do not respond well to CD3 ligation but stimulation with anti-CD2, with or without CD28 costimulation, elicits a strong proliferative and cytokine response. When the LPL-produced cytokines are analysed, the response seems to be dominated by IFNγ.[18,47,57] However, it has also been demonstrated that T cells from the lamina propria are very high producers of IL10 compared with BLs.[14] In addition, Taguchi et al.[131] revealed that LPLs had the highest number of cells spontaneously secreting IL5 compared with IELs and CD4+ cells isolated from Peyer's patches. Functionally it would seem that although both Th1- and Th2-type cytokines are produced by LPLs, the overall effect is Th2-predominant.

Immunoregulatory function

The immunoregulatory functions of the GALT are skewed in favour of tolerance induction to the gastrointestinal content and food. LPLs exert a regulatory influence (help/suppression) on immunoglobulin (Ig) synthesis and also play a role in regulating other lymphoid and non-lymphoid cells. Isolated human LPLs demonstrate both helper and suppressor activity. However, only modest suppressor activity is found unless the cells are activated by exposure to a mitogen such as ConA. The fact that LPLs are predominantly CD4+ indicates that their net functional capacity is significantly shifted toward helper function.

B cell help

As with other mucous membranes, the predominant isotype of Ig secreted by the lymphocytes of the gut is IgA, accounting for 70–90% of all Ig present in the normal intestinal mucosa.[13,127]

LPLs provide marked help during IgA production.[119] In the process of IgA antibody production, mucosal T cells and their derived cytokines play a crucial role during two major steps: the induction of μ to α isotype switching in the PP and the subsequent differentiation of surface IgA+ (sIgA+) B cells to IgA-secreting plasma cells in the lamina propria.[90] The generation of secretory IgA in the gut is driven by Th2 cytokines.

In rodents, Th1 cytokines support IgG2a synthesis in B cell cultures, while Th2 cytokines support IgA, IgG1 and IgE responses.[23,139] TGFβ[75] and IL5[6,120] derived from Th2 cells are involved in the isotype switch from IgM to IgA in mucosal B lymphocytes. Terminal differentiation of sIgA+ B cells into IgA-secreting plasma cells is predominantly regulated by IL5 and IL6, with a synergistic contribution by IL2 and IL4.[42,74] (For a detailed discussion on Ig regulation in the gut, see Chapter 11.)

Intestinal epithelial cells

LPLs, like IELs, also play a role in the regulation of IECs. In turn, LPL responses are regulated not only by ligand–receptor interactions with other lymphocytes but also by the IECs. In addition to the participation of IECs in antigen presentation, cytokines secreted by IECs have direct effects on the lymphocytes both in the epithelial and lamina propria compartment. The bidirectional regulation between IECs and the mucosal lymphocytes makes a complex but efficient communication network (Fig. 7.4).

ORAL TOLERANCE

The GALT immune system has the inherent property of not only providing protective cell-mediated and humoral responses against invading pathogens (danger signals) but also of preventing potential harmful host responses against innocuous dietary proteins and resident bacteria. Exposure of the gastrointestinal tract to

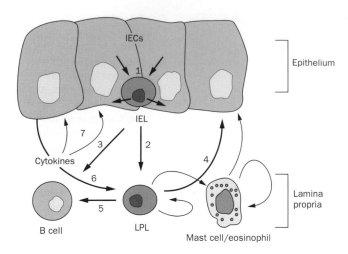

Fig. 7.4 Communication network between mucosal lymphocytes and intestinal epithelial cells. Intraepithelial lymphocytes (IEL) produce cytokines and other factors that influence epithelial cell growth and differentiation (1) as well as the function of underlying cells in the lamina propria (2). Via cytokine secretion IELs also have the ability to interact with B cells in the lamina propria (3). Lamina propria lymphocytes (LPL) activated by IELs and intestinal epithelial cells (IECs) release mediators which act on IECs (4), B cells (5) as well as on other cell populations within the lamina propria. In turn, cytokines produced by IECs can stimulate IELs (1) and LPLs (6) as well as having autocrine or paracrine effects on other epithelial cells (7).

soluble antigen leads to a state of antigen-specific systemic hyporesponsiveness upon antigen challenge. This phenomenon is termed oral tolerance and is a physiological mechanism for the prevention of hypersensitivity at mucosal surfaces. There have been many studies trying to elucidate the mechanisms of oral tolerance.[126,137] It now seems clear that oral tolerance is normally mediated by T cells through different mechanisms depending on the dose of fed antigen. Low-dose antigen favours the induction of regulatory T cells, which mediate active suppression of immune responses, and high-dose antigen induces T cell anergy or rarely clonal deletion.

Active suppression is mediated by the induction of regulatory T cells (T reg) in the GALT, which then migrate to other lymphoid organs.[113] A primary mechanism of active cellular suppression is the secretion of suppressive cytokines such as TGFβ, IL4 and IL10 following antigen-specific triggering.[21] Weiner *et al.* have demonstrated IL10 and TGFβ secretion in the Peyer's patches and lamina propria shortly after oral administration of antigen. TGFβ is produced by both CD4[+] and CD8[+] GALT-derived T cells and is an important mediator of the active suppression component of oral tolerance.[21,49]

The majority of reports of the T reg cells that are induced during oral tolerance induction have so far implicated CD4[+] TCRαβ[+] T cell subsets, but immune-suppressive CD8[+] T cells have also been described.[65,138] There is an indication that TCRγδ[+] T cells may be contained within this population, as oral tolerance is abrogated in mice lacking γδ T cells.[66] Other data also suggest that the TCRγδ[+] IELs play an important role in regulating responses to antigen encountered via the oral route.[44]

A characteristic of the T reg cells induced by a fed antigen is their ability to suppress immune responses stimulated by a dif-

ferent antigen as long as the fed antigen is present in the anatomical vicinity. This concept of linked or bystander suppression has recently been reviewed.[22] T reg cells' ability to inhibit both Th1 and Th2 responses makes them excellent targets for immune therapy in a diverse number of diseases, including allergy, transplantation and autoimmune diseases. Traditionally, antigen-specific approaches to immune therapy have been hampered by the fact that in many cases the precise antigen which triggers the disease is unknown. The ability of T reg to mediate antigen-driven bystander suppression may circumvent this problem, as T reg could be generated in response to antigens known to be present in the target organ. As the molecular events associated with the generation and modulation of oral tolerance are better understood, the ability to apply mucosal tolerance successfully for the treatment of human diseases is a distinct possibility.

GASTROINTESTINAL T LYMPHOCYTES AND CLINICAL DISEASES

The same effector mechanisms that have evolved to protect the host from invading microorganisms can, if inappropriately regulated, induce immune pathology. A number of diseases owe their aetiologies to the induction of aberrant immune responses or loss of 'tolerance'. The following disease examples are intended to highlight the underlying principles whereas a more detailed analysis of the aetiologies is provided in Section C of Part I of this book.

Inflammatory bowel disease
The intestine harbours an enormously complex microflora, which in any one individual may be composed of more than 400 bacterial species. Cells of the intestinal immune system reside in close proximity to this diverse enteric bacterial flora in a state of 'controlled' inflammation. The importance of an intact immune system for intestinal homeostasis has been revealed by the fact that a number of immune manipulations, including deletion of cytokine genes and alterations in T cell subsets, lead to the development of an inflammatory bowel disease (IBD)-like syndrome in mice.[32,106] In chronic IBD the number of inflammatory cells is increased in the mucosa, and in both Crohn's disease and ulcerative colitis (UC) there is an increase in the number of T cells in the epithelia and in the lamina propria, especially around the bases of the crypt (Fig. 7.5).

There have been many studies of cytokine production in Crohn's disease and UC in an effort to understand aetiological factors in human intestinal inflammation. It seems that IL2, IFNγ and TNFα are elevated in the gut of patients with Crohn's disease, but not in patients with UC.[15,96,114] These findings suggest that the activated T helper cells in Crohn's disease show a Th1-type profile compared with T cells in UC, which seem to have a Th2 predominance.

This skewed cytokine response is likely to be an important factor in the development of IBD. IL10 has accordingly been shown to play a pivotal role in intestinal immune regulation, as mice with a targeted disruption of the IL10 gene (IL10[-/-] mice) develop a Th1 cell-mediated colitis under conventional conditions.[10,71] Furthermore, systemic administration of recombinant IL10 prevents the development of colitis in several experimental models.[28,108]

Prevention of a damaging Th1-type response to enteric foreign antigens in mice seems to depend on the activity of regulatory T (T reg) cells contained within the CD4[+] CD45RB[lo] population,

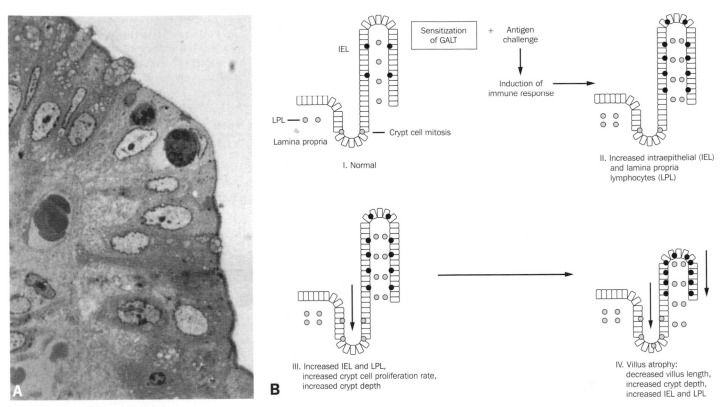

Fig. 7.5 Increased number of intraepithelial and lamina propria lymphocytes in both Crohn's disease and ulcerative colitis. A Semi-thin section of colonic mucosa from a child with Crohn's disease demonstrating intraepithelial granulocytes. Resin-embedded, basic fuchsin–toluidine blue–polychrome stain. Original magnification × 1000. **B** Hypothetical chain of events in the generation of mucosal damage in intestinal cell-mediated immunity (hypertrophic villus atrophy). This model is derived from a series of observations and formal studies in human food-related enteropathies and experimentally induced cell-mediated immunity in animals. Still unresolved are the influences of genetic and environmental features involved in the pathogenesis of mucosal damage. Steps II and III can occur independently and need not necessarily progress to a more severe state of mucosal injury.

and this subset of T cells controls inflammatory responses in the intestine.[91,107,108] Transfer of CD4+ CD45RB[hi] T cells from normal mice to severe combined immune-deficient (SCID) recipients leads to the development of Th1-mediated wasting disease and colitis that can be inhibited by cotransfer of the reciprocal CD4+ CD45RB[lo] population.[91,107] Immunosuppressive effects seem dependent on TGFβ.[105] The function of this T reg subset is also dependent on IL10, as transfer of CD4+ CD45RB[lo] cells from IL10[−/−] mice fails to inhibit colitis.[4] Taken together, studies in the SCID model of colitis suggest that both IL10 and TGFβ play non-redundant roles in the function of the T reg subset, which controls inflammatory responses to intestinal antigens, and thus the precarious balance that exists within the mucosal environment to continuously downregulate excessive or unbalanced Th1 and Th2 cytokine production.

Food-sensitive enteropathies

Hypersensitivity reactions to foods have been implicated in clinical diseases such as eczema, asthma, migraine, rheumatoid arthritis, behavioural disorders and others.[31,80] In a considerable number of these conditions, a clear immunological pathogenesis has not yet been established. Here we will briefly outline food-related hypersensitivities which cause gastroenteropathies with different degrees of mucosal pathology (Fig. 7.5B). Coeliac disease, with its persistent intolerance to gluten, has been studied most intensively. Similar mucosal abnormalities, although not as severe,

have been reported in hypersensitivity reactions to milk, soya, rice, fish, egg and chicken.[2,59,136] From an immunological point of view, however, any food antigen could potentially cause a similar hypersensitivity reaction and careful evaluation of enteropathies in the future will most likely demonstrate clinical syndromes caused by a wide variety of foods and other antigens.

As a permanent form of a food-sensitive gastroenteropathy the study of the aetiopathogenesis of coeliac disease has been facilitated through the identification of the antigenic trigger (gliadin), whereas the study of other possible food-related hypersensitivities and that of IBD have been hampered by the lack of clearly defined trigger antigens or allergens. In coeliac disease, the epithelium is characteristically densely infiltrated with T cells, many of which are γδ[+122] (Fig. 7.6); however, there is also a massive increase in lamina propria CD3+, αβ+, CD4+ T cells. A large number of the T cells invading the lamina propria seem to be CD25+,[55] and it has furthermore been reported that following gluten challenge *in vivo* there is a rapid increase in cells making IFNγ transcripts in the mucosa.[70] IL4 and IL10 transcripts are not elevated in active coeliac disease.[9] It thus seems that also in coeliac disease there is an exaggerated Th1-type response in the mucosa and that the imbalance between Th1 and Th2 cytokines is at least partly responsible for the gastrointestinal pathology seen in this condition. (See Chapter 40.)

Increased numbers of IELs and LPLs have also been demonstrated in cow's milk sensitive enteropathy syndrome.[56,72,102] This

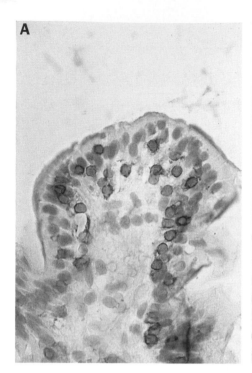

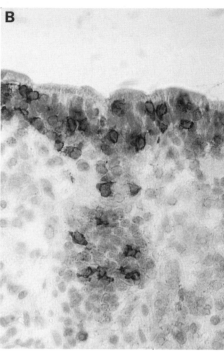

Fig. 7.6 Dense infiltration of an intestinal villus (A) and of crypt epithelium (B) with γδ-positive lymphocytes in gluten-sensitive dermatitis herpetiformis (coeliac disease). Immunoperoxidase staining of an intestinal biopsy of a patient with dermatitis herpetiformis and coeliac disease, demonstrating a dense infiltration of γδ-positive cells (magnification × 400). A gluten-free diet reduces this infiltration, but numbers may remain moderately increased, even on a strict elimination diet. The pathogenetic role of the γδ-lymphocytes remains unclear (with kind permission of Prof. E. Savilahti).

severe gastroenteropathy form of cow's milk allergy is now less frequently reported. Cow's milk, however, continues to cause a wide variety of gastrointestinal symptoms, including vomiting, diarrhoea and failure to thrive. Jejunal biopsies from children with this intestinal disease contain a dramatically increased frequency of CD4+ T cells secreting IFNγ.[57] In cow's milk sensitivity disease and most other food-sensitive enteropathies, the number of T lymphocytes in the gut returns to normal on an elimination diet and rises on subsequent challenge.

CONCLUSION

Intraepithelial cells represent a unique population of lymphoid cells intimately associated with the epithelial surfaces that constitute the interface between the external and internal environments. IELs are described in the skin (dendritic epidermal T cells), respiratory mucosa and genitourinary tract mucosa; however, the greatest numbers of IELs are found within the intestinal mucosa. IELs are interspersed between the mucosal columnar epithelial cells of the villi in the small and large intestine, and are considered to be the first cells of the immune system to encounter food antigens and pathogens that have passed the protective mucus layer that overlies the lumenal surface of the intestinal epithelium. They are a phenotypically and functionally distinct cell population from the lamina propria T cells and many may have a non-thymic origin.

LPLs reside in the highly vascular, loose connective tissue matrix between the muscularis mucosa and epithelium. T cells stimulated under various conditions in the Peyer's patches and other mucosal tissues leave the inductive sites and 'home' to the mucosal lamina propria, which is a dynamic process. In the lamina propria, T cells lie in a 'dormant' state as resting memory cells, and on re-encounter with antigen, express specific effector functions.

There is substantial evidence that both the IELs and LPLs are critical for maintaining normal host defence in the mucosal environment and that they differ from lymphocyte populations in the blood and in other tissue sites in a number of ways.

The immunoregulatory properties of these IEL and LPL populations are crucial for the induction of oral tolerance and may be used therapeutically in the oral treatment of autoimmune and allergic diseases.

REFERENCES

1 Abreu-Martin MT, Targan SR. Lamina propria lymphocytes: a unique population of mucosal lymphocytes. In: *Essentials of Mucosal Immunology* (Kagnoff MFKH, ed.) Academic Press, New York, 1996: 227–45.

2 Ament ME, Rubin CE. Soy protein – another cause of the flat intestinal lesion. *Gastroenterology* 1972; 62(2): 227–34.

3 Aranda R, Sydora BC, Kronenberg M. Intraepithelial lymphocytes: function. In: *Mucosal Immunology* (Ogra PL, Mestecky J, Lamm ME, Strober W, Bienenstock J, McGhee JR, eds.). Academic Press, New York, 1999: 429–37.

4 Asseman C, Mauze S, Leach MW, Coffman RL, Powrie F. An essential role for interleukin 10 in the function of regulatory T cells that inhibit intestinal inflammation. *J Exp Med* 1999; 190(7): 995–1004.

5 Bandeira A, Itohara S, Bonneville M *et al*. Extrathymic origin of intestinal intraepithelial lymphocytes bearing T-cell antigen receptor gamma delta. *Proc Natl Acad Sci USA* 1991; 88(1): 43–7.

6 Beagley KW, Eldridge JH, Kiyono H *et al*. Recombinant murine IL-5 induces high rate IgA synthesis in cycling IgA-positive Peyer's patch B cells. *J Immunol* 1988; 141(6): 2035–42.

7 Beagley KW, Fujihashi K, Lagoo AS *et al*. Differences in intraepithelial lymphocyte T cell subsets isolated from murine small versus large intestine. *J Immunol* 1995; 154(11): 5611–19.

8 Beagley KW, Husband AJ. Intraepithelial lymphocytes: origins, distribution, and function. *Crit Rev Immunol* 1998; 18(3): 237–54.

9 Beckett CG, Dell'Olio D, Kontakou M, Przemioslo RT, Rosen BS, Ciclitira PJ. Analysis of interleukin-4 and interleukin-10 and their

association with the lymphocytic infiltrate in the small intestine of patients with coeliac disease. *Gut* 1996; 39(96): 818–23.

10 Berg DJ, Davidson N, Kuhn R et al. Enterocolitis and colon cancer in interleukin-10-deficient mice are associated with aberrant cytokine production and CD4(+) TH1-like responses. *J Clin Invest* 1996; 98(4): 1010–20.

11 Boismenu R, Havran WL. Modulation of epithelial cell growth by intraepithelial gamma delta T cells. *Science* 1994; 266(5188): 1253–5.

12 Bonneville M, Itohara S, Krecko EG et al. Transgenic mice demonstrate that epithelial homing of gamma/delta T cells is determined by cell lineages independent of T cell receptor specificity. *J Exp Med* 1990; 171(4): 1015–26.

13 Brandtzaeg P, Halstensen TS, Kett K et al. Immunobiology and immunopathology of human gut mucosa: humoral immunity and intraepithelial lymphocytes. *Gastroenterology* 1989; 97(6): 1562–84.

14 Braunstein J, Qiao L, Autschbach F, Schurmann G, Meuer S. T cells of the human intestinal lamina propria are high producers of interleukin-10 [see comments]. *Gut* 1997; 41(2): 215–20.

15 Breese E, Braegger CP, Corrigan CJ, Walker SJ, MacDonald TT. Interleukin-2- and interferon-gamma-secreting T cells in normal and diseased human intestinal mucosa. *Immunology* 1993; 78(1): 127–31.

16 Camerini V, Panwala C, Kronenberg M. Regional specialization of the mucosal immune system. Intraepithelial lymphocytes of the large intestine have a different phenotype and function than those of the small intestine. *J Immunol* 1993; 151(4): 1765–76.

17 Carman PS, Ernst PB, Rosenthal KL, Clark DA, Befus AD, Bienenstock J. Intraepithelial leukocytes contain a unique subpopulation of NK-like cytotoxic cells active in the defense of gut epithelium to enteric murine coronavirus. *J Immunol* 1986; 136(5): 1548–53.

18 Carol M, Lambrechts A, Van-Gossum A, Libin M, Goldman M, Mascart LF. Spontaneous secretion of interferon gamma and interleukin 4 by human intraepithelial and lamina propria gut lymphocytes [see comments]. *Gut* 1998; 42(5): 643–9.

19 Cerf-Bensussan N, Guy-Grand D, Griscelli C. Intraepithelial lymphocytes of human gut: isolation, characterisation and study of natural killer activity. *Gut* 1985; 26(1): 81–8.

20 Cerf-Bensussan N, Jarry A, Brousse N, Lisowska-Grospierre B, Guy-Grand D, Griscelli C. A monoclonal antibody (HML-1) defining a novel membrane molecule present on human intestinal lymphocytes. *Eur J Immunol* 1987; 17(9): 1279–85.

21 Chen Y, Kuchroo VK, Inobe J, Hafler DA, Weiner HL. Regulatory T cell clones induced by oral tolerance: suppression of autoimmune encephalomyelitis. *Science* 1994; 265(5176): 1237–40.

22 Cobbold S, Waldmann H. Infectious tolerance. *Curr Opin Immunol* 1998; 10(5): 518–24.

23 Coffman RL, Seymour BW, Lebman DA et al. The role of helper T cell products in mouse B cell differentiation and isotype regulation. *Immunol Rev* 1988; 102: 5–28.

24 Collan Y. Characteristics of non-epithelial cells in the epithelium of normal rat ileum. A light and electron microscopical study. *Scand J Gastroenterol* 1972; 7 (Suppl 18): 1–66.

25 Comer GM, Ramey WG, Kotler DP, Holt PR. Isolation of intestinal mononuclear cells from colonoscopic biopsies for immunofluorescence analysis by flow cytometry. *Dig Dis Sci* 1986; 31(2): 151–6.

26 De-Maria R, Fais S, Silvestri M et al. Continuous *in vivo* activation and transient hyporesponsiveness to TcR/CD3 triggering of human gut lamina propria lymphocytes. *Eur J Immunol* 1993; 23(12): 3104–8.

27 Deusch K, Luling F, Reich K, Classen M, Wagner H, Pfeffer K. A major fraction of human intraepithelial lymphocytes simultaneously expresses the gamma/delta T cell receptor, the CD8 accessory molecule and preferentially uses the V delta 1 gene segment. *Eur J Immunol* 1991; 21(4): 1053–9.

28 Duchmann R, Schmitt E, Knolle P, Meyer-zum BK, Neurath M. Tolerance towards resident intestinal flora in mice is abrogated in experimental colitis and restored by treatment with interleukin-10 or antibodies to interleukin-12. *Eur J Immunol* 1996; 26(4): 934–8.

29 Ebert EC. Proliferative responses of human intraepithelial lymphocytes to various T-cell stimuli. *Gastroenterology* 1989; 97(6): 1372–81.

30 Ebert EC. Intra-epithelial lymphocytes: interferon-gamma production and suppressor/cytotoxic activities. *Clin Exp Immunol* 1990; 82(1): 81–5.

31 Egger J, Carter CM, Wilson J, Turner MW, Soothill JF. Is migraine food allergy? A double-blind controlled trial of oligoantigenic diet treatment. *Lancet* 1983; 2(8355): 865–69.

32 Elson CO, Sartor RB, Tennyson GS, Riddell RH. Experimental models of inflammatory bowel disease. *Gastroenterology* 1995; 109(4): 1344–67.

33 Enerbäck L. Mast cells in rat gastrointestinal mucosa. 2. Dye-binding and metachromatic properties. *Acta Pathol Microbiol Scand* 1966; 66(3): 303–12.

34 Ernst PB, Clark DA, Rosenthal KL, Befus AD, Bienenstock J. Detection and characterization of cytotoxic T lymphocyte precursors in the murine intestinal intraepithelial leukocyte population. *J Immunol* 1986; 136(6): 2121–6.

35 Farstad IN, Halstensen TS, Fausa O, Brandtzaeg P. Do human Peyer's patches contribute to the intestinal intraepithelial gamma/delta T-cell population? *Scand J Immunol* 1993; 38(5): 451–8.

36 Fell JM, Walker SJ, Spencer J, MacDonald TT. The distribution of dividing T cells throughout the intestinal wall in inflammatory bowel disease (IBD). *Clin Exp Immunol* 1996; 104(2): 280–5.

37 Ferguson A. Intraepithelial lymphocytes of the small intestine. *Gut* 1977; 18(11): 921–37.

38 Ferguson A, Parrott DM. Growth and development of 'antigen-free' grafts of foetal mouse intestine. *J Pathol* 1972; 106(2): 95–101.

39 Ferguson A, Parrott DM. The effect of antigen deprivation on thymus-dependent and thymus-independent lymphocytes in the small intestine of the mouse. *Clin Exp Immunol* 1972; 12(4): 477–88.

40 Ferguson A, Ziegler K, Strobel S. Gluten intolerance (coeliac disease). *Ann Allergy* 1984; 53(6 Pt 2): 637–42.

41 Fichtelius KE. The gut epithelium – a first level lymphoid organ? *Exp Cell Res* 1968; 49(1): 87–104.

42 Fujihashi K, McGhee JR, Lue C et al. Human appendix B cells naturally express receptors for and respond to interleukin 6 with selective IgA1 and IgA2 synthesis. *J Clin Invest* 1991; 88(1): 248–52.

43 Fujihashi K, Taguchi T, Aicher WK et al. Immunoregulatory functions for murine intraepithelial lymphocytes: gamma/delta T cell receptor-positive (TCR+) T cells abrogate oral tolerance, while alpha/beta TCR+ T cells provide B cell help. *J Exp Med* 1992; 175(3): 695–707.

44 Fujihashi K, Taguchi T, McGhee JR et al. Regulatory function for murine intraepithelial lymphocytes. Two subsets of CD3+, T cell receptor-1+ intraepithelial lymphocyte T cells abrogate oral tolerance. *J Immunol* 1990; 145(7): 2010–19.

45 Fujihashi K, Yamamoto M, McGhee JR, Kiyono H. Alpha beta T cell receptor-positive intraepithelial lymphocytes with CD4+, CD8– and CD4+, CD8+ phenotypes from orally immunized mice provide Th2-like function for B cell responses. *J Immunol* 1993; 151(12): 6681–91.

46 Fujihashi K, Yamamoto M, McGhee JR, Kiyono H. Function of alpha beta TCR+ and gamma delta TCR+ IELs for the gastrointestinal immune response. *Int Rev Immunol* 1994; 11(1): 1–14.

47 Fuss IJ, Neurath M, Boirivant M, Klein JS et al. Disparate CD4+ lamina propria (LP) lymphokine secretion profiles in inflammatory bowel disease. Crohn's disease LP cells manifest increased secretion of IFN-gamma, whereas ulcerative colitis LP cells manifest increased secretion of IL-5. *J Immunol* 1996; 157(3): 1261–70.

48 Gelfanov V, Gelfanova V, Lai YG, Liao NS. Activated alpha beta-CD8+, but not alpha alpha-CD8+, TCR-alpha beta+ murine intestinal intraepithelial lymphocytes can mediate perforin-based cytotoxicity, whereas both subsets are active in Fas-based cytotoxicity. *J Immunol* 1996; 156(1): 35–41.

49 Gonnella PA, Chen Y, Inobe J, Komagata Y, Quartulli M, Weiner HL. *In situ* immune response in gut-associated lymphoid tissue (GALT) following oral antigen in TCR-transgenic mice. *J Immunol* 1998; 160(10): 4708–18.

50 Goodman T, Lefrancois L. Expression of the gamma-delta T-cell receptor on intestinal CD8+ intraepithelial lymphocytes. *Nature* 1988; 333(6176): 855–8.

B

51 Guy-Grand D, Cerf-Bensussan N, Malissen B, Malassis SM, Briottet C, Vassalli P. Two gut intraepithelial CD8+ lymphocyte populations with different T cell receptors: a role for the gut epithelium in T cell differentiation. *J Exp Med* 1991; 173(2): 471–81.

52 Guy-Grand D, Griscelli C, Vassalli P. The gut-associated lymphoid system: nature and properties of the large dividing cells. *Eur J Immunol* 1974; 4(6): 435–43.

53 Guy-Grand D, Griscelli C, Vassalli P. The mouse gut T lymphocyte, a novel type of T cell. Nature, origin, and traffic in mice in normal and graft-versus-host conditions. *J Exp Med* 1978; 148(6): 1661–77.

54 Halstensen TS, Scott H, Brandtzaeg P. Human CD8+ intraepithelial T lymphocytes are mainly CD45RA-RB+ and show increased co-expression of CD45R0 in celiac disease. *Eur J Immunol* 1990; 20(8): 1825–30.

55 Halstensen TS, Scott H, Fausa O, Brandtzaeg P. Gluten stimulation of coeliac mucosa *in vitro* induces activation (CD25) of lamina propria CD4+ T cells and macrophages but no crypt-cell hyperplasia. *Scand J Immunol* 1993; 38(6): 581–90.

56 Harrison M, Kilby A, Walker-Smith JA, France NE, Wood CB. Cows' milk protein intolerance: a possible association with gastroenteritis, lactose intolerance, and IgA deficiency. *Br Med J* 1976; 1(6024): 1501–4.

57 Hauer AC, Breese EJ, Walker SJ, MacDonald TT. The frequency of cells secreting interferon-gamma and interleukin-4, -5, and -10 in the blood and duodenal mucosa of children with cow's milk hypersensitivity. *Pediatr Res* 1997; 42(5): 629–38.

58 Ibraghimov AR, Lynch RG. Heterogeneity and biased T cell receptor alpha/beta repertoire of mucosal CD8+ cells from murine large intestine: implications for functional state. *J Exp Med* 1994; 180(2): 433–44.

59 Iyngkaran N, Abidin Z, Meng LL, Yadav M. Egg-protein-induced villous atrophy. *J Pediatr Gastroenterol Nutr* 1982; 1(1): 29–33.

60 Jalkanen S. Lymphocyte traffic to mucosa-associated lymphatic tissues. *Immunol Res* 1991; 10(3–4): 268–70.

61 Jalkanen S, Nash GS, De-los-Toyos J, MacDermott RP, Butcher EC. Human lamina propria lymphocytes bear homing receptors and bind selectively to mucosal lymphoid high endothelium. *Eur J Immunol* 1989; 19(1): 63–8.

62 James SP, Fiocchi C, Graeff AS, Strober W. Phenotypic analysis of lamina propria lymphocytes. Predominance of helper-inducer and cytolytic T-cell phenotypes and deficiency of suppressor-inducer phenotypes in Crohn's disease and control patients. *Gastroenterology* 1986; 91(6): 1483–9.

63 James SP, Graeff AS. Spontaneous and lymphokine-induced cytotoxic activity of monkey intestinal mucosal lymphocytes. *Cell Immunol* 1985; 93(2): 387–97.

64 James SP, Strober W. Cytotoxic lymphocytes and intestinal disease. *Gastroenterology* 1986; 90(1): 235–7.

65 Ke Y, Kapp JA. Oral antigen inhibits priming of CD8+ CTL, CD4+ T cells, and antibody responses while activating CD8+ suppressor T cells. *J Immunol* 1996; 156(3): 916–21.

66 Ke Y, Pearce K, Lake JP, Ziegler HK, Kapp JA. Gamma delta T lymphocytes regulate the induction and maintenance of oral tolerance. *J Immunol* 1997; 158(8): 3610–18.

67 Klein JR. Ontogeny of the Thy-1–, Lyt-2+ murine intestinal intraepithelial lymphocyte. Characterization of a unique population of thymus-independent cytotoxic effector cells in the intestinal mucosa. *J Exp Med* 1986; 164(1): 309–14.

68 Klein JR, Mosley RL. Phenotypic and cytotoxic characteristics of intraepithelial lymphocytes. In: *Advances in Host Defense Mechanisms. Mucosal Immunology: Intraepithelial Lymphocytes* (Kiyono HMJR, ed). Raven Press, New York, 1993: 33–60.

69 Klein JR, Mosley RL, Kaiserlian D. Expression of the asialo GM1 determinant on murine intestinal epithelia. *Proc Soc Exp Biol Med* 1990; 195(3): 329–34.

70 Kontakou M, Przemioslo RT, Sturgess RP *et al*. Cytokine mRNA expression in the mucosa of treated coeliac patients after wheat peptide challenge. *Gut* 1995; 37(1): 52–7.

71 Kuhn R, Lohler J, Rennick D, Rajewsky K, Muller W. Interleukin-10-deficient mice develop chronic enterocolitis [see comments]. *Cell* 1993; 75(2): 263–74.

72 Kuitunen P, Visakorpi JK, Savilahti E, Pelkonen P. Malabsorption syndrome with cow's milk intolerance. Clinical findings and course in 54 cases. *Arch Dis Child* 1975; 50(5): 351–6.

73 Kummer JA, Kamp AM, Tadema TM, Vos W, Meijer CJ, Hack CE. Localization and identification of granzymes A and B-expressing cells in normal human lymphoid tissue and peripheral blood. *Clin Exp Immunol* 1995; 100(1): 164–72.

74 Kunimoto DY, Nordan RP, Strober W. IL-6 is a potent cofactor of IL-1 in IgM synthesis and of IL-5 in IgA synthesis. *J Immunol* 1989; 143(7): 2230–5.

75 Lebman DA, Lee FD, Coffman RL. Mechanism for transforming growth factor beta and IL-2 enhancement of IgA expression in lipopolysaccharide-stimulated B cell cultures. *J Immunol* 1990; 144(3): 952–9.

76 Lefrancois L. Phenotypic complexity of intraepithelial lymphocytes of the small intestine. *J Immunol* 1991; 147(6): 1746–51.

77 Lefrancois L, Fuller B, Olson S, Puddington L. Development of intestinal intraepithelial lymphocytes. In: *Essentials of Mucosal Immunology* (Kagnoff MF, Kiyono H, eds). Academic Press, New York, 1996: 183–93.

78 Lefrancois L, LeCorre R, Mayo J, Bluestone JA, Goodman T. Extrathymic selection of TCR gamma delta + T cells by class II major histocompatibility complex molecules. *Cell* 1990; 63(2): 333–40.

79 Lefrancois L, Olson S. A novel pathway of thymus-directed T lymphocyte maturation. *J Immunol* 1994; 153(3): 987–95.

80 Lessof M. *Clinical Reactions to Food*. John Wiley and Sons, Chichester, 1983.

81 Lin T, Matsuzaki G, Kenai H, Nakamura T, Nomoto K. Thymus influences the development of extrathymically derived intestinal intraepithelial lymphocytes. *Eur J Immunol* 1993; 23(8): 1968–74.

82 Lundqvist C, Baranov V, Hammarstrom S, Athlin L, Hammarstrom ML. Intra-epithelial lymphocytes. Evidence for regional specialization and extrathymic T cell maturation in the human gut epithelium. *Int Immunol* 1995; 7(9): 1473–87.

83 Lundqvist C, Baranov V, Teglund S, Hammarstrom S, Hammarstrom ML. Cytokine profile and ultrastructure of intraepithelial gamma delta T cells in chronically inflamed human gingiva suggest a cytotoxic effector function. *J Immunol* 1994; 153(5): 2302–12.

84 Lundqvist C, Melgar S, Yeung MM, Hammarstrom S, Hammarstrom ML. Intraepithelial lymphocytes in human gut have lytic potential and a cytokine profile that suggest T helper 1 and cytotoxic functions. *J Immunol* 1996; 157(5): 1926–34.

85 MacDonald TT, Ferguson A. Hypersensitivity reactions in the small intestine. III. The effects of allograft rejection and of graft-versus-host disease on epithelial cell kinetics. *Cell Tissue Kinet* 1977; 10(4): 301–12.

86 Marsh MN. Studies of intestinal lymphoid tissue. III. Quantitative analyses of epithelial lymphocytes in the small intestine of human control subjects and of patients with celiac sprue. *Gastroenterology* 1980; 79(3): 481–92.

87 Mayrhofer G. Fixation and staining of granules in mucosal mast cells and intraepithelial lymphocytes in the rat jejunum, with special reference to the relationship between the acid glycosaminoglycans in the two cell types. *Histochem J* 1980; 12(5): 513–26.

88 Mayrhofer G. Thymus-dependent and thymus-independent subpopulations of intestinal intraepithelial lymphocytes: a granular subpopulation of probable bone marrow origin and relationship to mucosal mast cells. *Blood* 1980; 55(3): 532–5.

89 Mayrhofer G, Whately RJ. Granular intraepithelial lymphocytes of the rat small intestine. I. Isolation, presence in T lymphocyte-deficient rats and bone marrow origin. *Int Arch Allergy Appl Immunol* 1983; 71(4): 317–27.

90 Mega J, Bruce MG, Beagley KW *et al*. Regulation of mucosal responses by CD4+ T lymphocytes: effects of anti-L3T4 treatment on the gastrointestinal immune system. *Int Immunol* 1991; 3(8): 793–805.

91 Morrissey PJ, Charrier K, Braddy S, Liggitt D, Watson JD. CD4+ T cells that express high levels of CD45RB induce wasting disease when transferred into congenic severe combined immunodeficient mice. Disease development is prevented by cotransfer of purified CD4+ T cells. *J Exp Med* 1993; 178(1): 237–44.

92 Mosley RL, Klein JR. A rapid method for isolating murine intestine intraepithelial lymphocytes with high yield and purity. *J Immunol Methods* 1992; 156(1): 19–26.

93 Mosley RL, Styre D, Klein JR. CD4+CD8+ murine intestinal intraepithelial lymphocytes. *Int Immunol* 1990; 2(4): 361–5.

94 Mowat AM, Ferguson A. Hypersensitivity in the small intestinal mucosa. V. Induction of cell-mediated immunity to a dietary antigen. *Clin Exp Immunol* 1981; 43(3): 574–82.

95 Mowat AM, Ferguson A. Intraepithelial lymphocyte count and crypt hyperplasia measure the mucosal component of the graft-versus-host reaction in mouse small intestine. *Gastroenterology* 1982; 83(2): 417–23.

96 Mullin GE, Lazenby AJ, Harris ML, Bayless TM, James SP. Increased interleukin-2 messenger RNA in the intestinal mucosal lesions of Crohn's disease but not ulcerative colitis. *Gastroenterology* 1992; 102(5): 1620–7.

97 O'Connell SM, Roberts AI, Ebert EC. The CD2 receptor regulates the proliferation of intraepithelial lymphocytes in response to phytohemagglutinin but not to staphylococcal enterotoxin B. *Gastroenterology* 1992; 102(4).

98 Otto HF. The interepithelial lymphocytes of the intestinum. Morphological observations and immunologic aspects of intestinal enteropathy. *Curr Top Pathol* 1973; 57: 81–121.

99 Pang G, Buret A, Batey RT *et al*. Morphological, phenotypic and functional characteristics of a pure population of CD56+ CD16– CD3– large granular lymphocytes generated from human duodenal mucosa. *Immunology* 1993; 79(3): 498–505.

100 Parrott DM, Tait C, MacKenzie S, Mowat AM, Davies MD, Micklem HS. Analysis of the effector functions of different populations of mucosal lymphocytes. *Ann NY Acad Sci* 1983; 409: 307–20.

101 Petit A, Ernst PB, Befus AD *et al*. Murine intestinal intraepithelial lymphocytes I. Relationship of a novel Thy-1–, Lyt-1–, Lyt-2+, granulated subpopulation to natural killer cells and mast cells. *Eur J Immunol* 1985; 15(3): 211–15.

102 Phillips AD, Rice SJ, France NE, Walker-Smith JA. Small intestinal intraepithelial lymphocyte levels in cow's milk protein intolerance. *Gut* 1979; 20(6): 509–12.

103 Poussier P, Edouard P, Lee C, Binnie M, Julius M. Thymus-independent development and negative selection of T cells expressing T cell receptor alpha/beta in the intestinal epithelium: evidence for distinct circulation patterns of gut- and thymus-derived T lymphocytes. *J Exp Med* 1992; 176(1): 187–99.

104 Poussier P, Teh HS, Julius M. Thymus-independent positive and negative selection of T cells expressing a major histocompatibility complex class I restricted transgenic T cell receptor alpha/beta in the intestinal epithelium. *J Exp Med* 1993; 178(6): 1947–57.

105 Powrie F, Carlino J, Leach MW, Mauze S, Coffman RL. A critical role for transforming growth factor-beta but not interleukin 4 in the suppression of T helper type 1-mediated colitis by CD45RB(low) CD4+ T cells. *J Exp Med* 1996; 183(6): 2669–74.

106 Powrie F, Leach MW. Genetic and spontaneous models of inflammatory bowel disease in rodents: evidence for abnormalities in mucosal immune regulation. *Ther Immunol* 1995; 2(2): 115–23.

107 Powrie F, Leach MW, Mauze S, Caddle LB, Coffman RL. Phenotypically distinct subsets of CD4+ T cells induce or protect from chronic intestinal inflammation in C. B-17 scid mice. *Int Immunol* 1993; 5(11): 1461–71.

108 Powrie F, Leach MW, Mauze S, Menon S, Caddle LB, Coffman RL. Inhibition of Th1 responses prevents inflammatory bowel disease in scid mice reconstituted with CD45RBhi CD4+ T cells. *Immunity* 1994; 1(7): 553–62.

109 Rocha B, Vassalli P, Guy GD. Thymic and extrathymic origins of gut intraepithelial lymphocyte populations in mice. *J Exp Med* 1994; 180(2): 681–6.

110 Rocha B, von-Boehmer H, Guy GD. Selection of intraepithelial lymphocytes with CD8 alpha/alpha co-receptors by self-antigen in the murine gut. *Proc Natl Acad Sci USA* 1992; 89(12): 5336–40.

111 Röpke C, Everett NB. Proliferative kinetics of large and small intraepithelial lymphocytes in the small intestine of the mouse. *Am J Anat* 1976; 145(3): 395–408.

112 Rudzik O, Bienenstock J. Isolation and characteristics of gut mucosal lymphocytes. *Lab Invest* 1974; 30(3): 260–6.

113 Santos LM, al-Sabbagh A, Londono A, Weiner HL. Oral tolerance to myelin basic protein induces regulatory TGF-beta-secreting T cells in Peyer's patches of SJL mice. *Cell Immunol* 1994; 157(2): 439–47.

114 Sartor RB. Cytokines in intestinal inflammation: pathophysiological and clinical considerations. *Gastroenterology* 1994; 106(2): 533–9.

115 Schieferdecker HL, Ullrich R, Hirseland H, Zeitz M. T cell differentiation antigens on lymphocytes in the human intestinal lamina propria. *J Immunol* 1992; 149(8): 2816–22.

116 Schieferdecker HL, Ullrich R, Weiss BA *et al*. The HML-1 antigen of intestinal lymphocytes is an activation antigen. *J Immunol* 1990; 144(7): 2541–9.

117 Senju M, Wu KC, Mahida YR, Jewell DP. Two-color immunofluorescence and flow cytometric analysis of lamina propria lymphocyte subsets in ulcerative colitis and Crohn's disease. *Dig Dis Sci* 1991; 36(10): 1453–8.

118 Shields JG, Parrott DM. Appearance of delayed-type hypersensitivity effector cells in murine gut mucosa. *Immunology* 1985; 54(4): 771–6.

119 Smart CJ. Trejdosiewiez LK, Badr-el DS, Heatley RV. T lymphocytes of the human colonic mucosa: functional and phenotypic analysis. *Clin Exp Immunol* 1988; 73(1): 63–9.

120 Sonoda E, Matsumoto R, Hitoshi Y *et al*. Transforming growth factor beta induces IgA production and acts additively with interleukin 5 for IgA production. *J Exp Med* 1989; 170(4): 1415–20.

121 Spencer J, Dillon SB, Isaacson PG, MacDonald TT. T cell subclasses in fetal human ileum. *Clin Exp Immunol* 1986; 65(3): 553–8.

122 Spencer J, Isaacson PG, Diss TC, MacDonald TT. Expression of disulfide-linked and non-disulfide-linked forms of the T cell receptor gamma/delta heterodimer in human intestinal intraepithelial lymphocytes. *Eur J Immunol* 1989; 19(7): 1335–8.

123 Spencer J, MacDonald TT, Isaacson PG. Heterogeneity of non-lymphoid cells expressing HLA-D region antigens in human fetal gut. *Clin Exp Immunol* 1987; 67(2): 415–24.

124 Strobel S, Ferguson A. Effects on neonatal antigen feeding on subsequent systemic and local CMI responses. *Gut* 1982; 23.

125 Strobel S, Miller HR, Ferguson A. Human intestinal mucosal mast cells: evaluation of fixation and staining techniques. *J Clin Pathol* 1981; 34(8): 851–8.

126 Strobel S, Mowat AM. Immune responses to dietary antigens: oral tolerance. *Immunol Today* 1998; 19(4): 173–81.

127 Strober W, Harriman GR. The regulation of IgA B-cell differentiation. *Gastroenterol Clin North Am* 1991; 20(3): 473–94.

128 Sydora BC, Habu S, Taniguchi M. Intestinal intraepithelial lymphocytes preferentially repopulate the intestinal epithelium. *Int Immunol* 1993; 5(7): 743–51.

129 Sydora BC, Mixter PF, Holcombe HR *et al*. Intestinal intraepithelial lymphocytes are activated and cytolytic but do not proliferate as well as other T cells in response to mitogenic signals. *J Immunol* 1993; 150(6): 2179–91.

130 Taguchi T, Aicher WK, Fujihashi K *et al*. Novel function for intestinal intraepithelial lymphocytes. Murine CD3+, gamma/delta TCR+ T cells produce IFN-gamma and IL-5. *J Immunol* 1991; 147(11): 3736–44.

131 Taguchi T, McGhee JR, Coffman RL *et al*. Analysis of Th1 and Th2 cells in murine gut-associated tissues. Frequencies of CD4+ and CD8+ T cells that secrete IFN-gamma and IL-5. *J Immunol* 1990; 145(1): 68–77.

132 Trepel F. Number and distribution of lymphocytes in man. A critical analysis. *Klin Wochenschr* 1974; 52(11): 511–15.

133 Ullrich R, Schieferdecker HL, Ziegler K, Riecken EO, Zeitz M. Gamma delta T cells in the human intestine express surface markers of activation and are preferentially located in the epithelium. *Cell Immunol* 1990; 128(2): 619–27.

134 Umesaki Y, Setoyama H, Matsumoto S, Okada Y. Expansion of alpha beta T-cell receptor-bearing intestinal intraepithelial lymphocytes after microbial colonization in germ-free mice and its independence from thymus. *Immunology* 1993; 79(1): 32–7.

135 Van-der-Heijden PJ, Stok W. Improved procedure for the isolation of functionally active lymphoid cells from the murine intestine. *J Immunol Methods* 1987; 103(2): 161–7.

136 Vitoria JC, Camarero C, Sojo A, Ruiz A, Rodriguez SJ. Enteropathy related to fish, rice, and chicken. *Arch Dis Child* 1982; 57(1): 44–8.

137 Weiner HL. Oral tolerance: immune mechanisms and treatment of autoimmune disease. *Immunol Today* 1997; 18(7): 335–43.

138 Weiner HL, Friedman A, Miller A *et al*. Oral tolerance: immunologic mechanisms and treatment of animal and human organ-specific autoimmune diseases by oral administration of autoantigens. *Annu Rev Immunol* 1994; 12: 809–37.

139 Xu AJ, Beagley KW, Mega J, Fujihashi K, Kiyono H, McGhee JR. Induction of T helper cells and cytokines for mucosal IgA responses. *Adv Exp Med Biol* 1992; 327: 107–17.

140 Zeitz M, Greene WC, Peffer NJ, James SP. Lymphocytes isolated from the intestinal lamina propria of normal nonhuman primates have increased expression of genes associated with T-cell activation. *Gastroenterology* 1988; 94(3): 647–55.

141 Zeitz M, Schieferdecker HL, Ullrich R, Jahn HU, James SP, Riecken EO. Phenotype and function of lamina propria T lymphocytes. *Immunol Res* 1991; 10(3–4): 199–206.

142 Agace WW, Roberts AI, Wu L, Greineder C, Ebert EC, Parker CM. Human intestinal lamina propria and intraepithelial lymphocytes express receptors specific for chemokines induced by inflammation. *Eur J Immunol* 2000; 30: 819–26.

Chapter 8

Natural killer cells and aspects of intestinal immunity

S. Strobel and J. Strid

INTRODUCTION

Considering the gut's ability to handle large amounts of foreign antigens as well as bacteria (commensal and pathogenic) and viruses, the complexity of the intestinal immune regulation and associated anti-inflammatory strategies is not surprising. The intestinal tract is equipped with a large number of specific immunological mechanisms and harbours unique cell populations, which contribute both to local defence and to immunopathological and inflammatory reactions. The gut and the gut-associated lymphoid tissues (GALT) also contain large numbers of non-specific effector cells, including macrophages, mast cells, eosinophils and cells of lymphocyte origin with direct and indirect (antibody-dependent) cytolytic activity.

Natural killer (NK) cells represent one cell population of the innate immune system, which has both direct and indirect effector and immunoregulatory properties. This chapter will mainly focus on the characteristics and possible roles of NK cells in the intestinal tract.

DEFINITION OF NK CELLS

NK cells are identified by their ability to kill susceptible lymphoid tumour cell lines *in vitro* without the need for prior immunization or sensitization. This property makes them particularly well suited to antiviral activities and effective immune surveillance. A large array of NK-associated cell surface markers have been identified, overlapping with those found on cells of other lineages, including T cells, macrophages and granulocytes, and are summarized in Table 8.1.

CHARACTERISTICS OF NK CELLS

Histologically NK cells belong to a subset of large granular lymphocytes which are characterized by distinct azurophilic cytoplasmic granules. Cells with an NK cell phenotype CD16 (Table 8.1) are detectable at 6 weeks of gestation in the fetal liver and comprise about 15% of blood lymphocytes (BLs) at birth and in adults. Due to the higher lymphocyte count of neonates, the total number of NK cells at that age is twice as high as in adults, although the cytolytic function of neonatal NK cells may only reach about 50% of those of adults.[10] The fraction of NK cells expressing the CD56 and CD57 surface antigen are lower at birth, and the reduced cytolytic activity seems to be due to this fact.[58,80]

Origin of NK cells

NK cells seem to belong to the lymphoid lineage.[79] Although the T and NK cell lineages are closely related to each other, NK cells can develop independently of the thymus.[1,71] CD3+ T cells expressing NK receptors (NK T cells) have been identified and may be of particular importance in recognizing glycolipid antigens in connection with the non-classical MHC antigen CD 1d.[16] Apart from the blood, cells with NK activity are predominantly found within the gut epithelium and within germinal centres, possibly indicating their role in immunoregulation.

Function of NK cells

NK cells that will bind to and kill sensitive targets can be isolated from uninfected individuals. This activity is increased up to 100-fold during infection, when NK cells are exposed to interferon α

CD antigens expressed on natural killer (NK) cells					
CD antigens	Cellular expression on NK and other cells	MW (kDa)	Functions	Other names	Family relationships
CD2	T cells, thymocytes, NK cells	45–58	Adhesion molecule, binding CD58 (LFA-3). Binds Lck intracellularly		
CD16	Neutrophils, NK cells, macrophages	50–80	Component of low affinity Fc receptor. FcγRIII mediates phagocytosis and antibody-dependent cell-mediated cytotoxicity	FcγRIII	Immunoglobulin superfamily
CD27	Medullary thymocytes, T cells, NK cells, some B cells	55	Binds CD70; can function as a costimulator for T and B cells		NGF receptor superfamily
CD30	Activated T, B and NK cells, monocytes	120	Binds CD30L; crosslinking CD30 enhances proliferation of B and T cells	Ki 1	NGF receptor superfamily
CD39	Activated B cells, activated NK cells, macrophages, dendritic cells	78	Unknown, may mediate adhesion of B cells		
CD57	NK cells, subsets of T cells, B cells and monocytes		Oligosaccharide, found on many cell surface glycoproteins	HNK 1, Leu-7	
CD56	NK cells	135–220	Isoform of neural cell adhesion molecule (NCAM), adhesion molecule	NKH 1	Immunoglobulin superfamily
CD62L	B cells, T cells, monocytes, NK cells	150	Leukocyte adhesion molecule (LAM), binds CD34, GlyCAM, mediates rolling interactions with endothelium	LAM 1, L-selectin, LECAM 1	C-type lectin, EGF and CCP superfamily
CD69	Activated T and B cells, activated macrophages and NK cells	28,32 homodimer	Unknown, early activation antigen	Activation inducer molecule (AIM)	C-type lectin
CD87	Granulocytes, monocytes, macrophages, T cells, NK cells, wide variety of non-haematopoietic cell types	35–59	Receptor for urokinase plasminogen activator	uPAR	Ly-6 superfamily
CD94	T cells subsets, NK cells	43	Unknown	KP43	
CD98	T cells, B cells, NK cells, granulocytes, all human cell lines	80,45 heterodimer	May be amino acid transporter	4F2, FRP 1	
CD122	NK cells, resting T cell subsets, some B cell lines	75	IL2 receptor β chain	IL2R	Cytokine receptor superfamily, fibronectin type III superfamily
CD158a	NK cell subsets	50 or 58	Inhibits NK cell cytotoxicity on binding HLA-C alleles, KIR	p50.1, p58.1	Immunoglobulin superfamily
CD158b	NK cell subsets	50 or 58	Inhibits NK cell cytotoxicity on binding HLA-Cw alleles, KIR	p50.2, p58.2	Immunoglobulin superfamily
CD161	NK cells, T cells	44	Regulates NK cytotoxicity	NKRP1	C-type lectin

B

Table 8.1 CD antigens expressed on natural killer (NK) cells. KIR = killer inhibitory receptor

Composition of human cytolytic granules

Name	Function	MW*
Granzyme 1	Protease	45 000
Granzyme 2	Protease	30 000
Granzyme 3	Protease	25 000
Perforin	Pore formation	70 000
Proteoglycan	Packaging	200 000
Nucleolysis triggering factor	DNA degradation	50 000

* Apparent molecular weight by SDS-PAGE (unreduced) (After Podack et al.[59])

Table 8.2 Composition of human cytolytic granules.

(IFNα), interferon β (IFNβ), or to the NK activating factor interleukin 12 (IL12) that is produced early during infection.

The cytoplasmatic granules of NK cells contain a number of very potent Ca-dependent enzymes (Table 8.2) which are efficiently used in target cell destruction by cytolytic lymphocytes (Fig. 8.2). This and other findings suggest that contact-dependent cytotoxic activity of large granular morphology is mediated by a secretory process of toxic products, which leads to membrane damage of the target cell and nuclear breakdown in a multistep process.[33,34]

IL12 together with tumour necrosis factor α (TNFα) also triggers production of IFNγ by NK cells. This secreted IFNγ is instrumental in controlling some infections before T cells are activated to produce IFNγ. The order of lymphocyte subset induction during infection of *Listeria monocytogenes* in mice has revealed activation of NK cells before activation of extrathymic and thymus-derived T cells. Elimination of NK cells results in death, due to an otherwise nonlethal infection,[55] before induction of protective adaptive immunity.

REGULATORY NK RECEPTORS

A fine balance of inhibitory and triggering signals controls the function of NK cells. NK cells are found in two functionally different forms – activatory and inhibitory – which differ in their cytoplasmic tail. Inhibitory receptors contain two conserved motifs called 'immunoreceptor tyrosine-based inhibition motifs' (ITIMS), which are missing in activatory receptors.[48,81] For most known receptors both forms exist, but there are exceptions. NK cell activity is suppressed through recognition of certain major histocompatibility complex (MHC) Class I molecules.[43] The group of surface receptors, which play this inhibitory role belong to the immunoglobulin superfamily[44] (Fig. 8.2a). NK cells do not rearrange their receptor and the nature of NK cell triggering by receptor–ligand interaction is not well defined.

Interestingly, some activating molecules are homologous to inhibitory molecules and have been demonstrated in humans and rodents. Receptors with a repressive function were defined as p58 and p70/p140 molecules or killer inhibitory receptors;[9,46] proteins triggering cytotoxicity were named p50 or killer activating receptors (Fig. 8.2b).[13,45,49] NK cells are known to be an important source of IFNγ and TNFα, cytokines that provide powerful activation signals for other cells, such as macrophages, to kill both intracellular and extracellular microorganisms.

Due to their antimicrobial effects, recent research has focused on the above cytokines, although NK cells produce other important mediators which may influence host resistance to infections; these include chemotactic proteins (IL8, MIP1α), haematopoietic

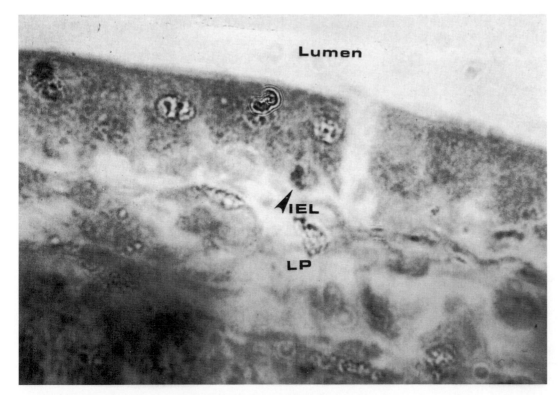

Fig. 8.1 Granulated intraepithelial lymphocyte.

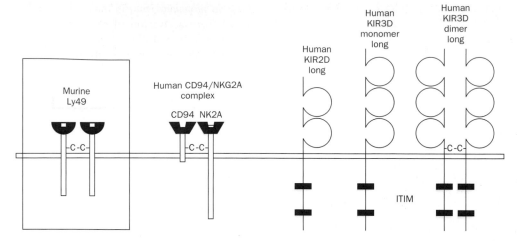

Fig. 8.2a Inhibitory NK cell receptor for MHC Class I. All family members (except CD94) contain immunoreceptor tyrosine-based inhibition motifs (ITIM) sequences in the cytoplasmic domain. KIR are members of the immunoglobulin (Ig)-superfamily and contain either two or three Ig domains in the extracellular region. CD94, NKG2 and Ly49 are members of the C-type lectin superfamily and possess carbohydrate recognition domains in the extracellular region. (Modified after Lanier.[43])

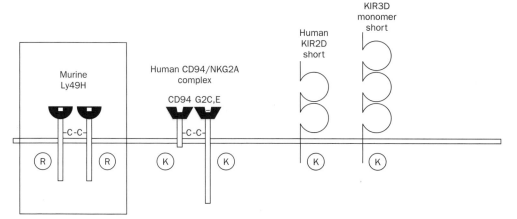

Fig. 8.2b Stimulatory NK cell receptors. Noninhibitory NK cell receptors of the Ly49, CD94/NKG2 and KIR families. Note the lack of ITIM in the cytoplasmic domains and the presence of charged amino acids in the transmembrane domains of Ly49H, KIR3DS, NKG2C, E and CD94. ITIM = immunoreceptor tyrosine-based inhibition motifs. (Modified after Lanier[43].)

factors (granulocyte–macrophage colony-stimulating factor (GM-CSF) and macrophage colony-stimulating factor (M-CSF)) and IL3.[14] A summary detailing known and presumed NK cell functions is provided in Table 8.3.

NK cell functions
Tumour immunity
inhibition of primary tumour development
inhibition of metastases
in vitro cytotoxicity
Transplantation immunity
hybrid resistance
graft-*versus*-host disease
organ transplant rejection
Cell regulation
up- or downregulation of antibody responses
up- or downregulation of cell-mediated responses
natural suppression
control of haematopoiesis
Infection
protection against viral, fungal, parasitic and bacterial infection

Table 8.3 NK cell functions.

NK CELL DEFICIENCY

Despite the clearly important functions of NK cells, it is intriguing that the clinical effects of isolated NK deficiency, possibly a very rare occurrence, are not as severe as anticipated.

One patient described[12] was asymptomatic until 13 years of age when she developed severe varicella and 4 years later a severe cytomegalovirus infection. Further siblings studied[42] were essentially asymptomatic. Studies in the rodent equivalent, the beige mouse strain, have provided conflicting results.[39,63,69] In other diseases where diminished or absent NK activity has been reported – as in Chédiak–Higashi syndrome,[38,61] lymphocyte adhesion deficiencies[66] and haemophagocytic lymphohistiocytosis[37,40] – deficiencies of other effector mechanisms due to the primary disease are likely to account for the clinical symptomatology.

OTHER EFFECTOR FUNCTIONS

The ability of NK cells to kill tumour cell targets *in vitro* has led to the concept that NK cells may act as an important nonspecific immune–surveillance mechanism in the defence against tumours (Fig. 8.3). This is supported by the accelerated growth of tumours in NK-cell-depleted animals and by the ability of an enriched population to mediate tumour resistance.[41] Experiments with transplanted tumour cell lines suggest that NK cells reject transformed cells that lack Class I expression,[2,47,57] although it remains speculative whether this is a mechanism of tumour

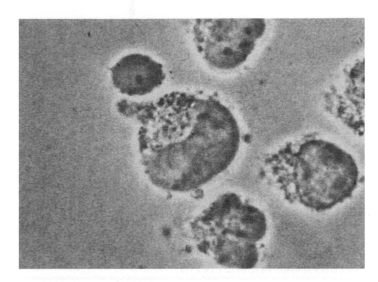

Fig. 8.3 Attack of target cell by an IL-2 activated cytotoxic killer cell. In this model, killing by NK cells depends on the intercellular adhesion molecule ICAM-2 and is regulated by the distribution of ICAM-2 on the cell surface. Cytotoxic killer cells recognize adhesion molecules that are present on normal cells but which may be concentrated into active regions by cytoskeletel reorganization in diseased cells. Phase contrast micrograph of an IL-2 activated lymphocyte adhering to the uropod (localized ICAM-2). (With kind permission of Dr T Helander, Helsinki, *Nature* 1996;382:265–8)

Innate cytokine and chemokine regulation of natural killer cell functions	
Cytokine	**Direct and indirect effects on NK cells**
Cytokines	
IFNα/β	Induces cell trafficking and cytotoxic activity: stimulates proliferation *in vivo*; inhibits IL12 production; elicits expression of IL15 mRNA
IL12	Stimulates IFNγ production; induces cytotoxicity and is critical for the response during certain non-viral infections; synergizes with IL15 to induce expression of MIP1α
TNF	Synergizes with IL12 for IFNγ production
IL1α/β	Synergizes with IL12 for IFNγ production
IL15	Promotes cell growth and maturation; synergizes with IL12 for induction of IFNγ production; synergizes with IL12 to induce expression of MIP 1α
IL18	Stimulates IFNγ production; synergizes with IL12 for IFNγ production and cytotoxic activity
IL10	Inhibits IL12 production
TGFβ	Inhibits IFNγ production; inhibits IL12 production; blocks proliferation and cytotoxicity
Chemokines	
MIP 1α	Induces chemotaxis in culture and following infection *in vivo*
MIP 1β	Induces chemotaxis *in vitro*
MCP 1,2,3	Induces chemotaxis *in vitro*
RANTES	Induces chemotaxis *in vitro*

(After Biron et al.[13])

Table 8.4 Innate cytokine and chemokine regulation of natural killer cell functions.

surveillance.[20,24] A further role as immune effector cell is in T-cell-mediated immune responses where NK cell activation has been described – for example, during hybrid resistance after bone marrow allografts, graft-versus-host reaction and in skin delayed hypersensitivity reactions.[70,76,82] The observation that inhibitory MHC Class I receptors are expressed on a subset of T lymphocytes suggests that they may regulate both NK and T cell responses, which supports earlier observations that lymphocytes with an NK phenotype could suppress antibody production.[53] NK cells secrete and respond to a number of innate cytokines and chemokines (summarized in Table 8.4).

INFLAMMATORY BOWEL DISEASE AND NK CELL FUNCTION

In ulcerative colitis, Crohn's disease and other inflammatory diseases of the bowel, the normally protective immune response is not appropriately downregulated, and highly activated effector cells produce prolonged and often severe inflammation. A number of genetically modified animal models have shown that T cells are generally required for the development and for the regulation of the disease.[60] Beige mice that lack NK activity do not have an increased incidence of inflammatory bowel disease.[62,68,72] Cytotoxic activity could be exerted via CD8 cytotoxic cells and an increased local level of IFNγ, which would also act on mucosal NK cells. Low NK activity in the blood of patients with both Crohn's disease[28,30,65] and ulcerative colitis has been reported,[28] although some of the differences may be treatment-related[4] or could be due to sequestration of effector cells in the mucosa. Studies investigating mucosal and peripheral blood NK activity have not been able to separate primary from secondary effects.

COELIAC DISEASE

In coeliac disease, defined as a permanent gluten sensitivity associated with particular major histocompatibility HLADR types (DR3, DR4, DR5/7), reduced numbers and reduced activity of NK and cytotoxic cells have been described in blood,[21] in the lamina propria[5,6] and in the epithelium.[54] It remains unclear whether the occurrence of intraepithelial large granular lymphocytes and NK cells is suited to distinguish between two distinct forms of gluten intolerance – the transient and permanent (coeliac disease) form – the latter being associated with a decrease in both cell populations.[31]

NEOPLASTIC DISEASE

The association of NK cells with immuno-surveillance against neoplastic disease has led to a large number of clinical studies of NK cell activity in tumour-bearing individuals. In many cases, clear-cut results have not been obtained, because it is difficult to determine whether abnormalities in NK activity precede the development of the tumour or are merely secondary to the disease. Furthermore, assays of peripheral NK activity may not reflect events in the affected tissues themselves. However, animal studies do indicate that NK cells are important in preventing

B

and regulating the progress of neoplasia[3,36] and thus it might be anticipated that NK cells are involved in local responses to intestinal tumours. Indeed, colonic cancer cells may be sensitive to NK cells[35] and it has been suggested that the low incidence of small intestinal tumours is related to the higher number of granular lymphocytes found in the upper gut compared with the colon.[78]

In general, assays of circulating NK cells are unhelpful in deciding whether low NK activity found in tumour-bearing intestine is causally related to the disease, and only prospective studies of individuals at risk will be able to answer this question.

INFECTIONS

Many authors[11,13,46] have reported a major role of the NK cell in the defence against viral infections. In humans, IL15 plays a pivotal role in the development, survival and function of NK cells. The IL15 receptor includes the IL2/15R β and γ C subunits, which are shared with the IL2 and an IL15 specific receptor subunit. Abnormal expression of these receptors has been described in patients with inflammatory bowel disease and in HIV disease,[77] which is in keeping with earlier reports of reduced

NK activities in inflammatory bowel disease and during intestinal HIV infection.[64]

The exact role of NK cells during intestinal infections has been studied in experimental models, where the available evidence points to a proactive role of NK cells in some conditions. Furthermore, it appears that IL12- and NK cell-derived IFNγ responses are critical to antiviral defence and must be tightly controlled to promote beneficial and to avoid detrimental effects.[11] Some viruses with a lifelong latency, e.g. the cytomegalovirus, have adapted to the body's NK and T cell defences by downregulating MHC Class I expression on infected cells, thus avoiding recognition by the immune system and killing by cytotoxic cells. As a further strategy, virally infected cells are also able to prevent a cytolytic attack by activating a killer inhibitory receptor (Fig. 8.4).[22]

INTESTINAL NK ACTIVITY

The study of intestinal NK cells and their *in vitro* functions has been limited by difficulties in obtaining pure populations of mucosal lymphoid cells, a lack of NK cell specific markers and the focus on the NK cell's role in tumour immunology. NK cells form

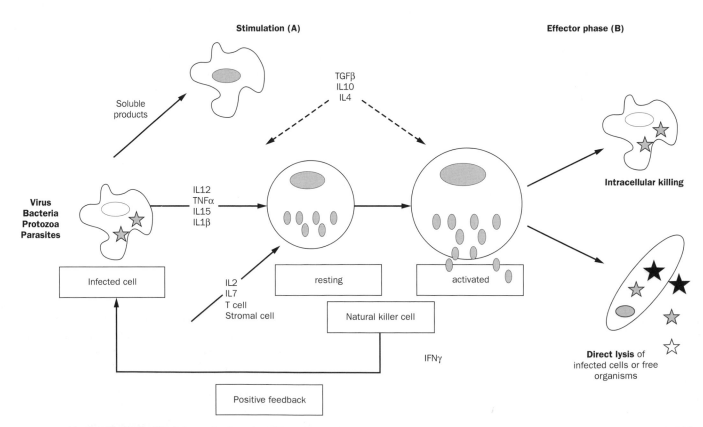

Fig. 8.4 Proposed pathway for the interaction between NK cells and infectious pathogens. In the stimulatory phase (A), intact pathogens or soluble parasite-derived products make contact with the appropriate host accessory cells (e.g. macrophages, dendritic cells) and trigger synthesis of IL12 and TNFα, which results in the activation of resting NK cells into effector cells. IL1β, IL2, IL7 and IL15 have been implicated as positive regulators of this process. In the effector phase (B), the activated NK cells control bacterial or parasite growth primarily through an indirect mechanism involving IFNγ-dependent macrophage activation and intracellular killing of the organism. NK cells may also limit replication of pathogens through direct lysis of infected host cells or of free organisms, although the physiological significance of this direct mechanism remains controversial. The IFNγ produced as a consequence of NK cell activation acts as a positive feedback loop by enhancing the synthesis of IL12, TNFα and other monokines by infection-stimulated accessory cells. In turn, the NK cell response can be downmodulated (broken arrows) by regulatory signals provided by TGFβ, IL10 and probably also IL4, which target both the stimulatory and effector phases of the pathway. (Modified after Scharton-Kersten 1997).

a large proportion of lymphocytes with azurophilic granules within the intestinal epithelium, which can exert spontaneous cytotoxicity[7,8] and lyse defined NK cells' targets.[74] Unlike T or B cells, NK cells develop normally in mice with a severe combined immunodeficiency (SCID) phenotype caused by disruption of the RAG gene complex.[50,67] Infants suffering from the human equivalent of these immunodeficiency diseases have normal NK cells, since gene rearrangement is not needed for their differentiation and function.[44] Infants with mutations or deletions of the IL2 receptor γ chain (SCIDX1) are characterized by a defect in T cell and NK differentiation (with poorly functioning B cells), indicating that the IL2 receptor γ chain (shared with IL4, IL7, IL9, IL15 and IL13 receptors) seems to be essential for NK development.[22] In these studies, the development of gut-associated intraepithelial lymphocytes was severely diminished and Peyer's patches were not detected. NK cell functions are regulated, directly and indirectly, by an array of innate cytokines and chemokines (Table 8.4).

Overall conflicting results have been obtained when assessing and comparing NK activity of cells isolated from the intestinal epithelium. This has been attributed to NK assays and isolation procedures,[51] the site of isolation and species used[17,29] and to different levels of endogenous IFNγ.[23] These studies would suggest that a significant proportion of IEL have NK characteristics and the potential for NK activity, but it remains unclear if and in which way this activity is expressed *in vivo*. In general, isolated lamina propria cells have little or no NK activity in a number of species investigated.[8,29,75]

NK cells in GALT

It seems that both Peyer's patches (PP) and mesenteric lymph nodes (MLN) have little or no NK activity in mice.[52,73,74] In humans, the apparent lack of NK activity[29] seems to reflect a reduced number of cells rather than a deficient lytic ability.

Regulation of intestinal NK cell activity

A better understanding of the regulation of intestinal NK activity has recently been gained by the discovery of families of NK cell inhibitory and stimulatory receptors[43,44] (Figs 8.2 and 8.3). Although these receptor families have been described mainly on blood-derived NK cells of humans and mice, it is likely that these structures are also active on site-specific NK cells.

Early reports describe enhanced NK activity in the intra-epithelial lymphocyte (IEL) population of mice rejecting allogeneic tumour cells and during a graft-*versus*-host reaction (GvHR).[15] NK-activating agents such as IFNα/β enhanced systemic and intestinal consequences of a GvHR induced in neonatal mice.[26] Direct administration of IFNα/β to normal mice could induce and reproduce intestinal lesions, which could be prevented by *in vitro* depletion of NK cells with anti-asialo-GM1 antibodies. This indicates a possible effector role of NK cells in immunologically mediated enteropathies,[25-27] although intestinal NK cells are less likely to play an important role during TNFα-induced enteropathies.[27] Selective modulation of NK activity of IEL by the neuropeptide substance P has been described in mice *in vitro*.[19]

Events associated with target cell lysis have not been defined on a molecular level, although contact-dependent lysis through cytolytic granules containing a number of proteases has been demonstrated.[32,59] The highly lytic granule proteases considered to contribute to NK functions are shown in Table 8.5.

Contribution of lytic granule proteases to NK functions
1 Cleavage of adherence proteins to facilitate cell recycling
2 Internalization into target cells, leading to nuclear breakdown of target
3 Degradation of matrix protein to facilitate cell migration
4 Interaction of Perforin to facilitate pore formation
5 Recruitment and activation of inflammatory cells

Table 8.5 Contribution of lytic granule proteases to NK functions.

CYTOTOXIC FUNCTION OF INTESTINAL LYMPHOCYTES

Cytotoxic T lymphocytes (CTL) may play an important effector role in the function of the GALT and contribute to the pathogenesis of intestinal disease. Under, as yet, ill-defined circumstances, these cytolytic cells are able to injure – directly or indirectly – infected cells, neoplastic cells and normal and altered epithelial cells of the gastrointestinal tract. Cytolytic cells may also have indirect effects through cytokine-mediated interactions and recruitment of other cells of the immune system of the intestinal tract. Furthermore, absence or inhibition of these cytolytic cells may lead to a local immunodeficiency state. A number of different lymphocyte-mediated cytotoxic mechanisms might potentially be active in the gut, including antibody-dependent cell-mediated cytotoxicity (ADCC), T-cell-mediated cytotoxicity and lymphokine-activated killer (LAK) cell cytotoxicity. Functional studies reported are consistent with the conclusion that NK and ADCC activity are infrequent in the intestinal lamina propria.[56]

CONCLUSIONS

Despite the rapidly increasing understanding of inhibitory and activatory molecules on NK and NK T cells, the precise role of the intestinal NK cell remains to be resolved.

NK cells represent a population of rapidly acting cells of lymphoid origin which exert their function in the absence of specific immunization, without the need to recognize targets via the classical antigen recognition (Class II) pathway. They do not exhibit memory functions and display a broad spectrum of receptors.

The NK cell's role in gastrointestinal diseases is still speculative. Increased numbers of IELs with NK cell functions have been described in hypersensitivity disease to foods such as cow's milk and gluten (coeliac disease), although there is no information about their effector roles. The lamina propria has very little NK activity and it seems that the intestinal immune system has evolved in a way that its nonspecific, regulatory and cytotoxic effector cells are concentrated in the most superficial layer, the mucosal epithelium, where recognition and surveillance functions are most needed.

Innate immune responses are likely to have immunoregulatory influences on the adaptive immune system, and NK cells could provide conditions – e.g. via cytokines – which promote and affect downstream adaptive responses (Fig. 8.5). The recent

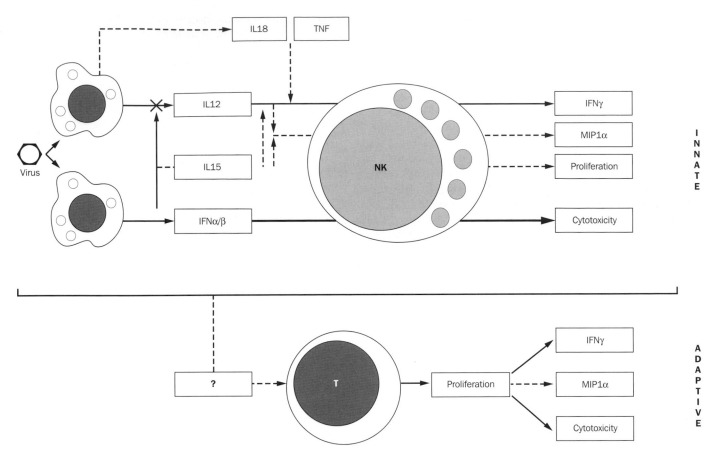

Fig. 8.5 Innate and adaptive immunity during viral infection. This figure illustrates known and hypothetical cytokine-mediated pathways operative during early NK cell activation and during downstream adaptive immunity. The secretion patterns of early cytokines are likely to be modified by the nature of the infecting agents. Many viral infections induce systemic and high levels of IFNα/β. These cytokines are good inducers of NK cell cytotoxicity, and elicit the proliferation of NK cell and memory T cells *in vivo*. An intermediary factor for proliferation is IL15. IL12 is induced in some viral infections. When present, it is tightly regulated and of short duration. It is required for NK cell IFNγ responses to viruses, and these responses contribute significantly to NK-cell-mediated antiviral functions. IL18 is an example of a cytokine with a synergistic effect with IL12 for the induction of NK cell IFNγ. Others with synergistic functions are TNF, IL1 and IL15. The IFNα/β responses suppress IL12 production during viral infections. Induction of NK cell migration through chemokines, and NK cell production of chemokines, are likely to play pivotal roles during viral infections. There are IL12-independent pathways for promoting T cell IFNγ responses during viral infections. *Solid arrows* represent known pathways or responses; *broken arrows* represent proposed pathways; the X represents inhibition. (After Biron *et al.*[13])

progress in unravelling novel regulatory pathways has led to better appreciation of the ways in which T and NK cells are able to communicate (cross-talk). Our understanding, however, of the exact roles and the links between innate and adaptive immunity through the enigmatic NK cell in the context of infections, autoimmunity and neoplastic diseases is still in its infancy.

REFERENCES

1 Abo T, Watanabe H, Sato K *et al.* Extrathymic T cells stand at an intermediate phylogenetic position between natural killer cells and thymus-derived T cells. *Nat Immun* 1995; 14(4): 173–87.

2 Agrawal S, Marquet J, Freeman GJ *et al.* Cutting edge: MHC class I triggering by a novel cell surface ligand costimulates proliferation of activated human T cells. *J Immunol* 1999; 162: 1223–6.

3 Altmann GG, Lala PK. Initiated stem cells in murine intestinal carcinogenesis: prolonged survival, control by NK cells, and progression. *Int J Cancer* 1994; 59(4): 569–79.

4 Aparicio-Pages MN, Verspaget HW, Hafkenscheid JC *et al.* Inhibition of cell mediated cytotoxicity by sulphasalazine: effect of *in vivo* treatment with 5-aminosalicylic acid and sulphasalazine on *in vitro* natural killer cell activity. *Gut* 1990; 31(9): 1030–2.

5 Arato A, Kosnai I, Gergely P. Natural killer cell activity in celiac disease in children on a gluten-free diet and after gluten challenge. *J Pediatr* 1988; 112(1): 44–6.

6 Arato A, Savilahti E, Tainio VM, Verkasalo M, Klemola T. HLA-DR expression, natural killer cells and IgE containing cells in the jejunal mucosa of coeliac children. *Gut* 1987; 28(8): 988–94.

7 Arnaud-Battandier F, Bundy BM, Nelson DL. Natural killer cells in guinea pig spleen bear Fc receptors. *Eur J Immunol* 1978; 8(6): 400–6.

8 Arnaud-Battandier F, Bundy BM, O'Neill M, Bienenstock J, Nelson DL. Cytotoxic activities of gut mucosal lymphoid cells in guinea pigs. *J Immunol* 1978; 121(3): 1059–65.

9 Bakker AB, Phillips JH, Figdor CG, Lanier LL. Killer cell inhibitory receptors for MHC class I molecules regulate lysis of melanoma cells

mediated by NK cells, gamma delta T cells, and antigen-specific CTL. *J Immunol* 1998; 160(11): 5239–45.

10 Baley JE, Schacter BZ. Mechanisms of diminished natural killer cell activity in pregnant women and neonates. *J Immunol* 1985; 134(5): 3042–8.

11 Biron CA. Activation and function of natural killer cell responses during viral infections. *Curr Opin Immunol* 1997; 9(1): 24–34.

12 Biron CA, Byron KS, Sullivan JL. Severe herpesvirus infections in an adolescent without natural killer cells [see comments]. *N Engl J Med* 1989; 320(26): 1731–5.

13 Biron CA, Nguyen KB, Pien GC, Cousens LP, Salazar-Mather TP. Natural killer cells in antiviral defense: function and regulation by innate cytokines. *Annu Rev Immunol* 1999; 17: 189–220.

14 Bluman EM, Bartynski KJ, Avalos BR, Caligiuri MA. Human natural killer cells produce abundant macrophage inflammatory protein-1 alpha in response to monocyte-derived cytokines. *J Clin Invest* 1996; 97(12): 2722–7.

15 Borland A, Mowat AM, Parrott DM. Augmentation of intestinal and peripheral natural killer cell activity during the graft-versus-host reaction in mice. *Transplantation* 1983; 36(5): 513–9.

16 Burdin N, Brossay L, Kronenberg M. Immunization with alpha-galactosylceramide polarizes CD1-reactive NK T cells towards Th2 cytokine synthesis. *Eur J Immunol* 1999; 29(6): 2014–25.

17 Chiba M, Bartnik W, ReMine SG, Thayer WR, Shorter RG. Human colonic intraepithelial and lamina proprial lymphocytes: cytotoxicity *in vitro* and the potential effects of the isolation method on their functional properties. *Gut* 1981; 22(3): 177–86.

18 Christ AD, Stevens AC, Koeppen H *et al.* An interleukin 12-related cytokine is up-regulated in ulcerative colitis but not in Crohn's disease. *Gastroenterology* 1998; 115(2): 307–13.

19 Croitoru K, Ernst PB, Bienenstock J, Padol I, Stanisz AM. Selective modulation of the natural killer activity of murine intestinal intraepithelial leucocytes by the neuropeptide substance P. *Immunology* 1990; 71(2): 196–201.

20 Dawson HD, Li NQ, DeCicco KL, Nibert JA, Ross AC. Chronic marginal vitamin A status reduces natural killer cell number and function in aging Lewis rats. *J Nutr* 1999; 129(8): 1510–17.

21 Di Sabatino A, Bertrandi E, Casadei Maldini M, Pennese F, Proietti F, Corazza GR. Phenotyping of peripheral blood lymphocytes in adult coeliac disease. *Immunology* 1998; 95(4): 572–6.

22 DiSanto JP, Muller W, Guy-Grand D, Fischer A, Rajewsky K. Lymphoid development in mice with a targeted deletion of the interleukin 2 receptor gamma chain. *Proc Natl Acad Sci USA* 1995; 92(2): 377–81.

23 Flexman JP, Shellam GR, Mayrhofer G. Natural cytotoxicity, responsiveness to interferon and morphology of intra-epithelial lymphocytes from the small intestine of the rat. *Immunology* 1983; 48(4): 733–41.

24 Foster PN, Heatley RV, Losowsky MS. Natural killer cells in coeliac disease. *J Clin Lab Immunol* 1985; 17(4): 173–6.

25 Garside P, Bunce C, Tomlinson RC, Nichols BL, Mowat AM. Analysis of enteropathy induced by tumour necrosis factor alpha. *Cytokine* 1993; 5(1): 24–30.

26 Garside P, Felstein MV, Green EA, Mowat AM. The role of interferon alpha/beta in the induction of intestinal pathology in mice. *Immunology* 1991; 74(2): 279–83.

27 Garside P, Mowat AM. Natural killer cells and tumour necrosis factor-alpha-mediated enteropathy in mice. *Immunology* 1993; 78(2): 335–7.

28 Giacomelli R, Passacantando A, Frieri G *et al.* Circulating soluble factor-inhibiting natural killer (NK) activity of fresh peripheral blood mononuclear cells (PBMC) from inflammatory bowel disease (IBD) patients. *Clin Exp Immunol* 1999; 115(1): 72–7.

29 Gibson PR, Dow EL, Selby WS, Strickland RG, Jewell DP. Natural killer cells and spontaneous cell-mediated cytotoxicity in the human intestine. *Clin Exp Immunol* 1984; 56(2): 438–44.

30 Ginsburg CH, Dambrauskas JT, Ault KA, Falchuk ZM. Impaired natural killer cell activity in patients with inflammatory bowel disease: evidence for a qualitative defect. *Gastroenterology* 1983; 85(4): 846–51.

31 Hadziselimovic F, Emmons LR, Schaub U, Signer E, Burgin Wolff A, Krstic R. Occurrence of large granular lymphocytes and natural killer cells in the epithelium of the gut distinguishes two different coeliac diseases. *Gut* 1992; 33(6): 767–72.

32 Hameed A, Lowrey DM, Lichtenheld M, Podack ER. Characterization of three serine esterases isolated from human IL-2 activated killer cells. *J Immunol* 1988; 141(9): 3142–7.

33 Hameed A, Olsen KJ, Cheng L, Fox WMd, Hruban RH, Podack ER. Immunohistochemical identification of cytotoxic lymphocytes using human perforin monoclonal antibody. *Am J Pathol* 1992; 140(5): 1025–30.

34 Hameed A, Olsen KJ, Lee MK, Lichtenheld MG, Podack ER. Cytolysis by Ca-permeable transmembrane channels. Pore formation causes extensive DNA degradation and cell lysis. *J Exp Med* 1989; 169(3): 765–77.

35 Helms RA, Bull DM. Natural killer activity of human lymphocytes against colon cancer cells. *Gastroenterology* 1980; 78(4): 738–44.

36 Herberman RB, Ortaldo JR. Natural killer cells: their roles in defenses against disease. *Science* 1981; 214(4516): 24–30.

37 Imashuku S, Hibi S, Sako M *et al.* Heterogeneity of immune markers in hemophagocytic lymphohistiocytosis: comparative study of 9 familial and 14 familial inheritance-unproved cases. *J Pediatr Hematol Oncol* 1998; 20(3): 207–14.

38 Introne W, Boissy RE, Gahl WA. Clinical, molecular, and cell biological aspects of Chédiak–Higashi syndrome. *Mol Genet Metab* 1999; 68(2): 283–303.

39 Johnson LL, Sayles PC. Strong cytolytic activity of natural killer cells is neither necessary nor sufficient for preimmune resistance to *Toxoplasma gondii* infection. *Nat Immun* 1995; 14(4): 209–15.

40 Kataoka Y, Todo S, Morioka Y *et al.* Impaired natural killer activity and expression of interleukin-2 receptor antigen in familial erythrophagocytic lymphohistiocytosis. *Cancer* 1990; 65(9): 1937–41.

41 Kiessling R, Wigzell H. Surveillance of primitive cells by natural killer cells. *Curr Top Microbiol Immunol* 1981; 92: 107–23.

42 Komiyama A, Kawai H, Yabuhara A *et al.* Natural killer cell immunodeficiency in siblings: defective killing in the absence of natural killer cytotoxic factor activity in natural killer and lymphokine-activated killer cytotoxicities. *Pediatrics* 1990; 85(3): 323–30.

43 Lanier LL. Follow the leader: NK cell receptors for classical and non-classical MHC class I. *Cell* 1998; 92(6): 705–7.

44 Lanier LL. NK cell receptors. *Annu Rev Immunol* 1998; 16: 359–93.

45 Lanier LL, Corliss B, Wu J, Phillips JH. Association of DAP12 with activating CD94/NKG2C NK cell receptors. *Immunity* 1998; 8(6): 693–701.

46 Leong CC, Chapman TL, Bjorkman PJ *et al.* Modulation of natural killer cell cytotoxicity in human cytomegalovirus infection: the role of endogenous class I major histocompatibility complex and a viral class I homolog [published erratum appears in *J Exp Med* 1998 Aug 3; 188(3): following 614]. *J Exp Med* 1998; 187(10): 1681–7.

47 Litwin V, Gumperz J, Parham P, Phillips JH, Lanier LL. NKB1: a natural killer cell receptor involved in the recognition of polymorphic HLA-B molecules. *J Exp Med* 1994; 180(2): 537–43.

48 Lopez-Botet M, Bellon T. Natural killer cell activation and inhibition by receptors for MHC class I. *Curr Opin Immunol* 1999; 11(3): 301–7.

49 Mandelboim O, Kent S, Davis DM *et al.* Natural killer activating receptors trigger interferon gamma secretion from T cells and natural killer cells. *Proc Natl Acad Sci USA* 1998; 95: 3798–803.

50 Mombaerts P, Iacomini J, Johnson RS, Herrup K, Tonegawa S, Papaioannou VE. RAG-1-deficient mice have no mature B and T lymphocytes. *Cell* 1992; 68(5): 869–77.

51 Mowat AM, Parrot DM. Immunological responses to fed protein antigens in mice. IV. Effects of stimulating the reticuloendothelial system on oral tolerance and intestinal immunity to ovalbumin. *Immunology* 1983; 50(4): 547–54.

52 Mowat AM, Tait RC, MacKenzie S, Davies MD, Parrott DM. Analysis of natural killer effector and suppressor activity by intraepithelial lymphocytes from mouse small intestine. *Clin Exp Immunol* 1983; 52(1): 191–8.

53 Nabel G, Allard WJ, Cantor H. A cloned cell line mediating natural killer cell function inhibits immunoglobulin secretion. *J Exp Med* 1982; 156(2): 658–63.

54 Oberhuber G, Vogelsang H, Stolte M, Muthenthaler S, Kummer AJ, Radaszkiewicz T. Evidence that intestinal intraepithelial lymphocytes are activated cytotoxic T cells in celiac disease but not in giardiasis. *Am J Pathol* 1996; 148(5): 1351–7.

55 Ohtsuka K, Sato K, Watanabe H, Kimura M, Asakura H, Abo T. Unique order of the lymphocyte subset induction in the liver and intestine of mice during *Listeria monocytogenes* infection. *Cell Immunol* 1995; 161(1): 112–24.

56 Pang G, Buret A, Batey RT *et al.* Morphological, phenotypic and functional characteristics of a pure population of CD56(+) CD16(–) CD3(–) large granular lymphocytes generated from human duodenal mucosa. *Immunology* 1993; 79(3): 498–505.

57 Pazmany L, Mandelboim O, Vales Gomez M, Davis DM, Reyburn HT, Strominger JL. Protection from natural killer cell-mediated lysis by HLA-G expression on target cells. *Science* 1996; 274(5288): 792–5.

58 Phillips JH, Hori T, Nagler A, Bhat N, Spits H, Lanier LL. Ontogeny of human natural killer (NK) cells: fetal NK cells mediate cytolytic function and express cytoplasmic CD3 epsilon, delta proteins. *J Exp Med* 1992; 175(4): 1055–66.

59 Podack ER, Konigsberg PJ. Cytolytic T cell granules. Isolation, structural, biochemical, and functional characterization. *J Exp Med* 1984; 160(3): 695–710.

60 Powrie F. T cells in inflammatory bowel disease: protective and pathogenic roles. *Immunity* 1995; 3(2): 171–4.

61 Roder JC, Haliotis T, Klein M *et al.* A new immunodeficiency disorder in humans involving NK cells. *Nature* 1980; 284(5756): 553–5.

62 Sartor RB, Rath HC, Lichtman SN, van Tol EA. Animal models of intestinal and joint inflammation. *Bailliére's Clin Rheumatol* 1996; 10(1): 55–76.

63 Schito ML, Barta JR. Nonspecific immune responses and mechanisms of resistance to *Eimeria papillata* infections in mice. *Infect Immun* 1997; 65(8): 3165–70.

64 Schneider T, Ullrich R, Jahn HU *et al.* Loss of activated CD4-positive T cells and increase in activated cytotoxic CD8-positive T cells in the duodenum of patients infected with human immunodeficiency virus. Berlin Diarrhea/Wasting Syndrome Study Group. *Adv Exp Med Biol* 1995; 21: 1019–21.

65 Senju M, Hulstaert F, Lowder J, Jewell DP. Flow cytometric analysis of peripheral blood lymphocytes in ulcerative colitis and Crohn's disease. *Gut* 1991; 32(7): 779–83.

66 Shibuya K, Lanier LL, Phillips JH *et al.* Physical and functional association of LFA-1 with DNAM-1 adhesion molecule [in process citation]. *Immunity* 1999; 11(5): 615–23.

67 Shinkai Y, Rathbun G, Lam KP *et al.* RAG-2-deficient mice lack mature lymphocytes owing to inability to initiate V(D)J rearrangement. *Cell* 1992; 68(5): 855–67.

68 Simpson SJ, Mizoguchi E, Allen D, Bhan AK, Terhorst C. Evidence that CD4+, but not CD8+ T cells are responsible for murine interleukin-2-deficient colitis. *Eur J Immunol* 1995; 25(9): 2618–25.

69 Solomon JB, Forbes MG, Solomon GR. A possible role for natural killer cells in providing protection against *Plasmodium berghei* in early stages of infection. *Immunol Lett* 1985; 9(6): 349–52.

70 Soulillou JP, Vie H, Moreau JF, Peyrat MA, Blandin F. Increased NK cell activity in rats rejecting heart allografts. *Transplantation* 1983; 36(6): 726–7.

71 Spits H, Blom B, Jaleco AC *et al.* Early stages in the development of human T, natural killer and thymic dendritic cells. *Immunol Rev* 1998; 16: 75–86.

72 Strober W, Ehrhardt RO. Chronic intestinal inflammation: an unexpected outcome in cytokine or T cell receptor mutant mice [comment]. *Cell* 1993; 75(2): 203–5.

73 Tagliabue A, Befus AD, Clark DA, Bienenstock J. Characteristics of natural killer cells in the murine intestinal epithelium and lamina propria. *J Exp Med* 1982; 155(6): 1785–96.

74 Tagliabue A, Luini W, Soldateschi D, Boraschi D. Natural killer activity of gut mucosal lymphoid cells in mice. *Eur J Immunol* 1981; 11(11): 919–22.

75 Targan S, Britvan L, Kendal R, Vimadalal S, Soll A. Isolation of spontaneous and interferon inducible natural killer like cells from human colonic mucosa: lysis of lymphoid and autologous epithelial target cells. *Clin Exp Immunol* 1983; 54(1): 14–22.

76 Tartof D, Curran JJ, Levitt D, Loken MR. The skin test antigen stimulated killer (STAK) cell mediating NK like CMC is OKM1 positive and OKT3 negative. *Clin Exp Immunol* 1983; 54(2): 561–6.

77 Waldmann TA, Tagaya Y. The multifaceted regulation of interleukin-15 expression and the role of this cytokine in NK cell differentiation and host response to intracellular pathogens. *Annu Rev Immunol* 1999; 17: 19–49.

78 Ward JM, Argilan F, Reynolds CW. Immunoperoxidase localization of large granular lymphocytes in normal tissues and lesions of athymic nude rats. *J Immunol* 1983; 131(1): 132–9.

79 Williams NS, Klem J, Puzanov IJ *et al.* Natural killer cell differentiation: insights from knockout and transgenic mouse models and *in vitro* systems. *Immunol Rev* 1998; 16: 47–61.

80 Yabuhara A, Kawai H, Komiyama A. Development of natural killer cytotoxicity during childhood: marked increases in number of natural killer cells with adequate cytotoxic abilities during infancy to early childhood. *Pediatr Res* 1990; 28(4): 316–22.

81 Yokoyama WM. HLA class I specificity for natural killer cell receptor CD94NKG2A: two for one in more ways than one. *Proc Natl Acad Sci USA* 1998; 95: 4791–4.

82 Yu YY, George T, Dorfman JR, Roland J, Kumar V, Bennett M. The role of Ly49A and 5E6(Ly49C) molecules in hybrid resistance mediated by murine natural killer cells against normal T cell blasts. *Immunity* 1996; 4(1): 67–76.

Chapter 9

The mucosal B cell and its functions

Per Brandtzaeg

INTRODUCTION

Secretory IgA

Secretory immunity is the best characterized part of the mucosal immune system, although the regulation of B cells forming its basis is poorly understood. The interest in specific immunity of secretions was significantly boosted in the 1960s when it was reported by several laboratories that the predominant immunoglobulin (Ig) class in various external body fluids is IgA rather than IgG.[155] This secretory IgA (SIgA) was, moreover, shown to have unique immunochemical and physicochemical properties because of its polymeric nature and association with the secretory component (SC), which is an epithelial glycoprotein previously called the 'secretory piece'.[382] Shortly afterwards, Crabbé et al.[97] demonstrated an isotype distribution of mucosal Ig-producing immunocytes (plasma blasts and plasma cells) strikingly different from that found in peripheral lymphoid organs; in the gut IgA cells were reported to be more than 20 times as numerous as the IgG counterparts. A general mucosal dominance of IgA immunocytes is now well established[51] despite its lacking immunoregulatory explanation. The first direct evidence showing that in the gut and other secretory tissues IgA immunocytes are peculiar, by producing dimers or larger polymers (collectively called pIgA) rather than monomers, was provided by our laboratory in 1973;[33] but again, the mechanism(s) driving this additional striking feature of mucosal B cells remains elusive.

Secretory IgM

In 1968 it was pointed out by our laboratory that pentameric IgM like pIgA is enriched in exocrine fluids because of active external transport.[64] Secretory IgM (SIgM) was later also shown to be associated with SC and to follow the same intracellular route through secretory epithelia as SIgA;[37,78] and in 1974 a common epithelial transport model was proposed for pIgA and pentameric IgM.[34,35]

J chain

The 'joining' (J) chain had been identified a few years earlier as a unique polypeptide of approximately 15 kDa shared by the two Ig polymers.[150,254] Our original suggestion that the J chain and transmembrane epithelial SC represent the 'lock and key' in receptor-mediated external translocation of pIgA and pentameric IgM[58] has recently been firmly established.[386,387] Furthermore, it has been shown that prominent production of J chain is a common feature of B cells subjected to terminal differentiation at secretory effector sites.[36,41] In teleological terms, one would like to think that this complex cooperation between the mucosal B cell system and secretory epithelia has developed in phylogeny and is preserved in mammals because secretory antibodies are necessary for survival.

The latter view is challenged by the fact that approximately two-thirds of subjects with selective deficiency of IgA remain healthy,[57] apparently even when living under poor hygienic conditions.[85] Therefore, nonspecific innate defence mechanisms together with T-cell-mediated immunity and SIgM antibodies often afford sufficient mucosal protection;[251] but lack of SIgA antibodies does predispose for allergic disorders, autoimmunity, coeliac disease and upper respiratory tract infections.[57] Importantly, gastrointestinal infections are more common in patients with generalized B cell deficiency than in selective IgA deficiency.[57] Altogether, it is difficult to evaluate the clinical role of secretory antibodies in the gut, especially in subjects with a completely normal immune system, because a superimposed protective effect of concurrent systemic cellular and humoral immunity must always be considered.[45]

GALT

The so-called gut-associated lymphoid tissue (GALT) is of central importance in the induction of secretory immunity. GALT includes organized lymphoepithelial structures such as the ileal Peyer's patches (Fig. 9.1) and numerous solitary lymphoid follicles scattered throughout the gastrointestinal tract, particularly in the large bowel. Some authors also consider the mesenteric lymph nodes to be part of GALT, which may be justified because, to some extent, they mirror the B cell biology of Peyer's patches, as discussed later. This chapter focuses on the functional characteristics of mucosal B cells and on their generation in GALT and other parts of mucosa-associated lymphoid tissue (MALT). Emphasis is placed on the human secretory immune system and on B cell alterations that take place in gut diseases. Initially, a brief outline of the complex interactions between the various compo-

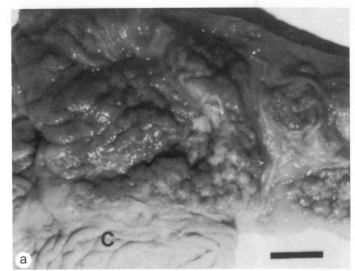

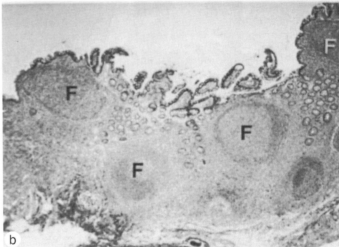

Fig 9.1 Peyer's patches. (a) Peyer's patches in the terminal ileum of a 10-year-old girl. Bar represents 1 cm; C = caecum. (b) Histology of normal human Peyer's patch (haematoxylin-eosin staining) containing several activated lymphoid follicles (F) with germinal centres beneath the specialized dome epithelium that lacks villi. ×25.

nents of the gastrointestinal humoral defence system is given as a basis for subsequent discussions.

HUMORAL DEFENCE OF THE GUT

Immune exclusion

This term is coined for mucosal surface protection mediated by antibodies in cooperation with innate nonspecific factors and thus refers to the 'first line' of defence (Fig. 9.2). Antibody activities in the mucus barrier (left panels in Fig. 9.3) and exocrine secretions are mainly provided by SIgA and SIgM, but there may be some contribution by serum-derived or locally produced IgG which can reach the surface of irritated mucosae quite rapidly by intercellular diffusion through the epithelium.[298]

Immune regulation

Regulation of secretory immunity takes place both in organized inductive MALT structures (on the left in Fig. 9.2) and in diffuse mucosal effector sites of the mucosa such as the intestinal lamina

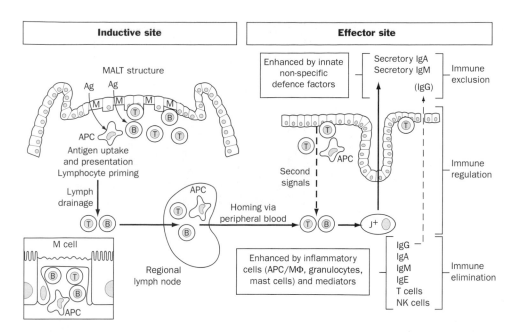

Fig 9.2 Three main components of mucosal immune defence: immune exclusion, immune regulation and immune elimination. Antigen stimulation in mucosa-associated lymphoid tissue (MALT) provides 'first signals' to B cells which migrate to glandular parts of the mucosa via lymph and peripheral blood. 'Second signals' (dashed heavy arrow) induce local proliferation and terminal differentiation of the extravasated B cells. Most plasma cells generated in this way produce J chain-containing (J+) dimeric IgA which is translocated to the lumen as stabilized secretory IgA. Also some IgM is actively transported by the crypt cells, whereas small amounts of IgG normally reach the lumen by passive diffusion (dashed thin arrow).

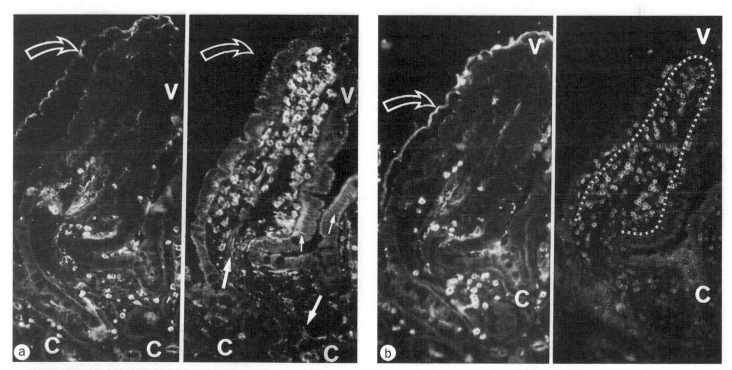

Fig 9.3 Two-colour immunofluorescence staining (same field) for IgA (left panels) and (a) human leukocyte antigen HLA-DR or (b) T cells (respective right panels) in two serial sections of normal ileal mucosa. Note that the IgA-containing mucus layer (open arrows) has become detached from the villus during tissue preparation. (a) There is striking apical DR expression on the villous epithelium (V) contrasting with the crypt epithelium (C) that contains mainly IgA. The enterocytes show additional diffuse cytoplasmic DR staining with intensification along basolateral membranes (small arrows). Note that the mucus is negative for DR (open arrow). Numerous DR-positive macrophages or dendritic cells occur in the luminal part of the villus, whereas only few such cells are intermingled with the IgA immunocytes in the crypt region. In addition, there are a few DR-positive vessel walls (large arrows) and some interstitial IgA. (b) Only few T lymphocytes are intermingled with the IgA immunocytes in the crypt (C) region, whereas numerous such cells occur in the villus (V) – partly within the epithelium (basement membrane zone indicated by dashed line). ×80.

propria and surface epithelium (on the right). Antigen appears to be primarily taken up by MALT through the follicle-associated epithelium (FAE) which contains 'membrane' (M) cells particularly designed for sampling and inward transport of luminal material. By cognate interactions with antigen-presenting cells (APCs), naive T and B lymphocytes are primed to become memory and effector cells for subsequent dissemination to effector sites.[62,63]

Antigen presentation

Antigen is usually presented to T lymphocytes by professional dendritic APCs or macrophages after intracellular processing to provide immunostimulatory peptides. In addition, luminal antigenic peptides may be presented directly to sub- and intraepithelial T lymphocytes by epithelial cells.[88] In humans, mucosal APCs, the FAE of GALT outside the M cells, and the small intestinal villous epithelium (right panel in Fig. 9.3a) express surface determinants encoded by loci present in the Class II region of the major histocompatibility complex (MHC), particularly the human leukocyte antigen HLA-DR,[61] and also classical and nonclassical MHC Class I molecules.[88] These gene products are required for an appropriate antigen-presenting function in immune responses. Class II-positive B lymphocytes that abound close to the M cells may also present antigens efficiently to T cells in cognate immunostimulatory or downregulatory interactions.[62]

T cells subjected to stimulation in MALT release immunological mediator substances (cytokines) which act on other lymphocytes in the microenvironment. The adjacent B cells primed by such 'first signals' migrate rapidly via lymphatics to regional lymph nodes where they may be subjected to further stimulation; they then mostly reach peripheral blood and are finally seeded into distant mucosal effector sites such as the intestinal lamina propria where they develop to Ig-producing plasma cells. This terminal differentiation requires 'second signals' (Fig. 9.2) which are modulated by available cognate antigen, various local cell-types expressing MHC Class II molecules (right panel in Fig. 9.3a), and regulatory T lymphocytes (right panel in Fig. 9.3b). Most B cells included in this traffic ('homing') from MALT to mucosal effector sites apparently belong to memory or effector clones of an early maturation stage; this is indicated by their proneness to express cytoplasmic J chain regardless of concomitant isotype production, although the IgA class is normally predominant.[62,63] J-chain-containing pIgA and pentameric IgM are finally translocated to the lumen as SIgA and SIgM by a regulated receptor-mediated (SC-dependent) epithelial transport mechanism (see later).

Immune elimination

This term refers to mechanisms involved in removal of foreign material that has penetrated the epithelial barrier; it represents a 'second line' of mucosal defence that depends partly on serum-derived or locally produced antibodies of various isotypes, probably often operating in combination with antibody-dependent cell-mediated cytotoxicity (ADCC), T cells and natural killer (NK) cells (Fig. 9.2). Immune elimination is enhanced by a variety of non-specific biological amplification systems of innate immunity which, however, may evolve into overt inflammation and immunopathology, thereby giving rise to mucosal disease if satisfactory removal of antigen is not rapidly achieved.[61] Such 'frustrated' immunological elimination mechanisms are apparently part of the evolving pathogenesis of various gut disorders such as coeliac disease and inflammatory bowel disease (IBD).

B CELLS IN NORMAL GUT MUCOSA

Distribution of Ig-producing immunocytes

All normal exocrine effector sites in adult humans contain a remarkable preponderance of IgA-producing immunocytes (plasma cells and their immediate precursors). This is particularly

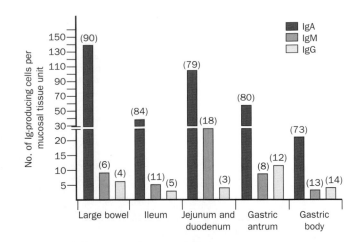

Fig 9.4 Numbers of IgA-, IgM- and IgG-producing cells in various segments of normal human gastrointestinal mucosa. The counts are related to a 'mucosal tissue unit' which constitutes a 6-μm-thick and a 500-μm-wide section area extending from the muscularis mucosae to the lumen. The percentage isotype distribution of the immunocytes is indicated above the columns. Based on published data from the author's laboratory.

true for the intestinal mucosa (Fig. 9.4), as first reported on the basis of immunohistochemical studies by Crabbé et al.[97] and Rubin et al.[328] There are approximately 10^{10} such cells per metre of adult bowel.[51] Absolute figures are difficult to obtain for other exocrine tissues where the cells are more heterogeneously distributed throughout the stroma than they are in the intestinal lamina propria, but it has been convincingly established that most ($\geq 80\%$) Ig-producing cells are located in the gut, both in mice[392] and men.[67] Moreover, the size of the adult human intestinal immunocyte population is quite impressive compared with the figure of 2.5×10^{10} estimated for the total number of Ig-producing cells present in bone marrow, spleen and lymph nodes.[384]

Phenotypes of intestinal B cells

Analyses of B cells isolated from the gut lamina propria of mice[383] indicated a fairly similar content of Ig-producing immunocytes and small B lymphocytes (22% versus 18%). Most of the latter expressed IgD and IgM on their surface (sIgD+IgM+) or only IgM (sIgD-IgM+), thus representing the naive and memory/effector phenotype, respectively.[221] The total fraction of B cells was found to equal that of T lymphocytes.[383] However, such studies are prone to underestimate the relative number of Ig-producing immunocytes because it is difficult to exclude circulating small lymphocytes from the tissue suspensions and, in addition, there may be a selective loss of large (stimulated) lymphoid cells during the isolation steps.[131] Indeed, earlier analyses of B cells isolated from human intestinal mucosa have provided highly discrepant results and are inconclusive in quantitative terms.[242] Moreover, preparation of mucosal mononuclear cell suspensions is jeopardized by the fact that various lymphoid cells have different compartmental distributions, and it is difficult if not impossible to exclude small GALT structures (solitary lymphoid follicles) when studying the lamina propria.

Distribution of B cells in GALT versus intestinal lamina propria

In our recent studies of human GALT (Peyer's patches and appendix), in comparison with normal small intestinal lamina propria,

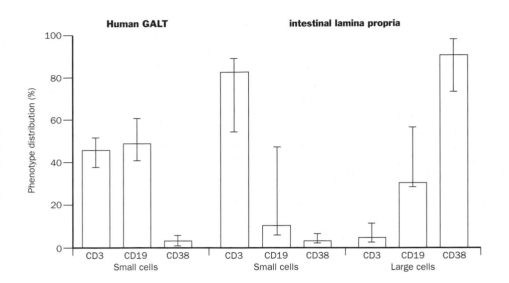

Fig 9.5 Human intestinal lymphocyte distribution. Phenotypic distribution (%) of T lymphocytes (CD3), B lymphocytes (CD19), and B cell blasts and plasma cells (CD38) obtained by flow cytometry with small mononuclear GALT (Peyer's patches and appendix) cells, or with normal intestinal lamina propria small and large mononuclear cells as indicated. Medians (columns) and observed ranges (vertical lines) are depicted. Adapted from Farstad et al.[123] and including our unpublished data representative for 10 additional samples.

we found striking differences in the phenotypic distribution of lymphoid cells.[123] Suspensions of GALT structures contained approximately equal proportions of small B lymphocytes (CD19[+]) and T lymphocytes (CD3[+]), but very few terminally differentiated (CD38[+]) B cells (Fig. 9.5). *In situ* paired immuno-fluorescence studies showed that the small naive B lymphocytes were mainly derived from the follicular mantle-zone population (CD19[+]CD20[+]sIgD[+]IgM[+]) surrounding the germinal centres (Fig. 9.6). Concersely, most small lymphoid cells in the lamina propria were T lymphocytes, and most large cells expressed B cell markers (Fig. 9.5) and were mainly of the terminally differentiated phenotype (CD38[+]) with IgA on the surface and/or in the cytoplasm (Table 9.1). This distribution was confirmed by *in situ* studies.[123]

Animal experiments have indicated that T lymphocytes become preferentially localized in the villi.[20] This is also where most IgA-producing cells are found in the mouse (unpublished observations), whereas in the rat they accumulate mainly around the crypt regions.[168] Likewise, in human jejunal mucosa approximately 65%

Flow cytometric analysis of the phenotypic B-cell distribution and associated marker expression		
Phenotypes	**Small cells[b]**	**Large cells[b]**
Organized GALT		
CD19[+]	50% ($\alpha 4\beta 7^{lo/int}$)	
	(25% L-sel[–])[c]	
CD19[+]sIgA[+]	10% ($\alpha 4\beta 7^{int}$)	
CD19[+/–]CD38[+]		<5% ($\alpha 4\beta 7^{int/hi}$)
Mucosal lamina propria		
CD19[+]	10% ($\alpha 4\beta 7^{int/hi}$ L-sel[–])	
	(>80% sIgA[+])[c]	
CD19[+/–]CD38[+]		90% ($\alpha 4\beta 7^{hi}$ L-sel[–])
		(>90% s/cIgA[+])[d]

[a] Adapted from Farstad et al.[123-125]
[b] Dispersed mononuclear cells gated according to size and analysed for fluorescence intensity (positive, +; negative, –; low, lo; intermediate, int; and high, hi).
[c] Percentage of B cells positive for L-selectin (L-sel) or surface IgA (sIgA) as indicated.
[d] Cytoplasmic IgA (cIgA) determined by immunohistochemistry.

Table 9.1 Flow cytometric analysis of the phenotypic B cell distribution and associated expression of adhesion molecules in mononuclear cell fractions obtained from two human gut compartments[a].

of all Ig-producing immunocytes are normally located in a zone including the luminal 100 μm of the crypt layer and the basal 100 μm of the villi.[8] In this zone, which constitutes less than one-third of the total mucosal height, Ig-producing cells are intermingled with relatively few T lymphocytes, whereas the latter often abound more apically in the villi (Fig. 9.7). However, this distribution of the memory/effector cells does not necessarily indicate the mucosal level where their extravasation takes place.[168]

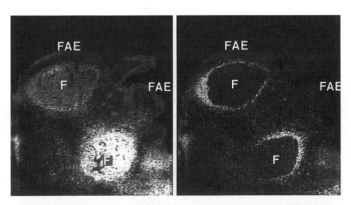

Fig 9.6 Two-colour immunofluorescence staining (same field) for B cells (CD20, left panel) and IgD (right panel) in a section from human Peyer's patch. Note that IgD as a marker of naive B cells is only expressed on the surface of B lymphocytes in the mantle zones surrounding the lymphoid follicle (F) centres and to some extent on B lymphocytes distributed in the extrafollicular areas. FAE = follicle-associated epithelium. ×25.

Disparate distribution of IgA subclass-producing cells

A relatively increased contribution of the IgA2 subclass (17–64%) has been reported for IgA immunocytes in gastrointestinal mucosa compared with that (7–25%) found in peripheral lymphoid tissue, tonsils and the airways,[6,62,80,98,179,186] although the IgA2

B

131

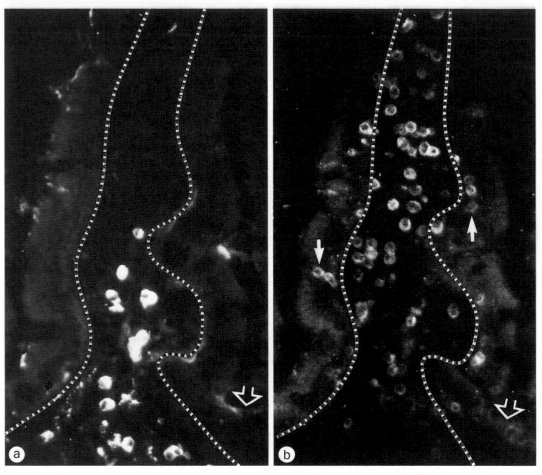

immunocytes are predominant only in the large bowel (Fig. 9.8). The concentration ratios of the two SIgA subclasses in various exocrine secretions[128,179,264] are quite similar to the relative distribution of IgA1 and IgA2 immunocytes at the corresponding effector sites, attesting to the fact that pIgA of both isotypes are equally well transported externally, as also suggested by their binding properties for SC.[39] The relative increase of pIgA2 in secretions may be important for the stability of secretory antibodies because SIgA2, in contrast to SIgA1, is resistant to several IgA1-specific proteases which are produced by a variety of bacterial species.[187]

The molecular events underlying preferential IgA1 or IgA2 responses remain elusive. Secretory antibodies to lipopolysac-charide (LPS) from Gram-negative bacteria generally occur in SIgA2, whereas protein antigens usually stimulate predominantly SIgA1.[253,374] The fact that jejunal IgA immunocytes are mainly of the IgA1 subclass (~77%), in contrast to the IgA2 dominance (~64%) in the colon,[186] may reflect the disparate distribution of food antigens *versus* Gram-negative bacteria in the normal gut. We have observed that bacterial overgrowth in bypassed jejunal segments alters the composition of the local immunocyte population with an increase of IgA2 and a decrease of IgM, suggesting LPS-induced direct isotype switching from Cμ (IgM) to Cα2 (IgA2) or progressive sequential downstream switching of the Ig heavy-chain constant region (C_H) genes.[62,184]

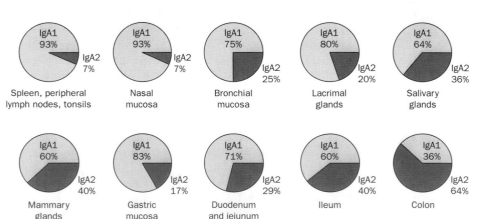

Fig 9.8 Average percentage subclass distribution of IgA-producing immunocytes in human lymphoid organs and normal secretory tissues. Based on published data from the author's laboratory, and from Burnett et al.[80] for bronchial mucosa.

Spleen, peripheral lymph nodes, tonsils — IgA1 93%, IgA2 7%

Nasal mucosa — IgA1 93%, IgA2 7%

Bronchial mucosa — IgA1 75%, IgA2 25%

Lacrimal glands — IgA1 80%, IgA2 20%

Salivary glands — IgA1 64%, IgA2 36%

Mammary glands — IgA1 60%, IgA2 40%

Gastric mucosa — IgA1 83%, IgA2 17%

Duodenum and jejunum — IgA1 71%, IgA2 29%

Ileum — IgA1 60%, IgA2 40%

Colon — IgA1 36%, IgA2 64%

IgM-producing cells

IgM immunocytes constitute a substantial but variable fraction of the normal gastrointestinal B cell population in adults (see Fig. 9.4). The reason for the relatively high proportion of this isotype in the proximal small intestine remains unknown, but may be related to the absence of LPS (see above); it is in striking contrast to the situation in the upper aerodigestive tract.[65,72] This disparity between the two regions is remarkably accentuated in patients with selective IgA deficiency (Fig. 9.9).

IgG-, IgD- and IgE-producing cells

IgG immunocytes constitute 3–5% in normal adult intestinal mucosa, but a considerably larger contribution is found in gastric mucosa (Figs 9.4 and 9.9), which often is affected by low-grade gastritis even in healthy subjects.[389] Only occasional IgD and IgE immunocytes are encountered in the gastrointestinal mucosa,[51] whereas IgD-producing cells constitute a significant fraction (3–10%) of the gland-associated immunocytes in the upper aerodigestive tract, including nasal mucosa and salivary and lacrimal glands.[65,72,198] In IgA deficiency, the disparity between the two regions is even more striking for IgD than for IgM immunocytes (Fig. 9.9).

Disparate distribution of IgG subclass-producing cells

Studies of mucosal IgG-producing cells have shown a distribution (56–69%) of IgG1 that generally makes it the predominating subclass.[23,62,161,272] In the distal gut, IgG2 cells are more frequent (20–35%) than IgG3 cells (4–6%), whereas the reverse is often true in the upper airway mucosa. This IgG subclass disparity supports the idea that the B cell isotype switching pathways differ in various mucosal regions (see above). Interestingly, the Cγ2 and Cα2 genes are located on the same DNA segment,[129] and many carbohydrate and bacterial antigens preferentially induce an IgG2 response in addition to IgA2, whereas proteins (T cell-dependent antigens) primarily generate an IgG1 (and IgG3) response together with IgA1,[289] such as seen in the proximal small intestine.[186,272]

J chain and nature of locally produced IgA and IgM

To support secretory immunity, MALT must favour the development and dissemination of B cells with prominent J chain expression, thereby allowing subsequent production of pIgA and pentameric IgM that can complex with SC and become externally transported at mucosal effector sites as SIgA and SIgM (see Fig. 9.2). The J chain gene is evolutionarily conserved to a remarkable degree,[372] suggesting that it has been acquired from the innate immune system. Its functional role in the adaptive immune system was an enigma until our laboratory obtained evidence that the presence of J chain in pIgA and pentameric IgM is crucial for the efficient non-covalent binding of these polymers to SC.[38,43,58] This notion has been supported by observations made in J chain knockout mice[162] and in transgenic plants expressing Ig, J chain and SC genes.[228] The actual pIg binding site for free SC[43] as well as transmembrane SC[386,387] can indeed be blocked by antibody to J chain. Moreover, experimental studies have suggested that the cellular amount of J chain determines the production ratio between pIgA and monomeric IgA.[43]

Expression of J chain and cytoplasmic SC affinity

IgA immunocytes at secretory effector sites clearly differ from those found in lymph nodes, spleen and bone marrow by showing a much more prominent synthesis of dimers and larger polymers than of monomers. The presence of pIgA in their cytoplasm becomes immunohistochemically apparent by incubating tissue sections with purified free SC.[33,41] The SC binding site (and therefore the polymeric structure) of pIgA as well as pentameric IgM can thus be shown to be generated at the cytoplasmic level by incorporation of J chain, and both IgA and IgM immunocytes in the gut produce abundant amounts of this polypeptide.[41,56]

Immunohistochemical staining of IgA-associated J chain is largely dependent on unmasking of antigenic determinants by acid urea treatment.[41] Conversely, intestinal IgM immunocytes seem to contain a substantial excess of free cytoplasmic J chain as indicated by 100% positivity even in untreated tissue sections. Likewise, studies of murine plasmacytomas showed that J-chain production was excessive in IgM cells compared with that in IgA cells.[290] Moreover, a five-fold molar excess of cytoplasmic over secreted J chain was found in IgM-producing rabbit spleen cells after mitogen stimulation.[324]

Mucosal production of IgA polymers

On average, 88% of IgA1 and 100% of IgA2 immunocytes in normal intestinal mucosa are engaged in pIgA production as suggested by their J chain expression,[185] but this does not exclude a variable

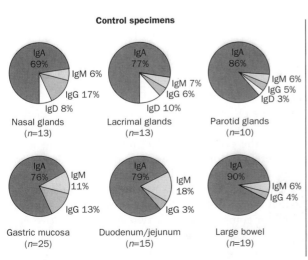

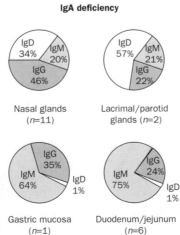

Control specimens

IgA deficiency

Nasal glands (n=13): IgA 69%, IgM 6%, IgG 17%, IgD 8%

Lacrimal glands (n=13): IgA 77%, IgM 7%, IgG 6%, IgD 10%

Parotid glands (n=10): IgA 86%, IgM 6%, IgG 5%, IgD 3%

Nasal glands (n=11): IgD 34%, IgM 20%, IgG 46%

Lacrimal/parotid glands (n=2): IgD 57%, IgM 21%, IgG 22%

Gastric mucosa (n=25): IgA 76%, IgM 11%, IgG 13%

Duodenum/jejunum (n=15): IgA 79%, IgM 18%, IgG 3%

Large bowel (n=19): IgA 90%, IgM 6%, IgG 4%

Gastric mucosa (n=1): IgG 35%, IgM 64%, IgD 1%

Duodenum/jejunum (n=6): IgG 24%, IgM 75%, IgD 1%

Fig 9.9 Average percentage distribution of immunocytes producing different Ig classes in various secretory tissues from controls and subjects with IgA deficiency. Based on published data from the authors' laboratory.

concurrent output of monomers.[41,43] The latter possibility was indicated by the finding that the venous effluent of perfused segments of human gut contained 20–30% monomeric IgA.[79] However, physicochemical analyses of the IgA spontaneously secreted by cultured mononuclear cells obtained from human gut mucosa have provided discrepant information: MacDermott et al.[230] reported 31% monomers, whereas Kutteh et al.[205] concluded that about equal proportions of monomeric IgA and pIgA were produced. Contamination with epithelial cells, which release preformed SIgA, is an inherent problem in such experiments.[205] It is also possible that free SC, released into the culture fluid from epithelial cells, may complex with pIgA and thereby partially mask its in vitro production. On the other hand, evidence suggests that the proportion of secreted pIgA may increase after prolonged incubation of lymphoid cells.[258] Altogether, therefore, no conclusive information is as yet available with regard to the proportion of monomers actually secreted by the intestinal pIgA-producing immunocytes.

Nature of intracellular IgA

There are discrepant opinions as to the nature of intracellular IgA in the mucosal immunocytes. We have maintained that the diffuse cellular in-vitro binding of free SC, along with the immunohistochemical requirement for unmasking of cytoplasmic J chain, constitutes direct evidence of a substantial intracellular polymerization in intestinal IgA immunocytes.[41,43] Our ultrastructural localization of J chain in such normal cells suggests that polymerization begins in the endoplasmic reticulum,[266] which is supported by similar studies performed on transformed normal lymphoid cells.[261] Conversely, pokeweed mitogen-stimulated human peripheral blood lymphoid cells, and an Epstein–Barr virus-transformed lymphoblastoid cell line, were reported to contain very little pIgA despite secreting mainly such polymers.[258] These results are in agreement with previous studies on murine tumour cells.[108]

It is difficult to know to what extent such in-vitro results reflect the normal situation in the gut. After B cell stimulation, there is increased intracellular expression of J chain,[255,324] and also induction of a sulphydryl oxidase catalysing the assembly of Ig polymer subunits.[325] Delamette et al.[107] suggested that this enzyme's activity is expressed only in the Golgi apparatus of Ig-producing tumour cells, whereas stimulation of normal immunocytes triggers its synthesis at the membranous elements of the rough endoplasmic reticulum. Thus, the amount and subcellular distribution of this enzyme may influence Ig polymerization. Therefore, direct analyses of single normal intestinal IgA immunocytes are required before their content of monomers and dimers can be defined in quantitative terms.

Nature of locally produced IgM

The SC-binding capacity of IgM immunocytes in various secretory tissues was 17–23% lower than the J chain positivity, and in some intestinal specimens the proportion of SC-binding IgM cells was below 40%.[41] Such disparity between J chain-expressing and SC-binding capacity was much smaller for the IgA immunocytes.[41] Intracellular polymerization of IgM can take place without initial incorporation of J chain, which may actually occur during the release process.[363] This might explain a lack of cytoplasmic SC affinity. Human IgM immunocytes may secrete varying proportions of J chain-positive pentamers and J chain-negative hexa-

mers,[252] the latter being produced mainly in T cell-independent responses, especially when LPS activates the B cells.[74] Teleologically, it might be advantageous to avoid SC-mediated external transport of hexameric antibodies, as their superior complement-activating properties (up to 20-fold more active than pentamers) could be useful to clear infectious agents from mucosae, although at the risk of acute inflammation and tissue damage. To what extent this type of putative IgM hexamer-dependent defence operates in the gut is unknown.

J-chain expression unrelated to IgA and IgM

Almost 90% of the IgG immunocytes in normal intestinal mucosa express J chain.[21,56,273] However, J chain does not combine with IgG and is therefore not secreted from IgG-producing cells but becomes degraded intracellularly.[262] The same is probably true for J chain in IgD immunocytes which are almost 100% positive for this polypeptide in secretory tissues.[41,56,65,198] J chain-positive mucosal IgG and IgD immunocytes probably represent 'spin-offs' from the MALT differentiation of relatively immature B cell effector clones on their way to pIgA expression (Fig. 9.10).

This notion is supported by the fact that IgA immunocytes show less than 50%, and IgG immunocytes less than 10%, J chain positivity in nonglandular tissues,[36] except in the MALT germinal centres.[62] Down-regulation of J chain expression in extrafollicular B cells appears to be a sign of clonal maturation according to the 'decreasing potential' hypothesis, involving enhanced tendency for local terminal differentiation and apoptosis.[4] Thus, B cells undergoing terminal differentiation in extrafollicular MALT compartments generally show reduced J chain and prominent IgG production,[22,24] suggesting that they belong to relatively exhausted effector clones that have been through several rounds of stimulation (Figs 9.10 and 9.11). Local retention of such putative mature clones increases in the order of GALT, mesenteric lymph nodes, peripheral lymph nodes and palatine tonsils from adults.[62] These differences might depend on the magnitude of persistent stimulation, which is probably much higher in the tonsils, with their antigen-retaining crypts, than in GALT.

J chain regulation

Little is known about cytokine profiles or other microenvironmental conditions that induce and maintain so strikingly the expression of J chain in B cells, giving rise to immunocytes at secretory effector sites. As discussed above, such expression is also seen, although to a lesser degree, in immunocytes associated with organized MALT structures (Figs 9.10 and 9.11), the highest levels being expressed by extrafollicular IgA- and IgD-producing cells in normal tonsils from children[56,62,199] and by IgA-producing cells retained around GALT follicles (right panels in Fig. 9.12).

Murine studies

The regulation of J chain expression has mainly been studied in mice,[200] and both positive and negative regulatory elements have been defined on the promoter of the murine J chain gene. A nuclear transcription factor, BSAP or Pax5, mediates silencing of the gene during early stages of B cell development, but this repression is relieved by interleukin 2 (IL-2) during antigen-driven differentiation that downregulates BSAP RNA expression.[317] BSAP apparently acts in competition with two adjacent positive elements, JA and JB; the activity of the latter has been shown to be mediated by PU.1, a transcription factor belonging to the Ets

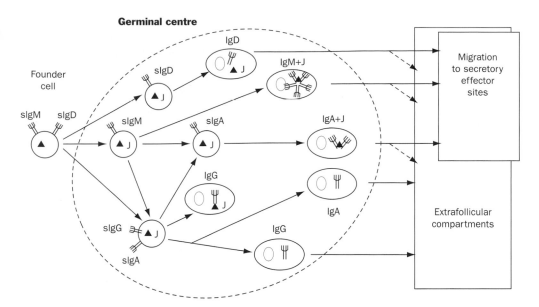

Fig 9.10 Putative B cell developmental stages in the germinal centre (outlined by broken line) of a MALT follicle. The pathways to terminal plasma cell differentiation may include coexpression of cytoplasmic J chain and any of the four Ig classes depicted, but the J chain can only combine with cytoplasmic IgA and IgM to form polymers (IgA+J, dimeric IgA; IgM+J, pentameric IgM). The J chain-expressing B cells may to some extent terminate their differentiation topically in extrafollicular compartments (broken arrows), but they preferentially migrate to distant secretory effector sites. sIg, surface Ig. Further details are discussed in the text.

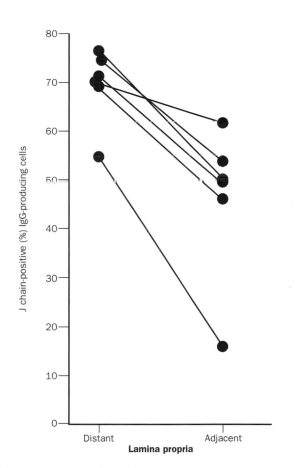

Fig 9.11 Comparison of J chain expression shown by IgG-producing immunocytes in the lamina propria of normal appendix mucosa distant from, and adjacent to, lymphoid follicles. Adapted from Bjerke and Brandtzaeg.[22]

In addition to IL-2 and IL-5, IL-6 has been suggested to contribute to upregulation of the murine J chain,[314,373] whereas IL-4 appears to have an opposing effect.[380]

Human studies

Immunohistochemical observations also suggest that the human J chain production increases as a function of plasma cell differentiation. However, molecular information concerning the regulation of J chain expression during B cell development in humans has been obtained mainly from leukaemic and EBV-transformed cell lines. Contrary to the situation in mice, however, these studies have suggested that transcription of the human J chain gene is initiated during early stages of B lineage differentiation, even before Ig production takes place.[148,203,240,247] Recent data on normal cells have supported the apparent difference in J chain regulation between the two species. Thus, J chain RNA could be detected in human fetal liver before μ-chain expression.[171] This result was confirmed and extended with haematopoietic subpopulations from human fetal and adult tissues.[19] In the bone marrow, transcripts for J chain were detected at all B lineage stages, including the progenitor (CD19−CD34+) and pro-B (CD19+CD34+) cell subsets. J chain RNA was also detected during fetal thymocyte development, including the double-negative (CD4−CD8−) and single-positive (CD4+ or CD8+) subpopulations, but the transcription was turned off in peripheral CD3+ T cells from either fetal or adult samples examined with the same molecular method.[19] Similar studies have apparently not been performed on the various inductive MALT compartments. Altogether, much remains to be learned about the regulation of the J chain gene.

STIMULATION OF B CELLS IN MUCOSA-ASSOCIATED LYMPHOID TISSUE

oncoprotein family.[347] A described zinc finger-containing putative transcription factor, Blimp-1, nuclear protein, has also been reported to be involved in murine B cell differentiation; it apparently acts as a target of IL-2 and IL-5 regulation, thereby contributing to the induction of J chain mRNA and Ig production.[385]

Mucosal immune responses are believed to be regulated primarily in the organized parts of MALT that lack afferent lymphatics but, instead, are designed to sample antigens from mucosal surfaces. In mechanistic terms, the best studied such mucosa-associated inductive sites are the GALT structures of various

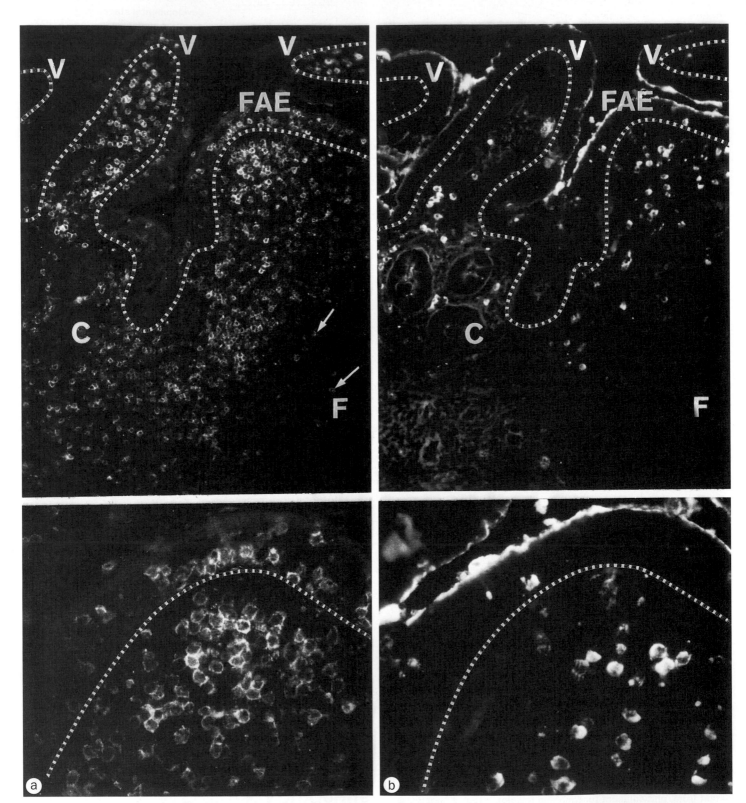

Fig 9.12 Two-colour immunoflourescence staining (same field) of T cells (left panels) and IgA (right panels) in a section of normal human Peyer's patch. (a) Numerous T lymphocytes are present in the dome area beneath the follicle-associated epithelium (FAE), in the T cell zone alongside a lymphoid follicle (F), and in the adjacent crypt (C) areas and villi (V). Note that more intraepithelial T lymphocytes are found in the FAE than in the villi (epithelial basement membrane zone indicated by dashed line). Note also that a few T cells (arrows) appear within the follicle (F). IgA-producing immunocytes occur in the dome area and at the base of the villi. The crypt epithelium shows uptake of IgA and the surface mucus layer contains IgA. (b) Larger magnification of the dome area. (a) ×150; (b) ×340.

experimental animals, including the ileal Peyer's patches and the appendix.[61,334] The chief function of GALT is protection of the gut, but its primed effector cells also migrate to other exocrine tissues such as the upper airway mucosae and the lacrimal, salivary and lactating mammary glands. Additional immune responses may be elicited in bronchus-associated lymphoid tissue (BALT), palatine tonsils and other organized lymphoid tissue of the Waldeyer's pharyngeal ring, including nasal-associated lymphoid tissue (NALT) – particularly the adenoids or nasopharyngeal tonsil.[44,55] Vaccine development can exploit the functional integration of the mucosal immune system, but accumulating evidence suggests that its regionalized or compartmentalized regulation must also be considered.[62,63,71] See also Chapter 10.

Generation of memory and effector B cells in germinal centres

A Peyer's patch consists by definition of five or more B cell follicles.[61] Primary intestinal follicles occur early in fetal life, but secondary follicles with germinal centres (see Fig. 9.1) depend on antigenic stimulation and do not appear until shortly after birth.[73] The primary follicles contain recirculating CD19+CD20+ lymphocytes with a naive phenotype (sIgD+IgM+), both sIg isotypes contributing to the same antigen specificity of the B cell receptor (BCR). The naive lymphocytes pass into the spaces of the network formed by the antigen-capturing follicular dendritic cells (FDCs), the origin of which remains obscure.[182]

One important signal for FDC clustering and the follicle development is known to be the soluble homotrimer lymphotoxin α (LT-α), previously termed tumour necrosis factor β (TNF-β).[86,375] Experimental evidence suggests that the B cell-derived type of

this cytokine is particularly important.[133] Among the known actions of LT-α is augmentation of B cell proliferation and adhesion molecule expression. Knockout mice deficient in LT-α (LT-α−/−) virtually lack lymph nodes and have no detectable Peyer's patches. A membrane-associated form of LT moreover exists as a heterotrimeric complex containing LT-α together with a transmembrane protein designated LT-β. Knockout mice deficient in LT-β have no detectable FDCs and they lack Peyer's patches, peripheral lymph nodes, as well as organized splenic germinal centres.[86]

The germinal centre reaction

In humans, this process has been most extensively studied in the tonsils.[220,221,232] Germinal centres are of vital importance for T cell-dependent generation of memory B cells, affinity maturation of the BCR and Ig isotype switching.[4] It is believed that naive B cells are initially stimulated in the extrafollicular area (on the left in Fig. 9.13) through cognate help by activated CD4+ T cells to which interdigitating APCs have presented processed foreign antigen. The B cells then produce unmutated IgM (and some IgG) antibody of low affinity that can bind circulating antigen; subsequently, the resulting soluble immune complexes become deposited on FDCs (on the right in Fig. 9.13), where antigen is retained for prolonged periods to maintain B cell memory.[4,217,220,232] The actual germinal centre 'founder cell' has been tentatively identified in human palatine tonsils as an sIgD+IgM+CD38+ proliferative lymphocyte subset;[220] animal experiments suggest that its attraction to the primary follicles is partially determined by certain chemokines that interact with the Burkitt's lymphoma receptor 1 (BLR1 or CXCR5), or other as yet undefined receptors on the B cells.[130,142,375]

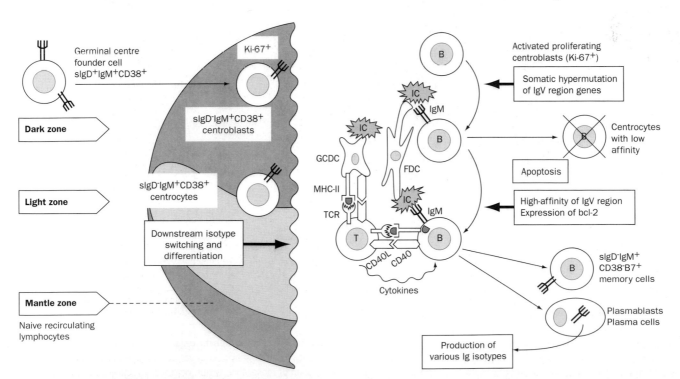

Fig 9.13 B cell developmental events believed to take place in the dark and light zones of germinal centres. These events lead to the generation of extrafollicular and distant plasma cells of various isotypes (see Fig. 9.10). The germinal centre founder cell is activated in the extrafollicular compartment and migrates to the dark zone, where it proliferates. The molecular cell–cell interactions and immune events taking place in the germinal centre reaction are depicted on the right. Further details are discussed in the text.

Molecular cell–cell interactions in germinal centres

A variety of adhesion molecules and other receptor proteins mediate the cellular interactions that lead to the germinal centre reaction (Fig. 9.13). Tonsillar FDCs express both intercellular adhesion molecule 1 (ICAM-1 or CD54) and vascular cell adhesion molecule 1 (VCAM-1 or CD106) that can bind B cells through the leukointegrins lymphocyte function-associated antigen 1 (LFA-1, αLβ2 or CD11a/CD18) and very late antigen 4 (VLA-4, α4β1 or CD49d/CD29), respectively.[217] This appears to be a general feature of GCs present in peripheral lymphoid tissue, whereas relatively high levels of mucosal addressin cell adhesion molecule 1 (MAdCAM-1) occur on dendritic GALT elements as observed in normal Peyer's patches of mice[370] and humans (T Yamanaka, IN Farstad, MJ Briskin and P Brandtzaeg, unpublished observations). This regional difference might be involved in GALT recruitment of memory B and T cells with high levels of the counter-receptor integrin α4β7 ('mucosal homing receptor', or LPAM-1), whereas a dominance of VCAM-1 in normal tonsils and peripheral lymph nodes could favour localization of α4β1^{high} (predominantly α4β7^{low}) cells (Fig. 9.14). Alternatively, such differential dendritic expression of MAdCAM-1 might, instead, induce the high levels of α4β7 expressed by memory/effector cells destined for the intestinal mucosa (see later).

The complement receptors CR2/CR1 (CD21/CD35) are considered among the cell surface molecules that play a crucial role in the germinal centre reaction. CD21 is expressed abundantly on both FDCs and B cells, thereby having a critical function either by localizing antigen to the FDC network and/or by lowering the threshold of B cell activation via recruitment of CD19 into the BCR.[375] Activation of complement occurs on FDCs when they retain immune complexes (on the right in Fig. 9.13) but generally without apparent harm to the germinal centres. Inhibition of C9 polymerization by associated S-protein (vitronectin), protectin (CD59) and decay accelerating factor (DAF or CD55) most likely dampens the lytic activity.[54,209] Nevertheless, release of inflammatory mediators may cause local oedema that facilitates dispersion of FDC-derived 'immune complex-coated bodies' or iccosomes, thereby enhancing the BCR-mediated uptake of their contained antigens by B cells.[55]

Positive and negative B cell selection in germinal centres

Secondary follicles resulting from the germinal centre reaction can be divided into different compartments in which antigen-dependent selection of B cells takes place.[232] Stimulation in the dark zone produces exponential growth of B cell blasts positive for the Ki-67 nuclear proliferation marker.[54] The resulting centroblasts somatically hypermutate their Ig variable (V) region genes

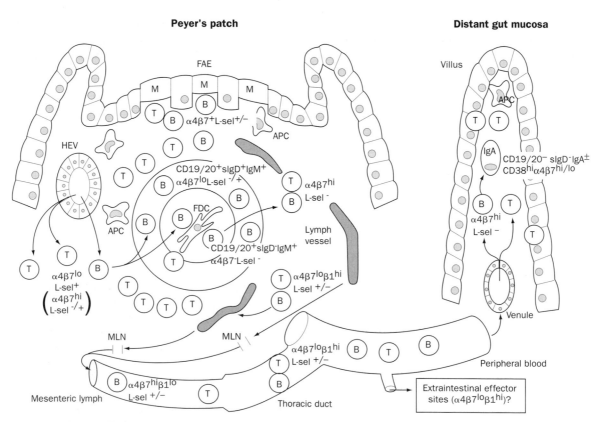

Fig 9.14 Distribution of leukocyte adhesion molecules in various human intestinal tissue compartments, mesenteric lymph, and peripheral blood. The predominant expression pattern (positive, +; high intensity, hi; low intensity, lo; or negative, –) of various surface molecules on B cells (B) is indicated. The phenotype given in parenthesis indicates low priority. MLN marks location of mesenteric lymph nodes, FDC represents follicular dendritic cells in germinal centre of secondary lymphoid follicle, HEV depicts high endothelial venule located in T cell (T) zone of Peyer's patch, and the parafollicular microlymphatics are shaded. L-sel = L selectin; APC = antigen-presenting cell. The migration routes of B and T cells are indicated by arrows, the heavy ones marking the GALT–lamina propria axis preferentially followed by the primed (memory or effector) α4β7^{hi} L-sel$^-$ subsets, most B cells terminating as IgA-producing mucosal plasma cells. Further details are discussed in the text.

and give rise to sIgD⁻IgM⁺CD38⁺ centrocytes (Fig. 9.13). This process changes the affinity as well as specificity of the BCR and will likely induce some self-reactivity. However, mechanisms exist to eliminate auto-reactive B cell clones.[309] Also centrocytes with foreign specificities die by apoptosis unless selected by high-affinity binding via their sIgM (BCR) to antigen on FDCs (Fig. 9.13). The centrocytes may actually pick up such antigen from iccosomes, process it and present foreign peptide to CD4⁺ T helper cells[217,220] that always are found scattered in the follicles (see left panel in Fig. 9.12a).

In addition to B cell adhesion to FDCs and antigen crosslinking of BCR, cognate costimulatory interaction takes place between the activated intrafollicular T cells, which express the CD40 ligand (CD40L, gp 39 or CD154), and memory B cells, which express CD40 (see Fig. 9.13); this appears to be an important event in rescuing centrocytes from CD95 (APO-1/Fas)-induced apoptosis and a key signal for their maintained survival.[91,197] The interaction may be enhanced by sustained activation of the T helper cells via specialized CD4⁺CD11c⁺ germinal centre dendritic cells which can also pick up foreign antigens by binding immune complexes.[146] Following immune activation, it is furthermore crucial that the positively selected centrocytes express Bcl-2 that prevents apoptosis (Fig. 9.13).

No germinal centres are formed when CD40–CD40L ligation is experimentally blocked, documenting the importance of cognate interaction between B and T cells.[217] Moreover, this ligation promotes switching of the C_H genes from C_μ (IgM) to downstream isotypes, while apparently representing a negative signal for terminal B cell differentiation within the follicles.[220] Separate signals probably contribute to the important decision as to whether B cells should continue along the memory pathway or differentiate along the effector pathway[4] to extrafollicular plasma cells or become distributed to distant effector sites (see Fig. 9.10).

Regionalized isotype development and emigration of primed B cells

Most memory B cells (sIgD⁻IgM⁺CD38⁻) apparently migrate rapidly out of the germinal centres to extrafollicular compartments, such as the tonsillar crypt epithelium[219] or Peyer's patch M-cell areas, where they may continue to present antigen.[62] Also, most of the precursors for plasma cells (CD20⁻CD38ʰⁱᵍʰ) rapidly exit to terminate at local (extrafollicular) or distant effector sites (see Fig. 9.10), after which their half-life varies from some days to several months:[4] those ending up in the gut mucosa may be particularly short-lived, which may explain why mucosal immune responses have a relatively limited memory.[350]

Local stimuli for isotype differentiation

As alluded to earlier, the cytokine profiles and other microenvironmental factors determining isotype differentiation and co-expression of J chain in B cells remain obscure. The fact that the IgA immunocytes of the tonsils and regional exocrine effector sites are mainly of the IgA1 subclass (see Fig. 9.8), supports the notion that effector cell differentiation in this mucosal region takes place mainly from sIgD⁻IgM⁺CD38⁺ centrocytes by sequential downstream C_H gene switching.[44] Conversely, the enhanced IgA2 development in the Peyer's patches[23] and the distal gut altogether (see Fig. 9.8), including the mesenteric lymph nodes,[21,23] might reflect direct switching from C_μ to Cα2 expression with

looping out of intervening C_H gene segments.[73] There is much evidence to suggest that B cells from murine Peyer's patches can undergo a direct switch from C_μ to Cα,[366] and in human B cells this pathway may preferentially lead to IgA2 production.[95]

The germinal centre reaction of human GALT structures (Peyer's patches and appendix) generates relatively more intra-follicular IgA immunocytes with J chain than seen in the tonsillar follicles; and in the adjacent intestinal lamina propria and dome zones, immunocytes producing IgA equal, or dominate over, those producing IgG[22,24] which is in contrast to the more than two-fold extrafollicular dominance of IgG immunocytes in the tonsils.[44] Thus, the drive for switching to IgA and expression of J chain is clearly much more pronounced in GALT than in tonsils and peripheral lymph nodes. Many explanations for this remarkable intestinal B cell regulation have been offered elsewhere.[62] Perhaps the continuous superimposition of new environmental and microbial stimuli in the gut enhances the development of early effector B cell clones with increased potential for IgA and J chain expression (see earlier). Alternatively, the GALT microenvironment may be at least partially distinct from that of other immune-inductive sites because of special accessory cells or a particular cytokine profile. Altogether, it is possible that molecular events in the GALT germinal centres promote the generation of a particular (and as yet incompletely characterized) B cell phenotype.

sIgM-negative B cells

In this context it is interesting that a unique sIgM-negative subset (sIgD⁺IgM⁻CD38⁺) of centroblasts has been identified in the dark zone of palatine tonsillar germinal centres; they show C_H gene deletion of the C_μ and switch (S_μ) region, therefore apparently giving rise selectively to IgD-producing plasma cells.[7] We have recently obtained molecular evidence for the regular existence of B cells with the same C_H gene deletion also in the adenoids and exocrine effector tissues of the upper aerodigestive tract, but virtually not in the small intestinal mucosa.[71] Our observations strongly support the notion that preferential B cell homing takes place from nasopharyngeal MALT structures to the upper aerodigestive tract;[55] such compartmentalized migration of sIgD⁺IgM⁻CD38⁺ centroblasts probably explains the relatively high frequency of the IgD isotype among mucosal plasma cells in this region normally, and particularly in selective IgA deficiency (see Fig. 9.9). It is possible that the upper airway microbiota contributes to this regional B cell regulation. Thus, most strains of *Haemophilus influenzae* and *Moraxella (Branhamella) catarrhalis*, which are frequent colonizers of this region, produce an IgD-binding factor (protein D) that can crosslink sIgD.[176,327] In this way, the sIgD⁺sIgM⁻CD38⁺ tonsillar B cell subset could be stimulated to proliferate and differentiate in a polyclonal manner. On the other hand, LPS that is abundantly present in the distal gut may inhibit the expression of IgD.[291]

Identified IgA-promoting stimuli

Dendritic cells from murine Peyer's patches and spleen were initially suggested to enhance IgA production in a microculture system based on cognate interactions between B and T cells.[340] A similar role for dendritic cells was later observed in a human *in vitro* test system not including T cells but employing CD40-activated naive B cells.[127] As reviewed elsewhere,[46] transforming growth factor β (TGF-β) has previously been reported to be a

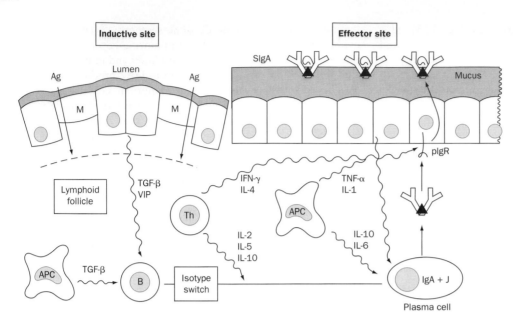

Fig 9.15 Regulatory aspects of secretory immunity that take place in inductive compartment (on the left) and at mucosal effector site (on the right). Various cytokines are apparently involved in isotype switching and terminal differentiation of mucosal B cells to promote the striking generation of plasma cells that produce dimeric IgA with J chain (IgA + J) at secretory effector sites. Some of these cytokines may be derived from antigen-presenting cells (APC), T helper cells (Th) or the epithelium, as indicated. In the gut, both TGF-β and vasoactive intestinal peptide (VIP) may act as IgA switch factors. Certain Th- and APC-derived cytokines also upregulate epithelial expression of transmembrane secretory component (or pIgR), thereby providing a regulatory link between the immunological activity at the effector site and the magnitude of local external transport of secretory IgA (SIgA). Ag, antigen; M, M cell.

crucial IgA 'switch factor', while IL-2, IL-5 and IL-10 are important cytokines for clonal expansion of activated B cells and their preferential IgA expression (on the left in Fig. 9.15). Terminal differentiation to IgA-producing plasma cells may additionally involve IL-6, IL-10 and, possibly, interferon γ (IFN-γ) (on the right in Fig. 9.15), all cytokines known to be produced by antigen-activated CD4[+] T cells cloned from human intestinal mucosa.[270] IL-6 preferentially enhances IgA production (IgA2>IgA1) by human appendix B cells,[135] and in mice this cytokine appears to be essential for terminal B cell maturation.[46] In humans, a central role for IL-10 is supported by the fact that this cytokine can release the differentiation block of IgA-committed B cells from IgA-deficient patients.[75] Moreover, human native B cells activated through CD40 require only TGF-β and IL-10 for IgA secretion.[106] Interestingly, dendritic cells enhance synergistically the effect of these two cytokines on IgA expression, and may, via unknown signals, be essential for IgA2 production *in vitro*.[127]

Gut hormones and other putative region-specific B cell stimuli

Human fetal B cells activated *in vitro* through CD40 were selectively induced by vasoactive intestinal peptide (VIP) to IgA1 and IgA2 production.[191] Similarly treated sIgM⁻CD19[+] pre-B cells from human fetal bone marrow were induced to produce IgM and both IgA subclasses.[191] These results suggested that VIP can act as a true switch factor (on the left in Fig. 9.15), which is interesting in view of its relatively high concentrations in gut mucosa. Furthermore, VIP was reported to promote the number of IgA precursors, together with increased IgA and decreased IgG synthesis, in cultures of intestinal mononuclear cells.[28] Finally, substance P has been shown to enhance IgA and IgM production by murine B cell lines, the latter isotype particularly in the presence of LPS.[293]

In mice, intestinal 'contrasuppressor cells' have been implicated as an additional mechanism selectively releasing IgA responses from T cell-mediated suppression (oral tolerance). This IgA-enhancing effect (probably cytokine-mediated) was ascribed to TCRγ/δ[+] intraepithelial lymphocytes (IELs). Support for this notion was subsequently obtained in TCRδ⁻/⁻ knockout mice that

showed a significantly reduced number of intestinal IgA-producing cells and a poor IgA antibody response after oral immunization, while IgM and IgG were intact.[134] If γ/δ T cells exert a similar effect in humans, this could contribute to the relatively large IgA production in the gut where TCRγ/δ[+] IELs are considerably more frequent than in the upper respiratory tract.[174] Additional region-specific differences may exist: for example microenvironmental levels of IL-7, a cytokine mainly produced by goblet cells in the gut and known to be a growth factor for human intestinal lymphocytes.[400]

HOMING MECHANISMS GUIDING MUCOSAL B CELLS

Migration of B cells through GALT

Extravasation of naive cells

As mentioned earlier, the organized MALT structures are considered as the chief inductive sites of the mucosal immune system in which naive lymphocytes initially are stimulated (Fig. 9.14). Certain adhesion molecules are more strongly expressed on the naive than on the primed (memory/effector) subsets, and vice versa, and some are relatively tissue-specific in their function. Such molecules expressed on endothelial cells may likewise show tissue specificity.[82] Thus, in GALT and mesenteric lymph nodes, but not in peripheral lymph nodes, high endothelial venules (HEVs) abundantly express MAdCAM-1, and the same is true for the ordinary flat venules in the intestinal lamina propria.[76] Indeed, this complex multidomain adhesion molecule appears to play a major role in intestinal extravasation of immune cells.[364] The human counterpart of MAdCAM-1 has recently been cloned and characterized,[348] but the microenvironmental factor(s) that induce its preferential expression on endothelial cells in the gut remains elusive.[110]

Studies in rodents have shown that when MAdCAM-1 is expressed by HEVs in organized GALT structures, the glycosylation of its mucin-like domain promotes binding of L-selectin (CD62L) that is strongly expressed on naive lymphocytes (Fig. 9.16a). This initial adherence, together with binding of

a GALT
Naive lymphocyte

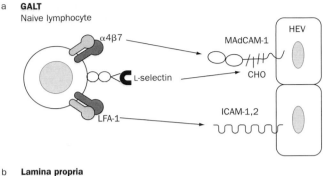

b Lamina propria
Memory lymphocyte

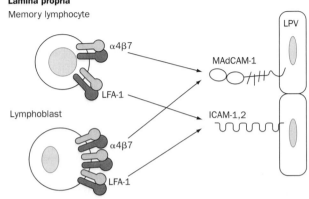

Fig 9.16 Adhesion molecules involved in lymphocyte-endothelial recognition directing (a) naive lymphocytes to organized GALT structures, and (b) primed T and B cells (memory lymphocytes and lymphoblasts) to the intestinal lamina propria. In GALT, high endothelial venule (HEV) in the parafollicular zone expresses MAdCAM-1 in which the membrane-near mucin-like domain (bottle brush symbol) contains L-selectin-binding O-linked carbohydrates (CHO); this interaction initiates emigration of naive lymphocytes into the inductive GALT structures. Interaction between unmodified MAdCAM-1 expressed by ordinary flat lamina propria venule (LPV) is most important for targetting primed lymphoid cells to the mucosal effector site.

leukointegrin α4β7 to the two N-terminal Ig-like domains of MAdCAM-1, apparently explains the preferential emigration of naive T and B cells into inductive sites such as the Peyer's patches and the appendix (on the left in Fig. 9.14). The less prominent extravasation of primed counterparts (α4β7[high]) in GALT is probably also mediated by MAdCAM-1. Regardless of tissue site, additional contribution to the emigration of both subsets is provided by other more generalized adhesion molecules such as leukointegrin LFA-1 (αLβ2) or (CD11a/CD18) that binds to ICAM-1 and ICAM-2 (CD120) on the endothelium.[82]

Distribution of lymphoid cells and their adhesion molecule profiles
These have recently been analysed in human Peyer's patches and the appendix.[123–125] As discussed earlier (see Fig. 9.5), approximately equal numbers of small T and B cells were present in the mononuclear cell suspensions, and in-situ studies showed that the naive B cells of the follicular mantle zones mostly expressed abundant L-selectin but variable levels of α4β7 and usually no β1 (CD29). Most lymphocytes expressing L-selectin around or within the parafollicular HEVs showed the naive T cell phenotype (CD3+CD45RA+) but some were B cells, again mainly of the naive (sIgD+) phenotype. The lymphocytes expressing L-selectin were usually only weakly positive or negative for α4β7.[125] Altogether, our

in-situ data accorded well with the flow–cytometric characteristics of dispersed human GALT cells (see Table 9.1) and were compatible with the adhesion molecule profile expected for lymphocytes at their site of entrance and accumulation in GALT (on the left in Fig. 9.14).

Microenvironmental migration
Very little knowledge exists about how immune cells after emigration are directed to and retained in the various microcompartments within organized lymphoid tissue. It is assumed that chemokines[142,375] as well as fibronectin and other extracellular matrix components play an essential role. As mentioned earlier, chemokines interacting with BLR1 (CXCR5) on B cells appear to contribute to their migration into lymphoid follicles.[130] Moreover, interactions between leukointegrins (α4β1 and α4β7) and fibronectin[307] or MAdCAM-1[370] may be particularly involved in GALT.[62] Consistent with this notion, reticular fibres with fibronectin, collagen and laminin have been found to be oriented parallel to the presumed migration pathway from HEVs to the domes of murine Peyer's patches.[282] Interestingly, cells from the monocyte/macrophage series may accompany the lymphocytes in their migration, as discussed elsewhere.[63]

Exit of primed B cells from GALT
The interfollicular zones of GALT are not only the site of entrance for lymphoid cells but also where they exit through microlymphatics (on the left in Fig. 9.14). These vessels were identified in human Peyer's patches and the appendix as thin-walled spaces lacking endothelial expression of von Willebrand factor.[125,126] Similar parafollicular microlymphatics have been described in human tonsils.[136] Such draining lymph vessels are believed to start blindly with a fenestrated endothelium, and it is possible that lymphoid cells enter the lymphatics by a passive process, although more selective mechanisms cannot, as yet, be disregarded. Within human GALT, memory B (sIgD−) and T (CD45R0+) cells with high expression of α4β7 were often found to be situated near the microlymphatics and were also present intraluminally together with some CD19+CD38[high]α4β7[high] B cell blasts.[125,126] However, these vessels mainly contained naive lymphocytes with low expression of α4β7. Cytochemical and flow cytometric analyses of human mesenteric lymph provided similar marker profiles; notably, the small fraction of identified B cell blasts (2–6%) contained cytoplasmic IgA, IgM and IgG in the proportions 5 : 1 : <0.5.[126]

Our studies suggested that the α4β7[high] subsets identified at exit in GALT reflect the first homing step to furnish mucosal effector sites with primed lymphoid cells (Fig. 9.14). Relatively few memory cells expressed high levels of L-selectin in intestinal and mesenteric lymph;[126] those that did could likely either re-enter GALT or extravasate in non-mucosal lymphoid tissue or tonsils from peripheral blood along with naive cells by binding to mucin-like peripheral lymph node addressin (PNAd) expressed on HEVs there.[31] A recent flow cytometric study of circulating human lymphocytes supported such a fundamental subdivision according to adhesion properties.[326]

The heterogeneity of GALT-derived B cells might explain systemic dissemination of IgG as well as IgA responses after oral immunization. Convincing evidence exists that the systemic and mucosal immune systems are not totally segregated;[61] it is quite possible to prime and boost local immune responses by parenteral immunization, and vice versa. Interestingly, we observed both B and T memory cells with high levels of $\alpha4\beta1$ at exit in GALT.[125] These subsets probably corresponded to the $\alpha4\beta7^{low}$ cells appearing in draining lymphatics,[126] perhaps destined to extravasate at extraintestinal mucosal effector sites by means of VCAM-1, which is the chief ligand for $\alpha4\beta1$ (see later). Conversely, regardless of origin, the $\alpha4\beta7^{high}$ subsets with little L-selectin would not be expected to adhere to PNAd and only subsidiarily to VCAM-1; they were therefore most likely destined primarily for the intestinal lamina propria (Fig. 9.14).

Migration of B cells from GALT to distant lamina propria
Lamina propria effector cells
After antigen-induced activation, proliferation and partial differentiation in GALT, it is assumed that primed lymphoid cells go rapidly to mesenteric lymph nodes, from which (after some further differentiation) they follow the lymph into the peripheral blood circulation (see Figs 9.2 and 9.14). In experimental animals, it has been directly shown that IgA-expressing plasmablasts mature as they migrate from Peyer's patches via mesenteric lymph nodes and thoracic duct lymph to the intestinal lamina propria because the relative fraction of cells with cytoplasmic IgA increases from initially around 2% through 50% and 75% to 90%, respectively.[292]

In mice, peritoneal B cells are composed of a special B-1 (CD5$^+$) subset than can repopulate the gut with IgA-producing immunocytes.[29] Kroese and co-workers have determined that approximately 50% of the murine intestinal lamina propria plasma cells are derived from this subset. It is generally believed that B-1 cells produce polyreactive ('natural') antibodies encoded by unmutated (germline) IgV region genes, but murine CD5$^+$ B cells often show hypermutation as a sign of selection.[29] Human intestinal plasma cells from the duodenum, ileum and colon have highly mutated IgV region genes, suggesting that their BCR is shaped by persistent antigenic challenge.[116] Interestingly, sequences of IgV$_H$ region genes from Peyer's patch germinal centre B cells were found to be clonally related to those of ileal plasma cells, thus substantiating the intestinal homing pattern of GALT-derived primed B cells.[115] Moreover, despite the presence of polyreactive SIgA antibodies in human exocrine secretions (see later), there is no evidence that these antibodies are produced by plasma cells originating from the peritoneal cavity.[224]

Extravasation of primed cells
As mentioned earlier, homing of primed lymphoid cells to the intestinal lamina propria appears to be determined mainly by their high levels of $\alpha4\beta7$ in the absence of L-selectin (Fig. 9.16b). This phenotype can bind to unmodified MAdCAM-1 expressed on the lamina propria microvasculature,[82] and fits with the predominant adhesion molecule profile of antibody-producing cells present in human peripheral blood after intestinal stimulation.[181,312,313] Conversely, circulating specific B cells generated by systemic immunization show preferential expression of L-selectin but relatively low $\alpha4\beta7$ levels.[181,312,313]

At present, interactions of human MAdCAM-1 with L-selectin have not been defined to the same extent as for the murine counterpart. Nevertheless, the virtual absence of lymphoid cells bearing the latter adhesion molecule in human intestinal lamina propria (see Table 9.1), strongly suggests that MAdCAM-1, when expressed outside organized GALT structures, does not bind L-selectin. Many large B cells retain high levels of $\alpha4\beta7$ after

extravasation in the human intestinal lamina propria, despite abundant coexpression of CD38 and cytoplasmic IgA as signs of terminal maturation (see Table 9.1, Fig. 9.14). It is possible that $\alpha4\beta7$, in addition to mediating homing of primed cells, contributes together with CD44 to retention of effector cells by showing affinity for extracellular matrix components.[202]

Second signals for proliferation and terminal differentiation
Little is known about factors triggering terminal B cell differentiation at various secretory sites (see Fig. 9.2), although IL-5, IL-6 and IL-10 have been suggested to be important as discussed above (Fig. 9.15). The immediate availability of antigens (and mitogens?) appears to be reflected by a density of Ig-producing cells that is about seven times higher in the colonic mucosa than in the parotid and lactating mammary glands.[42] Substantial antigen-driven proliferation of IgA precursor cells has been revealed in the intestinal lamina propria of various experimental animals,[167,210,302] especially in the crypt regions[168] where most IgA immunocytes are also found in the human jejunal mucosa.[8] Moreover, in the human secretory immune system, the role of topical antigens outside of Peyer's patches has been clearly demonstrated in terms of localization, magnitude and persistence of SIgA antibody responses.[281]

It is not so obvious that foreign material, live or dead, gains access to secretory effector sites remote from mucosal surfaces, and terminal B cell differentiation in these exocrine tissues may depend more on other types of stimulation. One possibility is epithelial expression of HLA-DR molecules, which are normally present on human parotid intercalated duct cells[379] and on alveolar cells of lactating mammary glands.[268] Because the magnitude of immune responses may be related to the density of such 'self-antigens',[175] one may assume that their abundant epithelial expression – in combination with only trace amounts of foreign antigens or anti-idiotypic antibodies – may elicit sufficient 'second signals' for some terminal B cell differentiation to take place. The epithelium may also mediate more non-specific stimulatory effects on the B cells. Thus, it has been reported that a soluble factor from bursal epithelial cells can induce IgA production,[118] perhaps representing one of the cytokines mentioned above (Fig. 9.15).

Extraintestinal migration of primed B cells
As reviewed elsewhere, migration to the gut lamina propria of B cells primed in the lymphoepithelial tissue of Waldeyer's ring (NALT) and BALT is probably negligible both in experimental animals and humans.[55,63] This has recently been substantiated by the apparent absence of the tonsillar sIgD$^+$sIgM$^-$CD38$^+$ subset in human small intestinal mucosa.[71] Conversely, there is considerable evidence to suggest that GALT can provide exocrine sites beyond the gut with primed B cells, although the molecular mechanisms directing this dissemination are poorly defined.[63] Such compartmentalization of the mucosal immune system is probably explained by disparity in adhesion molecules expressed by the local microvascular endothelium and by lymphoid cells primed in the regional MALT structures. The regional antigen repertoire may be of additional importance; although topical antigen exposure appears to play no direct role in the selectivity of B cell extravasation, it may clearly influence the apparent homing pattern by causing specific accumulation (retention and proliferation) of lymphoid cells.[61,82,167,168,210,280,302] Thus, primed cells tend to home preferentially to effector sites corresponding to the inductive sites where they were initially stimulated.

Mucosal homing molecules operating outside GALT

Both animal and human studies have demonstrated that MAdCAM-1 is shared between GALT structures and the intestinal lamina propria, and it also shows considerable expression on HEVs in mesenteric lymph nodes.[82,364] Other unidentified regional endothelial determinants may be shared between the immune inductive sites and exocrine effector sites in the upper aerodigestive tract. Interestingly, very little or no MAdCAM-1 can be detected on HEVs in normal human tonsils (T Yamanaka, IN Farstad, MJ Briskin and P Brandtzaeg, unpublished observations), and this molecule appears to be absent from regional exocrine tissues, such as the lungs and salivary glands, as well as from the human uterus, and usually also from mammary glands.[76] Moreover, there is some evidence suggesting that α4β7 is not an important homing receptor for lymphoid cells in the airways of humans,[301] mice[398] and sheep.[1] Indeed, circulating antibody-producing cells detected after intranasal immunization in humans have been reported to show considerable coexpression of α4β7 and L-selectin, in contrast to the results obtained after intestinal immunization.[181]

This compartmentalization of the mucosal immune system must be further evaluated and eventually taken into account in the development of effective mucosal vaccines to protect mucosae beyond the gut, such as the airways, the eyes, the oral cavity and the urogenital tract. Even without employing interactions between α4β7 and MAdCAM-1, preferential homing of putative early effector B cell clones with abundant expression of J chain and pIgA is just as remarkable to exocrine effector sites in the upper aerodigestive tract as to the intestinal lamina propria.[62,63] It is difficult to understand how L-selectin and its counter-receptors might contribute to such selectivity in B cell extravasation. Another possibility is a major involvement of α4β1 on mucosal B cells that home to exocrine effector sites outside the gut (Fig. 9.14). The chief counter-receptor for this integrin is VCAM-1, which is expressed both by bronchial and nasal microvascular endothelium.[16,172] However, no direct evidence exists to suggest that high expression of β1 integrin directs primed lymphoid cells to the upper aerodigestive tract and lungs. Therefore, the generalized homing preference for J chain-expressing B cells to exocrine tissues, and also the compartmentalization of the mucosal immune system, remains elusive.

COOPERATION BETWEEN LOCAL B CELLS AND SECRETORY EPITHELIUM

Receptor-mediated transport of polymeric immunoglobulins
Normal distribution of secretory component
Epithelial SC is clearly a key factor in the secretory immune system. In its transmembrane form, SC is expressed on the basolateral surface of normal columnar epithelial cells[40] as a receptor protein,[263] now usually called the polymeric Ig receptor (pIgR). In the human small intestine, it is produced by columnar cells of the crypts of Lieberkühn and decreases in concentration in the epithelium covering the villi.[52] In the large bowel it is generally present also in the surface epithelium (Fig. 9.17a). In the normal gastric mucosa, SC is produced mainly by cells of the antral glands and their isthmus zones.[388]

It is now well established that transmembrane SC acts as a pIgR in the selective external transport of J chain-containing pIgA and pentameric IgM.[38,46,58] After being formed on the basolateral

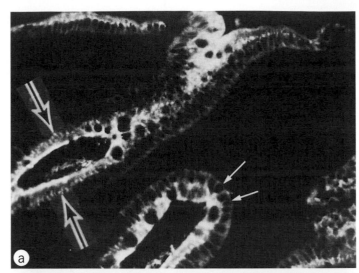

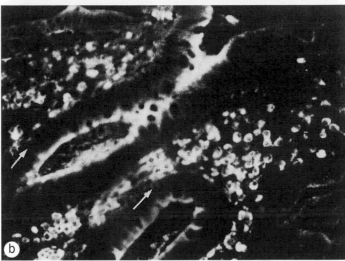

Fig 9.17 Immunofluorescence staining for (a) secretory component (SC) and (b) IgA in comparable fields from two serial sections of human colonic mucosa (lumen at the top) from a patient with ulcerative colitis. There is intense staining for IgA in the columnar cells of the crypts, while the surface epithelium contains less IgA. Note that SC is present in the Golgi regions (large arrows) which, by contrast, are devoid of IgA (see Fig. 9.18). Both SC and IgA are associated with the epithelial basolateral cell membranes (small arrows). Goblet cells are negative. ×250.

surface of the epithelial cell, the pIg–pIgR complexes are translocated by endocytosis and transcytosis to the lumen (Fig. 9.18). As a consequence, immunohistochemical staining reveals a cytoplasmic distribution of SC and the two pIg classes that is congruent except in the Golgi region (see Fig. 9.17) where pIgR accumulates selectively before it migrates basolaterally to meet its ligand.[35] The epithelial staining for IgA is normally stronger than that for IgM,[37] both because of the relatively abundant local pIgA production (see Fig. 9.4) and because the pIgR is less accessible to pentameric IgM (see later).

Mechanism and magnitude of pIgR-mediated transport
The pIgR consists of an approximately 100-kDa epithelial glycoprotein (transmembrane SC) which belongs to the Ig supergene family.[46] The first of its five extracellular Ig-like domains initiate the noncovalent ligand interaction at the basolateral epithelial

B

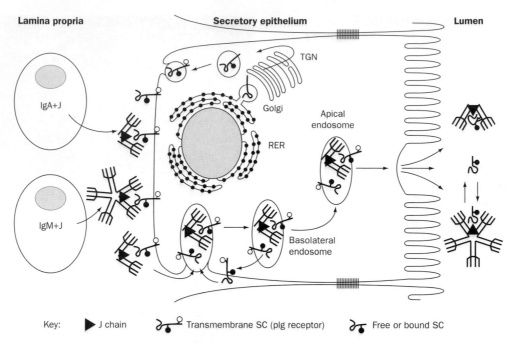

Fig 9.18 Various steps involved in the generation of human secretory IgA (right, top) and secretory IgM (right, bottom) via pIgR-mediated epithelial transport of J chain-containing dimeric IgA (IgA+J) and pentameric IgM (IgM+J) produced by mucosal plasma cells (left). Transmembrane secretory component (SC) is synthesized in the rough endoplasmic reticulum (RER) of secretory epithelial cell and matures by terminal glycosylation (–●) in the Golgi complex. After being sorted through the trans-Golgi network (TGN), it is phosphorylated (–o) and expressed as pIgR at the basolateral plasma membrane. Endocytosis of ligand-complexed and unoccupied pIgR is followed by transcytosis to apical endosomes and finally by cleavage and release of secretory Ig molecules with bound SC, as well as excess of free SC, at the luminal cell face. Some basolateral recycling may initially take place for unoccupied pIgR as indicated. During the external translocation, covalent stabilization of the IgA/SC complexes regularly occurs (disulphide bridge indicated in secretory IgA), whereas free SC in the secretion apparently serves to stabilize the noncovalent IgM/SC complexes (dynamic equilibrium indicated for secretory IgM).

membrane (Fig. 9.18). At the apical surface, SIgA and SIgM are released by cleavage of the pIgR, and only the C-terminal transmembrane and cytoplasmic part of the receptor remains for degradation in the epithelial cell. During transcytosis, the approximately 80-kDa extracellular part of pIgR is incorporated into the secretory antibody molecules as so-called bound SC, thereby conferring protection against non-specific proteolytic degradation, particularly to SIgA in which it becomes covalently linked.[43,46] More pIgA (~40 mg/kg body weight) is translocated to the adult gut lumen as SIgA by this mechanism every day than the total daily IgG (~30 mg/kg) production.[94] Therefore, the intestinal mucosa is quantitatively the most important effector organ of adaptive humoral immunity.

Excess of unoccupied pIgR is released apically by proteolytic cleavage in the same manner as SIgA and SIgM to form so-called free SC (Fig. 9.18). Variable amounts of this fragment (~80 kDa, identical to bound SC) are usually present in exocrine secretions;[32] by equilibrium with the bound component, free SC exerts a stabilizing effect on the quaternary structure of SIgM in which bound SC remains noncovalently linked.[37] In various ways, free SC in secretions may also contribute to innate mucosal defence (see later).

Different transport efficiency for pIgA and pentameric IgM
In normal adults, external secretions contain much more SIgA than SIgM,[32,141] which alone can not be accounted for by the striking predominance of local pIgA-producing cells (see Figs 9.4 and 9.9). Thus, in well-controlled quantitative studies of jejunal fluid and parotid saliva, the concentration ratio of IgA to IgM is found to be

2.4- to 4.9-fold higher than the corresponding local immunocyte class ratio.[32,64,128,264,308] This estimate is based on the observation of a fairly similar synthetic rate in IgA- and IgM-producing cells.[139] Moreover, as discussed above, mucosal IgA plasma cells release variable amounts of monomeric IgA in addition to pIgA, whereas IgM-producing cells normally are virtually restricted to pentamer secretion.[5] Altogether, our calculations suggest that external transfer of pIgA is favoured at least 6- to 12-fold over that of pentameric IgM on a molar basis. Significant biological variables of secretory immunity other than the local immunocyte distribution therefore appear to exist. Such variables could be differences in the ligand affinity for pIgR, in the efficiency of receptor-mediated epithelial transcytosis of the two ligands or in their diffusion properties across the stromal matrix and basement membrane.

We have examined the impact of these variables on the epithelial transport of pIgA and pentameric IgM by employing polarized Madin–Darby canine kidney (MDCK) cells transfected to express the human pIgR.[267] When the affinity of pIgA and pentameric IgM for free SC in solution was determined *in vitro*, the latter ligand bound with considerably higher avidity.[39,43] Conversely, we found that pIgR expressed by the MDCK cells interacted with pIgA and pentameric IgM with similar affinity, but nevertheless bound on average three times more molecules of the latter than the former ligand.[267] This difference might reflect that pIgA complexes with more than one receptor, which would accord with the possibility that this ligand induces dimerization of the pIgR upon binding.[164] Nevertheless, both pIgA and pentameric IgM were found to be internalized fast and with similar rates at 37°C, and endocytosis was completed within 5 min. Moreover, both ligands were handled with similar efficiency during transcytosis in our test system.[267]

Possible ligand-enhanced transport

The ability of human pIgA to stimulate epithelial transcytosis has been described in experiments employing rabbit pIgR; the increase in transcytotic rate was reported to be 2- to 3-fold in the presence of pIgA compared with Fab fragments of antibody to rabbit SC used as a substitute ligand.[356] A similar ability to stimulate transcytosis of pIgR was also reported for human tetrameric IgA.[357] We therefore measured the rate of pIgA and pentameric IgM transcytosis by pulse labelling with low and extremely high concentrations of the same ligands.[267] Both polymers were found to be transported across MDCK cells expressing the human pIgR with similar kinetics, and we did not observe enhanced transport rate when the ligand concentration was increased 20 times. This result suggested that different levels of receptor saturation did not influence the rate of epithelial transport mediated by the human pIgR.

Evolutionary significance of enhanced pIgA transport

IgM was the first Ig class to evolve and is found in external secretions of lower vertebrates.[306,359] All characterized mammalian species, and also chickens,[236] contain IgA in addition to IgM. The evolution of IgA as the major secretory antibody class has introduced interesting changes conducive to mucosal homeostasis. Although our in-vitro data showed that human pIgR-mediated transport of pentameric IgM is just as efficient as that of pIgA, we concluded that external translocation of the latter polymer is strikingly favoured in vivo because of its better diffusion through the extracellular matrix and basement membranes.[267] Therefore, the reduced size of pIgA may reflect a compromise between its advantageous external translocation and the number of antigen-binding sites carried to the secretions.

The pIgA molecule as such is well adapted to the proteolytic environment in external secretions.[141,315] In addition, its stabilization with covalently bound SC endows SIgA with increased resistance against non-specific bacterial proteases.[141] Moreover, pIgA's inability to activate the classical complement pathway[331] is desirable to avoid continuously altered mucosal homeostasis by inflammatory mediators at effector sites with persistent antigen exposure (see later). Altogether, pIgA appears to be a 'smaller and smarter' antibody molecule than pentameric IgM in terms of mucosal defence.

Regulation of pIgR expression

The pIgR is constitutively expressed even early in fetal life[73] and it can be upregulated postnatally by various cytokines, particularly interferon γ (IFN-γ) and IL-4,[46] which in some studies have been shown to act synergistically.[111,299] Also the proinflammatory cytokines TNF-α and IL-1 enhance SC expression in the HT-29 adenocarcinoma cell line,[46,159,206] especially together with IFN-γ and butyrate,[206] a bacterial fermentation product that abounds in the large bowel. Conversely, the stimulatory effect of IL4 is selectively decreased by butyrate.[206]

Transcriptional regulation of the human SC gene

Our recent molecular experiments with the same cell line have demonstrated that IFN-γ, IL-4 and TNF-α enhance SC expression by transcriptional activation,[269] and these cytokines can thus provide an immunoregulatory link between the level of local immune responses and the antibody transport function of pIgR (on the right in Fig. 9.15). We and others have cloned and characterized the SC gene, including its promoter region, and putative binding sites for various transcription factors as well as for glucocorticoid and androgen receptors have been identified.[178,180,201,393] A composite DNA element constituting an E box consensus motif (Fig. 9.19), which binds proteins of the basic helix loop helix leucine zipper family, was shown to be most important for constitutive SC transcription in a reporter gene assay.[178]

In a similar functional assay,[303] induction of the SC promoter by IFN-γ was mapped to a region that contains two consensus sequences for interferon-stimulated response element (ISRE), whereas binding of interferon regulatory factor 1 (IRF-1) after such stimulation of HT-29 cells was demonstrated to a different ISRE located in exon 1 (Fig. 9.20). Gel electrophoresis mobility shift assay accordingly demonstrated binding of nuclear proteins from HT 29 cells to this ISRE of the SC gene after IFN-γ stimulation, and also weakly after TNF-α stimulation, but the latter cytokine mainly produced involvement of a 5' promoter binding site for the nuclear factor (NF)-κB p50 subunit.[269] In a reporter assay (Fig. 9.20), exon 1 ISRE has nevertheless been shown to be functionally important for gene expression after TNF-α stimulation.[180] Furthermore, recent work in our laboratory has identified DNA elements in intron 1 that are involved in both TNF-α- and IL-4-mediated activation of the SC gene.[338,339]

Immunohistochemical observations in coeliac disease, chronic gastritis and Sjögren's syndrome harmonize with an immune response-associated enhancement of secretory immunity (Fig. 9.15); signs of upregulated SC expression and increased pIgR mediated uptake of IgA are seen in glandular epithelia in all these immunologically active lesions.[60] Nevertheless, the epithelial

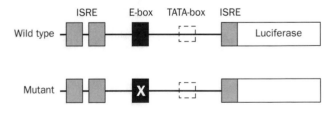

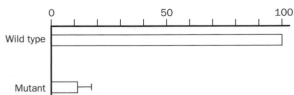

Fig 9.19 Dependency on E-box in the promoter of the human secretory component (SC) gene for its constitutive expression. Schematic diagram (top) of the proximal promoter region and reporter genes with a wild type and mutant (×) E-box as indicated. Results (bottom) of this mutation in SC gene promoter-driven reporter (luciferase) assay is given in percentage of wild type activity; it is reduced to that of the TATA-box alone (not shown). ISRE, Interferon-stimulated response element. Data from Johansen et al.[178]

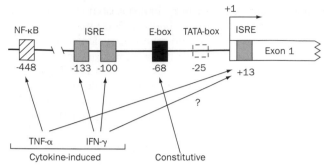

Fig 9.20 Regulatory elements in the human secretory component gene The diagram delineates DNA elements believed to be important for constitutive expression (see Fig. 9.19), IFN-γ-induced upregulation (all three ISREs included), and TNF-α-induced upregulation (an upstream NF-κB binding site in the promoter and an ISRE in exon 1), with central base positions in relation to transcription start site indicated. The broken arrow marked +1 denotes the transcription start site and the open box a consensus TATA sequence. Question marks indicate putative cytokine-mediated induction not yet shown by reporter gene assay. In addition, intron 1 contains regulatory elements stimulated by IL-4 and TNF-α. (See Refs 338 and 339.)

transport capacity may be insufficient in certain patients with an exceptionally expanded intestinal IgA immunocyte expansion, resulting in excessive amounts of pIgA in serum.[53]

PROTECTIVE FUNCTIONS OF SIgA ANTIBODIES AND FREE SC

Functional properties of SIgA

The main purpose of the secretory antibody system is, in cooperation with innate mucosal defence mechanisms, to perform immune exclusion (see Figs 9.2 and 9.21). Most important, SIgA inhibits colonization and invasion by pathogens,[141] and pIgA antibodies internalized by the pIgR may even inactivate viruses (e.g. rotavirus) inside epithelial cells.[81,243,244] Both the agglutinating and virus-neutralizing antibody effect of pIgA is superior to monomeric antibodies,[61,141,315] and SIgA antibodies may block microbial invasion quite efficiently.[165] Thus, individuals negative for human immunodeficiency virus (HIV) who live together with HIV-positive partners for several years often appear to be protected by specific SIgA antibodies in their genital tract.[245] A potentially important additional defence function is the ability of IgA antibodies to induce loss of bacterial plasmids that code for adherence-associated molecules and resistance to antibiotics.[305] Moreover, induction of SIgA responses has been shown to interfere significantly with mucosal uptake of macromolecules in experimental animals.[61]

Collectively, therefore, the functions of locally produced pIgA would be to inhibit mucosal colonization of microorganisms as well as penetration of soluble antigens (Fig. 9.21). Notably,

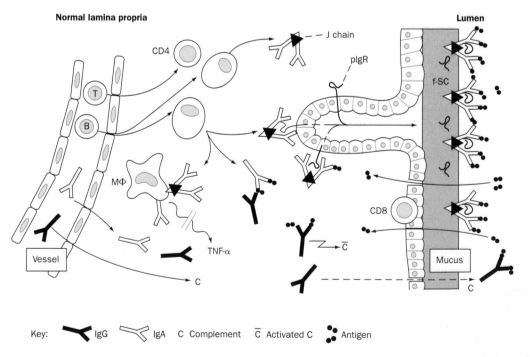

Key: IgG   IgA   C Complement   C̄ Activated C   Antigen

Fig 9.21 Normal mucosal homeostasis in the gut. Contributing biological variables are represented as a critical balance between available immunoglobulin classes (for simplicity, only IgG and IgA are indicated). Secretory IgA (to the right) is generated from dimeric IgA with associated J chain produced by lamina propria immunocytes and transported by the transmembrane secretory component (SC or pIgR) to the lumen, together with variable amounts of unoccupied cleaved receptor, called free SC (f-SC). Secretory IgA antibodies act in a first-line defence by performing antigen exclusion in mucus on the epithelial surface. Antigens circumventing this barrier meet corresponding serum-derived IgG antibodies in the lamina propria. The resulting immune complexes activate complement, and inflammatory mediators are formed within the mucosa, thus causing a temporarily increased external transfer of IgG antibodies by leakage between epithelial cells to the lumen (broken arrow). A persistent and adverse inflammatory development is normally inhibited by blocking antibody activities (competition for antigen depicted) exerted in the lamina propria by serum-derived monomeric IgA as well as by locally produced monomeric and especially dimeric IgA. Both types of IgA molecules may, independent of their antibody specificities, also inhibit mediator release (TNF-α depicted) from activated phagocytic cells such as macrophages (MΦ). Moreover, antigens may be returned in a non-inflammatory way to the lumen by the pIgR-mediated transport mechanism after being bound to J chain-containing dimeric IgA antibody, as indicated.

because of its stability, SIgA can retain its antibody activity for remarkably prolonged periods in a hostile environment such as the oral cavity.[229] This immune exclusion function is most likely reinforced by the relatively high levels of crossreacting SIgA antibodies present in external secretions.[311] Apparently, these polyreactive 'natural' antibodies are designed for urgent protection before an adaptive immune response is elicited; they are therefore reminiscent of innate immunity,[30] although their site and mechanism of induction remain unclear (see earlier).

In addition, it has been claimed that SIgA can perform ADCC and promote phagocytosis via FcαR (CD89) present on macrophages and granulocytes, enhance sticking of certain bacteria to mucus, interfere with growth factors (e.g. iron) and enzymes necessary for pathogenic bacteria and parasites[61,141] and exert positive influences on the inductive phase of mucosal immunity by promoting relevant antigen uptake in GALT.[45] The latter possibility adds to the importance of breast feeding in providing a supply of SIgA antibodies to the infant's gut.[47]

Interactions of SIgA and free SC

Eosinophils possess FcαR and apparently also a receptor for SC.[208] Therefore, SIgA exhibits particularly potent eosinophil-activating properties,[2] thus providing a proinflammatory potential of the secretory immune system when immune exclusion fails. However, free SC is able to block this activity,[208] and it can also inhibit epithelial adhesion of *Escherichia coli*.[140] Moreover, a pneumococcal surface protein (SpsA) has been shown to interact directly with both free and bound SC.[154] Altogether, these biological properties of SC suggest that, phylogenetically, it has originated from the innate defence system like many other proteins involved in specific immunity.

Non-inflammatory IgA-mediated immune elimination
Magnitude of mucosal uptake of soluble antigens

Intact antigenic material from the gut lumen has been shown to cross the mucosal barrier and enter the bloodstream even in normal adults, although the actual amount of uptake remains uncertain. Work performed in experimental animals with ^{125}I-labelled albumin has been difficult to interpret due to marker instability.[60] Both degradation of the protein molecule and release of the label can result in considerable overestimation of penetrability as determined by scintillation counting compared with data based on immunological quantification. However, several human studies have reported absorption of intact dietary antigens in healthy adults. Paganelli and Levinsky[284] found up to 3 ng/ml of β-lactoglobulin in peripheral blood after an intake of 1.2 litres of bovine milk. Kilshaw and Cant[189] often detected both β-lactoglobulin and ovalbumin in serum as well as in breast milk of lactating women, the levels ranging from 110 pg/ml to 6.4 ng/ml in the latter fluid. Husby *et al.*[169] detected up to 10 ng/ml of ovalbumin, which corresponds to about 10^{-5} of the amount consumed. Most of the antigen appeared in the circulation after 2–5 hours and was partly present in immune complexes (see later).

Routes of intestinal antigen uptake

Several routes may be visualized for the penetration of intact antigen through the normal intestinal epithelium: paracellular diffusion bypassing the tight junctions or via epithelial discontinuities such as the cell extrusion zones of the villus tips; translocation through enterocytes by endocytosis and subsequent exocytosis; or transport by M cells in GALT. The relative importance of these mechanisms for uptake of soluble antigens from the gut lumen in health and disease remains unknown; and the consequences in terms of sensitization or induction of oral tolerance probably depend on the route of uptake as well as on the nature of the antigen (soluble, lectin-like or particulate). A detailed discussion of these possibilities is given elsewhere.[48,61,333]

Putative mechanisms of immune elimination

It may be envisioned that IgA antibodies contribute to local homeostasis not only by performing immune exclusion on the mucosal surface but also by trapping of antigens in the lamina propria (Fig. 9.21). Both these IgA-mediated blocking mechanisms would be noninflammatory in competition with corresponding complement-activating IgG (and IgM) antibodies.[61,331] In addition, epithelial transport of pIgA-containing immune complexes may also be an efficient noninflammatory antigen clearance mechanism (Fig. 9.21) as suggested by *in-vitro* experiments; it was shown that pIgR-expressing polarized epithelial monolayers translocated undegraded antigen bound to pIgA antibody from the basolateral side to the apical medium.[243] Interestingly, monomeric IgA or IgG antibodies, when crosslinked via antigen to pIgA of the same specificity, could contribute to such pIgR-mediated external transcystosis of antigen.[243] The secretory epithelium may thus participate in the clearance of immune complexes directly at the mucosal site where they are most likely to be formed.

Additional IgA-mediated putative homeostatic mechanisms

Experimental evidence suggests that, in several ways, IgA may influence local homeostasis by its binding to FcαR on leukocytes. Firstly, monomeric IgA, and particularly pIgA or IgA-containing immune complexes, are able to suppress the attraction of neutrophils, eosinophils and monocytes, thereby reducing the availability of the numerous potent inflammatory mediators that may be released from these cells.[61] Secondly, IgA can downregulate the secretion of proinflammatory cytokines such as TNF-α from activated monocytes,[406] and perhaps also from lamina propria macrophages (Fig. 9.21). Thirdly, activation of neutrophils and monocytes that results in generation of reactive oxygen intermediates (respiratory burst) may also be inhibited by IgA.[407] On the other hand, pIgA or aggregated monomeric IgA can trigger resting monocytes to show increased activity, such as TNF-α secretion,[113] and can also cause eosinophil degranulation.[2] This proinflammatory potential of the local IgA system probably reflects a need for enhanced antigen elimination when immune exclusion fails, for example in parasitic mucosal infestations; but it is difficult to know how the balance between SIgA and free SC may influence eosinophils (see earlier). Altogether, the divergent *in-vitro* results emphasize that the contribution of IgA to normal mucosal homeostasis *in-vivo* must be remarkably fine-tuned.

Individual variations in the development of mucosal homeostasis

The postnatal development of the IgA-producing cell system shows large individual variations.[73] On the basis of IgA measurements in serum, it has been suggested that infants and children at hereditary risk of atopy have a retarded postnatal development of their IgA system.[358,376] Perhaps their SIgA-mediated immune exclusion and other noninflammatory mucosal antigen-handling mechanisms are transiently deficient. This notion was later supported by quantitation of jejunal immunocytes; a significantly reduced IgA response to luminal antigens, without any IgM compensation, was indicated in the mucosa of atopic children.[351] Another study showed an inverse relationship between the serum IgE concentration and the number of IgA-producing cells in jejunal mucosa of food-allergic children.[295] More recently it was reported that infants born to atopic parents have a significantly higher prevalence of salivary IgA deficiency than age-matched control infants.[391] Kilian *et al.*[188] found that the throats of 18-month-old infants with, presumably, IgE-mediated clinical problems, contained significantly higher proportions of IgA1 protease-producing bacteria than age-matched healthy controls. Therefore, a combination of reduced mucosal barrier function and hereditary elevated IgE responses might often underlie the pathogenesis of gastrointestinal allergy, at least in many of the atopic children.

PROINFLAMMATORY ANTIGEN HANDLING AS A POSSIBLE BASIS FOR MUCOSAL DISEASE

It is well known that circulating IgG antibodies to food antigens are often present in normal individuals, although with remarkably varying subclass contributions.[69] Because approximately 50% of the circulating pool of IgG is extravascularly distributed, these antibodies will be well represented locally in the intestinal mucosa. Parenteral immunization eliciting high levels of IgG antibodies may reduce mucosal antigen penetration,[61] although some studies have reported increased uptake.[17] Our *in-vitro* results showed that IgG antibodies could retard mucosal penetration of

the corresponding antigen; conversely, the penetration of an unrelated bystander macromolecule was significantly enhanced.[60] A similar detrimental side effect of IgG antibody has been observed *in vivo*.[216] This is probably explained by local formation of complement-fixing IgG-containing immune complexes[61] and activation of mast cells.[17] The proinflammatory potential of maternal IgG present in the intestinal mucosa of the newborn (see later), or of locally produced IgM and IgG antibodies, may be less important in infants who are breast-fed because milk SIgA antibodies, which have little or no complement-activating capacity,[331] will exert a noninflammatory blocking effect.[47]

As long as the mucosal homeostasis remains in control, IgG-mediated immune reactions occurring in the mucosa will not cause clinical symptoms and may be viewed as a 'second line' of defence (Fig. 9.21). However, in patients with pronounced regional IgE responses to dietary antigens, immune-mediated degranulation of mucosal mast cells and activation of eosinophils are likely to result in a massive release of potent inflammatory mediators overruling the IgA-mediated homeostatic mechanisms (see later). Such 'parasite-directed' pathotopic potentiation of the second line of mucosal defence is probably the basis of overt atopic allergy,[368] and may be considered as break of oral tolerance to food. In IBD (Crohn's disease and ulcerative colitis), mucosal homeostasis is severely altered with signs of immunological hyperactivation, downregulated J chain expression and substantial local overproduction of IgG;[70] together, these features are believed to signify break of oral tolerance to antigens from the indigenous bacterial flora accompanied by less restricted extravasation of leukocytes (Fig. 9.22).

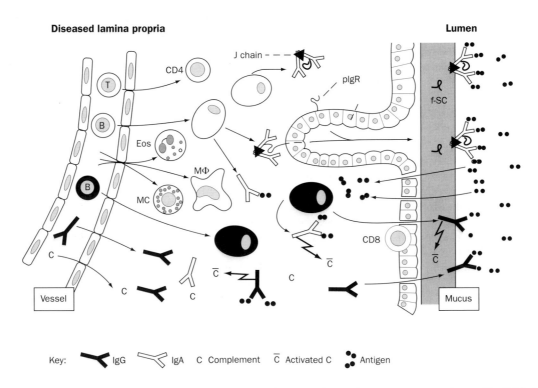

Fig 9.22 Altered mucosal homeostasis in inflammatory bowel disease. For comparison with normal homeostasis, see Fig. 9.21. An imbalance develops when there is distorted local B cell stimulation because of unselective leukocyte extravasation and increased mucosal permeability with excessive antigen exposure of the mucosal immune system. To limit dissemination of foreign material, a second line of defence is set up in the mucosa, including exudation and local production of IgG as well as ingress of inflammatory cells such as monocyte-derived macrophages (Mφ), mast cell (MC) precursors and eosinophils (Eos). Because IgG antibodies exhibit proinflammatory properties, such as complement activation, a vicious circle develops with further increase of antigen penetrability, massive attraction of inflammatory cells and release of lysosomal enzymes as well as other inflammatory mediators.

APPARENT EXTRAINTESTINAL MANIFESTATIONS OF PROINFLAMMATORY FOOD ANTIGEN HANDLING

Consequences of altered mucosal homeostasis

Although it is unknown to what extent circulating immune complexes with dietary antigens are formed in the gut mucosa or within the vascular system, the observation that food challenge in normal individuals often results in IgA-containing complexes suggests that they are indeed derived from the intestinal lamina propria.[288] The appearance in serum of SIgA-containing immune complexes has been related to the development of arthritis in patients with jejunoileal bypass disease.[92] Also, there are several case reports on ankylosing spondylitis in patients with selective IgA deficiency,[250,377] and it has been argued that this immune defect may aggravate the disease.[163] Importantly, IgA-deficient subjects show increased uptake of dietary antigens[61] and greatly expanded intestinal IgM and IgG immunocyte populations (see Fig. 9.9). When local immune exclusion of antigens is unsuccessful, the proinflammatory properties of these antibody classes, whether locally produced or serum-derived, will become dominating, and the selective leukocyte homing mechanisms may break down in the mucosa. In IBD there is convincing evidence that the adhesion properties of the mucosal vascular endothelium are more similar to those expressed in peripheral lymph nodes, thus probably allowing extravasation of B and T cells representing systemic instead of mucosal immunity.[70] As mentioned above, such altered mucosal homeostasis is reflected by a disproportionate increase in mucosal IgG-producing cells (even in individuals with an intact IgA system) and locally formed IgG-containing immune complexes (Fig. 9.22).

Dissemination of immune complexes

If penetrated luminal antigens and locally formed immune complexes escape trapping and degradation in the mucosa, they may reach peripheral blood via intestinal lymph, but (depending on their size and on the state of the vascular bed) a fraction may become absorbed into intestinal capillaries and enter the portal circulation directly. These two alternative routes will obviously influence the subsequent possibilities for retention and degradation in mesenteric lymph nodes, the spleen, the bone marrow and the liver.[61] The final fate of the immune complexes, for example deposition in synovium or musculature, will moreover be influenced by the tissue affinity of the contained antigen and the involved antibody isotypes.[61] As most immune complexes in a clinical context are mixed with regard to Ig isotypes (see later), their size, effector cell affinity and complement-activating properties will depend on the relative magnitude of the IgA, IgG, IgM and IgE immune responses. All these variables will probably influence the possible mucosal and/or extraintestinal hypersensitivity manifestations of gastrointestinal antigen uptake.[61]

RELATION OF INTESTINAL ALLERGY TO MUCOSAL IMMUNITY

Is food allergy a result of abrogated oral tolerance?

It is only possible to identify a small fraction of adverse reactions to food as immune-mediated: in children some 10–20% and in adults some 3–12%. One may assume that at least these cases represent abrogation of immunological tolerance to dietary antigens, but activated immune mechanisms also appear to be involved in many of the remaining patients as suggested by similarly increased intestinal permeability[13,193] and release to the gut lumen of mediators from mast cells and eosinophils[14] after intestinal challenge with relevant food. One unproven possibility is that unidentified mucosal immune reactions cause dietary hypersensitivity in these patients. Importantly, oral tolerance to luminal antigens will not be maintained when the epithelial barrier function is persistently compromised.[48] Increased antigen penetrability may be caused by humoral immune reactions with release of inflammatory mediators from the complement cascade (IgG and IgM: Type III hypersensitivity) or from mast cells (IgE: Type I hypersensitivity or atopy), it can be T cell-mediated (Th1: Type IV 'delayed type' hypersensitivity) or it can result from a combination of several immune mechanisms.[49] Moreover, the neuroendocrine network may be involved in an adverse development because an array of peptide hormones, neurotransmitters and receptors for such mediators are expressed by T and B lymphocytes as well as by immunological effector cells.[26] In particular, the mucosal mast cells may serve as 'relay stations' between the microenvironment and the nervous system because of their spatial relationship to nerve endings.[249]

Altered mucosal homeostasis in IgE-mediated food allergy

Only a small proportion of children (3–5%) and adults (1–2%) with apparent gastrointestinal food allergy can conclusively be shown to have IgE-mediated hypersensitivity to food, and the primary events in the pathogenesis of such atopic disease are poorly understood. As discussed above, it has been suggested that children at hereditary risk of atopy have a relatively slow postnatal development of their IgA system. SIgA-mediated immunological antigen exclusion may be transiently deficient in these individuals, and a combination of reduced mucosal barrier function and a genetically determined brisk IgE response may explain their gastrointestinal allergy. It also appears plausible that disorders such as gastrointestinal virus infections involving activation of NK cells may promote mucosal permeability with subsequent IgE sensitization in predisposed individuals. Although infections and NK cell activation generally cause release of IFN-γ that tends to downregulate Th2-dependent IgE production,[49] IFN-γ has a detrimental effect on the epithelial barrier, particularly in combination with TNF-α.[105,233] Moreover, both these cytokines can induce or enhance the expression of adhesion molecules on vascular endothelial cells.[70] Interestingly, enhanced IL-4 production in the presence of elevated IFN-γ has been reported in food-allergic children.[158] In addition, the epithelial cells may respond to many types of irritant by cytokine release as an 'early warning' system,[117] and several basic environmental factors are known to act directly on mast cells to cause degranulation.[237] Therefore, the mucosal cytokine profile resulting from a variety of initiating hits may act on the microvasculature and cause altered and less restricted leukocyte extravasation (Fig. 9.22) as an important component of apparently 'food-induced' mucosal inflammation.[49]

Nevertheless, the dominating pathogenic factor in overtly atopic patients appears to be a genetic impact on the tendency to elicit excessive IgE responses to protein antigens;[104] as a consequence of efficient immune-mediated mast cell degranulation, their gastrointestinal exclusion of dietary antigens and the gatekeeper function of their mucosal microvasculature is persistently compromised.[49] Thus, after food challenge of these individuals, there is an excessive uptake of antigens which for some time remain bound chiefly to IgG and IgE in the circulation.[83,287] Because such immune complexes often show C1q-binding properties, they are probably mixed – containing IgG-antigen-IgE and sometimes perhaps also IgA.[288] In many patients the development of symptoms such as skin itching and wheezing has been reported to be associated with the appearance of such circulating complexes. The systemic symptoms may therefore be due to both Type 1 and Type 3 hypersensitivity. By contrast, food challenge in normal non-atopic individuals results mainly in IgA-containing immune complexes in the circulation (and probably first in the mucosa; see Fig. 9.21), apparently as part of a safe non-inflammatory antigen-handling mechanism.[288]

Importance of IgE production and sensitization of mast cells in food allergy

Enhanced IgE production and IgE sensitization of mast cells, as well as a variety of other known mast cell stimuli, including IgG immune complexes,[369] may in different ways drive the mucosal immune response against food antigens towards a chronic inflammatory reaction (Fig. 9.22). Mast cells have been shown to produce an array of cytokines, of which IL-5 and TNF-α are known to induce rapid and prolonged priming of eosinophils, mast cells and basophils for increased mediator release when exposed to subsequent stimuli.[104,237] Activated mast cells also generate IL-4 and the lipid mediator leukotriene B$_4$ (LTB$_4$), both of which can significantly contribute to the development of a Th2 response.[409] The cytokine profile of CD4$^+$ Th2 memory cells tend to be polarized towards IL-4, IL-5, IL-10 and IL-13 secretion, whereas a Th1 response with prominent IFN-γ secretion (promoting cell-mediated Type IV hypersensitivity) is dominating in infections.[84] Such Th1

skewing appears to be determined mainly by macrophage-derived IL-12, although costimulatory molecules such as B7.1 (CD80) *versus* B7.2 (CD86) on mucosal APCs may also be of importance, as well as their LPS receptor CD14.[204,329]

A prominent Th2 response has also been associated with preferential extravasation of eosinophils, at least in the airways. Thus, cultured nasal polyp microvascular endothelium exposed to IL-4 and IL-13 shows increased expression of VCAM-1[173] – an adhesion molecule that binds integrin $\alpha 4\beta 1$ present on eosinophils but absent on neutrophils. We have demonstrated directly *in situ* an association between vascular VCAM-1 expression and mucosal eosinophilia in the human upper respiratory tract.[172] Moreover, eosinophils produce IL-4 that may further promote a local Th2 response.[276] Therefore, it appears that the late-phase allergic reaction generally has its origin in preferential activation of CD4$^+$ Th2 memory cells combined with triggering of mast cells and eosinophils, all as part of a vicious immunoregulatory circle.

The number of eosinophils has been reported to be significantly increased in the intestinal mucosa of children with cow's milk allergy,[405] suggesting an underlying extravasation and activation of mast cells on the basis of a Th2-dependent regional IgE response (Fig. 9.23). Also, reduced intestinal uptake of antigens after oral treatment of patients with cromoglycate, and the beneficial effect of this drug on their systemic and intestinal symptoms, further attest to the involvement of mast cells in the pathogenesis of food allergy.[103,285] However, this does not exclude a contributing pathogenic role of IgG antibodies, because complement activation gives rise to the split products C3a and C5a that may cause mast cell degranulation.[399] In addition, antibodies of the IgG4 subclass may sensitize mast cells, and IgG4 antibodies against food antigens (particularly gluten and β-lactoglobulin)

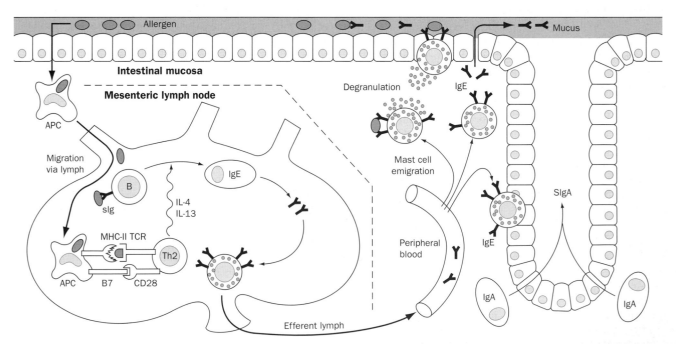

Fig 9.23 Regional induction of IgE antibody production, arming of mast cell precursors with IgE and mucosal homing of sensitized mast cells as a basis for atopic food allergy. Dietary allergen is carried by antigen-presenting cells (APC) to mesenteric lymph node where APC is activated to express costimulatory molecules (e.g. B7) enabling it to present antigenic peptides in an MHC Class II (MHC-II) restricted manner to Th2 cells. Their cytokine profile (IL-4 and IL-13) promotes IgE production and subsequent mast cell arming. When the sensitized mast cells, after emigration, meet specific allergen at the mucosal site, degranulation and release of inflammatory mediators will occur. IgE may leak into the gut fluid after shedding from mast cells or by an exudative process. sIg, surface Ig; SIgA, secretory IgA.

are often prominent.[69] It is unlikely, therefore, that a beneficial effect of cromoglycate in intestinal disorders makes a reliable distinction between IgE- and IgG-induced inflammation.[286]

IgE immunocytes or IgE-positive mast cells

Several early studies were made to relate 'IgE-containing' cells to gastrointestinal diseases. Some workers deemed an increased mucosal number of such cells to suggest ongoing local Type 1 hypersensitivity, whereas others based the same conclusion on a reduced number, implying IgE consumption by the atopic reaction. However, usually, no distinction was made between IgE-positive mast cells and IgE-producing immunocytes.[50] This was also true for the disease entities called allergic proctitis[160,323] and infantile allergic colitis,[177] which are both characterized by a high number of 'IgE-containing' cells in the mucosal lesions.

Early reports on the jejunal mucosa of patients with food allergy were likewise difficult to interpret. Rosekrans *et al.*[321]

observed a high number of 'IgE-containing' cells (up to 100 per mm² lamina propria section area), which probably represented mast cells because we[319] and others[335,362] have been unable to find a consistent increase in IgE-producing cells associated with cow's milk protein intolerance, whereas numerous IgE-bearing mast cells are usually present (see later). The latter cells are mainly located at the base of the crypts, but are also found among the IgA-producing immunocytes around the level of the crypt openings (Fig. 9.24). They may be quite numerous, even in the complete absence of local IgE-producing cells. According to our studies,[319] IgE immunocytes are just as sparse in the intestinal mucosa of patients with atopic food allergy as in non-specific chronic inflammatory lesions of different origins.[390] Others have likewise reported low and inconsistent numbers of jejunal and rectal IgE immunocytes in children with food allergy and atopic eczema[295] and in children with soya protein allergy.[297]

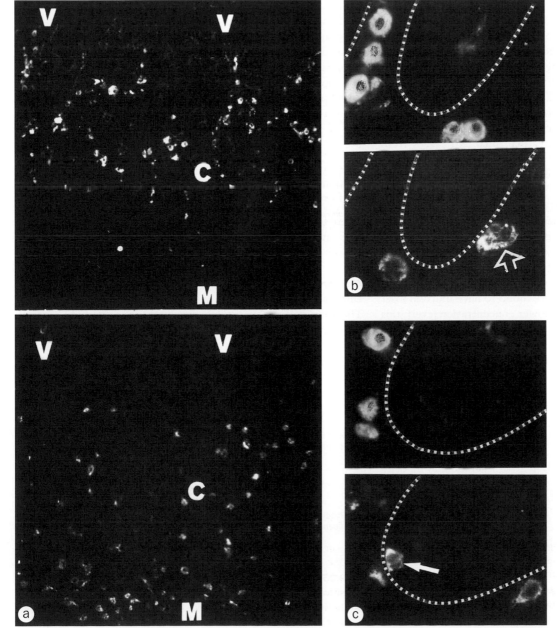

Fig 9.24 Two-colour immunofluorescence staining (same field) for IgA (top panels) and IgE (bottom panels) in a partly transverse section of jejunal mucosa from a patient with food allergy. (a) IgA-producing immunocytes are found in normal distribution, mainly in the upper crypt (C) region and at the base of some villi (V); IgE-positive mast cells are found mainly between the crypts and muscularis mucosae (M), but some are intermingled with IgA immunocytes. (b,c) Two fields adjacent to crypts (indicated by dashed lines) illustrate that IgA immunocytes and IgE-positive mast cells have different immuno-fluorescence appearances: the former show intense cytoplasmic staining, whereas the latter show mainly peripheral granular staining (open arrow). The mast cells occurring in the crypt region are often located near to or within (arrow in (c)) the epithelium. Note that the exposure times needed to display mast cells were much longer than that for immunocytes. (a) ×150, (b,c) ×600.

It seems justifiable to conclude that IgE-positive mast cells may be involved in the pathogenesis of certain gastrointestinal diseases despite concurrent mucosal synthesis of IgE being generally lacking or minimal. This notion accords with experimental immunohistochemical observations in parasite-infested rats that have disclosed that IgE is produced chiefly in the mesenteric lymph nodes and spleen rather than in the diseased intestinal mucosa.[218,241] Direct evidence for a major clonal expansion of IgE-producing cells in mesenteric lymph nodes of rats after infestation with the gut-dwelling helminth parasite *Nippostrongylus brasiliensis* has been obtained by an immunoplaque assay.[346]

Arming of intestinal mast cells with IgE in normal and food-allergic individuals

It follows from the experimental studies referred to above that mucosal mast cells acquire their IgE mainly in regional lymph nodes.[138] Therefore, the excess of free IgE reaching the blood from the production site probably reflects rather poorly the extent of regional mast cell arming; such sensitization will depend on the local availability of IgE and be reflected in the mucosal homing of mast cell precursors (see Fig. 9.22). A preferential regional sensitization harmonizes with the observation that distinctly IgE-positive mast cells were more often encountered in the bronchial mucosa than in the skin of allergic patients with recurrent pulmonary complaints.[397] The armed mast cells probably shed their IgE both within the mucosa and, after entering the epithelium, also directly into the gut lumen (see Fig. 9.23). This mechanism most likely explains the significantly raised levels of IgE (or rather IgE fragments) found in the intestinal juice and faeces from patients with different kinds of atopic disease, including food allergy, without any consistent relationship to the IgE concentrations in serum.[12,195,196]

Using immunohistochemistry, we have demonstrated that arming of mucosal mast cells with IgE is relatively prominent (92%) in the gut of patients with food-related diarrhoea suggested to be IgE-mediated by a positive skin prick test.[15] Intestinal atopic hypersensitivity reactions could therefore be of pathogenic significance in most of these patients. However, because half of the normal control individuals were found to have mucosal mast cells with IgE (albeit usually at a lower concentration level), this phenomenon presumably reflects a general defence mechanism of the gut. Subsequently, other have reached a similar conclusion.[147] Indeed, IgE fragments have been found in the faeces of normal children[196] and at substantially increased levels in patients with parasitic gut infection.[194] The concentration of IgA both in the intestinal lumen[195] and in the respiratory tract[294] apparently shows some relationship to the corresponding IgE level; perhaps IgE antibodies via mast cell degranulation increase mucosal penetrability for antigens, thereby enhancing the stimulation of the local IgA immunocyte system. In fact, IgA rather than IgE may mediate the eosinophil degranulation (see earlier) that occurs in IgE-associated mucosal disease.[294] Interestingly, the expression of receptors for IgA on eosinophils is increased in allergy.[259]

Mucosal extravasation of mast cells and eosinophils

It has been suggested that mast cells may employ the same homing receptor ($\alpha 4\beta 7$) as primed T and B cells to enter the gut mucosa.[352] As discussed earlier, this integrin binds to MAdCAM-1 expressed on the lamina propria microvasculature (see Fig. 9.16b). Moreover, the epithelial affinity of mast cells

(bottom panels in Fig. 9.24), like that of CD8[+] IELs, appears to be explained by a change of integrin expression from $\alpha 4\beta 7$ to $\alpha E\beta 7$ – the latter showing affinity for E-cadherin expressed basolaterally on the epithelium.[352] MAdCAM-1 may also contribute to the extravasation of eosinophils in the intestinal mucosa, because these cells are known to bear $\alpha 4\beta 7$ in addition to $\alpha 4\beta 1$.[120] This is probably of considerable importance in the gut because VCAM-1, for some unexplained reason, is poorly or not at all expressed *in situ* by the intestinal microvasculature even in IBD[70] and, surprisingly, IL-4 is unable to induce VCAM-1 on cultured human gut endothelium.[157] It would be of interest in the future to examine if increased expression of MAdCAM-1 is a feature of food allergy in the gut because this adhesion molecule has recently been found to be considerably upregulated in IBD.[76]

COELIAC DISEASE AS A MODEL FOR CELL-MEDIATED AND HUMORAL FOOD ALLERGY

Coeliac disease, or gluten-sensitive enteropathy, is a rather common malabsorption condition that represents an excellent model for studying the relationship between hypersensitivity to food and intestinal immunopathology. The complexity of the mucosal immune system is emphasized by the fact that, despite enormous efforts over several decades to unravel the nature of this intriguing enteropathy, it is still unclear how the 'flat' duodenal/jejunal lesion develops. Two major mechanisms may be visualized (Fig. 9.25):

- negative effect(s) on the surface epithelium causing damage and loss of enterocytes (villous atrophy) followed by compensatory crypt hyperplasia;
- positive effect(s) on the crypt cells directly inducing proliferation, with the villous atrophy being only 'apparent' as a result of crypt hyperplasia.

There is considerable immunological evidence for both possibilities, and a complex and variable interplay of many biological factors is probably the basis for the coeliac immunopathology.

Mechanisms of mucosal immune activation in gluten-sensitive enteropathy

The immunological basis of coeliac disease appears to be a poorly developed oral tolerance to gluten from wheat flour in the newborn period, or subsequent abrogation of such tolerance in genetically susceptible individuals. Oral tolerance clearly involves more than one immunoregulatory mechanism, and experiments in rodents based on feeding of soluble proteins have revealed an

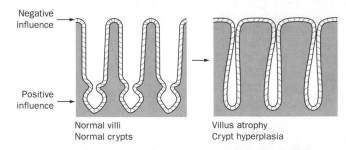

Normal villi
Normal crypts

Villus atrophy
Crypt hyperplasia

Fig 9.25 Mucosal alterations leading to the flat lesion in gluten-sensitive enteropathy may be caused by negative (damaging) effects on the villous enterocytes, positive (stimulatory) effects on the crypt cells or a combination of both.

overwhelming complexity. Identifiable biological variables are genetics, age, feeding dose and timing, antigenic structure, epithelial barrier integrity, and the degree of concurrent local immune activation, as reflected in the mucosal APCs and the microenvironmental cytokine profiles.[48]

Because professional APCs are central in immune responses, their function in the mucosa may likewise be crucial for induction and maintenance of oral tolerance.[394] Subepithelial macrophages in the normal human intestinal lamina propria express only low levels of costimulatory molecules such as B7[329] and they exhibit poor T cell stimulatory properties.[310] Therefore, it is possible that in the normal state they carry penetrating gluten peptides (and other dietary antigens) to regional lymph nodes, thus avoiding initiation of cell-mediated immunity in the mucosa. Conversely, in an activated state (due to infection or complement activation?), mucosal APCs may trigger gluten-reactive T cells in the lamina propria and thereby initiate coeliac disease and perhaps other types of food allergy (see earlier) in predisposed individuals.[344]

Signs of markedly enhanced cellular and humoral immunity are seen in the untreated coeliac lesion.[69,344] An early gluten-induced event appears to be activation of CD4[+] T cells,[151] which can be reproduced *in vitro* by exposing duodenal/jejunal biopsy specimens from patients to peptides obtained by peptic–tryptic digestion of gluten (or more specifically gliadin, the alcohol-soluble prolanin fraction of wheat flour). Such *in-vitro* re-stimulation increases strikingly the number of activated (CD25[+]) mucosal T cells,[153] thereby allowing their isolation and cloning.[225,256] In addition, there is extensive induction of CD25 on mucosal macrophages,[151,153] and the increased cellular expression of the costimulatory molecules ICAM-1,[367] B7.2 and CD40[330] is further evidence of local immune activation.

The most abundant cytokine secreted by activated gluten-reactive mucosal T cells in coeliac disease is IFN-γ.[270,271] This cytokine is most likely a major factor in the increased expression of SC (see earlier and Fig. 9.26a) and HLA-DR[68] seen in the flat lesion (left panels in Fig. 9.26). In particular, together with TNF-α[105] IFN-γ may also be involved in the increased epithelial permeability[233] and the marked expansion of the mucosal immunocyte populations,[69,344,345] Humoral immunopathology is signified by subepithelial complement activation, which may be an early event in the mucosal lesion.[152]

Immunogenetics of gluten-sensitive enteropathy

The TCRα/β of the gluten-reactive mucosal T cells generally shows a molecular restriction that matches the genetic predisposition to coeliac disease (and the related gluten-sensitive enteropathy, dermatitis herpetiformis or DH). In Europe, this susceptibility is mainly associated with a particular HLA-DQ2 (DQα1*0501, β1*0201) heterodimer, and to a smaller extent by an HLA-DQ8 (DQα 1*0302, β1*0301) heterodimer.[353] Other reported associations (e.g. HLA-B8, HLA-DR3, HLA-DR7) reflect linkage disequilibrium on an extended disease-related haplotype. However, identical twins show at least 25% discordance with regard to the clinical presentation of coeliac disease, which proves that there are pathogenic factors (environmental cotriggers?) in addition to the immunostimulatory gluten-derived prolamins. Moreover, although the disease activity depends mainly on the presence of gliadin peptides, prolamins from rye and barley

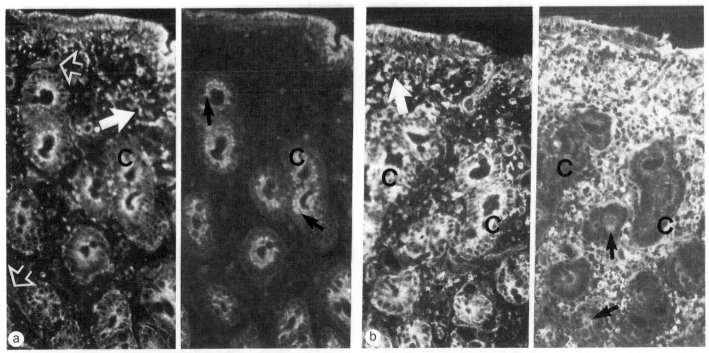

Fig 9.26 Two-colour immunofluorescence staining (same field) for HLA-DR (left panels) and (a) secretory component (SC) or (b) IgA (respective right panels) in two serial sections of jejunal mucosa from a patient with untreated coeliac disease. Both the surface epithelium (at the top) and the hyperplastic crypts (C) show bright apical and membrane-related DR staining and there are DR-positive macrophages or dendritic cells (solid arrows) and vascular endothelium (open arrows) in the lamina propria. (a) In contrast to the normal situation (see right panel in Fig. 9.3a), DR is expressed together with SC by both the surface and crypt epithelium. Note that the distribution of the two markers is not completely congruent, especially because of the accumulation of SC in the Golgi zones (small arrows). (b) Numerous IgA immunocytes are present between DR-positive crypts and there are large amounts of interstitial IgA in the lamina propria. Epithelial IgA staining signifies external transport (small arrows). ×150.

can also be pathogenic, but less likely avenin from the more distantly related oats.[49] Cereals from unrelated grass families (e.g. rice, maize and millet) are completely inactive in this respect.

Somewhat surprisingly, gluten-reactive CD4[+] T cell clones isolated from individual coeliac patients have been found to become stimulated by prolamin peptides derived not only from different wheats but also from rye.[226] There are apparently several similar (identical?) prolamin motifs recognized by the actual TCRα/β, probably comprising 10–15 amino acids, that can fit the polymorphic region of the disease-associated HLA-DQ molecule expressed by the mucosal APCs.[344] It may be relevant in this context that the prolamins of wheat, rye and barley are very rich in glutamine and proline, which occur in repetitive sequences (see later).

Involvement of the intestinal B cell system in gluten-sensitive enteropathy

Mucosal Ig-producing cells

In untreated adult coeliac disease, the average numbers of jejunal IgA, IgM and IgG immunocytes per mucosal tissue unit were found to be increased 2.4, 4.6 and 6.5 times, respectively.[8] Similar results were obtained in adult DH patients with flat jejunal lesions.[9] Our results in coeliac children were comparable but also some of the young histologically normal controls had a relatively high mucosal IgG immunocyte number.[343] Immunohistochemical findings published by others[322,362] are in keeping with our data, although a less prominent IgG cell response was revealed in tissue specimens subjected to crosslinking fixatives[322] than in our ethanol-fixed biopsy material, which is particularly well suited for detection of IgG immunocytes.[59] Interestingly, the jejunal IgA immunocyte population was shown to consist of 47% IgA2 in untreated adult patients[183] compared with 29% in the controls (see Fig. 9.8). In agreement with our observations,[8] virtually no IgD- and IgE-producing cells have been found in the coeliac lesion.[322,362]

Mucosal B cell response to gluten

Our immunohistochemical findings agree with studies of mucosal Ig synthesis in tissue cultures; when jejunal biopsy specimens from patients with coeliac disease were compared with normal control specimens, incorporation of [^{14}C] leucine was highly elevated for both IgA and IgM.[121,223] This result emphasizes the immunostimulatory effect of gluten in coeliac patients. Thus, when clinical symptoms reoccurred after 8–12 days with gluten challenge following treatment (gluten-free diet), the total mucosal IgA and IgM synthesis was increased two- to five-fold.[121,223] In children with coeliac disease, the jejunal immunocyte population was quite normal following treatment for 1.2–9 years, whereas in treated adult patients both the immunocyte numbers and isotype ratios fell between those of untreated patients and controls.[8] This difference suggested either that the adult jejunal mucosa does not have the same potential for improvement, or that a strict gluten-free diet is more difficult to achieve in adults than in children.

Isotypes of antibodies to gluten

The increase in mucosal tissue culture Ig synthesis observed after gluten challenge was apparently in the main due to antibodies against gliadin peptides (29–75%); although the isotypes of these antibodies were not stated, experiments in one patient indicated that only 60% was accounted for by IgA and IgM.[122] This figure agrees with the result obtained by the ELISPOT method performed on dispersed mononuclear cells from untreated coeliac

lesions, showing on average 68% of the anti-gliadin spot-forming cells to be of the IgA class, whereas up to approximately 30% was accounted for by IgG- or IgM-producing cells in some of the patients.[227] In a preliminary study of an untreated adult patient, we detected by indirect immunofluorescence staining directly in the lesion, a small fraction of jejunal immunocytes with specificity for gliadin peptides, and about 60% of these were of the IgA isotype;[51] interestingly, a much larger proportion of the total IgG than of the total IgA cell population was positive (5.7% *versus* 1.6%). Another preliminary immunofluorescence study based on mucosal specimens from children with coeliac disease indicated gliadin specificity in 11%, 10.5% and 6.5% of the jejunal IgG, IgM and IgA immunocytes, respectively.[361]

Increased mucosal production of IgG, IgM and IgA antibodies to both gliadin and other dietary antigens in coeliac disease has been supported by *in-vitro* studies of biopsy specimens[89] and dispersed intestinal lymphoid cells.[90] Moreover, in treated patients that were challenged with gluten, a significant inverse correlation appeared between the time to clinical relapse and the number of jejunal IgG immunocytes found after challenge (Fig. 9.27). This suggested that an imbalanced local immune response to gliadin (and probably also to other dietary antigens), with a shift towards IgG, is involved in the pathogenesis of coeliac disease. Because some 50% of the circulating IgG is extravascularly distributed, serum-derived antibodies may likewise have an immunopathological effect in the coeliac lesion. Most untreated patients with coeliac disease have relatively high levels of IgG1 (sometimes together with IgG3) antibodies to gliadin in serum,[69,170] and these two isotypes show complement-activating properties.[137] Therefore, they may cause epithelial permeability, which could explain that their relative level is related to a high IgA response to gliadin.[170] Also notably, although the mucosal IgG immunocyte response in coeliac disease shows some preference for IgG2 (of as yet unknown specificity), proinflammatory IgG1 is the dominating locally produced IgG isotype.[320] An even more

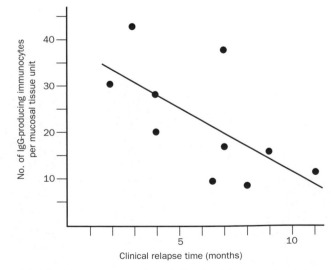

Fig 9.27 Scatter diagram of the relation in children with coeliac disease between time to clinical relapse and the number of jejunal IgG-producing immunocytes as revealed by biopsy after a completed period with gluten challenge. The relapse time was significantly shorter in patients with the brisker mucosal IgG response. ($r = -0.645$, $P < 0.05$.) Adapted from Scott et al.[343]

prominent proportion of mucosal IgG1 immunocytes occurs in patients with IgE-mediated food allergy.[320]

Secretory antibodies to gluten

In contrast to the situation in IBD,[70] J chain expression is well preserved in the expanded jejunal IgA-producing immunocyte population of the untreated coeliac lesion.[183] Because this expansion favours the IgA2 subclass, the estimated potential for local SIgA2 secretion is increased to approximately 50% in untreated coeliac patients compared with 30% in controls.[183] The marked increase of local IgM production, and the heightened epithelial SC expression (right panel in Fig. 9.26a), also contribute to enhanced secretory immunity in gluten-sensitive enteropathy.

With an enzyme-linked immunosorbent assay (ELISA), relatively high concentrations of IgA and IgM antibodies to gluten/gliadin (only the IgM class in IgA deficiency) have been detected in the jejunal fluid from untreated coeliac patients,[207,214,395] in agreement with the immunohistochemical observations and mucosal Ig synthesis data discussed earlier. As expected, the IgA antibodies were found to be mainly of the SIgA type[93,277] and to contain a greater proportion of IgA2 than comparable antibodies in serum.[239] Moreover, the IgA antibodies were shown to disappear more slowly from gut fluid than from serum during gluten restriction,[207] and the IgM antibodies persisted for prolonged periods in the jejunum of treated adults.[277]

In a group of DH patients on a normal diet, but without enteropathy ('latent coeliac disease'), intestinal IgA and IgM antibody levels to gliadin and other food proteins were found to match the levels in untreated coeliac disease.[278] The intestinal IgM antigliadin response was particularly disease-specific. These results agreed with our immunohistochemical studies that showed considerable expansion of the jejunal IgA and IgM (but not IgG) cell population in a group of similar DH patients who also showed no consistent increase of serum IgA and IgM levels.[9,69] Therefore, mucosal production of IgA and IgM antibodies to dietary antigens, and particularly to gliadin, appears to be an early event in gluten-sensitive enteropathy but does not initially cause a flat lesion. Conversely, the magnitude of the jejunal IgG cell response is closely related to the degree of histopathology[69] and is also indicative of the proneness to clinical relapse after gluten challenge (Fig. 9.27).

Humoral immunopathology

A putative immunopathological role of mucosal IgG, and perhaps IgM antibodies, has gained further support by the detection of activated complement beneath the surface epithelium in jejunal lesions of untreated coeliac and DH patients; this deposition was well correlated with the number of mucosal IgG cells and also with the serum levels of gliadin-specific IgG and IgM antibodies.[152] The latter observation suggested that gliadin peptides are part of these immune complexes. As mentioned above, 50% of circulating IgG is extravascularly distributed and a disproportionately high fraction of IgG immunocytes in the coeliac lesion sometimes appears to be specific for gliadin.[51,227] It has also been shown that antibodies to gliadin can mediate ADCC.[371]

The striking crypt hyperplasia of the coeliac lesion may therefore be partly compensatory, following antibody-mediated damage of the surface epithelium (on the left in Fig. 9.28). Also,

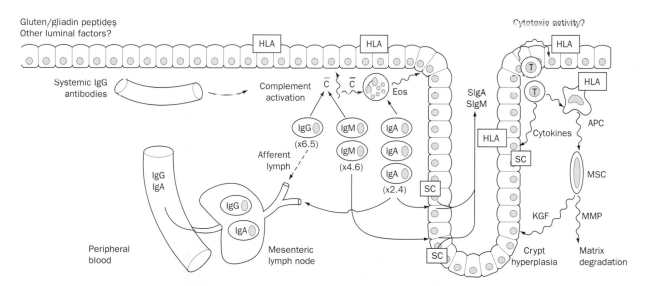

Fig 9.28 Hypothetical scheme for immunopathological mechanisms in coeliac disease, schematically depicting humoral immunity (on the left) with approximate relationship between IgG, IgM and IgA immunocyte subsets (relative numerical increase factor indicated) and features of cell-mediated immunity (on the right). The disease initiation is determined by gluten/gliadin peptides and other (unidentified) luminal factors on an HLA-associated genetic background. Complement activation C̄ induced by serum-derived or locally produced IgG (and perhaps IgM) antibodies may be an early pathogenic event by increasing the epithelial permeability. Complement split products may further activate eosinophils (Eos), causing release of their cytotoxic proteins, and these cells may also be degranulated by locally produced dimeric IgA. Despite enhanced external transport of secretory immunoglobulins (SIgA and SIgM), an excess of locally produced IgA antibodies to gluten/gliadin and other dietary antigens will reach peripheral blood and reflect the severity of the mucosal lesion, whereas IgG antibodies (probably produced mainly in the mesenteric lymph nodes) are usually a poor indicator of the activity in the lesion (see Fig. 9.29). Cell-mediated immunity with release of cytokines from activated T cells (T) and antigen-presenting cells (APC) may explain most of the immunopathological features of the lesion. Thus, cytokines induce enhanced expression of secretory component (SC) and epithelial HLA molecules (boxes) and stimulate mucosal stromal cells (MSC) to secrete keratinocyte growth factor (KGF) and matrix metalloproteinases (MMP) which contribute to the mucosal remodelling. Surface epithelial cells may, in addition, be directly harmed or eliminated by intraepithelial cytotoxic T cells.

complement split products, particularly the anaphylatoxins C3a and C5a, may cause mucosal oedema directly by increasing vascular permeability and indirectly by inducing mast cell degranulation with histamine release (see earlier). Furthermore, the activation fragment C5a is a potent chemotactic factor for neutrophils, eosinophils and monocytes and may, through leukocyte priming, initiate the release of various biologically potent products of arachidonic acid, including prostaglandin (PG). It has been shown that a single intraluminal challenge with gliadin in coeliac patients produces rapid mucosal permeability increase[213] and local release of histamine[211] and PGE$_2$.[212] Superficial mucosal deposition of eosinophil cationic protein has, moreover, been reported,[149] and its prominent cytotoxic properties may be involved in epithelial damage (on the left in Fig. 9.28). Perhaps immune complexes containing pIgA or SIgA antibodies are responsible for the degranulation of eosinophils in the lesion (see earlier). Activated eosinophils may play a central immunopathological role that, perhaps, is amplified by an autocrine and paracrine action of IL-5, which they apparently synthesize abundantly in the coeliac lesion.[112]

The involvement of humoral immunity in the pathogenesis of coeliac disease has been questioned on the basis of a single reported case with severe generalized B cell deficiency.[402] Nevertheless, it is difficult to exclude that an extremely sensitive effector mechanism such as the complement cascade operates in the intestinal mucosa also in hypogammaglobulinaemia. The complement system is usually intact in these patients and they are given gammaglobulin substitution therapy. The systemically administered IgG reaches the intestinal lamina propria[402] and contains antibodies to various dietary antigens, which might initiate subepithelial complement activation. It is also important that these patients often have some Ig-producing cells in their gut mucosa, particularly of the complement-activating IgM class,[77] and they show evidence of increased food protein uptake.[61]

Mucosal complement activation may thus be an initiating event in the pathogenesis of coeliac disease, perhaps by starting a cascade of cytokine release from epithelial and lamina propria cells. Chowers *et al.*[87] found that the mucosal mRNA levels for several proinflammatory cytokines increased many thousand-fold following *in-vivo* challenge of rectal mucosa with gluten in coeliac patients, while only little IFN-γ expression was seen initially. Therefore, the characteristic Th1 response to gliadin peptides and other prolamins (see earlier) may develop subsequently in genetically susceptible individuals;[344] via cell-mediated mechanisms. This response will promote crypt hyperplasia and contribute to the villous atrophy (on the right in Fig. 9.28).

Circulating IgA antibodies to gliadin as a probe of mucosal B cell activation

Excessive IgA production in the flat mucosal lesion probably explains the commonly increased serum IgA concentration characteristic of untreated or challenged coeliac patients;[69] a strong positive correlation has been found between serum levels of IgA antibodies to gliadin and the number of jejunal IgA immunocytes per mucosal tissue unit.[183] The fact that 57–61% of circulating IgA gliadin antibodies is pIgA in untreated coeliac disease,[93,238] in addition to the substantial enrichment of the IgA2 subclass in such antibodies,[283] further attests to a significant mucosal origin. Alternatively, gliadin antibodies may be released to serum from circulating primed IgA immunocyte precursor cells on their way from GALT to the intestinal lamina propria.[156] It is not surprising,

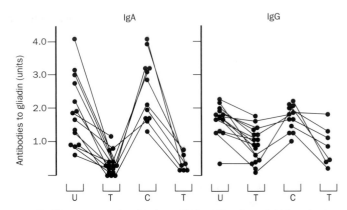

Fig 9.29 Measurements of IgA and IgG antibodies (ELISA optical density units) to gliadin peptides performed on two or three serum samples from 24 children with coeliac disease. Untreated (U), treated approximately 1 year with a gluten-free diet (T) or challenged for 4–19 months with a gluten-containing diet (C). Adapted from Scott *et al.*[345]

therefore, that ELISA determination of serum IgA antibodies to gliadin has become a useful adjunct in the diagnosis and follow-up of coeliac patients, particularly in childhood (Fig. 9.29). Such monitoring may be considered an indirect way of probing the level of disease-associated mucosal B cell activation (Fig. 9.28). Although serum IgG antibodies to gluten occur in fairly high titres, they do not show the same specificity for coeliac disease as the IgA counterparts.[345] These IgG antibodies are probably in the main produced in mesenteric lymph nodes and will hence only to a lesser extent reflect mucosal immunopathology (Figs 9.28 and 9.29).

Nature and diagnostic value of IgA endomysial antibodies (IgA-EMAs)

In patients with coeliac disease, ingestion of gluten induces IgA antibodies that, by indirect immunofluorescence staining, show binding to antigenic determinants present in the reticulin sheets (endomysium) surrounding the subepithelial smooth muscle bundles in monkey oesophagus.[342] The IgA-EMAs are autoantibodies with variable species crossreactivity; they apparently account also for the R1-type reticulin and jejunal IgA antibodies associated with gluten-sensitive enteropathy – the variable fluorescence staining pattern being a consequence of the choice of tissue substrate used for the testing. Dietrich *et al.*[114] recently identified the actual (or the major) antigen detected by IgA-EMAs as tissue transglutaminase (tTG, or EC 2.3.2.13), which is a ubiquitous enzyme abundantly released from cells during stress and tissue damage. It catalyses the formation of isopeptide bonds between glutamine (donor) and lysine (acceptor) residues, thereby promoting the crosslinking of certain extracellular matrix proteins. Interestingly, the glutamine-rich gliadin peptides are a preferred donor substrate.[341]

Circulating IgG antibodies to tTG have been detected in a variety of inflammatory and autoimmune disorders,[114] but the IgA-EMAs are nearly 100% specific for gluten-induced enteropathy. The reported sensitivity of this serological test in adult patients with untreated coeliac disease is 68–100% and in untreated children 85–100%, being notably reduced below 2 years of age.[342] In DH the sensitivity result depends on the severity of villous atrophy.[342] Because this test is not positive in all patients with gluten-induced enteropathy, combined determination of IgA gliadin antibodies and IgA-EMAs is recommended in a diagnostic setting. In our hands, the latter test and an ELISA

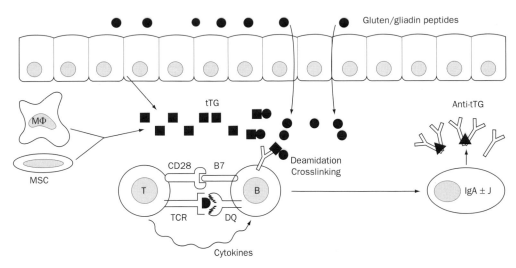

Fig 9.30 Putative reciprocal immune stimulation in intestinal mucosa of coeliac disease patient by cognate interactions between B cells specific for tissue transglutaminase (tTG) and T cells specific for gliadin. Gluten/gliadin peptides penetrate the epithelial barrier by transcytosis or paracellular diffusion (at the top) and become deamidated by, and crosslinked with, tTG, which is released from several cell types such as macrophages (Mφ) and mucosal stromal cells (MSC). The B cell endocytoses tTG–gliadin complexes via its tTG-specific surface receptor, and presents processed peptides in an HLA-DQ-restricted manner to the gliadin-specific receptor (TCR) of the T cell. If appropriate costimulation exists (e.g. CD28-B7 ligation), the T cell will become activated and secrete cytokines that stimulate the production of IgA autoantibodies to tTG, both dimeric and monomeric (IgA ± J).

based on recombinant human tTG as antigen coat, provide quite similar sensitivity and specificity results. Although the final coeliac diagnosis still depends on histological evaluation of duodenal/jejunal biopsies, the two serological tests combined are a most useful adjunct and can largely replace biopsies in the follow-up of diet compliance during treatment.

Mucosal production of IgA EMAs

The striking relationship between the severity of gluten-sensitive enteropathy and the presence of serum IgA-EMAs or IgA anti-tTG antibodies, suggests that such antibodies originate in the intestinal lesion as discussed above for circulating IgA antibodies to gliadin (see Fig. 9.28). However, while 31% of the latter belongs to the IgA2 subclass, therefore being compatible with a duodenal/jejunal origin (see earlier), only 6% of the IgA-EMAs is of this subclass – rather suggesting an extraintestinal production site.[283] However, even in coeliac disease, most (53%) jejunal IgA immunocytes actually produce the IgA1 subclass,[183] and IgA-EMAs occur in the intestinal juice of patients with gluten-sensitive enteropathy.[246] Importantly, culture fluid of mucosal biopsy specimens from untreated patients contains IgA-EMAs, and production of such antibodies can be induced in jejunal specimens from treated patients restimulated *in vitro* with gliadin peptides.[300]

It has been a puzzle how gluten can drive the IgA-EMA response in the gut. Important in this context is the fact that tTG is abundantly present in the subepithelial region of the intestinal lamina propria, and its expression appears to be increased in coeliac disease.[257] Therefore, one likely possibility is that tTG forms complexes with available gliadin peptides,[114] thereby allowing gluten-reactive T cells to provide help for tTG-specific B cells that have endocytosed and processed the tTG–gliadin complexes[354] and then presented gliadin peptides in an HLA-DQ-restricted fashion to the cognate T cells (Fig. 9.30). Of further importance is the recent discovery that tTG by deamidation of certain glutamine residues can enhance the DQ-binding properties of gliadin peptides and hence their T cell stimulatory capacity.[257] It is thus possible to visu-

alize that the induction of IgA-EMAs in the gut can be promoted in two ways by local interactions between tTG and gliadin (Fig. 9.30). This is apparently the first example of reciprocally induced or enhanced immune responses directed against an autoantigen and a dietary antigen, respectively.

Putative pathogenic role of IgA antibodies to tissue transglutaminase

Whether IgA-EMAs (or antibodies to tTG) represent an epiphenomenon in gluten-sensitive enteropathy, or are of pathogenic importance, is an issue of controversy. It should be kept in mind that coeliac disease occasionally occurs against a background of immunodeficiency: either a selective IgA defect (commonly; Ref. 57) or a generalized B cell defect (rarely; see earlier). These case reports provide evidence that IgA autoantibodies to tTG cannot be of primary pathogenic importance. Nevertheless, it is intriguing to speculate that such IgA-EMAs (or other isotypes of EMAs) are involved in the pathogenesis of villous atrophy, as recently proposed by Schuppan *et al.*[341] Thus, the development of absorptive enterocytes may partly depend on TGF-β, which is secreted by a variety of cell types as an inactive or 'latent' form in a protein complex. Degradation of the prosegments associated with the mature cytokine homodimer by proteases (e.g. plasmin) is necessary to release the active form. Because tTG apparently has a significant role in preparing latent TGF-β for such proteolytic activation, IgA-EMAs may inhibit enterocyte differentiation in the coeliac lesion (Fig. 9.31). This interesting hypothesis will need further work to become substantiated.

DEVELOPMENTAL ASPECTS OF THE MUCOSAL B-CELL SYSTEM

Perinatal immunity

Human exocrine fluids contain only variable trace amounts of IgA and IgM the first days after birth, whereas some IgG is usually present.[47,73] Its immediate source is interstitial tissue fluid which,

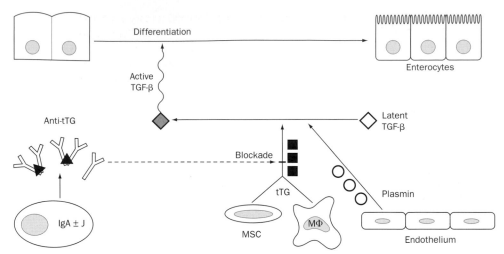

Fig. 9.31 Hypothetical scheme for a possible pathogenic action of IgA autoantibodies to tissue transglutaminase (tTG) produced in coeliac disease (see Fig. 9.30). Both tTG (released from various cell types) and proteolytic enzymes such as plasmin are necessary for activation of latent TGF-β. In its active form, this cytokine apparently promotes the differentiation of intestinal epithelial cells to absorptive enterocytes. Antibodies to tTG may exert a blockade on its beneficial enzymatic effect and thereby contribute to villous atrophy. Modified from Schuppan et al.[341]

after a gestational age of 18 weeks, contains maternal IgG in substantial amounts.[281] Thus, immunohistochemistry of fetal intestinal mucosa shows bright diffuse staining for IgG in the lamina propria, whereas IgA is totally lacking (Fig. 9.32).

Maternal IgG in the neonate's mucosa is unquestionably of value in protecting against infections, but IgG antibodies to dietary antigens may, in theory, adversely affect mucosal penetrability for macromolecules.[17,60,216] Mucosal integrity may be damaged by lysosomal enzymes released from polymorphonuclear granulocytes which are known to be attracted when complement-activating immune complexes are formed locally.[11] This proinflammatory mechanism may contribute to a greater influx of dietary antigens in newborns than in older infants, although the evidence for such a difference is rather circumstantial.[61,318] The proinflammatory potential of maternal IgG antibodies (and locally produced IgM in the newborn; see below) is probably dampened by blocking SIgA antibodies in breast milk.[47] Moreover, breast milk contains large

amounts of the soluble complement inhibitor CD59 or protectin.[25] Also, this factor and other complement regulatory proteins are expressed by the gastrointestinal epithelium.[18]

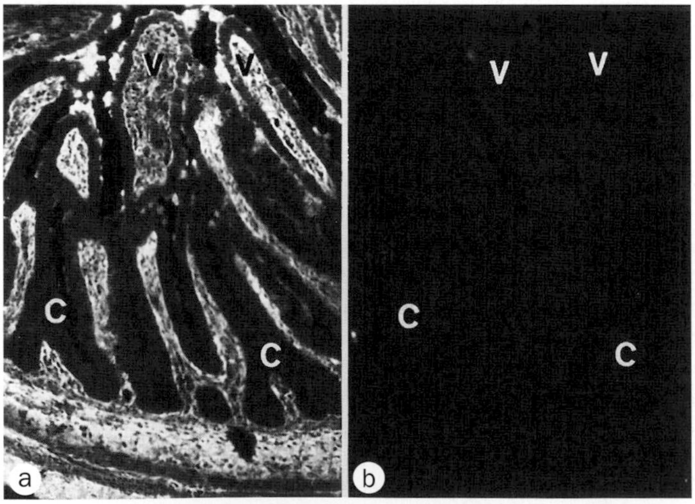

Scattered B and T lymphocytes are seen in fetal intestinal lamina propria from 14 weeks' gestation.[73,231] Occasional IgM- and IgG-producing plasma cells have been reported to appear somewhat later and they remain few until birth, whereas IgA-producing cells are either absent or extremely rare even until 10 days of age. By contrast, the salivary glands sometimes contain scattered J chain-expressing IgA immunocytes in addition to the IgM and IgG isotypes, especially after 30 weeks' gestation.[378] This apparent difference between the salivary glands and the gut mucosa with regard to low-grade fetal B cell activation is intriguing; perhaps it reflects oral stimulation by maternal anti-idiotypic antibodies, cytokines, or foreign protein antigens present in amniotic fluid.[73] However, GALT is certainly immunocompetent at least during the final trimester; numerous plasma cells can appear in the intestinal mucosa in response to intrauterine infection.[349]

Postnatal development

The literature contains highly discrepant information about the postnatal development of the human secretory immune system. This may be explained by methodological problems in quantifying SIgA in secretions, differences among various secretory sites and large individual variations.[47] Using immunohistochemistry, Ig-producing cells are not normally detectable in human intestinal mucosa before 2 weeks of age, except for rare IgM immunocytes.[73] Thereafter a rapid increase takes place, particularly for the IgM immunocytes, which usually dominate up to 1 month.[296] Thus, the average rectal number of IgA-producing cells in 1–3-month-old children is only about 20% of that seen after 2 years (Fig. 9.33). Likewise, SIgM responses have been found to be relatively predominant early in infancy,[73,215] and prominent development of IgM cells in the early phase of gut immune responses has been shown also in animal experiments.[381]

Blanco et al.[27] observed no significant increase of small intestinal IgA immunocytes in children after 1 year although IgM-producing cells decreased. A similarly decreasing trend for IgM immunocytes with age has been reported by others, but at the same time a continuing increase of IgA cells has been indicated, even after 2 years.[234] The early SIgM response is probably of protective value but it is known that the immune response to certain bacterial capsular polysaccharides is poor or lacking before 2 years

Fig. 9.32 Immunofluorescence staining for (a) IgG and (b) IgA in comparable fields from serial sections of the small intestinal mucosa from a 26-week-old fetus. The tissue was directly fixed in ethanol to retain diffusible proteins. IgG abounds diffusely in the lamina propria and submucosa but is absent from the crypt epithelium (C). The epithelium covering the villi (V) contains some intercellular IgG, indicating leakage of interstitial fluid to the gut lumen where IgG is associated with the mucus (a). Note complete lack of IgA (b). ×80.

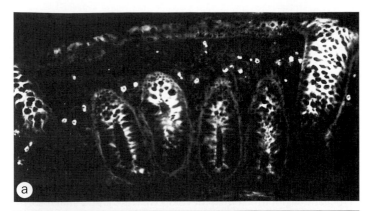

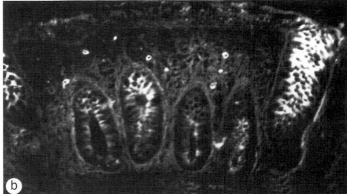

Fig 9.33 Immunofluorescence staining for (a) IgA and (b) IgM in comparable fields from two serial sections of histologically normal rectal mucosa from a 2-month-old infant (gut lumen at the top). Compared with normal adult mucosa, the number of Ig-producing cells is small; the ratio of IgA:IgM immunocytes is 2.5:1 compared with an adult large bowel isotype ratio of approximately 15:1 (see Fig. 9.9). Despite relatively few local immunocytes, large amounts of IgA and IgM are taken up by columnar crypt cells as a sign of external transport. The virtual absence of interstitial IgA staining reflects a low serum level of IgA. ×120.

of age. This creates a window of susceptibility at the time of disappearance of protective maternal IgG antibodies and weaning with deprivation of passively acquired SIgA from breast milk. The basis for the impaired response to polysaccharides is unclear, but reduced levels of CR2 expression on B cells and FDCs together with low complement activity in newborns may result in lack of CR2-BCR synergy (see earlier) and contribute to defective B cell activation.[145] There is compelling evidence that interaction of the complement split product C3d with CR2 is an extremely important link between innate immunity and specific B cell responses.[109]

Role of antigen exposure in the development of IgA-producing cells

The antigenic and mitogenic load on the mucosa is a decisive factor for the postnatal development of the secretory immune system. The indigenous microbial flora is probably of utmost importance, as indicated by the fact that the intestinal IgA system of germ-free or specific pathogen-free mice is normalized after about 4 weeks of conventionalization.[96,166] *Bacteroides* and *E. coli* strains seem to be particularly stimulatory for the development of intestinal IgA immunocytes.[222,260] Antigenic constituents of food exert an additional stimulatory effect, as suggested by fewer lamina propria IgA-producing cells in mice fed on hydrolysed milk proteins[332] as well as in parenterally fed babies.[192]

Reduced amounts of microbial and dietary antigens thus explain why the colonic numbers of IgA- and IgM-producing immunocytes were found to be decreased by about 50% after 2–11 months in children who had been subjected to defunctioning colostomies.[404] Postnatal and prolonged observations on defunctioned ileal segments in lambs have even more strikingly revealed a scarcity of immunocytes in the lamina propria; this result was explained by reduced local accumulation of B cell blasts and might involve both hampered migration from GALT to the mucosa and subsequently decreased local proliferation and differentiation.[316] It follows that the postnatal development of the mucosal IgA system is usually much faster in developing countries than in the industrialized world.[73] This difference apparently holds true even in malnourished children,[265] which reflects that mucosal immunity is highly adaptable to the antigenic load of the environment.

Nutrition and intestinal immunity

An early immunohistochemical study of children with low protein–calorie intake reported selective reduction of intestinal IgA-producing immunocytes.[144] This was supported by experiments in rodents with prolonged and severe malnutrition;[396] hampered homing of IgA-expressing B cells from GALT might be involved.[248] Severe vitamin A deficiency appears in particular to have a markedly adverse effect on mucosal IgA antibody responses,[403] with no consistent downregulation of epithelial IgA transport.[360] Interestingly, it has been reported that undernourished children respond to bacterial overgrowth in the gut with enhanced synthesis as well as upregulated external transfer of IgA.[10] It is of further great clinical importance that detrimental effects of severe malnutrition exerted on the SIgA system can be reversed with re-nutrition.[401]

IMPACT OF IMMUNODEFICIENCY ON THE MUCOSAL B CELL SYSTEM

Deficiency of IgA-producing cells

The activity of the secretory immune system in IgA-deficient subjects is fairly unpredictable on the basis of individual serum IgA levels.[57,73] A decreased intestinal IgA:IgM cell ratio reflects immaturity of the secretory immune system, and also appears to be a good indicator of a significant IgA deficiency after infancy. Thus, the intestinal IgA immunocyte population is commonly intact when serum IgA concentrations are above 18% of the normal average, whereas between 18% and 5%, the number of jejunal IgA cells is usually decreased but that of IgM cells increased.[336] A dichotomy between the immunocyte patterns in jejunal and rectal mucosa is seen in some subjects.[66,337]

Mucosal IgA cells and clinical problems in IgA-deficient subjects

In a group of 14 IgA-deficient patients (serum IgA<0.1 g/L) subjected to immunohistochemical studies of their jejunal mucosa in this laboratory, coeliac disease was diagnosed in two children and four adults;[273] a good response on a gluten-free diet was noted in four of them. A few patients suffered from other types of food intolerance, irritable colon, gastric ulcer, atopic eczema, asthmatic bronchitis or periodic depression. Autoimmune disease was observed in one patient with systemic lupus erythematosus (SLE) and in another with Raynaud's disease. Malignancies such as gastrointestinal non-Hodgkin's lymphoma occurred later on in one patient. Only a few of the patients suffered from chronic lung disease, except bronchitis, which was quite common; 12 of the patients suffered from recurrent infections, mostly of the respiratory tract.

One additional adult deficiency patient, with a tendency to respiratory tract infections, had quantitatively fully developed rectal and jejunal IgA immunocyte populations.[66] Nevertheless, an increased proportion of jejunal IgM cells, and an excess of free J chain in the intestinal IgA immunocytes, indicated some imbalance of his mucosal immune system. This case demonstrated that a general B cell maturation defect does not necessarily prevent the development of intestinal IgA-producing cells. The reason for such a dichotomy between systemic and local IgA is probably the heavy stimulatory antigen and mitogen load on GALT.

Replacement of IgA-producing cells

Interestingly, the total number of jejunal Ig-producing cells per defined mucosal tissue unit in subjects who completely lack IgA cells was found to be distributed within a range (40–227 cells/unit) that overlapped with values for the total local immunocyte population in normal controls (86–199 cells/unit) and adults with treated coeliac disease (144–335 cells/unit) examined in this laboratory.[65,273] Also, the immunocyte density in normal parotid tissue from an IgA-deficient subject was within the normal range (29 compared with 26–98 cells/mm²), and the same was true in the normal lacrimal gland of another IgA-deficient patient (432 compared with 307–789 cells/mm²). Thus, mucosal B cells without IgA-secreting capacity are able to migrate from MALT to secretory effector sites and undergo local terminal differentiation.

An important regional discrepancy appears when it comes to replacement of the IgA immunocytes that are lacking (Fig. 9.9): in the upper aeroalimentary tract, numerous IgD-producing cells (25–80%) are often found, whereas in the gastrointestinal tract such immunocytes usually make up less than 1% along with a regular predominance of IgM-producing cells (64–75%) and a varying fraction of IgG-producing cells.[56,65,72] Regardless of isotype, however, the 'compensatory' immunocytes show prominent J chain expression,[56,65,273] which attests to their differentiation from B cells generated in MALT (see earlier).

Intestinal compensation with mucosal IgM and IgG production

Enhanced intestinal production and secretion of IgM in selective IgA deficiency may partly explain the fact that most subjects with this disorder have no or few gastrointestinal symptoms;[57] their problems are rather related to the upper respiratory tract where compensation with IgM is often lacking.[72] However, immune exclusion in the intestine is clearly suboptimal in IgA-deficient individuals because more than half of them have raised levels of IgG antibodies to bovine milk proteins and circulating immune complexes containing such antigens.[101,102] It seems that these phenomena, which clearly reflect increased gastrointestinal permeability, may explain the relatively high incidence of autoimmunity seen in selective IgA deficiency.[99] Moreover, the incidence of this deficiency is considerably higher among patients with coeliac disease than in the general population,[57] and atopic food allergy may be associated with a defect of the mucosal IgA system in infancy (see earlier).

It is intriguing that up to 40% of the jejunal immunocytes may produce IgG without causing overt clinical signs of disturbed mucosal homeostasis.[273] Indeed, the jejunal IgG cells expand more than the IgM cells in response to oral cholera vaccination in IgA-

deficient subjects.[132,275] Therefore, intestinal SIgM and IgG antibodies usually afford satisfactory mucosal protection of the gut with preserved local homeostasis in IgA-deficient subjects as long as the innate defence mechanisms and cell-mediated immunity are functioning adequately.[251] One compensatory T cell-mediated mechanism may be an increased number of TCRγ/δ⁺ IELs.[274]

Generalized B cell deficiency

Still more intriguing is the fact that gastrointestinal disorders are quite rare in patients with infantile X-linked (Bruton-type) B cell deficiency leading to agammaglobulinaemia.[57,119,279] Conversely, 20–50% of the patients with common variable immunodeficiency (hypogammaglobulinaemia) develop diarrhoea and malabsorption. The intestinal lesions vary over a wide range, from showing more or less villous atrophy to mimicking Crohn's disease. The common diagnoses of intestinal diseases should probably not generally be used in these cases because immunodeficiency apparently by 'imitation' may result in a variety of lesions.

The intestinal mucosa of patients with generalized B cell deficiency contains no, or only very little, interstitial IgG unless substitution therapy has been given.[34,51] However, some mucosal plasma cells (mainly of the IgM isotype) are often seen in hypogammaglobulinaemia,[34,77] particularly associated with solitary lymphoid follicles (see below). SC occurs in a normal epithelial distribution,[51] so the small amounts of locally produced IgM can probably contribute to immune exclusion. It may seem paradoxical, therefore, that hypogammaglobulinaemic patients are usually found to have strikingly raised levels of bovine milk proteins in their blood, whereas the agammaglobulinaemic patients apparently do not have more than normal levels.[100]

Solitary lymphoid follicles

Some patients with hypogammaglobulinaemia who present with diarrhoea show a markedly increased number of solitary lymphoid follicles in their gastrointestinal mucosa, mainly in the small intestine.[100] These follicles contain a distinct mantle zone of sIgD⁺IgM⁺ naive B lymphocytes. The B cell maturation defect is to some extent overcome under the influence of antigens from the lumen, as indicated by the development of a few IgM-producing immunocytes between the follicles and the surface epithelium (Fig. 9.34). It is possible that nodular lymphoid hyperplasia reflects immune stimulation due to an excessive influx of antigens from the lumen,[100] but there is no apparent relationship between this mode of reaction and development of intestinal B cell (MALT) lymphoma.

CONCLUSIONS

Are intestinal IgA production and oral tolerance interrelated?

This chapter has mainly focused on the effector functions of terminally differentiated mucosal B cells (immunocytes). However, it is becoming increasingly evident that B cells can also exert important immunoregulatory activities both as efficient APCs[235] and by secreting a variety of cytokines.[304] In the mucosal immune system, such B cell characteristics remain elusive. Nevertheless, B cells located at the presumed sites of antigen entrance in GALT express the necessary costimulatory molecules to function as APCs, perhaps leading to enhanced diversification of mucosal immune responses, thereby explaining the observation that SIgA antibodies show broader specificity than comparable serum antibodies.[62,408]

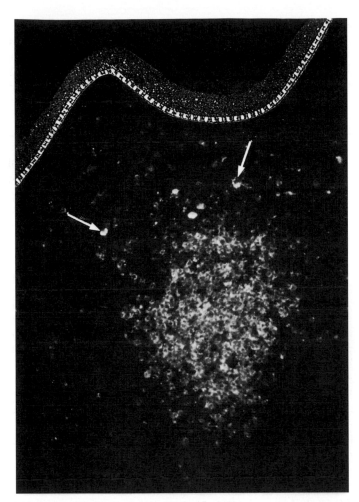

Fig 9.34 Immunofluorescence staining for IgM in a section of jejunal mucosa from a patient with hypogammaglobulinaemia. The biopsy specimen had been extensively washed in isotonic saline to remove diffusible Ig before fixation in ethanol. Note the solitary lymphoid follicle with IgM-bearing B lymphocytes (these naive cells also express surface IgD; not shown). A few immunocytes (arrows) with cytoplasmic IgM can be seen beneath the surface epithelium (basement membrane zone indicated by dashed line). ×150.

The relationship between induction of intestinal IgA responses and oral tolerance is also enigmatic.[48] Experiments in CD8 knock-out mice have suggested that this phenotype of T lymphocytes (the predominant IEL subset) is crucial for downregulation of the mucosal B cell system.[143] The tone of hyporesponsiveness in the intestinal immune system appears to be quite robust, because even a strong immunogen such as cholera toxin (CT) is unable to abrogate it although oral tolerance cannot be induced in the presence of CT.[143] On the other hand, TGF-β has been shown to be important in promoting IgA switching (see Fig. 9.15) also in mice immunized with CT[190] and in addition, this cytokine is believed to be one of the major mediators of oral tolerance in murine test systems.[365] It is not yet possible to extrapolate such apparently contradictory information to the human gut.

What do we know about the human intestinal B cell and its functions?

It is well established in the human gut that the muscosal immune system responds to infection with an IgA and IgM immunocyte response[355] and it appears that the level of this response may determine whether clinical symptoms will occur or not.[3] The following facts and open questions on the human intestinal B cell system can be summarized:

1. Humoral immunity in the gut depends on an intimate co-operation between mucosal B cells and the secretory epithelium. The obvious biological significance of the striking J chain expression shown by GALT-derived immunocytes is that IgA and IgM polymers with high affinity for SC can be produced locally and become readily available for external pIgR-mediated epithelial transport. This important functional goal, in terms of clonal differentiation, appears to be sufficient justification for the J chain to be also expressed by B cells terminating locally with IgG or IgD production; these immunocytes may be considered as 'spin-offs' from early effector clones that through isotype switching are on their way to pIgA expression.

2. There is considerable evidence to support the notion that human intestinal immunocytes are largely derived from B cells initially induced in GALT. However, insufficient knowledge exists concerning the relative importance of M cells, MHC Class II-expressing epithelial cells, B cells and other professional APCs in the transport, processing and presentation of luminal antigens that take place in GALT to accomplish the extensive and continuous priming and expansion of mucosal B cells. Also, it is not clear how the germinal centre reaction in GALT so strikingly promotes isotype switching to IgA and expression of J chain.

3. Although the B cell migration to the small intestinal lamina propria is guided by rather well-characterized adhesion molecules, the chemotactic stimuli involved in extravasation and microcompartmental distribution of various B cell subsets remain elusive.

4. Retention and accumulation of B cells extravasated in the intestinal mucosa are influenced by antigen-driven local proliferation and differentiation. However, the role of lamina propria T cells and IELs, MHC Class II-positive APCs and epithelial cells in providing the necessary stimulatory signals for proliferation and terminal differentiation of the local B cells is poorly defined.

5. The mucosal barrier normally allows some penetration of intact soluble antigens, so there is probably always a need for immune elimination in the lamina propria. If immune exclusion is impaired (e.g. in IgA deficiency), or if there is too large an antigen load on the epithelial barrier (e.g. in infection), activated non-specific amplication mechanisms involved in immune elimination may cause hypersensitivity, which is observed clinically as gut disease. This immunopathological development may be mediated by proinflammatory IgG, IgM and IgE antibodies as well as by hyperactivated APCs and T cells. Although these immunopathogenic mechanisms are rather well understood in several types of intestinal disorders such as atopic food allergy and coeliac disease, the cause of their initiation generally remains unexplained.

6. Clinical observations in immunodeficient patients have shown that SIgA, SIgM and IgG are not the only important components of the intestinal mucosal defence system. It is becoming increasingly evident that innate immunity is crucial and

much more complex than previously believed; the cooperation between innate and adaptive mucosal immunity needs exploration to better understand how homeostasis of mucous membranes is normally maintained.

Acknowledgements

This work was supported by the Norwegian Cancer Society, the Research Council of Norway, and Anders Jahre's Foundation. Ms. Hege Eliassen Bryne and Mr. Erik Kulø Hagen are gratefully acknowledged for excellent assistance with the manuscript.

REFERENCES

1 Abitorabi MA, Mackay CR, Jerome EH, Osorio O, Butcher EC, Erle DJ. Differential expression of homing molecules on recirculating lymphocytes from sheep gut, peripheral, and lung lymph. *J Immunol* 1996; 156: 3111–17.

2 Abu-Ghazaleh RI, Fujisawa T, Mestecky J, Kyle RA, Gleich GJ. IgA-induced eosinophil degranulation. *J Immunol* 1989; 142: 2393–400.

3 Agus SG, Falchuk ZM, Sessoms CS, Wyatt RG, Dolin R. Increased jejunal IgA synthesis *in vitro* during acute infectious non-bacterial gastroenteritis. *Am J Dig Dis* 1974; 19: 127–31.

4 Ahmed R, Gray D. Immunological memory and protective immunity: understanding their relation. *Science* 1996; 272: 54–60.

5 Alberini CM, Bet P, Milstein C, Sitia R. Secretion of immunoglobulin M assembly intermediates in the presence of reducing agents. *Nature* 1990; 347: 485–7.

6 André C, André F, Fargier MC. Distribution of IgA1 and IgA2 plasma cells in various normal human tissues and in the jejunum of plasma IgA-deficient patients. *Clin Exp Immunol* 1978; 33: 327–31.

7 Arpin C, de Bouteiller O, Razanajaona D *et al.* The normal counterpart of IgD myeloma cells in germinal center displays extensively mutated IgVH gene, Cμ-Cδ switch, and λ light chain expression. *J Exp Med* 1998; 187: 1169–78.

8 Baklien K, Brandtzaeg P, Fausa O. Immunoglobulins in jejunal mucosa and serum from patients with adult coeliac disease. *Scand J Gastroenterol* 1977; 12: 149–59.

9 Baklien K, Fausa O, Thune PO, Gjone E. Immunoglobulins in jejunal mucosa and serum from patients with dermatitis herpetiformis. *Scand J Gastroenterol* 1977; 12: 161–8.

10 Beatty DW, Napier B, Sinclair-Smith CC. Secretory IgA synthesis in Kwashiorkor. *J Clin Lab Immunol* 1983; 12: 31–6.

11 Bellamy JEC, Nielsen NO. Immune-mediated emigration of neutrophils into the lumen of the small intestine. *Infect Immun* 1974; 9: 615–9.

12 Belut D, Moneret-Vautrin DA, Nicolas JP, Grilliat JP. IgE levels in intestinal juice. *Dig Dis Sci* 1980; 25: 323–32.

13 Bengtsson U, Knutson TW, Knutson L, Dannaeus A, Hällgren R, Ahlstedt S. Increased levels of hyaluronan and albumin after intestinal challenge in patients with cow's milk intolerance. *Clin Exp Allergy* 1996; 26: 96–103.

14 Bengtsson U, Knutson TW, Knutson L, Dannaeus A, Hällgren R, Ahlstedt S. Eosinophil cationic protein and histamine after intestinal challenge in patients with cow's milk intolerance. *J Allergy Clin Immunol* 1997; 100: 216–21.

15 Bengtsson U, Rognum TO, Brandtzaeg P *et al.* IgE-positive duodenal mast cells in patients with food-related diarrhea. *Int Arch Allergy Appl Immunol* 1991; 95: 86–91.

16 Bentley AM, Durham SR, Robinson DS *et al.* Expression of endothelial and leukocyte adhesion molecules intercellular adhesion molecule-1, E-selectin, and vascular cell adhesion molecule-1 in the bronchial mucosa in steady-state and allergen-induced asthma. *J Allergy Clin Immunol* 1993; 92: 857–68.

17 Berin MC, Kiliaan AJ, Yang PC, Groot JA, Taminiau JA, Perdue MH. Rapid transepithelial antigen transport in rat jejunum: impact of sensitization and the hypersensitivity reaction. *Gastroenterology* 1997; 113: 856–64.

18 Berstad AE, Brandtzaeg P. Expression of cell membrane complement regulatory glycoproteins along the normal and diseased human gastrointestinal tract. *Gut* 1998; 42: 522–9.

19 Bertrand FE, Billips LG, Gartland GL, Kubagawa H, Schroeder HW. The J chain gene is transcribed during B and T lymphopoiesis in humans. *J Immunol* 1996; 156: 4240–4.

20 Bienenstock J, Befus D, McDermott M, Mirski S, Rosenthal K. Regulation of lymphoblast traffic and localization in mucosal tissues, with emphasis on IgA. *Fed Proc* 1983; 42: 3213–7.

21 Bjerke K, Brandtzaeg P. Terminally differentiated human intestinal B cells. J chain expression of IgA and IgG subclass-producing immunocytes in the distal ileum compared with mesenteric and peripheral lymph nodes. *Clin Exp Immunol* 1990; 82: 411–15.

22 Bjerke K, Brandtzaeg P. Immunoglobulin- and J-chain-producing cells associated with the lymphoid follicles of human appendix, colon and ileum, including the Peyer's patches. *Clin Exp Immunol* 1986; 64: 432–41.

23 Bjerke K, Brandtzaeg P. Terminally differentiated human intestinal B cells. IgA and IgG subclass-producing immunocytes in the distal ileum, including Peyer's patches, compared with lymph nodes and palatine tonsils. *Scand J Immunol* 1990; 32: 61–7.

24 Bjerke K, Brandtzaeg P, Rognum TO. Distribution of immunoglobulin producing cells is different in normal human appendix and colon mucosa. *Gut* 1986; 27: 667–74.

25 Bjørge L, Jensen TS, Vedeler CA, Ulvestad E, Kristoffersen EK, Matre R. Soluble CD59 in pregnancy and infancy. *Immunol Lett* 1993; 36: 233.

26 Blalock JE. The immune system. Our sixth sense. *Immunologist* 1994; 2: 8–15.

27 Blanco A, Linares P, Andion R, Alonso M, Sanchez Villares E. Development of humoral immunity system of the small bowel. *Allergol Immunopathol* 1976; 4: 235–40.

28 Boirivant M, Fais S, Annibale B, Agostini D, Delle Fave G, Pallone F. Vasoactive intestinal polypeptide modulates the *in vitro* immunoglobulin A production by intestinal lamina propria lymphocytes. *Gastroenterology* 1994; 106: 576–82.

29 Bos NA, Bun JC, Popma SH *et al.* Monoclonal immunoglobulin A derived from peritoneal B cells is encoded by both germ line and somatically mutated VH genes and is reactive with commensal bacteria. *Infect Immun* 1996; 64: 616–23.

30 Bouvet JP, Dighiero G. From natural polyreactive autoantibodies to a la carte monoreactive antibodies to infectious agents: is it a small world after all? *Infect Immun* 1998; 66: 1–4.

31 Bradley LM, Watson SR. Lymphocyte migration into tissue: the paradigm derived from CD4 subsets. *Curr Opin Immunol* 1996; 8: 312–20.

32 Brandtzaeg P. Structure, synthesis and external transfer of mucosal immunoglobulins. *Ann Inst Pasteur Immunol* 1973; 124C: 417–38.

33 Brandtzaeg P. Two types of IgA immunocytes in man. *Nature, New Biol* 1973; 243: 142–3.

34 Brandtzaeg P. Mucosal and glandular distribution of immunoglobulin components. Immunohistochemistry with a cold ethanol-fixation technique. *Immunology* 1974; 26: 1101–14.

35 Brandtzaeg P. Mucosal and glandular distribution of immunoglobulin components. Differential localization of free and bound SC in secretory epithelial cells. *J Immunol* 1974; 112: 1553–9.

36 Brandtzaeg P. Presence of J chain in human immunocytes containing various immunoglobulin classes. *Nature* 1974; 252: 418–20.

37 Brandtzaeg P. Human secretory immunoglobulin M. An immunochemical and immunohistochemical study. *Immunology* 1975; 29: 559–70.

38 Brandtzaeg P. Complex formation between secretory component and human immunoglobulins related to their content of J chain. *Scand J Immunol* 1976; 5: 411–19.

39 Brandtzaeg P. Human secretory component. VI. Immunoglobulin-binding properties. *Immunochemistry* 1977; 14: 179–88.

40 Brandtzaeg P. Polymeric IgA is complexed with secretory component (SC) on the surface of human intestinal epithelial cells. *Scand J Immunol* 1978; 8: 39–52.

41 Brandtzaeg P. Immunohistochemical characterization of intracellular J-chain and binding site for secretory component (SC) in human immunoglobulin (Ig) producing cells. *Mol Immunol* 1983; 20: 941–66.

42 Brandtzaeg P. The secretory immune system of lactating human mammary glands compared with other exocrine organs. *Ann NY Acad Sci* 1983; 409: 353–81.

43 Brandtzaeg P. Role of J chain and secretory component in receptor-mediated glandular and hepatic transport of immunoglobulins in man. *Scand J Immunol* 1985; 22: 111–46.

44 Brandtzaeg P. Immune functions and immunopathology of palatine and nasopharyngeal tonsils. In: *Immunology of the Ear* (Bernstein JM, Ogra PL, eds). Raven Press, New York, 1987: 63–106.

45 Brandtzaeg P. Immune responses to gut virus infections. In: *Viruses and the Gut* (Farthing MJG, ed.). Smith Kline & French Laboratories Ltd., London, 1989: 45–54.

46 Brandtzaeg P. Molecular and cellular aspects of the secretory immunoglobulin system. *APMIS* 1995; 103: 1–19.

47 Brandtzaeg P. Development of the mucosal immune system in humans. In: *Recent Developments in Infant Nutrition* (Bindels JG, Goedhart AC, Visser HKA, eds). Kluwer Academic Publishers, London, 1996: 349–76.

48 Brandtzaeg P. History of oral tolerance and mucosal immunity. *Ann NY Acad Sci* 1996; 778: 1–27.

49 Brandtzaeg P. Mechanisms of gastrointestinal reactions to food. *Environ Toxicol Pharmacol* 1997; 4: 9–24.

50 Brandtzaeg P, Baklien K. Inconclusive immunohistochemistry of human IgE in mucosal pathology. *Lancet* 1976; i: 1297–8.

51 Brandtzaeg P, Baklien K. Immunohistochemical studies of the formation and epithelial transport of immunoglobulins in normal and diseased human intestinal mucosa. *Scand J Gastroenterol* (Suppl. 36) 1976; 11: 1–45.

52 Brandtzaeg P, Baklien K. Intestinal secretion of IgA and IgM. a hypothetical model. *Ciba Found Symp* 1977; 46: 77–108.

53 Brandtzaeg P, Baklien K. Characterization of the IgA immunocyte population and its product in a patient with excessive intestinal formation of IgA. *Clin Exp Immunol* 1977; 30. 77–88.

54 Brandtzaeg P, Halstensen TS. Immunology and immunopathology of tonsils. *Adv Otorhinolaryngol* 1992; 47: 64–75.

55 Brandtzaeg P, Haneberg B. Role of nasal-associated lymphoid tissue in the human mucosal immune system. *Mucosal Immunol Update* 5 1997; No 1: 4 8.

56 Brandtzaeg P, Korsrud FR. Significance of different J chain profiles in human tissues: generation of IgA and IgM with binding site for secretory component is related to the J chain expressing capacity of the total local immunocyte population, including IgG and IgD producing cells, and depends on the clinical state of the tissue. *Clin Exp Immunol* 1984; 58: 709–18.

57 Brandtzaeg P, Nilssen DE. Mucosal aspects of primary B-cell deficiency and gastrointestinal infections. *Curr Opin Gastroenterol* 1995; 11: 532–40.

58 Brandtzaeg P, Prydz H. Direct evidence for an integrated function of J chain and secretory component in epithelial transport of immunoglobulins. *Nature* 1984; 311: 71–3.

59 Brandtzaeg P, Rognum TO. Evaluation of nine different fixatives. 1. Preservation of immunoglobulin isotypes, J chain, and secretory component in human tissues. *Pathol Res Pract* 1984; 179: 250–66.

60 Brandtzaeg P, Tolo K. Mucosal penetrability enhanced by serum-derived antibodies. *Nature* 1977; 266: 262–3.

61 Brandtzaeg P, Baklien K, Bjerke K, Rognum TO, Scott H, Valnes K. Nature and properties of the human gastrointestinal immune system. In: *Immunology of the Gastrointestinal Tract* (Miller K, Nicklin S, eds), Vol. I. CRC Press, Boca Raton, Florida, 1987: 1–85.

62 Brandtzaeg P, Baekkevold ES, Farstad IN, Jahnsen FL, Johansen FE, Nilsen EM, Yamanaka T. Regional specialization in the mucosal immune system: what happens in the microcompartments? *Immunol Today* 1999; 20: 141–51.

63 Brandtzaeg P, Farstad IN, Haraldsen G. Regional specialization in the mucosal immune system: primed cells do not always home along the same track. *Immunol Today* 1999; 20: 267–77.

64 Brandtzaeg P, Fjellanger I, Gjeruldsen ST. Immunoglobulin M: Local synthesis and selective secretion in patients with immunoglobulin A deficiency. *Science* 1968; 160: 789–91.

65 Brandtzaeg P, Gjeruldsen ST, Korsrud F, Baklien K, Berdal P, Ek J. The human secretory immune system shows striking heterogeneity with regard to involvement of J chain positive IgD immunocytes. *J Immunol* 1979; 122: 503–10.

66 Brandtzaeg P, Guy-Grand D, Griscelli C. Intestinal, salivary, and tonsillar IgA and J-chain production in a patient with severe deficiency of serum IgA. *Scand J Immunol* 1981; 13: 313–25.

67 Brandtzaeg P, Halstensen TS, Kett K *et al*. Immunobiology and immunopathology of human gut mucosa: humoral immunity and intraepithelial lymphocytes. *Gastroenterology* 1989; 97: 1562–84.

68 Brandtzaeg P, Halstensen TS, Huitfeldt HS *et al*. Epithelial expression of HLA, secretory component (poly-Ig receptor), and adhesion molecules in the human alimentary tract. *Ann NY Acad Sci* 1992; 664: 157–79.

69 Brandtzaeg P, Halstensen TS, Hvatum M, Kvale D, Scott H. The serologic and mucosal immunologic basis of celiac disease. In: *Immunophysiology of the Gut* (Walker WA, Harmatz PR, Wershil BK, eds). Bristol-Myers Squibb/Mead Johnson Nutrition Symposia, Vol. 11. Academic Press, London, 1993: 295–333.

70 Brandtzaeg P, Haraldsen G, Rugtveit J. Immunopathology of human inflammatory bowel disease. *Springer Semin Immunopathol* 1997; 18: 555–89.

71 Brandtzaeg P, Johansen F-E, Baekkevold ES, Farstad IN. Homing of human B cells with Cµ gene deletion reveals distinct compartmentalization of mucosal immunity. Submitted, 2002.

72 Brandtzaeg P, Karlsson G, Hansson G, Petruson B, Björkander J, Hanson LÅ. The clinical condition of IgA-deficient patients is related to the proportion of IgD- and IgM-producing cells in their nasal mucosa. *Clin Exp Immunol* 1987; 67: 626–36.

73 Brandtzaeg P, Nilssen DE, Rognum TO, Thrane PS. Ontogeny of the mucosal immune system and IgA deficiency. *Gastroenterol Clin North Am* 1991; 20: 397–439.

74 Brewer JW, Randall TD, Parkhouse RM, Corley RB. IgM hexamers? *Immunol Today* 1994; 15: 165–8.

75 Brière F, Bridon JM, Chevet D *et al*. Interleukin 10 induces B lymphocytes from IgA-deficient patients to secrete IgA. *J Clin Invest* 1994; 94: 97–104.

76 Briskin M, Winsor-Hines D, Shyjan A *et al*. Human mucosal addressin cell adhesion molecule-1 is preferentially expressed in intestinal tract and associated lymphoid tissue. *Am J Pathol* 1997; 151: 97–110.

77 Broom BC, de la Concha EG, Webster AD, Loewi G, Asherson GL. Dichotomy between immunoglobulin synthesis by cells in gut and blood of patients with hypogammaglobulinaemia. *Lancet* 1975; 2: 253–6.

78 Brown WR, Isobe Y, Nakane PK. Studies on translocation of immunoglobulins across intestinal epithelium. II. Immunoelectron-microscopic localization of immunoglobulins and secretory component in human intestinal mucosa. *Gastroenterology* 1976; 71: 985–95.

79 Bull DM, Bienenstock J, Tomasi TB. Studies on human intestinal immunoglobulin A. *Gastroenterology* 1971; 60: 370–80.

80 Burnett D, Crocker J, Stockley RA. Cells containing IgA subclasses in bronchi of subjects with and without chronic obstructive lung disease. *Clin Pathol* 1987; 40: 1217–20.

81 Burns JW, Siadat-Pajouh M, Krishnaney AA, Greenberg HB. Protective effect of rotavirus VP6-specific IgA monoclonal antibodies that lack neutralizing activity. *Science* 1996; 272: 104–7.

82 Butcher EC, Picker LJ. Lymphocyte homing and homeostasis. *Science* 1996; 272: 60–6.

83 Carini C, Brostoff J, Wraith DG. IgE complexes in food allergy. *Ann Allergy* 1987; 59: 110–17.

84 Carter LL, Dutton RW. Type 1 and type 2: a fundamental dichotomy for all T-cell subsets. *Curr Opin Immunol* 1996; 8: 336–42.

85 Castrignano SB, Carlsson B, Carneiro-Sampaio MS, Soderstrom T, Hanson LA. IgA and IgG subclass deficiency in a poor population in a developing country. *Scand J Immunol* 1993; 37: 509–14.

86 Chaplin DD, Fu Y. Cytokine regulation of secondary lymphoid organ development. *Curr Opin Immunol* 1998; 10: 289–97.

87 Chowers Y, Marsh MN, De Grandpre L, Nyberg A, Theofilopoulos AN, Kagnoff MF. Increased proinflammatory cytokine gene expression in the colonic mucosa of coeliac disease patients in the early period after gluten challenge. *Clin Exp Immunol* 1997; 107: 141–7.

88 Christ AD, Blumberg RS. The intestinal epithelial cell: immunological aspects. *Springer Semin Immunopathol* 1997; 18: 449–61.

89 Ciclitira PJ, Ellis HJ, Wood GM, Howdle PD, Losowsky MS. Secretion of gliadin antibody by coeliac jejunal mucosal biopsies cultured *in vitro*. *Clin Exp Immunol* 1986; 64: 119–24.

90 Ciclitira PJ, Hooper LB, Ellis HJ, Freedman AR. Gliadin antibody production by small intestinal lymphocytes from patients with coeliac disease. *Int Arch Allergy Appl Immunol* 1989; 89: 246–9.

91 Cleary AM, Fortune SM, Yellin MJ, Chess L, Lederman S. Opposing roles of CD95 (Fas/APO-1) and CD40 in the death and rescue of human low density tonsillar B cells. *J Immunol* 1995; 155: 3329–37.

92 Clegg DO, Zone JJ, Samuelson CO, Ward JR. Circulating immune complexes containing secretory IgA in jejunoileal bypass disease. *Ann Rheum Dis* 1985; 44: 239–44.

93 Colombel JF, Mascart-Lemone F, Nemeth J, Vaerman JP, Dive C, Rambaud JC. Jejunal immunoglobulin and antigliadin antibody secretion in adult coeliac disease. *Gut* 1990; 31: 1345–9.

94 Conley ME, Delacroix DL. Intravascular and mucosal immunoglobulin A: Two separate but related systems of immune defense? *Ann Intern Med* 1987; 106: 892–9.

95 Conley ME, Bartelt MS. *In vitro* regulation of IgA subclass synthesis. II. The source of IgA2 plasma cells. *J Immunol* 1984; 133: 2312–6.

96 Crabbé PA, Nash DR, Bazin H, Eyssen H, Heremans JF. Immunohistochemical observations on lymphoid tissues from conventional and germ-free mice. *Lab Invest* 1970; 22: 448–57.

97 Crabbé PA, Carbonara AO, Heremans JF. The normal human intestinal mucosa as a major source of plasma cells containing γ A-immunoglobulin. *Lab Invest* 1965; 14: 235–48.

98 Crago SS, Kutteh WH, Moro I *et al*. Distribution of IgA1-, IgA2-, and J chain-containing cells in human tissues. *J Immunol* 1984; 132: 16–8.

99 Cunningham-Rundles C, Brandeis WE, Pudifin DJ, Day NK, Good RA. Autoimmunity in selective IgA deficiency: relationship to anti-bovine protein antibodies, circulating immune complexes and clinical disease. *Clin Exp Immunol* 1981; 45: 299–304.

100 Cunningham-Rundles C, Carr RI, Good RA. Dietary protein antigenemia in humoral immunodeficiency. Correlation with splenomegaly. *Am J Med* 1984; 76: 181–5.

101 Cunningham-Rundles C, Brandeis WE, Good RA, Day NK. Bovine antigens and the formation of circulating immune complexes in selective immunoglobulin A deficiency. *J Clin Invest* 1979; 64: 272–9.

102 Cunningham-Rundles C. The identification of specific antigens in circulating immune complexes by an enzyme-linked immunosorbent assay: detection of bovine κ-casein IgG complexes in human sera. *Eur J Immunol* 1981; 11: 504–9.

103 Dannaeus A, Inganas M, Johansson SG, Foucard T. Intestinal uptake of ovalbumin in malabsorption and food allergy in relation to serum IgG antibody and orally administered sodium cromoglycate. *Clin Allergy* 1979; 9: 263–70.

104 de Vries JE. Atopic allergy and other hypersensitivities. Editorial overview. *Curr Opin Immunol* 1994; 6: 835–7.

105 Deem RL, Shanahan F, Targan SR. Triggered human mucosal T cells release tumour necrosis factor-α and interferon-γ which kill human colonic epithelial cells. *Clin Exp Immunol* 1991; 83: 79–84.

106 Defrance T, Vanbervliet B, Briere F, Durand I, Rousset F, Banchereau J. Interleukin 10 and transforming growth factor beta cooperate to induce anti-CD40-activated naive human B cells to secrete immunoglobulin A. *J Exp Med* 1992; 175: 671–82.

107 Delamette F, Marty MC, Panijel J. *In vitro* study of IgM polymerization. *Cell Immunol* 1975; 19: 262–75.

108 Della Corte E, Parkhouse RME. Biosynthesis of immunoglobulin A (IgA) and immunoglobulin M (IgM). Requirement for J-chain and a disulphide exchange enzyme for polymerization. *Biochem J* 1973; 136: 597–606.

109 Dempsey PW, Allison ME, Akkaraju S, Goodnow CC, Fearon DT. C3d of complement as a molecular adjuvant: bridging innate and acquired immunity. *Science* 1996; 271: 348–50.

110 Denis V, Dupuis P, Bizouarne N *et al*. Selective induction of peripheral and mucosal endothelial cell addressins with peripheral lymph nodes and Peyer's patch cell-conditioned media. *J Leukoc Biol* 1996; 60: 744–52.

111 Denning GM. IL-4 and IFN-γ synergistically increase total polymeric IgA receptor levels in human intestinal epithelial cells. Role of protein tyrosine kinases. *J Immunol* 1996; 156: 4807–14.

112 Desreumaux P, Janin A, Colombel JF *et al*. Interleukin 5 messenger RNA expression by eosinophils in the intestinal mucosa of patients with coeliac disease. *J Exp Med* 1992; 175: 293–6.

113 Devière J, Vaerman J-P, Content J *et al*. IgA triggers tumor necrosis factor α secretion by monocytes: a study in normal subjects and patients with alcoholic cirrhosis. *Hepatology* 1991; 13: 670–5.

114 Dieterich W, Ehnis T, Bauer M *et al*. Identification of tissue transglutaminase as the autoantigen of celiac disease. *Nat Med* 1997; 3: 797–801.

115 Dunn-Walters DK, Isaacson PG, Spencer J. Sequence analysis of human IgVH genes indicates that ileal lamina propria plasma cells are derived from Peyer's patches. *Eur J Immunol* 1997; 27: 463–7.

116 Dunn-Walters DK, Boursier L, Spencer J. Hypermutation, diversity and dissemination of human intestinal lamina propria plasma cells. *Eur J Immunol* 1997; 27: 2959–64.

117 Eckmann L, Kagnoff MF, Fierer J. Intestinal epithelial cells as watchdogs for the natural immune system. *Trends Microbiol* 1995; 3: 118–20.

118 Eerola E, Jalkanen S, Granfors K, Toivanen A. Immune capacity of the chicken bursectomized at 60 h of incubation. Effect of bursal epithelial cells and bursal epithelium-conditioned medium on the production of immunoglobulins and specific antibodies *in vitro*. *Scand J Immunol* 1984; 19: 493–500.

119 Eidelman S. Intestinal lesions in immune deficiency. *Hum Pathol* 1976; 7: 427–34.

120 Erle DJ, Briskin MJ, Butcher EC, Garcia-Pardo A, Lazarovits AI, Tidswell M. Expression and function of the MAdCAM-1 receptor, integrin α4β7, on human leukocytes. *J Immunol* 1994; 153: 517–28.

121 Falchuk ZM, Strober W. Increased jejunal immuno globulin synthesis in patients with nontropical sprue as measured by a solid phase immunoadsorption technique. *J Lab Clin Med* 1972; 6: 1004–13.

122 Falchuk ZM, Strober W. Gluten-sensitive enteropathy synthesis of antigliadin antibody *in vitro*. *Gut* 1974; 15: 947–52.

123 Farstad IN, Halstensen TS, Lazarovits AI, Norstein J, Fausa O, Brandtzaeg P. Human intestinal B-cell blasts and plasma cells express the mucosal homing receptor integrin α4β7. *Scand J Immunol* 1995; 42: 662–72.

124 Farstad IN, Halstensen TS, Lien B, Kilshaw PJ, Lazarovits AI, Brandtzaeg P. Distribution of β7 integrins in human intestinal mucosa and organized gut-associated lymphoid tissue. *Immunology* 1996; 89: 227–37.

125 Farstad IN, Halstensen TS, Kvale D, Fausa O, Brandtzaeg P. Topographic distribution of homing receptors on B and T cells in human gut-associated lymphoid tissue. Relation of L-selectin and integrin α4β7 to naive and memory phenotypes. *Am J Pathol* 1997; 150: 187–99.

126 Farstad IN, Norstein J, Brandtzaeg P. Phenotypes of B and T cells in human intestinal and mesenteric lymph. *Gastroenterology* 1997; 112: 163–73.

127 Fayette J Dubois B, Vandenabeele S *et al*. Human dendritic cells skew isotype switching of CD40-activated naive B cells towards IgA1 and IgA2. *J Exp Med* 1997; 185: 1909–18.

128 Feltelius N, Hvatum M, Brandtzaeg P, Knutson L, Hällgren R. Increased jejunal secretory IgA and IgM in ankylosing spondylitis: normalization after treatment with sulfasalazine. *J Rheumatol* 1994; 21: 2076–81.

129 Flanagan JG, Rabbitts TH. Arrangement of human immunoglobulin heavy chain constant region genes implies evolutionary duplication of a segment containing gamma, epsilon and alpha genes. *Nature* 1982; 300: 709–13.

130 Förster R, Mattis AE, Kremmer E, Wolf E, Brem G, Lipp M. A putative chemokine receptor, BLR1, directs B cell migration to defined lymphoid organs and specific anatomic compartments of the spleen. *Cell* 1996; 87: 1037–47.

131 Fossum S, Rolstad B, Tjernshaugen H. Selective loss of S-phase cells when making cell suspensions from lymphoid tissue. *Cell Immunol* 1979; 48: 149–54.

132 Friman V, Quiding M, Czerkinsky C et al. Intestinal and circulating antibody-forming cells in IgA-deficient individuals after oral cholera vaccination. Clin Exp Immunol 1994; 95: 222–6.

133 Fu YX, Huang G, Wang Y, Chaplin DD. B lymphocytes induce the formation of follicular dendritic cell clusters in a lymphotoxin α-dependent fashion. J Exp Med 1998; 187: 1009–18.

134 Fujihashi K, McGhee JR, Kweon MN et al. γ/δ T cell-deficient mice have impaired mucosal immunoglobulin A responses. J Exp Med 1996; 183: 1929–35.

135 Fujihashi K, McGhee JR, Lue C et al. Human appendix B cells naturally express receptors for and respond to interleukin 6 with selective IgA1 and IgA2 synthesis. J Clin Invest 1991; 88: 248–52.

136 Fujisaka M, Ohtani O, Watanabe Y. Distribution of lymphatics in human palatine tonsils: a study by enzyme-histochemistry and scanning electron microscopy of lymphatic corrosion casts. Arch Histol Cytol 1996; 59: 273–80.

137 Gallagher RB, Cervi P, Kelly J, Dolan C, Weir DG, Feighery C. The subclass profile and complement activating potential of anti-α-gliadin antibodies in coeliac disease. J Clin Lab Immunol 1989; 28: 115–21.

138 Gillon J. Where do mucosal mast cells acquire IgE? Immunol Today 1981; 2: 80–1.

139 Gitlin D, Sasaki T. Immunoglobulins G, A, and M determined in single cells from human tonsil. Science 1969; 164: 1532–4.

140 Giugliano LG, Ribeiro STG, Vainstein MH, Ulhoa CJ. Free secretory component and lactoferrin of human milk inhibit the adhesion of enterotoxigenic Esherichia coli. J Med Microbiol 1995; 42: 3–9.

141 Goldblum RM, Hanson LÅ, Brandtzaeg P. The mucosal defense system. In: Immunologic Disorders in Infants & Children (Stiehm ER, ed.) 4th edn. W.B. Saunders, Philadelphia, 1996: 159–99.

142 Goodnow CC, Cyster JG. Lymphocyte homing: the scent of a follicle. Curr Biol 1997; 7: R219–22.

143 Grdic D, Hörnquist E, Kjerrulf M, Lycke NY. Lack of local suppression in orally tolerant CD8-deficient mice reveals a critical regulatory role of CD8+ T cells in the normal gut mucosa. J Immunol 1998; 160: 754–62.

144 Green F, Heyworth B. Immunoglobulin-containing cells in jejunal mucosa of children with protein energy malnutrition and gastroenteritis. Arch Dis Child 1980; 55: 380–3.

145 Griffioen AW, Franklin SW, Zegers BJ, Rijkers GT. Expression and functional characteristics of the complement receptor type 2 on adult and neonatal B lymphocytes. Clin Immunol Immunopathol 1993; 69: 1–8.

146 Grouard G, Durand I, Filgueira L, Banchereau J, Liu YJ. Dendritic cells capable of stimulating T cells in germinal centres. Nature 1996; 384: 364–7.

147 Grove A, Poulsen LO, Fallingborg J, Teglbjærg PS. Immunoglobulin E-positive mast cells in the gastric and duodenal mucosa of healthy subjects. Eur J Gastroenterol Hepatol 1994; 6: 303–7.

148 Hadju I, Moldoveanu Z, Cooper M, Mestecky J. Ultrastructural studies of human lymphoid cells. μ and J chain expression as a function of B cell differentiation. J Exp Med 1983; 158: 1993–2006.

149 Hällgren R, Colombel JF, Dahl R et al. Neutrophil and eosinophil involvement of the small bowel in patients with celiac disease and Crohn's disease: studies on the secretion rate and immunohistochemical localization of granulocyte granule constituents. Am J Med 1989; 86: 56–64.

150 Halpern MS, Koshland ME. Novel subunit in secretory IgA. Nature 1970; 228: 1276–8.

151 Halstensen TS, Brandtzaeg P. Activated T lymphocytes in the celiac lesion: non-proliferative activation (CD25) of CD4 α/β cells in the lamina propria but proliferation (Ki-67) of α/β and γ/δ cells in the epithelium. Eur J Immunol 1993; 23: 505–10.

152 Halstensen TS, Hvatum M, Scott H, Fausa O, Brandtzaeg P. Association of subepithelial deposition of activated complement and immunoglobulin G and M response to gluten in celiac disease. Gastroenterology 1992; 102: 751–9.

153 Halstensen TS, Scott H, Fausa O, Brandtzaeg P. Gluten stimulation of coeliac mucosa in vitro induces activation (CD25) of lamina propria CD4+ T cells and macrophages but no crypt cell hyperplasia. Scand J Immunol 1993; 38: 581–90.

154 Hammerschmidt S, Talay SR, Brandtzaeg P, Chhatwal GS. SpsA, a novel pneumococcal surface protein with specific binding to secretory immunoglobulin A and secretory component. Mol Microbiol 1997; 25: 1113–24.

155 Hanson LÅ, Brandtzaeg P. The discovery of secretory IgA and the mucosal immune system. Immunol Today 1993; 14: 416–17.

156 Hansson T, Dannaeus A, Kraaz W, Sjoberg O, Klareskog L. Production of antibodies to gliadin by peripheral blood lymphocytes in children with celiac disease: the use of an enzyme-linked immunospot technique for screening and follow-up. Pediatr Res 1997; 41: 554–9.

157 Haraldsen G, Kvale D, Lien B, Farstad IN, Brandtzaeg P. Cytokine-regulated expression of E-selectin, intercellular adhesion molecule-1 (ICAM-1), and vascular cell adhesion molecule-1 (VCAM-1) in human intestinal microvascular endothelial cells. J Immunol 1996; 156: 2558–65.

158 Hauer AC, Breese EJ, Walker-Smith JA, MacDonald TT. The frequency of cells secreting interferon-γ and interleukin-4, -5, and -10 in the blood and duodenal mucosa of children with cow's milk hypersensitivity. Pediatr Res 1997; 42: 629–38.

159 Hayashi M, Takenouchi N, Asano M et al. The polymeric immunoglobulin receptor (secretory component) in a human intestinal epithelial cell line is up-regulated by interleukin-1. Immunology 1997; 92: 220–5.

160 Heatley RV, Calcraft BJ, Fifield R, Rhodes J, Whitehead RH, Newcombe RG. Immunoglobulin E in rectal mucosa of patients with proctitis. Lancet 1975; ii: 1010–12.

161 Helgeland L, Tysk C, Järnerot G et al. The IgG subclass distribution in serum and rectal mucosa of monozygotic twins with or without inflammatory bowel disease. Gut 1992; 33: 1358–64.

162 Hendrickson BA, Rindisbacher L, Corthesy B et al. Lack of association of secretory component with IgA in J chain-deficient mice. J Immunol 1996; 157: 750–4.

163 Herrero-Beaumont G, Armas JB, Elswood J, Will RK, Calin A. Selective IgA deficiency and spondyloarthropathy: a distinct disease? Ann Rheum Dis 1990; 49: 636–37.

164 Hirt RP, Hughes GJ, Frutiger S et al. Transcytosis of the polymeric Ig receptor requires phosphorylation of serine 664 in the absence but not the presence of dimeric IgA. Cell 1993; 74: 245–55.

165 Hocini H, Bélec L, Iscaki S et al. High-level ability of secretory IgA to block HIV type 1 transcytosis: contrasting secretory IgA and IgG responses to glycoprotein 160. AIDS Res Hum Retrovirus 1997; 13: 1179–85.

166 Horsfall DJ, Cooper JM, Rowley D. Changes in the immunoglobulin levels of the mouse gut and serum during conventionalisation and following administration of Salmonella typhimurium. Aust J Exp Biol Med Sci 1978; 56: 727–35.

167 Husband AJ, Monié HJ, Gowans JL. The natural history of cells producing IgA in the gut. Ciba Found Symp 1977; 46: 29–42.

168 Husband AJ. Kinetics of extravasation and redistribution of IgA-specific antibody-containing cells in the intestine. J Immunol 1982; 128: 1355–9.

169 Husby S, Jensenius JC, Svehag S-E. Passage of undegraded dietary antigen into the blood of healthy adults. Quantification, estimation of size distribution, and relation of uptake to levels of specific antibodies. Scand J Immunol 1985; 22: 83–92.

170 Hvatum M, Scott H, Brandtzaeg P. Serum IgG subclass antibodies to a variety of food antigens in patients with coeliac disease. Gut 1992; 33: 632–8.

171 Iwase T, Saito I, Takahashi T et al. Early expression of human J chain and mu chain gene in the fetal liver. Cell Struct Funct 1993; 18: 297–302.

172 Jahnsen FL, Haraldsen G, Aanesen JP, Haye R, Brandtzaeg P. Eosinophil infiltration is related to increased expression of vascular cell adhesion molecule-1 in nasal polyps. Am J Respir Cell Molec Biol 1995; 12: 624–32.

173 Jahnsen FL, Brandtzaeg P, Haye R, Haraldsen G. Expression of functional VCAM-1 by cultured nasal polyp-derived microvascular endothelium. Am J Pathol 1997; 150: 2113–23.

174 Jahnsen FL, Farstad IN, Aanesen JP, Brandtzaeg P. Phenotypic distribution of T cells in human nasal mucosa differs from that in the gut. Am J Respir Cell Molec Biol 1998; 18: 392–401.

B

175 Janeway CA, Bottomly K, Babich J *et al*. Quantitative variation in Ia antigen expression plays a central role in immune regulation. *Immunol Today* 1984; 5: 99–105.

176 Janson H, Heden LO, Grubb A, Ruan MR, Forsgren A. Protein D, an immunoglobulin D-binding protein of *Haemophilus influenzae*: cloning, nucleotide sequence, and expression in *Escherichia coli. Infect Immun* 1991; 59: 119–25.

177 Jenkins HR, Pincott JR, Soothill JF, Milla PJ, Harries JT. Food allergy: the major cause of infantile colitis. *Arch Dis Child* 1984; 59: 326–9.

178 Johansen F-E, Bosløven B, Krajči P, Brandtzaeg P. A composite DNA element in the promoter of the polymeric immunoglobulin receptor promoter regulates its constitutive expression. *Eur J Immunol* 1998; 28: 1161–71.

179 Jonard PP, Rambaud JC, Dive C, Vaerman JP, Galian A, Delacroix DL. Secretion of immunoglobulins and plasma proteins from the jejunal mucosa. Transport rate and origin of polymeric immunoglobulin A. *J Clin Invest* 1984; 74: 525–35.

180 Kaetzel CS, Blanch VJ, Hempen PM, Phillips KM, Piskurich JF, Youngman KR. The polymeric immunoglobulin receptor: structure and synthesis. *Biochem Soc Trans* 1997; 25: 475–80.

181 Kantele A, Kantele JM, Savilahti E *et al*. Homing potentials of circulating lymphocytes in humans depend on the site of activation: oral, but not parenteral, typhoid vaccination induces circulating antibody-secreting cells that all bear homing receptors directing them to the gut. *J Immunol* 1997; 158: 574–9.

182 Kapasi ZF, Qin D, Kerr WG *et al*. Follicular dendritic cell (FDC) precursors in primary lymphoid tissues. *J Immunol* 1998; 160: 1078–84.

183 Kett K, Scott H, Fausa O, Brandtzaeg P. Secretory immunity in celiac disease: cellular expression of immunoglobulin A subclass and joining chain. *Gastroenterology* 1990; 99: 386–92.

184 Kett K, Baklien K, Bakken A, Kral JG, Fausa O, Brandtzaeg P. Intestinal B-cell isotype response in relation to local bacterial load: evidence for immunoglobulin A subclass adaptation. *Gastroenterology* 1995; 109: 819–25.

185 Kett K, Brandtzaeg P, Fausa O. J-chain expression is more prominent in immunoglobulin A2 than in immunoglobulin A1 colonic immunocytes and is decreased in both subclasses associated with inflammatory bowel disease. *Gastroenterology* 1988; 94: 1419–25.

186 Kett K, Brandtzaeg P, Radl J, Haaijman JJ. Different subclass distribution of IgA-producing cells in human lymphoid organs and various secretory tissues. *J Immunol* 1986; 136: 3631–5.

187 Kilian M, Reinholdt J, Lomholt H, Poulsen K, Frandsen EV. Biological significance of IgA1 proteases in bacterial colonization and pathogenesis: critical evaluation of experimental evidence. *APMIS* 1996; 104: 321–38.

188 Kilian M, Husby S, Host A, Halken S. Increased proportions of bacteria capable of cleaving IgA1 in the pharynx of infants with atopic disease. *Pediatr Res* 1995; 38: 182–6.

189 Kilshaw PJ, Cant AJ. The passage of maternal dietary proteins into human breast milk. *Int Arch Allergy Appl Immunol* 1984; 75: 8–15.

190 Kim P-H, Eckmann L, Lee WJ, Han W, Kagnoff MF. Cholera toxin and cholera toxin B subunit induce IgA switching through the action of TGF-β1. *J Immunol* 1998; 160: 1198–1203.

191 Kimata H, Fujimoto M. Induction of IgA1 and IgA2 production in immature human fetal B cells and pre-B cells by vasoactive intestinal peptide. *Blood* 1995; 85: 2098–2104.

192 Knox WF. Restricted feeding and human intestinal plasma cell development. *Arch Dis Child* 1986; 61: 744–9.

193 Knutson TW, Bentsson U, Dannaeus A *et al*. Intestinal reactivity in allergic and nonallergic patients: an approach to determine the complexity of the mucosal reactions. *J Allergy Clin Immunol* 1993; 91: 553–9.

194 Kolmannskog S. Immunoglobulin E in feces of children with intestinal *Ascaris lumbricoides* infestation. *Int Arch Allergy Appl Immunol* 1986; 80: 417–23.

195 Kolmannskog S, Haneberg B. Immunoglobulin E in feces from children with allergy. Evidence of local production of IgE in the gut. *Int Arch Allergy Appl Immunol* 1985; 76: 133–7.

196 Kolmannskog S, Florholmen J, Flaegstad T, Kildebo S, Haneberg B. The excretion of IgE with feces from healthy individuals and from others with allergy and diseases affecting the intestinal tract. *Int Arch Allergy Appl Immunol* 1986; 79: 357–64.

197 Koopman G, Keehnen RM, Lindhout E, Zhou DF, de Groot C, Pals ST. Germinal center B cells rescued from apoptosis by CD40 ligation or attachment to follicular dendritic cells, but not by engagement of surface immunoglobulin or adhesion receptors, become resistant to CD95-induced apoptosis. *Eur J Immunol* 1997; 27: 1–7.

198 Korsrud FR, Brandtzaeg P. Quantitative immuno histochemistry of immunoglobulin- and J-chain-producing cells in human parotid and submandibular glands. *Immunology* 1980; 39: 129–40.

199 Korsrud FR, Brandtzaeg P. Immunohistochemical evaluation of J-chain expression by intra- and extrafollicular immunoglobulin-producing human tonsillar cells. *Scand J Immunol* 1981; 13: 271–80.

200 Koshland ME. The coming of age of the immunoglobulin J chain. *Annu Rev Immunol* 1985; 3: 425–53.

201 Krajči P, Kvale D, Taskén K, Brandtzaeg P. Molecular cloning and exon-intron mapping of the gene encoding human transmembrane secretory component (the poly-Ig receptor). *Eur J Immunol* 1992; 22: 2309–15.

202 Kremmidiotis G, Zola H. Changes in CD44 expression during B cell differentiation in the human tonsil. *Cell Immunol* 1995; 161: 147–57.

203 Kubagawa H, Burrows PD, Grossi CE, Mestecky J, Cooper MD. Precursor B cells transformed by Epstein–Barr virus undergo sterile plasma-cell differentiation: J-chain expression without immunoglobulin. *Proc Natl Acad Sci USA* 1988; 85: 875–9.

204 Kuchroo VK, Das MP, Brown JA *et al*. B7-1 and B7-2 costimulatory molecules activate differentially the Th1/Th2 developmental pathways: application to autoimmune disease therapy. *Cell* 1995; 80: 707–18.

205 Kutteh WH, Koopman WJ, Conley ME, Egan ML, Mestecky J. Production of predominantly polymeric IgA by human peripheral blood lymphocytes stimulated in vitro with mitogens. *J Exp Med* 1980; 152: 1424–9.

206 Kvale D, Brandtzaeg P. Constitutive and cytokine induced expression of HLA molecules, secretory component, and intercellular adhesion molecule-1 is modulated by butyrate in the colonic epithelial cell line HT-29. *Gut* 1995; 36: 737–42.

207 Labrooy JT, Hohmann AW, Davidson GP, Hetzel PA, Johnson RB, Shearman DJ. Intestinal and serum antibody in coeliac disease: a comparison using ELISA. *Clin Exp Immunol* 1986; 66: 661–8.

208 Lamkhioued B, Gounni AS, Gruart V, Pierce A, Capron A, Capron M. Human eosinophils express a receptor for secretory component. Role in secretory IgA-dependent activation. *Eur J Immunol* 1995; 25: 117–25.

209 Lampert IA, Schofield JB, Amlot P, Van Noorden S. Protection of germinal centres from complement attack: decay-accelerating factor (DAF) is a constitutive protein on follicular dendritic cells. A study in reactive and neoplastic follicles. *J Pathol* 1993; 170: 115–20.

210 Lange S, Nygren H, Svennerholm A-M, Holmgren J. Antitoxic cholera immunity in mice: influence of antigen deposition on antitoxin-containing cells and protective immunity in different parts of the intestine. *Infect Immun* 1980; 28: 17–23.

211 Lavö B, Knutson L, Loof L, Odlind B, Venge P, Hällgren R. Challenge with gliadin induces eosinophil and mast cell activation in the jejunum of patients with celiac disease. *Am J Med* 1989; 87: 655–60.

212 Lavö B, Knutson L, Loof L, Hällgren R. Gliadin challenge-induced jejunal prostaglandin E2 secretion in celiac disease. *Gastroenterology* 1990; 99: 703–7.

213 Lavö B, Knutson L, Loof L, Odlind B, Hällgren R. Signs of increased leakage over the jejunal mucosa during gliadin challenge of patients with coeliac disease. *Gut* 1990; 31: 153–7.

214 Lavö B, Knutson L, Sjöberg O, Hällgren R. Jejunal secretion of secretory immunoglobulins and gliadin antibodies in celiac disease. *Dig Dis Sci* 1992; 37: 53–9.

215 Lie SO, Fröland S, Brandtzaeg P, Vandvik B, Steen-Johnsen J. Transient B cell immaturity with intractable diarrhoea: a possible new immunodeficiency syndrome. *J Inherit Metab Dis* 1978; 1: 137–43.

216 Lim PL, Rowley D. The effect of antibody on the intestinal absorption of macromolecules and on intestinal permeability in adult mice. *Int Arch Allergy Appl Immunol* 1982; 68: 41–46.

217 Lindhout E, Koopman G, Pals ST, de Groot C. Triple check for antigen specificity of B cells during germinal centre reactions. *Immunol Today* 1997; 18: 573–7.

218 Lindsay MC, Blaies DB, Williams JF. *Taenia taeniaeformis*: immunoglobulin E-containing cells in the intestinal and lymphatic tissues of infected rats. *Int J Parasitol* 1983; 13: 91–9.

219 Liu YJ, Barthélémy C, de Bouteiller O, Arpin C, Durand I, Banchereau J. Memory B cells from human tonsils colonize mucosal epithelium and directly present antigen to T cells by rapid up-regulation of B7-1 and B7-2. *Immunity* 1995; 2: 239–48.

220 Liu Y-J, de Bouteiller O, Fugier-Vivier I. Mechanisms of selection and differentiation in germinal centers. *Curr Opin Immunol* 1997; 9: 256–62.

221 Liu Y-J, Banchereau J. The paths and molecular controls of peripheral B-cell development. *Immunologist* 1996; 4: 55–66.

222 Lodinova R, Jouja V, Wagner V. Serum immunoglobulins and coproantibody formation in infants after artificial intestinal colonization with *Escherichia coli* 083 and oral lysozyme administration. *Pediatr Res* 1973; 7: 659–69.

223 Loeb PM, Strober W, Falchuk ZM, Laster I. Incorporation of L-Leucine-^{14}C into immunoglobulins by jejunal biopsies of patients with celiac sprue and other gastrointestinal disease. *J Clin Invest* 1971; 50: 559–69.

224 Lue C, van den Wall Bake AW, Prince SJ et al. Intraperitoneal immunization of human subjects with tetanus toxoid induces specific antibody-secreting cells in the peritoneal cavity and in the circulation, but fails to elicit a secretory IgA response. *Clin Exp Immunol* 1994; 96: 356–63.

225 Lundin KEA, Scott H, Hansen T et al. Gliadin-specific, HLA-DQ(α1*0501, β1*0201) restricted T cells isolated from the small intestinal mucosa of celiac disease patients. *J Exp Med* 1993; 178: 187–96.

226 Lundin KE, Sollid LM, Anthonsen D et al. Heterogeneous reactivity patterns of HLA-DQ-restricted, small intestinal T-cell clones from patients with celiac disease. *Gastroenterology* 1997; 112: 752–9.

227 Lycke N, Kilander A, Nilsson LÅ, Tarkowski A, Werner N. Production of antibodies to gliadin in intestinal mucosa of patients with coeliac disease: a study at the single cell level. *Gut* 1989; 30: 72–7.

228 Ma JK, Hiatt A, Hein M et al. Generation and assembly of secretory antibodies in plants. *Science* 1995; 268: 716–19.

229 Ma JK, Hikmat BY, Wycoff K et al. Characterization of a recombinant plant monoclonal secretory antibody and preventive immunotherapy in humans. *Nat Med* 1998; 4: 601–6.

230 MacDermott RP, Nash GS, Bertovich MJ et al. Altered patterns of secretion of monomeric IgA and IgA subclass 1 by intestinal mononuclear cells in inflammatory bowel disease. *Gastroenterology* 1986; 91: 379–85.

231 MacDonald TT, Spencer J. Development of gastrointestinal immune function and its relationship to intestinal disease. *Current Opin Gastroenterol* 1993; 9: 946–52.

232 MacLennan ICM. Germinal centers. *Annu Rev Immunol* 1994; 12: 117–39.

233 Madara JL, Stafford J. Interferon-γ directly affects barrier function of cultured intestinal epithelial monolayers. *J Clin Invest* 1989; 83: 724–7.

234 Maffei HVL, Kingston D, Hill ID, Shiner M. Histopathologic changes and the immune response within the jejunal mucosa in infants and children. *Pediat Res* 1979; 13: 733–6.

235 Mamula MJ, Janeway CA. Do B cells drive the diversification of immune responses? *Immunol Today* 1993; 14: 151–2.

236 Mansikka A. Chicken IgA H chains. Implications concerning the evolution of H chain genes. *J Immunol* 1992; 149: 855–61.

237 Marshall JS, Bienenstock J. The role of mast cells in inflammatory reactions of the airways, skin and intestine. *Curr Opin Immunol* 1994; 6: 853–59.

238 Mascart-Lemone F, Cadranel S, Van den Broeck J, Dive C, Vaerman JP, Duchateau J. IgA immune response patterns to gliadin in serum. *Int Arch Allergy Appl Immunol* 1988; 86: 412–9.

239 Mascart-Lemone F, Colombel JF, Rambaud JC et al. Jejunal and serum IgA in adult coeliac disease. Abstract, *Gastroenterology* 1989; 96: A324.

240 Max EE, Korsmeyer SJ. Human J chain gene. Structure and expression in B lymphoid cells. *J Exp Med* 1985; 161: 832–49.

241 Mayrhofer G, Bazin H, Gowans JL. Nature of cells binding anti-IgE in rats immunized with *Nippostrongylus brasiliensis*: IgE synthesis in regional nodes and concentration in mucosal mast cells. *Eur J Immunol* 1976; 6: 537–45.

242 Mayrhofer G. Physiology of the intestinal immune system. In: *Local Immune Responses of the Gut* (Newby TJ, Stokes CR, eds). CRC Press, Boca Raton, Florida, 1984; 1–96.

243 Mazanec MB, Nedrud JG, Kaetzel CS, Lamm ME. A three-tiered view of the role of IgA in mucosal defense. *Immunol Today* 1993; 14: 430–5.

244 Mazanec MB, Coudret CL, Fletcher DR. Intracellular neutralization of influenza virus by immunoglobulin A anti-hemagglutinin monoclonal antibodies. *J Virol* 1995; 69: 1339–43.

245 Mazzoli S, Trabattoni D, Lo Caputo S et al. HIV-specific mucosal and cellular immunity in HIV-seronegative partners of HIV-seropositive individuals. *Nature Med* 1997; 3: 1250–7.

246 McCord ML, Hall RP. IgA antibodies against reticulin and endomysium in the serum and gastrointestinal secretions of patients with dermatitis herpetiformis. *Dermatology* 1994; 189: 60–3.

247 McCune JM, Fu SM, Kunkel HG. J chain biosynthesis in pre-B cells and other possible precursor B cells. *J Exp Med* 1981; 154: 138–45.

248 McDermott MR, Mark DA, Befus AD, Baliga BS, Suskind RM, Bienenstock J. Impaired intestinal localization of mesenteric lymphoblasts associated with vitamin A deficiency and protein-calorie malnutrition. *Immunology* 1982; 45: 1–5.

249 McKay DM, Bienenstock J. The interaction between mast cells and nerves in the gastrointestinal tract. *Immunol Today* 1994; 15: 533–8.

250 McLean IL, Kidd BL, Cawley MID. Ankylosing spondylitis and selective IgA deficiency. *Ann Rheum Dis* 1991; 50: 271.

251 McLoughlin GA, Hede JE, Temple JG, Bradley J, Chapman DM, McFarland J. The role of IgA in the prevention of bacterial colonization of the jejunum in the vagotomized subject. *Br J Surg* 1978; 65: 435–7.

252 Meng YG, Criss AB, Georgiadis KE. J chain deficiency in human IgM monoclonal antibodies produced by Epstein–Barr virus-transformed B lymphocytes. *Eur J Immunol* 1990; 20: 2505–8.

253 Mestecky J, Russell MW. IgA subclasses. *Monogr Allergy* 1986; 19: 277–301.

254 Mestecky J, Zikan J, Butler W. Immunoglobulin M and secretory immunoglobulin A: evidence for a common polypeptide chain different from light chains. *Science* 1971; 171: 1163–5.

255 Mestecky J, Winchester RJ, Hoffman T, Kunkel HG. Parallel synthesis of immunoglobulins and J chain in pokeweed mitogen-stimulated normal cells and in lymphoblastoid cell lines. *J Exp Med* 1977; 145: 760–5.

256 Molberg Ø, Kett K, Scott H, Thorsby E, Sollid LM, Lundin KE. Gliadin-specific, HLA-DQ2 restricted T cells are commonly found in small intestinal biopsies from coeliac disease patients, but not from controls. *Scand J Immunol* 1997; 46: 103–9.

257 Molberg O, Mcadam SN, Korner R et al. Tissue transglutaminase selectively modifies gliadin peptides that are recognized by gut-derived T cells in celiac disease. *Nat Med* 1998; 4: 713–7.

258 Moldoveanu Z, Egan ML, Mestecky J. Cellular origins of human polymeric and monomeric IgA: intracellular and secreted forms of IgA. *J Immunol* 1984; 133: 3156–62.

259 Monteiro RC, Hostoffer RW, Cooper MD, Bonner JR, Gartland GL, Kubagawa H. Definition of immunoglobulin A receptors on eosinophils and their enhanced expression in allergic individuals. *J Clin Invest* 1993; 92: 1681–5.

260 Moreau MC, Ducluzeau R, Guy-Grand D, Muller MC. Increase in the population of duodenal immunoglobulin A plasmocytes in axenic mice associated with different living or dead bacterial strains of intestinal origin. *Infect Immun* 1978; 121: 532–9.

261 Moro I, Iwase T, Komiyama K, Moldoveanu Z, Mestecky J. Immunoglobulin A (IgA) polymerization sites in human immunocytes: immunoelectron microscopic study. *Cell Struct Funct* 1990; 15: 85–91.

262 Mosmann TR, Gravel Y, Williamson AR, Baumal R. Modification and fate of J chain in myeloma cells in the presence and absence of immunoglobulin secretion. *Eur J Immunol* 1978; 8: 94–101.

263 Mostov KE, Blobel G. A transmembrane precursor of secretory component. The receptor for transcellular transport of polymeric immunoglobulins. *J Biol Chem* 1982; 157: 11816–21.

264 Müller F, Frøland SS, Hvatum M, Radl J, Brandtzaeg P. Both IgA subclasses are reduced in parotid saliva from patients with AIDS. *Clin Exp Immunol* 1991; 83: 203–9.

265 Nagao AT, Pilagallo MIDS, Pereira AB. Quantitation of salivary, urinary and faecal sIgA in children living in different conditions of antigenic exposure. *J Trop Pediatr* 1993; 39: 278–83.

266 Nagura H, Brandtzaeg P, Nakane PK, Brown WR. Ultrastructural localization of J chain in human intestinal mucosa. *J Immunol* 1979; 123: 1044–50.

267 Natvig IB, Johansen F-E, Nordeng TW, Haraldsen G, Brandtzaeg P. Mechanism for enhanced external transfer of dimeric IgA over pentameric IgM. Studies of diffusion, binding to the human polymeric Ig receptor, and epithelial transcytosis. *J Immunol* 1997; 159: 4330–40.

268 Newman RA, Ormerod MG, Greaves MF. The presence of HLA-DR antigens on lactating human breast epithelium and milk fat globule membranes. *Clin Exp Immunol* 1980; 41: 478–86.

269 Nilsen EM, Johansen F-E, Kvale D, Krajči P, Brandtzaeg P. Different regulatory pathways employed in cytokine-enhanced expression of secretory component and epithelial HLA class I genes. *Eur J Immunol* 1999; 29: 168–79.

270 Nilsen EM, Lundin KEA, Krajči P, Scott H, Sollid LM, Brandtzaeg P. Gluten-specific, HLA-DQ restricted T cells from coeliac mucosa produce cytokines with Th1 or Th0 profile dominated by interferon γ. *Gut* 1995; 37: 766–76.

271 Nilsen EM, Jahnsen FL, Lundin KEA *et al.* Gluten induces an intestinal cytokine response strongly dominated by interferon gamma in patients with celiac disease. *Gastroenterology* 1998; 115: 551–63.

272 Nilssen DE, Söderström R, Brandtzaeg P *et al.* Isotype distribution of mucosal IgG-producing cells in patients with various IgG subclass deficiencies. *Clin Exp Immunol* 1991; 83: 17–24.

273 Nilssen DE, Brandtzaeg P, Frøland SS, Fausa O. Subclass composition and J-chain expression of the 'compensatory' gastrointestinal IgG cell population in selective IgA deficiency. *Clin Exp Immunol* 1992; 87: 237–45.

274 Nilssen DE, Aukrust P, Frøland SS, Müller F, Fausa O, Halstensen TS, and Brandtzaeg P. Duodenal intraepithelial γ/δ T cells and soluble CD8, neopterin, and β2-microglobulin in serum of IgA-deficient subjects with or without IgG subclass deficiency. *Clin Exp Immunol* 1993; 94: 91–98.

275 Nilssen DE, Friman V, Theman K *et al.* B-cell activation in duodenal mucosa after oral cholera vaccination in IgA deficient subject with or without IgG subclass deficiency. *Scand J Immunol* 1993; 38: 201–8.

276 Nonaka M, Nonaka R, Woolley K *et al.* Distinct immunohistochemical localization of IL-4 in human inflamed airway tissues. IL-4 is localized to eosinophils *in vivo* and is released by peripheral blood eosinophils. *J Immunol* 1995; 155: 3234–44.

277 O'Mahony S, Arranz E, Barton JR, Ferguson A. Dissociation between systemic and mucosal humoral immune responses in coeliac disease. *Gut* 1991; 32: 29–35.

278 O'Mahony S, Vestey JP, Ferguson A. Similarities in intestinal humoral immunity in dermatitis herpetiformis without enteropathy and in coeliac disease. *Lancet* 1990; 23; 335: 1487–90.

279 Ochs HD, Ament ME. Gastrointestinal tract and immunodeficiency. In: *Immunological Aspects of the Liver and Gastrointestinal Tract* (Ferguson A, MacSween RNM eds). MTP Press, Lancaster, 1976: 82–120.

280 Ogra PL, Karzon DT. The role of immunoglobulins in the mechanism of mucosal immunity to virus infection. *Pediatr Clin North Am* 1970; 17: 385–400.

281 Ogra SS, Ogra PL, Lippes J, Tomasi TB. Immunohistologic localization of immunoglobulins, secretory component, and lactoferrin in the developing human fetus. *Proc Soc Exp Biol Med* 1972; 139: 570–2.

282 Ohtsuka A, Piazza AJ, Ermak TH, Owen RL. Correlation of extracellular matrix components with the cytoarchitecture of mouse Peyer's patches. *Cell Tissue Res* 1992; 269: 403–10.

283 Osman AA, Richter T, Stern M, Mothes T. The IgA subclass distributions of endomysium and gliadin antibodies in human sera are different. *Clin Chim Acta* 1996; 255: 145–52.

284 Paganelli R, Levinsky RJ. Solid phase radioimmunoassay for detection of circulating food protein antigens in human serum. *J Immunol Meth* 1980; 37: 333–41.

285 Paganelli R, Levinsky RJ, Brostoff J, Wraith DG. Immune complexes containing food proteins in normal and atopic subjects after oral challenge and effect of sodium cromoglycate on antigen absorption. *Lancet* 1979; 1: 1270–2.

286 Paganelli R, Fagiolo U, Cancian M, Sturniolo GC, Scala E, D'Offizi GP. Intestinal permeability in irritable bowel syndrome. Effect of diet and sodium cromoglycate administration. *Ann Allergy* 1990; 64: 377–80.

287 Paganelli R, Levinsky RJ, Atherton DJ. Detection of specific antigen within circulating immune complexes: validation of the assay and its application to food antigen–antibody complexes formed in healthy and food-allergic subjects. *Clin Exp Immunol* 1981; 46: 44–53.

288 Paganelli R, Atherton DJ, Levinsky RJ. Differences between normal and milk allergic subjects in their immune responses after milk ingestion. *Arch Dis Child* 1983; 58: 201–6.

289 Papadea C, Check IJ. Human immunoglobulin G and immunoglobulin G subclasses: biochemical, genetic, and clinical aspects. *Crit Rev Clin Lab Sci* 1989; 27: 27–58.

290 Parkhouse RMF, Della Corte E. Control of IgA biosynthesis. In: *The Role of Immunological Factors in Infections. Allergic, and Autoimmune Processes* (Beers RF, Bassett EG, eds). Raven Press, New York, 1976: 389–401.

291 Parkhouse RME, Cooper MD. A model for the differentiation of B lymphocytes with implications for the biological role of IgD. *Immunol Rev* 1977; 37: 105–26.

292 Parrott DM. The gut as a lymphoid organ. *Clin Gastroenterol* 1976; 5: 211–28.

293 Pascual DW, Xu-Amano JC, Kiyono H, McGhee JR, Bost KL. Substance P acts directly upon cloned B lymphoma cells to enhance IgA and IgM production. *J Immunol* 1991; 146: 2130–6.

294 Peebles RS, Liu MC, Adkinson NF, Lichtenstein LM, Hamilton RG. Ragweed-specific antibodies in bronchoalveolar lavage fluids and serum before and after segmental lung challenge: IgE and IgA associated with eosinophil degranulation. *J Allergy Clin Immunol* 1998; 101: 265–73.

295 Perkkiö M. Immunohistochemical study of intestinal biopsies from children with atopic eczema due to food allergy. *Allergy* 1980; 35: 573–80.

296 Perkkiö M, Svailahti E. Time of appearance of immunoglobulin-containing cells in the mucosa of the neonatal intestine. *Pediatr Res* 1980; 14: 953–5.

297 Perkkiö M, Savilahti E, Kuitunen P. Morphometric and immunohistochemical study of jejunal biopsies from children with intestinal soy allergy. *Eur J Pediatr* 1981; 137: 63–9.

298 Persson CG, Erjefält JS, Greiff L *et al.* Contribution of plasma-derived molecules to mucosal immune defence, disease and repair in the airways. *Scand J Immunol* 1998; 47: 302–13.

299 Phillips JO, Everson MP, Moldoveanu Z, Lue C, Mestecky J. Synergistic effect of IL-4 and IFN-gamma on the expression of polymeric Ig receptor (secretory component) and IgA binding by human epithelial cells. *J Immunol* 1990; 145: 1740–4.

300 Picarelli A, Maiuri L, Frate A, Greco M, Auricchio S, Londei M. Production of antiendomysial antibodies after *in-vitro* gliadin challenge of small intestine biopsy samples from patients with coeliac disease. *Lancet* 1996; 348: 1065–7.

301 Picker LJ, Martin RJ, Trumble A *et al.* Differential expression of lymphocyte homing receptors by human memory/effector T cells in pulmonary versus cutaneous immune effector sites. *Eur J Immunol* 1994; 24: 1269–77.

302 Pierce NF, Gowans JL. Cellular kinetics of the intestinal immune response to cholera toxoid in rats. *J Exp Med* 1975; 142: 1550–63.

303 Piskurich JF, Youngman KR, Phillips KM *et al.* Transcriptional regulation of the human polymeric immunoglobulin receptor gene by interferon-γ. *Mol Immunol* 1997; 34: 75–91.

304 Pistoia V. Production of cytokines by human B cells in health and disease. *Immunol Today* 1997; 18: 343–50.

305 Porter P, Linggood MA. Novel mucosal anti-microbial functions interfering with the plasmid-mediated virulence determinants of adherence and drug resistance. *Ann NY Acad Sci* 1983; 409: 564–78.

306 Portis JL, Coe JE. IgM the secretory immunoglobulin of reptiles and amphibians. *Nature* 1975; 258: 547–8.

307 Postigo AA, Sanchez-Mateos P, Lazarovits AI, Sanchez-Madrid F, de Landazuri MO. α4β7 integrin mediates B cell binding to fibronectin and vascular cell adhesion molecule-1: expression and function of α4 integrins on human B lymphocytes. *J Immunol* 1993; 151: 2471–83.

308 Prigent-Delecourt L, Coffin B, Colombel JF, Dehennin JP, Vaerman JP, Rambaud JC. Secretion of immunoglobulins and plasma proteins from the colonic mucosa: an *in vivo* study in man. *Clin Exp Immunol* 1995; 99: 221–5.

309 Pulendran B, van Driel R, Nossal GJ. Immunological tolerance in germinal centres. *Immunol Today* 1997; 18: 27–32.

310 Qiao L, Braunstein J, Golling M *et al*. Differential regulation of human T cell responsiveness by mucosal versus blood monocytes. *Eur J Immunol* 1996; 26: 922–7.

311 Quan CP, Berneman A, Pires R, Avrameas S, Bouvet JP. Natural polyreactive secretory immunoglobulin A autoantibodies as a possible barrier to infection in humans. *Infect Immun* 1997; 65: 3997–4004.

312 Quiding-Järbrink M, Lakew M, Nordström I *et al*. Human circulating specific antibody-forming cells after systemic and mucosal immunizations: differential homing commitments and cell surface differentiation markers. *Eur J Immunol* 1995; 25: 322–7.

313 Quiding-Järbrink M, Nordström I, Granström G *et al*. Differential expression of tissue-specific adhesion molecules on human circulating antibody-forming cells after systemic, enteric, and nasal immunizations. A molecular basis for the compartmentalization of effector B cell responses. *J Clin Invest* 1997; 99: 1281–6.

314 Randall TD, Parkhouse RM, Corley RB. J chain synthesis and secretion of hexameric IgM is differentially regulated by lipopolysaccharide and interleukin 5. *Proc Natl Acad Sci U S A* 1992; 89: 962–6.

315 Renegar KB, Jackson GD, Mestecky J. *In vitro* comparison of the biologic activities of monoclonal monomeric IgA, polymeric IgA, and secretory IgA. *J Immunol* 1998; 160: 1219–23.

316 Reynolds JD, Morris B. The influence of gut function on lymphoid cell populations in the intestinal mucosa of lambs. *Immunology* 1983; 49: 501–9.

317 Rinkenberger JL, Wallin JJ, Johnson KW, Koshland ME. An interleukin-2 signal relieves BSAP (Pax5)-mediated repression of the immunoglobulin J chain gene. *Immunity* 1996; 5: 377–86.

318 Roberton DM, Paganelli R, Dinwiddie R, Levinsky RJ. Milk antigen absorption in the preterm and term neonate. *Arch Dis Child* 1982; 57: 369–72.

319 Rognum TO, Brandtzaeg P. IgE-positive cells in human intestinal mucosa are mainly mast cells. *Int Arch Allergy Appl Immunol* 1989; 89: 256–60.

320 Rognum TO, Kett K, Fausa O *et al*. Raised number of jejunal IgG2-producing cells in untreated adult coeliac disease compared with food allergy. *Gut* 1989; 30: 1574–80.

321 Rosekrans PC, Meijer CJ, Cornelisse CJ, van der Wal AM, Lindeman J. Use of morphometry and immunohistochemistry of small intestinal biopsy specimens in the diagnosis of food allergy. *J Clin Pathol* 1980; 33: 125–30.

322 Rosekrans PCM, Meijer CJLM, Polanco I, Mearin ML, van der Wal AM, Lindeman J. Long-term morphological and immunohistochemical observations on biopsy specimens of small intestine from children with gluten-sensitive enteropathy. *J Clin Pathol* 1981; 34: 138–44.

323 Rosekrans PCM, Meijer CJLM, van der Wal AM, Lindeman J. Allergic proctitis, a clinical and immunopathological entity. *Gut* 1980; 21: 1017–23.

324 Roth R, Mather EL, Koshland ME. Intracellular events in the differentiation of B lymphocytes to pentamer IgM synthesis. In: *Cells of Immunoglobulin Synthesis* (Pernis B, Vogel HJ eds). Academic Press, London, 1979: 141–51.

325 Roth RA, Koshland ME. Identification of a lymphocyte enzyme that catalyzes pentamer immunoglobulin M assembly. *J Biol Chem* 1981; 256: 4633–9.

326 Rott LS, Briskin MJ, Andrew DP, Berg EL, Butcher EC. A fundamental subdivision of circulating lymphocytes defined by adhesion to mucosal addressin cell adhesion molecule-1. Comparison with vascular cell adhesion molecule-1 and correlation with β7 integrins and memory differentiation. *J Immunol* 1996; 156: 3727–36.

327 Ruan MR, Akkoyunlu M, Grubb A, Forsgren A. Protein D of *Haemophilus influenzae*. A novel bacterial surface protein with affinity for human IgD. *J Immunol* 1990; 145: 3379–84.

328 Rubin W, Fauci AS, Sleisenger MH, Jeffries GH. Immunofluorescent studies in adult celiac disease. *J Clin Invest* 1965; 44: 475–85.

329 Rugtveit J, Bakka A, Brandtzaeg P. Differential distribution of B7.1 (CD80) and B7.2 (CD86) co-stimulatory molecules on mucosal macrophage subsets in human inflammatory bowel disease (IBD). *Clin Exp Immunol* 1997; 110: 104–13.

330 Rugtveit J, Sollid LM, Fausa O, Scott H, Brandtzaeg P. Upregulation of the CD40 and CD86 on HLA-DQ⁺ mucosal macrophages in coeliac disease. Abstract 36, *Scand J Immunol* 1997: 437.

331 Russell MW, Reinholdt J, Kilian M. Anti-inflammatory activity of human IgA antibodies and their Fab alpha fragments: inhibition of IgG-mediated complement activation. *Eur J Immunol* 1989; 19: 2243–9.

332 Sagie E, Tarabulus J, Maeir DM, Freier S. Diet and development of intestinal IgA in the mouse. *Isr J Med Sci* 1974; 10: 532–4.

333 Sanderson IR, Walker WA. Uptake and transport of macromolecules by the intestine: possible role in clinical disorders (an update). *Gastroenterology* 1993; 104: 622–39.

334 Savidge TC. The life and times of an intestinal M cell. *Trends in Microbiology* 1996; 4: 301–6.

335 Savilahti E. Immunochemical study of the malabsorption syndrome with cow's milk intolerance. *Gut* 1973; 14: 491–501.

336 Savilahti E. Workshop on secretory immunoglobulins. In: *Progress in Immunology* (Brent L, Holborow J, eds.). North-Holland Publishing, Amsterdam; 1974; 2: 238–43.

337 Savilahti E, Pelkonen P. Clinical findings and intestinal immunoglobulins in children with partial IgA deficiency. *Acta Paediat Scand* 1979; 68: 513–19.

338 Schjerven H, Brandtzaeg P, Johansen F-E. Mechanism of IL-4-mediated up-regulation of the polymeric Ig receptor: role of STAT6 in cell type-specific delayed transcriptional response. *J Immunol* 2000; 165: 3898–906.

339 Schjerven H, Brandtzaeg P, Johansen F-E. A novel NF-κB/Rel site in intron 1 cooperates with proximal promoter elements to mediate TNF-α-induced transcription of the human polymeric Ig receptor. *J Immunol* 2001; 167: 6412–20.

340 Schrader CE, George A, Kerlin RL, Cebra JJ. Dendritic cells support production of IgA and other non-IgM isotypes in clonal microculture. *Int Immunol* 1990; 2: 563–70.

341 Schuppan D, Dieterich W, Riecken EO. Exposing gliadin as a tasty food for lymphocytes. *Nat Med* 1998; 4: 666–7.

342 Scott H, Brandtzaeg P. Endomysial autoantibodies. In: *Autoantibodies* (Peter JB, Shoenfeld Y, eds). Elsevier, Amsterdam, 1996; 237–44.

343 Scott H, Ek J, Baklien K, Brandtzaeg P. Immunoglobulin-producing cells in jejunal mucosa of children with coeliac disease on a gluten-free diet and after gluten challenge. *Scand J Gastroenterol* 1980; 15: 81–8.

344 Scott H, Nilsen E, Sollid LM *et al*. Immunopathology of gluten-sensitive enteropathy. *Springer Semin Immunopathol* 1997; 18: 535–53.

345 Scott H, Kett K, Halstensen T, Hvatum M, Rognum TO, Brandtzaeg P. The humoral immune system in coeliac disease. In: *Coeliac Disease* (Marsh MN, ed.). Blackwell Scientific Publications, Oxford; 1992: 239–82.

346 Sedgwick JD, Holt PG. Kinetics and distribution of antigen-specific IgE-secreting cells during the primary antibody response in the rat. *J Exp Med* 1983; 157: 2178–83.

347 Shin MK, Koshland ME. Ets-related protein PU.1 regulates expression of the immunoglobulin J-chain gene through a novel Ets-binding element. *Genes Dev* 1993; 7: 2006–15.

348 Shyjan AM, Bertagnolli M, Kenney CJ, Briskin MJ. Human mucosal addressin cell adhesion molecule-1 (MAdCAM-1) demonstrates structural and functional similarities to the α4β7-integrin binding domains of murine MAdCAM-1, but extreme divergence of mucin-like sequences. *J Immunol* 1996; 156: 2851–7.

349 Silverstein AM, Lukes RJ. Fetal response to antigenic stimulus. I. Plasmacellular and lymphoid reactions in the human fetus to intrauterine infection. *Lab Invest* 1962; 11: 918–32.

350 Slifka MK, Ahmed R. Long-lived plasma cells: a mechanism for maintaining persistent antibody production. *Curr Opin Immunol* 1998; 10: 252–8.

351 Sloper KS, Brook CG, Kingston D, Pearson JR, Shiner M. Eczema and atopy in early childhood: low IgA plasma cell counts in the jejunal mucosa. *Arch Dis Child* 1981; 56: 939–42.

352 Smith TJ, Weis JH. Mucosal T cells and mast cells share common adhesion receptors. *Immunol Today* 1996; 17: 60–3.

353 Sollid LM, Markussen G, Ek J, Gjerde H, Vartdal F, Thorsby E. Evidence for a primary association of celiac disease to a particular HLA-DQ α/β heterodimer. *J Exp Med* 1989; 169: 345–50.

354 Sollid LM, Molberg O, McAdam S, Lundin KE. Autoantibodies in coeliac disease: tissue transglutaminase – guilt by association? *Gut* 1997; 41: 851–2.

355 Söltoft J, Söeberg B. Immunoglobulin-containing cells in the small intestine during acute enteritis. *Gut* 1972; 13: 535–8.

356 Song W, Bomsel M, Casanova J, Vaerman JP, Mostov K. Stimulation of transcytosis of the polymeric immunoglobulin receptor by dimeric IgA. *Proc Natl Acad Sci USA* 1994; 91: 163–6.

357 Song W, Vaerman JP, Mostov KE. Dimeric and tetrameric IgA are transcytosed equally by the polymeric Ig receptor. *J Immunol* 1995; 155: 715–21.

358 Soothill JF. Some intrinsic and extrinsic factors predisposing to allergy. *Proc Roy Soc Med* 1976; 69: 439–42.

359 St. Louis-Cormier EA, Osterland CK, Anderson PD. Evidence for a cutaneous secretory immune system in rainbow trout (*Salmo gairdneri*). *Dev Comp Immunol* 1984; 8: 71–80.

360 Stephensen CB, Moldoveanu Z, Gangopadhyay NN. Vitamin A deficiency diminishes the salivary immunoglobulin A response and enhances the serum immunoglobulin G response to influenza A virus infection in BALB/c mice. *J Nutr* 1996; 126: 94–102.

361 Stern M, Dietrich R, Grüttner R. Gliadin-binding immunocytes in small intestinal lamina propria of children with coeliac disease. *Pediatr Res* 1981; 5: 1196.

362 Stern M, Dietrich R, Müller J. Small intestinal mucosa in coeliac disease and cow's milk protein intolerance: morphometric and immunofluorescent studies. *Eur J Pediatr* 1982; 139: 101–5.

363 Stott SI. Biosynthesis and assembly of IgM. Addition of J-chain to intracellular pools of 8S and 19S IgM. *Immunochemistry* 1976; 13: 157–63.

364 Streeter PR, Berg EL, Rouse BT, Bargatze RF, Butcher EC. A tissue-specific endothelial cell molecule involved in lymphocyte homing. *Nature* 1988; 331: 41–6.

365 Strobel S, Mowat AM. Immune responses to dietary antigens: oral tolerance. *Immunol Today* 1998; 19: 173–181.

366 Strober W, Sneller MC. Cellular and molecular events accompanying IgA B cell differentiation. *Monogr Allergy* 1988; 24: 181–90.

367 Sturgess RP, Macartney JC, Makgoba MW, Hung CH, Haskard DO, Ciclitira PJ. Differential upregulation of intercellular adhesion molecule-1 in coeliac disease. *Clin Exp Immunol* 1990; 82: 489–92.

368 Sutton BJ, Gould HJ. The human IgE network. *Nature* 1993; 366: 421–8.

369 Sylvestre DL, Ravetch JV. Fc receptors initiate the Arthus reaction: redefining the inflammatory cascade. *Science* 1994; 265: 1095–8.

370 Szabo MC, Butcher EC, McEvoy LM. Specialization of mucosal follicular dendritic cells revealed by mucosal addressin-cell adhesion molecule-1 display. *J Immunol* 1997; 158: 5584–8.

371 Saalman R, Wold AE, Dahlgren UI, Fallström SP, Hanson LA, Ahlstedt S. Antibody-dependent cell-mediated cytotoxicity to gliadin-coated cells with sera from children with coeliac disease. *Scand J Immunol* 1998; 47: 37–42.

372 Takahashi T, Iwase T, Takenouchi N *et al*. The joining (J) chain is present in invertebrates that do not express immunoglobulins. *Proc Natl Acad Sci USA* 1996; 93: 1886–91.

373 Takayasu H, Brooks KH. IL-2 and IL-5 both induce μ$_s$ and J chain mRNA in a clonal B cell line, but differ in their cell-cycle dependency for optimal signaling. *Cell Immunol* 1991; 136: 472–85.

374 Tarkowski A, Lue C, Moldoveanu Z, Kiyono H, McGhee JR, Mestecky J. Immunization of humans with polysaccharide vaccines induces systemic, predominantly polymeric IgA2-subclass antibody responses. *J Immunol* 1990; 144: 3770–8.

375 Tarlinton D. Germinal centers: form and function. *Curr Opin Immunol* 1998; 10: 245–51.

376 Taylor B, Norman AP, Orgel HA, Stokes CR, Turner MW, Soothill JF. Transient IgA deficiency and pathogenesis of infantile atopy. *Lancet* 1973; 2: 111–3.

377 Taylor HG, Dawes PT. Spondyloarthropathies and IgA deficiency. *Ann Rheu Dis* 1991; 50: 970.

378 Thrane PS, Rognum TO, Brandtzaeg P. Ontogenesis of the secretory immune system and innate defence factors in human parotid glands. *Clin Exp Immunol* 1991; 86: 342–8.

379 Thrane PS, Sollid LM, Haanes HR, Brandtzaeg P. Clustering of IgA-producing immunocytes related to HLA-DR-positive ducts in normal and inflamed salivary glands. *Scand J Immunol* 1992; 35: 43–51.

380 Tigges MA, Casey LS, Koshland ME. Mechanism of interleukin-2 signaling: mediation of different outcomes by a single receptor and transduction pathway. *Science* 1989; 243: 781–6.

381 Tlaskalova-Hogenova H, Cerna J, Mandel L. Peroral immunization of germfree piglets: appearance of antibody-forming cells and antibodies of different isotypes. *Scand J Immunol* 1981; 13: 467–72.

382 Tomasi TB, Tan EM, Solomon A, Prendergast RA. Characteristics of an immune system common to certain external secretions. *J Exp Med* 1965; 121: 101–24.

383 Tseng J. Expression of immunoglobulin isotypes by lymphoid cells of mouse intestinal lamina propria. *Cell Immunol* 1982; 73: 324–36.

384 Turesson I. Distribution of immunoglobulin-containing cells in human bone marrow and lymphoid tissues. *Acta Med Scand* 1976; 199: 293–304.

385 Turner CA, Mack DH, Davis MM. Blimp-1, a novel zinc finger-containing protein that can drive the maturation of B lymphocytes into immunoglobulin-secreting cells. *Cell* 1994; 77: 297–306.

386 Vaerman J-P, Langendries AE, Giffroy DA *et al*. Antibody against the human J chain inhibits polymeric Ig receptor-mediated biliary and epithelial transport of human polymeric IgA. *Eur J Immunol* 1998; 28: 171–82.

387 Vaerman JP, Langendries A, Giffroy D, Brandtzaeg P, Kobayashi K. Absence of SC/pIgR-mediated epithelial transport of a polymeric IgA devoid of J chain: in vitro and in vivo studies. *Immunology* 1998; 95: 90–6

388 Valnes K, Brandtzaeg P, Elgjo K, Stave R. Specific and nonspecific humoral defense factors in the epithelium of normal and inflamed gastric mucosa. Immunohistochemical localization of immunoglobulins, secretory component, lysozyme, and lactoferrin. *Gastroenterology* 1984; 86: 402–12.

389 Valnes K, Brandtzaeg P, Elgjo K, Stave R. Quantitative distribution of immunoglobulin-producing cells in gastric mucosa: relation to chronic gastritis and glandular atrophy. *Gut* 1986; 27: 505–14.

390 van Spreeuwel JP, Lindeman J, van Maanen J, Meyer CJ. Increased numbers of IgE containing cells in gastric and duodenal biopsies. An expression of food allergy secondary to chronic inflammation? *J Clin Pathol* 1984; 37: 601–6.

391 van Asperen PP, Gleeson M, Kemp AS *et al*. The relationship between atopy and salivary IgA deficiency in infancy. *Clin Exp Immunol* 1985; 62: 753–7.

392 van der Heijden PJ, Stok W, Bianchi AT. Contribution of immunoglobulin-secreting cells in the murine small intestine to the total 'background' immunoglobulin production. *Immunology* 1987; 62: 551–5.

393 Verrijdt G, Swinnen J, Peeters B, Verhoeven G, Rombauts W, Claessens F. Characterization of the human secretory component gene promoter. *Biochim Biophys Acta* 1997; 1350: 147–54.

394 Viney JL, Mowat AM, O'Malley JM, Williamson E, Fanger NA. Expanding dendritic cells *in vivo* enhances the induction of oral tolerance. *J Immunol* 1998; 160: 5815–25.

395 Volta U, Bonazzi C, Lazzari R *et al*. Immunoglobulin A antigliadin antibodies in jejunal juice: markers of severe intestinal damage in coeliac children. *Digestion* 1988; 39: 35–9.

396 Wade S, Lemonnier D, Alexiu A, Bocquet L. Effect of early postnatal under- and overnutrition on the development of IgA plasma cells in mouse gut. *J Nutr* 1982; 112: 1047–51.

397 Wagenaar SS, Peters A, Westermann CJJ, Oosting J. IgE bound to mast cells in bronchial mucosa and skin in atopic subjects. *Respiration* 1981; 41: 258–63.

398 Wagner N, Löhler J, Kunkel EJ *et al.* Critical role for β7 integrins in formation of the gut-associated lymphoid tissue. *Nature* 1996; 382: 366–70.

399 Warren SL. A new look at type I immediate hypersensitivity immune reactions. *Ann Allergy* 1976; 36: 337–41.

400 Watanabe M, Ueno Y, Yajima T *et al.* Interleukin 7 is produced by human intestinal epithelial cells and regulates the proliferation of intestinal mucosal lymphocytes. *J Clin Invest* 1995; 95: 2945–53.

401 Watson RR, McMurray DN, Martin P, Reyes MA. Effect of age, malnutrition and renutrition on free secretory component and IgA in secretion. *Am J Clin Nutr* 1985; 42: 281–8.

402 Webster AD, Slavin G, Shiner M, Platts-Mills TA, Asherson GL. Coeliac disease with severe hypogammaglobulinaemia. *Gut* 1981; 22: 153–7.

403 Wiedermann U, Hanson LA, Holmgren J, Kahu H, Dahlgren UI. Impaired mucosal antibody response to cholera toxin in vitamin A-deficient rats immunized with oral cholera vaccine. *Infect Immun* 1993; 61: 3952–7.

404 Wijesinha SS, Steer HW. Studies of the immunoglobulin-producing cells of the human intestine: the defunctioned bowel. *Gut* 1982; 23: 211–14.

405 Withrington R, Challacombe DN. Eosinophil-counts in duodenal tissue in cow's milk allergy. *Lancet* 1979; 1: 675.

406 Wolf HM, Vogel E, Fischer MB, Rengs H, Schwarz H-P, Eibl MM. Inhibition of receptor-dependent and receptor-independent generation of the respiratory burst in human neutrophils and monocytes by human serum IgA. *Pediatr Res* 1994; 36: 235–43.

407 Wolf HM, Fischer MB, Pühringer H, Samstag A, Vogel E, Eibl MM. Human serum IgA downregulates the release of inflammatory cytokines (tumor necrosis factor-α, interleukin-6) in human monocytes. *Blood* 1994; 83: 1278–88.

408 Yamanaka T, Straumfors A, Morton HC, Fausa O, Brandtzaeg P, Farstad IN. M cell pockets of human Peyer's patches are specialized extensions of germinal centers. *Eur J Immunol* 2001; 31: 107–17.

409 Yamaoka KA, Kolb JP. Leukotriene B4 induces interleukin 5 generation from human T lymphocytes. *Eur J Immunol* 1993; 23: 2392–8.

Chapter 10

The enterocyte

R. Mirakian and I.R. Sanderson

INTRODUCTION

The epithelium of the gastrointestinal mucosa is a key component of the gastrointestinal system as it provides a protective barrier against the potentially harmful external environment. The intestinal epithelial cell (iEC), which is mainly formed by enterocytes, is not a mere physical first line of defence[89,162] since it produces chemical agents such as the stomach acid and the digestive enzymes and antibacterial peptides, which provide chemical protection.[86] It physiologically associates with non-pathogenic microorganisms which compete with harmful microorganisms for attachment on epithelial cells and exerts an important ecological control.[13,86] In addition to protective mechanisms, the iEC carries out critical physiological functions as it constitutes the site for digestion and absorption of nutrients.[128]

Furthermore, the mucosal epithelial compartment is an integral component of the mucosal immune system which is primarily structured to respond to the continuous exposure to luminal antigens with a local secretory immunoglobulin (Ig) A antibody response[102] and an antigen-specific systemic hyporesponsiveness (oral tolerance).[109,179,185] In this context the iEC undertakes immunological regulatory functions through its antigen-presenting ability[20,116,127] and its ability to cross-talk and interact with luminal antigens and with the adjacent cells of the immune system.[141] These interactions, generally mediated through the release of cytokines, are required to maintain the mucosal integrity and prevent and/or contain mucosal injury[35,82,87,148].

This chapter describes briefly the morphological structure of the two main mucosal epithelial compartments of the gut, the enterocytes and the M cells, subsequently dealing with their non-immunological and immunological functions. Mention will also be given to apoptosis as a recognized mechanism in maintaining mucosal epithelial cell homeostasis.

STRUCTURE

Absorptive epithelial cell

The absorptive epithelial cell (the enterocyte) constitutes the major component of the mucosal intestinal epithelium.[128,162] This compartment is formed by columnar cells (25 μm long) the surface of which consists of a carpet of packed microvilli[125] which are relatively impermeable to the passage of macromolecules.[86] At the base of the microvilli is the plasma membrane, whose composition influences the antigen binding. The surface of the microvilli is covered with glycocalyx and a layer of mucus.[74,86,118,128,162,169] The glycocalyx, which firmly adheres to the microvilli, is formed mainly by a carbohydrate structure which allows the adherence to microorganisms and macromolecules, and which contains proteolytic enzymes and proteins responsible for the digestion and the absorption of nutrients. The mucus is resistant to digestion and functions as a barrier for mucosal protection as its viscous nature is able to entrap microorganisms and inhibit antigen and parasite attachment to the microvilli.[162,175]

The enterocytes are joined together by tight junctions, desmosomes and adhesion junctions, structures which form the junctional complex. The tight junctions constitute a barrier separating the outer from the inner environment which excludes peptides and macromolecules with antigenic potential, while the desmosomes and the adhesion junctions maintain cell–cell adhesions.[162] A 30-μm space separates the enterocyte basal membrane from the basal lamina, which contains mainly pores.[137] The basal lamina is thought to contribute to the polarity of the absorptive cell and to direct the enterocytes in their migration from the crypts to the desquamation sites.[86]

M cells

Scattered among enterocytes overlying the dome of the organized mucosal lymphoid follicles of the Peyer's patches (PP) and as a part of the follicle-associated epithelium (FAE) there are specialized cells, called M cells.[131,132] Their name was first derived from the 'microfolds' present over the luminal surface but more recently they have been renamed 'membranous' because the adjacent lymphoid cells push and reduce them into 'bands' which separate the lumen from the tissue compartments.[138–140] The M cells lie on the basal lamina and adhere to enterocytes. Because of their rarity throughout the gastrointestinal tract (0.1% of epithelial cells), it has not been possible to culture them *in vitro* to date, and no specific marker has yet been identified.[112,131] Their morphology has been investigated and characterized by ultrastructural analysis (Table 10.1).

M cells display a poorly developed brush border, a thin glycocalyx, the presence of variable microvilli, scanty lysosomes and a well developed microvesicular system, all critical features for their specialized function.[75,86,128] These cells are characterized by a unique structure, the 'pocket', which surrounds the underlying lymphoid cells and constitutes a 'sequestered' environment, independent from the control of the systemic immune system.[132,133] In the 'pocket' B cells expressing IgM, CD45RO+ T cells (mostly CD4+) and macrophages can be found.[86,132,133] The presence of these 'memory' phenotypes on the lymphoid cells is thought to reflect the active immunological function of these cells, which are ready to respond to incoming luminal antigens.[45,132] The lymphoid traffic in and out of the pockets is encouraged by the pores in the basal lamina. While the basolateral surface of M cells is involved in cell–cell adhesion, their basal portion interacts with the extracellular matrix and the basal lamina.

The M cell shape is maintained by a net of intermediate filaments of vimentin and its surface contains glycoproteins

Morphological features of M cells
Poorly developed brush border
Thin glycocalyx, variable microvilli
Well developed microvascular system
Scanty lysosomes
Pocket surrounding lymphoid cells

Table 10.1 Morphological features of M cells.

displaying glycosylation profiles different from those found on enterocytes.[50,131] These allow sampling of a broad range of microorganisms[75]. The exposure to microorganisms is critical for the development of the organized mucosal lymphoid tissue and the M cells.[27,174] There are indications that the lymphoid cell recruitment in turn promotes the differentiation of undifferentiated cells in adjacent crypts into specialized FAE and M cells.[27,52,131,165] Coculture experiments with Caco 2 intestinal cells have confirmed that B (but not T) lymphocytes can induce M cell differentiation. This local influence operates through the release of as yet unidentified factors and also through cell–cell contact.[75,90,131]

NON-IMMUNOLOGICAL FUNCTIONS

Uptake and transport of antigens by the absorptive epithelial cell

The most important functions of enterocytes are the digestion and absorption of nutrients into the bloodstream.[128] As the lumen is exposed to potentially harmful pathogens the epithelium limits the absorption of macromolecules and invading microorganisms, thus also acting as a protective barrier.[86,162] This function is carried out by non-immunological factors, such as mucus, the glycocalyx, pancreatic and gastric juices, and by the immunological properties of both the epithelium and mucosal immune system.[86] However, this barrier is not totally impermeable, and soluble antigens and critical macromolecules are allowed to enter. The access of luminal antigens into the gut mucosa occurs through three pathways: the path through the tight junctions (paracellular),[110] the route across the epithelial cell (transcellular),[32,37] and the most common route via the M cells.[81]

The transport of antigens is carried out in a controlled fashion and an efficient local and systemic immune response depends on an efficient transport.[128] To achieve an efficient intracellular transport the enterocyte polarity has to be maintained. This occurs by the presence of two subdomains in the cell basolateral surface. The lateral domain, which is rich in Na+, K+, ATPase and immunoglobulin receptors, is involved in cell–cell interactions via adhesion molecules; the basal subdomain contains receptors recognizing the extracellular matrix and the basal lamina.[128] An efficient diffusion of water and ions is ensured by the tight junctions which seal the apical poles of the cell and inhibit inconvenient lateral diffusion of substances. At the same time, these structures prevent the absorption of peptides and macromolecules.[86]

Endocytosis

In the iEC the endocytic uptake of macromolecules is carried out in mucosal sites located at the base of microvilli.[162] In these locations macromolecules can enter the enterocyte by binding to specific receptors or by non-specific binding. The plasma membrane invaginates to form vesicles. Clathrin is a protein which forms a lattice and controls the plasma membrane invaginations and promotes endocytosis.[29,95,136,172] The vesicles containing the macromolecules first fuse to form the 'early endosomes',[1,97] and then move to the tubulocysternae structures which primarily facilitate movement of the vesicles within the cell. In this acidic compartment the macromolecules are sorted[119] and are either transported to the lysosomes where they are destroyed or to the opposite basolateral membranes (transcytosis),[55,56,134] towards the lymphoid tissue of the lamina propria where they are ready for presentation.

Uptake and transport by M cells (Table 10.2)

Although M cells are in a minority in the intestinal epithelium, their location overlying PP is of paramount importance to ensure an efficient initiation of the immune response and a rapid transport of luminal antigens for processing or presentation to the underlying cells of the immune system.[134] Antigen uptake can involve a great range of antigens, such as macromolecules, viruses, bacteria and parasites,[86] which are concentrated effectively through an adherence mechanism before being endocytosed.[75,132] M cell adherence to these antigens is a critical step for induction of mucosal immunity and is mediated by a lectin–carbohydrate recognition system.[133,134]

Adherent antigens taken up by M cells are delivered to the well developed tubulovesicular structures that resemble the early endosomes of the enterocytes.[187] This material does not generally appear to enter the degradative compartment and the traffic is not directed toward lateral or basal surfaces as for the absorptive cell. Instead fusion of the vesicles occurs directly with the basolateral domain lying over the pocket. Non-adherent material can also be taken up by phagocytosis.[134,140] The efficiency of M cell function is the result of a fine balance between the efficient binding to M cells, the pathogenicity of pathogens and the macrophage phagocytic activity.

Stages in uptake and transport of antigens by M cells
1. Adherence of antigen to M cells by lectin–carbohydrate recognition
2. Delivery to tubulovesicular structures
3. Fusion of vesicles with basolateral domain

Table 10.2 Stages in uptake and transport of antigens by M cells.

IMMUNOLOGICAL FUNCTIONS

Intestinal epithelial cell effector functions

It is recognized that the first line of immunological defence against invading agents in the gut lumen is carried out by mucosal IgA which contributes to the prevention of potentially harmful antigens attaching to and penetrating the epithelium.[101]

Sampling of luminal antigens by the iEC induces the production of IgA from mucosal lamina propria plasma cells, particularly those belonging to the PP.[28] Dimeric IgA is taken up via a specific receptor-mediated binding mechanism expressed on the basolateral surface of the enterocyte. IgA is then transcytosed and secreted into the lumen (secretory IgA; sIgA), where it combines with the antigen to form complexes.[126] It has recently emerged that IgA interactions with antigens not only occur outside the cell but can also occur within the cell in an infected cell during IgA transit through the epithelium.[80,101,126] This mechanism aims to disrupt the production of new virus directly. Furthermore, IgA can also bind antigen in the lamina propria and the complex is transcytosed intact into the lumen. Upregulation of IgA receptor on infected iEC has been confirmed in vivo. iEC can also secrete soluble components such as C3 and C4 complement components[4] and cryptdins,[42] which are specifically produced by the Paneth cells of the small intestine. The func-

tion of these factors is to neutralize/inactivate harmful microorganisms. Finally, a further non-specific defence mechanism is provided by the secretion of the intestinal trefoil factor, which is secreted into the mucus and is involved in wound healing and mucosal integrity.[149]

Intestinal epithelial cell immunoregulatory functions
Conventional antigen-presenting function

Antigen recognition is classically mediated by HLA Class I and II/DR genes encoded for by the human chromosome 6 (Table 10.3) which display significant allelic polymorphism.[123,143] Class I products, which are expressed on the cell surface of most cells in the body (including the iEC), are formed by two polypeptide chains: the HLA-encoded heavy chain (or α chain) and the non-HLA-encoded β2 microglobulin (β2 m or β chain). The heavy chain is expressed as a 43–45-kDa glycoprotein containing three membrane distal domains, α1, α2 and α3 extracellular domains, a short transmembrane segment and a carboxyl terminal cytoplasmic tail. The α1 and α2 domains contain the majority of the allelic polymorphism[15] and form a groove for the binding site of nine amino acid short peptides.[14,43,176] The α3 domain is non-covalently associated with the fourth domain, the β2m, which is a 12-kDa non-glycosylated protein not directly attached to the cell.[113]

The function of the Class I molecules is to present endogenously generated peptides derived from invading bacteria and viruses to cytolytic CD8[+]-activated lymphocytes.[48] Peptides are generated in the cytosol by a processing mechanism operated by proteosomes. These peptides are subsequently transported by transporter (TAP) proteins into the endoplasmic reticulum, where they associate with HLA Class I molecules and move together to the cell surface.[59,76,171]

HLA Class II/DR products are mainly restricted to professional antigen-presenting cells (APC) such as dendritic cells, B cells or macrophages, although non-professional APC, such as

Classical and non-classical HLA molecule expression on enterocytes			
	HLA molecules	Function	Ligand
Classical HLA	HLA Class I	Bind to endogenous derived peptides	αβ+ CD8+
	HLA Class II	Bind to exogenous peptides	αβ+ CD4+
Non-classical HLA	CD1d	Binds to hydrophobic antigens (? lipids) (? peptides)	Intraepithelial lymphocytes (?CD8+)
	FcRn	Bind and transport IgG (through FcR)	IgG
	MICA/B	? Stress molecules	γδ+ Intraepithelial lymphocytes?

Table 10.3 Classical and non-classical HLA molecule expression on enterocytes.

endothelial cells, fibroblasts, activated T cells and mucosal epithelial cells also appear to express these determinants physiologically. HLA Class II/DR molecules are formed by a non-covalent complex of two transmembrane glycoprotein chains: the α (34 kDa) and the β (20 kDa) chains. Each chain expresses two extracellular domains.[49] The peptide-binding site is formed by an interaction between the α1 and β1 domains. The HLA Class II/DR function is to present exogenous antigens to activated CD4[+] helper/inducer T cells.[38,53] Exogenous luminal antigens are taken up into intracellular vesicles and then processed into peptides in the endosomal compartment[189,54]; In this cell location[3] they bind to HLA Class II products and are subsequently transported to the cell surface to be presented to the TCR of the activated CD4[+] T cells.[53,103]

Evidence for antigen presentation by intestinal epithelial cells

There is evidence that iEC are not passive players in the immune response but key regulators for maintaining the mucosal immunosuppressive state. They are candidates for antigen-presenting activity.[21,69,70,114] The epithelial cells in the small bowel and to some extent also of the colon express HLADR molecules[16,168] which have been shown to be functional as they are able to present antigens to primed T cells and to hybridomas *in vitro*.[17,83,117] It has been shown that iEC activate a lymphocyte subset with CD8αβ[+], IL2R[+], positive CD28[-] suppressor phenotype. Although the bulk of T cells stimulated to proliferate by enterocytes are CD8[+], a subset of HLA Class II-dependent CD4[+] cells proliferates as well and the T cell response is shown to be blocked by HLADR blocking antibodies. Functionally, CD8[+] T cells have been found to be non-cytolytic and to suppress the immune response in an antigen unrestricted fashion.[18] However, further *in vitro* studies have not been so successful. In experimental conditions using T84 and HT29 iEC lines transfected with DR4β cDNA, no antigen-presenting ability could be generated by these cells in the absence of interferon γ (IFNγ).

Furthermore, since the antigen processing ability of enterocytes is poor,[47] it is possible that their functional ability to induce an immune response is also reduced. There is also little evidence that enterocytes can express costimulatory molecules[163] which are prerequisites for an efficient immune response *in vivo*. It is clear that iEC are not professional APC as they constitutively express HLA Class II/DR molecules, do not express costimulatory products and are poor phagocytes. However, although the kinetics of antigen presentation are slow and the results depend on the cell system, enterocytes are known to be able to take up soluble antigens and to transport them, thus indicating that they have the potential immunological ability to present antigens. It is possible that the requirements for complete processing and presentation abilities may be different in the mucosal system in comparison with the systemic compartment.[115] On these grounds, it has been proposed that antigen presentation by enterocytes results in 'protective' anergy rather than proliferation. This issue is still open.

Non-conventional antigen-presenting function: the CD1 system

More recently, the original findings that *in vitro* presentation of luminal antigens by iEC preferentially stimulates CD8[+] cells but not CD4[+] cells (as one would expect in a Class II restricted context), have given rise to the suggestion that this stimulation is the result of an interaction of CD8[+] T cells with non-classical

HLA Class I molecules (Table 10.3) of the CD1-like family expressed on enterocytes.[19,22,116] CD1 molecules belong to a large family of products which present antigens to specific subsets of T cells in different anatomical locations.[23]

HLA Class I-like genes of the CD1 family have similarities with the exon–intron structures of the MHC Class I family. However, they also differ from classical HLA Class I genes as they show little polymorphism and therefore are thought to evolve for specialized and conserved functions.[22] In a similar manner to HLA Class I products, CD1 elements display an α1–α3 domain, a transmembrane domain and a cytoplasmic tail. They mostly share a dependence on β2m for function and contain many conserved contact sites for β2m.[194] In contrast to HLA Class I molecules, the CD1 family has a limited tissue distribution and binds non-peptide molecules in addition to peptide antigens.[151] The bound peptide on CD1 molecules displays a longer sequence than that recognized on classical HLA Class I products. Interestingly, the antigen-presenting pathway overlaps with that of HLA Class II molecules with which it shares homologies both in the nucleotide sequence and in the endosomal localization motif (YXXZ motif) in the cytoplasmic tail which is responsible for directing the antigen to the endocytic compartment.[12]

The human CD1 gene family contains five members mapping to the chromosome I CD1 A–E genes.[31,144] This family comprises two groups of molecules based on nucleotide and amino acid sequence homologies: CD1a–c and CD1d. CD1a–c antigens are restricted to professional antigen-presenting cells.[30] The CD1a–c determinants appear to present non-peptide antigens and the presentation involves an endocyte pathway (Table 10.4). In particular, CD1a presents lipids such as mycolic acid derived from bacterial antigens and CD1b,c non-peptide mycobacterial products to double negative (CD4[-] CD8[-]) αβ[+], γδ[+], αα[+] CD8[+] T cells.[78,150] These molecules could also be involved in the presentation of endogenous elements in autoimmune conditions as CD4[-] CD8[-] T cells can be raised in these diseases.

In addition to certain professional antigen-presenting cells such as B lymphocytes, CD1d products are mainly expressed on epithelial cells from a variety of locations. CD1d transcripts in the gut mucosa have been found in the lower portion of the crypts, whereas the protein expression is localized instead in the upper portions of the intestinal villi.[85]

iEC express two forms of CD1d: a cell surface and a cytoplasmic isoform which can be found either independently or associated with β2m. CD1d expressed on the cell surface independently of β2m is recognized by a subset of CD8[+] T cells. Antibody to CD1d can inhibit the T cell proliferation induced by iECs, but these antibodies do not have any effect on T cell activation by professional APC.[11,142] During immunoprecipitation studies of CD1d, a 180-kDa protein was found to be expressed

Human CD1 gene family
Five members CD1 A–E genes
Map to chromosome I
Two subgroups CD1a–c, CD1d
Present non-peptide antigens via endocyte pathway

Table 10.4 Human CD1 gene family.

on normal iEC.[193] A model has been proposed by which the expression of CD1d in association with gp180 on the surface of the iEC forms a HLA Class I-like complex able to present antigens to CD8+ non-specific T suppressor cells. This binding would signal through the activation of Src-like tyrosine kinase p56/lck.[107,116] The precise function of intracytoplasmic CD1d on iEC is, as yet, unknown.

It has recently been shown in peripheral blood that when CD1d is expressed in association with β2m, it functions as a ligand for an invariant TCRα chain present on double negative human T cells. This subset of T cells expresses a killer inhibitory receptor (KIR) phenotype and the ligation of CD1d with KIR cells induces the secretion of high concentrations of IL4 and IFNγ. It is not yet established whether this function is also performed by enterocytes.[24] As CD1d is expressed in various isoforms, it is envisaged that these may reflect different functions in iEC–IEL interactions.[144]

Fc receptor for immunoglobulin G

Other non-classical Class I HLA-related antigens have been found expressed in the human iEC in association with β2m. One of these, the Fc-Rn receptor (where n is neonatal), was originally identified in rodents as the protein that mediates transfer of maternal milk-borne IgG across rat neonatal gut.[79] Subsequently, it was found to be involved in regulating IgG catabolism and also serum IgG levels.[57] The isolation of a human homologue of Fc-Rn antigen from the syncytiotrophoblast of the placenta would represent its involvement in the passive acquisition of maternal IgG by the foetus. Using placenta cDNA as a probe, Fc-Rn messages have also been detected in the epithelium of the human adult intestine.[25,177] It is possible that Fc-Rn expression on human adult epithelium is involved in foreign antigen IgG complex sampling and subsequent delivery to immunocompetent cells in the lamina propria for appropriate presentation and initiation of the immune response.[25] However, its exact functional role on human epithelial cells requires further investigation.[20,73]

HLA Class I chain-related gene A/B (MICA/B)

The MICA family also belongs to the non-conventional HLA Class I genes; these molecules do not require β2m or conventional antigen-processing molecules to function.[9,10] MICB has greater than 80% homology to MICA. MICA/B products are expressed in gastrointestinal and thymus epithelial cells and have also been found in actively growing cells.

The exact function of these products is not yet known. Since the MICA gene is preceded by a heat-shock promoter and its expression may be induced by heat-shock, it is envisaged that these molecules are expressed after a stress signal.[62,63] It has been postulated that local T cells expressing ligands for MICA determinants may elicit cellular responses to epithelial cell injury.

GUT EPITHELIUM AS A T CELL EDUCATION SITE

Both thymus and gut epithelium are derived from endoderm and show similar immunological features.[105] Both compartments constitutively express HLA-DR molecules, which are susceptible to IFNγ upregulation and in both cases the epithelium is immunologically functional. Evidence has gradually emerged from experimental studies in rodents that the gastrointestinal epithelial microenvironment can also operate as an alternative primary lymphoid organ for a subset of IEL in an analogous method to that recognized for the thymic epithelium for T cell education and differentiation.[94,127,153,170] While most IEL are thymus-dependent, showing a CD8αβ+ phenotype and a conventional αβTCR, a proportion of CD8+ IEL and all γδ+ IEL express a non-conventional αα+ homodimeric form of CD8.[106] These CD8αα IEL also express a different CD3 signalling mechanism from that expressed by the peripheral blood lymphocytes as they exhibit a single CD3β chain linked to the γ chain rather than the CD3-linked ζζ chain homodimer. Furthermore, they also express the recombination activation gene 1 essential for the TCR rearrangement.[106] The presence of these unique phenotypes suggests that a proportion of IEL have gone through an extrathymic maturation in the gut epithelium.[64,65,94,170]

Experiments carried out in adult and neonatal mice having thymectomy and also in athymic mice reconstituted with bone marrow-derived stem cells have confirmed the existence of a gut-derived αβ and γδ+ TCR/CD8αα IEL.[106,127] Further confirmation of an intestinal cell source critical for the differentiation of a subset of IEL has emerged from the findings, showing that clusters of hundreds of immature T cells which are located under the gut epithelial cells (cryptoplasts) express IL7-R and c-*kit* (receptor for stem cell factor).[84,146] These differentiate after the influence of IL7 and stem cell factor secreted by the intestinal epithelium. Cryptoplasts would represent IEL precursors.[188]

ENTEROCYTES AS SOURCE AND TARGETS OF CYTOKINE ACTIVITY

The growth and functional differentiation of various compartments of the gastrointestinal mucosa are under the influence of cytokines and growth factors which operate with a paracrine and autocrine mechanism. A high degree of complexity and redundancy within the cytokine networks is present, as each cytokine can be produced by more than one cell type and each cell can produce a variety of cytokines.[148] This redundancy is necessary as a safety net to maintain the integrity and functional activity of all the structures of the mucosal system. Each cell type can function as a source of cytokine production and as a target of cytokine activity through bidirectional cross-talks occurring between lymphoid cells, both of the epithelium and of the lamina propria and the adjacent epithelium,[26,93,96,191] and also between the extracellular matrix and the epithelial compartment.[108] iEC have been shown to inhibit T cell proliferative reponse and Th1 and Th2 cytokine production of activated αβ and γδ IEL but not spleen T cells. This shows that specific 'intranets' are aimed at suppressing potential inflammatory responses at the mucosal surfaces.[191] In addition, since the iEC comes into contact with luminal microorganisms, this exposure results in an early cytokine response which induces the expression of immune activation molecules on epithelial cells[121] and contributes to the initiation of an inflammatory response in the mucosa (Table 10.5).[180]

For these complex networks to take place in an organized sequence the iEC–IEL biological unit must be maintained. The binding of tissue-specific adhesion molecules expressed on enterocytes, i.e. E-cadherin to its ligand, αEβ7 integrin, on IEL, ensures the localization of lymphocytes to the basolateral surface of the iEC.[33,41] This binding not only serves useful adhesive functions but also provides regulatory signals to activated IEL, inhibiting their proliferative responses and cytokine synthesis, and

Intestinal epithelial cells
Can inhibit T cell proliferative response
Can inhibit Th1 and Th2 cytokine protection of αβ and γd iEC
Cannot inhibit spleen T cell cytokine production
Cytokine response after contact with luminal microorganisms
E-cadherin adhesion molecule binds to αEβ7 integrin on IEL
iEC, intestinal epithelial cells; IEL, intraepithelial lymphocytes.

Table 10.5 Intestinal epithelial cells.

limiting possible antigen-mediated inflammatory response at the mucosal surface.[35]

The use of intestinal cell lines which allow the study of the kinetics of cytokine production in basal conditions, and after infection of iEC with bacterial agents or stimulation with various combinations of cytokines, provides useful information on possible physiological mechanisms of cytokines at the gut mucosal site.[82]

CONSTITUTIVE AND STIMULATED PRODUCTION OF PROINFLAMMATORY CYTOKINES BY INTESTINAL EPITHELIAL CELLS FOLLOWING AGONIST STIMULATION AND BACTERIAL INVASION

Constitutive expression of chemokines of the C-X-C and C-C families has been detected in human colon cell lines (Table 10.6). In particular, the detection of IL8 belonging to the C-X-C group is important as this cytokine is involved in polymorphonuclear (PMN) chemotaxis and activation.[39,111,121,167] Its secretion and mRNA transcription is upregulated not only by IL1β and TNFα but also by coculturing these cell lines with pathogenic (but not with non-pathogenic) bacteria.[39,46,121,] IL8 kinetics of production show an early response (2–4 h), followed by a decrease in spite of continuous stimulation. This reflects the IL8 involvement in acute inflammation as an initiator of PMN influx. In addition, monocyte chemotactic protein 1 (MCP 1), monocyte inhibiting proteins (MIPα and β) and RANTES, belonging to the C-C family, have also been found secreted, though at lower levels. These cytokines act on chemotaxis for monocyte/macrophages/eosinophils and T

Proinflammatory cytokines expressed by human intestinal epithelial cell lines		
C-X-C chemokines	C-C chemokines	Other cytokines
IL8	MCP 1	GM-CSF TNFα
GRO α, β, γ	MIP α,β RANTES	IL1β
IL8, interleukin 8; GRO, growth-related oncogene; MCP 1, monocyte chemotactic protein 1; MIP, monocyte inhibiting protein; GM-CSF, granulocyte–macrophage colony stimulating factor; TNFα, tumour necrosis factor α ;IL1β, interleukin 1β.		

Table 10.6 Proinflammatory cytokines expressed by human intestinal epithelial cell lines.

cells[159,191,192]. Since they are, in general, found expressed with delayed kinetics, they are thought to play a more complex role during inflammation.[82] Furthermore, traditional proinflammatory cytokines, including tumours necrosis factor α (TNFα) granulocyte–macrophage colony stimulating factors (GM-CSF) and IL1β[35,148,192] are secreted by iEC lines and their expression is further regulated by agonists such as TNFα and IL1β and also by bacterial infection.[40,82] Proinflammatory cytokine expression in the mucosal epithelium is critical because of these known cytokine autocrine effects on iEC, i.e. the upregulation of HLA Class II and ICAM 1 immune activation molecule expression.[72,88,145]

Interleukin 7 (Table 10.7)

IL7 has been found to be a particularly important cytokine involved in the interactions between the mucosal lymphocytes and iEC.[39,182] This cytokine is a known derived stromal growth factor, which was originally described as a growth factor for precursors of B cells.[60,130,] Subsequently, it has been found to have pleiotropic activities, acting as a potent costimulus for thymic T cell maturation,[186] for enhancing T cell activity,[5] as an inducer of proinflammatory cytokines and as a stimulator of proliferative and functional differentiation[183] of mucosal lymphocytes. IL7 transcripts have been detected in human intestinal mucosa, while the presence of IL7 protein in intestinal epithelium (particularly in the crypts and goblet cells) has been confirmed by immunochemistry and in situ hybridization techniques.[182] Conversely, IL7 receptor expression has been demonstrated in mucosal lymphocytes by a variety of methods in freshly isolated lymphocytes from the lamina propria but not from peripheral lymphocytes. This would indicate that the continuous antigenic stimulation within the intestinal microenvironment may stimulate the expression of mucosal lymphocyte receptors[182] and has prompted the suggestion that locally produced IL7 may serve as a critical regulating factor for intestinal mucosal lymphocytes.[182]

Following the recognition that human colonic epithelial cell lines express functional IL2 receptors,[36] it has been demonstrated that iEC lines and also primary human intestinal preparations express transcripts for a γc chain shared by IL2, IL4, IL7 and IL9 cytokines.[148,158] Indeed, the epithelial cells respond to the corresponding cytokine stimulation by activating intracellular signalling pathways. Interestingly, the tyrosine phosphorylation patterns in the intestinal epithelium are distinct from that found in stimulated lymphocytes.[148]

Unexpectedly, cytokines more commonly seen in association with antigen-specific acquired immune responses have not been identified in these cell lines. This possibly reflects the involvement of the mucosal epithelium in the regulation of innate rather than acquired antigen-specific immune responses.

Properties of interleukin 7
Costimulus for thymic T cell maturation
Enhances T cell activity
Induces proinflammatory cytokines from mucosal lymphocytes
Stimulates functional differentiation of mucosal lymphocytes
Stimulates proliferation of mucosal lymphocytes

Table 10.7 Properties of interleukin 7.

Among these regulatory mediators the detection of transforming growth factor (TGF) has been of great interest. TGFα and β have been found to modulate proliferation, differentiation and also transport of ions and nutrients across the epithelium.[51,147] TGFα transcripts and their products are found predominantly in the villus tips of the small intestine and in the surface epithelium of the colon, whereas TGFβ message is mainly detected in the mucosal lamina propria and also within a subset of crypt cells.[7,8] TGFα has been shown to stimulate the proliferation of iEC lines whereas TGFβ has been recognized as a potent inhibitor of cell proliferation and a promoter of epithelial cell differentiation.[100,148] In a more strictly immunological context, TGFβ is known to play a critical role in maintaining antigen-specific and non-specific systemic immune suppression[92,122,164,185] in association with IL10 and IL4, while stimulating local mucosal immune responses.[120,185]

Role of cytokines in epithelial repair

TGFβ production also appears to be increased after injury during the so-called process of 'epithelial restitution' or tissue repair which occurs via the migration of epithelial cells from areas adjacent to an injured/wounded epithelial surface.[58] Since TGFβ inhibits epithelial proliferation, it is clear that the process of restitution does not necessarily involve proliferation. A vast array of cytokines, including epidermal growth factor (EGF), IL1β, IL6, TNFα, IFNγ, TGFα and platelet-derived growth factor (PDGF), all increase repair *in vitro* by increasing TGFβ production.[58]

In addition, interactions between iEC and the underlying extracellular matrix have been shown to play a role in maintaining mucosal integrity. In particular, fibronectin[104,154] and collagen type IV[87,173] expressed in the basement membranes of crypts have been found to be produced not only by the stromal component but also by the small intestinal crypt cells. It has recently been proposed that fibronectin and type IV collagen increase the intestinal crypt epithelial restitution.[58]

APOPTOSIS

The rapid turnover rate of the mucosal epithelial cell (24–96 h) is controlled by programmed cell death (apoptosis), which is recognized by defined morphological and biochemical features.[77,184] This conserved evolutionary process, critical to maintain tissue homeostasis,[91,157] is known to be affected by dietary agents. In particular, dietary fibres which undergo anaerobic fermentation in the colon produce short-chain fatty acids (acetate, propionate and butyrate) and these account for an estimated 70% of the total energy consumption in the colon.[67,160] Sodium butyrate has been found to be associated with induction of apoptotic Bax in the colon and apoptosis.[68]

Apoptosis is also important in chronic inflammatory and neoplastic conditions where it is found dysregulated.[161,166]

Detection of apoptosis

Apoptosis, from the Greek (Apo, off; ptosis, falling), is characterized by cell shrinkage, chromatin condensation and nuclear fragmentation which appears on agarose gel electrophoresis as a ladder of 180–200 bp nucleosomal fragments.[190] These changes result in the formation of apoptotic bodies which are then phagocytosed by the cells of the immune system. Since apoptosis is a rapid process (only a few hours) and the apoptotic bodies are

cleared from the tissues, it is not always detectable by morphological means. Unfortunately, most of the techniques used for detection of apoptosis present with technical limitations. Therefore, when carrying out these studies more than one complementary technique must always be used. One of the most common methods is the terminal deoxynucleotidyl transferase (TdT) labelling technique which labels the 3' OH ends of the DNA. However, with this method not only apoptosis but also necrosis[61] can be detected, and the numbers of cell labelled in the intestine is highly dependent on the technical conditions.[77] Early apoptotic stages can also be detected by exploiting the externalization of phosphatidylserine, which in physiological conditions is located mainly on the inner plasma membrane.[44]

Control of apoptosis

Although the intracellular signalling pathways are not fully elucidated it is known that they are under the control of specific apoptotic/antiapoptotic regulatory genes, among which the *Fas/FasL*[6,129] and the *Bcl2* families,[99,135] respectively, are the most studied. The death signal triggers the binding of *Fas* to its receptor, *FasL*, and induces its trimerization. This activates a death domain responsible for the recruitment of a cascade of enzymes (called caspases). The last step of the cascade involves the activation of caspase 3, which induces the morphological alterations seen in apoptosis.[181]

Bcl2 was first described in B cell lymphomas and it is thought to be responsible for the neoplastic process because it prevents apoptosis. All the members of the *Bcl2* family (except for *Bad*) are predominantly located in the cell cytoplasm and the outer mitochondrial membrane.[2,129,135] The *Bcl2* family consists of antiapoptotic members (*Bcl2*, *Bcl-XL*, *Mcl-1*) and proapoptotic members (*Bax*, *BclX s*, *Bad*), which regulate each other through the formation of homodimers and heterodimers.[34] In particular, *Bad*, *Bak* and *Bax* can dimerize with *Bcl2* or *BclX*, thus inhibiting apoptosis. The fine balance between apoptotic and antiapoptotic regulatory genes of the *Bcl2* family is responsible for cell survival.[99,157]

Increased apoptotic rates in the villus tips of the small intestine and the luminal surface of the epithelial cells of the colon have been reported but these are unexpected and final confirmation is pending. However, stem cells in the small and large intestine have been shown to undergo apoptosis.[152,156] The documentation that the antiapoptotic Bcl2 molecule is expressed in proliferating colonic crypts and stem cells while the proapoptotic Bax molecule is expressed in the proximity of the lumen in the colon supports the involvement of apoptosis in iEC shedding. Conversely, in the crypts of the small intestine, *Bcl2* is not expressed while Bax protein is. It has been suggested that the differential expression of the Bcl2 family proteins may explain the higher frequency of colon cancer in comparison to the known low prevalence of cancer of the small intestine.[71,98,155]

The expression of *Fas/FasL* system has also been investigated. The Paneth cells of the small intestine express *FasL* and the normal colonic epithelial cells express *Fas* and are sensitive to *Fas* receptor crosslinking, thus indicating that they are potentially susceptible to apoptosis.[124,178] Studies are currently in progress to assess whether specific patterns of apoptotic/antiapoptotic gene expression can be identified in inflammatory bowel disease which can be targeted to devise possible therapeutic strategies. In animal models, the release of proinflammatory cytokines from activated small bowel IEL has been shown to play a role in the homeostasis of the villus epithelial cells and on the kinetics of epithelial renewal. It is possible that cytokine production could contribute to apoptosis through dysregulation of apoptotic/antiapoptotic gene expression.[66]

FUTURE DIRECTIONS

It is envisaged that, within the next decade, at least some of the questions still pending concerning enterocyte pleiotropic functions will be elucidated. In particular, an answer is expected about whether iEC are able to function *in vivo* as antigen-presenting cells; the functional role(s) of the novel non-conventional HLA-related molecules expressed on iEC; and the function of the gut epithelium as an alternative primary lymphoid organ for IEL subsets. Further clarification is also awaited on the complex interactions of the iEC–IEL biological unit both in physiological conditions and after bacterial exposure.

Finally, a clearer insight on the constitutive and cytokine-induced role of apoptotic and antiapoptotic regulatory genes involved in iEC homeostasis and disease-induced death should also be achieved.

REFERENCES

1 Abrahamson DR, Rodewald R. Evidence for the sorting of endocytic vesicle contents during receptor-mediated transport of IgG across newborn rat intestine. *J Cell Biol* 1981; 91: 270–80.

2 Adams JM, Cory S. The Bcl2 protein family: arbiters of cell survival. *Science* 1998; 281: 1322–6.

3 Amigorena S, Drake JR, Webster P, Mellman I. Transient accumulation of new class II MHC molecules in a novel endocytic compartment in B lymphoctes. *Nature* 1994; 369: 113–20.

4 Andoh A, Fujiama Y, Bamba T, Hasoda S. Differential cytokine regulation of complement C3, C4 and factor B synthesis in human intestinal epithelial cell line, CaCO$_2$. *J Immunol* 1993; 151: 4239–49.

5 Armitage RJ, Namen AE, Sassenfeld HM, Grabstein KH. Regulation of human T cell proliferation by IL7. *J Immunol* 1990; 144: 938–41.

6 Ashkenazi A, Dixit M. Death reception: signalling and modulation. *Science* 1998; 281: 1305–8.

7 Avery A, Paraskeva C, Hall P *et al*. TGFβ expression in the human colon. differential immunostaining along crypt epithelium. *Br J Cancer* 1993; 68: 137–9.

8 Babyatsky MW, Rossiter G, Podolski DK. Expression of transforming growth factor α and β in colonic mucosa in inflammatory bowel disease. *Gastroenterology* 1996; 100: 975–84.

9 Bahram S, Spies T. Nucleotide sequence of a human MHC Class I MICB cDNA. *Immunogenetics* 1996; 43: 230–3.

10 Bahram S, Bresnahan S, Geraghty DE *et al*. A second lineage of mammalian major histocompatibility complex class I genes. *Proc Natl Acad Sci USA* 1994; 91: 6259–63.

11 Balk SP, Ebert E, Blumenthal RL *et al*. Oligoclonal expansion and CD1 recognition by human intestinal intraepithelial lymphocytes. *Science* 1991; 253: 1411–15.

12 Beckman EM, Brenner MB. MHC Class I-like, Class II-like and CD1 molecules: distinct roles in immunity. *Immunology Today* 1995; 16: 349–52.

13 Bengmark S. Ecological control of the gastrointestinal tract. The role of probiotic flora. *Gut* 1998; 42: 2–7.

14 Bjorkman PJ, Saper MA, Samraoui B, Bennett WS, Strominger JL, Wiley DC. The foreign antigen binding site and T cell recognition region of class I histocompatibility antigens. *Nature* 1987; 329: 512–18.

15 Bjorkman PJ, Saper MA, Samroui B *et al*. Structure of the human class I histocompatibility antigen HLA-A2. *Nature* 1995; 329: 506–12.

16 Bland P. MHC Class II expression by the gut epithelium. *Immunology Today* 1988; 9: 174–8.

17 Bland PW, Warren LG. Antigen presentation by epithelial cells of the rat small intestine. I. Kinetics, antigen specificity and blocking by anti-Ia antisera. *Immunology* 1986; 58: 1–7.

18 Bland PW, Warren LG. Antigen presentation by epithelial cells of the rat small intestine II. Selective induction of suppressor T cells. *Immunology* 1986; 58: 9–14.

19 Bleicher PA, Balk SP, Hagen SJ, Blumberg RS, Flotte TJ, Terhorst C. Expression of murine CD1 on gastrointestinal epithelium. *Science* 1990; 250: 679–84.

20 Blumberg RS. Current concepts in mucosal immunity II. One size fits all: non-classical MHC molecules fulfil multiple roles in epithelial cell function. *Am J Physiol* 1998; 274: G227–31.

21 Blumberg RS, Balk SP. Intraepithelial lymphocytes and their recognition of non-classical MHC molecules. *Int Rev Immunol* 1994; 11: 15–30.

22 Blumberg RS, Terhost C, Bleicher P *et al*. Expression of a non-polymorphic MHC class I-like molecule, CD1d by human intestinal epithelial cells. *J Immunol* 1991; 147: 2518–24.

23 Blumberg RS, Gerdes D, Chott A, Porcelli SA, Balk SP. Structure and function of the CD1 family of MHC-like cell surface proteins. *Immunol Reviews* 1995; 147: 1–29.

24 Blumberg RS, Colgan SP, Balk SP. Cd1d. outside-in antigen presentation in the intestinal epithelium? *Clin Exp Immunol* 1996; 109: 223–5.

25 Blumberg RS, Simister N, Christ AD *et al*. MHC-like molecules on mucosal epithelial cells. In: *Mucosal Immunology* , (Kagnoff MF, Kiyono H eds). Academic Press, San Diego, CA 1996; 85–96.

26 Boismenu R, Havran WL. Modulation of epithelial cell growth by intraepithelial γδ cells. *Science* 1994; 266: 1253–5.

27 Borghesi C, Regoli M, Bertelli E, Niocoletti C. Modifications of the follicle-associated epithelium by short-term exposure to a non-intestinal bacterium. *J Path* 1996; 180: 326–32.

28 Brandtzaeg P. Distribution and characteristics of mucosal Ig producing cells. In: *Handbook of Mucosal Immunology* (Ogra PL *et al*., eds), Academic Press, San Diego, CA 1994, 251–62.

29 Brodsky FM. Living with clathrin: its role in intracellular membrane traffic. *Science* 1984; 242: 1396–402.

30 Brossay L, Jullien D, Cardell S, Sydora BC, Burdin N, Modlin RL, Kronenberg M. Mouse CD1 is mainly expressed on hemopoietic-derived cells. *J Immunol* 1997; 159: 1216–24.

31 Calabi F, Jarvis JM, Martin LH, Milstein C. Two classes of CD1 genes. *Eur J Immunol* 1989; 19: 285–92.

32 Carsley-Smith JR. The passage of ferritin into jejunal epithelial cells. *Experientia* 1967; 23: 370–1.

33 Cepek KL, Shaw SK, Parker CM *et al*. Adhesion between epithelial cells and T lymphocytes mediated by E-cadherin and the αεβ7 integrin. *Nature* 1994; 372: 190–3.

34 Chao DT, Korsemeyer SJ. Bc12 family; regulation of cell death. *Annu Rev Immunol* 1998; 16: 395–419.

35 Christ AD, Blumberg RS. The intestinal epithelial cell: immunological aspects. *Springer Semin Immunopathol* 1997; 18: 449–61.

36 Ciacci C, Mahida YR, Dignass A, Koizumi M, Podolski DK. Functional interleukin-2 receptors on intestinal epithelial cells. *J Clin Invest* 1993; 92: 527–33.

37 Cornell R, Walker WA, Isselbacher KJ. Small intestinal absorption of horseradish peroxidase. A cytochemical study. *Lab Invest* 1971; 25: 42–8.

38 Cresswell P. Assembly, transport and function of MHC Class II molecules. *Annu Rev Immunol* 1994; 12: 259–93.

39 Eckmann L, Jung HC, Schuerer-Maly CC, Panja A, Morzycka-Wrobleska E, Kagnoff MF. Differential cytokine expression by human intestinal cell lines; regulated expression of interleukin 8. *Gastroenterology* 1993; 105: 1689–97.

40 Eckmann L, Reed SL, Smith JR, Kagnoff MF. Entamoeba histolytical trophozoites induce an inflammatory cytokine response by cultured

human cells through the paraczine action of cytolytically released interleukin-1 alpha. *J Clin Invest* 1995; 96: 1269–79.

41 Efstathiou JA, Pignotelli M. Modulation of epithelial cell adhesion in gastrointestinal homeostasis. *Am J Path* 1998; 153: 341–7.

42 Eisenhaner PB, Harwig SS, Lehrer RI. Cryptdins: antimicrobial defensing of the murine small intestine. *Infect Immun* 1992; 60: 3556–62.

43 Engelhard VH. Structure of peptides associated with MHC class I molecules. *Curr Opin Immunol* 1994; 6: 13–23.

44 Fadok VA, Voelker DR, Campbell PA, Henson PM. Exposure of phosphatidylserine on the surface of apoptotic lymphocytes triggers specific recognition and removal by macrophages. *J Immunol* 1992; 148: 2207–16.

45 Farstad IN, Halstensen TS, Feusa O, Brandtzaeg P. Heterogeneity of M cell-associated B and T cells in human Peyer's Patches. *Immunology* 1994; 83: 457–64.

46 Fierer J, Eckmann L, Kagnoff MF. IL8 secreted by epithelial cells invaded by bacteria. *Infect Agents Dis* 1993; 2: 255–60.

47 Finzi G, Cornaggia M, Capeela C *et al.* Cathepsin E in follicle associated epithelium of intestine and tonsils. localization to M cells and possible role in antigen processing. *Histochemistry* 1993; 99: 201–11.

48 Fremont DH, Matsumura M, Stura EA, Peterson PA, Wilson I. Crystal structures of two viral peptides in complex with murine MHC class I H-2k^b. *Science* 1992; 257: 919–27.

49 Fremont DH, Hendrikson WA, Marrak P, Kappler J. Structure of an MHC Class II molecule with covalently bound single peptide. *Science* 1996; 272: 1001–4.

50 Gaidar YA. Vimentin-positive epithelial cells in the cupolas of the aggregated lymphoid noduli (Peyer's patches) of the rabbit. *Arch Anat Histol Embryol* 1989; 97: 84–8.

51 Gangarosa LM, Dempsey PJ, Damstrup L, Barnard JA, Coffey RJ. Transforming growth factor α. *Bailliére's Clin Gastroenterol* 1996; 10: 49–63.

52 Gebert A, Rothkotter HJ, Pabst R. M cells in Peyer's patches of the intestine. *Int Rev Cytol* 1996; 167: 91–159.

53 Germain RN. MHC dependent antigen processing and peptide presentation: providing ligands for T lymphocyte activation. *Cell* 1994; 76: 87–299.

54 Geuze HJ. The role of endosomes and lysosomes in MHC Class II functioning. *Immunology Today* 1998; 19: 282–7.

55 Geuze HJ, Slot JW, Strous GJAM *et al.* Intracellular receptor sorting during endocytosis: comparative immunoelectron microscopy of multiple receptors in rat liver. *Cell* 1984; 37: 195–204.

56 Geuze HJ, Slot JW, Schwartz AL. Membrane of sorting organelles displays lateral heterogeneity in receptor distribution. *J Cell Biol* 1987; 104: 1715–23.

57 Ghetie V, Ward ES. FcRN. the MCH class I-related receptor that is more than an IgG transporter. *Immunology Today* 1997; 18: 592–97.

58 Göke M, Podolski DK. Regulation of the mucosal barrier. *Bailliére's Clin Gastroenterol* 1996; 10: 393–405.

59 Goldberg AL, Rock KL. Proteolysis, proteosomes and antigen presentation. *Nature* 1992; 357: 375–9.

60 Goodwin RG, Lupton S, Schmierer A *et al.* Human interleukin 7: molecular cloning and growth factor activity on human and murine B-lineage cells. *Proc Natl Acad Sci (USA)* 1989; 86: 302–6.

61 Grasl-Kroupp B, Ruttkay-Nedecky H, Koudelka K, Bukowska K, Bursch W, Schulte-Hermann R. In situ detection of fragmented DNA (TUNEL assay) fails to discriminate among apoptosis, necrosis and antolytic cell death: a cautionary note. *Hepatology* 1995; 21: 1465–8.

62 Griffith E, Ramsburg E, Hayday A. Recognition by human gut γδ cells of stress inducible major histocompatibility molecules on enterocytes. *Gut* 1998; 43: 166–7.

63 Groh V, Bahram S, Bauer S, Herman A, Beauchamp M, Spies T. Cell stress related human histocompatibility complex class I gene expressed in gastrointestinal epithelium. *Proc Natl Acad Sci (USA)* 1996; 93: 12445–50.

64 Guy-Grand D, Vassalli P. Gut intraepithelial T lymphocytes. *Curr Opin Immunol* 1993; 5: 247–52.

65 Guy-Grand D, Cerf-Bensussan N, Malissen B, Malassis-Seris M, Briottet C, Vassalli P. Two gut intraepithelial CD8+ lymphocyte populations with different T cell receptors: a role of the gut epithelium in T cell differentiation. *J Exp Med* 1991; 173: 471–8.

66 Guy-Grand D, DiSanto JP, Henchoz P, MalAssis-Seris M, Vassalli P. Small bowel enteropathy: role of intraepithelial lymphocytes and of cytokines (IL-12, IFNα, TNF) in the induction of epithelial cell death and renewal. *Eur J Immunol* 1998; 28: 730–44.

67 Hague A, Singh B, Paraskeva C. Butyrate acts as a survival factor for colonic epithelial cells: further fuel for the in vivo versus in vitro debate. *Gastroenterology* 1997; 112: 1036–40.

68 Hass R, Busche R, Luciano L, Reale E, Engelhardt W. Lack of butyrate is associated with induction of Bax and subsequent apoptosis in the proximal colon of guinea pig. *Gastroenterology* 1997; 112: 875–81.

69 Hershberg RM, Framson PE, Cho DH *et al.* Intestinal epithelial cells use two abstract pathways for HLA Class II antigen processing. *J Clin Invest* 1997; 100: 204–15.

70 Hershberg RM, Cho DA, Yovakim A *et al.* Highly polarised HLA Class II antigen processing and presentation by human intestinal epithelial cells. *J Clin Invest* 1998; 102: 792–803.

71 Hockenberry DM, Zutter M, Hickey W, Nahm M, Korsmeyer S. Bc12 protein is topographically restricted in tissues characterised by apoptotic cell death. *Proc Natl Acad Sci (USA)* 1991; 88: 6961–5.

72 Huang GT, Eckmann L, Savidge TC, Kagnoff MF. Infection of human intestinal epithelial cells with invasive bacteria upregulates apical intercellular adhesion molecule-1 (ICAM-1) expression and neutrophil adhesion. *J Clin Invest* 1996; 98: 572–83.

73 Israel EJ, Taylor S, Wu Z *et al.* Expansion of the neonatal Fc receptor, FcRn, in human intestinal epithelial cells. *Immunology* 1997; 92: 69–74.

74 Ito S. Form and function of the glycocalyx on free cell surfaces. *Philos Trans R Soc London Ser* 1974; B268: 55–66.

75 Jepson MA, Clark MA. Studying M cells and their role in infection. *Trends in Microbiol* 1998; 6: 359–65.

76 Jondal M, Schrimbeck R, Reinmann J. MHC Class I-restricted CTL responses to exogenous antigens. *Immunity* 1996; 5: 295–300.

77 Jones BA, Gores GJ. Physiology and pathophysiology of apoptosis in epithelial cells of the liver, pancreas and intestine. *Am J Physiol* 1997; 273: G1174–88.

78 Jullien D, Stenger S, Ernst WA, Modlin RL. CD1 presentation of microbial non peptide antigens to T cells. *J Clin Invest* 1997; 99: 2071–4.

79 Junghans RP. Finally! The Brambell receptor (FcRB). mediation of transmission of immunity and protection from catabolism for IgG. *Immunol Res* 1997; 16: 29–57.

80 Kaetzel CS, Robinson JK, Chintalacharuvu KR, Vaeman JP, Lamm ME. The polymeric Ig receptor (secretory component) mediates transport of immune complexes across epithelial cells: a local defense function of IgA. *Proc Natl Acad Sci (USA)* 1991; 88: 8796–800.

81 Kagnoff MF. Immunology of the digestive system. In: *Physiology of the Gastrointestinal Tract*, 2nd ed. (Johnson LR, ed.) New York, Raven Press, 1987: 1699–728.

82 Kagnoff MF, Eckmann L. Epithelial cells as sensors for microbial infection. *J Clin Invest* 1997; 100 (Suppl): 551–5.

83 Kaiserlain D, Vidal K, Revillard JP. Murine enterocytes can present soluble antigen to specific class II restricted CD4+ T cells. *Eur J Immunol* 1989; 19: 1513–16.

84 Kanamori Y, Ishimaru K, Nanno M *et al.* Identification of novel lymphoid tissues in murine intestinal mucosa where clusters of c-kit+ IL7R+thy1+lymphopoietic progenitors develop. *J Exp Med* 1996; 184: 1449–59.

85 Kasai K, Matsuura A, Kikuchi K, Hashimoto Y, Ichimiya S. Localization of rat CD1 transcripts and protein in rat tissues: an analysis of rat CD1 expression by in situ hybridization and immunochemistry. *Clin Exp Immunol* 1997; 103: 317–22.

86 Kato T, Owen RL. Structure and function of intestinal mucosal epithelium. In: *Handbook in Immunology* (Ogra PL *et al.*, eds), Academic Press, San Diego, CA 1994: 11–24.

87 Kedinger M, Fritsch C, Evans GS *et al.* Role of stromal–epithelial cell interactions and of basement membrane molecules in the onset and maintenance of epithelial integrity. In: *Essentials of Mucosal Immunology* (Kagnoff MF, Kiyono H, eds). Academic Press, San Diego, CA 1996; 111–23.

88 Kelly CP, O'Keane JC, Ocellana J et al. Human colon cancer cells express ICAM-1 in vivo and support LFA-1 dependent lymphocyte adhesion in vitro. *Am J Physiol* 1992; 263: G864–70.

89 Kelsall BL, Strober W. Host defenses at mucosal surface. In: *Clinical Immunology* (Rich RR, Fleisher TA, Schwartz BD et al., eds), Mosby, St Louis, Missouri 1996; 299–332.

90 Kerneis S, Bogdanova A, Kraenhenbuhl JB, Pringault E. Conversion by Peyer's patch lymphocytes of human enterocytes into M cells that transport bacteria. *Science* 1997; 277: 949–53.

91 Kerr JRF, Wyllie AH, Curie AR. Apoptosis: a basic biological phenomenon with widespread implications in tissue kinetics. *Br J Cancer* 1972; 26: 239–257.

92 Khoury SJ, Hancock WW, Weiner HL. Oral tolerance to myelin basic protein and natural recovery from experimental autoimmune encephalomyelitis are associated with downregulation of inflammatory cytokines and differential upregulation of transforming growth factor β, interleukin 4 and prostaglandin E expression in the brain. *J Exp Med* 1992; 176: 1355–76.

93 Kiyono H, Fujihashi K, Yamamoto M et al. Intraepithelial γδ T cell and epithelial cell interactions in the mucosal immune system. In: *Essentials of Mucosal Immunology* (Kagnoff MF, Kiyono M, eds) Academic Press, San Diego, CA 1996; 195–203.

94 Klein JR. Whence the intestinal intraepithelial lymphocyte? *J Exp Med* 1996; 184: 1203–6.

95 Knutton S, Limbrick AR, Robertson JD. Regular structures in membranes: membranes in the endocyte complex of ileal epithelial cells. *J Cell Biol* 1974: 62: 679–94.

96 Komano H, Fujura Y, Kawaguchi M et al. Homeostatic regulation of intestinal epithelia by intra-epithelial lymphocytes. *Proc Natl Acad Sci (USA)* 1995; 92: 6147–51.

97 Kornfield S, Mellman I. The biogenesis of lysosomes. *Annu Rev Cell Biol* 1989; 5: 483–525.

98 Krajewski SM, Krajewska M, Shabaik A, Miyashita T, Wang HG, Reed JC. Immunohistochemical determination of in vivo distribution of Bax, dominant inhibitor of Bcl2. *Am J Path* 1994; 145: 1323–36.

99 Kroemer G. The protooncogene Bcl2 and its role in regulating apoptosis. *Nature Med* 1997; 3: 614–20.

100 Kurokawa M. Effects of growth factors on an intestinal epithelial cell line: Transforming growth factor β inhibits proliferation and stimulates differentiation. *Biochem Biophys Res Commun* 1987; 142: 775–82.

101 Lamm ME. Interaction of antigens and antibodies at mucosal surfaces. *Annu Rev Microbiol* 1997; 51: 311–40.

102 Lamm ME. Current concepts in mucosal immunity IV. How epithelial transport of IgA antibodies relates to host defense. *Am J Physiol* 1998; 274: G6 14–7.

103 Lanzabecchia A, Reid PA, Watts C. Irreversible association of peptides with Class II MHC molecules in living cells. *Nature* 1992; 357: 249–52.

104 Laurie GW, Lebond CP, Martin GR. Localization of type IV collagen, amin, heparan sulphate, proteoglycan and fibronectin to the basal lamina of basement membrane. *J Cell Biol* 1982; 95: 340–4.

105 Lefrancois L. Basic aspects of intraepithelial lymphocyte immunobiology. In: *Handbook of Mucosal Immunology* (Ogra PL, McGhee JR, Mestecky J et al., eds), Academic Press, San Diego, CA 1994: 287–97.

106 Lefrancois L, Puddington L. Extrathymic intestinal T cell development: virtual reality? *Immunology Today* 1995; 16: 16–21.

107 Li Y, Yio XY, Mayer L. Human intestinal epithelial cell induced CD8+ T cell activation is mediated through CD8 and the activation of CD8-associated p56lck. *J Exp Med* 1995; 182: 1079–88.

108 Luggering N, Kucharzik T, Gockel H, Sorg C, Stoll R, Domsche W: Human intestinal epithelial cells down-regulate IL8 expression in human intestinal microvascular endothelial cells; role of transforming growth factor-beta 1 (TGF.B1). *Clin Exp Immunol* 1998; 114: 377–84.

109 MacDonald TT. T cell immunity to oral allergens. *Curr Opin Immunol* 1998; 10: 620–7.

110 Madara JL. Pathobiology of the intestinal epithelial barrier. *Am J Pathol* 1990; 137: 1273–81.

111 Madara JL. Migration of neutrophils through epithelial monolayers. *Trends Cell Biol* 1994; 4: 4–7.

112 Madara JL. The chameleon within; improving antigen delivery. *Science* 1997; 227: 910–11.

113 Madden DR. The three-dimensional structure of peptide-MHC complexes. *Annu Rev Immunol* 1995; 13: 587–622.

114 Mayer L. Antigen presentation in the intestine. *Curr Opin Gastroenterol* 1991; 7: 446–9.

115 Mayer L. Regulation of mucosal immune responses: distinct antigens and antigen presenting cells. *J Clin Immunol* 1997; 17: 349–53.

116 Mayer L. Current concepts in mucosal immunity I. Antigen presentation in the intestine: new rules and regulations. *Am J Physiol* 1998; 274: G67–9.

117 Mayer L, Shilen R. Evidence for function of Ia molecules on gut epithelium in man. *J Exp Med* 1987; 166: 1471–83.

118 Maury J, Nicoletti C, Guzzo-Chambraud I, Maroux S. The filamentous brush border glycocalyx, a mucin-like marker of enterocyte hyperpolarization. *Eur J Biochem* 1995; 228: 323–31.

119 Maxfield FR, Yamashiro DJ. Acidification of organelles and the intracellular sorting of proteins during endocytosis. In: *Intracellular Trafficking of Proteins* (Steer CJ, Hanover JA, eds). Cambridge University Press, Cambridge, 1991: 157–82.

120 McCarthy-Francis NL, Wahl SM. Transforming growth factor β: a matter of life and death. *J Leuk Biol* 1994; 55: 401–9.

121 McCormack BA, Jung HC, Eckmann L et al. A distinct array of proinflammatory cytokines is expressed in human colon epithelial cells in response to bacterial invasion. *J Clin Invest* 1995; 95: 55–65.

122 Miller A, Lider O, Roberts AB, Sporn MB, Weiner HL. Suppressor T cells generated by oral tolerization to myelin basic protein suppress both in vitro and in vivo immune responses by the release of transforming growth factor β after antigen-specific triggering. *Proc Natl Acad Sci (USA)* 1992; 89: 421–6.

123 Moller G. Origin of major histocompatibility complex diversity. *Immunol Reviews* 1995; 143: 5–292.

124 Moller P, Walczak H, Riedl S, Strater J, Krammer PH. Paneth cells express high levels of CD95 ligand transcripts – a unique proprietary among gastrointestinal epithelia. *Am J Path* 1996; 149: 9–13.

125 Mooseker M. Organization, chemistry and assembly of the cytoskeletal apparatus of the intestinal brush border. *Annu Rev Cell Biol* 1985; 1: 209–41.

126 Mostov KE. Transepithelial transport of Igs. *Annu Rev Immunol* 1994; 12: 3–84.

127 Mowat A, Viney JL. The anatomical basis of intestinal immunity. *Immunol Reviews* 1997; 156: 145–66.

128 Murphy S, Walker WA. Antigen absorption. In: *Food Allergy. Adverse Reaction to Foods and Additives* (Metcalfe DD et al., eds). Blackwell, Oxford, UK 1997; 93–105.

129 Nagata S. Apoptosis by death factor. *Cell* 1997; 88: 355–65.

130 Namen AE, Lupton S, Hjerrild K et al. Stimulation of B-cell progenitors by cloned murine interleukin 7. *Nature* 1988; 331: 571–5.

131 Neutra MR. Current concepts in mucosal immunity V. Role of M cells in transepithelial transport of antigens and pathogens to the mucosal immune system. *Am J Physiol* 1998; 274: G785–91.

132 Neutra MR, Pringawlt E, Kraehenbuhl JP. Antigen sampling across epithelial barriers and induction of mucosal immune responses. *Annu Rev Immunol* 1996; 14: 275–300.

133 Neutra MR, Frey A, Kraehenbulh JP. Epithelial M cells: gateways from mucosal infection. *Cell* 1996; 86: 345–48.

134 Neutra MR, Kraehenbuhl JP. Cellular and molecular basis for antigen transport in the intestinal epithelium. In: *Handbook in Immunology* (Ogra PL et al., eds). Academic Press, San Diego, CA 1994; 27–35.

135 Newton K, Strasser A. The Bcl2 family and cell death regulation. *Curr Opin Genet Develop* 1998; 8: 68–75.

136 North RJ. Endocytosis. *Semin Hematol* 1970; 7: 161–71.

137 Ohtsuka A, Piazza AJ, Ermak TH, Owen RL. Correlation of extracellular matrix components with the cytoarchitecture of Peyer's patches. *Cell Tissue Res* 1992; 269: 403–10.

138 Owen RL. M cells – entryways of opportunity for enteropathogens. *J Exp Med* 1994; 180: 7–9.

139 Owen RL. Sequential uptake of horseradish peroxidase by lymphoid follicle epithelium of Peyer's patches in the normal unobstructed mouse intestine: an ultrastructural study. *Gastroenterology* 1997; 72: 440–51.

140 Owen RL, Jones AL. Epithelial cell specialisation within Peyer's patches: an ultrastructural study of human intestinal lymphoid follicles. *Gastroenterology* 1974; 66: 189–203.

141 Panja A, Mayer L. Antigen presentation in the intestine. *Baillière's Clin Gastroenterol* 1996; 10: 407–425.

142 Panja A, Blumberg RS, Balk SP, Mayer L. CD1d is involved in T cell epithelial cell interactions. *J Exp Med* 1993; 178: 1115–19.

143 Parham P, Adams EJ, Arnett KL. The origin of HLA-ABC polymorphism. *Immunol Reviews* 1995; 143: 141–80.

144 Park SH, Chiu Y-H, Jaryawardena J, Roark J, Kavita U, Bendelac A. Innate and adaptive functions of the CD1 pathway of antigen presentation. *Semin Immunol* 1998; 10: 391–8.

145 Parkos CA, Colgan SP, Diamond MS *et al.* Expression and polarization of intercellular adhesion molecule-1 a human intestinal epithelial: consequences for CD11b/CD18 mediated interaction with neutrophils. *Mol Med* 1996; 2: 489–505.

146 Peschon J, Morissey PJ, Grabstein KH *et al.* Early lymphocyte expansion is severely impaired in IL7R deficient mice. *J Exp Med* 1994; 180: 1955–60.

147 Pignatelli M, Gilligan CJ. Transforming growth factor β in GI neoplasia, wound healing and immune response. *Baillière's Clin Gastroenterol* 1996; 10: 65–81.

148 Podolski DK. Regulatory peptides and integration of the intestinal epithelium in mucosal responses. In: *Essential of Mucosal Immunology* (Kagnoff MF, Kiyono M, eds). Academic Press, San Diego, CA 1996: 101–9.

149 Podolski DK, Kindon H, Lynch-Devaney K, Dignass A, Babyatski M. Epithelium in inflammatory bowel disease: trefoil peptides at the interface. In: *Inflammatory bowel disease* (Tytgat GNJ *et al.*, eds). Falk Symposium 85, Kluwer, Dordrecht 1995: 360–65.

150 Porcelli S, Morita CT, Brenner MB. CD1b restricts the response of human CD4⁻8⁻ T cell lymphocytes to a microbial antigen. *Nature* 1992; 360: 593–7.

151 Porcelli SA, Morita CT, Modlin RL. T cell recognition of non-peptide antigens. *Curr Opin Immunol* 1996; 8: 510–16.

152 Potten CS. Epithelial cell growth and differentiation. II Intestinal apoptosis. *Am J Physiol* 1997; 273: G253–7.

153 Poussier P, Julius M. T cell development and selection in the intestinal epithelium. *Semin Immunol* 1995; 7: 321–334.

154 Quaroni A, Isselbacher KJ, Ruoshlathi E. Fibronectin synthesis by epithelial crypt cells of rat small intestine. *Proc Natl Acad Sci USA* 1978; 75: 5548–52.

155 Que F, Gores G. Cell death by apoptosis: basic concepts and disease relevance for the gastroenterologist. *Gastroenterology* 1996; 110: 1238–43.

156 Quiao L, Kozoni V, Trioulias GJ *et al.* Selected eicosanoids increase the proliferation rate of human colon carcinoma cell lines and mouse colonocytes in vivo. *Biochem Biophys Acta* 1995; 1258: 215–23.

157 Raff MC. Social controls on cell survival and cell death. *Nature* 1992; 356: 398–400.

158 Reinecker HC, Podolski DK. Human intestinal epithelial cells express functional cytokine receptors sharing the common γc chain of the interleukin 2-receptor. *Proc Natl Acad Sci USA* 1995; 92: 8353–60.

159 Reinecker HC, Loh EY, Ringler DJ, Mehta A, Rombeau JL, MacDermott RP. Monocyte-chemoattractant protein 1 gene expression in intestinal epithelial cells and inflammatory bowel disease mucosa. *Gastroenterology* 1995; 108: 40–50.

160 Roediger WEW. Role of anaerobic bacteria in the metabolic welfare of the colonic mucosa in man. *Gut* 1980; 21: 793–8.

161 Rudin CM, Thompson CB. Apoptosis and disease. *Annu Rev Med* 1997; 48: 267–81.

162 Sanderson IR, Walker WA. Mucosal barrier. In: *Handbook in Mucosal Immunology* (Ogra PL, McGhee JR, Mestecky J *et al*, eds). Academic Press, San Diego, CA 1994; 41–50.

163 Sanderson IR, Oullette AJ, Carter EA, Walker WA, Harmatz PR. Differential regulation of B7 mRNA in enterocytes and lymphoid cells. *Immunology* 1993; 79: 434–8.

164 Santos LMB, Al-Sabbagh A, Londono A, Weiner HL. Oral tolerance to myelin basic protein induces regulatory TGFβ secreting cells in Peyer's patches of SJL mice. *Cell Immunol* 1994; 157: 439–48.

165 Savidge TC, Smith MW. Evidence that membranous (M) cell genesis is immunoregulated. In: *Advances in Mucosal Immunology* (Mestecky J, ed.). New York, Plenum, 1995: 239–41.

166 Savill J. Apoptosis in disease. *Eur J Clin Invest* 1998; 281: 1317–22.

167 Schuerer-Maly CC, Eckmann L, Kagnoff MF, Felco MT, Maly FE. Colonic epithelial cell lines as a source of interleukin-8: stimulation by inflammatory cytokine and bacterial lipopolysaccharide. *Immunology* 1994; 81: 85–91.

168 Scott H, Solheim BG, Brandtzaeg P *et al.* HLADR like antigens in the epithelium of the human small intestine. *Scand J Immunol* 1980; 12: 77–82.

169 Semenza G. Anchoring and biosynthesis of stalked brush border membrane glycoproteins. *Annu Rev Cell Biol* 1986; 2: 255–314.

170 Shanahan F. A gut reaction: lymphoepithelial communication in the intestine. *Science* 1997; 275: 1897–8.

171 Shepherd JC, Schumacher TNM, Ashton-Rickardt PG *et al.* TAP-1-dependent peptide translocation in vitro is ATP-dependent and peptide-selective. *Cell* 1993; 74: 577–84.

172 Shibata Y, Arima T, Yamamoto T. Regular structures on the microvillar surface membrane of ileal cells in suckling intestine. *J Ultrastruct Res* 1983; 85: 70–81.

173 Simon-Assmann P, Bouziges F, Freund JN *et al.* Type IV collagen mRNA accumulates in the mesenchymal compartment at early stages of murine developing intestine. *J Cell Biol* 1990; 110: 849–57.

174 Smith MW, James PS, Tivey DR. M cell numbers increase after transfer of SPF mice to a normal animal house environment. *Am J Pathol* 1987; 128: 385–9.

175 Snyder JS, Walker WA. Structure and function of intestinal mucin: developmental aspects. *Int Arch Allergy Appl Immunol* 1987; 82: 351–56.

176 Stern LJ, Wiley DC. Antigenic peptide binding by class I and class II histocompatibility proteins. *Structure* 1994; 2: 245–51.

177 Story CM, Mikulska JE, Simister NE. A major histocompatibility complex class I-like Fc receptor cloned from human placenta: possible role in transfer of immunoglobulin G from mother to fetus. *J Exp Med* 1994; 180: 2377–81.

178 Strater J, Wellish I, Kiedl S *et al.* CD95 (APO-1/Fas) mediated apoptosis in colon epithelial cells: a possible role in ulcerative colitis. *Gastroenterology* 1997; 113: 160–7.

179 Strobel S, Mowat MCI. Immune responses to dietary antigens: oral tolerance. *Immunology Today* 1998; 19: 173–81.

180 Svanborg C, Agace W, Hedges S, Hedlund M, Svensson M. Bacterial activation of mucosal cytokine production. In: *Essentials of Mucosal Immunology* (Kagnoff MF, Kiyono M, eds.) Academic Press, San Diego, CA 1996: 73–81.

181 Thornberry NA, Lazebnick Y. Caspases: enemies within. *Science* 1998; 281: 1312–16.

182 Watanabe M, Veno Y, Yajima T. Interleukin 7 is produced by human intestinal epithelial cells and regulates the proliferation of intestinal mucosa lymphocytes. *J Clin Invest* 1995; 95: 2945–53.

183 Watanabe M, Veno Y, Hibi T. Intestinal epithelial cell-derived interleukin-7 as a regulatory factor for intestinal mucosal lymphocytes. In: *Essentials of Mucosal Immunology* (Kagnoff MF, Kiyono H, eds). Academic Press, San Diego, CA 1996: 279–89.

184 Watson AJM. Necrosis and apoptosis in the gastrointestinal tract. *Gut* 1995; 37: 165–7.

185 Weiner HL. Oral tolerance: immune mechanisms and treatment of autoimmune diseases. *Immunology Today* 1997; 18: 335–43.

186 Welch PA, Namen AE, Goodwin RG, Armitage R, Cooper MD. Human IL7: a novel T cell growth factor. *J Immunol* 1989; 143: 3562–7.

187 Weltzin RAP, Jandris L, Michetti P, Fields BN, Kraehenbul JP, Neutra MR. Binding and transepithelial transport of immunoglobulins by intestinal M cells: demonstration using monoclonal IgA Ab against enteric viral proteins. *J Cell Biol* 1989; 108: 1673–85.

188 Williams N. T cells on the mucosal frontline. *Science* 1998; 280: 198–200.

189 Wolf PR, Ploegh HL. How MHC Class II molecules acquire peptide cargo: biosynthesis and trafficking through the endocytic pathway. *Annu Rev Cell Dev Biol* 1995; 11: 167–306.

B

183

190 Wyllie AH, Harris RGK, Smith AL, Dunlop D. Chromatin cleavage in apoptosis in association with condensed chromatin morphology and dependence on macromolecular synthesis. *J Pathol* 1984; 142: 67–77.

191 Yamamoto M, Fujihashi K, Kawabata K, McGhee JR, Kiyono H. A mucosal intranet: intestinal epithelial cells down-regulate intraepithelial, but not peripheral, T lymphocytes. *J Immunol* 1998; 160: 2188–96.

192 Yang SK, Eckmann L, Panja A, Kagnoff MF. Differential and regulated expression of C-X-C- and C-chemokines by human colon epithelial cells. *Gastroenterology* 1998.113: 1214–23

193 Yio XY, Mayer L. Characterization of a 180 kDa intestinal epithelial cell membrane glycoprotein gp180. A candidate molecule mediating T cell–epithelial cell interactions. *J Biol Chem* 1997; 272: 12786–92.

194 Zheng ZH, Castano AR, Segelke B, Stura EA, Peterson PA, Wilson IA. The crystal structure of murine CD1: an MHC-like fold with a large hydrophobic antigen binding groove. *Science* 1997; 277: 39–45.

Chapter 11

Mucosal antibodies and induction of the immunoglobulin A response

J. Mestecky and M. W. Russell

INTRODUCTION

The daily production of immunoglobulins (Ig) in a human weighing 75 kg is estimated to be 8 g. When individual isotypes are considered, roughly 60% of all Ig produced is of the IgA isotype (70 mg/kg/day), 30% is IgG (35 mg/kg/day) 7% is IgM (8 mg/kg/day), and there are small amounts of IgD and IgE.[103] However, human sera contain relatively low levels of IgA as compared to IgG because more than half of the IgA produced does not enter the circulation but is directly and selectively transported by a receptor-mediated mechanism into external secretions[103] (Fig. 11.1). Furthermore, the half-life of human serum IgA is considerably shorter because of its fast catabolism (5–6 days for IgA and 20–24 days for IgG). Although Ig of all isotypes have been detected in various human external secretions, there is a pronounced preponderance of IgA, particularly in its secretory IgA (S-IgA) form, in tears, saliva, colostrum and milk, nasal and all intestinal fluids. In contrast, male and female genital tract secretions, bronchoalveolar fluid, and hepatic bile may contain equal or greater levels of IgG than IgA.[62] However, it should be emphasized that the levels of Ig in external secretions depend on the methods used in their collection and subsequent processing (because of proteolytic degradation, which is not the same for all

isotypes) the dilution inevitable in the collection of some fluids (e.g. vaginal washes), the techniques employed in Ig measurement, and the standard Ig used, the presence of local inflammation, and potential hormonal influences. All these variables may contribute to the variations in levels of total as well as antigen-specific Ig frequently reported from different laboratories (for review see reference 62).

Because most secretory Ig is produced in corresponding mucosal tissues and is selectively transported into secretions, the induction of specific and protective antibodies at various sites has been the subject of extensive studies on effective immunization. Such efforts[98] are predicated on the anatomical and functional division of the mucosal immune system into inductive and effector sites. Inductive sites, such as intestinal Peyer's patches, contain cell populations involved in the uptake, processing and presentation of luminal antigens, and induction of specific humoral and cellular immune responses. Most importantly, antigen-sensitized lymphoid cells exit from the inductive sites to populate remote effector sites (e.g., lactating mammary gland) where the terminal differentiation of such migrating cells occurs. In both inductive and effector sites, extensive functional interdependence of lymphoid and epithelial cells distinguishes the mucosal from the systemic immune compartment.[23] Epithelial

B

185

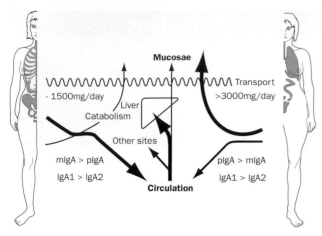

Fig. 11.1 Mucosal and circulatory compartments of the human IgA immune system. Circulating IgA is produced in the bone marrow, and consists mainly of mIgA and the IgA1 subclass; very little reaches the secretions, and it is mostly catabolized in the liver (a small fraction may escape catabolism and be transported into the bile). Mucosal IgA is produced in the effector sites of the mucosal immune system (e.g., the intestinal, respiratory and genital mucosae, and exocrine glands), and consists mainly of pIgA, with approximately similar amounts of both IgA1 and IgA2; little of this enters the circulation, and the majority is transported into secretions as S-IgA.

cells at the inductive site are necessary for the uptake, processing, and probably presentation of environmental antigen to resident lymphoid cells. At the effector sites the transport of locally produced Ig in external secretions is mediated by epithelial cells.

STRUCTURE OF MUCOSAL IMMUNOGLOBULINS

Although all external secretions contain Ig, there are considerable differences in levels and Ig isotype distribution among various secretions in addition to pronounced species differences. For example, human colostrum and milk contain IgA as the dominant isotype, while in pig and cow milks, IgG levels exceed those of IgA. Nevertheless, with the exception of genital tract secretions and hepatic bile, IgA is the dominant isotype in human secretions.

In contrast to almost all animal species that produce IgA, human IgA molecules are more heterogeneous: there are two subclasses, IgA1 and IgA2, and two molecular forms, monomers (m) and polymers (p), which display characteristic structural and functional properties as well as body fluid distribution[106] (Figs. 11.1 and 11.2). In pIgA, an additional glycoprotein, the J chain, is covalently linked to the Fc region. S-IgA contains another glycoprotein, the secretory component (SC), acquired during the transepithelial transport of pIgA.

Primary amino acid and glycan structures of human IgA of both subclasses, J chain and SC, are known.[106] However, the secondary, tertiary and quaternary structures of the component chains and the resultant S-IgA molecules have not yet been determined because of lack of crystallographic data.

Heavy (α) chains of IgA

The heavy (α) chains of IgA1 and IgA2 consist of one variable (VH) and three constant region (CH 1–3) domains (Figs 11.2 and 11.3). There are surprisingly few differences in the amino acid sequences in the C region of α1 and α2 chains, except for the

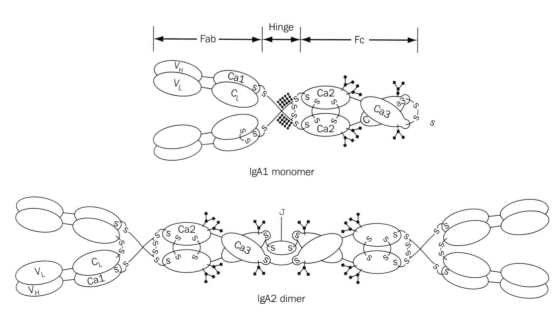

Fig. 11.2 Schematic diagrams of mIgA1 (top) and dimeric IgA2 (bottom). Small solid circles shown in mIgA1 represent the hinge region O-linked oligosaccharides which are absent from IgA2. Small solid squares on branched lines represent the N-linked oligosaccharides found on both subclasses, and these are shown in positions corresponding to their proposed relationships to the Ig domains; note that N-linked glycans are probably disposed differently in the two subclasses. The disulfide bonds shown in mIgA1 are the α-L interchain bond (also present in IgA2 of the A2m(2) allotype), α–α interchain bonds and two intrachain bonds (Cys196–Cys220 and Cys242–Cys299) not involved in Ig domain folding. In dimeric IgA2, the two monomer units are joined through opposing Fc regions with an interposed J chain that is attached by disulfide bonds to Cys471 of one α chain of each monomer, while the other Cys471 residues are directly bonded to each other. The two L chains in each monomer unit of IgA2 (of A2m(1) allotype) are joined by disulfide bonds to each other and not to the adjacent α chains.

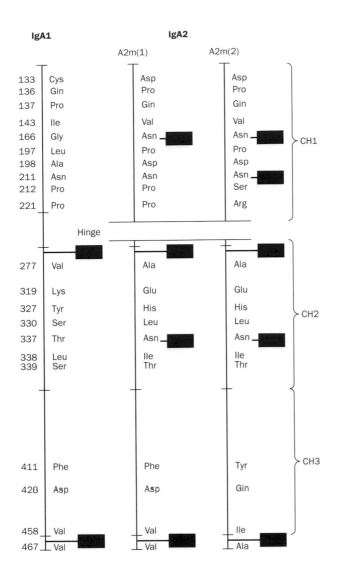

Fig. 11.3 Differences in amino acid sequences and glycan side chains between the constant domains of α1, α2m(1) and α2m(2) heavy chains. Solid boxes represent N-linked glycosylation sites. The hinge regions are shown in Fig. 11.4.

hinge region (Fig. 11.4), which is present in the α1 chain between Cα1 and Cα2 domains. It consists of some 20 amino acids with repeated proline, serine and threonine residues; the peptide bonds between Pro–Ser and Pro–Thr residues are susceptible to cleavage by bacterial IgA1 proteases produced by several bacterial species. The gene segment encoding the human α1 hinge region represents a recent insertion into the α chain gene.

It is generally assumed that the α chain domains are folded in a manner analogous to domains of the γ chain of IgG, with seven antiparallel β sheets typical of other members of the Ig superfamily. However, it is likely that the interdomain interactions, especially between the Cα2 domains of two adjacent α chains, are different from those of the Cγ2 interactions.[95] Crystallographic analyses of the Fcα will be necessary to determine the interaction of Cα domains.

The C terminus of the α chain extends by some 18 amino acid residues over C termini of γ, ε and δ H chains. This 'tail', also present in the μ chain, is required for binding of the J chain and for IgA and IgM to form polymers. The α chain contains 17 Cys residues involved in the formation of inter-H, H–L and H–J chain as well as several intra-H chain disulfide bridges.

The phylogenetically older IgA2 exists in two allotypic forms, A2m(1) and A2m(2). A major structural difference concerns the absence of the α–L chain disulfide bond in IgA2 of A2m(1) allotype.

Glycans contribute 6–10% of the total molecular mass of IgA. The higher carbohydrate content of IgA2 is the result of additional N-linked side chains. Analyses of IgA1 and IgA2 glycans reveal a

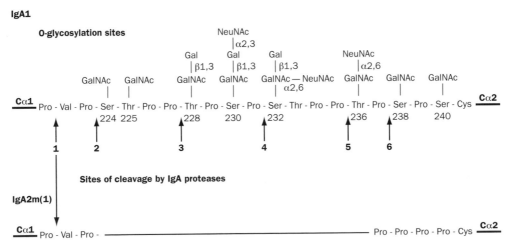

Fig. 11.4 Hinge regions of human IgA1 and IgA2. The hinge region of the α1 heavy chain encompasses approximately 20 amino acid residues consisting of proline, serine and threonine, and including an exact repeat of eight residues (223–230 and 231–238). The seryl and threonyl residues may bear O-linked oligosaccharide chains, and examples of the glycans known or proposed to occur are shown (not all sites shown are necessarily glycosylated in a single α chain; between three and seven, commonly five, sites may be glycosylated[95]) Peptide bonds cleaved by bacterial IgA proteases are shown (numbered 1–6); species known to cleave at the sites are: (1) *Clostridium ramosum* (cleaves both IgA1 and IgA2 of A2m(1) allotype); (2) *Prevotella* and *Capnocytophaga*; (3) *Streptococcus pneumoniae*, *S. sanguis*, *S. oralis* and *S. mitis*; (4) *Haemophilus influenzae*; (5) *Neisseria meningitidis*, *N. gonorrhoeae*, *H. influenzae* and *Ureaplasma urealyticum*; and (6) *N. meningitidis* and *N. gonorrhoeae*. The hinge region of the α2 heavy chain is much shorter, and lacks the IgA protease cleavage sites other than the Pro–Val site cleaved by *C. ramosum*.

marked variability in the total content of glycans, their composition and number of side chains.[34] N-linked glycans, present in both IgA1 and IgA2, comprise complex and high mannose (Man) types of chains (Figs 11.3 and 11.4). The hinge region of IgA1 contains from three to eight short chains linked by O-glycosidic bonds to Ser and Thr residues. These chains contain N-acetyl galactosamine (GalNAc), galactose (Gal) and N-acetyl neuraminic (sialic) acid (NeuNAc). Like the N-linked glycans, a considerable degree of heterogeneity has been described in O-linked chains with respect to the presence of galactose and sialic acid.

Joining (J) chain

A low molecular weight (15.6 kDa) glycoprotein is found in pIgA and IgM in serum and S-IgA and S-IgM in exocrine secretions. Because of its characteristic association with pIg, it was proposed that this polypeptide 'joins' component IgA and IgM monomers.[78] The J chain consists of approximately 130–140 amino acids, with a high content of acidic Asp and Glu residues: eight Cys residues are present, of which six participate in the formation of three intrachain disulfide bridges and two are linked to penultimate Cys residues of the α and μ chains. Primary structures of the J chains from various vertebrate species (e.g., human, rabbit and mouse) are remarkably conserved and thus display a high degree of sequence homology.[106] Interestingly, recent results indicate that a J chain highly homologous to that of vertebrates is also present in invertebrate species. The J chain apparently displays an Ig domain-like structure with a high content of β sheets. A single N-linked glycan side chain is attached to an Asn residue.

Immunohistochemical studies of Ig- and J chain-producing cells indicate that both are produced in plasma cells and their precursors. In humans, J chain synthesis precedes the production of Ig and thus may be detected in null, pro-B and pre-B cells devoid of fully assembled surface or intracellular Ig.

Although J chain may participate in the regulation of assembly of Igs, it is not absolutely required: pIgM totally devoid of J chain has been detected. A well established function of J chain concerns the binding of SC and assembly of S-IgA (see below).

Secretory component

SC is a heavily glycosylated protein with a molecular mass of approximately 70 kDa which is attached by disulfide bridges to the J chain-containing Fcα fragment of pIgA. SC is the extracellular part of the pIg receptor (pIgR) expressed on the surfaces of epithelial cells (and hepatocytes of some species, e.g., rabbit, rat, and mouse), and is acquired during the transcellular transport of pIgA or IgM.[114] In addition to the S-IgA-bound form, free SC is found in several exocrine secretions such as saliva and milk.

SC consists of five Ig-like domains each with one or two intradomain disulfide bridges (Fig. 11.5). The primary structures of human, mouse, cow, rat and rabbit SC have been determined; there is a marked sequence homology among SC from these species. Approximately 22% of the total molecular mass of SC is contributed by glycans; between five and seven N-linked side chains composed of N-acetyl glucosamine, fucose, mannose, galactose and sialic acid are present.[114]

Structural arrangement of polypeptide chains in secretory IgA molecules

In human external secretions, S-IgA occurs predominantly in a dimeric form; however, approximately 30–40% is present as

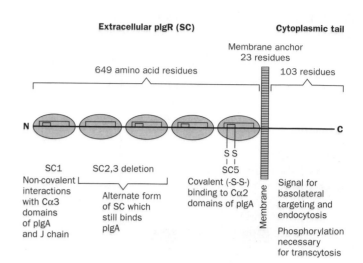

Fig. 11.5 Domain structure of pIgR and secretory component (SC). The extracellular part of pIgR, corresponding to SC, consists of five Ig-like domains. Domain 1 binds non-covalently to J chain-containing pIgA, and domain 5 contains a labile disulfide bridge that rearranges to form disulfide bonds with the Cα2 domain of one monomer unit of the pIgA. The remaining SC domains stabilize the interaction of SC with pIgA. The cytoplasmic tail of pIgR contains sequences necessary for targeting the receptor first to the basolateral surface of the epithelial cell and then, after phosphorylation, to the apical surface by vesicular transcytosis.

tetramers. Stoichiometric studies of component chains indicate that there is one molecule of each J chain and SC per dimer or tetramer. Both J chain and SC are attached by disulfide bonds to the Fcα fragment: SC to Cys residue 311 in the Cα2 domain, and J chain to the penultimate Cys of the α chain tail.[106] Although SC and J chain are not mutually connected by disulfides and are attached to different parts of the α chain, the ability of pIgA to interact with SC is highly dependent on the presence of J chain: pIgA molecules deficient in J chain do not bind SC and anti-J chain antibodies inhibit pIgA–SC interactions.[151] Results concerning the structures of IgA, SC and J chain suggest that all component chains display Ig domain-like structures and that their mutual interactions are likely to be based on the complementarities of their domains.

The L and α chains that become assembled intracellularly into mIgA molecules are synthesized on separate sets of polyribosomes and are assembled into the monomeric unit through several pathways.[49] Depending on the cell type studied, various types of pairings of H and L chains occur early on polyribosomes, but the final core-glycosylated molecule of mIgA is assembled in the Golgi apparatus. Additional carbohydrate residues are attached during the intracellular passage of mIgA from the Golgi apparatus to the cell surface and ultimate secretion into the medium.

Intracellular IgA

Early investigations of the biosynthetic pathways of mouse IgA suggested that, in cells secreting pIgA, most of the intracellular IgA was present as monomers and that polymerization occurred shortly before or at the time of secretion.[124] This hypothesis is supported by subsequent comparative biochemical studies of the molecular forms of intracellular *versus* secreted IgA in lysates and tissue culture supernatants of cells derived from various human tissues and lymphoblastoid cell lines, which indicated that, although small amounts of pIgA were detected in some cell lysates, most intracellular IgA occurred in a monomeric form even when the predominant form of secreted IgA was polymeric.[20,82,84,109] Nevertheless, the presence of intracellular polymers can easily be demonstrated by an SC-binding test performed on fixed IgA-producing cells.[11,12,112,127]

Binding of pIgR to pIgA begins with a high affinity non-covalent association followed by the formation of disulfide bonds through which SC links to only one of the IgA monomer subunits.[35,41,150] Several groups have reported association constants of the order of 10^8 M^{-1} for the non-covalent interaction, but these data in all likelihood underestimate the affinity.[136] More important, however, is the fact that dissociation of the complex is much slower than the time required (30 min) for the pIgA–pIgR complex to cross the epithelial cell, during which time pIgA must stay bound to its receptor to ensure that it reaches the apical face of the cell and is discharged into the lumen.[115]

Distribution of cells producing mIgA, pIgA, IgA1 and IgA2

Analyses of molecular forms of IgA in perfusates and supernatants of tissue explants cultured *in vitro*, as well as immunohistochemical studies of mucosal tissues and glands, clearly demonstrate separate populations of pIgA- and mIgA-secreting cells that display a characteristic tissue distribution (for reviews, see references 12,103,104). Typically, most of the IgA cells in normal human bone marrow produce mIgA (they do not express J chain and do not bind SC), whereas the majority of such cells in the intestinal lamina propria produce pIgA, express J chain, and bind SC. The spleen and lymph nodes from different locations display a variable proportion of pIgA- and mIgA-secreting cells. Under pathological conditions (e.g., IgA multiple myeloma), the bone marrow may contain predominantly J chain positive cells secreting pIgA.[107,127]

Using polyclonal and monoclonal antibodies specific for human IgA1 and IgA2, several groups of investigators have determined that serum IgA is represented primarily by the IgA1 subclass (about 85% of total serum IgA; for reviews see references 24,108,). This value mirrors the proportion of IgA1- and IgA2-secreting cells in the bone marrow[25,140] and, in conjunction with additional data[5,52] indicates that almost all serum IgA originates from this source.

The proportion of IgA1 to IgA2 varies in individual secretions. Currently available results obtained using polyclonal[29] or monoclonal anti-IgA1 and anti-IgA2 reagents[83,85] do not include all external secretions. Because most S-IgA in humans is of local origin, this IgA1:IgA2 ratio apparently reflects the distribution of IgA1- and IgA2-secreting cells in the corresponding tissue[25,70,81] (Fig. 11.6). Although IgA1-producing cells predominate in most mucosal tissues and glands, in the large intestine and in the female genital tract the IgA2 cells equal or outnumber IgA1-positive cells. Lymph nodes contain a mixed proportion of IgA1 and IgA2 cells, depending on their anatomical location.

SELECTIVE TRANSPORT OF IgA INTO EXTERNAL SECRETIONS AND IgA CATABOLISM

The distribution of IgA in human body fluids is dependent on the properties of the IgA molecules and their ability to interact with receptors expressed on a broad spectrum of morphologically and functionally different cell types. As a consequence of these interactions, several biologically significant functions are initiated, such

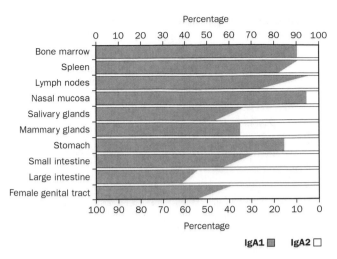

Fig. 11.6 Distribution of IgA1- or IgA2-producing cells in human systemic and mucosal tissues.

as the selective transport of pIgA through epithelial cells and hepatocytes into external secretions, removal of IgA-containing circulating immune complexes, hepatic catabolism of IgA, and binding and uptake of IgA-coated antigens by polymorphonuclear leukocytes, monocytes, macrophages and eosinophils. The receptors involved in IgA binding have been partially characterized with respect to their cell distribution, molecular properties, cytokine- and hormone-dependent regulation of their expression, and relative biological importance.

Selective epithelial transport of pIgA

The dominance of IgA in external secretions, as opposed to IgG in plasma, has been recognized since 1963.[149] The essential roles of pIgA and of epithelial cells expressing pIgR have been studied and the selective transport of pIgA has been elucidated at a molecular level (for review see reference 114).

The importance of the pIgA form and the presence of J chain in the selective binding and transepithelial transport has been documented in extensive structural studies of pIgA and S-IgA, in *in vitro* interactions of SC with IgA of various molecular forms, and by immunohistochemical studies of isolated plasma cells, epithelial cells and mucosal tissues (for reviews see references 106, 114). IgA-producing plasma cells adjacent to mucosal epithelial cells secrete pIgA associated with J chain (Fig. 11.7). During the secretion of IgA, mIgA, which is present as the dominant *intracellular* form, is polymerized, and J chain becomes incorporated shortly before externalization. Whether J chain is an absolute prerequisite for polymerization of immunoglobulins remains controversial, as disulfide-linked polymeric (mostly hexameric) IgM can be produced in the absence of J chain.[15] Nevertheless, only J chain-containing pIgA and IgM are capable of binding pIgR expressed on epithelial cells and hepatocytes.[14,151] In the absence of relevant crystallographic data concerning the three-dimensional arrangement of component chains in the Fc fragment of the IgA molecules, the structural basis for the exquisite specificity of pIgA–J chain–pIgR interactions remains elusive.

Binding of IgA to pIgR

In the first step, the first domain of pIgR (or SC) associates non-covalently with the $C\alpha2$ and/or $C\alpha3$ domains of one of the two monomeric subunits of a dimeric IgA molecule.[50,114] The fifth

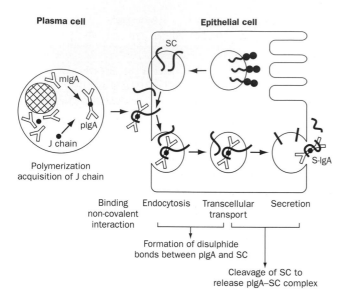

Fig. 11.7 Expression and transcytosis of pIgR (secretory component; SC) in the transport of pIgA to form S-IgA. In an epithelial cell, pIgR is synthesized on polyribosomes, inserted into a vesicular membrane, and shuttled to the basolateral surface. J chain-containing pIgA secreted by locally resident plasma cells binds to pIgR and is endocytosed into vesicles which are translocated through the cytoplasm of the epithelial cell to the apical surface. During transcytosis, the disulfide bridge between SC domain 5 and Cα2 of one of the monomer units of pIgA is formed, and pIgR is proteolytically cleaved between domain 5 and the transmembrane segment. On fusion of the vesicular membrane to the apical surface, S-IgA is released into the lumen. Thus pIgR acts as a 'sacrificial receptor' for the transport of pIgA, and remains associated with it as SC to form S-IgA.

SC domain, which contains a labile intrachain disulfide bond, interacts with Cα2 domain(s) on the other mIgA subunit, and the disulfide bond between Cys 467 of SC and Cys 311 of the α chain is formed. SC domains 2–4 apparently enhance and stabilize non-covalent associations between SC and pIgA; SC deletion mutants lacking these domains display considerably decreased pIgA binding. The essential contribution of J chain to SC binding (J chain-deficient pIgA and IgM do not bind SC) is probably related to molecular complementarities of J chain with SC domains 2–4, or to conformational change of the α chain induced by incorporation of the J chain, resulting in the exposure of additional SC-binding sites on Cα2 and Cα3 domains.

The pathways of pIgR movement from the intracellular site of synthesis to the basolateral surface of epithelial cells, and from the basolateral to the apical surface (with or without pIgA attached), are rather complex and depend on signals encoded in the intracellular (cytoplasmic) domain. Studies of deletion mutants of the 103-amino acid intracellular domain indicate specific segments that regulate initial basolateral targeting, endocytosis, surface re-expression, and transport to the apical surface.

Process of transepithelial transcytosis

It is estimated that the process of transepithelial transcytosis takes approximately 30 min; during this process, the pIgA–pIgR complex is stabilized by the formation of the disulfide bonds described above. These interactions occur within intracellular vesicles which are propelled by a microtubule-dependent mechanism to the apical surface, where the fusion of vesicles with the

membrane ultimately leads to the externalization of S-IgA molecules. The extracellular portion of pIgR (SC), whether free or pIgA-bound, is cleaved by specific proteases, thus releasing pIgA–J chain–SC complex or free SC into the external secretion; the intracellular domain of pIgR is mostly degraded. Individual events and transcytotic steps are regulated at multiple levels through phosphorylation of specific seryl residues in the cytoplasmic domain and activation of calmodulin.

The magnitude of pIgR expression, but probably not transcytosis, is regulated by cytokines and, in tissues of the genital tract, by hormones (for reviews see references 103, 114, 158). Interferon γ (IFNγ) is particularly effective in the upregulation of pIgR expression and, to a lesser degree, so are tumour necrosis factor (TNF) α, IL-4, TGFβ and IL-1. Although the biological effects of IFNγ and IL4 are usually antagonistic, a combination of these cytokines acts synergistically on pIgR expression.

Additional regulation of pIgR expression is mediated by hormones; estrogens (estradiol) and prolactin enhance, while progesterone decreases, pIgR expression[158] with pronounced tissue specificity (e.g., uterus, prostate, and mammary and lacrimal glands). The presence or absence of galactose or vitamin A in *in vitro* tissue culture fluids influences the level of pIgR expression.

Hepatic transport and catabolism of IgA

Hepatocytes of some species (e.g., rabbits, rats and mice) express pIgR on their cell membrane and are involved in a highly efficient transport of pIgA from plasma (in these species, pIgA is the dominant circulating form) into the bile and ultimately the intestinal fluid.[123] It is estimated that in these species most S-IgA found in the intestine is of plasma origin, and reinforces mucosal immunity in this organ. This is not the case in primates and other species in which hepatocytes do not express pIgR.[123]

Hepatocytes of all species examined (e.g. humans, monkeys, mice and chickens) express the asialoglycoprotein receptor (ASGP-R) which recognizes, in the presence of Ca^{2+}, terminal Gal and GalNAc residues on N- as well as O-linked glycan side chains of glycoproteins and glycolipids.[7] Although *not specific* for IgA, this receptor is nevertheless involved in the catabolism of plasma IgA, irrespective of the IgA subclass and molecular form.[144,148] Intravenously injected radiolabelled IgA1, mIgA1, or IgA2 or monkey and murine IgA are promptly removed from the circulation and taken up by the liver.[110] Analysis of cell-associated radioactivity has revealed that the hepatocytes internalize IgA; studies of the binding and catabolism of IgA by a human hepatic carcinoma cell line have demonstrated that IgA binding is mediated by ASGP-R and that most of the internalized IgA is degraded into low molecular mass fragments.[148]

Both selective transport and catabolism participate in the efficient removal of large quantities of IgA produced daily in mucosal tissues, bone marrow, lymph nodes and spleen (Fig. 11.1). Disturbances in these mechanisms (e.g., in J chain-deficient mice, or blockade of hepatic clearance) result in elevated levels of IgA in plasma and decreased levels of IgA in external secretions.[48,103]

FUNCTIONS OF SECRETORY IgA ANTIBODIES AT MUCOSAL SURFACES

Inhibition of adherence

Inhibition of adherence by S-IgA antibodies is recognized as a major protective mechanism against pathogens at mucosal surfaces.[1,157] S-IgA antibodies to microbial surface antigens have been demonstrated to inhibit adherence to pharyngeal, intestinal, and genitourinary tract epithelia, and to tooth surfaces (reviewed in reference 130). The hydrophilicity and negative charge of the Fc-SC part of S-IgA are thought to be important in surrounding a microbe with a hydrophilic shell that repels attachment to the mucosal surface. Agglutination may be an additional mechanism that allows clumped organisms to be swept away in flowing secretions: pIgA and S-IgA antibodies readily agglutinate microorganisms, but mIgA antibodies do not.[49] There is some evidence to suggest that human S-IgA, especially S-IgA, can bind bacteria by means of its carbohydrate chains and thereby interfere with their adherence. Thus mannose-rich glycans of IgA2 agglutinate *Escherichia coli* through type 1 (mannose-dependent) pili and inhibit type 1 pilus-dependent adherence of *E. coli* to epithelial cells *in vitro*.[159]

Mucus trapping

It was originally thought that S-IgA can associate specifically with mucins, so that S-IgA antibodies would be aligned at the surface of mucus layers to form an immunological flypaper or antiseptic paint. However, more recent findings suggest that S-IgA diffuses freely through mucus.[134] Nevertheless, microorganisms coated with S-IgA antibodies become less hydrophobic and readily entrapped in mucus.[32,92] High molecular weight mucin fractions of saliva contain S-IgA, suggesting an interaction between them, and S-IgA binds to salivary mucin MG2.[9] Interestingly, interaction of the Fc-SC region of S-IgA with mucus seems to occur in spermatozoa coated with S-IgA antibodies, which impair their ability to penetrate cervical mucus. Treatment of the spermatozoa with IgA1 protease restores this ability.[16]

Virus neutralization

S-IgA antibodies neutralize viruses through several mechanisms, including inhibition of binding to cellular receptors, internalization and intracellular replication.[6] S-IgA antibodies may be more effective than IgG in mediating cross-protective immunity against different antigenic variants of influenza virus,[90] and dimeric IgA antibody neutralizes transmissible gastroenteritis virus more effectively than monomeric IgG.[22] Although any isotype of antibody to Epstein–Barr virus (EBV) can neutralize its infectivity for B cells (via complement receptor CR2), pIgA antibodies may promote its uptake by pIgR-expressing epithelial cells.[139] Likewise, IgA antibodies can interfere with HIV infection of T cells,[18] but promote infection of FcαR-expressing monocytes.[63,79] Although these effects might alter the tissue tropism of viruses, the state of the cells is critical, as *polarized* epithelial cells or hepatocytes transport pIgA-coated EBV *in vitro* or *in vivo*.[40]

Viral neutralization may also occur during the SC-mediated transport of pIgA across epithelial cells if the vesicles interact with virus invading from the apical surface. Thus IgA antibodies have been shown to neutralize Sendai and influenza viruses in polarized pIgR-expressing epithelial cells *in vitro*,[96,97] and some evidence suggests that IgA antibodies can neutralize murine rotavirus or hepatitis viruses *in vivo* within intestinal epithelial cells or hepatocytes.[19,58]

Neutralization of enzymes and toxins

The ability of IgA antibodies to inhibit enzymes or toxins has been demonstrated in several systems (reviewed in reference 130). These effects are probably because of steric blocking of access to the substrate, or to conformational changes in the enzyme or toxin molecule induced by antibody binding, and are therefore independent of antibody isotype or even the presence of the Fc region. This has been shown for antibodies that inhibit bacterial IgA1 proteases, since Fab fragments of cleaved IgA1 antibodies continue to inhibit enzyme activity.[43]

Inhibition of antigen uptake

Intestinal uptake of food antigens is diminished by S-IgA antibodies induced by previous exposure,[154] and absorption of protein instilled into the trachea is inhibited by the simultaneous administration of IgA antibody.[145] Such intestinal immunity has potential applications in inhibition of the absorption of environmental carcinogens.[138] IgA-deficient subjects show increased absorption of food antigens and formation of circulating immune complexes[28] as well as statistically increased susceptibility to atopic allergies or autoimmune disease, thereby illustrating the importance of sIgA-mediated immune exclusion. The mechanisms probably include a combination of those described above, i.e., agglutination, hydrophilicity and mucus trapping. SC-mediated transport of pIgA by enterocytes may also serve to re-export absorbed antigens that become complexed with pIgA antibody in the lamina propria;[40,65] this process is analogous to hepatobiliary transport of pIgA-complexed antigens. Because of their non-inflammatory nature, IgA antibodies, in contrast to other Ig isotypes, can form immune complexes and participate in host defence functions without inducing inflammatory reactions that might cause collateral damage to nearby tissues.[17] This property of IgA may be especially important at mucosal surfaces, where the immune system continuously interacts with exogenous materials.

Interaction with innate antimicrobial factors

The secretions of most mucosal surfaces contain numerous innate defence factors that kill or inhibit microorganisms. Although few such interactions have been described in molecular detail, S-IgA may be able to interact synergistically with some of these systems (reviewed in reference 130). S-IgA may form complexes or act synergistically with lactoferrin.[142,155] Enhancement of the inhibitory effect of lactoperoxidase-H_2O_2-SCN^- on bacterial metabolism by IgA appears to be due to stabilization of enzyme activity.[147] However, the lytic activity reported against *E. coli* by human or pig colostral S-IgA antibody, complement and lysozyme[3,53] has not been confirmed in later studies.

BIOLOGICAL ACTIVITIES OF IgA IN TISSUES

Interaction with complement

IgA does not bind C1q or activate the classical complement pathway (CCP) as it does not have the C1q-binding motif found in IgG, but the concept that IgA activates the alternative complement pathway (ACP) under physiological conditions is not justified by experimental evidence. Artificially aggregated, chemically crosslinked, denatured or deglycosylated human IgA can activate the ACP *in vitro*,[10,44,51,131] and chimeric human IgA2/rat antibody shows ACP activation when complexed with a haptenated protein antigen.[152] However, human IgA antibody–antigen complexes fail to activate the ACP. Such conflicting results may be because of a number of factors, including the conformational integrity of IgA after exposure to denaturing conditions during purification, abnormal glycosylation of proteins produced in hybridoma or transfectoma cells, and direct activation of the ACP by heavily haptenated proteins (for review see reference 130). In contrast, IgA antibodies or their Fab fragments have been shown to inhibit IgG or IgM antibody-dependent complement-mediated cytolysis.[46,64,128,133] Thus, human IgA antibodies have poor or no complement-activating ability when bound physiologically to antigen, whereas ACP activation by IgA depends on some degree of denaturation or conformational change that does not ensue directly from binding to antigen, or possibly on abnormal structure, including the glycan chains. Such changes may occur under pathological circumstances *in vivo* as a result of either aberrant synthesis or microbial degradation, and thereby contribute to inflammatory conditions in which IgA is implicated. The anti-inflammatory property of IgA antibodies with respect to complement activation may be of physiological significance in controlling inflammation at mucosal surfaces where IgA is abundant, and where maintenance of the mucosal barrier is important.

Interaction with leukocytes

Most early experiments on the interaction of IgA with phagocytes used myeloma IgA proteins or colostral S-IgA regardless of antibody activity, but several instances of complement-independent opsonization or antibody-dependent cell-mediated cytotoxicity by IgA antibodies, including the postphagocytic respiratory burst and intracellular killing, have been reported (for review see reference 68).

Phagocytic cells

Phagocytic cells (PMN, eosinophils, and monocytes/macrophages) express a receptor specific for the Fcα region of IgA molecules;[69] the Fcα-R is now designated CD89 (for review see references 113 and 69). It is a member of the Ig superfamily and is extensively and variably glycosylated, having an observed M_r of 50 000–70 000 (90 000 on eosinophils), whereas the calculated M_r of the polypeptide chain is approximately 29 900. The neutrophil Fcα-R binds both subclasses of IgA and S-IgA equally, with an apparent affinity constant of $5 \times 10^7 \, M^{-1}$, and there are about 6000–7000 molecules per cell. The binding site on IgA has been located to the junction of the Cα2 and Cα3 domains.[21] Although constitutively expressed on neutrophils and monocytes, Fcα-R is upregulated on exudative neutrophils (e.g., from the gingival crevice) or by exposure of cells to activating agents, including phorbol esters, cytokines, bacterial lipopolysaccharide, chemotactic factors, or even IgA itself.[36,56,93] Among cytokines, TNFα, IL-8 and GM-CSF have been found to enhance the surface expression of FcαR on neutrophils, whereas IFNγ and TGFβ down regulate it (for review see reference 130).

Lymphocytes

The presence of IgA receptors on lymphocytes has been somewhat controversial, although several reports describe IgA (Fc) binding by T cells and B cells (reviewed in reference 130). However, the receptors have not been characterized biochemically or cloned, and their biological significance remains unclear. IgA, especially IgA2, was found to inhibit NK cell activity in a manner that suggested interaction with carbohydrate-specific receptors.[77] Subsequently, a minor subset of NK cells was found to express receptors for IgA, and this expression was increased by exposure to IgA complexed with IgG antibody. The receptor-positive cells were thought to have a role in isotype-specific regulation of Ig secretion by B cells.[75]

Phagocytosis

Despite some evidence to the contrary, human IgA can mediate phagocytosis and related processes by neutrophils, monocytes, or macrophages, and induce postphagocytic intracellular events (for review see reference 130). Although plasma IgA concentrations are sufficient to saturate neutrophil FcαR, the cells are not triggered unless the receptors are crosslinked,[143] and pIgA or S-IgA is more able to activate monocytes than mIgA.[38] As IgG antibodies strongly activate complement, whereas IgA antibodies inhibit IgG-mediated complement activation, the opsonizing effects of IgA and IgG antibodies in the presence of complement are different, and IgA antibodies have been shown to interfere with complement-dependent IgG-mediated opsonization.[117] In contrast, neutrophils activated by treatment with TNFα, IL-8 or GM-CSF display enhanced phagocytosis of IgA-opsonized particles consistent with enhanced surface expression of FcαR.[57,117,156] This effect may be physiologically relevant at mucosal surfaces such as the intestine, where inflammatory and chemotactic cytokines induced in epithelial cells by adhering or invading bacteria attract and activate neutrophils which must act in an IgA-rich environment.

IgA-mediated killing of bacteria by intestinal T cells has also been described[146] and, as activated murine γ/δ T cells appear to express an IgA receptor,[135] it is possible that γ/δ CD8+ intraepithelial cells are involved. Biphasic concentration-dependent effects of IgA have been observed on the chemotaxis or chemokinesis of neutrophils exposed to chemoattractants *in vitro*,[137] whereas others have reported inhibition of neutrophil chemotaxis by IgA.[61,67,153]

Regulation of cytokine release

A novel area of investigation is opened by the finding that IgA can downregulate the release of inflammatory cytokines and induce the production of IL-1 receptor antagonist in human monocytes stimulated with bacterial lipopolysaccharide.[160] As this effect is mediated through FcαR, it becomes important to determine the intracellular signalling mechanisms of FcαR in cells that naturally express this receptor, and how they differ from those mediated by Fcγ and complement receptors, which generally induce inflammatory responses. Meanwhile, the potential therapeutic application of this anti-inflammatory effect of IgA is suggested by the finding that oral administration of an IgA-IgG preparation may be beneficial in necrotizing enterocolitis.[33]

IgA also appears to be particularly effective in stimulating the degranulation of eosinophils[2] and in mediating the killing of schistosomes by eosinophils.[31,45] Human eosinophils are also reported to bind S-IgA and SC by a 15-kDa receptor that is distinct from FcαR and that mediates degranulation.[86] In contrast, IgA antibodies have been found to inhibit IgE-mediated hypersensitivity, which is sometimes associated with eosinophil responses.[60,129]

On most mucosal surfaces where S-IgA is the predominant Ig, however, functionally active complement and phagocytes are not normally present, and consequently S-IgA does not have the opportunity to activate either system. Where the mucosal barrier is breached or inflammation occurs, both luminal S-IgA and subepithelial pIgA secreted by resident plasma cells could have an important anti-inflammatory regulatory activity in a complex interplay of immunological effectors that may therefore provide not only immune defence, but also damage limiting capability. Other manifestations of this effect may be responsible for the observations that IgA antibodies to HLA Class I determinants enhance the survival of kidney allografts,[76] and that IgA antibodies block cytotoxicity against melanoma cells or antibody-dependent cellular cytotoxicity against EBV-related nasopharyngeal carcinoma.[94,119]

BACTERIAL IgA PROTEASES

Further evidence for the importance of IgA-mediated defence of the mucosal surfaces arises from the fact that several medically important bacteria produce highly specialized proteases that uniquely cleave human IgA1 at one of the proline–threonine or proline–serine bonds in the hinge region to yield Fab and Fc fragments (for reviews see references 73 and 74; Fig. 11.4). The Fab fragments retain antigen-binding activity but, lacking the Fc region, they lose many of their defensive properties, as discussed above. Bacteria known to produce IgA1 proteases include respiratory tract pathogens (*Haemophilus influenzae*, *Neisseria meningitidis* and *Streptococcus pneumoniae*), which are also the main causes of bacterial meningitis; urogenital pathogens (*Neisseria gonorrhoeae* and *Ureaplasma urealyticum*); several species of oral streptococci (*Streptococcus sanguis*, *S. oralis* and some strains of *S. mitis*), which are typically early colonizers of the tooth surfaces; and some subgingival organisms that have been implicated in periodontal disease (*Prevotella* and *Capnocytophaga* species).

Remarkably, the IgA1 proteases comprise at least three completely different types of enzyme: the *Haemophilus* and *Neisseria* enzymes are closely homologous serine proteases, the streptococcal enzymes are metalloproteases, the *Prevotella* and *Capnocytophaga* enzymes are thought to be thiol proteases, and the *U. urealyticum* enzyme is probably also a serine protease, but different from the *Haemophilus–Neisseria* enzyme (Table 11.1). Thus the same specialized catalytic activity has evolved independently in at least three or four quite separate groups of bacteria, a circumstance which argues strongly for the importance of IgA1 proteases as virulence factors. Another enzyme is produced by some strains of *Clostridium ramosum*, which is a colonizer of the large bowel but has uncertain pathological significance. This enzyme cleaves a proline–valine bond at the start of the hinge region in both IgA1 and IgA2 of allotype A2m(1).

Antigenic variation of proteases

Because of the exquisite specificity of IgA proteases for human IgA (only the chimpanzee, gorilla and orang-utan have IgA1 that is also susceptible to cleavage by IgA1 proteases), experimental investigation of IgA proteases as putative virulence factors is very difficult to accomplish. It has been proposed that the cleavage of pre-existing IgA1 antibodies to the capsular polysaccharide antigens of *H. influenzae*, *N. meningitidis* and *S. pneumoniae* by their respective IgA1 proteases allows the organisms to become coated with non-protective Fab fragments that block access of other intact antibodies and thereby facilitate colonization and invasion.[72] In support of this hypothesis, it has been shown that Fab fragments of IgA1 antibodies can effectively interfere with IgG antibody-mediated complement activation and bacteriolysis.[64,133] In addition, the IgA1 proteases, especially of *H. influenzae* and, to a lesser extent, those of the pathogenic *Neisseria* species, are antigenically variable. In the case of *H. influenzae*, over 30 antigenic types have been described on the basis of activity-inhibiting antibodies against IgA1 proteases. Thus, IgA1 proteases induce antibody responses to themselves, but have evolved an escape mechanism through antigenic variation. It seems likely that mucosal immunity to these pathogens may depend, in part, upon a balance between S-IgA1 antibodies to bacterial surface antigens, which form the critical substrate for IgA1 proteases, and enzyme-inhibitory antibodies against IgA1 proteases, or alternatively, the sequence in which these antibodies are generated. However, not all IgA1 protease-producing organisms seem to have developed the system to this extent, as the oral streptococcal IgA1 proteases generally do not appear to induce inhibitory antibodies and display little or no antigenic variation.

Since IgA1 proteases are extracellular enzymes, they are presumably able to cleave any available IgA1 molecule regardless of antibody activity, and thereby produce a local antibody deficiency, which may then permit bystander organisms or antigens to penetrate the mucosal epithelium. Evidence in support of this concept is provided by the finding that infants who develop atopic allergies have a significantly higher prevalence of IgA1 protease-producing organisms in their pharyngeal microbiota than non-atopic infants.[71] It is proposed that the diminution of mucosal protection by IgA1 proteases acting on IgA1, which is the most abundant Ig isotype in the upper respiratory tract, permits entry of allergens and sensitization for atopic responses.

INDUCTION OF IgA IMMUNE RESPONSES

The immune system can be divided into two compartments which display a considerable degree of mutual independence: the systemic immune system, represented by the bone marrow, spleen and lymph nodes; and the mucosal immune system, represented by lymphoid tissues in mucosae and in external secretory glands (Fig. 11.1). To understand the induction of immune responses, this concept of compartmentalization is essential: immunization in one of these systems may not necessarily be reflected in the other.[101] Generally, parenteral immunization induces poor mucosal immune responses; however, mucosal immunization offers the advantage that some routes of mucosal immunization (e.g., intranasal) induce both mucosal and systemic immunity.[98] Furthermore, these two systems do not display a parallel pattern of maturation and the lymphoid cells differ markedly in their phenotype and origin.[4] In general, the mucosal immune system

Bacterial IgA1 proteases	
Type	**Bacteria**
Serine proteases	*Haemophilus influenzae* *Neisseria meningitidis* *Ureaplasma urealyticum*
Metalloproteases	*Streptococcus sanguis* *Streptococcus oralis* *Streptococcus mitis*
Thiol proteases	*Prevotella* spp. *Capnocytophaga* spp.

Table 11.1 Bacterial IgA1 proteases.

matures earlier than its systemic counterpart[26] and mucosal immune responses are induced by commensal microbiota shortly after birth.

Inductive sites

Studies of the origin of antibody-producing cells in mucosal tissues indicate that a large proportion of such cells originates mainly in the organized lymphoepithelial structures found along the gastrointestinal and respiratory tracts. In the intestine, numerous lymphoid aggregates called Peyer's patches contain epithelial cells that can absorb soluble as well as particulate antigens, which are further processed and presented by resident macrophages and dendritic cells[99] to T cells (Fig. 11.8). The lymphoid aggregates comprise one or more lymphoid follicles with a germinal centre, and B and T cell zones; quantitatively, B cells predominate over T cells.

An important feature of cells in the Peyer's patches is that they consist of *precursor* rather than *effector* cells. Although Peyer's patches contain many B cells, few plasma cells are present despite intensive exposure to antigens taken up from the gut lumen. However, B cells in the Peyer's patches become committed under the influence of local T and dendritic cells[100] to the production of IgA with specificity to antigens absorbed from the gut lumen. Differentiating B cells leave Peyer's patches and migrate to remote effector sites, such as salivary and lactating mammary glands, or return to the lamina propria of the gut, where terminal maturation into IgA-producing plasma cells occurs (Fig. 11.9). Structures analogous to the Peyer's patches of the small intestine are also present in the large intestine, particularly in the rectum, and in the respiratory tract of some species (bronchus-associated lymphoid tissue, BALT). Mucosal tissues of the male and female genital tracts are devoid of Peyer's patches-like structures. However, antigen-processing and -presenting cells are found in these tissues, and immune responses which are usually restricted to the site of immunization may be induced (see below).

The well established fact that antigen-sensitized precursors of IgA plasma cells migrate from inductive sites (e.g., Peyer's patches) and populate remote effector mucosal tissues (e.g., salivary and lacrimal glands, intestinal lamina propria) led to the proposal of the common mucosal immune system (CMIS): stimulation of the inductive sites results in dissemination of humoral immune responses at several, anatomically remote, effector sites.[99]

The existence of the CMIS and its compartments in various animal models and in humans has had a profound impact on studies of humoral immune responses in external secretions and design and application of vaccines. In addition to stimulation of Peyer's patches-dependent immune responses by *oral immunization*, alternative inductive sites have been explored in recent experiments. Follicular structures analogous to Peyer's patches are

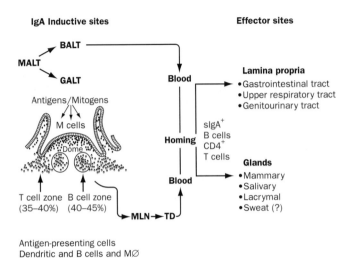

Fig. 11.8 Mucosa-associated lymphoid tissue (MALT) and the dissemination of IgA-committed B cells and corresponding T helper cells to effector sites of mucosal immunity. BALT, bronchus-associated lymphoid tissue; GALT, gut-associated lymphoid tissue; MLN, mesenteric lymph nodes; TD, thoracic duct.

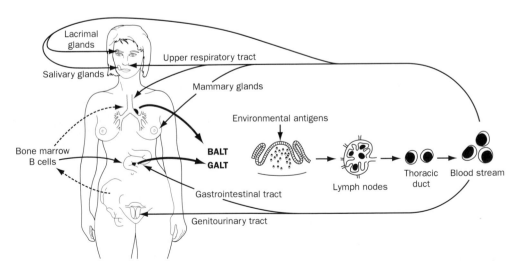

Fig. 11.9 The common mucosal immune system. Naïve B cells generated in the bone marrow migrate to the inductive sites of mucosal immunity represented by the gut-associated lymphoid tissues (GALT; Peyer's patches and lymphoid follicles of the large bowel) or bronchus-associated lymphoid tissue (BALT), where they are stimulated by antigens taken up and presented by antigen-presenting cells and cognate T helper cells. Antigen-stimulated B and T cells migrate out through the draining lymph nodes and lymphatics, enter the bloodstream, and finally relocate or 'home' to the effector sites including the lamina propria of the gastrointestinal, respiratory and genital tracts, and various exocrine glands.

also found in the large intestine, with especially pronounced accumulations in the rectum.[87,118] The potential importance of rectal lymphoid tissues as an inductive site is suggested from several studies performed in humans, monkeys and mice.

Rectal immunization

Rectal immunization of humans with a bacterial vaccine (*Salmonella typhi* Ty21a) induces specific antibodies not only at the site of immunization but also in saliva.[37,66]

The rectal route of immunization has also been evaluated in animal experimentation. Rhesus monkeys immunized intrarectally with simian immunodeficiency virus (SIV) displayed both T and B cell-mediated immune responses, including the induction of anti-SIV antibodies.[88,89] Mice immunized intrarectally with cholera toxin (CT) or recombinant vaccinia virus expressing gp120 of SIV also generated humoral immune responses in genital tract secretions as well as in serum; this immunization route was frequently superior to either the intragastric or intravaginal route.[47,111] Therefore, the rectal immunization route appears to be effective in the induction not only of local but also of generalized mucosal immune responses because of the presence of inductive site tissue. However, there are pronounced species differences with respect to the magnitude of the response induced: mice display a more vigorous response than humans. The type and dose of antigen, as well as the frequency of immunization, may be partially responsible for such observed differences. Further studies will be necessary to validate the limited results obtained thus far, and males will be included in future immunization attempts to determine whether specific immune responses are generated in male genital tract secretions.

Genital tract

In several recent studies, women who were rectally immunized with viral or bacterial vaccines[27,54,55,66,80,116] showed modest levels of vaginal IgA and IgG antibodies. Considered in the context of the common mucosal immune system, these results suggest a further subcompartmentalization that may be controlled by selective homing of IgA plasma cell precursors. Thus, certain IgA-inductive sites may provide precursor lymphocytes for a particular effector site. By extension, oral immunization may be less effective for the induction of S-IgA in the genital tract than rectal administration. For effective vaccines to be designed, further comparative studies will be necessary to determine how diverse mucosal immunization routes lead to specific sIgA antibodies in various external secretions.

Tonsils

Accumulations of lymphoid tissues, such as palatine, lingual and nasopharyngeal tonsils (Waldeyer's ring), are strategically positioned at the beginning of the digestive and respiratory tracts. They are continuously exposed to ingested and inhaled antigens and possess structural features similar to those of both lymph nodes and GALT,[13,120] including in the tonsillar crypts a lymphoepithelium containing M cells which are essential for selective antigen uptake. In addition, B and T cells, plasma cells and antigen-presenting cells (APCs) are also present. Several observations have suggested that these lymphoid tissues may serve as a source for precursors of IgA plasma cells found in the upper respiratory and digestive tracts. The immune response to the oral poliovirus vaccine in tonsillectomized children, who

display reduced levels of sIgA, is inferior to that induced in children with intact tonsils.[120] However, direct unilateral injection of antigens such as CT-B subunit and tetanus toxoid (TT) into the tonsils of human volunteers results in the induction of mainly local immune responses which manifest by the appearance of antigen-specific IgG-producing cells and, to a lesser degree, IgA-producing cells in the injected tonsil.[125] Although considerable numbers of anti-CT-B and anti-TT antibody-forming cells with a similar distribution of isotypes were detected in peripheral blood, the immune responses were not disseminated to various mucosal effector sites, as observed after oral immunization. Therefore, the tonsils appear to be autonomous and may serve as an inductive site that is effective in the stimulation of local mucosal immune responses.

Nasal immunization

Several recent studies have emphasized the importance of inductive sites in the nasal cavity for the generation of mucosal and systemic immune responses that may exceed in magnitude those induced by oral immunization.[8,30,39,91,122,132,141] When introduced into the nasal cavity, usually along with mucosal adjuvants such as CT and/or CT-B, viral and bacterial antigens induce superior immune responses in external secretions such as saliva and, surprisingly, in female genital tract secretions of rodents, rhesus monkeys, chimpanzees and humans. Because neither IgG nor IgA antibodies in vaginal washes correlated with serum antibody responses, it is assumed that antibodies of both isotypes are predominantly of mucosal origin. This finding may have important implications for the design of vaccines effective in the induction of immune responses in the genital tract. Although analogous studies with bacterial antigens have not been performed in humans, induction of genital tract immune responses by intranasal immunization would have profound implications for the prevention of sexually transmitted diseases, including AIDS.[102]

Thus, different immunization routes (intranasal and oral) can induce generalized mucosal immune responses, although the relative representation of dominant antibody isotypes may vary. Nevertheless, nasal immunization appears to induce S-IgA immunity in a broader range of mucosal tissues than oral vaccination. This may be explained by the recent observation that circulating IgA-secreting cells induced after nasal vaccination express a more promiscuous profile of homing receptors than their corresponding counterparts raised after oral or rectal immunization.[126] Whether such antibody responses are also induced in the male genital tract remains to be determined. Further studies using innovative approaches should be initiated to evaluate critically the role of nasally induced responses in human mucosal immunity.

Other sites

Mucosal immune responses restricted to the site of immunization can be induced in mucosal tissues that lack the inductive lymphoepithelial aggregates described above. Application of soluble or particulate antigens in the conjunctival sac or vaginal mucosa[121] (for review see reference 101) results in the induction of strictly local but not particularly vigorous immune responses at the site of immunization. Similarly, injection of antigens into the lactating mammary gland or salivary gland stimulates antibody production, often dominated by IgG rather than IgA, restricted to secretions of the immunized gland.[42,59]

Some studies suggest that a combination of several mucosal immunization routes (e.g., oral and rectal, or rectal and vaginal, etc.) in addition to repeated vaccination, may be the most effective approach for induction of efficient humoral immune responses in external secretions.[111] Furthermore, mucosal antigen delivery systems, including the incorporation of antigens into absorbable particles and expression in recombinant microorganisms or edible plants,[98,99,105] have been explored for induction of mucosal responses.

REFERENCES

1 Abraham SN, Beachey EH. Host defenses against adhesion of bacteria to mucosal surfaces. In: *Advances in Host Defense Mechanisms* Vol. 4. (Gallin JF, Fauci AS, eds), Raven Press, New York, 1985; 63–88.

2 Abu-Ghazaleh RI, Fujisawa T, Mestecky J, Kyle RA, Gleich GJ. IgA-induced eosinophil degranulation. *J Immunol* 1989; 142: 2393–400.

3 Adinolfi M, Glynn AA, Lindsay M, Milne CM. Serological properties of γA antibodies to *Escherichia coli* present in human colostrum. *Immunology* 1966; 10: 517–26.

4 Alley CD, Mestecky J. The mucosal immune system. In: *B Lymphocytes in Human Disease* (Bird G, Calvert JE, eds) Oxford University Press, Oxford, 1988; 222–54.

5 Alley CD, Nash GS, MacDermott RP. Marked *in vitro* spontaneous secretion of IgA by human rib bone marrow mononuclear cells. *J Immunol* 1982; 128: 2604–8.

6 Armstrong SJ, Dimmock NJ. Neutralization of influenza virus by low concentrations of hemagglutinin-specific polymeric immunoglobulin A inhibits viral fusion activity, but activation of the ribonucleoprotein is also inhibited. *J Virol* 1992; 66: 3823–32.

7 Ashwell G, Harford J. Carbohydrate-specific receptor of the liver. *Annu Rev Biochem* 1982; 52: 531–54.

8 Bergquist C, Johansson E-L, Lagergard T, Holmgren J, Rudin A. Intranasal vaccination of humans with recombinant cholera toxin B subunit induces systemic and local antibody responses in the upper respiratory tract and the vagina. *Infect Immun* 1997; 65: 2676–84.

9 Biesbrock AR, Reddy MS, Levine MJ. Interaction of a salivary mucin-secretory immunoglobulin A complex with mucosal pathogens. *Infect Immun* 1991; 59: 3492–7.

10 Boackle RJ, Pruitt KM, Mestecky J. The interactions of human complement with interfacially aggregated preparations of human secretory IgA. *Immunochemistry* 1974; 11: 543–8.

11 Brandtzaeg P. Two types of IgA immunocytes in man. *Nature New Biol* 1973; 243: 142–3.

12 Brandtzaeg P. Immunohistochemical characterization of intracellular J-chain and binding site for secretory component (SC) in human immunoglobulin (Ig)-producing cells. *Mol Immunol* 1983; 20: 941–66.

13 Brandtzaeg P. Immune functions of human nasal mucosa and tonsils in health. In: *Immunology of the Lung and Upper Respiratory Tract* (Bienenstock J, ed.), McGraw-Hill, New York, 1984; 28–95.

14 Brandtzaeg P, Prydz H. Direct evidence for an integrated function of J chain and secretory component in epithelial transport of immunoglobulins. *Nature* 1984; 311: 71–3.

15 Brewer JW, Randall TD, Parkhouse RME, Corley RB. IgM hexamers. *Immunol Today* 1994; 15: 165–8.

16 Bronson RA, Cooper GW, Rosenfeld DL, Gilbert JV, Plaut AG. The effect of an IgA1 protease on immunoglobulins bound to the sperm surface and sperm cervical mucus penetrating ability. *Fertil Steril* 1987; 47: 985–91.

17 Brown TA, Russell MW, Mestecky J. Hepatobiliary transport of IgA immune complexes: molecular and cellular aspects. *J Immunol* 1982; 128: 2183–6.

18 Burnett PR, VanCott TC, Polonis VR, Redfield RR, Birx DL. Serum IgA-mediated neutralization of HIV type 1. *J Immunol* 1994; 152: 4642–8.

19 Burns JW, Siadat-Pajouh M, Krishnaney AA, Greenberg HB. Protective effect of rotavirus VP6-specific IgA monoclonal antibodies that lack neutralizing activity. *Science* 1996; 272: 104–7.

20 Buxbaum JN, Zolla S, Scharff MD, Franklin EC. The synthesis and assembly of immunoglobulins by malignant human plasmocytes. III. Heterogeneity of IgA polymer assembly. *Eur J Immunol* 1974; 4: 367–9.

21 Carayannopoulos L, Hexham JM, Capra JD. Localization of the binding site for the monocyte immunoglobulin (Ig) A-Fc receptor (CD89) to the domain boundary between Cα2 and Cα3 in human IgA1. *J Exp Med* 1996; 183: 1579–86.

22 Castilla J, Sola I, Enjuanes L. Interference of coronavirus infection by expression of immunoglobulin G (IgG) or IgA virus-neutralizing antibodies. *J Virol* 1997; 71: 5251–8.

23 Christ AD, Blumberg RS. The intestinal epithelial cell: immunologic aspects. *Springer Semin Immunopathol* 1997; 18: 449–61.

24 Conley ME, Delacroix DL. Intravascular and mucosal immunoglobulin A: two separate but related systems of immune defense? *Ann Intern Med* 1987; 106: 892–9.

25 Crago SS, Kutteh WH, Moro I *et al*. Distribution of IgA1- and IgA2- and J chain-containing cells in human tissues. *J Immunol* 1984; 132: 116–8.

26 Cripps AW, Gleeson M. Ontogeny of mucosal immunity and aging. In: *Mucosal Immunology*, 2nd edn (Ogra PL, Mestecky J, Lamm ME, Strober W, Bienenstock J, McGhee JR., eds), Academic Press, New York 1999; 253–66.

27 Crowley-Nowick PA, Bell MC, Brockwell R *et al*. Rectal immunization for induction of specific antibody in the genital tract of women. *J Clin Immunol* 1997; 17: 370–9.

28 Cunningham-Rundles C, Brandeis WE, Good RA, Day NK. Milk precipitins, circulating immune complexes, and IgA deficiency. *Proc Natl Acad Sci USA* 1978; 75: 3387–9.

29 Delacroix DL, Dive C, Rambaud JC, Vaerman JP. IgA subclasses in various secretions and in serum. *Immunology* 1982; 47: 383–5.

30 Di Tommaso A, Saletti G, Pizza M *et al*. Induction of antigen-specific antibodies in vaginal secretions by using a nontoxic mutant of heat-labile enterotoxin as a mucosal adjuvant. *Infect Immun* 1996; 64: 974–9.

31 Dunne DW, Richardson BA, Jones FM, Clark M, Thorne KJI, Butterworth AE. The use of mouse/human chimaeric antibodies to investigate the roles of different antibody isotypes, including IgA2, in the killing of *Schistosoma mansoni* schistosomula by eosinophils. *Parasite Immunol* 1993; 15: 181–5.

32 Edebo L, Richardson N, Feinstein A. The effects of binding mouse IgA to dinitrophenylated *Salmonella typhimurium* on physicochemical properties and interaction with phagocytic cells. *Int Arch Allergy Appl Immunol* 1985; 78: 353–7.

33 Eibl M, Wolf HM, Fürnkranz H, Rosenkranz A. Prevention of necrotizing enterocolitis in low-birth-weight infants by IgA-IgG feeding. *New Engl J Med* 1988; 319: 1–7.

34 Endo T, Mestecky J, Kulhavy R, Kobata A. Carbohydrate heterogeneity of human myeloma proteins of the IgA1 and IgA2 subclasses. *Molec Immunol* 1994; 33: 1415–22.

35 Fallgren-Gebauer E, Gebauer W, Bastian A *et al*. The covalent linkage of the secretory component to IgA. *Adv Exp Med Biol* 1995; 371A: 625–8.

36 Fanger MW, Goldstine SN, Shen L. Cytofluorographic analysis of receptors for IgA on human polymorphonuclear cells and monocytes and the correlation of receptor expression with phagocytosis. *Molec Immunol* 1983; 20: 1019–27.

37 Forrest BD, Shearman DJC, La Brooy JT. Specific immune response in humans following rectal delivery of live typhoid vaccine. *Vaccine* 1990; 8: 209–12.

38 Furrie E, Bonner BC, Hutchings A, Lang ML, Kerr MA. Differential activation of peripheral blood monocytes using various forms of human IgA. *Biochem Soc Trans* 1997; 25: 332S.

39 Gallichan WS, Rosenthal KL. Specific secretory immune responses in the female genital tract following intranasal immunization with a recom-

binant adenovirus expressing glycoprotein B of Herpes simplex virus. *Vaccine* 1995; 13: 1589–95.

40 Gan YJ, Chodosh J, Morgan A, Sixbey JW. Epithelial cell polarization is a determinant in the infectious outcome of immunoglobulin A-mediated entry by Epstein–Barr virus. *J Virol* 1997; 71: 519–26.

41 Garcia-Pardo A, Lamm ME, Plaut AG, Frangione B. Secretory component is covalently bound to a single subunit in human secretory IgA. *Mol Immunol* 1979; 16: 477–82.

42 Genco RJ, Taubman MA. Secretory gamma-A antibodies induced by local immunization. *Nature* 1969; 221: 679–81.

43 Gilbert JV, Plaut AG, Longmaid B, Lamm ME. Inhibition of microbial IgA proteases by human secretory IgA and serum. *Molec Immunol* 1983; 20: 1039–49.

44 Götze O, Müller-Eberhard HJ. The C3-activator system: an alternative pathway of complement activation. *J Exp Med* 1971; 134: 90S–108S.

45 Grezel D, Capron M, Grzych J-M, Fontaine J, Lecocq J-P, Capron A. Protective immunity induced in rat schistosomiasis by a single dose of the Sm28GST recombinant antigen: effector mechanisms involving IgE and IgA antibodies. *Eur J Immunol* 1993; 23: 454–60.

46 Griffiss JM, Broud D, Bertram MA. Bactericidal activity of meningococcal antisera. Blocking by IgA of lytic antibody in human convalescent sera. *J Immunol* 1975; 114: 1779–84.

47 Haneberg B, Kendall D, Amerongen HM, Apter FM, Kraehenbuhl J-P, Neutra MR. Induction of specific immunoglobulin-A in the small intestine, colon-rectum, and vagina measured by a new method for collection of secretions from local mucosal surfaces. *Infect Immun* 1994; 62: 15–23.

48 Hendrickson BA, Rindisbacher L, Corthesy B et al. Lack of association of secretory component with IgA in J chain-deficient mice. *J Immunol* 1996; 157: 750–54.

49 Heremans JF. Immunoglobulin A. In: *The Antigens*, Vol. II. (Sela M, ed.), Academic Press, New York, 1974; 365–522.

50 Hexham JM, White KD, Carayannopoulos LN et al. A human immunoglobulin (Ig) A Cα3 domain motif directs polymeric Ig receptor-mediated secretion. *J Exp Med* 1999; 189: 747–51.

51 Hiemstra PS, Gorter A, Stuurman ME, van Es LA, Daha MR. Activation of the alternative pathway of complement by human serum IgA. *Eur J Immunol* 1987; 17: 321–6.

52 Hijmans W. Circulating IgA in humans. *Adv Exp Med Biol* 1987; 216B: 1169–74.

53 Hill IR, Porter P. Studies of bactericidal activity to *Escherichia coli* of porcine serum and colostral immunoglobulins and the role of lysozyme with secretory IgA. *Immunology* 1974; 26: 1239–50.

54 Hopkins S, Kraehenbuhl J-P, Schödel F et al. A recombinant *Salmonella typhimurium* vaccine induces local immunity by four different routes of immunization. *Infect Immun* 1995; 63: 3279–86.

55 Hordnes K, Tynning T, Kvam AI, Johnsson R, Haneberg B. Colonization in the rectum and uterine cervix with group B streptococci may induce specific antibody responses in cervical secretions of pregnant women. *Infect Immun* 1996; 64: 1643–52.

56 Hostoffer RW, Krukovets I, Berger M. Increased FcαR expression and IgA-mediated function on neutrophils induced by chemoattractants. *J Immunol* 1993; 150: 4532–40.

57 Hostoffer RW, Krukovets I, Berger M. Enhancement by tumor necrosis factor-α of Fcα receptor expression and IgA-mediated superoxide generation and killing of *Pseudomonas aeruginosa* by polymorphonuclear leukocytes. *J Infect Dis* 1994; 170: 82–7.

58 Huang DS, Emancipator SN, Lamm ME et al. Virus-specific IgA reduces hepatic viral titers in vivo on mouse hepatitis virus (MHV) infection. *Immunol Cell Biol* 1997; 75 (Suppl. 1): A12.

59 Hurlimann J, Lichaa M. Local immunization in the mammary glands of the rabbit. *J Immunol* 1976; 116: 1295–1301.

60 Ishizaka K, Ishizaka T, Hornbrook MM. Blocking of Prausnitz-Küstner sensitization with reagin by normal human β_{2A}globulin. *J Allergy* 1963; 34: 395–403.

61 Ito S, Mikawa H, Shiromiya K, Yoshida T. Suppressive effect of IgA soluble immune complexes on neutrophil chemotaxis. *Clin Exp Immunol* 1979; 37: 436–40.

62 Jackson S, Mestecky J, Moldoveanu Z, Spearman P. Collection and processing of human mucosal secretions. In: *Mucosal Immunology*, 2nd edn (Ogra PL, Mestecky J, Lamm ME, Strober W, Bienenstock J, McGhee JR, eds), Academic Press, New York 1999; 1567–76.

63 Janoff EN, Jackson S, Wahl SM, Thomas K, Peterman JH, Smith PD. Intestinal mucosal immunoglobulins during human immunodeficiency virus type 1 infection. *J Infect Dis* 1994; 170: 299–307.

64 Jarvis GA, Griffiss JM. Human IgA1 blockade of IgG-initiated lysis of *Neisseria meningitidis* is a function of antigen-binding fragment binding to the polysaccharide capsule. *J Immunol* 1991; 147: 1962–67.

65 Kaetzel CS, Robinson JK, Chintalacharuvu KR, Vaerman J-P, Lamm ME. The polymeric immunoglobulin receptor (secretory component) mediates transport of immune complexes across epithelial cells: a local defense function for IgA. *Proc Natl Acad Sci USA* 1991; 88: 8796–800.

66 Kantele A, Hakkinen M, Moldoveanu Z et al. Differences in immune responses induced by oral and rectal immunizations with *Salmonella typhi* Ty21a: Evidence for compartmentalization within the common mucosal immune system in humans. *Infect Immun* 1998; 66: 5630–35.

67 Kemp AS, Cripps AW, Brown S. Suppression of leucocyte chemokinesis and chemotaxis by human IgA. *Clin Exp Immunol* 1980; 40: 388–95.

68 Kerr MA. The structure and function of human IgA. *Biochem J* 1990; 271: 285–96.

69 Kerr MA, Woof JM. Fcα receptors. In: *Mucosal Immunology*, 2nd edn (Ogra PL, Mestecky J, Lamm ME, Strober W, Bienenstock J, McGhee JR, eds), Academic Press, New York 1999; 213–24.

70 Kett K, Brandtzaeg P, Radl J, Haaijman JJ. Different subclass distribution of IgA-producing cells in human lymphoid organs and various secreting tissues. *J Immunol* 1986; 136: 3631–35.

71 Kilian M, Husby S, Host A, Halken S. Increased proportions of bacteria capable of cleaving IgA1 in the pharynx of infants with atopic disease. *Pediatr Res* 1995; 38: 182–86.

72 Kilian M, Reinholdt J. A hypothetical model for the development of invasive infection due to IgA1 protease producing bacteria. *Adv Exp Med Biol* 1987; 216B: 1261–9.

73 Kilian M, Reinholdt J, Lomholt H, Poulsen K, Frandsen EVG. Biological significance of IgA1 proteases in bacterial colonization and pathogenesis; critical evaluation of experimental evidence. *APMIS* 1996; 104: 321–38.

74 Kilian M, Russell MW. Bacterial evasion of mucosal immune defenses. In: *Mucosal Immunology*, 2nd edn (Ogra PL, Mestecky J, Lamm ME, Strober W, Bienenstock J, McGhee JR, eds), Academic Press, New York 1999; 241–51.

75 Kimata H, Saxon A. Subset of natural killer cells is induced by immune complexes to display Fc receptors for IgE and IgA and demonstrates isotype regulatory function. *J Clin Invest* 1988; 82: 160–7.

76 Koka P, Chia D, Terasaki PI et al. The role of IgA anti-HLA class I antibodies in kidney transplant survival. *Transplantation* 1993; 56: 207–11.

77 Komiyama K, Crago SS, Itoh K, Moro I, Mestecky J. Inhibition of natural killer cell activity by IgA. *Cell Immunol* 1986; 101: 143–55.

78 Koshland ME. The coming age of the immunoglobulin J chain. *Annu Rev Immunol* 1985; 3: 425–53.

79 Kozlowski PA, Black KP, Shen L, Jackson S. High prevalence of serum IgA HIV-1 infection-enhancing antibodies in HIV-infected persons: masking by IgG. *J Immunol* 1995; 154: 6163–73.

80 Kozlowski PA, Cu-Uvin S, Neutra MR, Flanigan TP. Comparison of the oral, rectal, and vaginal immunization routes for induction of antibodies in rectal and genital tract secretions of women. *Infect Immun* 1997; 65: 1387–94.

81 Kutteh WH, Hatch KD, Blackwell RE, Mestecky J. Secretory immune system of the female reproductive tract: I. Immunoglobulin and secretory component-containing cells. *Obstet Gynecol* 1988; 71: 56–60.

82 Kutteh WH, Moldoveanu Z, Prince SJ, Kulhavy R, Alonso F, Mestecky J. Biosynthesis of J-chain in human lymphoid cells producing immunoglobulins of various isotypes. *Mol Immunol* 1983; 20: 967–76.

83 Kutteh WH, Prince SJ, Hammonds KR, Kutteh CC, Mestecky J. Variations in immunoglobulins and IgA subclasses of human uterine cervical secretions around the time of ovulation. *Clin Exp Immunol* 1996; 104: 538–42.

84 Kutteh WH, Prince SJ, Mestecky J. Tissue origins of human polymeric and monomeric IgA. *J Immunol* 1982; 128: 990–95.

85 Ladjeva I, Peterman JH, Mestecky J. IgA subclasses of human colostral antibodies specific for microbial and food antigens. *Clin Exp Immunol* 1989; 78: 85–90.

86 Lamkhioued B, Gounni AS, Gruart V, Pierce A, Capron A, Capron M. Human eosinophils express a receptor for secretory component. Role in secretory IgA-dependent activation. *Eur J Immunol* 1995; 25: 117–25.

87 Langman JM, Rowland R. The number and distribution of lymphoid follicles in the human large intestine. *J Anat* 1986; 194: 189–94.

88 Lehner T, Brookes R, Panagiotidi C *et al*. T- and B-cell functions and epitope expression in nonhuman primates immunized with simian immunodeficiency viral antigen by the rectal route. *Proc Natl Acad Sci USA* 1993; 90: 8638–42.

89 Lehner T, Panagiotidi C, Bergmeier LA, Ping T, Brookes R, Adams SE. A comparison of the immune response following oral, vaginal, or rectal route of immunization with SIV antigens in non-human primates. *Vaccine Res* 1992; 1: 319–30.

90 Liew FY, Russell SM, Appleyard G, Brand CM, Beale J. Cross protection in mice infected with influenza A virus by the respiratory route is correlated with local IgA antibody rather than serum antibody or cytotoxic T cell reactivity. *Eur J Immunol* 1984; 14: 350–6.

91 Lubeck MD, Natuk RJ, Chengalvala M *et al*. Immunogenicity of recombinant adenovirus-human immunodeficiency virus vaccines in chimpanzees following intranasal administration. *AIDS Res Hum Retroviruses* 1994; 10: 1443–9.

92 Magnusson K-E, Stjernström I. Mucosal barrier systems. Interplay between secretory IgA (SIgA), IgG and mucins on the surface properties and association of salmonellae with intestine and granulocytes. *Immunology* 1982; 45: 239–48.

93 Maliszewski CR, Shen L, Fanger MW. The expression of receptors for IgA on human monocytes and calcitriol-treated HL-60 cells. *J Immunol* 1985; 135: 3878–81.

94 Mathew GD, Qualtiere LF, Neel HB, Pearson GR. IgA antibody, antibody-dependent cellular cytotoxicity and prognosis in patients with nasopharyngeal carcinoma. *Int J Cancer* 1981; 27: 175–80.

95 Mattu RS, Pleass RJ, Willis AC *et al*. The glycosylation and structure of human serum IgA1, Fab and Fc regions and the role of N-glycosylation on Fcα receptor interactions. *J Biol Chem* 1998; 273: 2260–72.

96 Mazanec MB, Kaetzel CS, Lamm ME, Fletcher D, Nedrud JG. Intracellular neutralization of virus by immunoglobulin A antibodies. *Proc Natl Acad Sci USA* 1992; 89: 6901–5.

97 Mazanec MB, Coudret CL, Fletcher DR. Intracellular neutralization of influenza virus by immunoglobulin A anti-hemagglutinin monoclonal antibodies. *J Virol* 1995; 69: 1339–43.

98 McGhee JR, Czerkinsky C, Mestecky J. Mucosal vaccines – an overview. In: *Mucosal Immunology*, 2nd edn (Ogra PL, Mestecky J, Lamm ME, Strober W, Bienenstock J, McGhee JR, eds), Academic Press, New York 1999a: 741–58.

99 McGhee JR, Lamm ME, Strober W. Mucosal immune responses. In: *Mucosal Immunology*, 2nd edn (Ogra PL, Mestecky J, Lamm ME, Strober W, Bienenstock J, McGhee JR, eds), Academic Press, New York 1999b: 485–506.

100 McIntyre TM, Strober W. Gut-associated lymphoid tissue. In: *Mucosal Immunology*, 2nd. Ed. (Ogra PL, Mestecky J, Lamm ME, Strober W, Bienenstock J, McGhee JR, eds.), Academic Press, New York 1999; 319–56.

101 Mestecky J. The common mucosal immune system and current strategies for induction of immune responses in external secretions. *J Clin Immunol* 1987; 7: 265–76.

102 Mestecky J, Kutteh WH, Jackson S. Mucosal immunity in the female genital tract: Relevance to vaccination efforts against the human immunodeficiency virus. *AIDS Res Hum Retroviruses* 1994; 10: S11–20.

103 Mestecky J, Lue C, Russell MW. Selective transport of IgA: cellular and molecular aspects. *Gastroenterol Clin North Am* 1991; 20: 441–71.

104 Mestecky J, McGhee JR. Immunoglobulin A (IgA): molecular and cellular interactions involved in IgA biosynthesis and immune response. *Adv Immunol* 1987; 40: 153–245.

105 Mestecky J, Moldoveanu Z, Michalek SM *et al*. Current options for vaccine delivery systems by mucosal routes. *J Controlled Release* 1997; 48: 243–57.

106 Mestecky J, Moro I, Underdown BJ. Mucosal immunoglobulins. In: *Mucosal Immunology*, 2nd. Ed. (Ogra PL, Mestecky J, Lamm ME, Strober W, Bienenstock J, McGhee JR, eds.), Academic Press, New York 1999; 133–52.

107 Mestecky J, Preud'homme J-L, Crago SS, Mihaesco E, Prchal JT, Okos AJ. Presence of J chain in human lymphoid cells. *Clin Exp Immunol* 1980; 39: 371–85.

108 Mestecky J, Russell MW. IgA subclasses. *Monogr Allergy* 1986; 19: 277–301.

109 Moldoveanu Z, Egan ML, Mestecky J. Cellular origins of human polymeric and monomeric IgA: intracellular and secreted forms of IgA. *J Immunol* 1984; 133: 3156–62.

110 Moldoveanu Z, Moro I, Radl J, Thorpe SR, Komiyama K, Mestecky J. Site of catabolism of autologous and heterologous IgA in non-human primates. *Scand J Immunol* 1990; 32: 577–83.

111 Moldoveanu Z, Russell MW, Wu HY, Huang W-Q, Compans RW, Mestecky J. Compartmentalization within the common mucosal immune system. *Adv Exp Med Biol* 1995; 371: 97–102.

112 Moro I, Iwase T, Komiyama K, Moldoveanu Z, Mestecky J. Immunoglobulin A (IgA) polymerization sites in human immunocytes: immunoelectron microscopic study. *Cell Struct Funct* 1990; 15: 85–91.

113 Morton HC, Van Egmond M, Van de Winkel JGJ. Structure and function of human IgA Fc receptors (FcαR). *Crit Rev Immunol* 1996; 16: 423–40.

114 Mostov K, Kaetzel CS. Immunoglobulin transport and the polymeric immunoglobulin receptor. In: *Mucosal Immunology*, 2nd. Ed. (Ogra PL, Mestecky J, Lamm ME, Strober W, Bienenstock J, McGhee JR, eds.), Academic Press, New York 1999; 181–211.

115 Nagura H, Nakane PK, Brown WR. Translocation of dimeric IgA through neoplastic colon cells *in vitro*. *J Immunol* 1979; 123: 2359–68.

116 Nardelli-Haefliger D, Kraehenbuhl JP, Curtiss R *et al*. Oral and rectal immunization of adult female volunteers with a recombinant attenuated *Salmonella typhi* vaccine strain. *Infect Immun* 1996; 64: 5219–24.

117 Nikolova EB, Russell MW. Dual function of human IgA antibodies: inhibition of phagocytosis in circulating neutrophils and enhancement of responses in IL-8-stimulated cells. *J Leukocyte Biol* 1995; 57: 875–82.

118 O'Leary AD, Sweeney EC. Lympho-glandular complexes of the colon: structure and distribution. *Histology* 1986; 10: 267–83.

119 O'Niell PA, Romsdahl MM. IgA as a blocking factor in human malignant melanoma. *Immunol Commun* 1974; 3: 427–38.

120 Ogra PL. Effect of tonsillectomy and adenoidectomy on nasopharyngeal antibody response to poliovirus. *N Engl J Med* 1979; 284: 59–64.

121 Ogra PL, Ogra SS. Local antibody response to poliovaccine in the female genital tract. *J Immunol* 1973; 110: 1307–11.

122 Pal S, Peterson EM, de la Maza LM. Intranasal immunization induces long-term protection in mice against a *Chlamydia trachomatis* genital challenge. *Infect Immun* 1996; 64: 5341–48.

123 Peppard JV, Russell MW. Phylogenetic development and comparative physiology of IgA. In: *Mucosal Immunology*, 2nd. Ed. (Ogra PL, Mestecky J, Lamm ME, Strober W, Bienenstock J, McGhee JR, eds.), Academic Press, New York 1999; 153–62.

124 Parkhouse RME. Immunoglobulin A biosynthesis. Intracellular accumulation of 7S subunits. *FEBS Lett* 1971; 16: 71–3.

125 Quiding-Järbrink M, Granström G, Nordström I, Holmgren J, Czerkinsky C. Induction of compartmentalized B cell responses in human tonsils. *Infect Immun* 1995; 63: 853–7.

126 Quiding-Järbrink M, Nordström I, Granström G *et al*. Differential expression of tissue-specific adhesion molecules on human circulating antibody-forming cells after systemic, enteric and nasal immunizations: a molecular basis for the compartmentalization of effector B cell responses. *J Clin Invest* 1997; 99: 1281–6.

127 Radl J, Schuit HRE, Mestecky J, Hijmans W. The origin of monomeric and polymeric forms of IgA in man. *Adv Exp Med Biol* 1974; 45: 57–65.

128 Russell-Jones GJ, Ey PL, Reynolds BL. The ability of IgA to inhibit the complement-mediated lysis of target red blood cells sensitized with IgG antibody. *Molec Immunol* 1980; 17: 1173–80.

129 Russell-Jones GJ, Ey PL, Reynolds BL. Inhibition of cutaneous anaphylaxis and Arthus reactions in the mouse by antigen-specific IgA. *Int Arch Allergy Appl Immunol* 1981; 66: 316–25.

130 Russell MW, Kilian M, Lamm ME. Biological activities of IgA. In: *Mucosal Immunology*, 2nd edn (Ogra PL, Mestecky J, Lamm ME, Strober W, Bienenstock J, McGhee JR, eds), Academic Press, New York 1999; 225–40.

131 Russell MW, Mansa B. Complement-fixing properties of human IgA antibodies: alternative pathway complement activation by plastic-bound, but not by specific antigen-bound IgA. *Scand J Immunol* 1989; 30: 175–83.

132 Russell MW, Moldoveanu Z, White PL, Sibert GJ, Mestecky J, Michalek SM. Salivary, nasal, genital, and systemic antibody responses in monkeys immunized intranasally with a bacterial protein antigen and the cholera toxin B subunit. *Infect Immun* 1996; 64: 1272–82.

133 Russell MW, Reinholdt J, Kilian M. Anti-inflammatory activity of human IgA antibodies and their Fabα fragments: inhibition of IgG-mediated complement activation. *Eur J Immunol* 1989; 19: 2243–9.

134 Saltzman WM, Radomsky ML, Whaley KJ, Cone RA. Antibody diffusion in human cervical mucus. *Biophys J* 1994; 66: 508–15.

135 Sandor M, Houlden B, Bluestone J, Hedrick SM, Weinstock J, Lynch RG. *In vitro* and *in vivo* activation of murine γ/δ T cells induces the expression of IgA, IgM, and IgG Fc receptors. *J Immunol* 1992; 148: 2363–9.

136 Schiff JM, Endo Y, Kells DIC, Fisher MM, Underdown BJ. Kinetic differences in hepatic transport of IgA polymers reflect molecular size (abst.) *Fed Proc* 1983; 42: 1341.

137 Sibille Y, Delacroix DL, Merill WW, Chatelain B, Vaerman JP. IgA-induced chemokinesis of human polymorphonuclear neutrophils: requirement of their Fc-α receptor. *Molec Immunol* 1987; 24: 551–9.

138 Silbart LK, Keren DF. Reduction of intestinal carcinogen absorption by carcinogen-specific secretory immunity. *Science* 1989; 243: 1462–4.

139 Sixbey JW, Yao Q. Immunoglobulin A-induced shift of Epstein–Barr virus tissue tropism. *Science* 1992; 255: 1578–80.

140 Skvaril F, Morell A. Distribution of IgA subclasses in sera and bone marrow plasma cells of 21 normal individuals. *Adv Exp Med Biol* 1974; 45: 433–5.

141 Staats HF, Nichols WG, Palker TJ. Systemic and vaginal antibody response after intranasal immunization with the HIV-1 C4V3 peptide TISP10 MN(A). *J Immunol* 1996; 157: 462–72.

142 Stephens S, Dolby JM, Montreuil J, Spik G. Differences in inhibition of the growth of commensal and enteropathogenic strains of *Escherichia coli* by lactotransferrin and secretory immunoglobulin A isolated from human milk. *Immunology* 1980; 41: 597–603.

143 Stewart WW, Mazengera RL, Shen L, Kerr MA. Unaggregated serum IgA binds to neutrophil FcαR at physiological concentrations and is endocytosed but cross-linking is necessary to elicit a respiratory burst. *J Leukocyte Biol* 1994; 56: 481–7.

144 Stockert RJ, Kressner MS, Collins JC, Sternlieb I, Morell AG. IgA interactions with the asialoglycoprotein receptor. *Proc Natl Acad Sci USA* 1982; 79: 6229–31.

145 Stokes CR, Soothill JF, Turner MW. Immune exclusion is a function of IgA. *Nature* 1975; 255: 745–6.

146 Tagliabue A, Villa L, De Magistris MT *et al*. IgA-driven T cell-mediated anti-bacterial immunity in man after live oral Ty21a vaccine. *J Immunol* 1986; 137: 1504–10.

147 Tenovuo J, Moldoveanu Z, Mestecky J, Pruitt KM, Mansson-Rahemtulla B. Interaction of specific and innate factors of immunity: IgA enhances the antimicrobial effect of the lactoperoxidase system against *Streptococcus mutans*. *J Immunol* 1982; 128: 726–31.

148 Tomana M, Kulhavy R, Mestecky J. Receptor-mediated binding and uptake of immunoglobulin A by human liver. *Gastroenterology* 1988; 94: 762–70.

149 Tomasi TB Jr, Ziegelbaum SO. The selective occurrence of γ1A globulins in certain body fluids. *J Clin Invest* 1963; 42: 1552–60.

150 Underdown BJ, DeRose J, Plaut A. Disulfide bonding of secretory component to a single monomer subunit in human secretory IgA. *J Immunol* 1977; 118: 1816–21.

151 Vaerman J-P, Langendries AE, Giffroy DA *et al*. Antibody against the human J chain inhibiting polymeric Ig receptor-mediated biliary and epithelial transport of human polymeric IgA. *Eur J Immunol* 1998; 28: 171–82.

152 Valim YML, Lachmann PJ. The effect of antibody isotype and antigenic epitope density on the complement-fixing activity of immune complexes: a systematic study using chimaeric anti-NIP antibodies with human Fc regions. *Clin Exp Immunol* 1991; 84: 1–8.

153 Van Epps DE, Brown SL. Inhibition of formylmethionyl-leucyl-phenyl-alanine-stimulated neutrophil chemiluminescence by human immunoglobulin A paraproteins. *Infect Immun* 1981; 34: 864–70.

154 Walker WA, Isselbacher KJ, Bloch KJ. Intestinal uptake of macromolecules: effect of oral immunization. *Science* 1972; 177: 608–10.

155 Watanabe T, Nagura H, Watanabe K, Brown WR. The binding of human milk lactoferrin to immunoglobulin A. *FEBS Lett* 1984; 168: 203–7.

156 Weisbart RH, Kacena A, Schuh A, Golde DW. GM-CSF induces human neutrophil IgA-mediated phagocytosis by an IgA Fc receptor activation mechanism. *Nature* 1988; 332: 647–8.

157 Williams RC, Gibbons RJ. Inhibition of bacterial adherence by secretory immunoglobulin A: a mechanism of antigen disposal. *Science* 1972; 177: 697–9.

158 Wira CR, Kaushic C, Richardson J. Role of sex hormones and cytokines in regulating the mucosal immune system in the female reproductive tract. In: *Mucosal Immunology*, 2nd edn (Ogra PL, Mestecky J, Lamm ME, Strober W, Bienenstock J, McGhee JR, eds), Academic Press, New York 1999; 1449–61.

159 Wold AE, Mestecky J, Tomana M *et al*. Secretory immunoglobulin A carries oligosaccharide receptors for *Escherichia coli* type 1 fimbrial lectin. *Infect Immun* 1990; 58: 3073–7.

160 Wolf HM, Hauber I, Gulle H *et al*. Anti-inflammatory properties of human serum IgA: induction of IL-1 receptor antagonist and FcαR (CD89)-mediated down regulation of tumor necrosis factor-alpha (TNF-α) and IL-6 in human monocytes. *Clin Exp Immunol* 1996; 105: 537–43.

Chapter

12

The composition and function of the mucus barrier in the gastrointestinal tract

Anthony P. Corfield, Robert Longman, Tarek Shirazi, Sally Hicks, Neil Myerscough and Christopher Probert

INTRODUCTION

The mucosal surfaces of the body need to be well equipped to deal with aggressive elements in the external environment that they inevitably encounter while achieving their specific functions. This is a general phenomenon, exquisitely adapted for each mucosal surface throughout the body. Examination of these defensive systems shows that they share a number of fundamental characteristics that are built into the components of each mucosal defensive barrier. In order to create a stable defensive barrier and to allow exchange between the mucosal cells and the external environment for the purposes of nutrition, respiration, reproduction, etc., a protective layer is present. This consists of a layer of secreted mucus and a glycocalyx attached to the cell-surface membranes in contact with the secreted external mucus barrier. Both secreted mucus and glycocalyx contain mucins, which are very large carbohydrate-rich molecules. The mucins are multifunctional and are adapted to the particular requirements of the various mucosal surfaces throughout the body. In the gastrointestinal tract a number of major functions can be ascribed to the mucins and these are summarized in Table 12.1. Reference to these properties will appear throughout the chapter. A number of reviews on mucins have appeared in recent years and the reader is referred to these for additional detailed background information.[1–3,23,24,30,34,36,39,44,51,55,57,81,97]

THE MUCUS BARRIER AND THICKNESS

The gastrointestinal tract is coated by a layer of viscoelastic mucus in the form of an adherent gel (Fig. 12.1). The composition and thickness of this layer varies throughout the tract due to the secretions from different cells and glands at each location, but in general its viscoelastic properties are governed by the mucins, a family of very high molecular weight glycoproteins. A general classification has identified two main types of mucin:[97] (1) secreted,

gel-forming mucins, which are responsible for the viscoelastic gels present on the mucosal surface, and (2) membrane-associated mucins, which are usually located in the apical membranes of epithelial cells and form an important part of the carbohydrate-rich glycocalyx. These two groups of mucins each make a specific contribution to mucosal defence.[97] A further group of mucin-like molecules, which has been described, is largely represented in endothelial cells;[87,97] the significance of these molecules in epithelial cells is uncertain and they will not be discussed in this chapter.

The fundamental characteristics of the mucus barrier represent primary physiological indicators of the status of the barrier. The thickness of secreted mucus layer varies throughout the gastrointestinal tract (Table 12.2), but remains relatively constant at specific sites, indicating a functionally optimized secretion for each location.[52,75] The nature of the glycocalyx also varies throughout the tract in accordance with function; the dimensions of the extended mucin molecules in the glycocalyx have implicated a range of interactions with *secreted* mucin gels, secreted proteins and effector molecules, bacteria, viruses and other organisms.[65,70,97]

MUCUS-SECRETING CELLS IN THE GASTROINTESTINAL TRACT

The mucins are synthesized and secreted from surface epithelial cells and specialized glands throughout the gastrointestinal tract[32] (Table 12.3, Fig. 12.2). The distribution of these cells and the expression of different mucins at each location indicates the specific requirement for mucus at each site. A population of specialized, mucin-producing cells, the goblet cells, is present throughout the gastrointestinal tract and contains vesicles with stored mucin.[89] The proportion of goblet cells increases through the gastrointestinal tract, with maximum density in the rectum. The cells mature after propagation from stem cells and show characteristic maturation patterns at each location throughout the tract.

Some functions of mucins at the mucosal surface of the gastrointestinal tract
• Lubrication of mucosal surfaces
• Hydration and prevention of desiccation
• Structural interactions (e.g. anchoring) between membrane-associated and secreted mucin gels

• Functions of the unstirred gel layer:
  Formation of pH gradient
  Mucus fingering, passage of acid through the mucus gel to the lumen
  Diffusion barrier to nutrients, toxins, ions, drugs and macromolecules
  Medium for interaction with protective proteins

• Protective functions:
  Non-specific interactions – trapping of particles
  Specific binding – bacteria, viruses and parasites
                – mutagens, toxins, lipids
  Quenching of free radicals
  Detoxification – heavy metal binding
  Protection of the mucosal surfaces against proteolytic attack
  Interaction with the mucosal immune system

• Active mucosal response – mucus release stimulated by: Irritants, secretagogues, toxins, lectins, immune complexes, enzymes, cytokines, microorganisms and parasites
• Energy source for the enteric microflora

Table 12.1 Some functions of mucins at the mucosal surface of the gastrointestinal tract.

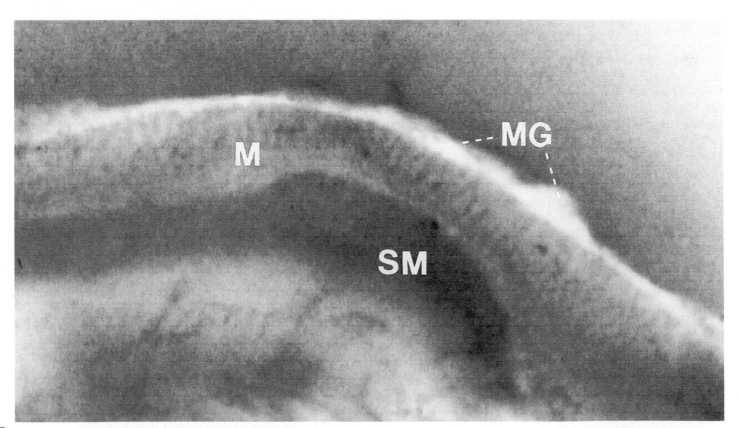

Fig. 12.1 Visualization of the adherent mucus gel layer in the human colorectum. Light microscopic image of a fresh 6 mm colorectal mucosal slice, without fixation, showing the mucus gel layer (MG), the mucosal cell layer (M) and the submucosa (SM). Magnification is ×19. Provided by Dr Cathryn Edwards, John Radcliffe Hospital, Oxford, UK.

Thickness of the adherent mucus layer in the human gastrointestinal tract		
Location	Thickness (µm)	Reference
Oesophagus	absent	A Allen, Newcastle, pers comm
Gastric antrum	144 ± 52	52
Duodenum	16 ± 5	65
Sigmoid colon	66 ± 47	52

Table 12.2 Thickness of the adherent mucus layer in the human gastrointestinal tract.

STRUCTURE OF MUCUS

Mucins

The mucins are a family of polydisperse glycoproteins of impressive complexity; they are designed to function at mucosal surfaces throughout the gastrointestinal tract, where they carry out many different tasks (see Table 12.1). The multiple functions are directly related to different levels of structural organization present within each molecule. To account for the biological action of mucins it is necessary to relate this structural organization to individual mucins and their proven functions. The properties of secreted and membrane-associated epithelial mucins are compared with the endothelial/leukocyte mucin-like molecules listed in Table 12.4. The *secreted* mucins are biological polymers

Cells expressing mucins in the human gastrointestinal tract					
Gastrointestinal organ	Site	Cells	Mucins*	Biochemistry	Reference
Salivary glands	Submandibular/ sublingual glands	Acini	MUC5B, 7 >1	MUC5B sulfated, MUC7 sialylated	67, 68
Oesophagus	Surface epithelium		MUC1, 4	?	4
	Submucosal glands	Acini	MUC5B	Mostly sulfated	4
		Ducts	MUC4	Mostly sulfated	4
Stomach	Fundus	Surface epithelium	MUC5B 5AC >1	Neutral with some sialo-sulfomucins	7, 32
		Glands	MUC6> 1	Neutral with some sialomucins>sulfomucins	7, 32
	Body and antrum	Surface foveolar cells	MUC5AC> 1, 3	Neutral mucins with, some sialo-sulfomucins	32, 78
		Mucous neck cells	MUC6> 1	Neutral mucins some sialomucins	32, 78
Small intestine	Duodenal Brunner's gland	Acini	MUC6	Neutral mucins	7, 32, 51
	Surface/villi	Goblet cells	MUC2> 3>, 1, 4	Sialomucins	7, 32, 51
		Enterocytes	MUC1, 3, 4	?	7
	Deep/crypts	Goblet cells	MUC2> 1, 4	Neutral mucins	7, 32, 51
		Enterocytes	MUC1, 4	?	6
Colorectum	Surface/villi	Goblet cells	MUC2, 4, 11 >12 >3, 1	Sulfated sialomucin, predominant in the right colon, non-sulfated mucin in the left colon	7, 32, 51
		Colonocytes	MUC3, 4 >1, 12	?	7
	Deep/crypts	Goblet cells	MUC2, 11 >4, 12 >5B, 1	Sulfated sialomucin predominant in the left colon, non-sulfated mucin in the right colon	7, 32, 51
		Colonocytes	MUC4> 12 >1	?	7

*The mucin gene expression is shown as the relative level reported. Other mucin genes have been described in the gastrointestinal tract; however, the levels are low and variable and only major mucin patterns are described here.

Table 12.3 Cells expressing mucins in the human gastrointestinal tract.

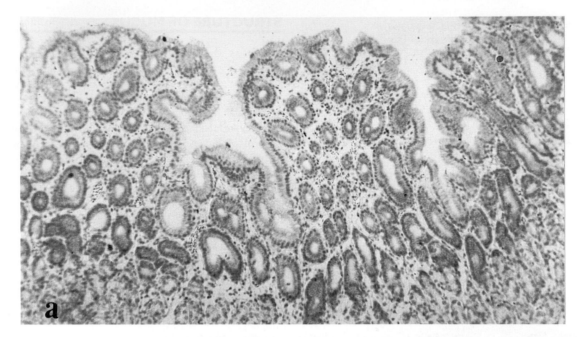

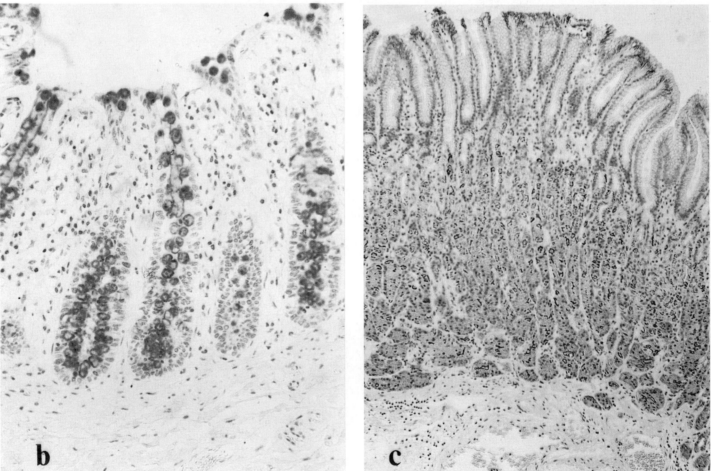

Fig. 12.2 Immunohistology of MUC genes in human gastrointestinal epithelial tissue. Antimucin antibodies were used to demonstrate the location of mucins in the following tissues: (a) Human gastric antrum stained for MUC5AC using the non-VNTR (non-variable number tandem repeat), antipeptide antibody 21M1 (Dr Jacques Bara, Paris, France). Staining is present in superficial epithelial cells but not in the deeper glands. (b) Human colon stained for MUC2 using the non-VNTR, antipeptide antibody LUM2–3 (Dr Ingemar Carlstedt, Lund, Sweden). Staining is seen in goblet cells throughout the colonic crypts. (c) Human gastric body stained for MUC1 using the VNTR, antipeptide antibody BC2 (Dr Mike McGuckin, Brisbane, Australia). Staining localized in the extreme superficial epithelial cells and in the deep gland cells. (d). Human colon stained for MUC4 using a mixture of the VNTR, antipeptide antibodies M4.171 and M.4.275 (Dr Mike McGuckin, Brisbane, Australia). The staining is found in both goblet and absorptive cells throughout the epithelial cells.

Fig. 12.2d see next page

Fig. 12.2 (*continued*)

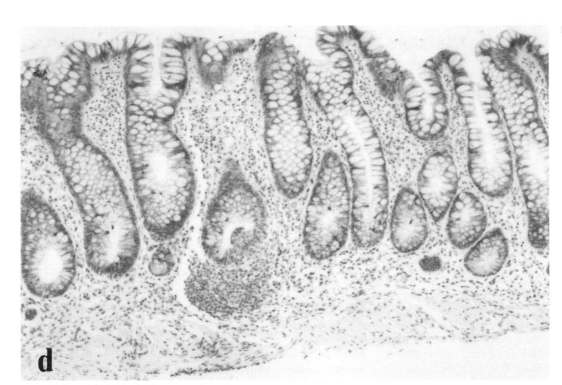

d

	General properties of secreted and membrane-associated mucins		
Property	**Epithelial MUC gene mucins**		**Endothelial/leucocyte mucin-like molecules**
	Secreted mucins	**Membrane-associated mucins**	
Examples	MUC2, 5AC, 5B, 6, 7 (8?), 9, 11	MUC1, 3, 4, 12	CD31, CD43, GlyCAM 1, MAdCAM 1, PSGL 1
Location	Mucous secretory cells, goblet cells and mucous gland cells	Mucous and non-mucous cells. Cell membrane and secretory forms	Leukocytes, endothelial cells, some epithelial cells. Transmembrane or membrane located
Mature product size	$>10^6$ Da, up to 40×10^6 Da in aggregates	$2-4 \times 10^5$ Da	$5-24 \times 10^4$ Da
VNTR	Yes	Yes	No
Polymorphism	Yes (except MUC5B)	Yes	Yes
Non-VNTR domains	Yes, von Willebrand type, cysteine knot type (except MUC7)	Yes, transmembrane domain, EGF type	Ig domains
Intra-molecular disulfide bridges	Yes (except MUC7)	No	No
Oligomerization	Yes	No, monomers	No, monomers and dimers only
Splice variants	Few	Yes	Yes
Function	Extracellular gel	Cell-surface glycocalyx	Cellular lectin ligands, cell–cell interactions

CD = cluster designation
EGF = epidermal growth factor
GlyCAM 1 = glycosylation-dependent cell adhesion molecule 1
MAdCAM 1 = mucosal addressin cell adhesion molecule 1
MUC1, 2, 3, etc. = family of mucin genes
PSGL 1 = P-selection glycoprotein ligand 1
VNTR = variable number tandem repeat.

Table 12.4 General properties of secreted and membrane-associated mucins.

characterized by their very high molecular weight and size, a high proportion of O-glycosidically linked carbohydrate (usually 50–80%) and their ability to form viscoelastic gels. *Membrane-associated* mucins belong to the same family of molecules, share many of the basic structural properties, but are adapted for functional roles as active membrane components. This means that they do not form gels, are monomeric and do not form polymers and possess membrane anchors (Tables 12.4 and 12.5).

The complex, polydisperse nature of the mucins resides in the natural variation built into the molecules at the levels of peptide and especially carbohydrate structure. Recent advances in the molecular biology of the MUC genes and the biochemistry of the mature products have contributed to a better understanding of the nature of this variation and have now indicated reasons why this polydispersity exists and the biological advantages associated with it.

The mucin genes

The family of mucin genes (MUC genes) comprises 12 members at present (Table 12.5).[10,29,36,38,40,41,58,65,85,92,102] The *secreted* mucins are represented by MUC2, MUC5AC, MUC5B, MUC6, MUC7, MUC8, MUC9 and MUC11. These genes code for mucins that are found as viscous secretions (MUC7) or viscoelastic gels at mucosal surfaces throughout the body. Four of them (MUC2, MUC5AC, MUC5B and MUC6) are clustered on chromosome 11p15.5. Complete sequence information is available for MUC2[38] and MUC5B,[29] most of MUC5AC is now known, but MUC6 is still incomplete.[93] All of the chromosome 11p15.5 MUC genes are expressed in the gastrointestinal tract, albeit at different locations (Tables 12.3 and 12.5). MUC2, MUC5AC and MUC6 show major expression in the epithelia from the stomach to the rectum,[7,18] while MUC5B shows major expression in salivary glands[101] and oesophageal glands,[4] but minor levels in gastric and colorectal epithelia.[7,95] MUC8 was originally identified in the tracheobronchial epithelium but has not been detected in the gastrointestinal tract. MUC9 is oviductin with limited tissue expression,[58] and MUC11 is largely found in the large intestine.[102]

The membrane-associated mucins comprise MUC1, MUC3, MUC4 and MUC12. Evidence for the involvement of these genes in membrane-associated events including signalling is now convincing. MUC1 has tyrosine residues in the cytoplasmic tail sequence which are phosphorylated and are thought to function in the regulation of signal transduction[9,107] and similar tyrosine phosphorylation sites have been identified in MUC3 and MUC12. MUC3, MUC4 and MUC12 all have epidermal growth factor (EGF)-like domains and have also been linked with signalling pathways.[16,66,103] The demonstration of these motifs in these membrane-associated mucins provides strong support for a regulatory role of these molecules in epithelial cells in addition to the cell-adhesion properties originally put forward.[44] In addition, MUC1, MUC3 and MUC4 have been shown to exist in soluble or 'shed' forms, which raises further questions of functional aspects that are as yet unexplored. Finally, a second cluster of MUC genes identified on chromosome 7q22 comprises MUC3, MUC11 and MUC12[102,103] and provides another focus of attention, as this is also a disease-susceptibility locus for inflammatory bowel disease.[56]

Mucin peptide structure

Variable number tandem repeat (VNTR) sequences

All of the MUC genes are characterized by the presence of variable number tandem repeat (VNTR) sequences, which contain high amounts of serine, threonine and proline (STP-rich regions).[34,36,39,81,90,102] As the carbohydrate side chains are attached to serine and threonine residues through O-glycosidic linkages, these regions represent the major site of glycosylation in the mucins.[20,57,81] Similar patterns are seen in the endothelial and leucocyte mucin-like molecules, except that there are only STP regions but no tandem repeats[97] (Tables 12.4 and 12.5). Most of the MUC genes show polymorphism at the VNTR level,[27,99] which results in real molecular size differences in the translated mature mucins. The presence of VNTR regions also has great relevance in the detection of mucins in general. As these regions

Characteristics of MUC genes						
Gene	**VNTR size**	**Chromosome**	**Gel forming**	**Von Willebrand domains**	**Membrane anchor**	**Reference**
MUC1	20	1q21	No	No	Yes	35
MUC2	23	11p15.5	Yes	Yes	No	37
MUC3	17/59/375	7q22	No?	No	Yes	26, 40, 103
MUC4	16	3q29	No?	No	Yes	65
MUC5A/C	8	11p15.5	Yes	Yes	No	41
MUC5B	29	11p15.5	Yes	Yes	No	31
MUC6	169	11p15.5	Yes	Yes	No?	92
MUC7	23	4q13-q21	No	No	No	10
MUC8	13/41	12q24.3	Yes?	?	No?	85
MUC9	16	1p13	No	No	?	58
MUC11	28	7q22	?	?	No?	102
MUC12	28	7q22	?	No?	Yes	102

Table 12.5 Characteristics of MUC genes. The properties of the mucin (MUC) genes are shown. Question marks (?) indicate the absence of direct experimental evidence in support of the statement. VNTR (variable number tandem repeat) size is given as the number of amino acid residues. Data for this table were complied from the literature listed.

were initially identified as unique mucin characteristics, antibodies to these peptide sequences were prepared as gene-specific reagents.[104] However, the glycosylation of these sequences during normal biosynthesis of the mucins blocks the binding of most of these reagents. The detection of mucins with these antibodies would be expected in the Golgi apparatus where the peptide is first translated but has not been O-glycosylated, and typical perinuclear–Golgi staining patterns have been reported. Recent efforts have focused on the preparation of reagents that are directed to the non-VNTR sequences in the MUC genes, as these have become available.[48,101]

Non-VNTR domains in secretory MUC genes

Investigation of the secretory genes MUC2, MUC5AC, MUC5B and MUC6 shows that, in addition to the VNTR, STP-rich regions, there are multiple cysteine-rich domains which show homology with the D domains of pre-pro-von Willebrand factor and carboxy-terminal, cystine-knot domains.[38,41] In other non-mucin proteins such as von Willebrand factor, these domains are required for oligomerization as the molecules are processed through the rough endoplasmic reticulum and the Golgi network.[82] The distribution of the domains at the N- and C-termini of the proteins is related to the initial formation of dimers and eventual polymerization to higher forms as two distinct stages in separate subcellular compartments. These domains also contribute to the mode of storage of the molecules before secretion.[82] The three-dimensional arrangement of the cysteine residues in these domains is highly conserved and the formation of intramolecular disulfide bridges, leading to dimerization and subsequent oligomerization, is analogous to the processes believed to occur for the mucins.[38,82] The presence of these domains with a similar molecular organization in the secreted mucins strongly suggests that they are fulfilling similar functions of oligomerization and storage. The absence of cysteine-rich domains in the secreted salivary mucin MUC7 supports this concept. Accordingly, it is smaller than the other secretory mucins and does not form viscoelastic gels.[10]

Peptide structure in membrane-associated mucins

MUC1, MUC3, MUC4 and MUC12 are mucins designed to fulfil a membrane function.[65,70,102,103] They have characteristics typical of membrane glycoproteins; they are monomeric, do not form polymers or gels, have membrane anchors and possess potential phosphorylation sites. All of these mucins are coded for by single genes that have typical mucin STP-rich VNTR sequences[36,65] and show polymorphism,[27,36,99] as described for the secreted mucins above. MUC1[70] and MUC4[65] have peptide cleavage sites, which generate two fragments: a peptide with a C-terminal cytoplasmic 'tail' region and hydrophobic membrane spanning anchor, and a larger 'mucin' fragment which may be released from the apical surface of the cells and may contribute to the extracellular mucus gel. As a result, both MUC1 and MUC4 may occur in the membrane as a complex of the two cleavage products, which remain associated by non-covalent forces.[65,70] MUC4 has been shown to be the human homologue of a well-documented rat sialomucin complex and proteolytic cleavage has been identified as a normal part of the biosynthetic pathway for this mucin.[16,49] In addition, both MUC1 and MUC4 genes show splice variants that could also result in the formation of soluble forms of these mucins.[65,66,70] The tissue distribution of

these two mucin genes is different to that of the secreted mucins. They are not limited to typical mucous cells but are also found, for example, in the absorptive cells of the colon (Table 12.4).[7,36]

MUC3 is now established as a membrane-associated mucin.[26,103] The gene is expressed in the small and large intestine and has a typical cellular distribution, appearing in the majority of surface epithelial cells and the upper-third of the colonic crypt cells, but is not restricted to the goblet cells alone. The human gene is complex, showing both VNTR and sequence polymorphism and a membrane anchor.[26,27,40,103] MUC3, MUC4 and MUC12 contain C-terminal EGF domains, which have not been found in other MUC genes to date. These mucin genes have thus been implicated in extracellular matrix and cell adhesion, chemotaxis, wound healing and cell signalling.[26,40,65,103]

The membrane mucins expressed in the gastrointestinal tract are thought to be integrated into the glycocalyx at the apical surface of epithelial cells. Here they may have multiple roles, including structural membrane properties, mucosal and bacterial cell–cell and cell–matrix interactions, the presentation of carbohydrate epitopes for identification and ligand interaction with growth factors, hormone and other signalling molecules. The structural properties of the membrane-associated mucins fit well with the range of functions required of glycoproteins in a protective and interactive surface glycocalyx.

Mucin glycosylation

The mucins located at each section of the gastrointestinal tract have a typical carbohydrate composition that reflects their site-specific functional requirements. As carbohydrate comprises the major part of the mature mucins and shows a bewildering structural complexity, it is important to know whether this complexity represents 'packaging' alone or has more precise structure–function relationships. By far the greatest contribution to the carbohydrate composition of mucins is made by the O-linked oligosaccharide chains. However, mucins also possess N-linked oligosaccharides linked to asparagine residues in the mucin polypeptide through an N-glycosidic bond to N-acetyl-D-glucosamine. The consensus peptide sequence asn-X-ser/thr acts as a potential N-glycosylation site and these have been detected in most mucins sequenced to date, mostly outside the VNTR regions.[29,36,40,57,65,93] The oligosaccharides have a common pattern, with a branched trimannosyl core attached to two N-acetyl-D-glucosamine units linked to the peptide. Various additions to this core structure lead to a family of oligosaccharides rich in mannose (high mannose) or with D-galactose, N-acetyl-D-glucosamine, L-fucose and terminal sialic acids (complex) and mixtures of the two (hybrid). The presence of mannose in these chains is in contrast to the O-linked chains and was at one time thought to be an indication of the impurity of mucin preparations. N-linked oligosaccharides are added early in mucin biosynthesis and have specific functions in subcellular compartment targeting through the Golgi complex and into secretory vesicles, folding of the mucin polypeptides and, perhaps, in recycling pathways for some of the membrane-associated mucins.[28,30,34,36,39,43,44]

The O-linked oligosaccharides in mucins are concentrated in the STP-rich VNTR regions. They are attached through the oxygen of serine and threonine residues to N-acetyl-D-galactosamine. There is no apparent amino acid consensus sequence for O-linkages, although a predictive system based on sequence context and surface accessibility was proposed recently.[42] The oligosaccharides

Table 12.6 Structure of oligosaccharide cores found in gastrointestinal mucins.

Structure of oligosaccharide cores found in gastrointestinal mucins			
Core	Structure	Occurrence	Reference
Core 1	GalNAc-α-O-peptide Galβ1–3	Meconium, saliva, gastric	57, 81, 84
Core 2	GlcNAcβ1–6 GalNAc-α-O-peptide Galβ1–3	Meconium, saliva, gastric	57, 81, 84
Core 3	GalNAc-α-O-peptide GlcNAcβ1–3	Meconium, saliva, gastric, colonic	57, 81, 84
Core 4	GlcNAcβ1–6 GalNAc-α-O-peptide GlcNAcβ1–3	Meconium, saliva, gastric, colonic	57, 81, 84

can be divided up into three regions.[57,84] All chains have a core, some have a backbone and most have peripheral additions. Up to eight different core units linked to the peptide have been identified; these are composed of di- or trisaccharides all containing N-acetyl-D-galactosamine.[84] Of these, four are commonly found in mucins throughout the gastrointestinal tract.[81,84] These are shown in Table 12.6.

Salivary and gastric mucins contain all four cores, while the colonic mucins are limited to core 3 only.[81] Meconium mucins have been found to contain additional core structures[81] and this implies a role for mucin glycosylation during the process of gastrointestinal development. Due to the specificity of the glycosyltransferases, only certain structures can be formed and the initiation of a chain with a particular core determines the nature of the final product[84] (see Fig. 12.5). Backbone regions are found in some mucins with elongated oligosaccharide chains. They are comprised of alternating D-galactose and N-acetyl-D-glucosamine residues in either β1–3 (type 1) or β1–4 (type 2) linkage and are known as poly N-acetyllactosamine units. Type 2 disaccharide units can be found in linear or branched forms, giving rise to the I/i antigens.[57,84]

The final additions to the oligosaccharide chains make up the peripheral regions; these are often the structures that donate characteristic identity and are implicated in specific binding characteristics – some examples are given in Table 12.7. They include sialic acids and sulfate, which donate negative charge, blood group and Lewis antigens, which are present on the glycoproteins found at mucosal surfaces of the gastrointestinal tract in secretor-positive individuals. These terminal residues are important in mucin antigenicity, mucin charge (neutral or acid properties), mucin rheology and in mucin degradation.

The sialic acids may occur in several different linkages in mucin oligosaccharides: α2–3, α2–6 in most chains and α2–8 in di-, tri- or polysialyl units. In man, the parent form of sialic acid, N-acetyl-D-neuraminic acid, is found; the N-glycolyl form, found in most other mammals, is antigenic in man and the gene for the hydroxylase which catalyses this conversion is suppressed.[20] The sialic acids are found only at the non-reducing oligosaccharide termini; furthermore, they exist as a family of modified monosaccharides. Most commonly detected are the O-acetylated sialic acids, which may be mono- or poly-O-acetylated and have a

tissue-specific distribution in gastrointestinal mucins. The presence of poly-O-acetylated sialic acid in colonic mucins gives these molecules a unique hydrophobic character and resistance to degradation.[20] Sulfate adds a further dimension to the mucins in the gastrointestinal tract.[79] It carries a double negative charge and is found in D-galactose and N-acetyl-D-glucosamine residues in oligosaccharide chains (Table 12.7).

Furthermore, there are a variety of peripheral structures that have significance as developmental antigens or are induced in response to inflammation. Many of these structures also appear during malignancy and other diseases.[81] Accordingly, the collection of data for mucins in well-defined disease conditions has led to the identification of disease-related glycosylation pathways and disease-related carbohydrate antigens.[20,81]

Non-mucin components

The mucus barrier contains many non-mucin components, which are essential factors of the physiological barrier and play different roles in the multifunctional nature of the whole supramucosal layer. These aspects have been reviewed elsewhere[1,8,34,60] and components of particular current interest are given more detailed attention here.

Electrolytes and bicarbonate

Total mucus contains fluid and electrolytes that contribute to the hydrated and viscoelastic properties of the whole secretion. The control of secretion and absorption of these components is vital to the normal function of mucus at each mucosal surface throughout the gastrointestinal tract. The secretion of mucins may be coupled with fluid and electrolyte secretion through a variety of mechanisms reviewed elsewhere[33,34] and briefly below. The secretion of bicarbonate is an important feature of the gastroduodenal mucosa. The interaction of bicarbonate with the unstirred mucus layer has been shown to ensure a neutral pH at the mucosal surface, give rise to a pH gradient across the mucus gel layer and combat the high acidity of the gastric and duodenal lumen.[1] The H+ ions present in the gastric lumen are able to diffuse through the mucus layer, but are effectively neutralized by the bicarbonate secreted from the mucosal cells, which also diffuses across the mucus gel. The presence of the mucus gel prevents dissipation of the secreted bicarbonate and provides an effective mechanism for the neutral-

Name	Structure	Comment
Blood group H Type 1 (Galβ1–3GlcNAc)	Fucα1–2Galβ1–3GlcNAcβ1-	Basic blood group structure, also found on Type 2 chains (Galβ1–4GlcNAc)
Blood group A Type 1 (Galβ1–3GlcNAc)	GalNAcα1–3(Fucα1–2)Galβ1–3GlcNAcβ1-	Terminal alpha-linked sugar, also found on Type 2 chain (Galβ1–4GlcNAc)
Blood group B Type 1(Galβ1–3GlcNAc)	Galα1–3(Fucα1–2)Galβ1–3GlcNAcβ1-	Terminal alpha-linked sugar, also found on Type 2 chain (Galβ1–4GlcNAc)
Lewis a	Galβ1–3(Fucα1–4)GlcNAcβ1-	Lewis antigen on Type 1 chain
Lewis b	Fucα1–2Galβ1–3(Fucα1–4)GlcNAcβ1-	Lewis antigen on Type 1 chain
Lewis x	Galβ1–4(Fucα1–3)GlcNAcβ1-	Lewis antigen on Type 2 chain
Lewis y	Fucα1–2Galβ1–4(Fucα1–3)GlcNAcβ1-	Lewis antigen on Type 2 chain
Sialyl Lewis a	Neu5Acα2–3Galβ1–3(Fucα1–4)GlcNAcβ1-	Sialylated Lewis antigen, also found for Lewis x
Sulfo Lewis a	SO^3-3Galβ1–3(Fucα1–4)GlcNAcβ1-	Sulfated Lewis antigen, also found for Lewis x
Sialyl-Tn	Neu5Acα2–6GalNAc-α-O-peptide	Cancer-associated antigen
Tn antigen	GalNAc-α-O-peptide	Commonly found as a tumour-associated antigen, normally substituted with sialic acid
Thomsen Friedenreich T-antigen	Galβ1–3GalNAc-α-O-peptide	Commonly found as a tumour-associated antigen, normally substituted with sialic acid

Table 12.7 Examples of peripheral units commonly found in mucin oligosaccharides. Terminal, non-reducing oligosaccharide structures commonly found in gastrointestinal mucins; note that many of these structures are substituted on Type 1 (Galβ1–3GlcNAc) and/or Type 2 (Galβ1–4GlcNAc) backbone units.

ization of acid to occur efficiently. The presence of a continuous and renewable mucus gel layer is fundamental to this process. The apparent paradox of both acid and bicarbonate secretion originating from the gastric mucosa without the acidification of the mucus gel layer and the mucosal surface may be explained by viscous fingering. This phenomenon depends on a physicochemical property of mucus whereby acid, a low-viscosity fluid, is secreted under pressure into the high-viscous mucus fluid. The low pH increases the viscosity of the mucus and gives rise to viscous fingers, which are maintained as single channels, emerge at the surface and do not re-enter the gel.[8] This is in contrast to the high-pH bicarbonate secretion.

Lipids and the hydrophobic barrier properties of mucus
It has long been known that lipids are associated with mucus throughout the gastrointestinal tract and that these can form complexes with the mucins. These complexes have more pronounced viscoelastic properties than the isolated lipid-free mucins.[60] Up to 20% of the organic material has been detected as lipid in isolated gastric mucus, although its origin remains conjectural and sloughed cells and shed membranes may contribute to the total. Lipids identified in association with mucins include phospholipids, ceramides and glyceroglucolipids, in addition to covalently linked fatty acids. Further support for a role of these lipids in mucosal protection has come from studies of gastric secretagogues which link both phospholipid and mucin secretion.

Proposed functions for the lipids are concerned with the mucus resistance to gastric acid attack,[60] the increased protection to degradation by bacterial mucinase activity and protection against mucin degradation by free radicals.

Defensive proteins
Mucus contains a number of proteins that contribute in different ways to the protective functions of the barrier. Many of these proteins, such as lysozyme, lactoferrin, secretory immunoglobulin A (sIgA) and protease inhibitors, have been known for some time, while others have only recently been identified. This section focuses in more detail on some of the novel proteins reported in mucus (Table 12.8).

Lysozyme
Mucosal cells throughout the gastrointestinal tract secrete the antibacterial protein lysozyme. In some cases, co-secretion with mucins has been identified. The protein has a positive charge and is often found bound to the negatively charged mucins. The general antibacterial properties of this protein make it an important participant in mucosal defence.

Lactoferrin
Lactoferrin is an iron-sequestering glycoprotein that predominates in mucosal secretions, where the level of free extracellular iron (10^{-18} mol/L) is not sufficient for bacterial growth. This

Defensive proteins in the gastrointestinal tract associated with mucus	
Lysozyme	Antibacterial protein
Lactoferrin	Iron-sequestering glycoprotein
Secretory IgA	Specific mucosal antibody
Protease inhibitors	e.g. pancreatic secretory trypsin inhibitor (PSTI)
Growth factors	e.g. transforming growth factor α (TGFα) PSTI, epidermal growth factor (EGF)
Defensins (α, β)	Antimicrobial peptides
β-Galectins	Carbohydrate-binding proteins
Trefoil factor peptides	Rapid response mucosal repair peptides

Table 12.8 Defensive proteins in the gastrointestinal tract associated with mucus.

represents a mechanism of resistance to bacterial infections by prevention of colonization of the host by pathogens. Lactoferrin is secreted by mucosal cells throughout the gastrointestinal tract and is found in mucus secreted at most locations.[106] As a result of the known protective roles of this protein, the benefits of orally administered bovine lactoferrin have been widely examined as a dietary factor, having an influence on bacteriostasis and the immune system.

Secretory IgA

Mucosal surfaces throughout the gastrointestinal tract produce and secrete immunoglobulins. Secretory IgA (sIgA) is the major mucosal defence immunoglobulin and is a part of the mucus secretion. In man, almost all intestinal antibodies are produced locally by plasma cells in the gut mucosa and are not derived to a significant degree from the circulation. Passive protection provided by effective prenatal transplacental transport of maternal antibodies, or postnatal consumption of milk antibodies in breast-fed newborns, is essential for the survival of neonates.[63] A full discussion of the roles and interactions of sIgA is given in Chapter 11.

Protease inhibitors

A range of peptides with antiprotease and antipeptidase activity has been identified in gastrointestinal tract mucosal cells. The most significant of these appear to be α_1-antitrypsin inhibitor and pancreatic secretory trypsin inhibitor (PSTI). PSTI is synthesized in gastrointestinal mucous cells and has a protective effect on gastric and colonic mucus. Its reduction in disease is associated with depletion of the mucus barrier.[73]

Growth factors

Many peptide growth factors and cytokines have been identified in the gastrointestinal tract and a variety of different functional roles of these agents have been described. A recent classification of the functions of these peptides has addressed the type of peptide, its sites of synthesis, its mechanism of action and fluctuations in its levels at damaged mucosal locations.[71] Under

this classification all peptides fall into one of three groups. First, mucosal integrity peptides, which are expressed throughout the gastrointestinal tract and act to preserve mucosal integrity; these include transforming growth factor α (TGFα) and PSTI. TGFα shows structural similarity to EGF and binds to EGF receptors. Its functions as a paracrine growth factor include stimulation of cellular DNA synthesis, induction of mucosal cell migration and inhibition of acid secretion. Its interactions with mucus are not well understood. PSTI is found in all gastrointestinal mucosae and is discussed under protease inhibitors above. Its anti-proteolytic action restricts the action of luminal proteases on gastrointestinal mucus. Secondly, luminal surveillance peptides, the best known example in this group is EGF. This peptide is continuously secreted, but appears to exert an action only when there is mucosal damage. Further evidence in favour of such a role has been suggested as the EGF receptors are found at the baso-lateral and not apical membranes of mucosal cells and would only be accessible to luminal EGF when the mucosal surface is disrupted.[73] The importance of EGF in binding to mucus and mucins remains unclear, and interactions of EGF with mucus have not been assessed. Furthermore, the presence of EGF domains on MUC3 and MUC4 peptides also awaits a functional explanation. Among various functions EGF has been shown to stimulate the release of mucus from jejunum,[50] making a contri-bution to intestinal cytoprotection. Finally, rapid response peptides provide an immediate response to mucosal damage and initiate the process of mucosal repair. Examples of such agents are the trefoil peptides, which are discussed below.

Defensins

The defensins are a family of antimicrobial peptides secreted by leukocytes and Paneth cells in the small intestine. In keeping with most antimicrobial peptides the defensins are amphiphatic and kill microorganisms by disruption of the microbial cell membrane.[69] The defensins consist of two genetically related peptide families, the α- and β-defensins; they are cationic and range in size from 3 to 4 kDa. They contain six cysteine residues, which form three disulfide bridges, and all have a very similar three-dimensional structure. The α-defensins, also termed cryptdins, have been studied in the small intestine, where they are found localized at the base of the crypts of Lieberkühn in Paneth cell granules. Other components of the granules are lysozyme and secretory phospho-lipase A_2, tumour necrosis factor α (TNFα), cysteine-rich intestinal polypeptide, matrilysin and α_1-antitrypsin. A synergistic action of defensins with these molecules in crypt defence has been pro-posed.[69] No influence on the secretion of mucins has been reported. This mechanism may ensure the distribution of the Paneth cell granules and their contents along the crypt lumen to the mucosal surface and more effectively combat microbial colonization. Defensins are believed to be part of an innate defen-sive system in man, as mRNA can be detected before birth corresponding with the maturation of Paneth cells in the first trimester of gestation.[69]

Beta-galectins

The β-galectins are a gene family of eight or more animal carbo-hydrate-binding proteins that were formerly called S-type lectins and that are discrete from the C-lectins, another large group of calcium-dependent carbohydrate-binding proteins.[53] They are soluble proteins and show a tissue selective distribution. Galectins

3 and 4 are expressed in gastrointestinal mucosal cell cytoplasm; they are secreted and are found associated with the apical surfaces and within the extracellular matrix.[53]

The binding of galectins to mucins secreted onto the mucosal surface and also to the glycocalyx has been demonstrated in several studies.[11,88,100] Normal colonic mucins are known to possess elongated oligosaccharides with poly-LacNAc structures and galectin 3 binds to native and desialylated human colonic mucin.[11] The ability of galectins to form crosslinkages between glycoconjugates may play a direct role at the mucosal surface. Carbohydrate chains are present in abundance in the glycocalyx anchored to the apical surfaces of epithelial cells and also in the macromolecules secreted on the mucosal surface. Furthermore, many interactions between basal lamina glycoconjugates (laminin, integrins) and the extracellular matrix rely on the recognition of oligosaccharide chains in these molecules. The galectins comprise a group of molecules which may operate as crosslinking binding partners in some of these interactions. Indeed, Wasano and Hirakawa have proposed that mucin–mucin and mucin–extracellular matrix interaction may be mediated by galectins 3 and 4 in the gastrointestinal tract.[100]

Trefoil factor peptides

Trefoil peptides are a family of three small cysteine-rich peptides that share a unique common structural motif characteristic of a '3-leafed clover' shape[73,83] (see Fig. 12.3), and in an attempt to standardize the nomenclature they are referred to as trefoil factor family (TFF) peptides. The trefoil peptides are normally expressed in a site-specific pattern within the human gastrointestinal epithelium. TFF1 is found throughout the stomach in foveolar epithelial surface cells, TFF2 in the distal stomach and in the lower portions of Brunner's glands in the duodenum and TFF3 along the length of the small and large intestine.[74,83] They are very durable molecules, being resistant to acid, proteases and heat degradation. Two significant functions of trefoil peptides have so far been identified in the gastrointestinal tract: namely, epithelial protection and mucosal healing. Trefoils are considered as 'rapid response' peptides to mucosal injury, with upregulation of expression in the early stages of mucosal repair.[71,72]

Trefoil peptides may enhance the protective capabilities of the supramucosal defence barrier of the gastrointestinal tract by interacting or crosslinking with mucin glycoproteins to form the viscoelastic mucus gel layer.[83] Recent evidence has been presented that both MUC2 and MUC5AC von Willebrand C-domains may interact with TFF1.[91] They may also have a role in controlling goblet cell vesicle packaging of mucin glycoproteins and thus affect mucin secretion and function. It has been shown that the trefoil peptides are co-localized with specific secreted mucins: TFF1 with MUC5AC, TFF2 with MUC6 and TFF3 with MUC2.[61] This co-expression of chromosome 11 mucin genes and trefoil peptides in normal and in diseased gastrointestinal mucosa indicates a possible synergistic action in protection and repair.

THE BIOSYNTHESIS OF MUCINS

The biosynthesis of mucins is an integrated process involving a series of interlinked pathways that ensure the production of the correct MUC gene, correct folding of the peptide, the appropriate glycosylation, polymerization and storage. Understanding of the regulation and integration of these processes in the gastrointestinal tract is still in its infancy. However, study of disease has made a contribution, through the identification of aberrant events and pathways. Although individual studies on the relationship of nutrition to mucin biosynthesis have been few, there are implications from host and microflora energy metabolism and mucosal biology that suggest how these may be linked.

The biosynthesis of secreted mucins can be summarized as shown in Fig. 12.4. The sequence of events in this scheme is not firmly established and may include concomitant processes. The biosynthesis of membrane-associated mucins occurs by another pathway where signal peptide recognition targets the molecules to the correct subcellular compartments for maturation and transport to the apical cell-surface membranes.

The early stages of MUC peptide biosynthesis include N-glycosylation after the recognition of consensus sites. The N-linked oligosaccharides may be instrumental in directing the precursor peptides to their correct subcellular compartments for dimerization, subsequent O-glycosylation and oligomerization.[5,28,96] In addition, the presence of core type, glucose-containing N-glycans may allow the correct folding of the mucin peptide through the action of the endoplasmic reticulum lectins calnexin and calreticulin in common with other glycoproteins.[43] This process would ensure the correct alignment for the formation of disulfide bridges in the von Willebrand D-domains, cystine knot and EGF domains.

The existence of MUC precursor forms with N-glycosylation but no O-glycosylation has been shown in experiments with specific antimucin peptide antibodies and metabolic labelling.[96]

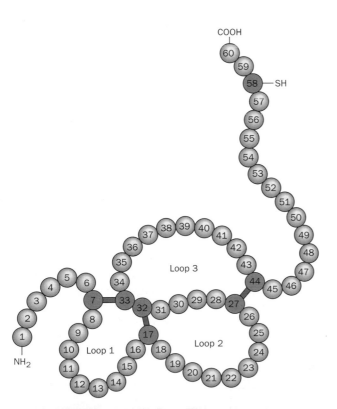

Fig. 12.3 Human trefoil family factor 1 (TFF1). Amino acid sequence and secondary structure of TFF1. The three-loop structure characteristic of a 'clover leaf' is maintained by three disulfide bonds (hatched) between three pairs of cysteine residues (dotted). A seventh cysteine residue at position 58 is probably important for dimerization. (Adapted from Ref. 74.)

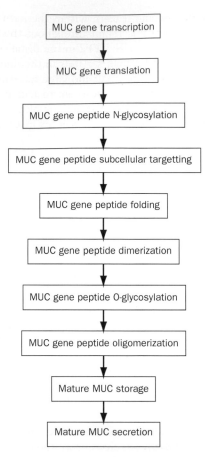

Fig. 12.4 General pathways of mucin biosynthesis. The scheme shows steps identified in the biosynthesis of secreted mucins. Some of these events may occur simultaneously and the sequence is not proven for all steps. Refer to the text for detailed discussion.

These techniques have also been employed to show the presence of dimerization and the movement of the maturing peptides through the rough endoplasmic reticulum and Golgi apparatus prior to O-glycosylation. Dimerization is believed to be an early stage in the biosynthesis of secreted mucins occurring in the rough endoplasmic reticulum. MUC2, MUC5AC, MUC5B and MUC6 have been shown to undergo this process in the gastrointestinal tract.[5,86,96] This process has been shown to involve the formation of reduction-sensitive disulfide bridges at the C-terminal of the molecules. Selectivity in the process for the mucins exists as no heterodimerization between different MUC subunits has been found. The continued oligomerization of the mucins is poorly understood. Both monomers and dimers are transferred to the Golgi apparatus and undergo O-glycosylation.[5,86,96] The mode of multimerization remains to be elucidated but is thought to take place in different subcellular compartments to dimerization,[86,96] and may involve the formation of non-SH-sensitive crosslinkages.

Pathways of mucin oligosaccharide biosynthesis (Fig. 12.5) have been determined as a result of detailed oligosaccharide structural analysis and identification of individual glycosyltransferase-catalysed steps using specific substrates.[12,81] The individual glycosyltransferases add monosaccharides sequentially to the growing oligosaccharide chain attached to the mucin peptide. The monosaccharides are activated through conjugation with nucleotides and the respective nucleotide sugars are the donors in these reactions.[12,15] It has now become apparent that the amino acid sequence in the tandem repeat structure of the different MUC genes has a bearing on the order of acceptor amino acid substitution by the action of the initial glycosyltransferase N-acetyl-galactosaminyl transferase. This activity is represented by a family of enzymes which carry out this initial transfer.[19] Further glycosylation follows to give sequences which are determined by the

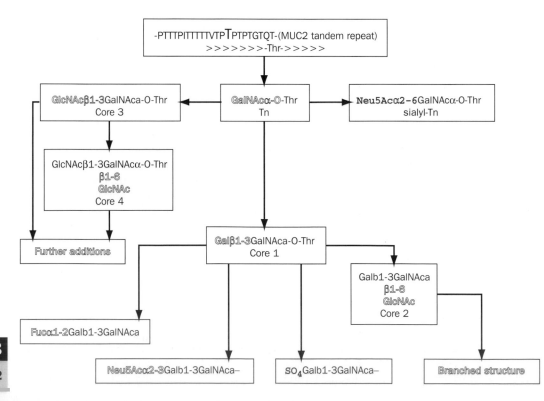

Fig. 12.5 Pathways of oligosaccharide formation. Initial steps of oligosaccharide formation on mucin tandem repeat peptides. Examples of known pathways in oligosaccharide biosynthesis are shown. This is a selection of pathways from many existing examples to illustrate the formation of oligosaccharide sequences during mucin biosynthesis.

strict substrate specificity and enzyme availability in the respective tissues. Thus the availability of a range of glycosyltransferases within a particular Golgi subcellular compartment will ensure the formation of defined oligosaccharide structures.[12,81] The loss of individual glycosyltransferase activity has highlighted the significance of changes in oligosaccharide sequence associated with disease structures,[12,81] and the formation of cancer-related carbohydrate antigens.

SECRETION OF MUCINS AND MUCUS

The range of mucus-secreting cells described earlier in the chapter (see Table 12.3) produce and store mucins in preparation for secretion to form and supplement the mucus barrier at the mucosal surface. The apical granules observed in goblet cells accumulate secretory vesicles at the apical pole and discharge the contents by exocytosis, which takes place with the fusion of the vesicle and plasma membranes and the formation of a fusion pore.[33,34] The process probably requires a force to expel the mucins and this may arise from the hydration of the stored mucins on contact with the external aqueous environment.[98] In addition, a washout secretion may be supplied from the base of the granules by the action of ion-channel proteins and ATP-dependent proton pumps.[33] In some cases rapid and extensive exocytosis may occur, leading to typical goblet cell cavitation with loss of cytoplasm and granule membranes.[89] Secretion takes place by two pathways in secretory cells. A constitutive pathway is responsible for a continuous secretion of mucins and proteins from vesicles that are not triggered by receptor-mediated secretagogues. These vesicles mature and discharge without any long-term residence at the apical pole of the goblet cells and are responsible for the continuous production and secretion of mucus. In addition to this continuous secretion, is the regulated pathway characterized by vesicles that are distended and accumulate at the apical pole of the goblet cells and are induced to exocytosis by receptor-mediated secretagogues. A large number of secretagogues have been tested, leading to the identification of cholinergic, purinergic and neurotensin receptors. These act by increasing intracellular calcium and activate the calcium-mediated and protein kinase C-mediated signal pathways.[33,34] Intestinal goblet cells operate both constitutive and regulated pathways and thus contain vesicles delivering the maintained secretion and those sensitive to the action of secretagogues.[33,34] Many possibilities for the release of mucus from goblet cells through dietary components exist on the basis of the identified receptors; however, it is difficult to assess the daily contribution of the diet to this process.

CATABOLISM AND TURNOVER OF MUCINS AND MUCUS

The degradation of mucus is a normal feature of the dynamic status of the adherent barrier. There is an equilibrium between mucosal synthesis and secretion and the degradation of the existing adherent gel layer by bacterial and host hydrolytic enzymes. It is clear that this equilibrium is under a regulation that ensures a continual protection of the mucosal surface against potentially damaging compounds entering in the diet. Chapter 21 contains further discussion of the impact of nutrition on the enteric bacterial flora.

The concept of a mucinase activity is well known and derives from observations of mucin carbohydrate loss and metabolic conversion by bacteria in the large intestine. Bacterial strains were identified which possess enzymes capable of specific and complete degradation of mucins.[45] The breakdown products were utilized for bacterial energy production ultimately leading to the production of short-chain fatty acids, the end products of bacterial metabolism and potential energy sources for the host mucosal epithelial cells.

As a result of the complex composition of the mucins, the pathways for their degradation are diverse and include many different degrading enzymes.[79] Activities are required that will act on the mucus gel to reduce it to a viscous fluid, enzymes to degrade the accessible peptide backbone and enzymes to cleave the individual sugars from the oligosaccharide chains. As many bacteria normally present in the gut do not possess all of these enzymes, it is clear that cooperation exists in this process and that this itself may constitute part of the regulative process in action in the colorectum.[79] Not only do the individual bacterial strains have their own battery of hydrolytic enzymes but the location of the enzymes in cell membranes, periplasmic space or as secreted forms needs to be correlated with substrate specificity and mode of action at the mucosal surface.

The large intestine is the main site of mucinase activity in the gut. Mucinase activity arises from the enteric gut flora; it is acquired at birth and accumulates over the first 2 years of life.[64] It has been measured in faecal samples using electrophoretic[64] and direct mucinase assays (Gill, Corfield and Millar, unpublished work). In adults, the mucinase potential comprises peptidases, glycosidases and sulfatases, which are present as secreted or membrane-bound enzymes in the gut flora.[46] Mucin-degrading enzymes are produced by the main groups of bacteria present in the large intestine in different proportions, depending on individual strains. One group of bacteria has been identified which possesses all enzymes necessary to completely degrade mucin oligosaccharide chains but which produces relatively little proteolytic activity.[21,46] The colorectum shows the same symbiotic relationship demonstrated for the human oral cavity, where different bacterial strains ensure total mucin degradation.

The initial step in mucus degradation is the destruction of the mucus gel, which is thought to occur as a result of the action of faecal bacterial protease activity. The enteric bacterial population produces a variety of cell-associated and secreted protease activities[62] that allow optimal interaction with the mucus gel to initiate its solubilization. Further degradation of the proteolytically cleaved mucin glycopeptides depends on glycosidases and sulfatases acting on the carbohydrate chains. The majority are exoenzymes that remove a single monosaccharide from the non-reducing oligosaccharide terminus. Endoglycosidases act at internal sites in the carbohydrate chain, releasing oligosaccharide fragments rather than monosaccharides. Exoenzyme degradation of the peripheral residues on oligosaccharides is linked to the overall rate of degradation. The enzymes which remove the peripheral sialic acids, sulfate and blood group antigens from oligosaccharides are important as they release the remainder of the chain to the action of other glycosidases. There is evidence that both the sialic acid esterases, sulfatases and blood group specific α-galactosidases and N-acetyl-α-D-galactosaminidases are rate-limiting in mucin oligosaccharide degradation.[79]

In more than 90% of Europeans and North Americans, colonic mucins contain sialic acids with O-acetyl esters on the C7–C9 hydroxyl groups of their sialic acids.[14] These O-acetyl esters protect the sialic acids against the action of sialidases (neuraminidases) present in high levels in many enteric bacteria.[25,79] The removal of sialic acids by sialidase is enabled by the action of a specific sialate O-acetyl esterase produced by many enteric bacteria.[21] This esterase is thought to act as a rate-limiting enzyme in the removal of sialic acids from mucin oligosaccharide chains, as its level of activity is considerably lower than that of the sialidases[21,22] (Fig. 12.6).

The secretion of sulfate-rich mucins in regions of the gastrointestinal tract suggests a similar protective role for terminal sulfate groups on mucin oligosaccharides which harbour the major bacterial communities. A family of carbohydrate sulfatases act on mucins.[80] These enzymes are specific for the sulfated monosaccharide and the position of the sulfate.[79,80] Sulfatase activities have been detected in faecal extracts[22,94] and individual bacterial strains.[80]

The final group of structures that impose a limit on the rate of oligosaccharide degradation are the A and B blood group antigens (see Table 12.7). The blood group antigens are expressed on

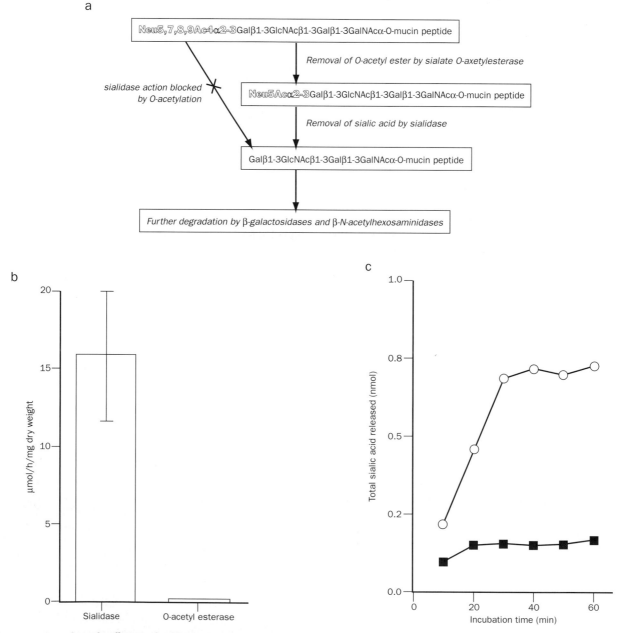

Fig. 12.6 Regulation of mucin oligosaccharide degradation. Oligosaccharide degradation by bacterial exoglycosidases. An example of regulated oligosaccharide degradation is given using the O-acetylated sialic acid residues commonly found on colorectal mucins. (a) The action of sialidase and sialate O-acetyl esterase on tri- (7, 8, 9)-O-acetyl-N-acetyl-D-neuraminic acid (Neu5,7,8,9,Ac4) as terminal residue on a colorectal mucin oligosaccharide chain. Arrows show the route of degradation through the action of the esterase as the O-acetylation of the sialic acid blocks the action of sialidase. (b) Assay of sialidase and sialate O-acetyl esterase enzymes shows the large difference in relative activities in normal faecal extracts. (c) Removal of O-acetyl esters by saponification (O) releases the block on sialidase activity with the native, O-acetylated colonic mucin (■).

the mucosal secretions of secretor-positive individuals throughout the gastrointestinal tract, except for the distal colon in adults, while the fetal colon shows expression throughout.[105] The enzymes required to remove the α-linked sugars are the N-acetyl-α-galactosaminidases (A activity) and α-galactosidases (B activity). The rate-limiting activity of these enzymes has been demonstrated in faecal extracts from secretor-positive individuals with either A, B or H blood group status acting on mucins with A, B or H blood group activity. The presence of the relevant enzyme activities correlates with the ability to completely degrade the mucins.

Faecal extracts from H individuals were incapable of degrading mucins with A or B activity, while the mucins with H activity were rapidly degraded by extracts from A and B individuals.[47] Apart from the enzymes acting on the peripheral residues of mucin oligosaccharides, the remaining chain structure is hydrolysed by a variety of glycosidases which show specificity for the glycosidic linkage, the neighbouring sugar and the region in the chain. High levels of β-galactosidases and N-acetyl-β-D-glucosaminidases have been detected which will act on mucin removing the poly N-acetyllactosamine backbone structures where present. Once the peripheral and backbone monosaccharides have been removed, the core units remain. O-glycanases, which remove the disaccharide Galβ1–3GalNAc (see core 1, Table 12.6) from mucin peptides have been described in the mucin oligosaccharide degrader and other strains. The existence of a similar enzyme acting on the core 3 structure GlcNAcβ1–3GalNAc has not been reported.

DEVELOPMENTAL ASPECTS OF MUCIN EXPRESSION

The expression of the mucin genes throughout human fetal development has been determined for the MUC1–8 and generally appear from the start of the mid-trimester.[17,76] These studies have been based on mRNA detection and no indication of translation into mature products has been systematically reported. In the stomach strong expression of MUC5AC and MUC6 was found at 23 weeks.[76] MUC5AC appeared in the surface epithelial mucus-secreting cells, while MUC6 was restricted to the mucous neck cells. These patterns agree well with the known adult location of these secreted mucin genes.[7] Throughout the intestine the MUC2 could be detected from as early as week 9 and correlates well with the known patterns of crypt and villus development in the small intestine.[13,76] MUC2 expression switches from a fetal to an adult pattern at week 23 of gestation in the small intestine and week 27 in the colon.[13,17] These results indicate that MUC2 is the major fetal and adult colonic mucin. Transitory expression of MUC5AC in the primitive gut at week 8[13] and in the colon at week 17[76] has been reported; both studies confirmed the disappearance of mRNA beyond this period and the absence in normal adult intestine. Apart from low levels of MUC6 from week 13 through to week 23,[76] no expression of the other mucin genes has been reported.

A clear difference in the expression of MUC1, MUC3 and MUC4 compared with MUC2 and other secreted mucins has been found in man.[13,76] MUC1 was detected in the colon at 18 weeks of gestation, earlier than MUC2.[17] MUC3 and MUC4 appear at 6.5 weeks, a very early gestational age when the epithelium is stratified and undifferentiated, as part of the primitive gut endoderm.[13] In adult intestine these three genes are found in mucus-secreting and non-mucus-secreting epithelial cells and are clearly implicated in cellular roles that reflect their association with membranes. The adult pattern of major MUC2 and MUC4 gene expression and low-to-background MUC1 and MUC3 was found in the neonatal period from birth to 3 months.[6]

Histochemical studies have shown that sulfation and sialic acid O-acetylation are present in mucins in the fetal colon already at week 12 and that the distribution of these carbohydrate-related structures follows the expected developmental pathways leading to the adult patterns.[59,77] These patterns also suggest that responses to development and nutrition are related more closely with glycosylation than with the mucin core peptide expression. Indeed, disease-related changes apparent in the fetus do not appear to relate to switches in mucin gene expression and are largely detected as changes in glycosylation.[32,54]

Mucin and mucus degradation is closely related to the biology and development of the mucus barrier, as outlined under mucin turnover above. There is a close link between nutrition, development and mucin metabolism at this early stage of life. The phases of lactation and weaning, together with the colonization of the gut with the normal enteric bacterial flora, play a vital role in the development of the intestinal mucosa and its protective barrier. They contrive to program a mucus barrier that is always adapting throughout this period, but which provides a continuous defence against the external environment.

SUMMARY

1. Mucus is a dynamic, multifunctional barrier interacting with dietary components while providing mucosal protection to the external environment.
2. The mucins are major components of the defensive barrier and are present as secreted and membrane-associated forms.
3. The mucins contain a high proportion of carbohydrate as oligosaccharides attached to variable number tandem repeat, serine/threonine-rich domains of the mucin peptides.
4. A family of mucin (MUC) genes code for the mucin peptides and show a tissue-specific expression throughout the gastrointestinal tract.
5. The mucins are synthesized in a regulated series of events involving dimerization, glycosylation and oligomerization, leading to mature products present in goblet cell vesicles and mucous gland cells.
6. The secretion of mucins occurs from goblet cells by constitutive and regulated pathways under the influence of a range of secretagogues.
7. Mucins interact with other mucosal proteins functioning in mucosal defence, such as lysozyme, lactoferrin, trefoil peptides and galectins.
8. The enzymatic degradation of mucins in the gastrointestinal tract follows a predicted pattern in a symbiotic relationship with enteric bacteria. Recycling of mucin carbohydrate is a feature of this relationship.

Acknowledgements

The authors wish to thank the following for support for the work presented in this chapter: The Wellcome Trust grants

046530/Z/96 and 0051586/Z/97; European Union consortium CEEBMH4-CT98-3222; Royal College of Surgeons, CM Matthews Fellowship and South and West NHS Executive Research and Development Research Studentship. We would also like to thank Dr C. Edwards for Fig. 12.1 and Professor A. Allen, University of Newcastle-upon-Tyne for data included in Table 12.2.

REFERENCES

1 Allen A. Gastrointestinal mucus. In: *Handbook of Physiology* (Forte JG, ed.), Vol. 3. American Physiological Society, 1989: 359–82.

2 Allen A, Cunliffe WJ, Pearson JP, Venables CW. The adherent gastric mucus gel barrier in man and changes in peptic ulceration. *J Intern Med* 1990; 228 (suppl 1): 83–90.

3 Allen A, Hutton DA, Pearson JP, Sellers LA. The colonic mucus gel barrier: structure, gel formation and degradation. In: *The Cell Biology of Inflammation in the Gastrointestinal Tract* (Peters TJ, ed.). Corners Publications, Hull, 1990: 113–25.

4 Arul GS, Moorghen M, Myerscough N, Alderson DA, Spicer RD, Corfield AP. Mucin gene expression in Barrett's oesophagus, an *in situ* hybridisation and immunohistochemical study. *Gut* 2000: 47: 753–8.

5 Asker N, Axelsson MAB, Olofsson SO, Hansson GC. Dimerization of MUC2 mucin in the endoplasmic reticulum is followed by a N-glycosylation dependent transfer of the mono- and dimers to the Golgi apparatus. *J Biol Chem* 1998; 273: 18857–63.

6 Aslam A, Spicer RD, Corfield AP. Histochemical and genetic analysis of colonic mucin glycoproteins in Hirschsprung's disease. *J Paediatr Surg* 1999; 34: 330–3.

7 Audié JP, Janin A, Porchet N, Copin MC, Gosselin B, Aubert JP. Expression of human mucin genes in respiratory, digestive and reproductive tracts ascertained by *in situ* hybridization. *J Histochem Cytochem* 1993; 41: 1479–85.

8 Bansil R, Stanley E, LaMont JT. Mucin biophysics. *Annu Rev Physiol* 1995; 57: 635–7.

9 Baruch A, Hartmann M, Yoeli M *et al.* The breast cancer-associated MUC1 gene generates both a receptor and its cognate binding protein. *Cancer Res* 1999; 59: 1552–61.

10 Bobek LA, Liu J, Sait SNJ, Shows TB, Bobek Y, Levine MJ. Structure and chromosomal localization of the human salivary mucin gene, MUC7. *Genomics* 1996; 31: 277–82.

11 Bresalier RS, Byrd JC, Wang L, Raz A. Colon cancer mucin: a new ligand for the beta-galactoside-binding protein galectin-3. *Cancer Res* 1996; 56: 4354–7.

12 Brockhausen I. Clinical aspects of glycoprotein synthesis. *Crit Rev Clin Lab Sci* 1993; 30: 65–151.

13 Buisine MP, Devisme L, Savidge TC *et al.* Mucin gene expression in human embryonic and fetal intestine. *Gut* 1998; 43: 519–24.

14 Campbell F, Appleton MAC, Fuller CE *et al.* Racial variation in the O-acetylation phenotype of human colonic mucosa. *J Pathol* 1994; 174: 169–74.

15 Carlstedt I, Sheehan JK, Corfield AP, Gallagher JT. Mucous glycoproteins: a gel of a problem. *Essays in Biochemistry* 1985; 20: 40–76.

16 Carraway KL, Price-Schiavi SA, Komatsu M *et al.* Multiple facets of sialomucin complex/MUC4, a membrane mucin and erbb2 ligand, in tumors and tissues (Y2K update). *Front Biosci* 2000; 5: D95–107.

17 Chambers JA, Hollingsworth MA, Trezise AE, Harris A. Developmental expression of mucin genes MUC1 and MUC2. *J Cell Sci* 1994; 107: 413–24.

18 Chang S-K, Dohrman AF, Basbaum CB *et al.* Localization of mucin (MUC2 and MUC3) messenger RNA and peptide expression in normal human intestine and colon cancer. *Gastroenterology* 1994; 107: 28–36.

19 Clausen H, Bennett EP. A family of UDP-GaINAc: polypeptide N-acetylgalactosaminyl-transferases control the initiation of mucin-type O-linked glycosylation. *Glycobiology* 1996; 6: 635–46.

20 Corfield AP, Myerscough N, Gough M, Brockhausen I, Schauer R, Paraskeva C. Glycosylation patterns of mucins in colonic disease. *Biochem Soc Trans* 1995; 23: 840–5.

21 Corfield AP, Wagner SA, Clamp JR, Kriaris MS, Hoskins LC. Mucin degradation in the human colon: Production of sialidase, sialate O-acetyl esterase, N-acetylneuraminate lyase, arylesterase and glycosulfatase activities by strains of fecal bacteria. *Infect Immun* 1992; 60: 3971–8.

22 Corfield AP, Wagner SA, O'Donnell LJD, Durdey P, Mountford RA, Clamp JR. The roles of enteric bacterial sialidase, sialate O-acetyl esterase and glycosulfatase in the degradation of human colonic mucin. *Glycoconj J* 1993; 10: 72–81.

23 Corfield AP, Longman R, Sylvester P, Arul S, Myerscough N, Pigatelli M. Mucins and mucosal protection in the gastrointestinal tract: new prospects for mucins in the pathology of gastrointestinal disease. *Gut* 2000; 47: 594–8.

24 Corfield AP, Warren BF. The modern investigation of mucus glycoproteins and their role in gastrointestinal disease. *J Pathol* 1996; 180: 8–17.

25 Corfield T. Bacterial sialidases – roles in pathogenicity and nutrition. *Glycobiology* 1992; 2(6): 509–21.

26 Crawley SC, Gum JR, Jr, Hicks JW *et al.* Genomic organization and structure of the 3' region of human MUC3: alternative splicing predicts membrane-bound and soluble forms of the mucin. *Biochem Biophys Res Commun* 1999; 263: 728–36.

27 Debailleul V, Laine A, Huet G *et al.* Human mucin genes MUC2, MUC3, MUC4, MUC5AC, MUC5B and MUC6 express stable and extremely large mRNAs and exhibit a variable length polymorphism. *J Biol Chem* 1998; 273: 881–90.

28 Dekker J, Strous GJ. Covalent oligomerization of rat gastric mucin occurs in the rough endoplasmic reticulum, is N-glycosylation dependent, and precedes initial O-glycosylation. *J Biol Chem* 1990; 265: 18116–22.

29 Desseyn J-L, Guyonet-Dupérat V, Porchet N, Aubert J-P, Laine A. Human mucin gene MUC5B, the 10.7-kb large central exon encodes various alternate subdomains resulting in a super-repeat. *J Biol Chem* 1997; 272: 3168–78.

30 Devine PL, McKenzie IFC. Mucins, structure, function and associations with malignancy. *BioEssays* 1992; 14: 619–25.

31 Dufossé J, Porchet N, Audié JP *et al.* Degenerate 87-base pair tandem repeats create hydrophilic/hydrophobic alternating domains in human mucin peptides mapped to 11p15. *Biochem J* 1993; 293: 329–37.

32 Filipe IM, Ramachandra S. The histochemistry of intestinal mucins; changes in disease. In: *Gastrointestinal and Oesophageal Pathology*, 2nd edn. (Whitehead R, ed.). Churchill Livingstone, Edinburgh, 1995: 73–95.

33 Forstner G. Signal transduction, packaging and secretion of mucins. *Annu Rev Physiol* 1995; 57: 585–605.

34 Forstner JF, Forstner GG. Gastrointestinal mucus. In: *Physiology of the Gastrointestinal Tract*, 3rd edn. (Johnson LR, ed.). Raven Press, New York, 1994: 1255–83.

35 Gendler S, Taylor-Papadimitriou J, Duhig T, Rothbard J, Burchell J. A highly immunogenic region of a human polymorphic epithelial mucin expressed by carcinomas is made up of tandem repeats. *J Biol Chem* 1988; 263: 12820–23.

36 Gendler SJ, Spicer AP. Epithelial mucin genes. *Annu Rev Physiol* 1995; 57: 607–34.

37 Gum JR, Hicks JC, Toribara NW, Lamport DTA, Kim YS. Molecular cloning of human intestinal mucin cDNAs. Sequence analysis and evidence for genetic polymorphism. *J Biol Chem* 1989; 264: 6480–87.

38 Gum JR, Hicks JW, Toribara NW, Siddiki B, Kim YS. Molecular cloning of human intestinal mucin (MUC 2) cDNA. Identification of the amino acid functions and overall sequence similarity to prepro-von Willebrand factor. *J Biol Chem* 1994; 269: 2440–46.

39 Gum JR, Jr. Human mucin glycoproteins: varied structures predict diverse properties and specific functions. *Biochem Soc Trans* 1995; 23: 795–9.

40 Gum JRJ, Ho JJL, Pratt WS *et al*. MUC3 human intestinal mucin. Analysis of gene structure, the carboxyl terminus, and a novel upstream repetitive region. *J Biol Chem* 1997; 272: 26678–86.

41 Guyonnet-Duperat V, Audie JP, Debailleul V *et al*. Characterization of the human mucin gene MUC5AC: a consensus cysteine-rich domain for 11p15 mucin genes? *Biochem J* 1995; 305: 211–19.

42 Hansen JE, Lund O, Tolstrup N, Gooley AA, Williams KL, Brunak S. NetOglyc: prediction of mucin type O-glycosylation sites based on sequence context and surface accessibility. *Glycoconjugate J* 1998; 15: 115–30.

43 Helenius A, Trombetta ES, Hebert DN, Simons JF. Calnexin, calreticulin and the folding of glycoproteins. *Trends Cell Biol* 1997; 7: 193–200.

44 Hilkens J, Ligtenberg MJL, Vos HL, Litvinov SV. Cell-membrane associated mucins and their adhesion-modulating property. *TIBS* 1992; 17: 359–63.

45 Hoskins LC. Human enteric population ecology and degradation of gut mucins. *Dig Dis Sci* 1981; 26: 769–72.

46 Hoskins LC, Agustines M, McKee WB, Boulding ET, Kriaris M, Niedermeyer G. Mucin degradation in human ecosystems. Evidence for the existence and role of bacterial subpopulations producing glycosidases as extracellular enzymes. *J Clin Invest* 1985; 75: 944–53.

47 Hoskins LC, Boulding ET, Gerken TA, Harouny VR, Kriaris M. Mucin glycoprotein degradation by mucin oligosaccharide – degrading strains of human faecal bacteria. Characterization of saccharide cleavage products and their potential role in nutritional support of larger faecal bacterial populations. *Microb Ecol Health Dis* 1992; 5: 193–207.

48 Hovenberg HW, Davies JR, Herrmann A, Linden CJ, Carlstedt I. MUC5AC, but not MUC2, is a prominent mucin in respiratory secretions. *Glycoconjugate J* 1996; 13: 839–47.

49 Hull SR, Sheng Z, Vanderpuye OA, David C, Carraway KL. Isolation and partial characterization of ascites sialoglycoprotein-2 (ASGP-2) of the cell surface sialomucin complex of 13762 rat mammary adenocarcinoma cells. *Biochem J* 1990; 265: 121–9.

50 Ishikawa S, Cepinskas G, Specian RD. Epidermal growth factor attenuates jejunal mucosal injury – induced by oleic acid – role of mucus. *Am J Physiol* 1994; 266: G1067–77.

51 Jass JR, Roberton AM. Colorectal mucin histochemistry in health and disease: A critical review. *Pathology International* 1994; 44: 487–504.

52 Jordan N, Newton J, Pearson J, Allen A. A novel method for the visualization of the *in situ* mucus layer in rat and man. *Clin Sci* 1998; 95: 97–106.

53 Kasai K, Hirabayashi J. Galectins. A family of animal lectins that decipher glycocodes. *J Biochem* 1996; 119: 1–8.

54 Kim YJ, Varki A. Perspectives on the significance of altered glycosylation of glycoproteins in cancer. *Glycoconj J* 1997; 14: 569–76.

55 Kim YS, Gum JJ, Brockhausen I. Mucin glycoproteins in neoplasia. *Glycoconjugate J* 1996; 13: 693–707.

56 Kyo K, Parkes M, Takei Y *et al*. Association of ulcerative colitis with rare VNTR alleles of the human intestinal mucin gene, MUC3. *Hum Mol Genet* 1999; 8: 307–11.

57 Lamblin G, Degroote S, Perini JM *et al*. Human airway mucin glycosylation: a combinatory of carbohydrate determinants which vary in cystic fibrosis. *BioLexis* 2000; 1: *www.biolexis.org/uk*.

58 Lepenseé L, Paquette Y, Bleau G. Allelic polymorphism and chromosomal localization of the human oviductin gene (MUC9). *Fertility and Sterility* 1997; 68: 702–8.

59 Lev R, Orlic D. Histochemical and radio autographic studies of normal human foetal colon. *Histochemistry* 1974; 39: 301–11.

60 Lichtenberger LM. The hydrophobic barrier properties of gastrointestinal mucus. *Annu Rev Physiol* 1995; 57: 565–83.

61 Longman RJ, Douthwaite J, Sylvester PA *et al*. Co-ordinated expression of mucin and trefoil peptide genes in the ulcer associated cell lineage and the gastrointestinal mucosa. *Gut* 2000; 47: 792–800.

62 Macfarlane GT, Macfarlane S. Human colonic microbiota: Ecology, physiology and metabolic potential of intestinal bacteria. *Scand J Gastroenterol* 1997; 32: 3–9.

63 Mestecky J, Russell MW. Passive and active protection against disorders of the gut. *Vet Quarterly* 1998; 20: S83–7.

64 Midtvedt AC, Carlstedt-Duke B, Midtvedt T. Establishment of a mucin-degrading intestinal microflora during the first two years of human life. *J Pediat Gastroenterol Nutr* 1994; 18: 321–6.

65 Moniaux N, Nollett S, Porchet N, Degand P, Laine A, Aubert J-P. Complete sequence of the human mucin MUC4: a putative cell membrane-associated mucins. *Biochem J* 1999; 338: 325–33.

66 Moniaux N, Escande F, Batra SK, Porchet N, Laine A, Aubert J-P. Alternative splicing generates a family of putative secreted and membrane-associated MUC4 mucins. *Eur J Biochem* 2000; 267: 4536–44.

67 Nielsen PA, Bonnet EP, Wandall HH, Therkildsen MH, Hannibal J, Clausen H. Identification of a major human high molecular weight salivary mucin (MG1) as tracheobronchial mucin MUC5B. *Glycobiology* 1997; 7: 413–19.

68 Nieuw Amerongen AV, Bolscher JGM, Veerman ECI. Salivary mucins: protective functions in relation to their diversity. *Glycobiology* 1995; 5: 733–40.

69 Ouellette AJ, Selsted ME. Enteric defensins. *Curr Opin Gastroenterol* 1997; 13: 494–9.

70 Patton S, Gendler SJ, Spicer AP. The epithelial mucin, MUC1, of milk, mammary gland and other tissues. *Biochem Biophys Acta* 1995; 1241: 407–24.

71 Playford RJ. Peptides and gastrointestinal mucosal integrity. *Gut* 1995; 37: 595–7.

72 Playford RJ, Marchbank T, Chinery R *et al*. Human spasmolytic polypeptide is a cytoprotective agent that stimulates cell migration. *Gastroenterology* 1995; 108: 108–16.

73 Playford RJ, Shaw-Smith C. Growth factors and ulcerative disease. In: *Cytokines and Growth Factors in Gastroenterology* (Goodlad RA, Wright NA, eds.), Vol. 10, No. 1. Baillière Tindall, London, 1996; 135–49.

74 Poulsom R. Trefoil peptides. In: *Baillière's Clinical Gastroenterology. International Practice and Research* (Goodlad RA, Wright NA, eds.), Vol. 10. No. 1. Baillière Tindall, London, 1996; 113–34.

75 Pullan RD, Thomas GAO, Rhodes M *et al*. Thickness of adherent mucus on colonic mucosa in humans and its relevance to colitis. *Gut* 1994; 35: 353–9.

76 Reid CJ, Harris A. Developmental expression of mucin genes in the human gastrointestinal system. *Gut* 1998; 42: 220–6.

77 Reid PE, Owen DA, Magee F, Park CM. Histochemical studies of intestinal epithelial goblet cell glycoproteins during the development of the human foetus. *Histochem J* 1990; 22: 81–6.

78 Reis CA, David L, Correa P *et al*. Intestinal metaplasia of human stomach displays distinct patterns of mucin (MUC1, MUC2, MUC5AC and MUC6) expression. *Cancer Res* 1999; 59.

79 Roberton AM, Corfield AP. Mucin degradation and its significance in inflammatory conditions of the gastrointestinal tract. In: *Medical Importance of the Normal Microflora* (Tannock GW, ed.). Kluwer Academic Publishers, Dordrecht, 1998; 222–61.

80 Roberton AM, Wright DP. Bacterial glycosulfatases and sulfo-mucin degradation. *Can J Gastroenterol* 1997; 11: 361–6.

81 Roussel P, Lamblin G. Human mucosal mucins in diseases. In: *Glycoproteins and Disease* (Montreuil J, Vliegenthart JFG, Schachter H, eds.). Elsevier Science BV, Amsterdam, 1996; 351–93.

82 Sadler JE. Biochemistry and genetics of von Willebrand factor. *Annu Rev Biochem* 1998; 67: 395–424.

83 Sands BE, Podolsky DE. The trefoil peptide family. *Annu Rev Physiol* 1996; 58: 253–73.

84 Schachter H, Brockhausen I. The biosynthesis of serine (threonine)-N-acetylgalactosamine-linked carbohydrate moities. In: *Glyoconjugates* (Allen HJ, Kisailus EC, eds.), Marcel Dekker, New York, 1992; 263–332.

85 Shankar V, Pichan P, Eddy RLJ *et al*. Chromosomal localization of a human mucin gene (MUC8) and cloning of the cDNA corresponding to the carboxy terminus. *Am J Respir Cell Mol Biol* 1997; 16: 232–41.

86 Sheehan JK, Thornton DJ, Howard M, Carlstedt I, Corfield AP, Paraskeva C. Biosynthesis of the MUC2 mucin: Evidence for a slow assembly of fully glycosylated units. *Biochem J* 1996; 315: 1055–60.

87 Shimizu, Y, Shaw S. Mucins in the mainstreams. *Nature* 1993; 366: 630–1.

88 Sparrow CP, Leffler H, Barondes SH. Multiple soluble β-galactoside-binding lectins from human lung. *J Biol Chem* 1987; 262: 7383–90.

89 Specian RD, Oliver MG. Functional biology of intestinal goblet cells. *Am J Physiol* 1991; 260: C183–C193.

90 Strous, GJ, Dekker J. Mucin-type glycoproteins. *Crit Rev Biochem Mol Biol* 1992; 27: 57–92.

91 Tomasetto C, Masson R, Linares JL *et al*. pS2/TFF1 interacts directly with the VWFC cysteine-rich domains of mucins. *Gastroenterology* 2000; 118: 70–80.

92 Toribara NW, Gum E, Lau P, Gum JR, Kim YS. Human gastric mucin (MUC6): Sequencing of the carboxy terminus and analysis of its structural features. *Gastroenterology* 1996; 110: A143.

93 Toribara NW, Ho SB, Gum E, Gum JRJ, Lau P, Kim YS. The carboxy-terminal sequence of the human secretory mucin, MUC6. *J Biol Chem* 1997; 272: 16398–403.

94 Tsai HH, Sunderland D, Gibson GR, Hart CA, Rhodes JM. A novel mucin sulphatase from human faeces: its identification, purification and characterization. *Clin Sci* 1992; 82: 447–54.

95 Van Klinken BJ-W, Dekker J, van Gool SA, Van Marle J, Büller HA, Einerhand AWC. MUC5B is the predominant mucin in the human gallbladder and is also expressed in a subset of colonic goblet cells. *Am J Physiol* 1998; 274: G871–78.

96 Van Klinken BJW, Einerhand AWC, Büller HA, Dekker J. The oligomerization of a family of four genetically clustered human gastrointestinal mucins. *Glycobiology* 1998; 8: 67–75.

97 van Klinken, BJW, Dekker J, Buller HA, Einerhand AWC. Mucin gene structure and expression: Protection vs. adhesion. *Amer J Physiol* 1995; 269: G613–27.

98 Verdugo P. Mucin exocytosis. *Am Rev Respir Dis* 1991; 144: S33–7.

99 Vinall LE, Hill AS, Pigny P *et al*. Variable number tandem repeat polymorphism of the genes located in the complex on 11p15.5. *Hum Genet* 1998; 102: 357–66.

100 Wasano K, Hirakawa Y. Recombinant galectin-1 recognizes mucin and epithelial cell surface glycocalyces of gastrointestinal tract. *J Histochem Cytochem* 1997; 45: 275–83.

101 Wickström C, Davies J, Eriksen G, Veerman ECI, Carlstedt I. MUC5B is the major gel-forming, oligomeric mucin from human salivary gland, respiratory tract and endocervix: identification of glycoforms and C-terminal cleavage. *Biochem J* 1998; 334: 685–93.

102 Williams SJ, McGuckin MA, Gotley DC, Eyre HJ, Sutherland GR, Antalis TM. Two novel mucin genes down-regulated in colorectal cancer identified by differential display. *Cancer Res* 1999; 59: 4083–9.

103 Williams SJ, Munster DJ, Quin RJ, Gotley DC, McGuckin MA. The MUC3 gene encodes a transmembrane mucin and is alternatively spliced. *Biochem Biophys Res Commun* 1999; 261: 83–9.

104 Xing PX, Prenzoska J, Layton GT, Devine PL, McKenzie IFC. Second generation monoclonal antibodies to intestinal MUC2 peptide reactive with colon cancer. *J Natl Cancer Inst* 1992; 84: 699–703.

105 Yuan M, Itzkowitz SH, Palekar A *et al*. Distribution of blood group antigens A, B, H, Lewis[x] and Lewis[y] in human normal, fetal and malignant colonic tissue. *Cancer Res* 1985; 45: 4499–511.

106 Zagulski T, Jarzabek Z, Zagulska A, Zimecki M. The main systemic, highly effective, and quickly acting antimicrobial mechanisms generated by lactoferrin in mammals *in vivo* – activity in health and disease. *Adv Exp Med Biol* 1998; 443: 247–50.

107 Zrihan-Licht S, Baruch A, Elroy-Stein O, Keydar O, Wreschner DH. Tyrosine phosphorylation of the MUC1 breast cancer membrane proteins. *FEBS Letts* 1994; 356: 130–6.

Chapter 13

Role of the mucosal barrier in antigen handling by the gut

Ian R. Sanderson and W. Allan Walker

INTRODUCTION

During the course of absorption of nutrients the intestine is exposed to a wide variety of antigens derived from foods, resident bacteria and invading microorganisms. The intestine acts as a barrier to prevent the indiscriminant passage of antigen into the body. Selective mechanisms exist to allow certain antigens access to the mucosal immune system and to the circulation. In addition, the intestine transports macromolecules that are important in growth and development; for example, epidermal growth factor (EGF)[14,140,141] and maternal immunoglobulin (Ig)G.[107,120] Thus any mechanism that acts as a barrier must also allow entry of physiologically important molecules whose size is comparable to many antigens.

The lumen of the intestine is capable of harbouring harmful microorganisms;[122] to mount an immune response against these potential pathogens, the mucosal immune system must survey antigens in the lumen. There is strong evidence that immuno-surveillance by the small intestine depends on transport of antigens across the gut.[145] However, such transport must occur in a controlled manner to avoid harmful immune responses. Nevertheless, there are times when the control of antigen entry breaks down and this may lead to an excessive influx of antigens which may ultimately cause disease.[111] Both Crohn's disease[75] and necrotizing enterocolitis[52] are associated with increased uptake of macromolecules. These two diseases remain among the most important problems facing those investigating diseases of the intestine in children.

Macromolecular absorption

To maintain immunosurveillance, antigens are transported across the intestine in physiological amounts, but pathological transport may occur when the mucosal barrier is breached. This barrier consists of two main components. Extrinsic mechanisms will limit the amount of antigen reaching the surface of the intestine; the intrinsic barrier consists of the structural and functional properties of the intestine itself.

There is both clinical and experimental evidence that antigens traverse the epithelium and enter the circulation,[93,140] but for the most part this transport is not harmful and may at times be beneficial.

Production of immunoglobulins directed towards luminal antigen depends on immunologically intact antigen interacting with membrane-bound immunoglobulins on the surface of B cells that are located beyond the intestinal epithelium.[56] Mechanisms that allow passage of antigen through the intestinal epithelium in controlled amounts are therefore an essential prelude to B cell activation.

T cell responses, on the other hand, are initiated by presentation of short peptides bound to major histocompatibility complexes (MHC).[134] As luminal antigen can activate mucosal T cells (as occurs, for example in coeliac disease)[76], the intestine processed luminal antigen to peptides of the correct size which can bind to MHC molecules and in turn interact with T cell receptors. Antigens could be processed in two ways by the intestine. First, peptide fragments could be generated during epithelial transport; second, antigen could be processed from whole antigen that has traversed the epithelium and reached antigen-presenting cells in the mucosal immune system. In either case uptake of antigen by the epithelium is essential. Moreover, the pathway by which the antigen or its products reach the immune system of the gut may critically affect the type of immune reaction that ensues. Thus an understanding of the mechanisms whereby antigen is handled is central to the study of the mucosal immune response.

PHYSIOLOGICAL TRANSPORT

Sampling of luminal antigen by the mucosa is likely to be a physiological phenomenon, which will result in appropriate immune responses by the gut. These will include the local production of secretory IgA and mechanisms that lead to oral tolerance.[130] Such reactions are beneficial and are described in other chapters of this book. There will be times, however, when excessive antigen crosses the intestine, causing more widespread immune reactions. These reactions could result in gastrointestinal disease,[110] or even systemic illness such as eczema.

Macromolecules cross intestinal epithelial cells in two ways of which we can be certain (Table 13.1). They can be shuttled through absorptive cells on specific receptors (in which case only those macromolecules that bind to a receptor will pass) or they can pass through specialized epithelial cells called M cells. A further possibility is that antigenic fragments cross epithelial cells for presentation by Class II MHC molecules at the basolateral surface. The definitive evidence for this mode of uptake is still awaited, but this would constitute a third form of macromolecular transport.

Receptor-bound transport

Most of the macromolecules required can be made *de novo*; however, this is not always the case. For example, certain growth factors, including EGF, transforming growth factor γ (TGFα) and nerve growth factor (NGF), are all polypeptides that are transported across the intestinal epithelial cells. IgG, also, can be transported across the intestine at times.[120]

The newborn makes very little immunoglobulin and most circulating antibody is IgG derived passively from the mother. For the most part, in humans IgG is transferred by the placenta during late gestation, whereas in many animals the transfer occurs from maternal milk through the proximal small intestine. The transfer of IgG across the gut is mediated by receptors that are similar to those present in human placenta.[114] They bind to the Fc portion of the immunoglobulin molecule.

Macromolecules are transferred by a mechanism that is altogether different from the transport of nutrients such as glucose and amino acids. Nutrient molecules enter the intestinal

cell cytoplasm at the apical membrane and exit the basolateral membrane. Macromolecules, on the other hand, traverse the cell (Fig. 13.1) in membrane-bound compartments that invaginate from the apical membrane. The first step in this process is attachment to receptors on the apical surface of enterocytes.

Enterocyte transport of IgG

In young mice maternal IgG absorption shows features characteristic of a membrane receptor transport: IgG is selectively absorbed[42,55] and its absorption shows saturation kinetics.[12] Binding is pH-dependent, occurring at pH 6.5, not at pH 7.4. As the contents of the upper jejunum are at low pH, the conditions are ideal for binding. Moreover, the intracellular membrane and components are acidic and so binding would be maintained after invagination of surface membrane and formation of vesicles.[1] The IgG receptor has now been isolated, its gene cloned and the nucleic acid sequence determined. From this the amino acid sequence has been deduced.[88] It is a molecule homologous to those of Class I MHC, and is bound in its active form to β_2 macroglobulin. Despite the homology the two molecules have very different functions and their assembly is different.

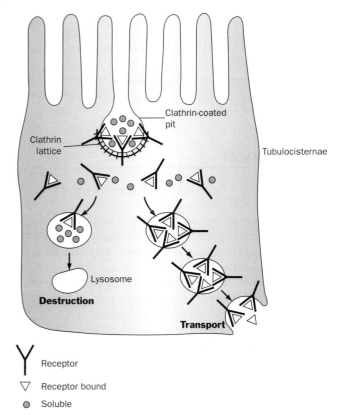

Fig. 13.1 **Macromolecular endocytosis in enterocytes**. Plasma membrane between microvilli invaginates to form vesicles. Clathrin, a protein which forms a membrane lattice, controls the curvature of the membrane. Macromolecules can enter the vesicle bound to surrounding membrane by its own receptor or by non-specific attraction; they can also enter free in solution. After entry they move to the tubulocisternae where they are sorted and pass either to vesicles which travel towards the lysosome or to vesicles which traverse the cell to the basolateral pole. Membrane-bound molecules are more likely than those in solution to traverse the cell. (Reproduced with kind permission of the Editors of *Gastroenterology*.)

Physiological transport of macromolecules across the intestinal epithelium
1 Receptor-bound transport across enterocytes
2 Passage across M cells
3 Uptake, processing and presentation in association with Class II MHC molecules

Table 13.1 **Physiological transport of macromolecules across the intestinal epithelium.**

Direct evidence of non-specific macromolecular transport through endocytic compartments of enterocyte has been demonstrated in ultrastructural studies of horseradish peroxidase (HRP) in mature intestine.[18] Macromolecules are taken up by the enterocyte in two ways: molecules may bind to receptors on the apical membrane in a non-specific manner and then enter the cell by endocytosis or, conversely, molecules in solution close to the apical membrane will be engulfed by the developing vesicle.[111] Within the enterocyte there is, therefore, scope for molecules from the lumen to be processed and leave from the basolateral membrane in a different form from that in which they enter.

Enterocyte processing of horseradish peroxidase

The ability of the enterocyte to process HRP has recently been examined.[129] In this study, HRP was placed on the apical membrane, and the fractions eluted from basolateral membrane were analysed. Approximately half the HRP given appeared at the basolateral membrane as individual amino acids. About 10% appeared as the intact whole molecule, and the remaining 40% were peptides of a wide range of molecular weights but with a median size of about 1 kD. Because the response of lymphocytes to antigens is highly dependent upon the size of proteins and polypeptides encountered, processing of food by the epithelial cell in this way will directly affect immune responses in the intestine. The mechanisms by which whole proteins are taken up by the epithelial cell and then processed within it are, therefore, an integral part of the epithelial–immune cell interaction. The intracellular proteases that digest molecules taken up by the epithelial cell, the cathepsins, are active in epithelial cells. Cathepsins B and D play a major role in the processing *in vitro* of antigens.[107] Such proteases are active in the intestinal epithelium.[25,129,135] The regulation of the activity of these enzymes is therefore important in generating mucosal immune responses. Alterations in cathepsin activity would result in different peptides being transported out of the cell.

Cathepsins and class II MHC molecules

At present, there is little work on the regulation of activity of cathepsins in the epithelial cell. It is not clear how much of their activity is regulated by interferon γ (IFNγ) secreted by activated T cells. Cathepsin activity does not alter in HT29 cells stimulated with this cytokine.[129] In addition, the fraction of antigenic peptides released by the epithelial cell was not altered by IFNγ. It did, however, induce the expression of Class II MHC molecules on the epithelial cell line HT29. These complexes are not normally expressed in these cell lines. Thus, the passage of antigenic peptides out of the cell in experiments performed in the absence of IFNγ did not depend on Class II MHC expression. Nevertheless, this may be an important factor in the fate of macromolecules taken up by the epithelial cell (see below).

The mechanisms involved in the transit of membrane-bound ligands to the basolateral pole of the enterocyte are still poorly understood. In electron microscopic studies, the apical membrane of absorptive cells invaginates to form endosomes (Fig. 13.1). On the inner aspect of these developing membrane compartments there appear to be regular arrays of clathrin,[40,59,116] a protein designed to form lattices around membrane vesicles. Clathrin has a central role in the budding and fusion of membrane vesicles.[13] In particular, clathrin assembly at the surface membrane of cells promotes the endocytosis of external receptors.[124]

Further transit into the cell may occur by the movement of separated vesicles (Fig. 13.1). Hopkins *et al.* (1990) have challenged this concept and favour a single transport compartment called the endosomal reticulum that extends from the cell surface.[49] The shape and movement of these intracellular compartments depend on the structural proteins that make up the cytoskeleton of the cell.

Transcytosis of Fc receptors

The Fc receptor is able to move across the epithelial cell. Transcytosis occurs in both directions. The receptor is carried with the membrane trafficking from lumen to serosa and returns by another membrane transport mechanism. Some membrane proteins contain specific amino acid sequences that direct the protein within the cell; for instance, the polymeric IgA receptor[15] that transports IgA from the basolateral membrane to the apical membrane. However, the amino acid sequences that determine the movement of Fc receptor have not been elucidated.

Transfer of maternal IgG in the neonatal rodent falls markedly at weaning (after 21 days of age), a phenomenon known as closure. This is now known to be due to the decrease in the expression of the Fc receptor gene.[88] Thus factors in breast milk may affect Fc receptor gene expression. The Fc receptor has been detected in humans. It is present in the placenta and transfers maternal immunoglobulin *in utero* during the later stages of gestation. Israel *et al.*[53] have shown that the Fc receptor may be present on small intestinal epithelium in the first trimester, and may possibly function early in the transfer of maternal IgG from amniotic fluid to the fetus.

Cells specialized for macromolecular transport

Generation of secretory immune responses by the intestinal mucosa depends on transfer of antigens across the epithelium. Any loss of the molecular structure of the antibody recognition sites, the epitopes, during transport would render them unrecognizable by B cells. The passage of intact macromolecules across the gut is at variance with the role of the gut as a macromolecular barrier. For macromolecules to cross the gut in a controlled manner, specialized epithelial cells have evolved that overlay lymphoid follicles.[11,92]

These microfold, or M, cells have few microvilli on their surface and correspondingly little of the glycocalyx that typifies enterocytes. There is also less mucus covering the cell surface. In addition, lysosomal enzymic activity within the cell is reduced. Thus, these components of normal barrier function are less well developed in M cells than in other epithelial cells. Furthermore, there is a deep invagination of their basal membrane into which cells of the immune system can intrude. This invagination is separated by only a narrow band of cytoplasm from the apical membrane. Thus lymphocytes and macrophages can position themselves close to the intestinal lumen.

Amerongen and colleagues[3] have reviewed microorganisms and other macromolecules known to be transported by M cells (Table 13.1). M cells also transport luminal antigen from the gut and therefore represent the primary physiological route for non-receptor transport of macromolecules. This has been shown by electron microscopy using antigens which include ferritin and HRP. Soluble macromolecules are incorporated into membrane-bound compartments, transferred across the cell, and extruded from the serosal surface into the interstitium containing lymphoid cells.

An important but as yet unanswered question is whether specific receptors exist on the surface of M cells which aid the transport of macromolecules across the epithelium. Some infectious agents, including reovirus[146] and *Escherichia coli* (strain RDEC-1),[50] bind selectively to M cells. The question of receptors is made more complex by the fact that different agents are taken up in different ways by M cells. For example, poliovirus[119] is taken into clathrin-coated pits by endocytosis, whereas reovirus is taken up in vesicles that do not contain clathrin.[146]

Enterocytes as antigen-presenting cells

Effective immune responses to antigenic proteins require the help of T lymphocytes. Stimulation of T cells in turn depends on exogenous antigen being presented by antigen-presenting cells (APC).[134] The APC must internalize, digest and link a small fragment of the antigen to a surface glycoprotein (the MHC Class II or HLA-D in man) that interacts with a T cell receptor. A number of cells of the immune system can act as APC, including B cells, macrophages and dendritic cells. The ability of these cells to present antigen depends on the expression of Class II MHC on their surface.[134] Class II MHC are also present in epithelia of the normal small intestine, particularly on villous cells, in both man[143] and rodents.[58] *In vitro* studies[8,57,80] have demonstrated that isolated enterocytes from rat and human small intestine can present antigens to appropriately primed T cells. This raises the possibility that, in the intestine, Class II MHC might present peptides from cellular membrane compartments to cells of the immune system that are localized below the epithelium. In support of this concept, Class II MHC molecules have been detected in adult rat jejunum villi in association with intracellular organelles.[84] Class II molecules have not been detected in microvillus brush border or vesicles at the base of microvilli. However, organelles below the terminal web and throughout the apical cytoplasm were stained specifically. Basolateral membranes clearly showed Class II MHC molecules. These molecules are therefore in an ideal position for binding with polypeptides that may have taken up and been processed within the epithelial cell (Fig. 13.2).

Interestingly, the expression of Class II MHC in the gastrointestinal epithelium is increased in a number of diseases. In Crohn's disease[83,115] there is enhanced expression on enterocytes in inflamed areas. Moreover, the effect of enterocytes from inflamed tissue is to stimulate helper T lymphocytes.[82] Increased expression of Class II MHC is also evident in the small intestine in patients with autoimmune enteropathy and in graft-*versus*-host disease.[77] Certain gastrointestinal infections increase Class II MHC expression; for example, in stomach infected with *Helicobacter pylori*[29] and in intestine infested with nematode parasites.[78] If Class II MHC molecules transport peptides derived from luminal macromolecules, then these diseases will lead to an increase in the presentation of these peptides to the gastrointestinal immune systems. This may cause further inflammation and further presentation of luminal antigens, leading to a vicious cycle. Some drugs used to treat inflammatory bowel disease reduce Class II MHC expression in epithelial cells. 5-ASA, for example, reduces expression that occurs in cultured cells that express Class II MHC in response to IFNγ.[19]

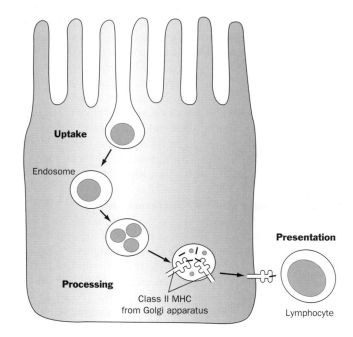

Fig. 13.2 Model of antigen presentation by enterocyte.
Macromolecules can enter membrane-bound organelles of the enterocyte. Instead of binding to the surrounding membrane or being destroyed in lysosomes, antigen is processed within the endosomal component into fragments that can bind to Class II MHC on the inner membrane of the components. From there they are presented on the basolateral surface of the cell. (Drawing prepared with the help of Dr L. Mayer and reproduced with kind permission of the Editors of *Gastroenterology*.)

T cell activation and B7 antigens

T cell activation depends not only on presentation of antigen by Class II MHC, but also on the attachment of separate surface molecules to molecules on the APC. The molecules on the surface of APC include ICAM 1 (which binds to LFA 1) on the T cell; the activation antigens B7 (now renamed B7-1) and the recently identified B7-2 (which both bind to CD28 and CTLA 4);[6,34–36,44,63] and heat-stable antigen (whose ligand on the T cell is still unknown and whose role as a costimulatory molecule is not as well defined as the B7s). There is probably[65] a functional distinction between the ICAM 1/LFA 1 bond and the other two bonds. ICAM 1 is thought to provide support for the weak[79] Class II MHC/TCR bond; whereas the B7s and heat-stable antigen (the so-called costimulatory molecules) transmit specific stimulatory signals through their ligands to T cells.[23] Lack of binding by B7s to CD28 may result in T cell tolerance[113] because blocking of CD28 during antigen presentation leads to clonal anergy in T cells,[43] with absence of T cell proliferation and IL2 production.

Cells of the small intestinal epithelium[10,111] do not express B7-1. It is tempting to speculate that epithelial cell presentation may therefore downregulate T cell responses under normal circumstances. Under these circumstances the epithelial cell's role as a barrier to antigen absorption would not only be passive; the epithelium could actively inhibit the immune responses initiated by the passage of antigen that has leaked through to professional APC in the lamina propria (which do express costimulatory molecules). In disease states, however, such an inhibition of T cell activation may be inappropriate. It is interesting, therefore, that *Helicobacter pylori* induces expression of costimulatory molecules on gastric epithelium.

BARRIERS PREVENTING PATHOLOGICAL TRANSPORT

Physiological passage of macromolecules is essential for the development of immune responses by the intestine, but uncontrolled penetration of antigens could initiate pathological processes that lead to gastrointestinal disease states. For antigen transport to be controlled, non-specific entry into the circulation must be limited. This is done in two ways. First, by restricting the amount of antigen reaching the surface of the intestine (extrinsic barrier); second, by the physical characteristics of the intestine itself (intrinsic barrier).

Many barrier mechanisms are not fully developed at birth and there is good evidence that antigen transport in the neonatal period is less restricted than in adults. In animals the changes in antigen absorption from the newborn to adults is particularly evident, a phenomenon known as closure. Initially, the phenomenon was applied to the transport of immunoglobulins,[12] but significant changes in absorption have been documented for antigens that do not have specific transport receptors. In one study designed to measure protein absorption, radiolabelled bovine serum albumin (BSA)[131] was fed in physiological amounts to rabbits at birth, 1 week, 2 weeks, 6 weeks and 1 year of age and the plasma radioactivity measured. From 1 week, there was a marked fall in the transport of BSA across the intestine. Moreover, in a later study[132] it was found that the development of the mucosal barrier depended on the type of feeding during the neonatal period. Naturally fed (breast fed) rabbits had lower plasma BSA levels than formula fed rabbits, suggesting that breast milk affects the development of the mucosal barrier.

These findings appear to be applicable to humans since a fall in antigen absorption has been demonstrated and milk proteins penetrate more readily in infancy than in adults. In one study α-lactalbumin absorption decreased with age in breast-fed babies.[5] In a second study, formula-fed neonates had greater levels of β-lactoglobulin than older infants.[106]

Extrinsic barrier
Proteolysis and gastrointestinal acidity
There are several ways by which antigen access to the epithelium is limited (Table 13.2). Proteolysis will destroy the structure of antigens and thus destroy epitopes for immunological recognition. Altering the proteolytic capacity of the gastrointestinal tract affects macromolecular uptake. In everted gut sacs[138] taken from rats who had previously undergone ligation of the pancreatic duct, transport of HRP was greater than in sacs made in sham-operated

animals. Furthermore, prior feeding of pancreatic extract decreased the uptake of HRP. The effects of digestion on macromolecular uptake have been elegantly confirmed by feeding rats aprotinin (a trypsin inhibitor) together with lysine vasopressin.[109] This peptide hormone is absorbed through the intestine in sufficient quantities to have a noticeable effect on fluid retention when fed orally. When given together with aprotinin, however, the effects of vasopressin are more marked, implying that more has reached the surface of the intestine because of reduced proteolysis.

Experiments to neutralize gastric acidity (which reduced the activity of gastric enzymes) also increase antigen transport. When oral feeds of sodium bicarbonate are given to rats at the same time as BSA, increased BSA is found in the gut.[138] These findings have important consequences because deficiencies of pancreatic enzymes occur in various diseases. In cystic fibrosis, where pancreatic activity is severely affected, there is an increased incidence of cows' milk allergy, presumably because of increased antigen uptake. Also, gastric acidity[48] and pancreatic activity[60] may be lower in the newborn and this may have consequences on development of the mucosal barrier.

In addition to the acid secreted into the stomach, the epithelial cells of the intestinal epithelium create an acid microclimate. Mucus and the outer glycocalyx of the intestinal epithelium are composed of negatively charged carbohydrate side chains. This negative charge reduces the diffusibility of hydrogen ions within the surface layer of the cell. Any pH at the apical surface of the epithelium will therefore be maintained in the region. Studies on the absorption of salicylic acid,[67] a weak electrolyte, indicate that its uptake is much greater than expected when the bulk phase of the intestine is alkaline. In fact, the absorption of salicylate in experiments was equivalent to that expected had the bulk phase been at a pH of 2 lower than in fact it was. Absorption of weak bases were altered in the opposite direction to weak acids in rat small intestine.[144] In a relationship of absorption against pH, the uptake of a weak electrolyte should be at 50% of its maximum when the pH of the absorptive surface is equal to the electrolyte's pK. These data have resulted in the proposal that the microclimate of the small intestinal surface is acidic. Direct experiments measuring the pH of the surface with microelectrodes have confirmed this prediction both in humans and in rodents.[24,66,103,104]

Microclimate
The microclimate changes during ontogeny. In the suckling rat the microclimate is even more acidic than in the adult. Weak acids (such as short chain fatty acids) are particularly well absorbed under these conditions. Said *et al.*[110] not only showed that age differences resulted in differences in the acid microclimate, but also that the microclimate was maintained by mucus.[110] The addition of a mucolytic agent (N-acetyl cysteine) reduced the acidity of the apical surface.

Although mucus impedes the free diffusion of hydrogen ions into the bulk phase, it does not generate acidity. Hydrogen ions are secreted by the epithelial cells in exchange for entry of sodium ions by a Na^+/H^+ antiporter in the intestinal apical membrane. Sodium passes readily into epithelial cells down its concentration gradient, causing hydrogen ions to be pumped into the apical space where they are trapped by the negatively charged mucopolysaccharide side chains, as discussed above. Removal of

Limiting antigen access to epithelium
Proteolysis – obliteration of antigen epitopes
Gastric acidity
Negative charges of mucins
Secretory IgA antibodies

Table 13.2 Limiting antigen access to epithelium.

sodium from the bulk phase causes a reduction in the micro-climate.[117] An investigation of how the microclimate might alter the uptake of antigens or invading organisms has never been undertaken. However, acidity has a marked effect on the absorption of smaller molecules. For weak electrolytes (such as short chain fatty acids), sodium removal would indirectly alter absorption by increasing the pH which maintains the weak acid in its more soluble form. The acid microclimate has a direct effect on dipeptide transport[64] which, unlike amino acids, are transported in to the cell in association with hydrogen ions. Based on work in rodents,[110] it appears that neonates produce a microclimate sufficient for these absorptive functions. However, little is known about the microclimate in the preterm neonate, and this remains an interesting area for further study.

Peristalsis

The time available for absorption depends on the speed of luminal contents through the bowel. It is a common experience in clinical gastroenterology that uptake of nutrients in patients with limited absorptive capacity (such as short bowel syndrome) is improved by reduced intestinal motility with agents such as loperamide.[105] There is good reason to believe that antigen absorption too will be limited by peristaltic action. An association between motility and antigen absorption has important implications. First, motility patterns change throughout development[7,86] and this may contribute to alterations in antigen uptake with age. Second, gastrointestinal disease can affect the motility of the intestine[81] and may result in changes in antigen absorption, although such changes may be small relative to the effect that a disease has on the physical barrier created by the intestine itself. Nevertheless, antibody–antigen complex formation in the mucus coat, coupled with peristalsis, causes rapid expulsion of antigens from small intestine.[121]

Mucus coat

Structure of mucus coat

The mucus coat lining the intestine is comprised of a solution of glycoproteins (mucin) of molecular weights ranging from one to several million daltons. Intestinal mucin molecules are made up of carbohydrate side chains (70–80%) bound to a protein skeleton. This protein core has a high proportion of serine, threonine and proline residues,[2,33] and carbohydrate moieties are attached to it by means of N-acetylgalactosamine. Five carbohydrate moieties (N-acetylgalactosamine, N-acetylglucosamine, fucose, galactose and sialic acid) are arranged in side chains of 2–22 sugars in length.

The exact composition of the molecules of mucin can vary greatly. There are clear differences between animal species. Even within localized regions of the intestinal tract, mucus molecules appear to be a heterogeneous group. At least six different mucin species have been identified following separation on diethylaminoethanol (DEAE)–cellulose chromatography from both rat and human.[100] Each species had distinct carbohydrate and amino acid composition. Marked changes in the composition of mucin occur with development. The mucin from the small intestine of newborn rats contains more protein than does adult rat mucin.[118] The carbohydrate content also changes as the animals grow. Not only does the total carbohydrate ratio increase with age, but the types of sugar moieties change also: newborn rat mucin has less fucose and N-acetylgalactosamine than mucin from adult rats.

Function of mucus coat

Viscous coat: there are a number of ways by which mucus offers protection to the intestinal wall. Firstly, it provides a mucus blanket. The physical characteristics of this blanket are determined by the chemical structure of the glycoprotein molecules themselves. The sticky quality of the mucus is an important mechanism for preventing penetration of organisms. The motility of *Entamoeba histolytica* trophozoites,[62] for example, is significantly decreased by mucus. The increased viscosity that mucus provides to the luminal solution enhances the depth of the unstirred layer overlying the surface of the intestine. This reduces the diffusion of molecules towards the intestinal surface.[128] The effect is most marked for larger molecules, and this limits absorption of antigens rather than nutrient molecules which are smaller.

Competitive binding: the carbohydrate moieties which comprise the major part of mucus are analogous to the glyco-protein and glycolipid receptors that exist on the enterocyte membrane.[39] They could, therefore, act as competitors to the binding of proteins and microorganisms at the enterocyte surface. Many infectious agents adhere to epithelial cells through cell surface appendages (fimbria, pili and flagella)[37] which have carbohydrate binding properties. Indeed, competition between salivary mucus glycoproteins and receptors on buccal epithelium has already been shown for binding of pathogenic streptococci.[142] Furthermore, it is possible that the invasiveness of *Shigella flexneri* in primates, in part, depends on the lack of barrier function of mucus.[26] Guinea pig colonic mucus inhibits invasion of HeLa cells by *Shigella*, whereas monkey colonic mucus (and, by implication, human mucus) does not.

Mucin release: release of mucus into the gastrointestinal tract acts as a barrier by generating a stream that draws luminal contents away from epithelial cells. Both non-specific and immunological agents can initiate mucus release. The role of non-immunological agents and their relationship to endogenous agents that alter mucus secretion are not well understood.[121] Cholinergic agents[123] and mustard oil[91] cause goblet cell release, but a number of regulatory peptides (including histamine, serotonin, α- and β-adrenergic agents) had no effect. Nevertheless, immunological phenomena cause goblet cells to release mucus (see below).

Immunological barrier

The adequacy of immune function in the gastrointestinal tract affects the attachment and penetration of bacteria and toxins. This has been elegantly shown[145] by implantation of IgA-secreting hybridomas under the skin of infant mice who are then inoculated with cholera. IgA appears in large amounts in the small intestine as secretory IgA (sIgA). When hybridomas are implanted that secrete IgA antibodies to *Vibrio cholerae*, mortality from cholera is dramatically reduced.

It is also likely that IgA prevents the transfer of antigens across the gut. This hypothesis is supported by studies of patients with selective IgA deficiency. These patients have increased circulating immune complexes and precipitating antibodies to absorbed bovine milk proteins,[21] peak concentrations occurring between 1 and 2 h after milk ingestion[22] (see Chapter 12).

Innate immunity encompasses appropriate defence responses that are not adaptive.[85] This definition excludes the involvement of lymphocytes, but includes other cell types which respond to molecular patterns. This concept is well developed in the macrophage, but enterocytes also recognize specific patterns, especially those derived from bacteria. For example, chemotactic cytokines are released from epithelial cells after invasion by *Salmonella*[28] or attachment of *Helicobacter*.[20] In addition, the metabolite of resident bacteria (butyrate) enhances chemokine secretion by epithelial cells stimulated by proinflammatory agents. Innate immunity has an older phylogeny than adaptive immunity. The epithelial cell's early evolution, compared to the lymphocyte, is consistent with its role in innate immunity.

Combined effects of immunological and non-immunological barriers

Both oral and parenteral immunization with specific antigens can reduce their uptake by the intestine.[136,137] These observations may well be a combined effect of immunological and non-immunological components of the mucosal barrier. Proteolysis of intestinal antigens is considerably greater in immunized animals than in non-immunized controls.[138] It is likely that this enhanced proteolysis is the result of interaction of immune complexes in the mucus coat.

Another example of combined protection is the increased discharge of goblet cell mucus occurring in intestinal anaphylaxis. Lake and colleagues[60] have shown, using radiolabelled goblet cell mucus to quantitate release, that IgE-mediated mast cell discharge of histamine results in enhanced mucus release into the intestinal tract. This may explain why parasites are eventually expelled from the intestine, together with mucus.[87]

Intrinsic barrier

Once antigens have negotiated the many components of the extrinsic barrier mechanism there is a considerable physical barrier to further penetration. This barrier is due to the surface of the enterocytes and the tight junctions that are formed between. However, this barrier is not impervious to the passage of antigens, as was once thought. The integrity of this barrier is often reduced in diseases of the gastrointestinal tract.

Microvillus structure

Microvilli could constitute a significant barrier because of their size and charge. In the intestinal epithelium of children[98] there are 40 microvilli every 5 µm, each having a diameter of 100 nm. Thus, if microvilli beat in unison the distance between them is only 25 nm, which is the same order of magnitude as some macromolecules: the dimensions of albumin, for example, are 3×13 nm. Microvilli are also negatively charged and therefore stain easily with ruthenium red;[54] a charged molecule may be significantly inhibited even if its diameter is well below 25 nm.

The site of invagination of the apical plasma membrane has been demonstrated as being between microvilli.[40,59,116] Thus, it is likely that antigens have to pass the microvillus barrier to enter the cell. This has direct relevance to disease processes, for any agent that strips off microvilli or affects their formation will alter the barrier function of the intestine. Microvillus structure is greatly altered by infections of cryptosporidia[99] or enteropathogenic *E. coli*.[133]

Further support for the concept of a microvillus barrier comes from morphological studies on M cells. The function of these cells is macromolecular transport. Unlike absorptive cells they do not have well developed microvilli. As every morphological feature of these cells is in keeping with their function, this would suggest that microvilli constitute a significant barrier.

Enterocyte surface membrane

At the base of the microvilli the surface of the enterocyte consists of plasma membrane. As in other cells, this is composed of a lipid bilayer through which are situated membrane-bound proteins. This bilayer presents a considerable barrier to antigen transport because of its physical structure. In fact it is very unlikely that antigens can cross this lipid bilayer into the enterocyte cytosol. However, invagination of apical membranes occurs regularly, allowing macromolecules to be carried into the cell within membrane-bound compartments (Fig. 13.1). Indeed, there are a large number of compartments beneath the apical surface of the enterocyte into which antigens can be transferred. Some of this activity is physiological and has been described in an earlier section; however, bystander molecules can be carried into the cell by this process. This has been clearly demonstrated in electron micrographs which show HRP inside membrane-bound compartments.[18] Stern and Walker[125] have shown that binding to the surface of the enterocyte is a prerequisite for transport of macromolecules across the cell. For both BSA and B-lactoglobulin (BLG), absorption was non-saturable and correlated with binding to the intestinal surface. Membrane-bound macromolecular transport can be distinguished from molecules moving freely in lumen of enterocyte compartments[40] in newborn rat ileum.

Surface binding of macromolecules

Binding to the surface of the cell depends on the structure of the antigen and the chemical composition of the microvillus membrane. Both these factors can vary. BSA binds less efficiently to the surface of the intestine than BLG and in consequence is transported less readily.[125] In addition, structural alterations in antigen caused by proteolysis might also affect its binding, as this will change the physiochemical characteristics of the molecule. For example, the gliadin fraction B3[126] binds less well to MVM protein than the pure gliadin peptide B3142.

Membrane composition

The composition of the microvillus membrane has a marked effect on antigen binding. Plasma membranes consist of both lipids and proteins, and changes in either will affect binding to antigen. Partial digestion of the microvillus membrane can alter binding to macromolecules.[126] Damage to the protein in membranes is unlikely to occur in healthy individuals as the intestinal surface is protected by mucus. However, if the mucus layer was affected by, for example, resident bacteria, some digestion of the surface membrane might occur, leading to increased antigen binding and transport, but this is probably rare. Changes in lipid composition, on the other hand, are regularly encountered because lipid composition alters with development. Differences in membrane composition can be detected by electron spin resonance (ESR). In this technique, the movements of the lipid-soluble probe can be followed by a spectrophotometer.[94] Movements of the probe in the membrane from the newborn rabbit have been found to be less confined than in adults, suggesting a more disorganized membrane structure. Indeed, chemical analysis of the membrane[16] demonstrates changes in the phospholipid headgroups with age as well as alterations in protein:lipid ratios.[94] Changes in membrane fluidity noted by ESR were found to correlate with an alteration in lectin binding.[95] These changes were noted to be under hormonal control since alterations in the fluidity were affected by both cortisone and thyroxine.[51]

Intracellular organelles and enzymes

Antigens that enter enterocytes from the lumen are affected by a number of different factors that will influence transport to the basolateral surface. Of primary importance is the rate of vesicular passage to the basolateral membrane. This will depend on the rate of endocytosis, the proportion of vesicles being divided towards the lysosome and the speed of travel of membrane-bound compartments. The rate of breakdown of products held in membrane compartments is determined by enzymes derived from lysosomes. These include proteases such as cathepsin B and D and those that catalyse carbohydrate breakdown such as acid phosphatase and mannosidase. It is the degree to which the organellar contents encounter such enzymes that determines the rate of intracellular destruction of macromolecules. This encounter can be in the lysosome or in endocytic vesicles.[27] We know that such enzymes are present in intestinal epithelial cells and at levels of activity that can influence macromolecular transport. In the rat,[25] cathepsin B and D activity can be found throughout the length of the intestine, particularly in the mid and distal thirds. Interestingly, this activity peaks in the second week of age and then progressively falls. The ontogeny of macromolecular transport[131] in no way reflects this pattern, emphasizing that it is the importance of interaction between membrane-bound compartment flow and enzyme activity which is of prime importance. This is more clearly seen in the piglet, where intestinal cathepsin B and D levels do not alter with age,[30] yet closure can be clearly demonstrated in the same animals in the second day of life.

While cathepsins are capable of destroying macromolecular biological activity, they may not completely digest the protein molecule, and the final steps in digestion of peptides may be by peptidases[135] in the cytoplasm.

Junctions between cells

The physical barrier that prevents penetration of antigen across the intestinal epithelium consists of two main components: the epithelial cells (the transcellular route) and the spaces between cells (the paracellular route). The pathophysiology of this latter pathway has been well reviewed in recent years.[41,72,74,101] The pathway consists of the tight junctions (or zonulae occludentes) and the subjunctional space.

Tight junctions

The subjunctional space does not act as a significant barrier as molecules as large as HRP can diffuse freely between the serosa and this space. However, the tight junctions offer a substantial barrier to diffusion of large molecules, although they are permeable to water and small ions.[38] Claude and Goodenough[17] have demonstrated a correlation between the structure of the tight junction as seen in freeze fracture preparations and passive electrical permeability in a number of epithelial preparations. When viewed under the electron microscope, the preparations show a network of characteristic anastomosing strands likely to be proteins of high tensile strength. In tight epithelia (such as the gallbladder) there are many such strands, whereas in more permeable epithelia (like mammalian proximal small intestine) there are few. The relationship between strand density and epithelial resistance has been confirmed in intestinal epithelial cells.[69] TE 84 cells grow as confluent monolayers in culture. In the first 10 days after passage, the junctions become increasingly

tight, as judged by transepithelial resistance. This resistance has been found to correlate with the number of strands formed between cells.

The barrier formed by tight junctions is preserved even when epithelial cells themselves are extruded at the villous tip. The bands from the tight junction move away from the apex down the lateral aspect of the cell as the cell is extruded.[74] Eventually, younger cells beneath the extruding cell form tight junctions at the very moment that the old cell is lost. Thus the preservation of the tight junction network is a function whose importance overrides that of epithelial cell viability.

Cell–cell adhesions

Cell–cell adhesions depend on a family of molecules, the cadherins, which bind either to β-catenins or to plakoglobin, which in turn binds to β-catenins.[47,90] These interactions not only preserve the epithelial cell barrier but also prevent epithelial cells from breaking away from their monolayer, as is seen in intestinal neoplasia. Interestingly, suppressing the normally expressed E-cadherin in the epithelia with a dominant negative N-cadherin (NCAD) disrupts cell–cell interactions.[45] Transgenic mice, in which distinct areas of the intestinal epithelium expressed NCAD, exhibited changes in the lamina propria only in those areas which expressed the NCAD gene.[46] Changes in the lamina propria included infiltration with lymphocytes and histiocytes, IgA- and IgG-secreting plasma cells and increased expression of Class II MHC. By 3 months of age, crypt distortion and crypt abscesses appeared. Chimeras expressing NCAD along the entire crypt–villus axis had greater disease than those with NCAD expression confined to the villous epithelium. This animal model exemplifies the importance of the epithelial barrier in the prevention of inflammatory bowel disease.

Opening of tight junctions

The tight junction is a dynamic structure in which resistance varies with events taking place in the epithelium and intestinal lumen. Changes in paracellular absorption occur during active transport of nutrients by epithelial cells, particularly in relation to smaller molecules. Pappenheimer and colleagues[70,96,97] have calculated that the rate of uptake of molecules smaller than 5500 D from the lumen was proportional to the rate of fluid absorption, a concept known as solvent drag. The application of an alternating current across isolated intestine, with and without mucosa, gave an estimate of the impedance of the intestinal mucosa. The impedance falls with the stimulation of sodium-coupled solute transport across the enterocyte. It is, therefore, possible that sodium-coupled solute transport triggers contraction of cytoskeletal elements of the enterocyte which in turn pull open tight junctions. These predictions have been confirmed by electron microscopy.[70] Sodium-dependent solutes such as glucose and amino acids induce expansion of intercellular spaces associated with condensation of microfilaments of the actinomycin ring associated with the tight junction. While these observations have enormous importance on the physiology of absorption of nutrients, their impact on our understanding of macromolecular transport has yet to be fully assessed. The calculated pore radius of the open tight junction (5 nm) is similar to that of small macromolecules: glucose–Na transport will in fact allow the passage of polypeptides 11 amino acids long (MP-1)[4] but larger immunogenic proteins may not pass through this route under physiological conditions. HRP, for example, does not pass the tight junctions[4] even when they have been rendered permeable to MP-1.

Pathological opening of tight junctions

On the other hand, pathological insults to the intestine may open these pores sufficiently to allow passage of antigens. The macromolecular permeability of the gut in disease models needs to be re-examined using Pappenheimer's methodology. Macromolecular markers of different sizes, charge and hydrophilicity have all been used independently *in vivo* in both animals and humans, but the physical characteristics of these molecules has not been used to predict pore size in disease. An important model of increased permeability because of intestinal inflammation is the effect of mast cell-dependent reactions in the rat intestine after *Nippostrongylus brasiliensis* infection. Increased amounts of BSA can be detected immunologically in the circulation after infection with the organism following mild systemic anaphylaxis.[9] Similarly, transfer of ^{51}Cr-labelled EDTA and ovalbumin is enhanced.[102] It should be possible to make an estimate of the physical characteristics of the paracellular pathway during inflammation.

The permeability of the tight junction can be examined *in vitro*. This enables workers to study the effects of epithelial events that are seen *in vivo*. Monolayers of epithelial cells (T 84), have effective tight junctions, producing a resistance of around 1500 cm^2. Application of IFNγ[72] reduces the resistance and allows easier permeation of large sugars. IFNγ levels are increased in the mucosa of patients with Crohn's disease because of T cell activation (see Chapter 24). Bowel inflammation is characterized by the transepithelial passage of polymorphoneutrophils (PMN). This phenomenon has been reproduced *in vitro* by putting chemotactic agents and PMN on different sides of the monolayer.[89] The passage of neutrophils opens tight junctions, reducing the monolayer's resistance and allowing transfer of large sugars.

CONCLUSIONS

The mucosal barrier, like the skin, defines the boundary between an animal and its environment. Unlike the skin, the mucosae of the gut and respiratory tract must absorb substances that are essential for life. To be selective, the intestinal mucosa has developed a complex network comprising elements that are extrinsic to the intestine itself, as well as those defined by intestinal structure.

The challenges for the future lie in defining the role of this barrier in the establishment of gastrointestinal disease. It will also be interesting to examine whether cellular elements in the mucosal immune system can recognize antigens without needing to penetrate the intestinal epithelium. The observations that members of the immunoglobulin superfamily are found on the surface of the epithelium and that lymphocytes can pass into the intestinal lumen make this a tantalizing possibility.

REFERENCES

1 Abrahamson DR, Rodewald R. Evidence for the sorting of endocytic vesicle contents during the receptor-mediated transport of IgG across the newborn rat intestine. *J Cell Biol* 1981; 91: 270–80.

2 Allan A. Structure and function of gastrointestinal mucus. In: *Physiology of the Gastrointestinal Tract*, Vol. 7; 1981: 617–39.

3 Amerongen MH, Weltzin RW, Mack JA *et al*. M-cell mediated antigen transport and monoclonal IgA antibodies for mucosal immune protection. *Ann N Y Acad Sci* 1992; 664: 18–26.

4 Atisook K, Madara JL. An oligopeptide permeates intestinal tight junctions at glucose-elicited dilatations. Implications for oligopeptide absorption. *Gastroenterology* 1991; 100: 719–24.

5 Axelsson I, Jakobsson I, Lindberg T, Poleberger S, Benediktsson B, Raiha N. Macromolecular absorption in preterm and term infants. *Acta Paediatr Scand* 1989; 78: 532–7.

6 Azuma M, Ito D, Yagita H *et al*. B70 antigen is a second ligand for CTLA-4 and CD28. *Nature* 1993; 366: 76–9.

7 Bissett WM, Watt JB, Rivers RPA, Milla PJ. The ontogeny of small intestinal motor activity. *Ped Res* 20: 692.

8 Bland PW, Warren LG. Antigen presentation by epithelial cells of the rat small intestine. I. Kinetics, antigen specificity and blocking by anti-Ia antisera. *Immunology* 1986; 58: 1–8.

9 Bloch KJ, Bloch DB, Sterns M, Walker WA. Intestinal uptake of macromolecules. VI. Uptake of protein antigen *in vivo* in normal rats and rats infected with *Nippostrongylus brasiliensis* or subjected to mild systemic anaphylaxis. *Gastroenterology* 1979; 77: 1038–44.

10 Bloom S, Simmons D, Jewell DP. Adhesion molecules intercellular adhesion molecule (ICAM-1), ICAM-3 and B7 are not expressed by epithelium in normal or inflamed colon. *Clin Exp Immunol* 1995; 101: 157–63.

11 Bockman DE, Cooper MD. Pinocytosis by epithelium associated with lymphoid follicles in the Bursa of Fabricus, appendix and Peyer's patches. An electron microscopic study. *Am J Anat* 1973; 136: 455–78.

12 Brambell FW. The transmission of immunity from mother to young and the catabolism of immunoglobulins. *Lancet* 1966; II: 1087–93.

13 Brodsky FM. Living with clathrin: its role in intracellular membrane traffic. *Science* 1984; 242: 1396–1402.

14 Carpenter G, Wahl MI. The epidermal growth factor family. In: *Peptide Growth Factors and Their Receptors I*, (MB Sporn, AB Roberts, eds), Springer-Verlag, New York; 1991: 69–171.

15 Casanova JE, Apdoaca G, Mostov KE. An autonomous signal for basolateral sorting in the cytoplasmic domain of the polymeric immunoglobulin receptor. *Cell* 1991; 66: 65–75.

16 Chu SW, Walker WA. Growth factor signal transduction in human intestinal cells. In: *Immunology of Milk and the Neonate* (J. Mestecky *et al*., eds). Plenum Press, New York, 1991; 107–12.

17 Claude P, Goodenough DA. Fracture faces of zonulae occludentes from 'tight' and 'leaky' epithelia. *J Cell Biol* 1973; 58: 390–440.

18 Cornell R, Walker WA, Isselbacher KJ. Small intestinal absorption of horseradish peroxidase. A cytochemical study. *Lab Invest* 1971; 25: 42–8.

19 Crotty B, Hoang P, Dalton HR, Jewell DP. Salicylates used in inflammatory bowel disease and colchicine impair interferon-induced HLA-DR expression. *Gut* 1992; 33: 59–64.

20 Crowe SE, Alvarez L, Dytoc M *et al*. Expression of interleukin 8 and CD54 by human gastric epithelium after *Helicobacter pylori* infection *in vitro*. *Gastroenterology* 1995; 108: 65–74.

21 Cunningham-Rundles C, Brandeis WE, Good RA, Day NK. Milk precipitin circulating immune complexes and IgA deficiency. *Proc Natl Acad Sci USA* 1978; 75: 3387–89.

22 Cunningham-Rundles C, Brandeis WE, Good RA, Day NK. Bovine antigens and the formation and the circulating immune complexes in selective immunoglobulin A deficiency. *J Clin Invest* 1979; 64: 272–79.

23 Damle NK, Klussman K, Linsley PS, Aruffo A. Differential costimulatory effects of adhesion molecules B7, ICAM-1, LFA-3, and VCAM-1 on resting and antigen-primed CD4+ T lymphocytes. *J Immunol* 1992; 148: 1982–85.

24 Daniel H, Neugebauer B, Kratz A, Rehner G. Localization of acid microclimate along intestinal villi of rat jejunum. *Am J Physiol* 1985; 248: G293–98.

25 Davies PH, Messer M. Intestinal cathepsin B and D activities of suckling rats. *Biol Neonate* 1984; 45: 197–202.

26 Denari G, Hale TL, Washington O. Effect of guinea pig or monkey colonic mucus on *Shigella* aggregation and invasion of HeLa cells by *Shigella flexneri* 1b and 2a. *Infect Immunity* 1986; 51: 975–78.

27 Dinsdale D, Healy PJ. Enzymes involved in protein transmission by the intestine of the newborn lamb. *Histochem J* 1982; 14: 811–21.

28 Eckmann L, Jung HC, Schurer-Maly C, Panja A, Morzycka-Wroblewska E, Kagnoff MF. Differential cytokine expression by human intestinal epithelial cell lines: regulated expression of interleukin 8. *Gastroenterology* 1993; 105: 1689–97.

29 Engstrand L, Scheynius A, Pahlson C, Grimelius L, Schwan A, Gustavsson S. Association of *Campylobacter pylori* with induced expression of class II transplantation antigen on gastric epithelial cells. *Infect Immun* 1989; 57: 827–32.

30 Ekstrom GM, Westrom BR. Cathepsin B and D activities in intestinal mucosa during postnatal development in pigs. Relation to intestinal uptake and transmission of macromolecules. *Biol Neonate* 1991; 59: 314–21.

31 Elson CO, Kagnoff MF, Fiocchi C, Befus AD, Targan S. Intestinal immunity and inflammation: recent progress. *Gastroenterology* 1986; 91: 746–68.

32 Field M, Frizell RA. Intestinal absorption and secretion. In: *The Gastrointestinal System* Vol. IV, (SG Schultz, ed.), American Physiology Society, Bethesda, Maryland, 1991.

33 Forstner J. Intestinal mucins in health and disease. *Digestion* 1978; 17: 234–63.

34 Freeman GJ, Freedman AS, Segil JM, Lee G, Whitman JF, Nadler LM. B7, a new member of the Ig superfamily with unique expression on activation and neoplastic B cells. *J Immunol* 1989; 143: 2714–22.

35 Freeman GJ, Gray GS, Gimmi CD *et al*. Structure, expression, and T cell costimulatory activity of the murine homologue of the human B lymphocyte antigen B7. *J Exp Med* 1991; 174: 625–31.

36 Freeman GJ, Gribben JG, Boussiotis VA *et al*. Cloning of B7-2: a CTLA-4 counter-receptor that costimulates human T cell proliferation. *Science* 1993; 262: 909–11.

37 Freter R. Mechanisms of association of bacteria with mucosal surfaces. In: *Elliott, O'Connor, Whelen, 80th CIBA Foundation Symposium*, Pitman Medical, London, 1981; 36–47.

38 Frizzell RA, Schultz SG. Ionic conductance of extracellular shunt pathway in rabbit ileum. *J Gen Physiol* 1982; 59: 318–46.

39 Gibbons RA. Mucus of the mammalian genital tract. *Br Med Bull* 1981; 34: 34–8.

40 Gonnella PA, Neutra MR. Membrane-bound and fluid-phase macromolecules enter separate prelysosomal compartments in absorptive cells of suckling rat ileum. *J Cell Biol* 1984; 99: 909–17.

41 Gumbiner B. The structure, biochemistry, and assembly of epithelial TJs. *Am J Physiol* 1987; 253: C749–58.

42 Guyer RL, Koshland ME, Knopf PM. Immunoglobulin binding by mouse intestinal epithelial cell receptors. *J Immunol* 1976; 117: 587–93.

43 Harding FA, McArthur JG, Gorss JA, Raulet DH, Allison JP. CD28-mediated signalling co-stimulates murine T cells and prevent induction of anergy in T cell clones. *Nature* 1992; 365: 607–9.

44 Hathcock KS, Laszlo G, Dickler HB, Bradshaw J, Linsley P, Hodes RJ. Identification of an alterative CTLA-4 ligand costimulatory for T cell activation. *Science* 1993; 262: 905–7.

45 Hermiston ML, Gordon JI. Analysis of cadherin function in the mouse intestinal epithelium. Essential roles in adhesion, maintenance of differentiation, regulation of programmed cell death. *J Cell Biol* 1995; 129: 489–506.

46 Hermiston ML, Gordon JI. Inflammatory bowel disease and adenomas in mice expressing a dominant mutant negative N-cadherin. *Science* 1995; 270: 1203–7.

47 Hinck L, Nathke IS, Papkoff J, Nelson WJ. Dynamics of cadherin/catenin complex formation: novel protein interactions and pathways of complex assembly. *J Cell Biol* 1994; 125: 1327–40.

48 Hyman PE, Clarke DD, Everett SL *et al*. Gastric acid secretory function in preterm infants. *J Ped* 1985; 106: 467–71.

49 Hopkins CR, Gibson A, Shipman M, Miller K. Movement of internalized ligand–receptor complexes along a continuous endosomal reticulum. *Nature* 1990; 346: 335–39.

50 Inman LR, Cantey JR. Specific adherence of *Escherichia coli* (strain RDEC-1) to membranous (M) cells of the Peyer's patch in *Escherichia coli* diarrhea in the rabbit. *J Clin Invest* 1983; 71: 1–8.

51 Israel EJ, Pang KY, Harmatz PR, Walker WA. Structural and functional maturation of rat gastrointestinal barrier with thyroxine. *Am J Physiol* 1987; 252: 762–6.

52 Israel EJ. Neonatal necrotizing enterocolitis, a disease of the immature intestinal mucosal barrier. *Acta Paediatr* 1994; Suppl. 396: 27–32.

53 Israel EJ, Simister N, Freiberg E, Caplan A, Walker WA. Immunoglobulin G binding sites on the human foetal intestine: a possible mechanism for the passive transfer of immunity from mother to infant. *Immunology* 1993; 79: 77–81.

54 Jacobs LR. Biochemical and ultrastructural characterization of the molecular topography of the rat intestinal microvillous membrane. Asymmetric distribution of hydrophilic groups and anionic binding sites. *Gastroenterology* 1983; 85: 46–54.

55 Jones EA, Waldmann TA. The mechanism of intestinal uptake and transcellular transport of IgG in the newborn rat. *J Clin Invest* 1972; 51: 2916–27.

56 Kagnoff MF. General characteristics and development of the immune system. In: *Immunology and Disease of the Gastrointestinal Tract*, 4th edn (MH Sleisenger, JS Fordtran, eds), 1989; 114–43.

57 Kaiserlian D, Vidal K, Revillard J-P. Murine enterocytes can present soluble antigen to specific class II-restricted CD4$^+$ T cells. *Eur J Immunol* 1989; 19: 1513–16.

58 Kirby WN, Parr EL. The occurrence and distribution of H-2 antigens on mouse intestinal epithelial cells. *J Histochem Cytochem* 1979; 27: 746–50.

59 Knutton S, Limbrick AR, Robertson JD. Regular structures in membranes: membranes in the endocytic complex of ileal epithelial cells. *J Cell Biol* 1974; 62: 679–94.

60 Lake AM, Bloch KJ, Sinclair KJ, Walker WA. Anaphylactic release of intestinal goblet cell mucus. *Immunology* 1980; 39: 173–78.

61 Lebenthal E, Lee PC. Alternate pathways of digestion and absorption in early infancy. *J Pediat Gastroenterol Nutr* 1982; 3: 1–3.

62 Leitch GJ, Dickey AD, Udezuler IA, Bailey GB. *Entamoeba histolytica* trophozoites in the lumen and mucus blanket of rat colons studied *in vivo*. *Infect Immunity* 1985; 47: 68–73.

63 Linsley PS, Brady W, Grosmire L, Aruffo A, Damle NK, Ledbetter JA. Binding of the B cell activation antigen B7 to CD28 costimulates T cell proliferation and interleukin 2 mRNA accumulation. *J Exp Med* 1991; 173: 721–30.

64 Lister N, Sykes AP, Bailey PD, Boyd CA, Bronk JR. Dipeptide transport and hydrolysis in isolated loops of rat small intestine: effects of stereospecificity. *J Physiol* 1995; 484: 173–82.

65 Liu Y, Jones B, Aruffo A, Sullivan KM, Linsley PS, Janeway CA. Heat-stable antigen is a costimulatory molecule for CD4 T cell growth. *J Exp Med* 1992; 175: 437–45.

66 Lucas ML. Determination of acid surface pH in vivo in rat proximal jejunum. *Gut* 1983; 24: 734–39.

67 Lucas ML. Weak electrolyte absorption and the acid microclimate. In: *Intestinal Absorption and Secretion* (Skadhauge and K. Heintze, eds) MTP, Lancaster UK, 1984; 39–54.

68 MacDonald TT, Hutchings P, Choy MY, Murch S, Cooke A. Tumor necrosis factor-alpha and interferon-gamma production measured at the single cell level in normal and inflamed human intestine. *Clin Exp Immunol* 1990; 81: 305.

69 Madara JL, Dharmsathaphorn K. Occluding junction structure–function relationships in a cultured epithelial monolayer. *J Cell Biol* 1985; 101: 2124–33.

70 Madara JL, Pappenheimer JR. Structural basis for physiological regulation of paracellular pathways in intestinal epithelia. *J Membr Biol* 1987; 100: 149–64.

71 Madara JL. Loosening TJs. Lessons from the intestine. *J Clin Invest* 1989; 83: 1089–94.

72 Madara JL, Stafford J. Interferon-γ directly affects barrier function of cultured intestinal epithelial monolayers. *J Clin Invest* 1989; 83: 724–27.

73 Madara JL. Maintenance of the macromolecular barrier at cell extrusion sites in intestinal epithelium: physiological rearrangement of tight junction. *J Membr Biol* 1990; 116: 177–84.

74 Madara JL. Pathobiology of the intestinal epithelial barrier. *Am J Pathol* 1990; 137: 1273–81.

75 Malin M, Isolauri E, Pikkarainen P, Karikoski R, Isolauri J. Enhanced absorption of macromolecules: a secondary factor in Crohn's disease. *Dig Dis Sci* 1996; 41. 1423–28.

76 Marsh MN. Gluten, major histocompatibility complex, and the small intestine. A molecular and immunobiologic approach to the spectrum of gluten sensitivity (celiac sprue). *Gastroenterology* 1992; 102: 330–54.

77 Mason DW, Dallman M, Barclay AN. Graft-versus-host disease induces expression of Ia antigen in rat epidermal cells and gut epithelium. *Nature* 1981; 293: 150–1.

78 Masson SD, Perdue MH. Changes in distribution of Ia antigen on epithelium of the jejunum and ileum in rats infected with *Nippostrongylus brasiliensis. Clin Immunol Immunopath* 1990; 57: 83–95.

79 Matsui K, Boniface JJ, Reay PA, Schild H, Frazekas-de-St Broth B, Davis MM. Low affinity interaction of peptide–MHC complexes with T cell receptors. *Science* 1991; 254: 1788–91.

80 Mayer L, Shlien R. Evidence for function of Ia molecules on gut epithelial cells in man. *J Exp Med* 1987; 166: 1471–83.

81 Mayer EA, Raybould H, Koelbel C. Neuropeptides, inflammation and motility. *Dig Dis Sci* 1988; 33: 71S–7S.

82 Mayer L, Eisenhardt D. Lack of induction of suppressor T cells by intestinal epithelial cells from patients with inflammatory bowel disease. *J Clin Invest* 1990; 86: 1255–60.

83 Mayer L, Eisenhardt D, Salomon P, Bauer W, Plous R, Piccinini L. Expression of class II molecules on intestinal epithelial cells in humans. Differences between normal and inflammatory bowel disease. *Gastroenterology* 1991; 100: 3–12.

84 Mayrhofer G, Spargo LDJ. Distribution of class II major histocompatibility antigens in enterocytes of the rat jejunum and their association with organelles of the endocytic pathway. *Immunology* 1990, 70. 11–19.

85 Medzhitov R, Janeway CA. Innate immunity: impact on the adaptive immune response. *Curr Opin Immunol*, 1997; 9: 4–9.

86 Milla PJ. Intestinal motility during ontogeny and intestinal pseudo-obstruction in children. *Pediatr Clin North America* 1996; 43: 511–32.

87 Miller HRP, Nawa Y. Immune regulation of intestinal goblet cell differentiation. *Nouv Revue Hemat* 1979; 21: 31–45.

88 Mostov KE, Simister NE. Transcytosis. *Cell* 1985; 42: 389–90.

89 Nash S, Stafford J, Madara JL. Effects of polymorphonuclear leukocyte transmigration of the barrier function of cultured intestinal epithelial monolayers. *J Clin Invest* 1987; 80: 1104–13.

90 Nathke IS, Hinck L, Swedlow JR, Papkoff J, Nelson WJ. Defining interactions and distributions of cadherin and catenin complexes in polarized epithelial cells. *J Cell Biol* 1994; 125: 1341–52.

91 Neutra MR, O'Malley LJ, Specian RD. Regulation of intestinal goblet cell secretion. II. A survey of potential secretagogue. *Am J Physiol* 1982; 242: G380–87.

92 Owen RL. Sequential uptake of horseradish peroxidase by lymphoid follicle epithelium of Peyer's patches in the normal unobstructed mouse intestine: an ultrastructural study. *Gastroenterology* 1977; 72: 440–51.

93 Paganelli R, Levinsky RJ, Brostoff J, Wraith DG. Immune complexes containing food proteins in normal and atopic subjects after oral challenge and effect of sodium cromoglycate on antigen absorption. *Lancet* 1979; I: 1270–72.

94 Pang KY, Bresson JL, Walker WA. Development of the gastrointestinal mucosal barrier: evidence for structural differences in microvillus membranes from newborn and adult rabbits. *Biochim Biophys Acta* 1983; 727: 201–8.

95 Pang KY, Newman AP, Udall JN, Walker WA. Development of the gastrointestinal mucosal barrier. VI. In utero maturation of the microvillus surface by cortisone. *Am J Physiol* 1985; 249: G85–91.

96 Pappenheimer JR, Reiss KZ. Contribution of solvent drag through intercellular junctions to absorption of nutrient by the small intestine of the rat. *J Membr Biol* 1987; 100: 123–36.

97 Pappenheimer JR. Physiological regulation of transepithelial impedance in the intestinal mucosa of rat and hamster. *J Membr Biol* 1987; 100: 137–48.

98 Phillips AD, France NE, Walker-Smith JA. The structure of the enterocyte in relation to its position on the villus in childhood: an electron microscopical study. *Histopathology* 1979; 3: 117–30.

99 Phillips AD, Thomas AG, Walker-Smith JA. Cryptosporidium, chronic diarrhoea and the proximal small intestinal mucosa. *Gut* 1992; 33: 1057–61.

100 Podolsky DK. Oligosaccharide structure of isolated human colonic mucin species. *J Biol Chem* 1985; 260: 15510–15.

101 Powell D. Barrier function of epithelia. *Am J Physiol* 1981; 231: G272–88.

102 Ramage JK, Stanisz A, Scicchitano R, Hunt RH, Perdue MH. Effect of immunologic reactions on rat intestinal epithelium. Correlation of increased permeability to chromium 51-labeled ethylenediaminetetraacetic acid and ovalbumin during acute inflammation and anaphylaxis. *Gastroenterology* 1988; 94: 1368–75.

103 Reckhemmer G. Transport of weak electrolytes. In: *Gastrointestinal system IV. Handbook of Physiology*. Washington DC, 1992; 371–88.

104 Rechkemmer G, Wahl M, Kuschinsky W, von Engelhardt W. pH-microclimate at the luminal surface of the intestinal mucosa of guinea pig and rat. *Pfluegers Arch* 1986; 407: 33–40.

105 Remington M, Malagelada JR, Zinsmeiste A, Fleming CR. Abnormalities in gastrointestinal motor activity in patients with short bowels: effect of a synthetic opiate. *Gastroenterology* 1983; 85: 629–36.

106 Roberton DM, Paganelli R, Dinwiddie R, Levinsky RJ. Milk antigen absorption in the preterm and term neonate. *Arch Dis Child* 1982; 57: 369–72.

107 Rodewald R, Kraehenbuhl JP. Receptor-mediated transport of IgG. *J Cell Biol* 1984; 99: 159S–64S.

108 Rodriguez GM, Diment S. Role of cathepsin D in antigen presentation of ovalbumin. *J Immunol* 1992; 149(9): 2894–8.

109 Saffron M, Franco-Saenz R, Kong A, Pepthadjopoulos D, Szoka F. A model for the study of oral administration of peptide hormones. *Can J Biochem* 1979; 57: 548–53.

110 Said HM, Smith R, Redha R. Studies on the intestinal surface acid microclimate: developmental aspects. *Ped Res* 1987; 22: 497–9.

111 Sanderson IR, Walker WA. Uptake and transport of macromolecules by the intestine: possible role in clinical disorders (an update). *Gastroenterology* 1993; 104: 622–9.

112 Sanderson IR, Ouellette AJ, Carter EA, Walker WA, Harmatz PR. Differential regulation of B7 mRNA in enterocytes and lymphoid cells. *Immunology* 1993; 79: 434–8.

113 Schwartz RH, Bogema S, Thorne MM. A cell culture model for T lymphocyte clonal anergy. *Science* 1990; 248: 1349–56.

114 Sedmak DD, Davis DH, Singh U, van de Winkel JG. Expression of IgG Fc receptor antigens in placenta and on endothelial cells in humans. An immunohistochemical study. *Am J Pathol* 1991; 138: 175–81.

115 Selby WS, Janossy G, Maso DY, Jewell DP. Expression of HLA-DR antigens by colonic epithelium in inflammatory bowel disease. *Clin Exp Immunol* 1983; 53: 614–18.

116 Shibata Y, Arima T, Yamamoto T. Regular structures on the microvillar surface membrane of ileal cells in suckling at intestine. *J Ultrastruct Res* 1983; 85: 70–81.

117 Shimada T. Factors affecting the microclimate pH in rat jejunum. *J Physiol* 1987; 392: 113–27.

118 Shub MD, Pang KY, Swann DA, Walker WA. Age-related changes in chemical composition and physical properties of mucus glycoproteins from rat small intestine. *Biochem J* 1983; 215: 405–11.

119 Sicinski P, Rowinski J, Wasrchol JB, *et al.* Poliovirus type 1 enters the human host through intestinal M cells. *Gastroenterology* 1990; 98: 56–8.

120 Simister NE, Rees AR. Isolation and characterization of an Fc receptor from neonatal rat small intestine. *Eur J Immunol* 1985; 15: 733–8.

121 Snyder JD, Walker WA. Structure and function of intestinal mucin: developmental aspects. *Int Arch Allergy Appl Immunol* 1987; 82: 351–6.

122 Snyder JD. Bacterial infections. In: *Pediatric Gastrointestinal Disease: Pathophysiology, Diagnosis, Management* (Walker WA *et al.*, eds.), 1991; 527–37.

123 Specian RD, Neutra MR. Mechanism of rapid mucus secretin in goblet cells stimulated by acetylcholine. *J Cell Biol* 1980; 85: 626–40.

124 Steinman RM, Mellman IS, Mueller WA, Cohn ZA. Endocytosis and the recycling of plasma membrane. *J Cell Biol* 1983; 96: 1–27.

125 Stern M, Walker WA. Food proteins and the gut mucosal barrier. I. Binding and uptake of cow's milk proteins by rat jejunum in vivo. *Am J Physiol* 1984; 246: G556–62.

126 Stern M, Gellermann B. Food proteins and maturation of small intestinal microvillus membranes (MVM). I. Binding characteristics of cow's milk proteins and concanavalin A to MVM from newborn and adult rats. *J Pediatr Gastroenterol Nutr* 1988; 7: 115–21.

127 Stern M, Gellermann B, Belitz HD, Wieser H. Food proteins and maturation of small intestinal microvillus membranes (MVM). II. Binding of gliadin hydrolysate fractions and of the gliadin peptide B3142. *J Pediatr Gastroenterol Nutr* 1988; 7: 122–7.

128 Strocchi A, Levitt MD. A reappraisal of the magnitude and implications of the intestinal unstirred layer. *Gastroenterology* 1991; 101: 843–7.

129 Terpend K, Boisgerault MA, Desjeux JF, Heyman M. Protein transport and processing by human HT29-19A intestinal cells: effect of interferon γ. *Gut* 1998; 42: 538–45.

130 Thompson HSG, Staines NA. Could specific oral tolerance be a therapy for autoimmune disease? *Immunology Today* 1991; 11: 396–9.

131 Udall JN, Pang K, Fritze L, Kleinman R, Walker WA. Development of gastrointestinal mucosal barrier. I. The effect of age on intestinal permeability to macromolecules. *Ped Res* 1981; 15: 241–4.

132 Udall JN, Colony P, Fritze L, Pang K, Trier JS, Walker WA. Development of gastrointestinal mucosal barrier. II. The effect of natural versus artificial feeding on intestinal permeability to macromolecules. *Ped Res* 1981; 15: 245–9.

133 Ulshen MH, Rollo JL. Pathogenesis of *Escherichia coli* gastroenteritis in man – another mechanism. *N Engl J Med* 1980; 302: 99–101.

134 Unanue ER. Antigen presenting function of the macrophage. *Ann Rev Immunol* 1984; 2: 395–428.

135 Vaeth GF, Henning SJ. Postnatal development of peptidase enzymes in rat small intestine. *J Pediatr Gastroenterol Nutr* 1982; 1: 111–17.

136 Walker WA, Isselbacher KJ, Bloch KJ. Intestinal uptake of macromolecules: effect of oral immunization. *Science* 1972; 177: 608–10.

137 Walker WA, Isselbacher KJ, Bloch KJ. Intestinal uptake of macromolecules. II. Effect of parenteral immunization. *J Immunol* 1973; 111: 221–6.

138 Walker WA, Wu M, Isselbacher JK, Bloch KJ. Intestinal uptake of macromolecules IV. The effect of duct ligation on the breakdown of antigen and antigen–antibody complexes on the intestinal surface. *Gastroenterology* 1975; 69: 1123–9.

139 Warshaw AL, Walker WA. Intestinal absorption of intake antigenic protein. *Surgery* 1974; 76: 495–9.

140 Weaver LT, Walker WA. Epidermal growth factor and the developing human gut. *Gastroenterology* 1988; 94: 845–7.

141 Weaver LT, Gonnella PA, Israel EJ, Walker WA. Uptake and transport of epidermal growth factor by the small intestinal epithelium of the fetal rat. *Gastroenterology* 1990; 98: 828–37.

142 Williams RC, Gibbons RJ. Inhibition of streptococcal attachment of receptors on human buccal epithelial cells by antigenically similar salivary glycoproteins. *Infect Immunity* 1975; 11: 711–15.

143 Wiman K, Curman B, Forsum U *et al*. Occurrence of Ia antigen on tissue of non-lymphoid origin. *Nature* 1978; 276: 711–13.

144 Winne D. Shift of pH–absorption curves. *J Pharmacokinet Biopharm* 1977; 5: 53–94.

145 Winner LS, Mack J, Weltzin RA, Mekalanos JJ, Kraehenbuhl JP, Neutra MR. New model for analysis of mucosal immunity: intestinal secretion of specific monoclonal immunoglobulin A from hybridoma tumors protects against *Vibrio cholerae* infection. *Infect Immun* 1991; 59: 977–82.

146 Wolf JL, Rubin DH, Finberg R *et al*. Intestinal M cells: a pathway for entry of reovirus into the host. *Science* 1991; 212: 471–2.

147 Ye G, Barrera C, Fan X *et al*. Expression of B7-1 and B7-2 costimulatory molecules by human gastric epithelial cells: potential role in CD4+ T cell activation during *Helicobacter pylori* infection. *J Clin Invest* 1997; 99: 1628–36.

Chapter 14

Immunodeficiency and antigen exclusion

C. Cunningham-Rundles

INTRODUCTION

In health, the secretory mucosa contains non-immunological factors such as acid and mucus, and immunological factors such as lymphocytes, macrophages and secretory immunoglobulin A (SIgA). This combination results in a remarkably effective barrier, eliminating excessive local immunological activation, and preventing excessive systemic absorption of dietary and other antigens. The exact role of each of these components has not been defined, although work on mucosal immunity indicates that SIgA is a central immune mechanism for exclusion of environmental antigens.[4,6,59] SIgA is produced in great quantities by the plasma cells in the lamina propria, perhaps as much as 3 g of SIgA per day.[13] The three congenital immunodeficiency diseases – IgA deficiency, common variable immunodeficiency and X-linked agammaglobulinaemia (Table 14.1) – present a range of naturally occurring immunological abnormalities; the unifying theme, the lack of secretory IgA, is common to all of them. This defect leads to a variety of infections and inflammatory conditions, but for each deficiency disease, the manifestations vary. In another medical condition, the chemotherapy and radiation regimens that have been used to precondition recipients for bone marrow transplantation, also lead to transient but substantial mucosal immune defects. The role of IgA in intestinal immunity has been clarified by a number of studies, but there is a mystery as to the compensatory mechanisms which can be brought to bear when IgA is lacking. The defective mucosal system in these diseases leads to an excessive absorption of various luminal antigens, the best studied being dietary proteins. While the medical consequences

of these events are largely unknown, the absorption of these antigens may produce systemic immunological events which are discussed in this chapter.

Mechanisms of failure of antigen exclusion

1 Immaturity

2 Congenital immune deficiency
   IgA deficiency
   Common varied immunodeficiency
   X-linked aggamaglobulinaemia

3 Allergic

4 Gastrointestinal disease
   Inflammatory bowel diseases
   Gluten-sensitive enteropathy
   Other gastrointestinal diseases

5 Bone marrow transplant recipients

6 Miscellaneous
   Protein malnutrition
   Surgery
   Drugs
   Radiation

Table 14.1 Mechanisms of failure of antigen exclusion.

SELECTIVE IgA DEFICIENCY

IgA deficiency is the commonest primary immune deficiency disease of man, affecting up to 1 in 400 individuals.[1,38] Although sIgA is known to be important in mucosal immunity, most people who are IgA deficient are healthy, suggesting that additional compensations are brought to bear in the absence of IgA. For example, healthy IgA-deficient individuals may have increased levels of secretory IgM in nasal and oral mucosa which compensate for secretory IgA,[5,7,59] while those who have the most illnesses may be also deficient in IgG_2.[65] Additional immunological deficits have been identified in IgA deficiency that could increase susceptibility to infection; these include a relatively poor response to bacterial carbohydrate antigens, even if IgG_2 subclass levels are normal,[37] and, in some, a deficiency of IgG_4 without IgG_2 deficiency.[33] However, the presence of, or level of, IgM in secretions is not well correlated with health in IgA deficiency, and IgG subclass or antibody deficits are not usually found in those who have more illnesses, suggesting that additional explanations are needed.

IgA secretion: *in vitro* studies

The essential characteristic of IgA deficiency is a greatly reduced number of IgA-bearing circulating B cells and a lack of IgA-secreting plasma cells in all mucosal locations.[8,16] IgA-deficient subjects have low but detectable numbers of circulating IgA+ B cells, but these are of a relatively immature phenotype, bearing both IgA and IgM isotypes.[14] In a number of early studies, B cells from IgA-deficient subjects were cultured with mitogens to determine their ability to secrete IgA *in vitro*. Pokeweed mitogen was reported to cause IgA secretion, but subsequent studies using various other stimulators found that little if any IgA was actually produced.[52] In fact, Islam *et al.*[42] showed that pokeweed mitogen-stimulated peripheral blood lymphocytes from IgA-deficient subjects have a significant decrease in switch μ to switch α junctions, and a profound decrease in C α membrane mRNA expression, suggesting a generalized failure of switching to IgA production.

In the last 25 years, a number of potential reasons for failure of terminal differentiation of B cells to IgA secretion in IgA deficiency have been described (Table 14.2), including inadequate or defective T helper cells,[46] the actions of IgA-specific T cell suppresser cells, intrinsic B cell defects[78] and, in some cases, the transplacental passage of maternal anti-IgA antibodies which might suppress fetal IgA development.[66] Many studies have emphasized T cell immunity because it has been tempting to suggest that a T cell regulatory abnormality could best explain the lack of terminal B cell differentiation. T cells of most IgA-deficient subjects do appear capable of supporting IgA production by normal B cells, suggesting that these T cells can provide the

necessary cellular factors for IgA differentiation; however, more subtle T cells defects have not been excluded.[21,71]

Cytokines and IgA production

Antigen-stimulated B cells undergo isotype switch and terminal differentiation into IgA-secreting plasma cells under the influence of a number of cytokines. CD4+ T cells, in particular, regulate IgA production in the mouse, and perhaps in man, involving secretion of interleukins IL2, IL5, IL6 and IL10.[30,53,72,80] A number of studies, especially in mouse systems, point to transforming growth factor β (TGFβ) as a key cytokine in this process, prompting isotype switch and committing antigen-primed B cells to secrete IgA.[61,76]

While these events have been more easily addressed in mouse models, the cytokines involved in the differentiation in human B cells has been more difficult to assess. Recent work has indicated that engagement of the CD40 receptor on B cells, coupled with TGFβ appear to be the crucial mediators.[81] B cells of IgA-deficient subjects have been tested under a number of conditions to assess the role of cytokines in IgA deficiency. In one study, B cells of IgA-deficient subjects were found capable of secreting IgA when stimulated by a combination of anti-CD40 antibody, *Staphylococcus aureus* and IL10: while IL10 was not absolutely required for IgA secretion for B cells of normal donors, for IgA-deficient subjects, it appeared necessary for IgA secretion.[9] In another study, it appeared that B cells of infection-prone IgA-deficient subjects had somewhat less production of IgA than B cells of healthy IgA-deficient subjects tested under the same conditions.[35] Another study indicated that IL10 and IL4, along with CD40 ligation, was a more effective system for stimulating IgA secretion.[54] TGFβ has also been investigated in IgA deficiency; serum levels of TGFβ in IgA-deficient sera were reduced compared with normal controls, but the biological meaning of this is unclear.[60] On the other hand, Islam *et al.*[42] found no difference in TGFβ mRNA in IgA-deficient subjects compared with controls. In another study, mitogen-stimulated mononuclear cells of IgA-deficient patients with the common MHC haplotype, HLA-B8, DR3 had significantly reduced IL5 production.[51]

IgA deficiency and the gastrointestinal tract
Role of secretory IgA

For many years it has been known that SIgA contains antibody directed to bacteria, viruses and proteins normally restricted to the intestinal tract (Table 14.3). The relative inability of IgA to fix complement suggests that secretory IgA serves to clear antigens while provoking little in the way of inflammation. Other roles for IgA in mucosal immunity have been identified. Dimeric IgA secreted by plasma cells is selectively transferred through epithelial cells with the polymeric immunoglobulin receptor by transcytosis. After cleavage of this receptor to release the secretory component, secretory IgA is excreted into the mucosal lumen. IgA can also complex other antigens which have escaped into the mucosal lamina propria, and transport them across epithelial cells to facilitate antigen exclusion.[44] Secretory IgA thus binds and excludes antigens present in the intestinal tract from the systemic system. Dimeric IgA transiting through cells in this way can impede the replication of intracellular antiviral viruses, and thus plays an additional intracellular antiviral role.[55]

Mucosal immunity in IgA deficiency

Since SIgA has both relevant antibody activity and the ability to exclude environmental antigens from the blood, a number of

Causes of failure of terminal differentiation of IgA B cells
Inadequate or defective T helper cells
Actions of IgA-specific T suppressor cells
Intrinsic B cell defects
Suppression of fetal IgA development by transplacental maternal anti-IgA antibodies

Table 14.2 Causes of failure of terminal differentiation of IgA B cells.

Specific secretory IgA antibodies				
Bacteria	**Viruses**	**Fungi**	**Protozoa**	**Others**
Escherichia coli	Rotavirus	Candida albicans	Giardia	Milk proteins
Salmonella	Poliovirus			Soy lectin
Shigella	Echovirus			Peanut lectin
Vibrio cholerae	Coxsackie virus			Wheat gluten
Bordetella pertussis	Respiratory syncytial virus			Ovalbumin
Streptococcus mutans	Influenzae			Galactosyl
Streptococcus mitis				Carbohydrates
Streptococcus salivarius				
Clostridium diphtheriae	Arbovirus			
Clostridium tetani	Semliki			
Lipoteichoic acid	Ross river			
Streptococcus pneumoniae	Japanese B			
	Dengue			
Endotoxin	Mumps			
Neisseria meningitidis	Human immunodeficiency virus			
Haemophilus influenzae b	Herpes simplex			
Tetanus toxoid	Herpes zoster			
	Coronavirus			
	Rubella			
	Cytomegalovirus			

Table 14.3 Specific secretory IgA antibodies.

studies have been done in the last few decades to determine what effect the lack of this immunoglobulin has on people who are IgA deficient. In IgA deficiency there is a striking paucity of IgA-secreting plasma cells in the submucosa of all secretory tissues, and little or no secretory IgA in mucosal fluids. On the other hand, there does appear to be a substitution of IgM-secreting plasma cells for the absent IgA-secreting cells in the intestinal tract in IgA deficiency.[5,6] There is also an increase in the concentration of secretory IgM in the saliva and other intestinal fluids in IgA deficiency.[5,6,57] Since IgM can bind to the secretory component, it has the capacity to transit through the epithelial layer, and thus the substitution of IgM for IgA would presumably be of biological importance.[3]

However the data for this are thin. First, secretory IgM is more easily degraded than secretory IgA in mucosal fluids. In addition, secretory IgM antibodies may be intrinsically less biologically efficient, resulting, for example, in more prolonged excretion of vaccine viruses than seen in normal subjects.[69] Whether IgM serves the same role as IgA is also challenged by another study; Mellander et al.[57] attempted to relate the number of respiratory tract infections in IgA-deficient subjects to the level of IgM in saliva, hypothesizing that an inverse relationship was likely to be present. These studies showed that there was no such relationship. On the other hand, Fernandes et al.[32] found that IgA-deficient children with increased levels of salivary antibodies of the IgM isotype to Streptococcus mutans had less dental caries, which suggests that the secretory IgM exerted a protective role in this circumstance.

It is also possible that there is a mucosal substitution of IgG, as well as IgM, in IgA deficiency. Oral vaccination of IgA-deficient subjects with cholera vaccine resulted in both increased IgG and IgM antibody responses, as judged by immunoglobulin-secreting cells retrieved from the intestine and peripheral blood; in normal individuals, an IgA response to this cholera is predominant.[34] Several investigators have analysed the intestinal tract of IgA-deficient subjects with and without IgG$_2$ deficiency to determine which IgG subclass would be provoked; after oral cholera vaccination, IgA-deficient subjects of both groups had an increased number of IgG$_1$-producing intestinal B cells.[34,63] Even though IgG-secreting mucosal cells might be important in local immunity in IgA deficiency, complement activation by immune complex associated IgG could lead to mucosal inflammation.

Other gastrointestinal immunological alterations

Probably the most common gastrointestinal abnormality in IgA deficiency is nodular lymphoid hyperplasia.[49] These lymphoid nodules are 5 mm or larger in size, and are found predominantly in the lamina propria and submucosa of the small intestine, but occasionally in the large intestine, rectum or stomach. These nodules may be focal, but are usually multiple in antibody deficiency syndromes. They can be associated with mucosal flattening and, if large, can cause obstruction; if the nodules are multiple and produce villous flattening, malabsorption may develop. Immunofluorescence studies of the nodules in IgA deficiency usually demonstrate a proliferation of IgM plasma cells.[5] This is in contrast to the lymphoid nodules found in the gastrointestinal tract of some hypogammaglobulinaemic patients; in the latter, plasma cells are often greatly reduced in number and the nodules tend to contain an expanded population of B lymphocytes, with few or no plasma cells.

The lamina propria of the normal intestinal mucosa contains numerous T lymphocytes, some of which enter the surface epithelium. In health, the majority of these intraepithelial T lymphocytes (IELs) are of the CD8 phenotype, with the remainder having a CD4 phenotype. While IgA-deficient individuals seem to have an increased number of IELs, most of these lymphocytes are also CD8 positive.[47] In contrast to normal subjects, an increased proportion of these T cells appear activated, bearing IL2 receptor (CD25). Klemola *et al.*[48] found that IgA-deficient and control subjects had the same number of γ/δ T cells, while Nilssen *et al.*[62] found that healthy IgA-deficient subjects appeared to have an increased number of γ/δ T cells. Increased numbers of activated IEL in IgA deficiency might serve as a useful check on lymphocyte proliferation and/or the amount of local antibody produced. IgA-deficient coeliac patients given gluten have a further increase in the number of CD8+ T cells in the epithelial compartment,[62] suggesting that a sensitizing antigen is necessary for the appearance of these suppressor lymphocytes.

Jejunal and crypt epithelial expression of the Class II major histocompatibility complex (MHC) antigen DR, is similar in IgA-deficient patients to that of normal controls.[47] For IgA-deficient coeliac patients with coeliac disease, DR expression is normal while on a wheat-free diet but enhanced after gluten challenge. The biological meaning of this is not certain; since the density of the DR antigen on antigen-presenting cells may dictate the magnitude of the immune response, enhanced DR expression might augment the hypersensitivity to food and/or microbial antigens. Mucosal inflammation due to any of these intestinal abnormalities could lead to increased intestinal permeability and absorption of dietary or other intestinal antigens.

Non-immunological mucosal abnormalities in IgA deficiency

While the best-described differences between normal and IgA-deficient individuals are those of the immunological system, non-immunological differences in mucosal architecture are also present. Goblet cells were found increased in the nasal mucosa in IgA deficiency,[45] but this was not found by another investigator who studied the intestinal tract. In the same study, the median percentage of crypt cells in mitosis was higher in IgA deficiency than in controls, suggesting chronic antigen stimulation.[47] Giorgi *et al.*[36] found that the small intestinal mucosa of children with IgA deficiency exhibited unusual pathological changes, some of which were only detectable at the ultrastructural level. These lesions included extensive alterations of the surface epithelium, areas of missing glycocalyx and enterocytes with 'frayed' microvilli. Since these abnormalities were found in the absence of ongoing disease, the authors believed these changes to be characteristic of 'normal' IgA-deficient individuals.

Giving various-sized polyethylene polymers to IgA-deficient subjects by mouth, we found that the urinary excretion of the larger polymers exceeded that expected for normal subjects, demonstrating that structural gastrointestinal tract lesions are present.[20,74] Gut permeability to lactulose and L-rhamnose is also increased, as demonstrated by an abnormally large urinary excretion of these compounds.[67] Since these substances are immunologically inert, these data tend to confirm the notion that structural gastrointestinal lesion(s) may be present, in addition to the lack of secretory IgA. The lesions described could also permit the absorption of antigens from the intestinal lumen, even in the presence of local compensations (such as increased IgM) for secretory IgA.

Absorption of dietary antigens

While most intestinal antigens are prevented from entering the systemic circulation, serum antibodies to dietary antigens are found in the sera of all immunocompetent humans, demonstrat-ing that these substances are absorbed in sufficient quantities to immunize. Antibodies to cow's milk proteins are present in 98% of infants between the age of 7 and 27 weeks, with the highest titres at ages 3–6 months. Antibodies of the IgG isotype predominate in serum of normal subjects, although Mestecky *et al.*[58] detected IgA antibodies to a number of dietary antigens in these sera. IgG_1, IgG_2 and IgG_4 antibodies were the predominant IgG isotypes; for IgA, antibodies of the IgA_1 isotype predominated in both serum and secretions.

One of the first demonstrations that secretory IgA constitutes an important barrier to the absorption of dietary proteins was the observation that sera of IgA-deficient patients are much more likely to contain precipitating antibodies to cow's milk than that of normal subjects.[10] We and others have shown that serum of IgA-deficient subjects contains increased amounts of antibody to a wide variety of food antigens, such as casein, bovine immunoglobulin, bovine albumin, α-lactalbumin, chicken ovalbumin and gliadin,[10,12,25,41] suggesting globally increased antigen absorption. For obscure reasons, IgA-deficient sera often have more antibody to bovine γ-globulin than other milk proteins, which is strange considering that this protein is only a very minor constituent compared with the other proteins in milk.[75]

Immune complexes and dietary antigens

Another measure of antigen absorption is detection of circulating immune complexes after eating. Circulating immune complexes, containing bovine proteins, appear in the sera of IgA-deficient subjects as early as 15–30 min after milk ingestion and remain for at least 2–4 hours.[24,25] Of 25 IgA-deficient patients, circulating immune complexes were found in the serum of 24 patients after milk ingestion over a period of 2 hours; 15 of these subjects had sufficient milk antigen in the serum to be detected by as an insensitive a method as agar diffusion (Fig. 14.1).

There did not appear to be any predictable relationship between the amount of immune complex formed and the amount of serum or salivary IgA.[18] Some IgA-deficient subjects with no serum or

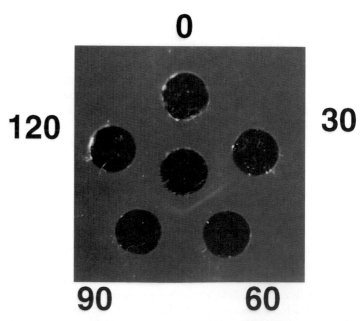

Fig. 14.1 Sera of IgA-deficient subjects given milk has enough bovine κ-casein in the serum to be detected by agar diffusion.

salivary IgA had no circulating immune complexes following milk ingestion, while other individuals with readily detectable serum and salivary IgA had large amounts of immune complexes after drinking milk. Some subjects who had only modest deficits of serum IgA (levels 30–60 mg/dl), had large amounts of bovine antigens detectable in their sera after drinking milk.

These data showed a relatively leaky intestinal tract to be present in individuals who have only a modestly reduced level of serum IgA; some of these individuals would not normally be classified as immune deficient. On the other hand, the level of immune complex in the circulation after drinking milk was closely related to the level of serum antibody to bovine milk proteins ($p<0.01$).[18]

Consequences of antigen absorption

The consequences of excessive antigen absorption in IgA deficiency remain unknown. However, the presence of circulating immune complexes in the serum of an IgA-deficient person is associated with an increased likelihood of autoimmune disease.[27] While a reason for this association has not been defined, the presence and/or degree of the intestinal permeability defect could lead to the excessive absorption of numerous exogenous antigens to which a variety of antibodies could then be raised. Some of these exogenous antigens could share antigenic crossreactivity with endogenous antigens and perhaps serve as a stimulus to autoantibody formation. In addition to the large amount of antibody to dietary proteins discussed above, IgA-deficient serum also contains antibodies to a bovine mucoprotein constituent of the fat globule membrane formed by the bovine mammary gland in the process of milk formation,[11] showing that unexpected bovine epithelial antigens can stimulate antibody production. Other dietary constituents could present additional unusual antigenic components to which an IgA-deficient subject could become sensitized. It is also possible that tissue damage by immune complexes could secondarily stimulate autoantibody production and provoke autoimmune disease.

Anti-idiotypic antibodies

Another effect of the absorbed gastrointestinal antigens appears to be the production of autologous anti-idiotypic antibodies, or antibodies directed to the variable regions of the absorbed antigens. Antibodies to anti-bovine-casein have been detected in the sera of IgA-deficient donors with large amounts of anti-casein antibodies[17] and participate in immune complex formation, along with the inciting antigen and original antibody. Since at least some anti-idiotypic antibodies made by the IgA-deficient individual were found directed at the binding site of the primary antibody, it seems likely that casein antigen and the anti-idiotypic antibody could bind alternatively to the primary antibody, depending upon the serum concentration of the antigen. After drinking milk, for example, a large amount of casein might be present, which would tend to displace the anti-idiotypic antibody from the anti-casein antibody. After a period of fasting, the amount of casein antigen in the blood might be lower, and the immune complex present would be more likely to contain idiotypic and anti-idiotypic antibodies.

The curious part of this phenomenon is the appearance of idiotypic and anti-idiotypic antibodies in the blood of IgA-deficient individuals at the same time.[29] One explanation could be that the continued absorption of dietary casein stimulates the production of anti-casein antibody, despite such controls as the

anti-idiotypic antibodies can supply. Another possibility is that the anti-idiotypic antibodies may serve to stimulate further anti-casein antibody production. While other anti-idiotypic antibodies (anti-anti-ovalbumin, for example) have not been sought, it seems probable that numerous additional anti-idiotypes related to gastrointestinal antigens are present in the sera of IgA-deficient patients.

COMMON VARIABLE IMMUNODEFICIENCY

Common variable immunodeficiency (CVI) is a primary immunodeficiency disease with an estimated incidence of 1:30 000 to 1:60 000. Serum levels of IgG, IgA and usually IgM are low, and there is little or no antibody production, which leads to recurrent infections, particularly of the sinopulmonary tracts.[19,68] While it is generally suspected that CVI is a genetic disease, the cause is unknown and indeed might be different among different subjects. Patients with CVI are more likely than controls to have inherited the major histocompatibility complex antigens HLA B8 and DR3, the same antigens found in increased prevalence in IgA deficiency. For this reason, and the fact that some families may have some members with CVI and others with IgA deficiency, these two diseases are considered genetically related abnormalities.[70,77]

Immunological defects

CVI has the phenotype of a humoral immune defect, since serum immunoglobulin levels are low and antibody production is severely impaired. Although some patients have low numbers of B cells, more than half of all patients also have significant T cell deficiencies, including poor proliferation to mitogens, lack of response to antigens and may have subnormal production of IL2, IL4, IL5, interferon γ and B cell differentiation factor.[73] As found for IgA-deficient subjects, stimulating B cells of CVI subjects with anti-CD40 and IL10 can elicit IgA production in some; the B cells of about half of these subjects can produce normal amounts of IgG and IgM,[64] demonstrating that the B cell defects in these subjects are not necessarily irreversible.

Mucosal immunological defects

In IgA deficiency, there is a lack of maturation of IgA-producing B cells, but in CVI the differentiation of all B cells to plasma cells is impaired. Although there are a considerable numbers of J chain-synthesizing early B cells in the intestinal tract, there is a generalized paucity of all immunoglobulin-staining cells and a severe depletion of plasma cells, IgA being the most affected isotype, and IgM the least affected isotype.[39] While plasma cells are scarce, for CVI patients with chronic or intermittent diarrhoea, mucosal biopsy samples are likely to show a mononuclear cell infiltrate, in some cases severe enough to resemble graft-versus-host disease. Granulomatous lesions are not uncommon, as has been found for CVI subjects in general.[19,56] While the numbers of IEL in IgA-deficient subjects is normal or somewhat increased, for patients with CVI, IEL are significantly increased, especially for patients with villous atrophy. There was no relationship between IEL and peripheral blood CD4:CD8 ratio.[62]

Gastrointestinal tract abnormalities (nodular lymphoid hyperplasia, malabsorption and inflammatory bowel disease)

As for IgA-deficient individuals, perhaps the commonest gastrointestinal abnormality in CVI is nodular lymphoid hyperplasia,

C

characterized by multiple discrete nodules of lymphoid tissue, located diffusely throughout the intestinal tract, but particularly in the small intestine.[79] Originally *Giardia* infections were believed to be the most likely cause of these lymphoid nodules, but this appears rarely to be the case. In most situations, no treatment is required, but nodular hyperplasia can be associated with malabsorption, diarrhoea and weight loss. Occasionally, severe diarrhoea and malabsorption occurs in CVI without nodular lymphoid hyperplasia or other explanation, even after a thorough gastrointestinal evaluation. When malabsorption occurs, it may include impaired absorption of fat, D-xylose, minerals and vitamin B[12]. Intestinal biopsy may reveal changes similar to those seen in coeliac sprue, but a more striking mononuclear infiltrate may develop, giving a nodular appearance to the mucosa.[40,73,79] Inflammatory bowel disease also occurs in CVI; in our group of 187 patients, 16 have had Crohn's disease and 4 ulcerative colitis.

Antigen absorption

Since patients with hypogammaglobulinaemia also lack sIgA, one might expect that patients with this defect could have an equally excessive gastrointestinal permeability compared with the IgA-deficient patients. In analysing a series of such patients, large amounts of bovine casein and bovine γ-globulin are found in the serum.[28] The amount of foreign protein in these sera could not be correlated with gastrointestinal disease nor with any specific immunological parameter; however, for still unknown reasons, higher level of these antigens in the blood were related to splenomegaly in particular and lymphadenopathy in general. Unlike IgA-deficient patients, hypogammaglobulinaemic patients produce antibodies poorly or not at all, and thus the ingested dietary proteins do not elicit antibody production. On the other hand, patients with CVI are given infusion of intravenous immunoglobulin which do contain high levels of antibodies to dietary antigens. After infusions, we found that CVI subjects do develop large amounts of immune complex in the serum.[22] To investigate this further, we developed a monoclonal antibody to bovine κ-casein, a constituent of cow's milk.[31] Using this antibody we showed that the immune complexes did contain this dietary protein, while at the same time the amount of free κ-casein in the serum fell (Fig. 14.2).[22]

X-LINKED AGAMMAGLOBULINAEMIA

X-linked agammaglobulinaemia (XLA), a more uncommon humoral immune defect than CVI, is due to an abnormality of an X chromosome encoded B cell cytoplasmic tyrosine kinase, BTK, necessary to B cell maturation.[15] The hallmark of the illness is very low to absent serum immunoglobulins and absent or nearly absent circulating B cells. Due to the lack of antibody, males with XLA usually become ill in the first year of life with respiratory or gastrointestinal tract infections.[50]

Mucosal immunity and disease

In classic cases of XLA, there are no lymphoid germinal centres in the mucosa, and nodular lymphoid hyperplasia does not develop. Plasma cells are lacking and there is no immunoglobulin secretion in mucosal fluids. While male infants may first present with gastrointestinal disease, chronic gastrointestinal disease appears less commonly in older subjects with XLA than in individuals with CVI. While on clinical presentation, 31 of 98 patients

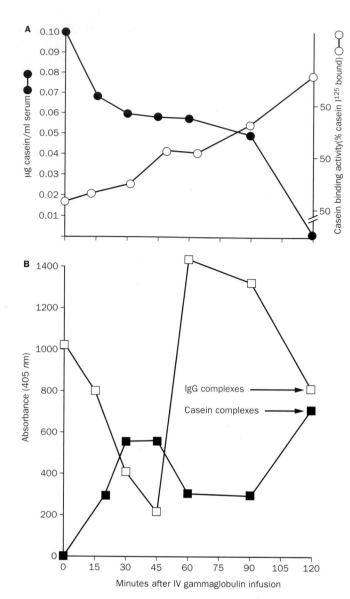

Fig. 14.2 A The serum of a hypogammaglobulinaemic patient who ingested milk the previous day was tested during the course of an infusion of intravenous (IV) immunoglobulin to determine if casein antigen decreased, as casein-binding activity (IgG antibody) increased. **B** Similarly, we also determined the level of IgG immune complex in the serum and the amount of casein containing immune complexes during this period. (From Ref. 77 with permission.)

in a large reported series of XLA patients had acute gastrointestinal infections, and 3 had perirectal abscesses, chronic gastrointestinal tract infections were found in only 10 of the 98 patients (10.2% as opposed to 32–80% in CVI).[50] Nine patients of the group were found to have infections with *Giardia lamblia*; there was one case each of *Salmonella* and enteropathogenic *Escherichia coli*.[50] *Campylobacter* infections also occur in XLA. For unclear reasons, typical inflammatory bowel disease, malabsorption and coeliac disease are quite uncommon in XLA. With the lack of antibody production, autoantibodies are not found.

Antigen absorption in XLA

While not studied in as much detail as patients with selective IgA deficiency or CVI, males with XLA also appear to have less gastrointestinal tract permeability to dietary antigens. Three subjects with XLA, for example, had very little detectable dietary protein antigen in their sera, in comparison with a group of subjects with CVI.[28]

BONE MARROW TRANSPLANT RECIPIENTS

The above sections describe data collected in the studies of patients with primary immunodeficiency who have an impaired immune system due to the congenital lack of IgA. However, in a number of other situations, the secretory immune system is weak due to other processes. One example of this is the defective mucosal immune system that develops in the wake of the chemotherapy and radiation procedures that have been used to precondition recipients of bone marrow transplantation. After transplantation, mucosal immunity is restored by the implantation of donor cells, but this occurs slowly. In patients in whom graft-*versus*-host disease develops, secretory immunity is further impaired.[2,43] sIgA-producing plasma cells appear more slowly post-transplantation in patients who develop graft-*versus*-host disease.[43] The reasons for this are complex and involve both delayed reconstitution by donor cells, and lower levels of sIgA due to injured epithelial surfaces.

We analysed the sera of bone marrow transplant recipients before and up to 1 year after transplantation to determine whether evidence of excessive gastrointestinal permeability could be linked to graft-*versus*-host disease.[23] Post-transplantation of bone marrow, sera of most patients contained increased levels of anti-casein antibody, and the sera of those who developed acute or chronic graft-*versus*-host disease were also more likely to contain circulating immune complexes containing bovine casein[23] (Fig. 14.3). One such case, with profound IgA deficiency and late stage graft-*versus*-host disease was found to have bovine casein deposits in skin.[26]

CONCLUSIONS

The immunodeficiency states discussed above present a range of naturally occurring, or induced, immunological abnormalities; the unifying theme, lack of sIgA, is common to all. The lack of IgA leads to a variety of infections and inflammatory conditions, but in each deficiency disease the manifestations vary. The role of IgA in intestinal immunity has been clarified by a number of studies, but what can be brought to bear when IgA is lacking is still not clearly understood. One clear biological risk for IgA is the exclusion of antigens, normally confined to the intestinal tract, from entering the systemic compartment. Macromolecular absorption of these antigens, in the absence of IgA leads to a

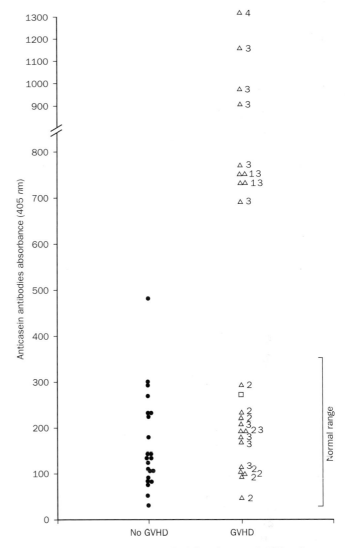

Fig. 14.3 Antibody to bovine casein (absorbance at 405 nm) was compared for 46 post-transplantation sera drawn from 19 patients. Patients who did not develop graft-*versus*-host disease (GVHD) are distinguished from those who did. The state of the graft-*versus*-host (GVH) reaction for the latter patients is indicated for each sample. The range for normal controls is indicated. (△) Acute; (□) chronic; (▲) acute and chronic. (From Ref. 83 with permission.)

number of events, including antigenaemia, immune complex formation, stimulation of anti-idiotypic antibodies and, most likely, still unexplored additional immunological events.

REFERENCES

1 Ammann AJ, Hong R. Selective IgA deficiency: Presentation of 30 cases and review of the literature medicine. *Medicine* 1971; 50: 223–9.

2 Beschorner WE, Yardley JH, Tutschka PJ, Santos GW. Deficiency of intestinal immunity with graft vs host disease in humans. *J Infect Dis* 1981; 114: 38.

3 Brandtzaeg P. Transport models for secretory IgA and secretory IgM. *Clin Exp Immunol* 1981; 44: 221–32.

4 Brandtzaeg P. Development and basic mechanisms of human gut immunity. *Nutr Rev* 1998; 56: 5–18.

5 Brandtzaeg P, Fjellanger J, Giruldsen ST. Immunoglobulin M: Local synthesis and selective secretion in patients with selective IgA deficiency. *Clin Exp Immunol* 1979; 35: 296–9.

6 Brandtzaeg P, Valnes K, Rognum TO, Bjerke K, Baklien K. The human gastrointestinal secretory immune system in health and disease. *Scand J Gastroenterol* 1985; 114: 17–38.

7 Brandtzaeg P, Karlsson G, Hansson G, Petrusson B, Björkander J, Hanson LA. The clinical condition of IgA deficient patients is related to the proportion of IgD and IgM producing cells in the nasal mucosa. *Clin Exp Immunol* 1987; 67: 626–36.

C

8 Brandtzaeg P, Nilssen DE, Rognum TO, Thrane PS. Ontogeny of the mucosal immune system and IgA deficiency. *Gastroenterol Clin North Am* 1991; 20: 397–439.

9 Briere F, Bridon JM, Chevet D *et al*. Interleukin 10 induces B lymphocytes from IgA deficient patients to secrete IgA. *J Clin Invest* 1994; 94: 97–104.

10 Buckley RH, Dees SC. The correlation of milk precipitins with IgA deficiency. *N Engl J Med* 1969; 231: 465–9.

11 Butler JE, Oskvig R. Cancer, autoimmunity and IgA deficiency, related by a common antigen-antibody system. *Nature* 1974; 249: 830–33.

12 Cardinale F, Friman V, Carlsson B, Björkander J, Armenio L, Hanson LA. Aberrations in titer and avidity of serum IgM and IgG antibodies to microbial and food antigens in IgA deficiency. *Adv Exp Med* 1995; 371: 713–16.

13 Clancy R, Bienenstock J. Secretion immunoglobulins. *Clin Gastroenterol* 1976; 5: 229–49.

14 Conley ME, Cooper MD. Immature IgA B cells in IgA deficient patients. *N Engl J Med* 1981; 305: 495.

15 Conley ME, Parolini O, Rohrer J, Campana D. X-linked agammaglobulinemia: new approaches to old questions based on the identification of the defective gene. *Immunol Rev* 1994; 138: 5–21.

16 Crabbé PA, Heremans JF. Selective IgA deficiency with steatorrhea. A new syndrome. *Am J Med* 1967; 42: 319–26.

17 Cunningham-Rundles C. Naturally occurring autologous anti-idiotypic antibodies: participation in immune complex formation in selective IgA deficiency. *J Exp Med* 1982; 155: 711–19.

18 Cunningham-Rundles C. Analysis of the secretory immune barrier in IgA deficiency. *Ann Allergy* 1986; 57: 31–5.

19 Cunningham-Rundles C, Bodian C. Common variable immunodeficiency: clinical and immunological features of 248 patients. *Clin Immunol* 1999; 92(1): 34–48.

20 Cunningham-Rundles C. Macromolecular antigen absorption from the gastrointestinal tract in primary immunodeficiency disease. In: *Nutrition and Immunity* (S Cunningham-Rundles, ed.). Marcel Dekker, New York, 1992: 339–58.

21 Cunningham-Rundles C. Selective, IgA deficiency. In: *Immunologic Disorders of Infants and Children* (H. Stiehm, ed.). Academic Press, New York, 1996.

22 Cunningham-Rundles C, Carr RI. Dietary bovine antigens and immune complex formation after intravenous immunoglobulin in common varied immunodeficiency. *J Clin Immunol* 1986; 6: 381–7.

23 Cunningham-Rundles C, O'Reilly R. Association of circulating immune complexes containing bovine proteins and graft-vs-host disease. *Clin Exp Immunol* 1986; 64: 323–9.

24 Cunningham-Rundles C, Brandeis WE, Good RA, Day NK. Milk precipitins, circulating immune complexes and IgA deficiency. *Proc Natl Acad Sci USA*, 1978; 75: 3386–9.

25 Cunningham-Rundles C, Brandeis WE, Good RA, Day NK. Bovine antigens and the formation of circulating immune complexes in selective IgA deficiency. *J Clin Invest* 1979; 64: 270–2.

26 Cunningham-Rundles C, Brandeis WE, Safai B, O'Reilly RJ, Day NK, Good RA. Selective IgA deficiency and circulating immune complexes containing bovine proteins in a child with graft-vs-host disease. *Am J Med* 1979; 67: 883.

27 Cunningham-Rundles C, Brandeis WF, Pudifin DJ, Day NK, Good RA. Autoimmunity in selective IgA deficiency: relationship to anti-bovine protein antibodies, circulating immune complexes and clinical disease. *Clin Exp Immunol* 1981; 45: 299–304.

28 Cunningham-Rundles C, Carr RI, Good RA. Dietary protein antigenemia in humoral immunodeficiency disease: correlation with splenomegaly. *Am J Med* 1984; 76: 181–5.

29 Cunningham-Rundles C, Feng ZK, Zhuo Z, Woods KR. Relationship between naturally occurring human antibodies to casein and autologous antiidiotypic antibodies: implications for the network theory. *J Clin Immunol* 1991; 11: 279–90.

30 Fayette J, Dubois B, Vandenabeele S *et al*. Human dentritic cells skew isotype switching of CD40-activated naïve B cells towards IgA1 and IgA2. *J Exp Med* 1997; 185: 1909–18.

31 Feng ZK, Cunningham-Rundles C. Production of a monoclonal antibody to bovine kappa casein. *Hybridoma* 1989; 8: 223.

32 Fernandes FR, Nagao AT, Mayer MP, Zelante F, Carneiro-Sampaio MM. Compensatory levels of salivary IgM anti-*Streptococcus mutans* IgA-deficient patients. *J Investig Allergol Clin Immunol* 1995; 5: 1515–18.

33 French MA, Denis KA, Dawkins R, Peter JB. Severity of infections in IgA deficiency: correlation with decreased serum antibodies to pneumococcal polysaccharides and decreased serum IgG2 and/or IgG4. *Clin Exp Immunol* 1995; 100: 47–53.

34 Friman V, Quiding M, Czerkinsky C *et al*. Intestinal and circulating antibody-forming cells in IgA-deficient individuals after oral cholera vaccination. *Clin Exp Immunol* 1994; 95: 226.

35 Friman V, Hanson LA, Bridon JM, Tarkowski A, Banchereau J, Briere F. IL-10 driven immunoglobulin production by B lymphocytes from IgA-deficient individuals correlates to infection proneness. *Clin Exp Immunol* 1996; 104: 432–8.

36 Giorgi PL, Catassi C, Sharbati A, Bearzi I, Cinti S. Ultrastructural findings in the jejunal mucosa of children with IgA deficiency. 3. *Pediatr Gastroenterol Nutr* 1986; 5: 92–390.

37 Hammarstrom L, Persson MAA, Smith CIE. Immunoglobulin subclass distribution of human anti-carbohydrate antibodies: aberrant pattern in IgA deficient donors. *Immunology* 1985; 54: 21–26.

38 Hanson LA. Selective IgA deficiency. In: *Primary and Secretory Immunodeficiency Disorders* (RK Chandra, ed.). Churchill Livingstone, Edinburgh, 1983: 62–84.

39 Herbst EW, Armbruster M, Rump JA, Buscher HP, Peter HH. Intestinal B cell defects in common variable immunodeficiency. *Clin Exp Immunol* 1994; 95: 215–21.

40 Hermans PE, Diaz-Buxo JA, Stobo JD. Idiopathic late-onset immunoglobulin deficiency, clinical observations in 50 patients. *Am J Med* 1976; 61: 221–37.

41 Husby S, Oxelius VA, Svehag SE. IgG subclass antibodies to dietary antigens in IgA deficiency quantification and correlation with serum IgG subclass levels. *Clin Immunol Immunopathol* 1992; 62: 85–90.

42 Islam KB, Baskin B, Nilsson L, Hammarström L, Sideras P, Smith CI. Molecular analysis of IgA deficiency. Evidence for impaired switching to IgA. *J Immunol* 1994; 152: 1442–52.

43 Izutsu KT, Sullivan KM, Schubert MM *et al*. Disordered salivary immunoglobulin secretion and sodium transport in human chronic graft-vs-host disease. *Transplantation* 1983; 35: 441.

44 Kaetzel CS, Robinson JK, Chintalacharuvu KR, Vaeman JP, Lamm ME. The polymeric immunoglobulin receptor (secretory component) mediates transport of immune complexes across epithelial cells: a local defense function for IgA. *Proc Natl Acad Sci USA* 1991; 88: 8796–800.

45 Karlsson G, Hansson HA, Petruson B, Björkander J, Hanson LA. Goblet cell number in the nasal mucosa relates to cell mediated immunity in patients with selective antibody deficiency syndromes. *Int Arch Allergy Appl Immunol* 1985; 78: 86–91.

46 King MA, Wells JV, Nelson DS. IgA synthesis by peripheral blood mononuclear cells from normal and selective IgA deficient subjects. *Clin Exp Immunol* 1979; 38: 306–10.

47 Klemola T. Immunohistochemical findings in the intestine of IgA deficient persons. *J Pediatr Gastroenterol Nutr* 1988; 7: 537–43.

48 Klemola T, Savilahti E, Arato A *et al*. Immunohistochemical findings in jejunal specimens from patients with IgA deficiency. *Gut* 1995; 37: 519–23.

49 Lai Ping So A, Mayer L. Gastrointestinal manifestations of primary immunodeficiency. *Semin Gastrointest Dis* 1997; 8: 220–32.

50 Lederman HM, Winkelstein JA. X-linked agammaglobulinemia: an analysis of 96 patients. *Medicine* 1985; 64: 145–6.

51 Lio D, DíAnna C, Gervasi F *et al*. *In vitro* impairment of interleukin 5 production in HLA-B8. DR3-positive individuals implications for immunoglobulin A synthesis dysfunction. *Hum Immunol* 1995; 44: 170–4.

52 Luzi G, Kabagawa H, Crain MJ, Cooper MD. Analysis of IgG subclass production in cell cultures from IgA deficient patients and normal controls as a function of age. *Clin Exp Immunol* 1986; 65: 434–42.

53 McIntyre TM, Kehry MR, Snapper CM. Novel *in vitro* model for high rate IgA class switching. *J Immunol* 1995; 154: 3156–60.

54 Marconi M, Plebani A, Avanzini MA *et al*. IL-10 and IL-4 co-operate to normalize *in vitro* IgA production in IgA deficient (IgAD) patients. *Clin Exp Immunol* 1988; 112: 528–32.

55 Mazanec MB, Kaetzel CS, Lamm ME, Fletcher D, Nedrud JG. Intracellular neutralization of virus by immunoglobulin A antibodies. *Proc Natl Acad Sci USA* 1992; 89: 6901–5.

56 Mechanic LJ, Dikman S, Cunningham-Rundles C. Granulomatous disease in common variable immunodeficiency. *Ann Intern Med* 1993; 118: 720–30.

57 Mellander L, Bjorkander J, Carlsson B, Hanson LA. Secretory antibodies in IgA deficient and immuno-suppressed individuals. *J Clin Immunol* 1986; 6: 284–91.

58 Mestecky J, Czerwinski C, Russell MW *et al*. Induction and molecular properties of secretory and serum IgA antibodies for environmental antigens. *Ann Allergy* 1987; 59: 54–9.

59 Mestecky J, Lue C, Russell MW. Selective transport of IgA. Cellular and molecular aspects. *Gastroenterol Clin North Am* 1991; 20: 441–71.

60 Muller F, Aukrust P, Nilssen DE, Froland SS. Reduced serum level of transforming growth factor-beta in patients with IgA deficiency. *Clin Immunol Immunopathol* 1995; 76: 203–8.

61 Nillson L, Islam KB, Olafsson O *et al*. Structure of TGF-β1 induced human immunoglobulin Cα1 and Cα2 germ-line transcripts. *Int Immunol* 1991; 3: 1107.

62 Nilssen DE, Aukrust P, Florland SS *et al*. Duodenal intraepithelial gamma/delta T cells and soluble CD8, neopterin, and beta 2-microglobulin in serum of IgA deficient subjects with or without IgG subclass deficiency. *Clin Exp Immunol* 1993; 94: 91–8.

63 Nilssen DE, Friman V, Theman K *et al*. B cell activation in duodenal mucosa after oral cholera vaccination in IgA deficient subjects with or without IgG subclass deficiency. *Scand J Immunol* 1993; 38: 201–8.

64 Nonoyama S, Farrington M, Ishida H, Howard M, Ochs H. Activated B cells from patients with common variable immunodeficiency proliferate and synthesize immunoglobulin. *J Clin Invest* 1993; 92: 1282–7.

65 Oxelius VA, Carlsson AM, Hammarström L, Björkander J, Hanson LA. Linkage of IgA deficiency to Gm allotypes: the influence of Gm allotypes on IgA–IgG subclass deficiency. *Clin Exp Immunol* 1995; 99: 211–15.

66 Petty RE, Sherry DD, Johannson J. Anti-antibodies in pregnancy. *N Engl J Med* 1985; 313: 1620–5.

67 Pignata C, Budillon G, Monaco G *et al*. Jejunal bacterial overgrowth and intestinal permeability in children with immunodeficiency syndromes. *Gut* 1990; 31: 879–82.

68 Report of an IUIS Scientific Committee. International Union of Immunological Societies. Primary immunodeficiency diseases. *Clin Exp Immunol* 1999; 118 (Suppl 1): 1–28.

69 Savilahti E, Klemola T, Hovit I *et al*. IgA deficient persons excrete attenuated vaccine viruses longer than controls. In: *Progress in Immunodeficiency Research and Therapy II*: (Vosser E, Griscelli C, eds). Elsevier Amsterdam, 1986: 231–60.

70 Schaffer FM, Palermos J, Zhu ZB, Barger BO, Cooper MD, Volanakis JE. Individuals with IgA deficiency and common variable immunodeficiency share polymorphisms of major histocompatibility complex class III genes. *Proc Natl Acad Sci USA* 1989; 86: 8015–19.

71 Schaffer FM, Monteiro RC, Volanakis JE, Cooper MD. IgA deficiency. *Immunodef Rev* 1991; 3: 15–44.

72 Shockett P, Stavnezer J. Effect of cytokines on switching to IgA and germline transcripts in B lymphoma 1.29μ: transforming growth factor β activates transcription of the unrearranged Cα gene. *J Immunol* 1991; 147: 4374.

73 Sneller MC, Strober W, Eisenstein E, Jaffe JS, Cunningham-Rundles C. NIH Conference. New insights into common variable immunodeficiency. *Ann Intern Med* 1993; 118: 720–30.

74 Sundvist T, Mangusson KE, Sjodahl R, Stjernstrom I, Tagesson C. Passage of molecules through the wall of the gastrointestinal tract. II. Application of low molecular weight polyethylene glycol and a deterministic mathematical model for determining the intestinal permeability in man. *Gut* 1980; 21: 208–14.

75 Tomasi TB, Katz L. Human antibodies against bovine immunoglobulin M in IgA deficient sera. *Clin Exp Immunol* 1971; 9: 3–10.

76 Van Vlasselaer P, Punnonen J, de Vries JE. Transforming growth factor β directs IgA switching in human B cells. *J Immunol* 1992; 148: 2062.

77 Vorechovsky I, Zetterquist H, Paganelli R *et al*. Family and linkage study of selective IgA deficiency and common variable immunodeficiency. *Clin Immunol Immunopathol* 1995; 77: 185–92.

78 Waldman TA, Broder S, Krakauer R *et al*. Defects in IgA secretion and in IgA specific suppressor cells in patients with selective IgA deficiency. *Trans Assoc Am Phys* 1976; 89: 215.

79 Washington K, Stenzel TT, Buckley RH, Gottfried MR. Gastrointestinal pathology in patients with common variable immunodeficiency and X-linked agammaglobulinemia. *Am J Surg Pathol* 1996; 10: 1240–52.

80 Whitmore ACD, Prowse M, Haughton G, Arnold L. Ig isotype switching in B lymphocytes: the effect of T cell-derived interleukin, cytokines, cholera toxin, and antigen on isotype switch frequency of a cloned B cell lymphoma. *Int Immunol* 1991; 3: 95–8.

81 Zan H, Cerutti A, Dramitinos P, Schaffer A, Casali P. CD40 engagement triggers switching to IgA1 and IgA2 in human B cells through induction of endogenous TGF-β: evidence for TGF-β but not IL-10 dependent direct Sμ–Sα and sequential Sμ–Sγ, Sγ–Sα DNA recombination. *J Immunol* 1998; 161: 5217–25.

Chapter

15

Causes and consequences of altered gut permeability

Ingvar Bjarnason and Ian S. Menzies

INTRODUCTION

It was demonstrated 27 years ago that recovery of non-metabolized oligosaccharides in the urine after oral administration could provide a reliable non-invasive measure of intestinal permeability in man.[132] Acceptance of the method was initially slow as its reliability depends upon detailed control of the test procedure, particularly the osmotic aspects of dose composition, the importance of which was not sufficiently appreciated. Subsequent introduction[46,47] of polyethylene glycol (PEG) 400 for estimation of intestinal permeability produced more confusion as the behaviour of these polymers was found to be quite different, suggesting permeability changes that were often the reverse of those indicated by oligosaccharide probes of similar molecular dimension. This, however, stimulated a more detailed investigation of the problem, with the introduction of differential permeability tests which employed combinations of non-metabolizable probes that cross the absorptive surface by different pathways. The theory behind the differential urinary excretion principles is illustrated in Table 15.1. The differential urinary excretion ratio of probes that differ with respect to the permeability pathways to which they have access, provides a more reproducible and specific method of expressing the state of intestinal permeability than the behaviour of a single probe, although the latter remains the best way to measure total intestinal uptake. The last few years have seen a proliferation of studies from different sources using these tests to assess permeability and other aspects of gastrointestinal dysfunction in disease.

Tests of intestinal permeability were introduced with a view to the investigation of intestinal barrier function; indeed, these terms are often regarded as synonymous. Such investigations may relate to at least four purposes. These include:

1. The detection of intestinal disease as clinical screening tests.
2. To assess the severity of intestinal dysfunction, particularly for monitoring response to therapy and confirmation of

Factors affecting the outcome of non-invasive permeability/absorption tests		
Variables	**Effect on probe**	
	Monosaccharide	**Disaccharide**
Delivery of test probes		
1. Content and formulation of test solution	Equal	
2. Ingestion (? Regurgitation)	Equal	
3. Gastric emptying/intestinal transit	Equal	
4. Gastric and intestinal dilution	Equal	
5. Degradation	Equal	
Intestinal permeation		
6. Area of absorptive surface	Equal	
7. State of mucosal permeability/transport	Differential effect on permeation	
Disposal		
8. Systemic distribution	Nearly equal	
9. Metabolic degradation	Equal or non-existent	
10. Renal clearance	Equal	
11. Urine collection	Equal	
Analytical		
12. Sample preservation	Equal	
13. Analytical estimation	Equal	

Simultaneous administration of two test probes, mono- and di-saccharide (lactulose and L-rhamnose for example), but in principle any 2 suitable compounds, which respond in an identical way to each variable except that selected for investigation, provides a non-invasive method for assessing specific aspects of intestinal function. Correctly devised the di-/mono-saccharide excretion ratio (of percentages recovered in urine) provides a specific index of the selected function (in this case intestinal permeability) unaltered by the other variables.

diagnosis (e.g. gluten withdrawal and challenge in coeliac disease).

3. To investigate the impact of non-intestinal factors on intestinal function. These may be exogenous, related to radiotherapy, drugs, alcohol, dietary or environmental factors; or endogenous, because of malnutrition, reduced blood flow, anaemia and other systemic conditions.

4. To assess the importance of intestinal barrier function in the aetiology, pathophysiology and pathogenesis of intestinal and systemic disease.

Unfortunately there has been a tendency to underestimate the complexity of factors affecting the outcome of these non-invasive procedures. The essential aspects of these techniques will therefore be discussed, together with modifications that allow different functions and regions of the gut to be assessed. Clinical applications, with special reference to the characterization of reaction to food constituents, drugs and other causes of intestinal dysfunction, will then be described.

NON-INVASIVE USE OF PROBES TO ASSESS INTESTINAL FUNCTION AND INTEGRITY

Sugars such as lactulose and other non-metabolized disaccharides (melibiose), trisaccharides (raffinose) or polysaccharides (dextran MW 3000 D)[111,132,203] and, more recently polysucrose (MW 1500 D),[145,146] in addition to isotopically labelled [51]CrEDTA[29,31] or [99m]TcDTPA,[45] were all employed initially as single markers. Physical and biochemical characteristics such as molecular dimension (possibly shape) and solubility, affinity for mucosal hydrolysis and mediated transport, and efficiency of renal clearance, provide a basis for selection.[30,52,80,134,190] Ideally, such probes should be non-toxic, resist digestion in the intestine and be fully recoverable in urine after absorption. Fig. 15.1 outlines the permeation pathways that some of the more clinically useful test markers use. Fig. 15.2 shows a more detailed schematic of saccharide digestion and absorption, with special reference to commonly used test sugars. Characterization of these probes follows in the next sections.

Large pore probes ($\geq$ 0.5 nm molecular radius)
Lactulose (β1–4 fructogalactoside, MW 342 D)
As with most oligosaccharides, lactulose adopts an extracellular distribution and is rapidly and almost completely excreted in urine after intravenous administration.[123,132] Like melibiose, raffinose, stachyose and fluorescein-labelled dextran (MW 342, 504, 666 and 3000 D, radii 0.5, 0.59, 0.62 and 1.25 nm, respectively), it also resists the action of human intestinal disaccharidases and is suitable for assessing large pore permeation in the small intestine. These sugars are, however, susceptible to rapid degradation by colonic bacteria.

Cellobiose (β1–4 diglucoside, MW 342 D)
Although it is used as a probe for assessing small intestinal permeability,[48] this disaccharide is susceptible to hydrolysis presumably by human intestinal lactase.[55]

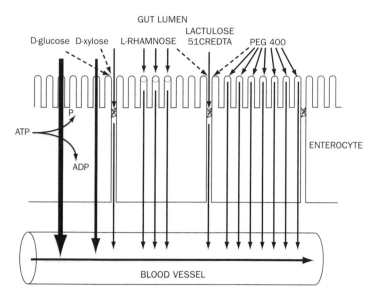

Fig. 15.1 The behaviour of intestinal absorption and permeability test probes can be explained on the basis of their differing permeation pathways. Absorption of 3-O-methyl-D-glucose and D-xylose are carrier-mediated, the former being Na-linked and ATP-driven (an active process), the latter by means of a facilitated route with lower capacity. L-rhamnose and mannitol are absorbed by non-mediated diffusion predominantly across aqueous pores in the brush border membrane, whereas lactulose and ^{51}CrEDTA being, like inulin, unable to pass across cell wall membranes, normally permeate very slowly through the 'tight' intercellular junctions. Although PEG 400 and the monosaccharides can also pass through tight junctions (broken lines), the diffusion rates observed suggest access to alternative high capacity pathways. PEG 400 may partition through the lipid bilayer of cell membranes, but this is a controversial issue.

^{51}CrEDTA (MW 340 D, but may bind some water molecules)
This probe was first introduced for the non-invasive estimation of human intestinal permeability in 1983[29,31] and has molecular dimensions (approximate molecular radius 0.5 nm) and physiological disposition almost identical to those of lactulose and melibiose. Resistance to bacterial degradation, however, also permits ^{51}CrEDTA to be used to assess colonic permeability. Recovery after oral administration to patients with ileostomy is quantitatively similar to that of lactulose, while in subjects with intact colons excretion of ^{51}CrEDTA becomes progressively greater than that of lactulose over a period of 24 h after ingestion.[92–95]

Small pore probes (≤ 0.4 nm molecular radius)
D-mannitol (D-mannose hexitol, MW 182 D)
Uptake of mannitol from human intestine is relatively slow, suggesting lack of affinity for biochemically mediated mucosal transport. Distribution after absorption is extracellular, and recovery in urine complete following intravenous instillation.[110] Mannitol of dietary (and possibly metabolic) origin is often present in human urine in trace amounts.[110]

L-rhamnose (6-deoxy-L-mannose, a 'methylpentose' sugar, MW 164 D)
The comparatively slow uptake of L-rhamnose from human small intestine suggests a low affinity for receptor-mediated transport.[126] The physiological behaviour of L-rhamnose is similar to that of

mannitol, but recovery in urine after intravenous instillation is somewhat less complete.

Mediated transport
3-O-methyl-D-glucose (MW 194 D)
This is a synthetic monosaccharide with affinity for the active intestinal Na-linked D-glucose transport system. It is not metabolized and renal clearance in the human is complete after intravenous administration.[71,134]

D-xylose (MW 150 D)
D-xylose is a pentose mainly of plant origin. In the human, absorption is mainly from the jejunum by a passive carrier-mediated system distinct from that used by 3-O-methyl-D-glucose. It is partially metabolized after reaching the circulation, about 50% being recovered in urine following intravenous administration.[71,134] During the last 50 years D-xylose has been widely used for assessing clinical malabsorption.[72,76]

Permeation pathway undetermined
Polyethylene glycol
PEG 400 has been used as a probe for estimating human intestinal permeability predominantly by three groups,[46,47,64,67,83,84,99,108,120–22,139,180] especially for assessing intestinal function in patients with food sensitivity or allergy. Intestinal permeation of the eight polymers (MW 194–502 D) that comprise PEG 400 is not only much more (20-fold) efficient than water-soluble probes of similar molecular dimension but is comparable with that of monosaccharides that have facilitated absorption mechanisms.[123,134] Recovery in urine after intravenous administration is in the range of 26–72% in 5 h, depending on polymer size.[123] Alterations in the permeation of PEG 400 recorded in various diseases do not accord in a logical fashion with the behaviour of other 'large pore' probes such as ^{51}CrEDTA, which are known to show a significant correlation with macromolecular permeation.[58,69,158] Since PEG 400 can pass into human erythrocytes, equilibrating within 60 min,[134] the explanation for this is probably related to an affinity for cell wall lipid that augments transmucosal permeation.[89] Although the controversy concerning the use of PEG polymers for assessment of intestinal function continues unabated,[53,83,89,108,109,117,134] the above reservations should be kept in mind, especially with respect to the recorded effects of food constituents on intestinal function, as most studies addressing this subject refer to the use of PEG 400.

EVALUATION OF DIFFERENT FUNCTIONS

Permeability
It is important to distinguish small aqueous channels with a high mucosal incidence (approximate radius 0.4 nm which can only accommodate probes of the size of mannitol and L-rhamnose or smaller) from larger, low frequency aqueous channels which can also accommodate lactulose, ^{51}CrEDTA, etc. The incidence of intestinal large/small aqueous channels (in reality large/large plus small channels) in normal UK residents, expressed as the differential urinary excretion of lactulose/L-rhamnose, is about 1/40 (0.025) and characteristically rises in the presence of mucosal damage owing to a variety of causes. Normal ranges vary from

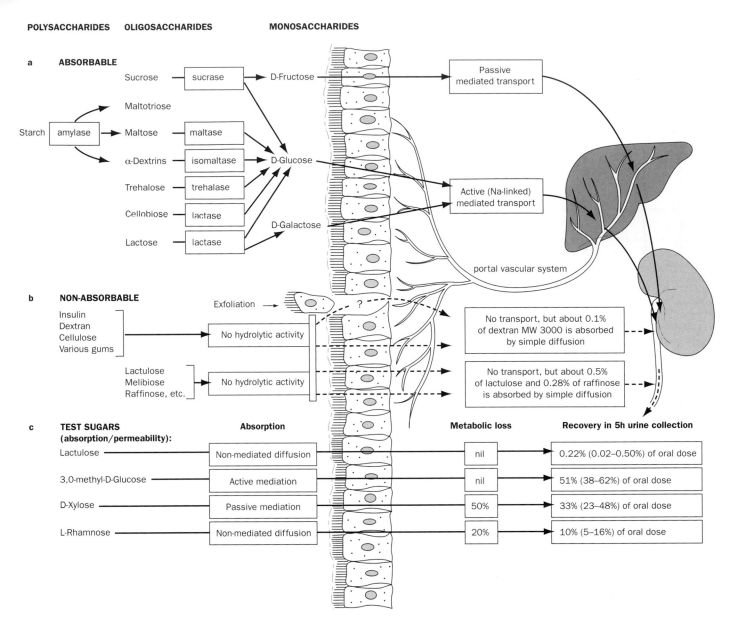

Fig. 15.2 Digestion and absorption of saccharides. (a) Ingested starch is broken down to the various disaccharides by salivary and pancreatic amylase. The disaccharides are cleaved by the various brush border disaccharidases to yield D-fructose, D-glucose and D-galactose. These in turn are transported across the brush border and the enterocytes, and into the circulation by specific transport systems. (b) Non-hydrolysable polysaccharides and disaccharides and trisaccharides are thought to be excluded from permeation across the brush border. The small quantities that do permeate the intestine appear to pass by a paracellular route or through areas of cell extrusion (apoptosis). (c) Four commonly used sugars used in a combined test of intestinal absorptive capacity and intestinal permeability use different transport routes across the intestine, which allows assessments of the various intestinal functions. This increases the discriminate value of the tests when assessing intestinal disease.

country to country, being higher in most tropical areas because of the presence of tropical enteropathy.[135]

Absorptive capacity

The greater uptake of 3-O-methyl-D-glucose and D-xylose compared with mannitol, L-rhamnose and oligosaccharides relates to biochemically defined receptor-mediated transport systems. As an indicator of absorptive capacity, 3-O-methyl-D-glucose is relatively insensitive, absorption not being significantly affected by mild mucosal disease on account of the large reserve for intestinal uptake of this sugar.[71] In contrast, because the normal intestine has no reserve capacity for the absorption of D-xylose, it is a

much more sensitive indicator. However, this applies only to the jejunum as uptake from ileum is minimal.[71]

Disaccharide hydrolysis

Uptake of intact disaccharide is influenced by the level of small intestinal disaccharidase activity. Being inversely related to the rate of hydrolysis,[21,124] uptake of intact disaccharide is very limited, contributed from stomach and upper small bowel, but increases, extending further down the small intestine, when disaccharidase activity is impaired. Comparison of timed urinary recovery of hydrolysable disaccharides such as lactose, sucrose and palatinose (substrates for intestinal lactase, sucrase and isomaltase, respectively) with that of non-hydrolysable lactulose can be used to assess the efficiency of small intestinal disaccharide hydrolysis.[21,124,143]

Multiple function tests
When required the above functions can be undertaken simultaneously by combining test procedures.[136]

Four-sugar differential absorption and permeability test
A test to assess small intestinal absorptive capacity and intestinal permeability simultaneously[50,74] has distinct advantages for routine purposes. The following is now a well tried procedure.

After overnight fast the following test sugars are ingested as an iso-osmolar solution dissolved in 100 ml drinking water (or 250 ml when larger doses of 3-O-methyl-D-glucose and D-xylose are given) to enable estimation of blood levels: 3-O-methyl-D-glucose (0.2 g) assesses active carrier-mediated glucose/galactose transport; D-xylose (0.5 g) assesses a passive carrier-mediated transport system; L-rhamnose (1.0 g) detects non-mediated permeation: there is a high incidence in small water channels; and lactulose (5.0 g) shows non-mediated permeation, with a low incidence in small water channels. Blood D-xylose/3-O-methyl-D-glucose estimations give excellent discrimination for the detection of villus atrophy. A complete 5-h urinary collection is made into a bottle containing preservative, the volume recorded and an aliquot stored for analysis.

INVESTIGATING DIFFERENT REGIONS OF THE INTESTINE

Tests that employ sugars, most of which are rapidly degraded by bacterial action in the colon, are usually considered to reflect the state of small intestinal uptake. Survival of sugars reaching the colon is probably brief enough to justify this assumption. On the other hand, permeation of ^{51}CrEDTA and PEG, which resist bacterial degradation, is contributed from both small and large intestine.

Localizing intestinal permeability changes
It is possible to define the levels at which intestinal permeation and absorption occur. This can be done by comparison of the plasma concentration/time profile of the constituent being investigated with those derived from simultaneously ingested markers, the uptakes of which are known to be related to defined regions of the intestine.[187] In the case of intestinal permeability, comparison of the uptake of ^{51}CrEDTA with that of simultaneously administered reference markers allows the site of increased intestinal permeability to be verified.

Substances suitable for reference include: 3-O-methyl-D-glucose, which is rapidly absorbed by the D-glucose carrier mechanism upon entering the small bowel and is absorbed predominantly from the jejunum by the glucose carrier (active mediated transport); [57]covitamin B[12]-intrinsic factor complex, absorbed by specific carriers from the terminal ileum; and sulfasalazine, which passes unchanged into the caecum where it is cleaved into five aminosalicylic acid and sulfapyridine groups by azoreductase-containing bacteria. Sulfapyridine is then rapidly absorbed and its appearance in serum indicates when the test solution enters the caecum.

Figure 15.3 shows representative results obtained from patients with untreated coeliac disease (increased serum levels of ^{51}CrEDTA correspond to the 3-O-methyl-D-glucose absorption curve), Crohn's disease (where the peak serum levels of ^{51}CrEDTA correspond to appearance of the ileal and colonic

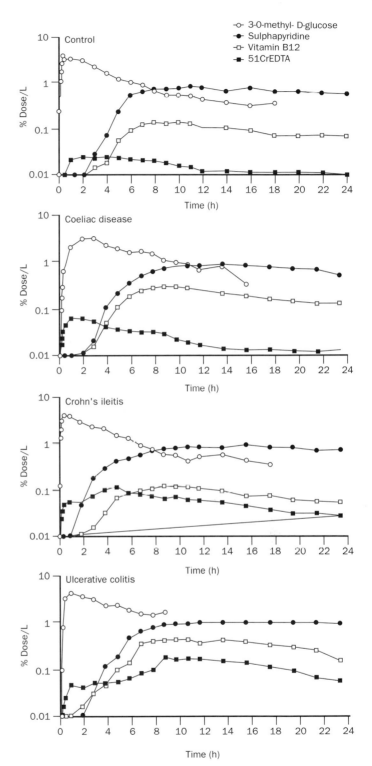

Fig. 15.3 Localization of increased permeability in coeliac, Crohn's disease and ulcerative colitis (see text for description of technical details). The figure demonstrates little or no permeation of ^{51}CrEDTA in normal subjects after 8 h. Increased permeation of ^{51}CrEDTA in a patient with coeliac disease coincides with the 3-O-methyl-D-glucose peak, and the ileal and colonic markers in a patient with Crohn's ileitis (the test also suggests increased colonic permeation of ^{51}CrEDTA). The permeability to ^{51}CrEDTA in ulcerative colitis is increased after the appearance of the ileal and colonic marker. Note that the serum levels (y axis) are on a logarithmic scale and that the ileal marker may appear at the same time as the caecal marker. The reason for this is that the absorption of vitamin B12 is somewhat delayed because of intracellular metabolism.

markers) and ulcerative colitis (increased serum levels of [51]CrEDTA appear some time after the appearances of vitamin B12 and sulfapyridine). This method provides the first *in vivo* evidence that the site of increased intestinal permeability in patients with coeliac and inflammatory bowel disease is indeed the diseased intestinal mucosa itself. The technique is clearly not suitable for routine use, being expensive and demanding on patient and investigator alike.

Further analysis of the test results allows other interesting information to be deduced. Because serial serum samples are obtained it is possible to calculate transit times using this technique. The time from ingestion of the test solution to the time of appearance of 3-O-methyl-D-glucose reflects gastric emptying time; the time to the appearance of sulfapyridine indicates orocaecal transit time; and the time of appearance of sulfapyridine less that of 3-O-methyl-D-glucose then becomes a specific measure of jejuno-to-caecal transit. It may be important to dissociate gastric emptying from jejuno-to-caecal transit especially in diseases such as diabetes mellitus and in advanced HIV disease, where gastric emptying time is delayed and small intestinal transit is accelerated. Figure 15.4 demonstrates this in a patient with AIDS. Also note that no sulfapyridine is detectable until there is a definite sharp rise. In patients with Crohn's disease and documented small bowel bacterial overgrowth (Fig. 15.4c), this sharp peak is also evident. However, shortly after ingestion of the test substance there are low levels of sulfapyridine, which are almost certainly because of the bacterial action. Hence the test appears to detect small bacterial overgrowth.

Colonic permeability

This involves combined administration of [51]CrEDTA with lactulose and L-rhamnose followed by urine collection at 0–5 and 5–24h for marker analyses.[94,95,157] The 5-h differential urinary excretion of lactulose:L-rhamnose provides an index of small intestinal permeability. However, when the test solution enters the colon both lactulose and L-rhamnose are rapidly degraded while [51]CrEDTA is not. The difference between the 24-h recovery of [51]CrEDTA and lactulose is considered to represent colonic permeation because the contribution of both probes from the small intestine is identical.[93] The test shows increased permeation of [51]CrEDTA (less that of lactulose) in severe colonic disease.[92,94,157] This relates to colonic permeation (total uptake of a single probe) rather than permeability (an index of porosity).

Assessment of gastric permeability

Sutherland *et al.*[181] present a method in which sucrose is employed for assessing gastric as opposed to small intestinal permeability. The validity of the test rests on the assumption that small intestine hydrolysis is so rapid and complete that uptake of sucrose after ingestion can be regarded as a specific feature of gastric permeability.[127,174,181] This is questionable, especially as increased urinary excretion of sucrose from the small intestine has been described in primary sucrase deficiency,[124] and is a well recognized feature of conditions such as coeliac disease[75] and tropical sprue[166] in which increased permeability and disaccharidase deficiency are both the consequences of small intestinal disease.[134]

Sucrose permeation is predictably increased in coeliac disease.[174,197] While this may be useful for diagnostic screening, as was suggested by Gryboski *et al.* over 30 years ago,[75] it does not provide reliable evidence of gastric hyperpermeability.[53] In the absence of any practical non-invasive way of confining a test probe to the stomach, measurement of gastric permeability remains a problem.

FORMULATION OF TEST SOLUTIONS

Apart from choice of probes, two different osmotic effects, the first related to osmolarity and the second to the poorly absorbed solute of test solutions, need careful consideration. Figure 15.5 shows the test dose composition from nine different published sources and summarizes the results in normal controls. The figure demonstrates the effect of test dose osmolarity on the permeation of lactulose and the mean differential urinary excretion of lactulose mannitol as well as the effect of poorly absorbed solute on the permeation of mannitol.

'Hyperosmolar stress' and osmotic fillers

Ingestion of hyperosmolar solutions (over 1500 mosm/l) cause a significant temporary increase of intestinal permeability to polar probes of molecular radius 0.5 nm and above in normal human subjects. Some workers have made their test solutions hyperosmolar (up to 1500 mosm/l) on purpose by addition of 'osmotic fillers' such as glycerol, glucose or sucrose (by itself or with lactose)[11,44,62,101,103,140,194,196,205] to facilitate the detection of villus atrophy in which the intestine becomes more sensitive to 'hyperosmolar' stress.[130,132,134,203] Although response to hyperosmolar solutions shows better discrimination for the detection of mild mucosal abnormalities, the quantitative relationship to severity of intestinal disease is unreliable because of individual variation both in susceptibility to the stress and the efficiency with which osmotic fillers are absorbed. On the other hand, iso-osmolar test solutions are more reliable for evaluating the impact of intestinal disease when assessing absorptive capacity and natural predisposition to macromolecular uptake or monitoring responses to therapy and gluten challenge. The 1500 mosm/l test dose was originally considered to be the average threshold osmolarity above which ingestion of a 100-ml solution significantly increased intestinal permeability to lactulose in healthy subjects.[111,134] However, the level of test solution osmolarity required to give optimal discrimination when screening patients with suspected small bowel disease has not been defined, and is likely to vary with the disease in question and the 'osmotic filler' employed.

Osmotic effect of poorly absorbed solute in test solutions

The solute content of test solutions, especially those which are poorly absorbed such as lactulose, mannitol and rhamnose, also needs to be carefully controlled as this influences the proportion of test probes absorbed by inducing accumulation of fluid in the intestine and acceleration of transit.[93,128] This effect has a much greater influence on the absorption of lactulose and L-rhamnose than that of D-xylose, and least influence on the absorption of 3-O-methyl-D-glucose.[128] To minimize such distortions it is desirable to keep the dose of poorly absorbed probes (and other solutes in the test solution) as low as reliable analysis of the urinary and plasma concentrations will allow.

ANALYSIS OF TEST MARKERS

Reliable separation and quantitation of these sugar markers in urine requires great care and experience. Quantitative thin-layer chro-

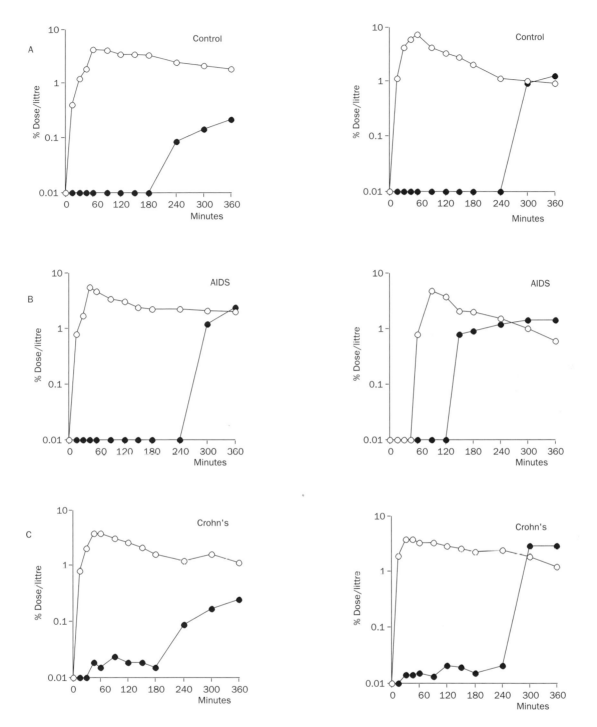

Fig. 15.4 Representative permeation profiles of 3-O-methyl-D-glucose and sulfapyridine after ingestion of the monosaccharide and sulfasalazine in two control subjects, two patients with AIDS and two patients with Crohn's disease associated with small bowel bacterial overgrowth. (a) In the control subjects 3-O-methyl-D-glucose (percentage dose/litre plotted on a logarithmic scale) was detected 15 min after ingestion of the test solution. There was no serum sulfapyridine evident until the obvious rise 4 h after ingestion of the solution. (b) One patient with AIDS does not differ from controls. The other patient with AIDS shows a 60-min interval between ingestion of the test solution and detectable 3-O-methyl-D-glucose levels. Sulfapyridine was detected at 150 minutes, which gives a jejunal-to-caecal transit time of 90 min. (c) These clearly differ from controls and patients with AIDS in that low levels of sulfapyridine were evident in serum before the characteristic and obvious increase which we take to indicate small intestinal bacterial metabolism of sulfasalazine and the arrival of the 'head of the solution' in the caecum, respectively. ○——○ = 3-O-methyl-D-glucose; ●——● = sulfapyridine.

matography (TLC),[129,133] enzyme analyses, radioisotope labelling, gas–liquid chromatography (GLC) and high-performance liquid chromatography (HPLC) all have their proponents and pitfalls, but detailed discussion of the techniques is outside the scope of this chapter. Analysis of PEG is by GLC or HPLC, while radiometric measurement of ^{51}CrEDTA is clearly the most simple.

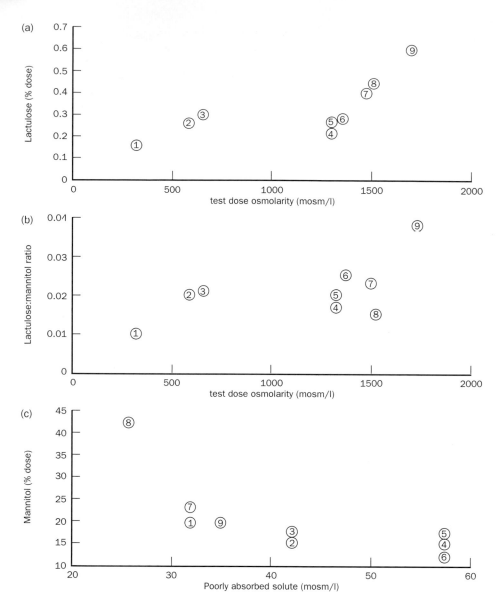

Fig. 15.5 Test dose composition and normal mean values quoted for the recovery of lactulose, mannitol and differential lactulose/mannitol ratio in human urine from nine different published sources. Number of controls varied from 12 to 100. (a) This demonstrates that the urinary excretion of lactulose increases with increasing osmolarity of the test solution. (b) This shows that the differential urinary excretion of lactulose/mannitol (intestinal permeability) is not significantly affected until test dose osmolarity reaches 1500 mosm/l, above which an increase in intestinal permeability is evident in normal subjects. Part (c) demonstrates the decline in mannitol absorption associated with increase in the amount of poorly absorbed solute in the test solution.

Oral test solution	Ukabam (195)	Murphy (140)	Andre (9)	Wyatt (205)	Elia (62)	Kapembwa(103)	V der Hulst (205)	Juby (101)	Blomquist (44)
Lactulose	10.0g	5.0g	5.0g	10.0g	10.0g	10.0g	10.0g	5.0g	10.0g
Mannitol	0.5g	5.0g	5.0g	5.0g	5.0g	5.0g	0.5g	2.0g	1.0g
Other solute	nil	nil	nil	glucose 22g	lactose 1.5g	nil	xylose 5.0g	glucose 22.3g	glycerol 2.0g
Reference in text	82	63	88	66	59	62	65	61	58

CONDITIONS ASSOCIATED WITH INCREASED INTESTINAL PERMEABILITY

Investigation of intestinal permeability can be used clinically for diagnostic screening and assessing response to therapy. Intestinal permeability has been found in a number of conditions, some of which are listed in Table 15.2. Research interest in the subject, however, has been largely concerned with the extent to which increased intestinal permeability might play a part in the aetiology of disease. Questions concerning the extent to which local and systemic associations represent the result as opposed to the cause of altered permeability present a familiar 'chicken and egg' problem.

The relevance of increased mucosal permeability assessed with probes such as lactulose, [51]CrEDTA and PEG to the uptake of macromolecules such as ovalbumin is controversial,[131] but some studies in man and experimental animals indicate that a correlation exists.[58,69,146,158] Speculation that a predisposition to the consequences of macromolecular entry may be justified under such circumstances, but the available evidence tends to be equivocal, especially with regard to induction of systemic effects.[199,200] As an example, it has recently been suggested that increased intestinal permeability following measles, mumps and rubella vaccination[198] might allow increased passage of exorphins, opiate-like substances, partially digested barley, rye, oats, casein, etc. that could give rise to behavioural abnormalities similar to those seen in patients with

Some conditions reported to be associated with increased intestinal permeability	
Non-steroidal anti-inflammatory drugs	Inflammatory bowel disease
Alcohol	Ankylosing spondylitis
Renal failure	Coeliac disease
Abdominal radiation	Intestinal ischaemia
Cytotoxic drug treatment	Hypogammaglobulinaemia
Abdominal surgery	HIV infection
Fasting	Endotoxinaemia
Total parenteral nutrition	Multiorgan failure
Food allergy	Diabetic diarrhoea
Multiple sclerosis	Scleroderma
Cystic fibrosis	Reactive arthritis
Recurrent abdominal pain of children	Intestinal infections/bacterial overgrowth
Neomycin	Whipple's disease
Acute and chronic liver disease	Sarcoidosis

Table 15.2 Some conditions reported to be associated with increased intestinal permeability.

schizophrenia.[59,204] A problem is that the increased intestinal permeability mentioned concerns water-soluble substances and may not therefore be relevant to the transfer of such constituents which, being in many cases lipid rather than water-soluble, would not be determined by the state of aqueous pathways across the intestinal and blood–brain barriers.

There would seem to be a much stronger case, however, for an aetiological relationship between increased intestinal permeability and local intestinal disease. Theories about the complex interrelationship between intestinal permeability and disease are best illustrated by references to some specific examples, for instance, whether or not increased intestinal permeability might play a pathogenic role in Crohn's disease.[32,84,85,173]

Inflammatory bowel disease

Most patients with small intestinal Crohn's disease and half of those with colonic involvement have increased intestinal permeability.[4,11,29,45,87,96,97,140,147,151,155,160,165,184,186,192,193,201] In magnitude this relates to the extent and activity of disease, and also to surgical intervention.

In patients with ulcerative colitis the uptake of [51]CrEDTA from the colon, estimated by measuring recovery in urine following a test enema, is reported to be markedly increased.[147,159] More recently, this finding has been supported by measuring recovery of [51]CrEDTA in urine for 24 h after ingestion, applying a lactulose correction to make allowance for small intestinal permeation[94] or by the localization technique described above.[188]

Permeability tests can be used to assess response to therapy in patients with Crohn's disease,[165,184] with a return of intestinal permeability to normal following elemental diet treatment predicting a remission in excess of 6 months, whereas persistence of hyperpermeability is associated with early relapse.[186] Wyatt et al.[205] also found that patients with Crohn's disease in whom intestinal permeability was normal did well, while the presence of increased intestinal permeability indicated that relapse was imminent. Although such observations might suggest that defective intestinal barrier function could play an important role in the relapse of inflammatory bowel disease,[25–28] increased

permeability could equally be regarded as providing a sensitive indication of the presence and progress of an established inflammatory lesion. However, indices of intestinal inflammation such as 4-day faecal [111]indium white cell excretion and tests of intestinal permeability do not have the same significance and provide different information in patients with Crohn's disease.[186]

Permeability in relatives of patients with Crohn's disease

Altered intestinal permeability has been reported by some authors in the relatives of patients with Crohn's disease and is quoted as evidence for the presence of subclinical disease, if not of a genetically determined factor of aetiological importance. However, the atypical behaviour of PEG 400[84] already discussed complicates the interpretation of early reports which relate to this probe of increased intestinal permeability in first degree relatives of patients with Crohn's disease.[139,164,185] However, intestinal permeability assessed by means of differential urinary excretion of sugar probes or [51]CrEDTA[5,185] has not been found to be significantly abnormal in the relatives of patients with Crohn's disease, although, as with most series of normal control subjects, occasional individuals may have a high reading.[5,86,104,185,206] Whether observations based upon the use of PEG merit the interest that they continue to receive is a matter of speculation. Perhaps the main importance of increased intestinal permeability in patients with inflammatory bowel disease is the possibility that it may be the central mechanism of clinical relapse.[26,28]

Neutrophil response and gut permeability

The severity of the neutrophil response in Crohn's disease, which is an order of magnitude greater than that seen in other conditions of enhanced intestinal permeability (such as acute bacterial enteritis, non-steroidal anti-inflammatory drug (NSAID) ingestion, etc.), could be because of an underlying immune derangement of the disease itself, representing evidence for an excessive response to some luminal factor. In this framework, relapse of Crohn's disease may not be due to an alteration in submucosal reactivity so much as to exposure to luminal factors, for instance normal intestinal flora, enhanced by a breach in the intestinal barrier. This notion is supported by the observation that intestinal permeability provides a much better prognostic index for relapse than faecal [111]indium leukocyte output[186,205] and that several recognized causes of relapse (infection, NSAID therapy, stress) are known to increase intestinal permeability or have the potential to do so.

In such a complex situation as Crohn's disease, unequivocal demonstration of an aetiological role for mucosal hyperpermeability (which must certainly be considered a result as well as a possible cause of the inflammatory lesion) is likely to be difficult unless it can be clearly shown that it precedes all other features of the pathological process. As with so many aspects of the study of intestinal permeability, ideas are plentiful but experimental support is scarce.

Coeliac disease

Untreated coeliac disease (or gluten-sensitive enteropathy) is associated with increased small intestinal permeability which improves and often returns to normal when response to a gluten-free diet has been satisfactory. Exposure to gluten fractions present in wheat and certain other cereals is an essential predisposing factor: presumably these produce the characteristic reaction after penetrating the intestinal mucosa of susceptible individuals. Although genetic predisposition is well recognized, with the condition having a familial incidence and being confined to certain ethnic groups, the presence of increased intestinal permeability has not hitherto been demonstrated or sought in relatives. In this condition, increased intestinal permeability is to be regarded as a consequence of the disease. However, the observation that symptomatic gluten-induced enteropathy frequently follows acute gastroenteritis and that toleration of dietary gluten is often prolonged provided the lesion is well healed, suggests the possibility that the state of mucosal permeability might also, by modifying penetration of the intestinal mucosa by gluten fractions, have a pathophysiological significance. The predisposition of the proximal jejunum to this enteropathy also suggests that mucosal uptake of gluten might be accentuated by exposure to dietary factors (hyperosmolar stress, etc.) which are capable of increasing permeability, and this is likely to be more intense in the upper small intestine.

Non-steroidal anti-inflammatory drug enteropathy

The effects of NSAIDs on intestinal permeability were first noticed when patients with rheumatoid arthritis were investigated to discover whether increased macromolecular permeation could be an aetiological factor.[24] Although increased permeability was demonstrated it turned out, somewhat ironically, to be iatrogenic! Following ingestion of NSAIDs there is a consistent increase in intestinal permeability occurring within 12 h. The increased permeability occurs in the immediate period after drug absorption because the enterocytes are then exposed to the highest concentration of the drug.[1–3,15,22,32,34–37,39,40,57,95,98] The effect of NSAIDs on the small intestine is often overlooked[24] because of the more acute and severe effect on the gastroduodenal mucosa. Perforation and bleeding from NSAID-associated ulcers contribute to the premature death of over 1000 people in the UK annually. Although the mechanism of initial damage is speculative and only adequately studied in experimental animals, a pathogenic framework for the damage is shown in Fig. 15.6 which recognizes 'topical' and 'systemic' phases of the damage.

Topical and systemic phases

The 'topical' phase refers predominantly to mucosal exposure directly after ingestion, which includes the question of re-exposure when NSAIDs (with the noticeable exception of aspirin and

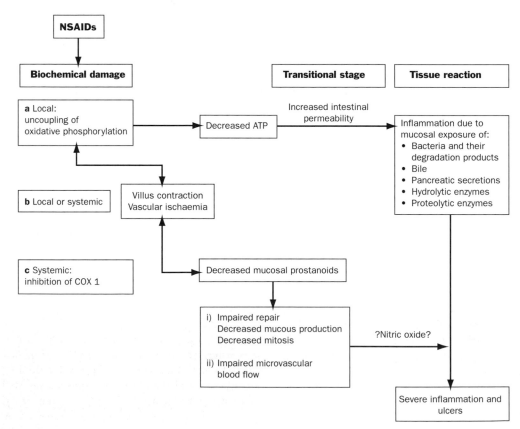

Fig. 15.6 Pathogenic framework for the development of NSAID-induced enteropathy. It is suggested that NSAIDs have a dual biochemical action, namely a non-prostaglandin-mediated 'topical' effect, which involves uncoupling of mitochondrial oxidative phosphorylation, and the better known effect of inhibiting cyclo-oxygenase 1 (COX 1). It is suggested that the mitochondrial effect leads to increased intestinal permeability and a low grade inflammatory reaction which is driven by the luminal aggressive factors gaining access to the mucosa (bacteria and their degradation product, etc.). A 'normal' response to such injury is an increase in mucosal prostaglandins which play a part in the healing of the damage, in part by increasing mucosal bloodflow and tissue oxygenation. However, the concomitant inhibition of COX 1 prevents this increase in prostaglandins. The consequence is, we suggest, that the low grade inflammation is converted to severe inflammation with ulcers. The precise role of villus-shortening and vascular ischaemia, both of which appear to be early pathogenic events in the enteropathy, requires further study. However, a distinct possibility is that this villus–vascular effect has its main effect on the microcirculation on the mesenteric side of the small bowel, where most of the ulcers are situated. This region of the bowel is supplied by a delicate system of end arteries.

nabumetone) are recycled in bile. The nature of the 'topical' damage may involve 'ionic trapping' by lipophobic conversion of NSAIDs within epithelial cells during drug absorption. This may allow sufficient drug concentrations to develop to uncouple mitochondrial oxidative phosphorylation (or inhibit the respiratory chain) which decreases cellular ATP levels. Resulting loss of control over the junctions between adjacent enterocytes is associated with increased intestinal permeability. Figure 15.7 shows a representative result of the effect of NSAIDs on intestinal permeability in normal human volunteers. Ingestion of indomethacin for 1 week increased intestinal permeability significantly while the non-acidic pro-NSAID, nabumetone, has no significant effect despite its metabolite, 6-methoxy-2-naphthylacetic acid, which is an effective inhibitor of cyclo-oxygenase. It is suggested that changes in permeability may lead to mild small intestinal inflammation. When reduced, mucosal prostaglandin levels are associated with the systemic phase of NSAID action; however, the inflammatory response is driven to an ulcerative process, presumably because of lack of vasodilatory prostaglandin action.

Small bowel inflammation

In patients taking NSAIDs small bowel inflammation can be demonstrated by means of the [111]indium-labelled leukocyte technique,[40,43,161,170] enteroscopy[138] or at post mortem.[6] Patients with untreated rheumatoid and osteoarthritis show no evidence of intestinal pathology but, depending on the method of detection used, 20–65% of those taking NSAIDs have small intestinal inflammation (NSAID enteropathy).[6,40,43,138] The clinical implications of NSAID enteropathy are clear. Patients bleed from the site of inflammation[24,41,81,183] and, although this is usually mild (2–10 ml/day), when combined with low iron absorption because of hypochlorhydria or inadequate diet, it may predispose to iron deficiency. Most patients with NSAID enteropathy also lose protein from the gut:[41] this is usually mild, but at times may lead to clinically significant hypoalbuminaemia.

Rheumatoid patients with the most severe NSAID enteropathy develop significant, but asymptomatic, malabsorption of [75]SeHCAT although absorption of vitamin B[12] remains normal.[43,176,177] Finally, development of septate strictures is a rare pathognomonic manifestation of NSAID pathology.[42,100,112,119,141,167,178,179] These thin (2–4 mm), concentric, septate projections are multiple, the number of small bowel strictures ranged from 3–70, and may narrow the diameter of the lumen to a few millimetres in most cases, sometimes causing complete obstruction. Representative pathology, termed 'diaphragm disease', is shown in Fig. 15.8. These strictures are, in most cases, localized to the mid or ileal region of the small bowel, but identical strictures have recently been described in the caecum and the ascending colon of patients receiving sustained release diclofenac sodium[68,77,88,137,172] (Voltarol Retard).

To summarize, NSAIDs have a specific biochemical action on enterocytes not evident in other tissues which are subject to lower drug exposure. Biochemically induced ultrastructural alterations lead to increased intestinal permeability and a low grade enteropathy, and the associated inhibition of prostaglandins may predispose to the development of ulcers. Although the above could be regarded as an example of intestinal pathology in which 'primary' disruption of the intestinal barrier leads to mucosal inflammation, it is not completely certain that the one is an aetiological consequence of the other, as both might represent independent consequences of the impact of NSAIDs on mucosal cell biochemistry.

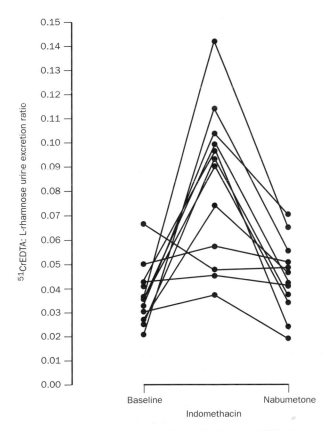

Fig. 15.7 Effect of NSAIDs on small intestinal permeability. Twelve volunteers underwent a [51]CrEDTA/L-rhamnose small intestinal permeability test as baseline, following ingestion of a conventional NSAID, indomethacin (150 mg/day) and a non-acidic NSAID, nabumetone (1.0 g/day) for 1 week. Intestinal permeability is significantly increased after indomethacin but there is no significant effect of nabumetone, presumably as it does not uncouple mitochondrial oxidative phosphorylation and thereby does not cause the 'topical' damage which is important for initiation of NSAID damage.

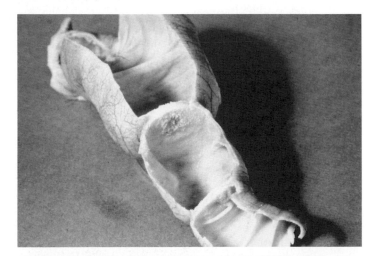

Fig. 15.8 'Diaphragm disease' of the small intestine caused by NSAIDs. This is a formalin-inflated small intestinal resection specimen from a patient with longstanding rheumatoid arthritis who had taken NSAIDs for 23 years. Symptoms included subacute intermittent small intestinal obstruction, but conventional investigation failed to provide a diagnosis. Four diaphragmatic strictures which progressively constrict the lumen are shown, but, in all, there were over 65 such lesions present in this patient.

Immunological incompetence

Patients with hypogammaglobulinaemia have been studied in some detail. Raised intestinal permeability is a constant feature and this is associated with a considerable increase in the faecal excretion of [111]indium leukocytes (mean (range) 6.9% (1.1–14.5%)).[189] In HIV infection, intestinal permeability remains normal, but increases with the onset of AIDS, regardless of subgrouping.[105,116] In AIDS, increased intestinal permeability is also associated with a low grade enteropathy, indicated by increased output of [111]indium leukocytes of similar severity to that found in NSAID enteropathy.[33]

Intestinal permeability in food intolerance and allergy

Studies reported of food allergy and intolerance suffer from a lack of agreed diagnostic criteria. Dermatological manifestations such as eczema are often considered in relation to food allergy because a genetically determined impairment of immunological responsiveness to dietary antigens may underlie both conditions.[14,115] This is in part supported by the prevalence of histological abnormalities in jejunal biopsies from eczematous and asthmatic children,[107] who either experience bronchospasm on challenge with specific foods or in whom properly performed exclusion diets may produce dramatic improvement of eczema.[13,73,82,102] The situation in adults appears to be different in that they do not respond to food exclusion. Such a distinction is not unique; for instance, children with Crohn's disease seem to respond to elemental diets better than adults, and this may be important when interpreting studies related to food allergy. Nevertheless, there are major discrepancies in findings which are difficult to resolve at this stage.

Atopic eczema

Adult patients with severe atopic eczema, of whom 50% had food intolerance, were demonstrated to have normal intestinal permeation of [51]CrEDTA using *in vivo* and *in vitro* techniques[17,23] and this was also the case in a further well defined group of patients with food intolerance without eczema.[168] Small, consistent increases in intestinal [51]CrEDTA permeation, however, followed challenge with the offending food.[168] Paganelli *et al.*, using β lactoglobulin as a probe,[149] also found that intestinal permeability was within the normal range in most food-intolerant subjects; nevertheless, treatment with hypoallergen diet or sodium chromoglycate was followed by a significant reduction. Hamilton *et al.* failed to find any consistent abnormalities in 62 adult patients with atopic eczema but did not comment on food sensitivity,[78] while Ukabam *et al.*[195] found an increase in lactulose, and Newton *et al.*[142] reported normal lactulose with reduced L-rhamnose permeation (and therefore a raised lactulose:L-rhamnose ratio) in adults with eczema.

At a busy gastroenterology outpatient clinic at King's College Hospital, where these tests are routinely available, a normal intestinal permeability test is thought to be characteristic of the 'irritable bowel syndrome' (Bjarnason *et al.*, unpublished observation) and usually contraindicates more invasive gastrointestinal investigation. In this context, food allergy and intolerance are infrequently diagnosed: this may, however, be misleading as there is at present no local specialist interest in this aspect. In France, experience of the situation reported by Andre *et al.* is different, food allergy being a prevalent condition associated with increased lactulose:mannitol permeation.[7–10,12] In the UK Dumont *et al.*[60] found that intestinal lactulose:L-rhamnose was normal in food-allergic eczematous children, although Barau *et al.*[16] and Dupont

et al.[61] demonstrated that food provocation increased intestinal permeability in paediatric irritable bowel syndrome and atopic dermatitis, respectively. Alternatively, Pike *et al.*[153] found lactulose:mannitol permeation to be significantly raised in 26 atopic children, many of whom were on a restricted diet as part of their treatment, but curiously they subsequently state that only four of 26 atopic children were found to have abnormal lactulose:L-rhamnose excretion ratios.[154]

The possibility that some food additives may increase intestinal permeability, however, deserves further consideration.[182]

Children with cow's milk intolerance have markedly increased permeation of [51]CrEDTA and raised lactulose:mannitol.[79,91,169] One study demonstrated a difference in intestinal permeability between breast fed infants and those receiving cow milk formulae, all of whom were symptomless and thriving.[202] It needs to be remembered, however, that some commercial milk preparations may contain lactulose.[18] Troncone *et al.*[191] showed that nine of ten children (median age 13 months) who developed symptoms after milk challenge had a coincident rise in cellobiose:mannitol permeation, whereas this occurred in only one of 22 without symptoms. Dupont *et al.*[61] found normal intestinal permeability in children being treated for milk sensitivity, but demonstrated that this increased following a challenge with cow's milk.

Food allergy

Changes of intestinal PEG permeation recorded in food allergy have, despite anticipated differences in behaviour compared with oligosaccharide and [51]CrEDTA, been more consistent, possibly because most studies with this probe have been undertaken by the same group of workers. Jackson *et al.*[90] found that patients with eczema had increased permeation of PEG 4000 regardless of concomitant food allergy, but permeation of simultaneously administered PEG 600 was normal. Falth-Magnusson *et al.*[65] record the permeation of PEG 400 and 1000 to be normal in children with a diagnosis of food allergy and in a large number of women with atopic eczema.[67] Furthermore, children with cow's milk allergy, even with a challenge, were also normal.[66] As an explanation for these apparently conflicting findings, it is possible that the uptake of ethylene glycol polymers which, at a corresponding molecular dimension (PEG 400) is vastly greater than that of oligosaccharide and [51]CrEDTA, may diminish in the higher range (PEG 4000) to correspond more closely with that of other macromolecular probes.

Miscellaneous

Intestinal permeability has been demonstrated in a number of diverse conditions, including alcohol misuse,[38,132,175] antineoplastic agents,[150,152,156,171] in diabetes mellitus,[51] patients undergoing major surgery or experiencing intestinal ischaemia,[144,148,162] after major burns and abdominal radiation,[49,157,163,207] in small bowel bacterial overgrowth or infections,[70,180] in cystic fibrosis,[56,63,113,114] asthma[19], birch allergy[106] 'stress'[54,118] which may relate to cholinergic stimulation,[20] etc. However, to a large extent it remains to be determined whether increased intestinal permeability in these situations leads to an inflammatory response within the intestine.

PATHOGENIC IMPORTANCE OF INCREASED INTESTINAL PERMEABILITY

Intestinal barrier function, along with immunological mechanisms, has been taken to be of central importance to the protection of the intestinal mucosa from 'luminal aggressive factors'. It has been suggested that when disruption of this barrier of sufficient severity and duration disturbs the balance between factors of mucosal protection and aggression, a non-specific mucosal reaction (intestinal inflammation – enteropathy) may be induced by increased access of neutrophil chemoattractants from the intestinal lumen.[24,28] Furthermore, increased permeation from the lumen of macromolecular constituents with allergenic or other tissue-damaging potential might also predispose to systemic pathology.

In the majority of instances described, increased intestinal permeability accompanies the development of inflammation and other features of intestinal mucosal disease, and is therefore likely to be a secondary phenomenon. However, for intestinal permeability to be regarded as a significant primary factor requires, at the least, demonstration that its appearance pre-dates all other features of pathology. Of the conditions discussed this requirement seems most likely to apply to NSAID enteropathy; even so, it is difficult to decide to what extent other features of the enteropathy (inflammation, etc.) could truly be a consequence of increased mucosal permeability rather than a further manifestation of NSAID exposure. Although allocation of systemic consequences remote from the intestine should not present such a difficult problem, demonstration of increased permeability in the absence of intestinal pathology does not yet appear to have been confirmed in any systemic disease.

CONCLUSIONS

Tests of intestinal permeability have come a long way in the 27 years since they were introduced. They are simple to use, accurate and sensitive, and provide information which cannot be obtained by other non-invasive methods. The test procedures exploiting the principle of 'differential' oral absorption described, in which renal excretion of several test markers is measured after oral administration, allow specific assessment of regional changes in permeability and absorption. Nevertheless, there are many practical aspects of their use which require special attention. These have, in part, been outlined, but it seems likely that a wider range of applications has yet to emerge. A recent advance which involves an integrated approach to the study of intestinal permeability and inflammation in various diseases, especially in classic inflammatory bowel disease, is providing insight into the existence of a common final pathway for an intestinal inflammatory response. The idea that increased intestinal permeability could predispose to, or modify the course of, intestinal or systemic pathology is very attractive, but this difficult question remains to be resolved. Nevertheless, provided that the techniques are adequately controlled, measurements of intestinal permeability make a valuable contribution to the detection and monitoring of intestinal abnormality in clinical medicine and research.

REFERENCES

1 Aabakken L, Larsen S, Osnes K. Sucralfate for prevention of naproxen-induced mucosal lesions. *Scand J Rheumatol* 1989; 18: 361–8.

2 Aabakken L, Larsen S, Osnes M. Cimetidine tablets or suspension in the prevention of gastrointestinal mucosal lesions caused by non-steroidal anti-inflammatory drugs. *Scand J Rheumatol* 1989; 18: 647–55.

3 Aabakken L, Osnes M. ^{51}Cr-ethylenediaminetetraacetic acid absorption test. Effects of naproxen, a non-steroidal, antiinflammatory drug. *Scand J Gastroenterol* 1990; 25: 917–24.

4 Adenis A, Colombel JF, Lecouffe P, Wallaert BBH, Marchandise X, Cortot A. Increased pulmonary and intestinal permeability in Crohn's disease. *Gut* 1992; 33: 678–82.

5 Ainsworth M, Eriksen J, Rasmussen JW, Schaffalitzkydemuckadel OB. Intestinal permeability of ^{51}Cr-labelled ethylenediaminetetraacetic acid in patients with Crohn's disease and their first degree relatives. *Scand J Gastroenterol* 1989; 24: 993–8.

6 Allison MC, Howatson AG, Torrance CJ, Lee FD, Russell RI. Gastrointestinal damage associated with the use of nonsteroidal anti-inflammatory drugs. *N Engl J Med* 1992; 327: 749–54.

7 Andre C, Andre F, Colin LSC. Measurement of intestinal permeability to mannitol and lactulose as a means of diagnosing food allergy and evaluating therapeutic effectiveness of disodium chromoglycate. *Ann Allergy* 1987; 59: 127–30.

8 Andre C, Andre F, Colin L. Effect of allergen ingestion challenge with and without cromoglycate cover on intestinal permeability in atopic dermatitis, urticaria and other symptoms of food allergy. *Allergy* 1989; 9: 47–51.

9 Andre C, Collin L, Descos L, Daniere S. Non-invasive evaluation of intestinal permeability in food allergy, coeliac disease and inflammatory bowel disease. *Gut* 1984; 25:A1189–90.

10 Andre C. Diagnostic objectif et test l'efficacite therapeutique par measure de la permeabilite intestine. *Presse Med* 1986; 15: 105–8.

11 Andre F, Andre C, Emery Y. Assessment of the lactulose-mannitol test in Crohn's disease. *Gut* 1988; 29: 511–15.

12 Andre F, Andre C, Feknous M, Colin L, Cavagna S. Digestive permeability to different-sized molecules and to sodium cromoglycate in food allergy. *Allergy Proc* 1991; 12: 293–8.

13 Atherton DJ, Sewell M, Soothill JF, Wells RS, Chivers CD. A double blind, controlled, crossover trial of antigen avoidance diet in atopic eczema. *Lancet* 1978; i: 401–3.

14 Atherton DJ. Allergy and atopic eczema II. *Clin Exp Dermatol* 1981; 6: 317–25.

15 Auer IO, Habscheid W, Hiller S, Gerhards W, Eilles C. Nicht-steroidale antiphlogistika erhohen die darmpermeabilitat. *Deut Med Wochensch* 1987; 112: 1032–7.

16 Barau E, Dupont C. Modifications of intestinal permeability during food provocation procedures in pediatric irritable bowel syndrome. *J Pediatr Gastroenterol Nutr* 1990; 11: 72–7.

17 Barba A, Schena D, Andreaus MC *et al*. Intestinal permeability in patients with atopic eczema. *Br J Dermatol* 1989; 120: 71–5.

18 Beach R, Menzies IS. Lactulose and other non-absorbable sugars in infant milk. *Lancet* 1983; i: 425–6.

19 Benard A, Desreumeaux P, Huglo D, Hoorelbeke A, Tonnel AB, Wallaert B. Increased intestinal permeability in bronchial asthma. *J Allergy Clin Immunol* 1996; 97: 1173–8.

20 Bijlsma PB, Kiliaan AJ, Scholten G, Heyman M, Groot JA, Taminiau JAJM. Carbacol, but not forskolin, increases mucosal-to-serosal transport of intact protein in rat ileum in vitro. *Am J Physiol* 1996; 271:G147–55.

21 Bjarnason I, Batt R, Catt S, Macpherson A, Maxton D, Menzies IS. Evaluation of differential disaccharide excretion in urine for non-invasive assessment of intestinal disaccharidase activity caused by α-glucosidase inhibition, primary hypolactasia and coeliac disease. *Gut* 1996; 39: 374–81.

22 Bjarnason I, Fehilly B, Smethurst P, Menzies IS, Levi AJ. The importance of local versus systemic effects of non-steroidal anti-inflammatory drugs to increase intestinal permeability in man. *Gut* 1991; 32: 275–7.

23 Bjarnason I, Goolamali SK, Levi AJ, Peters TJ. Intestinal permeability in patients with atopic eczema. *Br J Dermatol* 1985; 112: 291–7.

24 Bjarnason I, Hayllar J, Macpherson AJ, Russell AS. Side effects of non-steroidal anti-inflammatory drugs on the small and large intestine. *Gastroenterology* 1993; 104: 1832–47.

25 Bjarnason I, Macpherson A, Menzies IS. Intestinal permeability: the basics. In: *Inflammatory Bowel Disease. Basic research, clinical*

implications and trends in therapy (Sutherland LR, Collins SM, Martin F, McLeod RS, Targan SR, Wallace JL, Williams CN, eds), Kluwer Academic Press, Dordrecht, 1994; 53–70.

26 Bjarnason I, Macpherson AJ, Somasundaram S, Teahon K. Nonsteroidal anti-inflammatory drugs and inflammatory bowel disease. *Can J Gastroenterol* 1993; 7: 160–9.

27 Bjarnason I, Macpherson AJM, Hollander D. Intestinal permeability: an overview. *Gastroenterology* 1995; 108: 1566–81.

28 Bjarnason I, Macpherson AJS, Somasundaram S, Teahon K. Non-steroidal anti-inflammatory drugs and Crohn's disease. In: *Inflammatory Bowel Diseases: Pathophysiology as basis of treatment* (Scholmeric J, Kruis W, Goebbell H, Hohenberger W, Gross V, eds) Falk Symposium No 67. Kluwer Academic Publishers, Lancaster, 1993: 8208–22.

29 Bjarnason I, O'Morain C, Levi AJ, Peters TJ. The absorption of ^{51}Cr EDTA in inflammatory bowel disease. *Gastroenterology* 1983; 85: 318–22.

30 Bjarnason I, Peters TJ, Levi AJ. Intestinal permeability: clinical correlates. *Dig Dis* 1986; 4: 83–92.

31 Bjarnason I, Peters TJ, Veall N. A persistent defect of intestinal permeability in coeliac disease as demonstrated by a ^{51}Cr-labelled EDTA absorption test. *Lancet* 1983; i: 323–5.

32 Bjarnason I, Peters TJ. Helping the mucosa make sense of macromolecules. *Gut* 1987; 28: 1057–61.

33 Bjarnason I, Sharpstone D, Francis N *et al*. Intestinal inflammation, ileal structure and function in HIV. *AIDS* 1996; 10: 1385–91.

34 Bjarnason I, Smethurst P, Clarke P, Menzies IS, Levi AJ, Peters TJ. Effect of prostaglandins on indomethacin induced increased intestinal permeability in man. *Scand J Gastroenterol* 1989; 29(Suppl 164): 97–103.

35 Bjarnason I, Smethurst P, Fenn GC, Lee CF, Menzies IS, Levi AJ. Misoprostol reduces indomethacin induced changes in human small intestinal permeability. *Dig Dis Sci* 1989; 34: 407–11.

36 Bjarnason I, Smethurst P, Macpherson A *et al*. Glucose and citrate reduce the permeability changes caused by indomethacin in humans. *Gastroenterology* 1992; 102: 1546–50.

37 Bjarnason I, Smethurst P, Menzies IS, Peters TJ. The effect of polyacrylic acid polymers (carbopol) on small intestinal function and permeability changes caused by indomethacin. *Scand J Gastroenterol* 1991; 26: 685–8.

38 Bjarnason I, Ward K, Peters TJ. The leaky gut of alcoholism: possible route of entry for toxic compounds. *Lancet* 1984; i: 179–82.

39 Bjarnason I, Williams P, Smethurst P, Peters TJ, Levi AJ. The effect of NSAIDs and prostaglandins on the permeability of the human small intestine. *Gut* 1986; 27: 1292–7.

40 Bjarnason I, Williams P, So A *et al*. Intestinal permeability and inflammation in rheumatoid arthritis; effects of non-steroidal anti-inflammatory drugs. *Lancet* 1984; ii: 1171–4.

41 Bjarnason I, Zanelli G, Prouse P *et al*. Blood and protein loss via small intestinal inflammation induced by nonsteroidal anti-inflammatory drugs. *Lancet* 1987; ii: 711–4.

42 Bjarnason I, Zanelli G, Smethurst P *et al*. Clinico-pathological features of nonsteroidal antiinflammatory drug induced small intestinal strictures. *Gastroenterology* 1988; 94: 1070–4.

43 Bjarnason I, Zanelli G, Smith T *et al*. Nonsteroidal antiinflammatory drug induced intestinal inflammation in humans. *Gastroenterology* 1987; 93: 480–9.

44 Blomquist L, Bark T, Hedenborg G, Svenberg T, Norman A. A comparison between the lactulose/mannitol and ^{51}CeEDTA/^{14}C-mannitol methods for intestinal permeability. *Scand J Gastroenterol* 1993; 28: 274–80.

45 Casellas F, Aguade S, Soriano B, Accarino A, Molero J, Guarner L. Intestinal permeability to ^{99m}Tc diethylene-tetraaminopentaacetic acid in inflammatory bowel disease. *Am J Gastroenterol* 1986; 81: 767–70.

46 Chadwick VS, Phillips SF, Hofman AF. Measurements of intestinal permeability using low molecular weight polyethylene glycols (PEG 400). I. Chemical analysis and biological properties of PEG 400. *Gastroenterology* 1977; 73: 241–6.

47 Chadwick VS, Phillips SF, Hofman AF. Measurements of intestinal permeability using low molecular weight polyethylene glycols (PEG

400). II. Application to study of normal and abnormal permeability states in man and animals. *Gastroenterology* 1977; 73: 247–51.

48 Cobden I, Dickinson RJ, Rothwell J, Axon ATR. Intestinal permeability assessed by excretion ratios of two molecules: results in coeliac disease. *BMJ* 1978; ii: 1060.

49 Coltart RS, Howard GC, Wraight EP, Bleehen NM. The effect of hyperthermia and radiation on small bowel permeability using ^{51}Cr EDTA and ^{14}C mannitol in man. *Int J Hyperthermia* 1988; 4: 467–77.

50 Cook CG, Menzies IS. Intestinal absorption and unmediated permeation of sugars in post-infective tropical malabsorption (tropical sprue). *Digestion* 1986; 33: 109–16.

51 Cooper BT, Ukabam SO, O'Brien IAD, Hara JPO, Corrall RJM. Intestinal permeability in diabetic diarrhoea. *Diabetic Medicine* 1987; 4: 49–52.

52 Cooper BT. The small intestinal permeability barrier. In: *Gut Defences in Clinical Practice* (Losowski MH, Heatley RV, eds) Churchill Livingstone, Edinburgh, 1986: 117–32.

53 Cox MA, Iqbal TH, Lewis KO, Cooper BT. Viewpoints in intestinal permeability. *Gastroenterology* 1997; 112: 669–70.

54 Crowe SE, Sestini P, Perdue MH. Allergenic reactions of rat jejunal mucosa. *Int Arch Allergy Appl Immunol* 1990; 91: 270–7.

55 Dahlqvist A. Specificity of human intestinal disaccharidases and implications for hereditary disaccharide intolerance. *J Clin Invest* 1962; 41: 463–70.

56 Dalzell AM, Freestone NS, Billington D, Heaf DP. Small intestinal permeability and orocaecal transit time in cystic fibrosis. *Arch Dis Child* 1990; 65: 585–8.

57 Davies GR, Rampton DS. The pro-drug sulindac may reduce the risk of intestinal damage associated with the use of conventional non-steroidal anti-inflammatory drugs. *Aliment Pharmacol Ther* 1991; 5: 593–8.

58 Davin JC, Forget P, Mahieu PR. Increased intestinal permeability to (^{51}Cr)EDTA is correlated with IgA immune complex-plasma levels in children with IgA-associated nephropathies. *Acta Pediatr Scand* 1988; 77: 118–24.

59 Dohan FC. Coeliac disease and schizophrenia. *Lancet* 1970; i: 897–8.

60 Dumont GCL, Beach RC, Menzies IS. Gastrointestinal permeability in food-allergic eczematous children. *Clin Allergy* 1984; 14: 55–9.

61 Dupont C, Barau E, Molkhou P, Raynaud F, Barbet JP, Dehennin L. Food-induced alteration in intestinal permeability in children with cow's milk-sensitive enteropathy and atopic dermatitis. *J Pediatr Gastroenterol Nutr* 1989; 8: 459–65.

62 Elia M, Beherens R, Northrop C, Wraight P, Neale G. Evaluation of mannitol, lactulose and ^{51}Cr labelled ethylenediaminetetraacetate as markers of intestinal permeability in man. *Clin Sci* 1987; 73: 197–204.

63 Escobar H, Perdomo M, Vasconez F, Camarero C, del Olmo MT, Suarez L. Intestinal permeability to 51Cr-EDTA and orocecal transit time in cystic fibrosis. *J Pediatr Gastroenterol Nutr* 1992; 14: 204–7.

64 Falth-Magnusson K, Jansson G, Stenhammar L, Sundquist T, Magnusson KE. Intestinal permeability assessed with different-sized polyethylene glycols in children undergoing small-intestinal biopsy for suspected coeliac disease. *Scand J Gastroenterol* 1989; 24: 40–6.

65 Falth-Magnusson K, Kjellman NIM, Magnusson KE, Sundquist T. Intestinal permeability in healthy and allergic children before and after sodium-chromoglycate treatment assessed with different sized polyethylene glycols (PEG 400 and 1000). *Clin Allergy* 1984; 14: 277–86.

66 Falth-Magnusson K, Kjellman NIM, Odelram H, Sundquist T, Magnusson KE. Gastrointestinal permeability in children with cow's milk allergy: effect of milk challenge and sodium chromoglycate as assessed with polyethylene glycols (PEG 400 and PEG 1000). *Clin Allergy* 1986; 16: 543–51.

67 Falth-Magnusson K, Kjellman NIM, Sundquist T, Magnusson KE. Gastrointestinal permeability in atopic and non-atopic mothers, assessed with different sized polyethylene glycols (PEG 400 and PEG 1000). *Clin Allergy* 1985; 15: 565–70.

68 Fellows IW, Clarke JM, Roberts PF. Non-steroidal anti-inflammatory drug-induced jejunal and colonic diaphragm disease: a report of two cases. *Gut* 1992; 33: 1424–26.

69 Ferry DM, Butt TJ, Broom MF, Hunter J, Chadwick VS. Bacterial chemotactic oligopeptides and the intestinal mucosal barrier. *Gastroenterology* 1989; 97: 61–7.

70 Ford RPK, Menzies IS, Phillips AD, Walker-Smith JA, Turner MW. Intestinal sugar permeability: relationship to diarrhoeal disease and small bowel morphology. *J Pediatr Gastroenterol Nutr* 1985; 4: 568–74.

71 Fordtran JS, Clodi PH, Soergel KH, Ingelfinger FJ. Sugar absorption tests, with special reference to 3-O-methyl-D-glucose and D-xylose. *Ann Int Med* 1962; 57: 883–91.

72 Fourman LPR. The absorption of xylose in steatorrhoea. *Clin Sci* 1948; 6: 289–94.

73 Goldsborough J, Francis DEM. Dietary management: In: *Proceedings of the Second Fission's Food Allergy Workshop* (Coombes RAA, ed.) The Medicine Publishing Foundation, Oxford 1983: 89–95.

74 Griffiths CEM, Menzies IS, Barrison IG, Leonard JN, Fry L. Intestinal permeability in dermatitis herpetiformis. *J Invest Dermatol* 1988; 91: 147–9.

75 Gryboski JD, Thayer WR, Gabrielson IW, Spiro HM. Disacchariduria in gastrointestinal disease. *Gastroenterology* 1963; 45: 633–7.

76 Haeney MR, Culank LS, Montgomery RD, Sammonds HG. Evaluation of xylose absorption as measured in blood and urine: a one hour blood xylose screening test in malabsorption. *Gastroenterology* 1978; 75: 393–400.

77 Halter F, Weber B, Huber T, Eigenmann F, Frey M, Rutchi C. Diaphragm disease of the ascending colon associated with sustained release diclofenac. *J Clin Gastroenterol* 1993; 16: 74–80.

78 Hamilton I, Fairris GM, Rothwell J, Cunliffe WJ, Dixon MF, Axon ATR. Small intestinal permeability in dermatological disease. *Q J Med* 1985; 56: 559–67.

79 Hamilton I, Hill A, Rose B, Boucher IAD, Forsyth JS. Small intestinal permeability in pediatric clinical practice. *J Pediatr Gastroenterol Nutr* 1987; 6: 697–701.

80 Hamilton I. Small intestinal permeability. In: *Recent Advances in Gastroenterology 6* (Pounder RE, ed.) Churchill Livingstone, Edinburgh, 1986: 73–91.

81 Hayllar J, Price AB, Smith T, Macpherson A, Gumpel MJ, Bjarnason I. Nonsteroidal antiinflammatory drug-induced small intestinal inflammation and blood loss: effect of sulphasalazine and other disease modifying drugs. *Arthr Rheum* 1994; 37: 1146–50.

82 Hill DJ, Lynch BC. Elemental diet in the management of severe eczema in childhood. *Clin Allergy* 1982; 12: 313–5.

83 Hollander D, Rickets D, Boyd CAR. Importance of 'probe' molecular geometry in determining intestinal permeability. *Can J Gastroenterol* 1988; 2(Suppl. A): 35A–38A.

84 Hollander D, Vadheim C, Brettholz E, Pattersen GM, Delahunty T, Rotter JI. Increased intestinal permeability in patients with Crohn's disease and their relatives. *Ann Int Med* 1986; 105: 883–5.

85 Hollander D. Crohn's disease – A permeability disorder of the tight junctions? *Gut* 1988; 26: 1621–4.

86 Hollander D. Permeability in Crohn's disease – altered barrier function in healthy relatives? *Gastroenterology* 1993; 104: 1848.

87 Howden CW, Robertson C, Duncan A, Morris AJ, Russell RI. Comparison of different measurements of intestinal permeability in inflammatory bowel disease. *Am J Gastroenterol* 1991; 86: 1445–9.

88 Huber T, Ruchti C, Halter F. Nonsteroidal antiinflammatory drug-induced colonic strictures: a case report. *Gastroenterology* 1992; 100: 1119–22.

89 Iqbal TH, Lewis KO, Cooper BT. Diffusion of polyethylene glycol-400 across lipid barriers in vitro. *Clin Sci* 1993; 85: 111–5.

90 Jackson PG, Baker RWR, Lessof HM, Ferrett J, MacDonald DM. Intestinal permeability in patients with eczema and food allergy. *Lancet* 1981; i: 1285–6.

91 Jalonen T. Identical intestinal permeability changes in children with different clinical manifestations of cow's milk allergy. *J Allergy Clin Immunol* 1991; 88: 737–42.

92 Jenkins AP, Bjarnason I, Nukajam WS, Menzies IS, Creamer B. Effect of colitis on intestinal permeation of ^{51}CrEDTA and lactulose. *Gut* 1990; 31:A36.

93 Jenkins AP, Menzies IS, Nukajam WS, Creamer B. The effect of ingested lactulose on absorption of L-rhamnose, D-xylose and 3-O-methyl-D-glucose in subjects with ileostomies. *Scand J Gastroenterol* 1994; 29: 820–5.

94 Jenkins AP, Nukajam WS, Menzies IS, Creamer B. Simultaneous administration of lactulose and ^{51}Cr-ethylenediaminetetraacetic acid. A test to distinguish colonic from small-intestinal permeability change. *Scand J Gastroenterol* 1992; 27: 769–73.

95 Jenkins AP, Trew DR, Nukajam WS, Crump BJ, Menzies IS, Creamer B. Do nonsteroidal anti-inflammatory drugs increase colonic permeability? *Gut* 1991; 32: 66–9.

96 Jenkins RT, Jones DB, Goodacre RL *et al*. Reversibility of increased intestinal permeability to ^{51}CrEDTA in patients with gastrointestinal inflammatory bowel disease. *J Rheumatol* 1987; 82: 1159–64.

97 Jenkins RT, Ramage JK, Jones DB, Collins SM, Goodacre RL, Hunt RH. Small bowel and colonic permeability to ^{51}CrEDTA in patients with active inflammatory bowel disease. *Clin Invest Med* 1988; 11: 151–5.

98 Jenkins RT, Rooney PJ, Jones DB, Bienenstock J, Goodacre RL. Increased intestinal permeability in patients with rheumatoid arthritis. A side effect of nonsteroidal antiinflammatory drug therapy. *Br J Rheumatol* 1987; 26: 103–7.

99 Johansen K, Stintzing G, Magnusson KE *et al*. Intestinal permeability assessed with polyethylene glycols in children with diarrhoea due to rotavirus and common bacterial pathogens in a developing country. *J Pediatr Gastroenterol Nutr* 1989; 9: 307–13.

100 Johnson F. Recurrent small bowel obstruction with piroxicam. *Br J Surg* 1987; 74: 654.

101 Juby LD, Rothwell J, Axon ATR. Lactulose/mannitol test. An ideal screening test for coeliac disease. *Gastroenterology* 1989; 96: 79–85.

102 Juto P, Engberg S, Winberg J. Treatment of infantile atopic dermatitis with a strict elimination diet. *Clin Allergy* 1978; 8: 493–500.

103 Kapembwa MS, Fleming SC, Sewankambo N *et al*. Altered small-intestinal permeability associated with diarrhoea in human-immuno-deficiency-virus-infected Caucasian and African subjects. *Clin Sci* 1991; 81: 327–34.

104 Katz KD, Hollander D, Vadheim CM *et al*. Intestinal permeability in patients with Crohn's disease and their healthy relatives. *Gastroenterology* 1989; 97: 927–31.

105 Keating J, Bjarnason I, Somasundaram S *et al*. Intestinal absorptive capacity, intestinal permeability and jejunal histology in HIV infected patients and their relation to diarrhoea. *Gut* 1995; 37: 623–9.

106 Knutson TW, Bengtson U, Ahlstedt S, Knutson L. Effects of luminal antigen on intestinal albumin and hyaluronan permeability and ion transport in atopic patients. *J Allergy Clin Immunol* 1996; 97: 1225–32.

107 Kokkonen J, Simila S, Herva R. Gastrointestinal findings in atopic children. *Eur J Pediatr* 1980; 134: 249–52.

108 Krugilak P, Hollander D, Ma TY *et al*. Mechanism of polyethylene glycol 400 permeability of perfused rat intestine. *Gastroenterology* 1989; 97: 1164–70.

109 Krugliak P, Hollander D, Le K, Ma T, Dadufalza VD, Katz KD. Regulation of polyethylene glycol 400 intestinal permeability by endogenous and exogenous prostanoids. Influence of non-steroidal anti-inflammatory drugs. *Gut* 1990; 31: 417–21.

110 Laker MF, Bull HJ, Menzies IS. Evaluation of mannitol for use as a probe marker of gastrointestinal permeability in man. *Eur J Clin Invest* 1982; 12: 485–91.

111 Laker MF, Menzies IS. Increase in human intestinal permeability following ingestion of hypertonic solutions. *J Physiol (London)* 1977; 265: 881–94.

112 Lang J, Price AB, Levi AJ, Burk M, Gumpel JM, Bjarnason I. Diaphragm disease: the pathology of non-steroidal anti-inflammatory drug induced small intestinal strictures. *J Clin Path* 1988; 41: 516–26.

113 Leclercq-Foucart J, Forget P, Sodoyez-Gouffaux F, Zappitelli A. Intestinal permeability to ^{51}CrEDTA in children with cystic fibrosis. *J Pediatr Gastroenterol Nutr* 1986; 5: 384–87.

114 Leclercq-Foucart J, Forget P, Van Cutsem JL. Lactulose-rhamnose intestinal permeability in children with cystic fibrosis. *J Pediatr Gastroenterol Nutr* 1987; 6: 66–70.

115 Lessof MH, Wraith DG, Merrett J, Buisseret PD. Food allergy and intolerance in 100 patients – local and systemic effects. *Q J Med* 1980; 195: 259–71.

116 Lim SG, Menzies IS, Lee CA, Johnson MA, Pounder RE. Intestinal permeability and function in patients infected with human immunodeficiency virus. *Scand J Gastroenterol* 1993; 28: 573–80.

117 Ma TY, Hollander D, Krugliak P, Katz K. PEG 400, a hydrophyllic molecular probe for measuring intestinal permeability. *Gastroenterology* 1990; 98: 39–46.

118 MacQueen G, Marshall J, Perdue M, Siegel S, Bienenstock J. Pavlovian conditioning of rat mucosal mast cells to protease II. *Science* 1989; 243: 83–5.

119 Madhok R, Mackenzie JA, Lee FD, Bruckner FE, Terry TR, Sturrock RD. Small bowel ulceration in patients receiving NSAIDs for rheumatoid arthritis. *Q J Med* 1986; 58: 53–8.

120 Magnusson KE, Sundquist T, Sjodahl R, Tageson C. Altered intestinal permeability to low-molecular-weight polyethylene glycols (PEG 400) in patients with Crohn's disease. *Acta Chir Scand* 1983; 149: 323–27.

121 Magnusson M, Magnusson KE, Sundqvist T, Denneberg T. Reduced intestinal permeability measured by differently sized polyethylene glycols in acute uremic rats. *Nephron* 1992; 60: 193–98.

122 Magnusson M, Magnusson KE, Sundqvist T, Denneberg T. Urinary excretion of differently sized polyethylene glycols after intravenous administration in uremic and control rats: effects of low- and high-protein diets. *Nephron* 1990; 56: 312–16.

123 Maxton DG, Bjarnason I, Reynolds AP, Catt SD, Peters TJ, Menzies IS. Lactulose, ^{51}CrEDTA, L-rhamnose and polyethylene glycol 400 as probe markers for 'in vivo' assessment of human intestinal permeability. *Clin Sci* 1986; 71: 71–80.

124 Maxton DG, Catt SD, Menzies IS. Combined assessment of intestinal disaccharidases in congenital asucrasia by differential urinary disaccharide excretion. *J Clin Pathol* 1990; 43: 406–9.

125 May GR, Sutherland LR, Meddings JB. Is small intestinal permeability really increased in relatives of patients with Crohn's disease? *Gastroenterology* 1993; 104: 1627–32.

126 McCance RA, Madders K. The comparative rates of absorption of sugars from human intestine. *Biochem J* 1930; 24: 795–804.

127 Meddings JB, Sutherland LR, Byles NI, Wallace JL. Sucrose: a novel permeability marker for gastroduodenal disease. *Gastroenterology* 1993; 104: 1619–26.

128 Menzies IS, Jenkins AP, Heduan E, Catt SD, Segal MB, Creamer B. The effect of poorly absorbed solute on intestinal absorption. *Scand J Gastroenterol* 1990; 25: 1257–64.

129 Menzies IS, Mount JN, Wheeler MJ. Quantitative estimation of clinically important monosaccharides in plasma by rapid thin layer chromatography. *Ann Clin Biochem* 1978; 15: 65–76.

130 Menzies IS, Pounder R, Heyer S *et al.* Abnormal intestinal permeability to sugars in villus atrophy. *Lancet* 1979; ii: 1107–9.

131 Menzies IS, Turner MW. Intestinal permeation of molecules in health and disease. In: *Immunology of Gastrointestinal Disease* (MacDonald TT, ed.), Kluwer Academic Publishers, Dordrecht, 1992: 173–91.

132 Menzies IS. Absorption of intact oligosaccharide in health and disease. *Biochem Soc Transact* 1974; 2: 1042–47.

133 Menzies IS. Quantitative estimation of sugars in blood and urine by paper chromatography using direct densitometry. *J Chromatogr* 1973; 81: 109–27.

134 Menzies IS. Transmucosal passage of inert molecules in health and disease. In: *Intestinal Absorption and Secretion* (Skadhauge E, Heintze K, eds) MTP Press, Lancaster: Falk Symposium 36, 1984: 527–43.

135 Menzies IS, Zuckerman MJ, Nukajam WS *et al.* Geography of intestinal permeability and absorption. *Gut* 1999; 44: 483–9.

136 Menzies IS, Crane R. Assessing intestinal absorptive capacity and permeability *in vivo.* In: *Methods in Disease: Investigating the Gastrointestinal Tract* (Preedy VR, Watson RR, eds), Greenwich Medical Media, London, 1998: 41–64.

137 Monahan W, Starnes EC, Parker AL. Colonic strictures in a patient on long-term non-steroidal anti-inflammatory drugs. *Gastroint Endosc* 1992; 38: 385–6.

138 Morris AJ, Wasson LA, Mackenzie JF. Small bowel enteroscopy in undiagnosed gastrointestinal blood loss. *Gut* 1992; 33: 887–9.

139 Munkholm P, Langholz E, Hollander D *et al.* Intestinal permeability in patients with Crohn's disease and ulcerative colitis and their first degree relatives. *Gut* 1994; 35: 68–72.

140 Murphy MS, Eastham EJ, Nelson R, Pearson ADJ, Laker MF. Intestinal permeability in Crohn's disease. *Arch Dis Child* 1989; 64: 321–5.

141 Neoptolemos JP, Locke TJ. Recurrent small bowel obstruction associated with phenylbutazone. *Br J Surg* 1983; 70: 244–5.

142 Newton JA, Maxton DG, Bjarnason I, Reynolds AP, Menzies IS. Intestinal permeability in atopic eczema. *Clin Sci* 1984; 67: 64P.

143 Noone C, Menzies IS, Banatvala JE, Scopes JW. Intestinal permeability and lactulose hydrolysis in human rotaviral gastroenteritis assessed simultaneously by non-invasive differential sugar permeation. *Eur J Clin Invest* 1986; 16: 217–25.

144 Ohri SK, Somasundaram S, Koak Y *et al.* The effect of intestinal hypoperfusion during cardiopulmonary bypass surgery on saccharide permeation and intestinal permeability in man. *Gastroenterology* 1994; 106: 318–23.

145 Oman H, Akerblom E, Richter W, Johansson SGO. Chemical and physiological properties of polysucrose, a new marker of intestinal permeability to macromolecules. *Int Arch Allergy Immunol* 1992; 98: 220–6.

146 Oman H, Blomquist L, Henriksson AEK, Johansson SGO. Comparison of polysucrose 15000, ^{51}Cr-labelled ethylenediaminotetraacetic acid, and 14C-mannitol as markers of intestinal permeability in man. *Scand J Gastroenterol* 1995; 30: 1172–7.

147 O'Morain C, Abelon AC, Chervli LR, Fleischner GM, Das KM. ^{51}CrEDTA a useful test in the assessment of inflammatory bowel disease. *J Lab Clin Med* 1986; 108: 430–5.

148 Otamiri T, Sjodahl R, Tagesson C. An experimental model for studying reversible intestinal ischemia. *Acta Chir Scand* 1987; 153: 51–6.

149 Paganelli R, Fagiolo U, Cancian M, Sturniolo GC, Scala E, D'Offizi GP. Intestinal permeability in irritable bowel syndrome. Effect of diet and sodium chromoglycate administration. *Ann Allergy* 1990; 64: 377–80.

150 Parrilli G, Iaffaioli RV, Martorano M *et al.* Effects of anthracycline therapy on intestinal absorption in patients with advanced breast cancer. *Cancer Res* 1989; 49: 3689–91.

151 Pearson AD, Eastham EJ, Laker ME, Craft AW, Nelson R. Intestinal permeability in children with Crohn's disease and coeliac disease. *BMJ* 1982; 285: 20–21.

152 Pearson ADJ, Craft AW, Pledger JV, Eastham EJ, Laker MF, Perason CS. Small bowel function in acute lymphoblastic leukemia. *Arch Dis Child* 1984; 59: 460–5.

153 Pike MG, Heddle RJ, Boulton P, Turner MW, Atherton DJ. Increased intestinal permeability in atopic eczema. *J Invest Dermatol* 1986; 86: 101–4.

154 Pike MG, Riches P, Atherton DJ. Fecal al-antitrypsin concentration and gastrointestinal permeability to oligosaccharides in atopic dermatitis. *Pediatr Dermatol* 1989; 6: 10–12.

155 Pironi L, Miglioli M, Ruggeri E *et al.* Relationship between intestinal permeability to (^{51}Cr)EDTA and inflammatory activity in asymptomatic patients with Crohn's disease. *Dig Dis Sci* 1990; 35: 582–8.

156 Pledger JV, Pearson ADJ, Craft AW, Laker MF, Eastham EJ. Intestinal permeability during chemotherapy for childhood tumors. *Eur J Pediatr* 1988; 147: 123–7.

157 Qvist H, Somasundaram S, Macpherson A, Menzies IS, Giercksky K, Bjarnason I. The effect of pelvic radiation on small and large intestinal absorption and permeability in man. *Gastroenterology* 1994; 106:A430.

158 Ramage JK, Stanisz A, Scicchitano R, Hunt RH, Perdue MH. Effects of immunologic reactions on rat intestinal epithelium. Correlation of increased intestinal permeability to chromium 51-labelled ethylenediaminetetraacetic acid and ovalbumin during acute inflammation and anaphylaxis. *Gastroenterology* 1988; 94: 1368–75.

159 Rask-Madsen J, Schwartz M. Absorption of ^{51}CrEDTA in ulcerative colitis following rectal instillation. *Scand J Gastroenterol* 1979; 5: 361–8.

160 Resnick RH, Royal H, Marshall W, Barron R, Werth T. Intestinal permeability in gastrointestinal disorders. *Dig Dis Sci* 1990; 35: 205–11.

161 Rooney PJ, Jenkins RT, Smith KM, Coates G. 111-Indium-labelled polymorphonuclear scans in rheumatoid arthritis – an important clinical cause of positive results. *Br J Rheumatol* 1986; 15: 167–70.

162 Roumen RM, van der Vliet JA, Wevers RA, Goris RJ. Intestinal permeability is increased after major vascular surgery. *J Vasc Surg* 1993; 17: 734–7.

163 Ruppin H, Hotze A, During A *et al*. Reversible funktionsstorungen des intestinaltraktes durch abdominelle strahlentherapy. *Zeitschrift fur Gastroenterologie* 1987; 25: 261–9.

164 Ruttenberg D, Young GO, Wright JP, Isaacs S. PEG 400 excretion in patients with Crohn's disease, their first degree relatives, and healthy volunteers. *Dig Dis Sci* 1992; 37: 705–8.

165 Sanderson IR, Boulton P, Menzies IS, Walker-Smith JA. Improvement of abnormal lactulose/rhamnose permeability in active Crohn's disease of the small bowel by an elemental diet. *Gut* 1987; 28: 1073–6.

166 Santini R, Perez-Santiago E, Martinez-De-Jesus J, Butterworth CE. Evidence of increased intestinal absorption of molecular sucrose in sprue. *Am J Dig Dis* 1957; 2: 663–8.

167 Saverymuttu SH, Thomas A, Grundy A, Maxwell JD. Ileal stricturing after long term indomethacin treatment. *Postgrad Med J* 1986; 62: 267–8.

168 Scadding C, Bjarnason I, Brostoff J, Levi AJ, Peters TJ. Intestinal permeability to ^{51}Cr-labelled ethylenediaminetetraacetate in food-intolerant subjects. *Digestion* 1989; 42: 104–9.

169 Schrander JJP, Unsalan-Hooyen RWM, Forest PP, Jansen J. [^{51}Cr]EDTA intestinal permeability in children with cow's milk intolerance. *J Pediatr Gastroenterol Nutr* 1990; 10: 189–92.

170 Segall AW, Isenberg DA, Hajirousow V, Tolfree S, Clark J, Snaith ML. Preliminary evidence for gut involvement in the pathogenesis of rheumatoid arthritis? *Br J Rheumatol* 1986; 25: 162–6.

171 Selby PJ, Lopes N, Mundy V, Crofts M, Millar JL, McElwain TJ. Cyclophosphamide priming reduces intestinal damage in man following high dose melphalan chemotherapy. *Br J Cancer* 1987; 55: 531–3.

172 Sheers R, Williams WR. NSAIDs and gut damage. *Lancet* 1989; ii: 1154.

173 Shorter RG, Huizenga GA, Spencer RJ. A working hypothesis for the etiology and pathogenesis of nonspecific inflammatory bowel disease. *Dig Dis Sci* 1972; 17: 1024–31.

174 Smecuol E, Bai JC, Vazques H *et al*. Gastrointestinal permeability in coeliac disease. *Gastroenterology* 1997; 112: 1129–36.

175 Smethurst P, Menzies IS, Levi AJ, Bjarnason I. Is alcohol directly toxic to the small bowel mucosa? *Clin Sci* 1988; 75: 50–51P.

176 Smith T, Bjarnason I, Hesp R. Critical analysis of a combined test ([75]SeHCAT and [58]CoB12) of ileal function using a whole body counter. *Clin Phys Physiol Meas* 1987; 8: 159–71.

177 Smith T, Bjarnason I. Experience with the use of a gastrointestinal marker ([51]CrCl3) in a combined study of ileal function using [75]SeHCAT and [58]CoVitB12 measured by whole body counting. *Gut* 1990; 31: 1120–25.

178 Sturges HF, Krone CL. Ulcers and strictures of the jejunum in a patient on long term indomethacin therapy. *Am J Gastroenterol* 1973; 59: 162–9.

179 Sukumar L. Recurrent small bowel obstruction with piroxicam. *Br J Surg* 1987; 74: 186.

180 Sundquist T, Magnusson KE, Larsson L, Tageson C, Backman L, Nordenvall B. Reduced intestinal permeability to low-molecular-weight polyethylene glycols (PEG400) in patients with jejunoileal bypass. *Acta Chir Scand* 1984; 150: 567–71.

181 Sutherland LR, Verhoef M, Wallace JL, Rosendaahl GV, Crutcher R, Meddings JB. A simple, non-invasive marker of gastric damage: sucrose permeability. *Lancet* 1994; 343: 998–1000.

182 Tageson C, Edling C. Influence of surface-active food additives on the integrity and permeability of rat intestinal mucosa. *Fd Chem Toxic* 1984; 22: 861–4.

183 Teahon K, Bjarnason I. Comparison of leukocyte excretion and blood loss in inflammatory disease of the bowel. *Gut* 1993; 34: 1535–8.

184 Teahon K, Smethurst P, Levi AJ, Bjarnason I. The effect of elemental diet on intestinal permeability and inflammation in Crohn's disease. *Gastroenterology* 1991; 101: 84–9.

185 Teahon K, Smethurst P, Levi AJ, Menzies IS, Bjarnason I. Intestinal permeability in patients with Crohn's disease and their first degree relatives. *Gut* 1992; 33: 320–3.

186 Teahon K, Smethurst P, Macpherson AJ, Levi AJ, Menzies IS, Bjarnason I. Intestinal permeability in Crohn's disease and its relation to disease activity and relapse following treatment with elemental diet. *Eur J Gastroenterol Hepatol* 1993; 5: 79–84.

187 Teahon K, Smith T, Smethurst P, Bjarnason I. A technique for localizing alterations of intestinal permeability in man. *Gastroenterology* 1991; 100:A251.

188 Teahon K, Somasundaram S, Smith T, Menzies I, Bjarnason I. Assessing the site of increased intestinal permeability in coeliac and inflammatory bowel disease. *Gut* 1996; 38: 864–9.

189 Teahon K, Webster AD, Price AB, Bjarnason I. Studies of gastrointestinal structure and function in patients with primary hypogammaglobulinaemia. *Gut* 1994; 35: 1244–9.

190 Travis S, Menzies IS. Intestinal permeability: functional assessment and significance. *Clin Sci* 1992; 82: 471–88.

191 Troncone R, Caputo N, Florio G, Finelli E. Increased intestinal sugar permeability after challenge in children with cow's milk allergy or intolerance. *Eur J Allergy Clin Immunol* 1994; 49: 142–6.

192 Turck D, Ythier H, Maquet E *et al*. Increased intestinal permeability to [51]CrEDTA in children with Crohn's disease and coeliac disease. *J Pediatr Gastroenterol Nutr* 1987; 6: 535–7.

193 Ukabam SO, Clamp JR, Cooper BT. Abnormal intestinal permeability to sugars in patients with Crohn's disease of the terminal ileum and colon. *Digestion* 1982; 27: 70–4.

194 Ukabam SO, Homeda MA, Cooper BJ. Small intestinal permeability in Sudanese subjects: evidence of tropical enteropathy. *Trans Roy Soc Trop Med Hyg* 1986; 40: 204–7.

195 Ukabam SO, Mann RJ, Cooper BT. Small intestinal permeability to sugars in patients with atopic eczema. *Br J Dermatol* 1984; 110: 649–52.

196 van der Hulst PRWJ, Kreel BK, Meyenfelt MF *et al*. Glutamine and the preservation of gut integrity. *Lancet* 1993; 341: 1363–65.

197 Vogelsang H, Oberhuber G, Wyatt J. Lymphocytic gastritis and gastric permeability in patients with coeliac disease. *Gastroenterology* 1996; 111: 73–7.

198 Wakefield AJ, Murch SH, Anthony A *et al*. Ileal-lymphoid-nodular hyperplasia, non-specific colitis, and pervasive developmental disorder in children. *Lancet* 1998; 351: 637–41.

199 Walker AW, Isselbacher KJ. Uptake and transport of macromolecules by the intestine. Possible role in clinical disorders. *Gastroenterology* 1974; 67: 531–50.

200 Walker WA. Mechanisms of antigen handling by the gut. *Clin Immunol Allergy* 1982; 2: 15–34.

201 Wallaert B, Colombel JF, Adenis A *et al*. Increased intestinal permeability in active pulmonary sarcoidosis. *Am Rev Respir Dis* 1992; 145: 1440–45.

202 Weaver LT. The impact of milk and weaning diet on gastrointestinal permeability in English and Gambian infants. *Transact Roy Soc Trop Med Hyg* 1988; 82: 784–89.

203 Wheeler PG, Menzies IS, Creamer B. Effect of hyperosmolar stimuli and coeliac disease on the permeability of the human gastrointestinal tract. *Clin Sci Mol Med* 1978; 54: 495–501.

204 Wood NC, Hamilton I, Axon ATR *et al*. Abnormal intestinal permeability. An aetiological factor in chronic psychiatric disorders? *Br J Psychiatr* 1987; 150: 853–6.

205 Wyatt J, Vogelsang H, Hubl W, Waldhoer T, Lochs H. Intestinal permeability and the predictor of relapse in Crohn's disease. *Lancet* 1993; 341: 1437–9.

206 Yacyshyn BR, Meddings JB. CD45RO expression on circulating CD19+B cells in Crohn's disease correlates with intestinal permeability. *Gastroenterology* 1995; 108: 132–7.

207 Yeoh EK, Horowitz M, Russo A, Muecke T, Robb T, Chatterton BE. Gastrointestinal function in chronic radiation enteritis – effects of loperamide-N-oxide. *Gut* 1993; 34: 476–82.

Chapter 16

Oral tolerance: probable mechanisms and possible therapeutic applications

S.J. Challacombe and C. Czerkinsky

INTRODUCTION

The mucosal immune system is constantly exposed to an immense number and variety of food and microbial antigens. Indeed the majority of the contacts of the human body with foreign antigenic materials occur at mucosal surfaces. The total area of the mucosae is approximately 400 m² compared with 1.8 m² for skin. In addition, whereas the skin is covered by keratin and a stratified squamous epithelium, the gut surface is a thin unicellular layer of epithelial cells characterized by absorptive properties. Approximately 1 ton (1000 kg) of food proteins reaches the human intestine per year and between 130 and 190 g of these proteins are absorbed daily in the gut.[4] Although most dietary antigens are degraded by the time they reach the small intestine, much undergraded or partially degraded antigen can be absorbed into the systemic circulation.[5] Bacteria in the gut provide an additional source of antigen stimulation in both the small and large bowel and the number of bacteria colonizing the colon is as much as 10^{12} microorganisms per gram of stool.[31]

One striking feature of the gut is the abundance of lymphoid tissue (see Chapter 4). There are approximately 10^{10} lymphoid cells per metre of human small intestine and the number of immunoglobulin-secreting cells in the gut is several fold greater than the number of immunoglobulin secreting cells in all other lymphoid organs together.[36,58]

Major features of the mucosal immune system

The consequences of antigen challenge in the gut can be (a) a local non-inflammatory humoral immune response of secretory immunoglobulin (IgA); (b) a specific systemic inflammatory response with the generation of serum antibodies; and (c) a systemic state of hypo-responsiveness to the antigen, i.e. oral tolerance. Since the amount of antigen in or transversing the gut is several times greater than the number of cells or quantity of antibody produced per day, it is likely that immunological non-responsiveness predominates over immune responsiveness. It is possible that oral tolerance allows the mucosal immune system to focus on antigens or pathogens representing a threat to the host. However, the context in which an antigen is encountered usually determines the resulting immune response. Oral tolerance is thus not simply the absence of a response but one end of a spectrum of responses to exogenous antigens and is accepted as an active process.

HISTORY OF ORAL TOLERANCE (Table 16.1)

The first reported reference to what can be interpreted as oral tolerance appears to be in 1829 when the French physician R Dakin reported that an inflammatory cutaneous reaction provoked by poison oak and poison ivy might be prevented or even cured by allowing the forbidden leaves to be eaten.[14] The first experimental approach was reported in 1909 by the Russian scientist Alexandra Besredka, who showed that guinea pigs treated with milk by the oral route became refractory to an anaphylactic reaction.[2] H. G. Wells in 1911 confirmed and expanded this work in a large series of experiments in guinea pigs, showing that anaphylaxis to hen's egg as well as to vegetable protein could be prevented by prior feeding of these proteins.[63]

The immunological basis of these observations were investigated by Chase in 1946 who showed that guinea pigs fed a skin-sensitizing agent were rendered non-allergic to a normal sensitizing dose. He also established the specific nature of the inhibition and showed that while suppression was easily induced, feeding worked poorly as a therapy for already sensitized animals.

Systemic tolerance after feeding re-emerged as a subject to be investigated nearly 30 years later and was renamed oral tolerance[56] and began to be extensively investigated.[1,52,59] In recent

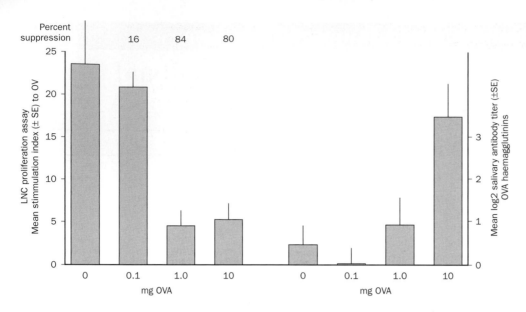

Fig. 16.1 Salivary antibodies and systemic suppression after intragastric administration of OVA in CBA/J mice. Results show mean +/– SE of four to six mice groups. Animals were given OVA or PBS IG, and 7 days later challenged with 100 µg OVA in H37 Ra complete adjuvant; 8 days later (day 15), samples of serum and saliva were taken and the proliferative assay performed. Salivary antibody titres were assayed by haemagglutination. No serum antibodies were detected.

History of oral tolerance	
1677	Peyer's patches – Johann Conrad Peyer 1653–1712
1911	Tolerance after feeding egg proteins to guinea-pigs (H. G. Wells[63])
1946	Tolerance to skin reactivity to DNCB in guinea-pigs after feeding (Chase M[8a])
1975–85	Oral tolerance to SRBC and protein antigen in many models
1980	Term 'oral tolerance' (Tomasi et al.[56])
1980	Demonstration that secretory immunity and oral tolerance could be induced by same feeding (Challacombe & Tomasi[6])
1994	Experimental oral tolerance in man (Husby et al.[25])

Table 16.1 History of oral tolerance

Aspects of the immune system susceptible to oral tolerance
IgM and all IgG isotypes
Serum but not salivary IgA
IgE antibody responses
All aspects of cell mediated responses, including proliferation and cytokine production
Cytokines IL2, 3, 4, 5, 10
IFNγ *in vivo*
Delayed hypersensitivity and contact sensitivity *in vivo*
CD[8+] CTL responses (either CD4-dependent or independent)

CD, cluster designation (cell surface markers); CTL, cytotoxic T lymphocytes; IFNγ, interferon γ; Ig, immunoglobulin; IL, interleukin.

Table 16.2 Aspects of the immune system susceptible to oral tolerance.

years, oral tolerance has begun to attract considerable attention since it was realized that it was a phenomenon demonstrable in humans[25] and it might be applied for the treatment of human autoimmune diseases.[62] The mechanisms of oral tolerance have provided insight into the function and complexity of the mucosal immune system, especially since it has been demonstrated that systemic tolerance and secretory antibodies can be induced by the same antigenic challenge (Fig. 16.1).[6]

MAJOR FEATURES OF ORAL TOLERANCE

The major and most important feature of oral tolerance is antigen specificity – the tolerance induced is specific for the antigen that is fed – and this applies to both cellular and humoral immune responses.[41] Oral tolerance appears to be more effective for cellular immunity than for humoral. Thus, in humans, the feeding of KLH resulted in decreased cellular proliferative responses with little effect on the humoral responses.[25] However, in animals, significant reduction, though not total abrogation, of antibodies has been reported.[6,8]

Oral tolerance has been described in most animal systems and with a wide variety of soluble antigens. Feeding antigen can provide stable and long-lasting tolerance. A wide range of immune responses has been demonstrated to be affected (Table 16.2) and, in general, the induction phase of immunity is much more susceptible than the effector phase: in other words, it is more difficult to tolerize an already sensitized individual than to prevent sensitization. The mechanisms controlling oral tolerance are complex and not fully understood; the major factors influencing mechanisms are still controversial, especially in humans (see below).

Humoral tolerance

Hyporesponsiveness of systemic antibody production has been demonstrated in several studies after enteric immunization. Many authors have examined plaque-forming cells and have shown that animals given oral antigen have reduced numbers of splenic IgM and IgG antibody producing cells.[1,26] Hyporesponsiveness of serum IgA responses has also been demonstrated[7] and suppression of serum IgA concurrent with the induction of salivary IgA has been reported.[7] IgE responses can also be suppressed.[42]

Suppression of systemic antibody responses can also be demonstrated by suppression of circulating antibody-secreting cells.[12]

Cellular tolerance

In general, cellular responses can be profoundly suppressed by feeding antigen, and this has been demonstrated with delayed-type hypersensitivity reactions,[55] proliferative assays and production of Th1 cytokines (for review see Refs 19 and 51).

Duration of oral tolerance

Oral tolerance can sometimes be detected in animal models within days of a single feed and can be demonstrated for at least 18 months in laboratory mice. This suggests that the response may be long-lived in humans, but this has not been demonstrated. It is also possible that the duration of tolerance may differ depending on the sites of its induction.

Parameters for the induction of oral tolerance

Many different factors can affect the induction and degree of oral tolerance, and these are listed in Table 16.3. The types of antigen that have been demonstrated to induce oral tolerance include various protein antigens, contact allergens, allo- and xenogenic cells and certain viruses.[15] Tolerance has also been demonstrated after the feeding of multiple proteins. Most tolerogenic antigens induce T-cell-dependent immune responses when given parenterally and most are good immunogens. Oral tolerance does not appear to be effectively induced by T-cell-independent antigens.[55] However, it should not be assumed that feeding of all proteins, especially bacterial proteins, would result in oral tolerance. The dose of antigen to induce tolerance via the gut is usually in milligram quantities but it is not known how much of this is actually taken up across the gut wall.[20] The age of the animal modifies the response,[49] as does the genetic background and species.[94]

SITE OF INDUCTION OF ORAL INTOLERANCE

It should be noted that presentation of antigen via the enteric route is not the only way in which antigen present at mucosal surfaces can induce tolerance. Oral (mucosal) tolerance can be induced by stimulation of the bronchial-associated lymphoid tissue (BALT)[24] in a manner analogous to gut-associated lymphoid tissue (GALT) (Fig. 16.2). Similarly, nasal application of certain antigens has also been reported to lead to systemic tolerance.[13]

Irrespective of effector mechanism(s) involved, a major question that arises is where and how oral tolerance is induced, be it suppression, anergy, deletion, ignorance and/or anatomical deviation. To date, very little is known regarding the mechanisms governing induction of mucosal tolerance, and especially the intracellular pathways of entry of tolerogens, the nature of antigen-presenting cell (APC) elements involved, their tissue localization, and the characteristics of signals transduced from such cells to responding T cells. At vari-

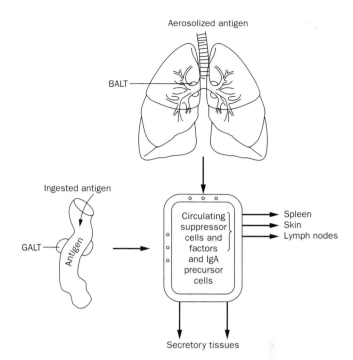

Fig. 16.2 Similarity of tolerance induction by bronchial-associated lymphoid tissue (BALT) and gut-associated lymphoid tissue (GALT).

ance with systemically administered antigens, antigens handled in mucosal tissues have already been subject to a variety of innate factors such as, e.g. proteases, acids, salts, mucins, that have altered their form prior to uptake. As a result of this extratissular processing different epitopes may be exposed and their uptake and/or processing may involve many different cell types.

Role of Epithelial Cells

The observation that mucosally induced systemic tolerance depends on an intact epithelial barrier (Strobel et al, 1983; Bruce and Ferguson, 1986) suggests a central role for the epithelium. Specialized epithelial M cells overlying organized lymphoid aggregates such as the Peyer's patches or the tonsils, have been shown to uptake a variety of particulate antigens such as viruses and bacteria, and to allow direct entry of invasive microorganisms to mucosal inductive sites. Such a pathway is thought to result in the induction of secretory IgA immune responses. Although the ability of M cells to serve as antigen-presenting cells (APCs) appears to be poorly supported, these cells could still theoretically be involved in an abortive form of antigen presentation leading to tolerance induction.

The role of absorptive epithelial cells, such as intestinal enterocytes, in tolerance induction has been underscored by several studies and in particular by elegant experiments reported by Rubin and co-workers (1981). Reovirus type III enters M cells and elicits a protective IgA response, whereas reovirus type I infects enterocytes and induces tolerance. Most of the currently available data indicate that antigens sampled from the lumen by intestinal enterocytes are preferentially presented to CD8+ suppressor cells (Mayer et al, 1996). Epithelial enterocytes express co-stimulatory molecules such as non-classical MHC class I (CD1d) molecules involved in antigen presentation to subpopulations of T cells and abnormal forms or levels of MHC class II molecules (Kaiserlian, 1995), leading to selective triggering of suppressive CD8+ T cells and/or abortive presentation to CD4+ T cells. In addition, epithelial enterocytes

Parameters for the induction of oral tolerance	
Type of antigen	Species
Dose of antigen	Genetic background
Frequency of feeding	Age
Mucosal route	Delivery system/adjuvant
Immunogenicity of the antigen	

Table 16.3 Parameters for the induction of oral tolerance.

have also been shown to produce cytokines, such as IL-10 and TGF β, which are particularly efficient at suppressing the inductive phase of CD4+ T cell-mediated responses.

Role of Antigen Presenting Cells

All known types of classical APCs, including dendritic cells, macrophages and B cells, have been shown to populate mucosal tissues but, because of their heterogeneity and of the difficulty in isolating pure subpopulations of APCs from mucosal tissues, their respective roles in inducing or maintaining tolerance has not yet been elucidated. Although activated B cells and tissue macrophages are powerful APCs for memory T helper cells, evidence suggests that antigen presentation by resting B cells results in T cell tolerance (Eynon and Parker, 1992, Fuchs and Matzinger, 1992). Resting B cells lack critical co-stimulatory molecules but are efficient at internalizing specific antigens. It should be noted however, that B cells activated in vitro with bacterial lipopolysaccharide, a prominent component of the normal mucosal microflora, are capable of inducing tolerance when injected into naïve hosts (Fuchs and Matzinger 1992).

Although functional dendritic cells have been identified in mucosal tissues such as the Peyer's patches (Kelsall and Strober, 1996), the mesenteric lymph (Liu and MacPherson, 1993), the intestinal lamina propria (Pavli et al, 1990) and the airway mucosa (McWilliam et al, 1994), their role in activating rather than suppressing naïve T cells has received strongest support. Interestingly, LPS, which is known to cause the rapid exit of dendritic cells, has also been shown to enhance tolerance induction (Khoury et al, 1990). However, Holt (1994) has proposed that a subpopulation of dendritic cells in the airway mucosa may leak out immunogenic peptides from MHC class II to MHC class I molecules or to non-classical restriction elements resulting in subsequent presentation to CD8+ γδ T cells. The latter could secrete immunosuppressive cytokines (IFN-γ) that would prevent the proliferation of CD4+ T cells, especially Th2 cells. Such a hypothesis has been proposed to explain the suppressive effect of airborne antigens on induction of respiratory type I allergic responses.

The above strongly suggests that both the site of entry and the intracellular pathway of processing of antigens administered to a mucous membrane have a major influence in the induction of tolerance and/or immunity and emphasises the need for the development of vaccine formulations with intrinsic immuno-modulating and cellular targeting properties.

With regard to the gut, the exact site of tolerance induction for any given antigen has not been clearly established. Peyer's patches, mesentenial lymph nodes or lymphoid follicles, the epithelial layer or the systemic lymphoid compartment exposed to antigenic fragments may all be involved. However, Peyer's patches certainly represent one site of tolerance induction.[47] In common with BALT and GALT it seems that each of the mucosal surfaces at which tolerance can be induced contain lymphoid follicles. However, there has been increasing recognition that the intestinal cell layer is an active component of the mucosal immune system.[16] Epithelial cells respond to and produce a wide variety of cytokines and are part of an epithelial lymphoid cell network in the mucosa since epithelial cells express both MHC Class I and Class II molecules and can process and present soluble antigens. Interestingly, antigen presentation by gut epithelial cells *in vitro* seems to preferentially induce suppressor cells[3,32] and, as speculated by Elson and Zivny,[19] this may be because epithelial cells lack

Experimental oral tolerance in humans
Korenblat *et al*:[29] Compared oral and parenteral exposure to bovine serum albumin
Lowney:[30] Suppression of contact sensitization by dinitrochlorobenzene (DNCB)
Husby *et al*: Fed humans KLH and suppression of T- but not B-cell immunity

Table 16.4 Experimental oral tolerance in humans.

costimulatory molecules such as B7.[46] This appears a fruitful area for further investigation.

Experimental oral tolerance in humans

Three studies appear to have induced experimental oral tolerance in humans (Table 16.4). Korenblat *et al*.[29] compared oral and parenteral exposure to bovine serum albumin (BSA) and, in a possible incidental finding, showed that those given BSA orally were then unresponsive. Suppression of contact sensitization by dinitrochlorobenzene (DNCB) was carefully shown by Lowney[30] in volunteers fed DNCB. The most comprehensive study has been that of Husby *et al*.[25] Eight adult volunteers ingested 0.5 g of keyhole limpid haemocyanin and were then challenged with subcutaneous immunization. A marked reduction in KLH T-cell proliferation and in skin delayed hypersensitivity reactions was demonstrated; surprisingly, there was an increase in circulating IgG or IgM antibody cells and an increase in serum and secretory IgA antibody. These results suggested that T-cell but not B-cell tolerance was found after antigen feeding and also confirmed that systemic tolerance could occur in the presence of a concurrent induction of secretory antibody first demonstrated in mice.[6]

MECHANISMS OF ORAL TOLERANCE

Multiple mechanisms of oral tolerance have been identified, perhaps consistent with its importance to the functioning of the mucosal immune system but also reflecting a composite immune response as the net result of several interactive components. There are three major mechanisms identified:

1. the induction of suppressor T cells[45]
2. clonal deletion.[9]
3. clonal anergy.[34]

However, these mechanisms are not mutually exclusive and more than one could be operative simultaneously.

Suppressor T cells

Adoptive transfer studies demonstrated that cells obtained from antigen-fed donors could transfer to a recipient animal tolerance to subsequent parenteral administration of an antigen which would otherwise evoke a strong immune response. These cells appear to be T cells originating in Peyer's patches and later appearing in other tissues as a result of cell migration.[53]

In early studies the cells were assumed to be CD8+ rather than CD4+,[43] but in more recent studies the evidence is in favour of active CD4+ cells.[60] Oral tolerance can be induced in CD8+ T-cell deficient mice,[10] but it is possible or even probable that both cell types could play a role in oral tolerance via different mechanisms. More recently it has become clear that while the suppressor cell requires specific antigens to become activated, the suppression is actually mediated by antigen non-specific cytokines including transforming growth factor β (TGF-β).

However, evidence against regulatory TH2 CD4⁺ cells is that oral tolerance to OVA can suppress both TH1 and TH2 responses,[21] and oral tolerance can be induced in the absence of TH2 cells in interleukin 4 (IL4) knockout mice. Evidence in favour of acts of modulation by CD8⁺ T cells includes the observations that tolerance is transferable to naïve recipients with CD8⁺ cells and is prevented by pre-treatment with cyclophosphamide. In addition, transfer of CD8⁺ T cells can suppress experimental autoimmune encephalomyelitis.

Other evidence suggests that CD8⁺ cells may not be needed, since oral tolerance can be induced and maintained in mice depleted of CD8⁺ cells either by monoclonal antibody treatment[21] or in CD8⁺ knockout mice.[22]

Clonal anergy or clonal deletion

Evidence for clonal deletion as one mechanism contributing to oral tolerance includes the demonstration *in vivo* that following oral administration of OVA to T-cell receptor deficient transgenic mice, very large doses of antigen were required and that there may have been transient activation before deletion.[9] By analogy with peripheral tolerance, antigen-reactive lymphocytes are absent in many models of oral tolerance, but antigen reactivity can be restored *in vitro* with IL-2. Clonal anergy could also explain the capacity of oral tolerant cells to retain the ability to produce IL4 and TGF-β. High-dose antigen appears to give rise to deletion or anergy of TH1 and perhaps of TH2 cells.[28,48,51] In these studies oral administration of antigen was followed by the rapid appearance in the circulation of a form of intact antigen that was tolerogenic on passive transfer.

Thus, a general scheme is shown in Fig. 16.3 for mechanisms of oral tolerance in relation to dose.

Bystander suppression

Feeding of an antigen can be manipulated in such a way as to induce antigen-specific suppressor cells. Once induced in the gut, such cells will circulate widely in the body and, upon re-encounter with antigen in lesions, release various inhibitory cytokines.[39] Thus, theoretically, oral tolerance could be used as a novel potential therapy, since such cytokines produced are themselves non-specifically inhibitory and will downregulate cells in inflammatory lesions that recognize other antigens. Candidate cytokines would include TGFβ with a wide inhibitory spectrum, produced from CD8 or CD4⁺ T cells and IL4 or IL10 from CD4⁺ cells. The latter cytokines exhibit potent inhibition of macrophages and TH1 cells.

With regard to IL4, suppression can be transferred by IL4-secreting clones, and depletion of IL4 can reverse the active suppression. However, no upregulation of the IL4 has been detected and oral tolerance can be induced in IL4 knockout mice using both high- and low-dose antigen challenge. IL10 is produced normally only by TH3 cells although IL10 TH3 clones have been found in mice fed myelin basic protein (MBP). However, oral tolerance can be induced in IL10 knockout mice.

TGFβ is abundant in normal intestine and regulates epithelial homeostasis and IgA switching. However, it is suppressive on many immune responses and protection against experimental allergic encephalomyelitis (EAE) can be transferred with CD8⁺ TGFβ-producing cells. Interestingly, bystander suppression can be blocked by anti TGFβ, but few studies have examined TGFβ *in vivo*.

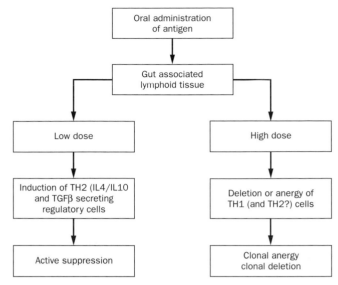

Fig. 16.3 Mechanisms of oral tolerance.

It is possible that interferon γ (IFNγ) may have a role, since CD8⁺ γδ T cells, which produce IFNγ, can transfer oral tolerance but, conversely, oral tolerance can be induced in IFNγ-deficient mice.[22]

The most compelling evidence for bystander suppression comes from the work of Miller *et al.*[38] in which rats fed OVA and tolerant to OVA were challenged with MBP with or without OVA. Those challenged with MBP and adjuvant with OVA were protected from EAE, while those challenged with MBP without OVA developed EAE. This protection could be transferred with CD8⁺ T cells.

A possible role for γδ⁺ T cells

Recently, it has been shown that oral tolerance cannot be induced in γδ T-cell depleted mice.[35] In addition, transfer of as little as 500 antigen-specific γδ T cells has been shown to suppress CD4⁺ responses and IgE.[33] It is possible, though not yet proven, that they are the CD8⁺ IFNγ-producing regulatory T cells.

Can oral tolerance be enhanced by adjuvants?

A few studies have addressed this question. Feeding bacterial lipopolysaccharide along with a protein antigen-enhanced oral tolerance to MBP.[27] Oral administration of antigens covalently bound to recombinant cholera toxin B subunit (CTB) resulted in enhancement of tolerance although the mechanisms remain unclear (Sun *et al*, 1994). CTB-driven oral tolerance was shown to affect both Th1- and Th2-driven responses but suppression of the latter responses., including IgE antibody responses, appeared to be dependent on the frequency rather than the dose of fed antigen (Rask *et al*, 2000). Elson *et al.*[17] demonstrated that BSA given as a multiple emulsion with a bacterial protein resulted in enhanced oral tolerance. It seems that this would be a fruitful area for further investigation.

A summary of the factors which have been shown to augment or decrease oral tolerance is shown in Table 16.5.

ORAL TOLERANCE AND EXPERIMENTAL AUTOIMMUNE AND ALLERGIC DISEASES

Since mucosally induced immunological tolerance is exquisitely specific of the antigen initially ingested or inhaled, and thus does not influence the development of systemic immune responses

Modulation of oral tolerance	
Augments	**Decreases**
IL2	IFNγ
IL4/IL10a	IL12
Anti-IL12	CT
CTB antigens	Anti-MCP-1
LPS	Anti-γδ-Ab
IFNβ	GVHR
Multiple emulsions	CY
	2'-dGuo
	Oestradiol

Table 16.5 Modulation of oral tolerance.

Suppression of autoimmunity by oral tolerance	
Animal models	**Protein fed**
EAE	MBP, PLP
Arthritis (CII, AA, Ag, Pris)	Type II collagen
Uveitis	S-Antigen, IRBP
Diabetes (NOD mouse)	Insulin, glutamate decarboxylase
Myasthenia gravis	AChR
Thyroiditis	Thyroglobulin
Transplantation	Alloantigen, MHC peptide
Human diseases trials	**Proteins**
Multiple sclerosis	Bovine myelin
Rheumatoid arthritis	Chicken type II collagen
Uveoretinitis	Bovine S-antigen
Type 1 diabetes	Human insulin

Table 16.6 Suppression of autoimmunity by oral tolerance.

against other antigens, its manipulation has become an increasingly attractive strategy for preventing and possibly treating illnesses associated with or resulting from the development of adverse immunological reactions against self and non-self antigens. This approach had earlier been proposed as a strategy to prevent or to reduce the intensity of allergic reactions to chemical drugs (Chase, 1946). Later, the same rationale was followed in attempts to prevent or treat allergic reactions to common allergens (Wortmann 1977; Rebien *et al*, 1982). More recently, nasal administration of a synthetic peptide (Der P1) entailing a dominant T cell epitope of house dust mite allergen could inhibit T cell and reaginic antibody responses in mice (Hoyne *et al*, 1993).

The feeding of autoantigens has been established in animal models as an effective way to suppress autoimmunity.[54] What these systems, summarized in Table 16.6, have in common is the induction of disease by immunization with an autoantigenic protein or peptide, and most are mediated by TH1-type CD4 T cells. Thus, in these models, prior feeding of the same antigen that is used to induce the disease can abrogate the disease induction. In some models the disease can be modified by feeding the antigen to animals with already established disease. EAE is perhaps the best example of the use of oral tolerance to treat experimental autoimmune disease.[23] The inhibition of type 2 collagen-induced arthritis by prior feeding has been established[54] and may be associated with CD8[+] suppressor T cells. Interestingly, in the nonobese diabetic (NOD) mouse model of type 1 diabetes, the feeding of porcine insulin to young prediabetic mice appears to be an effective method of delaying the onset of this disease but was inefficient in mice when initiated during the post-wearing period.[64]

ORAL TOLERANCE AS A THERAPY FOR HUMAN DISEASE

The experiments of Husby *et al*.[25] in humans established that oral tolerance, at least of the cell-mediated arm of the immune response, could be demonstrated in humans. The rabbit seems to be one of the few species in which it has been difficult to demonstrate oral tolerance.[44] The encouraging results from animal models have allowed a number of human disease trials to be undertaken. These are shown in Table 16.6, and include multiple sclerosis feeding bovine myelin, rheumatoid arthritis feeding chicken type II collagen, uveoretinitis using bovine S-antigen and type 1 diabetes using human insulin. The multiple sclerosis patients with relapsing remitting disease were fed 300 mg/day of bovine myelin in a double blind trial.[61] No toxicity was observed and there did appear to be some reduction in the number of major attacks in patients fed myelin.

Similar results were found with the feeding of chicken type II collagen at between 0.1 and 0.5 mg/day for 3 months to patients with severe active rheumatoid arthritis.[57] No toxicity was observed, and some patients showed a significant reduction in some parameters of arthritic activity. These promising observations have led to the initiation of larger clinical trials in patients with recent onset diabetes and in relatives from subjects with type 1 diabetes (preventive trial). The outcome of these two trials are expected in the next few years. In addition, two phase 3 clinicals trials of oral tolerance have been completed recently in patients with multiple sclerosis and in patients with rheumatoid arthritis fed heterologous myelin and collagen type II respectively. The results of these two latter trials have been rather disappointing with unusual placebo effects. The nature and origin (animal) of the autoantigens fed, the dose and frequency of their administration and the clinical status (by analogy woth animal models, oral tolerance may be more effective if induced earlier in the disease) may explain these results. Clearly, much remains to be done in this area.

CONCLUSION

Oral tolerance has developed from a phenomenon induced by feeding antigen in animal models to a biological mechanism applicable to humans. It is assumed that it is one mechanism by which unwanted and possibly damaging reactions to food and environmental antigens are suppressed while allowing mucosal responses to unusual or pathogenic antigens. As the mechanisms underlying oral tolerance become better understood, the prospects for the application of oral tolerance to the control of autoimmune and allergic diseases in humans are enhanced.

KEY POINTS

- Oral tolerance is defined as a state of immunological unresponsiveness to an antigen induced by the feeding of that antigen.

- It is accepted that oral tolerance can now be induced by application of antigen to other mucosal induction sites such as the nose.
- Oral tolerance is the immunological mechanism by which the mucosal immune system maintains unresponsiveness to the myriad of antigens in the mucosal environment which might otherwise induce damaging immune responses.
- Oral tolerance appears to be mediated by several distinct but interacting mechanisms, which include the antigen-specific generation of T cells producing antigen non-specific cytokines and the induction of clonal deletion and/or anergy.
- A lack of oral tolerance may be associated with the occurrence of mucosal inflammation. It is now realistic to assume that the induction of oral tolerance may be used to treat certain autoimmune diseases and allergic disorders.

REFERENCES

1 Andre C, Heremans JF, Vaerman JP, Cambiaso CL. A mechanism for the induction of immunological tolerance by antigen feeding: antigen–antibody complexes. *J Exp Med* 1975; 142: 1509–19.

2 Besredka A. De l'anaphylaxie. Sixiéme memoire de l'anaphylaxie lactique. *Ann Inst Pasteur* 1909; 23: 166–74.

3 Bland PW, Warren LG. Antigen presentation by epithelial cells of the rat small intestine. II. Selective induction of suppressor T cells. *Immunology* 1986; 58: 9–14.

4 Brandtzaeg P. Development and basic mechanisms of human gut immunity. *Nutr Rev* 1998; 56: S5–18.

5 Bruce MG, Ferguson A. Oral tolerance to ovalbumin in mice: studies of chemically modified and 'biologically filtered' antigen. *Immunology* 1986; 57: 627–30.

6 Challacombe SJ, Tomasi TB, Jr. Systemic tolerance and secretory immunity after oral immunization. *J Exp Med* 1980; 152: 1459–72.

7 Challacombe SJ. Salivary antibodies and systemic tolerance in mice after oral immunization with bacterial antigens. *Ann NY Acad Sci* 1983; 409: 177–93.

8 Challacombe SJ, Rahman D, Jeffery H, Davis SS, O'H DT. Enhanced secretory IgA and systemic IgG antibody responses after oral immunization with biodegradable microparticles containing antigen. *Immunology* 1992; 76: 164–8.

8a Chase MW Inhibition of experimental drug allergy by prior feeding of the sensitizing agent. *Pro Soc Exp Biol Med* 1946; 61: 257–259.

9 Chen Y, Inobe J, Marks R, Gonnella P, Kuchroo VK, Weiner HL. Peripheral deletion of antigen-reactive T cells in oral tolerance [published erratum appears in *Nature* 1995 Sep 21; 377(6546): 257]. *Nature* 1995; 376: 177–80.

10 Chen Y, Inobe J, Weiner HL. Induction of oral tolerance to myelin basic protein in CD8-depleted mice: both CD4+ and CD8+ cells mediate active suppression. *J Immunol* 1995; 155: 910–16.

11 Czerkinsky C, Prince SJ, Michalek SM *et al*. IgA antibody-producing cells in peripheral blood after antigen ingestion: evidence for a common mucosal immune system in humans. *Proc Nat Acad Sci USA* 1987; 84: 2449–53.

12 Czerkinsky C, Holmgren J. The mucosal immune system and prospects for anti-infectious and anti-inflammatory vaccines. *Immunologist* 1995; 3: 97–193.

13 Czerkinsky C, Anjuere F, McGhee JR *et al*. Mucosal immunity and tolerance: relevance to vaccine development. [Review, 265 refs]. *Immunol Rev* 1999; 170: 197–222.

14 Dakin R. Remarks on a cutaneous affection produced by certain poisonous vegetables. *Am J Med Sci* 1829; 4: 98–100.

15 Elson CO. Induction and control of the gastrointestinal immune system. [Review, 92 refs]. *Scand J Gastroenterol – Suppl* 1985; 114: 1–15.

16 Elson CO, Beagley KW, Sharmanov AT *et al*. Hapten-induced model of murine inflammatory bowel disease: mucosa immune responses and protection by tolerance. *J Immunol* 1996; 157: 2174–85.

17 Elson CO, Tomasi M, Dertzbaugh MT, Thaggard G, Hunter R, Weaver C. Oral-antigen delivery by way of a multiple emulsion system enhances oral tolerance. *Ann NY Acad Sci* 1996; 778: 156–62.

18 Elson C, Zivny J. Oral tolerance: a commentary. *Essentials of Mucosal Immunology*. Academic Press, New York, 1996: 543–54.

18a Eynon EE, Parker DC. Small B cells as antigen-presenting cells in the induction of tolerance to soluble protein antigens. *J Exp Med* 1992; 175: 131–138.

19 Faria AM, Weiner HL. Oral tolerance: mechanisms and therapeutic applications [Review, 566 refs]. *Adv Immunol* 1999; 73: 153–264.

20 Friedman A, Weiner HL. Induction of anergy or active suppression following oral tolerance is determined by antigen dosage. *Proc Nat Acad Sci USA* 1994; 91: 6688–92.

20a Fuchs EJ, Matzinger P. B cells turn off virgin but not memory T cells. *Science* 1992; 258: 1156–1159.

21 Garside P, Steel M, Liew FY, Mowat AM. CD4+ but not CD8+ T cells are required for the induction of oral tolerance. *Int Immunol* 1995; 7: 501–4.

22 Grdic D, Hornquist E, Kjerrulf M, Lycke NY. Lack of local suppression in orally tolerant CD8-deficient mice reveals a critical regulatory role of CD8+ T cells in the normal gut mucosa. *J Immunol* 1998; 160: 754–62.

23 Higgins PWHL. Suppression of experimental autoimmune encephalomyelitis by oral administration of myelin basic protein and its fragments. *J Immunol* 1988; 140: 440–5.

23a Holt PG. A potential vaccine strategy for asthma and allied atopic diseases during early childhood. *Lancet* 1994; 344: 456–458.

24 Holt PG, Leivers S. Tolerance induction via antigen inhalation: isotype specificity, stability, and involvement of suppressor T cells. *Int Arch Allergy & Appl Immunol* 1982; 67: 155–60.

24a Hoyne GF, O'Hehir RE, Wraith DC, Thomas WR, Lamb JR. Inhibition of T cell and antibody responses to house dust mite allergen by inhalation of the dominant T cell epitope in naive and sensitized mice. *J Exp Med* 1993; 178: 1783–1788.

25 Husby S, Mestecky J, Moldoveanu Z, Holland S, Elson CO. Oral tolerance in humans. T cell but not B cell tolerance after antigen feeding. *J Immunol* 1994; 152: 4663–70.

26 Kagnoff MF. Oral tolerance. *Ann NY Acad Sci* 1982; 392: 248–65.

26a Kaiserlian D, Lachaux A, Grosjean I, Graber P, Bonnefoy JY. CD23/FC epsilon RII is constitutively expressed on human intestinal epithelium, and upregulated in cow's milk protein intolerance. *Adv Exp Med Biol* 1995; 371B: 871–874.

26b Kelsall BL, Strober W. The role of dendritic cells in antigen processing in the Peyer's patch. *Ann N Y Acad Sci* 1996: 778: 47–54.

27 Khoury SJ, Lider O, al-Sabbagh A, Weiner HL. Suppression of experimental autoimmune encephalomyelitis by oral administration of myelin basic protein. III. Synergistic effect of lipopolysaccharide. *Cellular Immunol* 1990; 131: 302–10.

28 King C, Davies J, Mueller R *et al.* TGF-beta1 alters APC preference, polarizing islet antigen responses toward a Th2 phenotype. *Immunity* 1998; 8: 601–13.

29 Korenblat PE, Rothberg RM, Minden P, Farr RS. Immune responses of human adults after oral and parenteral exposure to bovine serum albumin. *J Allergy* 1968; 41: 226–35.

29a Liu LM, MacPherson GG. Antigen processing: cultured lymph-borne dendritic cells can process and present native protein antigens. *Immunology* 1995; 84: 241–246.

30 Lowney ED. Suppression of contact sensitization in man by prior feeding of antigen. *J Invest Dermatol* 1973; 61: 90–3.

31 Macfarlane GT, Macfarlane S. Human colonic microbiota: ecology, physiology and metabolic potential of intestinal bacteria [Review, 66 refs]. *Scand J Gastroenterol* – Suppl 1997; 222: 3–9.

32 Mayer L, Eisenhardt D, Shlien R. Selective induction of antigen nonspecific suppressor cells with normal gut epithelium as accessory cells. *Monographs in Allergy* 1988; 24: 78–80.

32a Mayer L, So LP, Yio XY, Small G. Antigen trafficking in the intestine. *Ann N Y Acad Sci* 1996; 778: 28–35.

33 McMenamin C, Pimm C, McKersey M, Holt PG. Regulation of IgE responses to inhaled antigen in mice by antigen-specific gamma delta T cells. *Science* 1994; 265: 1869–71.

33a McWilliam AS, Nelson D, Thomas JA, Holt PG. Rapid dendritic cell recruitment is a hallmark of the acute inflammatory response at mucosal surfaces. *J Exp Med* 1994; 179: 1331–1336.

34 Melamed D, Friedman A. Direct evidence for anergy in T lymphocytes tolerized by oral administration of ovalbumin. *Eur J Immunol* 1993; 23: 935–42.

35 Mengel J, Cardillo F, Aroeira LS, Williams O, Russo M, Vaz NM. Anti-gamma delta T cell antibody blocks the induction and maintenance of oral tolerance to ovalbumin in mice. *Immunol Lett* 1995; 48: 97–102.

36 Mestecky J. The common mucosal immune system and current strategies for induction of immune responses in external secretions [Review, 117 refs]. *J Clin Immunol* 1987; 7: 265–76.

37 Mestecky J, Husby S, Moldoveanu Z *et al.* Induction of tolerance in humans: effectiveness of oral and nasal immunization routes [Review, 25 refs]. *Ann NY Acad Sci* 1996; 778: 194–201.

38 Miller A, Lider O, Weiner HL. Antigen-driven bystander suppression after oral administration of antigens. *J Exp Med* 1991; 174: 791–8.

39 Miller A, Lider O, al-Sabbagh A, Weiner HL. Suppression of experimental autoimmune encephalomyelitis by oral administration of myelin basic protein. V. Hierarchy of suppression by myelin basic protein from different species. *J Neuroimmunol* 1992; 39: 243–50.

40 Miller CC, Cook ME. Evidence against the induction of immunological tolerance by feeding antigens to chickens. *Poultry Sci* 1994; 73: 106–12.

41 Miller SD, Hanson DG. Inhibition of specific immune responses by feeding protein antigens. IV. Evidence for tolerance and specific active suppression of cell-mediated immune responses to ovalbumin. *J Immunol* 1979; 123: 2344–50.

42 Ngan J, Kind LS. Suppressor T cells for IgE and IgG in Peyer's patches of mice made tolerant by the oral administration of ovalbumin. *J Immunol* 1978; 120: 861–5.

43 Nussenblatt RB, Caspi RR, Mahdi R *et al.* Inhibition of S-antigen induced experimental autoimmune uveoretinitis by oral induction of tolerance with S-antigen. *J Immunol* 1990; 144: 1689–95.

43a Pavli P, Woodhams CE, Doe WF, Hume DA. Isolation and characterization of antigen-presenting dendritic cells from the mouse intestinal lamina propria. *Immunology* 1990; 70: 40–47.

44 Peri BA, Rothberg RM. Circulating antitoxin in rabbits after ingestion of diphtheria toxoid. *Infection & Immunity* 1981; 32: 1148–54.

44a Rask C, Holmgren J, Fredriksson M, Lindblad M, Nordstrom I, Sun JB, Czerkinsky C. Prolonged oral treatment with low doses of allergen conjugated to cholera toxin B subunit suppresses immunoglobulin E antibody responses in sensitized mice. *Clin Exp Allergy* 2000; 30: 1024–1032.

44b Rebien W, Puttonen E, Maasch HJ, Stix E, Wahn U. Clinical and immunological resonse to oral and subcutaneous immunotherapy with grass pollen extraxts. A prospective study. *Eur J Pediatr* 1982; 138: 341–344.

45 Richman LK, Chiller JM, Brown WR, Hanson DG, Vaz NM. Enterically induced immunologic tolerance. I. Induction of suppressor T lymphocytes by intragastric administration of soluble proteins. *J Immunol* 1978; 121: 2429–34.

45a Rubin D, Weiner HL, Fields BN, Greene MI. Immunologic tolerance after oral administration of reovirus: requirement for two viral gene products for tolerance induction. *Journal of Immunology* 1981; 127: 1697–701.

46 Sanderson IR, Walker WA. Uptake and transport of macromolecules by the intestine: possible role in clinical disorders (an update) [Review, 199 refs]. *Gastroenterology* 1993; 104: 622–39.

47 Santos LM, al-Sabbagh A, Londono A, Weiner HL. Oral tolerance to myelin basic protein induces regulatory TGF-beta-secreting T cells in Peyer's patches of SJL mice. *Cellular Immunol* 1994; 157: 439–47.

48 Strobel S, Mowat AM, Drummond HE, Pickering MG, Ferguson A. Immunological responses to fed protein antigens in mice. II. Oral tolerance for CMI is due to activation of cyclophosphamide-sensitive cells by gut-processed antigen. *Immunology* 1983; 49: 451–6.

49 Strobel S, Ferguson A. Immune responses to fed protein antigens in mice. 3. Systemic tolerance or priming is related to age at which antigen is first encountered. *Ped Res* 1984; 18: 588–94.

50 Strobel S, Mowat AM. Immune responses to dietary antigens: oral tolerance [Review, 115 refs]. *Immunol Today* 1998; 19: 173–81.

51 Strober W, Kelsall B, Marth T. Oral tolerance [Review, 135 refs]. *J Clin Immunol* 1998; 18: 1–30.

51a Sun JB, Holmgren J, Czerkinsky C. Cholera toxin B subunit: an efficient transmucosal carrier-delivery system for induction of peripheral immunological tolerance. *Proc Natl Acad Sci* 1994; 91: 10795–10799.

52 Thomas HC, Parrott MV. The induction of tolerance to a soluble protein antigen by oral administration. *Immunology* 1974; 27: 631–9.

53 Thomas HC, Ryan CJ, Benjamin IS, Blumgart LH, MacSween RN. The immune response in cirrhotic rats. The induction of tolerance to orally administered protein antigens. *Gastroenterology* 1976; 71: 114–17.

54 Thompson HS, Staines NA. Could specific oral tolerance be a therapy for autoimmune disease? [Review, 57 refs]. *Immunol Today* 1990; 11: 396–9.

55 Titus RG, Chiller JM. Orally induced tolerance. Definition at the cellular level. *Int Arch Allergy & Appl Immunol* 1981; 65: 323–38.

56 Tomasi TBJ, Larson L, Challacombe S, McNabb P. Mucosal immunity: the origin and migration patterns of cells in the secretory system. *J Allergy & Clin Immunol* 1980; 65: 12–19.

57 Trentham DE, Dynesius-Trentham RA, Orav *et al.* Effects of oral administration of type II collagen on rheumatoid arthritis [see comments]. *Science* 1993; 261: 1727–30.

58 van der Heijden PJ, Stok, Bianchi AT. Contribution of immunoglobulin-secreting cells in the murine small intestine to the total 'background' immunoglobulin production. *Immunology* 1987; 62: 551–5.

59 Vaz NM, Maia LC, Hanson DG, Lynch JM. Inhibition of homocytotropic antibody responses in adult inbred mice by previous feeding of the specific antigen. *J Allergy & Clin Immunol* 1977; 60: 110–15.

60 Vistica BP, Chanaud NP, Felix N *et al.* CD8 T-cells are not essential for the induction of 'low-dose' oral tolerance. *Clinic Immunol & Immunopathol* 1996; 78: 196–202.

61 Weiner HL, Mackin GA, Matsui M *et al.* Double-blind pilot trial of oral tolerization with myelin antigens in multiple sclerosis [see comments]. *Science* 1993; 259: 1321–4.

62 Weiner HL. Oral tolerance: immune mechanisms and treatment of autoimmune diseases [Review, 143 refs]. *Immunol Today* 1997; 18: 335–43.

63 Wells HG. Studies on the chemistry of anaphylaxis (III). Experiments with isolated proteins, espically those of the hen's egg. *J Infect Dis* 1911; 8: 147–71.

63a Wortmann F. Oral hyposensitization of children with pollinosis or house-dust asthma. *Allergol Immunopathol* 1977; 5: 15–26.

64 Zhang ZJ, Davidson L, Eisenbarth G, Weiner HL. Suppression of diabetes in nonobese diabetic mice by oral administration of porcine insulin. *Proc Nat Acad Sci USA* 1991; 88: 10252–6.

Chapter 17

Intestinal pathogenetic correlates of clinical food allergic disorders

Michael N Marsh

ADVERSE REACTIONS TO FOOD AND FOOD ADDITIVES

The public is showing an increasing interest in diet, nutrition and health, as witnessed by the growing trend towards high-fibre, low-fat diets and organically produced dairy products and meat. On the other hand, some degree of public apprehension and distrust abounds because of what is loosely termed 'allergy' and with it, the notion that many foods, food additives, drinks and even water are the culprits behind a mystifyingly large array of physical and psychological problems, if not other chronic disabling diseases of our era. This corner of the 'fringe' market is being exploited by an increasing medley of food allergists, immunologists, reflexologists, aromatherapists and biopathologists, all wanting to apply their particular beliefs and specific techniques. This is another trend that is not particularly helped by public ignorance and incomprehension of the various causes of food allergy and intolerance.[45]

We all, of course, experience adverse or unpleasant reactions to food. The clinical manifestations may be minimal, like simple distaste for a particular delicacy, or a sense of discomfort some hours after a very large meal. There may be more specific, and regularly occurring, symptoms that suggest an organic cause. In certain instances a specific food will be directly responsible for morbidity, such as gluten protein in a coeliac sprue patient or milk, perhaps, in someone who is severely lactase deficient. Note the 'severely' here: milk intolerance is a notable example blamed for many ills, and it is important to read what Suarez et al.[106] have to say on this subject. Clearly the mechanisms underlying these

reactions are multiple and hence incapable of being viewed solely as allergies, with the implied immunological basis.

In 1984, the report of the joint committee of the Royal College of Physicians and the British Nutrition Foundation (1984)[94] issued the following category definitions:

(i) *Food intolerance* – unpleasant, but reproducible, reaction to a specific food (or ingredient) which lacks either psychological or known physical basis.
(ii) *Food allergy* – a specialized form of (i) in which an aberrant immune reaction to a food or component occurs.
(iii) *Food aversion* – psychological problem with ingesting particular foods, which would not occur if presented in disguised form.

Intolerances that are reproducible, but not true aversions or immunologically driven allergic phenomena, are based on other defined mechanisms or factors (Table 17.1), such as pharmacological (caffeine), non-specific histamine release (strawberries), enzyme deficiency (lactase, sucrase, etc.).[7,41]

Despite such apparent clear-cut definitions, diagnosis at clinical level is far more difficult to establish. Hence there are dangers in accepting claims that food allergic reactions are on the increase, whether supposedly due to agricultural or industrial food processes; the use of substances (including antibiotics) that promote animal growth, preserve and stabilize raw foodstuffs and products for distribution; or beverages, other drinks, and even domestic tap water. Thus, we are in danger of proving what is, in effect, a circular argument, derived from a series of unproven hunches and speculations.

Table 17.1 Common non-allergic factors in food intolerance.

Common non-allergic factors in food intolerance	
Chemicals	**Toxins**
Caffeine	Ethanol
Salicylates	Quinine
Tartrazine dyes	Fava beans
Benzoates	Fungal (aflatoxins)
Sodium metabisulfite	Microbial (botulinum, staphylococcal)
Monosodium glutamate	Mushroom (amanitine)
Nitrites, nitrates	Shellfish (saxitoxin)
Tyramine	
Hexachlorobenzene	**Psychological**
Pesticides (cholinesterase inhibitors)	Phobias
	Anxiety state
Irritants	Hysterical
Onions	Food-fads
Phenylethylamine	
Histamine	**Miscellaneous GI disorders**
Spices	Irritable bowel syndrome
Curries	Gall bladder disease
	Gastro-oesophageal reflux
	Gastroduodenal ulceration
Specific enzyme deficiencies	Eosinophilic gastroenteritis
Lactase	Mast cell disease
Sucrase–isomaltase	C'1-esterase deficiency (angio-oedema)

CHARACTERIZATION OF FOOD REACTIONS AT THE MUCOSAL LEVEL

Many food-provoked symptoms such as nausea, vomiting, abdominal cramps, distension and diarrhoea[62,63] are presumed to arise from the gastrointestinal tract. The difficulty in ascribing such common, generalized gastrointestinal symptoms to a specific immunological response is obvious, particularly as the same set of features typify two common conditions confronting gastroenterologists in the West; i.e. non-ulcer dyspepsia and the irritable bowel syndrome (IBS). While the latter may, in some individuals, be due to immediate-type allergic mechanisms, other causes may be related to lifestyle, coupled with dietary habits comprising a predominance of wheat-based carbohydrate whose ultimate salvage is performed by the colon and its resident bacterial flora.[6] This often leads to painful stretching and distension of the bowel from gas formation, and will be relieved by use of either a wheat- or gluten-free diet. Many such individuals who discover this for themselves invariably consider themselves to be 'wheat sensitive' or even to have gluten sensitivity, which is unlikely to be the case. Physicians must recognize this and in offering a carbohydrate-reduced diet should explain the *biochemical* reason for the symptoms;[6,82,95] this is not a food allergy.[13] One also needs to be aware of rare syndromes that may apparently simulate some of the features of food-allergic disease, such as eosinophilic gastroenteritis, mast cell disease, and C'1 esterase deficiency (Table 17.2).

Post-dysenteric irritable bowel syndrome

The post-dysenteric form of irritable bowel syndrome (IBS) must be recognized. This is perhaps becoming more common because of the effects of increased travel to remote and comparatively unsanitized parts of the world, and exposure to *Salmonella*, *Campylobacter*, *Giardia* and *E. coli* spp. In a small proportion of cases, the diarrhoea may persist for up to 2 years although ultimately a normal bowel action will be restored.[3,117] But prospectively, this kind of problem requires extensive investigation to exclude many other forms of organic disease, as well as the knowledge and confidence to make this diagnosis and reassure the patient.

In this respect, it is difficult to work with a patient who is already convinced that his symptoms, or illness, are due to 'food allergy', or who has already thus been diagnosed as having an allergy. In what way can the overworked physician deal with such difficult problems within the context of a busy outpatient clinic and address the real nature of the underlying problem, whether immunological, non-immunological or other?

Although it is possible, theoretically, to conceive a variety of possible immunopathogenetic mechanisms to account for food allergic reactions[25,42,43,86] in our present state of knowledge, two mechanisms seen most plausible: intestinal (Type I) anaphylactic reactions, and presumptive T lymphocyte-based (Type IV) conditions associated with defined and recognizable mucosal reactions.

ANAPHYLACTIC (TYPE I) HYPERSENSITIVITY REACTIONS

Superficially, it would seem reasonable to suppose that phenomena such as pyloric spasm, hypermotility and spasm in the large and small intestine, mural oedema, increased mucus secretion and rectal spasm could be construed in terms of immediate-type allergic responses to ingested immunogens.[25] However, we may be in some difficulty in assuming that such reactions are necessarily IgE-mediated.

Uncommon disorders resembling food allergy		
Eosinophilic gastroenteritis	**Mast cell disease**	**C′1 esterase deficiency**
Long history: Episodes of colicky abdominal pain, vomiting or diarrhoea May be drug-induced Some cases due to dog worm (*Ancylostoma canis*) *X-ray*: upper GI series reveals diffuse/localized swelling of mucosal folds, dilated loop(s), oedematous areas *Biopsy*: Mucosal oedema, with marked eosinophilia. Variable architectural disturbances *Treatment*: steroids, merbendazole(parasite), ?cromoglycate	*Long, variable history:* Flushing, rash, Headache, Pruritus, Precipitate, uncontrollable diarrhoea, Abdominal pain, nausea, vomiting with severe prostration after attack *X-ray*: Non-specific changes – swollen mucosal folds, nodular pattern or filling defects *Treatment*: Cromoglycate – use may be diagnostic. Exclude myeloproliferative disease	Intermittent attacks of facial, glossal and pharyngeal oedema: severe attacks, abdominal pain, accompanied by watery diarrhoea or recurrent vomiting *X-ray*: non-specific change: constricted loop: stacked-coin appearance suggesting mucosal oedema *Protein studies*: Low level of complement C2, C4 and C1–1NH levels
Note: These are uncommon conditions which may initially, and even for some time, masquerade under other diagnoses, especially if dealt with by practitioners of 'alternative medicine'. In long-standing cases where diagnostic doubt exists, they should be considered if only for the reason that they are capable of effective treatment.[22,35,43,83,105,107,110]		

Table 17.2 Uncommon disorders resembling food allergy.

Although we have little sound evidence to draw on in the human, there is now a growing body of data from animal experiments from which we might extract some meaningful information.

Several groups have devised models of immediate-type anaphylaxis in animals previously sensitized to egg albumin, β-lactoglobulin, Trichinella or Nippostrongylus antigen, whose intestinal mucosa was subsequently challenged *in vivo* or *in vitro*, either from the serosal or luminal side in Ussing chambers.[9–12,21,25,88–91]

Central role of the intestinal mast cell

Despite variations in technique, tissue used (jejunum, ileum or proximal colon) and side from which secondary challenge was performed, there appears to be an underlying consistency in interpretation (Table 17.3) that the mucosal mast cell is central to much of the ensuing pathophysiological responses such as (i) release of mediator (histamine; 5HT, PGE_2 and their inhibition by appropriate 'blocking' agents), (ii) secondary effects on epithelium (increased chloride secretion and reduced absorption of Na, K ions), (iii) alterations in permeability from lumen-to-serosa or serosa (or blood)-to-lumen, (iv) contraction of smooth muscle, (v) involvement of mucosal nerves and interplay with adjacent cells, especially mast cells and (vi) morphological changes.

Morphological changes

These are the least impressive or uniform aspects of these reactions (Fig. 17.1) which, in the other respects noted above, seem to be rapid (20–120 min) antigen-specific events which are (i) subject to tachyphylaxis and (ii) evidently transferable by immune serum.[27,28,47,87,88] Animal tissues giving a weak passive cutaneous anaphylaxis (PCA) reaction, presumed to correlate with low IgE titre antibody, respond poorly under challenge conditions, although in one instance, activity appeared to reside in an enriched IgG fraction.[10]

The formation of subepithelial 'blebs' may occur following challenge accompanied by partial stripping of surface epithelium from subadjacent basal lamina: this is an inconstant phenomenon,

Features of Type 1 Anaphylactic Intestinal Reactions
Antigen-specific – IgE (IgG_1) mediated
Rapid onset (20–120 min: depending on conditions of re-challenge)

Mast cell discharge (loss of granules)
    mucosal histamine reduced
  – luminal histamine increased

Enterocyte/epithelial involvement:
  – increased Cl^- secretion
  – reduced brush border membrane hydrolase activity
  – increased enterocyte shedding into lumen ('blebbing')

Reduced ionic transport – Na: K: Cl: H_2O

Increased macromolecular permeability
  – blood to lumen
  – no villous/crypt alteration in mucosal architecture
  – ? loss of enterocytes (enzyme matrix disruption)
  – ? contraction of villous musculature
  – inconstant subepithelial blebbing
  – goblet cell discharge (? artefact)

Table 17.3 Features of Type 1 Anaphylactic Intestinal Reactions.

even throughout the intestinal tract of the same animal. Furthermore, it is not entirely clear whether such responses are largely due to substantial contraction of axial smooth muscle within the villi and subjacent lamina propria, or possibly to enzyme-mediated disruption of basement membrane, and hence cell–matrix adhesion, through possible mast-cell-derived enzymes, such as RMCP II, or neutrophil-derived proteases. In some studies counts both of mucosal mast cells stained with azure blue and their contained granules were reduced in challenged animals but retained in animals blocked specifically by doxantrazole but interestingly not cromoglycate. Some evidence for ultrastructural change in basement membrane of ovalbumin-challenged rats has also been noted, and in such animals, an increase in intraluminal

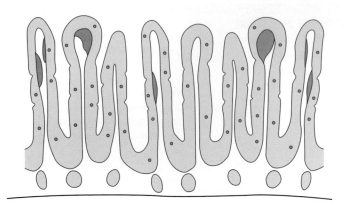

Fig. 17.1 The intestinal morphology of an acute Type I hypersensitivity reaction is inconstant and hardly 'diagnostic'. Subepithelial fluid blebs may be evident but areas of such abnormality may lie adjacent to apparently normal areas. Evidence of cellular activation, or discharge, may require the use of specialized histological techniques, or morphometric analysis applied either at the level of light, or electron, microscopy.

debris consisting largely of discarded enterocytes, is present together with losses of enterocyte sucrase, Na, K, ATPase and alkaline phosphatase activity.

Worm-derived antigen

It should be noted that in the more complicated reactions following challenge with Trichinella or Nippostrongylus worm-derived antigen, the mucosal lesions are considerably more difficult to interpret, because additional T-cell influences are likely to be present,[76] causing observable reductions in villous height as part of a T-cell-mediated local immune response (see below). The discharge of goblet cells may, or may not, be antigen-induced: this phenomenon can also easily be evoked artefactually merely by handling, stripping and mounting of tissues.

Intestinal anaphylaxis and mast cells

There are more data which further strengthen the relationship of true intestinal anaphylaxis to mast cell physiology. Importantly, an explanation for the remarkable rapidity of onset of these reactions is provided in the study[14] where re-challenge of intestinal tissue sensitized with horseradish peroxidase resulted in very rapid transcellular (endocytic) and paracellular (widened tight junctions) passage of the large electron-dense marker horseradish peroxidase – the antigen – within a few minutes of the second application, followed after 30 min, by the expected modulation of epithelial barrier function. Moreover, once subepithelial mast cells have been triggered, further increases in epithelial permeability are to be expected.

Chronic low-dose antigen administration results in mucosal mast cell hyperplasia[26,72] but, in the long term, mast cell responsiveness appears to be blunted,[93] a feature also demonstrated in operative mucosa obtained from patients undergoing surgery for ulcerative colitis or Crohn's disease.[25]

Epithelial response to cell activation

Other recent advances have shown the extent to which the epithelium itself responds to the subepithelial activation of lymphocytes and mast cells, but also actively contributes to

that response by elaborating its own cell-derived brew of co-inflammatory molecules,[74] including IL1, IL2, IL4, IL6, IL10, IL12, GM-CSF and IFNγ,[23,34,67,92] in addition to the important role of epithelial cell antigen-presentation to adjacent immuno-competent cells.[19,50] These advances, hopefully, might also lead to further understanding of other important advances in this field in respect of (i) psychological stress and life trauma episodes and (ii) the recently recognized importance of a previous (naturally occurring) intestinal infection in exaggerating subsequent colonic reactions.[24] This is a field ripe for further innovative investigation.

Which antibody is involved?

From all this, it is clear that anaphylactic-type responses can, on an acute timescale, be evoked in animals suitably primed by low-dose inoculation of antigen. Such reactions depend on systemic primary immunization (subcutaneous or intraperitoneal) in young rats and guinea pigs which are most easily primed for presumptive IgE-mediated responses. Some antigens appear not to prime for IgE, but result in IgM/IgA local mucosal responses. It would be reassuring to know (i) what species of antibody is involved (IgE/G) rather than implied in these reactions, (ii) in what part of the molecule such activity resides and (iii) whether specific anaphylactic antibody could be eluted out, labelled and then reinjected for radioautographic localization before and after subsequent challenge with specific, and control, antigens. In many experiments, while the secretory and pharmacological aspects have been performed elegantly, the morphological/immunopathological descriptions have been largely visual, and sometimes very poorly documented in terms of numerical or quantitative aspects.

The clinical perspective

There are problems, however, as viewed from the clinical perspective. While these laboratory experiments clearly implicate mast cells and mucosal neural tissues as basic ingredients of acute anaphylactic-type mucosal responses following antigen challenge, they do not necessarily illuminate the mechanism of reactions in the patient with supposed food 'allergy', despite use of elemental diets, mast cell stabilizing compounds (cromoglycate), and so on. It would also be necessary to distinguish critically between a true allergic response, and pseudo-allergic responses occasioned by very non-specific (low-threshold) discharge of mast cells through a variety of possible stimuli.

Finally, but most importantly, the mode of sensitization of the experimental animal is *not* how natural sensitization might be expected to occur in the human. Further experiments are required to determine the conditions for *intraluminal* priming for presumptive IgE responses. In addition, because some investigators have found it difficult, or impossible, to re-challenge from the luminal side, as opposed to serosal side, it would now be useful to perform further experiments with breakdown products of sensitizing protein (? peptic–tryptic digests) rather than whole molecules, in order to secure a greater chance of penetration and access to deeper tissue cells, as well as to identify actual epitopes and their structural features. Use of a wider range of sensitizing/challenging antigens would also provide a more useful means of exploring these phenomena to better advantage.[104]

Although this type of research will advance our understanding of integrated responses of the intestinal mucosa to antigen sensitization, its translation to the clinical scene, to the benefit of the food-allergic patient, seems a long way off.

CELL-MEDIATED (TYPE IV) HYPERSENSITIVITY REACTIONS OF THE SMALL INTESTINAL MUCOSA

Many experiments on cell-mediated ('delayed') reactivity have involved alloantigens intrinsic to the tissue under study, or antigens derived from infecting organisms (helminths or protozoa). Poor results have accrued with soluble antigens such as ovalbumin and bovine serum albumin. The pathogenesis of cell-mediated reactions in intestinal mucosa has been extensively investigated and found to be related to cytokine release by activated T lymphocytes: there is no evidence that cytotoxicity (T or NK cells), or antibody, play any major role in tissue remodelling or injury.

Some of the most successful and enlightening data have been with heterotopically transplanted allografts of fetal mouse intestine, and with the graft versus host (GVH) reaction in neonatal and adult hosts.[44,80] More recently, the approach of challenging fetal material in organ culture has likewise proved to be a valuable tool.[66] Although villous flattening and crypt hypertrophy can be produced, the earliest effects on mucosal architecture comprise crypt hyperplasia, which precedes any demonstrable villous effacement. An even earlier phenomenon in allograft rejection[44] is lymphocytic infiltration of lamina propria, followed by an increase in the intraepithelial lymphocyte (IEL) population. In neonatal mice with GVH reactions, induced on the sixth day of life by injection of parental spleen cells, IEL counts became elevated within 24 hours of inoculation, together with increased IEL mitotic activity and crypt enlargement, but no architectural derangement of villi.

These experiments, and many like them, were important in establishing two principles concerned with mucosal cell-mediated reactions:

(i) T cells are necessary for their induction, and
(ii) that the mature architecture of the adult intestinal mucosa is susceptible to change, via mesenteric T-lymphocyte influences.

The spectrum of the resultant mucosal changes and injury (Fig. 17.2) is detailed elsewhere.[44,66,69]

T-cell-mediated reactions

These reactions to food antigens should not normally occur because of oral tolerance, but by analogy with these experimental observations, their occurrence leads to what are now recognized as the typical hallmarks of a host-driven, intestinal mucosal reaction to the offending antigen, i.e. infiltration of epithelium by lymphocytes, crypt hyperplasia and, finally, villous effacement, accompanied by migration of mast cells and neutrophils into lamina propria with resultant oedema and microvascular hyperpermeability.[44,68]

Thus, in contrast to acute (Type I) anaphylactic reactions, where mucosal pathology is not a significant finding, Type IV cell-mediated reactions are characterized by the constancy of mucosal injury such that they are instantly recognizable by histological and immunohistological examination. This rule applies irrespective of the inciting antigen (Fig. 17.2) whether that be food-derived, microbial, parasitic or drug-related.[70]

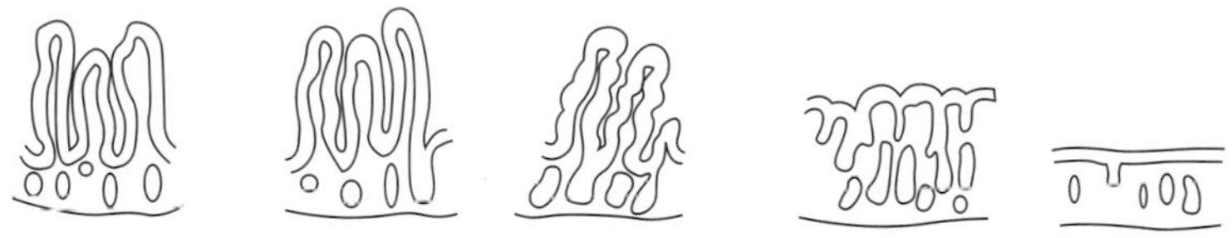

	Pre infiltrative (Type 0)	Infiltrative (Type 1)	Infiltrative hyperplastic (Type 2)	Flat destructive (Type 3)	Atrophic hyperplastic (Type 4)
1. Prolamine hypersensitivities: wheat, barley, rye, oats	+	+	+	+	+
2. Infective/parasitic: giardiasis/cryptosporidiosis infective enteritis AIDS enteropathy	+	+	+	+	
3. Tropical diarrhoea malabsorption syndrome: (tropical sprue and tropical enteropathy)	+	+	+	+	
4. Graft versus host disease:		+	+	+	
5. Transient food sensitivities: milk proteins, egg, soya, chicken, fish		+	+	+	

Fig. 17.2 The morphology of cell-mediated mucosal changes is represented by a spectrum of recognizable lesions, as illustrated. Characteristically, in the earlier phases of the reaction, there is lymphocytic infiltration of villous epithelium. The crypts may or may not be hypertrophic at this stage, but as the lesion progresses, crypt hypertrophy develops before substantial villous attrition occurs. The absence of villi characterizes the typical flat-destructive lesion of gluten sensitivity. The literature reveals similar host-directed responses to a variety of environmental antigens, derived from food, bacteria, parasites or tissue histoincompatibilities. In most of these, the development of a truly flat lesion is less commonly observed. Thus, there is a pathological differential diagnosis for infiltrative, as well as for flat-destructive lesions. The irreversible atrophic lesion that is rarely seen in gluten sensitivity is due, not to continued gluten ingestion, but to an entirely different pathological process.

BACKGROUND TO FOOD ALLERGIC DISEASE IN HUMANS

The prevalence of reliably documented food allergy in the general population is not known with certainty.[75] Prevalence rates clearly reflect the age of the population studied, being much higher for babies and toddlers[58] than in adults, where rates are ~1%.[100,113] Symptoms are more likely to appear in individuals with an atopic background. In two relevant studies, it is interesting that only approximately 50% or less subjects reporting an adverse reaction to food were confirmed by either positive skin prick tests with the offending allergen(s),[8,46] or controlled double-blind placebo/food challenges.[16]

Other features, in addition to the commoner symptoms of abdominal cramps, diarrhoea, nausea or vomiting, are encountered. Importantly, the oropharynx may be involved, with tingling and pruritus around the lips, buccal skin, on the tongue and within the mouth and throat. This is a common and rapid type of response that is seen in codfish allergy[49] and in the oral allergy syndrome where there is a strong association between Silver Birch allergic rhinitis and allergic reactions in the oropharynx to fruits and vegetables. Experience reveals that such a syndrome may not be accompanied by other symptomatology. Other complaints include swelling of lips and adjacent tissues and facial flushing. These latter oropharyngeal symptoms may very occasionally be seen in C'1-esterase deficiency and mast cell disease. Similar symptoms may precede the onset of acute anaphylactic reactions in which wheezing, cyanosis, hypotension and circulatory collapse may rapidly follow the oropharyngeal prodrome; peanuts, nuts, fish and crustacea are most likely to precipitate systemic anaphylaxis.[5,75]

Other skin manifestations comprise blotches (urticaria), atopic dermatitis, eczema and chronic urticaria, while more remote symptoms include headache, fits and irritability.[16] Interestingly, in this last study, double-blind controlled food challenges signally failed to reproduce the often expected, and alleged, response in the nose (rhinitis, otitis media) or chest (asthmatic reactions). Even behavioural disturbances, after provocation, were not impressive. Nevertheless, there seems to be general agreement[75] that the most commonly documented foods causing symptoms are milk, eggs, wheat, soya, chicken, turkey, fish, shrimp, peanuts, nuts, bananas, peas and rye.[18,98] The role of exercise-induced anaphylaxis should not be overlooked.[59,73]

THE CHEMISTRY OF FOOD ALLERGENIC PROTEINS

Given that food ingestion results in reproducible symptomatology in appropriately studied individuals, it is next important to consider the pathogenetic role of food-derived macromolecules. In the early literature, evidence for the absorption of whole protein was offered, based on the technique of passive cutaneous sensitization. With this methodology, serum from a known allergic person is injected intracutaneously into a test subject who then ingests the same antigen. The development of erythematous wheals at the cutaneous sites of injection indicates the presence of antibody and thus confirms the sensitivity, but also provides information on the timing of, and factors affecting, antigen absorption.[20,109,111] These are fascinating studies, which, today, would be totally unethical! Moreover, they perhaps lack the degree of sophistication that nowadays would provide certainty that such reactions were always due to absorption of whole, unaltered protein.

Rapid onset of allergic reactions

However, these early studies do emphasize the rapidity of onset (within a few minutes of ingestion) of some reactions, as also occurs after double-blind oral challenge.[84,98] In 65 control patients,[109] aged 15–70 years, who were tested, only 4 failed to react at the site where the hyperallergic serum was inoculated: in non-fasted individuals, reactions tended to be fewer or absent, but oral administration of dilute hydrochloric acid before the antigen was ingested resulted in diminished responses, while bicarbonate caused enhancement.[20] These observations reflect on current tests of 'intestinal permeability', indicating that an abnormal sugar ratio does not necessarily affirm that primary mucosal defects underlie food-induced anaphylaxis.[36,65] However, allergen challenge can lead to increased intestinal permeability.

A series of specific allergens has been extracted from various plant and mammalian food tissues (Table 17.4; see also Chapter 26). It is difficult to draw specific conclusions, although their resistance to acid hydrolysis and peptidase degradation has been noted.[75] Two peptides have been characterized from shrimps: the 8.2 kDa Sa-l protein, and the 34 kDa, 301 amino acid Sa-l protein, the latter rich in glutamine and asparagine residues. These revealed 54% cross-reactivity on in-vitro testing: both were specific against specific IgE-antisera from affected patients.[81] In Scandinavian countries where fish consumption is particularly high, fish hypersensitivity is common.[1] These researchers[1,2] and others[37] have isolated proteins from cod muscle, the latter being a relatively large peptide of 113 amino acid residues.

DIAGNOSIS, CLINICAL ASPECTS AND TREATMENT

By far the most consistent approach to diagnosis is the double-blind, placebo-controlled food challenge performed under standard conditions.[18,101] The conduct of such trials requires organization and adherence to strict protocols, and hence should be performed in a hospital-based setting that is dedicated to such work. The results of such tests may also be compared with prick tests (intracutaneous) which seem to be the most reliable monitors of immediate-type reactions. RAST tests, using solid-phase antigen, may not be totally reliable, in correlating with the clinical condition. The differential diagnosis must also be considered, as well as other non-allergic factors (see Table 17.1).

Treatment

In terms of treatment, exclusion of the offending food(s) is the safest and most logical way to proceed, whether performed in an 'open' or 'blind' manner.[17] Other forms of treatment – desensitization, immunotherapy etc. – have not been proven, despite their use by various food allergists. Since children predominate in food-allergic conditions, attempts have been made to reduce the allergenic content of the diet during pregnancy, or throughout the pre-weaning period. This has been difficult to document because of many other environmental variables, the discipline of maintaining the diet throughout pregnancy and the social and nutritional deprivation that may ensue.[40] Nevertheless,

Chemistry of Known Allergic Species			
Source	**Allergen**	**Molecular size**	**Reference**
Shrimp	Sa-I	8.2 kDa Antigen I (20.4 kDa) Antigen II (36.8 kDa)	Nagpal et al.[81] Hoffman et al.[53]
Cod	DS22 M peptide	18 kDa 12.3 kDa (113 residues) TM-1 (1–75) TM-2 (26–113)	Aas and Jebsen[2] Elsayed and Bennich[37] Elsayed and Apold[38]
Peanut	Conarchin α-conarchin Arachin (Peanut-1)	14–30 kDa 18–33 kDa	Sachs et al.[97]
Soybean	Globulins (85%) 15 S 11 S 7 S 2 S SBT1 (20–21 kDa) Whey (15%) urease trypsin inhibitor haemagglutin		Shibaski et al.[103] Kunitz[61] Moroz and Young[79]
Cow's milk:	Casein (80%) α₁ casein α₂ casein β casein κ casein Whey (20%) β-lactoglobulin α-lactoglobulin lactoferrin transferrin	 23.6 kDa 25.2 kDa 24 kDa 19 kDa 36 kDa P(Tr) 2–11 kDa 67 kDa 77 kDa 77 kDa	Huang et al.[54]
Egg:	Ovalbumin Ovomucoid Lysozyme	36 kDa 27 kDa 14.8 kDa	

Table 17.4 Chemistry of known allergic species.

success in reducing food allergy[116] as well as atopic disease[115] has been claimed during the first 2 years of life. This is still a controversial area, about which consensus is still lacking.

Anaphylaxis

Finally, it is important to be aware of acute anaphylaxis, and the risk to life implied by such an occurrence.[99,114] In the event, adrenaline (epinephrine) is the treatment of choice, and must be repeated if signs of continued systemic collapse persist: hospitalization is mandatory to achieve a sufficient level of care necessary to preserve life.[85] In this respect, there is a potential risk of ingesting a forbidden ('masked') antigen if its presence is not declared by the manufacturer.[77] Clearly, this is another difficult and contentious issue,[78] which may prove fatal.[15] Luckily, this form of complication is uncommon, despite some recent fatalities following unexpected exposure to peanut allergens.[39]

COW'S MILK PROTEIN INTOLERANCE

Although not entirely easy to compartmentalize, true allergies to cow's milk protein do commonly appear to induce reaginic-type responses in susceptible infants and children. The almost universal decrease in breast feeding in most developed countries seems to have made cow's milk protein intolerance an important cause of infant morbidity.[102] Since most infants develop antibodies to milk proteins without adverse effect, diagnosis is dependent on clinical response to cow's milk ingestion, or challenge. Its true incidence is about 2%.[57] Those affected will react within the first few months of life.[52] Symptoms due to (or concurrent with) lactose intolerance, resulting from absence or low levels of the brush border membrane hydrolase β-galactosidase, should be excluded by giving breast milk which has a high content of lactose.

The problem arises as to the role of concurrent infection to which all neonates and young children are subject as they slowly mature and respond to environmental microbial challenge. Some clinicians[55] argue that the milk allergy is precipitated by a specific infective event, whereas others indicate that removal of cow's milk from the feed permits resolution of infection and diarrhoea. However, this train of events is reminiscent of latent gluten sensitivity and tropical enteropathies, both of which may become clinically apparent as a result of acute infection (Fig. 17.3): thus, in terms of individuals predestined to develop intestinal cell-mediated responses, recurrent episodes of diarrhoea may awaken a latent susceptibility and result in the onset of clinical symptoms. Thus, where milk sensitivity appears to follow an acute gastro-intestinal illness, its diagnosis is only valid after exclusion of persistent bacterial gastroenteritis, giardiasis or secondary lactase deficiency (by biopsy enzyme assay).[52]

Clinical features

Intestinal symptoms, such as acute diarrhoea, colic, vomiting, acidosis and dehydration, predominate, which may simulate an

Cow's milk protein intolerance

Constitutional syndrome
- failure to thrive
- Vomiting
- Weight loss

Diarrhoeal syndrome
- Weight loss
- Steatorrhoea
- Abdominal distension

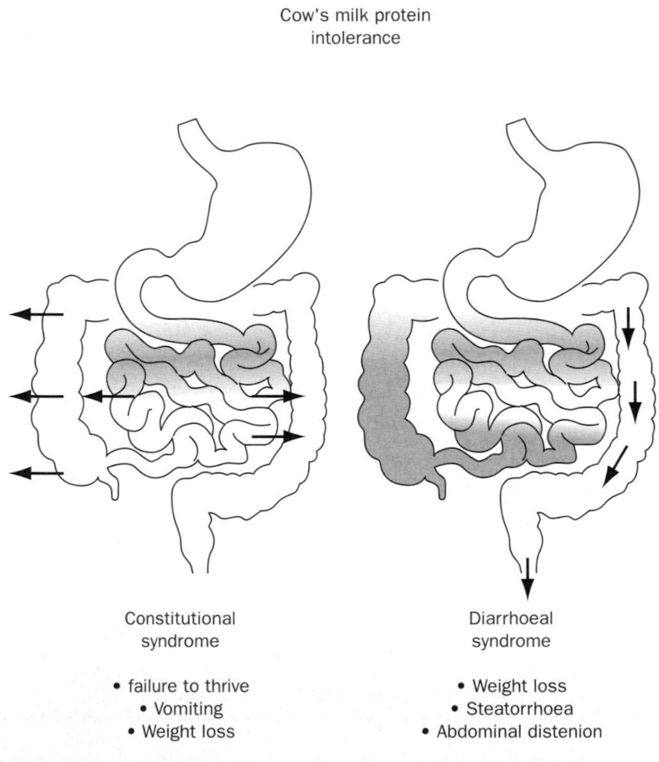

Fig. 17.3 In cow's milk protein intolerance, the mucosal lesion, as in gluten sensitivity, is severe proximally but becomes progressively attenuated distally, so that only 30–50% of the entire small intestine is involved. Adaptive hyperplasia of the distal jejunum and ileum may therefore compensate for the upper segmental defect, leading to a state of latent compensation. Children with cow's milk protein intolerance may either (i) never be diagnosed, (ii) present with a constitutive syndrome of vomiting and failure to thrive or (iii) develop a severe malabsorption syndrome in which the distal compensating segment is itself destabilized through microbial action (via toxins, cytotoxicity or cytopathogenicity). The latter is probably the most common presentation, because it is during the first 2 years of life, when children gradually developing immunity to a wide range of pathogenic organisms which invade the gastrointestinal tract, usually succumb to these effects.

infective entity in young infants, or chronic diarrhoea with vomiting and failure to thrive in older infants. These may also be associated with faecal blood loss, failure of weight gain, abdominal protuberance and hypotonia.

In a computerized analysis of symptoms developing after application of a strict challenge protocol, Hill and colleagues[52] divided their 100 patients into three cohorts.

Immediate reactions

(i) 26 infants reacted within 45 min of challenge. A large proportion developed circumoral or other cutaneous eruptions, while 1 in 3 developed respiratory symptoms like wheezing, coughing or rhinitis: rarely stridor occurred. The mean age of this group of infants was 15 months and all had positive skin reactions to cow's milk proteins.

Late reactions

(ii) 57 children developed symptoms within 20 hours of challenge, which were largely confined to the gastrointestinal tract, with skin pallor, vomiting and diarrhoea. Review of these individuals although of similar age (12 months) revealed evidence of instability and failure to thrive: skin reactivity in this group was negligible.

Delayed reactions

(iii) The remaining 17 patients developed symptoms >20 hours after challenge, of which >50% developed diarrhoea, or respiratory symptoms. Eczema was also more common to this reactive group, whose mean age was 30 months. Patients with eczema had positive skin tests.

Mechanisms of reactions

Although mechanisms for reactivity in each of the three groups identified were not addressed in this study, it seems likely that the response (group (i)), which occurred within 1 hour of challenge was due to IgE-mediated allergic sensitization, as has been noted by other previous investigators.[31,48,51,102]

T-cell reactivity

By contrast, in the intestinal form of cow's milk allergy, reaginic antibody levels are low, or absent.[29,30,51] This suggests that slower, evolving reactions of intestinal type (group (ii)) develop through other mechanisms, and are probably associated with the cellular and architectural changes characteristic of local T-cell-mediated reactivity.[56,60] These could also lie dormant and be awakened by infection; the infective process is associated with enterocyte damage, reductions in membrane hydrolase activity and involvement in other parts of the intestine beyond that damaged directly by the milk protein sensitivity. Walker-Smith[108] has suggested the occurrence of primary (immunological), and secondary (post-infectious/mucosal damage), forms of cow's milk protein intolerance. The other possibility is that the (infective) insult merely awakened what was already present in the upper intestine (even though latent) (see Fig. 17.3). After all, if several children with life-long gluten sensitivity can escape detection in early life because their lesion remains latent, why not those with cow's milk hypersensitivity as well? Indeed, the symptomatic children may merely represent the small tip of yet another intestinal hypersensitivity iceberg induced by milk protein.

Complement activation

The evidence for complement activation[112] and consumption is least convincing and not well represented in the literature regarding cow's milk allergy. Such a mechanism could, however, underlie the morbilliform and eczematous skin reactions observed in reactions of intermediate/late timing (groups (ii) and (iii) above).

Given the rather broad and differing rates of presentation of cow's milk protein intolerance, it is not surprising that diagnosis cannot be made by any single test, but only by reproducible responses to milk challenge under suitably controlled conditions, as indicated by other studies.[33,48]

Most children with cow's milk protein intolerance tolerate milk satisfactorily by 3 years of age, but a small number continue to have symptoms beyond this age and require continued milk restriction. When elimination diets are used in children it is vitally important that the diet is nutritionally adequate for the growing child. Elimination diets can be hazardous[32] and it is essential that a paediatrician and/or dietician regularly supervises them.

Non-immune causes of milk intolerance

The exclusion of common non-immune causes of gastrointestinal milk intolerance is very important and this can be done by following the protocol of Davidson *et al.*[33] Stool microscopy, culture and electron microscopy exclude most infectious causes. The initial small bowel biopsy further excludes giardiasis and sucrase–isomaltase deficiency and provides a basis for interpreting post-challenge mucosal changes.

Soya sensitivity

Sensitivity to soya protein, which also causes cell-mediated-type mucosal lesions of the intestinal tract[4] is often associated with cow's milk hypersensitivity.[57] Although it is usual for these syndromes to spontaneously revert by the age of 2–3 years, it is reasonable to recommend avoidance of all foods that may give rise to similar forms of short-term sensitization, including gluten, fish, eggs and soya. Since these conditions recover spontaneously, they are clearly different from the lifelong, genetically determined form of gluten sensitivity: their origin may be thus related to a transient failure of the intestinal immune system to tolerize the individual to these dietary proteins.[71]

CONCLUSIONS

This chapter briefly surveys the field of food 'allergic' reactivity, its presumptive pathogenetic mechanisms and the intestinal lesions that might be expected, in particular, within the jejunal mucosa. In general, it will be appreciated that our knowledge and understanding of cell-mediated intestinal pathology and of reaginic-(IgE)-mediated mucosal reactions has progressed considerably over the last few decades.

Nevertheless, precise details of all the cellular and molecular events that are recruited, and why they should occur in only some individuals, still require elucidation. These are important questions that need to be addressed in the future in order to further dissect pathogenesis in molecular–genetic terms. Nevertheless, in these conditions, there are now several specific features within target tissues that can be evaluated and perhaps utilized as precise diagnostic aids.

There can be no doubt that ingestion of a food antigen sometimes sensitizes the individual for potentially harmful immune responses to foods, so that food allergic syndromes result when the food is subsequently encountered. The mechanisms whereby active immunity and/or tolerance are induced and maintained are not completely understood either, even for the much-investigated inbred mouse. However, while a variety of mechanisms is likely to be involved in the creation and modulation of the state of oral tolerance, their manipulation in the clinical situation could provide entirely new approaches to the effective management of gastrointestinal allergic disease.

Our understanding of other presumed allergic responses in the infantile and adult human intestine, whether IgE-mediated or not, is less secure. This difficulty is compounded by the lack of data on IgE plasma cells in the human intestinal mucosa and by the fact that 'IgE-positive cells' may include mast cells in addition to IgE-secreting plasma cells. Secondly, it is difficult to measure local release of mast cell products discharged by cross-linking of IgE. At present, therefore, we are still only able to operate at the clinical level by conducting rigid double-blind challenges with the likely offending foods. The prevalence of food reactions, however, is increasing and thus in order to combat this rising epidemic, further stringent methodologies will have to be used in the future. These will include sophisticated chemical technology to isolate, and identify, the provoking antigens from allergenic foodstuffs. Furthermore, it may be necessary to replace crude tests (skin-prick, RAST) by more specific and reproducible in-vitro techniques in affected individuals, in order to improve the diagnostic precision which, at present, we lack at clinical level. But this is another 'challenge' for the clinical scientist of tomorrow.

REFERENCES

1   Aas K. Studies of hypersensitivity to fish. *Int Arch Allergy* 1966; 29: 346–63.

2   Aas K, Jebsen JW. Studies of hypersensitivity to fish: partial purification and crystallization of a major allergenic component of cod. *Int Arch Allergy* 1967; 32: 1–20.

3   Afzalpurkar R, Schiller L, Little K, Santangelo W, Fordtran JS. The self-limited nature of chronic idiopathic diarrhoea. *N Engl J Med* 1992; 327: 1849–1952.

4   Ament ME, Rubin C. Soy protein – another cause of the flat lesion. *Gastroenterology* 1972; 62: 227–34.

5   Amlot PL, Kemeny DM, Zachary C, Parkes P, Lessof MH. Oral allergy syndrome (OAS): symptoms of IgE-mediated hypersensitivity to foods. *Clin Allergy* 1987; 17: 33–42.

6   Anderson IH, Levine AS, Levitt MD. Incomplete absorption of the carbohydrate in all-purpose wheat flour. *N Engl J Med* 1981; 304: 891–2.

7   Anderson JA. The establishment of common language concerning adverse reactions to food and food additives. *J Allergy Clin Immunol* 1986; 78: 140–4.

8   Atkins FM, Steinberg SS, Metcalfe DD. Evaluation of immediate adverse reactions to foods in adult patients. I – Correlation of demographic, laboratory, and prick skin test data with response to controlled oral food challenge. *J Allergy Clin Immunol* 1985; 75: 348–55.

9   Baird AW, Barclay WS, Blazer-Yost BL, Cuthbert AW. Affinity purified immunoglobulin G transfers immediate hypersensitivity to guinea pig colonic epithelium in vitro. *Gastroenterology* 1987; 92: 635–42.

10 Baird AW, Cuthbert AW. Neuronal involvement in type 1 hypersensitivity reactions in gut epithelium. *Br J Pharmacol* 1987; 92: 647–55.

11 Baird AW, Cuthbert AW, Pearce FL. Immediate hypersensitivity reactions in epithelia from rats infected with *Nippostrongylus braziliensis*. *Br J Pharmacol* 1985; 85: 787–95.

12 Barron DA, Baird AW, Cuthbert AW, Margolius HS. Intestinal anaphylaxis: rapid changes in mucosal ion transport and morphology. *Am J Physiol* 1988; 254: G307–14.

13 Bengsston U, Nilsson-Balknäs, Hanson LÅ, Ahlstedt S. Double blind, placebo controlled food reactions do not correlate to IgE allergy in the diagnosis of staple food related gastrointestinal symptoms. *Gut* 1996; 39: 130–5.

14 Berin CM, Kilian AJ, Yang P, Groot J, Taminiau J, Perdue MH. Rapid transepithelial antigen transport in rat jejunum: impact of sensitization and the hypersensitivity reaction. *Gastroenterology* 1997; 113: 856–64.

15 Bidat E, Tannery B, Lagardere B. Choc anaphylactique par allergie alimentaire: issue fatale malgré l'injection très précoce d'adrénaline. *Arch Fr Pediatr* 1993; 50: 361.

16 Bock SA. A critical evaluation of clinical trials in adverse reactions to foods in children. *J Allergy Clin Immunol* 1986; 78: 165–74.

17 Bock SA. Prospective appraisal of complaints of adverse reactions to food in children during the first three years of life. *Pediatrics* 1987; 79: 683–8.

18 Bock SA. Food challenges in the diagnosis of food hypersensitivity. In: de Weck AL, Sampson HA (eds) *Intestinal Immunology and Food Allergy*, Nestle Nutrition Workshop Series No 34. Vevey/Raven, New York, 1995; 105–17.

19 Brandeis J, Sayegh M, Gallon L. Rat intestinal epithelial cells present MHC complex allopeptides to primed T cells. *Gastroenterology* 1994; 107: 1537–42.

20 Brunner M, Walzer M. Absorption of undigested proteins in human beings: the absorption of unaltered fish proteins in adults. *Arch Int Med* 1928; 42: 172–9.

21 Castro GA, Harari Y, Russell DA. Mediators of anaphylaxis-induced ion transport changes in small intestine. *Am J Physiol* 1987; 253: G540–8.

22 Cherner JA, Jensen RT, Dubois A, O'Dorisio T, Gardner JD, Metcalfe DD. Gastrointestinal dysfunction in systemic mastocytosis. *Gastroenterology* 1988; 95: 667–75.

23 Colgan SP, Resnick M, Parkos C *et al.* IL-4 directly modulates function of a model human intestinal epithelium. *J Immunol* 1994; 153: 2122–9.

24 Collins SP, McHugh K, Jacobson K *et al.* Previous inflammation alters the response of the rat colon to stress. *Gastroenterology* 1996; 111: 1509–15.

25 Crowe SE, Perdue MH. Gastrointestinal food hypersensitivity: basic mechanisms of pathophysiology. *Gastroenterology* 1992; 103: 1075–95.

26 Curtis G, Patrick M, Catto-Smith A, Gall DG. Intestinal anaphylaxis in the rat. Effect of chronic antigen exposure. *Gastroenterology* 1990; 98: 1558–66.

27 D'Inca R, Ramage JK, Hunt RH, Perdue MH. Antigen-induced damage and restitution in the small intestine of the immunized rat. *Int Arch Allergy Appl Immunol* 1990; 91: 270–7.

28 D'Inca R, Hunt RH, Perdue MH. Mucosal damage during intestinal anaphylaxis in the rat. Effect of betamethasone and disodium and disodium cromoglycate. *Dig Dis Sci* 1992; 37: 1704–8.

29 Dannaeus A, Johansson SGO, Foncard T, Ohman S. Clinical and immunological aspects of food allergy in childhood. I – Estimation of IgG, IgA and IgE antibodies to food antigens in children with food allergy and atopic dermatitis. *Acta Paediatr Scand* 1977; 66: 31–7.

30 Dannaeus A, Johansson SGO, Foncard T, Ohman S. Clinical and immunological aspects of food allergy in childhood. II – Development of allergic symptoms and humoral immune response to foods in infants of atopic mothers during the first 24 months of life. *Acta Paediatr Scand* 1978; 67: 497–504.

31 Dannaeus A, Johansson SGO. A follow-up study of infants with adverse reactions to cow's milk. I – Serum IgE, skin test reactions and RAST in relation to clinical course. *Acta Paediatr Scand* 1979; 68: 377–82.

32 David TJ, Waddington E, Stanton RH. Nutritional hazards of elimination diets in children with atopic eczema. *Arch Dis Child* 1984; 59: 323–5.

33 Davidson GP, Hill DJ, Townley RRW. Gastrointestinal milk allergy in childhood: a rational approach. *Med J Austr* 1976; 1: 945–7.

34 Dignass A, Podolsky D. Cytokine modulation of intestinal epithelial cell restitution: central role of transforming growth factor beta. *Gastroenterology* 1993; 105: 1323–32.

35 Dolovich J, Punthakee ND, MacMillan AB et al. Systemic mastocytosis: control of lifelong diarrhoea by ingested disodium cromoglycate. *Canad Med Assoc J* 1974; 111: 684–5.

36 Dupont C. Evaluation of intestinal permeability in food hypersensitivity disorders. In: de Weck AL, Sampson HA (eds) *Intestinal Immunology and Food Allergy*, Nestle Nutrition Workshop Series No 34. Vevey/Raven, New York, 1995; 73–91.

37 Elsayed S, Bennich H. The primary structure of allergen M from cod. *Scand J Immunol* 1975; 4: 203–8.

38 Elsayed S, Apold J. Immunochemical analysis of cod fish allergen M: locations of the immunoglobulin binding sites as demonstrated by the native and synthetic peptides. *Allergy* 1983; 38: 449–59.

39 Evans S, Skea D, Dolovitch J. Fatal reaction to peanut antigen in almond icing. *Canad Med Assoc J* 1988; 139: 231–2.

40 Fälth-Magnusson K. Dietary restrictions during pregnancy. In: de Weck AL, Sampson HA (eds) *Intestinal Immunology and Food Allergy*, Nestle Nutrition Workshop Series No 34. Vevey/Raven, New York, 1995; 191–201.

41 Farah DA, Calder J, Benson L, Mackenzie JF. Specific food intolerances: its place as a cause of gastrointestinal symptoms. *Gut* 1985; 26: 164–8.

42 Ferguson A, Mowat A, Strobel S, Barnetson R. T-cell mediated immunity in food allergy. *Ann Allergy* 1983; 51: 246–8.

43 Ferguson A. Food-allergic disorders. In: Booth CC and Neale G (eds) *Disorders of the Small Intestine*. Blackwells, Oxford, 1985; 118–34.

44 Ferguson A. Models of immunologically-driven small intestinal damage. In: Marsh MN (ed.) *The Immunopathology of the Small Intestine*. Wiley, Chichester, 1987; 225–52.

45 Ferguson A. Adverse reactions to food. *Human Toxicol* 1987; 6: 339–341.

46 Fiorini G, Rinaldi G, Bigi G, Sironi D, Cremonini LM. Symptoms of respiratory allergies are worse in subjects with co-existing food sensitization. *Clin Exp Allergy* 1990; 20: 689–92.

47 Forbes D, Patrick M, Perdue M, Buret A, Gall DG. Intestinal anaphylaxis: in vivo and in vitro studies of the rat proximal colon. *Am J Physiol* 1988; 255: G201–5.

48 Goldman AS, Anderson DW, Sellers W, Saperstein S, Knilar W, Halpern SR. Milk allergy. I – Oral challenge with milk and isolated milk proteins in allergic children. *Pediatrics* 1963; 32: 425–43.

49 Hansen TK, Bindslev-Jansen C. Codfish allergy in adults: identification of diagnosis. *Allergy* 1992; 47: 610–17.

50 Hershberg R, Nepom GT. Regulation of antigen presentation by an intestinal epithelial cell line. *J Clin Invest* 1997; 100: 204–15.

51 Hill DJ, Davidson GP, Cameron DJ, Barnes GL. The spectrum of cow's milk allergy in childhood. *Acta Paediatr Scand* 1979; 68: 847–52.

52 Hill DJ, Ford RPK, Shelton MJ, Hosking CS. A study of 100 infants and young children with cow's milk allergy. *Clin Rev Allergy* 1984; 2: 125–42.

53 Hoffman DR, Day ED, Miller JS. The major heat stable allergen of shrimp. *Ann Allergy* 1981; 47: 17–22.

54 Huang Q, Coleman JW, Stanworth DR. Investigation of the allergenicity of β-lactoglobulin and its cleavage fragments. *Int Arch Allergy & Appl Immunol* 1985; 78: 337–44.

55 Hutchins P, Walker-Smith JA. The gastrointestinal system. In: Brostoff J, Challacombe SJ (eds) *Food Allergy*. Saunders, London, 1982; 43–76.

56 Iyngkaran N, Yadav M. Food allergy. In: Marsh MN (ed) *Immunopathology of the Small Intestine*. Wiley, Chichester, 1987; 415–49.

57 Jakobsson I, Linberg T. A prospective study of cow's milk protein intolerance in Swedish infants. *Acta Paediatr Scand* 1979; 68: 853–8.

58 Kajosaari M. Food allergy in Finnish children aged 1 to 6 years. *Acta Paediatr Scand* 1982; 71: 815–19.

59 Kidd JM, Cohen SH, Sosman AJ, Fink JN. Food-dependent exercise-induced anaphylaxis. *J Allergy Clin Immunol* 1983; 71: 407–11.

60 Kuitenen P, Rapola J, Savilahti E, Visakorpi J. Response of the jejunal mucosa to cow's milk in the malabsorption syndrome with cow's milk intolerance. *Acta Paediatr Scand* 1973; 62: 585–95.

D

61 Kunitz M. Crystalline soybean and inhibitor. II – General principles. *J Gen Physiol* 1946; 30: 290–310.

62 Lessof MH. Food intolerance and allergy – A review. *Quart J Med* 1983; 206: 111–19.

63 Lessof MH, Wraith DG, Merrett TG, Buisseret PD. Food allergy and intolerance in 100 patients – local and systemic effects. *Quart J Med* 1980; 49: 259–71.

64 Lloyd-Still JD. Chronic diarrhoea of childhood and misuse of elimination diets. *J Paediatr* 1979; 95: 10–13.

65 Lovegrove JA, Osman DL, Morgan JB, Hampton SM. Transfer of cow's milk β-lactoglobulin to human serum after a milk load: a pilot study. *Gut* 1993; 34: 203–7.

66 MacDonald TT. T cell mediated intestinal injury. In: Marsh MN (ed). *Coeliac Disease*. Blackwell Scientific Publications, Oxford, 1992; 283–304.

67 Madara JL, Stafford J. Interferon gamma directly affects barrier junction of cultured intestinal epithelial cell monolayers. *J Clin Invest* 1989; 83: 724–7.

68 Marsh MN. Studies of intestinal lymphoid tissue. XI – The immunopathology of cell-mediated reactions in gluten-sensitivity and other enteropathies. *Scanning Microsc* 1988; 2: 1663–84.

69 Marsh MN. The mucosal pathology of gluten-sensitivity. In: Marsh MN (ed) *Coeliac Disease*. Blackwell Scientific Publications, Oxford; 1992; 136–91.

70 Marsh MN Coeliac disease. In: Marsh MN (ed) *Immunopathology of the Small Intestine*. Wiley, Chichester, 1987; 371–99.

71 Marsh MN, Cummins A. The interactive role of mucosal T lymphocytes in intestinal growth, development and enteropathy. *J Gastroenterol Hepatology* 1993; 8: 270–8.

72 Marshall J. Repeated antigen challenges in rats induces a mucosal mast cell hyperplasia. *Gastroenterology* 1993; 105: 391–8.

73 Maulitz RM, Pratt DS, Shocket AL. Exercise-induced anaphylactic reaction to shellfish. *J Allergy Clin Immunol* 1979; 63: 433–4.

74 Mayer L. Putting up a different front for food hypersensitivity. *Gastroenterology* 1997; 113: 1034–6.

75 Metcalfe DD. Food allergy. In: Ogra PL, Strober W, Mestecky J et al (eds) *Handbook of Mucosal Immunology*. Academic Press, London, 1994; 493–504.

76 Miller HRP. Immunopathology of nematode infestation and expulsion. In: Marsh MN (ed) *Immunopathology of the Small Intestine*. Wiley, Chichester, 1987; 177–208.

77 Miller JB. Hidden food ingredients, chemical food additive and incomplete food labels. *Ann Allergy* 1978; 41: 93–8.

78 Moneret-Vautrin DA. Masked food allergens. In: de Weck AL, Sampson HA (eds) *Intestinal Immunology and Food Allergy*, Nestle Nutrition Workshop Series No 34. Vevey/Raven, New York; 1995: 249–57.

79 Moroz LA, Yang WH. Kunitz soybean trypsin inhibitor: a specific allergen in food anaphylaxis. *N Engl J Med* 1980; 302: 1126–8.

80 Mowat AM, Felstein MV. Intestinal graft-versus-host reactions in experimental animals. In: Burakoff SJ, Ferrara J (eds), Dekker, New York, 1989; 205–44.

81 Nagpal S, Rajappa L, Metcalfe DD, Subba Rao P. Isolation and characterisation of heat-stable allergens from shrimp (*P endens indicus*). *J Allergy Clin Immunol* 1989; 83: 26–36.

82 Nanda R, James R, Smith H, Dudley CRK, Jewell DP. Food intolerance and irritable bowel syndrome. *Gut* 1989; 30: 1099–1104.

83 Neale G, Booth CC. Infiltrative lesions. In: Booth CC, Neale G (eds) *Disorders of the Small Intestine*. Blackwells, Oxford, 1985; 218–30.

84 Nøgaard A, Bindslev-Jensen C. Egg and milk allergy in adults. *Allergy* 1992; 47: 503–9.

85 Nordlee J, Atkins F, Bush R, Taylor S. Anaphylaxis from undeclared walnut in commercially pressed cookies. *J Allergy Clin Immunol* 1993; 91: 154 (Abstr 56).

86 Paganelli R, Cavagni G, Pallone F. The role of antigenic absorption and circulating immune complexes in food allergy. *Ann Allergy* 1986; 57: 330–6.

87 Patrick MK, Dunn IJ, Buret A *et al*. Mast cell protease release and mucosal ultrastructure during intestinal anaphylaxis in the rat. *Gastroenterology* 1988; 94: 1–9.

88 Perdue MH, Forstner JF, Roomi NW, Gall DG. Epithelial response to intestinal anaphylaxis in rats: goblet cell secretion and enterocyte damage. *Am J Physiol* 1984; 247: G632–7.

89 Perdue MH, Chung M, Gall DG. Effect of intestinal anaphylaxis on gut function in the rat. *Gastroenterology* 1984; 86: 391–7.

90 Perdue MH, Gall DG. Intestinal anaphylaxis in the rat: jejunal response to in vitro antigen exposure. *Am J Physiol* 1986; 250: G427–31.

91 Ramage JK, Stanisz A, Scicchitano R, Hunt RH, Perdue MH. Effect of immunologic reactions on rat intestinal epithelium. Correlation of increased permeability to ^{51}Cr-EDTA and ovalbumin during acute inflammation and anaphylaxis. *Gastroenterology* 1988; 94: 1367–75.

92 Reinecker H-C, Podolsky D. Human intestinal epithelial cells express functional cytokine receptors sharing the common gamma chain of the IL-2 receptor. *Proc Natl Acad Sci USA* 1995; 92: 8353–7.

93 Rioux KP, Wallace JL. Long-term antigen challenge results in progressively diminished mucosal mast cell degranulation in rats. *Gastroenterology* 1996; 111: 1516–23.

94 Royal College of Physicians/British Nutrition Foundation. A report on Food Intolerance and Food Aversion. *J Roy Coll Phys (Lond)* 1984; 18: (No. 2).

95 Rumessen JJ, Gudmand-Høyer E. Functional bowel disease: malabsorption and abdominal distress after ingestion of fructose, sorbitol, and fructose–sorbitol mixtures. *Gastroenterology* 1988; 95: 694–700.

96 Russell DA, Castro GA. Anaphylactic-like reaction of small intestinal epithelium in parasitized guinea pigs. *Immunology* 1985; 54: 573–9.

97 Sachs MI, Jones RT, Yunginger JW. Isolation and partial characterization of a major peanut allergen. *J Allergy Clin Immunol* 1981; 67: 27–34.

98 Sampson HA. Role of immediate food hypersensitivity in the pathogenesis of atopic dermatitis. *J Allergy Clin Immunol* 1983; 71: 473–80.

99 Sampson HA, Mendelson L, Rosen JP. Fatal and near fatal anaphylactic reactions to food in children and adolescents. *N Engl J Med* 1992; 327: 380–4.

100 Sampson HA, Metcalfe DD. Food allergies. *J Am Med Assoc* 1992; 268: 2840–4.

101 Sampson HA. Nonintestinal manifestations of food hypersensitivity. In: de Weck AL, Sampson HA (eds) *Intestinal Immunology and Food Allergy*, Nestle Nutrition Workshop Series No 34. Vevey/Raven, New York, 1995; 119–29.

102 Savilahti E. Cow's milk allergy. *Allergy* 1981; 36: 73–88.

103 Shibaski M, Suzuki S, Tajima S, Nemoto H, Kuroume T. Allergenicity of major component proteins of soybean. *Int Arch Allergy Appl Immunol* 1980; 61: 441–8.

104 Sjölander A, Magnusson K-E. Effects of antigen challenge on intestinal permeability and morphology in rats immunized with gliadin or ovalbumin. *Int Arch Allergy Appl Immunol* 1987; 84: 284–90.

105 Soter NA, Austen F, Wasserman SI. Oral disodium cromoglycate in the treatment of systemic mastocytosis. *New Engl J Med* 1979; 301: 465–9.

106 Suarez F, Saviano DA, Levitt MD. The treatment of lactose intolerance. *Aliment Pharmacol Ther* 1995; 9: 589–97.

107 Talley NJ. Eosinophilic gastroenteritis. In: Feldman M, Scharsschmidt B, Sleisenger MH (eds) *Gastrointestinal and Liver Disease*, 6th edn, Vol. 2. Saunders, Philadelphia, 1998; 1679–88.

108 Walker-Smith JA. *Diseases of the Small Intestine in Childhood*, 3rd edn. Blackwell, London, 1988.

109 Walzer M. Absorption of allergens. *J Allergy* 1992; 13: 554–62.

110 Webster ADB. Immune deficiency. In: Booth CC, Neale G (eds) *Disorders of the Small Intestine*. Blackwells, Oxford; 1985; 218–30.

111 Wilson SJ, Walzer M. Absorption of undigested proteins in human beings. IV – Absorption of unaltered egg protein in infants and in children. *Am J Dis Child* 1935; 50: 49–54.

112 Yadav M, Iyngkaran N. Immunological studies in cow's milk protein-sensitive enteropathy. *Archiv Dis Child* 1981; 56: 24–30.

113 Young E, Patel S, Stoneham M, Rona R, Wilkinson JD. The prevalence of reaction to food additives in a survey population. *J R Coll Phys (Lond)* 1987; 21: 241–7.

114 Yunginger JW, Sweeney K, Sturner WQ *et al*. Fatal food-induced anaphylaxis. *J Am Med Assoc* 1988; 260: 1450–2.

115 Zeiger RS, Heller S, Mellon MH *et al*. Effect of combined maternal and infant food-allergen avoidance on development of atopy in early infancy: a randomised study. *J Allerg Clin Immunol* 1989; 84: 72–89.

116 Zeiger RS. Breast-feeding and dietary avoidance. In: de Weck AL, Sampson HA (eds) *Intestinal Immunology and Food Allergy*, Nestle Nutrition Workshop Series No 34. Vevey/Raven, New York, 1995; 203–22.

117 Zoppi G, Deganello A, Gaburro D. Persistent post-enteritis diarrhoea. *Eur J Paediat* 1977; 126: 225–36.

Chapter 18

Animal models of food sensitivity

Christopher R. Stokes, Michael Bailey and Paul W. Bland

INTRODUCTION

During the course of a lifetime it has been calculated that an individual may consume between 100 and 700 tons of food. For the average British citizen this is likely to include some 550 poultry, 36 pigs, 36 sheep, eight oxen, 10 000 eggs, and dairy products (milk, butter, cheese, etc.) equivalent to 18 tonnes of milk. As if that were not sufficient a challenge, the homeostasis within the intestine is further complicated by the presence of 10^5–10^{11} bacteria (pathogenic and non-pathogenic) per gram of mucus and the constant turnover of gut epithelial cells. Add to that the fact that this complicated interaction is required to take place over a vast surface area (upward of 400 m²), and one can hardly be surprised at the high incidence of inappropriate responses to dietary components and the resultant food allergic reactions. Despite the obvious morbidity associated with food allergic reactions and the heightened public awareness of their importance, progress in unravelling the mechanisms involved since the first edition of this book has been painfully slow. In an

attempt to start to determine the mechanisms responsible for damaging responses to food antigens, the use of a number of animal models has been explored. The authors of many of these studies have restricted themselves to the analysis of systemic humoral (often immunoglobulin E; IgE) and cellular responses, but for the purpose of this chapter we have chosen to focus almost exclusively on models which have clearly been shown to result in gut pathology.

For any food-derived allergen to cause pathology it must first pass through the mucosal barrier, a process which is discussed in detail elsewhere in this volume (Chapters 9 and 13). Briefly, it has been shown that, after feeding, a small proportion (less than 0.005%) of any feed is absorbed intact and can be detected in mesenteric blood.[96] Significantly, it has been shown that, whereas serum collected from mice 1 h after feeding ovalbumin was capable of transferring suppression to naïve mice, serum collected after 5 min was non-tolerogenic. Recent biochemical analysis of these sera has revealed that in the 1-h sera, in addition to native ovalbumin, it was possible to detect two additional fragments with apparent molecular weights of 21 000 and 24 000 daltons.[29] The precise cellular mechanisms whereby this antigen is taken up from the gut lumen have not been established. While there is substantial evidence to document the uptake of antigen via M cells in the Peyer's patches, the route involving enterocytes and uptake into the lamina propria is unclear.

The mucosal immune system associated with the gastrointestinal tract is capable of recognizing and responding to antigens presented via the gastrointestinal tract. Moreover, it is able to recognize and distinguish between potential pathogens and harmless dietary antigens, and mount a response that is appropriate. An understanding of this recognition process is critical, for not only will it hold the key to the control and prevention of food allergic reactions but also to the development of vaccines that will protect against a whole range of enteric pathogens.

RODENTS

For reasons both of economy and the availability of an impressive armoury of well defined reagents (antibodies, nucleotide probes, inbred, transgenic and 'knock out' strains), the majority of studies of animal models have been focused on rodents. Experimental regimes have been described for rats and mice to show that both humoral and cellular mechanisms may be involved in gut pathology.

Humoral-mediated damage
While in a number of rodent systems methods of immunization have been developed to stimulate the production of IgE antibodies,[55,77] few have attempted to demonstrate whether such responses lead to intestinal anaphylaxis. Similarly, many models have involved parenteral immunization with adjuvants and only rarely has sensitization been achieved by the oral route.[13,37,39,48] Whilst the difficulty in achieving sensitivity via this route is explainable by the induction of oral tolerance (for review see reference 93 and Chapter 14), the physiological relevance of studies involving 'unnatural' routes of immunization must always be questioned.

Reaginic (IgE) antibody
The increase in leakage of plasma proteins into the gut in association with subepithelial oedema[67] has been used as an indicator of intestinal anaphylaxis. Thus, Byars and Ferraresi[20] showed that rats sensitized by injection of ovalbumin and *Bordetella pertussis* adjuvant and subsequently injected intra-venously with ^{125}I-labelled bovine serum albumin (BSA) immediately before oral challenge with ovalbumin had greatly increased levels of radioactivity in intestinal tissue compared with non-sensitized controls. Since the sera from sensitized rats gave positive 24-h passive cutaneous anaphylaxis (PCA) tests, reaginic antibody was the likely effector mechanism. Similar studies showed that homologous radiolabelled serum albumin (RSA) could also be used to demonstrate the accumulation of plasma proteins in intestinal secretions and gut segments.[52]

Recently, Ito *et al.*[37] have shown that simple feeding of casein to mice induces raised systemic IgE levels. This induction is accompanied by Th2 cytokine profiles in spleen, liver and MLN, suggesting that this may be a valuable model for defining local and systemic T cell control of IgE responses induced by dietary antigen. This model also highlights the differences between dietary proteins in their capacity to overcome tolerance mechanisms and induce hypersensitivity – feeding of ovalbumin, for example, induces tolerance.

The feeding regime (daily, ad lib, etc.) also appears to be important to the generation of sytemic reaginic antibodies. For example, in a recently described BN rat model, although both IgG and IgE responses were generated by daily feeding of Ova, ad lib feeding induced only an IgG anti-Ova response.[48] Confirmation that IgE antibody could lead to intestinal anaphylaxis was provided by passive transfer studies; serum from rats containing high levels of IgE anti-ovalbumin being able to promote release of intestinal goblet cell mucus upon intraduodenal challenge.[52] A further indicator of intestinal anaphylaxis is histamine levels in intraluminal contents which rise 15 min after antigen challenge and continue to increase for up to 1 h.[50] Further similar studies[76] have demonstrated a reduction of absorption of water, sodium, potassium and calcium within 10 min of intraluminal perfusion of ovalbumin in parenterally sensitized rats. There was also a reduction in gut tissue histamine content and in the numbers of granulated mucosal mast cells. Mucosal oedema was observed but there were no changes in villus height or crypt depth, and mucosal permeability was unchanged (Table 18.1). Other, more recent, studies[99] using intragastric challenge of mice with Ova after systemic priming with alum-precipitated Ova – a model widely used in rats in the 1970s – have shown mucosal mast cell activation, which was blocked, after challenge, by anti-IL-4 or anti-IL-10. It is important that older data on IgE induction and local mast cell activation after oral challenge are readdressed in the light of more recent advances in cytokine control mechanisms.

Comparison of the features of immediate type hypersensitivity reactions and cell-mediated immune (CMI) reactions described in rodent models of food allergy	
Humoral-mediated (immediate) reactions	**Cell-mediated reactions (CMI)**
Subepithelial oedema	Crypt hyperplasia
Histamine content: gut lumen ⇑	Villus atrophy
Histamine content: gut tissue ⇓	Intraepithelial lymphocytes ⇑
Leakage of plasma proteins	Changes in brush border enzymes
Goblet cell mucus release	Goblet cell number ⇑
Malabsorption: H_2O, K^+, Na^+, Cl^-	Xylose absorption ⇓
	Secretory epithelial cells ⇑
	Absorptive epithelial cells ⇓

Table 18.1 Comparison of the features of immediate type hypersensitivity reactions and cell-mediated immune (CMI) reactions described in rodent models of food allergy.

Other immunoglobulin isotypes

In addition to damage mediated by IgE, other isotypes have also been implicated. Instilling immune complexes (presumably IgG) in antibody excess into the duodenum of rats has been shown to result in goblet cell mucus discharge.[102] However, it has been shown[51] that, while rats orally immunized with 100 mg of BSA on 5 consecutive days and then weekly for 5 weeks, showed enhanced release of goblet cell mucus upon intestinal challenge, those immunized by intraperitoneal injection in complete Freund's adjuvant and having high levels of serum antibodies did not. Such studies emphasize not only the importance of the type of adjuvant but also the route of immunization, in determining the clinical outcome.

Cell-mediated hypersensitivity

Most of the evidence that feeding soluble antigen may lead to a cell-mediated immune reaction capable of causing changes in gut morphology is based on work carried out using contact sensitizing agents. It has been shown[19] that feeding a contact sensitizing agent resulted in xylose malabsorption and changes in intestinal morphology in guinea pigs and pigs (Table 18.1), but others have failed to replicate this in mice,[32] despite there being clear evidence that such regimes can sensitize for delayed type hypersensitivity reactions at other sites.[4,70] Of particular interest in this respect, Czerkinsky and colleagues[1-3] have described a recent series of experiments in which either oral or systemic priming with contact sensitizers caused a delayed type hypersensitivity (DTH) response in oral mucosa on oral challenge. Although no reference was made to change in cell-mediated immunity (CMI) in other regions of the gastrointestinal (GI) tract, careful analysis in this model may reveal more details of the balance between hypersensitivity and tolerance induction at mucosal sites in general. The question as to whether oral immunization can lead to local CMI and the manifestation of food allergy is not related to any doubt that feeding can stimulate a systemic DTH. This has been shown by feeding a wide range of antigens, including those from infectious agents,[28,31] contact sensitizing agents,[4,70] particulate antigens such as sheep red blood cells[40] and dietary antigens such as ovalbumin.[89] Where doubt remains it relates to whether such responses occur to common dietary components and, if so, whether they have local effects within the GI tract. The major suggestion put forward to explain lack of local reactivity is the development of oral tolerance.

Strain differences in delayed type hypersensitivity

Inbred strains of mice differ in their ability to mount DTH skin responses following ovalbumin feeding at a dose rate of 20 mg/day. CBA mice skin tested 2, 3 or 4 days after feeding with ovalbumin gave a positive 24-h response, whereas similarly treated balb/c mice did not respond at that time[90] (Table 18.2). It remains to be determined whether such differences are reflected locally in response to feeding soluble protein antigens, and the effect that this might have on gut morphology. That this might be so is indicated by the altered ability of mice to respond to a new dietary antigen introduced 2 days after the start of feeding with another unrelated antigen. CBA male mice fed a single tolerizing dose of HSA 2 days after commencing oral immunization with ovalbumin failed to become tolerant to HSA. In contrast, those fed the HSA 4 days after commencing feeding with ovalbumin gained tolerance. No differences were observed in the responses to ovalbumin,[89] with both groups developing tolerance (Table 18.3).

The mechanism underlying this change is not clear but since it occurs at a time when DTH reactions can be elicited at distant sites it has been suggested that it may be a consequence of a local CMI reaction to the first oral immunogen (ovalbumin). It is postulated that such reactions cause an 'altered presentation' of antigens.[69] Whatever the mechanism, it does indicate that the manner in which new dietary antigens are introduced can profoundly influence the response and even prevent the induction of oral tolerance and, as such, have significant consequences on the development of food allergy.

Oral tolerance (see Chapter 16)

In common with humoral antibody responses it is clear that prior feeding can suppress an animal's specific ability to mount DTH reactions to erythrocytes[41] and to a wide range of protein antigens (reviewed in reference 93). To allow expression of local CMI to fed antigens, studies have attempted to abrogate oral tolerance before immunizing for active intestinal immunity. Early studies of feeding high doses of antigen, have implicated suppressor T cells in the resulting tolerance,[73,78,79] and such cells can be inhibited by cyclophosphamide.[5,81] In an attempt to prevent tolerance induction, ovalbumin has been fed to cyclophosphamide-treated mice. In these mice both systemic and local DTH was observed. In the intestine following ovalbumin challenge there was an increase in

			Change in footpad thickness at 24 h (10^{-3} cm)			
Mean (range) 24-h increase in skin thickness following the injection of 30 μl ovalbumin into the footpad of two strains of mice						
	ip sensitized	**Negative control**	**Oral ovalbumin**			
			2 day	**3 day**	**4 day**	**7 day**
CBA	6.4 (5–7)	1.5 (1–3)	3.0 (2–5)	3.0 (2–5)	3.0 (1–4)	1.4 (1–2)
Balb/c	nd	0.9 (0–2)	nd	1.0 (0–3)	nd	nd

Table 18.2 Mean (range) 24-h increase in skin thickness following the injection of 30 μl ovalbumin into the footpad of two strains of mice. Control mice were either unsensitized (negative control) or sensitized by intraperitoneal (ip) injection of ovalbumin in complete Freund's adjuvant. The effect of feeding ovalbumin for 2, 3, 4 or 7 days on the ability to mount delayed type hypersensitivity (DTH) reactions is compared. Significant responses after feeding were found only in the CBA mice. nd, not determined.

Sequential effects of the introduction of ovalbumin (25 mg/day) into the diet of mice on responsiveness to ovalbumin and other non-related antigens							
	Days after start of oral immunization with 25 mg/day ovalbumin						
	1	**2**	**3**	**4**	**5**	**6**
Responses to ovalbumin						
Antibody tolerance	No	No	No	No	Yes	Yes	Yes
DTH skin test	–ve	–ve	+ve	+ve	+ve	–ve	–ve
Responses to unrelated antigen						
Antibody response to ip antigen	⇔	⇔	⇑	⇑	⇑	⇑	⇔
Oral tolerance to 50 mg HSA		No	No	Yes	Yes		

Table 18.3 Sequential effects of the introduction of ovalbumin (25 mg/day) into the diet of mice on responsiveness to ovalbumin and other non-related antigens. Tolerance to ovalbumin was tested after injection (ip) with Ova in adjuvant. Delayed type hypersensitivity (DTH) 24-h skin test responses were measured after footpad challenge. Responses to unrelated antigens were measured following injection (ip) with sheep red blood cells, or a single feed of 50 mg HSA. The results show that, following the introduction of ovalbumin into the diet, the mice showed a transient sensitivity to that antigen before becoming tolerant. The period of sensitivity was associated with a period during which the responses to unrelated antigens were altered. (For experimental details see reference 89).

the rate of crypt cell division and in the numbers of intraepithelial lymphocytes (IELs). Cells isolated from the mesenteric lymph node produced macrophage migration inhibition factor (MIF), indicating that in these mice feeding could result in local CMI reactions to dietary antigens and that these led to an altered gut morphology.[64] A recent revisit of this model[74] has shown enhanced proliferative responses to Ova by both IEL and lamina propria lymphocytes (LPL). Other studies have indicated that cyclophosphamide, while having no effect on the intestinal absorption of ovalbumin,[95] acts to eliminate the generation of suppressor cells in the local lymph node.[33] In experimental models, a number of factors have been shown to influence the development of oral tolerance. These include genetic differences,[91] age,[34,94] liver function,[21] bacterial lipopolysaccharide[70,104] and protein malnutrition.[97] By using these observations, it has been possible to delay the induction of oral tolerance and allow the expression of local CMI even in the absence of immunosuppressive drugs.

Oral immunization with erythrocytes

In contrast to ovalbumin and other soluble dietary proteins where the period of tolerance induction is relatively short, feeding erythrocytes can lead to a longer period of DTH sensitivity (of approximately 1 week)[40,71] before the development of the protected state of tolerance. This model therefore provides a method for assessing the effects of a local CMI reaction on gut integrity. Groups of eight CBA male mice sensitized by feeding 3×10^9 sheep red blood cells (SRBC) daily for 2 days and then challenged 10 days later on 3 consecutive days with fed SRBC show a significantly impaired capacity to absorb fed xylose compared to unsensitized control animals and those sensitized with the non-crossreacting horse red blood cells (HRBC). Interestingly, in mice that have been fed SRBC for 14 days (and which are tolerant, as judged by their inability to mount DTH skin tests), the ability to absorb xylose was not impaired (Fig. 18.1). This indicates that a phase of sensitivity during which gut damage can occur precedes the development of the protected state of tolerance.

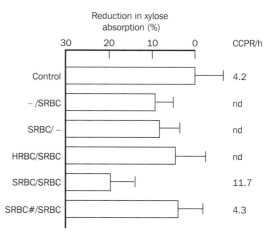

Fig. 18.1 Percentage reduction (SD) in the ability to absorb xylose and in the rate of production of crypt cells (CCPR/h) in groups of eight male CBA mice. Plasma xylose levels were measured 30 min after a single feed of 10 mg of xylose. Mice had been previously sensitized by feeding sheep red blood cells (SRBC) for 2 days (SRBC/–), followed 10 days later by challenge on 3 consecutive days with SRBC (SRBC/SRBC). Xylose tests were performed on the following day and compared to those in unsensitized mice (–/SRBC), mice orally tolerized by feeding SRBC for 14 days (SRBC#/SRBC) and those sensitized with the non-crossreacting antigen, horse red blood cells (HRBC/). Crypt cell production rates were measured on the same day. nd, not determined.

Histological studies have indicated that the malabsorption was associated with an increase in the rate of production of crypt cells and in the number of IEL. In the SRBC-fed mouse model it is clear that the gut damage is immune-mediated. While detailed studies of the mechanism involved remain to be completed, the evidence that damage only occurs during the period when positive skin tests can be elicited would suggest that it is likely to be cell-mediated. Preliminary cell transfer studies with mesenteric lymph node and Peyer's patch cells isolated from the intestine of mice fed SRBC for 2 days would support this view.

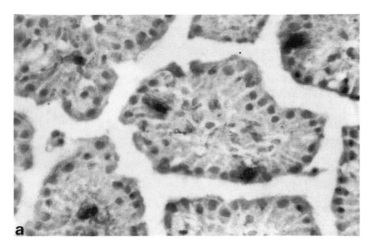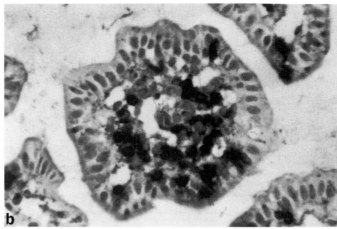

Fig. 18.2 Colonization of the neonatal pig intestine with T cells. Intestinal tissue was taken from newborn, unsuckled (a) and 1 week old (b) piglets. Transverse sections were stained using a monoclonal antibody recognizing pig CD2 and staining visualized with peroxidase plus substrate. Very few CD2+ cells are present in newborn intestine: within 1 week the number of cells increase markedly.

Inflammatory bowel disease and oral tolerance

Over the past 5 years, several mouse models employing targeted deletion of cytokine, TCR and signalling molecule genes, or selective reconstitution of severe combined immunodeficient mice, have been introduced for the analysis of local mechanisms involved in inflammatory bowel disease (IBD) and oral tolerance. The IBD-inducing models have concentrated on the inflammatory pathology in the large bowel. The emphasis in this research is now shifting towards examination of bacterial antigens of possible aetiological consequence. However, following initial breakdown of the epithelial barrier, it is just as likely that an individual develops inappropriate responses to dietary antigens, and examination of dietary hypersensitivity in these models could be extremely productive.

THE PIG AS A LARGE ANIMAL MODEL

Immune development and functional specialization

The young piglet has been extensively used for studies of the interaction between diet, intestinal microflora and the mucosal immune system. The initial stimulus to these studies was the observation that, unlike humans or rodents, the pig placenta does not transport maternal immunoglobulin. Newborn piglets acquire maternal antibody entirely during the first 24 h or so of life, by uptake from colostrum. The newborn piglet thus provides a model in which environmental and maternally derived factors (antigen, antibody, anti-idiotype) can be controlled in gnotobiotic conditions.[98]

Recently, however, it has also become apparent that the T cell component of the intestinal mucosa of the newborn piglet is much more poorly developed than that of human infants (Fig. 18.2).

Peyer's patches organize in the first few days, while the T cell component of the intestinal lamina propria develops slowly during the first 9 weeks of life.[18,59,82,101] This development occurs in distinct phases. Within 1 week, lymphocytes expressing the CD2 surface molecule characteristic of T cells enter the lamina propria (Fig. 18.2b). However, these early cells coexpress neither CD4 nor CD8. Conventional T cells expressing CD4 do not appear until 3–4 weeks of age, while CD8+ cells begin to appear after 5 weeks (Fig. 18.3).

The final distribution of T cells in the lamina propria shows a high degree of spatial organization, the tissue deep to the capillary plexus containing predominantly CD4+ T cells while CD8+ cells occur luminally and in the epithelium.[106] This is paralleled by functional specialization, demonstrated by a highly polarized cytokine profile biased towards IL-4 rather than IL-2.[7] Interestingly, this development does not occur in germfree piglets, indicating that it is driven by exposure to luminal antigens, presumably from commensal microorganisms.[82]

Function of antigen-driven T cells

Clearly there are two possible functions for these antigen-driven T cells; firstly they could be involved in surveillance and expression of active responses to potential pathogens;[38] secondly, however, they may be involved in the regulation and maintenance of mucosal tolerance.[10] In this department activation of isolated pig lamina propria cells has been shown to result in high levels of cell death when compared with similarly isolated splenic lymphocytes (Fig. 18.4), suggesting that the primary function of this environment may be to prevent the expression of active T cell responses to antigens normally present in the intestinal lumen.

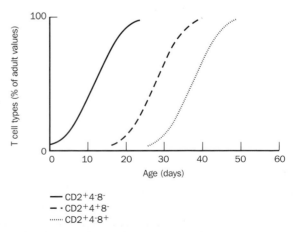

Fig. 18.3 Rates of colonization of neonatal pig intestine with different T cell types. The first cells to appear are CD2+4-8-; CD4+ cells appear around 3 weeks and CD8+ cells afterwards.

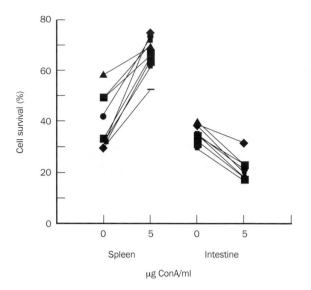

Fig. 18.4 The effect of polyclonal activation on survival of splenic and lamina propria lymphocytes. Cells are cultured with and without concanavalin A for 40 h, recovered and counted to determine the percentage survival of the starting population over this time. Each line is the result from an individual pig. Activation increases the survival of splenic cells but decreases survival of lamina propria lymphocytes.

Effect of weaning

Thus, exposure to environmental antigens derived from food and from commensal bacteria occurs during, and influences, the development of a highly specialized, and possibly tolerogenic, immunological architecture. This is most marked during the process of weaning. Under natural conditions, weaning occurs gradually and is not complete until 10–12 weeks old. However, abrupt weaning of piglets aged 3–5 weeks is routine husbandry practice. Postweaning diarrhoea commonly occurs, but is not associated with a particular age of pig, rather with the specific event of weaning. It may be controlled by dietary management, such as a reduction in food intake or protein content of the diet.[17] Such practices reduce the severity and incidence of disease.

Characteristics of postweaning diarrhoea

The initial and characteristic lesion of the disease is severe villus atrophy (Fig. 18.5) in the small intestine which is associated with a fall in levels of the disaccharidases sucrase and lactase in the enterocyte brush border and with malabsorption. These changes occur within 3–4 days of weaning and partial recovery occurs after 7–10 days. The enteropathic changes can occur in the complete absence of microbial involvement,[40] and have been hypothesized to be a consequence of transient expression of hypersensitivity reactions to the novel protein antigens in the diet.

Soya-based diets

The impact of abrupt weaning of piglets onto soya-based diets is particularly severe and this model has been used to study the interaction between diet and the mucosal immune system. It is clear that the feeding of soya diets to young piglets does result in absorption of intact protein from the intestine and in an active, primary response to major storage proteins of the soya bean.[107] The level of serum IgG anti-soya antibody produced was comparable in 3-week old piglets fed soya diets or immunized

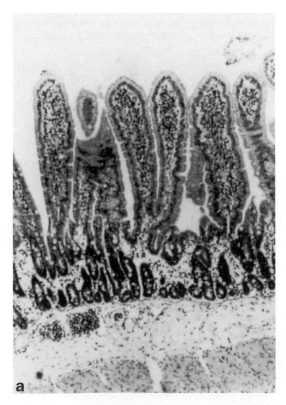
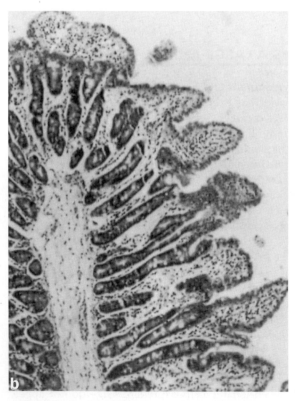

Fig. 18.5 Section of piglet small intestine stained with haematoxylin and eosin. (a) Tissue taken from an unweaned piglet, 26 days old. (b) Tissue taken from a piglet 5 days after weaning at 3 weeks of age on to a soya-containing diet.

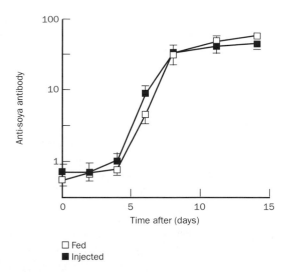

Fig. 18.6 Serum IgG anti-soya antibody in piglets exposed to soya proteins by feeding or injection. Three-week-old piglets were left with the sow and immunized (ip) 2 mg soya proteins plus saponin adjuvant (filled squares) or weaned onto diets containing 22% soya protein (open squares). All piglets were bled at the time points shown. Each line represents the mean (+/- SEM) of 12–14 animals.

intraperitoneally (ip) with soya proteins in adjuvant (Fig. 18.6).[8] Despite the similarity of the initial, primary response, there were clear, qualitative differences between the responses generated by feeding and injection. Continued feeding did result in systemic tolerance, as determined by subsequent ip challenge,[8] while priming by injection resulted in strong secondary responses to challenge. Importantly, a single, oral dose of soya proteins given to piglets at birth reduced the level of antibody produced after feeding soya proteins at weaning but had no effect on the response to injected antigen.[9]

These results demonstrate that the response to fed soya protein can be regulated independently of the response to systemic antigen, suggesting that it reflects inappropriate triggering of a mucosal immunological compartment. It is tempting to suggest that active, primary sensitization in young piglets occurs as a result of exposure of the poorly developed mucosal immunological architecture to high doses of antigenic protein. Studies in piglets reared in more natural, family pen systems in which weaning occurs gradually, have shown that systemic tolerance to soya proteins is established by 12 weeks of age and that this develops in the absence of an initial, primary antibody response.[63]

Mechanisms of gut damage

Although serum IgG anti-soya antibody is present after weaning, it is not clear whether this is involved in the pathogenesis of post-weaning diarrhoea. Deposition of antigen–antibody complexes can cause mucosal damage. Isolated gut loops were prepared in pigs which had been immunized parenterally with BSA and had a high level of circulating antibody. After challenge with BSA into the intestine, there was an influx of neutrophils into the lumen, epithelium and subepithelial capillaries within 4 h.[16] Interestingly, however, the neutrophil infiltration into the intestine was not accompanied by haemorrhage, oedema or thrombosis – features typical of an Arthus reaction that could be observed after intra-

cutaneous inoculation of BSA into similarly prepared pigs.[15] No significant effects on fluid and electrolyte movements were caused by the neutrophil response.[14] The ability to mount such responses would appear to be age-related, since attempts to repeat these studies in animals over 8 weeks of age have been unsuccessful.[42] Thus, antigen–antibody interaction and its consequences are unlikely to account for all the pathology observed in postweaning diarrhoea.

Role of T cells

Some lines of evidence support an involvement of T cells in the pathological changes. Vega-Lopez et al.[101] demonstrated an increase in the numbers of T cells present in the intestinal lamina propria of piglets 4 days after weaning compared to litter-matched controls. Splenic T cells from weaned animals produced less IL-2 than did controls, although both populations expressed the IL-2 receptor to the same degree.[6] Given previous observations that resident T cells from normal, stable pigs produce IL-4 but little IL-2, this might suggest relocalization of IL-2 producing Th1-type cells to the intestinal lamina propria following weaning with resulting local inflammation. However, direct evidence for this has not been obtained, and depression of IL-2 production could also be a result of activation of the hypothalamus/pituitary/adrenal axis associated with stress after weaning.

There is evidence that local T cell activation can be detected in the intestine of pigs following oral immunization with both infectious agents[28] and soluble protein antigens.[36] In the latter study, pigs were fed with dinitrophenylated bovine γ-globulin (DNP-BGG) and the immune response assessed using an indirect macrophage migration assay. Two days after the start of oral immunization, cultures of cells from the intestine, but not the mesenteric lymph node or spleen, could be stimulated by antigen to produce MIF. By day 7 all three sites produced MIF, indicating that the antigen-reactive cell response was now generalized. In this early study the effect of local CMI on mucosal pathology was not examined, but subsequent studies would suggest that it would have been present.

Effect of introduction of new dietary antigens on gut flora

At weaning the withdrawal of maternal milk is followed by a period in which a vast array of different dietary components are presented, possibly for the first time in large amounts. In the pig, postweaning diarrhoea commonly occurs, but it is not associated with a particular age of pig, rather with the specific event of weaning. It may be controlled by dietary management, such as a reduction in food intake or protein content of the diet.[17] Such practices reduce the severity and incidence of disease.

The initial and characteristic lesion of the disease is a severe villus atrophy (Fig. 18.5) in the small intestine which is associated with a fall in levels of the disaccharidases sucrase and lactase in the enterocyte brush border and with malabsorption. These changes occur within 3–4 days of weaning and a partial recovery occurs after 7–10 days. These enteropathic changes can occur in the complete absence of microbial involvement.[43] The commonly observed proliferation of *Escherichia coli* is subsequent to such change, suggesting therefore that it is acting as an opportunist rather than a primary pathogen.[61]

Manipulation of responses to dietary antigens

We have, over the past few years, attempted to investigate the possibility that a transient hypersensitivity reaction to antigens in

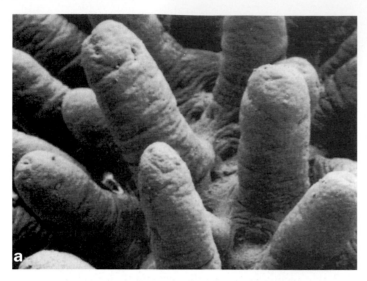
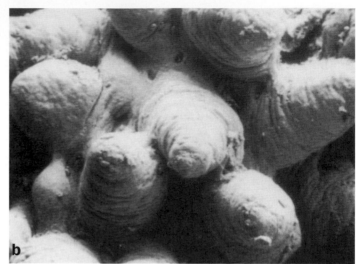

Fig. 18.7 Scanning electron micrographs of piglet small intestine. (a) Tissue taken from an unweaned piglet 26 days of age. (b) Tissue taken from a piglet 5 days after weaning at 3 weeks of age on to a soya-containing diet.

the postweaning diet may be the cause of the morphological changes described during this period. To test this hypothesis a number of approaches to manipulating the response to dietary antigens have been employed.

In the first group of experiments pigs were weaned at 3 weeks of age on to a conventional postweaning diet. Before weaning, piglets were assigned into three experimental groups so as to receive no supplementary feed, a small amount of feed of the postweaning diet or a large amount of the postweaning diet, such groups in immunological terms being equivalent to naive animals, sensitized animals and orally tolerized animals, respectively. Upon weaning, the incidence of *E. coli* proliferation and diarrhoea was greatest in the primed group, least in the tolerized group, with an intermediate incidence occurring in the naive animals; unweaned animals by comparison showed no change. Reduction in ability to absorb xylose was greatest in the primed group, and in all cases there was a degree of recovery by day 14 after weaning.[61] If such findings have an immunological basis then it should be possible to reduce the incidence of the disease by lowering the antigenicity of the postweaning diet. To this end animals were weaned on to a diet in which the protein source was either hydrolysed casein or antigenic casein. No increase in faecal water or *E. coli* proliferation was observed in the pigs weaned on to the minimally antigenic diet.[61,62] In these experiments disease was associated with increased crypt depth, villus atrophy and decreased sucrase activities in the brush borders.

Postweaning allergic reactions: effect of different feeds

To characterize the effect and significance of allergic reactions to antigens in the postweaning diet further, a series of experiments was performed in pigs weaned at 3 weeks of age on to diets containing soya (Fig. 18.7), such pigs having received no prior supplementary feed. Pigs weaned on to a diet in which the sole protein source was a soya protein (which had been treated to remove antinutritional factors) were highly susceptible to an enteritis immediately after weaning. Measurement of absorptive function *in vivo* by uptake of xylose showed a severe malabsorption by 5 days after weaning, which had substantially recovered

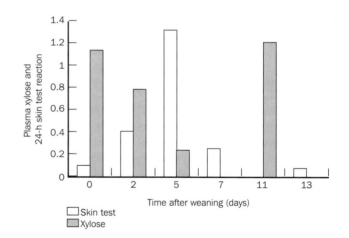

Fig. 18.8 Changes in skin test sensitivity and ability to absorb xylose following weaning. Increase in skin thickness at 24 h (cm^{-5}) after intradermal challenge with an extract of soya (open bars) in unweaned pigs and those weaned on to a soya-based diet 2, 5, 7 or 13 days earlier. Closed bars show levels of plasma xylose (mMol) in pigs 60 min after a single feed of xylose (100 mg/kg). Pigs were examined sequentially, preweaned, and on days 2, 5 and 11 postweaning on to a soya-based diet.

by 2 weeks postweaning (Fig. 18.8). During this period a DTH response to the soya antigen could be demonstrated by skin test which was at a maximum on day 5 and which had disappeared by day 13 (Fig. 18.8). As in the previous experiments with casein, adequate feeding of the soya antigen before weaning completely abrogated any malabsorption or diarrhoea, thus supporting the suggestion that a transient immune response to the dietary antigens may predispose to clinical disease. This indicates that orally induced hyporesponsiveness may protect against changes in gut morphology and therefore disease susceptibility.

Morphological and physiological consequences

The consequences of feeding such diets are profound. There is marked crypt hyperplasia and villus atrophy throughout the small intestine. The crypt hyperplasia can occur before the villus atrophy, as early as day 2 after weaning. Increased numbers of both goblet cells and IEL were also present from day 5. Thus the morphological picture is similar to both that observed in rodent models of food allergy and in children with cow's milk allergy.[103] In the soya-weaned pig there is a marked malabsorption of carbohydrates, which is accompanied by a reduction in the ability of enterocytes to transport amino acids (alanine and lysine) (Fig. 18.9) and to absorb fluid. The weaning procedure also influences brush border disaccharidase development, with maltase, isomaltase, sucrase and trehalase activities being reduced, reflection that enzyme development is disturbed.

The changes observed in gut physiology can be explained by a change in the relative maturity of enterocytes present on the villi. Enterocytes arise by division of precursors in the crypts and migrate from the crypt to the tip of the villus. During this migration there is a change from secretory to absorptive function and an increase in the activity of brush border enzymes. Severe changes in the rate of division and migration or length of villi can influence the physiological role of the enterocyte and alter crypt:villus ratios. Water and electrolytes are continuously secreted into the lumen of the small intestine by crypt enterocytes, mainly in the upper and middle small intestine and predominantly by the villi in the posterior ileum (Fig. 18.10). This movement may account for up to 30% of total body water each day,[58] and thus any shift in enterocyte maturity could on its own be severe enough to result in diarrhoea.

Mechanism of cell-mediated hypersensitivity to dietary antigen

The precise mechanism whereby cell-mediated hypersensitivity reactions to dietary antigens within the gut lead to the morphological changes is not clear but it has been postulated to be lymphokine-mediated (for detailed reviews see references 65 and 93). Microbial agents such as rotavirus may also bring about a similar morphological change;[54] however, they are unlikely to be significant in the pig model described here since, when found, they were exclusive to the upper small intestine, and maximum immune-mediated damage was found in the lower small intestine. Furthermore, it is difficult to envisage how dietary manipulation before weaning could influence the growth of a virus after weaning.

Interaction between diet and bacteria

The interaction between diet and bacteria in the gut should, however, not be discounted. Following weaning, bacteria can be seen adhering (Fig. 18.11) to the villi on days 5 and 7 after weaning but are absent by day 13. Withdrawal of milk antibody is clearly a factor that can influence proliferation, but the delay between weaning and when they appear and the complete lack of appearance in pigs orally tolerized before weaning, suggests that dietary factors are also important. It is possible that a shift in the relative maturity of enterocytes might influence either bacterial adhesion in a manner similar to that shown for the binding of lectins[26] or by altering luminal nutrition for the bacteria as a result of maldigestion. It has also been shown that during the first weeks of life there is a decline in susceptibility of the intestine to the hypersecretory effects of *E. coli* enterotoxin, but immediately after weaning there is a transient, abrupt increase in susceptibility to the levels seen in the neonatal pig.[87] Similarly, it has been shown that in parasite-induced villus atrophy the intestine is also more susceptible to enterotoxin.[57]

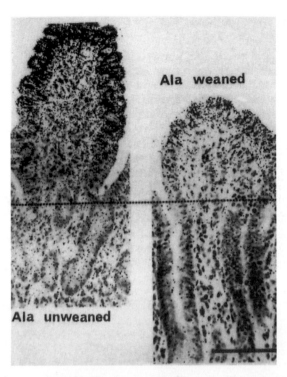

Fig. 18.9 Autoradiographic localization of titrated alanine in small intestinal villi of unweaned and weaned piglets. The horizontal dotted line indicates the crypt–villus junction. The weaned animals show a reduced uptake of alanine, as indicated by the number of grains on the villi. The reduced villus height and increased crypt depth is also clearly shown.

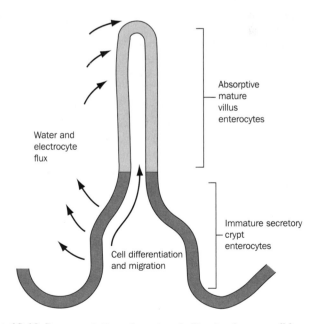

Fig. 18.10 Representation of crypt and villus to show possible function effects of changes in crypt cell production rate. Enterocytes arise from division of cells in the crypt and then migrate up the villi and are shed at the tips. During this migration they mature and differentiate, changing from immature secretory cells to mature absorptive cells. It has been suggested that an increase in the rate of division of crypt cells will lead to a reduction in the relative maturity of the enterocytes. Such a change would lead to an excess of secretory cells and water imbalance.

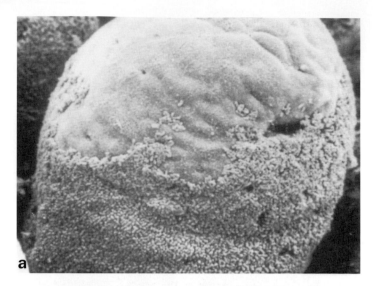

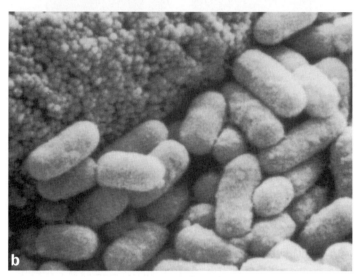

Fig. 18.11 Scanning electron micrographs of piglet small intestine taken 5 days after weaning. (a) Low power showing *E. coli* covering most of the available surface of a villus. (b) High power showing the bacteria adhering to the brush border, microvillus surface.

While the mechanism of increased susceptibility has not been determined in either case, the change towards a higher proportion of immature (secretory) cells relative to mature (absorptive) cells would accentuate the effect of enterotoxin by increasing the number of target cells available (enterotoxin acts on secretory cells) and by reducing the capacity of the small intestine to reabsorb. Finally, an interaction whereby bacterial lipopolysaccharide can modulate the response to dietary protein[70] will be discussed in detail later.

RUMINANTS

Secretory immunoglobulin G and tolerance
The ruminant GI immune system differs markedly from that of monogastric animals. For example, IgG in cattle is a major secretory immunoglobulin.[68] Furthermore, unlike most other species which are hyporesponsive to skin test challenge with dietary antigens that they 'tolerate', adult cattle give positive skin test reactions to grass extracts even though they have shown no clinical sensitivity throughout their period of being fed.[92] Since evidence would suggest that gastric secretions have important effects in reducing the antigenicity of fed antigen,[47,49] one might expect that, in ruminants with their complex rumen digestive processes, this protective effect would be greatest. This is because considerable protein degradation occurs within the rumen itself and, by acting as a reservoir for ingesta, it can ensure that the rate of delivery of food into the true stomach is optimal for the digestive process. It is not surprising therefore that problems related to food intolerance are in general restricted to the preruminant period.

Preruminant calves: allergy to soya
Raw soya bean meal contains a variety of antinutritional factors, most of which can be readily inactivated by modern industrial processing.[108] Despite this treatment, feeding preruminant calves with milk replacers containing more than 30% soya can lead to diarrhoea, weight loss and even death.[22,86] This is associated with the presence of high titres of circulating antibody specific for soya bean antigens,[11,12,44,85] and evidence has been put forward to link the changes in GI function motility with an allergic response.[86] Morphological changes in gut architecture observed include a broadening and shortening of the villi, a lymphocytic infiltration and an increase in the number of goblet cells.[11] These changes are occasionally associated with small haemorrhages although mucosal thickness generally remain unchanged. Changes in mucosal integrity have also been indicated by functional studies.

Increased intestinal permeability and altered motility
In soya-sensitized calves, intestinal permeability to β-lactoglobulin increased 1–2 h after ingestion of soya bean proteins and was greatly elevated at 4–6 h, returning to normal by 24 h.[46] Feeding soya led to increased ileal flow rates,[45] which were attributable partly to a decrease in transit time[85] but also to the very large volume of fluid which has been suggested to result from leakage of body fluids into the intestinal lumen.[46] Recent studies have shown that, in hypersensitive calves, disturbances in the myoelectric activity patterns in the duodenum and mid-jejunum could be related to the antigenicity and level of particular soya antigens fed,[53] suggesting a close link between the allergic response to food and gut motor function.

Mechanisms of hypersensitivity
Antibodies found in the sera of soya bean-fed calves include those specific to glycinin and β-conglycinin.[45] While the increased sensitivity of the gut is accompanied by rising IgG, IgA and IgM antibodies in serum, the precise immunological mechanisms responsible for the intestinal changes are uncertain. Both complement-fixing IgG1[11] and IgE[12,44] antibodies have been detected, but the appropriate passive transfer studies have not been made to determine the relative importance of each. Similarly, the possibility of cell-mediated damage has not been evaluated but the kinetics of change are consistent with a type I hypersensitivity. Interestingly, gut hypersensitivity in preruminant calves is not restricted to those fed on soya, since antibody production and GI reactions have also been noted in ovalbumin-fed animals.

OTHER ANIMAL MODELS

The rabbit has been used extensively to study the immune response to fed antigens, but little is known of the effect of such responses upon clinical symptoms. In the guinea pig, gut pathology has been associated with antigen feeding and these effects have been augmented by secondary intestinal inflammation.[27] Besides local gut changes, prolonged antigen feeding has been found to have immunopathological effects at distal sites such as the respiratory tract[23] and within joints.[24] Interestingly, unlike most monogastric species, feeding of ovalbumin to guinea pigs leads to a persistent serum antibody response and, even after 11 weeks of feeding, responsiveness is not fully suppressed, indicating that in this species tolerance is difficult to induce.[35]

Allergic reactions to dietary antigens are often implicated as a cause of skin reactions and GI disturbance in both cats and dogs. Recently, an inbred colony of dogs with high IgE antibody titres to specific food antigens has been described.[25] Local challenge with allergenic extracts of food resulted in mucosal swelling, erythema, petechiae and occasional generalized gastric erythema and hyperperistalsis. Examination of biopsy specimens collected immediately after challenge revealed oedema but few inflammatory cells, whereas the later biopsy specimens revealed increased eosinophil and mononuclear cell infiltrates typical of late-phase allergic inflammatory reactions.

FUTURE USE OF ANIMAL MODELS

The justification for developing any animal model of human disease must be to bring about an understanding of the pathogenesis of the disease and then to provide indicators for successful treatment or, even better, the prevention of the disease. On this basis, how successful have models of food allergy been and what might they provide in the future?

Immune-mediated gut damage following feeding

The evidence that ingestion of food can lead to immune-mediated gut damage is convincing. As to the immune effector mechanisms involved, both type I and type IV hypersensitivity reactions have been clearly implicated and the morphological changes detailed above. The role of immune complex (type III)-mediated hypersensitivity is, however, less convincing; the pathological changes induced in animals are both difficult to reproduce and bear little resemblance to the condition in man.

Non-physiological routes of immunization

In general, animal models of food allergy have required the use of both non-physiological routes of antigen presentation (intraperitoneal) and injection of adjuvants. While such models are of use in the listing of drugs that can prevent or reduce symptoms, they provide little useful information as to how or why an individual becomes hypersensitive to dietary antigens. Similarly, they do not indicate how the disease may be prevented. It is perhaps churlish to criticise such models as unphysiological, as it is likely that the same mechanisms that protect in man necessitate the use of parenteral antigen presentation in animal models. The protection afforded by the development of immune exclusion and oral tolerance is discussed in detail elsewhere in this volume (see Chapters 12 and 14).

Maintenance of tolerance

From studies investigating the mechanisms responsible for the maintenance of tolerance it has become clear that, before the induction of the protected state, animals pass through a brief phase of sensitivity. This sequence has been shown after feeding contact sensitizing agents[4,70] and erythrocytes.[41,89] With soluble protein dietary antigens, a serum antibody response may also be stimulated[56] which is subsequently suppressed,[96] although the local mucosal antibody response persists. In the case of cell-mediated responses after feeding ovalbumin to balb/c mice, Mowat and Ferguson[66] showed that tolerance resulted, and to generate DTH responses it was necessary to administer cyclophosphamide. In contrast, in other species such as the pig, feeding DNP-BGG resulted in the appearance of lymphokine-producing lymphocytes in the gut, mesenteric lymph node and spleen.[36]

Further, it has subsequently been shown that, in other inbred strains of mice, transient sensitivity, as assessed by the ability to mount 24-h skin test responses, does occur.[89] If a similar pattern of responsiveness occurs in man, one could argue that virtually all individuals pass through a food allergic phase upon introduction to a new dietary antigen and those who fail subsequently to downregulate the response develop the clinical manifestations of food allergy.

Mechanisms of tolerance

The feeding of contact sensitizing agents stimulates both the appearance of effector T cells and cells capable of transferring suppression.[4] Similarly, after feeding soluble proteins, effector cells[84] and suppressor cells[73,79] can be demonstrated in populations of gut lymphocytes. The spleens of mice fed SRBC can be shown by passive transfer studies to contain both effectors and suppressors of DTH reactions.[71,92] Early on in the feeding regime the former predominated, and mice fed SRBC for less than 8 days readily show DTH reactions to SRBC upon challenge. Passive transfer of spleen cells of mice fed for longer periods indicated that subsequently cells capable of mediating predominated. It is tempting to suggest, therefore, that agents that enhance the development of cell that can downregulate allergic responses might influence the development of allergy. To this end, results in laboratory animals have shown that adjuvants given either systemically or orally can accelerate the 'tolerization' process[104] and convert what was a sensitizing oral dose of antigen into one that induced tolerance.[70]

Development of tolerance

Many factors have been shown to influence the development of oral tolerance (for reviews see references 92 and 93 and Chapter 14), including dietary manipulation and bacterial lipopolysaccharide. In the former context it has been shown that in the immediate postweaning period mice cannot be tolerized.[34,94] Further, it has been shown that even a minor change, such as the introduction of 20 mg of a new protein into the diet of mice, can prevent the induction of tolerance to a second antigen added to the diet a few days following the first.[89] At weaning, in addition to the introduction of new dietary antigens, milk is withdrawn and the controlling influence of maternal antibody upon gut flora with it. Since bacterial lipopolysaccharides can influence the induction of tolerance,[70] this further emphasizes the importance of weaning on subsequent food allergy. The observation that rats reared on 'infant feed formulations' are more readily sensitized with ovalbumin than conventionally reared animals[80] would support this view. The importance of this link between gut flora and the regulation of responses to dietary antigens cannot be over emphasized. For example, while it has been shown that feeding cholera toxin or the heat labile enterotoxin of *E. coli* can abrogate the induction of oral tolerance,[105] it has also been shown that the duration of this potentially harmful effect could be reduced by an 'appropriate gut flora'.[30]

Allergenicity and pathology

The type of studies described above, and those in which denatured or chemically modified antigens[75] have been fed, clearly illustrate how the specific allergenicity associated with a particular antigen can be directly related to gut pathology. The complexity of the range of antigens presented to the gut has shown that these responses can be modified by the simultaneous introduction of other totally unrelated dietary and microbial antigens. Besides those modulators already discussed there is a growing interest in determining the effects of feeding specific types of polyunsaturated fatty acids on a wide range of immunological responses. For example, it has been shown that feeding fish oil can diminish the antigen presenting cell activity of dendritic cells migrating from the gut[83] and it has been suggested that this may start to explain the possible beneficial effects of n-3 polyunsaturated fatty acids on a host of immunological responses such as graft survival and chronic inflammation. The possibility of a similar 'control' of food allergic responses has yet to be systematically evaluated.

KEY FACTS

- Following the introduction of a new dietary antigen all animals pass through a brief phase of sensitivity to that antigen.
- Transient sensitivity to a new dietary antigen is associated with crypt hyperplasia, villus atrophy and an altered ability to respond to unrelated antigens.
- In the pig the T cell compartment develops over the first 2–3 months of life, corresponding with the period of suckling under natural conditions.
- T cell development is antigen-driven and *in vitro* data suggest that the T cell component is directed at maintaining tolerance.
- Common weaning practice results in massive mucosal antigenic challenge before a mature (tolerogenic) immunological architecture develops.
- Weaning onto soya proteins results in a strong primary immune response, apparently regulated by the mucosal immune system. Concurrent alterations in mucosal function indicate that this response is harmful.
- Despite the magnitude of the primary response, tolerance does ultimately occur.

REFERENCES

1. Ahlfors E, Czerkinsky C. Suppression of delayed-type contact sensitivity in the murine oral mucosa by prior intragastric administration of hapten. *Scand J Immunol* 1997; 46: 268–73.

2. Ahlfors E, Czerkinsky C. Contact sensitivity in the murine oral mucosa. I. An experimental model of delayed-type hypersensitivity reactions at mucosal surfaces. *Clin Exp Immunol* 1991; 86: 449–56.

3. Ahlfors E, Jonsson R, Czerkinsky C. Experimental T cell-mediated inflammatory reactions in the murine oral mucosa. 2. Immunohistochemical characterization of resident and infiltrating cells. *Clin Exp Immunol* 1996; 104: 297–305.

4. Asherson GL, Zembalan M, Perera MACC *et al*. Production of immunity and unresponsiveness in the mouse by feeding contact sensitising agents and the role of suppressor cells in the Peyer's patches, mesenteric lymph nodes and other lymphoid tissues. *Cell Immunol* 1977; 33: 145–55.

5. Attallah AM, Ahmed A, Sell KW. In vivo induction of carrier-specific cyclophosphamide sensitive suppressor cells for cell mediated immunity in mice. *Int Arch Allergy Appl Immunol* 1979; 60: 178–85.

6. Bailey M, Clarke CJ, Wilson AD, Williams NA, Stokes CR. Depressed potential for IL-2 production following early weaning of piglets. *Vet Immunol Immunopathol* 1992; 34: 197–207.

7. Bailey M, Hall L, Bland P, Stokes CR. Production of cytokines by lymphocytes from spleen mesenteric lymph node and intestinal lamina propria. *Immunology* 1994; 82: 577–83.

8. Bailey M, Miller BG, Telemo E, Stokes CR, Bourne FJ. Specific immunological unresponsiveness following active primary to proteins in the weaning diets of piglets. *Int Arch Allergy Immunol* 1993; 101: 266–71.

9. Bailey M, Miller BG, Telemo E, Stokes CR, Bourne FJ. Altered immune response to protein antigens fed after neonatal exposure of piglets to the antigen. *Int Arch Allergy Immunol* 1994; 103: 183–7.

10. Bailey M, Plunkett F, Clarke A *et al*. Activation of CD4+ cells from the intestinal lamina propria. *Scand J Immunol* 1998; 48: 177–82.

11. Barratt MEJ, Strachan PJ, Porter P. Antibody mechanisms implicated in digestive disturbances following ingestion of soya protein in calves and piglets. *Clin Exp Immunol* 1978; 31: 305–12.

12. Barrett MEJ, Porter P. Immunoglobulin classes implicated in intestinal disturbances of calves associated with soya protein antigens. *J Immunol* 1979; 123: 676–80.

13. Bazin H, Platteau B. Production of circulating reaginic (IgE) antibodies by oral administration of ovalbumin to rats. *Immunology* 1976; 30: 679–84.

14. Bellamy JEC, Hamilton DL. Effects of immune mediated enteroluminal neutrophil emigration on intestinal function in pigs. *Can J Comp Med* 1977; 41: 36–40.

15. Bellamy JEC, Nielsen NO. Immune mediated emigration of neutrophils into the lumen of the small intestine. *Infect Immun* 1974; 9: 615–19.

16. Bellamy JEC, Nielsen NO. A comparison between the active cutaneous Arthus reaction and immune mediated enteroluminal neutrophil emigration in pigs. *Can J Comp Med* 1974; 38: 193–202.

17. Bertshinger HU, Eggenberger E, Jucker H, Pfirter HP. Evaluation of low nutrient, high fibre diets for the prevention of porcine *Escherichia coli* enterotoxaemia. *Vet Microbiol* 1979; 3: 281–90.

18. Bianchi AT, Zwart RJ, Jeurissen SH, Moonen-Lensen HW. Development of T and T cell compartments in porcine lymphoid organs from birth to adult: an immunohistological approach. *Vet Immunol Immunopathol* 1992; 33: 201–21.

19. Bicks RO, Azar MM, Rosenberg EW *et al*. Delayed hypersensitivity reactions in the intestinal tract. 1. Studies of 2,4-dinitrochlorobenzene caused guinea pig and swine colon lesions. *Gastroenterology* 1967; 53: 422–36.

20. Byars NE, Ferraresi RW. Intestinal anaphylaxis in the rat as a model for food allergy. *Clin Exp Immunol* 1976; 24: 352–6.

21. Cantor HM, Dumont AH. Hepatic suppression of sensitisation to antigen absorbed into the portal system. *Nature* 1967; 215: 744–5.

22. Colvin BM, Ramsey HA. Soy flour in milk replacers for young calves. *J Dairy Sci* 1968; 51: 899–904.

23. Coombs RRA, Devey ME, Anderson KJ. Refractoriness to anaphylactic shock after continuous feeding of cow's milk to guinea pigs. *Clin Exp Immunol* 1978; 32: 263–71.

24. Coombs RRA, Oldham G. Early rheumatoid like joint lesions in rabbits drinking cows' milk. *Int Arch Allergy Appl Immunol* 1981; 64: 287–92.

25. Ermel RW, Kock M, Griffey SM *et al*. The atopic dog: a model for food allergy. *Laboratory Animal Science* 1997; 47: 40–9.

26. Etzler ME. Lectins as probes in studies of intestinal glycoproteins and glycolipids. *Am J Clin Nutr* 1979; 32: 133–8.

27. Fargeas MJ, Theodorou V, More J *et al*. Boosted systemic immune and local responsiveness after intestinal inflammation in orally sensitized guinea pigs. *Gastroenterol* 1995; 109: 53–62.

28. Frederick GT, Bohl EH. Local and systemic cell mediated immunity against transmissible gastroenteritis and intestinal viral infection of swine. *J Immunol* 1976; 116: 1000–4.

29. Furrie E, Turner MW, Strobel S. Partial characterisation of a circulating tolerogenic moiety which, after a feed of ovalbumin, suppresses delayed-type hypersensitivity in mice. *Immunology* 1995; 86: 480–6.

30. Gaboriaurouthiau V, Moreau MC. Gut flora allows recovery of oral tolerance to ovalbumin in mice after transient breakdown mediated by cholera toxin or *Escherichia coli* heat labile enterotoxin. *Pediatric Research* 1996; 39: 625–9.

31. Gadol N, Waldmann RH, Clem WL. Inhibition of macrophage migration by normal guinea pig intestinal secretions. *Proc Soc Exp Biol Med* 1976; 151: 654–8.

32. Glaister JR. Some effects of oral administration of oxazolone. *Int Arch Allergy Appl Immunol* 1973; 45: 828–43.

33. Hanson DG, Miller, SD. Inhibition of specific immune responses by feeding protein antigens. V. Induction of the tolerant state in the absence of specific suppressor T cells. *J Immunol* 1982; 128: 2378–81.

34. Hanson DG. Ontogeny of orally induced tolerance to soluble proteins in mice. 1. Priming and tolerance in newborns. *J Immunol* 1981; 127: 1518–24.

35. Heppell LM, Kilshaw PJ. Immune responses in guinea pigs to dietary protein. 1. Induction of tolerance by feeding ovalbumin. *Int Arch Allergy Appl Immunol* 1982; 68: 54–9.

36. Huntley JH, Newby TJ, Bourne FJ. The cell mediated immune response of the pig to orally administered antigen. *Immunology* 1979; 37: 225–30.

37. Ito K, Inagaki Ohara K, Murosaki S *et al*. Murine models of IgE production with a predominant Th2 response by feeding protein antigen without adjuvants. *Eur J Immunol* 1997; 27: 3427–37.

38. James SP, Zeitz M. Human gastrointestinal mucosal T cells. In: *Handbook of Mucosal Immunology*, (Ogra P, Lamm ME, McGhee JR *et al*. eds), Academic Press, San Diego, Ca, 1994: 275–83.

39. Jarrett EEE, Haig D, McDougal W, McNulty E. Rat IgE production, II. Primary and booster reaginic antibody responses following intradermal or oral immunisation. *Immunology* 1976; 30: 671–7.

40. Kagnoff ME. Effects of antigen feeding on intestinal and systemic immune responses. III. Antigen-specific serum mediated suppression of humoral antibody responses after antigen feeding. *Cell Immunol* 1978; 40: 186–203.

41. Kagnoff ME. Effects of antigen-feeding on intestinal and systemic immune responses. 2. Suppression of delayed type hypersensitivity reactions. *J Immunol* 1978; 120: 1509–13.

42. Keirby JL. *Aspects of the local immune system of the gut and mammary gland*. Bristol: University of Bristol, 1983: 176 pp. PhD thesis.

43. Kenworthy R, Allen WD. Influence of diet and bacteria on small intestinal morphology, with special reference to early weaning on *Escherichia coli*. Studies with germ free and gnotobiotic pigs. *J Comp Pathol* 1966; 76: 291–6.

44. Kilshaw PJ, Sissons JW. Gastrointestinal allergy to soya bean protein in preruminant calves. Antibody production and digestive disturbances in calves fed heated soya bean flour. *Res Vet Sci* 1979; 27: 361–5.

45. Kilshaw PJ, Sissons JW. Gastrointestinal allergy to soya bean protein in preruminant calves. Allergenic constituents of soya bean products. *Res Vet Sci* 1979; 27: 366–71.

46. Kilshaw PJ. Gastrointestinal hypersensitivity in the preruminant calf. In: *The Mucosal Immune System*. (Bourne FJ, ed.), The Hague: Martinus Nijhoff 1981: 203–19.

47. Klipstein FA, Engert RF. Protective effect of active immunisation with purified *Escherichia coli* heat labile enterotoxin in rats. *Infect Immun* 1979; 23: 592–9.

48. Knippels LMJ, Penninks AH, Spanhaak S *et al*. Oral sensitization to food proteins: a brown Norway rat model. *Clin Exp Allergy* 1998; 28: 368–75.

49. Kraft SC, Rothberg RM, Knauer CM *et al*. Gastric acid output and circulating anti-bovine serum albumin in adults. *Clin Exp Immunol* 1967; 2: 321–30.

50. Lake AH, Block KJ, Neutra MR, Walker WA. Intestinal goblet cell mucus release. II. In vivo stimulation by antigen in the immunised rat. *J Immunol* 1979; 122: 834–7.

51. Lake AM, Bloch KJ, Sinclair KJ, Walker WA. Anaphylactic release of intestinal goblet cell mucus. *Immunology* 1980; 39: 173–8.

52. Lake AM. Experimental models for the study of gastrointestinal food allergy. *Ann Allergy* 1983; 51: 226–8.

53. Lalles JP, Benkredda D, Toullec R. Influence of soya antigen levels in milk replacers on the disruption of intestinal motility patterns in calves sensitive to soya. *J Veterinary Medicine Series A* 1995; 42: 467–78.

54. Lecce JG, Clare DA, Balsbaugh RK, Collier DV. Consequences of maternal exposure to porcine parvovirus at different times during gestation. *J Clin Microbiol* 1983; 17: 689–95.

55. Levine BB, Vaz NM. Effect of combinations of strain, antigen dose on reagin production in the mouse. A mouse model for human atopy. *Int Arch Allergy* 1969; 39: 156–71.

56. Lippard VW, Schloss OM, Johnson PA. Immune reactions induced in infants by intestinal absorption of incompletely digested cows milk protein. *Am J Dis Child* 1936; 51: 562–74.

57. Ljungstrom I, Holmgren J, Huldt G *et al*. Changes in intestinal fluid transport and immune response to enterotoxins due to concomitant parasitic infection. *Infect Immun* 1980; 30: 734–40.

58. Low AG, Partridge IG, Sambrook IE. Studies on digestion and absorption in the intestines of growing pigs. 2. Measurements of the flow of dry matter, ash and water. *Br J Nutr* 1978; 39: 515–26.

59. Makala LHC. *Isolation and characterization of pig Peyer's patch dendritic cells*. Bristol: University of Bristol, 1996; 219 pp. PhD thesis.

60. Miller B, Newby TJ, Stokes CR *et al*. The role of dietary antigen in the aetiology of post weaning diarrhoea. *Ann Rech Vet* 1983; 14: 487–92.

61. Miller BG, Newby TJ, Stokes CR, Bourne FJ. Influence of diet on post-weaning malabsorption and diarrhoea in the pig. *Res Vet Sci* 1984; 36: 187–93.

62. Miller BG, Newby TJ, Stokes CR *et al*. The importance of dietary antigen in the cause of postweaning diarrhoea in pigs. *Am J Vet Res* 1984; 45: 1730–3.

63. Miller BG, Whittemore CT, Stokes CR, Telemo ET. The effect of delayed weaning on the development of oral tolerance to soya bean protein in pigs. *Br J Nutrition* 1994; 71: 615–25.

64. Mowat A Mcl, Ferguson A. Hypersensitivity reactions in the small intestine. VI. Pathogenesis of the graft-versus-host reaction in the small intestinal mucosae of the mouse. *Transplantation* 1981; 32: 238–43.

65. Mowat A Mcl. The immunopathogenesis of food sensitive enteropathies. In: *Local Immune Responses of the Gut*. (Newby TJ, Stokes CR, eds), Roca Baton: CRC Press, 1984; 199–225.

66. Mowat AM, Ferguson A. Hypersensitivity in the small intestinal mucosa. V. Induction of cell mediated immunity to a dietary antigen. *Clin Exp Immunol* 1981; 43: 574–82.

67. Murray M, Jarrett EE, Jennings FW. Mast cells and macromolecular leak in intestinal immunological reactions. The influence of sex of rats infected with *Nippostrongylus brasiliensis*. *Immunology* 1971; 21: 14–31.

68. Newby TJ, Bourne FJ. The nature of the local immune system of the bovine small intestine. *Immunology* 1976; 31: 475–80.

69. Newby TJ, Stokes CR, Bourne FJ. Altered polyvinyl pyrrolidone clearance and immune responsiveness caused by small dietary changes. *Clin Exp Immunol* 1980; 39: 349–54.

70. Newby TJ, Stokes CR, Bourne FJ. Effects of feeding bacterial lipopolysaccharide and dextran sulphate on the development of oral tolerance to contact sensitizing agents. *Immunology* 1980; 41: 617–21.

71. Newby TJ, Stokes CR, Bourne FJ. The effect of orally administered or intraperitoneally injected adjuvant on the generation of oral tolerance in mice. In: *Adjuvants, Interferon and Non-specific immunity*. (Cancellotti FM, Galassi D, eds), Luxembourg: CEC, 1984: 87–94.

72. Newby TJ, Stokes CR, eds. *Local Immune Responses of the Gut*. Boca Raton: CRC Press, 1984.

73. Ngan J, Kind LS. Suppressor T cells for IgE and IgG in the Peyer's patches of mice made tolerant by oral administration of ovalbumin. *J Immunol* 1978; 120: 861–5.

74. Ohtsuka Y, Yamashiro Y, Maeda M *et al*. Food antigen activates intra-epithelial and lamina propria lymphocytes in food-sensitive enteropathy in mice. *Pediatric Res* 1996; 39: 862–6.

75. Peng HJ, Chang ZN, Han SH *et al*. Chemical denaturation of ovalbumin abrogates the induction tolerance of specific IgG antibody and DTH responses in mice. *Scand J Immunol* 1995; 42: 297–304.

76. Perdue MH, Chung M, Gall DG. Effect of intestinal anaphylaxis on gut function in the rat. *Gastroenterology* 1984; 86: 391–7.

77. Revoltella R, Ovary Z. Reaginic antibody production in different mouse strains. *Immunology* 1969; 17: 45–54.

78. Richman LK, Chiller JM, Brown WR *et al*. Enterically induced immuno-logic tolerance. 1. Induction of suppressor T-lymphocytes by intragastric administration of soluble proteins. *J Immunol* 1978; 121: 2429–34.

79. Richman LK, Graeff AS, Yarchoan R, Strober W. Simultaneous induction of antigen specific IgA helper T cells and IgG suppressor T cells in murine Peyer's patch after protein feeding. *J Immunol* 1981; 126: 2079–83.

80. Roberts S, Soothill JF. Provocation of allergic response by supplementary feeds of cows milk. *Arch Dis Child* 1982; 57: 127–30.

81. Rollinghoff M, Starzinski-Powitz A, Pfizenmaier K, Wagner H. Cyclophosphamide-sensitive T-lymphocytes suppress the in vivo generation of antigen specific cytotoxic T-lymphocytes. *J Exp Med* 1977; 145: 455–9.

82. Rothkotter HJ, Ulbrich H, Pabst R. The postnatal development of gut lamina propria lymphocytes: numbers, proliferation and T and B cell subsets in conventional and germ-free pigs. *Pediatr Res* 29: 237–42.

83. Sanderson P, MacPherson GG, Jenkins CH, Calder PC. Dietary fish oil diminishes the antigen presentation activity of rat dendritic cells. *J Leucocyte Biol* 1997; 62: 771–7.

84. Shields JG, Parrott DMV. Appearance of delayed-type hypersensitivity effector cells in murine gut mucosa. *Immunology* 1985; 54: 771–6.

85. Sissons JW, Smith RH. The effect of different diets including those containing soya bean products, on digesta movement and water and nitrogen absorption in the small intestine of the preruminant calf. *Br J Nutr* 1976; 36: 421–38.

86. Smith RH, Sissons JW. The effect of different feeds, including those containing soya bean products, on the passage of digesta from the abomasum of the preruminant calf. *Br J Nutr* 1975; 33: 329–49.

87. Stevens JB, Gyles CL, Barum DA. Production of diarrhoea in pigs in response to *Escherichia coli* enterotoxin. *Am J Vet Res* 1972; 33: 2511–26.

88. Stokes CR, Newby TJ, Bourne FJ. Altered immune function associated with dietary factors. In: *The Mucosal Immune System*. (Bourne FJ, ed.), The Hague: Martinus Nijhoff, 1981: 224–39.

89. Stokes CR, Newby TJ, Bourne FJ. The influence of oral immunisation on local and systemic immune responses to heterologous antigens. *Clin Exp Immunol* 1983; 52: 399–406.

90. Stokes CR, Newby TJ, Miller BG, Bourne FJ. The immunological significance of transient cell-mediated immune reactions to dietary anti-gens. In: *Cell Mediated Immunity*. (Quinn PJ, ed.), Luxembourg: CEC, 1984: 249–59.

91. Stokes CR, Swarbrick ET, Soothill JF. Genetic differences in immune exclusion and partial tolerance to ingested antigens. *Clin Exp Immunol* 1983; 52: 678–84.

92. Stokes CR. Induction and control of intestinal immune responses. In: *Local Immune Responses of the Gut*. (Newby TJ, Stokes CR, eds), Boca Raton: CRC Press, 1984: 97–141.

93. Strobel S, Mowat A Mcl. Immune responses to dietary antigens: oral tol-erance. *Immunology Today* 1998; 19: 173–81.

94. Strobel S, Ferguson A. Immune responses to fed protein antigens in mice. III. Systemic tolerance or priming is related to the age at which antigen is first encountered. *Paediatr Res* 1984; 18: 588–94.

95. Strobel S, Mowat A Mcl, Drummond HE *et al*. Immunological responses to fed protein antigens in mice. II. Oral tolerance for CMI is due to activation of cyclophosphamide-sensitive cells by gut processed antigen. *Immunology* 1983; 49: 451–6.

96. Swarbrick ET, Stokes CR, Soothill JF. Absorption of antigens after oral immunisation and the simultaneous induction of specific systemic tolerance. *Gut* 1979; 20: 121–5.

97. Swarbrick ET, Stokes CR. The immune effects of ingested antigens in mice. In: *Protein Transmission Through Living Membranes*. (Hemmings WA, ed.), Amsterdam: Elsevier/North-Holland, 1979: 309–18.

98. Telemo E, Bailey M, Miller BG, Stokes CR, Bourne FJ. Dietary antigen handling by mother and offspring. *Scand J Immunol* 1991; 43: 689–96.

99. vanHalteren AGS, van der Cammen MJF, Biewenga J *et al*. IgE and mast cell responses on intestinal allergen exposure. A murine model to study the onset of food allergy. *J Allergy Clin Immunol* 1997; 99: 94–9.

100. Vega-Lopez MA, Telemo E, Bailey M, Stevens K, Stokes CR. Immune cell distribution in the small intestine of the pig: immunohistological evidence for an organised compartmentalisation in the lamina propria. *Vet Immunol Immunopathol* 1993; 37: 49–60.

101. Vega-Lopez MA, Bailey M, Telemo E, Stokes CR. Effect of early weaning on the development of immune cells in the pig small intestine. *Vet Immunol Immunopathol* 1995; 44: 319–27.

102. Walker WA, Wu M, Bloch KJ. Stimulation by immune complexes of mucus release from goblet cells of the rat small intestine. *Science* 1977; 197: 370–2.

103. Walker-Smith JA. Cow's milk intolerance as a cause of postenteritis diarrhea. *J Paediatr Gastroenterol Nutr* 1982; 1: 163–73.

104. Wannemuehler MJ, Kiyono H, Babb JL *et al*. Lipopolysaccharide (LPS) regulation of the immune response: LPS converts germ-free mice to sensitivity to oral tolerance induction. *J Immunol* 1982; 129: 959–65.

105. Williams NA, Hirst TR, Nashar TO. Immune modulation by the cholera-like enterotoxins: from adjuvant to therapeutic. *Immunol Today* 1999; 20: 95–101.

106. Wilson AD, Haverson K, Southgate K *et al*. Expression of MHC class II antigens on normal porcine intestinal endothelium. *Immunology* 1996; 88: 98–103.

107. Wilson AD, Stokes CR, Bourne FJ. Effect of age on absorption and immune responses to weaning or introduction of novel dietary anti-gens. *Res Vet Sci* 1989; 46: 180–9.

108. Wolf WJ, Cowan JC. *Soya Beans as a Food Source*. Boca Raton: CRC Press, 1971.

Chapter 19

Immunologically mediated damage of the gut

William E. Fickling and Duncan A. F. Robertson

INTRODUCTION

The gastrointestinal tract is exposed to an enormous load of potentially antigenic foreign material, and it is a measure of the efficient exclusion and handling of these antigens that damaging reactions to food are so uncommon. However, adverse reactions to food do occur, and some of these are thought to have an allergic basis. In this chapter possible local mechanisms of food allergy are discussed.

This is a controversial area, and little is known for certain about the mechanisms of food allergic reactions in man. For example, in the best studied and commonest food allergy in children, cow's milk allergy, the immunopathogenesis remains unclear. Similarly, in coeliac disease it is not clear whether the abnormal immunological phenomena demonstrated in this condition are of primary importance, or secondary to a mucosal enzyme deficiency.[29] Much progress has been made in the understanding of leukocyte recruitment to the gut with subsequent damaging reactions in other diseases, and these mechanisms will be reviewed.

THE NORMAL SYSTEMIC IMMUNE RESPONSE

After systemic exposure to an antigenic stimulus, the individual responds by the primary immune reaction, which may involve the development of specific antibody, the development of cell-mediated immunity or both. Alternatively, the specific state of non-responsiveness known as tolerance may be induced.

Humoral response

In the humoral response, B lymphocytes differentiate into plasma cells, producing specific antibody which combines with soluble antigen such as bacterial toxins to produce immune complexes. These are then phagocytosed by polymorphonuclear leukocytes or macrophages/monocytes with or without the fixation of complement. Complexes with excess antigen will not activate complement and will utilize the Fc receptor mechanism. Cellular antigens such as bacteria will be coated with antibody (opsonized) to enhance phagocytosis (Fig. 19.1).

In the gut antigens are 'sampled' by membranous epithelial cells or 'M' cells which allow macromolecules to traverse the epithelial barrier and initiate an appropriate immune response. The secretory immune system can be stimulated independently from the systemic system and leads to a local immune response with production of specific IgA-producing plasma cells in the lamina propria. Dimeric IgA combines with the mucin layer to provide a mucosal immune barrier to limit further antigen absorption. Gastrointestinal IgA synthesis is quantitatively the largest immunoglobulin production in the body.

Cell-mediated response

The cell-mediated response is directed primarily towards intracellular microorganisms, such as viruses and mycobacteria, and to foreign cells (allografts). Sensitized T cells proliferate and differentiate to produce two major effector mechanisms – cytotoxic cells and cells which release lymphokines (Table 19.1). These polypeptides modulate the behaviour of other cells, enhancing phagocytosis non-specifically and activating

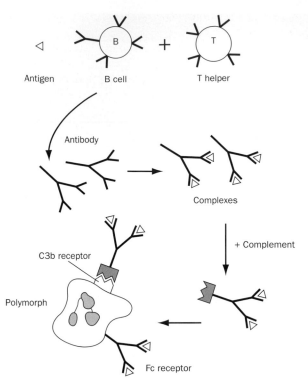

Fig. 19.1 The humoral antigen elimination system. B lymphocytes differentiate into plasma cells, producing specific antibodies. T helper cells are important at this stage. Immune complexes are formed which fix complement if there is antibody excess, or are phagocytosed using the Fc receptor mechanism if there is antigen excess.

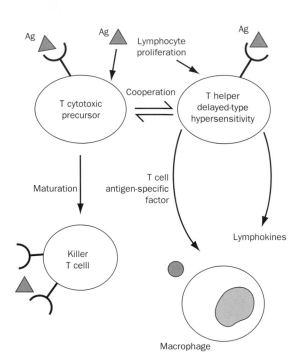

Fig. 19.2 The cellular antigen (Ag) elimination system. Sensitized T cells differentiate into cytotoxic cells, or cells releasing lymphokines and antigen-specific factors, which activate macrophages.

Table 19.1 Lymphokines: polypeptides of molecular weight 20 000 to 80 000.

Lymphokines: polypeptides of molecular weight 20 000 to 80 000	
Mononuclear phagocyte chemotactic factor Migration inhibition factor (MIF)	Increase local macrophage population
Macrophage activating factor α-Interferon	Synonymous. Stimulates killing of intracellular organisms and inhibits viral replication
Interleukin 2	T cell proliferation
Lymphocyte inhibitory factor (LIF)	T suppressor function
Others, of uncertain function	

macrophages with T cell antigen-specific factors (Fig. 19.2). Helper T cells recognize antigen in association with class II major histocompatible molecules and express the CD4 surface marker; cytotoxic T cells express CD8 and recognize antigen with class I molecules.

After effective elimination of the antigen, the systemic immune system remains primed and able to respond promptly should the antigen be encountered once more.

The humoral and cell-mediated responses do not operate in isolation and are interdependent at several levels.

Chemokines and cell recruitment

The extravasation of leukocytes from the blood into the tissues underlies all immunological reactions, and is a highly regulated sequence of events which involves specific interactions between leukocytes and the endothelium (Fig. 19.3). These are controlled by families of molecular regulators, including selectins, integrins, adhesion molecules and chemokines. Selectins aid movement of leukocytes along the endothelial cell surface by forming low-affinity interactions that dissociate if not amplified. Chemokines (chemotactic cytokines – see Table 19.2) provide the signals to convert these into high-affinity integrin-dependent interactions that lead to migration of cells into tissues. The main stimulus for chemokine production is the presence of bacterial products, viral infection, pro-inflammatory cytokines such as interleukin 1, tumour necrosis factor-alpha (TNFα), but activated TH-1 and TH-2 lymphocytes will induce chemokine secretion, and this may be the mechanism in food allergic diseases.

There is differential expression of chemokine receptors on helper lymphocytes: for example, CXCR receptors are expressed on TH-1-type cells in response to bacterial infection and elicit a neutrophil response, but CCR3 is expressed on TH-2-type cells

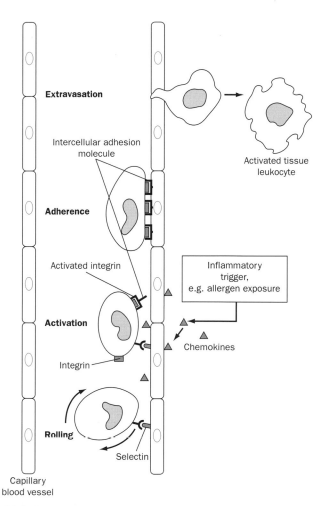

Fig. 19.3 Chemokines regulate leukocyte movement into tissues.

Chemokines and their cellular targets	
Chemokine	**Cell type**
Monocyte chemoattractant protein 3 (MCP 3) Eotaxin 1	Eosinophil
Macrophage inhibitory protein (MIP) Secondary lymphoid tissue chemokine (SLC) regulated upon activation, normal T cell expressed and secreted (RANTES)*	Activated T cell
Lymphotactin	Resting T cell
Interleukin 8 (IL8) Epithelial cell-derived neutrophil, activating peptide (ENA-78)	Neutrophil
MCP 1–5	Natural killer cell
MCP-5	Basophil
Fractalkine Stromal cell-derived factor 1 (SDF-1)	Monocyte

* RANTES, Regulated upon activation, normal T cell expressed and secreted.

Table 19.2 Chemokines and their cellular targets.

as well as eosinophils and basophils and this will trigger an allergic-type reaction.[31]

Chemokine expression will determine the nature of the allergic reaction: eotaxin and interleukin 5 will result in a tissue eosinophilia,[9] whereas IL5 and IL3 prime basophils to release histamine and leukotrienes after stimulation by monocyte chemoattractant protein.[4]

Specific tolerance

The alternative to specific immunization is the development of specific tolerance, where further exposure to an antigen leads to a state of non-responsiveness: activated T and B cells being rendered unresponsive by antigen-specific suppressor T cells is thought to be one of the major mechanisms involved. Anergy[24] or clonal deletion may also be involved, or all strategies may be employed depending on the timing and dose of antigen. (See also Chapter 16, Oral Tolerance.)

CONTROL OF THE IMMUNE RESPONSE

The magnitude and quality of the immune response is highly specific and under control at a variety of levels. Immune response genes are closely linked to the HLA genes and provide a genetic level of control, and high and low responders to a specific antigenic stimulus can be identified. The monocyte/macrophage series is important in processing of antigens and presenting them to the lymphocyte in such a way that an appropriate immune response is triggered. There are interactions between T cells and B cells, such that certain antibody responses are T cell-dependent. Helper and suppressor T cells regulate the immune response: helper cells amplify the system; suppressor cells, which may be antigen-specific or non-specific, apply a brake to the system. Control is exerted by other factors, including the feedback inhibition of specific antibody.

Antigenic exclusion

Despite the enormous antigenic load present in the gut, the systemic immune response is relatively small. This is because the majority of antigens are excluded by non-immune means (Chapter 13). Most of the antigens that do stimulate a response are effectively contained within the mucosa and the systemic response is more likely to involve the development of specific tolerance to the antigen.[8] However, under certain circumstances an immunizing reaction may occur, which normally leads to the effective elimination of the antigen without tissue damage. If the antigen is present in sufficiently large amounts or if the cellular or humoral response is excessive, then host tissue damage can occur. This is called hypersensitivity and forms the basis of food allergic reactions.

The nature of food antigens

Antigenic determinants are defined by the quaternary structure of small areas of the surface of proteins, glycoproteins or polypeptides, and may be sequential, where the antigen is made up of amino acids in linear sequence, or conformational, where the antigen is formed by the three-dimensional convolutions of the protein. Conformational antigens are usually readily denatured by cooking or luminal digestion, whereas sequential antigens are more resistant. Some antigenic proteins have been well characterized and the epitope found to be a simple tetrapeptide.[13]

D

HYPERSENSITIVITY REACTIONS

Coombes and Gell[10] describe four groups of hypersensitivity reactions. This remains a useful classification, but it is not clear whether all types of reaction are involved in the pathogenesis of food allergy, either in the gut itself or in remote organs. The four groups are not intended to be mutually exclusive and more than one mechanism may operate in any allergic reaction.

TYPE I. ANAPHYLACTIC SENSITIVITY (Fig. 19.4)

Type I hypersensitivity occurs when antigen combines with reaginic antibody (usually IgE) bound by its Fc piece to the surface of tissue and blood mast cells or basophils. The bound antibodies are cross-linked by antigen, the mast cell degranulates and releases large amounts of stored, pharmacologically active substances including histamine, 5-hydroxytryptamine and heparin; other substances are synthesized, such as leukotrienes, prostaglandins and thromboxanes. The combined effect of these agents is to constrict smooth muscle, dilate capillaries and induce cell infiltration (Table 19.3). This mechanism underlies the common problem of atopic allergy, which affects approximately 20% of the population. Following intradermal injection of antigen in a sensitized subject, a local wheal and flare reaction occurs, and it is this that forms the basis of intradermal skin testing. In the nasal mucosa, the reaction causes the rhinorrhoea and congestion typical of hay fever. In the bronchial tree, bronchial constriction and a clinical asthmatic attack may be precipitated. Rarely, systemic anaphylaxis with bronchoconstriction, hypotension and

Mediators released by mast cell triggering	
Mediator	**Effects**
Granule release (pre-formed mediators)	
Histamine	Vasodilatation; Increased vascular and gut permeability Chemotaxis Bronchoconstriction
Heparin	Anticoagulant
Tryptase Chymase Carboxypeptidase	Inactivates fibrinogen Activates complement and collagenase
Platelet activating factor	Pro-thrombotic
Eosinophil/neutrophil chemotactic factors	Cell recruitment
Newly synthesized	
Lipoxygenase pathway leukotrienes	Histamine-like
Cyclo-oxygenase pathway prostaglandins	Platelet aggregation Vasodilatation
Overall effects of mast cell triggering	
1. Primary effect – Anaphlaxis 2. Induction of chronic inflammation 3. Proteolytic enzyme release	

Table 19.3 Mediators released by mast cell triggering.

death can occur following exposure to antigens such as a bee sting or after ingestion of tiny amounts of a food allergen.[3]

Atopic food sensitivity

In atopic food hypersensitivity, shortly after ingestion of the offending food the subject may develop a local reaction such as swelling of the tongue or oral mucosa. Diarrhoea and vomiting may occur within a few minutes or a more generalized reaction may occur, such as urticaria or, rarely, anaphylaxis. Such food allergies are well recognized. On the whole, the subject correctly identifies the offending foodstuff and avoids it thereafter. There is evidence that less obvious symptoms can be attributed to Type I reactions to food. IgE-producing plasma cells are distributed throughout the gastrointestinal tract and are present in increased numbers in the jejunal mucosa of patients with food allergy.[30] Mast cells are also widely distributed throughout the gut[2] (Chapter 6) (Fig. 19.5), so the potential for Type I reactions is present in the gut in healthy individuals. Mast cell, basophil and eosinophil products have been demonstrated in the intestine in food allergic individuals on challenge.[20]

Type I-mediated damage: hypotheses

There are two main hypotheses to explain how certain predisposed individuals develop IgE antibodies and Type I hypersensitivity reactions. The first suggests that atopy is a consequence of

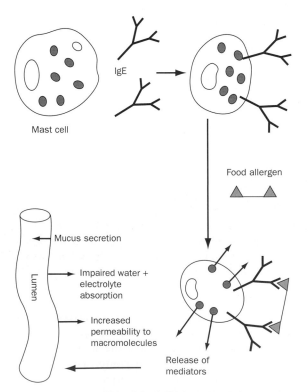

Fig. 19.4 Type I hypersensitivity. A food allergen cross-links two mast-cell-bound IgE molecules, causing local release of mediators. These cause increased mucus secretion, impaired absorption and increased permeability.

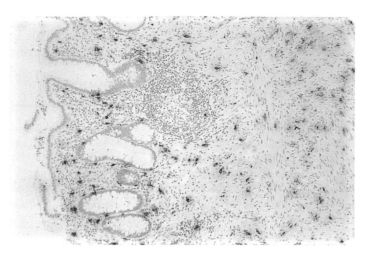

Fig. 19.5 Mast cells in normal colonic mucosa (anti-tryptase stain).

overstimulation by antigens during early life. In infants there is a relative IgA deficiency in the gut, resulting in an increased capacity to absorb macromolecules.[36] Events such as gastroenteritis can further disrupt intestinal integrity and lead to further antigen exposure and uptake. The alternative hypothesis suggests that antigen stimulation results in T suppressor cell activation, which suppresses IgE synthesis and the atopic individual has a specific suppressor T cell deficiency.[17]

Gut changes following type I reactions

Large changes in gut physiology can be demonstrated in sensitized experimental animals undergoing exposure to antigen. Thus, large changes in water and electrolyte transport,[27] goblet cell mucus release[21] and enterocyte turnover and differentiation[25] can be demonstrated following gut challenge, and it is proposed that IgE-mediated mast-cell release of chemical mediators, in particular histamine, accounts for the functional abnormalities demonstrated. A similar sequence of events in man may account for a variety of gastrointestinal symptoms, such as abdominal pain, distension and diarrhoea. Figure 19.6(A) shows mucosal oedema in the ileum in a patient with urticaria and abdominal pain. The ileum appears normal between attacks of pain (Fig. 19.6(B)).

TYPE II. ANTIBODY-DEPENDENT CYTOTOXIC HYPERSENSITIVITY

The best-recognized example of a Type II reaction occurs when an antigen present on a cell surface combines with antibody, either IgG or IgM, to cause cellular destruction by one of a number of pathways

1. Antibody-dependent cell-mediated cytotoxicity can occur. Non-sensitized lymphoreticular cells bind to the antibody by specific receptors. Polymorphs, macrophages and killer cells may be involved and killing occurs by an extracellular mechanism (Fig. 19.7).
2. The antibody-coated (opsonized) cell will be phagocytosed, e.g. hyperimmune graft rejection reaction.
3. Complement is activated as far as C3: C3A has an anaphylatoxic activity causing mast cell degranulation and release of chemotactic factors. There are specific receptors to C3B on

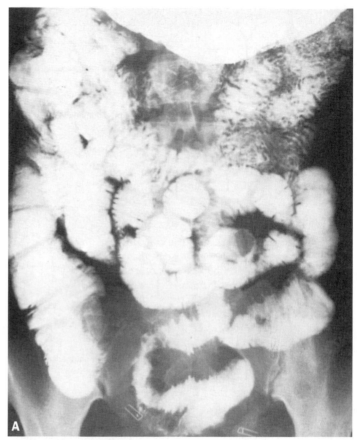

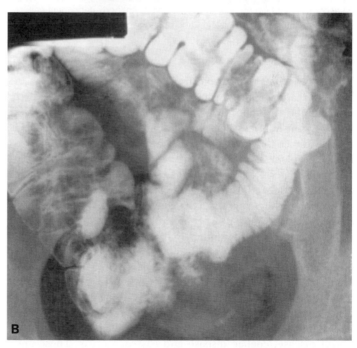

Fig. 19.6 Barium follow-through examination in a patient with urticaria and abdominal pain. During an acute attack of abdominal pain there is gross mucosal oedema (A), which is not present between attacks (B).

polymorphs and macrophages, permitting immune adherence and facilitating phagocytosis.
4. Complement is activated through to C8, C9 and cell lysis occurs.

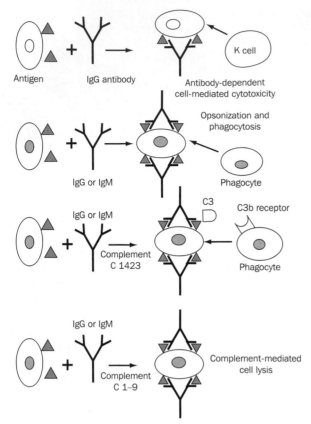

Fig. 19.7 Type II hypersensitivity. Destruction of antigen-bearing cells may be accomplished by a number of mechanisms. Antibody-dependent cell-mediated cytotoxicity, opsonization and phagocytosis, or complement activation.

Type II reactions and autoimmunity

Type II reactions form the basis of autoimmune haemolytic anaemia and thrombocytopenia. In other autoimmune diseases, the mechanism is less clear. In Goodpasture's syndrome there is good evidence that antiglomerular basement membrane antibodies fix complement and are directly responsible for the glomerulonephritis. In pernicious anaemia, gastric parietal cell antibodies are cytotoxic to isolated parietal cells,[12] but in other conditions where autoantibodies are common, e.g. Hashimoto's thyroiditis, the evidence for a pathogenic role of the antibody is less clear and it may represent an epiphenomenon.

Non-IgE antibodies to food

Non-IgE antibodies to food can be readily demonstrated in low concentrations in health and in an increased prevalence and concentration in a variety of groups of individuals such as normal infants and people with selective IgA deficiency, inflammatory bowel disease, coeliac disease and gastroenteritis. These antibodies do not appear to be of pathological significance and reflect the normal response to impaired exclusion of antigen. Antibody titres fall with appropriate treatment of the underlying condition.[19] Theoretically, tissue damage might occur if food antigens cross-react with host tissue antigens, initiating an autoimmune process. For example, there are reports of antibodies to *Escherichia coli* (a gut bacterial antigen but not a food antigen) cross-reacting with human colon in ulcerative colitis,[28] and it has been suggested that these antibodies are cytotoxic, but it is now

widely held that *E. coli* antibodies are not of pathogenic significance and may occur in a variety of other disease states.[37] There is therefore no evidence that Type II reactions are an important mechanism in food allergy.

TYPE III. IMMUNE-COMPLEX MEDIATED

Food antigens are often absorbed from the gut in small amounts and encounter specific antibodies in the circulation with the formation of immune complexes. These are normally cleared rapidly by the reticuloendothelial system and they are of no pathological significance. Tissue damage will result, however, if there are high concentrations of complexes and the nature of the damage depends upon whether antigen or antibody is present in excess (Fig. 19.8).

Antigen excess (serum sickness reaction)

These are usually generalized reactions associated with circulating complexes. When large doses of foreign antigens, e.g. horse serum, are given therapeutically, a specific antibody response is provoked with the formation of immune complexes in the presence of gross antigen excess. If the complexes are of an appropriate size, they are deposited in vessel walls and an inflammatory reaction is provoked in the endothelium with exposure of the basement membrane to which the complexes attach. Deposition in skin, kidney and joints leads to the clinical features of urticaria, albuminuria and arthritis, together with fever and lymphadenopathy.

Antibody excess (Arthus-type reaction)

These are usually local reactions. By injecting hyperimmune rabbits intradermally with the appropriate antigen, Arthus

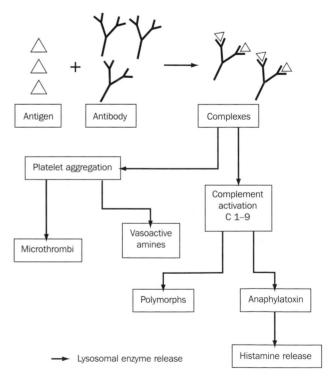

Fig. 19.8 Type III hypersensitivity. Complexes formed in antigen excess are deposited in vessel walls with aggregation of platelets and local release of inflammatory mediators. In antibody excess there is local precipitation of complexes with fixation of complement and release of inflammatory mediators.

induced a characteristic skin lesion with erythema and induration. There is a local deposition of complexes with fixation of complement, anaphylatoxin release, mast cell degranulation and local intravascular reactions. This type of reaction occurs in man in the lungs, in farmer's lung and aspergillosis, in the lymphatics in response to filarial worm infestation, and Type III reactions are implicated in the joints of patients with rheumatoid arthritis.

Immune complexes and food allergy

In food allergy, circulating immune complexes are demonstrable after ingestion of antigen, but are quantitatively and qualitatively different from the small amounts found in normal subjects.[26] In animal studies, the secondary development of immune complexes following increased absorption of antigen as the result of intestinal anaphylaxis (Type I) reaction may be important in the pathogenesis of the intestinal lesion.[38]

Animal models of Type III reactions

In animal models, Type III reactions can cause gastrointestinal abnormalities. In immunized pigs, ingestion of high levels of antigen leads to polymorph migration to the epithelium but no tissue damage or functional derangement.[3] In hyperimmune animals, there is a deposition of immune complexes in the gut, with only minor histological damage.[1] Major histological damage can be induced in the colon by injecting immune complexes into an animal where the colon has previously been traumatized by exposure to formalin,[16] and it has been suggested that the immune complexes found inconstantly in inflammatory bowel disease may be important in initiating a relapse of disease activity or perpetuating the disease.

TYPE IV. DELAYED HYPERSENSITIVITY (Fig. 19.9)

The classic reaction is the Mantoux reaction, where 1–3 days after injection of tuberculin into a sensitized subject (previously exposed to TB), an indurated erythematous lesion appears. Histologically, there is perivascular cuffing with mononuclear cells and later extensive exudation of monocytes and polymorphs. The predominant cell type is the macrophage/monocyte. If the reaction continues because of continuing antigen exposure (persistent infection), the macrophages differentiate to form epithelioid cells and fuse to form giant cells. This is a CD4+ T cell-dependent mechanism. Some of the stimulated T cells produce soluble factors mediating the hypersensitivity reaction (Fig. 19.9), while others develop cytotoxicity. Tissue damage occurs as a result of persisting antigenic stimulation, either because of continuing infection or because of autoimmunization. Macrophages with bacterial antigens on the surface will be destroyed by K cells and other cells are killed as innocent bystanders by non-specifically activated macrophages.

Type IV reactions and food antigens

There is evidence that Type IV reactions can cause intestinal damage, including villus atrophy, in a variety of animal models, including parasitic infections and graft-versus-host disease, and in man.[22] The importance of cell-mediated hypersensitivity reactions in the pathogenesis of food allergy is not clear. It is widely held that the enteropathy of coeliac disease is due to a local cell-mediated immune response to dietary gluten. Cell-mediated immunity to gluten in coeliac disease can be demonstrated by

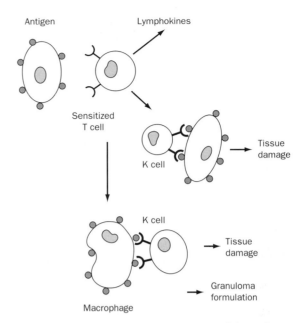

Fig. 19.9 Type IV hypersensitivity. In response to a cellular antigen, sensitized T cells differentiate to produce lymphokines and cytotoxic cells. Antigens are expressed on the surface of macrophages, and tissue damage results from continued infection or autoimmunization.

inhibition of leukocyte migration,[6] which persists despite a gluten-free diet. However, cell-mediated immunity to food antigens other than gluten can be demonstrated in coeliac disease[35] and this may be the result rather than the cause of villus atrophy.

Assessment of cell-mediated reactions

One of the major problems encountered in the assessment of cell-mediated immunity to food allergens is the inadequacy of the immunological methods available. For example, the phenomenon of leukocyte migration inhibition is thought to be due to macrophage migration inhibitory factor (MIF) production, a lymphokine. Studies in patients with coeliac disease have shown that the marked migration inhibition that occurs in the presence of gluten is not due to lymphokine release but may reflect cytophilic antibody, implying an entirely different mechanism, probably unrelated to the pathogenesis of coeliac disease.[34]

Mechanisms operating simultaneously

As emphasized previously, the hypersensitivity reactions Type I–IV of Gell and Coombs are not intended to be mutually exclusive and one might expect two or more mechanisms to operate simultaneously on occasion. Furthermore, these mechanisms were elucidated in the systemic immune response and have not been shown unequivocally to be operative in the gut. One might expect reactions to vary from tissue to tissue and indeed from time to time in the same tissue. The varied clinical features that can occur in cow's milk protein intolerance suggest different mechanisms in different patients.[14] Blood T cells from patients with rapid onset symptoms produce less interferon than late-onset patients, suggesting a Type IV reaction in the latter.[15]

It is not surprising, therefore, that clear immunogenic pathways of food allergy have not yet been defined. Even in the best-studied example, cow's milk protein intolerance, evidence is indirect and often conflicting and the distinction between primary pathogenic events and immunological phenomena secondary to mucosal damage is often difficult to assess. One of the best understood examples of food allergy is described here to illustrate the mechanisms involved.

THE MECHANISMS OF COW'S MILK INTOLERANCE

There is evidence to implicate all four types of reaction in cow's milk protein intolerance. In Type I reactions there is often a family or personal history of atopy. There are elevated titres of IgE specific for cow's milk protein, and skin testing may be positive.[11] There is an increase in IgE plasma cell numbers in the small bowel

mucosa following challenge.[33] Type II reactions are considered to be rare, but may account for the occasional thrombocytopenia seen in cow's milk protein intolerance,[18] particularly in association with the absent radius syndrome.[39] Type III reactions may well be important. Immune complexes of IgE, IgG and IgM with cow's milk proteins, such as beta-lactalbumin, are present after feeding.[5] Reduced complement levels[23] may be the result of clearance of immune complexes after challenge. Type IV reactions are suggested by studies demonstrating *in vitro* milk-induced lymphoblast transformation[32] and reduced neutrophil chemotaxis.[7] However, none of the above phenomena are specific for cow's milk protein intolerance, and there are many false-positive and false-negative reactions.

REFERENCES

1 ÄAccini L, Brentjens JR, Albini B, *et al*. Deposition of circulating antigen–antibody complexes in the gastrointestinal tract of rabbits with chronic serum sickness. *Am J Dig Dis* 1978; 23: 1098–1106.

2 Befus AD, Pearce FL, Gauldie J, *et al*. Mucosal mast cells. I. Isolation and functional characteristics of rat intestinal mast cells. *J Immunol* 1982; 128: 2475–80.

3 Bellamy JEC, Nielsen NO. Immune mediated emigration of neutrophils into the lumen of the small intestine. *Infect Immun* 1974; 9: 615.

4 Bischoff SC, Brunner T, De Weck AL, *et al*. Interleukin-5 modifies histamine release and leukotriene generation by human basophils in response to diverse agonists. *J Exp Med* 1990; 172: 1577–82.

5 Brostoff J, Carinii C, Wraith DG, Johns P. Production of IgE complexes by allergic challenge in atopic patients and the effect of sodium cromoglycate. *Lancet* 1979; ii: 1268–9.

6 Bullen A, Losowsky MS. Cell-mediated immunity to gluten fraction III in adult coeliac disease. *Gut* 1978; 19: 126–31.

7 Butler HL, Byrne WJ, Mammer DJ, *et al*. Depressed neutrophil chemotaxis in infants, with cow's milk intolerance and/or soy protein intolerance. *Pediatrics* 1981; 67: 264–8.

8 Challacombe SJ, Tomasi TB. Systemic tolerance and secretory immunity after oral immunisation. *J Exp Med* 1980; 152: 1459–72.

9 Collins PD, Marleau S, Griffiths-Johnson DA, *et al*. Cooperation between interleukin-5 and the chemokine eotaxin to induce eosinophil accumulation *in vivo*. *J Exp Med* 1995; 182: 1169–74.

10 Coombs RRA, Gell PGH, Lachmann PJ. *Clinical Aspects of Immunology*, 3rd edn. Blackwell Scientific, Oxford, 1974.

11 Dannaeus A, Johansson SGO. A follow-up study of infants with adverse reactions to cow's milk. I. Serum test, skin test reactions and RAST in relation to clinical course. *Acta Paediatr Scand* 1979; 68: 377–82.

12 De Aizpurua JH, Cosgrove LJ, Ungar B, Toh B-H. Autoantibodies cytotoxic to gastric parietal cells in serum of patients with pernicious anaemia. *N Engl J Med* 1983; 309: 625–9.

13 Elsayed S, Sornes S, Apold J *et al*. The immunological reactivity of the three homologous tetrapeptides in the region 41–64 of allergen M from the cod. *Scand J Immunol* 1982; 16: 77–82.

14 Firer MA, Hosking CS, Hill DJ. Cow's milk allergy and eczema: patterns of the antibody response to cow's milk in allergic skin disease. *Clin Allergy* 1982; 12: 385–90.

15 Hill DJ, Ball G, Hoskings CS, Wood PR. Gamma interferon production in cow milk allergy. *Allergy* 1993; 48: 75–80.

16 Hodgson HJF, Potter BJ, Skinner J, Jewell DP. Immune complex mediated colitis in rabbits. An experimental model. *Gut* 1978; 19: 225–31.

17 Jarrett E. Activation of IgE regulatory mechanisms by transmucosal absorption of antigen. *Lancet* 1977; ii: 223–5.

18 Jones RHT. Milk induced thrombocytopenia. *Arch Dis Child* 1977; 52: 744–5.

19 Kendrick KG, Walker-Smith JA. Immunoglubulins and dietary protein antibodies in childhood coeliac disease. *Gut* 1970; 11: 635–40.

20 Knutson TW, Bengtsson U, Dannaeus A, *et al*. Intestinal reactivity in allergic and nonallergic patients: an approach to determine the complexity of the mucosal reaction. *J Allergy Clin Immunol* 1993; 91: 553–9.

21 Lake AM, Bloch KJ, Walker WA. Anaphylactoid release of intestinal goblet cell mucus. *Immunology* 1980; 39: 1–6.

22 MacDonald TT, Spencer J. Cell-mediated immune injury in the intestine. *Gastroenterol Clin North Am* 1992; 21: 367–86.

23 Matthews TS, Soothill JE. Complement activation after milk feeding in children with cow's milk allergy. *Lancet* 1970; ii: 893–5.

24 Melamed D, Friedman A. Direct evidence for anergy in T lymphocytes tolerized by oral administration of ovalbumin. *Eur J Immunol* 1993; 151: 5752–61.

25 Nagata S, Yamashiro Y, Ohtsuka Y, *et al*. Quantitative analysis and immunohistochemical studies on small intestinal mucosa of food sensitive enteropathy. *J Paediat Gastro Nutr* 1995; 20: 40–48.

26 Paganelli R, Levinsky RJ, Brostoff J. Detection of specific antigen within circulating immune complexes. Validation of the assay and its application to food antigen–antibody complexes found in healthy and food allergic subjects. *Clin Expl Immunol* 1981; 46: 44–53.

27 Perdue MH, Chung M, Grantgall D. Effect of intestinal anaphylaxis on gut function in the rat. *Gastroenterology* 1984; 86: 391–7.

28 Perlmann P, Hammarstrom S, Lagercrantz R, Campbell D. Autoantibodies to colon in rats and human ulcerative colitis: cross-reactivity with *E. coli* 014 antigen. *Proc Soc Expl Biol* 1967; 125:975–80.

29 Peters TJ, Bjarnason I. Coeliac syndrome: biochemical mechanisms and the missing peptidase hypothesis revisited. *Gut* 1984; 28: 913–8.

30 Rosekrans PCM, Meijer CJLM, Cornellise CJ, *et al*. Use of morphometry and immunohistochemistry of small intestinal biopsy specimens in the diagnosis of food allergy. *J Clin Pathol* 1980; 33: 125–30.

31 Sallusto F, Mackay CR, Lanzavecchia A. Selective expression of the eotaxin receptor CCR3 by human helper T cells. *Science* 1997; 277: 2005–7.

32 Scheinmann P, Genorel D, Charlas J, Paupe J. Value of lymphoblast transformation test in cow's milk protein intolerance. *Clin Allergy* 1976; 6: 515–21.

33 Shiner M, Ballard J, Smith ME. The small intestinal mucosa in cow's milk allergy. *Lancet* 1975; i: 136–40.

34 Simpson FG, Field MP, Howdle PD, *et al*. Leukocyte migration inhibition test in coeliac disease – a reappraisal. *Gut* 1983; 24: 311–7.

35 Simpson FG, Robertson DAF, Howdle PD, Losowsky MS. Cell-mediated immunity to dietary antigens in coeliac disease. *Scand J Gastroenterol* 1982; 7: 671–6.

36 Taylor B, Norman AP, Orgel HA, *et al*. Transient IgA deficiency and pathogenesis of infantile atopy. *Lancet* 1973; ii: 111–3.

37 Triger DR, Alp MH, Wright R. Bacterial and dietary antibodies in liver disease. *Lancet* 1972; i: 60–3.

38 Walker WA, Wu M, Isselbacher KJ, Bloch KJ. Intestinal uptake of macromolecules. III. Studies on the mechanism by which immunisation interferes with antigen uptake. *J Immunol* 1975; 119: 854–61.

39 Whitfield MF, Barr DGD. Cow's milk allergy in the syndrome of thrombocytopenia with absent radius. *Arch Dis Child* 1976; 51: 337–43.

Chapter 20

Non-immune damage to the gut

William E. Fickling and Duncan A. F. Robertson

INTRODUCTION

Adverse organic reactions to food which do not involve the immune system are described as food intolerances rather than allergies. Gastrointestinal reactions can be classified into three main groups (Table 20.1).

The first group involves predictable reactions to food where adverse effects would be expected to occur in any individual exposed to that food, although there may be individual variations in susceptibility. Examples include the toxic effect of non-nutrients contained in foods, microbial contamination causing gastroenteritis, or the pharmacological effect of foods containing, for example, caffeine or alcohol.

The second group of disorders is rather rare and is attributable to a specific inborn or acquired error of metabolism, and symptoms occur after ingestion of a food that in most people would not cause adverse effects.

The final group includes idiosyncratic reactions where the mechanism of intolerance may be unclear but does not involve the immune system.

Diagnosis

Some reactions, particularly the predictable ones, are easily recognized as being associated with the ingested food, but the nature of the illness does not suggest an allergic mechanism. Other responses may closely resemble an allergic response; indeed they may share a common pathway, such as anaphylactoid reactions, where histamine release is brought about by such foods as shellfish, which cause symptoms and signs of a Type 1 reaction without involving IgE.

Classification of non-immunological mechanisms of damage	
Type	**Example**
1. Predictable reactions	Microbial contamination Alcohol
2. Errors of metabolism	Enzyme deficiencies Hypolactasia
3. Idiosyncratic reactions	Non-IgE mast cell degranulation

Table 20.1 Classification of non-immunological mechanisms of damage.

In addition to these acute reactions there are a large number of chronic gastrointestinal diseases where diet is an important pathogenic factor. These include ingestion of smoked foods in the development of gastric cancer and the role of alcohol consumption in oesophageal cancer.

PREDICTABLE REACTIONS

FOOD TOXICITY

Man's diet contains many thousands of chemical compounds, only a few of which are of nutritional significance.[28] Many of the others are not characterized chemically and may be toxic under certain circumstances, although centuries of use suggests these

Some naturally occurring toxic substances contained within foods		
Toxic substance	**Food source**	**Toxic effect**
Proteases	Legumes	Impaired growth
Lectins	Seeds	Haemagglutination Stimulation of mitosis Inflammation
Aflatoxins	Fungal contamination of cereals	Hepatotoxic Carcinogenic
Mycotoxins	Fungal contamination	Ergotism, alimentary toxic aleukia
Cyclopeptides	Mushrooms *Aminita phalloides*	Vomiting, diarrhoea Liver and renal necrosis
Muscarin	Mushrooms *Aminita muscaria*	Salivation, vomiting Abdominal pain, diarrhoea
Methyl mercury	Fish	Minamata disease
Lead	Environmental contaminant	Neuropathy Encephalopathy
Cadmium	Environmental contaminant and shellfish	Vomiting, diarrhoea Nephrotoxic Osteomalacia

Table 20.2 Some naturally occurring toxic substances contained within foods.

reactions are not common (Table 20.2). Some foods contain high levels of toxicants and are therefore avoided but may be consumed in error. Other foods may become contaminated either in their natural state or during processing and packaging.

Lectins

Leguminous plants contain biologically active substances that can cause marked gastrointestinal symptoms, particularly if ingested in a raw state. Substances such as phytohaemagglutinins or lectins have a number of biological properties, including agglutination of red cells, intense stimulation of mitosis and inflammation. Examples of such substances are ricin from the castor bean, concanavalin A from the jack bean and phytohaemagglutinin from the red kidney bean.[14] Ingestion of these beans can cause intense epithelial inflammation, producing diarrhoea and abdominal pain.

Mushrooms

Many species of mushrooms are poisonous, containing a variety of toxins that have been classified according to their physiological effects.[33,35] The cyclopeptides, amatoxin and phallotoxin, produced by *Amanita phalloides* or death cap mushroom are the most hazardous, interfering with ribonucleic acid synthesis to produce nausea, vomiting, abdominal pain and diarrhoea with liver and renal failure following in severe cases. Muscarine, originally isolated from *Amanita muscaria* but found in greater quantity in species of *Clitocybe* and *Inocybe*, affects the autonomic nervous system, causing increased salivation, abdominal pain and diarrhoea with hypotension and bradycardia.

PHARMACOLOGICAL EFFECTS

Caffeine

Caffeine (a methylxanthine) is the most widely used stimulatory drug, pharmacologically active effects becoming apparent after ingestion of approximately 200 mg or two strong cups of coffee. The effects are predictable and include stimulation of the central nervous system, diuresis, gastric acid secretion and tachycardia. Some susceptible individuals develop severe symptoms such as abdominal pain, supraventricular tachycardia and depression, which respond to withdrawal of the drug.[9] Such patients usually drink large amounts of coffee, and it is possible that all the effects are not due to caffeine but to some of the many other organic substances contained in coffee. Caffeine is a drug of addiction: withdrawal symptoms such as irritability, lassitude and headache may be anticipated.

Salt

Ingestion of large amounts of salt may lead to symptoms of headache, thirst and bloating. These occur particularly after eating Chinese takeaway meals which may contain up to 200 mmol of sodium and cause an elevation of the serum sodium of approximately 5 mmol per litre.[21] Some of the sodium is in the form of monosodium glutamate (MSG) and in the susceptible individual this can give rise to the 'Chinese restaurant syndrome',[32] where, 10–20 minutes after eating the food, the subject develops chest pain, facial flushing and headache. Some authors have questioned the role of MSG in this condition and suggested symptoms are related to the histamine content of Chinese food.[5,34] The mechanism of chest pain is uncertain, but it seems likely to be due to oesophageal spasm. A high prevalence of vitamin B_6 deficiency has been noted in sufferers, and pyridoxine treatment can prevent the reaction.[7,10]

Natural laxatives

Natural laxatives contained within foods or taken in the form of proprietary purgatives or tonics may cause gastrointestinal symptoms, usually cramp and diarrhoea. Magnesium, sulfate or phosphate, as naturally occurring laxatives, will cause osmotic diarrhoea. Senna and rhubarb increase intestinal secretions and motility. Castor oil, containing ricolinic acid, has a structure similar to that of bile acids and stimulates colonic secretion.[4]

Vasoactive amines

Vasoactive amines are commonly found in small amounts in normal foods and can cause a wide variety of symptoms, particularly affecting the gastrointestinal tract and central nervous system (Table 20.3). Adrenaline, noradrenaline, serotonin and histamine are all present in cheeses, cooked meats and sausages. Tyramine is produced by bacterial activity from tyrosine in fermented cheeses. Dihydrophenylalanine occurs in broad beans. Normally, ingested amines are rapidly metabolized by the monoamine oxidase enzymes, but if large quantities of food are eaten, symptoms can result. These include erythema, headaches, hypotension and migraine. The food additive sodium nitrite causes similar symptoms in susceptible individuals.[17,29]

BACTERIAL EFFECTS

Enterotoxins

After ingestion of food or water contaminated by pathogenic bacteria or their enterotoxins, diarrhoea and vomiting is a common

Vasoactive amines in foods		
Amine	**Food source**	**Approximate concentration (μg/g)**
Serotonin	Cheese	
Histamine	Fermented cheese Smoked herring roe Tinned tuna	up to 1300 350 20
Tyramine	Cheddar cheese Camembert	1500 50
Octopamine	Citrus fruits	
Phenylethylamine	Chocolate	60
Dopamine	Chocolate	
Dopa (Dihydroxyphenylalanine)	Broad beans	

Table 20.3 Vasoactive amines in foods.

sequel and can involve a variety of mechanisms. One of the best studied mechanisms is shared by the enterotoxins of cholera, *Staphylococcus aureas* and *Escherichia coli* (heat-labile enterotoxin). After penetrating the non-specific defences of the gastric acid barrier and the mucous coating of the small intestine, the protein subunit B of the enterotoxin adheres to a receptor on the epithelial cell of the small intestine and permits entry of subunit A, which is the active toxin. Subunit A binds irreversibly to the enzyme adenylate cyclase and stimulates production of cyclic adenosine monophosphate (AMP). This produces active secretion of chloride and bicarbonate ions and inhibits absorption of sodium and chloride. The colon is unaffected, but its absorptive capacity is exceeded by the massive small bowel secretion and copious diarrhoea results. Adenylate cyclase is permanently damaged by the toxin and recovery occurs only after replacement of the affected cell.[37]

Toxic changes induced by bacteria
Other bacteria, such as *Shigella*, cause invasive bacterial infection of the epithelial mucosa. Bacteria can produce toxic changes in food, even though the bacteria themselves are not responsible for infection. Bacterial decarboxylation of histidine accounts for very high levels of histamine in certain cheeses and sausages, which can lead to diarrhoea and nausea, rashes, flushing and headaches. Scombrotoxic fish poisoning occurs after eating poorly prepared mackerel or tuna, the characteristic illness produced being due to bacterial generation of histamine from histidine.[12] Toxicity can occur because of toxins ingested by foodstuffs lower in the food chain. Nausea, vomiting, diarrhoea and occasionally paralysis are produced by ingestion of shellfish which have themselves ingested planktonic dinoflagellates which produce curare-like neurotoxins.[6,35] These reactions are predictable and would occur in many normal people exposed to the same food. There are considerable individual variations in response. This variation may be accentuated by other factors such as drug ingestion and bacterial flora of the gastrointestinal tract. The rapid hepatic metabolism of histamine is inhibited in patients taking isoniazid, and patients taking monoamine oxidase inhibitors develop headache and hypertensive crises after ingestion of foods containing tyramine, which can normally be ingested without ill-effects.

ADVERSE FOOD REACTIONS ASSOCIATED WITH METABOLIC DEFECTS

The majority of these rather rare disorders are inherited, systemic, single enzyme deficiencies, but the commonest cause of symptoms is hypolactasia, an acquired defect of lactose digestion confined to the gastrointestinal tract (Table 20.4). In biological terms, lactose is an important foodstuff only during childhood and in adult life there is no advantage to maintaining an enzyme system with no substrate. It is not surprising, therefore, that lactase activity diminishes with age.

HYPOLACTASIA

Hypolactasia is found in 5–10% of Caucasians and in up to 90% of some other races.[8] Most individuals are able to tolerate moderate quantities of lactose, such as 25 g contained within 1 pint of cow's milk daily, without symptoms, but the lactase-deficient subject may develop bloating, abdominal pain and diarrhoea. The mechanism is that of an osmotic diarrhoea: 25 g of lactose retain 250 ml of water in the small intestine to preserve isotonicity and bacterial metabolism in the colon leads to the formation of lactic acid, short-chain fatty acids, carbon dioxide and hydrogen, with further osmotic and cathartic effects. If bacteria containing beta-galactosidase, such as the lactobacilli in yoghurt, are present, then this enzyme may substitute in part for the deficient brush border enzyme and permit lactase-deficient subjects to ingest lactose in the form of yoghurt without symptoms and with nutritional benefit.[18]

Hypolactasia is not uncommon in inflammatory bowel disease and may contribute to the diarrhoea,[27] but does not occur in increased frequency in patients with the irritable bowel syndrome.[20,36]

PRIMARY ENZYME DEFICIENCIES

Primary deficiencies of sucrase-isomaltase can occur, causing symptoms in childhood which can improve in adult life.[15] In

Enzyme deficiencies giving gastrointestinal reactions to food
Hypolactasia
Sucrase-isomaltase deficiency
Trehalase deficiency
Trypsinogen deficiency
Lipase deficiency
Glucose-6-phosphate (G6P) dehydrogenase deficiency

Table 20.4 Enzyme deficiencies giving gastrointestinal reactions to food.

D

trehalase deficiency, exposure to trehalose contained in certain species of mushroom leads to severe symptoms which may be mistaken for toxic effects or food allergy.[22] Inherited disorders of protein digestion, such as trypsinogen deficiency, are rare and lead to failure to thrive in infancy. Fat malabsorption, leading to steatorrhoea, occurs rarely as a result of isolated deficiency of lipase or colipase or, more commonly, in cystic fibrosis or Schwachmann's syndrome. See also Chapter 25 on Enzyme deficiency.

Food ingestion may precipitate symptoms in other metabolic disorders. A carbohydrate meal may precipitate symptoms in periodic familial hypokalaemic paralysis, where the insulin response to a meal leads to an intracellular shift of potassium and flaccid paralysis.[25] Ingestion of broad beans in glucose-6-phosphate dehydrogenase-deficient subjects may lead to haemolysis (favism).[3]

IDIOSYNCRATIC REACTIONS

Mast cells may be degranulated other than by antigen cross-linked IgE. Mediator release may follow contact with endogenous proteins on neutrophils and eosinophils or the anaphylatoxins generated by activation of the complement cascade. Exogenous polypeptides in foodstuffs which may bind to receptors for IgE include egg-white, lectins in legumes,[16] nuts and cereals, proteolytic enzymes in pineapple and polypeptides present in shellfish, strawberries, tomatoes and fish[24] (Fig. 20.1). Small amounts of

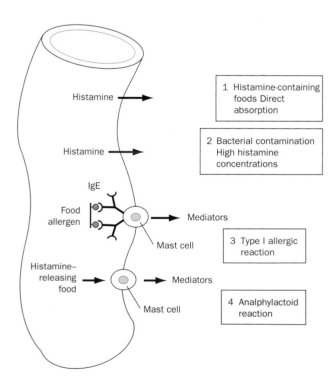

Fig. 20.1 Histamine may be absorbed directly from foods that contain large quantities either naturally or as a result of bacterial contamination. Alternatively, histamine and other mediators may be absorbed as a result of mast cell degranulation, either immunologically or non-immunologically mediated.

naturally occurring salicylates in food can cause symptoms such as wheeze, urticaria or angioedema, and the response of aspirin-sensitive subjects to the tiny doses contained in foods might suggest an allergic reaction. However, sensitivity to aspirin and related substances usually occurs in otherwise non-atopic individuals and often in middle life, suggesting a non-atopic mechanism.[31]

IRRITABLE BOWEL SYNDROME

The development of symptoms in the irritable bowel syndrome is often related by the patient to the ingestion of specific foods, including bran, widely used in the treatment of the condition.[11] Evidence for food intolerance has been sought in patients with the irritable bowel syndrome with conflicting results. Alun Jones *et al.*[1] found that symptoms could be produced in 14 of 21 patients on double-blind reintroduction of foods, and that relapse was associated with an increase in rectal levels of prostaglandin E_2, suggesting that prostaglandins were implicated in the pathogenesis of diarrhoea in this condition. This is supported by evidence suggesting that drugs inhibiting prostaglandin synthesis may reduce the incidence of food intolerance.[19] Bentley *et al.*[2] found evidence of food intolerance in 3 of 27 patients, each of whom had a previous history of atopic disease. A high prevalence of minor psychiatric disorders was found in this group of subjects, and it seems likely that psychological factors are most important in the pathogenesis of the irritable bowel syndrome. Very real changes in gastrointestinal motility occur under stress, and diarrhoea, nausea and abdominal pain can be provoked by telling patients that they have been given a food to which they believe themselves allergic.[13]

PSEUDO-FOOD ALLERGY

Pseudo-food allergy,[26] where the patient falsely believes he or she is allergic to a particular food, has become increasingly common in the last decade, and can lead to severe dietary restriction, which should not be encouraged unless there is good evidence for intolerance to a specific food. Food intolerance has been reported in one-sixth of patients with chronic fatigue syndrome and is particularly prevalent in those with a high prevalence of somatization disorder.[23] Treatment of the underlying psychiatric problems, such as chronic hyperventilation or depression, may be more appropriate.[30]

SUMMARY

Food intolerance is an adverse reaction to food not involving the immune system. There are three main groups: first, toxic or pharmacological, where an adverse reaction would be expected in any individual, are reactions that are very common and predictable; secondly, subjects with an error of metabolism such as hypolactasia, will react to foods that would not cause an effect normally; and thirdly, reactions where the mechanism is non-immune but unidentified.

REFERENCES

1 Alun Jones V, Shorthouse M, McLaughlan P, *et al*. Food intolerance: a major factor in the pathogenesis of the irritable bowel syndrome. *Lancet* 1982; ii: 115–8.

2 Bentley SJ, Pearson DJ, Rix KJB. Food hypersensitivity in irritable bowel syndrome. *Lancet* 1983; ii: 295–7.

3 Beuler E. Glucose-6-phosphate dehydrogenase deficiency. In: Stanbury JB, Fredrichson DS, *et al*. (eds) *The Metabolic Basis of Inherited Disease*, 3rd edn. McGraw-Hill, New York; 1972: 1629–53.

4 Binder MJ. Pharmacology of laxatives. *Annu Rev Pharmacol Toxicol* 1977; 17: 355–67.

5 Chin KW, Garriga MM, Metcalfe DD. The histamine content of oriental foods. *Food Chem Toxic* 1989; 27: 283–7.

6 Clarke RB. Biological causes and effects of paralytic shellfish poisoning. *Lancet* 1968; ii: 770–1.

7 Editorial. Possible B6 deficiency uncovered in patients with the Chinese Restaurant Syndrome. *Nutr Rev* 1982; 40: 15–6.

8 Ferguson A, McDonald DM, Brydon WG. Prevalence of lactase deficiency in British adults. *Gut* 1984; 25: 163–7.

9 Finn R, Cohen MN. 'Food allergy'. Fact or fiction? *Lancet* 1978; i: 426–8.

10 Folkers K, Shizukuishi S, Willis R, *et al*. The biochemistry of vitamin B6 is basic to the cause of the Chinese Restaurant Syndrome. *Hoppe Seylers Z Physiol Chem* 1984; 365(3): 405–14.

11 Francis CY, Whorwell PJ. Bran and irritable bowel syndrome: time for reappraisal. *Lancet* 1994; 344(8914): 39–40.

12 Gilbert RJ, Hobbs G, Murray CK, *et al*. Scrombotoxic fish poisoning; features of the first 50 incidents to be reported in Britain (1976–1979). *Br Med J* 1980; 281: 71–3.

13 Graham DT, Wolf S, Wolff HG. Changes in tissue sensitivity associated with varying life situations and emotions: their relevance to allergy. *J Allergy* 1950; 21: 478–86.

14 Grant G, More L, McKenzie NH, *et al*. A survey of the nutritional and haemagglutination properties of legume seeds generally available in the U.K. *Br J Nutr* 1983; 50: 207–14.

15 Gray GM. Intestinal disaccharidase deficiencies and glucose–galactase malabsorption. In: Stanbury JB, Wyngaarden JB, Fredrichson DS, *et al*. (eds) *The Metabolic Basis of Inherited Disease*, 3rd edn. McGraw-Hill, New York; 1983: 1729–42.

16 Helm RM, Froese A. Binding of the receptors for IgE by various lectins. *Intern Arch Allergy, Suppl Immunol* 1981; 65: 81–4.

17 Henderson WR, Raskin NH. Hot dog headache; individual susceptibility to nitrite. *Lancet* 1972; i: 1162–3.

18 Kolars JC, Levitt MD, Aouji M, Savaiano DA. Yoghurt – an autodigestive source of lactose. *N Engl J Med* 1984; 310: 1–3.

19 Lessof MH, Anderson JA, Youlten LJ. Prostaglandins in the pathogenesis of food intolerance. *Ann Allerg* 1983; 51(2 pt 2): 249–50.

20 Lisker R, Solomons NW, Perez Briceno R, Ramirez Mata M. Lactase and placebo in the management of the irritable bowel syndrome: a double-blind cross-over study. *Am J Gastroenterol* 1989; 84(7): 756–62.

21 MacGregor GA. New or old Chinese restaurant syndrome. *Br Med J* 1982; 285: 1205.

22 Madrazarovova-Nohhejlova J. Trehalase deficiency in a family. *Gastroenterology* 1973; 65: 130–3.

23 Manu P, Matthews DA, Lane TJ. Food intolerance in patients with chronic fatigue. *Int J Eat Disord* 1993; 13(2): 203–9.

24 Moneret-Vautrin DA. False food allergies: non-specific reactions to foodstuffs. In: Lessof M (ed.) *Clinical Reactions to Food*. John Wiley, Chichester; 1973.

25 Pearson CM, Kalyanaraman K. The periodic paralyses. In: Stanbury JB, Wyngaarden JB, Fredrichson DS, *et al*. (eds) *The Metabolic Basis of Inherited Disease*, 3rd edn. McGraw-Hill, New York; 1983: 1181–203.

26 Pearson DJ. Food allergy, hypersensitivity and intolerance. *J R Coll Physicians Lond* 1983; 19: 154–62.

27 Pena AS, Truelove SC. Hypolactasia and ulcerative colitis. *Gastroenterology* 1973; 64: 400–4.

28 Rampton RF, Charlesworth FA. Occurrence of natural toxins in food. *Br Med Bull* 1975; 31: 209–13.

29 Rice SL, Eitenmiller RR, Koehler PE. Biologically active amines in food: a review. *J Milk Food Technol* 1976; 39: 353–8.

30 Rix KJB, Pearson DJ, Bentley SJ. A psychiatric study of patients with supposed food allergy. *Br J Psychiatry* 1984; 145: 121–6.

31 Samter M, Beers RF. Intolerance to aspirin. Clinical studies and consideration of the pathogenesis. *Ann Intern Med* 1968; 68: 975–82.

32 Schaumberg HH, Byck R, Gerstl R, Mashman JH. Monosodium glutamate; its pharmacology and role in the Chinese Restaurant Syndrome. *Science* 1969; 826–8.

33 Spoerke DG Jr. Mushrooms. epidemiology and medical management. In: Hui YH, Gorham JR, Murrell KD, Cliver DO (eds) *Foodborne Disease Handbook, Vol. 3. Diseases Caused by Hazardous Substances*. Marcel Dekker, New York: 1994; 433–62.

34 Tarasoff L, Kelly MF. Monosodium L-glutamate: a double blind study and review. *Food Chem Toxicol* 1993; 31(12): 1019–35.

35 Taylor SL, Schantz EJ. Naturally occurring toxicants. In: Cliver DO, (ed.) *Foodborne Diseases*. Academic Press, San Diego, 1990: 67–84.

36 Tolliver BA *et al*. Does lactose intolerance really play a role in the irritable bowel. *J Clin Gastroenterol* 1996; 23(12):15–17.

37 Van Heyningen WE, Seal JR (eds). The biochemistry of cholera. In: *Cholera, the American Scientific Experience*. Westview Press, Boulder, Colorado; 1983: 249–84.

D

Chapter 21

Mediators in food allergy

C. H. Little

INTRODUCTION

If it is accepted that food allergy implies an adverse reaction to foods mediated by immunological mechanisms, then the mediators released during an allergic reaction will depend on the type of reaction involved.

At least three types of reaction have been identified:

1. IgE-based hypersensitivity
2. immune complex reactions
3. cell-mediated immunity.

In some cases, more than one type of reaction may be involved. Also, there may be additional processes to those listed above.

In each type of reaction, mediators will be released, some specific to that type, but others may be non-specific. The mediators can be derived from a variety of cellular sources, including macrophages, lymphocytes and effector cells such as mast cells, eosinophils, platelets, basophils and neutrophils.

Some of these mediators are only locally active with a short half-life. Demonstration of their release during an allergic reaction may only be possible using *in vitro* methods or staining tissue samples. Other mediators may be released into the circulation in significant amounts and are detectable in blood samples. The timing of blood collection may be critical, particularly if the half-life of the mediator is brief or its release is phasic. Studies on histamine[7,36] and serotonin[24,29] demonstrate these points well.

Although blood sampling is the most usual form of collection, in some cases samples of faecal fluid,[3] nasal secretions[31] and sputum can be studied.

The establishment of a suitable baseline is important in demonstrating a meaningful pattern of *in vivo* mediator release. Preliminary studies may be necessary to define the optimal time of sampling. Because allergies may be multiple, to study the changes associated with a particular antigen, other allergies must be controlled. If such care is not taken, 'background' release of mediators can obscure any meaningful pattern of change in mediator levels in response to an antigenic challenge. Observing patients in an Environmental Control Unit, where exposure to other allergens can be prevented, provides a unique opportunity to overcome this problem.

TYPES OF MEDIATOR PRODUCED

The mediators associated with particular types of immune reaction are listed in Table 21.1. Some of these mediators are unique to one type of reaction, but others may be released in more than one type. To define the immunological processes involved, attention has focused on determining whether the cytokines released *in vitro* or detectable in tissue samples are typical of a TH1 or TH2 type of response. TH1 cells produce IL2, lymphotoxin and IFNγ and TH2 cells produce IL4, IL5 and IL10.[28] Measurements of cytokines shared by both subsets, for example TNFα, do not distinguish between the two types of response. IL4 is critical for IgE synthesis[15] and IL5 is a cytokine selective for eosinophils.[16]

Earlier studies providing evidence of T-cell activation did not necessarily demonstrate cell-mediated immunity. This type of response involves the production of interferon-γ by TH1 cells.[28] Less-specific assays, e.g. the lymphocyte stimulation test (LST), are a measure of lymphocyte activation but do not indicate the

Mediators/cytokines produced during food allergy reactions

1. *IgE-based hypersensitivity*
- Vasoactive mediators: histamine, leukotrienes (C, D and E), platelet aggregating factor (PAF), serotonin, prostaglandins (PG)
- Chemotactic mediators: eosinophilic chemotactic factor (ECF), neutrophil chemotactic factor (NCF), leukotriene B, prostaglandin D_2
- Enzymes: tryptase, arylsulfatase, chymase, β-glucuronidase, β-hexosaminidase, heparin, kininogenase
- *Cytokines*: tumour necrosis factor-α, (TNFα) IL5, IL8, transforming growth factor-β (TGFβ)

2. *Immune complex reactions*
- Platelets: serotonin
- Neutrophils: lysosomal enzymes, PAF, cationic protein
- Macrophages: TNFα, IL1
- Mast cells: C-reactive protein, histamine, leukotrienes, prostaglandins

3. *Cell-mediated immunity*
- T cells (TH1) IL2, interferon-γ (INFγ), lymphotoxin
- Macrophages: macrophage inhibitory factor (MIF), TNFα, IL1

Table 21.1 Mediators/cytokines produced during food allergy reactions. Many of these mediators (e.g. TNFα) are released in more than one type of reaction.

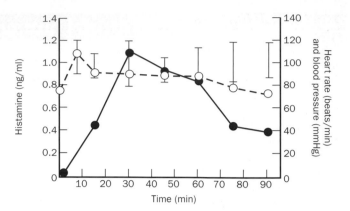

Fig. 21.1 Plasma histamine levels (●), heart rate (○) and blood pressure (I) after oral food challenge in a patient. From Atkins et al.,[7] with permission.

particular type of response: a variety of T cells could be activated, including helper T-cells (TH1 and TH2), effector T cells or other types of regulatory T cell.

Recent research has shown that a TH2 response to foods is associated with a population of T cells which produce the cytokine TGFβ.[11] This cytokine is thought to be pivotal in suppressing the cell-mediated immune response to foods.[37] The presence of this cytokine in the gut wall may exert direct or indirect effects on tissue function.

Increased production of cytokines in the gut wall as a result of an immune response to food may potentially activate afferent nerve endings. Watkins *et al.*[18] have demonstrated that IL1 may activate specialized vagal afferent nerve endings and TNFα can elicit firing in nociceptive afferent fibres.[38] They propose a cytokine–brain communication based on activation of afferent nerve endings by cytokines and the propagation of neural signals to the central nervous system.[39] The vagal nucleus (nucleus tractus solitarius), hypothalamus and nucleus raphe magnus are activated by this mechanism. Activation of vagal afferent fibres by cytokines could account for some of the cerebral symptoms and constitutional complaints reported in food allergy.

MEDIATORS IN IgE-BASED HYPERSENSITIVITY

IgE-based reactions are both more readily defined and easier to identify clinically than other types. As a result most studies have been done on this type of immune response.

HISTAMINE

A series of studies has been performed on *in vivo* release of histamine after a food challenge. Atkins *et al.*[7] studied a group of patients in whom reactions were immediate and relatively mild

in most instances. No significant rise in plasma histamine after food challenge was observed except in one patient (Fig. 21.1). Also there were no significant changes in urinary histamine (Fig. 21.2). The doses of food used in the study may have been insufficient to produce a significant rise in histamine post challenge or the principal mediators of the reaction may not have included histamine. In this study most of the patients were skin test positive to the foods producing a clinical reaction.

A study on histamine release was performed on a group of eczema patients.[36] These patients were atopic and developed skin reactions within 90 min of ingestion of the test food. Positive food challenges were associated with a significant rise in mean plasma histamine for this group; no such rise occurred with negative challenges or challenge with placebo. Of 35 positive challenges, 28 showed a significant rise in the plasma histamine level after challenge. In all but one case, positive clinical reactions were associated with positive prick tests to the food.

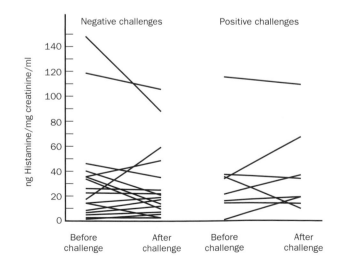

Fig. 21.2 Urinary histamine levels obtained before and during oral food challenges. There was no significant difference between prechallenge and postchallenge urinary histamine levels obtained during challenge procedures scored as negative or positive by use of the paired sample *t*-test. From Atkins et al.,[7] with permission.

GASTRIC CHALLENGE

Local histamine release has been detected on intragastric provocation.[35] There was associated mast-cell degranulation and visible changes including oedema and erythema. Not only was there a reduction in tissue histamine content in positive reactions (Fig. 21.3) but in most cases a rise in plasma histamine levels. The local histamine release showed a good correlation to a history of clinical reaction to the food.

Bankler and Lux demonstrated antigen-induced histamine release from duodenal biopsy specimens in patients allergic to foods.[8] Histamine release correlated better with food allergy than either skin tests or specific IgE. Specific IgE was demonstrated in only about two-thirds of the patients and not all reactions were clinically typical of immediate hypersensitivity. In some cases histamine release was presumably the result of mechanisms not involving IgE.

TRYPTASES RELEASED ALONG WITH HISTAMINE IN IMMEDIATE HYPERSENSITIVITY REACTIONS

One study[32] has shown a rise in both plasma histamine and tryptase in patients with immediate reactions to foods. (Figs 21.4 and 21.5). In patients with non-immediate reactions there was an elevation of plasma histamine only. The author proposed in the latter case that histamine was released from basophils. The possibility of histamine release from mast cells by neuropeptides was not considered. Although RAST scores were positive to the foods used for challenge, in some cases they were relatively low.

The release of tryptase and eosinophilic cationic protein (ECP) from the gut mucosa has been demonstrated in response to double-blind placebo-controlled food challenge positive (DBPCFC+)[34] foods, but not to foods that are tolerated in patients with gastrointestinal allergy (Figs 21.6 and 21.7). Little information was provided as to the levels of specific IgE against the foods.

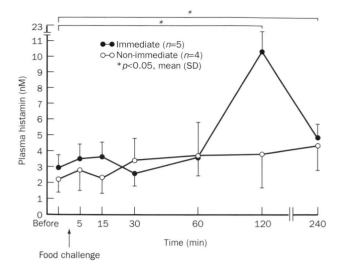

Fig. 21.4 Rise in plasma histamine in patients with immediate and non-immediate reactions to foods after food challenge. From Otsuka et al.,[32] with permission.

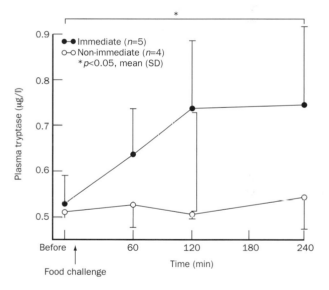

Fig. 21.5 Rise in plasma tryptase in patients with immediate and non-immediate reactions to foods after food challenge. From Otsuka et al.,[32] with permission.

THROMBOXANE

In a group of nine children who demonstrated immediate reactions to foods, the mean plasma thromboxane B2 level, a marker of thromboxane A2 activity, rose significantly at 2 and 3 hours after the challenge.[33] There was a significant rise in the mean plasma histamine level at the same times.

NEUTROPHIL CHEMOTACTIC FACTOR (NCF-A)

The release of this mediator has been demonstrated during both early and late phases of asthmatic reactions. Papageorgiou and co-workers[4] studied its release in four milk-sensitive subjects. In three subjects, a characteristic early asthmatic response developed which was accompanied by a rise in NCF-A (Fig. 21.8). However,

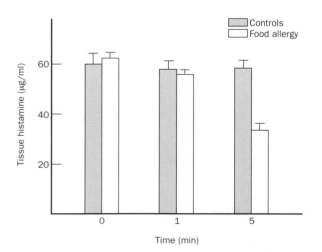

Fig. 21.3 Tissue histamine content of corpus mucosa at different time intervals after intragastral provocation in patients with food allergy ($n = 14$) and normal controls ($n = 10$). There was a significant ($P < 0.01$) decrease in tissue histamine content 5 min after allergen challenge in food-allergic patients. From Reiman et al.,[35] with permission.

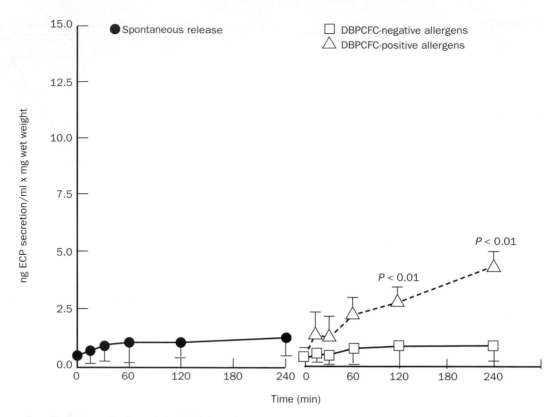

Fig. 21.6 Release of eosinophilic cationic protein (ECP) from human gut mucosa in response to double-blind placebo-controlled food challenge (DBPCFC)-positive and DBPCFC-negative allergens in patients with gastrointestinal allergy. From Raithel *et al.*,[34] with permission.

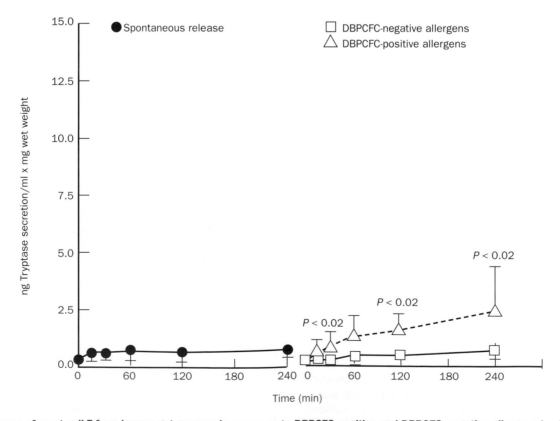

Fig. 21.7 Release of mast cell T from human gut mucosa in response to DBPCFC-positive and DBPCFC-negative allergens in nine patients with gastrointestinal allergy. From Raithel *et al.*,[34] with permission. For abbreviations, see text.

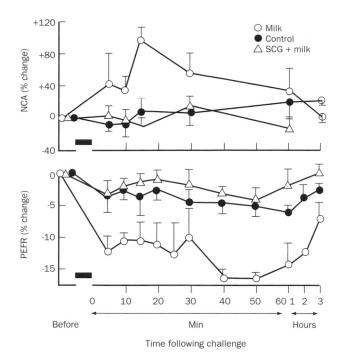

Fig. 21.8 Mean percentage change in NCA and PEFR in three asthmatics during the control day after milk ingestion. The effect of prior administration of oral sodium cromoglycate (SCG) on the changes in PEFR and NCA has also been shown. Each point represents the mean ± SEM. The mean prechallenge NCA on the control day was 121 neutrophils/10 hpf, milk day 101.5 neutrophils/10 hpf and SCG + milk day, 126.2 neutrophils/10 hpf. Solid bar = period of challenge. From Papageorgiou et al., with permission.

skin tests, specific IgE, basophil histamine release and precipitins against milk extracts were all negative. The chemotactic activity was associated with a protein with a molecular weight of about 600 000.

Comment: Histamine release may occur in association with non-IgE reactions to foods. In such cases IgG antibody (i.e. immune complexes) or neuropeptides may be involved.

LYMPHOCYTE STIMULATION TEST

Studies relying on the production of LIF or a positive LST are less conclusive. However, an earlier study[23] of infants and children with cow's milk allergy did suggest a cell-mediated immune response to the milk protein, β-lactoglobulin. In this study lymphocytes were cultured *in vitro* with β-lactoglobulin, and the production of LIF was measured. All the patients showed significant LIF production in response to β-lactoglobulin in comparison with controls. In the group of patients studied, manifestations of cow's milk allergy were quite severe with diarrhoea, vomiting, rashes, bloody stools and weight loss. At least some of these patients may have had milk-induced enteropathy. A similar study was also performed on patients with coeliac disease[5] with comparable results.

More recently it has been shown[25] that T cells from patients with coeliac disease secrete large amounts of IFNγ in response to gluten. In another study[20] peripheral blood mononuclear cells (PBMC) from infants with cow's milk allergy produced more TNFα when cultured in the presence of cow's milk proteins in comparison with control infants. These infants with cow's milk

allergy had a clinical presentation suggestive of cow's milk enteropathy with a positive history of digestive symptoms related to cow's milk ingestion, including vomiting, diarrhoea, failure to thrive and anaemia. However, the production of IFNγ in the presence of cow's milk proteins was not increased. Perhaps the PBMC contained too few T cells specific for cow's milk protein to show a significant increase in the production of IFNγ.

Cell-mediated immunity in atopic eczema
A number of studies[2,22] have indicated a role for cell-mediated immunity in eczema. Kondo *et al.*[23] demonstrated that the production of IL2 and IFNγ in response to ovalbumin by PBMC from patients with atopic dermatitis who were sensitive to egg were significantly higher than healthy children or patients who had immediate hypersensitivity to egg. A further study has demonstrated the presence of casein-specific T cells in the blood of patients with milk-induced atopic dermatitis.[40] The majority of casein-specific T cell clones produce IFNγ on stimulation with casein.[41] T cells from patients with milk-induced eczema express cutaneous lymphocyte antigen. It is possible that the skin of patients with food-induced eczema becomes infiltrated with TH1 cells reactive to specific foods. In milk or gluten enteropathy, a population of TH1 cells may infiltrate the gut.

MEDIATORS IN FOOD REACTIONS NOT ATTRIBUTABLE TO IgE OR CELL-MEDIATED IMMUNITY

There may be other immune responses to foods involving TH2 cells or perhaps another poorly defined T cells (see below). TH2 cells are associated with the production of IgG antibody. Immune complexes may form following ingestion of particular foods. As a consequence, mediators are released from mast cells and platelets, e.g. serotonin, histamine and prostaglandins. A demonstration of histamine release in adverse reactions to foods not mediated by IgE can be the result of mast-cell activation by other immune mechanisms: for example, by complement split products (C3a and C5a) or by neuropeptides.

Type 3 reactions have been implicated in food allergy. Suggested examples include coeliac disease, dermatitis herpetiformis, idiopathic nephrotic syndrome and Henoch–Schönlein purpura. Food allergy may be also involved in some cases of migraine[17,30] and rheumatoid arthritis,[24] with the formation of immune complexes. Serotonin release from platelets occurs with immune complex formation. Changing levels in whole blood serotonin or in the blood levels of its metabolite 5-HIAA (5-hydroxyindoleacetic acid) may be measurable after the ingestion of particular foods.

PROSTAGLANDINS

Prostaglandin release during food reactions was demonstrated by Buisseret *et al.*[9] who measured prostaglandins E_2 and F_2 in blood and stool samples of several patients developing acute gastrointestinal symptoms after the ingestion of specific foods. A rise in the level of these mediators was noted following food challenge, and the use of prostaglandin synthetase inhibitors blocked the reactions on subsequent challenge. The onset of symptoms was usually within 1–2 hours and skin tests were negative (Fig. 21.9).

D

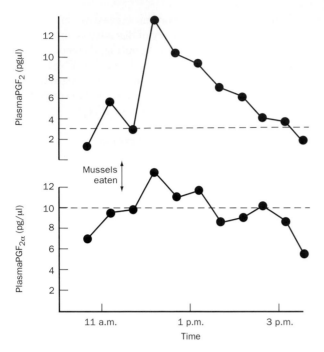

Fig. 21.9 Peripheral venous blood plasma PGE₂ and F₂ **concentrations during unprotected challenge with mussels.** Dashed lines indicate upper limits of normal. From Buisseret et al.,[9] with permission.

Food intolerance has been implicated in the irritable bowel syndrome.[3] In a study by Alun Jones et al., PGE₂ was measured in the rectal fluid after food challenge. In those patients developing diarrhoea after the challenge, significant and sustained elevations of PGE₂ were demonstrated; the prostaglandin level correlated well with faecal wet weight. However, patients who experienced pain rather than diarrhoea did not show such elevations. In this group of patients, there was no change in plasma histamine levels after challenge or evidence of histamine release from basophils after incubation with a test food.

SEROTONIN IN MIGRAINE

Several studies have demonstrated changing serotonin levels in migraine. In particular, a fall in whole blood serotonin and a subsequent rise in 5HIAA has been repeatedly observed during the headache phase.[4,29] This may be the result of immune complex formation. We have performed measurements of whole blood serotonin and 5HIAA in migraine patients before and after food challenge along with serial measurements of immune complexes (unpublished observations).

Case study; cow's milk allergy

In one particular patient there was a fall in whole blood serotonin, a rise in 5HIAA and the phasic appearance of immune complexes following the ingestion of 1 litre of milk (Figs 21.10 and 21.11). In the course of the challenge, the patient developed classic migraine with visual scotomata, paraesthesia, chills and restlessness; rhinitis and conjunctivitis were also observed. A drop in specific IgE antibody against milk was shown (Fig. 21.12). Perhaps both IgE- and IgG-containing immune complexes were formed during the migraine attack.

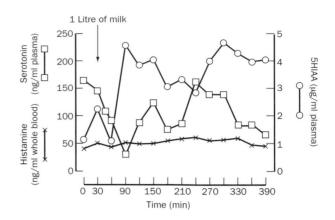

Fig. 21.10 Fall in 5-HT and rise in 5-HIAA following ingestion of 1 litre of milk.

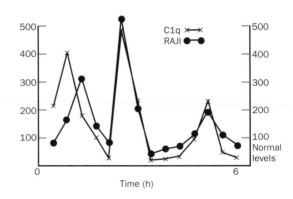

Fig. 21.11 Circulating immune complexes following milk challenge.

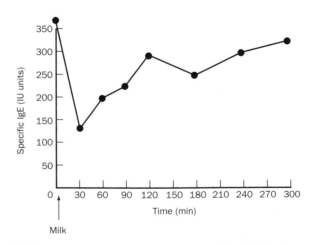

Fig. 21.12 Drop in specific IgE antibody following milk challenge.

There are other studies[26] demonstrating the presence of circulating immune complexes in food-induced migraine (Fig. 21.13). Also the serum level of IFNγ has been shown to rise and the levels of both IL4 and IL6 to fall[27] following ingestion of a food-provoking migraine (Fig. 21.14). Interpretation of these findings is difficult. Immune complex formation would suggest involvement

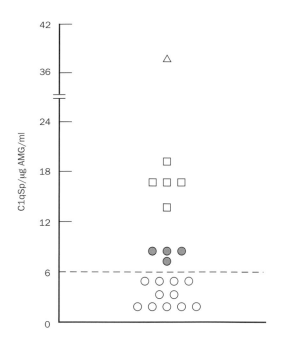

Fig. 21.13 Occurrence of circulating immune complexes in two food-induced migraine patients by the C1qSp assay (values ○ = negative; ● = borderline; □ = positive 1+; △ = positive 3+). From Martelletti et al.,[26] with permission.

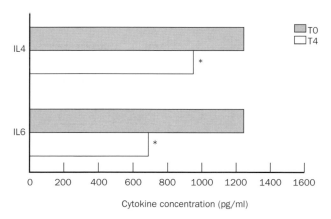

Fig. 21.14 Time-course of IL4 and IL6 serum levels before (T0) and after (T4) a specific challenge test in 20 patients suffering from dietary migraine. The concentration values (pg/ml) of both cytokines are decreased 4 hours after the administration of offending foods when compared to the values obtained at the baseline. (* = P <0.001). From Martelletti et al.,[27] with permission.

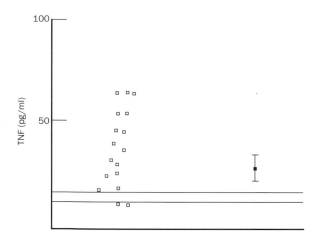

Fig. 21.15 TNF-alpha/cachectin serum concentrations in 20 patients with migraine without aura. ⊤ mean ± SE. = mean ± SE of TNF-alpha/cachectin serum concentrations in 16 normal donors. From Covelli et al.,[14] with permission.

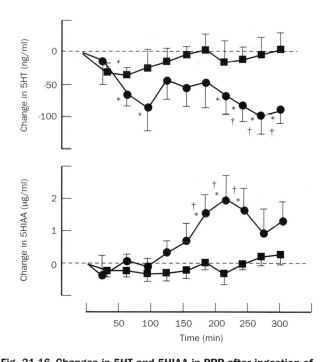

Fig. 21.16 Changes in 5HT and 5HIAA in PRP after ingestion of positive foods in food-intolerant patients (●) and healthy controls (■). Results are expressed as mean of changes from control levels (average of two estimations on samples taken before food ingestion) and 1 SEM. There were seven subjects in each group. *P <0.05, Student's paired t-test, compared with control concentrations. † P <0.05, Student's unpaired t-test, indicates a difference in magnitude of mean changes from concentrations in controls compared with patients at certain times after food ingestion. From Little et al.,[24] with permission.

of TH2 cells rather than TH1 cells. Perhaps measurement of serum levels of cytokines may be too indirect to reflect the specific immune process. A further study[14] has shown increased levels of TNFα in the blood of migraine patients. (Fig. 21.15). This cytokine is not specific for a particular type of immune response, but indicates immune activation.

Rheumatoid arthritis
We studied serotonin release in patients with rheumatoid arthritis whose condition was clearly exacerbated by the ingestion of certain foods.[24] There was a fall in whole blood serotonin and subsequent increase in 5HIAA following positive food challenges

in these patients (Fig. 21.16). In some patients the change in blood levels was particularly striking, as shown in Fig. 21.17.

Aside from the disorders mentioned above, we have observed a fall in whole blood serotonin and a rise in 5HIAA following a positive food challenge in a number of other conditions. Figure 21.18 shows changes that occurred in a patient who developed bronchospasm after milk challenge.

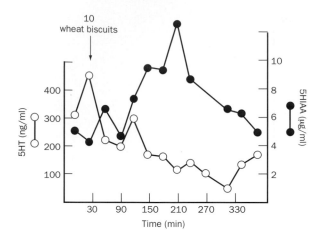

Fig. 21.17 5HT and 5HIAA in PRP after ingestion of wheat at 30 min.
Control samples were taken before ingestion of wheat followed by
sampling every 30 min for 330 min.

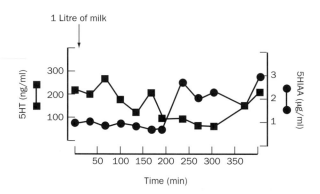

Fig. 21.18 Fall in blood serotonin (5HT) and rise in 5-hydroxyindoleacetic acid (5HIAA) following positive food challenge in patient.

NEW DIRECTIONS

Recent research on food tolerance to food proteins has indicated
three possible outcomes:

1. cell-mediated immunity (TH1 response)
2. humoral immunity (TH2 response)
3. absence of immune response with either anergy or deletion
   of reacting cells.

Accompanying humoral immunity is the production of the
cytokine TGFβ, which plays a central role in suppressing the cell-
mediated immune response.[37] The cellular source of this cytokine
is not known but may represent a separate type of T cell.[11,12]

T-CELL ANTIGEN-BINDING MOLECULES

We have studied a group of patients showing delayed reactions to
cow's milk who developed symptoms such as fatigue, headache
and musculoskeletal pain after milk ingestion[24a]. In this group,
there were significantly higher levels of circulating T-cell-derived
antigen-specific molecules (TABM), which bind to milk proteins
such as casein and β-lactoglobulin (Figs 21.19 and 21.20).

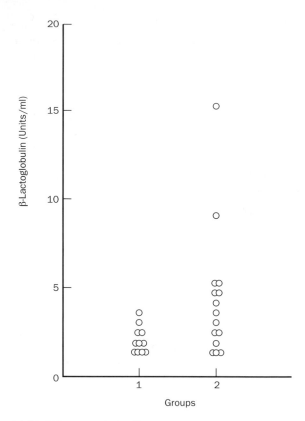

Fig. 21.19 TABM specific for β-lactoglobulin. Group 1 = controls.
Group 2 = patients. $P = 0.016$.

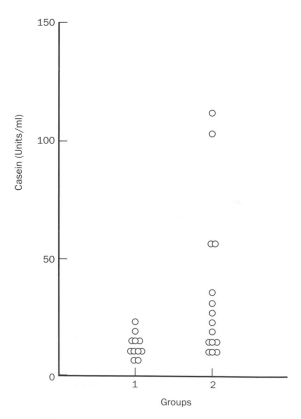

Fig. 21.20 TABM specific for casein. Group 1 = controls.
Group 2 = patients. $P = 0.011$.

TABM share epitopes with the T-cell receptor, are antigen specific and are linked to cytokines. They are thought to be important in the suppression of cell-mediated immunity to specific antigens[13] and may be produced in association with a TH2 response.

TABM specific for β-lactoglobulin (BL-TABM) was purified from a patient who showed a high titre of this molecule in the serum, as measured with anti-TABM antibody. This BL-TABM was shown to bind β-lactoglobulin using an ELISA assay. It was also demonstrated to contain TGFβ-1 and TGFβ-2 (Fig. 21.21)[24a].

The BL-TABM enhanced the release of TNFα from PBMC stimulated with lipopolysaccharide (LPS) (Fig. 21.22). This is attributable to the action of TGFβ. This finding is reminiscent of the study by Heyman *et al*.[20]

In further studies (unpublished observations) we have shown that, of the three principal antigenic proteins, α-lactalbumin is the major antigen for TBAM .IgGantibody is produced mainly to β-lactoglobulin and casein. In addition, we have found that TABM are produced to numerous other foods, including egg, wheat, apple, orange and chocolate.

In an extensive paper, published last year,[21a] we demonstrated that TGFβ enhances the release of neuropeptides from sensory nerve endings. (Fig. 21.23). Purified TABM specific to benzoic acid (BA-TABM), also associated with TGFβ, enhanced the release of neuropeptides.

(Fig. 21.24) This effect was blocked by anti-TGFβ antibody (Fig. 21.25). The addition of antigen to this purified BA-TABM caused the activation of the associated TGFβ, this effect depending on the ratio between the TABM and antigen (Fig. 21.26). Finally, the purified BA-TABM is associated with the enzyme elastase, presumably the acivator of the TGFβ (Figs 21.27 and 21.28)

In summary, TABM, although binding to nominal antigen, may be associated with cytokines such as TGFβ and elastase as a high molecular weight aggregate. The linking of TGFβ to antigen may ensure this cytokine is focused to where antigen is located, in order to suppress the cell-mediated response to the antigen. In the

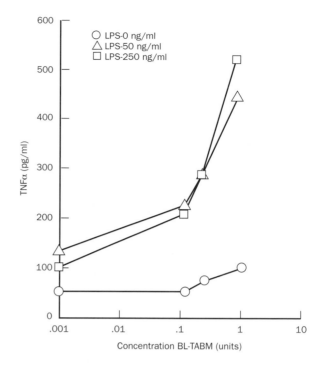

Fig. 21.22 TNFα production by PBMC incubated with LPS and BL-TABM.

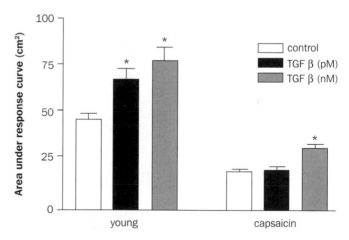

Fig. 21.23 Dose–response effect of TGF-β (10 pM & 10 nM concentrations) on the relative blood flow induced by 1 μM substance P(SP) in control and capsaicin-pretreated rats. SP was measuring the surface area under the blood flux curve obtained for 30 min after perfusion of SP alne or after 10 min perfusion of TGF-β. Columns represent the mean ± standard error of the mean (*n* = 8 in each group). An asterisk denotes a significant diference from SP alone.

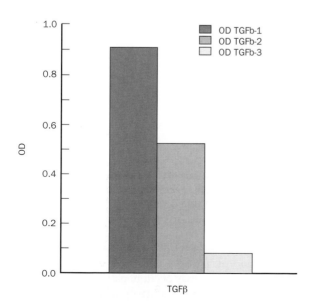

Fig. 21.21 ODs from ELISA assay for TGFβ on BL-TABM purified from a milk-sensitive patient.

case of food proteins, TABM may prevent a destructive cellular immune response, via the action of TGFβ.

However, the local activation of TGFβ in the gut wall may have untoward effects. TGFβ is a pleiotropic cytokine with many actions. It suppresses the release of cytokines such as IFNγ[21] and TNFα,[10] attracts mastcells[19] and enhances the release of neuropeptides from sensory nerves.[21a] As a consequence, there may be local inflammation, changes in gut motility and the relay of

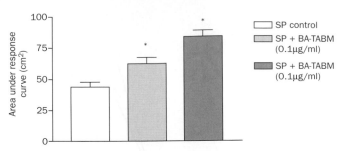

Fig. 21.24 Dose–response effect of purified TABM(BA-TABM) (0.1 and 1.0 mg/ml) on the relative blood flow induced by 1 µg/ml substance P(SP) in controls rats. SP was perfused over the base of blisters induced in naïve skin. Responses were calculated by measuring the surface area under the blood flux curve obtained for 30 min perfusion for SP alone or after 10 min perfusion of TABM. Columns represent the mean ± standard eror of the mean (*n* = 8 in each group). An asterisk denotes a significant diference from SP alone.

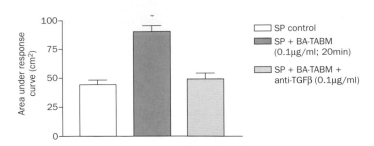

Fig. 21.25 Effect of 0.1 µg/ml anti TGFβ antibody on the effect of 0.1 µg/ml purified TABM in modulating the relative blood flow induced by 1µMSP in control rats. Responses were calculated by measuring the surface area under the blood flux curve obtained for a 30 min perfusion of SP alone or after a 10 min perfusion of TABM. Columns represent the mean ± standard error of the mean (*n* = 8 in each group). An asterisk denotes a significant difference from SP alone.

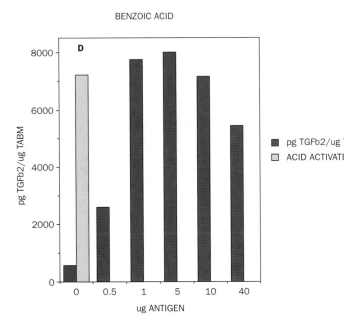

Fig. 21.26 A total of 100 ng of purified TABM (BA-TABM) was incubated for 1 hr at room temperature with benzoic acid. After incubation, the mixture was added to micro titre plates of a TGFβ ELISA Kit. TGFβ was quantified in the samples via comparison with the optical densities of TGFβ standards.

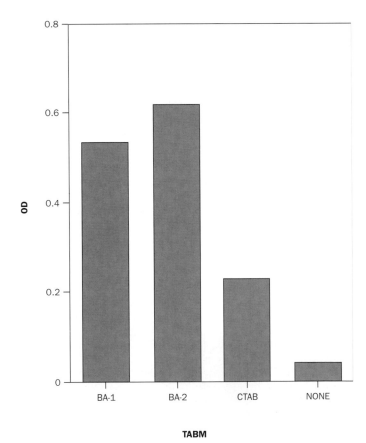

Fig. 21.27 ODS from ELISA assay for elastase on two purified preparations of benzoic acid specific TABM(BA-1 and BA 2)and Candida mannan specific TABM (CTAB).

neural signals to brain centres via vagal afferent nerves.[18a,3a] Such processes may be implicated in the production of symptoms associated with food intolerance.

The 'physiological' immune response to food proteins may be anergy.[31a] Indeed, anergic T cells are thought to have a regulatory function in maintaining peripheral tolerance.Immune deviation–humoral immunity with suppression of cellular immunity via the action of TGFβ – may have adverse effects. This immune response pattern may occur in patients who have adverse reactions to foods which are not attributable to IgE antibody or cellular immunity. In such patients TABM and/or IgG antibody to food proteins may play a central role.

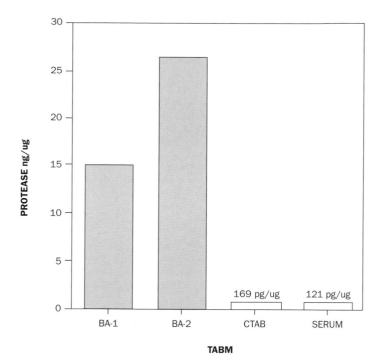

Fig. 21.28 Measurement of elastase from ELISA assay on benzoic acid specific TABM (BA-1 and BA-2), Candida mannan specific TABM and serum.

REFERENCES

1 Abernathy-Carver K, Sampson H, Picker L, Leung D. Milk-induced eczema is associated with the expansion of T cells expressing cutaneous lymphocyte antigen. *J Clin Invest* 1995; 95: 913–18.

2 Agata H, Kondo N, Fukutomi O, Shinoda S, Orii T. Interleukin-2 production of lymphocytes in food sensitive atopic dermatitis. *Arch Dis Childhood* 1992; 67: 280–4.

3 Alun Jones V, Laughlan P, Shorthouse M *et al*. Food intolerance. a major factor in the pathogenesis of irritable bowel syndrome. *Lancet* 1982; 1: 115–7.

4 Anthony M, Hinterberger H, Lance J. Plasma serotonin in migraine and stress. *Arch Neurol* 1967; 16: 544–52.

5 Ashkenazi A, Idar D, Handzel ZT *et al*. An in vitro immunological assay for diagnosis of coeliac disease. *Lancet* 1978; 1: 627.

6 Ashkenazi A, Levin S, Idar D *et al*. In vitro cell-mediated immunological assay for cow's milk allergy. *Paediatrics* 1980; 66: 399–402.

7 Atkins F, Steinberg S, Metcalf D. Evaluation of immediate adverse reactions to foods in adult patients. *J Allergy Clin Immunol* 1985; 75: 356–63.

8 Bankler H, Lux G. Antigen-induced histamine-release from duodenal biopsy in gastro-intestinal food allergy. *Ann Allergy* 1989; 62: 449–52.

9 Buisseret P, Youlten L, Heinzelmann D, Lessof M. Prostaglandin-synthetase inhibitors in prophylaxis of food intolerance. *Lancet* 1978; I: 906–8.

10 Chantry D, Turner M, Abney E, Feldmann M. Modulation of cytokine production by transforming growth factor-β 1. *J Immunol* 1989; 142: 4295–4300.

11 Chen Y, Weiner H. Dose-dependent activation and deletion of antigen-specific T cells following oral tolerance. *Ann NY Acad Sci* 1996; Vol. 778, Oral tolerance: mechanism and applications, pp. 111–21.

12 Chen Y, Kuchroo V, Inobe J, Hafler D, Weiner N. Regulatory T cell clones induced by oral tolerance: suppression of auto-immune encephalomyelitis. *Science* 1994; 265: 1237–40.

13 Cone R, Malley A. Soluble antigen-specific T-cells proteins: T-cell based humoral immunity? *Immunol Today* 1996; 17: 318–22.

14 Covelli V, Munno I, Pelligrino N, Venere A, Jirillo E, Buscaino G. Exaggerated spontaneous release of tumour necrosis factor-α/cachectin in patients with migraine without aura. *Acta Neurologica* 1990; 12: 257–63.

15 Del Prete GF, Maggi F, Parronchi P *et al*. IL-4 is an essential factor for the IgE synthesis induced *in vitro* by human T-cell clones and their supernatants. *J Immunol* 1988; 140. 4193–8.

16 Egan RW, Umland SP, Cuss FM, Chapman RW. Biology of interleukin-5 and its relevance to allergic disease. *Allergy* 1996; 51: 71–81.

17 Egger J, Carter C, Wilson J *et al*: Is migraine food allergy? *Lancet* 1983; ii: 863–9.

18 Goehler LE, Relton J, Mauer SF, Watkins LR. Biotinylated interleukin-1 receptor antagonist (IL-lra) labels paraganglia in the rat liver hilus and hepatic vagus. *Proc Soc Neurosci* 1994; 20: 956.

18a Goehler 1, Gaykema R, Hansen M, Anderson K, Maier S, Watkins L. Vagal immune-to brain communication:a visceral chemosensory pathway. *Neuroscience: Basic and Clinical* 2000;85:49–59.

19 Gruber BL, Marchese MJ, Keo RR. Transforming growth factor-β 1 mediates mast cell chemotaxis. *J Immunol* 1994; 152: 5860–7.

20 Heyman M, Darmon N, Dupont C *et al*.Mononuclear cells from infants allergic to cows milk secrete tumour necrosis factor α, altering intestinal function. *Gastroenterology* 1994; 106: 1514–23.

21 Holter W, Kalthoff F, Picki W, *et al*. Transforming growth factor-β inhibits IL-4 and IFN-γ production by stimulated human T-cells. *Int Immunol* 1994; 6: 469–75.

21a Khalil Z, Georgiou G, Cone R, Simpson F, Little C. Immunological and in-vivo neurological studies on a benzoic acid-specific T cell derived antigen-binding molecule from the serum of a toluene sensitive patient. *Arch Environ Health* 2000;55: 304–18.

22 Kondo N, Agata H, Fukutomi O, Motoyoshi F, Orii T. Lymphocyte responses to food antigens in patients with atopic dermatitis who are sensitive to foods. *J Allergy Clin Immunol* 1990; 86: 253–60.

23 Kondo N, Fukutomi O, Agata H *et al*. The role of T lymphocytes in patients with food sensitive atopic dermatitis. *J Allergy Clin Immunol* 1993; 91: 658–68.

24 Little C, Stewart A, Fennessy M. Platelet serotonin release in rheumatoid arthritis: a study in food-intolerant patients. *Lancet* 1983; 297–9.

24a Little C, Georgiou G, Shelton M, Cone R. Production of serum immunoglobulins and T cell antigen binding molecules specific for cows' milk antigens in adults intolerant to cows' milk. *Clin Immunol Immunopathol* 1998;89:160–70.

25 Lundin K, Scott H, Hansen T *et al*. Gliadin-specific HLA-DQ (α 1*0501, β 1*0201) restricted T cells isolated from the small intestinal mucosa of coeliac disease patients. *J Exp Med* 1993; 78: 187–96.

26 Martelletti P, Sutherland J, Anastasis E, Di Mario U, Giocavazzo M. Evidence for an immuno-mediated mechanism in food-induced migraine from a study on activated T-cells, IgG4 subclass, anti-IgG antibodies and circulating immune complexes. *Headache* 1989; 29: 664–70.

27 Martelletti P, Stirparo G, Rinaldi C, Frati L, Giocavazzo M: Disruption of the immunopeptidergic network in dietary migraine. *Headache* 1993; 33: 524–7.

28 Mosmann TR, Coffman RL. TH1 and TH2 cells: different patterns of lymphokine secretion lead to different functional properties. *Am Rev Immunol* 1989; 7: 145–73.

29 Muck-Seler D, Deanovic Z, Dupely M. Serotonin-releasing factors in migrainous patients. *Adv Neurol* 1983; 33: 257–64.

30 Munro J, Carini C, Brostoff J. Migraine is a food allergic disease. *Lancet* 1984; ii: 719–21.

31 Naclario R, Proud D, Togias A *et al*. Inflammatory mediators in late antigen-induced rhinitis. *N Eng J Med* 1985; 313: 65–70.

31a Nagler-Anderson C. Tolerance and immunity in the intestinal immune system. *Crit Rev Immunol* 2000;20:103–20.

32 Ohtsuka T, Matsumaru S, Uchida K *et al*. Time course of plasma histamine and tryptase following food challenges in children with suspected food allergy. *Ann Allergy* 1993; 71: 139–46.

33 Ohtsuka T, Matsumaru S, Uchida K *et al*. Pathogenic role of thromboxane A2 in immediate hypersensitivity reactions in children. *Am Allergy Asthma Immunol* 1996; 77: 55–9.

34 Raithel M, Pacurar A, Winterkamp S, Dalbay S, Ell C, Hahn E. Analysis and characteristics of mast cell tryptase and eosinophilic cationic protein from human gut mucosa in gastro-intestinal allergy. In: Wurich B, Ortolanic (eds), *Highlights in Food Allergy Manages Allergy*. Karger, Basel, Vol 32, 143–56.

35 Reiman H, Ring J, Utsch B, Wendt P. Intragastric provocation under endoscopic control in food allergy: mast cell and histamine changes in gastric mucosa. *Clin Allergy* 1985; 15: 195–202.

36 Sampson H, Jolie P. Increased plasma histamine concentrations after food challenges in children with atopic dermatitis. *N Eng J Med* 1984; 311: 372–6.

37 Strober W, Kelsall B, Fuss I *et al*. Reciprocal IFN-γ and TGF-β responses regulate the occurrence of mucosal inflammation. *Immunol Today* 1997; 18: 61–4.

38 Watkins LR, Goehler LE, Relton J, Brewer M, Mauer SF. Mechanisms of tumour necrosis factor α (TNF-α) hyperalgesia. *Brain Res* 1995; 692: 244–50.

39 Watkins LR, Mauer SF, Goehler LE. Cytokine-to-brain communications: a review and analysis of alternative mechanisms. *Life Sci* 1995c; 57: 1011–26.

40 Werfel T, Ahlers G, Schmidt P, Boeker M, Kapp A. Detection of a casein-specific lymphocyte response in milk-responsive atopic dermatitis. *Clin Exp Allergy* 1996; 26: 1380–6.

41 Werfel T, Ahlers G, Schmidt P, *et al*. Milk-responsive atopic dermatitis is associated with a casein-specific lymphocyte response in adolescent and adult patients. *J Allergy Clin Immunol* (in press)

Chapter 22

Diet and the metabolism of intestinal bacteria

G. T. Macfarlane and J. H. Cummings

INTRODUCTION

The human large bowel is a highly specialized digestive organ in which the activities of its resident microbiota affect human physiology in a multiplicity of ways (Table 22.1). Through fermentation, the bacteria of the hindgut complete the digestive process and contribute to metabolism. The colonic epithelium has an obligate requirement for bacterial fermentation products, while the maintenance of colonization resistance to microbial pathogens, the activation or destruction of genotoxins and mutagens, and modulation of the immune system,[97] are all dependent on the flora. Host tissues and other endogenous substrates such as mucins, pancreatic and other secretions are constantly broken down and recycled by intestinal bacteria, but the species composition and metabolic activities of the microbiota are primarily determined by diet. What we eat, therefore, particularly carbohydrate and protein, controls ecological, physiological and metabolic events in the bowel.

Large bowel function

Human large intestinal contents mainly comprise bacteria. Average daily faecal output in the United Kingdom is around 100 g, of which 25 g is solid matter. In addition to diet, the length of time digestive material spends in the large intestine is an important determinant of bacterial metabolism. Long colonic transits affect the metabolism of carbohydrates, proteins and xenobiotic substances, and have been linked to the occurrence of large bowel cancer.[50] Moreover, a significant correlation exists between transit time and bacterial mass in the large intestine. Stephen *et al.*[203] used the drug Senokot to speed up gut transit time from 64 to 25 h in human volunteers. This increased mean stool weight from 148 to 285 g/day, with bacterial mass increasing from 18.9 to 20.3 g/day.

Factors affecting development of the human colonic microbiota and its metabolic and health significance to the host	
Host, environmental and microbiological factors affecting microbiota development	**Health significance of the colonic microflora**
Diet, colonic transit time, epithelial cell turnover rates	Salvages energy from undigested carbohydrate by fermentation and SCFA production
Geographical residence/cultural factors associated with host	Barrier to invading pathogenic microorganisms, through colonization resistance
Disease, drugs, antibiotic therapy, rates of mucus production and its chemical composition	Bacterial cell mass stimulates peristalsis, colonic motility and affects bowel habit
pH and redox potential	Modulates activity of the immune system
Bacterial competition for limiting nutrients. Biofilm development on food particles, in mucus and at the epithelial surface. Cooperative interactions between microorganisms	Production and/or inactivation of toxic, mutagenic or carcinogenic substances from dietary constituents, or host tissues and secretions
Generic and species composition of microbiota	Enterohepatic circulation of steroids, drugs and xenobiotic metabolites
Bacterial inhibition by fermentation products including HS⁻, SCFA, phenolic compounds, deconjugated bile salts, etc. Microbial secretion of antagonistic substances	Control of growth and differentiation of colonic epithelium due to SCFA, especially butyrate
Synergistic effects of bacterial antagonism and local immunity and other defences in the mucus layer and at the mucosal surface	Vitamin production

Table 22.1 Factors affecting development of the human colonic microbiota and its metabolic and health significance to the host.

In contrast, treatment with codeine/loperamide increased colonic transit times from 47 to 88 h and reduced bacterial cell mass from 18.9 to 16.1 g/day.

Ecology of intestinal bacteria

The large intestine is a complex microbial ecosystem in which bacteria exist in a multiplicity of microhabitats and metabolic niches. The microbiota comprises several hundred bacterial species, subspecies and biotypes. Some organisms occur in higher numbers than others do, and about 40 species make up approximately 99% of all isolates. Due to their high numbers and frequency of detection, they are viewed as being autochthonous to the colon, but many other transient microorganisms are routinely detected in faeces. Species belonging to the genera *Bacteroides*, *Bifidobacterium* and *Eubacterium*, together with a variety of anaerobic Gram-positive rods and cocci predominate.[73]

Although many different types of relationship exist between intestinal bacterial populations, the ability to compete for limiting nutrients and adhesion sites on food particles, or on the colonic mucosa, is particularly important and effectively determines the composition of the microbiota. Biofilm communities growing on the surfaces of food particles in the colon form metabolically distinct assemblages in gut microbiota in relation to polysaccharide breakdown and metabolism, but at present there is insufficient evidence to determine whether they are genotypically different to non-adherent populations.[138]

While large inter-individual variations exist in intestinal bacterial populations at species level,[73] molecular studies show that only a small fraction of bacterial species in natural communities can be cultivated.[63,102] Consequently, we know surprisingly little

about the extent of microbial diversity in the large gut, or of the metabolic relationships that exist between individual bacterial communities, their ecology or the multicellular organization of the microbiota. However, increasing species diversity in a microbiota such as the large intestine is known to enforce metabolic homeostasis and structural stability,[81] while degenerative changes in species composition, through for example, antibiotic administration, reduce the ability of the ecosystem to resist invading pathogens. In animals, food deprivation leads to major changes in gut bacterial populations, and renders them more susceptible to enterobacterial infections.[208]

CARBOHYDRATE METABOLISM

Carbohydrates and bacterial growth

The principal determinant of species diversity in the colonic ecosystem is the multiplicity of different carbon sources to which intestinal microorganisms have access. The great majority of gut bacteria are saccharolytic,[132] but most simple sugars in the diet are absorbed in the small gut, the exceptions being the non-digestible oligosaccharides (NDO), for example fructooligosaccharides, galactooligosaccharides (see later), raffinose and stachyose, disaccharides such as lactose in many populations, lactulose, and the sugar alcohols sorbitol and xylitol.

The main sources of carbon and energy for the microbiota are resistant starches, plant cell wall polysaccharides (fibre) and host mucopolysaccharides, together with various proteins and peptides.[127] These complex molecules are depolymerized by bacterial polysaccharidases, glycosidases, proteases and peptidases to smaller oligomers and their component sugars and amino acids,

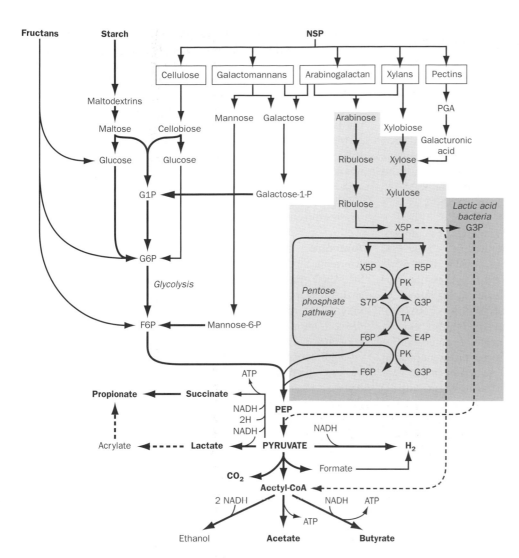

Fig. 22.1 Major pathways of polysaccharide fermentation in the large intestine.

which can be assimilated and fermented by the microbiota. Because the majority of carbohydrates entering the colon occur as polysaccharides, the rate at which these substances are depolymerized controls the availability of fermentable substrate, which in turn, affects end-product formation.[130] Carbohydrate fermentation is the major force driving the metabolic activities of the microbiota, and is quantitatively more important than amino acid catabolism, particularly in the proximal bowel where substrate availability is greatest. Figure 22.1 shows the principal pathways of carbohydrate utilization in colonic microorganisms.

Regulation of carbohydrate metabolism

Many different types of carbohydrates are present in the colon. Consequently, nutritionally versatile bacteria that can grow on a variety of carbon sources and adapt rapidly to changing substrate availability have a competitive advantage in the ecosystem. Carbohydrate utilization is controlled by catabolite regulatory mechanisms, which determine the synthesis of hydrolytic enzymes and substrate transport systems, as well as their physiological activities.[128]

Catabolite regulatory mechanisms enable colonic microorganisms to use certain substrates selectively to the exclusion of others, allowing some organisms to compete more efficiently for a restricted range of preferred substrates in relatively specialized metabolic niches. Because different bacteria form distinct patterns of metabolic end products, catabolite regulatory mechanisms ultimately affect the types and amounts of these substances that can be produced from individual substrates.[132,137] Consequently, these control processes are ecologically important, and are also of physiological significance to the host, since different fermentation products are metabolized at various sites in the body (see later).

Carbohydrate fermentation

Although many different carbohydrates are fermented by gut bacteria, they are catabolized in a relatively small number of metabolic pathways (see Fig. 22.1). Anaerobic metabolism is controlled by the requirement to maintain redox balance, mainly through the reduction and oxidation of ferredoxins, flavins and pyridine nucleotides. This affects the flow of carbon through the bacteria, the energy yield obtained from the substrate, and the fermentation products that are formed. Synthesis of chemically reduced metabolic products such as lactate, succinate, H_2, butyrate and ethanol is used to control redox balance during fermentation, whereas production of more oxidized substances, such as acetate, is linked to ATP generation. Conversely, more reduced fermentation products result in comparatively low ATP yields.[126]

NITROGEN METABOLISM

Substrates

Analysis of residues in different regions of the large bowel shows large amounts of soluble protein and peptides.[200] Approximately 13 g of proteins and peptides from diet and pancreatic secretions enter the colon daily, where they serve as nitrogen and energy sources for the microbiota.[33,134] Mucous secretions, urea and shed colonic epithelial cells also contribute to the pool of organic N-containing compounds.[49] Figure 22.2 provides an overview of the ways in which intestinal bacteria utilize these substances.

Proteolysis

The colon is strongly proteolytic due to the activities of a complex mixture of bacterial and pancreatic endopeptidases.[134] Microbial enzymes contribute considerably to overall protease activity, especially in the distal gut, and play an important role in digesting pancreatic enzymes which are the preferred organic nitrogen sources for some intestinal bacteria.[133] Faecal proteolysis differs both qualitatively and quantitatively from that in the small bowel. Gibson et al.[86] compared the ability of pancreatic proteases in ileal effluent and the proteolytic activity in faeces to digest different protein substrates. While there was a substantial reduction in protease activity in faeces compared with small intestinal contents, different proteins were seen to be digested in different ways. For example, casein was broken down more rapidly than collagen by both faecal and small intestinal proteases, whereas bovine serum

albumin (BSA) was not hydrolysed by pancreatic enzymes at all, but was digested by faecal proteases. This suggested that pancreatic endopeptidases may not be particularly efficient at breaking down some highly globular proteins in the small gut.

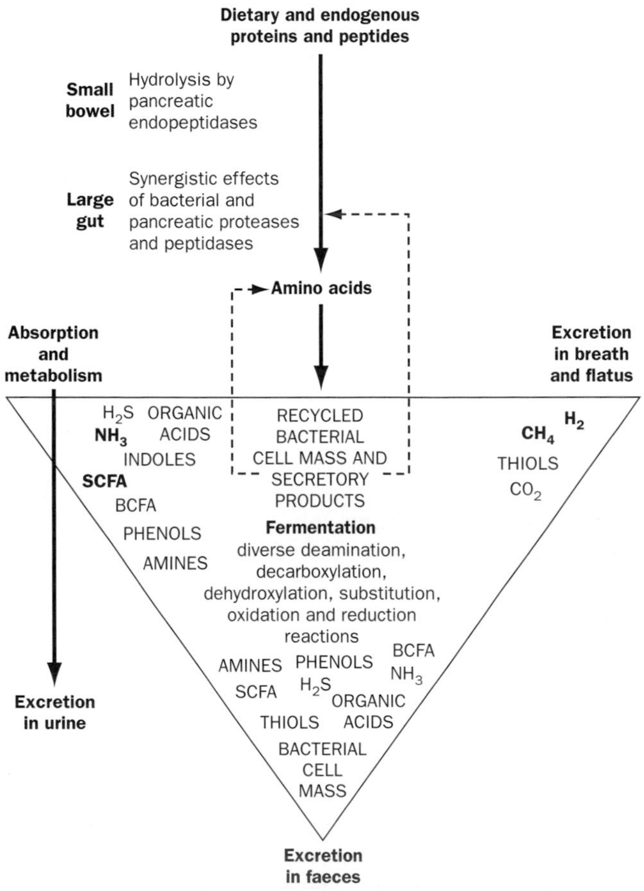

Although quantitatively less important than saccharolytic species, large numbers of amino acid fermenting bacteria exist in the large bowel.[200] The acidic end products of bacterial protein fermentation are varied and include short-chain fatty acids (SCFA), branched-chain fatty acids (BCFA), and a range of other non-volatile organic acids (see later). Other metabolites of amino acid fermentation include ammonia, CO_2, H_2, phenols, hydrogen sulphide, indoles and amines. Many of these substances are absorbed from the bowel, and are toxic to host tissues.

Ammonia

Ammonia alters the morphology and intermediary metabolism of intestinal epithelial cells, increases DNA synthesis and affects their lifespan,[216] while high concentrations in the colonic lumen may select for neoplastic growth.[37,148] In patients with liver disease, ammonia contributes to the onset of portal-systemic encephalopathy.[215,220]

High concentrations of ammonia are often found in human faeces,[46] and it was originally thought that this metabolite was primarily a product of bacterial ureolysis.[206] However, urea is not detected in significant amounts in ileal effluent,[38] indicating that protein breakdown and amino acid fermentation accounts for the majority of ammonia in the colon. This notion supports work by Cummings et al.[45] who observed a doubling in faecal ammonia excretion when daily protein intake was increased from 63 to 136 g in volunteers. This work also showed that faecal nitrogen excretion increases while ammonia levels fall when fermentation is stimulated by addition of fibre to the diet, with active carbohydrate fermentation routing nitrogen into bacterial protein.

This principle has been exploited in the treatment of patients with liver cirrhosis, where ammonia accumulates in body fluids, contributing to the onset of hepatic coma. Administration of the non-absorbable disaccharide lactulose reduces ammonia recycling by stimulating fermentation by the gut microflora.[152,220] Ammonia concentrations in the colon therefore represent a balance between deamination of amino acids by some organisms, subsequent uptake by bacterial cells as a nitrogen source for protein synthesis, and colonic absorption.

Fermentation of aromatic amino acids

Free tyrosine, tryptophan and phenylalanine are poorly assimilated by intestinal bacteria in comparison to other amino acids,[200] reflecting the hydrophobic character of these substances. However, their fermentation generates a wide range of phenolic and indolic metabolites in a series of deamination, transamination, decarboxylation and dehydrogenation reactions.[198] Phenol, p-cresol and hydroxylated phenol-substituted fatty acids are the principal products of tyrosine fermentation in the large intestine, while phenylacetate and phenylpropionate are produced from phenylalanine. Indole, ammonia, and pyruvate are formed from tryptophan by tryptophanase. A wide range of taxonomically diverse intestinal bacteria produce indole, and its excretion in urine as indican has often been used to provide an index of bacterial metabolism in the gut, especially in bacterial overgrowth syndromes,[91,212] although its lack of specificity led to it being abandoned for routine clinical use.

Fig. 22.2 Metabolism of organic nitrogen containing compounds in the large intestine.

Many intestinal microorganisms ferment aromatic amino acids, including clostridia,[68] bifidobacteria,[7] bacteroides,[147] lactobacilli[225] and anaerobic Gram-positive cocci,[57a] but few data are available concerning the physiological and nutritional factors that control these processes. However, distinct contrasts exist in the amounts and types of phenolic metabolites in digestive material in different regions of the large bowel. Concentrations of phenolic compounds are approximately four-fold greater in the distal colon. Moreover, phenol-substituted fatty acids predominate in the proximal large intestine, while simple phenols are the major products of aromatic amino acid fermentation in the distal gut.[198] This may result from differences in the absorptive capacities of the proximal and distal colons, variations in rates of protein breakdown and hence amino acid availability in different parts of the gut, as well as direct effects of pH and carbohydrate availability, on bacterial growth, substrate transport and metabolism.

Effect of diet

Production of phenols and indoles by gut bacteria is dependent on many factors, including diet, the secretory activities of the gastrointestinal tract and exocrine pancreas, as well as the species composition of an individual's microbiota. Studies on diet and amino acid fermentation showed that urinary phenol and p-cresol excretion was strongly reduced when 18 volunteers changed from a conventional Western diet to an uncooked vegan diet. When the volunteers reverted to their original lifestyle, phenol excretion returned to the original level after 4 weeks.[122]

Reduction of urinary excretion of phenolic compounds in volunteers consuming high-fibre diets has been related to the increased requirements of intestinal bacteria for tyrosine for use in biosynthetic processes consequent upon greater carbohydrate availability and cell growth.[45] In in vitro studies, starch and low pH strongly affected dissimilatory aromatic amino acid metabolism.[198] These investigations showed that the formation of phenolic compounds was inhibited at pH 5.5, which is characteristic of the proximal large bowel,[47] and indicated that carbohydrate availability is an important factor determining the metabolic fates of aromatic amino acids in the colon. In human feeding studies the addition of 39 g/day of resistant starch to the diet led to an increase in faecal total nitrogen excretion, presumably as a result of increased bacterial cell mass, and decreased faecal ammonia and phenol concentrations.[17]

Other investigations have demonstrated that increased production of phenolic and indolic compounds in the colon is related to slow transit times of material through the bowel.[45,104] While many of these putrefactive substances can elicit toxic effects on the host, evidence shows that their production can be lowered by either reducing the amount of protein in the diet, or by increasing fermentable carbohydrate, either as starch, or dietary fibre. The beneficial effects of increasing bacterial amino acid requirements for growth would be augmented by reduced colonic pH resulting from carbohydrate fermentation, as well as faster transit of material through the bowel due to increased laxation.

Detoxification

Phenolic and indolic metabolites are usually detoxified by either glucuronide or sulphate conjugation in the gut mucosa and liver.[176,177] However, phenol and indole production is implicated in several disease states. Phenols are believed to act as co-carcinogens in bladder cancer,[21] and have been implicated in schizophrenia,[53]

while p-cresol acts as a growth depressant in young pigs.[226] Other physiological manifestations include hyperactivity in children, where high levels of p-cresol are excreted in the faeces.[2] The importance of phenolic metabolites in cancer is unclear, but it is known that N-nitrosation of dimethylamine by nitrite is enhanced by phenol, while chemical reactions between phenol and nitrite produce the mutagen diazoquinone.[109] Indole and other tryptophan fermentation products have also been linked to cancer,[27,229] although they are not directly carcinogenic, but appear to be promoters of the disease.[65]

Amine formation

A wide range of amines are formed in varying amounts by colonic bacteria, including the simple aliphatic compounds such as methylamine, dimethylamine, propylamine, butylamine and 2-methybutylamine, the polyamines putrescine and cadaverine, and their heterocyclic oxidation products pyrrolidine and piperidine, as well as histamine and the aromatic amines tyramine, tryptamine and phenylethylamine.[199] Dimethylamine, together with methylamine, pyrrolidine and piperidine are major urinary excretory products[1,9] A number of intestinal anaerobes produce amines, including species belonging to the genera Clostridium, Bifidobacterium and Bacteroides,[5,59] but clostridia in particular, seem to form large amounts of these metabolites.[25a]

Amines produced in the large gut are detoxified by monoamine and diamine oxidases in the mucosa and liver, but in some circumstances they can enter the circulation.[168] A number of studies indicate that intestinal amine production may be detrimental, since these metabolites participate in N-nitrosation reactions,[195] which are dependent on pH, and on the availability of nitrite and amines. Many colonic microorganisms form N-nitroso compounds from secondary amines, which are detectable in stools.[31,72]

Pharmacological action

Amines are pharmacologically active, and their formation by intestinal bacteria affects the host in many ways. They have been associated with migraine[6] and the onset of hypertensive symptoms,[24] while amines formed in the bowel can induce portal-systemic encephalopathy in patients with liver disease.[168] Moreover, N-acyl and acetoxy derivatives of putrescine and cadaverine produced by intestinal bacteria are increased in the blood of schizophrenics, while patients with colon cancer excrete more of these fermentation products than healthy individuals.[155] Some amines, including histamine, cadaverine, tyramine and putrescine, are pressor or depressor substances, and may act as stimulators of gastric secretion or as vasodilators.[59] Increased amine excretion occurs in diarrhoea in pigs, especially putrescine and cadaverine,[172] while in humans, children with gastroenteritis have significantly higher levels of tyramine and phenylethylamine in their stools.[154]

Amines produced by bacteria in the large gut can be further metabolized, especially in the presence of a fermentable carbohydrate source. In vitro studies showed that during starch fermentation net amine production by faecal bacteria was reduced by 80%.[199]

Amines are major, though highly variable, products of bacterial amino acid metabolism in the human large intestine. A direct relationship exists between dietary protein intake and amine excretion and this may in part explain epidemiological findings that relate high levels of dietary protein to increased incidence of gut disease.[60] While the main nutritional determinant affecting amine formation in the large intestine is substrate availability (organic nitrogen-containing compounds), the formation of these potentially toxic metabolites can be reduced by increasing the supply of fermentable carbohydrate to the colon. As with the production of phenolic and indolic metabolites, control of amine formation in the large bowel may be readily achievable through the diet.

Amino acid metabolism and colorectal cancer

Epidemiological studies indicate that meat consumption is the principal risk factor for large bowel cancer. There are a number of possible mechanisms to explain this, including the occurrence of pro-carcinogens such as heterocyclic amines in cooked meat, the cancer-promoting effect of fat in meat, or that a proportion of meat protein reaches the large bowel where it is metabolized by the colonic microflora to provide precursors for genotoxic compounds.

G to A transitions in the second G of a GG pair at codon 12 of 13 of K-*ras* are common in colorectal cancer and are characteristic of alkylating agents such as N-nitroso compounds (N-NOC). Human faeces contain NOC and alkylated DNA adducts of O^6-methylguanine have been detected in colonic tissue. Inducible nitric oxide synthase produces NO from arginine, and high protein diets might increase nitrosation through amino acid fermentation producing amine precursors which are nitrosated by mucosally produced NO. Furthermore, dissimilatory reduction of nitrate in the diet to nitrite might contribute to N-NOC synthesis and elevated NOC levels have been shown in human faeces during dietary supplementation with nitrate.

In human feeding studies, an increase in meat intake leads to a corresponding increase in (N-nitroso excretion in faeces,[16] producing levels of N-NOC exposure in faeces similar to that from tobacco-specific N-NOC in cigarette smoke. These findings were developed in a further series of studies in which change from a low to a high meat diet led to a three-fold increase in N-NOC excretion in faeces and a doubling of faecal ammonia.[197] However, when 37 g of resistant starch was added to the subjects' diets an increase in faecal weight occurred from 118 to 153 g/day, faecal pH fell from 7.2 to 6.6, but there was no significant change in N-NOC excretion. Whole gut transit time remained the same.

SHORT-CHAIN FATTY ACIDS

Sources

Both carbohydrate and protein fermentation give rise to SCFA, although protein is a minor contributor. SCFA are the principal products of fermentation and, through their absorption and metabolism, the host can salvage energy from food not digested in the upper intestine. SCFA affect colonic epithelial cell transport, colonocyte metabolism, growth and differentiation, hepatic control of lipid and carbohydrates and provide energy to muscle, kidney, heart and brain. Already there are clinical uses suggested for SCFA in the management of ulcerative colitis and diversion colitis, and in enteral feeding.[41,51]

Occurrence in hindgut

Acetate is always the dominant SCFA, and propionate is usually equal to or greater than butyrate. Total concentrations are around 60–120 mmol/kg contents with average molar ratios of 60:20:20

for acetate : propionate : butyrate. In regional studies of colonic contents, SCFA concentrations are higher in the right side of the colon, including the caecal area. It is here that colonic bacteria first encounter carbohydrate substrates leaving the small intestine and it is thus the area of highest fermentative activity. However, the molar ratios of acetate : propionate : butyrate are similar in both right and left colon.[47]

In vitro studies of fermentation

Although it is not easy to compare experiments done in different laboratories, Table 22.2 summarizes 11 *in vitro* studies which have reported SCFA yields using human faecal inocula. Total yields (g SCFA per 100 g substrate) vary considerably, from as low as 10 g SCFA per 100 g from fibre preparations such as corn bran, pea fibre, oat fibre and from cellulose, to over 60 g SCFA per 100g for starch. Low yields may equate with incomplete fermentation, as is the case with bran NSP, or may mean other intermediates are being formed. In all cases, acetate is the major anion, comprising 67% overall of total SCFA. Pectin is a particularly good source of acetate (80% in 7 studies) while arabinogalactan (54%, $n = 3$) and guar (59%, $n = 3$) are the poorest sources. By contrast, guar and arabinogalactan are good sources of propionate (27 and 34%, respectively). Butyrate production varies over a wide range. Starch almost always gives high amounts of butyrate (62:15:22, acetate:propionate:butyrate, $n = 7$) followed closely by oat and wheat bran (60:16:20, $n = 5$). Pectin is the poorest source (80:12:8, $n = 8$) along with some of the very non-digestible corn, soya, sugar beet, pea and oat sources used. With regard to overall production of butyrate, starch yields both relatively high molar proportions (23%) and has a high yield per g substrate fermented (about 50%).

SCFA and diarrhoea

Diarrhoea, whether due to antibiotic administration or not, leads to reduced SCFA concentrations in faeces although total daily excretion may increase in proportion to rises in stool output. Studies which show increased SCFA outputs in faeces in relation to normal stool weight include the effects of bran,[43] a variety of

Molar ratios of fermentation products formed from different carbohydrates					
Substrate	**Acetate**	**Propionate**	**Butyrate**	**Yield***	**N†**
Starch	62	15	23	49	7
Pectin	80	12	8	39	8
Brans	64	16	20	40	5
Other NSP‡	63	22	8	38	24
Mixed diets	63	22	8	38	24
Overall mean	67	18	11	37	57

* Yield = g SCFA per 100 g substrate fermented.
† N = Number of studies.
‡ NSP = non-starch polysaccharide.
From Cummings (unpublished results).

Table 22.2 Molar ratios of fermentation products formed from different carbohydrates.

vegetables and cereal foods[222,223] and cellulose, xylan, corn bran or pectin.[75] Similarly, in diarrhoea due to mannitol, lactulose or raffinose,[191] magnesium sulphate[92] and intestinal resection,[42] increased excretion with increased stool output is seen, but generally with lower concentrations.

In diarrhoea, the underlying mechanism is failure of the colon to absorb water, whether because of increased volume and solute load from the small bowel, failure of solute absorption by a diseased mucosa, or the presence of bacterial toxins or non-absorbable ions. In any event, fermentation continues until total gut transit time falls to about 18 h below which SCFA levels decline to very low levels.[42] Provided SCFA are being produced, and the mucosal surface is normal, the amount excreted each day will depend directly on stool weight because SCFA are the principal anion in colonic contents. Thus, measurement of their output or concentration in faeces in diarrhoea will reflect stool weight, but their molar ratios can sometimes give useful information.

Diet

At least 95% of SCFA produced in the colon are absorbed, so it is not surprising if faecal SCFA measurements prove an insensitive guide to events going on more proximally in the large bowel. This has proved to be the case particularly when studying dietary change. In Fleming's review of 42 published studies of the effect of dietary fibre on faecal SCFA, the majority of human studies show no effect, although in the rat, pig and monkey, some differences are seen.[74] In a study of starch malabsorption, induced by the α-glucosidase inhibitor acarbose, an increase in the relative and absolute amounts of butyrate in faeces was seen.[192] Similarly, faecal butyrate concentrations increased on feeding resistant starch in the form of Hylon VII to healthy volunteers[153,169] although did not in other studies.[52] In *in vitro* studies, summarized in Table 22.2, starch seems to be a good source of butyrate. Moreover starch, not NSP, is probably the principal substrate for fermentation in the hindgut of many human populations, especially those with starchy staples as the main component of their diet and may be important in the prevention of large bowel cancer.[32]

Amino acids as substrates

Amino acid fermentation also gives rise to SCFA. Dissimilatory amino acid metabolism yields not only SCFA but the branched-chain fatty acids (BCFA) isobutyrate, isovalerate and 2-methyl-

butyrate, which arise, respectively, from valine, leucine and isoleucine. Although the amounts of BCFA are much lower than the three major SCFA, the presence of branched-chain fatty acids indicates that amino acid fermentation is taking place. A fraction of total SCFA must therefore come from protein breakdown. Macfarlane *et al.*[135] have shown, using batch culture studies of human faecal inocula, that SCFA are the principal end products formed during the degradation of protein by human colonic bacteria. Approximately 30% of protein is converted to SCFA. BCFA constitute 16% of SCFA produced from BSA and 21% of SCFA generated when casein is the substrate. BCFA concentrations in gut contents taken from the human proximal and distal colons were, on average, 4.6 and 6.3 mmol/kg, respectively, corresponding to 3.4% and 7.5% of total SCFA. These results suggest that protein fermentation could potentially account for about 17% of the SCFA found in the caecum, and 38% of the SCFA produced in the sigmoid/rectum (Fig. 22.3). Measurements of BCFA in portal and arterial blood taken from individuals undergoing emergency surgery indicated that net production of branched-chain fatty acids by the gut was in the region of 11 mmol/day, which would require the fermentation of about 12 g of protein. These data show that protein is a significant source of SCFA, and, with the known amounts of carbohydrate entering the colon, we have enough substrate available to account for 300–400 mmol SCFA production each day.

Cell metabolism and growth

Probably the single most important interaction between bacteria in the large intestine and their host lies in the metabolic effects of SCFA in the colonic epithelial cell. All three major SCFA are metabolized to some extent by the epithelium to provide energy, but butyrate is especially important as a fuel for these cells and may also play a critical role in moderating cell growth and differentiation.

The colonic epithelium derives 60–70% of its energy from bacterial fermentation products.[8,184,185] Studies of CO_2 production using mixtures of SCFA indicate that cellular activation is in the order butyrate > propionate > acetate. SCFA are metabolized to CO_2 and ketone bodies and are precursors for mucosal lipid synthesis. The human colonocyte also metabolizes glucose and glutamine. However, more than 70% of oxygen consumption in isolated colonocytes is due to butyrate oxidation, although there are regional differences. Carbon dioxide production from butyrate

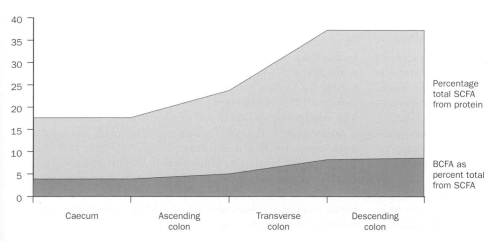

Fig. 22.3 Short-chain fatty acid (SCFA) and branched-chain fatty acid (BCFA) production from proteins and peptides in the proximal and distal colons.

is similar in both proximal and distal colon in man, but ketone body appearance is less in the distal gut. This implies that more butyrate enters the tricarboxylic acid (TCA) cycle in the distal colon and is more important in this region. Conversely, glutamine metabolism is greater proximally, as is glucose oxidation. Thus, the proximal colon resembles more the small bowel, while the distal colon relies on butyrate as a primary energy source.

Uptake and utilization of butyrate by the colonic epithelium *in vivo* can be demonstrated from study of levels of SCFA in portal and arterial blood and in colonic contents. In sudden death victims the molar proportion of butyrate falls from 21% within the colonic lumen to 8% in portal blood, indicating substantial butyrate clearance by the mucosa (assuming no production of acetate and propionate by the mucosa).[47] The fall to 8% in portal blood indicates a clearance of 65% of the butyrate by the mucosa. If either acetate or propionate are also metabolized by the mucosa, then 65% is a minimum estimate of clearance. However, surgical data[48,166] show that portal blood butyrate molar ratio is 17%, whereas in colostomy contents of patients from an identical population in the same hospital, butyrate is only 13% of total SCFA. This means that either the mucosa of this population is selectively metabolizing acetate and propionate – an unlikely event, producing butyrate – which is equally unlikely, or that all three acids are being taken up. These data all point to substantial butyrate, and probably some propionate and acetate, utilization by the mucosa in humans.

The trophic effect of SCFA on the large bowel mucosa has led to the suggestion that it may be a factor favouring tumour development.[79,107,219] However, Scheppach and colleagues[192,193] have shown, with colonic biopsy material, that this is unlikely to be the case. Using [³H] thymidine and bromodeoxyuridine to label incubated crypts, they calculated the labelling index (a measure of crypt cell growth rate) in whole crypts and five equal compartments of the crypt. Butyrate and propionate both increased proliferation rates, whereas acetate did not. Cell growth was stimulated only in the basal three compartments, not those near the surface as is characteristic of pre-neoplastic conditions.[123] Moreover, butyrate is well established as a growth inhibitor and inducer of differentiation in many cell lines (see later).

Differentiation, gene expression and large bowel cancer

Butyrate has remarkably diverse properties in a wide range of cells (Table 22.3). These include the arrest of cell growth early in G_1, induction of differentiation, stimulation of cytoskeletal organization and alteration in gene expression. The effects of butyrate on the cell were first highlighted in 1976 in a review by Prasad and Sinha.[173,174] Subsequently, much has been written about various mechanisms of action.[80,93,94,114,116]

The slowing or arrest of cell growth is seen in many cell lines and is associated with differentiation. The effect of butyrate on differentiation is related to the control of gene expression. Butyrate alters the expression of many genes, including the induction of haemoglobin synthesis in murine erythroleukaemia cells, epithelial growth factors (EGF) receptors in hepatocytes, plasminogen activator synthesis in endothelial cells, thyroid hormone receptors in the pituitary, metallothionein in hepatoma cells, oestrogen, prolactin and EGF receptors in breast tissue cells and many others. In colorectal cancer cells a number of changes in gene expression have been observed, including induction of *c-fos*, *PLAP* and carcinoembryonic antigen, inhibition of urokinase

Properties of butyrate in colonic epithelial cells
Effects
Arrest of cell growth in G_1
Differentiation
Modulation of gene expression (*PLAP*, *c-fos*, *c-myc*, *CEA*, ...)
Mechanisms
Inhibits histone deacetylase – increases histone acetylation
Apoptosis
Transcriptional proteins – 5′ region, SAR, HLH
Other
Energy source
Membrane lipid synthesis

Table 22.3 Properties of butyrate in colonic epithelial cells.

and release of plasminogen activator inhibitor, expression of brush border glycoprotein and P-glycoprotein. The induction of differentiation in tumour cell lines is associated with changes in cytoskeletal architecture and adhesion properties of cells.[224]

Cellular mechanisms

Kruh suggested a number of cellular mechanisms for the action of butyrate.[115,116] The best known is the effect on histone acetylation which has been shown in many cell types. Smith[201] has demonstrated that by inhibiting histone deacetylase, butyrate allows hyperacetylation of histones to occur. In turn, this 'opens up' the DNA structure, facilitating access of DNA repair enzymes. In an animal study in which wheat bran was fed, Boffa *et al.*[19] demonstrated that butyrate levels in the colonic lumen are positively related to colonic epithelial cell histone acetylation and inversely related to cell proliferation. Butyrate thus appears to be able to modulate DNA synthesis *in vivo*.

Other possible mechanisms of action include inhibition of chromatin protein phosphorylation, hypermethylation of DNA and chromatin structure. Paraskeva and colleagues[93,94] suggested that butyrate selects cells for apoptosis. In cell lines from colorectal cancers and polyps, sodium butyrate in 1–4 mmol/l concentrations induced apoptosis, while TGFα did not. Apoptosis in the colon may therefore be triggered as cells migrate up the crypt and are exposed to lumenal growth factors.

Does all this convert into a mechanism whereby anaerobic bacteria in the gut produce, from dietary carbohydrate, factors that lead to protection from large bowel cancer? Butyrate can induce transformed cells to acquire the phenotype of more differentiated cells, but it has paradoxical effects on normal and transformed colon epithelial cells. Some of the conflicting results in the literature may be related to the concentration of butyrate used in the *in vitro* studies. The most effective concentrations for inducing differentiation are usually no more than 5 mmol/l, while high concentrations lead to cell death. However, lumenal butyrate concentrations in the colon can exceed 20 mmol/l, and are usually in the range 10–30 mmol/l. It is difficult to believe that a naturally occurring fatty acid, ubiquitous in the mammalian hindgut, could promote or select for tumour growth. Its origin from fermentation of dietary carbohydrate does, however, provide a link between epidemiological studies, which show these carbohydrates to be protective against large bowel cancer, and the cellular mechanisms that occur. Ever since it was first proposed[46] that butyrate was the link between fibre and protection against large bowel cancer, it has remained the most likely candidate to fulfil this role.

LACTATE

Lactate formation by intestinal bacteria

Lactate is a major product of fermentation in many colonic bacteria. Both D- and L-enantiomers are formed, although the generic distribution of bacteria that make D-lactate in the large intestine is limited. In healthy adults, lactate concentrations seldom exceed more than a few mmol/kg of faeces, but measurements in material taken directly from the bowel suggest that it is mainly produced in the caecum and ascending colon.[136] Lactate is well absorbed by the large gut, but concentrations are also kept low by bacteria that ferment it to SCFA and other products. Many different species are able to do this, including desulfovibrios, propionibacteria, enterobacteria, bacteroides, clostridia and some anaerobic cocci. *In vitro* fermentation experiments demonstrate the capacity of faecal bacteria to ferment lactate. This is particularly evident in starch fermentations where lactate formation is initially rapid and is of a similar magnitude to the production of acetate, propionate and butyrate. However, as the fermentation progresses, lactate concentrations plateau and then decline, as it is taken up by the bacteria.[129]

Although lactate is a minor product of dissimilatory amino acid metabolism, it is primarily an electron sink in carbohydrate fermentation. The process is not directly coupled to energy generation, but like H_2 production, is used to oxidize reduced pyridine nucleotides which are in short supply in bacterial cells. Reduced pyridine nucleotides are produced in the early stages of fermentation and must be oxidized for fermentation reactions to continue.

Lactate production appears to be associated with the breakdown of certain substrates. For example, feeding studies with human volunteers showed that lactate was mainly formed from starches,[70] and that the fermentation of non-starch polysaccharides (NSP) or dietary fibre, produced little of this metabolite. Measurements of lactate and residual carbohydrate in gut contents taken at autopsy, show a positive correlation of lactate concentration with starch availability.[137] These observations may be partly explained on the basis that lactate-producing bacteria play an important role in starch breakdown, but not in the metabolism of NSP. However, the situation is probably more complex than this, since substrate concentration significantly affects the way in which bacteria ferment carbohydrates[56] and therefore, complex substrates that are rapidly depolymerized are more likely to serve as precursors of lactate.

D-Lactic acidosis

D-Lactate is produced continuously in the human large intestine but microbiological studies (described above) indicate that it is a minor product of fermentation, except during rapid breakdown of carbohydrate, where it serves as an electron sink. D-Lactate is readily absorbed from the colon[140] and metabolized in the kidney and liver to pyruvate by D-2-hydroxyacid dehydrogenase. Infusion studies with D-lactate in humans by Oh *et al.*[156] showed that 75–90% was metabolized, with little appearing in urine. After oral ingestion of mixtures of D-and L-lactate plasma half-life is 28–40 min and less than 2% appears in urine. Blood levels reach 0.3–0.4 mmol/l.[58] Healthy subjects do not suffer any significant symptoms during chronic ingestion of D-lactate.

D-Lactate is a metabolic product almost entirely from fermentation in the gut with very small quantities formed *in vivo* through the methylglyoxal pathway. Its use as a possible indicator of colonic carbohydrate breakdown has been investigated. In a study of healthy humans, Etterlin *et al.*[70] measured the classic fermentation products of breath hydrogen, methane and blood acetate following ingestion of resistant starch and non-starch polysaccharide containing test meals and compared the results with blood D-lactate levels. Hydrogen and acetate provided reliable markers of fermentation, as has been shown previously.[35,171] Resistant starch from potato produced a definite rise in blood D-lactate to around 20 µmol/l about 12 h after the meal, while a similar amount of NSP from soya did not. The peak of D-lactate in blood occurred about 3 h before the peak in breath hydrogen and blood acetate. D-lactate may therefore be a specific marker of resistant starch fermentation, or of more rapidly fermented substrates, although H_2 and acetate remain more robust and universal markers in practice.

On occasions D-lactate may reach toxic levels in blood, of the order of 5–20 mmol/l, and be dangerous to health.[214] D-Lactic acidosis occurs in patients who have had intestinal bypass or resections and the primary mechanism is the dumping into the caecum of large amounts of carbohydrate, rapid fermentation and probably some systemic impairment of D-lactate metabolism. Patients present with drowsiness, slurred speech, ataxia, weakness and nausea. Symptoms are typically episodic and the diagnosis may be overlooked without a high degree of clinical suspicion. Metabolic acidosis is a characteristic feature of the condition with an anion gap ($[Na^+] - [Cl^-] + [HCO_3^-]$) in plasma of usually greater than 10 mmol/l.

Bacteriology of faeces in patients with D-lactic acidosis usually shows a predominance of Gram-positive anaerobes, including lactobacilli, bifidobacteria and eubacteria[204] with low levels of bacteroides. Faecal pH is often very acid, below 5.0[30] and may favour development of the condition. The accumulation of D-lactate may possibly be contributed to by inhibition of lactate metabolism by bacteria. Oxalate is a known competitive inhibitor of D-2-hydroxyacid dehydrogenase[213] and concentrations may be high in association with malabsorption. A similar mechanism may operate systemically.[214] However, faecal DL-lactate is often increased in inflammatory bowel disease and malabsorption[101] without symptoms of lactic acidosis.

Treatment of D-lactic acidosis usually includes antibiotics, of which those most commonly used are metronidazole, ampicillin, vancomycin, kanamycin and neomycin. Diet can be modified to reduce fermentable carbohydrates and attempts may be made to correct acidosis.

HYDROGEN

Hydrogen production by intestinal bacteria

Hydrogen gas is a major fermentation product in the large bowel. Colonic bacteria use protons as electron sinks in catabolic reactions involving both sugars and amino acids, but carbohydrates, particularly low molecular mass, rapidly fermentable molecules, are quantitatively more important sources of gas production. Pyruvate has a central role in H_2 production in the large gut, because it is energetically most efficient for microorganisms to form the gas from this fermentation intermediate.[209] As shown in

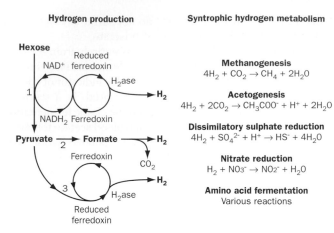

Fig. 22.4 Pathways of hydrogen formation from carbohydrates in the colon, and mechanisms of its consumption in different groups of syntrophic microorganisms.

Fig. 22.4, H_2 production from carbohydrate occurs in three main ways: through (1) cleavage of pyruvate to formate, which is then metabolized to H_2 and CO_2 by formate hydrogen lyase (enterobacteria); (2) generation from pyruvate through pyruvate–ferredoxin oxidoreductase and hydrogenase, as occurs in some clostridia; and (3) formation from the oxidation of pyridine and flavin nucleotides (ruminococci, some clostridia), where production of reduced ferredoxin from NADH–ferredoxin oxidoreductase occurs. Considerable potential for H_2 generation exists in the colon, as shown in calculations made by Cummings:[41]

$$59 \ C_6H_{12}O_6 + 38 \ H_2O \rightarrow 60 \ \text{acetate} + 96 \ CO_2 + 256 \ H^+ +$$
$$22 \ \text{propionate} + 18 \ \text{butyrate}$$

The composition of normal flatus gas is shown in Fig. 21.5. Theoretically, daily production of H_2 can be well in excess of 1 litre from an average dietary input of 40–50 g carbohydrate into the colon;[120] however, total flatus volume in normal healthy adults seldom exceeds this value.[111,117,118] Studies with healthy volunteers using whole body calorimeters show that ingestion of non-absorbable carbohydrate results in excretion of only 2.5–14% of predicted H_2 production.[36] This apparent discrepancy between theoretical and actual levels of H_2 excretion results from the activities of a variety of H_2-consuming microbial communities, as indicated in Fig. 22.4.

These observations make the interpretation of breath H_2, a widely used test in gastroenterological clinical practice, difficult

to interpret. The amount of H_2 that appears in breath in relation to the grams of substrate fermented will vary depending on the type of substrate, on the disposition of H_2 excretion between breath and flatus, and on the activity of the different microbial pathways of gas disposal. Breath H_2 is also used as a transit marker in gastrointestinal studies, using lactulose as the fermentable carbohydrate source.[20] The interval between ingestion of lactulose and first appearance of H_2 varies between 30 and 100 min and is related to the dose used; larger doses give faster mean transit times (MTT).[20,26] Similarly, higher molecular weight substances also give slower apparent MTT.[207] It is not, therefore, a true measure of transit time, and other methods are required to determine the average rate of passage for complete meals to the caecum.[178,180] A small proportion (about 5%) of subjects do not produce any detectable H_2 in breath following ingestion of fermentable carbohydrate[18,183] and this may be related to changes in colonic lumenal pH during fermentation[165] or bacterial gas utilization.

Clinical disorders of gas production

Gas production in the gut is frequently a cause for concern of patients. Two clinical syndromes are particularly associated with this: irritable bowel and pneumatosis cystoides intestinalis (PCI). Clear evidence exists for a disorder of H_2 metabolism in some irritable bowel patients.[110] PCI is an uncommon condition characterized by the presence of multiple gas-filled cysts in the mucosal lining of the large intestine that contain H_2, N_2 and CO_2.[66,78] Patients complain of diarrhoea with mucus and of passing excessive amounts of gas. Breath H_2 concentrations are usually elevated in these patients compared with normal subjects.[89,179]

Accumulation of H_2 in the colon may be caused by either an increase in production during fermentation, or by a reduction in removal of the gas. To determine the mechanism in PCI, Christl et al.[36] measured total H_2 excretion in a calorimeter in two patients, and breath H_2 concentrations in three patients with PCI, while they were taking a diet free of fermentable carbohydrates, and then in response to a dose of lactulose. The presence and metabolic activity of the major H_2-consuming bacteria in faeces were also determined and the data were compared with results from 10 healthy volunteers.

Hydrogen excretion rates were grossly elevated both in the fasting state and in response to lactulose in the PCI patients. Total H_2 excretion was 383–420 ml/day on the basal diet and 1430–1730 ml/day after lactulose administration, compared with 35 ± 6 ml/day and 262 ± 65 ml/day respectively, in controls. Basal breath H_2 levels in controls were 27 ± 6 vs. 214 ± 27 ml/day in patients and, after lactulose ingestion, 115 ± 18 vs. 370 ± 72 ml/day. Four controls were methanogenic. The other controls had high counts of sulphate-reducing bacteria and sulphate reduction rates. All PCI patients were non-methanogenic and had low sulphate reduction rates. These studies demonstrated that PCI patients excrete considerably more H_2 than a healthy population and have inactive H_2-metabolizing bacteria in their intestines, while the high pH_2 in colonic gas is sufficient to explain the accumulation of gas-filled cysts in the colonic wall.[76,119]

SULPHUR

Sulphur in diet and consequences for health

The major sources of sulphur in the human diet are sulphur-containing amino acids and inorganic sulphate. Sulphur also occurs

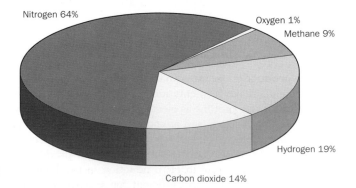

Fig. 22.5 Major components of intestinal gas.

naturally in brassica vegetables as glucosinolates and in volatile oils characteristic of the odour of garlic and onion. Endogenous host secretions such as mucus may also contribute to overall sulphur metabolism.

Sulphide is produced during fermentation of the amino acids cysteine and methionine by a wide range of intestinal bacteria. Any protein can contribute these amino acids to fermentation and studies in ileostomy subjects have shown that the amount of protein in the diet is the key to determining how much gets into the large bowel, rather than the type.[33,196] *In vitro*, in a model system of the gut, protein is a major source of sulphide.[182] In human feeding studies, the concentration of sulphide in faeces can be increased in a dose-dependent manner in relation to the amount of meat in the diet.[141] In this *in vitro* model, addition of carbohydrate to the system lowers sulphide levels by stimulating bacterial protein synthesis and growth. Whether this occurs *in vivo* in response to the addition of fermentable carbohydrates to the diet remains to be shown.

Inorganic sulphur, in the form of sulphur dioxide, sulphite, bisulphite, metabisulphite and sulphate, is widely used as a food additive (E220–227 and 514–518). Collectively known as S(iv) these additives are used in hundreds of foods primarily as a preservative, antioxidant and bleaching agent. They are mostly found in dried and pickled foods, bread, wine, beer and cider and preserved meats (Table 22.4). Intakes of sulphur from these sources are unknown. Addition of food containing high levels of S(iv) to the diet of healthy individuals increases faecal sulphide levels.[142] Sulphide production in the large intestine is undesirable, because it is toxic to the colonic epithelium.[10] However, potential mechanisms for sulphide disposal in the large intestine include its utilization in amino acid biosynthesis, conversion into less toxic forms in the intestinal mucosa such as volatile mercaptides or methanethiol,[221] oxidation by colonocytes, or conversion to thiocyanate in the colonic mucosa.[186,187]

Sulphate-reducing bacteria (SRB)

Studies on 87 healthy people living in the United Kingdom demonstrated that SRB occur in high numbers, up to 10^{11} per gram wet weight faeces, in non-methane excreting individuals.[87] Three broad population groupings were identified in these subjects: group 1 consisted of 21 persons who were strong CH_4 producers in whom SRB were completely absent from their stools. In group 2 (nine people) methanogenesis occurred and low numbers of SRB (10^5 per g wet weight faeces) were detected, although their metabolic activities were negligible. The final group consisted of 57 persons who had high faecal SRB and complete absence of methanogenesis.

The activities of SRB are controlled largely by the availability of oxidized sulphur compounds, especially the sulphates and sulphites used as food preservatives. SRB outcompete methanogenic microorganisms for the mutual growth substrate H_2 in the large intestine, which explains the absence of significant levels of methanogenesis in some individuals.[84,85] This was demonstrated in faecal slurries (Fig. 22.6), where methane was only a significant H_2 sink when SRB were either absent or inhibited with sodium molybdate.[85]

Because H_2-utilizing SRB have an obligate growth requirement for sulphate, variations in its availability may select for methanogenesis (limiting sulphate) or sulphate reduction (excess sulphate). Studies with ileostomists show that dietary sulphate reaching the colon ranges from 2 to 9 mmol/day.[77] Moreover, depolymerization and fermentation of host glycoproteins that are high in sulphate content, such as mucins and chondroitin sulphate, strongly stimulate sulphide production in faecal cultures containing SRB.[85]

Ulcerative colitis
Bacterial sulphur metabolism

The coincidence of the distribution of ulcerative colitis (UC) with the area of the gut most highly populated with bacteria

Sulphate in food		
High sulphate foods	**(mmol/kg)**	**Low sulphate foods (0–2 mmol/kg)**
Bread	13–15	Flour, maize, rice
Dried fruit	10–50	Beans
Sausage	10	Carrots
Broccoli	9	Onions
Brussels sprouts	9	Most fruit
Cabbage	8	Fresh fish
Shellfish	7	Meat
Nuts	3–9	Milk
Beer/wine	0–4	Most potable water

Table 22.4 Sulphate in food.

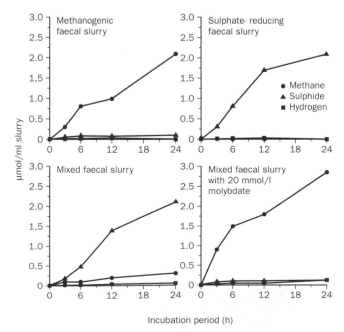

Fig. 22.6 Competition for hydrogen gas between sulphate-reducing bacteria and methanogenic microorganisms in faecal slurries. Data are from Gibson *et al.*[85]

points to a role for intestinal microorganisms in its aetiology. Moreover, since there are no animal models of UC that work in the germ-free state, it would be surprising if bacteria were not involved in the initiation and maintenance of inflammation in this condition. However, in no study has a specific species or mechanism yet been identified.[69,160–162,167]

Despite this, a number of lines of evidence point to bacterial sulphur metabolism being involved in the disease. In experimental animals a number of sulphated agents, such as degraded carrageenan, sodium lignosulphonate and sulphated amylopectin, when fed orally in drinking water to guinea pigs and rabbits, induce an acute attack of colitis.[144–146] The clinical and pathological features closely resemble human UC, except that the lesions extend distally from the caecum. The severity of the colitis is related to the amount of sulphate present in the polymer.

Role of antibiotics

Other investigations using antibiotics[112,161,217] or germ-free animals[162] show that intestinal bacteria are essential mediators of the disease process. Contrary observations have been described in germ-free rats, but these have been ascribed to species differences in the biological effect of degraded carrageenan.[100] Recently, there has been a resurgence in interest in experimental acute and chronic colitis in mice and hamsters using the dextran sulphate (DSS) model, in which the pathology is largely confined to the mucosa of the distal colon.[158,159] Populations of intestinal anaerobes increased significantly after administration of DSS, an effect nullified with metronidazole pre-treatment with attendant protection from colonic ulceration.[158] It is conceivable that in the carrageenan and DSS models the processing of sulphate by colonic bacteria yields a product, as yet undefined, that causes immune activation and resultant gastrointestinal damage. This would place UC in the category of an immune disorder. An alternative possibility is that a product of bacterial metabolism is directly affecting intracellular metabolism in the colonocyte, leading to a defect in butyrate oxidation. This metabolite could be sulphide, produced by sulphate-reducing bacteria amongst others.

Studies by Pitcher and colleagues[170] in 39 UC patients have shown that, while 95% carry SRB in the active phase of the illness, only 55% do so in quiescent disease. The mean counts of viable SRB were 3 logs higher in the active disease group than those in remission. Faecal sulphide concentration was higher in UC patients who were not taking 5-aminosalicylic acid (5-ASA) than in healthy controls.

Protective effect of salicylate

In animal models of UC a protective effect of salicylates has been observed. Sulfasalazine reduced the numbers of animals with carrageenan-induced mucosal inflammation by 50%, yet appeared to have no impact on the intestinal microflora.[162] More recently, sulfasalazine and olsalazine have both been found to be effective in preventing deaths in athymic mice, a strain more sensitive to DSS-induced distal colitis than the conventional rat, and a dose–response effect was observed in terms of survival.[11,12] A clinical response to sulfasalazine treatment has also been demonstrated in DSS-induced colitis in conventional BALB/c mice,[29] although two studies of chronic DSS-induced colitis using conventional rats have reported opposite findings with both attenuation and no effect on colonic inflammation with sulfasalazine.[34,228] In studies of sulphide generation *in vitro* using human faecal inocula, 5-ASA reduces sulphide levels in a dose-dependent manner.[170]

Colonocyte metabolism

So does HS^-, or other reduced sulphur compounds, produce the observed metabolic defect in UC cells? Roediger's group have shown that fatty acid oxidation can be inhibited by a range of sulphur-containing compounds.[64,186,187] Of these, sulphide, methanethiol and mecaptoacetate at levels of 1–5 mmol/l selectively diminished fatty acid oxidation by 30–50% without substantially altering glucose oxidation, which reflects the metabolic changes in UC. Selective impairment of butyrate uptake and oxidation to CO_2 and acetoacetate has been demonstrated with sodium sulphide in rat colonocytes at concentrations as low as 0.1–0.5 mmol/l NaHS.[186,202]

Preliminary attempts to define the site of sulphide-induced inhibition of butyrate oxidation in the colonocyte have localized a metabolic block at the level of FAD-linked oxidation by butyryl-CoA dehydrogenase (Roediger *et al*.[187]). No effect is seen on NAD-linked oxidation, which is supported by recent mRNA analysis for mitochondrial NAD/NADH-dependent dehydrogenases in colonic biopsies from patients with acute UC in which no evidence of enzyme deficiency was found.[149]

Thus, on present evidence, it may be concluded that reducing sulphur compounds are detrimental to colonic metabolism: first, by impairing the transport of *n*-butyrate into the colonocyte; and, secondly, by inhibition of *n*-butyrate oxidation within mitochondria. These mechanisms point to reducing sulphur compounds within the colonic lumen, and hydrogen sulphide in particular, being candidates for the initiation of ulcerative colitis.

CANDIDA, OTHER YEASTS AND BOWEL DISEASE

Candida albicans is a normal commensal found in all regions of the human gut and a well-recognized opportunistic pathogen. The majority of faecal specimens contain yeasts, with *C. albicans* being the most frequent isolate. However, counts are usually very low, 10^2–10^3/g of stool.[14,38] The transformation from commensal to pathogen is only usually seen in patients who have some predisposing factor such as AIDS, or other immunodeficiency syndrome; in association with prescription of corticosteroids, or other immunosuppressives, especially in transplant patients; following broad-spectrum antibiotic use; in very ill patients such as those on total parenteral nutrition; in association with underlying malignant disease; and in some less severe illnesses such as diabetes. Other fungi occasionally cause intestinal disease, such as *Aspergillus*, *Cryptococcus*, *Histoplasma* and *Blastomyces*, but these are not normal commensals of the gut and are therefore acquired from the environment.

The most common clinical presentation of fungal infection of the gut is that of oral or oesophageal infection. These patients have a sore mouth, painful swallowing and retrosternal chest pain. Systemic infection may rarely ensue. Oral candida infection, or thrush, can be recognized by the white patches of curd-like material that appear against a background of reddened inflamed mucosa.

More problematic is assigning a role to *Candida* spp. in the large intestine. Since candida is commonly isolated from faeces of healthy adults, it will also be isolated from stools during episodes of diarrhoea. Counts of candida in faeces increase during the use of broad-spectrum antibiotics in humans[210] and, in a murine model fed a chow containing C. *albicans*, both antibiotics and cytotoxic drugs increased gut colonization by the yeast, although methylprednisolone did not.[143,189] In a group of 24 elderly patients with antibiotic-associated diarrhoea who were negative for *Clostridium difficile* toxin, seven had counts of candida over 10^5 per ml faeces, and of these, five were given nystatin and promptly recovered.[54] In acute pruritis ani, which usually complicates other perianal disorders such as fissure, haemorrhoids, diarrhoea, diabetes, etc., candida is often found in scrapings from the perianal region. If the appearances are typical of candida infection, with excoriation, reddening and sometimes a white exudate, then it is worth a trial of antifungal powder or cream. However, in chronic states, candida is not thought to be primarily pathogenic, since these organisms grow readily on moist warm surfaces.

In Crohn's disease, candida is not thought to play a role,[139] but both IgG- and IgA-circulating antibodies to *Saccharomyces cerevisiae* are raised.[55] In this latter study there was no increase in antibody levels in UC or irritable bowel syndrome, although IgG levels were also raised in patients with chronic liver disease. The authors do not suggest that *S. cerevisiae* is pathogenic in Crohn's disease but rather that this finding might provide the basis for a diagnostic test.

Many patients with irritable bowel syndrome have food intolerance, and their symptoms can be controlled by diet. It has been suggested that food intolerance may be a consequence of intestinal overgrowth with candida. However, candida has not been found in excess in the stools of patients with irritable bowel syndrome[150] and the pathogenic mechanism proposed seems unlikely.[103] It has been suggested that candida, being a yeast, will ferment carbohydrate in the large intestine to alcohol, which is then absorbed and may give rise to a feeling of ill-health. Alternatively, enteric bacteria convert alcohol to acetaldehyde, which is undoubtedly metabolically toxic. Many bacterial species in the gut produce alcohol, and it is found normally in concentrations ranging from 2.1 to 16.4 mmol/kg contents in the large intestine.[136] Moreover, candida is not known to produce an enterotoxin, and it becomes pathogenic in the mouth and oesophagus by firstly proliferating, usually because the natural barrier due to the commensal flora is impaired, and then invades the epithelium by means of an advancing border of hyphae and pseudohyphae. While the aetiology of irritable bowel syndrome remains largely unknown, a role for fungi remains possible. As with many aspects of this condition, the decisive experiments have yet to be done.

PROBIOTICS AND PREBIOTICS

As we have seen, the metabolic activities of the microbiota are wide ranging and may affect health, and it is increasingly being recognized that many physiological traits can be modified by diet. However, while the metabolic activities of intestinal microorganisms can be modulated in this way,[142a] most studies on the effects of dietary fibre,[62] meat[98] or fat[44] on the bacterial composition of the colonic microbiota have failed to demonstrate consistent changes through dietary manipulation. Despite this, studies with probiotics and prebiotics are beginning to show that certain of these products can be used to improve health. Probiotics are live microbial feed supplements whose beneficial properties are expressed through ecological, physiological and immunological interactions with the hosts resident microflora and the body's mucosal surfaces. Probiotics are allochthonous organisms that in effect invade, and may transiently colonize the intestinal ecosystem, while prebiotics promote the growth of indigenous, or autochthonous intestinal bacteria.

Probiotics

Lactic acid bacteria (lactobacilli, streptococci) and bifidobacteria predominate in commercially available probiotic products. These organisms do not permanently colonize the host, and continuous administration is usually required for any health-promoting properties to persist. Large bifidobacterial populations are normally present in the colon, although their numbers are believed to decrease with age.[61] *Bifidobacterium adolescentis* and *B. longum* predominate in adults,[150a] while *B. infantis* and *B. breve* seem to be more important in infants.[61] Bifidobacteria predominate in the colons of breast-fed babies, accounting for up to 95% of all culturable bacteria, and it is thought that colonization by these organisms is a protective factor in relation to infection.[15,28,227] While the majority of adults also harbour bifidobacteria in their colons, they do not occur in such high numbers.[73] These organisms, together with some lactobacilli play an important role in the ecophysiology of the colonic microbiota,[83,218] resistance to infection[90,211] and cancer,[181,194] stimulation of immune system activity,[71] and other direct interactions with host metabolism.[88] Bifidobacteria also excrete a variety of water-soluble vitamins, but marked species and strain differences occur: high levels of folate, thiamine and nicotinic acid are formed by *B. bifidum* and *B. infantis* strains, in comparison to *B. breve* and *B. longum*, but these vitamins are not produced by *B. adolescentis*. Vitamin B_{12} and pyridoxine are also synthesized by *B. bifidum*, *B. breve*, *B. longum*, *B. infantis* and *B. adolescentis*, but not excreted by the organisms.[57] For these reasons, there is currently much interest in determining ways to increase numbers of these bacteria in the large bowel.

Used as probiotics, bifidobacteria pass into the large bowel, and may be excreted in large numbers in faeces, although they are rapidly expelled from the colon when oral dosing is stopped.[22] Bifidobacteria and lactobacilli are now widely used in fermented milks and have been tested in other dairy products such as ice cream.[96] Colonoscopic studies have shown that *Lactobacillus rhamnosus* strain GG administered in fermented whey drinks adhered to the colonic mucosa, and became the dominant faecal lactobacillus.[3]

Because the majority of studies using probiotic microorganisms have been observational rather than mechanistic, the processes that govern the majority of probiotic effects are not known with certainty, but competition for nutrients and adhesion on the mucosal surfaces, secretion of anti-microbial agents[82] and immunostimulation by Gram-positive cell wall components such as lipoteichoic acids[163] may all be involved.

Prebiotics

Prebiotics are food ingredients that stimulate selectively the growth and activity of specific species of bacteria in the gut, usually bifidobacteria and lactobacilli, with benefit to health. In practice they are short-chain carbohydrates (SCC) that are not hydrolysed by human digestive enzymes and have been called resistant SCC.[175] They are also referred to as non-digestible oligosaccharides (NDO). However, NDO are not strictly oligosaccharides and their non-digestibility is largely assumed and not proven.

Chemical compositions and characteristics of oligosaccharides with potential prebiotic properties	
Oligosaccharide	**Chemical composition**
Fructooligosaccharides (e.g. Raftilose P95)	87% oligosaccharides β(2-1) fructan. 60% Gfn, 40% Fn (DP 2–8, average 4–5)
Inulin	>99% oligosaccharides β(2-1) fructan (inulin). Average dp 10–12
Galactooligosaccharides	Oligogalactose (85%), small amounts of glucose, galactose and lactose
Transgalactosylated oligosaccharides (e.g. Oligomate 55)	Mainly 6'-galactosyllactose, DP of oligosaccharide fraction 2–5 (primarily DP 3). 55% pure
Soya oligosaccharides	Stachyose (F, gal, gal, glu) and raffinose (F, gal, glu), DP 3–4
Xylooligosaccharides	β(1–4) linked xylose. 29% pure, DP of oligosaccharide fraction 2–4
Pyrodextrins	Complex mixture of glucose containing oligosaccharides
Isomaltooligosaccharides	Mixture of α(1–6) linked glucose oligomers (isomaltose, panose, isomaltotriose)

DP, degree of polymerization; F, fructose; G, glucose; gal, galactose; Fn, (fructose)$_n$; Gfn, glucose-(fructose)$_n$.

Table 22.5 Chemical compositions and characteristics of oligosaccharides with potential prebiotic properties.

Table 22.5 lists some of the short-chain carbohydrates currently available for human consumption that are candidate prebiotics. They are best defined as 'carbohydrates with a degree of polymerization (DP) of two or more, which are soluble in 80% ethanol and are not susceptible to digestion by pancreatic and brush-border enzymes'.[175] The accepted definition of an oligosaccharide[106] is '… a molecule containing a small number (2 to about 10) of monosaccharide residues connected by glycosidic linkages.' Some of the current carbohydrates which are potential prebiotics clearly fall outside this definition, in that a number have a degree of polymerization (DP) greater than 10. What does distinguish them chemically, however, is their solubility in 80% ethanol, together with their *in vitro* resistance to pancreatic and brush-border enzymes.

Analysis of these preparations indicates that while some are very pure, containing 86–87% oligosaccharide, e.g. inulin and oligofructose (OF), for others the oligosaccharide content is a minor fraction, around 20–30%, the rest comprising free monosaccharides, starch and non-starch polysaccharides. For example, xylooligosaccharide (Suntory, Japan) contains 29% oligosaccharide, 41% starch and 15% monosaccharides. It is important to bear this in mind when interpreting human or animal feeding studies.

Digestibility

To be effective, prebiotics need to reach the caecum in some form. While it is more than likely, because of their chemical structure, that a fraction of the substances listed in Table 22.5 does escape digestion by pancreatic and small bowel enzymes in the human gut, and therefore arrives in the large bowel, the experimental proof of this is difficult and time consuming. Such studies as have been reported (Table 22.6) show that when either inulin or OF are fed to ileostomy subjects, average recovery at the terminal ileum lies between 86 and 89% of the material fed.[13,67] Similarly, when aspiration of gut contents is performed from the terminal ileum, after test meals containing OF, 89% is recovered.[151] Other evidence of non-digestibility is rather more circumstantial. A number of studies have shown that after intake of prebiotics breath hydrogen excretion increases. While this is evidence of their fermentability, it does not provide information on the true extent of their non-digestion (see below).

Fermentability

Any carbohydrate that reaches the caecum is a potential substrate for fermentation, and there is considerable evidence showing that current prebiotics are fermented. In a small number of human

Digestibility of prebiotics in human upper intestine					
Source	**Model system**	**Intake (g)**	**Recovery (g)**	**% Recovered**	**Reference**
Inulin	Ileostomy	7.07	6.1	86	Bach-Knudsen
Inulin		21.2	18.4	87	*et al.*[13]
Inulin	Ileostomy	17.0	15.0	88	Ellegard *et al.*[67]
Oligofructose		15.5	13.8	89	
Oligofructose	Aspiration from ileum	20.1	6.0	89	Molis *et al.*[151]
			Average recovery 88%		

Table 22.6 Digestibility of prebiotics in human upper intestine.

feeding studies, faecal recovery of inulin or fructooligosaccharides (FOS) has been measured and found to be zero.[4,121,151]

Gas

Carbon dioxide and H_2 are inevitable products of fermentation, but also provide the major clinical disincentive to consumption of prebiotics. Unwanted symptoms relating to gas production in the gut are widely reported in human prebiotic feeding studies.[83,95,105,164,188,205] In Stone-Dorshow and Levitt's study,[205] 12 subjects took 15 g FOS daily for 12 days. When compared with a group of five subjects taking sucrose, symptoms of abdominal pain, eructation, flatulence and bloating were all significantly more severe in the FOS group. There was no adaptation over the 12-day period, but symptoms were all reported as no more than mild. Breath H_2 after a 10 g challenge of FOS showed no difference between the groups at 12 days and was not statistically different from breath H_2 following a similar dose of lactulose. Other FOS studies at doses of 5 and 20 g/day show dose-related increases in breath H_2 and mild flatulence and borborygmi in general, with isolated individuals experiencing somewhat more discomfort.[88,108,125] Paradoxically, eight healthy subjects taking 10 g/day transgalactooligosaccharides (TOS) reported no digestive symptoms and a decrease in breath H_2 excretion.[23]

Inulin similarly leads to increased breath H_2.[25,88] At a dose of 14 g/day highly significant increases in flatulence, rumbling, stomach and gut cramps, together with bloating, were seen in a group of 64 women taking the inulin in a double-blind crossover study over 4-week periods. Twelve per cent of the volunteers considered the flatulence severe and unacceptable. No adaptation in symptoms occurred over time.[164]

An explanation of these various and idiosyncratic effects of prebiotics on symptomatology and H_2 metabolism is difficult to find. Wide individual variation is know to occur in response to fermentation of prebiotics[95] and it is likely that the stoichiometry of fermentation differs from carbohydrates of varying chain length and monosaccharide composition.[35] Using breath H_2 excretion alone it has been shown that lactitol, isomaltose and polydextrose each increase breath H_2 by 112, 73 and 11%, respectively, when given at equal doses to healthy subjects.[124] These findings were broadly reflected by in vitro fermentation studies and suggest that molecules with longer chain length are fermented more slowly and with less net H_2 excretion. A similar result was obtained by Brighenti et al.[25] when comparing lactulose, inulin and resistant starch (RS) in healthy subjects. Breath H_2 was only 4.7ppm/h/g fed with RS, compared with 19.1 for inulin and 26.6 for lactulose at a similar dose.

Bowel habit

Carbohydrates that reach the colon such as NSP and RS, have a laxative effect on bowel habit due to stimulation of microbial growth, resulting in increased bacterial cell mass, which leads to stimulation of peristalsis from the increased amount of bowel content.[40] It can be predicted therefore that prebiotics will be laxative. However, current evidence is patchy, largely because of study design and the type of volunteers used.

The clearest demonstration of a laxative effect is in the controlled diet study of Gibson et al.[88] which showed that 15 g FOS increased stool output significantly from 136 to 154 g/day ($n = 8$) and in a smaller group of subjects 15 g inulin was also laxative; 92 g/day control, 123 g/day inulin ($n = 4$). Three other human

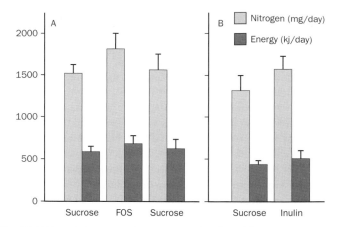

Fig. 22.7 Faecal nitrogen and energy excretion from (a) eight healthy volunteers fed 15 g/day fructooligosaccharides (FOS) for 15 days compared with two control periods, and (b) from four healthy volunteers fed 15 g/day inulin for 15 days compared to a single control period.[88]

experiments have not shown an increase[4,23,105] but diet was not controlled, which would tend to mask a small effect. In the study of Alles et al.,[4] subjects started with unusually high faecal weights on the control diet, 272 ± 26 g/day. Bouhnik et al.[23] gave volunteers 10 g TOS daily for 21 days without effect on bowel habit. Ito et al.,[105] who fed 4.8–19.2 g/day oligomate (52% galactooligosaccharides) to 12 healthy subjects were also unable to demonstrate a change in bowel habit, despite showing bifidogenicity and the subjects reporting an increase in abdominal symptoms. In three studies reporting only qualitative data, either FOS or inulin 'improved' constipation in small groups of hospitalized subjects.[99,113,190]

FOS and inulin are probably laxative, but because the effect is small it is difficult to detect except in carefully controlled studies. In terms of the magnitude of this effect, in the study of Gibson et al.[88] it was 1.3 g and 2.0 g increase in wet stool weight per gram of prebiotic fed. This is less than that seen with NSP sources such as wheat bran (5.4 g), or fruit and vegetables (4.7 g), but similar to that produced by more rapidly fermented polysaccharides such as pectin (1.2 g).[39]

The increase in faecal output is likely to be due to an increase in bacterial cell mass. Alongside the increase in dry matter excretion is a significant increase in nitrogen (Fig. 22.7). In the study of Gibson et al.,[88] the additional excretion of 0.32 g/day nitrogen when FOS was added to the diet is equivalent to 5 g of bacterial solids[201a] which, at the moisture content of faeces, is equivalent to 20–25 g of wet stool. This is exactly the change in stool output seen in this investigation.

CONCLUSIONS

The ability to target specific organisms in the large intestine, for defined health-promoting purposes, offers exciting possibilities for modulating the composition and metabolic activities of the colonic microbiota. However, many of the beneficial characteristics associated with usage of prebiotics and probiotics are hard to identify or quantitate in vivo, while putatively harmful long-term effects may as yet be unrecognized. While there is now a substantial literature dealing with the use of probiotics in humans, the information available on prebiotics is more limited, and many of the health claims made in relation to these functional foods require further study.

KEY FACTS

1. The normal colonic microbiota plays an important role in host health and disease.
2. Diet affects species composition and metabolic activities of the microbiota.
3. SCFA are the principal products of microbial digestion of carbohydrates and proteins.
4. Butyrate has a major nutritional and regulatory role in many host cellular processes.
5. Protein breakdown and amino acid fermentation is quantitatively more important in the distal large intestine.
6. Many products of protein breakdown, including sulphides, amines and ammonia, are genotoxic or mutagenic substances.
7. Hydrogen gas is produced during fermentation. Normally it is disposed of in breath and flatus, or used as an energy source by syntrophic organisms such as methanogens, acetogens or sulphate-reducing bacteria.
8. Sulphate-reducing bacteria use dietary sulphates and sulphites as terminal electron acceptors in metabolism. Their major end product is sulphide, which is toxic to mammalian cells.
9. Sulphide formation by intestinal bacteria may play a role in some inflammatory bowel disease.
10. New developments in probiotics and prebiotics provide significant opportunities to regulate the microbiota through relatively simple changes in diet.

REFERENCES

1 Abraham A, Radonich Z, Jones CT. Lysine absorption in the small intestine. The relevance of faecal cadaverine as an index of lysine malabsorption. *Clinica Chimica Acta* 1968; 22: 619–22.

2 Adams RF, Murray KE, Earl JW. High levels of faecal *p*-cresol in a group of hyperactive children. *Lancet* 1985; ii: 1313.

3 Alander M, Korpela R, Saxelin M, Vilpponen-Salmela T, Mattila-Sandholm T, von Wright A. Recovery of *Lactobacillus rhamnosus* GG from human colonic biopsies. *Lett Appl Microbiol* 1997; 24: 361–4.

4 Alles MS, Hautvast JGVA, Nagengast FM, Hartemink R, van Laere KMJ *et al.* Fate of fructo-oligosaccharides in the human intestine. *Br J Nutr* 1996; 76: 211–21.

5 Allison C, Macfarlane GT. Influence of pH, nutrient availability, and growth rate on amine production by *Bacteroides fragilis* and *Clostridium perfringens*. *Appl Environ Microbiol* 1989; 55: 2894–8.

6 Anon. Headache, tyramine, serotonin and migraine. *Nutr Rev* 1968; 26: 40–4.

7 Aragozzini F, Ferrari A, Pacini N, Saulandris R. Indole-3-lactic acid as a tryptophan metabolite produced by *Bifidobacterium* spp. *Appl Environ Microbiol* 1979; 38: 544–6.

8 Ardawi MSM, Newsholme EA. Fuel utilisation in colonocytes of the rat. *Biochem J* 1985; 231: 713.

9 Asatoor AM, Simenhoff ML. The origin of urinary dimethylamine. *Biochim Biophys Acta* 1965; 111: 384–92.

10 Aslam M, Batten JJ, Florin THJ, Sidebotham RL, Baron JH. Hydrogen sulphide induced damage to the colonic mucosal barrier in the rat. *Gut* 1992; 33:S69.

11 Axelsson L-G, Landstrom E, Bylund-Fellenius A-C. Sulfasalazine and olsalazine are effective for the treatment of dextran sulfate induced colitis in athymic mice. *Gastroenterology* 1994; 106:A648.

12 Axelsson L-G, Lundstrom L, Bylund-Fellenius AC, Midtvedt T. Dextran sulphate sodium induced colitis and sulfasalazine treatment in bacteria-free mice. *Gastroenterology* 1995; 108:A775.

13 Bach-Knudsen KE, Hessov I. Recovery of inulin from Jerusalem artichoke (*Helianthus tuberosus* L.) in the small intestine of man. *Br J Nutr* 1995; 74: 101–3.

14 Bernhardt H, Knoke M. Mycological aspects of gastrointestinal flora. *Scand J Gastroenterol* 1997; 32(suppl 222): 102–6.

15 Bezkorovainy A. Ecology of bifidobacteria. In: Bezkorovainy A, Miller-Catchpole R (eds) *Biochemistry and Physiology of Bifidobacteria*. CRC Press, Boca Raton, Florida; 1989; 29–72.

16 Bingham SA, Pignatelli B, Pollock JRA, Ellul A, Mallaveille C *et al.* Does increased endogenous formation of N-nitrosocompounds in the human colon explain the association between red meat and colon cancer? *Carcinogenesis* 1996; 17: 515–23.

17 Birkett A, Muir J, PhillipsJ, Jones G, O'Dea K. Resistant starch lowers fecal concentrations of ammonia and phenols in humans. *Am J Clin Nutr* 1996; 63: 766–72.

18 Bjorneklett A, Jenssen E. Relationships between hydrogen (H_2) and methane (CH_4) production in man. *Scand J Gastroenterol* 1982; 17: 985–92.

19 Boffa LC, Lupton JR, Mariani MR *et al.* Modulation of colonic epithelial cell proliferation, histone acetylation, and luminal short chain fatty acids by variation of dietary fiber (wheat bran) in rats. *Cancer Res* 1992; 52: 5906–12.

20 Bond JH, Levitt MD. Investigation of small bowel transit time in man utilising pulmonary H measurements. *J Lab Clin Med* 1974; 85: 546–59.

21 Bone E, Tamm A, Hill MJ. The production of urinary phenols by gut bacteria and their possible role in the causation of large bowel cancer. *Am J Clin Nutr* 1976; 29: 1448–54.

22 Bouhnik Y, Pochart P, Marteau P, Arlet G, Goderel I, Rambaud J-C. Fecal recovery in humans of viable *Bifidobacterium* sp. ingested in fermented milk. *Gastroenterology* 1992; 102: 875–8.

23 Bouhnik Y, Flourie B, D'Agay-Abensour L *et al.* Administration of transgalacto-oligosaccharides increases fecal bifidobacteria and modifies colonic fermentation metabolism in healthy humans. *J Nutr* 1997; 127: 444–8.

24 Boulton AA, Cookson B, Paulton R. Hypertensive crisis in a patient on MAOI antidepressants following a meal of beef liver. *Can Med Assoc J* 1970; 102: 1395.

25 Brighenti F, Casiraghi MC, Pellingrini N *et al.* Comparison of lactulose and inulin as reference standard for the study of resistant starch fermentation using hydrogen breath test. *Italian J Gastroenterol* 1995; 27: 122–8.

25a Brookes JB, Moore WEC. Gas chromatographic analysis of amines and other compounds produced by several species of clostridium. *Can J Microbiol* 1969; 15: 1433–47.

26 Brooy LSJ, Male PJ, Beavis AK, Misiewicz JJ. Assessment of the reproducibility of the lactulose H_2 breath test as a measure of mouth to caecum transit time. *Gut* 1983; 24: 893–6.

27 Bryan GT. The role of bacterial tryptophan metabolites in the etiology of bladder cancer. *Am J Clin Nutr* 1971; 24: 841–7.

28 Bullen CL, Willis AT. Resistance of the breast-fed infant to gastroenteritis. *Br Med J* 1971; 3: 338–43.

29 Bylund-Fellenius AC, Landstrom E, Axelsson L-G. Sulfasalazine ameliorates colitis induced by oral administration of dextran sulfate in mice. *Gastroenterology* 1994; 106:A659.

30 Caldarini MI, Pons S, D'Agostino D *et al.* Abnormal faecal flora in a patient with short bowel syndrome. An *in vitro* study on effect of pH on D-lactic acid production. *Dig Dis Sci* 1996; 41: 1649–52.

31 Calmels S, Ohshima H, Vincent P, Gounot AM, Bartsch H. Screening of microorganisms for nitrosation catalysis at pH 7 and kinetic studies on nitrosamine formation from secondary amines by *E. coli* strains. *Carcinogenesis* 1985; 6: 911–15.

32 Cassidy A, Bingham SA, Cummings JH. Starch intake and colorectal cancer risk: an international comparison. *Br J Cancer* 1994; 69: 937–42.

33 Chacko A, Cummings JH. Nitrogen losses from the human small bowel: obligatory losses and the effect of physical form of food. *Gut* 1988; 29: 809–15.

34 Chen Y, Conner EM, Grisham MB. Dextran sulfate sodium induces colitis in rats by enhancing mucosal permeability: effects of sulfasalazine. *Gastroenterology* 1995; 108:A796.

35 Christl SU, Murgatroyd PR, Gibson GR, Cummings JH. Production, metabolism and excretion of hydrogen in the large intestine. *Gastroenterology* 1992; 102: 1269–77.

36 Christl SU, Gibson GR, Murgatroyd PR, Sheppach W, Cummings JH. Impaired hydrogen metabolism in pneumatosis coli. *Gastroenterology* 1993; 104: 392–7.

37 Clausen MR, Mortensen PB. Fecal ammonia in patients with adenomatous polyps and cancer of the colon. *Nutr Cancer* 1992; 18: 175–80.

38 Cohen R, Roth FJ, Delgado E, Ahearn DG, Kalser MH. Fungal flora of the normal human small and large intestine. *New Engl J Med* 1969; 280: 638–41.

39 Cummings JH. The effect of dietary fiber on fecal weight and composition. In: *CRC Handbook of Dietary Fiber in Human Nutrition*, 2nd edn. CRC Press, Boca Raton, Florida; 1993; 263–349.

40 Cummings JH. Constipation. In: Misiewicz JJ, Pounder RE, Venables CW (eds) *Diseases of the Gut and Pancreas* 2nd edn. Blackwell Scientific Publications, Oxford;1994; 51–70.

41 Cummings JH. Short chain fatty acids. In: Gibson GR, Macfarlane GT (eds) *Human Colonic Bacteria: Role in Nutrition, Physiology and Health*. CRC Press, Boca Raton, Florida; 1995: 101–130.

42 Cummings JH, James WPT, Wiggins HS. Role of the colon in ileal resection diarrhoea. *Lancet* 1973; i: 344–7.

43 Cummings JH, Hill MJ, Jenkins DJA, Pearson JR, Wiggins HS. Changes in faecal composition and colonic function due to cereal fibre. *Am J Clin Nutr* 1976; 29: 1468–73.

44 Cummings JH, Wiggins HS, Jenkins DJA *et al*. Influence of diets high and low in animal fat on bowel habit, gastrointestinal transit time, fecal microflora, bile acid and fat excretions. *J Clin Invest* 1978; 61: 953–63.

45 Cummings JH, Hill MJ, Bone ES, Branch WJ, Jenkins DJA. The effect of meat protein and dietary fiber on colonic function and metabolism. Part II. Bacterial metabolites in feces and urine. *Am J Clin Nutr* 1979; 32: 2094–101.

46 Cummings JH, Stephen AM, Branch WJ. Implications of dietary fiber breakdown in the human colon. In: Bruce WR, Correa P, Lipkin M, Tannenbaum SR, Wilkins TD (eds) *Banbury Report 7: Gastrointestinal Cancer-Endogenous Factors*. Cold Spring Harbor Laboratory, New York, 1981; 71–81.

47 Cummings JH, Pomare EW, Branch WJ, Naylor CPE, Macfarlane GT: Short chain fatty acids in human large intestine, portal, hepatic and venous blood. *Gut* 1987; 28: 1221–7.

48 Cummings JH, Gibson GR Macfarlane GT. Quantitative estimates of fermentation in the hind gut of man. International Symposium on Comparative Aspects of the Physiology of Digestion in Ruminant and Hindgut Fermenters. *Acta Veterinarea Scandinavica*, 1989; 76–82.

49 Cummings JH, Macfarlane GT, Drasar BS. The gut microflora and its significance. In: Whitehead R (ed) *Gastrointestinal and Oesophageal Pathology*. Churchill Livingstone, Edinburgh, 1989; 201–19.

50 Cummings JH, Bingham SA, Heaton KW, Eastwood MA. Fecal weight, colon cancer risk, and dietary intake of nonstarch polysaccharides (dietary fiber). *Gastroenterology* 1992; 103: 1783–9.

51 Cummings JH, Rombeau JL, Sakata T (eds) *Physiological and Clinical Aspects of Short Chain Fatty Acids*. Cambridge University Press, Cambridge; 1995.

52 Cummings JH, Beatty ER, Kingman SM, Bingham SA, Englyst HN. Digestion and physiological properties of resistant starch in the human large bowel. *Br J Nutr* 1996; 75: 733–47.

53 Dalgliesh CE, Kelley W, Horning EC. Excretion of a sulphatoxyl derivative of skatole in pathological studies in man. *Biochem J* 1958; 70: 13P.

54 Danna PL, Urban C, Bellin E, Rahal JJ. Role of candida in pathogenesis of antibiotic-associated diarrhoea in elderly inpatients. *Lancet* 1991; 337: 511–14.

55 Darroch CJ, Barnes RMR, Dawson J. Circulating antibodies to *Saccharomyces cerevisiae* (bakers'/brewers' yeast) in gastrointestinal disease. *Clin Pathol* 1999; 52: 47–53.

56 Degnan BA, Macfarlane GT. Effect of dilution rate and carbon availability on *Bifidobacterium breve* fermentation. *Appl Microbiol Biotechnol* 1994; 40: 800–5.

57 Deguchi Y, Morishita T, Mutai M. Comparative studies on synthesis of water-soluble vitamins among human species of bifidobacteria. *Agric Biol Chem* 1985; 49: 13–19.

57a DeMoss RD, Moser K. Tryptopharase in diverse bacterial species. *J Bacteriol* 1969; 167–71.

58 de Vrese M, Koppenhoefer B, Barth CA. D-lactate acid metabolism after an oral load of DL-lactate. *Clin Nutr* 1990; 9: 23–8.

59 Drasar BS, Hill MJ. *Human Intestinal Microflora*. Academic Press, London, 1974.

60 Drasar BS, Irving D. Environmental factors and cancer of the colon and breast. *Br J Cancer* 1973; 27: 167–72.

61 Drasar BS, Roberts AK. Control of the large bowel microflora. In:Hill MJ, Marsh PD (eds) *Human Microbial Ecology*. CRC Press; Boca Raton. 1990: 87–101.

62 Drasar BS, Jenkins DJA, Cummings JH. The influence of a diet rich in wheat fibre on the human faecal flora. *J Med Microbiol* 1976; 9: 423–31.

63 Dunbar J, White S, Forney L. Genetic diversity through the looking glass: Effect of enrichment bias. *Appl Environ Microbiol* 1997; 63: 1326–31.

64 Duncan A, Kapaniris O, Roediger WEW. Measurement of mercaptoacetate levels in anaerobic batch culture of colonic bacteria. *FEMS Microbiol Ecol* 1990; 74: 303.

65 Dunning WF, Curtis MR. The role of indole in incidence of 2-acetylaminofluorene induced bladder cancer in rats. *Proc Soc Experim Biol Med* 1958; 99: 91–5.

66 Ecker JA, Williams RG, Clay KL. Pneumatosis cystoides intestinalis-bullous emphysema of the intestine. *Am J Gastroenterol* 1971; 56: 125–36.

67 Ellegard L, Andersson H, Bosaeus I. Inulin and oligofructose do not influence the absorption of cholesterol, or the excretion of cholesterol, Ca, Mg, Zn, Fe, or bile acids but increases energy excretion in ileostomy subjects. *Euro J Clin Nutr* 1997; 51: 1–5.

68 Elsden SR, Hilton MG, Walker JM. The end products of the metabolism of aromatic amino acids by clostridia. *Arch Microbiol* 1976; 107: 283–8.

69 Elson CO, Sartor RB, Tennyson GS, Riddell RH. Experimental model of inflammatory bowel disease. *Gastroenterology* 1995; 109: 1344–67.

70 Etterlin C, McKeown A, Bingham SA, Elia M, Macfarlane GT, Cummings JH. D-lactate and acetate as markers of fermentation in man. *Gastroenterology* 1992; 102:A551.

71 Famularo G, Moretti S, Marcellini S, De Simone C. Stimulation of immunity by probiotics. In: Fuller R (ed.) *Probiotics: Therapeutic and Other Beneficial Effects*. Chapman and Hall, London; 1997; 133–61.

72 Fine DH, Ross R, Roonbehler DP, Silvergleid A, Song L. Formation *in vivo* of volatile nitrosamines in man after ingestion of cooked bacon and spinach. *Nature* 1977; 265: 753–55.

73 Finegold SM, Sutter VL, Mathisen GE. Normal indigenous intestinal flora. In Hentges DJ (ed) *Human Intestinal Microflora in Health and Disease*. Academic Press, London; 1983; 3–31.

74 Fleming SE. Influence of dietary fiber on the production, absorption, or excretion of short chain fatty acids in humans. In Spiller GA (ed) *CRC Handbook of Dietary Fiber in Human Nutrition*, 2nd edn. CRC Press, Florida; 1992; 387–412.

75 Fleming SE, Rodriguez MA. Influence of dietary fibre on faecal excretion of volatile fatty acids by human adults. *J Nutr* 1983; 113: 1613–26.

76 Florin THJ, Hills BA. Does counterperfusion supersaturation cause gas cysts in pneumatosis cystoides coli, and can breathing heliox reduce them? *Lancet* 1995; 345: 1220–2.

77 Florin THJ, Neale G, Gibson GR, Christl SU, Cummings JH. Metabolism of dietary sulphate: absorption and excretion in humans. *Gut* 1991; 32: 766–73.

78 Forgacs P, Wright PH, Wyatt AP. Treatment of intestinalis gas cysts by oxygen breathing. *Lancet* 1973; 1: 579–82.

79 Freeman HJ. Effects of differing concentrations of sodium butyrate on 1,2-dimethylhydrazine-induced rat intestinal neoplasia. *Gastroenterology* 1986; 91: 596–602.

80 Fregeau CJ, Helgason CD, Bleackley RC. Two cytotoxic cell proteinase genes are differentially sensitive to sodium butyrate. *Nucleic Acids Res* 1992; 20: 3113–19.

81 Freter R. Mechanisms that control the microflora in the large intestine. In: Hentges DJ (ed) *Human Intestinal Microflora in Health and Disease*. Academic Press, London; 1983; 33–54.

82 Fuller R. Probiotics in human medicine. *Gut* 1991; 32: 439–42.

83 Gibson GR, Wang X. Regulatory effects of bifidobacteria on the growth of other colonic bacteria. *J Appl Bacteriol* 1994; 77: 412–20.

84 Gibson GR, Macfarlane GT, Cummings JH. Occurrence of sulphate-reducing bacteria in human faeces and the relationship of dissimilatory sulphate reduction to methanogenesis in the large gut. *J Appl Bacteriol* 1998a; 65: 103–111.

85 Gibson GR, Cummings JH, Macfarlane GT. Competition for hydrogen between sulphate-reducing bacteria and methanogenic bacteria from the human large intestine. *J Appl Bacteriol* 1988b; 65: 241–47.

86 Gibson SAW, McFarlan C, Hay S, Macfarlane GT. Significance of the microflora in proteolysis in the colon. *Appl Environ Microbiol* 1989; 55: 679–83.

87 Gibson GR, Macfarlane GT, Cummings JH. Sulphate-reducing bacteria and hydrogen metabolism in the human large intestine. *Gut* 1993; 34: 437–9.

88 Gibson GR, Beatty ER, Wang X, Cummings JH. Selective stimulation of Bifidobacteria in the human colon by oligofructose and inulin. *Gastroenterology* 1995; 108: 975–82.

89 Gillon T, Tadesse K, Logan RFA, Holt S, Sircus W. Breath hydrogen in pneumatosis cystoides intestinalis. *Gut* 1979; 20: 1008–11.

90 Gorbach SL, Chang T, Goldin B. Successful treatment of relapsing *Clostridium difficile* colitis with *Lactobacillus* GG. *Lancet* 1987; ii: 1519.

91 Greenberger NJ, Saegh S, Ruppert RD. Urine excretion in malabsorptive disorders. *Gastroenterology* 1968; 55: 204–11.

92 Grove EW, Olmsted WH, Koenig K. The effect of diet and catharsis on the lower volatile fatty acids in the stools of normal men. *J Biol Chem* 1929/30; 85: 127–36.

93 Hague A, Manning AM, Hanlon KA *et al*. Sodium butyrate induces apoptosis in human colonic tumour cell lines in a p53-independent pathway: implications for the possible role of dietary fibre in the prevention of large bowel cancer. *Int J Cancer* 1993; 55: 498.

94 Hague A, Elder DJE, Hicks DJ, Paraskeva C. Apoptosis in colorectal tumour cells: induction by the short chain fatty acids butyrate, propionate and acetate and by the bile salt deoxycholate. *Int J Cancer* 1995; 60: 400–6.

95 Hartemink R, Rombouts FM. Gas formation from oligosaccharides by the intestinal microflora. *International Symposium on Pro and Prebiotics*, Wageningen Graduate School, Wageningen, Netherlands; 1997; 57–66.

96 Hekmat S, McMahon DJ. Survival of *Lactobacillus acidophilus* and *Bifidobacterium bifidum* in ice cream for use as a probiotic food. *J Dairy Sci* 1992; 75: 1415–22.

97 Hentges DJ (ed). *Human Intestinal Microflora in Health and Disease*. Academic Press, London, 1983.

98 Hentges DJ, Maier BR, Burton GC, Flynn MA, Tsutkawa R. Effect of high beef on the fecal flora of humans. *Cancer Res* 1977; 37: 568–75.

99 Hidaka H, Hirayama M. Useful characteristics and commercial applications or fructo-oligosaccharides. *Biochem Soc Trans* 1991; 19: 561–5.

100 Hirono I, Sumi Y, Kuhara K, Miyakawa M. Effect of degraded carrageenan on the intestine in germfree rats. *Toxicology Lett* 1981; 8: 207–12.

101 Hove H, Nordgaard-Andersen I, Mortensen PB. Faecal DL-lactate concentration in 100 gastrointestinal patients. *Scand J Gastroenterol* 1994; 29: 255–9.

102 Hugenholtz P, Pace NR. Identifying microbial diversity in the natural environment: a molecular phylogenetic approach. *Trends Biotechnol* 1996; 14: 190–7.

103 Hunnisett A, Howard J, Davies S. Gut fermentation (or the 'auto-brewery') syndrome: a new clinical test with initial observations and discussion of clinical and biochemical implications. *J Nutr Med* 1990; 1: 33–8.

104 Ikeda N, Saito Y, Shimizu J, Ochi A, Watabe J. Variations in concentrations of bacterial metabolites, enzyme activities, moisture, pH and bacterial composition between and within individuals in faeces of seven healthy adults. *J Appl Bacteriol* 1994; 77: 185–94.

105 Ito M, Deguchi Y, Miyamori A *et al*. Effects of administration of galacto-oligosaccharides on the human faecal microflora, stool weight and abdominal sensation. *Microb Ecol Health Dis* 1990; 3: 285–92.

106 IUB–IUPAC Joint Commission on Biochemical Nomenclature. Abbreviated terminology of oliaosaccharide chains. Recommendations 1980. *J Biol Chem* 1982; 257: 3347–51.

107 Jacobs LR, Lupton JR. Relationship between colonic luminal pH, cell proliferation and colon carcinogenesis in 1,2-dimethylhydrazine-treated rats fed high fiber diets. *Cancer Res* 1986; 46: 1727.

108 Kawaguchi M, Tashiro Y, Adachi T, Tamura Z. Changes in intestinal condition, fecal microflora and composition of rectal gas after administration of fructooligosaccharide and lactulose at different doses. *Bifidobacteria Microflora* 1993; 13: 57–68.

109 Kikugawa K, Kato T. Formation of a mutagenic diazoquinone by interaction of phenol with nitrite. *Food Chem Toxicol* 1986; 26: 209–14.

110 King TS, Elia M, Hunter JO. Abnormal colonic fermentation in irritable bowel syndrome. *Lancet* 1998; 352: 1187–89.

111 Kirk E. The quantity and composition of human colonic flatus. *Gastroenterology* 1949; 12: 782–94.

112 Kitano A, Kobayashi K, Oshiumi H *et al*. Studies of experimental ulcerative colitis induced by carrageenan in rabbits. *Jpn J Gastroenterol* 1981; 78: 2104–111.

113 Kleessen B, Sykura B, Zunft H-J, Blaut M. Effects of inulin and lactose on fecal microflora, microbial activity, and bowel habit in elderly constipated persons. *Am J Clin Nutr* 1997; 65: 1397–1492.

114 Kruh J. Effects of sodium butyrate, a new pharmacological agent, on cells in culture. *Mol Cell Biochem* 1982; 42: 65–82.

115 Kruh J, Defer N, Tichonicky L. Action moleculaire et cellulaire du butyrate. *CR Soc Biol* 1992; 186: 12–25.

116 Kruh J, Defer N, Tichonicky L. Effects of butyrate on cell proliferation and gene expression. In Cummings JH, Rombeau JL, Sakata T *Physiological and Clinical Aspects of Short Chain Fatty Acids*. (eds) Cambridge University Press, Cambridge; 1995; 275–88.

117 Levitt MD: Production and excretion of hydrogen gas in man. *New Engl J Med* 1969; 281: 122–7.

118 Levitt MD. Volume and composition of human intestinal gas determined by means of an intestinal washout technique. *New Engl J Med* 1971; 284: 1394–8.

119 Levitt MD, Olsson S. Pneumatosis cystoides intestinalis and high breath H_2 excretion: insights into the role of H_2 in this condition. *Gastroenterology* 1995; 108: 1560–5.

120 Levitt MD, Gibson GR, Christl SU. Gas metabolism in the large intestine. In: Gibson GR, Macfarlane GT (eds) *Human Colonic Bacteria: Role in Nutrition, Physiology and Health*. CRC Press, Boca Raton, Florida; 1995; 131–54.

121 Lewis HB. The value of inulin as a foodstuff. *J Am Med Assoc* 1912; LVIII: 1176–7.

122 Ling WH, Hanninen O. Shifting from a conventional diet to an uncooked vegan diet reversibly alters fecal hydrolytic activities in humans. *J Nutr* 1992; 122: 924–30.

123 Lipkin M, Blattner WA, Fraumeni JFJ *et al*. Tritiated thymidine labeling distribution in the identification of hereditary predisposition to colon cancer. *Cancer Res* 1983; 43: 1899–1904.

124 Livesey G, Johnson IT, Gee JM *et al*. 'Determination' of sugar alcohol and polydextrose absorption in humans by the breath hydrogen (H_2) technique: the stoichiometry of hydrogen production and the interaction between carbohydrates assessed *in vivo* and *in vitro*. *Eur J Clin Nutr* 1993; 47: 419–30.

125 Luo J, Rizkalla SW, Alamovitch C *et al*. Chronic consumption of short-chain fructooligosaccharides by healthy subjects decreased basal hepatic glucose production but had no effect on insulin-stimulated glucose metabolism. *Am J Clin Nutr* 1996; 63: 939–45.

126 Macfarlane GT. Fermentation reactions in the large intestine. In. Cummings JH, Rombeau JL, Sakata T (eds) *Short Chain Fatty Acids: Metabolism and Clinical Importance*. Ross Laboratories Press, Columbus; 1991; 5–10.

127 Macfarlane GT, Cummings JH. The colonic flora, fermentation, and large bowel function. In: Phillips SF, Pemberton JH, Shorter RG (eds) *The Large Intestine, Physiology, Pathophysiology and Disease*. Raven Press, New York; 1991: 51–92.

128 Macfarlane GT, Degnan BA. Catabolite regulatory mechanisms in relation to polysaccharide breakdown and carbohydrate utilization. In: Malkki Y, Cummings JH (eds) *Dietary Fibre and the Human Colon*. Office for Official Publications of the European Communities, Luxembourg; 1996; 117–29.

129 Macfarlane GT, Englyst HN. Starch utilization by the human large intestinal microflora. *J Appl Bacteriol* 1986; 60: 195–201.

130 Macfarlane GT, Gibson GR. Co-utilization of polymerized carbon sources by *Bacteroides ovatus* grown in a two-stage continuous culture system. *Appl Environ Microbiol* 1991; 57: 1–6.

131 Macfarlane GT, Gibson GR. Metabolic activities of the normal colonic flora. In: Gibson SAW (ed) *Human Health: The Contribution of Microorganisms*. Springer Verlag, London, 1994; 17–52.

132 Macfarlane GT, Gibson GR. Carbohydrate fermentation, energy transduction and gas metabolism in the human large intestine. In: Mackie RI, White BA (eds) *Ecology and Physiology of Gastrointestinal Microbes Vol 1: Gastrointestinal Fermentations and Ecosystems*. Chapman and Hall, New York; 1996; 269–318.

133 Macfarlane GT, Macfarlane S. Utilization of pancreatic trypsin and chymotrypsin by proteolytic and non-proteolytic *Bacteroides fragilis*-type bacteria. *Curr Microbiol* 1991; 23: 143–8.

134 Macfarlane GT, Cummings JH, Allison C. Protein degradation by human intestinal bacteria. *J Gen Microbiol* 1986; 132: 1647–56.

135 Macfarlane GT, Cummings JH, Macfarlane S, Gibson GR. Influence of retention time on degradation of pancreatic enzymes by human colonic bacteria grown in a 3-stage continuous culture system. *J Appl Bacteriol* 1989; 67: 521–7.

136 Macfarlane GT, Gibson GR, Cummings JH. Comparison of fermentation reactions in different regions of the human colon. *J Appl Bacteriol* 1992; 72: 57–64.

137 Macfarlane GT, Gibson GR, Macfarlane S. Short chain fatty acid and lactate production by human intestinal bacteria grown in batch and continuous culture. In: Binder HJ *et al.* (eds) *Short Chain Fatty Acids*. Kluwer Publishing, London; 1994: 44–60.

138 Macfarlane S, McBain AJ, Macfarlane GT. Consequences of biofilm and sessile growth in the large intestine. *Adv Dental Res* 1997; 11: 59–68.

139 McKenzie H, Main J, Pennington CR, Parratt D. Antibody to selected strains of *Saccharomyces cerevisiae* (baker's and brewer's yeast) and *Candida albicans* in Crohn's disease. *Gut* 1990; 31: 536–8.

140 McNeil NI. The absorption of lactate from the human large intestine. In: Kasper H, Goebell H (eds) *Colon and Nutrition*. MTP Press, Boston; 1982; 141–3.

141 Magee EAM Cummings JH. Fecal sulfide levels generated in response to changes in meat intake. *Gastroenterology* 1997; 112:A891.

142 Magee EAM, Rochardson CJ, Cummings JH. The contribution of dietary protein and sulphur food additives to faecal sulphide in humans. *Digestion* 1998; 59: 53.

142a Mallett AK, Rowland IR. Factors affecting the gut microflora. In Rowland IR (ed) *Role of the Gut Flora in Toxicity and Cancer*. Academic Press, London, 1988; 347–82.

143 Maraki S, Bafaloukos D, Chatzinikolaou I, Datseris G, Samonis G: Gut colonisation of mice by yeast. effects of methylprednisolone and antibiotics. *Hepato-Gastroenterol* 1998; 45: 119–122.

144 Marcus R, Watt J. Seaweeds and ulcerative colitis in laboratory animals. *Lancet* 1969; August: 489–490 (Letters).

145 Marcus R, Watt J, Path MRC. Ulcerative disease of the colon in laboratory animals induced by pepsin inhibitors. *Gastroenterology* 1974; 67: 473–83.

146 Marcus SM, Marcus AJ, Watt J. Chronic ulcerative disease of the colon in rabbits fed native carageenans. *Proc Nutr Soc* 1983; 42: 155A.

147 Maryand D, Bourgeau G. Production of phenylacetic acid by anaerobes. *J Clin Microbiol* 1982; 16: 747–50.

148 Matsui T, Matsukawa Y, Sakai T, Nakamura K, Aoike A, Kawai K. Effect of ammonia on cell-cycle progression of human gastric cancer cells. *Eur J Gastroenterol Hepatol* 1995; 7:S79–S81.

149 Mayall T, MacPherson A, Bjarnason I, Forgacs I, Peters T. Mitochondrial function of colonic epithelial cells in inflammatory bowel disease. *Gut* 1992; 33:S24.

150 Middleton SJ, Coley A, Hunter JO. The role of faecal *Candida albicans* in the pathogenesis of food-intolerant irritable bowel syndrome. *Postgrad Med J* 1992; 68: 543–54.

150a Mitsuoka T. Taxonomy and ecology of bifidobacteria. *Bifid Microf* 1984; 3: 11–28. Scardovi V (ed): Genus Bifidobacterium. *Bergey's Manual of Systematic Bacteriology*, Williams & Wilkins, New York.

151 Molis C, Flourie B, Ouarne F *et al*. Digestion, excretion and energy value of fructooligosaccharides in healthy humans. *Am J Clin Nutr* 1996; 64: 324–8.

152 Mortensen PB, Holtug K, Bonnen H, Clausen MR. The degradation of amino acids, proteins, and blood to short-chain fatty acids in colon is prevented by lactulose. *Gastroenterology* 1990; 98: 353–60.

153 Munster IPV, Tangerman A, Nagengast FM. The effect of resistant starch on colonic fermentation, bile acid metabolism and mucosal proliferation. *Digest Dis Sci* 1994; 39: 834–42.

154 Murray KE, Adams RF, Earl J, Shaw KJ. Studies of the free amines of infants with gastroenteritis and of healthy infants. *Gut* 1986; 27: 1173–80.

155 Murray KE, Shaw KJ, Adams RF, Conway PL. Presence of N-acyl and acetoxy derivatives of putrescine and cadaverine in the human gut. *Gut* 1993; 34: 489–93.

156 Oh MS, Uribarri J, Alveranga D, Lazar I, Bazilinski N, Carroll H. Metabolic utilisation and renal handling of D-lactate in men. *Metabolism* 1985; 34: 621–5.

157 Ohkusa T. Production of experimental ulcerative colitis in hamsters by dextran sulfate sodium and change in intestinal microflora. *Jpn J Gastroenterol* 1985; 82: 1327–36.

158 Ohkusa T, Yamada M, Takenaga T. Protective effect of metronidazole in experimental ulcerative colitis induced by dextran sulfate sodium. *Jpn J Gastroenterol* 1987; 84: 2337–46.

159 Okayasu I, Hatakeyama S, Yamada M *et al*. A novel method in the induction of reliable experimental acute and chronic ulcerative colitis in mice. *Gastroenterology* 1990; 98: 694–702.

160 Onderdonk A, Hermos J, Bartlett J. The role of the intestinal microflora in experimental colitis. *Am J Clin Nutr* 1977; 30: 1819–25.

161 Onderdonk AB, Hermos JA, Dzink JL, Bartlett JG. Protective effect of metronidazole in experimental ulcerative colitis. *Gastroenterology* 1978; 74: 521–6.

162 Onderdonk AB, Bartlett MD. Bacteriological studies of experimental ulcerative colitis. *Am J Clin Nutr* 1979; 32: 258–65.

163 Op den Camp HJM, Oosterhof A, Veerkamp JH. Interaction of bifidobacterial lipoteichoic acid with human intestinal epithelial cells. *Infection and Immunity* 1985; 47: 332–34.

164 Pedersen A, Sandstrom B, Van Amelsuoort JMM. Effects of ingestion of inulin on blood lipids and gastrointestinal symptoms in healthy females. *Br J Nutr* 1997; 78: 215–22.

165 Perman JA, Modler S, Olson AC. Role of pH in production of hydrogen from carbohydrates by colonic bacterial flora. *J Clin Invest* 1981; 67: 643–50.

166 Peters SG, Pomare EW, Fisher CA. Portal and peripheral blood short chain fatty acid concentrations after caecal lactulose instillation at surgery. *Gut* 1992; 33: 1249–52.

167 Pfeiffer CJ. Animal models of colitis. In: Pfeiffer CJ (ed) *Animal Models for Intestinal Disease*. CRC Press; Boca Raton, Florida; 1985; 147–60.

168 Phear EA, Ruebner B. The *in vitro* production of ammonium and amines by intestinal bacteria in relation to nitrogen toxicity as a factor in hepatic coma. *Br J Exp Pathol* 1956; 37: 253–62.

169 Phillips J, Muir JG, Birkett A *et al*. Effect of resistant starch on fecal bulk and fermentation-dependent events in humans. *Am J Clin Nutr* 1995; 62: 121–30.

170 Pitcher MCL, Beatty ER, Cummings JH. The contribution of sulfate-reducing bacteria and 5-ASA to fecal sulphide in patients with ulcerative colitis. *Gut* 2000; 46: 64–72.

D

171 Pomare EW, Branch WJ, Cummings JH. Carbohydrate fermentation in the human colon and its relation to acetate concentration in venous blood. *J Clin Invest* 1985; 75: 1448–54.

172 Porter P, Kenworthy R. A study of intestinal and urinary amines in pigs in relation to weaning. *Res Vet Sci* 1969; 10: 440–7.

173 Prasad KN. Butyric acid. a small fatty acid with diverse biological functions. *Life Sci* 1980; 27: 1351–8.

174 Prasad KN, Sinha PK. Effect of sodium butyrate on mammalian cells in culture: a review. *In Vitro* 1976; 12: 125–32.

175 Quigley ME, Hudson GJ, Englyst HN. Determination of resistant short-chain carbohydrates (non-digestible oligosaccharides) using gas liquid chromatography. *Food Chem* 1999; 65: 381–90.

176 Ramakrishna BS, Gee D, Weiss A, Pannall PR, Roberts-Thomson IC, Roediger WEW. Estimation of phenolic conjugation by colonic mucosa. *J Clin Pathol* 1989; 42: 620–3.

177 Ramakrishna BS, Roberts-Thomson IC, Pannall PR, Roediger WEW. Impaired sulphation of phenol by the colonic mucosa in quiescent and active ulcerative colitis. *Gut* 1991; 32: 46–9.

178 Read NW, Miles CA, Fisher D. Transit of a meal through the stomach, small intestine, and colon in normal subjects and its role in the pathogenesis of diarrhoea. *Gastroenterology* 1980; 79: 1276–82.

179 Read NW, Al-Janabi MN, Cann PA. Is raised breath hydrogen related to the pathogenesis of pneumatosis coli? *Gut* 1984; 25: 839–45.

180 Read NW, Al-Janabi MN, Bates TE. Interpretation of the breath hydrogen profile obtained after ingesting a solid meal containing unabsorbable carbohydrate. *Gut* 1985; 26: 834–42.

181 Reddy BS, Rivenson A. Inhibitory effect of *Bifidobacterium longum* on colon, mammary, and liver carcinogenesis induced by 2-amino-3-methylimidazo [4,5-*f*] quinoline, a food mutagen. *Cancer Res* 1993; 53: 3914–18.

182 Richardson CJ, Cummings JH. Protein fermentation and sulphide production by human colonic bacteria: studies using an *in vitro* model. *Digestion* 1998; 59: 153.

183 Robb TA, Goodwin DA, Davidson GP. Faecal hydrogen production *in vitro* as an indicator for *in vivo* hydrogen producing capability in the breath hydrogen test. *Acta Paediatr Scand* 1985; 74: 942–4.

184 Roediger WEW. The colonic epithelium in ulcerative colitis: an energy-deficiency disease? *Lancet* 1980; 2: 712–15.

185 Roediger WEW. Short chain fatty acids as metabolic regulators of ion absorption in the colon. *Acta Vet Scand* 1989; 86: 116–25.

186 Roediger WEW, Duncan A, Kapaniris O, Millard S. Reducing sulfur compounds of the colon impair colonocyte nutrition: implications for ulcerative colitis. *Gastroenterology* 1993; 104: 802–9.

187 Roediger WEW, Duncan A, Kapaniris O, Millard S. Sulphide impairment of substrate oxidation in rat colonocytes: a biochemical basis for ulcerative colitis? *Clin Sci* 1993; 85: 623–7.

188 Rumessen JJ, Bode S, Hamberg O, Gudmand-Hoyer E. Fructans of Jerusalem artichokes: intestinal transport, absorption, fermentation and influence on blood glucose, insulin and C-peptide responses in healthy subjects. *Am J Clin Nutr* 1990; 52: 675–81.

189 Samonis G, Karyotakis NC, Anaissie EJ, Maraki S, Tselentis Y, Bodey GP. Effects of cyclophosphamide and ceftriaxone on gastrointestinal colonisation of mice by *Candida albicans*. *Antimicrobial Agents and Chemotherapy* 1996; 40: 2221–3.

190 Sanno T. Effects of Neosugar on constipation, intestinal microflora and gallbladder contraction in diabetics. *Proceedings of Third Neosugar Research Conference*, Tokyo, 1986; 109–117.

191 Saunders DR, Wiggins HS. Conservation of mannitol, lactulose and raffinose by the human colon. *Am J Physiol* 1981; 241:G397–G402.

192 Scheppach W, Fabian C, Sachs M, Kasper H. The effect of starch malabsorption on fecal short chain fatty acid excretion in man. *Scand J Gastroenterol* 1988; 23: 755–9.

193 Scheppach WM. Short chain fatty acids are a trophic factor for the human colonic mucosa *in vitro*. In: Silverman E (ed.) *Short Chain Fatty Acids: Metabolism and Clinical Importance*. Ross Laboratories, Columbus, Ohio, 1991; 90–93.

194 Sekine K, Watanabe-Sekine E, Ohta J, Toida T, Tatsuki T, Kawashima T. Induction and activation of tumoricidal cells *in vitro* and *in vivo* by the bacterial cell wall of *Bifidobacterium infantis*. *Bifidobacteria Microflora* 1994; 13: 65–77.

195 Shephard SE, Schlatter C, Lutz WK. N-Nitrosocompounds: relevance to human cancer. In: Bartels H, O'Neill IK, Herman RS (eds) IARC Scientific Publications No 57. International Agency for Research on Cancer Scientific Publications, Lyons; 1987; 328–32.

196 Silvester KR, Cummings JH. Does digestibility of meat protein help explain large bowel cancer risk? *Nutrition and Cancer* 1995; 24: 279–88.

197 Silvester KR, Bingham SA, Pollock JRA, Cummings JH, O'Neill IK. Effect of meat and resistant starch on fecal excretion of apparent *N*-nitroso compounds and ammonia from the human large bowel. *Nutrition and Cancer* 1997; 29: 13–23.

198 Smith EA, Macfarlane GT. Enumeration of human colonic bacteria producing phenolic and indolic compounds: effects of pH, carbohydrate availability and retention time on dissimilatory aromatic amino acid metabolism. *J Appl Bacteriol* 1996; 81: 288–302.

199 Smith EA, Macfarlane GT. Studies on amine production in the human colon: enumeration of amine forming bacteria and physiological effects of carbohydrate and pH. *Anaerobe* 1996; 2: 285–97.

200 Smith EA, Macfarlane GT. Enumeration of amino acid fermenting bacteria in the human large intestine: effects of pH and carbohydrate availability on peptide and dissimilatory amino acid metabolism. *FEMS Microbiol Ecol* 1998; 25: 355–68.

201 Smith PJ. *n*-Butyrate alters chromatin accessibility to DNA repair enzymes. *Carcinogenesis* 1986; 7: 423–9.

201a Stanier RY, Adelberg EA, Ingraham JL. *General Microbiology*. MacMillan, London; 1979.

202 Stein J, Schroder O, Milovic V, Caspary WF. Mercaptoproprionate inhibits butyrate uptake in isolated apical membrane vesicles of the rat distal colon. *Gastroenterology* 1995; 108: 673–9.

203 Stephen AM, Wiggins HS, Cummings JH. Effect of changing transit time on colonic microbial metabolism in man. *Gut* 1987; 28: 601–9.

204 Stolberg L, Rolfe R, Gitlin N *et al*. D-Lactic acidosis due to abnormal gut flora. Diagnosis and treatment of two cases. *New Engl J Med* 1982; 306: 1344–8.

205 Stone-Dorshow T, Levitt MD. Gaseous response to ingestion of a poorly absorbed fructo-oligosaccharide sweetener. *Am J Clin Nutr* 1987; 46: 61–5.

206 Summerskill WHJ, Wolpert E. Ammonia metabolism in the gut. *Am J Clin Nutr* 1970; 23: 633–9.

207 Tadesse K, Eastwood MA. Metabolism of dietary fibre components in man assessed by breath hydrogen and methane. *Br J Nutr* 1978; 40: 393–6.

208 Tannock GW, Savage DC. Influence of dietary and environmental stress on microbial populations in the murine gastrointestinal tract. *Infection and Immunology* 1974; 9: 591–8.

209 Thauer R, Jungermann K, Decker K. Energy conservation in anaerobic bacteria. *Bacteriol Rev* 1977; 41: 100–80.

210 Thomakos N, Maraki S, Liakakos T *et al*. Effect of cefamandole, cefuroxime and cefoxitin on yeast fecal flora of surgical patients. *Chemotherapy* 1998; 44: 324–7.

211 Tojo M, Oikawa T, Morikawa Y, Yamashita N, Iwata S, Satoh Y. The effects of *Bifidobacterium breve* administration on *Campylobacter enteritis*. *Acta Pediatrica Japan* 1987; 29: 160–7.

212 Tomkin GH, Weir DG. Indicanuria after gastric surgery. *Quart J Med* 1972; 41: 191–203.

213 Tubbs PK. The metabolism of d-alpha hydroxy acids in animal tissues. *Ann NY Acad Sci* 1965; 119: 920–6.

214 Uribarri J, OH MS, Caroll HJ. D-lactic acidosis. A review of clinical presentation, biochemical features and pathophysiologic mechanisms. *Med Baltimore* 1998; 77: 73–82.

215 Vince AJ. Metabolism of ammonia, urea, and amino acids, and their significance in liver disease. In: Hill MJ (ed) *Microbial Metabolism in the Digestive Tract*. CRC Press, Boca Raton, Florida; 1986; 83–105.

216 Visek WJ, Clinton SK, Truex CR. Nutritional and experimental carcinogenesis. *Cornell Veterinarian* 1978; 68: 3–39.

217 Waaij DVD, Cohen BJ, Anver MR. Mitigation of experimental inflammatory bowel disease in guinea pigs by selective elimination of the aerobic gram-negative intestinal microflora. *Gastroenterology* 1974; 67: 460–72.

218 Wang X, Gibson GR. Effects of the *in vitro* fermentation of oligofructose and inulin by bacteria growing in the human large intestine. *J Appl Bacteriol* 1993; 75: 373–80.

219 Watanabe K, Reddy BS, Weisburger JH Kritchevsky D. Effect of dietary alfalfa, pectin and wheat bran on azoxymethane- or methylnitrosourea-induced colon carcinogenesis in F344 rats. *J Nat Cancer Inst* 1979; 63: 141.

220 Weber FL, Banwell JG, Fresard KM, Cummings JH. Nitrogen in fecal bacteria, fiber and soluble fractions of patients with cirrhosis: effects of lactulose and lactulose plus neomycin. *J Lab Clin Med* 1987; 110: 259–63.

221 Weiseger RA, Pinkus LM, Jakoby WB. Thiol S-methyltransferase: suggested role in detoxication of intestinal hydrogen sulfide. *Biochem Pharmacol* 1980; 29: 2885–7.

222 Williams RD, Olmsted WH. The effect of cellulose, hemicellulose and lignin on the weight of the stool: a contribution to the study of laxation in man. *J Nutr* 1936; 11: 433.

223 Williams RD, Olmsted WH. The manner in which food controls the bulk of faeces. *Ann Int Med* 1936; 10: 717.

224 Wilson JR, Weiser MM. Colonic cancer cell (HT29) adhesion to laminin is altered by differentiation: adhesion may involve galactosyltransferase. *Exp Cell Res* 1992; 201: 330.

225 Yokoyama MT, Carlson JR. Production of skatole and para-cresol by a rumen *Lactobacillus* sp. *Appl Environ Microbiol* 1981; 41: 71–6.

226 Yokoyama MT, Tabori C, Miller ER, Hogberg MG. The effects of antibiotics in the weanling pig diet on growth and excretions of volatile phenolic and aromatic bacterial metabolites. *Am J Clin Nutr* 1982; 35: 1417–24.

227 Yoshioka M, Fujita K, Sakata H, Murono K, Iseki K. Development of the normal intestinal flora and its clinical significance in infants and children. *Bifidobacteria Microflora* 1991; 10: 11–17.

228 Yoshizumi M, Hirata I, Sasaki Sea. Effects of various drugs on chronic colitis induced by dextran sulfate sodium in rats. *Gastroenterology* 1995; 108:A947.

229 Zuccato E, Venturi M, Colombo L *et al*. Role of bile acids and metabolic activity of colonic bacteria after cholecystectomy. *Dig Dis Sci* 1993; 38: 514–19.

Chapter 23

Infections of the gastrointestinal tract and food intolerance

J. O. Hunter

INTRODUCTION

The mechanism of true food allergy is well understood. Small doses of an allergen combine with circulating IgE antibodies to produce unpleasant symptoms, such as rhinitis or urticaria. Patients often have high concentrations of IgE in their blood and allergies can accurately be diagnosed by skin prick or radioallergoabsorbent tests. A number of conditions however, including migraine, irritable bowel syndrome (IBS), Crohn's disease, eczema, hyperactivity and rheumatoid arthritis, have been shown in well-designed, carefully controlled trials to respond to exclusion diets in which certain food items are forbidden.[1,3,4,18,20,21] In these conditions, however, there is no evidence of a classical IgE-mediated allergic response[34] and this discrepancy has led some investigators to conclude that patients with this type of reaction do not have genuine food intolerance.[23]

An alternative explanation however, might be that food intolerance in these conditions is mediated by different mechanisms which need not necessarily be immunological.[28] It is well known that chemicals in foods can produce toxic effects. For example, tyramine in chocolate and cheese provokes bouts of migraine in susceptible people.[27] Milk may cause abdominal pain, flatulence and diarrhoea in subjects intolerant of lactose. In none of these examples is there any evidence of an immunological cause. Many people, however, can eat tyramine and lactose without ill effect. Clearly there must be an inherent difference between subjects who are intolerant of these chemicals and those who are not. Lactose intolerance is known to be caused by low concentrations of the enzyme lactase in the jejunal mucosa. Alactasia is frequently inherited, but acquired enzyme deficiencies may also occur and lead to food intolerance. Monamine oxidase inhibitor drugs depress hepatic concentrations of the enzyme monoamine oxidase, and patients receiving these drugs are therefore instructed to avoid foods such as cheese, yeast, pickles and red wine, which will provoke headaches and hypertension because the vasoactive amines that they contain pass unchanged through the liver to reach the systemic circulation.

Reduced enzyme concentrations, however, cannot be the sole cause of food intolerance because many patients report its onset in adult life and are upset by foods that they had eaten previously without ill-effect. The bacterial flora of the gut may also have an important role; encephalopathy develops in patients with cirrhosis after meals rich in protein, which is broken down by the gut flora producing amino compounds, which are absorbed from the gut and, bypassing the liver, act as false transmitters in the brain.

The suggestion that toxic products might be derived by bacterial malfermentation in the colon is far from new. Indeed it was first proposed by Metchnikoff.[38] He suggested that constipation led to disease because of autointoxication by chemicals which were not eliminated sufficiently rapidly. This theory is no longer accepted. However, a modern refinement of Metchnikoff's theory suggests that constipation or the rate of transit through the gut is itself unimportant but that specific foods may be metabolized to yield toxic chemicals if damage occurs to the healthy colonic flora. This theory has been investigated in most detail in patients suffering from food intolerance causing IBS.

IRRITABLE BOWEL SYNDROME AND FOOD INTOLERANCE

The evidence for the importance of food intolerance in the pathogenesis of IBS is discussed in more detail in Chapter 41. However, it is now clear that in every study which has been published, a proportion of patients with IBS has been found to suffer from food intolerance. The percentage involved varies from 6 to 67%[1,22] but the largest studies suggest that food intolerance is the cause of IBS in approximately 50% of cases.[41,42] The foods concerned are primarily wheat and other cereals such as maize and rye, dairy products, caffeine, yeast and citrus fruit. These foods have also been implicated as the most important in the food intolerances associated with migraine, Crohn's disease, eczema and rheumatoid arthritis.[1,3,4,18,20,21]

COLONIC MALFERMENTATION IN IBS

Levitt[35] reported a patient with alactasia who produced excessive volumes of rectal flatus. The gas was shown to comprise largely hydrogen and carbon dioxide. The hydrogen in particular could only have been produced by bacterial action, and dietary studies confirmed that it was a result of bacterial fermentation of undigested milk sugar. Subjects with normal levels of small intestinal lactase may also produce colonic gas by colonic fermentation. The same workers published reports of increased hydrogen production in normal volunteers after ingestion of gluten-containing foods but not after foods such as rice and sucrose, which were completely digested and absorption in the small intestine.[36] The presence of gluten in foods led to incomplete absorption of carbohydrate in the small intestine with the result that some reached the caecal bacteria and was fermented with the production of hydrogen.

It is now appreciated that as much as 40 g of starch, 4 g of fat and 14 g of protein, together with 20 g of fibre enter the caecum each day in normal individuals.[46] This provides a rich substrate for fermentation and it is known that short-chain fatty acids and ammonia may be produced by bacteria, along with soluble waste products and hydrogen.

Other food components that enter the caecum in substantial amounts include sugars such as sucrose,[9] fructose[44] and sorbitol.[30] Marked malabsorption of fructose and sorbitol but not of sucrose has been reported in IBS. In 7 out of 13 patients the fructose absorption capacities were below 15 g and mixtures of 25 g of fructose with 5 g of sorbitol caused significant abdominal distress.[43] Starch malabsorption may be increased in normal subjects by the glucosidase inhibitor acarbose (BAY g 5421) which is now used in the management of diabetes mellitus. This may also lead to increases in stool weight and abdominal symptoms.[45]

Whole body calorimetry

Evidence of abnormal colonic fermentation in patients with IBS itself has until recently been lacking. The simplest products of fermentation to measure in man are hydrogen and methane, which form a significant percentage of the total colonic gas. Previous studies using intubation or radiological techniques[14,33] have revealed no differences in the amount of colonic gas between patients and controls, nor was there any difference in the amounts of hydrogen excreted on the breath.[26] However, new information on fermentation in IBS has been provided by recent studies involving whole body calorimetry (Fig. 23.1).

Six female patients with IBS and six healthy female volunteers followed an identical protocol (Fig. 23.2). A standard diet of fixed composition was ingested for 2 weeks, and then after 2 weeks of *ad libitum* feeding, a fixed 'exclusion diet' was ingested for a further 2 weeks. On the last day of both fixed dietary periods, subjects entered a whole body calorimeter and received meals at 1000, 1400 and 1900 hours. Each diet provided three isocaloric meals totalling 8 MJ/day, adjusted to achieve near energy balance [estimated energy expenditure – 1.5 × basal metabolic rate (BMR)] with a starch- and fibre-free increment in which all carbohydrate was available for small bowel digestion. Energy was provided as 45% carbohydrate, 40% fat and 15% protein.

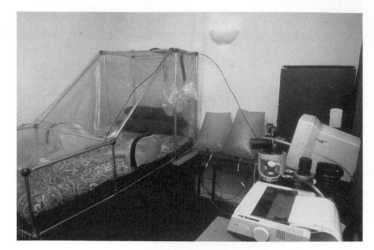

Fig. 23.1 Whole body calorimeter. The patient is nursed on the bed under the plastic tent through which air is drawn at 100 L/min. To the right of the bed are two Douglas bags into which air from the tent and the surrounding room is sampled every 30 minutes.

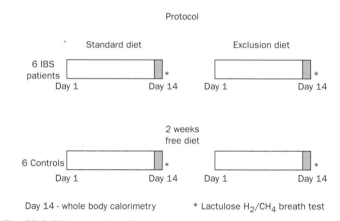

Fig. 23.2 Dietary protocol.

Both diets provided 12.5 g NSP (non-starch polysaccharide), 120 g starch and 3.5 g resistant starch daily. Food was provided from a metabolic kitchen and compliance assessed by daily contact and food diary. Total hydrogen and methane excretion was determined at 30-min intervals throughout the 24-h period. In addition, measurements of breath excretion of both gases were made during waking hours.

Hydrogen and methane excretion

On the standard diet IBS patients excreted significantly more hydrogen than controls (mean 389 ± 161 ml/ 24 h vs. 174 ± 84 ml/ 24 h). The maximum rates of excretion of hydrogen together with methane were considerably higher in the patients and in four out of six patients abdominal symptoms occurred when gas excretion was rapid. In contrast, in controls there were no symptoms, even at the highest rates of excretion. The exclusion diet reduced total gas excretion in patients by two-thirds, especially hydrogen (mean 302 ± 145 ml 24 h vs. 85 ± 66 ml/24 h). The maximum rate of gas excretion fell by over 80% in patients but no change occurred in controls (Fig. 23.3).

Immediately after completing 24 hours in the calorimeter, subjects were given an oral dose of 20 g lactulose. Hydrogen excretion on the breath was measured for the following 3 hours.

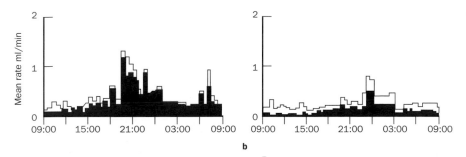

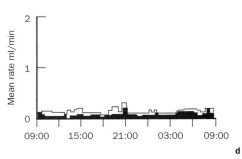

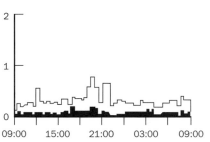

Fig. 23.3 Area charts showing median rate of total excretion (hydrogen: filled; methane: unfilled; ml/min (standard temperature and pressure) at 30 min intervals during 24 h measurement on standard and exclusion diets. (a) IBS patients on standards diet, (b) controls on standards diet, (c) IBS patients on an exclusion diet, (d) controls on exclusion diet. Taken with permission from King *et al. Lancet* 1998; 352: 1187–98.

Breath hydrogen excretion was reduced on the exclusion diet and breath methane excretion was greater (Fig. 23.4).[32]

This study provides strong evidence that the symptoms of IBS are linked to fermentation and that the exclusion diet is effective because of its dramatic effects upon this process. Increased rates of gas excretion are probably not solely the cause of symptoms but the local effects of fermentation products such as short-chain fatty acids or bioactive amines may also be important. The study suggests that the changes produced by the exclusion diet were associated with alterations in the activity of the colonic flora.

This is the reason for the changes on the two diets in the production of breath hydrogen and methane after an identical lactulose challenge. In one patient, lactose hydrogen breath tests were repeated after the patient had reintroduced foods which had been forbidden on the exclusion diet. Not until the patient had reintroduced wheat, the food which was found to be responsible for provoking her symptoms, did the hydrogen production revert to its original level (Fig. 23.5).

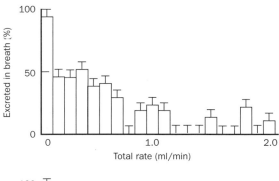

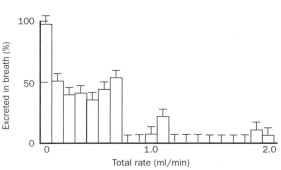

Fig. 23.4 Percentage of total excretion of hydrogen plus methane (breath + flatus) excreted via breath at each rate of total gas excretion. (a) IBS patients, (b) controls. Taken with permission from King *et al. Lancet* 1998; 1187–98.

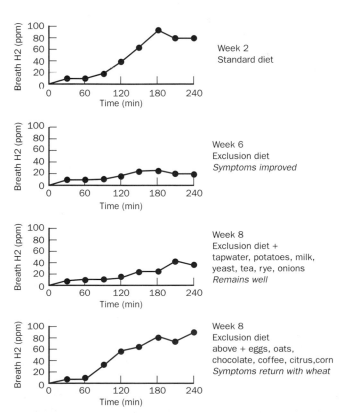

Fig. 23.5 Breath hydrogen excretion after ingestion of 20 g lactulose in a patient with irritable bowel syndrome caused by food intolerance after various dietary modifications.

THE COLONIC MICROFLORA IN IBS

Thus, it is clear that sufficient substrate may enter the caecum from the small intestine to provide a basis for both bacterial fermentation and for the provocation of symptoms in susceptible individuals. Normal people, however, do not suffer significant symptoms as a result of bacterial fermentation. As food residues pass into the caecum in both those subjects who develop symptoms and those who do not, it would seem likely that there are differences in the bacterial flora of the two groups.

Studies of the faecal flora in patients with food intolerances have supported this hypothesis. In preliminary experiments[6] six patients were hospitalized and microbiological analysis of the faecal flora was carried out for 48 h before and up to 72 h after challenge with wheat (five patients) or sugar (one patient). Similar studies were carried out in six age- and sex-matched controls. Higher numbers of aerobes were found in faecal samples from patients and, in two patients, a 100-fold increase in the number of aerobes occurred during challenge (Table 23.1). There were noticeable changes in the predominant aerobic flora of four patients and anaerobic flora of three patients as judged by colony morphology and microscopy. Much lower numbers of bifidobacteria were isolated than expected.[17]

Excretion of aerobic bacteria in faeces (viable bacteria/g dry weight faeces)				
	n	Samples	Mean	Range
Patients	6	30	2.2×10^9	2.9×10^7–1.1×10^{10}
Controls	6	6	9.8×10^7	3.9×10^6–2.7×10^8

Table 23.1 Excretion of aerobic bacteria in faeces (viable bacteria/g dry weight faeces).

Subsequently, three detailed studies were carried out. A large-scale blind study was performed in which levels of facultative bacteria, moisture content, pH and volatile fatty acids (VFAs) were determined on 103 stool samples from 101 patients.[7] These included a group of patients who had received antibiotics, a group of patients with IBS presenting at medical outpatients before any dietary therapy, and a control group drawn from healthy hospital employees. Freshly passed stools were collected at home and transported under cool conditions to the laboratory within 5 h. The increased viable aerobic bacterial count discovered in the previous study was not confirmed as a significant difference in patients with IBS, as the counts were similar for both IBS and control categories (Table 23.2).

Escherichia and *Streptococcus* were the common genera in the stools. Other genera isolated were *Staphylococcus*, *Proteus*, *Klebsiella*, *Enterobacter* and *Micrococcus*. Genera other than *Escherichia* and *Streptococcus* were isolated from 17 out of 38 patients from the IBS group and four out of 16 controls. There was a decrease in the percentage of Gram-positive aerobic bacteria in the stools in the patient groups, although the decrease was not statistically significant.

Change in gut flora related to diet and symptoms

These changes are similar to those observed by Balsari *et al.*[5] who showed that with a group of IBS patients faecal coliforms were significantly reduced and that *Pseudomonas* and *Enterobacter* appeared in the stool. The changes in the flora of the patients studied supported the idea that in some patients with functional bowel disorders the state of the aerobic gut flora may be an indicator of the disease state, although further work is required to elucidate the full significance of these findings.

In a second study, two patients with food-related IBS were admitted to hospital and the faecal microbial flora examined while they underwent double-blind food challenges.[50] Both patients displayed symptoms following challenge, and faecal

Faecal properties in food-related irritable bowel syndrome (IBS)	Log₁₀ aerobic bacteria/g wet weight		Moisture content (%)		pH		Total VFA† (mol/g wet weight)		
	n	Mean	SE	Mean	SE	Mean	SE	*n*	Mean	SE

	n	Mean	SE	Mean	SE	Mean	SE	*n*	Mean	SE
All categories										
IBS	56	7.62	0.14	75.0	1.0	7.10	0.08	38	118	6
Control	35	7.47	0.16	72.2	1.0	7.10	0.08	34	112	5
'Naturally arising'										
IBS	38	7.65	0.14	74.4	1.2	7.09	0.10	26	125	7
Control	16	7.42	0.17	73.8	1.5	7.01	0.14	16	115	8
Three months' post-hysterectomy placebo only	5	7.04*	0.32							
Prophylaxis	10	6.80*	0.47							
Antibiotic treatment	18	7.82*	0.16							

*Coefficient of contrast, $P = 0.018$.
†VFA, volatile fatty acid.

Table 23.2 Faecal properties in food-related irritable bowel syndrome (IBS). No change in the aerobic bacteria count was seen between IBS patients and controls but a significant increase in the count occurs in post-hysterectomy patients who had received antibiotic treatment compared to those who had not.

			Mean (SE) log$_{10}$ cfu/g*		Anaerobe:	Short-chain fatty acids [mean (SE) μmol/g*]			Moisture
Patient	**Diet**	**Number of samples tested**	**Aerobes**	**Anaerobes****	**aerobe ratio**	**Acetic**	**Propionic**	**n-Butyric**	**content [mean (SE) %]**
P3	Normal	7	9.16 (0.27) NS	11.38 (0.11) NS	166:1	374 (62.1) $P < 0.05$	15.0 (2.5) $P < 0.05$	18.1 (3.4) NS	71.3 (1.8) NS
	Challenge	7	8.42 (0.15)	11.25 (0.05)	676:1	653§ (75.6)	30.9§ (4.5)	33.4§ (6.8)	74.7 (2.6)
P7	Normal	10	8.7† (0.08) NS	11.27† (0.06) NS	372:1	289 (33.6) NS	42.2 (5.8) NS	69.2 (15.9) NS	79.6 (0.71) NS
	Challenge	10	8.98†† (0.13)	11.38†† (0.04)	251:1	292 (21.3)	38.5 (4.6)	89.2 (13.9)	80.1 (0.71)

Changes in faecal parameters in two patients during challenge with symptom-provoking food

NS = no significant difference; values were compared by Student's t test; cfu = colony-forming units.
*Dry weight; **includes facultative anaerobes; †9 samples tested; ††7 samples tested; § 6 samples tested.

Table 23.3 Changes in faecal parameters in two patients during challenge with symptom-provoking food.

output increased on the challenge diet although fibre content was kept constant. No significant diet-related differences in bacterial viable counts were seen in either patient (Table 23.3). The major short-chain fatty acids present in both patients were acetic, propionic and n-butyric acids and in one patient the concentrations of all three increased markedly during the challenge diet. Both patients had a lower than usual ratio of anaerobic to aerobic bacteria in their faeces.

A third patient suffering from severe IBS related to food intolerances was also studied at various stages during her clinical course.[11] Eight separate faecal samples were studied over an 18-month period. During this time the level of facultative organisms ranged from 72% to 0.7% and this seemed to correlate with the patient's clinical state. The flora was very variable, and there was an unusual incidence of *Clostridium* species.

These studies show that, although no pathogenic organisms are present in IBS, changes in some aspects of the gut flora may be associated with food-related diarrhoea, particularly the metabolic activity of the flora or the presence of increased numbers of aerobic species. These changes may move in different directions in different individuals and it is not certain whether they are the cause of the symptoms or just reflect other biological alterations. However, enough abnormalities have been discovered in the faecal flora of these patients to suggest that changes in the flora may indeed be the crucial factor in the pathogenesis of these conditions, even though the precise abnormality related to the bacteria concerned has still to be pinpointed.

Antibiotics and *Candida*

The administration of antibiotics may lead to overgrowth of *Candida*. It has been suggested that such overgrowth may persist and that food intolerance in IBS and other conditions may be due to excess numbers of *Candida* in the faecal flora. However, in a study in which *Candida albicans* was sought in stool samples of 38 patients with IBS and 20 healthy controls, this suggestion was not confirmed. In only three patients with IBS was C. *albicans* dis-

covered and all these patients had either recently received antibiotics or the stool sample had been delayed more than 24 h in transit. *Candida albicans* was isolated from none of the control stool samples and it is therefore difficult to believe that this organism is involved in the aetiology of IBS.[39]

COLONIZATION RESISTANCE AND THE STABILITY OF THE BACTERIAL FLORA

Anaerobic bacteria outnumber aerobes by a factor of 10 to 100 000 in the colon and appear to be of crucial importance in maintaining a stable bacterial flora. If extraneous organisms such as *E. coli* or *Pseudomonas* are ingested in healthy people, the organisms disappear completely during intestinal passage, as long as a normal anaerobic flora is present. Larger doses may persist in the faecal flora for a few days, but permanent colonization rarely occurs.[12,16] This phenomenon is known as colonization resistance.[48] Apart from the anaerobic flora, other factors in the gut, such as swallowing saliva, peristalsis, mucus secretion, cell desquamation and the secretion of IgA, may also be important in the maintenance of colonization resistance. However, after the administration of antibiotics, colonization resistance may be severely damaged. Overgrowth with species resistant to the antibiotic, such as *Candida* or other microorganisms may follow.[49] The relationship between the number of bacteria swallowed by an individual and that required for subsequent colonization often changes dramatically during treatment with those antibiotics that have an inhibitory effect on anaerobic bacteria, and intestinal colonization may occur following exposure to relatively small numbers of organisms.[8,47]

EVENTS LEADING TO THE DEVELOPMENT OF IBS

The bacterial flora may be damaged and colonization resistance reduced by a number of factors including infection, antibiotics, surgery, radiation and anaesthesia.[98] It is therefore of great interest that strong evidence exists that IBS may develop after such events in susceptible people. The development of IBS after attacks of gastroenteritis has been a well-known clinical phenomenon for many years.[15] More recent evidence has documented this progression in more detail.

Of 38 patients involved in two well-documented outbreaks of food poisoning due to *Salmonella enteritidis* phage type 4, 12 were discovered a year later to have persisting bowel symptoms consistent with IBS.[37] None of these had suffered bowel symptoms before their infection and all had become culture negative for *Salmonella*. There were five times as many women as men in the group with persistent symptoms and the severity of the acute illness had been greater in those who developed IBS, with a significantly greater proportion suffering vomiting or sustaining a weight loss greater than 7 lb (3.15 kg) during the acute infection. None of these patients had been given antibiotics.

A second study from the same group confirmed the link between acute gastroenteritis and IBS.[25] Seventy-five patients with acute gastroenteritis were studied and 6 months later 20 of these still had symptoms compatible with IBS. In this study, a series of psychometric tests was performed in patients who were hospitalized during their acute illness and it was found that those who subsequently developed IBS had higher scores at this early stage for anxiety, depression, somatization and neurotic trait than those who returned to normal bowel function. This finding was presented as evidence that psychological factors are important in the pathogenesis of IBS, but other interpretations may be equally valid. Those with higher psychometric scores may have suffered more severe gastroenteritis, or previous damage to the gut flora may have begun to undermine their health before the attack of gastroenteritis finally precipitated clinical IBS.[31]

Antibiotics and IBS

A prospective study of the role of antibiotics in the aetiology of IBS was performed in women undergoing hysterectomy.[2] Eighty-two patients previously free of gastrointestinal symptoms were randomized to receive either metronidazole or placebo suppositories to prevent postoperative infection, and 36 of these subsequently received further courses of other antibiotics. The women were assessed 3 months later: 7 out of the 62 patients who had received antibiotics developed IBS, while none did so from the 20 who did not receive antibiotics. However, assessment by questionnaires of the symptoms related to IBS in the hysterectomy patients showed that there was a significantly greater increase in symptom score in patients who had received postoperative courses of antibiotics than those receiving placebo or metronidazole prophylaxis ($P<0.04$). Furthermore, stools from the former group of patients showed higher viable counts of aerobes. There was a significant correlation between the 3-month postoperative symptom score and aerobic bacterial count, irrespective of drug treatment (Spearman's $p=0.469$, $P=0.009$).[7]

MODIFICATION OF THE GUT FLORA

As colonic fermentation is abnormal in some cases of food intolerance, it is logical to seek to influence the condition by manipulating the colonic flora. The use of bacterial preparations, such as fermented milks and bio yoghurts, is now widespread, although in most cases these products are promoted as likely to improve health in an ill-defined way, rather than as specific therapies for food intolerance. Nevertheless, the market for these products in Western Europe is growing rapidly.

As we have seen, colonization resistance is an important factor preventing the introduction of new species of bacteria into the faecal flora. Although this phenomenon acts as a valuable defence mechanism against pathogenic bacteria, it also considerably hinders attempts to recolonize the gut with organisms which are intended to be beneficial. Studies in which harmless probiotic bacteria were ingested by healthy volunteers or patients with IBS[10,29] confirm the organisms are cleared within a few days of administration.

Probiotics and IBS

When harmless probiotic bacteria are administered daily, benefits may follow. PR88 is a strain of *Enterococcus faecium* which does not possess markers of pathogenicity, such as haemolysin, hyalouronidase or thermonuclease, and which is sensitive to vancomycin. It has been shown to prevent villous atrophy and malabsorption in piglets after early weaning and it prevents the release of cyclic-AMP after treatment of K-1 cells from the Chinese hamster ovary after administration of *E. coli* heat-labile enterotoxin. When 10^{10} PR88 per day were administered for 12 weeks to 28 patients with the high-volume diarrhoea form of IBS caused by food intolerance, PR88 was identified in the stools of all the subjects in counts of 10^8/g. As PR88 counts rose, there was a corresponding drop in *Streptococcus faecalis* excretion, which reversed when PR88 feeding stopped when the organism was lost from the stools of virtually all subjects within 2 weeks. Symptoms improved in 19 out of 28 subjects and mean faecal weight for the whole group fell from 912 ± 679 g/3 days to 610 ± 400 g/3 days ($P=0.0005$).[29] Unfortunately, to date, no controlled studies of PR88 or of any other probiotic bacterium have been reported and although a number of commercial probiotic preparations are available in health food shops, their clinical value remains unproven.

In view of the difficulty in introducing new species into the bacterial flora, it has been suggested that a more promising approach might be to increase the numbers of those species already resident in the colon which are perceived to be beneficial, such as *Bifidobacter* and *Lactobacilli*. Substances which increase the growth of indigenous bacteria are called prebiotics. An example is fructose oligosaccharide which has been shown to promote the growth of *Bifidobacter* in normal volunteers.[24] To date, no information is available as to whether this approach is beneficial in patients with IBS or other forms of food intolerance.

CONCLUSION

In summary, 50% of IBS patients have symptoms which can be corrected by exclusion of certain foods, many of which contain residues which pass undigested from the small bowel to the caecum. Patients with IBS often develop their symptoms after damage to the gut flora has occurred following gastrointestinal infection or the use of antibiotics and the faecal flora is usually unstable, often with an overgrowth of facultative anaerobes. Fermentation is abnormal, with excessive hydrogen production coinciding with the development of abdominal symptoms. Exclusion diets not only relieve symptoms but also dramatically reduce hydrogen production.

Whether changes in fermentation are also important in the pathogenesis of food intolerance causing other conditions is not known. However, abnormalities in the bacterial flora have been reported in Crohn's disease[13] and the bacterial flora may also be abnormal in rheumatoid arthritis and ankylosing spondylitis. It has been claimed that in these conditions a molecule similar to HLA B27 is synthesized by the faecal flora and associated with the presence of facultative anaerobes – *Klebsiella* – in the stools.[19] See also chapter 55 on Ankylosing spondylitis and diet. Furthermore, inflammation of the gut may be present in a high proportion of patients with spondyloarthropathies.[40] It seems probable that food intolerance caused by abnormal fermentation may play an important part in the pathogenesis of diseases whose clinical manifestations arise far from the gastrointestinal tract.

REFERENCES

1 Alun Jones V, McLaughlan P, Shorthouse M *et al*. Food intolerance: a major factor in the pathogenesis of irritable bowel syndrome. *Lancet* 1982; ii: 1115–17.

2 Alun Jones V, Wilson AJ, Hunter JO, Robinson RE. The aetiological role of antibiotic prophylaxis with hysterectomy in irritable bowel syndrome. *J Obstet Gynaecol* 1984; 5: S22–23.

3 Alun Jones V, Dickinson RJ, Workman E *et al*. Crohn's disease: maintenance of remission by diet. *Lancet* 1985; ii: 177–80.

4 Atherton DJ, Sewell M, Soothill JF *et al*. A double blind crossover trial of an antigen avoidance diet in atopic eczema. *Lancet* 1978; i: 401–3.

5 Balsari A, Ceccarelli A, Dubini F, Fesce E, Poli G. The faecal microbial population in the irritable bowel syndrome. *Microbiologica* 1982; 5: 185–94.

6 Bayliss CE, Houston AP, Alun Jones V, Hishon S, Hunter JO. Microbiological studies on food intolerance. *Proc Nutr Soc* 1984; 43:16A.

7 Bayliss CE, Bradley HK, Alun Jones V, Hunter JO. Some aspects of colonic microbial activity in irritable bowel syndrome associated with food intolerance. *Ann Inst Super Sanita* 1986; 22(N3): 959–64.

8 Bernstein CA, McDermott W. Increased transmissibility of staphylococci to patients receiving an antimicrobial drug. *New Engl J Med* 1960; 262: 637–42.

9 Bond JH, Currier BE, Buchwald H, Levitt MD. Colonic conservation of malabsorbed carbohydrate. *Gastroenterology* 1980; 78: 444–7.

10 Bouhnik Y, Pochart P, Marteau P, Flourie B, Goderel I, Rambaud JC. Survival and kinetics in the human colon of bifidobacterium SP ingested in a fermented dairy product (FDP). *Gastroenterology* 1991; 100(5):A516.

11 Bradley HK, Wyatt GM, Bayliss CE, Hunter JO. Instability in the faecal flora of a patient suffering from food-related irritable bowel syndrome. *J Med Microbiol* 1986; 22: 1–4.

12 Buck AC, Cooke EM. The fate of ingested *Pseudomonas aeruginosa* in normal persons. *J Med Microbiol* 1969; 2: 521–5.

13 Burke DA, Axon ATR. Adhesive *Escherichia coli* in inflammatory bowel disease and infective diarrhoea. *Br Med J* 1988; 297:102–4.

14 Chami TN, Schuster MM, Bohlman ME, Pulliam TJ, Kamal N, Whitehead WE. A simple radiological method to estimate the quantity of bowel gas. *Am J Gastroenterol* 1991; 86: 599–602.

15 Chaudhury NA, Truelove SC. The irritable colon. *Quart J Med* 1962; 31: 307–22.

16 Cooke E, Hettiaratchy ICT, Buck AC. Fate of ingested *Escherichia coli* in normal persons. *J Med Microbiol* 1972; 5: 361–9.

17 Croucher SC, Houston AP, Bayliss CE, Turner RJ. Bacterial populations associated with different regions of the human colon wall. *Appl Env Microbiol* 1983; 45(3): 1025–33.

18 Darlington LG, Ramsey NW, Mansfield JR *et al*. Placebo controlled blind study of dietary manipulation therapy in rheumatoid arthritis. *Lancet* 1986; i: 236–38.

19 Ebringer RW, Cawdwell DR, Cowling P *et al*. Sequential studies in ankylosing spondilitis. Association of *Klebsiella pneumoniae* with active disease. *Ann Rheum Dis* 1978; 37: 145–51.

20 Egger J, Carter CM, Wilson J *et al*. Is migraine food allergy? A double-blind controlled trial of oligoantigenic diet treatment. *Lancet* 1983; ii: 865–69.

21 Egger J, Carter CM, Graham PJ *et al*. Controlled trial of oligoantigenic diet treatment in the hyperkinetic syndrome. *Lancet* 1985; i: 540–5.

22 Farah DA, Calder I, Benson L, Mackenzie JF. Specific food intolerance: its place as a cause of gastrointestinal symptoms. *Gut* 1985; 26: 164–8.

23 Gerrard JW. The diagnosis of the food-allergic patient. In. Pepys J, Edwards AM (eds) *The Mast Cell: Its Role in Health and Disease*. Pitman Medical, Bath; 1979; 416–21.

24 Gibson GR, Beatty EB, Wang X, Cummings JH. Selective stimulation of bifidobacteria in the human colon by oligofructose and inulin. *Gastroenterology* 1995; 108: 975–82.

25 Gwee KA, Graham JC, McKendrick MW *et al*. Psychometric scores and persistence of irritable bowel after infectious diarrhoea. *Lancet* 1996; 347: 150–3.

26 Haderstorfer B, Psycholgin D, Whitehead WE, Schuster MM. Intestinal gas production from bacterial fermentation of undigested carbohydrate in irritable bowel syndrome. *Am J Gastroenterol* 1989; 84: 375–8.

27 Hanington E. Migraine. In. Lessof MH (ed), *Clinical Reactions to Food*. Wiley, Chichester; 1983; 155–80.

28 Hunter JO. Food allergy – or enterometabolic disorder? *Lancet* 1991; 338: 495–96.

29 Hunter JO, Lee AJ, King TS, Barratt MEJ, Linggood MA, Blades JA. *Enterococcus faecium* strain PR88 – an effective probiotic. *Gut* 1996; 38:F246.

30 Hyams JS. Sorbitol intolerance: an unappreciated cause of functional gastrointestinal complaints. *Gastroenterology* 1983; 84: 30–3.

31 King TS, Hunter JO. Anxiety and the irritable bowel syndrome. *Lancet* 1996; 347: 617.

32 King TS, Elia M, Hunter JO. Abnormal colonic fermentation in irritable bowel syndrome. Lancet 1998; 352: 1187–9.

33 Lasser RB, Bond JH, Levitt MD. The role of intestinal gas in functional abdominal pain. *N Engl J Med* 1975; 293: 524–6.

34 Lessof MH, Wraight DG, Merrett TG *et al*. Food allergy and intolerance in 100 patients. *Q J Med* 1980; 195: 259–71.

35 Levitt MD. Studies of a flatulent patient. *New Engl J Med* 1976; 295: 260–2.

36 Levitt MD, Hirsh P, Fetzer CA, Sheahan M, Levine AS. H_2 excretion after ingestion of complex carbohydrates. *Gastroenterology* 1986; 92: 383–9.

37 McKendrick MW, Read NW. Irritable bowel syndrome – post salmonella infection. *J Infection* 1994; 29: 1–3.

38 Metchnikoff E. *The Prolongation of Life*. Heinemann, London, 1907.

39 Middleton SJ, Coley A, Hunter JO: The role of faecal *Candida albicans* in the pathogenesis of food-intolerant irritable bowel syndrome. *Postgrad Med J* 1992; 68: 453–4.

40 Mielants H, Veys E, Cuvelier C *et al*. The evolution of spondyloarthropathies in relation to gut histology. II Histological aspects. *J Rheumatol* 1995; 22: 2273–8.

41 Nanda R, James R, Smith H, Dudley CRK, Jewell DP. Food intolerance and the irritable bowel syndrome. *Gut* 1989; 30: 1099–1104.

42 Parker TJ, Naylor SJ, Riordan AM, Hunter JO. Management of patients with food intolerance in irritable bowel syndrome – the development and use of an exclusion diet. *J Human Nutrition and Dietetics* 1995; 8: 159–66.

43 Rasmussen JJ, Gudmand-Hoyer RT. Functional bowel disease: malabsorption and abdominal distress after ingestion of fructose, sorbitol and fructose sorbitol mixtures. *Gastroenterology* 1988; 95(3): 694–700.

44 Ravich WJ, Bayless TM, Thomas M. Fructose: incomplete intestinal absorption in humans. *Gastroenterology* 1983; 84: 26–9.

45 Scheppach W, Fabian C, Ahrens F, Spengler M, Kasper H. Effect of starch malabsorption on colonic function and metabolism in humans. *Gastroenterology* 1988; 95: 1549–55.

46 Stephen AM. Effect of food on the intestinal microflora. In: Hunter JO, Alun Jones V (eds) *Food and the Gut*. Bailliere Tindall, Eastbourne; 1985; 57–77.

47 Van der Waaij D, Berghuis-de Vries JM, Lekkerkerk-van der Wees JEC. Colonization resistance of the digestive tract in conventional and antibiotic treated mice. *J Hygiene* 1971; 69.405–11.

48 Wan der Waaij D. Colonization resistance of the digestive tract: clinical consequences and implications. *J Antimicrob Chemother* 1982; 10: 263–70.

49 Weinstein L. The spontaneous occurrence of new bacterial infections during the course of treatment with streptomycin or penicillin. *Am J Med Sci* 1947; 214: 56–63.

50 Wyatt GM, Bayliss CE, Lakey AF, Bradley HK, Hunter JO, Alun Jones V. The faecal flora of two patients with food-related irritable bowel syndrome during challenge with symptom-provoking foods. *J Med Microbiol* 1988; 26: 295–9.

Chapter 24

Is there an allergic and fermentative gut condition, and does it relate to *Candida*?

Keith Eaton

BACKGROUND

INTRODUCTION

Medical progress tends to be fitful: a novel diagnosis may appear, gain credibility and support, but then subsequently lose general acceptance and disappear. Subsequently it is reinvented and the cycle may be repeated with variations. When there is sufficient evidence this chain may be broken. The current topic is an example (see Box 24.1). This chapter discusses research done to date. However, there is a long way to go and we are still dealing with many unanswered questions.

At the present time the only cogent justification for a discussion of this topic is that there is a condition characterized by a number of symptoms which improves on a diet low in refined carbohydrate and mould-related foods with or without antifungal therapy. It does not seem to cause death, but its chronicity makes the lives of sufferers a misery and induces a very high and con-

---

Box 24.1 A brief historical note

- In the early 1900s there were descriptions of *germ carbohydrate fermentation*.[62]
- In the 1930s writers such as Sir Arthur Hurst espoused the concept of *intestinal carbohydrate dyspepsia*[32] which by the 1950s was being dismissed as of psychological causation.[5]
- Holti[29] and James and Warin[35] in 1966 and 1971, respectively, linked eczema and urticaria to yeast activity.
- In 1978 Truss described what he considered to be a new entity, and linked it with *Candida albicans*.[59]
- From the 1980s biochemical measurements have been reported.[4]

---

tinuing consumption of health service time. If managed conventionally the patients continue to seek help over a long period of time and form a significant part of those described as 'thick folder' or 'heartsink' patients.

The symptom complex is a ragbag which cannot logically be separated from other conditions on purely clinical grounds except by response to a management programme. Although laboratory tests are being developed they are not yet reliable (see below).

Patients with this condition often have had symptoms for years, and been subject to a number of different treatments without benefit. They become for the first time well when treated with a diet low in fermentable, yeasty and mould-containing foods, with or without antifungal drugs. Both the speed of improvement (within 1 month) and its degree (many stating that they have not felt so fit for many years) are often spectacular and the patients remain well in the long term on the regime (see below). Doctors experience few revolutions during their working lives. For the present author, food intolerance was one such, but this problem, accepted with initial extreme reluctance only as a result of the dramatic success of a colleague's intervention in a most difficult case, has been another of equal importance. Currently, there is little research to back up what we do (although there is some, and it is increasing). Our daily clinical experience reinforces the conviction that this is a highly important part of medical practice for the relief its good management brings to sufferers.

The condition needs a name until its cause is known. When in 1978 Truss formulated his theory he linked the condition with *Candida albicans*: in doing so he appears to consider that both the syndrome and the attribution are new. Table 24.1 however demonstrates the parallels between the work of Hurst and these later authors. In the first edition of this book Kroker used the term *chronic candidiasis sensitivity syndrome*:[39] we cannot justify it. Not only do we lack proof of *Candidal* involvement, we have yet to show that any fungus or yeast is causal, or that a sensitivity is

Old and new treatment protocols	
Hurst (1931)	**Truss and Crook (1978)**

Diet:
  low carbohydrates
  low legumes
	Diet:
	  low carbohydrates
	  low yeasts and moulds

Betaine hydrochloride	Betaine hydrochloride
Pancreatic enzymes	Pancreatic enzymes
Lactobacillus	*Lactobacillus*
Vitamin supplements	Vitamin supplements
	Antifungals

Table 24.1 Old and new treatment protocols.

present. Positive reactions to antifungals do not prove that fungi cause the condition as both nystatin[58] and amphotericin[51] have non-specific gut wall stabilizing properties which may be beneficial to the host independent of any antifungal effects. However Brostoff's term *'that syndrome which responds to diet and the use of antifungal drugs'* is unmanageable. The term *gut fermentation* was introduced in 1990 but almost instantly lost credence as the importance of normal gut fermentation was appreciated, and for a while the term *abnormal gut fermentation* was used. This too had to be discarded as it was realized that the assumption that all patients with the condition had abnormal fermentation was unproven and might not be true (see below). At a workshop in 1994 a further name – *dysfunctional gut syndrome* – was adopted,[19] representing a considerable compromise. This was not widely accepted as it is too much of an umbrella term and could be applied with equal validity to many other gut conditions. In the latest text, this has been replaced with the term *fungal-type dysbiosis*.[4] There is general agreement that gut flora are disturbed, justifying the term dysbiosis and circumstantial evidence of fungal involvement. Until research replaces surmise we hope that this term will serve.

This chapter considers the symptom complex and follows with a review of the published research studies and a section on patient management, worth trying on difficult cases, even if the current state of knowledge leaves questions open.

THE SYMPTOM COMPLEX

Almost all sufferers are polysymptomatic, but they suffer from a miscellany of symptoms and it is not possible to give a list of those which separate patients with fungal-type dysbiosis from those with related conditions. The majority have symptoms of irritable bowel, but not all do. Among those who do, bloating is often more troublesome than change of bowel habit or abdominal discomfort. Mucous membrane catarrhal symptoms are common and may include non-bacterial cystitis (mainly in females), vaginitis, rhinitis and asthma. Sinusitis seems common, as does otitis externa, often clearly fungally related. Anal itch is particularly prevalent.

It is also common to find complaints of musculoskeletal pain: this may be secondary to an accompanying magnesium deficiency.[22] Some patients mainly present with dermatological problems, including eczema and chronic urticaria.

However perhaps the most important symptoms are psychoneurological, predominantly minimal brain dysfunction. Gross fatigue is very frequent. A subset of patients presenting with chronic fatigue syndrome, whether apparently post-viral or not, will respond well to appropriate intervention. Characteristic findings are 'brain fog', where the process of logical thought is difficult, sometimes described as 'trying to think through treacle' and 'brain fag' where concentration is rapidly lost. However, confusion as to the names of common objects is not generally as common a finding as in other causes of chronic fatigue syndrome.

Much emphasis has been laid by previous writers[9,39,59] on a past history of fungal infections, repeated courses of broad-spectrum antibiotics usage and of oral steroids and long courses of the contraceptive pill: the latter has now become so ubiquitous that it is difficult to find women who have never taken it.[27] The range of symptoms which may respond varies from patient to patient and may include those generally associated with classical allergies such as asthma and rhinitis: here, an above average use of steroid drugs is to be expected. (On the other hand, when non-gut symptoms respond there may be residual symptoms which may respond to a food intolerance regime.) As yet, any association with heavy antibiotic usage remains anecdotal, although the clinical experience of clinicians who regularly treat the condition suggests that this is a true bill. However, triggering of what may be parts of the complex by antibiotics has been reported in a prospective double-blind trial by Alun-Jones *et al.*[1] When patients were given metronidazole or placebo in a random trial they found none of 20 who had not been given antibiotics developed postoperative irritable bowel syndrome (IBS). In those who had ($n = 62$: some patients had been given additional antibiotics on an open basis) 7 out of 62 developed IBS. Danna *et al.*[12] examined antibiotic induced diarrhoea in the elderly and found positive cultures of *Candida* spp. in 7 out of 24 who had received antibiotics. None of the matched control group of 24 had positive yeast cultures. Earlier writers[9] laid great stress on a past history of fungal diseases. This has proved difficult to evaluate as no lifetime prevalence studies exist for the general population.[20] A further study[33] found thrush but not athlete's foot to be positively correlated.

However the pattern of food craving in fungal-type dysbiosis differs from that in food intolerance, where any food may be craved – usually mildly. In fungal-type dysbiosis, cravings are severe and are usually for foods with high sugar levels and for refined starches and occasionally yeasts, but not normally to others.[18] Although the patient is aware of their ability to cause illness, the craving is such that they have not been given up.

Experienced physicians know that they see patients with this combination of problems and get good results from appropriate management. The question is whether the syndrome warrants separate status, and whether the cause is organic?

REVIEW OF THE RESEARCH STUDIES

Biochemical studies
The clinical picture cannot prove the existence of an organic syndrome or disprove Berk's[5] statement in 1944 about *intestinal carbohydrate dyspepsia*:

> These are essentially unhappy individuals ... Any suggested panacea and therapeutic straw is grasped. No regime is too severe, and no program too forbidding. With the tenacity of the

faithful they grope their way from one physician to the next in a relentless search for a permanently successful remedy.

The implication here is clear: the condition is of psychological origin.

One of the seminal studies looked at the spontaneous production of ethanol in whole blood after a fasting sugar challenge.[30] This has been developed into a test which is clinically useful, as an aid to diagnosis and as an index to response to treatment. Normal subjects do not produce any detectable ethanol after this challenge: however, a margin is allowed and tests are currently regarded as positive if ethanol exceeds 22 µmol/l. Patients who were symptomatic and later responded to diet with or without antifungals had positive tests which became negative after the symptoms were relieved.[17]

The symptoms of the condition are not characteristic of the effects of alcohol and the levels detected are much too low (2–3 mg/dl of whole blood) to cause the symptoms directly: in most countries people are considered to be safe to drive at levels 10 times higher than this. The production of alcohol must therefore be regarded as a marker: it is assumed, but not yet proven, that it is produced by the microflora of the gut.

The syndrome is distinct from a condition described in Japan and called *mitei-sho* ('drunk disease'). In this condition, endogenous alcohol production leads to very high alcohol levels and the patients are clinically extremely drunk. In one instance the cause was attributed to a severe gut infection with *C. albicans*.[34] It should be noted that cure on antifungals alone took only a few days.

In fungal-type dysbiosis, blood sampling for ethanol is taken at 1 hour after a sugar challenge (see Box 24.2) and the presence of alcohol in such early samples points to its origin in the upper gut, most likely in the jejunum.

Other products of fermentation must be considered. When testing was first introduced, the laboratory technique involved a modification of a standard commercial enzyme kit (Sigma-Aldrich Co. Ltd., Poole, Dorset). Subsequently, gas–liquid chromatography has replaced this, a technique which enables the profile to be extended to produce levels for a range of higher alcohols and short-chain fatty acids (SCFAs), known to be involved in bacterial fermentation.[43] As a result, it has now become clear that in newly diagnosed untreated patients with fungal-type dysbiosis the abnormality is chiefly of excess ethanol, with no or minimal changes in higher alcohols or SCFAs. In some patients, excesses of higher alcohols and/or raised or lowered SCFAs may be found in the absence of ethanol. Clinically, this group cannot be recognized prior to testing. Patients who have been previously and unsuccessfully treated often show increases in both elements, in our experience (Table 24.2). As ethanol suggests a yeast and the others bacterial fermentation, the process may be more complex than a single organism.

Not all patients with the syndrome produce alcohol. In some, this may be because they have achieved a partial therapeutic response by using a diet.[20] Others show excess urinary β-alanine, but not ethanol, after glucose challenge. β-Alanine is an amino acid which is an excretion product that results from normal colonic bacterial fermentation (Fig. 24.1).[21] Some *Candida* spp. generate ethanol but others methyl, amyl and iso-amyl alcohols[40,44,54] and Truss[60] suggested that the main fermentation product might be acetaldehyde.

Box 24.2 Laboratory technique for gut fermentation profile

Challenge procedure. Patients abstain from alcoholic beverages for 24 hours pre-test and from all food and drink (mineral water excepted) for 3 hours. They then swallow 2 g of dextrose in enteric gelatine capsules, washed down with 50 g of dextrose in approximately 100 ml of water. Blood is then drawn for analysis 60 min later. No pre-test sample is now taken: in earlier work these were all negative.

Alcohol estimations. Aliquots of plasma (250 µl) are measured into 5 ml glass vials containing 300 ml sodium chloride. Most of the air is expelled with argon using a 20 ml syringe filled from a cylinder. The vials are sealed with a rubber septum and an aluminium seal, and held at 60°C in a water bath for 30 min. Gas samples are removed from the headspace using a prewarmed gas-tight syringe and injected into the gas chromatograph. Alcohols are measured using the following analytical method: Capillary column 10 m × 0.32 mm fixed silica Poroplot Q (10 µm) (Perkin-Elmer cat. no. 0497-8376). Carrier gas is hydrogen at 5 psi. The initial column temperature is 120°C, increasing by 10°C/min to 200°C.

The flame ionization detector is adjusted for maximum sensitivity and then the hydrogen flow rate is slightly increased. This gives the highest precision.

The full range of alcohols, including ethanol and methanol, can be measured using the capillary column.

Short-chain fatty acids. These are measured in a separate chromatography technique. It is a modification of the classical alkaline transesterification procedure of Christopherson and Glass[8] and is essentially that given by Christie.[7] Plasma aliquots of 50 µl are used and formic acid is used in place of the acetic acid in the reaction mixture.

Recovery of alcohols prior to the headspace procedure averaged 93%, ranging from 97±2% for ethyl alcohol to 86±3% for butanol. The detector sensitivity was determined for each individual alcohol and a linear response was found up to 350 µmol/l. Only ethyl alcohol has been found above that level and such samples are diluted and reanalysed.

In the case of ethanol, sensitivity was met such that 1.9 µmol/l gave at least twice the noise width of the glass column. Pre-sensitivity was better than 0.3 µmol/l for the capillary column. The recovery of added short-chain fatty acids (SCFAs) was 94±5% and the linearity exceeded 500 µmol/l. The detector sensitivity is determined for each analyte.

Standardization of both gas chromatography proceedures is by standard addition. Day-to-day precision is checked using aliquots of a pooled sample. The pre-measured aliquots are stored at –20°C.

Measurement by enzyme technique. The enzyme technique uses a standard kit from Sigma Diagnostics (Poole, Dorset) who are able to supply full instructions. The sensitivity is increased by increasing the dilution of the specimen.

Other studies which have been performed have shown significant micronutrient changes in these patients. Measurement of B vitamin status (by functional analysis), zinc and magnesium (by sweat mineral profiles assessed by flame atomic absorption or

Raised levels of higher alcohols	
Ethanol	**Number of raised bacterial ferments**
4	10
8	8
12	13
14	11
14	8
14	10
20	7
12	9

Table 24.2 Raised levels of higher alcohols.

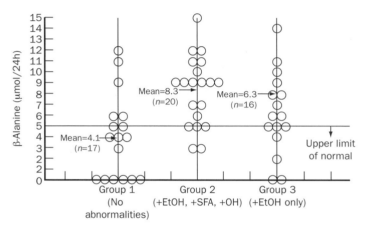

Fig 24.1 Ethanol and β-alanine production.

plasma emission spectrophotometry) reveals widespread deficiencies (Table 24.3). In one study[22] all subjects had had deficits of at least two of the nutrients examined; most had multiple abnormalities. Galland has also reported vitamin and mineral deficiencies.[26] Of the B vitamins, B_6 was the commonest deficiency in both studies. Magnesium status (by red cell magnesium) was low in 50% of patients. Analysis of the diets of some of our patients indicates that this is not due to poor diet. Possible other causes are excessive metabolic need (for which we have no biochemical evidence) or an absorptive failure, which is supported by a study revealing increased gut permeability[23] (Fig. 24.2), the 'leaky gut', in which there is an increased absorption of macromolecules, because of incompetence of the tight junctions, which may be made worse if other aspects of digestion are working poorly. Thus, for example, if proteins are not broken down into amino acids or peptides, they may be able to enter the body intact and might, by competitive inhibition, diminish the absorption of micronutrients.

Deficiency of essential fatty acids was identified in the study by Galland,[26] both from clinical and laboratory findings. Clinical signs (two or more of dry hair, dry scaly skin, brittle nails and follicular dermatitis) were found in 66% of patients. On laboratory assay by functional analysis, no patient had a normal profile: Ω-6 series were worse affected than Ω-3, as one might expect if part of the failure is metabolic. Dietary linoleic acid is metabolized to γ-linolenic acid by the enzyme delta-6-desaturase, which is itself dependent on adequate levels of zinc, magnesium and B vitamins: failure of this system has immunological consequences.

Aspects of amino acid metabolism in this condition have been considered in a number of studies. Truss in 1983 examined urinary excretion patterns for 25 amino acids in a group of 24 patients.[60] The measurements were performed using a Beckman amino acid

Table 24.3 Vitamin and mineral study.

Vitamin and mineral study				
	Group A (normal values for adults not able to produce alcohol)		**Group B (abnormal values for adults able to produce alcohol)**	
Parameter	***n***	**Mean (SD)**	***n***	**Mean (SD)**
Age	50	35 (7.20)	30	39.8 (9.50)
Blood B_1 (%)	50	9.14 (3.82)*	30	18.4 (5.80)*
Blood B_2 (%)	50	8.66 (3.93)*	30	14.23 (4.08)*
Blood B_6 (%)	50	8.32 (3.66)*	30	22.07 (7.53)*
Sweat Mg (mmol/l)	50	0.23 (0.03)*	30	0.19 (0.03)*
Sweat Zn [M] (μmol/l)	25	7.37 (1.37)*	6	4.96 (1.06)*
Sweat Zn [F] (μmol/l)	25	8.52 (2.64)*	24	5.35 (0.80)*
Sweat Zn [M+F] (μmol/l)	50	8.02 (2.18)*	30	5.28 (0.85)*
Blood EtOH (μmol/l)	50	8.4 (4.9)*	30	640 (181)*

*Wilcoxon and *t*-test, P<0.001.

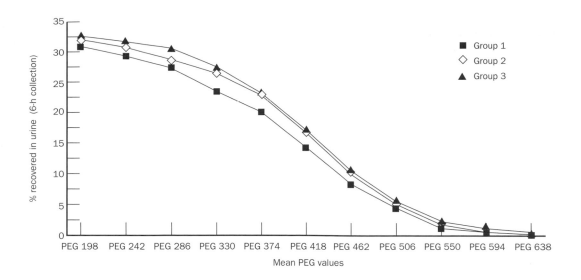

Fig 24.2 Gut permeability study.

	PEG198	PEG242	PEG286	PEG330	PEG374	PEG418	PEG462	PEG506	PEG550	PEG594	PEG638	TOTAL
r	0.3487	0.4611	0.3834	0.5162	0.4626	0.4033	0.3077	0.1437	0.0355	0.0175	0.0117	
p	<0.001	<0.001	<0.001	<0.001	<0.001	<0.001	0.001	0.138	0.715	0.858	0.904	
Group 1 mean (SD)	30.9 (2.1)	29.3 (1.7)	27.4 (1.3)	23.5 (1.3)	20.1 (1.2)	14.3 (1.1)	8.6 (1.3)	4.8 (0.7)	1.6 (0.4)	0.7 (0.4)	0.3 (0.2)	
Group 2 mean (SD)	31.7 (2.2)	30.8 (2.9)	28.5 (5.2)	26.4 (4.2)	22.9 (4.1)	16.7 (4.4)	10.6 (4.1)	5.8 (3.2)	2.4 (2.7)	1.3 (2.1)	0.6 (1.6)	13.5 (3.3)
Group 3 mean (SD)	32.6 (0.8)	31.7(1.4)	30.4 (1.8)	27.3 (2.9)	23.3 (2.6)	17.3 (3.2)	10.5 (2.4)	15.4 (1.0)	1.6 (0.5)	0.7 (0.4)	0.3 (0.3)	13..6 (1.8)

Group 1, normals (n=50);

Group 2, GFP-negative and FI (n=29)

Group 3, GFP-negative FI (n=29).

r, Pearson's correlation between the group numbers and the PEG recovered in urine.

analyser: laboratory normals were said to have been established for the 25 reported, although not for the remaining 16. However no details are given in this study as to how the laboratory (Bio-Science Laboratories, Los Angeles, California), arrived at their normal ranges. The original data are reported in an unusual order, which is presumably the sequence in which they come off the analyser. Here they have been redrawn to the usual convention. Truss analysed his data to show percentages of individual amino acids which were abnormal and this is the form reproduced here as Table 24.4. We have examined a parallel group from our patients, whose records were stored on computer (Biolab Medical Unit, London). Records for 28 patients, all with symptoms, positive ethanol tests, and having had urinary amino acid excretion patterns measured by high-performance liquid chromatography before the start of treatment. We measured 39 amino acids, shown in a similar summary to the same format as the Truss data as Table 24.5. There are of course differences between the US and UK figures: the patient selection may be different and the laboratory procedures certainly are. In view of these factors, it seems more appropriate to draw readers' attention to the many similarities.

β-Alanine which is normally regarded as a marker of normal colonic bacterial fermentation,[21] was frequently elevated in fungal-type dysbiosis – in some patients without excess ethanol it was the only marker – but raised urinary levels are also seen in patients who do produce ethanol: this is a useful diagnostic laboratory marker. Some recent findings suggest an explanation for these results.

Bacterial fermentation is known to result in excess hydrogen production, which is excreted in the breath.[56] However, the conventional opinion is that yeast fermentation does not generate hydrogen.[37] When ethanol production in newly diagnosed patients was compared with lactulose breath hydrogen estimations[25] the expectation was that those with fungal-type dysbiosis would generate ethanol (used as the diagnostic criterion for inclusion) but not hydrogen, whereas the bacterial dysbiosis group would. In the event, the only way the two groups could be distinguished was by ethanol production: there were no statistical differences between the two groups on hydrogen production. There are several possible explanations. Sampling for ethanol was at 60 min and for hydrogen at 90 min, so the results may not relate to the same segment of the gut. Yeasts may produce hydrogen, although this has not been reported. Lastly, fungal-type dysbiosis may involve bacterial elements as well as, or instead of, yeasts. Some moulds in the International Mycological Institute Culture Collection require the presence of 'contaminating' bacteria for their healthy growth.[37] If bacterial dysbiosis contributes to the condition, this would explain the increased β-alanine production.

Microbiological studies

Microbiological studies have not proved useful in diagnosis. *Meitei-sho* ('drunk disease') (see earlier) has the characteristics of a fungal infection and is distinct from fungal-type dysbiosis.

Endeavours have been made to detect *Candida* in fungal-type dysbiosis. Holti[29] studied 57 patients with IBS where stool yeast

D

Amino acid analysis (from Truss 1983)			
	High (%)	Low (%)	Normal (%)
Essential			
Threonine	0	75	25
Valine	0	50	50
Methionine	0	70.8	29.2
Leucine	0	54.2	45.8
Isoleucine	0	79.2	20.8
Phenylalanine	12.5	33.3	54.2
Lysine	4.2	33.3	62.5
Protein			
Histidine	0	16.7	83.3
Aspartic acid	4.2	0	95.8
Serine	4.2	45.8	50
Glutamic acid	0	95.8	4.2
Glutamine	0	62.5	37.5
Glycine	4.2	0	95.8
Alanine	4.2	4.2	91.7
Asparagine	0	100	0
Cystine	16.7	0	83.3
Tyrosine	0	50	50
Metabolic			
D-amino-adipic acid	0	91.7	8.3
Phosphoethanolamine	0	70.8	29.2
Methyl histidine	4.2	75	20.8
3-Methyl histidine	16.7	0	83.3
Taurine	0	12.5	87.5
α-Amino-*n*-butyric acid	0	37.5	62.5
Ethanolamine	41.7	4.2	54.2
Cystathionine	0	91.7	8.3

Table 24.4 Amino acid analysis (from Truss 1983).

Amino acid analysis: Biolab figures			
	High (%)	Low (%)	Normal (%)
Essential			
Threonine	18	0	82
Valine	0	0	100
Methionine	0	4	96
Leucine	4	0	96
Isoleucine	11	4	85
Phenylalanine	0	0	100
Lysine	0	4	96
Tryptophan	0	0	100
Protein			
Arginine	0	0	100
Histidine	4	11	85
Aspartic acid	0	0	100
Serine	0	11	89
Glutamic acid	4	0	96
Glutamine	21	0	79
Glycine	0	0	100
Alanine	7	0	93
Asparagine	0	21	79
Cystine	0	4	96
Tyrosine	11	0	89
Proline	0	0	100
Metabolic			
Phosphoethanolamine	54	0	46
α-Amino adipic acid	0	0	100
Homocysteine	0	0	100
Phosphoethanolamine	4	0	96
Methyl histidine	0	4	96
Citrulline	0	0	100
Carnosine	4	0	96
3-methyl histidine	39	0	61
β-Alanine	50	0	50
Taurine	0	4	96
β-Amino isobutyric acid	4	0	96
γ-Amino butyric acid	11	0	89
α-Amino butyric acid	0	0	100
Ethanolamine	11	0	89
Cystathionine	11	0	89
Hydroxylysine	0	0	100
Ornithine	0	0	100
Hydroxyproline	0	0	100
Methionine sulphoxide	7	0	93

Table 24.5 Amino acid analysis: Biolab figures.

cultures were positive. Nystatin was curative in 17 (30%), and partially so in 31 (54%), but 23 (40%) also required a yeast-free diet to produce cure. If it were a simple infection, diet would surely be unnecessary. Over the past 17 years repeated attempts have been made to justify a diagnosis of fungal-type dysbiosis by stool culture for *Candida*. In 1987 Kroker[39] concluded that this is not helpful in distinguishing patients with the syndrome from normal controls. Hauss[28] who sets some store by the technique, combined with culture from tongue smears, admits that 'a semi-quantative analysis does not seem to provide a useful answer.' Middleton *et al.*[48] performed faecal cultures in a group of 38 patients with food-intolerant IBS, as compared with 20 healthy controls. Some of these subjects could well have had a missed diagnosis of fungal-type dysbiosis. However they only achieved positives in 3, and in each instance the patient had either had recent broad-spectrum antibiotics or the stool sample had been delayed for more than 24 hours in transit.

Allergic and immunological studies

Intradermal skin testing with fungal allergens has been used in attempts to establish the cause of the syndrome. In most instances, allergists failed to observe the tests for delayed hyper-sensitivity;[16] which is curious since DHS reactions to *Candida* antigens have been used as a routine method of assessing immuno-logical competence because of the high incidence of sensitization in communities such as the UK. Purified *Candida* allergens are less effective at provoking DHS reactions.[3] It is clear that fungal-type dysbiosis is not a type 1 hypersensitivity response to C. *albicans*. As Kroker concluded, such skin tests do not distinguish patients from normal controls.[39,61] Because of mucosal exposure, the generation of candidal antibodies is a normal phenomenon:[41] the antibodies can be IgA, IgG, IgM and IgE classes, but in recur-rent vaginal candidiasis it is mainly secretory IgA.[46] Consequently, it remains possible that targeted specific antibody profiles might at some stage be shown to be relevant. As yet, however, their role is not established, and indeed the involvement of *Candida* is still unsubstantiated.

Holti[29] performed skin prick tests to C. *albicans* and to brewers' and bakers' yeast in chronic urticaria. Only immediate reactions were considered but, out of 255 patients, 49 (19%) responded to *Candida* and 27 (11%) to yeasts: this means that at least 70% responded to neither. James and Warin[35] found 36% of patients positive to *Candida* on prick testing: again 64% were not. They found that they could clear only 3 out of 36 patients with nystatin alone; 23 required a yeast-free diet as well. It should be remembered that inactivation of living yeast cells in the gut is effected by gastric acid: if this low, as it may be in fungal-type dysbiosis, then these organisms will pass down the gut in a viable form. Both of these trials therefore suggest a potential role for *Saccharomyces cerevisiae* (bakers' yeast) in the condition.

Urinary histidine excretion has been compared in patients with fungal-type dysbiosis, classical allergies and food intolerance.[24] All showed significant decreases from normal, but not from each other. Histidine is the precursor of histamine. Subsequent metabolites are not bioavailable; hence, allergics lose histamine and need more histidine, which is not available from blood (homeostasis) or muscle (not bioavailable). The increased requirements are mainly met by increasing renal reabsorption. That low levels of histidine excretion, expected in classical allergy, are also seen in fungal-type dysbiosis suggests allergy is involved.

THE DIAGNOSIS AND MANAGEMENT OF THE CLINICAL CONDITION

There is currently no way in which a reliable diagnosis can be made in all patients. The symptoms revealed by the history are often non-specific. Cases will only be detected if the possibility is regularly borne in mind, especially when dealing with patients with a multiplicity of symptoms. Patients who combine IBS, especially when bloating is the main complaint, with anal itch, brain 'fog' and 'fag' and who admit to marked sugar, starch and perhaps yeast craving are often dysbiotic. A most useful pointer is the complaint that a very modest alcohol intake leaves the patient feeling acutely drunk, so that alcohol has been given up. It is also important to consider this diagnosis when assessing progress in patients where other diagnoses have been made initially, but improvement on treatment has been disappointing. It can be a factor even in patients who appear to suffer from a simple allergic rhinitis with no apparent complicating factors and should always feature in the differential diagnosis of causes of chronic urticaria.

A positive ethanol gut fermentation test confirms the diagnosis although it is not ruled out by a negative test. Although the procedure for this test has been published on a number of occasions[18,22,54] and reproduced in other laboratories in the UK, Norway and the United States, it is currently only available from one laboratory (Biolab Medical Unit, London); it is carried out at other sites, the sample being sent by post. With easy access to this test, we prefer to test the majority of referrals and believe that to do so is a cost-effective policy. However, most doctors have to rely on a trial of the response to therapy,[34] which should include the diet, with or without antifungals. A single study examined the

effect of nystatin therapy on its own and failed to find positive results.[14] Although this trial has methodological flaws, which were criticized at the time in an editorial which accompanied it,[2] we are not aware of any evidence that antifungals alone are effective and the conclusion may well be true.

A possible diagnostic feature may be the existence of mould allergies in these patients. Currently, we do not know how common this is, nor whether we are considering a concurrent but unconnected diagnosis or one which is an intrinsic part of the condition: defining this might illuminate the aetiology. In the meantime, many experienced physicians have noted in the course of clinical work that both fungal-type dysbiosis and mould allergies may coexist and, possibly more significantly, treatment for the fungal-type dysbiosis can also reduce the severity of the mould problem without any other specific therapeutic measures.

TREATMENT

Diet

As a treatment, diet tends to be underrated by doctors, possibly as they conventionally have not been trained in nutrition and often have an irrational fear that it may cause malnutrition. The result is that where there is a choice between a purely dietary and a medication-based system, physicians generally prefer the latter.

Treatment diets for fungal-type dysbiosis started from the premise that the way the condition behaves suggests that a fungal or yeast factor is involved. Such organisms ferment simple sugars to produce ethanol.[55] Many brewing processes use complex starches as their substrates: beer and malt whisky use barley; maize is used for bourbon; rice is the basis of sake.[45] Thus, for our predecessors, limiting these foods in any dietary regime appeared logical. They also limited the consumption of foods which contained yeasts and moulds, arguing that such foods would have similar metabolic processes to the C. *albicans* yeast (thought to be the putative cause) and that any metabolite of yeast or fungal metabolism might supply nutritional support to the growth of the *Candida*. The diets were therefore based on theory: almost 20 years on, the dietary prescription needs to be re-examined to ensure that any restrictions we impose are justified. A number of questions must be answered:

1. How well do the diets work at controlling the problem?
2. Are the diets we use elimination diets by proxy?
3. Can each of the restrictions be justified?
4. Are they safe and nutritionally balanced?
5. Are some foods actively beneficial in this condition?
6. What research supports the procedures?

The original diets varied, some being more restrictive than others. We now have more information about some of these food elements and can, in part, assess their validity. First, strict carbohydrate restriction would also involve all fruits, some vegetables and all milks. Even if all known sources of free sugars were eliminated from the diet, they would be synthesized in the body from soluble vegetable fibre via SCFAs and gluconeogenesis.[11] It is therefore impossible, even if using a specially formulated elemental diet, to prepare a regime which is entirely sugar-free. Equally, starches (polysaccharides) are made up of sugars, which are released on digestion. It is not desirable on general nutritional terms to remove all polysaccharide foods, as this would involve removing all legumes for example. Interestingly, the diets used in the 1930s by Hurst did restrict the legumes.[32] Further, complete removal of milk and, for example, wheat, which are extremely common food allergens, turns the diet into an elimination diet as well, which would give false positive responses in many patients with food intolerance. Removing sugars also gives false positives in some patients with food intolerance.

The regimes developed by the early pioneers such as Crook[9] also addressed the questions of yeasts and moulds. Since then, there has been more experience and the practical effects of different interventions. In the UK, the Allergy Dieticians Group has undertaken a scrutiny of both the inclusions and exclusions of the diet, with a view to providing a sound baseline, looking at the role of starches as opposed to sugars and whether some traditionally excluded foods are produced by fermentation (spirit vinegars are not) and, whether other ferments actually cause problems.

Sugars seem to have an adverse effect on all these patients, but there are reports that the other foods which provoke symptoms differ between individuals.[20,33] Sugars are widespread in the diet (see above), but the complaints relate to free sugars, sweets and the like. Leavened bread, alcoholic drinks, yeast extract and mould-containing cheeses were used to challenge recovered patients in one study:[20] each of the food groups caused relapses and all but one of the patients relapsed on challenge with one or more of the foods. This may justify their removal from the initial treatment diet. Using larger numbers, but a different questionnaire approach. Hyland and Sodergren[33] found that patients tend to fall into one of two groups, according to the pattern of foods provoking symptoms, giving two separate clusters of health complaint.

In one of the groupings, sugar and sweets, chocolate and canned drinks were associated with adverse effects and blue cheese, green vegetables, yogurt, peas, beans and lentils were beneficial. In the other grouping, sugar, tea and raw mushrooms were adverse and canned drinks, beer, oranges and bread were not. Sugar caused symptoms in both groups of patients and this would include sweets and chocolate. The finding about beer conflicts with dietary practice and two new foods emerge: tea and raw mushrooms. Tea may be divided into green and black tea. Green tea involves plucking, rapid heat inactivation of enzymes (by steam or dry heat), rolling and a final air drying at high temperature. This is unlikely to allow significant mould contamination. However, black tea, which is the form largely consumed in the Western world, involves plucking, withering, maceration and drying, and is likely to engender mould growth – possibly *Aspergillus niger*.[36] It is not clear whether patients do in fact find differences in symptom generation between these two beverages, especially as the antioxidant properties of green tea might conceivably be beneficial[36] and tea should be excluded at least initially. Hyland and Sodergren's data on mushrooms may be new. Only raw mushrooms were considered. Are cooked mushrooms different? At present, both are excluded, which should continue, but the possibility that cooking renders them safe should be explored.

A proposed initial diet is shown as Box 24.3. Experimentally based comments on this would be welcome. For children, where many will wish to show greater liberality, Table 24.6, modified from Tettenborn is reproduced. The Allergy Dieticians Group considers diets on these principles to be nutritionally safe, at least for initial use, in those who have previously been adequately nourished, and when employed with an appropriate supplement programme (see below).

Most would agree management should start with the diet, with or without antifungal drugs. Shortly after starting, many patients will show an increase in the severity of symptoms. This only seems to happen in patients for whom the intervention has been relevant. The process has been termed 'die back' and attributed to a Herxheimer reaction to yeast cells, killed by the intervention,[9] but this cannot be justified: the non-pejorative term 'temporary worsening' is more appropriate. Clear-cut benefit can usually be assessed 1 month after the start of treatment. If effective, the initial diet should be continued for 3–6 months, although some may be allowed a more liberal diet. Some practitioners bring in yeast and mushrooms after the first month. If wheat, all milk products and all fruit are also avoided, the diet amounts to an elimination diet and false positive responses from patients with food intolerance are likely and the diet may not be safe for moderate long-term use. In that case, after 1 month some of the foods could be restored one after another to improve the nutritional qualities of the regime. If symptoms are provoked, this may point to food intolerance; repeated challenges might be needed.

Fungal-type dysbiosis diet for children (modified from Tettenborn)	
Avoid	**Allow**
All sugars, including glucose (dextrose), sucrose, honey, syrup, treacle and maple syrup, and foods containing them.	Unlimited vegetables, salads, meat, fish, milk and yoghurt.
Yeast extracts – Marmite, Oxo, stock-cubes etc., fermented products including vinegar (except 'spirit vinegar'), pickles, ketchups, soy sauces and mouldy cheeses.	Fresh fruit, up to twice a day (but not too many grapes or other really sweet fruits) and *small* amounts of sorbitol, isomaltose or artificial sweetener.
Any other foods that you already think cause problems.	Bread in moderate amounts: no more than two slices a day.
	Hard cheese in small amounts.

Table 24.6 Fungal-type dysbiosis diet for children (modified from Tettenborn). The aim is to avoid the foods that are very sweet and easily fermented, and also to avoid yeasty foods because they are such a common cause of symptoms in people who have problems with yeasts in their intestines. Foods that you already know upset the child should also be avoided. If you have been using sweets as treats, it is important to give instead some other small treat such as a toy or a comic so that the child does not feel punished.

Box 24.3 Basic diet for fungal-type dysbiosis

This diet is suitable only for patients with this problem. It does not help those with bacterial dysbiosis. It is also not intended as an elimination diet, used for the diagnosis of food intolerance. As far as possible it cuts out three classes of foods:

- Refined carbohydrates, especially sugar
- Foods containing yeasts
- Foods containing moulds.

None of these are removed absolutely: that is not practicable. You have to do the best you can. Vegetarians may have problems because most vegetable protein foods also include starch. The problem is eased if you are prepared to eat fish. If not ask for guidance.

Freely allowed
All vegetables (leaves, stalks and roots). Fresh herbs. You should increase the amounts of these to compensate for what you reduce. All 'fruits' classed as vegetables (tomatoes, peppers, cucumber, etc.). Onion, garlic, fresh herbs and turnip may help to control fermentation.

All fresh meats, fish and shellfish and *naturally* smoked fish. Green bacon, but not ham. Eggs.

All milks, other than sweetened condensed. Yogurts, especially well made bio-yogurts, are helpful.

Not allowed
Refined carbohydrates: sugar, fructose, glucose, maple syrup and honey and any made up food that has them in it. Dried fruits (e.g. raisins) may be 80% sugar.

Yeasts. Apart from Marmite we don't generally eat yeast on its own. It is in bread (but not proper soda bread), yeast pastries, pizza and natural vinegars (white spirit vinegar is purely chem-

ical). All alcoholic drinks involve a yeast fermentation and must be omitted. Cheaper vitamin supplements may contain yeast. Selenium supplements are often yeast based. Selenomethione isn't. Soy sauce is a different ferment and we don't yet know. Miss out at first.

Moulds. All cheese contains moulds: blue, brie and very mature hard cheeses have the most. Left-overs grow moulds, less in a freezer than a fridge. Edible fungi (mushrooms) are moulds. They may not be a problem cooked. Omit altogether at first.

Eat with caution
All fruit contains sugar. Maximum two pieces/day. Some patients may be better without any at first. If so, further increase vegetable intake. Fruit juice lacks the fibre in whole fruit and is relatively sweeter. Not too much and not too often.

Grains can be relatively easily fermented. We have no proof of problems with white wheat flour, but prefer wholemeal. We also believe that these are best in moderation. Watch for malt (higher sugar content) and yeast in biscuits and crispbread. Ryvita (some varieties), some oatcakes and rice cakes are safe. Always check the label.

Pulses, nuts and seeds can easily get mouldy. Always buy from an outlet with a rapid turnover. It is probably better not to have too much.

Tea as black tea, the usual kind, involves fermentation. Green tea doesn't. In practice 2–3 cups a day don't seem to be a problem. Coffee is allowed.

The artificial sweeteners, saccharine and aspartame, are not banned, but it is better to get used by degrees to the natural tastes of foods. Sorbitol is in a different category: it may increase levels of prebiotics in the large bowel which may be helpful. However excess will give you diarrhoea.

If adequate control of symptoms has been achieved the diet may be reviewed after 3 months' treatment. Those who enter the consulting room in sparkling good health are probably ready to start a broader diet, but still restricting the amounts of sugars, yeasts and moulds consumed. In older, or previously sicker patients, or those who have been untreated for longer, reassurance, support and encouragement are often the appropriate medical response at this point and the programme is continued for a further 3 months, reintroducing omitted foods – reintroduced preferably one after the other (see Table 24.7). In patients who are well, the supplement programme may be progressively reduced to a single regular daily supplement of a good yeast-free vitamin/mineral complex. Many can then assume responsibility for their own affairs and will no longer need regular medical support. However, not all do as well, and further action may be needed when there is only a partial response.

Drug treatment
There are two schools of thought about the use of antifungal drugs. Some believe that the initial therapy should be as minimal as possible: others, that recovery is quicker and that there are less long-term failures where drugs are used *ab initio* in addition to the diet. As yet, no firm conclusions may be drawn as to which view

is right. However, in one study, 84% of patients were rendered asymptomatic by diet alone:[20] if drug and diet are started simultaneously, it will not be clear whether an equally good response would have been seen by diet alone. While the drugs of choice are normally antifungals, in an early study it was noted that 5% of those with positive ethanol tests lost both symptoms and alcohol positivity when given broad-spectrum antibiotics.[17] This was apparently an antibiotic-responsive subgroup, since these normally worsen the complaint.

How do antifungals work? The fact that clinical benefit can result from both systemic and non-systemic antifungals does not prove that a fungal infection is the cause. The beneficial response could be the result of some property of the drug which is separate from its function as a polyene antibiotic. It is known that both nystatin and amphotericin can act as gut cell wall stabilizers[51,58] and clinical benefit may result from this property. The systemic conazoles are known to inhibit the cytochrome-mediated fungal enzyme lanosterol C-14 demethylase, which deprives the fungal cell wall of ergosterol, an essential constituent.[38] Ergosterol is unique to fungi, and manufacturers claim that it is highly unlikely that these agents will be active against bacteria. On the other hand, activity against *Blastocystis hominis* has been reported for ketoconazole both *in vitro* and *in vivo*.[10,15] Other actions, not

Table 24.7 Reintroduction diet.

Reintroduction diet

This step follows gaining acceptable recovery after a treatment regime. This will always involve a diet and a nutritional programme. For some patients, antifungal drugs will also be needed. In this group we need to get you off the antifungal before changing the diet. However, once this has been done, or if you are not on antifungals now, we can, if you are well, try to broaden the diet. Please note that while we are doing this any nutritional supplement programme should not be changed.

Step 1 Starches. If you have not already done so, try to increase modestly and by degrees your total starch intake.

Step 2 Cheese. The production of all cheeses involves yeasts but some are more of a problem than others. First, try cottage cheese (for 1 week). If no problems, try cream cheese. If this too is trouble free for 1 week, try mild hard cheeses like Edam or mild cheddar. The stronger flavoured ones like mature cheddar are possible for some: the final group if you wish are Brie/Camembert and the blue cheeses like Stilton. Note that in this group some can take one but not the other. There is no rule about it.

Step 3 Yeast. This includes:
(a) *yeast extract (Marmite)*: If this is clear, use foods which contain small amounts like gravy browning and packet soups and many other prepared foods. However, you might get away with the latter, but not Marmite itself. Try, if you wish.
(b) *alcoholic beverages*. For most, a small intake of wine (for most patients, white seems better). Some find that vodka seems safest. Try also.
(c) *genuinely fermented vinegars* like a malt or wine vinegar. Spirit vinegars are chemical products and are not fermented. Try.
(d) *ordinary leavened bread*. Most find at this stage that this is safe for use at about 1–2 slices/day once or twice / week. Note that not all these yeasts are the same. You may be able to take one but not another.

Step 4 Mushrooms. These are of course, fungi and thus theoretically must be a problem. However, this may in practice only occur for a subgroup. Try them first cooked, and then if you wish raw.

Step 5 Sugar. What we are concerned with here are the foods which contain lots of free (and therefore instantly fermentable) sugars. This includes sugar, glucose, fructose and honey. From the nutritional viewpoint no one actually needs these and over the months you may have grown used to not having them. If, however, you can take all the above you may wish to see if you can include some sugar in your diet (perhaps for occasional use) without major difficulties. If so, now is the time to do it. Try CAUTIOUSLY.

---

specifically antifungal, have not been reported, but this may be because they have not been looked for. Nevertheless, the fact that both the systemic and non-systemic drugs are marketed to combat fungal infections does suggest a fungal/yeast involvement of some sort.

The choice of antifungal drugs is between those which are not significantly absorbed from the gut and those with systemic activity. Since antifungal therapy may be required for some months, there is an advantage in using drugs which are not absorbed for maintenance, although some physicians initiate therapy with one of the conazoles, which are absorbed. Nystatin is not absorbed to any significant extent, and amphotericin B is very poorly absorbed from the gut and thus, in practice, may be considered non-systemic.[42] Other non-systemic compounds, such as natamycin could be considered theoretically: in practice, so far they have not. Commercially available preparations of nystatin include an oral suspension of low dosage and intended for children and sugar-coated tablets which are generally avoided because of the coating. If nystatin is used, topical preparations for dermatological use and vaginal pessaries will be needed in addition when fungal reactions outside the gut are noted, as oral dosage will not reach these sites. The usual form in which nystatin is used is as the pure BP powder, available in the UK from Becpharm Ltd. (Harlow, Essex) or Bristol-Myers Squibb (Hounslow, Middlesex). This is dispensed in 25 g canisters containing approximately 5000 IU/mg and must be kept refrigerated. It is normally taken mixed by the patient with water, or as it frequently causes nausea and has a most unpleasant taste, with 50% water and 50% glycerol BP, which cloaks the flavour. A childrens' formula using this mix has been devised by Tettenborn (Box 24.4) which is generally well tolerated.

The normal initial adult dosage is 1/4 teaspoon x4 daily, increasing to 1/2 teaspoon at the same intervals. It is given before food, as taking it with food may block vitamin absorption. The dosage is adjusted, subsequently, depending on clinical response: a correct level relieves symptoms, without side-effects other than possibly nausea. An underdose leads to worsening symptoms, whereas an overdose – while relieving symptoms – may cause the patient to become very mildly hypomanic. We know of no other instance where the appropriate dosage of an antibiotic is decided in this way. This variability suggests that, perhaps, response depends on non-specific rather than antifungal properties.

Box 24.4 Tettenborn paediatric nystatin formula

Becpharm pulv. in 50% purified water and 50% glycerol BP at 100 000 units/ml.
Dose: 50 000 units daily or twice daily initially, increasing as needed up to 300 000 units four times a day.

Some physicians have used very high doses and claim that this converts most failures into successes, but if a dose of 1/2 teaspoon four times a day does not relieve symptoms many prefer to use a different drug. With Amphotericin, a BP powder is available from Bristol-Myers Squibb, and this has been used in the same way as, and at similar doses to, Nystatin. It is, however, also marketed as Fungilin 100 mg tablets (Bristol-Myers Squibb), and these are generally used as 100–200 mg tds or qds, both ac, for the same reason as Nystatin. In France, oral capsules of 250 mg are marketed as Fungizone. As with nystatin, non-gut symptoms require additional prescriptions.

An alternative is the use of the conazoles, which act systemically and may not need topical support. The oldest of these, ketoconazole, is not recommended, since it is associated with liver damage in approximately 1:10 000 patients[63] and the risk may increase with length of use. Fluconazole and itraconazole may theoretically carry some risk of liver toxicity, but as yet this has not seemed to be a problem. Itraconazole capsules (100 mg, once daily) have been frequently used with clinical success continuously for periods of several months, but with prolonged use it might be wise to check liver function. When fluconazole has been used, probably because of cost implications, it has generally been at 50 mg daily and for short periods. It seems to be effective, especially where higher doses have been used, but relapse may follow quickly if the course is too short.

If some element of infection is implicated, can antibiotic resistance develop, and if so how should this prospect influence our treatment philosophy? So far, neither bacteriological witness nor clinical experience suggests that this is a significant problem. Some physicians do use a combined approach with, for example, fluconazole (systemic) and nystatin or amphotericin (non-systemic) together at first, subsequently discontinuing the fluconazole, usually after 2–4 weeks.

Nutritional supplementation

The case for supplementation is clear: most patients with the syndrome are reported to have a leaky gut[23] and to show nutrient deficiencies.[22] Malabsorption of micronutrients is common, increased gut permeability reflects damage, which may affect digestion and low levels of essential fatty acids,[26] the B vitamins, zinc and magnesium and have been reported.[22] No subject in this study had normal levels for all these nutrients and indeed many did not show normal levels for a single one of them. It is therefore easy to justify the use of a good multivitamin/mineral supplement, which should be yeast free. Even on the diet, nutrient levels for most micronutrients will be above recommended nutritional intake (RNI) levels but this may not provide adequate levels in disease. In a double-blind controlled population study Chandra and co-workers examined a well elderly group who were on good diets. They had fewer infections if they received a vitamin/mineral supplement and their immune systems functioned better.[6] It has also been reported that, because of biodiversity, optimum intakes for some individuals may be well in excess of RNI levels:[50] as yet, we do not know at what levels individuals will be repleted from the use of a good multivitamin/mineral supplement – we can only study laboratory test results. At responsible levels, there are no reports of serious toxic reactions. Additional preparations should be given when there is laboratory evidence of deficiency.

Garlic has long been recognized as having health benefits and seems to be helpful in fungal-type dysbiosis. The active principle, allicin, derives from the action of the enzyme allinase on the alliin component. The process is initiated by crushing a clove. Allicin is highly evanescent and probably best taken as the natural food and preferably raw: most supplements have poor allicin levels.[49] A similar reservation applies to supplements of *Bacillus acidophilus* and any other organisms. These may be found in a highly palatable form in live yogurts, especially those marketed as 'bioyogurts', although the strains in yogurts may not be human ones, whereas the best *B. acidophilus* supplements will be. The use of the supplements is most appropriate in milk-sensitive subjects who cannot take yogurts; the supplement should be milk free – most are not. There is no evidence about how effectively these replete deficiency of gut commensals when administered by mouth. *Lactobacilli* have also been proposed for use at very high doses for a shorter time, 30 billion in comparison with the normal of 4 billion organisms per day (Biocare Ltd, Birmingham). No comparative data about effectiveness have been published.

Bacteria need substrates which support their growth, which include butyrates, N-acetyl-glucosamine and fructo-oligosaccharides which have been termed prebiotics.[57] It has been suggested that these may stimulate recolonization.

Relapses and treatment failures

Since the recognition of the condition depends heavily on the response to therapy, difficulties exist about what to describe as treatment failure. If, however, a simple definition of cure: 'no symptoms on no treatment' is used, then any patients with residual symptoms or dependent on continuing therapy would be partial failures. In one study of patients referred to the author,[20] 84% of patients cleared on diet and a simple nutritional programme. Because of the scale of self-treatment,[20] there may well be many patients who follow published regimes and get better, about whom we have no data. Partial failures may be due to concurrent food intolerance, in which case an elimination diet may help, or to undetected nutritional deficiencies. There are some indications that immunotherapy can help.

LONG-TERM OUTLOOK

Some treated patients resume a totally normal lifestyle, but for most some restrictions will have to be continued. Most do not consume sugars to any significant extent, which may be regarded as an improvement on the average diet. Many, however, have to limit yeasts and mould-containing foods. Excess may be followed by a relapse, usually managed by a brief period of dietary rigour. In our experience, even after some years, relapses may follow the prescription of broad-spectrum antibiotics: this is again usually resolved by careful self-management. These episodes show that the condition is in remission, rather than cured. No figures can be put on these data and a long-term prospective audit is clearly required.

CONCLUSIONS

This chapter sets out to provide answers to two questions: Is the condition genuine and does it relate to *Candida*?

Fungal-type dysbiosis remains controversial. However, there is enough evidence to justify the view that the condition is genuine;

D

that it is organic rather than of psychological origin; and, finally, and most important, that it responds well to a specific treatment regime. It deserves our attention.

The evidence suggests that the condition is dysbiotic but we have not found evidence that establishes a causal role for *C. albicans* although this cannot be excluded. An absence of positive proof is not negative proof and *Candida* may be the cause, or one of the causes.

What is the cause of fungal-type dysbiosis? It is in the nature of medical training that we are only happy about a condition if we know the cause, but from the patient's viewpoint they are more interested in our ability to get them better. In this case, the cause or causes remains to be established but hypotheses may be cautiously offered to stimulate thought and research.

First, it remains possible that the important event in fungal-type dysbiosis is not the type of organism present but the way in which the gut responds to it, either by changes in permeability or in allergic reaction. If this were the case, the syndrome might result from a number of different organisms in different individuals.

Secondly, it might result not from the effects of the organisms that overgrow but from a deficiency of the commensals they displace.

Thirdly, if the organisms themselves cause the condition directly, this may involve fungi, but not necessarily *Candida*, and not necessarily alone.

There are some features of the condition which suggest a fungal involvement, particularly in cases of dysbiosis responding to antifungal drugs. However, nystatin and amphotericin are both known to have non-specific gut cell wall stabilizing actions[51,58] and, of the conazoles, ketoconazole has been reported to be active both in *vitro*[15] and *in vivo*[10] against *Blastocystis hominis*. The pharmaceutical companies do not hold any data suggesting any actions other than antifungal for the other conazoles[13] but this may be merely because no-one has looked. Thus, the antifungals might be effective because of other properties. The presence of bacterial fermentation products, hydrogen[25] and β-alanine[54] suggests a bacterial fermentation is involved.

With these conflicting data, might the answer be not one or the other, but both? Some fungi seem to depend upon bacterial 'contamination' for healthy growth.[37] A lichen is a commensal state between a fungal partner and a photobiont, usually a cyanobacterium (blue-green alga).[52] Is it not therefore possible that in fungal-type dysbiosis the causal mechanism involves some possibly symbiotic state between a fungal/yeast form and a bacterium? If so, this syndrome may not be easy to unravel. Our ignorance of bowel flora is profound. We do not know yet what is normal. Until recently, we were unaware of *Helicobacter pylori*. More recent discoveries, including *Mycoplasma fermentans incognitus*[53] and cell-wall deficient bacteria[47] have not been studied in this context.

Fungal-type dysbiosis continues to provide difficult and stimulating intellectual challenges. It is worthy of our best endeavours, both as a problem of pathology/aetiology and for the sake of the patients who can be helped.

REFERENCES

1. Alun-Jones V, Wilson AJ, Hunter JO, Robinson RE. The aetiological role of antibiotic prophylaxis with hysterectomy in irritable bowel syndrome. *J Obs Gyn* 1984; 5(Suppl. 1): 522–3.

2. Anonymous. *N Engl J Med* 1990; 323: 1693–4.

3. Anthony HM. Airedale Allergy Centre, Airedale, W. Yorks. Personal communication 1997.

4. Anthony HM, Birtwistle S, Eaton KK, Maberly J. *Environmental Medicine in Clinical Practice*. BSAENM Publications, Southampton; 1997: 141–57.

5. Berk JE. Intestinal carbohydrate dyspepsia. In: Bockus HL (ed.) *Gastroenterology*, Vol. 2, 1st edn. Saunders, Philadelphia; 1944: 248–57.

6. Chandra RK. Effect of vitamin and trace-element supplementation on immune responses and infection in elderly subjects. *Lancet* 1992; 340: 1124–7.

7. Christie WW. Gas chromatography and lipids. The Oily Press, Ltd, Ayr; 1989: 71–2.

8. Christopherson SW, Glass KL. Transesterification of short-chain fatty acids for analysis by gas chromatography. *J Diary Sci* 1969; 52: 1289–90.

9. Crook WG. *The Yeast Connection*, 2nd edn. Professional Books, Jackson, Tennessee, 1984.

10. Cohen AN. Ketoconazole and resistant *Blastocystis hominis* infection. *Ann Int Med* 1985; 103: 480–1.

11. Cummings JH, Rombeau JL, Sakata T. *Physiological and Clinical Aspects of Short-Chain Fatty Acids*. Cambridge University Press, Cambridge; 1995.

12. Danna PL, Urban C, Bellin E, Rahal JJ. Role of candida in pathogenesis of antibiotic-associated diarrhoea in elderly inpatients. *Lancet* 1991; 537: 511–14.

13. Dasmahapatra J. Personal communication (data on file, Pfizer Ltd.), 1997.

14. Dismukes WE, Wade JS, Lee JY *et al*. A randomised double-blind trial of nystatin therapy for the candidiasis sensitivity syndrome. *N Engl J Med* 1990; 323: 1717–23.

15. Dunn LA, Boreham PFL. The in-vitro activity of drugs against *Blastocystis hominis*. *J Antimicrobial Chemother* 1991; 27: 507–16.

16. Eaton KK. The prick skin test: studies on the duration of response. *Newsletter Soc Environ Ther* 1987; 7: 2–6.

17. Eaton KK. Gut fermentation: a reappraisal of an old clinical condition with diagnostic tests and management: discussion paper. *J Roy Soc Med* 1991; 84: 669–71.

18. Eaton KK. Sugars in food intolerance and abnormal gut fermentation. *J Nutr Med* 1992; 3: 295–301.

19. Eaton KK. Gut fermentation. *J Nutr Med* 1995; 5: 206–7.

20. Eaton KK, Howard M. Fungal-type dysbiosis of the gut: the occurrence of fungal diseases and the response to challenge with yeasty and mould-containing foods. *J Nutr Environ Med* 1998; 8: 247–55.

21. Eaton KK, Howard M, Hunnisett A. Urinary B-alanine is a marker of abnormal as well as normal gut fermentation. *J Nutr Med* 1994; 4: 157–63.

22. Eaton KK, McLaren HJ, Hunnisett A, Harris M. Abnormal gut fermentation: laboratory studies reveal deficiency of B vitamins, zinc and magnesium. *J Nutr Biochem* 1994; 4: 157–63.

23. Eaton KK, Howard M, McLaren Howard J. Gut permeability measured by polyethylene glycol absorption in abnormal gut fermentation as compared with food intolerance. *J Roy Soc Med* 1995; 88: 63–6.

24. Eaton KK, Howard M, Hunnisett A. Urinary histidine excretion in patients with classical allergy (type A allergy), food intolerance (type B allergy) and fungal-type dysbiosis. *J Nutr Biochem* 1998; 9: 586–90.

25. Eaton KK, Chan R, Howard J, McLaren-Howard J. A comparison of lactulose breath hydrogen measurements with gut fermentation profiles in patients with fungal-type dysbiosis. *J Nutr Environ Med* 2001; 11: 33–42.

26. Galland L. Nutrition and candidiasis. *J Orthomol Psych* 1985; 15: 50–60.

27. Grant E. Oral contraceptives and risk of breast cancer. *Lancet* 1994; 344: 1364.

28. Hauss R. Gastrointestinal mycoses: Insights and clinical pearls from the German perspective. 31st Annual meeting. *Am Acad Environ Med* 1996 (abstracts): 281–5.

29 Holti G. *Candida* allergy. In: Winner HI, Hurley R (eds) *Symposium on Candida infections*. Churchill Livingstone, Edinburgh; 1966: 74–81.

30 Hunnisett A, Howard J, Davies S. Gut fermentation (or the 'autobrewery' syndrome): a clinical test with initial observations and discussion. *J Nutr Med* 1990; 1: 33–38.

31 Hunnisett A. PhD thesis. Micronutrient interactions in the management of bone marrow transplant recipients. Oxford Brooks University, Oxford, 1996.

32 Hurst AF, Knott FA. Intestinal carbohydrate dyspepsia. *Quart J Med* 1930–31; 24: 171–80.

33 Hyland ME, Sodergren SC. Relationship between lifestyle and minor health complaints: evidence for two different types of dysfunctional gut microflora. *J Nutr Environ Med* 1998; 7: 253–65.

34 Iwata K. A review of the literature on drunken symptoms due to yeasts in the gastrointestinal tract. In: Iwata K (ed) *Yeasts and Yeast-like Microorganisms in Medical Science*. International Specialised Symposium on Yeasts. University of Tokyo Press, Tokyo, 1976: 184–90.

35 James J, Warin RP. An assessment of the role of *Candida albicans* and food yeasts in chronic urticaria. *Br J Dermatol* 1971; 84: 227–37.

36 Katiyar SK, Mukhtar H. Tea consumption and cancer. In: Simopoulos AP (ed) *Metabolic Consequences of Changing Dietary Patterns*. World Review of Nutrition and Dietetics, Vol. 79. Karger, Basel: 1996: 154–84.

37 Kelley J. International Mycological Institute, Egham, Personal communication, 1997.

38 Kritchevsky D. Phytosterols. In: Kritchevsky D, Bonfield C (eds) *Dietary Fiber in Health & Disease*. Plenum Press, New York; 1997: 235–43.

39 Kroker GF. Chronic candidiasis and allergy. In: Brostoff J, Challacombe SJ (eds). *Food Allergy and Intolerance*. Balliere-Tindall, London: 1986: 850–70.

40 Lehninger AL. *Biochemistry*. Worth Publishing, New York; 1970 (6th reprinting, 1981): 59, 110, 205, 210, 438.

41 Longbottom JL, Murray IG, Pepys J. Diagnosis of fungal diseases. In: Gell PGH, Coombs RRA (eds) *Clinical Aspects of Immunology*, (2nd edn.). Blackwell, Oxford; 1868; 80–4.

42 Louria DB. Some aspects of the absorption, distribution, and excretion of amphotericin B in man. *Antibiotic Med* 1958; 5: 295–300.

43 McNeil NI, Cummings JH, James WPT. Short-chain fatty acid absorption by the human large intestine. *Gut* 1978; 19: 818–22.

44 Markus H, Finck H. *Candida*, der entfesselte Hefepilz. Ratgeber Ehrenwirth, 1995.

45 Marrison LW. *Wines and Spirits* (revised edn). Penguin Books, Harmondsworth; 1958: 227–52.

46 Mathur S, Virella G, Koistinen J *et al*. Humoral immunity in vaginal candidiasis. *Infect Immun* 1977; 15: 287–94.

47 Mattman LH. *Cell Wall Deficient Forms: Stealth Pathogens*, 2nd edn. CRC Press, Baton Rouge, Florida, 1993: 222–4.

48 Middleton SJ, Coley A, Hunter JO. The role of faecal *Candida albicans* in the pathogenesis of food-intolerant irritable bowel syndrome. *Postgrad Med J* 1992; 68: 453–4.

49 Minney S, Garlic – the forgotten aid to modern medicine. *BioMed Newsletter* 1990; 1: 7.

50 Molloy AM, Daly S, Mills JL *et al*. Thermolabile variant of 5,10-methylenetetrahydrofolate reductase associated with low red cell folates: implications for folate intake recommendations. *Lancet* 1997; 349; 9065: 1591–3.

51 Mponaminga M, Culon J, Bonaly R. Effects of sub-inhibitory dose Amphotericin B on cell wall biosynthesis in *Candida albicans*. *Res Microbiol* 1989: 95–105.

52 Nash TH. (ed.) *Lichen Biology*. Cambridge University Press, Cambridge; 1996: 1–7.

53 Nicholson NL, Nicholson GL. The isolation, purification and analysis of specific gene-containing nucleoprotein complexes. *Meth Mol Genet* 1994; 5: 281–98.

54 Nolting S, Guzek B, Hauss R. *Mykosen des Verdauungstraktes*. Max Seimen, Hamburg; 1994.

55 Nout MJR. Useful role of fungi in food processing. In: Samson RA, Hoekstra ES, Frisvad JC, Filtenborg O (eds) *Introduction to Food Borne Fungi*. Centraalbureau voor Schimmelcultures, Baarn; 1996: 295.

56 Rhodes JM, Middleton P, Jewell DP. The lactulose hydrogen breath test as a diagnostic test for small-bowel bacterial overgrowth. *Scan J Gastroent* 1979; 14: 333–36.

57 Roberfroid MB. Health benefits of non-digestible oligosaccharides. In: Kritchevsky D, Bonfield C (eds) *Dietary Fiber in Health and Disease*. Plenum Press, New York; 1997: 211–19.

58 Shepherd MG. The pathogenesis and host defence mechanisms of oral candidosis. *NZ Dent J* 1986; 82(369): 78–81.

59 Truss CO. Tissue injury induced by *Candida albicans*: mental and neurologic manifestations. *J Orthomol Psychiatry* 1978; 7: 17–37.

60 Truss CO. Metabolic abnormalities in patients with chronic candidiasis: the acetaldehyde hypothesis. *J Orthomol Psych* 1984; 13: 66–93.

61 Truss CO. Restoration of immune competence to *Candida albicans*. *J Orthomol Psych* 1980; 9: 287–301.

62 Turner JG. Germ-carbohydrate fermentation. In: *A Discussion on Alimentary Toxaemia; its Sources, Consequences and Treatment*. Champneys FH(ed.) *Proc Roy Soc Med* 1913; 6: 160–3.

63 Van Tyle JM. Ketoconazole. Mechanism of action, pharmokinetics, drug interactions, adverse reactions and therapeutic use. *Pharmacotherapy* 1984; 4: 343–73.

Contents

SUMMARY

Abnormal reactions to foods and other ingested agents result from inherited defects of enzymes that participate in the metabolic incorporation of nutrients and in complex biosynthetic reactions. Similarly, defects in related proteins that affect the cellular transport of nutrient molecules and their metabolites also cause idiosyncratic reactions to foods. These constitutional variations may be incorrectly attributed to allergy or immune hypersensitivity; clear recognition of their nature is important for diagnosis and for definitive treatment. Dietary modification and specific supplementation with vitamins or other co-factors in most instances greatly improves symptoms and outcome.

Here are described:

- *Maldigestion syndromes* resulting from lack of specific digestive enzymes that lead to post-prandial abdominal symptoms and diarrhoea: specific deficiencies of the intestinal disaccharidases, lactase, sucrase-isomaltase, trehalase; pancreatic digestive enzymes (lipase, co-lipase, trypsinogen) and intestinal enterokinase.
- *Malabsorption syndromes* resulting from disordered transport of the monosaccharides – glucose (galactose) and fructose.
- *Metabolic disturbances* related to enzymatic deficiencies of fructose assimilation and breakdown; primary and secondary defects of urea formation (urea cycle defects and lysinuric protein intolerance).
- *Biosynthetic abnormalities* of reducing equivalents (NADPH-glucose 6-phosphate dehydrogenase deficiency) and of the formation of haem (acute hepatic porphyrias).

These disorders individually give rise to diverse intolerance syndromes with idiosyncrasy to lactose, glucose, galactose, fructose, starch, sucrose, trehalose, protein-rich or fat-rich meals, fava beans, alcohol as well as frequently prescribed drugs (Table 25.1).

INTRODUCTION

This section principally concerns the scientific basis for *idiosyncrasy* rather than allergy or hypersensitivity to foods. Idiosyncrasy represents a qualitatively abnormal reaction to a food, drug or other agent: it is a state that represents part of the *chemical individuality* of a person with, implicitly, a genetic basis. Here are described those idiosyncrasies that result from defined *enzymatic deficiencies* or defects in specific *carrier proteins* responsible for the transport of nutrients across cell membranes. Not only do these defects determine the tolerance of a person to individual constituents in the diet but they illustrate how adverse metabolic phenomena contribute to the development of taste preferences. The genetic disorders outlined here are important for clinical practice, since they often respond to *dietary manipulation* with or without specific *nutritional or enzymatic supplementation*: such treatment may dramatically improve the patient's symptoms and may also prevent long-term injurious effects. Enzymatic and related genetic disorders associated with food intolerance are classified into (1) those caused by *maldigestion* of nutrients; (2) those caused by *impaired metabolism* of nutrients and (3) *other enzymatic deficiencies* associated with dietary idiosyncrasies. For completeness, several rare disorders associated with idiosyncrasy to particular food components or gastrointestinal disturbances resulting from selective defects of digestion and absorption are described (Table 25.2).

Enzymatic and transport defects that cause intolerance of nutrients and drugs
Disorders of digestion and absorption
Disaccharidases
Lactase deficiency
Sucrase-isomaltase deficiency
Trehalase deficiency
Transport defects
Glucose/galactose malabsorption
Fructose malabsorption
Pancreatic enzyme defects
Lipase
Co-lipase
Trypsinogen
Enterokinase*
Disorders of metabolism
Fructose metabolism
Hereditary fructose intolerance (fructose-1-phosphate aldolase)
Fructose-1,6-bisphosphatase deficiency
Urea cycle defects (ammonia metabolism)
Carbamoyl phosphate synthetase deficiency
Argino succinate synthetase deficiency
Argino succinic acid lyase deficiency
Ornithine transcarbamoylase deficiency
Arginase deficiency
Lysinuric protein intolerance (transport defect)
Other enzymatic defects
Glucose-6-phosphate dehydrogenase deficiency (favism)
Haem biosynthesis – acute porphyrias
δ-Aminolaevulinate dehydratase deficiency
Porphobilinogen deaminase deficiency (acute intermittent porphyria)
Coproporphyrinogen III oxidase deficiency (hereditary coproporphyria)
Protoporphyrinogen IX oxidase deficiency (variegate or South African porphyria)

*Enterokinase is synthesized by the small intestinal mucosa but is required for activation of pancreatic enzymes.

Table 25.1 Enzymatic and transport defects that cause intolerance of nutrients and drugs.

MALDIGESTION

Absorptive physiology

The digestion and assimilation of nutrients involves the physical and enzymatic degradation of food constituents as well as their absorption through defined mechanisms for uptake and transport across the epithelial layer of the small intestinal mucosa.[46] The *enzymatic phase* of digestion is initiated in the stomach by pepsin at acid pH and continues in the lumen of the upper small intestine through the action, primarily, of pancreatic enzymes including lipase, amylase and proteases. Since most of the ingested carbohydrate consists of complex polysaccharides including starch and glycogen, only partial digestion is achieved in the lumen;

Guide to frequency of food and drug intolerance syndromes
Frequent
Lactose intolerance
Fructose malabsorption
Glucose-6-phosphate dehydrogenase deficiency
Uncommon
Hereditary fructose intolerance (1 in 18 000 in the UK)
Acute porphyrias (~ 1 in 50 000; up to 1 in 1–10 000 in certain populations) e.g. Lapps, South Africans
Urea cycle defects
Lysinuric protein intolerance (Finns)
Rare or very rare
Glucose/galactose malabsorption
Isolated pancreatic deficiencies/enterokinase deficiency
Fructose-1,6-bisphosphatase deficiency

Table 25.2 Guide to frequency of food and drug intolerance syndromes.

disaccharidases present on the microvillus membrane cleave the oligosaccharides and disaccharides into their component sugars for transport across the epithelium into the portal blood stream.

Pancreatic *lipase* binds to its co-factor, co-lipase, at the surface interface of the triglyceride droplet in combination with bile salts to form a lipolytic complex. Intraluminal digestion in the micellar phase releases fatty acids and monoglycerides, which penetrate the primary micelles to form mixed micelles containing fatty acids, monoglycerides and bile salts that are maintained in a clear solubilized phase. At the junction with the cell surface, fatty acids and monoglycerides are released from the micelles and enter the cell by diffusion where they are re-esterified to triglycerides and assembled into chylomicrons and very low density lipoproteins for secretion into the lymph or, in the case of medium-chain triglycerides, the portal venous system, where they are bound to plasma albumin.

Transport mechanisms
Several mechanisms of transport are involved in the absorptive process for the assimilation of digested luminal products: these include *active transport* across an electrical or chemical gradient (an energy-requiring process involving specific membrane carriers); *facilitated diffusion*, which involves transport down a concentration gradient facilitated by a specific carrier; *passive diffusion*, which resembles facilitated diffusion but occurs at a slower rate owing to the absence of a specific mediator; and, finally, *endocytosis*, which principally involves the uptake of antigens and immunoglobulins in the neonatal period but may persist to a limited extent in adult life.

Proteolysis is initiated in the stomach by pepsin but is usually completed within the lumen of the upper small intestine by the concerted action of pancreatic trypsin, chymotrypsin and other *endopeptidases* as well as *exopeptidases* such as carboxypeptidase. The final products are oligopeptides, dipeptides and free amino acids. Further digestion is completed at the brush-border surface of the mucosal cells by membrane-bound oligopeptidases. Dipeptides and amino acids are taken up by several *generic transport proteins* or mucosal carriers for neutral amino acids (including cysteine); distinct transport mechanisms also exist for

dicarboxylic acids and the imino acids as well as glycine, which can be transported by both neutral and imino acid carriers. Specific mucosal carriers in the small intestine include the sodium/hexose co-transporter for D-glucose and D-galactose transport across the brush-border membrane and the dibasic amino acid transporter for ornithine, arginine and lysine (not cysteine) on the basolateral rather than luminal membrane of renal tubular and intestinal epithelia.

DISACCHARIDASE DEFICIENCY – CARBOHYDRATE MALABSORPTION

Genetically determined deficiency of single disaccharidases or generalized loss of disaccharidase activity on the lumenal surface of the small intestine causes a characteristic syndrome of dietary carbohydrate intolerance.[3,64]

Pathophysiology (Fig. 25.1)
Disaccharides and oligosaccharides are derived from the luminal hydrolysis of starch and glycogen catalysed by salivary and pancreatic α-amylase. This enzyme cannot cleave the α-1,6-branching linkages and their vicinal 1,4-α-bonds so that the initial products of starch digestion are branched oligosaccharides containing at least one 1,6-α bond.[46] Free disaccharides also occur in the diet in the form of lactose (glucose–galactose), sucrose (glucose–fructose) and trehalose (glucose–glucose).

Site of enzyme activity
Distinct disaccharidases are present on the microvillar (luminal) epithelial surface of the intestine: maltase-glucoamylase is an α-glucosidase that removes glucose moieties sequentially from the non-reducing terminus of oligosaccharides. α-Dextrinase (isomaltase) continues the hydrolysis of branched oligosaccharides by cleaving the 1,6-α-glycosidic bond of the limit dextrins. This enzyme is a component of the bi-functional enzyme complex, sucrase-isomaltase. Sucrase hydrolyses glycosidic bonds in sucrose to yield fructose and glucose; the isomaltase subunit splits the 1,6-α-glycosidic bond in isomaltose and palatinose and in branched limit α-dextrins.[65] Lactase-glycosyl ceramidase is part of a β-glycosidase complex: it cleaves several β-glycosides including lactose into galactose and glucose as well as certain hydrophobic substrates such as phlorizin and glucosyl β-ceramides.[71] The disaccharidase trehalase is also a brush border α-glycosidase that cleaves the unusual 1α–1α glycosidic linkage of trehalose into its component glucose moieties.

Digestion of disaccharides
The disaccharides sucrose, lactose and trehalose like the α-dextrins are poorly absorbed, so that digestion is absolutely dependent upon the activity of the mucosal disaccharidases. These are present principally in the upper reaches of the small intestine and are optimally active at pH ~6. For most carbohydrates hydrolysis in the lumen and at the mucosal surface is sufficiently active to saturate the pathways for glucose and fructose transport across the microvillus membrane. However, the rate of hydrolysis of lactose is the limiting step for absorption of the glucose and galactose components; the specific activity of lactase in the intestinal mucosa is lower than that of all other disaccharidase activities. Once released, the component monosaccharides released by the activity of mucosal glycosidases are rapidly absorbed by the

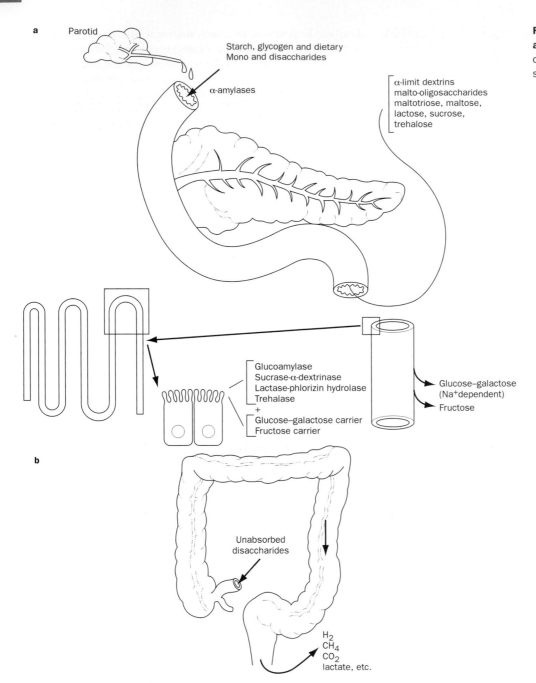

a

Parotid

Starch, glycogen and dietary
Mono and disaccharides

α-amylases

α-limit dextrins
malto-oligosaccharides
maltotriose, maltose,
lactose, sucrose,
trehalose

Glucoamylase
Sucrase-α-dextrinase
Lactase-phlorizin hydrolase
Trehalase
+
Glucose–galactose carrier
Fructose carrier

Glucose–galactose
(Na⁺dependent)

Fructose

b

Unabsorbed
disaccharides

H_2
CH_4
CO_2
lactate, etc.

Fig. 25.1 Carbohydrate digestion and absorption. Pathophysiology of carbohydrate/disaccharide intolerance syndrome.

specific carriers – the glucose–galactose carrier (SGLT1) (a sodium-dependent carrier system) and the fructose carrier (GLUT5).[9] The GLUT2 protein is localized to the basolateral membrane (anti-luminal) surface of the epithelial cells and is probably responsible for mediating efflux of glucose and fructose into the portal blood stream as well as the uptake of fructose by the liver.[14]

Disaccharidases

The disaccharidases are surface glycoproteins on the microvillus membrane and their synthesis continues throughout the active life of the mature absorptive cell. The complex process of biosynthesis and membrane entering of the mucosal disaccharides is not fully understood but it is clear that most of the enzyme complexes are heterodimers composed of non-identical subunits, only one of which is anchored in a trans-membrane domain close to the

N-terminus. Mature enzymes are highly glycosylated, with a mean residence time of only 6–8 hours within the microvillus membrane.

Intestinal lactase

Unlike in other mammals, α- and β-glucosidase activities in humans appear in the fetal intestine, so that the newborn infant is able to digest lactose and sugars containing α-glycosidic bonds so that weaning can be introduced very early. Intestinal lactase activity undergoes an unusual developmental programme that appears to be genetically determined. Mucosal lactase activity is greatest in full-term neonates but falls to about 25% of this value within the first year of life. By contrast, α-glucosidase activities of the other disaccharidases appear at around 10 weeks of gestation and remain at comparable levels throughout adult life.[22,23,69] Two adult human lactase phenotypes are recognized: a rare dominant allele is responsible for the persistence of lactase activity after childhood in most individuals of North European ancestry.[69] However, in most adult humans, inheritance of a recessive allele is responsible for a decline of lactase activity after childhood. Only low levels of lactase activity remain but this is normally without any consequence because the consumption of dairy products is minimal (see below). The genetic basis for lactase expression and the mechanism of its decline after weaning and especially after childhood, in humans, is not yet completely understood.[3,22,71]

Colonic (bacterial) digestion

Epithelial cells of the lower intestine and colon do not express appreciable disaccharidase activity; any unabsorbed carbohydrate resulting from maldigestion of disaccharides proximally thus provides fuel for colonic bacteria, which break down luminal oligosaccharides to generate short-chain organic acids, hydrogen, methane and carbon dioxide. Maldigestion of the osmotically active sugars and incomplete absorption of short-chain organic acids derived from them induce fluid retention within the luminal cavity of the lower intestine. Thus, ingestion of carbohydrate under circumstances where disaccharidase activity is reduced, distends the bowel with acidic fluid and gas, causing pain and a watery and gaseous diarrhoea.

The syndrome of carbohydrate intolerance

The abdominal symptoms may be noticed within 1 hour of ingesting foods containing the particular carbohydrate (Table 25.3). These symptoms include increased bowel sounds, abdominal distension and nausea followed by colicky pain. Watery diarrhoea associated with the passage of flatus may occur rapidly. Depending on the carbohydrate load and the nature of the disaccharidase deficiency, the onset of the diarrhoea varies from 1 hour to several hours after ingestion of the offending food or drink. For some individuals the symptoms occur after the consumption of only a few grams of the carbohydrate.

There is great variation in the amount of carbohydrate normally ingested, but typically 400–500 g of carbohydrate are consumed daily. About half of this consists of starch; the remainder comprises the disaccharides sucrose and lactose as well as the monosaccharides glucose and fructose. Given the ubiquity of these sugars in the Western diet, especially in confectionery as well as in many processed foods and drinks, it may be very difficult to identify particular dietary components that are responsible for the carbohydrate intolerance syndrome. However, deficiency of particular disaccharidases induces dietary intolerance of specific foods and drinks: milk products in the case of

Symptoms of carbohydrate intolerance syndrome
Increased bowel sounds
Distension
Nausea
Colicky pain
Watery diarrhoea
Greatly increased flatus

Table 25.3 Symptoms of carbohydrate intolerance syndrome.

lactase deficiency; table starch and sugar in a sucrose-isomaltase deficiency; and mushrooms (and possibly shellfish) in trehalase deficiency.[64,65]

LACTOSE INTOLERANCE

Most patients that suffer from lactose intolerance have lactase deficiency acquired as a result of generalized intestinal disease (especially postinfective gastroenteritis) or as a result of genetically programmed restriction of lactase expression in adulthood.

Congenital deficiency of lactase[41,62]

Congenital deficiency of lactase is a rare autosomal recessive disorder that causes infantile diarrhoea after the first feed with breast milk. The syndrome is distinct from congenital glucose–galactose malabsorption. In glucose–galactose malabsorption, introduction of a lactose-free formula feed corrects the diarrhoea of congenital lactase deficiency, whereas congenital lactose intolerance is caused by a profound genetically determined deficiency of mucosal lactase and is a lifelong condition.

Lactase deficiency in premature infants[44]

β-Galactosidase in the intestine is not fully expressed until after the 28th week of gestation and transient intolerance of milk feeds may occur in premature infants born before this age. Digestion of incompletely absorbed lactose is usually achieved in the large bowel by colonic bacteria but in very premature infants recessive enteral feeding with lactose-containing formulae and maternal milk disposal of lactose by this route may become dominant. Abdominal distress due to distention of the intestine with gas and diarrhoea requires careful attention to the diet and may have implications for fluid balance in premature infants.

Lactase restriction in children and adults[69]

Only a minority of adults retain the considerable capacity of the infant's intestine to digest and absorb dietary lactose. In most populations in Africa and Asia and elsewhere, 90% of individuals experience a genetically determined and physiological decline in mucosal lactase activity after weaning; restriction of lactase activity is observed in about 5% of adults and adolescents in peoples of Northern European origin. Since the consumption of dietary products decreases normally after weaning, low levels of lactase activity in the adult intestine are normally without any consequence unless the individual is challenged with milk, dairy products and many processed and ready-to-eat foods offered in modern Western-style diets.[3]

The selective pressures that maintain the physiological reduction in mucosal lactase deficiency in childhood are not fully understood but it is clear that lactase persistence is the least frequent physiological variant in the human population. However, because of increased international travel and migration, this physiological loss of lactase activity is a common cause of abdominal distress in those that adopt Western-style diets when they reach adult life. A proportion of patients considered to have irritable bowel disease or spastic colon may prove to have a component of lactase deficiency. Individuals who undergo partial gastrectomy and other surgical intervention in the upper intestine may develop symptomatic lactase malabsorption because of enhanced delivery of the offending carbohydrate to the mucosal epithelium of the jejunum.

Secondary lactase deficiency[30,35,57]

Infective gastroenteritis due to viral infection, e.g. rotavirus, is a frequent cause of transient lactase deficiency in the intestinal mucosa. It occurs principally in infants and causes continuing symptoms of lactose intolerance for days or weeks. The carbohydrate intolerance syndrome may induce or aggravate dehydration and is typically accompanied by prominent bloating and the passage of acidic sour-smelling stools. These symptoms are ameliorated by exclusion of dairy products from the diet. Long-standing mucosal inflammation such as that accompanying coeliac disease, intestinal giardiasis, cryptococcidosis or even intestinal Crohn's disease is often complicated by reduced lactase activity and dietary intolerance of lactose. Although all disaccharidases may be reduced by mucosal disease, the critical relation between lactase activity and the hydrolysis of lactose usually results in a syndrome in which lactose intolerance predominates. However, in patients with intestinal disease and generalized nutritional disturbances the use of high-calorie supplements containing oligosaccharides rich in maltose or sucrose may also contribute to the abdominal syndrome of carbohydrate intolerance.

Sucrase-isomaltase (α-dextrinase) deficiency[2,64,65,71]

Inherited deficiency of mucosal sucrase-isomaltase is rare in all populations except in Inuits.[32] Several genetic defects result in aberrant glycosylation and defective biosynthetic targeting of a translated enzyme to the brush border membrane. The disorder is inherited as an autosomal recessive trait.

Intolerance of dietary sucrose is responsible for most of the symptoms which develop as table sugar and sugar-containing foods are introduced during weaning. Intolerance of starch also occurs but is less conspicuous because the osmotic effect of retained partially digested α-dextrins in the gut lumen is less significant. However, ingestion of large, starchy meals may induce abdominal cramps with flatulent diarrhoea. Patients with sucrase-isomaltase deficiency develop persistent diarrhoea with a passage of frothy acid stools when they take a diet containing appreciable quantities of sucrose.

The diagnosis may be suspected on the basis of the history, diarrhoea at weaning and on the description of the stools. The condition must be differentiated from cow's milk allergy, infective or postinfective gastroenteritis, coeliac disease, pancreatic failure and other intestinal disorders. Biopsy of the jejunal mucosa and enzymatic assay is required for a definitive diagnosis and offers the opportunity for histological examination of the mucosa which is normal in inherited sucrase-isomaltase deficiency. Hydrogen breath tests after ingestion of sucrose and isomaltose may also prove useful in the operational diagnosis of this disorder.[48]

Trehalase deficiency[10,11,45]

A few patients have been reported with marked intolerance of mushrooms due to the absence of the mucosal disaccharidase trehalase – a brush border α-glycoprotein that cleaves the 1α–1α bond of trehalose, thus releasing glucose. The presence of this sugar in the haemolymph of arthropods poses the theoretical possibility of dietary intolerance of crustaceans but this has not been reported in trehalase deficiency. Since intolerance of mushrooms and other fungi is frequently reported, trehalase deficiency may underlie this dietary intolerance syndrome more frequently than hitherto suspected.[12]

Treatment of disaccharidase deficiency syndromes[65]

The mainstay of treatment involves strict dietary exclusion of the offending sugar(s). In severe functional deficiency of mucosal disaccharidases, the advice of a professional dietitian may be needed, particularly since sucrose and lactose are almost ubiquitous in Western-style diets (Tables 25.4 and 25.5). In adult-type hypolactasia, complete elimination is not usually required because some lactase activity is usually retained, but if symptoms are troublesome all potential sources of the offending sugars should be investigated.

Lactose-containing foods
Fresh, dried, skimmed, 'non-fat' and condensed milks
Cream
Yogurt
Cheese
Processed meats and sausages
Sauces, stuffings, salad dressings
Custard powder
Canned and dried soups
Biscuits, cakes, cookies, pancakes, waffles
Dried cereals
Confectionery
Frozen and canned fruits
Instant coffee
Lactose is frequently employed as a filler or stabilizer in powdered medicines and tablets.

Table 25.4 Lactose-containing foods.

Foods excluded in fructose and sucrose-free diets*
Table sugar (cane and beet origin)
Corn syrup
Fruit sugar, all fruit and fruit products, purées, etc., including tomatoes
Sorbitol (excipient of medicines, diabetic foodstuffs)
Honey, treacle
Molasses
Chocolate, sherbet and sugar-containing sweetmeats and confectionery
Preserves, jams and marmalade
Frankfurters, honey-roast and sweet-cured ham
Processed cheese spreads
Cream and cottage cheeses with chives, pineapple, etc.
Flavoured milks and yogurts; condensed milk; some infant milk formulae
Wheatgerm, brown rice, bran
Breakfast cereals
Coffee essence, powdered milk
Carbonated sweet drinks
Allspice, nuts, coconut, carob, peanut butter
Mayonnaise, pickles, salad dressings, sauces
Most legumes, some potatoes (especially stored 'new' potatoes)
Wines, sherries and liqueurs
Beers and stouts
*Sorbitol, sucrose and fructose are frequently employed as fillers and stabilizers in tablets, drug suspensions and syrups (especially for paediatric use).

Table 25.5 Foods excluded in fructose and sucrose-free diets.*

Diagnostic features of disaccharidase deficiency
Typical symptoms after ingestion of food/drink containing free disaccharides
Increased stool osmolality, lactate and acidic pH
Symptoms and positive breath hydrogen test after ingestion of pure disaccharide (e.g. 50 g lactose)
Absence of symptoms on introduction of strict exclusion diet
Deficiency of mucosal disaccharidase activity (intestinal mucosal biopsy)

Table 25.6 Diagnostic features of disaccharidase deficiency.

Recently, β-galactosidase prepared commercially from yeast or from *Aspergillus oryziae* has been shown to reduce symptoms. In some cases the enzymes may be added to milky foods before consumption to reduce the concentration of fermentable lactose.[59] In other instances, the enzymes are taken in tablet form for ingestion with lactose-containing foods, but this strategy is not usually indicated when dietary exclusion can be introduced.

Sucrase-isomaltase activity presents a particular challenge: reduction of starchy foods often improves the symptoms of starch intolerance but complete exclusion of sucrose-containing foodstuffs can be difficult. Recently, ingestion of dried brewer's yeast that is rich in invertase, which hydrolyses sucrose, has proved to be effective in controlling the symptoms of sucrase-isomaltase deficiency.[3]

Diagnosis of disaccharide malabsorption (Table 25.6)

Disaccharidase deficiency may be suspected from the dietary history, particularly in relation to changes in circumstances: for example, after immigration to countries where a Western-style diet is the rule. The diarrhoeal stool has an acid pH (<6.0), in increased osmolality of stool water (>350 mOsmol/kg) due to the presence of organic anions and lactate. Hydrogen excretion determined by rebreathing 2 hours after ingestion of 50 g[3,38,48] lactose may identify patients with lactase deficiency and, if necessary, may be later confirmed by assay of jejunal mucosa for enzymatic activity – the definitive, but rarely indicated, diagnostic investigation.

MALABSORPTION SYNDROMES CAUSING DIETARY INTOLERANCE[20]

Glucose-galactose malabsorption[21]

This very rare syndrome presents with torrential watery diarrhoea and failure to thrive in the neonatal period. Diarrhoea follows the onset of breast feeding or the introduction of artificial feeds, both of which contain the disaccharide lactose. When broken down to the constituent monosaccharides, glucose and galactose, the failure of the glucose–galactose transporter system (a sodium-dependent, active carrier) results in osmotic diarrhoea because of the absolute failure of glucose and galactose uptake. The condition responds to withdrawal of milk and artificial feeding; a partial response to the introduction of sucrose may be observed but elimination of all dietary carbohydrate except fructose – which is absorbed through a separate carrier system (GLUT5) – is necessary to prevent death from dehydration and malnutrition. Prompt parenteral rehydration is nearly always required at the same time as feeding a glucose–galactose and lactose-free diet. The definitive diagnosis and treatment of glucose–galactose malabsorption presents a major challenge.[20,42] The disorder must be distinguished from other inherited disorders including congenital lactase deficiency, sucrase-isomaltase deficiency, chloridorrhoea and sodium malabsorption as well as acquired monosaccharide intolerance induced by infective or inflammatory intestinal disease. Glucose–galactose malabsorption has been found to respond optimally to a completely carbohydrate-free formula supplemented with 70 g/litre D+ fructose.[42]

Diagnosis

The diagnosis may be suggested by the presence of glycosuria, resulting from the simultaneous defect of the reabsorption of glucose in the glomerular filtrate by carriers normally present on the microvillus border of the proximal renal tubular epithelium. The presence of reducing substances in acid stool water that tests positively for glucose together with the characteristic dietary history are indications for further systematic studies.

Glucose–galactose malabsorption is a severe disorder inherited as an autosomal recessive trait. Consanguinity may be observed in the parents. The diagnosis is suspected in children with marked intolerance of all dietary carbohydrate. Colonic bacteria may ferment undigested glucose and galactose partly to lactate and other organic acids; the stools are acid but contain appreciable quantities of unabsorbed monosaccharide. Perfusion studies and studies of the unidirectional uptake of radiolabelled glucose or galactose by biopsy specimens of small intestinal mucosa confirm selective loss of the intestinal glucose transporter SGLT1 in this disorder;[21] recently, inactivating mutations have been identified in the gene encoding the carrier protein. Patients suffering from this severe disorder should be distinguished from congenital deficiency of specific mucosal disaccharidases.[42]

DEFICIENCY OF ISOLATED PANCREATIC ENZYMES

Lipase

Isolated deficiency of pancreatic lipase,[24,67] and co-lipase,[34] have been reported. These deficiencies induce marked postprandial steatorrhoea after ingestion of fat-containing foods. Co-lipase is an essential protein for the activation of pancreatic lipase in the micellar phase of intralumenal digestion where it catalyses the activating interaction between bile salts and pancreatic lipase. Both syndromes are autosomal recessive disorders that present with severe diarrhoea with the characteristics of postfeeding steatorrhoea shortly after birth. Analysis of duodenal contents reveals normal amylase and proteolytic activity but a selected deficiency of pancreatic lipase: treatment with preparations of supplemental pancreatic enzymes reduces the diarrhoea and promotes normal growth and development. In the untreated state, only about 50% of ingested fat is absorbed; in co-lipase deficiency, malabsorption of vitamin B_{12} (with full-blown megaloblastic anaemia) has been observed as well as precocious gallstones that probably result from the reduced bile acid pool as a consequence of the incomplete resorption of intraluminal bile salts.[34]

Deficiency of trypsinogen[72]

This disorder presents with diarrhoea and anaemia in the newborn period, associated with failure to thrive and severe hypoproteinaemia leading to oedema. Analysis of duodenal contents shows a deficiency of proteolytic activity but addition of exogenous tryptic extracts allows activation of chymotrypsin and carboxy-peptidase activity. This is because of a failure of autoactivation of endogenous trypsin. Treatment of the condition consists of enteral or parenteral nutrition with amino acid supplements and later the introduction of pancreatic extracts.

Enterokinase deficiency[27]

Deficiency of the activating protease of the intestinal mucosa, enterokinase, leads to a failure of proteolytic activation of pancreatic proteases in luminal fluid of the duodenum and upper small intestine. Postprandial diarrhoea and failure to thrive are prominent features that might suggest food sensitivity. Enterokinase is present in the upper small intestinal mucosa and can be assayed in small intestinal biopsy specimens.

This disorder presents with severe diarrhoea and anaemia with failure to thrive and hypoproteinaemia shortly after birth. The diarrhoea results from the failure to digest proteins present in the diet. The infant is often dwarfed unless properly treated. Diagnosis may be made by studying the proteolytic activity of duodenal contents with or without the addition of exogenous enterokinase extracted from human or porcine intestinal mucosa. Enterokinase cleaves a specific bond in trypsinogen to form active trypsin, which then activates the other pancreatic proenzymes in their zymogen form. The disorder responds rapidly to the introduction of exogenous pancreatic enzyme supplements which contain tryptic, chymotryptic and carboxypeptidases that have already been activated during the extraction and purification process.

DISORDERS OF FRUCTOSE ABSORPTION

Fructose malabsorption

Many individuals complain of bloating, diarrhoea and flatulence on the ingestion of large quantities of fructose-rich foods. Given that transport of fructose across the mucosal epithelium of the small intestine occurs by facilitated transport rather than by an active carrier transport mechanism, it is easy to see why the capacity for fructose absorption can easily be exceeded, thus inducing a typical carbohydrate intolerance syndrome (see above).[58]

Studies in several patients with long-standing intolerance of dietary fructose indicate an improvement in symptoms after dietary fructose exclusion, suggesting that these patients may suffer from a partial defect of fructose absorption.[58] No evidence for a genetic basis for this disorder has been adduced, but studies using the breath hydrogen test after ingestion of an oral load of 50 g of D-fructose suggested that there may be a physiological basis for fructose-induced gastrointestinal symptoms.[73] Such *in vivo* studies, however, do not control for colonic flora or other physiological variables in the intestinal tract. However, studies in children systematically examined either with glucose or with sucrose or fructose loads suggests that those with symptoms do show excess breath hydrogen when given dietary fructose in the form of undiluted apple juice.[7,40]

One or two cases of possible fructose malabsorption have been studied in more detail, and suggest that there is indeed a mucosal defect in the absorption of fructose by its specific carrier. Clearly the treatment of this complaint will be dependent on clear identification of symptoms and a positive breath hydrogen test after a fructose load. Further studies are indeed required to identify the genetic and molecular basis for the putative fructose

malabsorption syndrome. After evaluation by a breath hydrogen test, a modified diet, in which fructose-rich foods and those containing sorbitol are reduced, should be recommended. Glucose appears to stimulate the absorption of fructose in healthy subjects.[73]

IMPAIRED METABOLISM OF NUTRIENTS

Deficiency of several protein moieties responsible for the *transport of nutrients* and for their *metabolic assimilation* is associated with food intolerance syndromes. The accumulation of metabolic intermediates under these circumstances induces cellular injury and consequential metabolic disturbances that cause symptoms. Disturbances in the metabolic assimilation of dietary fructose and primary or secondary defects in the disposal of amino nitrogen in the urea cycle result in a characteristic syndrome. In the survivors, specific dietary aversions develop. These disorders thus provide vivid examples of interactions between genetic makeup and environmental factors presented in the diet, i.e. sugar or protein.

Metabolism of fructose[19,28,36] (Fig. 25.2)

Fructose 6-phosphate and fructose-1,6-bisphosphate are key intermediates in glycolysis and gluconeogenesis. Fructose, a major dietary nutrient, occurs as the free monosaccharide in fruits, nuts, honey and some vegetables and is released by the hydrolysis of sucrose by α-dextrinase in the brush border membrane of the intestinal mucosa (see foregoing section). Other minor sugars may be converted to fructose but an additional source of fructose is the sugar alcohol sorbitol. Sorbitol, which is often used in diabetic foods and as an excipient in tablets and other medicines, is converted to fructose in the liver and intestine. In these forms, 50–150 g equivalents are ingested daily by most individuals in developed countries.

Absorption of dietary fructose

Fructose present in the intestinal lumen is absorbed rapidly by a carrier mechanism, GLUT5, that facilitates transport across the intestinal epithelium without a requirement for electrochemical energy. The monosaccharide is conveyed via the portal bloodstream to the liver, the principal site of assimilation. The jejunal mucosa and proximal tubule of the kidney are subsidiary sites of metabolism. The metabolic assimilation of fructose requires the combined activities of the enzymes fructokinase (ketohexokinase), aldolase B (liver aldolase) and triokinase, which are specifically expressed in these tissues.

Metabolic assimilation of fructose

Uptake of fructose occurs independently of insulin and its metabolic incorporation involving phosphorylation at the 1-carbon position and thus bypasses regulation of glycolytic fluxes at the level of phosphofructokinase-1. Phosphorylation of free fructose occurs rapidly through the agency of fructokinase, which has a high affinity for its substrate; in tissues not specialized for the assimilation of fructose, hexokinase brings about phosphorylation in the 6-carbon position. The specific pathway for fructose metabolism thereafter involves a specific aldolase isozyme, aldolase B, which has activity towards the fructose-1-phosphatase ester, in contrast to aldolase A (muscle aldolase), whose natural substrate is fructose-1,6-bisphosphate. Cleavage of fructose-1-phosphate generates glyceraldehyde and dihydroxyacetone phosphate which

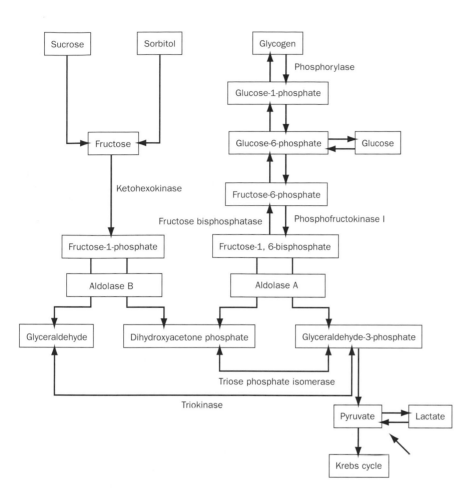

Fig. 25.2 Metabolism of fructose. The interrelation between exogenous sources of fructose and the glycolytic–gluconeogenic intermediary pathways.

enter the intermediary pools of carbohydrate metabolism and, through the agency of triokinase, yield glyceraldehyde-3-phosphate. This allows condensation by aldolase A to form fructose-1-6,bisphosphate, which participates in the gluconeogenic and glycolytic pathways (see Fig. 25.2).

Generation of glucose from lactate, glycerol, amino acids and Krebs cycle intermediates involves the specific hydrolysis of fructose-1,6-bisphosphate by the gluceoneogenic enzyme fructose-1,6-bisphosphatase to yield the glucose precursor fructose-6-phosphate. Fructose-1,6-bisphosphatase is active in the liver, kidney and intestine and is an essential component of the gluconeogenic pathway; it also allows exogenous fructose to serve as the source of glucose or glycogen when the normally thermodynamically favourable reactions of glycolysis are reversed by the concerted action of the sequence of gluconeogenic enzymes, including fructose-1,6-bisphosphatase.

Hereditary fructose intolerance[1,19]

This disorder provides a classical example of the role of enzymatic deficiency in interactions between heredity and the dietary environment. This disorder, first identified in 1956 in an adult, occurs in the UK with an estimated frequency of 1 in 18 000 live births.[37] Hereditary fructose intolerance is inherited as an autosomal recessive defect and first presents during weaning in infancy. However, the clinical disease may not be recognized until late childhood or adult life. The condition is very important because, provided the diagnosis is made before tissue injury is established, introduction of a strict exclusion diet ameliorates the metabolic disturbance and cures the symptoms.

The principal features of the illness are vomiting, diarrhoea and severe upper abdominal pain combined with hypoglycaemia (Table 25.7). These disturbances are induced by the ingestion of foods, drinks or medicines that contain fructose, sucrose or sorbitol. The metabolic disturbance is also characterized by lactic acidosis, hyperuricaemia, hyperkalaemia, hypophosphataemia and hypermagnesaemia. Hypoglycaemia itself causes trembling, irritability and impairment of higher mental functions and consciousness. Attacks are associated with pallor and sweating; severe attacks are associated with generalized convulsions. The attacks occur within 30 min of ingesting the harmful foods or drinks, but continued ingestion of the toxic sugars is associated with the

Principal clinical features of fructose intolerance and fructose-1,6-bisphosphatase deficiency
Vomiting – rejection or distaste for sweet-tasting foods (HFI only)
Diarrhoea
Hypoglycaemia – pallor, sweating, drowsiness, irritability after ingesting noxious foods and drinks
Acidosis
Failure to thrive
Hepatomegaly
Jaundice, wasting, bleeding tendency, aminoaciduria, rickets (in advanced cases)

Table 25.7 Principal clinical features of fructose intolerance and fructose-1,6-bisphosphatase deficiency.

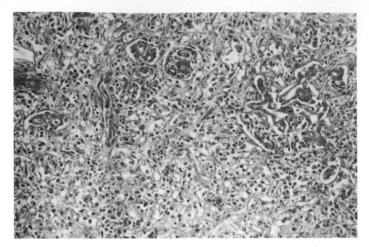

Fig. 25.3 Photomicrograph showing histological appearances of the liver of a 16-year-old patient who suffered acute hepatorenal failure after the accidental infusion of a sorbitol-containing solution following minor surgery in Germany. No surviving hepatic parenchymal cells are present in the specimen; only macrophages, sinusoidal cells and bile duct epithelium remain. The patient died 5 days after the infusion of 100–150 g of fructose equivalents. Retrospective diagnosis of hereditary fructose intolerance was confirmed after molecular analysis of the aldolase B gene obtained from archival tissue and after further investigations of the patient's family. The proposita and one surviving brother had suffered lifelong intolerance of sweet-tasting foods and drinks: subsequently, they were shown to have inherited two null alleles of the aldolase B gene (see Ali *et al. Quart J Med* 1993; 86: 25–30).

development of renal tubular disease, liver injury (with jaundice and coagulopathy), failure to thrive and growth retardation. Liver injury progresses to cirrhosis, coagulopathy and coma associated with marked aminoaciduria[18,28,53] (Fig. 25.3).

The first attack
The first attacks result from the *transfer from breast milk* to artificial feeds containing noxious sugars, and survival of the young infant is dependent on the recognition that certain foods containing fruit or sugar induce the symptoms, including vomiting. In later life, provided the child survives the stormy challenge at the period of weaning, a strong aversion to all sweet-tasting foods as well as vegetables and certain fruits develops. This protects against the more serious effects of fructose and sucrose. The risk of illness related to ingestion of inappropriate foods and drinks remains throughout life; many adults with the condition lack dental caries. Older children and adolescents with hereditary fructose intolerance may survive the stormy period of infancy but develop long-term illness due to the consumption of a low level of fructose and related sugars. Although episodes of symptomatic hypoglycaemia are not apparent, developmental retardation, lack of vigour and hepatosplenomegaly sometimes complicated by renal tubular acidosis with or without rickets due to phosphaturia, occur. At this stage, dietary treatment may improve growth and bring about regression of the other disease manifestations.[50]

Nature of the metabolic disturbance
Aldolase B activity is deficient in the liver, small intestinal mucosa and proximal renal tubular epithelium of patients with hereditary

fructose intolerance; it is these tissues that suffer injury as a result of persistent exposure to fructose. Deficiency of fructose-1-phosphate aldolase activity leads to depletion of the intracellular pool of inorganic phosphate and intracellular sequestration of fructose monoester as demonstrated by studies *in vivo* using ^{31}P magnetic resonance spectroscopy.[28]

Many of the metabolic disturbances induced by a fructose challenge are caused by accumulation of fructose-1-phosphate in a setting where free inorganic phosphate is also reduced. The ubiquitous aldolase A is subject to competitive inhibition and phosphorylase cannot be activated; as a result glycogenolysis and gluconeogenesis are impaired. Thus, hypoglycaemia occurs rapidly and is refractory to the infusion of glucagon or of gluconeogenic metabolites such as glycerol or dihydroxyacetone. Feedback inhibition of fructokinase limits the further incorporation of fructose by the liver and fructosaemia with an attendant fructosuria accompanies the ingestion of fructose. Ultimately, the fructose can be metabolized by adipose tissue and muscle, where it is phosphorylated at the sixth carbon position to fructose-6-phosphate – a reaction catalysed by hexokinase, which has a low affinity for ketosugars (see Fig. 25.2).

Patients with hereditary fructose intolerance who are challenged with fructose develop disturbances of blood electrolytes: hypokalaemia results from acute renal impairment with defective urinary acidification in the proximal tubule; this is accompanied by bicarbonate wasting and acidosis. Serum magnesium concentration may rise acutely as a result of the breakdown of the Mg^{2+} ATP complexes resulting from degradation of ATP by adenosine deaminase, which is itself activated under conditions of intracellular inorganic phosphate depletion. Breakdown of purine nucleotides also results in fructose-induced hyperuricaemia.

Pathology
Continued inadvertent ingestion of fructose and related sugars in patients with hereditary fructose intolerance causes hepatic injury. Histological examination reveals hepatocyte necrosis, with intralobular and periportal fibrosis; there is diffuse fatty change and increased deposition of glycogen.[53] Ultrastructural studies indicate a florid lysosomal reaction to the intracellular deposits of fructose-1-phosphate. Tragic instances have been observed when patients with hereditary fructose intolerance have been infused with fructose or sorbitol intravenously – fructose has now been withdrawn from most parenteral nutrition regimens, but instances are still reported in Germany and German-speaking countries where fructose solutions are still in occasional use[18] (see Fig. 25.3) Parenteral administration of fructose in a patient with hereditary fructose intolerance causes acute hepatorenal failure associated with a bleeding diathesis and widespread hepatic necrosis. This condition is usually fatal but at least one patient has been treated successfully by orthotopic liver transplantation.

The severe upper abdominal pain that accompanies ingestion of fructose and related sugars has never been satisfactorily explained. Stimulation of visceral nerves by local release of lactate (as a result of impaired gluconeogenesis), or by local release of purine degradation products, may be responsible.

Genetics[1,18]
Molecular analysis of the aldolase B gene has revealed numerous mutations responsible for the enzymatic deficiency in hereditary fructose intolerance. Several point mutations affecting the func-

tion of the enzyme occur in several populations and have diagnostic significance, since they may be detected directly by analysis of genomic DNA in samples of blood, buccal mucosal cells or other tissue. The severity of the disease phenotype appears to be independent of the nature of the mutation so far identified. One particular mutation, in which the amino acid alanine at position 149 of the protein is replaced by a proleni residue, is the most frequent mutant allele responsible for hereditary fructose intolerance in populations of European origin. In the UK more than 1% of neonates harbour one copy of this disease allele. There may be a case for introducing neonatal mass screening for this mutation, and certainly there is a case for introducing an investigative profile for molecular lesions in the aldolase B gene to identify persons with hereditary fructose intolerance in whom the diagnosis is suspected (see below).[37]

Diagnosis[70]

In infants and children the occurrence of persistent vomiting, failure to thrive, acidosis, hypoglycaemia and jaundice in association with liver enlargement raises the suspicion of hereditary fructose intolerance. The onset of symptoms at weaning and the effect of sugar-containing foods is very suggestive. A nutritional history paying particular attention to specific feeding difficulties may suggest the diagnosis. A history of postprandial abdominal pain and faintness, particularly in relation to specific foods, may be provided by adults and children with the condition who, on examination, may show little or no evidence of dental caries. Specific dietary preferences may be elicited. The presence of reducing sugar in the urine may also indicate fructosuria, which may be accompanied by aminoaciduria.

Given the severity of the disease, if fructose intolerance is considered then it is prudent to withdraw sucrose, sorbitol and fructose from the diet until diagnostic tests can be conducted. A differential diagnosis includes pyloric stenosis, galactosaemia, hepatitis, renal tubular disease, tyrosinosis and Wilson's disease.[28,70]

Once recovery has occurred, an intravenous fructose tolerance test will provide confirmatory information. This test should be conducted in the presence of medical personnel and involves the infusion of 20% w/v solution of fructose intravenously over 5 min at a total dose of 0.25 g/kg bodyweight (0.2 g/kg bodyweight in young infants). *Note: Given the extreme danger of large doses of parenteral fructose or sorbitol in patients with suspected fructose intolerance, great care must be taken in calculating the dose of fructose to be given in the intravenous fructose tolerance test.* Samples of blood are monitored for potassium, magnesium and phosphate iron concentrations as well as glucose at regular intervals over 2 hours after the infusion. Glucose should be available for a parenteral injection to treat hypoglycaemia, which may ensue in a positive fructose tolerance test. All challenges with fructose or sucrose may produce severe pain and shock and the patient may never return for further studies. A positive fructose tolerance test is given by induction of hypoglycaemia and marked hypophosphataemia within the first hour of infusion. Negative or normal response to fructose infusion at this dosage involves a mild, transitory reduction in phosphate concentrations, with slight rise in blood glucose concentration. In adults, the hypoglycaemic response is usually milder than in young infants and, for this reason, a reduced dose of fructose in the challenge test is recommended in infants.[28,70]

A definitive diagnosis may be obtained by enzymatic analysis of biopsy samples obtained from the liver or small intestinal mucosa. The material has to be frozen fresh for such a study: a biochemical assay demonstrates markedly reduced (<10% of normal) fructose-1-phosphate cleavage activity, with a partial deficiency of fructose-1,6-bisphosphate aldolase activity. Since deficiency of aldolases may accompany other parenchymal diseases of the liver, enzymatic analysis of liver tissue is of limited value in the acutely ill patient. It may be possible to avoid liver biopsy in patients with suspected hereditary fructose intolerance in whom it may be possible to identify mutations in the aldolase B gene by molecular analysis of DNA. Several common mutations responsible for the disease can be screened for by laboratories that specialize in molecular diagnostic work. The importance of a definitive diagnosis cannot be overemphasized, especially in infants at risk, because of the benefit of dietary adjustment before significant exposure to fructose occurs.[28] A definitive diagnosis clearly has implications for other family members, including siblings.

Treatment

The manifestations of hereditary fructose intolerance usually respond completely in the early stages to the withdrawal of sucrose, fructose and sorbitol from the diet[53] (see Table 24.5). All three sugars represent a threat to patients with this condition since sorbitol and sucrose are converted to fructose in the liver and intestine, respectively. The daily consumption of sugar should be reduced to less than 40 mg of fructose equivalent per kg bodyweight, i.e. only 2–3 g for an adult daily compared with the normal of 50 100 times this amount.[50] It has been shown that dietary exclusion of fructose to this level is required for the establishment of normal growth in children affected by hereditary fructose intolerance.

Since fructose and other sugars are almost ubiquitous as components of the Western diet, strict dietary exclusion may present serious difficulties; particular attention is required to exclude fructose present in sugar-coated pills and, especially, drug suspensions formulated for paediatric use which may contain large quantities of toxic sugar. The advice of a professional dietitian may be needed to develop an appropriate diet schedule for a patient with hereditary fructose intolerance and, although patients are occasionally unable to tolerate foods thought to be safe, it is advisable for them to avoid the offending item or to have it analysed. Strict avoidance of fruit and vegetables may lead to a diet deficient in folic acid and vitamin C. Clearly, vitamin supplements are desirable, especially if pregnancy is under consideration in an adult, but care must be taken to avoid harmful sugars contained in vitamin preparations. Ketovite™ (supplied by Paines & Byrne, Surrey, England) provides a satisfactory non-toxic source of these vitamin supplements.

Fructose bisphosphatase deficiency[6,28,36]

Deficiency of this key gluconeogenic enzyme causes an extremely rare, severe metabolic disorder in early infancy. Impaired gluconeogenosis results in metabolic acidosis and fasting hypoglycaemia. Although hypoglycaemia with a fall in organic phosphate concentration may follow administration of fructose in patients with fructose-1,6-bisphosphatase deficiency, there is no abdominal pain and aversion for sweet-tasting foods does not develop. Nonetheless, the condition is frequently fatal and represents a specific food intolerance syndrome; it is inherited as an autosomal recessive trait.

D

Metabolic defect

Failure of gluconeogenesis is due to enzymatic deficiency of fructose-1,6-bisphosphatase in the liver, intestinal mucosa and kidney.[6] The muscle isozyme of fructose-1,6-bisphosphatase is unaffected but, unlike hereditary fructose intolerance, the enzymatic defect may be identified in cultured mononuclear cells from peripheral blood.

Between meals, glucose homeostasis is maintained by glycogenolysis and the onset of symptoms in fructose bisphosphatase deficiency is, therefore, dependent on the stores of hepatic glycogen. During infections and other febrile illnesses, particularly those with diminished food intake, liver glycogen may be depleted. Such intercurrent illnesses frequently precipitate episodes of acidosis in patients with fructose bisphosphatase deficiency. This is accompanied by hypoglycaemia that is unresponsive to glucagon and is associated with exhaustion of the glycogen stores. Infusion of fructose, sorbitol, dihydroxyacetone and amino acid solutions only aggravates the acidosis and hypoglycaemia.

It appears, as in fructose intolerance, that the accumulation of phosphorylated sugar intermediates that cannot be further metabolized in this disorder, associated with reduced intracellular free inorganic phosphate, leads to a secondary defect of glycogenolysis, so that the hypoglycaemia is unresponsive to glucagon. Failure to utilize glucogenic amino acids as well as ketone bodies and glycerol leads to lactic acidosis hypophosphataemia, hyperuricaemia and hypoglycaemia. Triglyceride formation in the liver is increased, leading to hepatic steatosis. Neither renal tubular acidosis nor hepatic failure develop in fructose bisphosphatase deficiency.

Diagnosis

The diagnosis is suggested in newborn infants with severe metabolic disturbances characterized by acidotic hyperventilation, irritability, disturbed consciousness or coma. There is an unusual combination of ketonaemia, lactic acidaemia and hypoglycaemia induced by fasting as well as the administration of fructose, sorbitol, glycerol or by the ingestion of a diet enriched in fat.[54] Deterioration is often associated with episodes of infection and it is the combination of ketosis and lactic acidosis with hypoglycaemia which signals the gluconeogenesis. The differential diagnosis includes deficiency of glucose-6-phosphatase, pyruvate carboxylase, pyruvate dehydrogenase and phosphoenol pyruvate carboxykinase. The absence of abdominal distress, haemolysis, jaundice, coagulopathy and renal tubular disorders helps to differentiate the condition from hereditary fructose intolerance, Wilson's disease and tyrosinosis. The condition may be confused with disorders of long-, medium- and short-chain acyl coenzyme A dehydrogenase activities as well as defects of carnitine metabolism since these may be associated with secondary defects in gluconeogenesis.

Biochemical analysis of urine, and plasma samples show lactate, pyruvate and ketone bodies as well as other organic acids; glycerol excretion may be prominent because of the failure to convert this during starvation to glucose. This may suggest the diagnosis of fructose-1,6-bisphosphatase deficiency in some individuals. A definitive diagnosis is dependent on the demonstration of the enzyme defect in the tissue biopsy sample, particularly of the liver, which also allows other metabolic disorders and gluconeogenic defects to be excluded with confidence.[6] The enzyme defect may also be demonstrated in biopsy samples of jejunal mucosa and in cultured mononuclear cells obtained from peripheral blood; it is unusual, however, for the primary diagnosis in a propositus to be identified by these means, and biochemical analysis of liver tissue by an experienced metabolic biochemical laboratory is the usual pathway to the diagnosis.

Treatment and progress[28]

The severity of this disorder is such that a first affected infant may succumb from acidosis before the diagnosis can be made. However, the response to correct dietary management is favourable and the disorder is compatible with a benign course and restoration of normal growth.

Avoidance of starvation and prompt treatment of infections is as important as dietary adjustment. Attacks of acidosis should be managed with the early introduction of intravenous glucose therapy; parenteral infusions of bicarbonate may be required in severe cases. Breast milk, which is rich in lactose, is readily assimilated but difficulties may arise on transfer to artificial feeds during weaning. Sorbitol, sucrose and fructose must be strictly avoided, since these do aggravate hypoglycaemia in patients with fructose bisphosphatase deficiency (see Table 25.5). Dietary fats should be reduced and a diet containing 56% calories as carbohydrate with 32% calories as fat and 12% as protein has allowed normal growth and metabolic control to be established in patients with this disorder. Emphasis should be placed on the avoidance of fasting by the use of frequent meals containing appropriate carbohydrate supplements.[54]

PRIMARY AND SECONDARY UREA CYCLE DEFECTS: PROTEIN INTOLERANCE SYNDROMES[13,18]

Amino acids released during digestion in excess of requirements for protein synthesis are used as a source of energy: the carbon frameworks are degraded to either gluconeogenic intermediates (glucogenic amino acids) or ketone bodies (ketogenic amino acids). The amino groups are released for metabolic incorporation into urea, which is the principal form in which excess nitrogen is excreted. The ammonium ion (NH^+_4) is not the only source of waste nitrogen, since the α-amino nitrogen of aspartate (derived by transamination reactions from other amino acids) also provides nitrogen for the synthesis of urea. Deamination reactions, principally in the liver but also in the intestine and kidneys, provide a source of ammonium ions. Five enzymes participate in the catalytic cycle that leads to the net synthesis of urea from CO_2 (bicarbonate ions) and ammonia (ammonium ions) as well as aspartate (Fig. 25.4).

The mitochondrial matrix enzyme, carbamoyl phosphate synthase I catalyses the formation of the first committed precursor of the urea synthesis, carbamoyl phosphate from ammonium and bicarbonate ions. This enzyme is subject to allosteric regulation by N-acetyl glutamine; this reaction requires two molecules of ATP and is highly energy-dependent. Ornithine combines with carbamoyl phosphate in a reaction catalysed by ornithine transcarbamoylase (OTC) to form citrulline which also takes place within the mitochondrion. After extrusion into the cytosol, citrulline combines with aspartate under the influence of arginosuccinate synthase to form arginosuccinate, which is cleaved by arginosuccinate lyase to release fumarate and arginine. Arginase in the cytosol cleaves arginine to release urea and regenerate

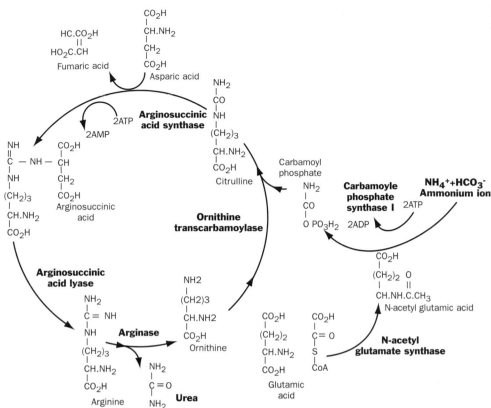

Fig. 25.4 The urea cycle, showing the disposal of ammonium ions.

ornithine, which can subsequently be taken up into the mitochondrion by a specific transporter, once again to combine with carbamoyl phosphate in the cyclic mechanism. Excess carbamoyl phosphate can be converted to the pyrimidine precursor, orotate, thus bypassing carbamoyl phosphate synthase II.

Clinical presentation[13]

All the defects are recessively transmitted inborn errors, but OTC is inherited as an X-linked trait in which disease expression may be observed in heterozygous females.[60] Deficiencies of four of the five enzymatic steps of the urea cycle have identical presentations, characterized by a neonatal hyperammonaemia syndrome after the first feeds. Intrauterine growth and metabolism are normal as a result of maternal urea disposal, but an encephalopathy associated with cerebral oedema and astrocyte swelling (attributed to intracellular accumulation of glutamine) results from ingestion of the first protein meal.

Milder enzymatic defects may be associated with presentations in infancy and childhood or even adult life, with episodic changes of mental status including behavioural abnormalities, lethargy and cognitive impairment. In the milder forms of four urea cycle defects – OTC deficiency, carbamoyl phosphate synthase deficiency, arginosuccinate synthase deficiency and arginosuccinic acid lyase deficiency – treatment is very challenging. It is not only necessary to reduce protein intake but also to improve the disposal of ammonium ions that prevent excess protein catabolism associated with febrile illnesses and starvation. Survivors of the neonatal period suffer profound intellectual impairment and other neurological damage. Complicity with dietary management and ingestion of ammonia-scavenging agents, including gram amounts of the distasteful phenyl acetate or phenyl butyrate (with or without benzoic acid), is limited. However, heterozygous females

with OTC deficiency and individuals with urea cycle defects in childhood or adult life presenting with episodic hyperammonaemic encephalopathy may show only trivial mental disturbances between attacks.

The first episode

The first episodes may be manifest at the time of weaning from breast milk or on conversion from the low-protein milk formulas, including breast milk, to cow's milk. Milder episodes may result from intercurrent infections of febrile episodes, often in combination with fasting. Patients with late-onset urea cycle defects, associated drowsiness, headache and malaise as well as disturbances of consciousness with the ingestion of protein-rich foods particularly those containing meat, fish or eggs involuntarily select low-protein foods from a vegetarian base. Slow onset of hyperammonaemia leads to neurological impairment, disorientation, ataxia, irritability and occasionally seizures, and this can lead to great difficulties in diagnosis.[8] An adult onset is recorded in all the urea cycle disorders but is particularly common in women heterozygous for defects in the OTC gene.

The restriction of protein intake occurs at a subconscious level: preliminary studies conducted in asymptomatic heterozygous carriers showed excretion of only 70% of the urinary nitrogen compared with their unaffected female relatives, thus indicating the degree to which a spontaneous restriction in protein intake occurs.

Arginase deficiency

The clinical features of deficiency of the last enzyme of the urea cycle, arginase, are quite distinct. This enzyme is expressed specifically in erythroid cells and in the liver. The disease presents with a distinct neurological syndrome including spastic quadriparesis, growth failure, epilepsy and psychomotor retardation.

Hyperammonaemia is less marked than with the other defects and although hyperammonaemic coma may result from heavy ingestion of protein foods, especially after prolonged fasting or infection, the principal manifestations relate to progressive neurological disease in early childhood. The explanation for this is quite unknown. Children with arginosuccinic acid lyase deficiency show a characteristic defect of their cranial hair – trichorrhexis nodosa – which appears to be unique to this disorder.

Pathology

In children dying from hyperammonaemic coma, cerebral oedema with astrocytic changes in the cortex and brain stem are observed as in any hyperammonaemic syndrome. Occasionally, neuronal abnormalities develop. Measurement of plasma ammonia concentrations is useful diagnostically and certainly correlates with the degree of coma observed. In carbamoyl phosphate synthase deficiency and OTC deficiency, plasma ammonia may be elevated 20–30 times above normal (approximately 40 µmol/l). Citrulline is greatly elevated in arginosuccinic acid synthase deficiency and arginosuccinic acid lyase deficiency is normal or low in the other defects. Plasma arginine is greatly elevated in arginase deficiency but low in the other defects.

Molecular defects have been described in all of the human genes encoding the urea cycle enzymes. Most mutations appear to be private, but molecular analysis of the implicated genes may benefit affected families who request antenatal diagnosis. Attempts have been made to introduce neonatal screening for urea cycle defects by the analysis of urinary orotic acid. The role of neonatal screening in the outcome of rare urea cycle defects has yet to be demonstrated. Nonetheless, vigilant suspicion of the diagnosis in full-term newborn infants that develop lethargy, vomiting, hypothermia and hyperventilation in the first few days of birth may have a critical influence on outcome. Of key importance has been the study of pedigrees affected by OTC deficiency – a sex-linked disorder. Such studies are based on pedigree analysis and subsequent biochemical testing of possible female heterozygotes. Many female heterozygotes who are asymptomatic for orinithine OTC deficiency excrete excess orotic acid and have greatly elevated plasma glutamine levels. Further exclusion of heterozygosity for a mutation at the OTC locus, once an index case has been identified in the pedigree, involves challenge with the agent allopurinol. The allopurinol challenge test has now replaced the outdated protein tolerance test, where a high protein meal is administered to carriers. Not only may this induce hyperammonaemia but is often unacceptable to asymptomatic carriers who have unconsciously reduced their consumption of protein-rich foods considerably throughout life. In the allopurinol test administration of a test dose of allopurinol induces increased excretion of orotidine and orotic acid and has a high sensitivity in known OTC heterozygotes.

Enzymatic analysis of liver samples remains the principal means for definitive diagnosis once hyperammonaemia and plasma amino acid and citrulline levels have been determined. Electroencephalographic changes in hyperammonaemic coma show specific slow-wave appearances that correlate with plasma ammonia concentrations and clinical status.

Treatment[13]

Treatment of the acute hyperammonaemic syndrome presenting in the neonatal period needs only cursory description here.

Diagnostic delays are catastrophic for ultimate outcome. There is evidence that elevation of plasma glutamine occurs before frank hyperammonaemia and may thus have predictive value for patient monitoring during risk periods.

Diet

The overall goal of therapy is to provide a diet sufficiently rich in arginine and protein and energy to allow growth and normal development while minimizing hyperammonaemic disturbances (Table 25.8). Thus, nitrogen intake should be reduced to the minimum by providing low-protein diets in combination with essential amino acids. However, if amino acid intake is insufficient to maintain slightly positive nitrogen balance, protein degradation will exceed protein synthesis and growth failure will occur with intermittent overproduction of ammonium ions for disposal through the urea pathway. In arginosuccinic acid lyase deficiency, attempts can be made to maximize the disposal of nitrogen by promoting excretion of arginosuccinic acid itself by provision of excess arginine. Studies in patients indicate that neither high-dose arginine therapy nor high-plasma arginosuccinate are toxic. Indeed, the hair abnormality of arginosuccinic acid lyase deficiency may be corrected by arginine supplementation. Arginosuccinic acid synthase deficiency may be treated by exploiting citrulline as a waste product for disposal of nitrogen. Supplementation also with phenyl butyrate allows disposal of glutamine nitrogen in the adduct phenyl acetyl glutamine and citrulline synthesis may be stimulated also by provision of supplements of arginine. Carbamoyl phosphate synthase and OTC deficiency require supplementation with citrulline, which serves as a source of arginine, provision of benzoate complexes serine- and glycine-derived nitrogen in the form of urinary hippurate. At the same time, phenyl acetate and phenyl butyrate can be utilized for disposal of glutamine nitrogen.

Mildly affected patients with urea cycle defects of late onset can often be controlled by dietary means alone, but the addition of phenyl butyrate has been found to provide an additional pathway for nitrogen excretion. Balance studies indicate that net urea nitrogen synthesis is suppressed.

Treatment of arginase deficiency

Despite dietary and pharmacological measures, patients with urea cycle defects remain at risk from episodes of life-threatening hyperammonaemia, and vigilance is required to reduce their frequency. Arginase deficiency appears to be very difficult to treat, but reduction in plasma arginine levels results from restriction of protein intake and the addition of sodium benzoate and high-

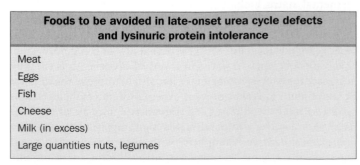

Foods to be avoided in late-onset urea cycle defects and lysinuric protein intolerance
Meat
Eggs
Fish
Cheese
Milk (in excess)
Large quantities nuts, legumes

Table 25.8 Foods to be avoided in late-onset urea cycle defects and lysinuric protein intolerance.

dose phenyl butyrate. Adjustment and monitoring of dietary control and use of agents to activate other pathways of waste nitrogen excretion is a specialized area of metabolic medicine, the conduct of which requires intensive expertise. The reader is referred to contemporary protocols as a guide to therapy.[13] The late-onset urea cycle disorders represent a classical problem in the field of food intolerance syndromes and their management requires attention to many aspects of human metabolism.

Lysinuric protein intolerance[68]

This represents an intermediate syndrome caused by a primary defect of membrane transport with secondary enzymatic deficiencies leading to features of a urea cycle disorder. Lysinuric protein intolerance is a rare autosomal recessive disorder with a high frequency in Finns. The disorder is manifest as a familial protein intolerance syndrome with deficient transport of basic amino acids, leading to functional deficiency of the key catalytic urea cycle intermediates arginine and ornithine. Ingestion of high-protein foods leads to a classical hyperammonaemic presentation. Other unexplained features include respiratory deficiency, membraneous or mesangeal proliferative glomerulonephritis, liver injury leading to cirrhosis, hypertension and osteoporosis.[15,55,56,68]

Underlying defect

There is functional deficiency of a cationic amino acid transporter for the amino acids ornithine, lysine and arginine in the proximal renal tubular and upper intestinal mucosa; minor defects of cystine transport occur.[56] Mutations in a gene, mapping to chromosome 14q 11.2, designated SLC 7A7 (member 7 of solute carrier family 7) have been identified in Finnish and non-Finish patients with this disease. The gene encodes a transporter subunit with the expected efflux properties for cationic amino acid and influx of neutral amino acids (with sodium) when expressed in Xenopus oocytes.[68] Analysis of plasma shows deficiency of these amino acids but increased concentrations of citrulline, arginine and glutamine. Urine clearance of lysine is greatly increased with less conspicuous excretion of ornithine and arginine. The primary transport defect in the intestine leads to plasma concentrations of lysine and arginine that fail to rise after ingestion of the lysine load because of the failure of transport to cross the basolateral rather than the brush border membrane of the intestinal epithelium. A similar defect has been identified in the renal tubule. Because of an inability to transfer ornithine across the mitochondrial membrane to participate in the urea cycle, a secondary hyperammonaemia and orotic aciduria occurs, with decreased tolerance of dietary protein.

Clinical presentation

Most infants present within the neonatal period after a normal pregnancy. They usually remain well while being fed on human breast milk, which has a relatively low protein content. On weaning or on transfer to cow's milk or formula feeds, there is a failure to thrive, delayed growth with hypotonia and postprandial vomiting. On occasion, the diagnosis may be delayed until school age or adult life.[66] Dietary-induced hyperammonaemia causes headache, malaise, confusion, ataxia and disturbances of consciousness. In childhood, the affected individual rapidly recognizes the relationship between protein-rich foods and the development of hyperammonaemic episodes. Spontaneously, the development of food aversions reduces the overall intake of non-essential protein nitrogen.

Protein restriction largely improves the hyperammonaemia. There may be difficulties in sustaining sufficient calorie intake to secure normal growth; moreover, protein restriction does not correct the deficiency of cationic amino acids, particularly lysine.[60] It may be that lysine deficiency contributes to collagen instability and ultimately to osteoporosis.[15] Supplementation with citrulline, which is absorbed through the activity of a carrier system distinct from that responsible for the transfer of cationic amino acids, provides a source of ornithine and arginine and lowers plasma ammonia.

Associated disorders

Survival through childhood to adult life is not without coincidental illnesses, including alveolar proteinosis (which may respond to oral prednisone), severe respiratory failure and unexplained glomerulonephritis, which may lead to renal failure, hypertension and cirrhosis.[60,68] The explanation for these complications is not obvious, but it is possible that deficiency of arginine, a key substrate for the synthesis of nitric oxide, reduces the capacity of macrophages to mount effective inflammatory and immune responses which are dependent on their complement of inducible nitric oxide synthase.

Treatment

Protein restriction and oral citrulline (5–10 g per day) may be supplemented[15] during acute hyperammonaemic crises with intravenous glucose and sodium benzoate. Phenyl butyrate will also stimulate alternative pathways of nitrogen disposal.

OTHER ENZYME DEFICIENCIES ASSOCIATED WITH DIETARY TOXICITY

Favism: deficiency of glucose-6-phosphate dehydrogenase[43]

The observation that Black American soldiers developed an acute haemolytic syndrome when treated with the prophylactic antimalarial agent primaquine led to the discovery of genetic variants of the red cell enzyme, glucose-6-phosphate dehydrogenase (G6PD).[16] This enzyme catalyses the oxidation of glucose-6-phosphate to 6-phosphogluconate with the generation of reduced NADP – the first reaction in the oxidation of glucose by the pentose phosphate pathway. Glucose-6-phosphate dehydrogenase thus maintains a high intracellular concentration of the reduced co-enzyme NADPH that is required for the maintenance of reduced glutathione. When G6DP-deficient individuals receive primaquine or other oxidizing agents, haemolysis occurs, associated with free radical-mediated intracorpuscular damage and Heinz body formation. The haemolytic response thus represents an intrinsic red cell abnormality.[5]

Malaria and fava beans

Glucose-6-phosphate dehydrogenase is encoded by a gene that maps to the X-chromosome. Thus, deficiency states which may show themselves in the form of chronic haemolysis, neonatal jaundice or favism (see below) occur particularly in men – although homozygous females occur with appreciable frequency in many ethnic groups. The disorder occurs particularly in those members of the population that have had an environmental exposure to malaria for which G6PD deficiency appears to exert a protective effect. Although many drugs besides primaquine induce haemolysis in G6PD-deficient individuals, it is also recognized that an acute haemolytic anaemia follows the ingestion of fava beans, which are widespread in the diet of the peoples of Italy, North Africa and the Middle East and Greece. Thus, favism is a classical example of an inherited enzymatic deficiency associated with a phenotype that is conditioned strictly by the nutritional environment. Fava beans are a critical factor, but favism occurs solely in individuals with an inherited deficiency of the enzyme in their red cells.

Pathogenesis[4]

Favism results from the ingestion of the broad bean or fava bean (*Vicia faba*). Extensive studies indicate that the active principles are the pyrimidine aglycones divicine and isouramil that appear to exert their toxicity in combination with ascorbic acid. After ingestion, the parent glycosides present in the beans are acted upon by β-glycosidases present in the membrane of the upper small intestinal mucosa (see above). Release of the active principle is dependent upon absorption and exposure to circulating erythrocytes in the bloodstream.[4] Many determinants, including composition of the beans and individual factors including physiological conditions in the gastrointestinal tract as well as the amount and composition of the individual beans, appear to determine the extent of the haemolytic damage. However, in the full-blown case there is a sudden onset of haemolytic anaemia within 48 hours of ingestion. Haemoglobinuria, pallor and jaundice occur as a result of intravascular haemolysis. The anaemia may be severe and acute renal failure may occur. Blood transfusion may be required, especially in affected children. Favism typically occurs after ingestion of fresh, young broad beans but has been recorded after eating dried or frozen beans even in male infants who have been breast-fed by a mother who has ingested appreciable quantities of the bean.

Favism appears to be most common in male children between the ages of 2 and 6 years, but it has been recorded in girls and it is well documented that heterozygous females may be affected although the haemolysis is generally milder. This occurs because of the lyonization and presence in the individual heterozygous female of two populations of erythrocytes, those expressing G6PD and those deficient in the enzyme as a result of the inactivation of the wild-type X-linked allele in the progenitor erythroid cell.

Mechanism of haemolysis

Historical studies indicate that favism has been recorded since classical times and the stricture issued by Pythagorus in the second century BC against the dangers of eating fava beans may well owe its origin to early observations of the frequent incidence of toxicity. The demonstration in Italy that patients with favism have a severe deficiency of erythrocyte G6PD quickly followed the original studies that demonstrated this enzymatic deficiency as the basis of primaquine-induced haemolysis. Although for many years it was suspected that haemolysis that accompanied favism resulted from chemical injury due to the presence of a toxin in the beans, it was many years before isouramil and divicine were identified as the agents in which the toxicity was invested.[17] It appears that the isouramil and glutathione interact to form a semiquinone with the release of superoxide. Further oxidation of glutathione occurs, so that superoxide dismutase is used to generate hydrogen peroxide in the disposal of the oxygen free radical. Hydrogen peroxide in turn oxidizes more glutathione via glutathione peroxidase, thus leading to overall intracorpuscular depletion of reduced glutathione.[25,74] In this setting there is no defence against the oxidation of haemoglobin, which becomes denatured to form the Heinz bodies characteristic of the condition and ultimately results in the lysis of the red cell that characterizes the attack.[4,5]

Clearly, many components are involved in maintaining the steady state of reduced glutathione in red cells and other factors may influence the release of the toxic aglycones but *in vitro* studies demonstrate even in normal erythrocytes exposure to isouramil and divicine induces a profound, although transient, deficiency of reduced glutathione. In G6PD-deficient erythrocytes, however, the effect is prolonged. However, this indicates that the enzyme is essential for the recovery of reduced glutathione after its consumption by a glutathione peroxidase – itself consequent upon the action of superoxide dismutase, which produces the hydrogen peroxide intermediate.

Genetics

Glucose-6-phosphate dehydrogenase maps to the tip of the X-chromosome at Xq28. Since X-inactivation occurs at this site, heterozygous females express two red cell populations as a result of lyonization; in them, the G6PD-deficient red cells are as susceptible to oxidative damage as are the universally deficient erythrocytes of a hemizygous male carrying a mutant G6PD allele on the only expressed X-chromosome. Since favism occurs in heterozygous females, it is not strictly correct to state that favism behaves as an X-linked recessive condition since there is clear expression in the heterozygous female.

The human G6PD locus is the most polymorphic genetic locus outside the human leucocyte antigen (HLA) region in humans. Many hundred variants of G6PD, resulting from mutations in the structural gene, have been identified and characterized by molecular analysis of the gene. Glucose-6-phosphate dehydrogenase deficiency results from extreme genetic heterogeneity, with the existence of numerous mutant alleles at the same locus. Many alleles are associated with favism. Most G6PD-deficient individuals are technically susceptible to favism, providing the additional dietary component related to the ingestion of fava beans is present.

The almost certain evolutionary advantage of G6PD deficiency in heterozygous females that results in favourable selection in environments where malaria is prevalent thus has other consequences, including the dietary idiosyncrasy, favism. Many of the defined G6PD variants are indeed known to be involved in the development of favism, but in practice the regions with the highest prevalence of favism are currently Greece, Italy (including Sardinia and Sicily), Israel, the Middle East and South-East Asia. Individuals of African origin in countries where fava beans are popular also are at risk from favism if they are G6PD-deficient.[26]

Prevention and treatment[43]

Full-blown favism is a medical emergency and requires meticulous attention to fluid balance, with prompt use of transfusion and the avoidance of precipitating drugs and fava beans.[25] Health education programmes in Sardinia linked to mass neonatal screening for G6PD deficiency appear to have been promising in reducing the frequency of severe favism on that island. Although blood transfusion is the primary therapeutic instrument, it has been suggested that treatment with the iron-chelating drug desferrioxamine as a single intravenous bolus may reduce the consequential effects of free radical-mediated erythrocyte injury. It probably interferes with iron-dependent formation of further oxidant radicals, such as hydroxyl ions, that may be formed in glutathione-depleted cells in which superoxide formation is stimulated.

A list of drugs that should be forbidden to patients who have had favism is provided in Table 25.9. Although the severity of the

Drugs that precipitate haemolysis in patients with glucose-6-phosphate dehydrogenase deficiency
Primaquine
Nitrofurantoin
Sulfonamides, including Dapsone and co-trimoxazole
Quinolone antimicrobials, e.g. ciprofloxacin, norfloxacin
Aspirin (large doses)
Chloroquine, quinine, quinidine (can be used in acute malaria)
Water-soluble vitamin K analogues
Probenecid

Table 25.9 Drugs that precipitate haemolysis in patients with glucose-6-phosphate dehydrogenase deficiency.

haemolytic reaction upon eating fava beans is very variable and some G6PD-deficient individuals appear to be able to eat some preparations of fava beans without serious consequences, this insensitivity is not constant. Clearly, inter-individual factors as well as variation in the content of the toxic component in the particular preparations of bean always pose a risk to the G6PD-deficient subject.[4,25] On the whole, therefore, it is wise to recommend a complete dietary exclusion of fava beans and their derivatives, cooked or uncooked, for affected families.

Diagnosis

The diagnosis of favism depends on a suspicious history and may be confirmed by either the direct slide test for G6PD deficiency or by formal measurement of G6PD activity in red cells. Corrections may have to be made during recovery from a haemolytic episode, since young red cells have a proportionately greater activity of G6PD than senescent erythrocytes. These issues are well dealt with in the diagnostic haematological literature.[43] It has been suggested that all newborn infants in endemic areas at risk should be screened for G6PD deficiency and that dietary advice should be provided to the parents of male hemizygotes and most female heterozygotes, particularly in relation to exposure to fava beans.

ACUTE (HEPATIC) PORPHYRIAS – DISORDERS OF HAEM BIOSYNTHESIS[51]

Porphyria is caused by inherited defects in the pathway of haem biosynthesis due to inherited single enzyme defects of the nine catalysed steps that lead to the production of ferroprotohaem: deficiency of eight enzymes leads to clinical porphyria, while deficiency of four causes acute neurovisceral attacks.[52] Since the haem biosynthetic pathway in erythroid cells and hepatic cells is subject to feedback regulation, partial deficiency of any of the enzymatic steps leads to the overproduction of the preceding metabolic intermediates – these porphyrin and haem precursors appear in the blood, urine and occasionally stool where they may be detected and thus contribute to diagnosis. It cannot be overemphasized that between attacks, these biochemical abnormalities may be undetectable.

Acute porphyrias

The acute porphyria syndromes are important because the attacks may be very severe and are induced by many commonly pre-

scribed drugs as well as fasting, ingestion of alcohol and typically during periods of rapidly changing reproductive hormone secretion, especially at puberty and during pregnancy. Although the syndromes are principally induced by drugs or may occur spontaneously, especially in women as a result of hormonal influences, the porphyrias are described here because an awareness of the drug hazard is important in their management. However, in the context of food allergy and intolerance there is an additional purpose: recently, some advocates have put forward porphyria as a form of generalized sensitivity syndrome to many chemicals, medications and environmental agents, including those that occur at work, scents and newsprint. It has been suggested that individuals who bitterly complain of chronic fatigue syndrome or of the *multiple chemical sensitivity* syndrome are indeed patients with unrecognized latent porphyria. In most cases, however, the proposed relationship between an acute porphyric attack and the multiple chemical sensitivity syndrome has not been supported by scrupulous laboratory tests.[33]

'Devonshire colic'

Despite the reservations given above it is clear that many toxic substances can alter flux through the haem biosynthetic pathway, leading to porphyria. Lead poisoning is a well-known example and since the 18th century has been recognized as a cause of severe abdominal symptoms and psychological disturbance in those who ingest cider stored in vessels containing lead glaze.[31,75] The Royal Physician Sir Henry Baker was the first to recognize cider as a source of lead poisoning in 'Devonshire colic'. Furthermore, in the 1960s, another environmental toxin induced a porphyric syndrome. This was hexachlorabenzene, which induced epidemic porphyria cutanea tarda (a non-neurovisceral form of porphyria) in Turkish villages where wheat exposed to the insecticide was consumed as food instead of being sown as a potential crop.[63]

Genetic transmission

In most instances the acute porphyrias are inherited as dominant traits with partial expression in the heterozygote carrier. Only about 10% of individuals carry a single mutant gene for acute intermittent porphyria (porphobilinogen deaminase deficiency[29]); hereditary coproporphyria (coproporphyrinogen III oxidase deficiency[47]) and variegate porphyria (protoporphyrinogen IX oxidase deficiency[39]) suffer acute attacks – they are thus described as suffering from *latent porphyria*. However, the acute neurovisceral symptoms that develop in aminolaevulinic acid dehydratase deficiency – the most rare form of acute porphyria – arise principally in homozygotes or compound heterozygotes from missense mutations in the δ-aminolaevulinate dehydratase gene.[61] There is some evidence, however, that the more common heterozygotes for δ-aminolaevulinate dehydratase deficiency show increased susceptibility to environmental lead toxicity.

Clinical presentations[52]

Neurovisceral manifestations of acute hepatic porphyrias include vomiting, neuralgic pain in the legs and upper arms and neuropathic features usually exacerbated by mental strain, starvation, alcohol use or decreased food intake. Constipation is the rule and abdominal pain, often colicky but without any abdominal signs, develops rapidly. The patient may become confused, alienated or extremely anxious. In about 10% of individuals with acute porphyric attacks, seizures occur and present a major difficulty for

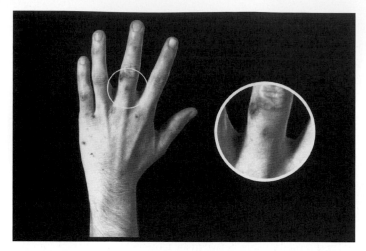

Fig. 25.5 Variegate porphyria. The hands of a 30-year-old woman suffering from recurrent disabling attacks of abdominal pain, mental confusion and neuralgia are shown. She had noticed continued blistering of the extremities on exposure to light, even through glass windows. Marked facial hirsutes was present and increased hair can be seen on the dorsum of the hands and wrist: the diagnosis of protoporphyrinogen IX oxidase deficiency was made on the basis of urine, stool and plasma porphyrin analysis.

treatment, since most accepted anticonvulsant drugs are highly porphyrinogenic and severely aggravate the condition. In two of the acute porphyrias – hereditary coproporphyria and the more frequent variegate porphyria that is prevalent in South Africa – skin photosensitivity occurs as a result of overproduction of photoactive porphyrins. These porphyrins circulate in the plasma and bind to skin components, characteristically causing light-sensitive bullous eruptions with pain, local hirsutes and increased skin fragility (Fig. 25.5). The appearance of such skin lesions in exposed areas may provide an important diagnostic clue to the cause of recurrent abdominal pain in a porphyric subject.

Many of the other manifestations of acute porphyria reflect changes in autonomic tone and have been ascribed to an autonomic neuropathy: hypertension is frequent and in the acute attack tachycardia and excessive sweating are prominent features. Careful studies have revealed clinical signs of disturbed autonomic innervation, especially in terms of abnormal cardiovascular reflexes. Ultimately a peripheral neuropathy, with striking asymmetrical weakness, may occur, and is usually reflected in distal muscle weakness with foot drop or wrist drop. The cranial nerves may be affected. Sensory changes tend to be milder, with areas of parasthesiae or loss of sensation. *Psychiatric symptoms* are complex and involve anxiety, sleeplessness, hallucinations, agitation and sometimes frank paranoia. Many relatives of patients with acute porphyria who are latent carriers have been identified in psychiatric institutions. Further evidence of an acute autonomic neuropathy is shown by rapid onset of hyponatraemia, which is due to inappropriate secretion of antidiuretic hormone and may be severe. Management of hyponatraemia in the acute porphyric attack may be in conflict with the use of parenteral glucose solutions to suppress the overproduction of haem precursors.

Pathogenesis
The cause of the neurovisceral symptoms in the acute porphyrias is not clear. Direct neurotoxicity has been invoked. Suggestion has been that aminolaevulinic acid has a similar 5-carbon chain

structure to the inhibitory neurotransmitter γ-aminobutyric acid as well as the excitatory neurotransmitter L-glutamate.[49] Contemporary studies of the action of clinical concentrations of aminolaevulinic acid on nervous tissue are lacking. The other principal hypothesis for the effects of porphyria is that many of the consequences of the attack result from a critical deficiency of haem proteins, including cytochromes and tryptophan dioxygenase. It is not clear, however, whether neuronal haem deficiency actually occurs, even though studies in whole patients indicate elevated blood levels of tryptophan and 5-hydroxytryptamine in patients with acute intermittent porphyria; these abnormalities reverted on repletion with haem arginate infusions. It seems likely that some of the psychiatric manifestations of porphyria, especially those in the central autonomic nervous system with central effects on mood, result from increased serotoninergic activity. The recent generation of a genetically modified mouse as a first animal model of an acute hepatic porphyria due to porphobilinogen deaminase deficiency promises to address some of the questions as to the pathogenesis of acute porphyric attacks.[49,51]

Diagnosis
Diagnosis of acute porphyria is dependent on suspicious clinical features.[29,39,51,52,61] There is often a family history of unexplained neurovisceral attacks occurring under conditions known to provoke the acute porphyric syndrome. It is critically important to realise, however, that between attacks of porphyria there may be no clinical abnormalities and, in particular, *no* abnormal excretion of porphyrins or other haem precursors in urine or stool. In many instances, patients with acute porphyric syndromes overproduce porphobilinogen (in lead poisoning and δ-aminolaevulinate dehydratase deficiency, this does not occur). Use of Ehrlich's aldehyde reagent provides a simple screening test for porphobilinogen excess and a positive result with the development of the cherry-red diazo adduct which is insoluble in organic solvents, unlike that of urobilinogen, provides good evidence for overproduction of porphyrins in the suspected case (Fig. 25.6). Specific confirmatory and quantitative tests of aminolaevulinate and porphobilinogen are required in the urine and further studies of stool and blood porphyrins may confirm the pattern of porphyrin excretion in biochemically manifest porphyrias. Later, specific enzymatic and molecular analysis of the appropriate gene can be carried out for the presence of *de novo* mutations and, ultimately, for diagnostic screening in first-degree relatives at risk.

Management[52]
The mainstay of treatment of acute porphyria is the avoidance of precipitating factors such as starvation, diverse drugs (including anaesthetic agents and hormones) and alcohol – a dietary constituent in many cultures (Table 25.10). Psychological stress, infections and pregnancy also predispose to acute attacks. In pedigrees affected by acute porphyria, identification of latent carriers of disease who are at risk is critical for the strategic avoidance of precipitating factors. In the acute attack, vigorous administration of carbohydrate improves outcome and suppresses the overproduction of putatively toxic biosynthetic intermediates. Intravenous or enteral supplements of >400 g glucose equivalents daily is required – parenteral administration of D-glucose solutions may be dangerous, however, in patients with acute hyponatraemia as a result of established inappropriate secretion of antidiuretic hormone since it may induce fatal cerebral oedema. In severe porphyric attacks,

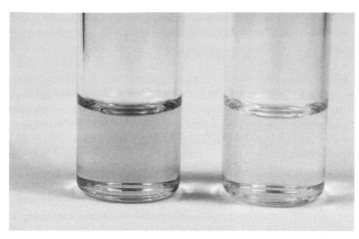

Fig. 25.6 Acute intermittent porphyria. Appearance of the urine tested for excess porphobilinogen using Ehrlich's diazo reagent (left), compared with urine sample from a healthy control subject (right). This 22-year-old woman complained of severe episodes of colicky abdominal pain after starting the oral contraceptive pill. Her younger brother had been diagnosed with acute porphyria many years earlier after suffering epileptic attacks that had been induced by the use of proprietary cough medicine. The urine test was conducted at the time of her outpatient visit to a gastroenterology clinic; subsequently, acute intermittent porphyria was diagnosed in the proband and other affected family members by enzymatic analysis of red cell porphobilinogen deaminase activity.

Agents and conditions that induce attacks of acute porphyria*
Starvation
Appetite suppressants
Alcohol
Anabolic steroids
Contraceptive steroids and replacement sex hormones
Antimicrobials, including cephalosporins, flucloxacillin, erythromycin, doxycycline, sulfonamides
Sulfonylureas
Barbiturates
Benzodiazepines
Many anticonvulsants
Antihistamine
Diuretics
Tricyclic antidepressants
Gold salts
Ergot derivatives

*This list is incomplete: for a complete list see *The British National Formulary (BNF)*, or *British Porphyria Association Handbook* (14 Mollison Rise, Gravesend, Kent, DA12 4QJ, UK).

Table 25.10 Agents and conditions that induce attacks of acute porphyria.*

parenteral administration of haem arginate ('Normosang' Leiras, Helsinki – available from Orphan Europe Ltd.), at a dose of 3 mg/kg body weight in physiological saline daily for 3 days, is effective in arresting the symptoms. Haem arginate therapy rapidly reduces the production of haem biosynthetic precursors.[29,52]

Management of the acute attack

Acute attacks of porphyria require treatment in hospital and scrupulous attention to precipitating factors such as drugs, intercurrent infection, starvation, hormonal changes and alcohol ingestion. Seizures present a particular challenge for treatment, since most anticonvulsant drugs precipitate porphyric attacks; diazepam, which theoretically may aggravate porphyria, can be used to control epilepsy under these circumstances. Menstrual attacks can be incapacitating in some women and when regularly severe may be controlled by the administration of high-dose synthetic gonadotrophins, e.g. goserelin or buserelin, as depôt preparations that in effect induce chemical castration. In some women, prophylactic infusions of haem arginate ameliorate or prevent porphyric attacks that can be predicted to occur in the luteal or premenstrual phase of their cycle. Acute porphyric attacks are associated with tachycardia and hypertension: β-blockers such as propanolol can be used safely to control these manifestations. Agitation and mania with accompanying hallucinations require the administration of psychotropic agents – chlorpromazine and haloperidol are safe drugs for controlling these disturbing features of the attack.

REFERENCES

1   Ali M, Rellos P, Cox TM. Hereditary fructose intolerance. *J Med Gen* 1998; 35: 353–65.
2   Ament ME, Perera DR, Esther LJ. Sucrose-isomaltoase deficiency, a frequently misdiagnosed disease. *J Pediatr* 1973; 83: 721–7.
3   Anonymous. Lactose intolerance. *Lancet* 1991; 338: 663–4.
4   Arese P, Mannuzzu L, Turrini F. Pathogenesis of favism. *Folia Haematologia* 1989; 116: 745–52.
5   Arese P, De Flora A. Pathophysiology of haemolysis in glucose 6-phosphate dehydrogenase deficiency. *Sem Haematol* 1990; 27: 1–40.
6   Baker L, Winegrad AI. Fasting hypoglycaemia and metabolic acidosis associated with a deficiency of hepatic fructose-1,6-diphosphatase activity. *Lancet* 1970; ii:13–16.
7   Barnes G, McKellar W, Lawrence S. Detection of fructose malabsorption by breath hydrogen test in a child with diarrhoea. *J Pediatr* 1983; 103: 575–7.
8   Batshaw ML, Roan Y, Jung AL, Rosenberg LA, Brusilow SW. Cerebral dysfunction in asymptomatic carriers of ornithine transcarbamoylase deficiency. *New Engl J Med* 1980; 302: 482–5.
9   Bell GI, Fukumoto H, Burant CF, Seino S. Genetics of glucose transporters. In: Randle PJ, Bell J, Scott J (eds) *Genetics and Human Nutrition*. John Libbey, London; 1990: 121–31.
10 Bergoz R. Trehalose malabsorption causing intolerance to mushrooms. *Gastroenterology* 1971; 5:909–12.
11 Bergoz R, Vallotton MC, Loizeau E. Trehalase deficiency. Prevalence and relation to single-cell protein food. *Ann Nutr Metabol* 1982; 26: 291–5.
12 Birch JB. Trehalose. *Adv Carbohydr Chem* 1963; 18: 201–25.
13 Brusilow SW, Horwich AL. Urea cycle enzymes. In: Scriver CR, Beaudet AL, Sly WS, Valle D (eds) *The Metabolic and Molecular Bases of Inherited Disease*, 8th edn. McGraw-Hill, New York; 2001; Vol. II; 1909–63.
14 Burrant CF, Takeda J, Brot-Laroche E, Bell GI, Davidson NO. Fructose transporter in human spermatazoa and small intestine is GLUT5. *J Biochem Chem* 1992; 267: 14523–6.
15 Carpenter TO, Levy HL, Holtrop ME, Shih V, Anast CS. Lysinuric protein intolerance presenting as childhood osteoporosis: clinical and skeletal response to citrulline therapy. *New Engl J Med* 1985; 312: 290–4.

16 Carson PE, Flanagan CL, Ickes CE, Alving A. Enzymatic deficiency in primaquine-sensitive erythrocytes. *Science* 1956; 124: 484–5.

17 Chevion M, Novak T, Glaser G, Mager J. The chemistry of favism-inducing compounds. The properties of isouramil and divicine and their reaction with glutathione. *Eur J Biochem* 1982; 127: 405–9.

18 Cox TM. Iatrogenic deaths in hereditary fructose intolerance. *Arch Dis Childhood* 1993; 69: 413–15.

19 Cox TM. Aldolase B and fructose intolerance. *FASEB J* 1994; 8: 62–71.

20 Desjeux J-F. Congenital transport defects. In: Walker WA, Durie PR, Hamilton JR, Walker-Smith JA, Watkins JB (eds) *Pediatric Gastrointestinal Disease*. BC Decker, Philadelphia; 1991: 668–88.

21 Desjeux J-F, Turk E, Wright E. Congenital selective Na+D-glucose cotransport defects leading to renal glycosuria and congenital selective intestinal malabsorption of glucose and galactose. In: Scriver CR, Beaudet AL, Sly WS, Valle D (eds) *The Metabolic and Molecular Bases of Inherited Disease*, 7th edn. McGraw-Hill, New York; 1995: 3563–80 (Vol. III).

22 Escher JC, de Koning ND, van Engen CGJ *et al.* Molecular basis of lactose levels in adult humans. *J Clin Invest* 1992; 89: 480–3.

23 Flatz G. The genetic polymorphism of intestinal lactase activity in adult humans. In: Scriver CR, Beaudet AL, Sly WS, Valle D (eds) *The Metabolic and Molecular Bases of Inherited Disease*, 7th edn. McGraw-Hill, New York; 1995: 4441–50 (Vol. III). See also: Swallow DM, Hollox EJ(2001) Genetic polymorphism of intestinal lactase activity in adult humans. In: Scriver CR, Beaudet AL, Sly WS, Valle D(eds) *The Metabolic and Molecular Bases of Inherited Disease*, 8th edition. McGraw-Hill, New York; 2001; 1651–63 (Vol.I).

24 Figarella C, DeCaro A, Leupold D, Poley JR: Congenital pancreatic lipase deficiency. *J Pediatr* 1980; 96: 412–16.

25 Gaetani GF, Luzzatto L. Haemolytic reactions induced by drugs and other agents: the role of red cell enzyme abnormalities and of abnormal haemoglobins. In: Dukor P, Kallos P, Schlumberger HD, West GB (eds) *Pseudo-Allergic Reactions – Involvement of Drugs and Chemicals*. Karger, Basel; 1980; 1–19 (Vol. 2).

26 Galiano S, Gaetani G-F, Barbino A *et al.* Favism in the African type of glucose-6-phosphate dehydrogenase deficiency (A). *Br Med J* 1990; 300: 236.

27 Ghisham FK, Lee PC, Lebenthal E, Johnson P, Bradley CA, Greene HL. Isolated congenital enterokinase deficiency: recent findings and review of the literature. *Gastroenterology* 1983; 85: 727–31.

28 Steinmann B, Gitzelmann R, Ven den Berghe G. Disorders of fructose metabolism. In: Scriver CR, Beaudet AL, Sly WS, Valle D (eds) *The Metabolic and Molecular Bases of Inherited Disease*, 8th edn. McGraw-Hill, New York; 2001: 1489–1520 (Vol.I).

29 Grandchamp B. Acute intermittent porphyria. *Sem Liver Dis* 1998; 18: 17–24.

30 Gray GM, Waler WM, Colver EH. Persistent deficiency of intestinal lactase in apparently cured tropical sprue. *Gastroenterology* 1968; 54: 552–8.

31 Grazinano JH, Blum C. Lead exposure from lead crystal. *Lancet* 1991; 337: 141–2.

32 Gudmand-Hoyer E. Sucrose malabsorption in children: a report of thirty-one Greenlanders. *J Pediatr Gastoenterol Nutr* 1985; 4: 873–7.

33 Hahn M, Bonkovsky HL. Multiple chemical sensitivity syndrome and porphyria. *Arch Intern Med* 1997; 157: 281–5.

34 Hildebrand H, Borgström B, Békássy A, Erlanson-Albertsson C, Helin I. Isolated co-lipase deficiency in two brothers. *Gut* 1982; 23: 243–6.

35 Hirschhorn N, Molla A. Reversible disaccharidase deficiency in cholera and other diarrhoeal diseases. *Johns Hopkins Med J* 1969; 125: 291–300.

36 Hommes FA. Inborn errors of fructose metabolism. *Am J Clin Nutr* 1993; 58: (supplement): 7885–955.

37 James CL, Rellos P, Ali M, Heeley AF, Cox TM. Neonatal screening for hereditary fructose intolerance: frequency of the most common mutant aldolase B allele (A149P) in the British population. *J Med Gen* 1996; 33: 837–41.

38 King CE, Toskes PP. The use of breath tests in the study of malabsorption. *Clin Gastroenterol* 1983; 12: 591–610.

39 Kirsch RE, Meissner PN, Hift RJ. Variegate porphyria. *Sem Liver Dis* 1998; 18: 33–41.

40 Kneepkens CMF, Jakobs C, Douwes AC. Apple juice, fructose and non-specific diarrhoea. *Eur J Pediatr* 1989; 148: 571–3.

41 Launiala K, Kuitnnen P, Visakorpe J. Disaccharidases and histology of duodenal mucosa in congenital lactose malabsorption. *Acta Paediatrica Scand* 1966; 55: 257–63.

42 Lloyd-Still JD, Listernick R, Buentello G. Complex carbohydrate intolerance: diagnostic pitfalls and approach to management. *J Pediatr* 1988; 112: 709–13.

43 Luzzatto L, Mehta A, Vulliamy T. Glucose 6-phosphate dehydrogenase deficiency. In: Scriver CS, Beaudet AL, Sly WS, Valle D (eds) *The Metabolic and Molecular Bases of Inherited Disease*, 8th edn. McGraw-Hill, New York; 2001: 4517–53 (Vol. III).

44 MacLean WL Jr, Fink BB. Lactose malabsorption by premature infants: magnitude and clinical significance. *J Pediatr* 1980; 97: 383–8.

45 Madzarovová-Nohejilová J. Trehalase deficiency in a family. *Gastroenterology* 1973; 65: 130–3.

46 Marsh MN, Riley SA. Digestion and absorption of nutrients and vitamins; Idem: Maldigestion and malabsorption. In: Feldman M, Scharshmidt BF, Sleisengher MH (eds) *Gastrointestinal and Liver Disease*, 6th edn, Vol. 2. WB Saunders, Philadelphia; 1998; 1471–1500; 1501–22.

47 Martásek P. Hereditary coproporphyria. *Sem Liver Dis* 1998; 18: 17–24.

48 Metz G, Jenkins DJA, Newman A, Blendis LM. Breath hydrogen in hyposucrasia. *Lancet* 1976; i: 119–20.

49 Meyer UA, Schuurmans MM, Lindberg RL. Acute porphyrias: pathogenesis of neurological manifestations. *Sem Liver Dis* 1998; 18: 43–52.

50 Mock OM, Perman JA, Thaler MM, Morris RC. Chronic fructose intoxication after infancy in children with hereditary fructose intolerance: a cause of growth retardation. *New Engl J Med* 1983; 309: 764–70.

51 Moore MR, McColl KEL, Rimington C, Goldberg A. *Disorders of Porphyrin Metabolism*. Plenum, New York; 1987.

52 Nordmann Y, Deybach J-C. Human hereditary porphyrias. In: Dailey HA (ed) *Biosynthesis of Heme and Chlorophylls*. McGraw-Hill, New York; 1990: 491–542.

53 Odièvre M, Gentil C, Gautier M, Alagille D. Hereditary fructose intolerance in childhood: diagnosis, management and course in 55 patients. *Am J Dis Children* 1978; 132: 605–8.

54 Pagliara AS, Karl IE, Keating JP, Brown BI, Kipnis DM. Hepatic-1,6-diphosphatase deficiency. A cause of lactic acidosis and hypoglycaemia in infancy. *J Clin Invest* 1972; 51: 2115–23.

55 Parto K, Svedström E, Majurin ML, Härkönen R, Simell O. Pulmonary manifestations in lysinuric protein intolerance. *Chest* 1993; 104: 1176–82.

56 Perheentupa J, Visakorpi JK. Protein intolerance with deficient transport of basic amino acids. *Lancet* 1965; ii: 813–16.

57 Plotkin GR, Isselbacher KJ. Secondary disaccharidase deficiency in adult celiac (non-tropical sprue) and other malabsorption states. *New Engl J Med* 1964; 271: 1033–7.

58 Ravich J, Boyless T, Thomas M. Fructose-incomplete intestinal absorption in humans. *Gastroenterology* 1983; 84: 26–9.

59 Rosado JL, Solomons NW, Lisker R *et al.* Enzyme replacement therapy for primary adult lactase deficiency. Effective reduction of lactose malabsorption and milk intolerance by direct addition of beta-galactosidase to milk at mealtime. *Gastroenterology* 1984; 87: 1072–82.

60 Rowe PC, Newman SL, Brusilow SW. Natural history of symptomatic partial ornithine transcarbamylase deficiency. *New Engl J Med* 1986; 314: 541–7.

61 Sassa S. ALAD porphyria. *Sem Liver Dis* 1998; 18: 95–101.

62 Sacilathi E, Launiala K, Kuitunen O. Congenital lactase deficiency: a clinical study on 16 patients. *Arch Dis Childhood* 1983; 58: 246–52.

63 Schmid R. Cutaneous porphyria in Turkey. *New Engl J Med* 1960; 263: 397–8.

64 Semenza G, Auricchio S, Mantei N. Small intestinal disaccharidases. In: Scriver CR, Beaudet AL, Sly WS, Valle D (eds) *The Metabolic and Molecular Bases of Inherited Disease*, 8th edn. McGraw-Hill, New York; 2001: 1623–50 (Vol. I).

65 Semenza G, Auricchio S. 1995; idem, Vol.III, 7th edn.,4451–53.

66 Shaw PJ, Dale G, Bates D. Familial lysinuric protein intolerance presenting as coma in two adult siblings. *J Neurol Neurosurg Psych* 1989; 52.648–51.

67 Sheldon W. Congenital pancreatic lipase deficiency. *Arch Dis Childhood* 1964; 39: 268–71.

68 Simell O. Lysinuric protein intolerance and other cationic aminoacidurias. In: Scriver CR, Beaudet AL, Sly WS, Valle D (eds) *The Metabolic and Molecular Bases of Inherited Disease*, 8th edn. McGraw-Hill, New York; 2001: 4933–56.(Vol. III).

69 Simoons FJ. The geographic hypothesis of lactose malabsorption. A weighing of the evidence. *Am J Dig Dis Sci* 1978; 23: 963–80.

70 Steinmann B, Gitzelmann R. The diagnosis of hereditary fructose intolerance. *Helvetica Paediatrica Acta* 1981; 36: 297–316.

71 Sterchi EE, Lentze MJ, Naim HY. Molecular aspects of disaccharidase deficiencies. *Bailliere's Clin Gastroenterol* 1990; 4: 79–96.

72 Townes PL. Trypsinogen deficiency and other proteolytic deficiency diseases. *Birth Defects (original article series)* 1972; VIII (2): 95–101.

73 Truswell AS, Seach JM, Thorburn AW. Incomplete absorption of pure fructose in healthy subjects and the facilitating effects of glucose. *Am J Clin Nutr* 1988; 48: 1424–30.

74 Winterborn C. Inhibition of autoxidation of divicine and isouramil by the combination of superoxide dismutase and reduced glutathione. *Arch Biochem Biophys* 1989; 271: 447–55.

75 Zuckerman MA, Savory D, Rayman G. Lead encephalopathy from an imported toby mug. *Postgrad Med J* 1989; 65: 307–9.

Chapter 26

Nutritional effects on human immune function

David A. Hughes

NUTRITIONAL IMMUNOLOGY

A relationship between malnutrition and increased disease susceptibility has been appreciated for centuries. As early as 5000 BC, the scriptures of India noted the association between diet and health, and church records in medieval England described how pestilence and epidemics of infectious diseases were preceded by consecutive years of crop failure and famine. Sadly, even today, malnutrition and infection play a major role in the causation of preventable deaths and disabilities that occur within the developing world, particularly among children. Immunization programmes have helped, but the World Health Organization (WHO) estimates that at least 2 million children per year die from diseases for which vaccines already exist, mainly as a result of malnutrition.

The realization that a marked reduction in food intake is usually associated with vitamin and mineral deficiencies led scientists to explore the effects of single nutrient deficiencies on the immune system. Over the last 30 years we have gained a considerable understanding of how dietary components interact with the immune system and identified several mechanisms by which diet can affect an individual's susceptibility to a variety of both infectious and chronic diseases. Of course, the interaction between nutrition and the immune response to infection is bidirectional: nutritional status influences host immune function and the ability to fight infection; conversely, infectious disease, whether acute or chronic, has a detrimental influence on the nutritional state. It is now appreciated that the interaction between diet and immunity is important to the health of people in the Western world as well as in less developed countries. Indeed, 'overnutrition' has also been shown to adversely modulate immune function, as well as, of course, being associated with obesity and type 2 diabetes.

One exciting area of current research is the possibility that immune function within certain vulnerable groups, such as the elderly, or those with chronic infections, can be enhanced by dietary means. For example, as described later, vitamin E supplementation has been shown to improve various parameters of immune function in the elderly and, it is hoped, might increase their ability to fight off infections. It is also hoped, in the future, that the course of other immune-related disorders, such as allergy, cardiovascular disease and cancer, might be modulated in a beneficial way by dietary intervention.

This chapter will concentrate on describing some of the major dietary components known to influence human immune function that are relevant to Western populations. However, it will begin by describing perhaps the most important area in which our growing knowledge of the relationship between nutrition and immunity can be applied: to help in reducing the global burden of malnutrition and infection in the developing world.

EFFECTS OF UNDERNUTRITION

In developing countries food allergy is not a major concern; the more pressing need is to achieve adequate nutrition, to prevent the development of impaired immune function and the associated increased risk of childhood morbidity and mortality from infection. Low birth weight is an indicator of fetal undernutrition and the WHO estimates that 25 million low birth babies are born each year, 95% of which are born within the developing world.[94] In addition, because approximately 50% of the transfer of some nutrients from mother to fetus occurs within the last 8 weeks of gestation, premature birth, which is also common in the developing world, often results in striking nutrient deficiencies of trace minerals such as iron, copper and zinc.[17]

Protein–energy malnutrition

Protein–energy malnutrition (PEM) covers a wide spectrum of disorders between the two polar entities of kwashiorkor (a major cause of ill health and death among children in the tropics, due

Changes in immune response observed in protein–energy malnutrition	
Parameter or test	**Response**
Weight of thymus, spleen, tonsils	↓
Delayed-type hypersensitivity response	↓
White blood cell counts	↔
T lymphocyte numbers	↓
CD4+ numbers	↓
CD8+ numbers	↓
Lymphocyte proliferation	↓
Cytokine production, e.g. IL1, IL2, IL6, TNFα, IFNγ	↓
Antibody production	↔
Bactericidal capacity	↓
Susceptibility to infection	↑

Table 26.1 Changes in immune response observed in protein–energy malnutrition.

to a diet deficient in protein and essential fatty acids) and marasmus (a progressive wasting, especially in young children, generally associated with defective feeding). Since proteins are essential for both cell replication and production of biologically active immune molecules (e.g. cytokines, antibodies, complement components) it is not surprising that nearly all forms of immunity are affected by PEM (Table 26.1). The thymus is the most vulnerable organ in this situation and the degree of atrophy can be used to gauge the severity of malnutrition.

Assessing delayed-type hypersensitivity

One of the few means of assessing immune function *in vivo* is to use the delayed-type hypersensitivity (DTH) response. This gives a measure of the individual's ability to mount a cell-mediated immune response when challenged with a subcutaneous injection of a group of antigens to which they have been previously exposed. The response consists of a T lymphocyte-mediated local inflammatory reaction that develops over 24–72 hours. The response is mediated by inflammatory type-1 helper T cells that enter the site of antigen injection, recognize complexes of peptide and major histocompatibility complex (MHC) Class II molecules on antigen-presenting cells, and release inflammatory cytokines that increase local blood capillary wall permeability. This results in an influx of fluid and protein into the tissue, producing a characteristic red weal and skin swelling. The lack of a DTH response, particularly in the elderly, is associated with an increased risk of morbidity and mortality,[92] and poor DTH responses are often observed in individuals suffering from malnutrition. An example of this is the study of Baqui *et al.*,[6] who observed that a poor DTH response and malnutrition were independent risk factors for persistent diarrhoea in Bangladeshi children.

Non-specific host defence

Anatomical barriers (skin, mucous membranes, epithelial surfaces) act as non-specific host defence mechanisms. Alterations to these barriers, such as skin lesions found in children with kwashiorkor, favour the penetration of microorganisms in an already compromised host. Adherence of bacteria to epithelial cells is a first step before invasion and infection can occur and it has been shown that the number of bacteria adhering to respiratory epithelial cells is increased in PEM.[21] An alteration to the surface of the gut by PEM also facilitates its invasion and colonization by pathogens. This has a further worsening effect on the health of the malnourished child, by further impairing the absorption of essential nutrients and by inducing more alterations in immune responses. Decreased secretory immunoglobulin (IgA) in malnutrition may further facilitate the colonization of the gastrointestinal (GI) tract by pathogens.[81] In addition, there is impairment in the maturation of B and T lymphocytes in gut-associated lymphoid tissue (GALT), resulting from malnutrition during lactation.

White blood cell counts

In contrast to lymphoid organs, the total white blood cell counts are normal or increased in PEM, although this is not due to an increase in lymphocytes, but rather to neutrophils. The absolute and relative numbers of total lymphocytes, helper (CD4+) and suppressor (CD8+) T cells are reduced in malnourished children. The degree of reduction in the mean per cent T cells is proportional to the degree of wasting. The proliferative responses of T cells to antigens and mitogens are reduced in malnourished individuals but can return to normal following dietary supplementation for 4 weeks.[53] Possible mechanisms for this reduced proliferative response include an inhibitory effect caused by an increase in the proportion of null cells in the blood, increased levels of free cortisol found in sera from malnourished children and altered cell function resulting from a defect in cell membrane composition.

Monocyte function

Mononuclear phagocyte function is altered in malnourished children. During the process of phagocytosis, monocyte-derived tissue macrophages release large amounts of oxygen intermediates, including superoxide anion ($O_2^{\cdot-}$) and hydrogen peroxide (the 'respiratory burst'), which are important for killing microorganisms. Resident peritoneal macrophages from weaning female mice subjected to PEM release larger amounts of $O_2^{\cdot-}$ after stimulation than those fed a normal diet.[85] In spite of this, macrophages from protein-deficient mice do not show any acceleration of phagocytosis of *Candida albicans* when cultured in the presence of normal serum (which normally increases phagocytosis through Fc or C3b receptor mediated pathways). Macrophages from protein-depleted mice also show a reduced expression of Ia antigen (the murine equivalent of human MHC Class II molecules), required for antigen presentation, when stimulated with interferon (IFN)-γ. Therefore, it seems likely that functional alterations to macrophages may be involved in the failure to develop strong immune responses under PEM and that the enhanced production of oxygen intermediates by macrophages may augment tissue damage under PEM.

Nutritional deprivation during gestation

The consequences of this can be very pervasive and may persist for many years, possibly compromising immune function permanently. This phenomenon of 'fetal programming' also appears to apply to long-term effects on postnatal growth, relative organ size and lipid metabolism of the offspring. For example, Chandra observed a significant correlation between low birth weight and serum immunoglobulin levels. In a 1-year follow up of very low birth weight infants, serum IgG_1 levels remained low and these low levels correlated with an increased susceptibility to bacterial infection.[19] Opsonic activity of plasma against yeast, and neutrophil migration and bactericidal capacity are also reduced in low birth weight infants. A further indication that cell-mediated immunity is impaired is the poor response to DTH response tests seen in low birth weight infants. Many of these infants fail to respond to any skin test antigens and this poor responsiveness can persist for many years.

The idea of an early, *in utero*, sensitivity of the immune system to malnutrition is supported by the observation that babies born up to 2–3 months after the peak of the hungry season in rural Gambia remain vulnerable in later life, having a greater incidence of premature mortality from the age of 15 years.[56] The authors of these findings suggest that fetal growth impairment in mid-pregnancy may have a carry-over effect even when the maternal nutrition improves in late pregnancy.

Malnutrition extending beyond the first generation

There is also evidence, from animal models, that intrauterine malnutrition can result in a persistence of a depressed cell-mediated immune response beyond the first-generation offspring. Chandra[18] showed a reduced immune response (numbers of IgG producing splenocytes) in the F1 generation offspring of starved female mice mated with healthy well-nourished males, even when the offspring were given free access to food. The F2 generation offspring also had a reduced antibody response.

Subsequently, it has been shown that individual nutrient deficiencies can also produce a persistent immunodeficiency. For example, female mice fed a diet moderately deficient in zinc from day 7 of gestation until parturition produced offspring with depressed immune function until 6 months of age. The second and third filial generations, all of which were fed the normal control diet, continued to exhibit a reduced immunocompetence, although not as significantly as the first generation.[7] The mechanism whereby zinc or other nutrients influence immune ontogeny in subsequent generations remains uncertain, but these findings have important implications for public health and human welfare, since the damaging effects of fetal nutritional deficiencies may persist despite generations of nutritional supplementation.

Vitamin A deficiency

Vitamin A deficiency is second to protein malnutrition in terms of the most serious nutritional deficiency diseases in the world today. It is strongly associated with increased morbidity and mortality in children and there is a particularly increased risk of respiratory disease.[17] This is related in part to the role of vitamin A in maintaining the functional integrity of epithelial and mucosal surfaces and the production of mucus secretion.

Production of lysozyme, an enzyme secreted at epithelial surfaces that lyses certain bacteria, is also vitamin A-dependent. Other aspects of immune function that are impaired include phagocytosis, natural killer (NK)-mediated cytolysis, mitogen-induced lymphocyte proliferation, interleukin (IL2) production and DTH responses.[30] Replenishment of vitamin A in depleted or deficient individuals leads to a restoration of immune function: increased phagocytosis, normal T cell proliferation and an intact resistance to pathogenic infections. Several studies have shown a decline in measles-related deaths in vitamin A-deficient children supplemented with vitamin A, and the WHO recommends that, in areas where the measles fatality rate is greater than 1%, children with measles should be supplemented with vitamin A.[17] Unfortunately, infections themselves (e.g. measles, chickenpox and human immunodeficiency virus (HIV)) can also lead to the development of vitamin A deficiency, and persistent infections in children can prevent a return to normal vitamin A status in spite of supplementation.[67]

Mineral deficiencies and the effects of supplementation

Minerals serve key roles in cell function, mainly because they are essential constituents of metalloenzymes; it is, therefore, not surprising that mineral deficiencies are associated with several detrimental changes in immune function. For example, copper deficiency, observed in the rare congenital disorder, Menkes' syndrome, is associated with an increased susceptibility to infections, pneumonia and diarrhoea.[26] The reduced immune function seen in these patients is related to a deficiency in several copper-containing proteins and enzymes, such as ceruloplasmin and cytochrome oxidase, the terminal oxidase of the electron transport chain from which adenosine triphosphate is synthesized. An excess of zinc in the diet can result in low copper status, because of competition for the same carrier molecule in the gut mucosa, but short-term zinc supplementation (as referred to below) is unlikely to result in copper depletion.

Zinc

Zinc deficiency is extremely rare in the Western world, but the condition acrodermatitis enteropathica, which is associated with a reduced ability to absorb dietary zinc, illustrates the changes in immune function that can occur. Thymic atrophy, impaired lymphocyte development and a reduced lymphocyte proliferative responsiveness are common features of the condition, but improvements in immune function and in DTH responses can be achieved by zinc administration.[78] Zinc is an essential cofactor for the thymus hormone thymulin, which has intrathymic and immunoregulatory properties and is necessary for an intact thymus. In the developing world, zinc administration to pre-term low birth weight infants increases T lymphocyte numbers and their ability to proliferate, and can greatly reduce the incidence of respiratory and GI infections.

In the Western world, many elderly individuals are marginally zinc deficient and some immunological dysfunctions seen in the elderly can be restored by zinc supplementation *in vitro*. There has been some interest in the possibility that zinc supplementation can reduce the duration of symptoms of the common cold. This idea is supported by results of a recent study that emphasizes that benefits were obtained when the patient started taking zinc acetate lozenges (12.8 mg every 2–3 hours while awake) within 24 hours of symptoms appearing. Average duration of symptoms was 4.5 days in the zinc group compared with 8.1 days in a placebo-treated control group.[65] It is thought that zinc might help defend against viral infections by stabilizing cell membranes (preventing viral penetration), increasing production of the interferon IFNα, or by inhibiting proteases involved in viral capsid formation.[93]

Iron

Iron deficiency is another cause of depressed immune function, but the relationship to infection is more complex than that of other minerals, since although an efficient immune response requires iron, microbes also need iron for multiplication. It has therefore been argued that the decline in circulating iron levels that accompany an infection is the host's attempt to starve the invading organism of iron. Iron-binding proteins such as lactoferrin are involved in immune responses and iron-containing enzymes are released by immune cells and exhibit destructive activity against microorganisms.

Anaemic individuals often exhibit normal humoral immunity, with normal serum and salivary levels of antibodies, but many parameters of cell-mediated immunity are impaired. There is a decrease in T cell numbers, a reduced DTH response to tetanus toxoid and *Candida albicans*, and a reduced T cell proliferative response to *in vitro* stimulation by mitogens.[79] The bactericidal capacity of neutrophils from iron-deficient children is also reduced, but can be restored following 2–6 weeks of iron supplementation. Although caution must be given in providing iron supplements during periods of infection,[14] it appears that supplementation of poorly nourished individuals with low amounts of iron (up to 100 mg/day for adults and proportionately less for children) can reduce the frequency and severity of infection.[22] Iron deficiency has repeatedly been shown to decrease NK cell function, suggesting that this may result in impaired tumour surveillance within the immune system, and it is thought that moderate iron deficiency may be a risk factor for tumorigenesis, since the immune system might be impaired while iron availability for tumour cell growth is not greatly reduced. Although animal studies support this suggestion, it has not been confirmed in human studies.[79]

EFFECTS OF DIETARY ANTIOXIDANTS

Free radicals and the immune system

Free radicals are highly reactive molecules containing one or more unpaired electrons. Examples of free radicals are the previously mentioned superoxide anion ($O_2^{·-}$) and the hydroxyl ion (OH·). The term 'reactive oxygen species' is a collective one that includes not only oxygen-centred radicals but also some non-radical derivatives of oxygen, such as hydrogen peroxide (H_2O_2), singlet oxygen and hypochlorous acid (HOCl). Hydrogen peroxide can very easily break down, particularly in the presence of transition metal ions (e.g. ferrous [Fe^{2+}] iron), to produce the hydroxyl radical, the most reactive and damaging of the oxygen free radicals:

$$H_2O_2 + Fe^{2+} \rightarrow OH· + OH^- + Fe^{3+}$$

Free radicals are generated during normal cellular metabolism and are also made deliberately. As mentioned earlier, $O_2^{·-}$ plays an essential role in the intracellular killing of microorganisms by activated phagocytes. Exogenous sources of free radicals include ozone, exposure to ultraviolet radiation in sunlight and cigarette smoke.

Free radicals can cause damage to all of the major classes of biomolecules. They cause strand breaks in DNA,[35] which can potentially lead to subsequent misrepair and tumour cell formation. An example of free radical-mediated damage to proteins is the formation of cataracts, resulting from the damage to the crystallins

in the lens of the eye. However, lipids are probably most susceptible to free radical attack, particularly long-chain polyunsaturated fatty acids (PUFA) that contain several double bonds. The oxidative destruction of PUFA, known as lipid peroxidation, can be extremely damaging, since it proceeds as a self-perpetuating chain reaction.

Since reactive oxygen species (ROS) are produced *in vivo*, organisms have evolved antioxidant defence systems to either prevent the generation of ROS or to intercept any that are generated. They exist in both the aqueous and membrane compartments of cells and can be enzymes or non-enzymes. Catalase and glutathione peroxidase are enzymes that can safely decompose peroxides, particularly hydrogen peroxide produced during the 'respiratory burst', while superoxide dismutase intercepts or 'scavenges' free radicals. However, the food we eat provides a large amount of our body's total supply of antioxidants.

Viewed from the perspective of a two-pan balance, with ROS in one pan and antioxidants in the other, tipping the balance in favour of the ROS is thought to be a major contributor to several degenerative disorders such as cancer and cardiovascular diseases (Table 26.2) and to the ageing process in general. Striking improvements in immune function have been observed in elderly individuals following supplementation with antioxidant nutrients,[48] but there is growing evidence that effects can also be observed in younger, healthy individuals. Strong associations between diets rich in antioxidant nutrients and a reduced incidence of cancer have been observed in numerous epidemiological studies and it has been suggested that a boost to the body's immune system by antioxidants might, at least in part, account for this. Indeed, it is probably crucial to attempts to keep the balance of ROS to antioxidants as level as possible, ideally by dietary means rather than by taking supplements, from as early an age as possible, to prolong the onset of, if not prevent, many age-related disorders.

The immune system appears to be particularly sensitive to oxidative stress. Immune cells rely heavily on cell–cell communication, particularly via membrane-bound receptors, to work effectively. Cell membranes are rich in PUFA, which, if peroxidized, can lead to a loss of membrane integrity and altered membrane fluidity,[5] and can result in alterations in intracellular signalling and cell function. It has been shown that exposure to ROS can lead to a reduction in cell membrane receptor expression.[34] In addition, the production of ROS by phagocytic immune cells can damage the cells themselves if they are not sufficiently protected by antioxidants.

Degenerative disorders associated with oxidative damage
Cancer
Cardiovascular disease
Stroke
Cataract
Degeneration of the macula region of the retina
Immunosenescence
Ageing

Table 26.2 Degenerative disorders associated with oxidative damage.

Sources of dietary antioxidants

Many free radical scavengers are obtained through the diet: in cell membranes the most important of these is α-tocopherol, the major member of the vitamin E family. This molecule acts as a 'chain-breaking antioxidant', intercepting lipid peroxyl radicals and so terminating lipid peroxidation chain reactions. Another group of lipid-soluble compounds that can act as antioxidants is the carotenoids, such as β-carotene, lycopene and lutein, found in highly pigmented fruits and vegetables.[49] The major water-soluble free radical scavenger is ascorbic acid (vitamin C), which also plays a role in 'sparing' vitamin E, by regenerating α-tocopherol from the oxidized tocopheroxyl radical.[11] More recently, attention has also focused on the antioxidant properties of plant polyphenols, found in tea and red wines,[70] but considerably more information on the absorption, metabolism and excretion of these compounds in humans is required before their relative contribution to preventing oxidative damage can be assessed.

Table 26.3 identifies dietary sources of minerals and antioxidants required by the immune system.

Selenium

Selenium is concentrated in tissues involved in the immune response, such as lymph nodes, spleen and liver,[82] and various components of the immune system have been shown to be impaired if dietary intake of selenium is inadequate (reviewed in Ref. 52). A major deficiency is seen in the microbicidal activity of phagocytes,[77] which is due to selenium being an integral component of glutathione peroxidase. Once a microorganism has been engulfed into a phagocytic cell, the phagocytic vesicle fuses with lysosomes and the pathogen is destroyed by the 'respiratory burst', which generates ROS from molecular oxygen. It has been suggested that a lack of glutathione peroxidase can lead to damage of lysosomal membranes by lipid hydroperoxides, resulting in the release of various hydrolytic enzymes into the cytoplasm with a subsequent reduction in cell function. Supplementation with selenium appears to boost cell-mediated immune responses and, as well as protecting against oxidative damage, selenium can upregulate the expression of IL2 receptors on T cells.[74] This may, at least in part, explain the stimulatory effect of selenium on B cell antibody production, since this is regulated by T cells.

In passing, it is also worth highlighting the work of Beck and colleagues,[9] who have demonstrated that selenium-deficient mice infected with the coxsackievirus B3 (CVB3) develop an increased myocarditis compared with adequately fed mice. The deficiency in selenium was associated with a change to the viral genotype, converting the virus from a benign to a virulent strain (which involved six nucleotide changes). It is thought that this resulted from an enhanced ability of the virus to replicate in deficient hosts, thereby increasing the chances of a mutation occurring. This finding has worrying implications for populations containing individuals with poor nutritional status since, once the mutations have occurred, even nutritionally adequate hosts will be susceptible to viral-induced disease.

Vitamin C

Vitamin C appears to affect most aspects of the immune system. It is found in high concentrations in white blood cells; it is rapidly utilized during infection, and reduced plasma levels are often associated with reduced immune function. Animal and human studies have suggested that the dietary requirements for vitamin C are increased in cancer, surgical trauma and infectious diseases. However, the belief that high intakes of vitamin C will prevent the onset of the common cold has not been scientifically substantiated, although the associated symptoms following infection appear to be reduced by a moderate intake.[24] Pauling's claims regarding the effects of vitamin C on the common cold[63] certainly inspired a great deal of research into its effect on immune function in the 1970s and early 1980s (reviewed in Refs 80 and 87), but research in this area has subsequently declined and there have been few recent studies examining the effects of vitamin C on the immune system in healthy individuals.

Vitamin C has been used to treat some clinical phagocytic cell dysfunctions. In Chédiak–Higashi syndrome, which is characterized in part by defective neutrophil functions, vitamin C supplementation has been shown to increase neutrophil chemotaxis, improve bactericidal activity and reduce the length of clinical illness. Vitamin C also appears to be beneficial in the treatment of chronic granulomatous disease[2] and in recurrent pyogenic infections.[69]

Ascorbate provides important antioxidant protection to plasma lipids and lipid membranes[29] and can also neutralize phagocyte-derived oxidants released extracellularly, thereby preventing oxidant-mediated tissue damage, particularly at sites of inflammatory activity. Other mechanisms which have been proposed for the immunostimulatory effects of vitamin C include modulation of intracellular cyclic nucleotide levels, modulation of prostaglandin synthesis, enhancement of cytokine production, antagonism of the immunosuppressive interaction between histamines and white blood cells and the protection of 5′-lipoxygenase.[3] There is a need for further research, not only into the mechanisms

Dietary sources of minerals and antioxidants required by the immune system
Carotenoids   β-carotene: carrots, broccoli, watercress, apricots   lycopene: tomatoes   lutein: peas
Copper   Meat, vegetables, milk, water
Iron   Red meat, fortified cereals, dark green vegetables, beans
Vitamin A   Liver, egg yolk, milk
Vitamin C   Vegetables and fruits, especially blackcurrants and citrus fruits
Vitamin E   Whole grains, vegetable oils, wheat germ
Selenium   Meat, fish, egg, whole grains
Zinc   Meat, dairy products, cereals, vegetables, oysters

Table 26.3 Dietary sources of minerals and antioxidants required by the immune system.

by which vitamin C can enhance immune cell function but also to define the optimal levels of intake required to maintain an optimal immune responsiveness throughout life and to reduce the incidence of degenerative disorders in later life. Indeed, one of the major present challenges within the field of nutritional immunology is to define markers of immune function in younger individuals that can predict long-term health.

Vitamin E

Studies of humans and animals in either states of deficiency or at supra-dietary levels suggest strongly that vitamin E is involved in maintaining immune cell function. Since vitamin E is the most effective chain-breaking, lipid-soluble antioxidant present in cell membranes, it is considered likely that it plays a major role in maintaining cell membrane integrity by limiting lipid peroxidation by ROS. Vitamin E deficiency states are associated with depressed B cell antibody production and T cell proliferation to mitogenic stimulation and an increased rate of infection.

A marked improvement in immune parameters can be seen in the elderly following supplementation with vitamin E. One study, providing 800 mg vitamin E/day for 30 days, showed a significant elevation in IL2 production, DTH responses and antibody titres to hepatitis B and tetanus vaccine. In another study, young and elderly individuals were supplemented with 800 mg vitamin E/day for 48 days before being asked to run downhill. Vitamin E supplementation was found to eliminate the age-associated difference in exercise-induced neutropenia, to prevent the exercise-induced increase in IL1 production and to inhibit IL6. Since these cytokines are involved in the inflammatory process and in exercise-induced muscle damage, their inhibition by vitamin E during damaging exercise might have practical implications.[54]

Recently, a beneficial effect of vitamin E in reducing pulmonary influenza virus titre in old mice has been reported.[36] Hopefully, future clinical trials will establish the efficacy of vitamin E in reducing the burden of influenza infection in the elderly. However, on a cautious note, one study has reported that prolonged high-dose intakes of vitamin E (1600 mg/day) can lead to inhibition of neutrophil phagocytosis,[13] suggesting that perhaps vitamin E supplements should only be taken in moderation to prevent an increased susceptibility to infection. Further research is needed to assess the optimal intake of this nutrient required to provide benefit for different groups of individuals (e.g. the young, elderly, smokers etc.).

Inhibition of the inflammatory response by antioxidants

It is possible that vitamin E and, indeed, other antioxidant nutrients can influence a variety of inflammatory processes by inhibiting the activity of a transcription factor called nuclear factor (NF)-κB. Transcription factors are intracellular regulators of gene expression. Once activated, the transcription factor binds to the promotor region of a specific gene within the DNA in the nucleus, resulting in that gene being 'turned on'. NF-κB is required for maximal transcription of many proteins that are involved in inflammatory responses, including several cytokines, such as IL1β, IL2 and tumour necrosis factor (TNF)-α. NF-κB is a redox-sensitive transcription factor and it is thought that the generation of ROS is a vital link in mediating NF-κB activation by a variety of stimuli.[47]

Vitamin E levels in smokers

Several studies have examined the effect of vitamin E in cigarette smokers. Cigarette smoke contains millions of free radicals per puff, and other compounds present can stimulate the formation of other highly reactive molecules.[66] Serum levels of vitamin E (as well as vitamin C and β-carotene) and lung vitamin E concentrations are significantly lower in smokers compared with non-smokers,[10] and even supplementation with 2400 IU/day for 3 weeks failed to restore lung vitamin E levels to that found in non-smokers.[60] Circulating phagocytes from smokers produce high levels of free radicals, which probably in part accounts for the depressed immune function observed in smokers,[44] and there is some evidence that vitamin E supplementation can reduce the overproduction of ROS by phagocytic cells from smokers.[71]

Effect of vitamin E supplementation in HIV

Reduced levels of vitamin E have also been reported in HIV-infected individuals. Passi et al.[62] found that plasma vitamin E levels were significantly lower in a group of 200 HIV-positive individuals compared with controls, but whether this is related to an inadequate intake of this vitamin is unclear. Dietary diaries from a group of 100 HIV-infected asymptomatic men did not indicate an inadequate intake of vitamin E, but plasma levels were low or marginally low in 74% of the men.[8] In a study of patients who had developed AIDS, an inverse relationship was observed between serum vitamin E levels and severity of disease.[27] A recent study of 49 HIV-infected subjects, provided with vitamin E and vitamin C, observed a significant reduction in oxidative stress and a trend towards a reduction in viral load after 3 months.[1] These studies suggest that larger trials of these and other antioxidant nutrients in the treatment of HIV-infected persons are worthwhile, since there is a need to find alternative, cheaper treatments than the combination therapies currently employed.

Carotenoids

The carotenoids are a group of over 600 naturally occurring coloured pigments that are widespread in plants, but of which only about 24 commonly occur in human foodstuffs. In nature they serve two essential functions: as accessory pigments in photosynthesis and in photoprotection. These two functions are achieved through the chemical structure of carotenoids (Fig. 26.1), which allows the molecules to absorb light and to quench singlet oxygen and free radicals.

Many epidemiological studies have shown an association between diets rich in carotenoids and a reduced incidence of many forms of cancer, and it has been suggested that the antioxidant properties of these compounds are a causative factor.[12] In recent years, principally since the review article in *Nature* by Peto et al.,[64] a great deal of attention has focused on the potential role of one particular carotenoid, β-carotene (found in high amounts in carrots, broccoli and watercress), in preventing cancer. Numerous publications have described *in vitro* experiments, animal studies and clinical trials that suggest that this carotenoid cannot only protect against cancer but also against other oxidative damage-associated disorders, listed in Table 26.2 (reviewed in Ref. 51). Because the immune system plays a major role in the prevention of cancer, it has been suggested that β-carotene may enhance immune cell function.

Supplements that reduce infection-related morbidity

Apart from the DTH response test, another of the few methods of assessing the *in vivo* effects of a compound on the human

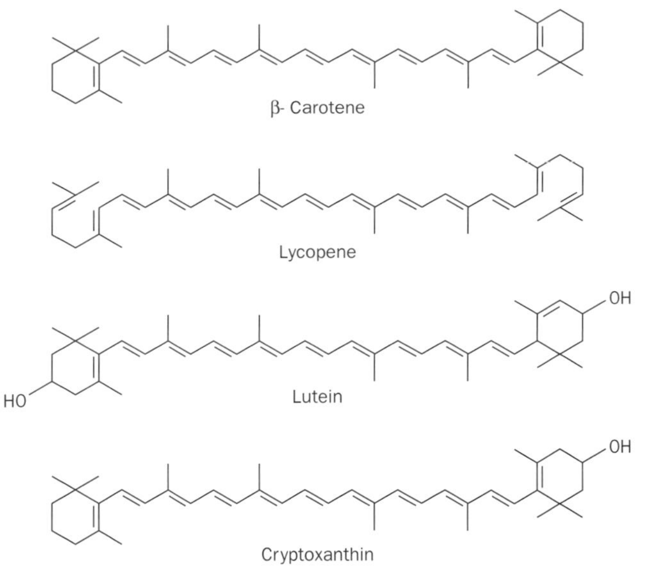

Fig. 26.1 Chemical structure of some common carotenoids found in the diet.

immune system is to measure the incidence of infection within a group of individuals given either the compound or placebo. Chandra[20] compared two groups of elderly volunteers given either a placebo or a multivitamin capsule, which contained 16 mg β-carotene, daily for 1 year. There was a marked reduction in infection-related morbidity (days of infection) in the vitamin-supplemented group, suggesting that the supplement had boosted immune defence in these elderly individuals. However, there have been no comparable studies undertaken to examine the effects of individual carotenoids on this measure of immune function. It has to be noted that it would be difficult to undertake similar studies in younger subjects, since they are more likely to have a lower incidence of infection than the elderly, dictating that much larger groups of individuals would be needed to provide sufficient statistical power.

β-Carotene protection against UV immune suppression

Individuals who are repeatedly exposed to ultraviolet (UV) light show suppression of immune function.[73] Because carotenoids can provide photoprotection, several studies have assessed the ability of β-carotene to protect the immune system from UV-induced free radical damage. In one study a group of young males were placed on a low-carotenoid diet (<1.0 mg/day total carotenoids) and given either placebo or 30 mg β-carotene/day for 28 days prior to periodic exposure to UV light. DTH responses were significantly suppressed in the placebo group after UV treatments and the suppression was inversely proportional to plasma β-carotene concentrations in this group,[32] but no significant suppression of DTH responses was seen in the β-carotene-treated group. The ability of β-carotene to protect against the harmful effects of natural UV – sunlight – has also been demonstrated by exposing healthy female students to time- and intensity-controlled sunlight exposure; a Berlin-based study, which involved taking volunteers to the Red Sea![33]

Several studies have examined the effect of β-carotene on immune function by measuring changes in the numbers of lymphocyte subpopulations and on the expression of cell activation markers. Various doses of β-carotene have been employed in these

studies, ranging from dietary achievable levels of 15 mg/day up to pharmacological doses of 180 mg/day, provided over periods of 14–365 days. There have been reported increases in the numbers of CD4+ cells or in the ratio of CD4+ to CD8+ cells, and in the percentages of lymphocytes expressing IL2 receptors and transferrin receptors (Refs 57 and 89), particularly in elderly subjects. The potential for increasing the numbers of CD4+ cells led to the suggestion that β-carotene might be useful as an immuno-enhancing agent in the treatment of HIV infection. Preliminary studies have shown a slight but insignificant increase in CD4+ numbers in response to β-carotene (60 mg/day for 4 weeks) in patients with AIDS,[31] but long-term effectiveness has not been reported.

No effect of β-carotene on T cell-mediated immunity

Other investigators have been unable to confirm the increase in T cell-mediated immunity in healthy individuals following β-carotene supplementation. Santos et al.[75] have recently reported the results of two studies in the elderly: a short-term, high-dose study (90 mg/day for 21 days) in women; and a longer-term, lower-dose trial (50 mg/alternate days for 10–12 years) in men. Both studies concluded that there was no significant difference in T cell function, as assessed by DTH response, lymphocyte proliferation, IL2 and prostaglandin E_2 production, and composition of lymphocyte subsets. However, these workers also examined the effect of β-carotene supplementation on NK cell activity in the longer-term trial with male volunteers. Supplementation resulted in significantly greater NK cell activity compared with subjects of a similar age given placebo treatment.[76] The study also highlighted the reduction in NK cell activity that is observed with age but, interestingly, the increase in NK cell activity observed in older males (65–86 years old) following β-carotene supplementation restored it to the level seen in a group of younger males (51–64 years old).

Enhancement of cell-mediated immunity by carotene

Since antigen-presenting cells initiate cell-mediated immune responses, we investigated whether β-carotene supplementation can influence blood monocytes, the main antigen-presenting cell type in the blood. A prerequisite for this function is the expression of MHC Class II molecules (HLADR, HLADP and HLADQ),[4] which are present on the majority of human monocytes. The antigenic peptide is presented to the helper T lymphocyte within a groove of the MHC Class II molecule (Fig. 26.2). Since the degree of immune responsiveness of an individual has been shown to be proportional to both the percentage of MHC Class II-positive monocytes and the density of these molecules on the cell surface,[43] it is possible that one mechanism by which β-carotene may enhance cell-mediated immune responses is by enhancing the cell surface expression of these molecules. In addition, cell-to-cell adhesion is critical for the initiation of a primary immune response, and it has been shown that the intercellular adhesion molecule-1 (ICAM–1)-leukocyte function associated antigen-1 (LFA 1) ligand–receptor pair is also capable of co-stimulating an immune response,[83] enhancing T cell proliferation and cytokine production. Therefore, we examined the effect of β-carotene supplementation, given for 26 days at a dietary achievable level (15 mg/day; equivalent to 150 g carrots), on monocyte surface expression of these molecules. Following dietary supplementation, there were significant increases in plasma levels of β-carotene and in the percentages of monocytes expressing the

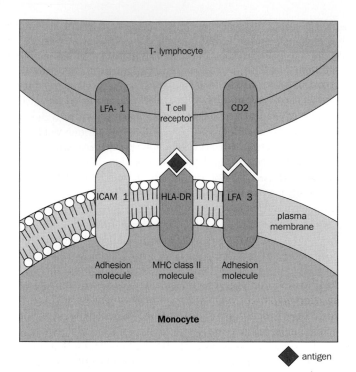

Fig. 26.2 Some of the cell surface molecules involved in antigen presentation: LFA, leukocyte function-associated antigen; ICAM 1, intercellular adhesion molecule-1; HLA, human leukocyte-associated antigen; MHC, major histocompatibility complex.

MHC Class II molecule HLADR, and the adhesion molecules ICAM 1 and LFA 3.[41] These results suggest that moderate increases in the dietary intake of β-carotene can enhance cell-mediated immune responses within a relatively short period of time, providing a potential mechanism for the anti-carcinogenic properties attributed to this compound. The increase in surface molecule expression may also, in part, account for the ability of β-carotene to prevent the reduction in DTH response following exposure to UV radiation, since the latter can inhibit both HLADR and ICAM 1 expression on human cell lines. This finding could certainly be relevant to the preventative action of β-carotene on the formation of skin cancer,[50] since immunosuppressed individuals, such as renal transplant patients, have an increased risk of skin cancer.

Very little is known about the influence of other carotenoids on human immune function, even though there is also strong epidemiological evidence to suggest that lycopene (found in tomatoes) and lutein (found in peas, watercress and other vegetables) can protect against prostate and lung cancer, respectively. We have also looked at the effect of dietary supplementation with lycopene and lutein on monocytes' surface molecule expression, and found that they appear to be less influential than β-carotene, when given at the same level of supplementation.[42] Another group has shown that enriching the diet with lycopene (by drinking 330 ml of tomato juice daily) for 8 weeks does not appear to modify cell-mediated immune responses in the elderly.[90] Other investigators have shown an opposing effect of β-carotene and lutein in regard to human lymphocyte proliferation,[91] emphasizing further that different carotenoids can affect immune function in different ways. Therefore, the influence of the combination of carotenoids contained in fruits and vegetables, on immune func-

tion may represent the sum total of these different effects and, indeed, the potential for synergistic effects remains to be investigated.

Effects of different carotenoids
One possible factor to explain the different effects seen with different carotenoids might be the preferred location of these compounds within the cell and within the body. Carotenoids are lipid soluble, and thus it is thought that most will be concentrated in the lipid-rich membranes of the cell. However, their exact location may influence their effectiveness in modulating specific cellular events. Within the body, lycopene appears to be selectively taken up within the prostate, a finding that may help explain the association between higher intakes of lycopene and a reduction in prostate cancer. So, it is possible that tests on peripheral blood cells to determine immune function will not detect any localized effects, suggesting that there might be 'hidden' benefits associated with certain dietary components that we have yet to discover.

Beneficial effects of carotenoids in preventing cancer
The strongest epidemiological evidence supporting a beneficial effect of carotenoids in preventing cancer is the protective effect of β-carotene intake in reducing the incidence of cancer of the lung. Carotenoid intake has been associated with a reduced lung cancer risk in 8 of 8 prospective studies and in 18 of 20 retrospective studies.[95] As a result, three major intervention trials were initiated, examining the efficacy of β-carotene in the prevention of lung cancer.[38,59,86] The failure of these trials to show a protective effect, with two of the studies showing an increase in lung cancer in smokers receiving β-carotene supplementation, has been widely publicized. The mechanism for the increased lung cancer risk associated with the supplementation is unclear, but several suggestions have been made. Since the participants in these studies could be classified as 'high risk' for developing lung cancer (long-term smokers or individuals previously exposed to asbestos), it is possible that many of them had undetected tumours prior to the commencement of supplementation. The stage (or stages) of carcinogenesis at which β-carotene might be effective is unclear, but if the effect is mediated via the immune system it is likely to occur during the promotional stages preceding the formation of a malignant tumour.

Can β-carotene 'protect' tumours?
The worrying possibility is that β-carotene might actually provide a protective effect to already established tumours. Tumour cells have an impairment in their antioxidant defences compared with normal cells[88] and so they might particularly benefit from an increased supply of antioxidants. It has recently been shown that *in vitro* pre-incubation of tumour cells with various antioxidants, including β-carotene, can increase their resistance to lysis by NK cells.[72] One of the major unresolved dilemmas of research into β-carotene is what intake is required for optimal immune function and other healthy properties? Most studies of this compound have been undertaken at levels that are not achievable within a normal healthy diet. It is still unclear whether different intakes are associated with different outcomes or, in mechanistic studies, with different effects on various aspects of immune function. In addition, there remains the potentiality that, at higher intakes, β-carotene may exhibit pro-oxidant activity, particularly in the presence of high oxygen tensions, as occurs in the lungs (reviewed in

Ref. 61). Of course, the probability remains that the apparent protection of consuming a diet rich in fruits and vegetables is the result of a multifactorial effect of a number of components of these foods. Greater emphasis should be placed on studying the effects of enriching the diet with antioxidants via real foodstuffs rather than by supplementation.

EFFECTS OF DIETARY FATS

Fatty acids and the immune system

Many studies have investigated the effects of the amounts and types of fat in the diet on immune function. Obesity, associated with a high fat intake, is often accompanied by an impaired immune response, with a particular decline in T cell function and NK cell activity. Changes in total fat intake can influence immune function. A reduction of fat intake (from 40 to 25% of total energy) resulted in a greatly enhanced T cell proliferative response to ConA (concanavalin A) stimulation,[45] and a similar study showed an increase in NK cell function, supporting the suggestion that high fat diets might suppress T cell function.

Fatty acids can be divided into distinct families that differ in structure and dietary origin (Table 26.4). Saturated fatty acids contain no double bonds in their structure; fatty acids that contain one double bond are described as monounsaturated, while those that contain more than one are termed polyunsaturated. The latter can be further classified by the position of the first double bond into n-6 or n-3 (sometimes referred to as ω-6 or ω-3) fatty acids. They are particularly important in the functioning of the immune system because of their structural role in cell membranes. The chain length of the fatty acids and their degree of unsaturation affects the fluidity of the membrane; membranes rich in long-chain polyunsaturated fatty acids are more fluid, and this influences the expression of surface receptors that play a crucial role in immune cell responsiveness and interaction. A great deal of research has been undertaken to examine the influence of n-6 and n-3 fatty acids on immune function.

Most of this work has been undertaken in animals and *in vitro* models, but the general finding is that diets rich in n-6 fatty acids tend to promote immune responses which lead to inflammation, while those rich in n-3 fatty acids tend to inhibit immune responses. The increasing use of n-6 fatty acid-rich vegetables oils in the Western world during the last century, particularly in spreads, has led to a high ratio of intake of n-6:n-3 fatty acids (about 5.6:1 in the UK, currently). It is thought that during mankind's evolution, when fish made up a substantial part of the diet, we had physiologically adapted to a considerably lower ratio

of n-6:n-3 fatty acids. Research is currently examining whether an optimal n-6:n-3 fatty acid ratio exists, to inform future dietary guidelines on this aspect of nutrition. Currently, it is recommended that we should eat at least one portion of oily fish, such as salmon, mackerel or sardines, a week.

n-3 fatty acids and immune function

Populations that have high dietary intakes of n-3 fatty acids, such as Greenland Inuits who consume large quantities of oily fish and seal meat, have a low incidence of inflammatory and autoimmune disorders and cardiovascular disease. This observation led to a growing interest in the potential use of n-3 fatty acid-rich fish oil in the treatment of disorders involving over-reactive immune responses, such as rheumatoid arthritis and psoriasis. Subsequently, a number of double-blind studies have reported that dietary fish oil supplementation in patients with rheumatoid arthritis is associated with mild to moderate improvement in symptoms, including reductions in morning stiffness and the number of tender joints.[28] Although it is unlikely that dietary modulation of chronic inflammatory reactions could replace conventional therapy, such as corticosteroids, it is possible that their combined usage would allow the dose of immunosuppressants to be reduced, thus lowering the severity of the side effects commonly associated with these treatments.

The cardiovascular disease risk and mortality lowering effect of ingesting n-3 fatty acids has been recognized from both population studies[46] and prospective trials,[23] at least in part because of reduced atherosclerosis.[58] There is now firm evidence of a chronic immune and inflammatory involvement in the formation of atherosclerotic lesions.[84] The presence of chronically stimulated T cells within lesions, together with the expression of MHC Class II molecules on lesional monocytes–macrophages, indicates that these cells are actively participating in the local immune response occurring during atherogenesis.[37] Supplementation studies have shown that n-3 fatty acids are incorporated into the lipids of atherosclerotic plaques in man,[68] and it is possible, if this incorporation results in a localized reduction in inflammatory activity, that this might retard, if not prevent, further lesion development.

Suppression of immune function by n-3 fatty acids

Most studies of the effects of n-3 fatty acids have been undertaken *in vitro* or in animal models and have been extensively reviewed.[15,16,39] The common finding in most of these studies is a suppression of immune cell function. T cell proliferative responses and NK cell function are reduced, cytokine production is inhibited and the expression of cell surface adhesion molecules is diminished. Dietary studies in humans have now confirmed several of these findings, although the levels of fish oil supplementation and length of supplementation varies considerably (1–6 g n-3 fatty acid/day, for between 4 weeks and 4 months). Levels of n-3 fatty acids remain elevated in the blood plasma several weeks after a period of supplementation and some researchers have observed a more striking effect on immune function after the supplementation has ceased. For example, Endres *et al.* demonstrated that fish oil supplementation for 6 weeks (18 g fish oil/day) inhibited the ability of mononuclear cells to produce the proinflammatory cytokines IL1 and TNFα when stimulated *in vitro* with endotoxin,[25] but that the effect was most pronounced 10 weeks after stopping the supplementation. Cytokine production only returned to presupplementation levels

The different types of fat in the diet	
Fatty acids	**Dietary sources**
Saturated fatty acids	Beef fat, palm oil
Unsaturated fatty acids	
Monounsaturated fatty acids	Olive oil, rapeseed oil
Polyunsaturated fatty acids	
n-6 (ω-6)	Most vegetable oils
n-3 (ω-3)	Fish oil, flaxseed oil

Table 26.4 The different types of fat in the diet.

20 weeks after the supplementation was ended. Fish oil supplementation also reduces the surface expression of monocyte MHC Class II molecules and adhesion molecules, required for antigen presentation,[40] providing another mechanism for the suppression of cell-mediated immunity associated with n-3 fatty acids.

Mechanisms of immune suppression by n-3 fatty acids

Several possible mechanisms have been suggested to explain the inhibitory effects of n-3 fatty acids on immune function. One of the main effects of enriching the diet with n-3 fatty acids is that they provide an alternative precursor to the n-6 fatty acid, arachidonic acid, for the production of eicosanoids, a group of messenger molecules that can have a potent effect on a variety of metabolic processes and cell types. Ingestion of fish oil will result in a decrease in cell membrane arachidonic acid levels, resulting in a decreased ability to synthesize eicosanoids from arachidonic acid. Figure 26.3 illustrates the different groups of derivatives from arachidonic acid and from eicosapentaenoic acid (EPA), one of the major n-3 fatty acids found in fish oil. The derivatives from EPA have different effects on immune cells to those derived from arachidonic acid and it is thought that the less proinflammatory effects of the former are, at least in part, responsible for the reduced immune responsiveness observed following fish oil supplementation.

Another possibility is that increasing the polyunsaturated fatty acid content of the cell membrane may render it more susceptible to lipid peroxidation (unsaturated fatty acids are more vulnerable than are saturated fats). Free radical-induced damage will result in a reduction in the membrane's integrity, which may cause various physical and biochemical changes. For instance, free radicals can suppress the expression of HLADR, and a reduced expression of this molecule is seen following increased fish oil consumption.[40] The fact that dietary supplementation with antioxidants such as β-carotene can enhance the expression of this molecule on blood monocytes[41] suggests that antioxidants might be reducing oxidative stress within the cell membrane.

A further possibility is that fatty acids can have a direct or indirect influence on gene expression, inhibiting immune function by reducing the switching on of genes encoding for proteins required to mount an immune response. For example, the transcription factor, NF-κB, referred to earlier (regarding vitamin E), can be activated by protein kinase C (PKC). Since it has been shown that n-3 fatty acids can reduce the activation of PKC isoforms,[55] it is possible that this will result in the suppressed synthesis of a number of proinflammatory proteins encoded by genes whose expression is under this transcription factor's control. Further studies are being undertaken to investigate these potential mechanisms.

Obviously, a greater understanding of the mechanisms by which dietary lipids – and indeed all dietary components – modulate immune function will aid in designing diets to prevent, prolong the development of and treat immune-related chronic disorders.

KEY FACTS

1. The connection between famine and death from infections has been appreciated since biblical times, but it is only in recent years that the influence of diet on our immune system has been appreciated. This led to many studies examining the influence of deficiencies of individual dietary components on immune function. It is now becoming increasingly clear that it is the 'sum of the parts' of the diet that affects the way our immune system is modulated by what we eat.

2. Protein–energy malnutrition and single nutrient deficiencies are still significant problems in the developing world, but can also occur in the Western world, sometimes secondary to disease states. These deficiencies affect cell-mediated immune responses (reduced DTH response, T cell numbers, lymphocyte proliferation and cytokine production), non-specific immune responses (reduced NK cell function and neutrophil bactericidal capacity) and, to a lesser extent, humoral immunity. These alterations severely weaken the individual's resistance to infection and result in an increased incidence of morbidity and mortality. Fortunately, dietary improvement in nutritional status often results in a restoration of immune function.

3. The immune system is highly reliant on accurate cell–cell communication for optimal function, and any damage to the signalling systems involved will result in an impaired responsiveness. Oxidant-mediated tissue injury is a particular hazard

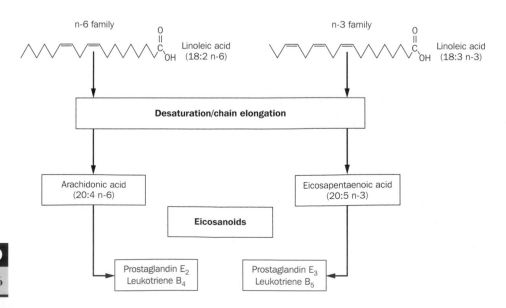

Fig. 26.3 Simplified diagram of polyunsaturated fatty acid metabolism and examples of different eicosanoids synthesized from arachidonic acid and eicosapentaenoic acid.

to the immune system, since phagocytic cells produce reactive oxygen species as part of the body's defence against infection. Therefore, adequate amounts of neutralizing antioxidants are required to prevent damage to the immune cells themselves. Many antioxidants can be obtained directly from the diet (e.g. vitamins C and E, carotenoids and polyphenolic flavonoids) or require micronutrients as integral components (e.g. selenium in the metalloenzyme, glutathione peroxidase).

4. Numerous epidemiological studies have found strong associations between diets rich in antioxidant nutrients and a reduced incidence of cancer and it has been suggested that a boost to the body's immune system by antioxidants might, at least in part, account for this. Although more striking effects have been observed in the elderly, there is evidence that antioxidant nutrients can also modify cell-mediated immune responses in younger individuals. It might be essential to have adequate intakes of antioxidant nutrients from an early age to help prevent, or at least delay the onset of, several degenerative disorders.

5. To try to maintain a healthy immune system, eat plenty of foods rich in antioxidants, particularly fruits and vegetables rich in vitamin C and carotenoids, and whole grains containing vitamin E.

6. Although there is increasing evidence that certain supplements such as vitamin E might be beneficial, especially in boosting immune function in the elderly, there are still concerns regarding their safety when taken at levels above their recommended daily allowances. More research needs to be done to assess the safety of long-term supra-dietary achievable levels of supplementation.

7. Since the strongest evidence in support of the benefits of consuming high intakes of many nutrients comes from epidemiological studies of populations eating real foodstuffs, it would still seem to be safer to increase ones intake of fruits and vegetables rather than to rely on supplements. After all, there are still many compounds present in plants whose identity, and biological effects on the immune system, we have still to discover.

8. Because high fat diets are associated with reduced immune function, it seems advisable to reduce total fat intake to below 35% of total energy. This is also a current recommendation in terms of reducing the risk of cardiovascular disease. It has also been suggested that we should eat at least one portion of oily fish, such as salmon, mackerel, herring or tuna, a week. However, tinned tuna is often low in n-3 fatty acids, due to the processing used.

REFERENCES

1 Allard JP, Aghdassi E, Chau J et al. Effects of vitamin E and C supplementation on oxidative stress and viral load in HIV-infected subjects. AIDS 1998; 12: 1653–9.

2 Anderson R. Effects of ascorbate on normal and abnormal leucocyte functions. Int J Vit Nutr Res 1982; 23 (suppl): 23–34.

3 Anderson R, Smit MJ, Joone GK, Van Straden AM. Vitamin C and cellular immune functions. Protection against hypochlorous acid-mediated inactivation of glyceraldehyde-3-phosphate dehydrogenase and ATP generation in human leukocytes as a possible mechanism of ascorbate-mediated immunostimulation. Ann N Y Acad Sci 1990; 587: 34–48.

4 Bach FH. Class II genes and products of the HLA-D region. Immunol Today 1985; 6: 89–94.

5 Baker KR, Meydani M. Beta-carotene in immunity and cancer. J Optim Nutr 1994; 3: 39–50.

6 Baqui AH, Sack RB, Black RE, Chowdhury HR, Yunus M, Siddique AK. Cell-mediated immune deficiency and malnutrition are independent risk factors for persistent diarrhea in Bangladeshi children. Am J Clin Nutr 1993; 58: 543–8.

7 Beach RS, Gershwin ME, Hurley LS. Gestational zinc deprivation in mice: persistence of immunodeficiency for three generations. Science 1982; 218: 469–71.

8 Beach RS, Mantero-Atienza E, Shor-Posner G et al. Specific nutrient abnormalities in asymptomatic HIV-1 infection. AIDS 1992; 6: 701–8.

9 Beck MA. The influence of antioxidant nutrients on viral infection. Nutr Rev 1998; 56: S140–6.

10 Bendich A. Recent advances in clinical research involving carotenoids. Pure Appl Chem 1994; 66: 1017–24.

11 Bendich A, Machlin LJ, Scandurra O, Burton GW, Wayner DDM. The antioxidant role of vitamin C. Free Radicals Biol Med 1986; 2: 419–44.

12 Block G, Patterson B, Subar A. Fruit, vegetables, and cancer prevention: a review of the epidemiological evidence. Nutr Cancer 1992; 18: 1–29.

13 Boxer LA. Regulation of phagocyte function by alpha-tocopherol. Proc Nutr Soc 1986; 45: 333–4.

14 Brock JH. Benefits and dangers of iron during infection. Curr Opin Clin Nutr Metab Care 1999; 2: 507–10.

15 Calder PC. Immunomodulatory and anti-inflammatory effects of n-3 polyunsaturated fatty acids. Proc Nutr Soc 1996; 55: 127–50.

16 Calder PC. Dietary fatty acids and the immune system. Nutr Rev 1998; 56: S70–83.

17 Calder PC, Jackson AA. Undernutrition, infection and immune function. Nutr Res Rev 2000; 13: 3–29.

18 Chandra RK. Antibody formation in first and second generation offspring of nutritionally deprived rats. Science 1975; 190: 289–90.

19 Chandra RK. Nutrition as a critical determinant in susceptibility to infection. World Rev Nutr Diet 1976; 25: 166–88.

20 Chandra RK. Effect of vitamin and trace element supplementation on immune responses and infection in elderly subjects. Lancet 1992; 340: 1124–7.

21 Chandra RK, Gupta SP. Increased bacterial adherence to respiratory and buccal epithelial cells in protein–energy malnutrition. Immunol Infect Dis 1991; 1: 55–7.

22 Chwang LC, Soemantri AG, Pollitt E. Iron supplementation and physical growth of rural Indonesian children. Am J Clin Nutr 1988; 47: 496–501.

23 Connor SL, Connor WE. Are fish oils beneficial in the prevention and treatment of coronary artery disease? Am J Clin Nutr 1997; 66: S1020–31.

24 Coulehan JL, Reisinger KS, Rogers KD, Bradley DW. Vitamin C prophylaxis in a boarding school. N Engl J Med 1974; 290: 6–10.

25 Endres S, Ghorbani R, Kelley VE et al. The effect of dietary supplementation with n-3 polyunsaturated fatty acids on the synthesis of interleukin-1 and tumour necrosis factor by mononuclear cells. N Engl J Med 1989; 320: 265–71.

26 Failla ML, Hopkins RG. Is low copper status immunosuppressive? Nutr Rev 1998; 56: S59–64.

27 Favier A, Sappey C, Leclerc P, Faure P, Micoud M. Antioxidant status and lipid peroxidation in patients infected with HIV. Chem Biol Interact 1994; 91: 165–80.

28 Fortin PR, Lew RA, Liang MH et al. Validation of a meta-analysis: the effects of fish oil in rheumatoid arthritis. J Clin Epidemiol 1995; 48: 1379–90.

29 Frei B, England L, Ames BN. Ascorbate is an outstanding antioxidant in human blood plasma. Proc Natl Acad Sci USA 1989; 86: 6377–81.

30 Friedman A, Sklan D. Vitamin A and immunity. In: Human Nutrition – A Comprehensive Treatise, Volume 8: Nutrition and Immunology (Klurfeld DM ed.). Plenum Press, New York, 1993: 197–216.

31 Fryburg DA, Mark RJ, Griffith BP, Askenase PW, Patterson TF. The effect of supplemental beta-carotene on immunological indices in patients with AIDS: a pilot study. *Yale J Biol Med* 1995; 68: 19–23.

32 Fuller CJ, Faulkner H, Bendich A, Parker RS, Roe DA. Effect of beta-carotene supplementation on photosuppression of delayed-type hypersensitivity in normal young men. *Am J Clin Nutr* 1992; 56: 684–90.

33 Gollnick PM, Hopfenmuller W, Hemmes C et al. Systemic beta-carotene plus topical UV-sunscreen are an optimal protection against harmful effects of natural UV-sunlight: results of the Berlin-Eilath study. *Eur J Dermatol* 1996; 6: 200–5.

34 Gruner S, Volk HD, Falck P, Baehr RV. The influence of phagocytic stimuli on the expression of HLA-DR antigens; role of reactive oxygen intermediates. *Eur J Immunol* 1986; 16: 212–15.

35 Halliwell B, Aruoma OI. DNA damage by oxygen-derived species: its mechanisms and measurement in mammalian systems. *FEBS Lett* 1991; 281: 9–19.

36 Han SN, Meydani SN. Antioxidants, cytokines, and influenza infection in aged mice and elderly humans. *J Infect Dis* 2000; 182(Suppl 1): S74–80.

37 Hansson GK, Holm J, Jonasson L. Detection of activated T lymphocytes in the human atherosclerotic plaque. *Am J Pathol* 1989; 135: 169–75.

38 Hennekens CH, Buring JE, Manson JE, Stampfer M. Lack of effect of long term supplementation with beta carotene on the incidence of malignant neoplasms and cardiovascular disease. *N Engl J Med* 1996; 334: 1145–9.

39 Hughes DA. *In vitro* and *in vivo* effects of n-3 polyunsaturated fatty acids on human monocyte function. *Proc Nutr Soc* 1998; 57: 521–5.

40 Hughes DA, Pinder AC, Piper Z, Johnson IT, Lund EK. Fish oil supplementation inhibits the expression of major histocompatibility complex class II molecules and adhesion molecules on human monocytes. *Am J Clin Nutr* 1996; 63: 267–72.

41 Hughes DA, Wright AJA, Finglas PM et al. The effect of beta-carotene supplementation on the immune function of blood monocytes from healthy male non-smokers. *J Lab Clin Med* 1997; 129: 309–17.

42 Hughes DA, Wright AJA, Finglas PM et al. Effects of lycopene and lutein supplementation on the expression of functionally associated surface molecules on blood monocytes from healthy male non-smokers. *J Infect Dis* 2000; 182(Suppl 1): S11–15.

43 Janeway CA, Bottomly K, Babich J et al. Quantitative variation in Ia antigen expression plays a central role in immune regulation. *Immunol Today* 1984; 5: 99–104.

44 Johnson JD, Houchens DP, Kluwe WM, Craig DK, Fisher GL. Effects of mainstream and environmental tobacco smoke on the immune system in animals and humans: a review. CRC *Crit Rev Toxicol* 1990; 134: 356–61.

45 Kelley DS. Nutritional modulation of human immune status. *Nutr Res* 1989; 9: 965–75.

46 Kromann N, Green A. Epidemiological studies in the Upernavik district, Greenland. *Acta Med Scand* 1980; 208: 401–6.

47 Lavrovsky Y, Chatterjee B, Clark RA, Roy AK. Role of redox-regulated transcription factors in inflammation, aging and age-related diseases. *Exp Gerontol* 2000; 35: 521–32.

48 Lesourd B, Mazari L. Nutrition and immunity in the elderly. *Proc Nutr Soc* 1999; 58: 685–95.

49 Mangels AR, Holden JM, Beecher GR, Forman MR, Lanza E. Carotenoid content of fruits and vegetables: an evaluation of analytical data. *J Am Diet Assoc* 1993; 93: 284–96.

50 Mathews-Roth MM. Beta-carotene: clinical aspects. In: *New Protective Roles for Selected Nutrients* (Spiller GA, Scala J eds). Alan R. Liss, New York, 1989: 17–38.

51 Mayne SM. Beta-carotene, carotenoids, and disease prevention in humans. *FASEB J* 1996; 10: 690–701.

52 McKenzie RC, Rafferty TS, Beckett GJ. Selenium: an essential element for immune function. *Immunol Today* 1998; 19: 342–5.

53 McMurray DN, Watson RR, Reyes MA. Effect of renutrition on humoral and cell-mediated immunity in severely malnourished children. *Am J Clin Nutr* 1981; 34: 2117–26.

54 Meydani SN, Santos MS, Wu D, Hayek MG. Antioxidant modulation of cytokines and their biologic function in the aged. *Z Ernahrungswiss* 1998; 37 Suppl 1: 35–42.

55 Miles EA, Calder PC. Modulation of immune function by dietary fatty acids. *Proc Nutr Soc* 1998; 57: 277–92.

56 Moore SE, Cole TJ, Poskitt EM et al. Season of birth predicts mortality in rural Gambia. *Nature* 1997; 388: 434.

57 Murata T, Tamai H, Morinobu T et al. Effect of long-term administration of beta-carotene on lymphocyte subsets in humans. *Am J Clin Nutr* 1994; 60: 597–602.

58 Newman W, Middaugh J, Propst M, Rogers D. Atherosclerosis in Alaska natives and non-natives. *Lancet* 1993; 341: 1056–7.

59 Omenn GS, Goodman GE, Thornquist MD. Effects of a combination of beta carotene and vitamin A on lung cancer and cardiovascular disease. *N Engl J Med* 1996; 334: 1150–5.

60 Pacht ER, Kasek H, Mohammad JR, Cromwell DG, Davis WB. Deficiency of vitamin E in the alveolar fluid of cigarette smokers: influence on alveolar macrophage cytotoxicity. *J Clin Invest* 1986; 77: 789–96.

61 Palozza P. Prooxidant actions of carotenoids in biological systems. *Nutr Rev* 1998; 56: 257–65.

62 Passi S, Picardo M, Morrone A. Study on plasma polyunsaturated phospholipids and vitamin E, and on erythrocyte glutathione peroxidase in high risk HIV infection categories and AIDS patients. *Clin Chem Enzymol Commun* 1993; 5: 169–77.

63 Pauling L. *Vitamin C and the Common Cold*. WH Freeman, San Francisco, 1970.

64 Peto R, Doll R, Buckley JD, Sporn MB. Can dietary beta-carotene materially reduce human cancer rates? *Nature* 1981; 290: 201–8.

65 Prasad AS, Fitzgerald JT, Bao B, Beck FW, Chandrasekar PH. Duration of symptoms and plasma cytokine levels in patients with the common cold treated with zinc acetate. A randomized, double-blind, placebo-controlled trial. *Ann Intern Med* 2000; 133: 245–52.

66 Pryor WA, Stone K. Oxidants in cigarette smoke. *Ann N Y Acad Sci* 1993; 686: 12–28.

67 Rahman MM, Mahalanabis D, Alvarez JO et al. Acute respiratory infections prevent improvement of vitamin A status in young infants supplemented with vitamin A. *J Nutr* 1996; 126: 628–33.

68 Rapp JH, Connor WE, Lin DS, Porter JM. Dietary eicosapentaenoic acid and docosahexaenoic acid from fish oil. Their incorporation into advanced human atherosclerotic plaques. *Arterioscler Thromb* 1991; 11: 903–11.

69 Rebora A, Dallegri F, Patrone F. Neutrophil dysfunction and repeated infections: influence of levamisole and ascorbic acid. *Br J Dermatol* 1980; 21: 49–56.

70 Rice-Evans C. Plant polyphenols: free radical scavengers or chain-breaking antioxidants? *Biochem Soc Symp* 1995; 61: 103–16.

71 Richards GA, Theron AJ, Van Rensburg CEJ et al. Investigation of the effects of oral administration of vitamin E and beta-carotene on the chemiluminescence responses and the frequency of sister chromatid exchanges in circulating leukocytes from cigarette smokers. *Am Rev Respir Dis* 1990; 142: 648–54.

72 Riondel J, Glise D, Fernandez-Carlos T, Favier A. *In vitro* comparative study of cytolysis mediated by natural killer cells towards malignant cells preincubated with antioxidants. *Anticancer Res* 1998; 18: 1757–64.

73 Rivers JK, Norris PG, Murphy GM et al. UVA sunbeds: tanning, photoprotection, acute adverse effects and immunological changes. *Br J Dermatol* 1989; 120: 767–77.

74 Roy M, Kiremidjian-Schumacher L, Wishe HI, Cohen MW, Stotzky G. Supplementation with selenium and human immune functions. I. Effect on lymphocyte proliferation and interleukin-2 receptor expression. *Biol Trace Elem Res* 1994; 41: 103–14.

75 Santos MS, Leka LS, Ribaya-Mercado JD et al. Short- and long-term beta-carotene supplementation do not influence T cell-mediated immunity in healthy elderly persons. *Am J Clin Nutr* 1997; 66: 917–24.

76 Santos MS, Meydani SN, Leka L et al. Natural killer cell activity in elderly men is enhanced by beta-carotene supplementation. *Am J Clin Nutr* 1996; 64: 772–7.

77 Serfass RE, Ganther HE. Defective microbicidal activity in glutathione peroxidase-deficient neutrophils of selenium-deficient rats. *Nature* 1975; 255: 640–1.

78 Shankar AH, Prasad AS. Zinc and immune function: the biological basis of altered resistance to infection. *Am J Clin Nutr* 1998; 68: 447S–63S.

79 Sherman AR, Spear AT. Iron and Immunity. In: *Human Nutrition – A Comprehensive Treatise, Volume 8: Nutrition and Immunology* (Klurfeld DM ed.). Plenum Press, New York, 1993: 285–307.

80 Siegel BV. Vitamin C and the immune response in health and disease. In: *Human Nutrition – A Comprehensive Treatise, Volume 8: Nutrition and Immunology* (Klurfeld DM, ed.). Plenum Press, New York, 1993: 167–96.

81 Sirinsinha S, Suskind RM, Edelman R, Asvapaka C, Olson RE. Secretory IgA in Thai children with protein-calorie malnutrition. In: *Malnutrition and the Immune Response* (Suskind RM ed.). Raven Press, New York, 1977: 195–9.

82 Spallholz JE, Boylan LM, Larsen HS. Advances in understanding selenium's role in the immune system. *Ann N Y Acad Sci* 1990; 587: 123–39.

83 Springer TA. Adhesion receptors of the immune system. *Nature* 1990; 346: 425–34.

84 Sullivan GW, Sarembock IJ, Linden J. The role of inflammation in vascular diseases. *J Leukoc Biol* 2000; 67: 591–602.

85 Teshima S, Rokutan K, Takahashi M, Nikawa T, Kido Y, Kishi K. Alteration of the respiratory burst and phagocytosis of macrophages under protein malnutrition. *J Nutr Sci Vitaminol* 1995; 41: 127–37.

86 The Alpha-tocopherol Beta-carotene Cancer Prevention SG. The effect of vitamin E and beta-carotene on the incidence of lung cancer and other cancers in male smokers. *N Engl J Med* 1994; 330: 1029–35.

87 Thomas WR, Holt PG. Vitamin C and immunity: An assessment of the evidence. *Clin Exp Immunol* 1978; 32: 370–9.

88 Toyokuni S, Okamoto K, Yodoi J, Hiai H. Persistent oxidative stress in cancer. *FEBS Lett* 1995; 358: 1–3.

89 Watson RR, Prabhala RH, Plezia PM, Alberts DS. Effect of beta-carotene on lymphocyte subpopulations in elderly humans: evidence for a dose–response relationship. *Am J Clin Nutr* 1991; 53: 90–4.

90 Watzl B, Bub A, Blockhaus M *et al.* Prolonged tomato juice consumption has no effect on cell-mediated immunity of well-nourished elderly men and women. *J Nutr* 2000; 130: 1719–23.

91 Watzl B, Bub A, Rechkemmer G. Modulation of T-lymphocyte functions by the consumption of carotenoid-rich vegetables. *Br J Nutr* 1999; 82: 383–9.

92 Wayne SJ, Rhyne RL, Garry PJ, Goodwin JS. Cell-mediated immunity as a predictor of morbidity and mortality in subjects over 60. *J Gerontol Med Sci* 1990; 45: M45–M48.

93 Wellinghausen N, Kirchner H, Rink L. The immunobiology of zinc. *Immunol Today* 1997; 18: 519–21.

94 World Health Organization. *World Health Report: Life in the 21st Century. A Vision for All.* World Health Organization, Geneva, 1998.

95 Zeigler RG, Mayne ST, Swanson CA. Nutrition and lung cancer. *Cancer Causes Contr* 1996; 7: 157–77.

Chapter 27

Foods as allergens

S. L. Taylor and S. L. Hefle

DEFINITIONS AND DISTINGUISHING FEATURES OF FOOD ALLERGY AND FOOD INTOLERANCE

Food allergies and intolerances, sometimes referred to as food sensitivities, are adverse reactions to otherwise harmless foods or food components that are experienced by certain individuals in the population upon ingestion of one or more specific foods.[74,116] True food allergies involve abnormal immunological responses to substances in foods. True food allergies can be further subdivided into immunoglobulin E (IgE)-mediated and cell-mediated hypersensitivities. Food intolerances are individualistic adverse reactions to foods that are not known to involve immunological mechanisms, but include metabolic food disorders, e.g. lactose intolerance, and idiosyncratic reactions, e.g. sulphite-induced asthma.

The severity of IgE-mediated reactions

IgE-mediated food allergies are the most worrisome, because they can elicit very serious and life-threatening reactions.[103,133] IgE-mediated food allergies affect an estimated 1–2% of adults and 4–8% of young children.[74,101,121] The percentage of individuals with IgE-mediated food allergies who are at risk of severe, life-threatening reactions is unknown. In IgE-mediated food allergies, mast cells and basophils become 'armed' with allergen-specific IgE antibodies during the sensitization process.[82] Subsequent exposure of a sensitized individual to the offending food results in allergen interaction with the IgE bound to mast cells and basophils stimulating the release of potent mediators of the allergic reaction, including histamine, prostaglandins and the leukotrienes, from the sensitized cells (see Chapter 21). Exposure to small amounts of allergen can elicit the release of comparatively large quantities of these mediators. Thus, in IgE-mediated food allergies, the tolerance for the offending food is quite low. The foods involved in IgE-mediated allergic reactions will be the major focus of this chapter.

The role of cell-mediated hypersensitivity

The premier example of this is probably coeliac disease, also known as gluten-sensitive enteropathy[34,123] (see also Chapter 40). This illness is provoked in certain individuals by ingestion of the gluten proteins of wheat, rye, barley and oats and is characterized by a cell-mediated, localized inflammatory reaction in the intestinal tract that results in villous atrophy, other inflammatory changes and impaired absorptive function.[34]

The symptoms of untreated coeliac disease are associated with the adverse effect on intestinal absorption, and include body wasting, diarrhoea, bloating, anaemia, bone pain, chronic fatigue, weakness, various nutritional deficiencies and muscle cramps.[34] Coeliac disease does not elicit life-threatening reactions. The prevalence of coeliac disease seems to vary from one part of the world to another for unexplained reasons, but the highest degree of prevalence approaches 1 in 250 individuals.[123] Coeliac patients are advised to eliminate gluten-containing foods for life.

The role of cell-mediated, delayed hypersensitivity in other types of food sensitivities remains uncertain. Food-induced, cell-mediated immune mechanisms may be involved in several intestinal illnesses, including allergic eosinophilic gastroenteritis, Crohn's disease and ulcerative colitis (see Chapter 41), but further

A

research will be needed to confirm this possibility. With the exception of coeliac disease, the specific foods involved in food-induced, cell-mediated hypersensitivities can only be determined by elimination diet, and subsequent oral challenge.

Metabolic food disorders

These result from defects in the ability to metabolize a food component, such as lactose due to enzyme deficiencies. Metabolic food disorders are often inherited traits. Lactose intolerance is the best known of the metabolic food disorders and results from an inherited deficiency of the enzyme, β-galactosidase, in the intestinal tract.[113] As a result of this deficiency, lactose, the primary sugar in milk, cannot be metabolized into its two constituent monosaccharides, galactose and glucose. Undigested lactose cannot be absorbed, and thus passes from the small intestine into the colon where bacteria ferment lactose to CO_2 and H_2O.

The symptoms include abdominal cramping, flatulence and frothy diarrhoea. Lactose intolerance affects almost 75% of individuals on a worldwide basis. Additionally, most lactose-intolerant individuals can tolerate some quantities of lactose.

Idiosyncratic reactions

These consist of food intolerances that occur through unknown mechanisms. The role of foods and food additives in these reactions has not been well established. The symptoms involved can range from very minor to life-threatening. The best example is sulphite-induced asthma.[118] Sulphites are used as food additives in a variety of foods, as shown in Table 27.1. About 1% of asthmatic individuals are sensitive to ingested sulphite.[30] While sulphite-induced asthma can be quite serious and deaths have been reported,[131] sulphite-sensitive individuals do have definite, though variable, tolerances for sulphite in foods.[119]

FOODS CAUSING IgE-MEDIATED FOOD ALLERGIES

The eight foods or food groups which are thought to be responsible for the vast majority of IgE-mediated food allergies are shown in Table 27.2.[47] However, some regional differences may exist. For example, celery allergy appears to be fairly prevalent in Europe,[18,129] sesame seed allergy appears to be fairly prevalent in many parts of the world[18,56,110] and buckwheat allergy is quite common in South Korea.[90] These regional differences may relate to patterns of food preferences in the diet and, in some cases such as celery, to coexistent pollen allergies. In addition to the eight major foods or food groups, over 160 other foods have been implicated as causing IgE-mediated food allergies in the medical

Foods containing sulphites
Dehydrated fruits and vegetables
Wine
Shrimp
Cured meats (not allowed in some countries)
Foods containing added sulphite as a preservative. Quantities range from <10 ppm to >2000 ppm in dried fruit.[118]

Table 27.1 Foods containing sulphites.

Foods commonly causing IgE-mediated reactions
Cow's milk
Egg
Fish
Wheat
Peanut*
Soybean
Crustacea (shrimp, crab, lobster, etc.)
Tree nuts (almond, hazel, walnut, etc.)
The eight foods or food groups are responsible for the majority of IgE-mediated food allergy.[48]
* Peanut is not a nut but a member of the legume family.

Table 27.2 Foods commonly causing IgE-mediated reactions.

literature.[53] Since food allergens are proteins, any food that contains protein residues can trigger allergic sensitization on at least some occasions. The eight most common foods or food groups involve foods with comparatively high protein content that are also fairly common in the diet. However, several other commonly consumed foods with high protein content, namely beef, pork, chicken and turkey, are rarely allergenic.

Peanuts

Peanut allergy is clearly one of the most common types of food allergy.[17,23,46,101] However, the few studies that have been conducted on the specific prevalence of peanut allergy within an unselected population suggest that it is among the most common of food allergies among infants.[56,115] The prevalence in adults is not known, but peanut allergy is often not outgrown.[14,16,102] Recently, population surveys have indicated that 0.6% of the US population and 0.5% of the British population believe that they have peanut allergies.[44,109] Although the accuracy of these perceptions was not confirmed with challenge testing, peanut allergy is sufficiently striking that misconceptions would be infrequent. Severe allergic reactions to peanuts, including fatal reactions, are well documented.[69,93,103,133] The threshold dose needed to elicit an allergic reaction in peanut-allergic individuals is not precisely known but is likely to be very small and variable from patient to patient. In a recent study among a small group of peanut-allergic individuals, the most sensitive individual suffered a mild allergic reaction from ingestion of 2 mg of peanut protein, while several subjects with impressive histories and positive oral challenge tests failed to react to the highest dose included in the trial, 50 mg.[62]

Soybean

Soybean allergy is less common than peanut allergy. However, among allergic infants referred to allergy clinics, soybean allergy is among the most common reactions to a food.[17,20,23,79,101,125] In a study of the prevalence of specific food allergies within unselected paediatric patients, soybean was again one of the most common offenders.[56] The prevalence of soybean allergy among adults is unknown. Soybean allergy is sometimes outgrown.[14,102] However, soybean allergy has been well described among adults.[54] Severe reactions, including several deaths, to soybeans have also been reported among soybean-allergic individuals.[15,54,70,132] The threshold dose for soybeans in soy-allergic individuals is not known.

Tree nuts

The tree nuts that can cause allergic reactions are shown in Table 27.3. While these tree nuts are from several different genera, all have been found to cause allergic reactions. Tree nut allergies are among the most common causes of food allergy among infants referred to specialty medical care[17,35,46,110] and also the most common in clinical studies on unselected populations.[56,115] The prevalence of tree nut allergies among adults is unknown but have been well described.[3,6,50,86] A recent population survey revealed that the perceived prevalence of tree nut allergy in the United States was approximately 0.4%.[109] The natural history has not been carefully investigated but it is thought that the allergy responses are persistent. The prevalence of individual tree nut allergies is not known, but the more frequently consumed tree nuts are the more common offenders. Unusual tree nuts such as coconut, kola nut and shea nut are rarely allergenic. Severe allergic reactions to tree nuts, including several deaths, have been documented.[19,70,71,93,103,133] The threshold dose needed to elicit adverse reactions to tree nuts in sensitive individuals is not known.

Wheat

Wheat is a common cause of food-allergic reactions among infants and young children referred to specialty practices,[17,20,23,101,125] and appears to be one of the most common allergenic foods among infants evaluated from an unselected population.[56] In infants and young children, wheat allergy is much more common than allergies to other grains such as barley, rye and oats[65] and can be outgrown.[102] The prevalence of wheat allergy among the general population is unknown. Allergic reactions to wheat are rarely severe, although a few severe cases have been described.[91,127] No deaths from allergic reactions to wheat have been recorded. True wheat allergy is thought to be relatively uncommon among adults.

Cow's milk

Cow's milk allergy is the most common type of food allergy among infants (see Chapter 30). The prevalence of cow's milk allergy among infants in the general population under the age of 2 was approximately 2% in several large clinical trials[56,59,63,104] and is of course also a common allergenic food among infants and young children referred to specialty medical practices.[13,17,20,23,35,101,125] Cow's milk allergy is frequently outgrown,[11,13–15,55,60,66,102] although cow's milk allergy has been described among teenagers and adults.[85,96,106] Many allergy reactions to cow's milk are comparatively mild; however, severe reac-

tions and deaths have been reported following inadvertent ingestion of cow's milk by sensitive individuals.[32,70,93,96,103,105,106,114]

Egg

Among infants and young children referred to paediatric allergy practices, eggs are among the most common allergenic foods.[13,17,20,23,35,101,125] The comparatively high prevalence of egg allergy in unselected paediatric populations has also been established[56] although the prevalence among adults is not known but has been well documented.[85,93] Egg allergies among infants are frequently outgrown[14,15,48,66,102] and although typically mild, severe reactions and deaths have been described.[70,93,103]

Fish

The prevalence of fish allergy is not quite so well established as are some of the other commonly allergenic foods (see Chapter 29). Among infants and young children referred to paediatric allergy practices, fish allergy is comparatively common[1,17,23,35,42,98,101] and also reasonably prevalent among an unselected paediatric population in Australia.[56] The prevalence in children appears to be somewhat higher in countries where fish are commonly eaten. Fish allergy has also been described among adult patients.[52,87] However, the prevalence of fish allergy in the general population is not known. Severe allergic reactions, including deaths, to fish are well documented.[93,133] In a study with a small group of cod-allergic patients, the threshold dose for eliciting allergic reactions was several grams for the majority of these patients.[52]

Crustacea

Crustacea include shrimp, prawns, crabs, lobsters and crayfish. The prevalence of crustacea allergy is unknown. However, crustaceans are well accepted as common causes of allergic reactions, especially among adults.[37,39,128] Shellfish allergy appears to be common in Asia, but the distinction between crustacea and molluscs was not made in the relevant study.[56] The prevalence of crustacean allergy among children appears lower than among adults, but crustacean allergy has been described in children[14] and is rarely outgrown.[14,38,66] Severe allergic reactions and deaths from inadvertent ingestion of crustacean products by allergic individuals have been described.[70,93,133]

Sesame seed

Several cases of sesame seed allergy have been documented in the medical literature.[64,67,68,72,77,122] However, virtually no information exists on the prevalence of sesame seed allergy among the general population or within referral populations. A recent study from Australia provides the first evidence that sesame seed may be an allergenic food of increasing importance.[56] Recently, a large number of cases of sesame seed allergy have been noted in Australian infants[110] but clinical information from other parts of the world is lacking. Further studies on the prevalence of sesame seed allergy are needed. Severe reactions to sesame seeds have been reported[64,67,82] but no deaths have occurred. Ultimately, sesame seeds may need to be added to the list of the most commonly allergenic foods established by the FAO in 1995.

Buckwheat

While buckwheat is infrequently consumed and rarely allergenic in most parts of the world, it may be an important allergenic

Members of the tree nut families
Walnut
Pecan
Almond
Hazel
Brazil
Cashew
Pistachio
Pine
Macadamia

Table 27.3 Members of the tree nut families.

food in southeast Asia where it is eaten in quantity. Buckwheat is a common ingredient in certain pastas eaten in South Korea and other southeast Asian countries. Although the prevalence of buckwheat allergy has not been documented in these countries, multiple cases of severe allergic reactions to buckwheat have been reported among these consumers.[90,130]

Cottonseed

Cottonseed protein clearly has the potential to be highly allergenic. Cottonseed protein or meal is rarely incorporated into human foods, and is instead relegated primarily for animal feeding. However, when cottonseed protein or meal is incorporated into foods, severe allergic reactions have been reported[80,88] and, clearly, its use should be approached with considerable caution.

Oral allergy syndrome

The foods mentioned thus far can cause severe systemic reactions in some allergic individuals. At the other end of the spectrum, the oral allergy syndrome primarily involves the oropharyngeal region where the symptoms include urticaria, angioedema, pruritis and flushing.[91] Only in rare instances does this syndrome include systemic reactions. Oral allergy syndrome most frequently occurs among individuals with pollen allergies. The foods associated with oral allergy syndrome are shown in Table 27.4. The cross-reacting foods contain structurally related allergens to those in the pollens. These allergens are sensitive to digestion and are heat labile, so that affected individuals are primarily affected by the ingestion of fresh fruits and vegetables.

ALLERGENS IN FOODS

The allergens in foods are almost always naturally occurring proteins. Although foods contain numerous individual proteins, only a comparative few have been documented as being allergens.[29] Some foods contain multiple allergenic proteins including peanuts, cow's milk and eggs.[29] However, in other foods such as codfish and Brazil nuts, one specific protein seems to be predominantly responsible for the allergic reactions.[29] Even among the foods that contain multiple allergens, not all of the proteins in these foods are capable of eliciting IgE production.

With the exception of the fresh fruits and vegetables noted above in the discussion of oral allergy syndrome, the most common allergenic foods are good sources of protein. As noted earlier, some common, protein-rich foods, such as beef, are rarely

allergenic. The allergens in the commonly allergenic foods are usually proteins that are comparatively abundant in that particular food. For example, with cow's milk, the major allergens are casein, β-lactoglobulin and α-lactalbumin, the principal proteins found in milk. These allergens possess certain properties that tend to enhance their allergenicity: namely, they are stable to digestion, acid and to heat denaturation.[117] Thus, these proteins can survive food processing operations and human digestive processes and still arrive in the intestinal tract in immunologically intact form. While it is beyond the scope of this chapter to provide detailed information on all of the well-described food allergens, the allergens in shrimp and peanuts will be discussed below as examples.

Shrimp allergens

In early allergen characterization work, identified allergens were named at the authors' preference. As the research progressed and recombinant techniques made it much easier to identify and isolate these proteins, a nomenclature system was adopted. Allergens are designated as to their source, with the first three letters of the genus name, followed by the first letter of the species name, and then an Arabic number to represent the order of their identification. For example, the major shrimp allergen discussed below was isolated from *Penaeus aztecus*, the brown shrimp and, hence, its designation is Pen a 1. The homologous molecule from Indian shrimp, *Penaeus indicus*, is Pen i 1.

Shrimp is the most thoroughly studied of the crustacea allergens. Hoffman *et al.*[57] were the first to partially characterize IgE-binding proteins from shrimp. Antigen I was isolated from raw shrimp and was found to be an acidic, heat-labile protein composed of two noncovalently bound polypeptide chains with a molecular weight of 21 kDa. Of the 11 serum samples from shrimp-allergic patients tested in the study, 7 had IgE specific for Antigen I which had an isoelectric point of 4.75–5 and contained 189 amino acid residues and 0.5% carbohydrate. In native form, it was 45 kDa in molecular weight, suggesting that it exists as a dimer. Antigen II, isolated from cooked shrimp, was found to be an acidic heat-stable glycoprotein with a molecular weight of 38 kDa and an isoelectric point of 5.4–5.8. Antigen II bound IgE from all 11 shrimp-allergic serum samples and, therefore, was a major allergen for the subjects in this study. Antigen II was composed of 341 amino acid residues and 4% carbohydrate. Antigens I and II were considered to be unrelated, based on amino acid composition and immunological studies. Nagpal *et al.*[84] described the identification of two allergenic proteins from cooked shrimp. One IgE-binding protein, designated SA-I, had a molecular weight of 8.2 kDa and was not further characterized. The second IgE-binding protein, SA-II, was composed of 301 amino acid residues, had a molecular weight of 34 kDa and appeared to be similar to Antigen I isolated by Hoffman *et al.*[57] However, it was reported not to contain carbohydrate.

Daul *et al.*[41] identified, isolated, and characterized the definitive major shrimp allergen, named Pen a 1, from boiled brown shrimp. Pen a 1 has a molecular weight of 36 kDa and is readily isolated from the boiling water and meat of cooked shrimp. It has been determined to be tropomyosin, a muscle protein. The allergen is composed of 312 amino acid residues and 2.9% carbohydrate, and constitutes 20% of the soluble protein in crude cooked shrimp extract. IgE from 28 of the 34 shrimp-allergic subjects in the study bound to Pen a 1. Monoclonal antibodies directed

Association of pollen allergy with foods causing the oral allergy syndrome
Ragweed pollen: Melon, banana[45]
Silver birch pollen: Apple, peach (and stone fruits) including cherry, hazelnut, etc.[43,93]
Mugwort pollen: Celery, carrot, fennel, parsley, certain spices[124,129]

Table 27.4 Association of pollen allergy with foods causing the oral allergy syndrome.

against Pen a 1 also recognized a 36 kDa protein in crayfish, crab and lobster extracts,[40] and Pen a 1-like proteins (tropomyosins) have been shown to be responsible for most of the allergenicity of these related crustacea.[76] Antigen I, SA-II and Pen a 1 appear to be the same protein, as the molecular weights, IgE-reactivity and amino acid composition are similar. In 1993, Shanti et al.[107] determined that SA-II was indeed tropomyosin. Further work has determined that tropomyosin is the major allergen for two additional shrimp species; the allergens were named Pen f 1 (Parapenaeus fissurus)[78] and Met e 1 (Metapenaeus ensis).[75] Met e 1 had 281 amino acid residues and a molecular weight of 34 kDa; the isoelectric point was not reported. Par f 1 was 39 kDa in size and had an isoelectric point of 5.1–5.6 kDa. The amount of carbohydrate contained in these latter two allergens was not determined.

Shanti et al.[107] reported that shrimp-specific IgE bound to two tryptically derived peptide sequences from Pen i 1, in regions 50–66 and 153–161. Region 50–66 is M-Q-Q-L-E-N-D-L-D-Q-V-Q-E-S-L-L-K and 153–161 is F-L-A-E-E-A-D-R-K. Leung et al.[75] found that Met e 1, also has both of these IgE-binding sequences. Reese et al.[97] described 13 peptide sequences, derived by recombinant and synthetic means, that bound IgE from shrimp-allergic patients. Three major IgE-binding regions occurred at residues 119–148, 153–179 and 241–282, suggesting that the centre and C-terminus contain most of the IgE-binding. There was apparently no binding to the 50–66 region, as was found in the other studies. However, shrimp-specific IgE did bind to a peptide of residues 157–169, containing E-A-D-R-K, confirming what was observed in the other studies.

Minor shrimp allergens

There are other IgE-binding allergens in shrimp that have been described. A minor allergenic tRNA moiety from cooked prawns (P. indicus) was described by Nagpal et al.[83] However, the researchers were not able to isolate a preparation completely devoid of protein, so it is possible that trace RNA-associated proteins were responsible for the allergenicity. Lin et al.[78] has identified a 74 kDa component in shrimp that bound IgE from 40% of their shrimp-allergic patients. Minor IgE-binding components of 41, 47, 50 and 86 kDa bound IgE from 10–20% of the sera. Characterization of these allergens has not been done to date.

Peanut allergens

Peanuts contain multiple allergenic proteins. Not all peanut-allergic individuals react to the same peanut proteins, but peanuts contain several major allergens that bind IgE from the serum of the majority of peanut-allergic patients.

Peanut-1

Sachs et al.[99] were the first to isolate and partially purify a peanut allergen, designated Peanut-1, from raw peanuts. Peanut-1 contained two major bands with molecular weights of 20 and 30 kDa and several minor bands whose molecular weights were reported to be above and below these. The allergen contained 8.7% carbohydrate, and had an isoelectric point of approximately 5.25–5.75. Peanut-1 elicited positive skin test results and histamine release from basophils in peanut-allergic subjects. The authors concluded that Peanut-1 is a major acidic glycoprotein with non-identical subunits, but was not the only allergenic moiety present in peanuts.

Concanavalin A reactive glycoprotein

Gleeson & Jermyn[51] first described the isolation of a concanavalin A reactive glycoprotein (CARG) from raw peanuts. The isolated protein had a molecular weight of 69 kDa and contained 12% carbohydrate. Barnett & Howden[7] later identified CARG as an allergen and subsequently purified and further characterized it. CARG appeared to be a major allergen of peanut, since approximately 50% of the serum samples from peanut-allergic patients in the latter study had specific IgE for it. CARG constituted approximately 1% of the total protein in peanut,[51] had an isoelectric point of 4.6 and contained 2.4% carbohydrate. CARG was also remarkably stable, withstanding temperatures at and above 100°C, and pH changes over the range 2.8–10.0. Barnett and Howden[7] also found that removing the carbohydrate portion of CARG slightly decreased but did not completely eliminate the allergenic activity.

Ara h 1

A 63.5 kDa molecular weight glycoprotein peanut allergen was identified by Burks et al.[27] using serum from peanut-allergic atopic dermatitis patients. The allergen has an isoelectric point of 4.55 and is a major allergen for peanut-allergic individuals in most studies to date. The allergen was named Ara h 1, and it appears that CARG and Ara h 1 are the same protein. Ara h 1 has been cloned and its amino acid sequence deduced. It was found to contain multiple IgE-binding sites (Fig. 27.1) and has significant sequence homology with the vicilin storage proteins,[22] showing 62–66% homology to broad bean, pea and soybean vicilin-like proteins. Burks et al.[22] also found that linear sequences in recombinant Ara h 1 bound IgE; while all 11 patients in the study had IgE that bound to native Ara h 1, 8 of the 11 bound to recombinant Ara h 1 (without carbohydrate). Burks et al.[25] found that there were at least 23 different IgE-binding epitopes along the entire length of Ara h 1; the epitopes ranged from 6–10 amino acids in length, and no obvious composition was shared by the epitopes. Four epitopes appeared to be immunodominant, as greater than 80% of the IgE from peanut-allergic subjects in the study bound to them. A single amino acid substitution in the immunodominant epitopes could obliterate IgE binding. The hydrophobic residues located in the centre of the molecule were found to be most critical for IgE-binding,[108] in contrast to previous observations of IgE binding occurring along the whole length of the molecule.[25] The position of these critical epitopes in a tertiary model showed that they were clustered in two areas of the molecule, and not, in fact, all along the entire molecule.

Ara h 2

The second major peanut allergen to be identified was Ara h 2,[26] which has a molecular weight of 17.5 kDa, an isoelectric point of 5.2 and contains 20% carbohydrate. The allergen is also a major allergen for peanut-sensitive patients, as most of them have specific IgE for it.[112] Ara h 2 has been cloned and the nucleotide sequence determined; it has 39% homology with conglutin-δ from lupin, 32–35% with mabilin I from caper, 34% and 30% with 2S albumins from sunflower and castor, respectively, 29% with α-amylase inhibitor from wheat and 27% with the CM3 protein from wheat.[112] The authors determined that Ara h 2 is a conglutin-like seed storage protein. The IgE-binding epitopes of Ara h 2 were investigated using synthetic overlapping peptides of the protein.[112] Ten IgE-binding epitopes were found, along the

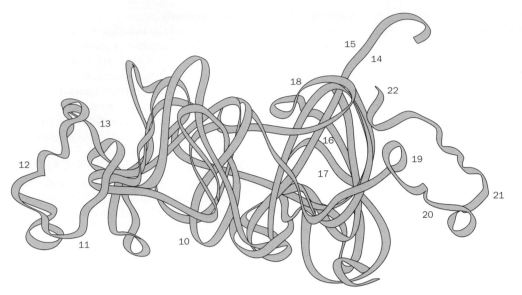

Fig. 27.1 The majority of the Ara 1 h IgE-binding epitopes are clustered in two regions of the allergen. The numbered dark areas are IgE-binding epitopes 10–22. Epitopes 13 and portions of 14 and 15 lie in an area of structural uncertainty.

complete length of the molecule, and were 6–10 amino acids in length. Three of these were recognized by all peanut-allergic sera tested, indicating the immunodominance of these moieties. No amino acid sequences were shared between the epitopes. Within the epitopes, 63% of the amino acids represented with either polar uncharged or apolar residues. As in the case of Ara h 1, a single amino acid change in the immunodominant epitopes could obliterate IgE-binding. This finding is important in that it may allow for improved diagnostic and therapeutic approaches to peanut hypersensitivity. In another study, Burks *et al.*[24] found that three of four T-cell binding sites in Ara h 2 did not map to the immunodominant IgE-binding regions. This could allow for development of an immunotherapeutic reagent where IgE-binding sites are altered so that IgE binding is prevented but the T-cell binding sites remaining intact.

Ara h 3

A third major allergen from peanuts was described by Bannon *et al.*,[5] with a molecular weight of 14 kDa. The allergen has been named Ara h 3, and amino acid sequencing showed 61% homology with a soybean glycinin subunit G3. Ara h 3 has been cloned and DNA sequencing revealed 70–80% homology to the glycinin family of seed storage proteins. Recombinant Ara h 3 was recognized by 8 of 18 (45%) of the sera from peanut-allergic patients in this study. One immunodominant epitope has been found and, again, a single amino acid change can affect or obliterate IgE binding.[95] The 14 kDa is a part of a larger 60 kDa molecular weight glycinin. Ten IgE-binding sites have been identified, with lengths of 6–10 amino acid residues. Although the subjects in these studies were not clinically allergic to soy, Ara h 3 has high homology to soy glycinin.[94] Clarke *et al.*[33] have found that in their peanut-allergic patient pool, specific IgE to Ara h 3 is correlated to a tendency to experience more severe reactions to peanut.[33]

Minor peanut allergen – peanut agglutinin

Burks *et al.*[21] have identified a minor allergen for which 5 of 10 (50%) peanut-allergic individuals in the study possessed specific IgE. The allergen had a molecular weight of 35 kDa and subsequent amino acid sequencing showed that it was peanut agglu-

Peanuts contain multiple allergenic proteins: a summary of their properties			
Peanut	**Molecular weight (kDa)**	**Carbohydrate (%)**	**Isoelectric point**
Peanut 1 An acidic glycoprotein with non-identical subunits	20,30	8.7	5.25–5.75
Ara h 1 (CARG) This protein contains 23 different IgE-binding epitopes along its entire length. Ara h 1 and CARG have been shown to be identical molecules	63.5	12	4.55
Ara h 2 A conglutin-like seed storage protein with 10 IgE-binding epitopes. One of the four T-cell binding epitopes does map with an IgE binding epitope	17.5	20	5.2
Ara h 3 Ten IgE-binding sites have been identified with lengths of 6–10 amino acid residues	14		
Minor peanut allergen Amino acid sequencing has shown this to be peanut agglutinin that exhibits specific (not non-specific) IgE binding	35		

Table 27.5 Peanuts contain multiple allergenic proteins: a summary of their properties.

tinin. The researchers found that IgE did not exhibit non-specific binding to this lectin, as had been previously theorized. A comparison of these allergens is shown in Table 27.5.

CROSSREACTIONS

Crossreactions sometimes occur between related foods. However, such crossreactions do not occur with all individuals and for all groups of related foods. Crossreactions are much more likely with certain food groups than with others.

Crustacea

The crustacean family serves as an excellent example of a food group where crossreactions are frequent. Most individuals with such allergies are allergic to all of the crustacea species, including shrimp, prawn, crab and lobster.[40] However, these same individuals can often eat other seafoods, including molluscan shellfish and finfish.

Milk and eggs

Crossreactions are also common with other food groups. Cow's milk-allergic individuals are also likely to be reactive to goat's milk and the milk of other non-human species.[111] Egg-allergic individuals are likely to react to eggs of all avian species.[73]

Legumes

The legume family serves as an excellent example of a food group where crossreactions are less frequently encountered. Among the legumes, peanuts are definitely the most commonly allergenic food. For most individuals with peanut allergy, peanuts are the only legume that elicits allergic reactions. These individuals can ingest other legumes without incident.[8] Many peanut-allergic individuals have positive skin prick tests to extracts of other legumes,[10] but are able to eat these other legume foods safely. Thus, the oral challenge test may be the only reliable method to establish the existence of crossreactions among related foods. Allergic reactions can occur, though less frequently, to other legumes including soybeans. Some of these individuals will also be allergic to peanuts.[54]

Foods and pollens

As noted earlier, crossreactions have been observed between common pollen allergies such as birch, ragweed and mugwort and allergic sensitivity to certain fresh fruits and vegetables (the oral allergy syndrome).

Other crossreactions

Similarly, crossreactions are less commonly encountered with other food groups. With fish, the situation seems quite complicated. Many fish-allergic individuals seem to experience allergic reactions with more than one species of fish.[9] However, at least some of these individuals can eat some fish species safely.[9] Of course, there is considerable taxonomic diversity within the fish group. Crossreactions between closely related species such as salmon and trout or cod and haddock may be more common. Crossreactions among the various fish species will require much more clinical study before any general recommendations can be made. The tree nut group is another assemblage of rather diverse species. Despite the genetic diversity, many tree nut-allergic individuals seem to have crossreactions with many, if not all, of the tree nuts.[50] Some of this crossreactivity would be expected because of close relationships between certain of the tree nuts, such as walnuts and pecans. However, the nature and frequency of crossreactions among the various tree nuts merits much closer study before attempting to reach any conclusions. With respect to IgE-mediated food allergies, little crossreactivity seems to occur among the grains. As noted earlier, wheat is the most commonly allergenic grain. Although barley and rye are closely related to wheat, IgE-mediated allergies to these grains are less commonly encountered. Of course, the situation is quite different with coeliac disease (see Chapter 40).

Crossreactions can also occur between latex allergies and allergic reactions to certain foods such as bananas, kiwis, avocados and chestnuts.[12] Several more unusual crossreactions have also been noted, including between snails and dust mites[126] and between cockroaches and shrimp.[36]

FOOD-DEPENDENT, EXERCISE-INDUCED ANAPHYLAXIS

Exercise-induced anaphylaxis (EIA) is a form of physical allergy involving urticaria, angioedema or shock occurring after vigorous exercise.[2] EIA is not always associated with foods. However, eating any food or, in some cases a specific food, is apparently involved in the development of EIA in over half of the cases.[58] Foods associated with F-EIA include celery, wheat, shrimp, oyster, chicken and peach. Some cases of F-EIA can be quite severe, as described in a recent series on wheat-associated EIA.[89]

ALLERGIC REACTIONS TO INGREDIENTS DERIVED FROM SPECIFIC FOODS

Edible oils

Individuals with specific food allergies will need to avoid all forms of that food that contain protein.[121] However, some ingredients derived from commonly allergenic foods do not contain detectable protein residues and may be safe for allergic individuals to ingest. For example, edible oils are often derived from commonly allergenic foods, including peanuts and soybeans. Although highly refined peanut and soybean oils contain extremely low levels of protein and have been demonstrated by double-blind, placebo-controlled food challenges to be safe for individuals with peanut and soybean allergies,[31,61,120] some caution must be exercised with edible oils. Less highly refined oils may not always be safe[61] and, if the oils have been used to fry foods, they may become contaminated with the allergens from those foods.

Lecithin, starch and gelatin

Other food ingredients may also be derived from commonly allergenic sources. Lecithin can be derived from soybeans or, less often, from eggs. Lecithin contains residues of proteins from either soybeans or eggs. Allergists vary in their advice to individuals with allergies to soy and eggs regarding the avoidance of lecithin, and few reactions have been reported. Starch is most commonly derived from corn, a rarely allergenic food. However, starch may also be derived from wheat. Wheat starch does contain trace residues of wheat protein, but allergic reactions to wheat starch have not been reported. Gelatin is most often derived from beef and pork, which are uncommon allergenic foods. Gelatin is itself a protein and may induce allergic sensitization on occasion, especially when used intravenously.[100] However, gelatin may occasionally be derived from fish, although the allergenicity of fish gelatin has not been established.

Food labels may contain collective terms that may include sources of commonly allergenic foods. Flavours are infrequently derived from allergenic sources and do not often contain protein residues; however, flavours can occasionally contain protein residues from allergenic foods that would not necessarily be divulged on the ingredient statement. Several allergic reactions have occurred to foods that contained flavours that had residues of milk or peanut proteins.[49,81] Another collective term is spices. Although spices rarely cause allergic reactions, sesame seeds may occasionally be included on food ingredient statements under the collective term spices.

REFERENCES

1 Aas K. Studies of hypersensitivity to fish: a clinical study. *Int Arch Allergy Appl Immunol* 1966; 29: 346–63.

2 Anderson JA. Allergic reactions to foods. *Crit Rev Food Sci Nutr* 1996; 36: S19–S38.

3 Arshad SH, Malmberg E, Krapf K, Hide DW. Clinical and immunological characteristics of Brazil nut allergy. *Clin Exp Allergy* 1991; 21: 373–6.

4 Atkins FM, Wilson M, Bock SA. Cottonseed hypersensitivity: new concerns over an old problem. *J Allergy Clin Immunol* 1988; 82: 242–50.

5 Bannon GA, Li XF, Rabjohn P *et al. Ara h* 3, a peanut allergen identified by using peanut sensitive patient sera absorbed with soy proteins. *J Allergy Clin Immunol* 1997; 99: S141.

6 Bargman TJ, Rupnow JH, Taylor SL. IgE-binding proteins in almonds (*Prunus amygdalus*): identification by immunoblotting with sera from almond-allergic adults. *J Food Sci* 1992; 57: 717–20.

7 Barnett D, Howden MEH. Partial characterization of an allergenic glycoprotein from peanut (*Arachis hypogaea* L.). *Biochim Biophys Acta* 1986; 882: 97–105.

8 Bernhisel-Broadbent J, Sampson HA. Cross-allergenicity in the legume botanical family in children with food hypersensitivity. *J Allergy Clin Immunol* 1989; 83: 435–40.

9 Bernhisel-Broadbent J, Scanlon SM, Sampson HA. Fish hypersensitivity. I. *In vitro* and oral challenge results in fish-allergic patients. *J Allergy Clin Immunol* 1992; 89: 730–7.

10 Bernhisel-Broadbent J, Taylor S, Sampson HA. Cross-allergenicity in the legume botanical family in children with food hypersensitivity. II. Laboratory correlates. *J Allergy Clin Immunol* 1989; 84: 701–9.

11 Bishop JM, Hosking CS, Hill DJ. Natural history of cow milk allergy. Clinical outcome. *J Pediatr* 1990; 116: 862–7.

12 Blanco C, Carrillo T, Castillo R *et al.* Latex allergy: clinical features and cross-reactivity with fruits. *Ann Allergy* 1994; 73: 309–14.

13 Bock SA. Prospective appraisal of complaints of adverse reactions to foods in children during the first three years of life. *Pediatrics* 1987; 79: 683–8.

14 Bock SA. The natural history of food sensitivity. *J Allergy Clin Immunol* 1982; 69: 173–7.

15 Bock SA. Natural history of severe reactions to foods in young children. *J Pediatr* 1985; 107: 676–80.

16 Bock SA, Atkins FM. The natural history of peanut allergy. *J Allergy Clin Immunol* 1989; 83: 900–4.

17 Bock SA, Atkins FM. Patterns of food hypersensitivity during sixteen years of double-blind, placebo-controlled food challenges. *J Pediatr* 1990; 117: 561–7.

18 Bousquet J, Bjorksten B, Bruijnzeel-Koomen CAFM *et al.* Scientific criteria and selection of allergenic foods for labeling. *Allergy* 1998; 53 (Suppl. 47): 3–21.

19 Boyd, GK. Fatal nut anaphylaxis in a 16-year-old male: case report. *Allergy Proc* 1989; 10: 255–7.

20 Bruno G, Cantani A, Ragno V *et al*: Natural history of IgE antibodies in children at risk for atopy. *Ann Allergy Asthma Immunol* 1995; 74: 431–6.

21 Burks AW, Cockrell GE, Connaughton CA *et al.* Identification of peanut agglutinin and soybean trypsin inhibitor as minor legume allergens. *Int Arch Allergy Immunol* 1994; 105: 143–9.

22 Burks AW, Cockrell G, Stanley JS *et al.* Recombinant peanut allergen *Ara h* 1 expression and IgE binding in patients with peanut hypersensitivity. *J Clin Invest* 1995; 96: 1715–21.

23 Burks AW, Mallory SB, Williams LW, Shirrell MA. Atopic dermatitis: clinical relevance of food hypersensitivity reactions. *J Pediatr* 1988; 113: 447–51.

24 Burks AW, Sampson HA, Bannon GA. Peanut allergens. *Allergy* 1998; 53: 725–30.

25 Burks AW, Shin D, Cockrell G *et al.* Mapping and mutational analysis of the IgE-binding epitopes on Ara h 1, a legume vicilin protein and a major allergen in peanut hypersensitivity. *Eur J Biochem* 1997; 245: 334–9.

26 Burks AW, Williams LW, Connaughton C *et al.* Identification and characterization of a second major peanut allergen, *Ara h* II, with use of the sera of patients with atopic dermatitis and positive peanut challenge. *J Allergy Clin Immunol* 1992; 90: 962–9.

27 Burks AW, Williams LW, Helm RM *et al.* Identification of a major peanut allergen, *Ara h* 1, in patients with atopic dermatitis and positive peanut challenges. *J Allergy Clin Immunol* 1991; 88: 172–9.

28 Burks AW, Williams LW, Mallory SB *et al.* Peanut protein as a major cause of adverse food reactions in patients with atopic dermatitis. *Allergy Proc* 1989; 10: 265–9.

29 Bush RK, Hefle SL. Food allergens. *Crit Rev Food Sci Nutr* 1996; 36: S119–S63.

30 Bush RK, Taylor SL, Holden K *et al.* Prevalence of sensitivity to sulfiting agents in asthmatic patients. *Am J Med* 1986; 81: 816–21.

31 Bush RK, Taylor SL, Nordlee JA *et al.* Soybean oil is not allergenic to soybean-sensitive individuals. *J Allergy Clin Immunol* 1985; 76: 242–5.

32 Businco L, Cantani A, Longhi MA *et al.* Anaphylactic reactions to a cow's milk whey protein hydrolysate (Alfa-Re Nestle) in infants with cow's milk allergy. *Ann Allergy* 1989; 62: 333–5.

33 Clarke MCA, Kilburn SA, Hourihane JO'B *et al.* Serological characteristics of peanut allergy. *Clin Exp Allergy* 1998; 28: 1251–7.

34 Cornell HJ. Coeliac disease: a review of the causative agents and their possible mechanisms of action. *Amino Acids* 1996; 10: 1–19.

35 Crespo JF, Pascual C, Burks AW *et al.* Frequency of food allergy in a pediatric population from Spain. *Pediatr Allergy Immunol* 1995; 6: 39–43.

36 Crespo JF, Pascual C, Helm R *et al.* Cross-reactivity of IgE-binding components between boiled Atlantic shrimp and German cockroach. *Allergy* 1995; 50: 918–24.

37 Daul CB, Morgan JE, Hughes J, Lehrer SB. Provocation-challenge studies in shrimp-sensitive individuals. *J Allergy Clin Immunol* 1988; 81: 1180–6.

38 Daul CB, Morgan JE, Lehrer SB: The natural history of shrimp hypersensitivity. *J Allergy Clin Immunol* 1990; 86: 88–93.

39 Daul CB, Morgan JE, Waring NP *et al*: Immunologic evaluation of shrimp-allergic individuals. *J Allergy Clin Immunol* 1987; 80: 716–22.

40 Daul CB, Morgan JE, Lehrer SB. Hypersensitivity reactions to crustacea and mollusks. *Clin Rev Allergy* 1993; 11: 201–22.

41 Daul CB, Slattery M, Reese G *et al.* Identification of the major brown shrimp (*Penae aztecus*) allergen (*Pen a* 1) as the muscle protein tropomyosin. *Int Arch Allergy Immunol* 1994; 105: 49–55.

42 De Martino M, Peruzzi M, de Luca M *et al.* Fish allergy in children. *Ann Allergy* 1993; 71: 159–65.

43 Dreborg S, Foucard T. Allergy to apple, carrot, and potato in children with birch pollen allergy. *Allergy* 1983; 38: 167–72.

44 Emmett SE, Angus FJ, Fry JS, Lee PN. Perceived prevalence of peanut allergy in Great Britain and its association with other atopic conditions and with peanut allergy in other household members. *Allergy* 1999; 54: 380–5.

45 Enberg RN, McCullough J, Ownby DR. Antibody responses in watermelon sensitivity. *J Allergy Clin Immunol* 1988; 82: 795–800.

46 Ewan PW. Clinical study of peanut and nut allergy in 62 consecutive patients: new features and associations. *Br Med J* 1996; 312: 1074–8.

47 Food and Agriculture Organization of the United Nations, Report of the FAO Technical Consultation on Food Allergies, Rome, Italy, 13–14 November 1995.

48 Ford RPK, Taylor B. Natural history of egg hypersensitivity. *Arch Dis Child* 1982; 57: 649–52.

49 Gern JE, Yang E, Evrard HM, Sampson HA. Allergic reactions to milk-contaminated 'nondairy' products. *N Engl J Med* 1991; 324: 976–9.

50 Gillespie DN, Nakajima S, Gleich GJ. Detection of allergy to nuts by radioallergo-sorbent test. *J Allergy Clin Immunol* 1976; 57: 302–9.

51 Gleeson PA, Jermyn MA. Leguminous seed glycoproteins that interact with concanavalin A. *Aust J Plant Physiol* 1977; 4: 25–37.

52 Hansen TK, Bindslev-Jensen C. Codfish allergy in adults. Identification and diagnosis. *Allergy* 1992; 47: 610–7.

53 Hefle SL, Nordlee JA, Taylor SL. Allergenic foods. *Crit Rev Food Sci Nutr* 1996; 36: S69–S89.

54 Herian AM, Taylor SL, Bush RK. Identification of soybean allergens by immuno-blotting with sera from soy-allergic adults. *Int Arch Allergy Appl Immunol* 1990; 92: 193–8.

55 Hill DJ, Firer MA, Ball G, Hosking CS. Natural history of cow's milk allergy in children: immunological outcome over 2 years. *Clin Exp Allergy* 1993; 23: 124–31.

56 Hill DJ, Hosking CS, Zhie CY *et al*. The frequency of food allergy in Australia and Asia. *Environ Toxicol Pharmacol* 1997; 4: 101–10.

57 Hoffman DR, Day ED, Miller JS. The major heat stable allergen of shrimp. *Ann Allergy* 1981; 47: 17–22.

58 Horan RF, Sheffer AL. Food-dependent exercise-induced anaphylaxis. *Immunol Allergy Clinics N Am* 1991; 11: 757–66.

59 Host A, Halken S. A prospective study of cow milk allergy in Danish infants during the first three years of life. *Allergy* 1990; 45: 587–96.

60 Host A, Jacobsen HP, Halken S *et al*. The natural history of cow's milk protein allergy/intolerance. *Eur J Clin Nutr* 1995; 49(Suppl. 1): S13–8.

61 Hourihane JO'B, Bedwani SJ, Dean TP *et al*. Randomised, double-blind, crossover challenge study of allergenicity of peanut oils in subjects allergic to peanut. *BMJ* 1997; 314: 1084–8.

62 Hourihane JO'B, Kilburn SA, Nordlee JA *et al*. An evaluation of sensitivity of peanut allergic subjects to very low doses of peanut protein: a randomized, double-blind, placebo-controlled food challenge study. *J Allergy Clin Immunol* 1997; 100: 596–600.

63 Jakobbson I, Lindberg T. A prospective study of cow's milk protein intolerance in Swedish infants. *Acta Pediatr Scand* 1979; 68: 853–9.

64 James C, Williams-Akita A, Rao YAK *et al*. Sesame seed anaphylaxis. *NY State J Med* 1991; 91: 457–8.

65 Jones SM, Magnolfi CF, Cooke SK, Sampson HA. Immunologic cross-reactivity among cereal grains and grasses in children with food hypersensitivity. *J Allergy Clin Immunol* 1995; 96: 341–51.

66 Juchet A, Dutau G. Evolution naturelle de l'allergie alimentaire. *Rev Fr Allergol* 1993; 33: 49–53.

67 Kagi MK, Wuthrich B. Falafel-burger anaphylaxis due to sesame seed allergy. *Lancet* 1991; 338: 582.

68 Kanny G, de Hauteclocque C, Moneret-Vautrin DA. Sesame seed and sesame seed oil contain masked allergens of growing importance. *Allergy* 1996; 51: 952–7.

69 Kemp SF, Lockey RF. Peanut anaphylaxis from food cross-contamination. *JAMA* 1996; 275: 1636–7.

70 Kjelkevik R, Edberg U, Yman IM. Labelling of potential allergens in foods. *Environ Toxicol Pharmacol* 1997; 4: 157–62.

71 Koepke JW, Williams PB, Osa SR, Dolen WK, Selner JC. Anaphylaxis to pinon nut. *Ann Allergy* 1990; 65: 473–6.

72 Kolopp-Sarda M, Moneret-Vautrin D, Gobert B *et al*. Specific humoral immune responses in 12 cases of food sensitization to sesame seed. *Clin Exp Allergy* 1998; 27: 1285–91.

73 Langeland T. A clinical and immunological study of allergy to hen's egg white. VI. Occurrence of proteins cross-reacting with allergens in hen's egg white as studied in egg white from turkey, duck, goose, seagull, and in hen egg yolk, and hen and chicken sera and flesh. *Allergy* 1983; 38: 399–412.

74 Lemke PJ, Taylor SL: Allergic reactions and food intolerances. In: *Nutritional Toxicology* (Kotsonis FN, Mackey M, Hjelle J eds). Raven Press, New York, 1994: 117–37.

75 Leung PSC, Chu KH, Chow WK *et al*. Cloning, expression, and primary structure of *Metapenaeus ensis* tropomyosin, the major heat-stable shrimp allergen. *J Allergy Clin Immunol* 1994; 94: 882–90.

76 Leung PSC, Chow WK, Duffey S *et al*. IgE reactivity against a cross-reactive allergen in crustacea and mollusca: evidence for tropomyosin as the common allergen. *J Allergy Clin Immunol* 1996; 98: 954–61.

77 Levy Y, Dannon YL. Allergy to sesame seed in infants. *Allergy* 2001; 56: 193–4.

78 Lin RY, Shen HD, Han SH. Identification and characterization of a 30 kD major allergen from *Parapenaeus fissurus*. *J Allergy Clin Immunol* 1993; 92: 837–44.

79 Magnolfi CF, Zani G, Lacava L *et al*. Soy allergy in atopic children. *Ann Allergy Asthma Immunol* 1996; 77: 197–201.

80 Malanin G, Kalimo K. Was the candy really responsible for the anaphylaxis in a cottonseed-sensitive patient? *J Allergy Clin Immunol* 1990; 86: 277–8.

81 McKenna C, Klontz KC. Systemic allergic reaction following ingestion of undeclared peanut flour in a peanut-sensitive woman. *Ann Allergy* 1997; 79: 234–6.

82 Mekori YA. Introduction to allergic disease. *Crit Rev Food Sci Nutr* 1996; 36: S1–S18.

83 Nagpal S, Metcalfe DD, Rao PV. Identification of a shrimp-derived allergen as tRNA. *J Immunol* 1987; 138: 4169–74.

84 Nagpal S, Rajappa L, Metcalfe DD *et al*. Isolation and characterization of heat-stable allergens from shrimp (*Penaeus indicus*). *J Allergy Clin Immunol* 1989; 83: 26–36.

85 Norgaard A, Bindslev-Jensen C. Egg and milk allergy in adults. Diagnosis and characterization. *Allergy* 1992; 47: 503–9.

86 Nordlee JA, Taylor SL, Townsend JA *et al*. Identification of a Brazil nut allergen in transgenic soybeans. *N Engl J Med* 1996; 334: 688–92.

87 O'Neil C, Helbling AA, Lehrer SB. Allergic reactions to fish. *Clin Rev Allergy* 1993; 11: 183–200.

88 O'Neil C, McCants M, Gutman A *et al*. Anaphylaxis following ingestion of candy: identification of the etiologic agent. *N Engl Reg Allergy Proc* 1988; 9: 279.

89 Palosuo K, Alenius H, Varjonen E *et al*. A novel wheat gliadin as a cause of exercise-induced anaphylaxis. *J Allergy Clin Immunol* 1999; 103: 912–7.

90 Park JW, Kang DB, Kim CW *et al*. Identification and characterisation of the major allergen of buckwheat. *Allergy* 2000; 55: 1035–41.

91 Pastorello E, Ortolani C. Oral allergy syndrome. In: *Food Allergy – Adverse Reactions to Foods and Food Additives*, 2nd edn. (Metcalfe DD, Sampson HA, Simon RA eds). Blackwell Scientific, Boston; 1997: 221–33.

92 Pastorello EA, Incorvaia C, Pravettoni V *et al*. New allergens in fruits and vegetables. *Allergy* 1998; 53(Suppl. 46): 48–51.

93 Pumphrey RSH. Lessons from management of anaphylaxis from a study of fatal reactions. *Clin Exp Allergy* 2000; 30: 1144–50.

94 Rabjohn P, West CM, Helm E *et al*. Glycinin, a third major peanut allergen identified by soy-adsorbed serum IgE from peanut sensitive individuals. *J Allergy Clin Immunol* 1998; 101: S240.

95 Rabjohn P, Helm EM, Stanley JS *et al*. Molecular cloning and epitope analysis of the peanut allergen Ara h 3. *J Clin Invest* 1999; 103: 535–42.

96 Rao YK, Chiaramonte LT. Anaphylaxis to cow's milk: a case report. *Ann Allergy* 1978; 41: 113–5.

97 Reese G, Ayuso R, Carle T *et al*. IgE-binding epitopes of shrimp tropomyosin, the major allergen Pen a 1. *Int Arch Allergy Immunol* 1999; 118: 300–1.

98 Saarinen UM, Kajosaari M. Does dietary elimination in infancy prevent or only postpone a food allergy? A study of fish and citrus allergy in 375 children. *Lancet* 1980; 1: 166–7.

99 Sachs MI, Jones RT, Yunginger JW. Isolation and partial characterization of a major peanut allergen. *J Allergy Clin Immunol* 1981; 67: 27–34.

100 Sakaguchi M, Hori H, Ebihara T *et al*. Reactivity of the immunoglobulin E in bovine gelatin-sensitive children to gelatins from various animals. *Immunol* 1999; 96: 286–90.

101 Sampson HA, McCaskill CC. Food hypersensitivity and atopic dermatitis. Evaluation of 113 patients. *J Pediatr* 1985; 107: 669–75.

102 Sampson HA, Scanlon SM. Natural history of food hypersensitivity in children with atopic dermatitis. *J Pediatr* 1989; 115: 23–27.

103 Sampson HA, Mendelson L, Rosen J. Fatal and near-fatal anaphylactic reactions to foods in children and adolescents. *N Engl J Med* 1992; 327: 380–4.

104 Schrander JJP, van den Borgart JPH, Forget PP *et al*. Cow's milk protein intolerance in infants under 1 year of age: a prospective epidemiological study. *Eur J Pediatr* 1993; 152: 640–4.

105 Schwartz RH. IgE-mediated allergic reactions to cow's milk. *Immunol Allergy Clin N Am* 1991; 11: 717–41.

106 Schwartz RH, Peers LB. IgE-mediated cow's milk allergy (IgE-CMA) in adults. *J Allergy Clin Immunol* 1996; 97: 237.

107 Shanti KN, Martin BM, Nagpal S *et al*. Identification of tropomyosin as the major shrimp allergen and characterization of its IgE-binding epitopes. *J Immunol* 1993; 151: 5354–63.

108 Shin DS, Compadre CM, Maleki SJ *et al*. Biochemical and structural analysis of the IgE binding sites on Ara h 1, and abundant and highly allergenic peanut protein. *J Biol Chem* 1998; 273: 13753–9.

109 Sicherer SH, Munoz-Furlong A, Burks AW, Sampson HA. Prevalence of peanut and tree nut allergy in the U.S. determined by a random digit dial telephone survey. *J Allergy Clin Immunol* 1999; 103: 559–62.

110 Sporik R, Hill D. Allergy to peanuts, nuts, and sesame seed in Australian children. *Br Med J* 1996; 313: 1477–8.

111 Spuergin P, Walter M, Schiltz E *et al*. Allergenicity of α-caseins from cow, sheep, and goat. *Allergy* 1997; 52: 293–8.

112 Stanley JS, King N, Burks AW *et al*. Identification and mutational analysis of the immunodominant IgE binding epitopes of the major peanut allergen *Ara h* 2. *Arch Biochem Biophys* 1997; 342: 244–53.

113 Suarez FL, Savaiano DA. Diet, genetics, and lactose intolerance. *Food Technol* 1997; 51: 74–6.

114 Tarim O, Anderson VM, Lifshitz F. Fatal anaphylaxis in a very young infant possibly due to a partially hydrolyzed whey formula. *Arch Pediatr Adolesc Med* 1994; 148: 1224–8.

115 Tariq SM, Stevens M, Matthews S *et al*. Cohort study of peanut and tree nut sensitization by age of 4 years. *Br Med J* 1996; 313: 514–7.

116 Taylor SL. Allergic and sensitivity reactions to food components. In: (Hathcock JN ed) *Nutritional Toxicology*, Vol. II. Academic Press, New York, 1987: 173–98.

117 Taylor SL, Lehrer SB. Principles and characteristics of food allergens. *Crit Rev Food Sci Nutr* 1996; 36: S91–S118.

118 Taylor SL, Bush RK, Nordlee JA. Sulfites. In: *Food Allergies – Adverse Reactions to Foods and Food Additives*, 2nd edn (Metcalfe DD, Sampson HA, Simon RA eds). Blackwell Scientific, Boston 1997: 485–97.

119 Taylor SL, Bush RK, Selner JC *et al*. Sensitivity to sulfited foods among sulfite-sensitive asthmatics. *J Allergy Clin Immunol* 1988; 81: 1159–67.

120 Taylor SL, Busse WW, Sachs MI *et al*. Peanut oil is not allergenic to peanut-sensitive individuals. *J Allergy Clin Immunol* 1981; 68: 372–5.

121 Taylor SL, Hefle SL, Munoz-Furlong A. Food allergies and avoidance diets. *Nutr Today* 1999; 34: 15–22.

122 Torsney PJ. Hypersensitivity to sesame seed. *J Allergy* 1964; 35: 514–9.

123 Troncone R, Greco L, Auricchio S. Gluten-sensitive enteropathy. *Pediatr Clin N Am* 1996; 43: 355–73.

124 Vallier P, Dechamp C, Vial O *et al*. A study of allergens in celery with cross-sensitivity to mugwort and birch pollens. *Clin Allergy* 1988; 18: 491–500.

125 Van Bever HP, Docx M, Stevens WJ. Food and food additives in severe atopic dermatitis. *Allergy* 1989; 44: 588–94.

126 Van Ree R, Antonicelli L, Akkerdaas JH *et al*. Asthma after consumption of snails in house-dust-mite-allergic patients: a case of IgE cross-reactivity. *Allergy* 1996; 51: 387–93.

127 Vichyanond P, Visitsuntorn N, Tuchinda M. Wheat-induced anaphylaxis. *Asian Pac J Allergy Immunol* 1990; 8: 49–52.

128 Waring NP, Daul CB, deShazo RD *et al*. Hypersensitivity reactions to ingested crustacea: clinical evaluation and diagnostic studies in shrimp-sensitive individuals. *J Allergy Clin Immunol* 1985; 76: 440–5.

129 Wuthrich B, Stager J, Johannson SGO. Celery allergy associated with birch and mugwort pollenosis. *Allergy* 1990; 45: 566–71.

130 Yamada K, Urisu A, Morita Y *et al*. Immediate hypersensitivity reactions to buckwheat ingestion and cross allergenicity between buckwheat and rice antigens in subjects with high levels of IgE antibodies to buckwheat. *Ann Allergy Asthma Immunol* 1995; 75: 56–61.

131 Yang WH, Purchase ECR, Rivington RN. Positive skin tests and Prausnitz–Kustner reactions in metabisulfite-sensitive subjects. *J Allergy Clin Immunol* 1986; 78: 443–9.

132 Yunginger JW, Nelson DR, Squillace DL *et al*. Laboratory investigation of deaths due to anaphylaxis. *J Forensic Sci* 1991; 36: 857–65.

133 Yunginger JW, Sweeney KG, Sturner WQ *et al*. Fatal food-induced anaphylaxis. *J Am Med Assoc* 1988; 260: 1450–2.

Section A Examples of Foods as Allergens

Chapter 28 Acute allergic reactions to foods and crossreactivity between foods

A. W. Frankland and R. S. H. Pumphrey

ANAPHYLAXIS IN RELATION TO FOOD ALLERGY

Definition

Acute allergic reactions to foods may cause local symptoms on the lips, the tongue, the pharynx, oesophagus, stomach or gut, leading to itching and swelling, hypersecretion and altered motility with vomiting or diarrhoea. When severe, even these local symptoms may be life threatening because of occlusion of the upper airway. Sometimes the allergen is easily destroyed by the low pH in the stomach, preventing the development of more generalised symptoms; for example, protein allergens in some fresh fruit are of this type and cause oral allergy. Other allergens may be easily absorbed through the oral mucosa or sufficiently stable to survive digestion and therefore can cause more generalised symptoms – small proteins related to lipid transfer factor found in various fruit and nuts are of this type and commonly cause systemic allergic reactions. The severity of these reactions may vary from transient urticaria to severe angioedema, from mild wheeze to severe bronchospasm, from itching in the throat to asphyxia due to laryngeal oedema, and from slight faintness to severe shock with pulseless electrical activity. Which of these symptoms predominate depends on the allergen, its presentation (concentration and mass having independent effects), the sever-

ity of the allergy and other genetic factors that determine whether the subject has an asthmatic tendency, a predisposition to shock and so on. When allergic reactions to foods have been fatal, the commonest cause of death has been severe asthma that caused respiratory arrest with a modal incidence at 30 minutes after ingestion. Less commonly, there has been asphyxia due to angioedema of the mucosa of the upper airway, and occasionally shock has contributed significantly to the cause of death.

Acute severe generalised allergic reactions to foods have commonly been associated with a history of previous milder reactions, and it is usually possible to demonstrate IgE antibodies specific for the supposed cause. There will usually be positive skin prick tests. Negative tests in those with a clear history should lead to enquiry about the quality of the reagents used for the tests, or the nature of the allergic epitope and whether the food needs cooking or digesting before the epitope is available.

Acute severe reactions following eating foods containing a putative allergen are commonly called anaphylactic reactions, but the pattern of such reactions caused by foods is different from that following stings, where shock is more commonly a major factor in fatalities. Histidine can be converted into histamine particularly in serombroid fish such as tuna and mackerel, if not stored properly. The serombroid fish poisoning due to histamine

A

413

Clinical reactions of acute anaphylaxis
Initial symptoms
Faint
Oral swelling
Pruritis
Feeling of doom
Cutaneous
Erythema
Urticaria
Angioedema
Respiratory
Upper airways obstruction (stridor)
Lower airways obstruction (asthma, cyanosis)
Cardiovascular
Tachycardia
Circulatory shock

Table 28.1 Clinical reactions of acute anaphylaxis.

presents as anaphylaxis. The excessive intake of biogenic amines and histamine may therefore give rise to non-immunological food reactions (see Chapters 23 and 48).

It is of some interest that the first research in immunology was carried out by a food (fish)-sensitive individual. Küstner had been highly sensitive to fish since the age of 6 years. What is strange about Küstner's fish allergy was that he was sensitive to cooked fish but not to raw fish. Usually cooking destroys, or partially destroys, the allergenicity of foods for many of those patients allergic to foods. Küstner's serum, when injected into the non-fish-sensitive Prausnitz's skin, sensitized the skin locally by passive transfer of fish antibodies. Strangely, they were unable to do the reverse, i.e. passively sensitize Küstner's skin with Prausnitz's pollen allergy.[41]

There are many triggering factors besides foods (drugs, insect stings) that can cause anaphylaxis and in any one patient the clinical symptoms of anaphylaxis (see Table 28.1) are very varied.

Most food anaphylactic reactions are classical Type I immediate IgE reactions. However, many food reactions that will be discussed are not immediate and are not IgE mediated. It is unfortunate that there is no experimental model that compares exactly to anaphylaxis in man. Some of the problems in investigating and treating anaphylaxis in man have been reviewed.[20]

REACTIONS THAT ARE NOT IgE-MEDIATED

Not all acute reactions after eating are due to an IgE-based process. Adverse reactions to foods may be divided into those triggered by sensory triggers (sight, smell, taste and so on) and those that occur even when these cues are masked in a double blind challenge. Sensory pathways may be involved for example in gustatory flushing and sweating (acute attacks of these symptoms affecting the blush area – the face and upper chest). These responses depend on autonomic innervation and are commonly mild; if severe, they may present as a supposed allergic reaction. The trigger is usually strong alcohol or highly spiced, strong tasting or acid food rather than food containing a specific allergen.

Responses that occur reproducibly even when sensory input is masked in a double blind challenge may be due to:

- toxic ingredients (these will affect the majority of the population)
- non-immune intolerance (affecting the minority of the population and often due to the inherited or acquired lack of an enzyme that alters the digestion of the food, causing adverse effects)
- immunological process causing an adverse effect (hypersensitivity, including IgE-mediated reactions, complex mechanisms such as gluten sensitivity, and probably other less well defined pathways).

Case history 1: Fructose intolerance

Allergists are often asked to see patients with possible food intolerances causing many different kinds of symptoms, but it must be very unusual to be asked to see a patient with 'food anaphylaxis' who was not anaphylactic and whose symptoms had nothing to do with allergy. The lady, when first seen aged 33, knew that she had not been able to eat puddings, fruit or sweets since early infancy without severe abdominal pain followed by vomiting and diarrhoea. On a few occasions she had become unconscious at the end of the attacks – from hypoglycaemia. She was suffering from hereditary fructose intolerance which, strangely, had never been diagnosed.[11]

Idiopathic urticaria/angioedema is a heterogeneous group of conditions with superficially similar symptoms, and attacks may sometimes occur after eating or with exercise, leading to confusion if it is supposed that the attack is due to food allergy. The confusion is increased when these conditions coincide with atopy, and the patient has positive allergy tests. There may be synergy between these conditions, and between aspirin and food allergy, leading for example to aspirin-dependent food-allergic reactions or even aspirin-dependent, exercise-induced food-allergic reactions.[25] There are many agents that can induce an acute 'attack', which is clinically similar to anaphylaxis. The agents and the clinical reactions they induce are summarized in Table 28.2.

Alcoholic drinks

Alcohol, especially the preprandial drink, allows rapid passage of foods across the intestinal mucous membrane. Ethanol is also a potent histamine releaser and many red and white wines are themselves rich in histamine. There are, therefore, many reasons why alcoholic drinks in some people may potentiate or cause not only mild, but sometimes severe, pseudo-allergic reactions.

Food additives and preservatives

When someone has a severe, and often unexpected, anaphylactic reaction during or just after a meal, particularly a restaurant meal, it is easy to say that the reaction was 'allergic'. However, this may often be impossible to prove and it is better to limit the use of the term 'allergic' to those reactions that are immunologically mediated or can be presumed to be. Very often anecdotal accounts with no documented proof have blamed serious reactions on various food additives. Food additives and preservatives are examples of substances that have been used for years but have recently been recognized as being hazardous to some people. Metabisulphate may cause anaphylaxis.[42] It may be that sulphur

Some causes of anaphylactoid reactions		
Anaphylactoid	**Mediator**	**Similarity to anaphylaxis**
opioid sensitivity	mast cells	complete
contrast media	mast cells (non-mast cell pathway?)	complete
autonomic	mast cells or direct vascular effects	complete
modified gelatines	basophils?	complete
NSAID reactions	leukotrienes	rashes, asthma, angioedema
scombrotoxin poisoning	histamine	vomiting, flushing, bronchospasm
ACE inhibitors or acquired C 1 inh deficiency	bradykinin	angioedema
dextran reactions	complement	shock, rashes, bronchospasm
cremophore (epoxylated castor oil used as solvent for vitamin K, taxol etc).	complement	shock, rashes, bronchospasm
vancomycin	not histamin	rash (red man)

Table 28.2 Some causes of anaphylactoid reactions.

dioxide, rather than the bisulphate, is what causes the acute symptoms. This is known to occur in some asthmatics who use aerosols that contain bisulphate. The asthma may become worse or anaphylaxis may occur.[56]

Normally the ubiquitous tissue enzyme sulphite oxidase converts sulphite (HSO_3) into the inactive sulphate (SO_4). It seems that 5 mg of sulphite orally may induce asthma in those patients who are very sensitive to sulphate or sulphur dioxide. It would seem that the sulphite oxidase enzyme is substantially reduced in the sulphite-sensitive asthmatic.[26] It may be, but it has yet to be proved, that it is this group that is particularly liable to have an anaphylactic response after eating in restaurants. It will be the large amount of preservatives in the food rather than an individual food that causes the reaction. It has been found that the patients shown to be most sensitive to oral challenge were not the same patients most sensitive to inhalation challenge. It has been shown[39] that all asthmatic subjects have bronchoconstriction after inhalation exposure of 1–5 ppm of sulphur dioxide. The mechanism for this reaction has been demonstrated to be a direct stimulation of different receptors in the bronchi by inhaled sulphur dioxide. A lot more work remains to be done to find out whether sulphite preservatives in food may not cause both asthma and food anaphylaxis.

FOOD-DEPENDENT EXERCISE-INDUCED ANAPHYLAXIS

This syndrome has also been called postprandial exercise-induced anaphylaxis.[38] In the original description of 16 patients[50] it was realized that because anaphylaxis did not always follow exercise it was likely that there was some other factor in addition to the exercise required for the reaction to occur. In this account only three of the patients thought the symptoms occurred after eating food. In subsequent accounts it has been realized that a specific food or foods must first be ingested for anaphylaxis to occur.

Serum IgE concentrations were not elevated in four of the five atopic patients assessed. Five of the patients who had ingested aspirin before the exercise, and two who had taken caffeine, had symptoms induced out of proportion to the modest exercise, whereas normally, without exercise, these substances did not produce symptoms. It seems important that anyone with this syndrome must be warned against taking aspirin at any time because, in some patients, the exercise that produced the attack was not at all strenuous – for example, a mild tennis warm-up or while jogging, particularly when it was warm. The hallmark of the syndrome is exercise-induced urticaria which generally progresses to angioedema involving face, palms and soles. Twelve of the 16 patients collapsed. Choking developed in 10 patients but wheezing was mild. Nausea, colic and diarrhoea may occur. Late sequelae are headaches persisting for 24–72 hours.

The relationship between aspirin and good ingestion is not always clear at a clinical level but has been validated by Double-Blind, Placebo-Controlled, Food-Exercise Challenge (DBPCF + EC) testing.[15b]

Role of skin tests

It may be that when an offending food is recognized, a positive skin test will be obtained to this food, which perhaps would not normally be tested. In an account of food-dependent exercise-induced anaphylaxis,[32] three of the four cases produced anaphylaxis only if celery had been eaten prior to the exercise. The patients gave positive skin-prick tests to celery. In the other case, a meal had to be eaten within 2 hours before exercise – no specific food seemed to be important.

Patients who have this rare form of anaphylaxis are advised not to take any strenuous exercise within 2 (and preferably 4) hours of a meal. Obviously, they would not partake of a food known to be a possible precipitating factor but, quite often, more than one – or no known food – is involved; rather, the anaphylaxis seems to be related to a meal. It is for this reason that the syndrome has been called postprandial exercise-induced anaphylaxis. The different types of exercise producing the symptoms can be very varied.

Perhaps exercise-induced anaphylaxis is not such a rare complaint as originally thought because from France comes an account of 159 patients reviewed with anaphylaxis: 19 gave a history of life-threatening exercise-induced anaphylaxis and in 12 patients the cause was wheat flour.[23] Sensitization to putative food antigens was identified by skin testing and screening for specific serum IgE antibodies. High levels of serum IgE were often found.

Exercise-induced anaphylaxis
Case history 2
A patient aged 30 was taken to hospital before half-time when playing his first game of football for 3 years. His next attack occurred when playing strenuous table tennis; his third attack when taking part in old-time dancing. He was atopic in that he had mild seasonal hayfever but there were no obvious food allergies, although these may be very difficult to find even when present.

The foods that may give rise to exercise-induced anaphylaxis are very varied. An athlete only had a reaction if he ate shellfish before going on a long-distance run.[34]

Case history 3
A 40-year-old banker, very keen on keeping fit, had been admitted to hospital on three occasions with severe anaphylaxis each time after jogging. He usually jogged without any difficulty. It was found from the history that anaphylaxis with exercise only occurred if he had, within 3 hours of exercise, taken his favourite drink of rum. His last attack was at Kennedy Airport when he had to change planes and had time for lunch – unfortunately with rum. He forgot the time and had to run to catch his plane – instead, he was admitted to hospital with anaphylaxis.

INVESTIGATING REACTIONS TO FOODS

Although acute allergic reactions to foods cause symptoms that are easy to recognise, it has proved curiously difficult to recognise anaphylactic reactions. Other conditions may cause similar symptoms: panic attacks can cause a feeling of difficulty breathing or choking, hyperventilation leading to faintness or dizziness, and a sense of impending doom that is also characteristic of anaphylactic reactions. A mild reaction that is accompanied by panic may appear to be a severe reaction. Idiopathic angioedema/urticaria following eating may be mistaken for food allergy. Scombrotoxin may cause flushing, vomiting and wheezing. Because it is important to verify the cause of a reaction in order to give appropriate advice about future management, care should be taken to make an accurate diagnosis.

Acute severe allergic reactions to foods are due to mediators released from mast cells. Some of these mediators can be measured directly, such as mast cell tryptase. Others such as histamine are unstable; their measurement in the serum presents practical problems but the metabolite methyl histamine can be measured in the first urine voided after a reaction. The histamine may have a dietary origin, but mast cell tryptase has no other source and if a rise in its serum concentration at the time of a reaction can be established, an allergic reaction is very likely.

If an allergic cause seems probable, the next difficulty is to identify the allergen. The most helpful allergy tests are skin prick tests and measurement of IgE antibodies in the serum. Both depend on the quality of the extracts used as reagents in the test – for example a recent investigation demonstrated that only one out of five commercial walnut skin prick test solutions contained significant quantities of walnut protein. Interpretation of specific IgE antibody levels is fraught with difficulty. For example, fol-

lowing fatal asthma attacks triggered by milk in milk allergic children the level of anti-milk IgE has usually been extremely high (500 to over 1000 kU_A/L measured by the Pharmacia cap system). A 52-year-old who died with laryngeal oedema after drinking tea with milk (which she usually avoided because of her milk allergy) had only 1 kU_A/L. Her total IgE was 50 kIU/L, and even though low, this specific IgE antibody to milk was the highest recorded out of 500 adults with total IgE in the normal range. Conversely, some children who eat peanuts without reacting have had peanut-specific IgE as high as 500 kU_A/L. It has been suggested that these antibodies may be directed against cross-reactive carbohydrate determinants that are unable to trigger the mast cells.

Because of the deficiencies of allergy tests, the double blind food challenge has been promoted as the "gold standard" for evaluating food allergy. This has proved invaluable in demonstrating the role of food allergy in childhood eczema, but there are problems in using this type of challenge for acute allergic reactions to foods. The intrinsic hazard of challenging someone who has had a life threatening reaction can be avoided by challenging only when the patient is well, their asthma well-controlled, and starting the challenge with trace quantities of the allergen under study. Unfortunately this may give a negative result in someone whose symptoms depend on a variety of cofactors such as tiredness, exercise or aspirin, or an increase in sensitivity of their asthma due to poor control of daily symptoms. One can only arrive at the most likely diagnosis by an intelligent assessment of the clinical history combined with allergy tests and when appropriate, a challenge test.

CLINICAL ASPECTS OF FOOD-INDUCED ANAPHYLAXIS

Age of onset
Allergy to each food has a characteristic age of onset: the first allergic reaction to milk is usually in infancy, to eggs at weaning, to nuts age 2–4 and the fresh fruit syndrome as an adult. The occasional occurrence of positive allergy tests and immediate allergic symptoms following breast-feeding in the first few days of life suggests that even intra-uterine allergic reactions might be possible when the mother eats food the fetus has become sensitized to. One mother, whose infant reacted (screaming, vomiting and urticaria) to breast-feeding after the mother had eaten peanuts, reported she experienced increased fetal movements after eating peanuts in the last few weeks of her pregnancy.

Acute allergic reactions to foods are common in infancy – particularly to undercooked white of hen's egg and more recently, peanut butter. These may be unpleasant, often with widespread urticaria and vomiting, facial angioedema and conjunctivitis. Life-threatening reactions are uncommon and caution is needed in interpreting accounts of fatal reactions, which in some cases may have been due to overenthusiastic treatment.

Case history 4
A patient became acutely allergic to sesame seed at the age of 50. In the past, she had often had bread with sesame seed on it and had used sesame in soups and biscuits. She noticed that a biscuit she was eating seemed to cause tingling of the buccal mucous membrane and irritation of the throat. In a few minutes she had developed a mild urticaria which disappeared in 1 hour. Two

weeks later, she had another sesame biscuit. In 5 min, she realized her lips and eyelids were becoming swollen; she then developed a gross generalized urticaria, felt very ill and phoned for her husband to come immediately. He found her unconscious on the floor. She gave a positive wheal and flare response to a sesame skin-prick test.

Case history 5

In a family who suffered from acute peanut anaphylaxis, two daughters became allergic under the age of 2. Their mother had become allergic to peanut at the age of 10 years but her father did not become anaphylactically allergic until the age of 68 years. It would seem therefore that, very occasionally, a specific food allergy to peanut may occur genetically.[21] Four members anaphylactically allergic to the same food in three generations must be very rare.

Some people after many years can become anaphylactically allergic to a food in the same way that the bee keeper, after many stings, becomes anaphylactically allergic to the venom. This contrasts to most food anaphylactic responses which may begin in infancy and generally, but not always, disappear. Death in infancy from food anaphylaxis is rare but was described by Finkelstein.[15] Children under the age of 7 if anaphylactically sensitive to a food which by mistake they swallow will usually vomit. This may be a life-saving protective mechanism. Adults may have a very delayed onset of symptoms and may collapse or develop severe asthma over 1 hour after eating the offending food. A hot curry containing a potent allergen may cause no symptoms in the mouth and throat and is swallowed. These patients have lost their protective mechanisms and warning of untoward symptoms in the mouth.

Severity of response

There are varying grades of severity of anaphylaxis. These have been described in patients who are venom allergic,[19] and similar grades occurs in food anaphylactic reactions. Because severe anaphylaxis and death may occur in the severely sensitized food allergic patient, the news media, describing such events, undoubtedly make many parents overanxious about a child's food reaction which may be very mild. Too many children are seen who have only had mild local swelling of the lips or face after eating some foods, but the parents seem to think that their child is at risk of anaphylaxis. In its mildest form, the responses are entirely cutaneous, with erythema, pruritis, urticaria and angioedema. The latter may be amazingly unilateral on the face. Only half of the upper or lower lip may be involved or only one eyelid. But both eyelids may be so swollen that the patient cannot see. Beside lip swelling, which is easily seen, there is often gross oedema of the buccal mucosa. The tongue may become so swollen that the patient has to keep the mouth open and the tongue protrudes through the teeth. The soft palate and particularly the uvula may become very swollen, speaking becomes difficult and it is about this time that there is difficulty in breathing, not only from the oedematous throat but because asthma has supervened. The respiratory difficulty can be made worse by acute abdominal pain and vomiting, which may be followed by diarrhoea. When there is an associated generalized urticaria, hypotension with loss of consciousness may occur. The treatment depends on the severity of the reaction and this will be considered when dealing with treatment below.

Development

Quite often the acute reaction occurs the first time the child eats some food containing eggs or drinks some milk. Perhaps a more common mechanism of sensitization occurs *in utero*. Warner and her co-workers[27] have shown that the fetus during the middle trimester of pregnancy may be sensitized to a food, especially if taken in excess during this time by the mother. Maternal dietary antigens can cross the placenta to enter the fetal circulation so that IgE specific for food antigens can be detected in newborn infants.[28,36] But we know that food antigens such as egg and cow's milk are also found in human milk and this may be the more likely way that babies are sensitized.

Food antigens in breast milk

Over 80 years ago Shannon[49] demonstrated the presence of food antigens in breast milk by inducing anaphylactic reactions in guinea pigs sensitized to egg protein by challenging them with breast milk from a woman taking eggs in her diet. We know that cow's milk and other food proteins may be detectable in breast milk, and this may explain not only why breast feeding may not protect the infant from allergic disease, but also why an infant may have an anaphylactic response the first time it receives such foods as milk or eggs. There may be other reasons that explain why a child reacts to a food the first time it ever attempts to eat it. A few million molecules of peanut butter which become airborne when a parent eats it may be enough to sensitize a young child to the food, so that the first time it eats a peanut (groundnut), it will experience an allergic reaction. This could manifest itself as gross facial oedema followed by diarrhoea, vomiting and shock. We must use the word anaphylaxis when we can demonstrate that the reaction is mediated by IgE antibodies but may use the word anaphylactoid when antigen–antibody reactions cannot be demonstrated.

The smell of food can provoke rhinitis and asthma in someone sensitized to the food and inhalation may be one of the ways a patient becomes sensitized. Parents or other children eating peanut butter could sensitize the baby if it repeatedly inhales a few million molecules of peanut from peanut butter.

The clinical spectrum of anaphylaxis has remained largely undefined, but a recent 3-year study of anaphylaxis seen at one emergency centre in the USA[61] as well as an analysis of 700 reactions occurring in 172 patients in the UK[43] found that foods were the commonest cause and peanut was the commonest food. Peanut allergy and anaphylaxis have been recently reviewed.[16,33] But while peanut anaphylaxis is common in the USA, France and the UK where 20 000 children may be sensitized to nuts, in many countries it is not described or perhaps not recognized.

Natural history

Anaphylaxis occurs equally in males and females and there is often a multiple pattern of food anaphylaxis, but there was no evidence[43] that reactions become progressively more severe since a comparable number of patients reported that their worst reaction was either the first, last or mid-sequence. This observation is important from a medicolegal point of view. What is impossible to evaluate is the quantity of the allergen that is taken. Quite often, especially in children, none of the offending food is swallowed but immediately spat out or, if swallowed, immediately vomited.

Once anaphylaxis has occurred to a food, the commonly held view that reactions become more severe is not therefore borne out

Foods suspected of triggering 58 recent fatal allergic reactions in UK		
Allergen	Confirmed	Suspected
Uncertain		7
Milk	4	3
Fish	2	1
Shellfish	2	0
Snail	0	1
Banana	1	0
Nectarine	0	1
Chickpea	1	1
Peanut	9	1
Nut	17	7
Totals	36	22

Table 28.3 Foods suspected of triggering 58 recent fatal allergic reactions in UK.

when studying large numbers.[44] Moreover, the worst reaction, although it often occurs under the age of 10 years, may not occur until the fourth or fifth decade. The age at which people die from food allergy seems to depend on which food they are allergic to – thus milk allergy has predominated in young children, peanut allergy from age 13–26, other nuts from 18–36. There have been too few deaths from other causes to discern a pattern. It has been more difficult to confirm a food-allergic cause in those over 40 years old and in most cases, there remains some doubt about the relation between food allergy, the food eaten and the cause of dead (Table 28.3). Deaths from acute attacks of asthma have been 60 times as common as those recognised as allergic reactions to food. It is likely that among them were some where the attack of asthma had been triggered by food allergy: unfortunately, asthma is regarded by pathologists and coroners as a natural cause of death and so an allergic cause has seldom been sought.

Most, but not all, children seem to grow out of their reaction after a few years.[43] Unfortunately, some patients retain their acute food allergy throughout life. One such patient, aged 76, who has had lifelong eczema and severe asthma, still retained her acute fish sensitivity.

However, the natural history of anyone with an IgE-mediated food allergy is unknown. Although most IgE reactions to food disappear with increasing age,[43] those that do not remain a social rather than a medical problem. Many adult patients who have food anaphylaxis react to the food that has always caused an immediate reaction. These patients nearly always retain the atopic stigmata of eczema and asthma that have been present since early childhood. Adults, not children, develop shellfish anaphylaxis. This is perhaps because children have not eaten shellfish and it may take two or three decades or more before shellfish reactions suddenly appear. It must be remembered that patients may not necessarily be atopic for them suddenly to develop, at any age, an acute food allergy.

Common food allergens

The basic treatment for all IgE-proven reactions is, without doubt, to identify the allergen that produces the reaction and avoid it. This may be possible with inhalant allergens, but can be very difficult on occasions when a common food allergen is involved.

Case history 6: Acute mustard allergy

A patient aged 18 knew that a minute amount of mustard, when ingested, would cause immediate anaphylactic shock. As a result of bitter experience, with many hospital admissions, she had decided never to eat away from home. To celebrate her birthday she had dinner at a restaurant and ate some salmon with mayonnaise which, she was assured, contained no mustard. Unfortunately, the waiter who served her and who had said he double-checked with the chef, was not speaking the truth. The mustard in a very small amount of mayonnaise caused immediate anaphylactic symptoms requiring emergency hospital treatment.

An infant under the age of 1 year will instinctively spit out egg that is causing an immediate reaction in the mouth. But egg, fish, nuts (including peanut which is a pulse) and, occasionally, milk can all cause immediate and severe anaphylactic shock with gross oedema of the face, abdominal pain, vomiting and diarrhoea, wheezing and urticaria. Skin-prick tests with the appropriate food allergen that causes anaphylaxis are safe and confirm the diagnosis, even in an infant aged 6 months. If a child has more than one acute food allergy, it might be prudent to prick test only one food at a session. The individual response may be very specific so that patients sensitive to one nut are not necessarily allergic to all nuts or, if to fish, to all fish. Peanut, which is a common allergen in very young children, may be the only food allergen causing acute anaphylaxis. Measles vaccine appears safe in the egg-sensitive child,[28] but influenza vaccines produced in ova have caused anaphylactic reactions in people with egg allergy.[8] Virtually any food can cause anaphylaxis.

Case history 7: Cow's milk allergy

A female, followed up for 25 years, remains anaphylactically sensitive to cow's milk. She is an interesting patient because the first time cow's milk was spilt on her leg, when she was 4 months old, the mother thought she had scalded her infant. She then realized that the local response was only urticarial, as it disappeared quickly. When still breast feeding her 14-month-old child, she put a drop of milk from a pipette into a glass of water and gave a teaspoonful of this very diluted milk to her daughter to drink. The child had an immediate anaphylactic response. This patient, at the age of 16, was successfully hyposensitized but, on discontinuing the injections, she relapsed and still cannot eat any dairy product. Socially, she finds her acute allergy to a common ingredient of the diet very embarrassing.

Chinese food

Although the same clinical conditions can be induced by immunological mechanisms, the pathways which also lead to the non-immunological causal event often remain to be established. Chinese food has been reported to cause many allergic reactions and monosodium glutamate seems in some established asthmatic individuals to produce asthmatic attacks.[1]

Case history 8: Anaphylaxis to Chinese food

An important component in Chinese food is tangeh, a sprouted small green bean which makes up a typical Chinese egg-roll. A patient is described[54] who had reactions to various inhalant and food allergens as well as exercise-induced urticaria and angioedema, and who developed generalized urticaria and angioedema within 15 min of eating tangeh in a Chinese restaurant. She gave a specific positive skin-prick test to tangeh as well as showing a specific histamine release and RAST (radioallergo-absorbent test). Some patients with IgE to peanut also have IgE antibodies against tangeh. As peanut is one of the commonest foods causing some IgE-related symptoms, it may be that this group of patients is especially liable to have an allergic reaction after eating Chinese food. In general it is wise to make sure when taking a medical history involving peanut anaphylaxis to find out whether other pulses such as lentils, peas and beans can be eaten.

Anaphylaxis to antibiotics in food

Beef cattle may be treated with antibiotics before being sold for the market. Moreover, antibiotics, particularly penicillin and streptomycin, are readily available in feed stores or obtainable from veterinary surgeons for various reasons. Different countries have various laws to deal with the potential hazard of antibiotics in food. It is recommended that there is a withdrawal of all antibiotics for a stated interval prior to slaughter for market. Milk must not be sold from a cow receiving penicillin for mastitis.

Case history 9: Antibiotic allergy

A 14-year-old girl had four anaphylactic reactions from beef over a period of 1 year. This was puzzling because she could often eat beef without difficulty. It was found from prick and Prausnitz–Küstner tests that she was allergic to streptomycin. She had had an injection of streptomycin at the age of 3 years. The authors make the point that 'idiopathic' anaphylaxis is not always idiopathic.[52]

Penicillin has been estimated to be responsible for 75% of anaphylactic deaths.[12] Anaphylaxis has been reported[59] from penicillin added to soft drinks and from hidden sources of penicillin in foods. Anaphylaxis has been described in a patient known to be allergic to penicillin who had a severe anaphylactic reaction after eating a frozen steak dinner which was shown to contain penicillin or penicilloyl groups.[47]

Penicillin in milk

Legal requirements are that milk should not be sold which might contain more than 0.02 iu/ml penicillin. A farmer may treat one infected udder of a cow with penicillin and he may not want to stop selling the milk from this cow for a week or longer. So quite large amounts of penicillin would be in the milk from the treated cow. The large milk distributors in a city such as London will carry out daily penicillin estimations on their bulk supplies. This is not to protect the potential penicillin-allergic individual but because, if penicillin is present, any unsold milk cannot be made into cheese or yoghurt. The whole subject of the supposed reactions – usually urticaria, and not anaphylaxis – has been reviewed.[13] It was pointed out that cases of so-called penicillin allergy due to milk as reported in the literature are very poorly documented and do not seem to pose a significant public health problem, although anaphylaxis due to penicillin in milk occurred in the patient who also reacted to penicillin in soft drinks.[59]

PEANUT ANAPHYLAXIS

Food-induced anaphylaxis is commonly due to nuts, and peanuts cause many of the fatalities.[62] Sampson et al.[45] found that three of six fatal cases of food anaphylaxis were due to peanuts and all the patients were asthmatic. 33 out of the 34 thought of have died from nut allergy took daily treatment for asthma. Many of those who died with a mainly asthmatic reaction had discontinued taking their inhaled steroids, suggesting that poor control of asthma may predispose to severe reactions. In a postal survey of nut anaphylaxis in which 1000 replies have been analysed, 40% of the sufferers were allergic before the age of 2 years and 70% before the age of 5 years. Some did not develop the peanut allergy before the age of 20 or 30 years and one developed it at the age of 68 years. Peanut anaphylaxis, *if severe*, is rarely outgrown.[30]

Peanut allergy was responsible for 60% of all nut allergic patients evaluated. Thirteen different tree nuts were responsible for 40% of other anaphylactically nut allergic patients. Cashews, brazil and walnuts have all caused anaphylactic deaths in the last 5 years in the UK. Most patients, except the very young, have multiple nut allergies. Many patients will know which nuts cause the most severe symptoms and which can be eaten with impunity. Not all tree nut allergic patients are peanut allergic. Crossreactions in the peanut allergic patient may occur with pulses such as peas, beans, lentils and also to soya which should always be tested for in the peanut allergic patient. Infants may also be milk allergic and it is not realized why soya is not helpful.

Patients often have unrelated food allergies. In this country sesame seed is not uncommon in the nut allergy group and accounts for 15% of anaphylactic reactions but in Australia it was the commonest food causing allergic reactions after peanut.[50]

ALLERGY TO PLANT PROTEINS

The most allergenic plant proteins belong to a relatively small number of protein types, and within each protein type, there is often cross-reactivity between plants even when they are only distantly related.[9b] For example, profilins (actin binding proteins) are common allergens, such as in peanuts (Ara h 5), soybeans (Gly m 3), celery (Api g 4), pear (Pyr c 4), hazelnut, apple, carrot, lychee, tomato, pumkin seeds and so on. Pathogenesis-related (PR) proteins are induced in plants by wounding, environmental stress and pathogens. Fourteen different families of PR protein have been recognised – some of these include the most potent plant allergens. Examples include PR-10 type proteins (Bet v 1 homologues) [Table 28.4], or PR-5 type proteins (thaumatin-like proteins) such as cherry (Pru av 2), apple (Mal d 2), bell pepper (P23).

It is important to recognise that allergy to fuit such as peaches can be of different types. In those allergic to the PR-14 type protein (lipid transfer protein Pru p 1, a small heat- and acid-stable protein), reactions may be generalised and severe: fatal anaphylaxis has been recorded due to peaches and nectarines. Alternatively, those with early season hay fever due to birch pollen allergy who have IgE antibodies to Bet v 1 may develop oral allergy symptoms (itching with urticaria on the lips, tongue and palate) after eating peaches due to cross-reactivity between Bet v 1 and the peach PR-10 homologue. Similarly, with birch pollen allergy there may be adult-type hazelnut allergy with oral allergy symptoms, contrasting with the childhood pattern of hazelnut allergy and systemic symptoms.

There is geographical partitioning of these allergies, with the PR10-related peach allergy commoner in northern Europe and

A

Table 28.4 Examples of cross-reactive food allergy.

Examples of cross-reactive food allergy		
Reference allergen	**Protein type**	**Cross-reactive allergens**
Birch Bet v 1	PR-10	Apple (Mal d 1), cherry (Pru av 1), apricot (Pru ar 1), pear (Pyr c 1), hazel (Cor a 1)
Birch Bet v 2	Profilin	Celery, potato, hazelnut, apple, pear, tomato, cherry
Mugwort	PR-14?	Celery heat stable antigen
Latex Hev b 6	PR-3, PR-4	Avocado (Pers a 1), banana, chestnut
Peach LTP	PR-14	Apricot, almond, cherry, maize LTP
House dust mite Der p 10	Tropomyosin	Shrimp, snail (cross-reactive antibodies to tropomyosin have been demonstrated, but oher proteins may be more important in this cross-allergy)

PR-14-related peach allergy in southern Europe. This has been attributed to different pollen exposure and eating preferences in these regions. The pattern of latex-crossreactive food allergy reported from different countries suggests that there is geographical variation here too, and while celery allergy is very common in Switzerland and France, it is rarely seen in the UK despite the widespread prevalence of mugwort species in the UK.

The proteins causing PR-10-related fruit allergy are commonly so unstable that extracts are no use for skin prick testing: prick-prick testing (where the lancet is inserted into the skin of the fruit and then into the patient's skin) can be used to evaluate sensitivity to these proteins. The PR-14-related proteins are also concentrated just under the skin of the fruit and allergy to them will be detected by prick-prick testing.

Natural rubber latex

This contains several allergenic proteins and rubber goods made from latex have caused an increasing incidence of (mostly minor) allergic problems such as contact urticaria from latex gloves in health care. Severe latex allergy is less common although there has been a small number of fatal reactions. The proteins in latex causing the allergy very according to the cause: thus children who have had multiple surgical operations have been reported to have IgE specific for Hev b 1 (rubber elongation factor) and Hev b 3 (small rubber particle protein) whereas the more common adult sensitisation pattern includes IgE to Hev b 6.

It has been found in the 'latex fruit syndrome' that 52% of latex allergic patients had allergy to fruits, and systemic anaphylaxis occurred in 36%.[9] Avocado, banana and chestnuts are commonly the fruits that crossreact with latex, but potato, tomato, kiwi and other fruits may also crossreact.[7] It must be remembered that a banana allergic subject may not be allergic to latex when first seen.[45] Recently, two nurses have been referred, one with avocado anaphylaxis and the other with banana, avocado and chestnut anaphylaxis which occurred 5 and 8 years, respectively, after the onset of latex allergy, which almost strangely they found a medical nuisance rather than a disability. However, it must be remembered that latex can be the cause of anaphylaxis and death.

TREATMENT OF FOOD INDUCED ANAPHYLACTIC REACTIONS

Consensus guidelines for treating anaphylactic reactions have recently been published,[42b,52b] and other sources of guidance such as the BNF are coming into line with these recommendations. This new guidance emphasises the need for early intramuscular adrenaline, and gives a revised dose according to the age of the patient (Table 28.4). It explains that while slow intravenous injection of adrenaline, titrated against the response may be the ideal treatment for anaphylaxis in a fully monitored patient, its use by unskilled personnel or on unmonitored patients is not recommended. A recent audit showed that one in five junior hospital doctors would have given a 1 mg intravenous bolus of adrenaline to treat an anaphylactic reaction.[27b]

Although appropriate for resuscitation following cardiac arrest, intravenous adrenaline has commonly had severe adverse consequences when given to a conscious patient, including fatal pulmonary oedema, cerebral infarction with paralysis or blindness, and cardiac arrhythmias.

An audit of treatment given to those attending A&E because of acute allergic symptoms suggests that doctors do not treat anaphylaxis: they treat symptoms such as urticaria, asthma and shock separately – urticaria/angioedema with hydrocortisone and antihistamines, and bronchospasm with inhaled salbutamol. Shock is not often a dominant feature in food-allergic reactions treated in

New consensus doses (mL of 1:1000 dilution) for intramuscular adrenaline for use in suspected anaphylactic reactions	
Adults and children over 12 years old	0.5
Children 6–12 years old	0.25
Children 6 months to 6 years old	0.12
Infants under 6 months	0.05

Table 28.5 New consensus doses (mL of 1:1000 dilution) for intramuscular adrenaline for use in suspected anaphylactic reactions.

A&E – when it is, adrenaline has commonly been given, usually with volume replacement with saline or colloid. Acute allergic reactions without shock are rarely given adrenaline unless the patient had their own adrenaline for self-treatment.

In addition to adrenaline, an antihistamine such as chlorpheniramine will help suppress the effects of histamine. In the most severe reactions, histamine may not be the dominant mediator and antihistamines alone are unlikely to prevent asthma – the main cause of fatality from food allergy. Steroids such as hydrocortisone should also be given to prevent later recurrence or progression of bronchospasm.

MANAGEMENT OF PATIENTS THOUGHT TO BE AT RISK OF A LIFE-THREATENING REACTION

For those whose diagnosis of food anaphylaxis has been established by detailed history, physical examination and allergy investigations, the best strategy is optimal daily management of asthma combined with allergen avoidance. Successful avoidance needs recognition of cross-reactivity such as between different types of nuts. As avoidance will never be wholly successful, some thought must be given to rescue from the effects of accidental exposure.

Over 30,000 patients in the UK, many of them children, have self-injectable adrenaline because of a fear that food allergy might be fatal, and in the hope that the kit will save a life. The logic of this is not clear: each year 4–5 people die from food allergy but only one of these has had a previous allergic reaction severe enough to suggest that adrenaline might be needed. It is interesting that the spectrum of severity of the previous worst reaction is similar in the population of older patients attending clinic and in the population of those that have died – the main difference being a subpopulation of fatal cases that had no previous reaction or reactions so mild that they were unlikely to have prompted referral to the clinic (Fig. 28.2).

One might conclude that if all patients who may die from their allergy should carry adrenaline, then everyone with the slightest allergy to the main fatal allergens (nuts, milk, fish and shellfish) should be given adrenaline. This implies 0.5–1% of the UK population – 3–6 million people – or a million if this is restricted to those at the age of greatest risk. Anaphylactic deaths have occurred in 8–16 year-olds from milk, 13–26 year-olds for peanuts and 18–36 year-olds for tree nuts. Increasingly, those who have had a previous severe reaction have had adrenaline, but have either not had it with them when it was needed, or have forgotten to use it in the panic of the reaction – or more worryingly, have used it but it did not work. The strategy of optimal daily asthma treatment with adequate steroids and minimal daily use of short-acting β_2-agonists, would have prevented 60–80% of deaths due to food allergy – as opposed to the maximum of 25% that might be saved by the current strategy for recommending self-injection of adrenaline to those who have had a previous life-threatening reaction.

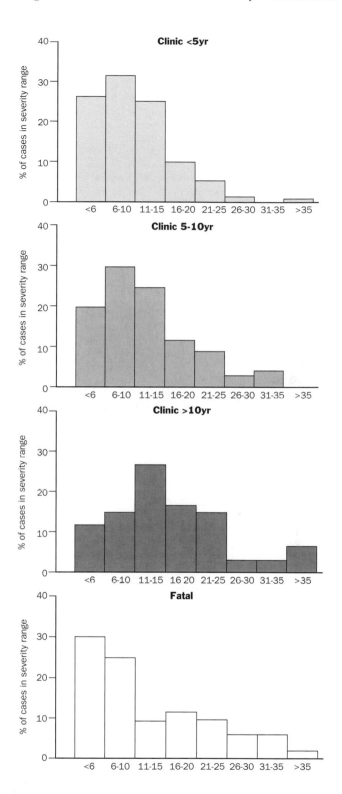

Fig. 28.2 The severity (calculated by a weighted index of symptoms) of the previous worst reaction in those dying from food allergy compared with patients of different ages seen in clinic for assessment of need for adrenaline for emergency self treatment

REFERENCES

1 Allen DH, Baker GJ. Asthma and MSG. *Med J Aust* 1981; 2: 576.

2 Almeida MM, Marta CS, Pratess A *et al*. Peach allergy with no pollen sensitization in children. *J Allergy Clin Immunol* 1996; 97 abs: 608.

3 Anderson KJ, McLaughlan P, Devey ME *et al*. Anaphylactic sensitivity of guinea pigs drinking different preparations of cows milk and infant formulae. *Clin Exp Immunol* 1979; 35: 454.

4 Atkins FM, Steinberg SS, Metcalf PD. Evaluation of immediate adverse reactions to foods in adults. A detailed analysis of reaction patterns during oral food challenge. *J Allergy Clin Immunol* 1985; 75: 356–63.

5 Austen KF. The anaphylactic syndrome. In: Samter M (ed.) *Immunological Diseases*. Little Brown, Boston; 1978; 2: 885–9.

6 Bauer L, Ebner C, Hirschwehr R *et al*. IgE cross-reactivity between birch pollen, mugwort pollen and celery is due to at least three distinct cross-reacting allergens: immunoblot investigation of birch–mugwort–celery syndrome. *Clin Exp Allergy* 1996; 26: 1161–70.

7 Beezhold DH, Sussman GL, Liss GM *et al*. Latex allergy can induce clinical reactions to specific foods. *Clin Exp Allergy* 1996; 26: 416–22.

8 Bierman CW, Shapiro G, Pierson WE *et al*. Safe influenza vaccination in allergic children. *J Infect Dis* 1977; 136(suppl): 652.

9 Blanco C, Carrillo T, Castillo *et al*. Latex allergy: clinical features and cross-reactivity to fruit. *Ann Allergy* 1994; 73: 309–414.

9b Breitender H, Ebner C. Molecular and biochemical classification of plant-derived food allergens. *J Allergy Clin Immunol* 2000; 106: 27–36.

10 Coombs RRA, Gell RGH, Lachmann PJ. *Clinical Aspects of Immunology*, 3rd edn. Blackwell Scientific, Oxford, 1974.

11 Cox TM, O'Donnell MW, Camilleri M. Allergic heterogeneity in adults hereditary fructose intolerance. *Mol Biol Med* 1983; 1: 393–400.

12 Delage C, Grey ND. Anaphylactic deaths: A clinic study of 43 cases. *J Forensic Sci* 1972; 17: 525.

13 Dewdney JM, Edwards MG. Penicillin hypersensitivity – is milk a significant hazard? A review. *J Roy Soc Med* 1984; 77: 866–77.

14 Escribano MM, Munoz FJ, Velazquez E *et al*. Anaphylactic reaction caused by cherry ingestion. *Allergy* 1995; 51: 756–7.

15 Finkelstin H. Kuhmilch als Ursach Akuter Ernahrungsstoerungen beir Sauglingen. *Monatssch Kinderheilk* 1905; 4: 65–72.

15b Fiocchi A, Mirri GP, Santini I, Bemardo L, Ottoboni F, Riva E. Exercise-induced anaphylaxis after food contaminant ingestion in double-blinded, placebo-controlled, food-exercise challenge. *J Allergy Clin Immunol* 1997 Sep; 100(3): 424–5.

16 Fries JH. Peanuts. allergic and other untoward reactions. *Ann Allergy* 1982; 48: 220–6.

17 Frankland AW. Peanut allergy. *Current Medical Literature* 1996; 2: 35–42.

18 Frankland AW. Food reactions in pollen and latex allergic patients. *Clin Exp Allergy* 1995; 25: 885–6.

19 Frankland AW. Chapter 25 Anaphylaxis in relation to food allergy. In: Brostoff J, Challacombe SJ (eds) *Food Allergy and Intolerance*. Ballière Tindall, London, 1987; 456–66.

20 Frankland AW. Allergy to insects and arachnids. In: Lessof MH (ed.) *Allergy: Immunological and Clinical Aspects*. John Wiley, Chichester, 1984: 425–45.

21 Frankland AW. Anaphylaxis – past and present. In: Molina C (ed.) *Proceedings of the Tenth Annual Meeting of the European Academy of Allergology and Clinical Immunology*. Technique and Documentation Laviosier, Paris; 1981; 1: 417–23.

22 Garcia Ortez JC, Cosmes Martin P, Lopez-Azunsolo A. Allergy to foods in patients monosensitized to *artemisia* pollen. *Allergy* 1996; 51: 927–31.

23 Guinnepain MT, Eloit C, Raffard M *et al*. Exercise-induced anaphylaxis: Useful screening of food sensitization. *Ann Allergy Asthma Immunol* 1996; 77: 491–6.

24 Hannaway PJ, Hopper GDK. Severe anaphylaxis and drug induced beta-blockage. *New Engl J Med* 1983; 308: 1536.

25 Harada S, Horikawa T, Ashida M, Kamo T, Nishioka E, Ichihashi M. Aspirin enhances the induction of type I allergic symptoms when combined with food and exercise in patients with food-dependent exercise-induced anaphylaxis. *Br J Dermatol* 2001 Aug; 145(2): 336–9.

26 Jacobson DW, Simon RA, Singh M. Sulphite oxidase deficiency and cobalamine projection in sulphite-sensitive asthma. *J Allergy Clin Immunol* 1984; 73: 135.

27 Jones AC, Miles EA, Warner JO *et al*. Fetal peripheral blood mononuclear cell proliferative responses to mitogenic and allergenic stimuli during gestation. *Ped Allergy Immunol* 1996; 7: 109–16.

27b Jowett NI. Speed of treatment affects outcome in anaphylaxis. *BMJ* 2000; 321: 571

28 Kalogeromitos D, Aremenaka M, Galatas I *et al*. Anaphylaxis induced by lentils. *Ann Allergy Asthma Immunol* 1996; 77: 480–82.

29 Katz SL. Safety of measles vaccine in egg sensitive individuals. *J Pediatr* 1978; 92: 859.

30 Kaufmann HS, Hobbs JR. Immunoglobulin deficiencies in an atopic population. *Lancet* 1971; 2: 1061.

31 Kemp ST, Lockey MD. Peanut anaphylaxis: An Allergist–Immunologist's personal experience with food cross-contamination. *J Allergy Clin Immunol* 1996; 97: abs 581.

32 Kidd JM, Cohen SH, Sosman AH *et al*. Food-dependent exercise-induced anaphylaxis. *J Allergy Clin Immunol* 1983; 71: 407–11.

33 Loza C, Brostoff J. Peanut Allergy: a review. *Clin Exp Allergy* 1995; 25: 493–502.

34 Maulitz RH, Pratt DS, Schirbet AL. Exercise-induced anaphylactic reaction to shellfish. *J Allergy Clin Immunol* 1979; 63: 433–4.

35 Maurer D, Ebner C, Reinieger B *et al*. The high affinity IgE receptor (FceR1) mediates IgE-dependent allergen presentation. *J Immunol* 1995; 154: 6285–90.

36 Michel FB, Bousquet J, Greillier P *et al*. Comparison of cord blood immunoglobulin E concentrations and maternal allergy for prediction of atopic diseases in infancy. *J Allergy Clin Immunol* 1980; 65: 422–30.

37 Mowbray JF, Brostoff J. Allergic urticaria and hereditary angioedema. *Clin Allergy* 1984; 14: 589–92.

38 Noveg HS, Fairshter R, Salness K *et al*. Post-prandial exercise-induced anaphylaxis. *J Allergy Clin Immunol* 1983; 71: 498–504.

39 Parish WE, Richards CB, France AE *et al*. Further investigations on the hypothesis that some cases of cot deaths are due to a modified anaphylactic reaction to cow's milk. *Int Arch Allergy* 1964; 24: 215.

40 Peppard D, Wong WS, Uepara CF *et al*. Lower threshold and greater bronchomotor responsiveness of asthmatic subjects to sulphur dioxide. *Am Rev Respir Dis* 1980; 122: 873.

41 Prausnitz C, Küstner H. Studien über die Überempfindlichkeit. *Zentralbl Bakteriol Parasitknd* 1921; 86: 160–9.

42 Prenner BM, Stevens JJ. Anaphylaxis after ingestion of sodium bisulphate. *Ann Allergy* 1976; 37: 18.

42b Project team of the Resuscitation Council (UK). Emergency medical treatment of anaphylactic reactions. *J Accid Emerg Med* 1999; 16: 243–7.

43 Price JF. Allergy in infancy and childhood. In: Lessof MH (ed.) *Allergy: Immunological and Clinical Aspects*. John Wiley, Chichester; 1984: 161.

44 Pumphrey RSH, Stanworth SJ. The clinical spectrum of anaphylaxis in north-west England. *Clin Exp Allergy* 1996; 26: 1364–70.

45 Sampson HA, Mendelson Z, Rosen JP. Fatal and near fatal anaphylactic reactions to food in children and adolescents. *New Engl J Med* 1992; 327: 38–84.

46 Savonious B, Venevra Z. Anaphylaxis caused by banana. *Allergy* 1993; 48: 215–16.

47 Schwartz HL, Sher PH. Anaphylaxis to penicillin in a frozen dinner. *Ann Allergy* 1984; 53: 342–3.

48 Schwartz LB, Metcalf DD, Miller JS *et al*. Tryptase levels as an indicator of mast cell activation in systemic anaphylaxis and mastocytosis. *New Engl J Med* 1987; 316: 1622–66.

49 Shannon WR. Demonstration of food proteins in human breast milk by anaphylactic experiments on guinea pigs. *Am J Dis Child* 1921; 22: 223.

50 Sheffer AL, Austen KF. Exercise-induced anaphylaxis. *J Allergy Clin Immunol* 1980; 66: 106–11.

51 Sporik R, Hill D. Allergy to peanuts, nuts and sesame seed in Australian children. *Brit Med J* 1996; 313: 1477–8.

52 Stanworth DR, Jones VM, Lewin IV *et al.* Allergy treatment with a peptide vaccine. *Lancet* 1990; 336: 1274–82.

52b Statement from the Resuscitation Council (UK) and the Joint Royal Colleges Ambulance Service Liaison Committee. The use of Adrenaline for anaphylactic shock (for ambulance paramedics). Ambulance UK 1997; 12: 16.

53 Tenkelman DG, Brock SA. Anaphylaxis presumed to be caused by beef containing streptomycin. *Ann Allergy* 1984; 53: 243–4.

54 Toorenberger AW, Diegers PH. IgE-mediated hypersensitivity to tangeh (sprouted small green beans). *Ann Allergy* 1984; 53: 239–42.

55 Turjanmaa K. Diagnostics of food allergy. New visions. *Allergy Supplement 32* 1996; 51: 16–17.

56 Twarog FJ, Leung PK. Anaphylaxis to a component of Isoetharine (sodium bisulphate). *JAMA* 1982; 248: 2030.

57 Valenta R, Kraft D. Type I allergic reactions to plant derived food: A consequence of primary sensitisation to pollen allergens. *J Allergy Clin Immunol* 1996; 97: 893–5.

58 Valenta R, Duchene M, Ebner C *et al.* Profilins constitute a novel family of functional plant pan-allergies. *J Exp Med* 1992; 175: 377–85.

59 Wicher K, Reisman RE. Anaphylactic reaction to penicillin (or a penicillin-like substance) in a soft drink. *J Allergy Clin Immunol* 1980; 66: 155–7.

60 Wicher K, Reisman RE. Anaphylactic reactions to penicillin in milk. *JAMA* 1969; 208: 143.

61 Yocum MD, Khan DA. Assessment of patients who have experienced anaphylaxis: a 3-year study. *Mayo Clin Proc* 1994; 69: 16–23.

62 Yunginger JW, Sweeny KG, Sturner WQ *et al.* Fatal food-induced anaphylaxis. *JAMA* 1988; 260: 1450–2.

Chapter 29

Fish allergy and the codfish allergen model

Said Elsayed

INTRODUCTION

Fish are a large group of animals represented by a variety of cold-blooded aquatic vertebrates of several evolutionary lines describing a life form rather than a taxonomic group. As members of the phylum *Chordata*, they share certain features with other vertebrates. The major class of fish is the teleosts (infraclass *Teleostei*) or bony fishes, a group that includes most of the world's important commercial edible sorts.

There are many reasons why fish are of interest to humans: the most important is their relationship with and dependence on the environment. Another more obvious reason for interest in fish is their role as an important part of the world's food supply.[30] The most edible fish belong to only a few orders and are shown in Table 29.1[61] These are a huge variety of edible fish (more than 20 000 sorts), the most commonly consumed of which are shown in Table 29.2. Despite the great advantages obtained by eating fish, several fish proteins are unfortunately highly potent allergens, playing important roles in the pathogenesis of many allergic manifestations, such as gastrointestinal, airway, and skin allergy. In industrial countries, e.g. France and Switzerland, fish hypersensitivity forms 15.4% of the food allergic population.[39,58]

During the last two decades the consumption of marine products has universally increased and allergic reactions to fish have consequently, became more frequent. The average world annual fish consumption is calculated to be 13.1 kg per capita in 1991 vs. 15.3 kg per capita in 1995 (in the United States annual fish consumption is 15.5 kg per capita).[6,71]

Fish hypersensitivity has an outstanding historical association with the field of allergy. As far back as 1921, serum from Küstner, who was allergic to fish, was intradermally injected into the skin

The commonly consumed (most edible) fish belong to few orders[30]	
Examples of Edible Fish	
Order	**Example**
Salmoniformes	Salmon, trout, whitefish
Perciformes	Perch, snapper, tuna
Gadiformes	Codfish, pollack, hake
Pleuronectiformes	Flounder
Clupeiformes	Herring, anchovy
Cypriniformes	Carp, catfish
Scorpaeniformes	Rock fish

Table 29.1 The commonly consumed (most edible) fish belong to few orders.[30]

of a non-allergic colleague Prausnitz. The injected and control sites were later challenged by injecting a minute amount of fish extract. Large wheal and flare reactions were clearly seen at the sites where the serum was injected but not the control ones. The experiment clearly demonstrated the passive transfer of a serum substance from the allergic to the non-allergic individual. This was later termed reagin, and shown to be specific for fish extract. This observation introduced the first scientific thinking to the field of allergy.[62]

The most consumed fish found in fresh, salt or deep waters of the world		
Salmon	Atlantic salmon	Fresh water and ocean
Trout	Salmo trutta	Freshwater and sea lakes
Mackerel	Scomber scombrus	North Sea and Skagerrak
Herring	Clupea harengus	North Sea and Skagerrak
Sprat	Sprattus sprattus	East Skagerrak
Eel	Anguilla anguilla	Saragasso Ocean, Florida
Atlantic halibut	Hippoglossus hippoglossus	Deepwater, fjord
Greenland halibut	Reinhardtius hippoglossoides	Arctic cold deepwater
Turbot	Scopthalmus maximum	North Sea
Carrelet	Pleuromectes platessa	North Sea, deepwater
Wolfish	Anarhichas sp.	Arctic, North Sea
Redfish	Sebastes sp.	Norwegian Sea
Angler fish	Lophuis piscatorius	W. British Isles deepwater
Codfish	Gadus callarius L	Saltwater fish, Arctic
Saithe	Pollachius veirens	North Arctic sea fish
Ling	Mova molva	Deepwater fish
Pollack	Pollachuys pollachius	North Sea
Haddock	Melanogrammus aeglefinus	North Sea
Tusk	Bromse bromse	Deepwater
Picked dogfish (!)	Squalus acanthias	Shark family, Deepwater

Table 29.2 The most consumed fish found in fresh, salt or deep waters of the world. Most fish that inhabit surface or mid-water regions are streamlined or flattened side-to-side while most deepwater bottom-dwellers are flattened top-to-bottom.

THE ALLERGENS OF CODFISH

Baltic cod allergen M (*Gad c1*), model

Fish hypersensitivity is frequently encountered in countries bordering the sea, such as Norway, where a large number of people work daily in fishing, fish-processing and manufacturing.[1] Food allergens are proteins or glycoproteins with molecular weights between 10 and 40 kDa.[20,22,56,66] In contrast, fish, egg and milk allergic reactions are elicited by low molecular weight peptides.[4,23,24,41] Despite the large variety of fish species, Baltic cod (Gadiformes), Atlantic salmon (Salmoniformes), flounder (Pleuronectiformes) and herring, anchovy (Clupeiformes) are the most consumed species in Europe (see Table 29.1).

PARVALBUMINS

Parvalbumins are generally found in other vertebrates than fish: for example, chicken muscle and thymus, human brain, cat, gerbil and monkey, are just some examples.[31,51] Two distinct phylogenetic lineages of parvalbumin, named α and β, were inferred after comparing many amino acid sequences. Allergen M belongs to the β-lineage (parvalbumin β-lineage, *Gadus callarias* L, *Gad c1*) and is the major allergen of Baltic codfish. It belongs to a large group of muscle calcium-binding proteins – namely, the parvalbumins. It is a 12.328 kDa protein composed of 113 amino acids.[25,34,50] It is composed of three homologous domains AB, CD and EF, each comprising one-third of the chain and consisting of helices interspaced by one loop. The loops of the CD and EF domains coordinate one Ca^{2+} each.[50] X-ray crystallographic studies have provided informative views of the calcium-binding mode (as shown in Figs 29.1 and 29.2). The Ca^{2+}-binding CD domain of allergen M is composed of negatively charged oxygen at G101 and D90, D 92 and D94 (Fig. 29.3), which is tightly bound to calcium and appears to be the critical residue for the conformational changes induced by the molecule.[27]

The capacity of Ca^{2+} to be coordinated to multiple ligands – six to eight oxygen atoms – enables it to crosslink different systems and

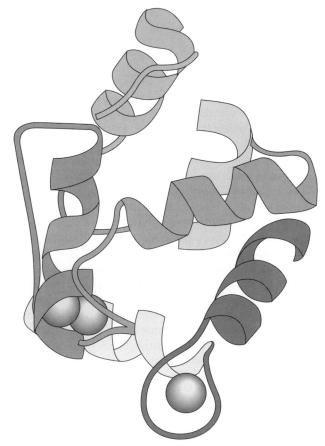

Fig. 29.1 X-ray crystallographic studies provide informative views of the calcium-binding proteins folding pattern proposed by Robert Kretsinger.[50] This view shows the structure of parvalbumin 12 kDa protein, which serves as a high-affinity calcium buffer in fish muscle (allergen M is one member of this group). (The image is produced by the free ware program Swiss PdP viewer.)

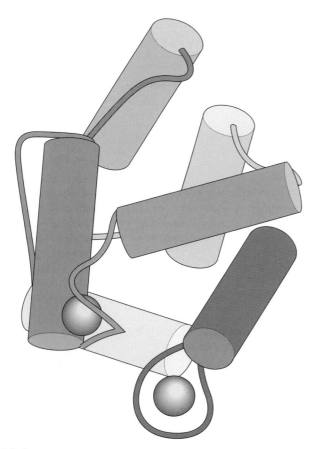

Fig. 29.2 Parvalbumin, the calcium-binding protein model, showing the domains EF, CD and AB: two calcium ions are bound in the CD and EF loops. (Image produced by free ware program Swiss PdP viewer.)

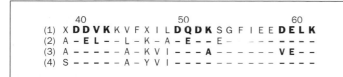

```
        40              50              60
(1) X D D V K K V F X I L D Q D K S G F I E E D E L K
(2) A - E L - - L - K - A - E - - E -   - - - - - - -
(3) A - - - - - A - K V I - - - A - - - - - - V E - -
(4) S - - - - - A - Y V I - - - - - - - - - - - - - -
```

Fig. 29.3 The amino acid (AA) sequence of the region 41–64 of the CD domain of parvalbumin. (1) Consensus AA sequence for the different studied vertebrate species; (2) Allergen M (parvalbumin-β) AA sequence; (3) Parvalbumin-β Atlantic salmon AA sequence; (4) Parvalbumin-α Atlantic salmon AA sequence. The boxes show the B cell motifs investigated. Hyphens represent indentities with the consensus sequence while gaps are indicated by dots. The bold residues represent the IgE-binding motifs.

induce large conformational changes.[16] Further confirmation of the importance of Ca^{2+} for IgE binding was reported at 1979 and later.[5,10] The second calcium-binding site is formed by the loop between the EF helix; a motif termed the 'EF hand' (Fig. 29.4).[60]

From the primary structure homology it is clear that the two Ca^{2+} binding sites of parvalbumin arose by triplication of a primordial gene encoding a main calcium-binding loop.[50] The EF hand is present in more than 100 parvalbumins belonging to many species and is the second motif for fish allergen cross-immunogenicity (Fig. 29.4).[60]

The cDNA encoding parvalbumin from Baltic cod and Atlantic salmon as identified and recombinant parvalbumins of these

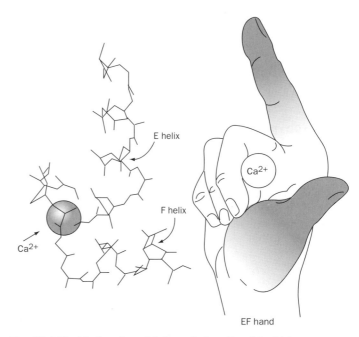

Fig. 29.4 The binding sites of Ca^{2+} are helices E and F, which are positioned like the forefinger and thumb of the right hand (the EF hand motif). (From Stryer, Lubert, *Biochemistry*, 4th edn. WH Freeman & Company, New York, 1995, p. 348).

species were expressed.[54,68–70] B cell epitope screening of allergen M from Baltic cod was elucidated.[27–29]

The native B cell epitopes of allergen M

THE susceptibility of allergen M to trypsin is limited to 14 lysyl (K) and 1 arginyl (R) peptide bonds. Blocking the amino groups of K leaves the molecule with only one R available as a cleavage site. This enabled the isolation of two allergenically active segments (PVA TM1 75 AA & PVA TM2 38AA).[23]

R-75 is one of the consensus amino acids in all the parvalbumins studied (Fig. 29.5). PVA/TM2 is considered to be a reasonable size, monovalent, natural allergenic fragment. It is easily available from many fish species and is a useful tool for experimental immunotherapy and for studies on the mechanisms of cross-immunogenicity of food allergens (Figs 29.5 and 29.6).

THE SYNTHETIC PEPTIDES OF THE CD LOOP

Allergen M synthetic peptides were derived by solid phase synthesis for studying the specific antibody binding to low molecular weight epitopes (Fig. 29.7). Two have been extensively studied: namely, sequence 49–64 of the CD loop and sequence 88–103 of the EF loop.[23,26,27]

Peptide 49–64 was purified by reversed phase/high-performance liquid chromatography (RP/HPLC) and its IgE and IgG bindings have been demonstrated (Fig. 29.8).[26]

The site is shown to be capable of inhibiting cod-specific IgE antibodies and was similarly reactive *in vivo*. The same peptide is also represented in Atlantic salmon (*Sal s 1*) α and β lineage (Fig. 29.3). The tetrapeptides 41–44 DELK, 51–54 DEDK and 61–64 DELK are consensus sequences present in more than 100 parvalbumins and are critical residues for antibody binding. In conclusion, the repetitive sequences of region 41–64 show that

```
       1          10          20          30          40          50          60          70          80
(1) X X T X X L X A X D I X X X A L X A X X A A D S F X H K X F F X X V G L  X X K S X D D V K K V F X  I LDQDKSGF I EEDELK L F L K X F S X X A R X T D X E T K A
(2) A F K G I - S N A - - K A - E A - C F K E G - - D E D G - Y A K - - - D A F - A - E L - - L - K - A-E- - E- - - - - - - - - - - - - - I A - A A D L - A - - A - - - -
(3) A C A H L C K E A - - K T - - E - C K - - - T - S F - T - - H T I - F A S - - A - - - - - A - K V I - - - A - - - - - - V E - - - - - I N - C P K - - E - - A - - - -
(4) S F A G . - N D A - V A A - - A R C T - - - - - N - - A - - A K - - - A S - - S - - - - - A - Y V I - - - - - - - - - - - - - - - - - - - Q N - - A S - - A - - A - - - -


      90         100        108
(1) F L A A GDXDGDGK IGVDE FX X L V X X
(2) - - K - - - S - - - - - - - - - - - G A - - D K W G A K G
(3) - - K - - - A - - - - M - - I - - - A V - - K I
(4) - - - D - - K - - - - M - - - - - - A A M I K D K
```

Fig. 29.5 The amino acid (AA) sequence of parvalbumins: (1) Consensus AA sequence for the different studied vertebrate species; (2) allergen M (parvalbumin-β) AA sequence; (3) parvalbumin-β Atlantic salmon AA sequence; (4) Parvalbumin-α Atlantic salmon AA sequence. The boxes show the B cell motifs investigated. Hyphens represent identities with the consensus sequence while gaps are indicated by dots. The bold residues represent the IgE-binding motifs.

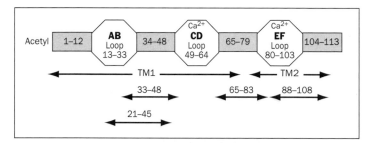

Fig. 29.6 Allergen M *Gad cl* schematic diagram. The molecule is composed of three domains, AB, CD and EF, of which the two last are the Ca^{2+}-binding sites. The locations of the peptides studied are indicated on the arrows. Two fragments, POVA/TM1 and TM2, are also shown.

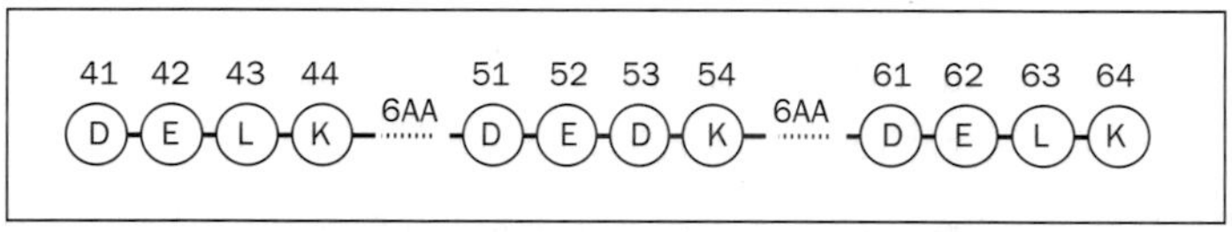

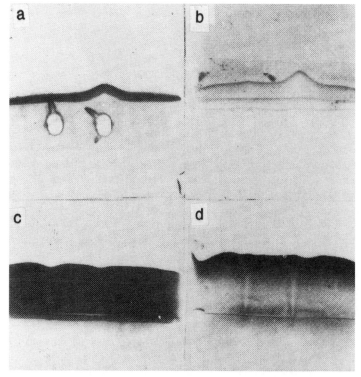

Fig. 29.7 A schematic drawing of the region 41–64 of allergen M showing the three tetrapeptide arrangement interspaced by six amino acids (6AA) in a segment of 24 residues.

Fig. 29.8 Rocket line immunoelectrophoresis patterns of octapeptide 57–64, in the first well and hexadecapeptide 49–64 in the second well of the plate (a) using allergen M line in the secondary gel and polyclonal antibodies against allergen M in the secondary gel. In plate (b) birch pollen extract BV line was applied in the secondary gel and rabbit anti *Bet vl* in the antibody gel. In plates (c) and (d) four different serum proteins were applied in the wells using anti-allergen M or anti-birch extract in the antibody gels. A deflection of allergen M line by peptide 49–64 is illustrated in plate (a). The same peptide could deflect one of the four lines of birch extract. No deflection was seen for the control-unrelated proteins, emphasizing the specificity of the reaction.

the immunogenicity of this region is determined by the three tetrapeptides DELK, DEDK and DELK (Fig. 29.7).[28,54]

The Ca²⁺-binding motif of the EF loop

The second Ca^{2+} coordination loop [88–103] of the EF domain (Fig. 29.5) was synthesized and purified to homogeneity by RP/HPLC. Both the *in vivo* and *in vitro* tests show that the immunological reactivity of the site is compatible with a monovalent haptenic function, blocking but not eliciting the allergic reaction. In the *in vivo* IgE binding inhibition test only minor reaction is elicited in the sites using a preincubated serum with the peptide upon challenge with the intact allergen.[27]

THE MINOR ALLERGENS OF CODFISH

The antigenic and allergenic profiles of codfish extract have been examined and a comparison made of the specificity of the deter-

minants defined by mouse monoclonal *Gad c1* antibodies (mAbs) and human IgE antibodies. By gel electrophoresis, codfish extract was found to comprise a heterogeneous mixture of proteins, in which the principal component and allergen was *Gad c1* (Fig. 29.9).

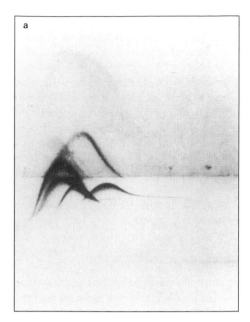

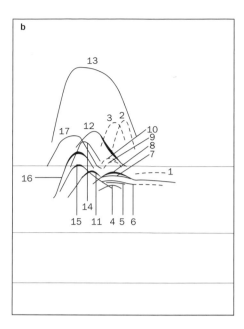

Fig. 29.9 Crossed immunoelectrophoretic reference pattern of cod parvalbumins: (a) Coomasie brilliant blue stained and (b) drawing with the numbers of the precipitates.

Using mAbs and sera from human codfish allergic subjects as immunological probes, common antigenic and allergenic determinants were demonstrated on some codfish proteins. It was also established that although two mAbs recognized the same determinant on *Gad c1*, there was no crossreactivity between this determinant and those specified by IgE antibodies in the sera of cod allergic patients. The specificity of IgE populations directed against *Gad c1* was found to vary from patient to patient, and was indicative of the existence of two types of allergenic determinant: those unique to a particular allergen and those shared by other proteins in the extract. These studies promote speculation regarding the relative immunogenicity of antigenic and allergenic determinants and the size and diversity of the IgE repertoire, given the potential immunogenicity of the entire protein surface.[38] This study shows that there could be a possibility that *Gad c1* is found in two isoforms belonging to the same β-lineage.

Further, a 41 kDa protein has been obtained by different chromatographic and electrophoretic techniques. This protein bound cod-specific IgE from sera of allergic patients and to mAbs against cod parvalbumin. This was assumed to contain a calcium-binding site corresponding to that of parvalbumin *Gad c1*.[33] This is in disagreement with other findings, since all the known parvalbumins have two distinct proteins belonging to either α- or β-lineage of 12 kDa (Fig. 29.10), with no known homology to any 41 kDa proteins.[19,28] Several other protein bands have been identified: 60, 67, 104 and 130 kDa. It was suggested that the new bands may correspond to aggregates and could be detected by specific IgE against *Gad c1*.[14]

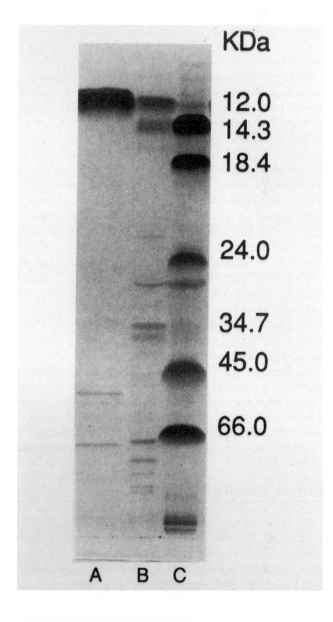

Fig. 29.10 SDS-PAGE analysis of cod and salmon parvalbumins. Parvalbumin for Baltic cod allergen M is shown in (A), next to parvalbumin from Atlantic salmon in (B) and a molecular weight marker in (C). Parvalbumin from salmon showed two bands (12 kDa and 14 kDa) while those of cod were located at 12 kDa.[54]

CROSSREACTIVITY WITH OTHER FISH

Most fish-allergic subjects suffer allergy reactions to multiple fish species. Species specificity and patterns of crossreactivity are still to be defined. Other studies to characterize crossreactive specific IgE-binding proteins in six different fish species (cod, tuna, salmon, perch, carp and eel) have been examined. IgE-binding components were characterized by immunoblotting, and crossreactive epitopes were studied by IgE-immunoblot inhibition experiments. Sera from 30 patients allergic to fish displayed IgE reactivities to parvalbumin from six different species.[9]

Immunological crossreactivity

The immunological reactivity of codfish-allergic adults to four species of fish – cod, mackerel, herring and plaice – were investigated. Eight codfish-allergic adult patients were defined by double-blind, placebo-controlled challenges with fresh raw codfish. Control subjects ($n=30$) were defined by means of 30 codfish-tolerant control subjects, using a skin-prick test (SPT), histamine release (HR), serum (s-) specific IgE, sodium dodecyl sulphate polyacrylamide gel electrophoresis (SDS-PAGE) and immunoblotting. The study confirmed that serologic crossreactivity to different fish species in clinically codfish-allergic adults exists, and that cod, mackerel, herring and plaice share a common antigenic structure.[35]

s-Specific IgE

The binding of s-specific IgE from children and adults to fish allergens was investigated. The clinical history of fish allergy is confirmed by SPT, RAST and with blinded oral food challenges. Five children with severe allergic reactions to catfish (4/5), cod (1/5) and tuna (1/5) and five adults with severe allergic reactions to catfish (5/5), cod (2/5), snapper (3/5) and tuna (2/5) were compared. Allergen extracts from catfish, cod, snapper and tuna were run on SDS-PAGE. IgE immunoblot and immunoblot inhibition were performed using serum samples from these 10 patients. Multiple fish proteins ranging from 12 to 45 kDa from the four fish extracts were identified by SDS-PAGE. *Gad c1* homologous protein (12 kDa) was present in all fish extracts (Fig. 29.10). Immunoblot using the 10 sera revealed that the major IgE-binding was to the 12 kDa protein from catfish, cod and snapper. Similar to previous studies of codfish, the authors confirmed that children and adult patients have specific IgE binding to the 12 kDa allergen M from different types of fish.[40]

Mono-allergic reactions

It is not often that fish-allergic patients react only towards one sort of fish. However, a patient specifically mono-allergic to swordfish and not to other fish was of interest. The sera did not recognize the *Gad c1* parvalbumin β-analogue (12 kDa) but demonstrated IgE directed against a 25 kDa protein. Both serological and clinical data demonstrate that the patient has monospecific allergy towards swordfish.[44]

CLINICAL MANIFESTATION

Fish allergy can be the cause of urticaria and other allergic skin manifestations, including flushing and angioedema; ocular conjunctivitis and gastrointestinal disorders, including oropharyngeal pruritus, nausea, vomiting, diarrhoea and abdominal cramping, are usually encountered. Although avoidance is effective and the most accepted treatment for food allergy, fish allergens are often difficult to eliminate. They may occasionally occur as inhalant allergens, vapours from cooking of marine products and sometimes as contaminants of other food items.[7,52]

Evidence that fish, compared with other food allergens, play some role in the pathogenesis of atopic dermatitis (AD) is not conclusively established. In a recent study it was found that approximately one-third of a number of children ($n=63$) with refractory, moderate or severe AD had IgE-mediated clinical reactivity to fish among other food proteins. The prevalence of food allergy in this AD population seems significantly higher than that in the general population.[18]

Other mechanisms involving autoimmune pathogenesis in atopic dermatitis are also gaining acceptance.[8]

Anaphylactic reactions

Symptoms of fish allergy can sometimes be serious and may lead to anaphylactic reactions. Generally fatal food-induced anaphylaxis is rarely reported.[11,53] In one study, seven victims with multiple allergies, including fish, crab, peanut and pecan, were reported.[72] Furthermore, a recently performed multicentre study has investigated the frequency of food-induced anaphylaxis in 794 cases, where food was the cause of anaphylactic reactions represented as 10.2% of aetiologies.[59]

Six children and adolescents who died of anaphylactic reactions to other foods than fish and seven others who nearly died and required intubation were reported by Sampson.[67] Further, an epidemiological study of anaphylaxis was recently reported by Yunginger.[73] The increase in frequency of anaphylaxis might also be explained by the general rise of food allergy. In a study of 44 children (aged 2 months to 15.5 years) who were admitted to the paediatric emergency in Rouen, France, 42.5% had food allergy; of those 75% were suffering serious anaphylactic reactions due to one of the following food items: fish, milk, egg and nuts.[55]

Hyposensitization therapy in food allergy is usually not recommended, since the patient may spontaneously outgrow their disease.[1] Others who favour immunotherapy have suggested it for treatment of fish allergy, since it may decrease the symptoms though not entirely suppress them.[11,13]

Airborne fish allergens may induce Type I reactions: studies from our laboratory showed that fish allergens were detectable at relatively high levels in dust collected from many school classrooms.[17]

Occupational hypersensitivity such as immediate contact urticaria caused by herring and occupational asthma in connection with handling salmon, trout and other marine products, has been reported.[12,15] Allergic reactions in seafood workers usually develop after occupational exposure and in consumers after preparation or ingestion of seafood.[52]

Histamine is often present in dietary fish and is attributed to microorganisms' by-products, which may act as endotoxins, in addition to its known pharmacological activity on smooth muscle.[43] Such inflammatory mediators in fish muscle would intensify the allergic response.

Fish allergy in children

For obvious reasons, most of the studies on fish hypersensitivity have been focused on children, mainly using codfish reactions as standard. Two main reasons could explain this: (a) food allergy induced by IgE and mast cells or basophils is rapid and often experienced in childhood and young adults:[1,2] (b) codfish includes the major and most potent and characterized fish allergen (parvalbumin), widely represented in almost all vertebrates.[20,22]

Studies of fish hypersensitivity in children were initiated more than three decades ago in Norway by Aas and co-workers.[3,19] At that time, the prevalence of fish allergy was estimated to be approximately 1 in 1000 children. In a series of trials on 825 children with asthma or urticaria, Aas demonstrated that ingestion of fish or inhalation of fish vapours from cooking provoked asthmatic attacks in 50 (6.9%) children with asthma ($n=725$) and 76 (10.3%) with urticaria patients. Fish was the only cause in 5 asthma and 32 urticaria children.[1,2]

Fish odours

Decades ago, fish 'odour' was reported to be a triggering cause of allergy.[3] The definition of 'fish odour' is far from clear. However, in this context, odour is not meant to include any olfactory chemoreceptor signals, only intrinsic fish allergenic proteins. Those proteins are the result of extremely minute fish particles from the steam of cooking fish. The airborne components should be considered as a totally different exposure to that of conventional ingestion of fish. In this context, the psychological effects that may cause histamine release from the perception of fish odour (trimethylamine) or sulphur (dimethyl sulphide) do not belong to this chapter. To exclude the psychological effects, a challenge with the odour of fish and subsequently to the ingestion of fish may be required.

From 197 children diagnosed with Type I allergy to fish, approximately 10% showed allergic reactions upon exposure to fish steam and ingestion of fish caused IgE-mediated reactions in 86%. Upon elimination of fish from the diet, inhalation of fish fumes still elicited an intense allergic reaction.[11,12] More basic studies on the characterization of allergens in cooking steam would be rewarding.

Fish allergy in adults

Food-allergic diseases in children are often IgE-mediated; in adults in addition to IgE-mediated allergy, other mechanisms involving subclasses of IgG, IgA, complement, Ig-complex formation or cellular reactions are possible.

In adult patients with food allergy based on suggestive history (geographical variability of 0.1–0.5% of the whole population), fish was implicated in 4.2% of the cases.[42]

Significant crossreactivity among fish, e.g. pollack, salmon, trout and tuna, and between mackerel and anchovy, means that complete exclusion of all fish in the relevant group is necessary for adequate treatment. Positive skin-prick tests to fish alone are not adequate criteria for the confirmation of a clinically relevant fish allergy. Double-blind placebo-controlled food challenge (DBPCFC) may be needed to confirm the sensitization status.[37] Strict overall elimination of fish in the diet is usually recommended, although some patients can tolerate some species of fish without suffering reaction. However, a pre-evaluation of the patient's tolerance towards one or another fish sort to include in the diet can be considered.

Occupational asthma due to fish inhalation, confirmed by specific bronchial challenge, has been shown in two patients whose asthma was induced by occupational exposure to fish. The results suggested that fish inhalation can elicit IgE-mediated occupational asthma.[64]

DIAGNOSIS OF FISH ALLERGY

The current increase in the prevalence of fish and other food allergies appears to have several causes, including better screening, improved diagnosis and changes in both the techniques used by food manufacturers and eating habits. Of note is the increasing risk of processed food contamination with allergenic food proteins. The establishment of an animal model for screening the allergenicity of food products is important for identifying potential IgE-binding contaminants.[57,65]

The diagnosis of fish allergy is not different from other food allergies and should include: clinical history; SPT, total and specific IgE, histamine release and allergen specific T lymphocyte stimulation test (LST); and DBPCFC, which is gaining wide acceptance as the most reliable test to confirm fish hypersensitivity and to identify putative allergens and their derivation.[35,61] The demonstration of the specificity of strong binding of IgE to a 12 kDa protein which completely matches with the DBPCFC results in many cases of fish allergy seems a sufficient test for establishing the diagnosis of fish allergy.[36] SPT and RAST are sensitive indicators of specific IgE. Previous studies suggested that high concentrations of fish-specific IgE antibody were predictive of food-induced clinical symptoms.[32]

The peripheral blood mononuclear cell proliferation test is used as a supplemental diagnostic test of adult food allergy in our laboratory, but is mainly used as research tool in other laboratories.[45–49]

Labial food challenge (LFC) is reported to be associated with only low risks of systemic reaction. It may be an alternative test to the oral food challenge (OFC) for paediatric use.[63]

CONCLUSION

1. Fish are a large group of animals represented by a variety of cold-blooded aquatic vertebrates of several evolutionary lines.
2. Despite the great advantages obtained from a fish diet, several fish proteins are unfortunately highly potent allergens, playing important roles in the pathogenesis of many allergic manifestations that affect the gastrointestinal tract, airways and skin.
3. Two distinct phylogenetic lineages of parvalbumin, named α and β, were identified after amino acid sequences were compared; allergen M belongs to the β-lineage.
4. Allergen M belongs to a large group of muscle calcium-binding proteins called 12.3 kDa parvalbumins composed of 113 AA.
5. The cDNA encoding parvalbumin from Baltic cod and Atlantic salmon were performed and recombinant parvalbumins of these species were expressed; B cell epitope screening of allergen M from Baltic cod was elucidated; long-term T cell lines and allergen-specific T cell clones were generated.
6. Two allergenically active segments (PVA TM1 75 AA & PVA TM2 38 AA) are available.
7. The tetrapeptides 41–44 DELK, 51–54 DEDK and 61–64 DELK of allergen M are consensus sequences present in more than 100 parvalbumins and are critical residues for antibody binding. The repetitive sequences of region 41–64 show that the immunogenicity of this region is determined by the three tetrapeptides DELK, DEDK and DELK.

8. Serological crossreactivity to different fish species in allergic adults exists. This can be defined by: double-blind, placebo-controlled challenges with fresh raw codfish, skin-prick test, histamine release, specific IgE, SDS-PAGE and immunoblotting.

9. Serologic crossreactivity to different fish species in clinically codfish-allergic adults exists, and cod, mackerel, herring and plaice share a common antigenic structure.

10. Allergic reactions to fish begin in most patients within the first 24 months of life.

11. Fish inhalation can elicit IgE-mediated occupational allergy.

12. Strict overall elimination of fish in the diet of fish-allergic patients is usually recommended. A pre-evaluation of the patient's clinical tolerance towards one or another type of fish to include in the diet can be considered.

13. A patient allergic to swordfish only demonstrated IgE directed against a 25 kDa protein and not to bind the 12.3 kDa band. Both serological and clinical data confirmed that the patient has monospecific allergy towards swordfish.

14. Hyposensitization therapy (allergen specific immunotherapy) in fish allergy is usually not recommended since the patient may spontaneously outgrow the disease. Others favour immunotherapy and have suggested it for treatment of fish allergy, since it may decrease the symptoms although not suppressing them.

15. The diagnosis of fish allergy comprises: clinical history; SPT, total and specific IgE, HR and LST; and DBPCFC, which is gaining wide acceptance as the most reliable means of confirming fish hypersensitivity and of identifying putative species.

16. Regarding the increasing risk of processed food contamination with allergenic food proteins, the establishment of an animal model for screening the allergenicity of food products is necessary to identify IgE-binding contaminants.

REFERENCES

1 Aas K. Thesis, Studies of hypersensitivity to fish. In: Department of Paediatrics, University of Oslo, Oslo, 1967.

2 Aas K. Studies of hypersensitivity to fish. A clinical study. *Int Arch Allergy* 1966; 29: 346–63.

3 Aas K, Jebsen JW: Studies of hypersensitivity to fish partial purification and crystallization of a major allergenic component of cod. *Int Arch Allergy* 1967; 32: 1–20.

4 Adams S, Barnett D, Walsh B *et al.* Human IgE-binding synthetic peptides of bovine beta-lactoglobulin and alpha-lactalbumin. *In vitro* crossreactivity of the allergens. *Immunol Cell Biol* 1991; 69(Pt3): 191–7.

5 Apold J, Elsayed S. The effect of amino acid modification and polymerization on the immunochemical reactivity of cod allergen M. *Molec Immunol* 1979; 16: 559–64.

6 Bernhisel-Broadbent J, Scanlon S, Sampson HA. Fish hypersensitivity. I. *In vitro* and oral challenge results in fish-allergic patients. *J Allergy Clin Immunol* 1992; 89: 730–7.

7 Bruijnzeelkoomen C: Food induced skin diseases. *Environ Toxicol Pharmacol* 1997; 4: 39–41.

8 Bruijnzeel-Koomen C. Pathophysiology of eczema. In: *VVII Congress of the European Academy of Allergology & Clinical Immunology*, Birmingham, 1998; MS3/40.

9 Bugajskaschretter A, Elfman L, Fuchs T *et al.* Parvalbumin, a cross-reactive fish allergen, contains IgE-binding epitopes sensitive to periodate treatment and Ca^{2+} depletion. *J Allerg Clin Immunol* 1998; 101: 67–74.

10 BugajskaSchretter A, Pastore A, Vangelista L *et al.* Molecular and immunological characterization of carp parvalbumin, a major fish allergen. *Int Arch Allergy Immunol* 1999; 118: 306–8.

11 Casimir G, Cuvelier P, Allard S *et al.* Life-threatening fish allergy successfully treated with immunotherapy. *Pediatr Allergy Immunol* 1997; 8: 103–5.

12 Crespo J, Pascual C, Dominguez C *et al.* Allergic reactions associated with airborne fish particles in IgE-mediated fish hypersensitive patients. *Allergy* 1995; 50: 257–62.

13 Dannaeus A, Inganas M. A follow-up study of children with food allergy. Clinical courses in relation to serum IgE and IgG antibody levels to milk, egg, and fish. *Clin Allergy* 1981; 11: 533–9.

14 Dory D, Chopin C, Aimonegastin I *et al.* Recognition of an extensive range of IgE-reactive proteins in cod extract. *Allergy* 1998; 53: 42–50.

15 Douglas J, McSharry C, Blaikie L *et al.* Occupational asthma caused by automated salmon processing. *Lancet* 1995; 346: 737–40.

16 Dreessen J, Lutum C, Schäfer BW *et al.* α-Parvalbumin reduces depolarization-induced elevations of cytosolic free calcium in human neuroblastoma cells. *Cell Calc* 1996; 19: 527–33.

17 Dybendal T, Wedeberg WC, Elsayed S. Dust from carpeted and smooth floors. IV. Solid material, protein and allergens collected in the different filter stages of vacuum cleaners after ten days of use in schools. *Allergy* 1991; 46: 427–35.

18 Eigenmann PA, Sicherer SH, Borkowski TA *et al.* Prevalence of IgE-mediated food allergy among children with atopic dermatitis. *Pediatrics* 1998; 101: E81–6.

19 Elsayed S. Four linear and two conformational epitopes of the major allergenic molecule of egg (*Gal d 1*, ovalbumin). CRC Press, Vienna; 1992.

20 Elsayed S. Allergens. In: Van Regenmortel MHV (ed.) *Structure of Antigens*. CRC Press, London; 1993: 293–316.

21 Elsayed S, Aas K. Isolation of purified allergen (cod) by isoelectric focusing. *Int Arch Allergy Appl Immunol* 1971; 40: 428–38.

22 Elsayed S, Apold J. Immunochemical analysis of cod fish allergen M: location of the immunological binding sites as demonstrated by the native and synthetic peptides. *Allergy* 1983; 38: 449–59.

23 Elsayed S, Aas K, Sletten K *et al.* Tryptic cleavage of a homogenous cod fish allergen and isolation of two active polypeptide fragments. *Immunochemistry* 1972; 9: 647–61.

24 Elsayed S, Sletten K, Aas K. The primary structure of a major allergen (Cod): NH_2-terminal amino acid sequence of fragment TM2. *Immunochemistry* 1973; 10: 701–5.

25 Elsayed S, Bennich H. The primary structure of allergen M from cod. *Scand J Immunol* 1975; 4: 203–8.

26 Elsayed S, Titlestad K, Apold J *et al.* A synthetic hexadecapeptide derived from Allergen M imposing allergenic and antigenic reactivity. *Scand J Immunol* 1980; 12: 171.

27 Elsayed S, Ragnarsson U, Apold J *et al.* Allergenic synthetic peptides corresponding to the second calcium binding loop of cod allergen M. *Scand J Immunol* 1981; 14: 207–11.

28 Elsayed S, Sørnes S, Apold J *et al.* The immunological reactivity of the three homologous repetitive tetrapeptides in the region 41–64 of Allergen M from cod. *Scand J Immunol* 1982; 16: 77–82.

29 Elsayed S, Ragnarsson U, Netteland B. Solid-phase synthesis of the non-calcium-binding loop of cod allergen M. Direct evidence of the reactivity of the amino-terminal segment. *Scand J Immunol* 1983; 17: 291–5.

30 Encyclopedia Britannica. *Fish Taxonomy*, 1998.

31 Føhr U, Weber B, Müntener M *et al.* Human α and β parvalbumins. Structure and tissue-specific expression. *Eur J Biochem* 1993; 215: 719–27.

32 Foucard T, Aas K, Johansson S. Concentration of IgE antibodies. PK titers, and chopped lung titers in sera from children with hypersensitivity to cod. *J Allergy Clin Immunol* 1973; 51: 39–44.

33 Galland AV, Dory D, Pons L *et al.* Purification of a 41 kDa cod-allergenic protein. *J Chromatogr B* 1998; 706: 63–71.

34 Gerday C. *Calcium and calcium binding proteins. Molecular and functional aspects*. Springer, Heidelberg 1988.

35 Hansen T, Bindslev-Jensen C. Codfish allergy in adults. Identification and diagnosis. *Allergy* 1992; 47: 610–7.

36 Hansen T, Bindslev-Jensen C, Skov P *et al*. Codfish allergy in adults: Specific tests for IgE and histamine release vs double-blind, placebo-controlled challenges. *Clin Exp Allergy* 1996; 26: 1276–85.

37 Helbing A, McCants M, Musmand J *et al*. Immunopathogenesis of fish allergy: identification of fish-allergic adults by skin test and radioallergosorbent test. *Ann Allergy Asthma Immunol* 1996; 77: 48–54.

38 Hemmens V, Baldo B, Underdown P *et al*. Common antigenic and allergenic determinants of cod fish proteins detected with mouse monoclonal IgG and human IgE antibodies. *Molecul Immunol* 1989; 26: 477–84.

39 Hoffer I. Food allergy. II – Prevalence of organ manifestations of allergy inducing food. A study on the basis of 173 cases 1978–1982. *Schweiz med Wocheschr* 1985; 115: 1437–42.

40 James J, Helm R, Burks A *et al*. Comparison of pediatric and adult IgE antibody binding to fish proteins. *Ann Allergy Asthma Immunol* 1997; 79: 131–7.

41 Johnsen G, Elsayed S. Antigenic and allergenic determinants of ovalbumin. III. MHC Ia-binding peptide (OA 323–339) interacts with human and rabbit specific antibodies. *Mol Immunol* 1990; 27: 821–7.

42 Joral A, Villas F, Garmendia J *et al*. Adverse reactions to food in adults. *J Invest Allergolog Clin Immunol* 1995; 5: 47–9.

43 Kalligas G, Kaniou I, Zachariadis G *et al*. Thin layer and high pressure liquid chromatography determination of histamine in fish tissues. *J Liq Chromatograph* 1994; 17: 2457–68.

44 Kelso J, Jones R, Yunginger J. Monospecific allergy to swordfish. *Ann Allergy Asthma Immunol* 1996; 77: 227–8.

45 Kondo N, Agata H, Fukutomi O *et al*. Lymphocyte responses to food antigens in patients with atopic dermatitis who are sensitive to foods. *J Allergy Clin Immunol* 1990; 86: 253–60.

46 Kondo N, Kobayashi Y, Shinoda S *et al*. Reduced interferon gamma production by antigen-stimulated cord blood mononuclear cells is a risk factor of allergic disorders – 6-year follow-up study. *Clin Experiment Allergy* 1998; 28: 1340–4.

47 Koning H, Baert M, Oranje A *et al*. Development of immune functions related to allergic mechanisms in young children. *Pediatr Res* 1996; 40: 363–75.

48 Koning H, Neijens HJ, Baert MRM *et al*. T cell subsets and cytokines in allergic and non-allergic children. 1. Analysis of IL-4, IFN-gamma and IL-13 mRNA expression and protein production. *Cytokine* 1997; 9: 416–26.

49 Koning H, Neijens HJ, Baert MRM *et al*. T cell subsets and cytokines in allergic and non-allergic children 2. Analysis of IL-5 and IL-10 mRNA expression and protein production. *Cytokine* 1997; 9: 427–36.

50 Kretsinger RH. *Calcium Binding Proteins and Natural Membrane*. Academic Press, New York, 1974.

51 Kuster T, Staudenmann W, Hughes G *et al*. Parvalbumin isoforms in chicken muscle and thymus. Amino acid sequence analysis of muscle parvalbumin by tandem mass spectrometry. *Biochemistry* 1991; 30: 8812–16.

52 Lehrer S. Hypersensitivity reactions in seafood workers. *Allergy Proc* 1990; 11: 67–8.

53 Lin HY, Shyur SD, Fu JL *et al*. Fish induced anaphylactic reaction: report of one case. *Chung Hua Min Kuo Hsiao Erh KO I Hsueh Hui Tsa Chih* 1998; 39: 200–2.

54 Lindstrøm CD, van Do T, Hordvik I *et al*. Cloning of two distinct cDNAs encoding parvalbumin, the major allergen of Atlantic salmon (*Salmo salar*). *Scand J Immunol* 1996; 44: 335–44.

55 Marguet C, Couderc L, Blanc T *et al*. Anaphylaxis in children and adolescents: apropos of 44 patients aged 2 months to 15 years. *Arch Pediatr* 1999; 6(Suppl 1): 72S–8S.

56 Metacalfe D. Allergic reactions to foods. Little Brown & Company, Boston, 1995.

57 Miller K, Matthews GS, Smyth M *et al*. The establishment of an animal model for the screening of food products with potentially allergenic constituents. *Biochem Soc Trans* 1997; 25: S376.

58 Moneret-Vautrin DA: Food antigens and additives. *J Allergy Clin Immunol* 1986; 78:1039–46.

59 Moneret-Vautrin DA, Kanny G. Food-induced anaphylaxis. A new French multicenter study. *Bull Acad Natl Med* 1995; 179: 161–72.

60 Nakayama S, Kretsinger RH. Evolution of the EF-hand family of proteins. *Annu Rev Biophys Biomol Struct* 1994; 23: 473–507.

61 O'Neil C, Helbling A, Lehrer S. Allergic reactions to fish. *Clin Rev Allergy* 1993; 11: 183–200.

62 Prausnitz C, Kustner H. Studien uber die Ueberempfindliehkeit. *Zentralbl Bakteriol Parasitenlzd Infektionskr Hyg* 1921; 86: 160.

63 Rannce F, Dutau G. Labial food challenge in children with food allergy. *Pediatr Allergy Immunol* 1997; 8: 41–4.

64 Rodriguez J, Reano M, Vives R *et al*. Occupational asthma caused by fish inhalation. *Allergy* 1997; 52: 866–9.

65 Rogstad A, Weng B. Extraction and analysis by high-performance liquid chromatography of antibiotics in a drug delivery system for farmed fish. *J Pharm Sci* 1993; 82: 518–20.

66 Sampson HA. Immunopathogenic role of food hypersensitivity in infancy. *Acta Derm Venerol Suppl (Stockholm)* 1992; 176: 34–7.

67 Sampson HA, Mendelson L, Rosen JP. Fatal and near-fatal anaphylactic reactions to food in children and adolescents [see comments]. *New Engl J Med* 1992; 327: 380–4.

68 Van Do T, Hordvik I, Endresen C *et al*. Recombinant salmon fish allergens. Further purification and characterization. *Allergy* 1999; 54: 182.

69 Van Do T, Hordvik I, Endresen C *et al*. Expression and analysis of recombinant salmon parvalbumin, the major allergen in Atlantic salmon (*Salmo salar*). *Scand J Immunol* 1999; 50: 619–25.

70 van Do T, Hordvik I, Endresen C *et al*. Cloning and expression of Baltic cod Allergen M and Alaska pollack parvalbumins. *Eur J Biochem* Submitted 2001.

71 Willman E. Personal-communication, Norwegian Ministry of Fisheries, Department of Aquaculture, Industry and Export, 1999.

72 Yunginger JW. Anaphylaxis. *Ann Allergy* 1992; 69: 87–96.

73 Yunginger J, Sweeney K, Sturner W *et al*. Fatal food-induced anaphylaxis. *JAMA* 1988; 260: 145–2.

A

Chapter 30

Cow's milk and breast milk

John W. Gerrard

INTRODUCTION

Adverse reactions to cow's milk were first reported more than 2000 years ago when Hippocrates[1] (460–70 BC) noted that cow's milk could cause gastric upset and urticaria. The subject, however, began to attract greater attention after the Second World War when, for the first time, most babies were being brought up on formula feeds. The switch from breast to formula feeding had been associated with an increase in the prevalence of infantile eczema[33] and in mortality rates due to gastroenteritis and pneumonia.[34,72] With the better understanding of the management of electrolyte disturbances, and appropriate use of antibiotics, mortality rates fell. It then became apparent that not all the gastrointestinal and respiratory problems were infectious in origin; some were due to adverse reactions to cow's milk itself. It was at this juncture that Goldman and his colleagues[31] carried out their now classical studies on cow's milk allergy (CMA). These studies indicated that cow's milk could cause many problems and that the only sure way of determining in any one case whether cow's milk was or was not responsible was the avoidance and reintroduction of cow's milk; to what extent reactions were due to allergy and to what extent they were due to other factors was not and still is not certain.

There are several reasons which make it difficult for physicians to recognize or realize that some adverse reactions are being precipitated by cow's milk. Firstly, many of the symptoms caused by cow's milk resemble those caused by infections; recurrent rhinorrhoea, a persistent nasal stuffiness and repeated spells of wheezy bronchitis resemble infectious colds and bronchiolitis rather than hay fever and asthma. Secondly, skin prick tests and RAST (radioallergosorbent test) are usually negative and this suggests that the child is not allergic to cow's milk when in point of fact he may be. Thirdly, with classical food allergy the patient usually comes to the doctor with the diagnosis already made, knowing that traces of egg cause vomiting or that strawberries cause urticaria. This rarely applies to CMA, for the mother does not suspect that the cow's milk which she is giving her child daily may be making him ill.

Although the nature of the reactions, allergy or intolerance has not yet been entirely resolved, the presence of adverse reactions to cow's milk is not difficult to confirm, for cow's milk can be excluded from and reintroduced into the diet relatively easily. The prevalence of adverse reactions in any given infant population is also easy to determine,[10,30,35,39,42] always provided the manifestations of CMA are recognized for what they are. Almost all children are given cow's milk, usually on a daily basis, and those whose symptoms clear when cow's milk is avoided and return when it is reintroduced can be readily determined.

SYMPTOMS PRODUCED BY CMA IN INFANCY

The symptoms most commonly produced by CMA in infancy are indicated in Table 30.1. The data are derived from three very different sources: Clein[10] was a general paediatrician with a special interest in CMA; Goldman,[31] an immunologist whose cases were culled from the practices of many different paediatricians, the diagnosis being confirmed in all instances by three separate

Manifestations of CMA in percentages as seen in a general paediatric practice			
Symptom	Clein	Goldman	Gerrard
Eczema	43	42	45
Vomiting	38	27	22
Colic	31	31	20
Diarrhoea	23	40	40
Irritability	19	13	
Bronchitis	17		20
Asthma	15	13	12
Constipation	3		
Refusing milk	3	4	
Apathy, cyanosis and collapse	2	8	
Urticaria and angioedema	2		
	(n = 209)	(n = 89)	(n = 787)

Table 30.1 Manifestations of CMA in percentages as seen in a general paediatric practice (Clein[10]), in a group of children with CMA proven by three repeated challenges (Goldman[31]) and in a series of newborns (Gerrard[30]).

challenges; while Gerrard[30] followed an unselected series of normal newborns in order to determine the incidence of CMA in the infant population. Their findings suggest that the manifestations of CMA are relatively uniform.

Eczema

The commonest manifestation of CMA is eczema and though eczema can be precipitated by contact with soaps, wool, diapers, etc., foods are important in infancy and cow's milk is probably the commonest precipitating factor. Typically, the eczema first starts on the cheeks, chin and forehead, spreading at times to the trunk and limbs, particularly to the flexures, often becoming more severe with the introduction of cereals and fruits.

Gastrointestinal problems

Vomiting, diarrhoea and colic can all be precipitated by cow's milk although they can also be precipitated by other factors such as pyloric stenosis and infections. Care should be taken to exclude these before incriminating cow's milk. Infants with diarrhoea due to cow's milk may fail to thrive, have wasted limbs and buttocks and abdominal distension (Fig. 30.1). They may also have scalded buttocks (Fig. 30.2) which clear as soon as cow's milk is avoided and the diarrhoea has subsided. CMA can also cause hypoalbuminaemia and generalized oedema (Fig. 30.3) due to a protein-losing gastroenteropathy[67] as well as an iron-deficiency anaemia (Fig. 30.4) due to occult or overt blood loss in the stools.[65]

The awareness that cow's milk could cause diarrhoea first surfaced at a time when attention was being focused on inborn errors of metabolism and enzyme deficiencies. Infants with diarrhoea due to cow's milk were nearly always placed on formulae containing neither cow's milk protein nor lactose. Their stools often contained reducing substances[19] and lactose tolerance tests were abnormal; it was therefore assumed by many that lactase deficiency was primarily responsible for the diarrhoea.[16] We ourselves felt that this was unlikely because many of the children continued to have diarrhoea on lactose-free soya formulae. In addition, when babies were found to be intolerant of most or all prepared formulae they frequently tolerated breast milk, a food rich in lactose. The usefulness of breast milk in the management of babies with diarrhoea due to cow's milk and other food intolerances has recently been emphasized by MacFarlane and Miller.[50]

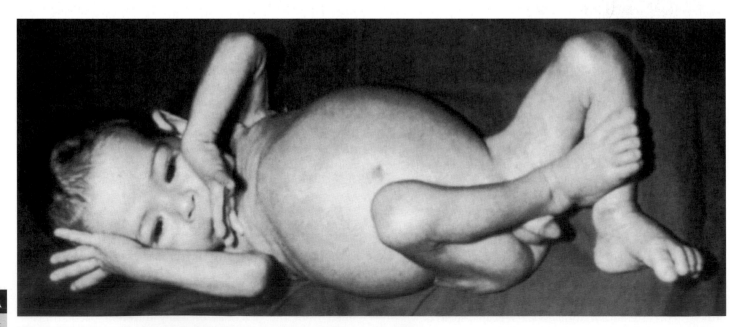

Fig. 30.1 An infant with abdominal distension and muscular wasting due to CMA.

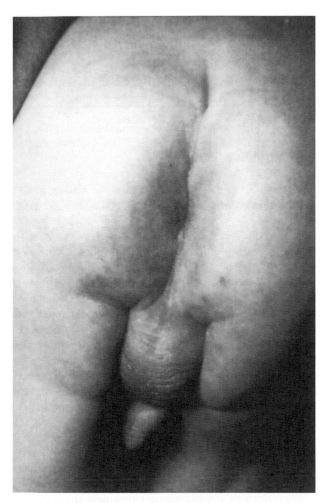

Fig. 30.2 Redness of perianal skin associated with diarrhoea due to CMA.

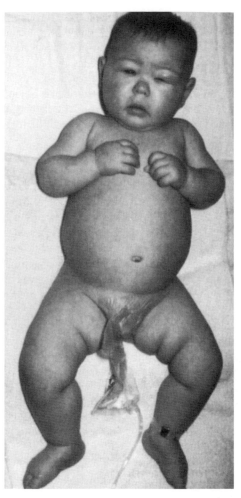

Fig. 30.3 Generalized oedema due to protein-losing gastroenteropathy.

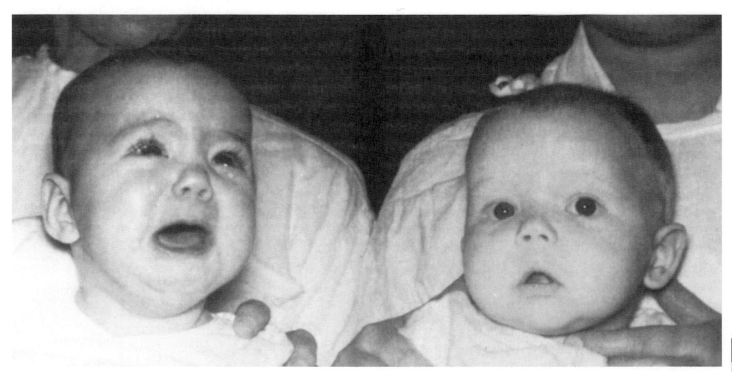

Fig. 30.4 Iron-deficiency anaemia due to CMA.

This finding confirms what Liu[48] demonstrated; namely, that babies with cow's milk protein intolerance often tolerate lactose as soon as cow's milk proteins have been excluded from the diet. Lactase activities in the jejunal mucosa of babies with CMA, though often diminished,[68] are not always absent.[49] Such deficiencies seen in these babies may therefore be secondary to CMA[36] and, in this respect, differ from the lactase deficiencies seen in ethnic groups that do not ordinarily drink milk after weaning.

Respiratory allergies

A recurrent or persistent rhinorrhoea or nasal stuffiness,[40] recurrent croup and recurrent bronchitis with or without (see also Chapter 35 by Zdenek Pelikan) wheezing are all common manifestations of CMA. Symptoms are sometimes persistent; at other times they are recurrent or episodic, the child appearing to recover from one attack of pneumonia or bronchiolitis only to develop another in spite of the fact that he has remained on his cow's milk formula all along. The most severe manifestation of respiratory CMA is Heiner's syndrome[34] – the child having repeated attacks of pneumonia associated with pulmonary infiltrates, haemosiderosis, anaemia and failure to thrive. Multiple precipitin bands to cow's milk proteins are present in the serum. The disease is not IgE mediated and skin prick and RAST tests to milk are negative.[46] There are more than 25 different proteins in cow's milk and the proteins which most commonly cause allergic reactions are β-lactoglobulin, casein, α-lactalbumin and bovine serum albumin.[31]

Neurological manifestations

Irritability and restlessness in babies are not usually thought of as being due to an adverse reaction to a food but they certainly can be, and in infancy cow's milk is the commonest offender.[10,31] Irritability would appear to be the counterpart in infancy of the tension fatigue syndrome in the child and depression in the adult.

Babies with CMA commonly have more than one symptom, the majority having several, e.g. eczema and rhinorrhoea or recurrent diarrhoea and recurrent bronchitis. Many are also often sensitive to more than one food for they tend to become sensitive to foods which they are given repeatedly. It is probably for this reason that babies sensitive to cow's milk when placed on soya formulae often become sensitive to the latter. Concomitant sensitivities to egg, citrus fruits and tomato are also common.[30]

Age at onset of symptoms

One might expect symptoms to start soon after the introduction of cow's milk, sometimes even after the first feed, but this is not always the case. In one series[25] symptoms started in just over a quarter (28%) within 3 days of the baby starting to take cow's milk or a cow's milk formula, in 41% within 7 days and in 68% within 1 month. Why it is that in some infants symptoms start almost immediately and in others later we do not know, but the later development of allergy seems often to be triggered by infections. This has been shown to be the case by Harrison *et al.*[37] We, too, have noticed that measles and even ordinary inoculations may trigger the development of an allergy to cow's milk. Viral infections in infancy are often associated with a rise in IgE levels.[24] We would speculate that such infections may act as adjuvants in initiating the development of new allergies. If the patient is seen

when older and the history indicates that symptoms first started soon after commencing a formula feed and have persisted, milk should be considered a potential cause of these problems.

SYMPTOMS DUE TO CMA IN THE OLDER CHILD AND ADULT

There are no hard and fast data regarding the incidence of CMA in the older child[39b,c] and adult but the following disorders can be milk related, although cow's milk is not necessarily the commonest precipitating factor in any one patient.

Respiratory symptoms
Allergic rhinitis
Cow's milk in our experience is as common a precipitating factor of perennial allergic rhinitis in childhood as it is in the infant. It is also common in the adult[21] and should be suspected if symptoms date from infancy, if they are not seasonal and if skin-prick tests to common inhalant allergens are negative. Although symptoms usually are perennial, they are often more severe in winter than in summer, possibly because of a concomitant house dust allergy, which increases the allergic load during the winter months. Another possible reason is because children often prefer juices and carbonated beverages to milk in the summer. Whatever the reason, there appear to be some children who are sensitive to cow's milk in the winter months but not in the summer.

Recurrent bronchitis
Recurrent bronchitis, like a recurrent nasal stuffiness, may be milk related both in children and in adults[25] and should be suspected in the adult if there is a child in the family with a respiratory milk sensitivity, if symptoms are perennial and if the patient is fond of and drinks much milk.

Asthma
Asthma, if seasonal, or by history or prick test is obviously due to inhalants, will probably not have a dietary component. Milk allergy should be considered as a cause when symptoms are perennial, if skin prick tests are negative to common inhalant allergens, if the patient is fond of and drinks much milk together with ice cream and cheese, and if a close relative is known to be allergic to milk (Table 30.2). Under these circumstances the patient should be asked to avoid milk and dairy products for at least 2 weeks. If the symptoms clear milk should be given in abundance to see if they return. If they do, milk, and dairy products should thereafter be avoided. If the patient's asthma is severe or 'brittle', such challenge studies should be undertaken under supervision.

Symptoms indicating milk may be a cause of asthma
Symptoms are perennial
Skin-prick tests negative
A family history of milk allergy is present
Patient likes and drinks much milk

Table 30.2 Symptoms indicating milk may be a cause of asthma.

Wraith[73] studying 119 food-allergic patients of whom 100 had asthma (34 with eczema), 7 had allergic rhinitis and 12 had urticaria, found that symptoms were precipitated by milk in 16 instances (wheat with 24 cases was the commonest food to precipitate a reaction). In no instance did milk cause an immediate reaction, clearly differing in this respect from classical IgE-mediated allergy. In only 4 cases was the RAST positive, indicating that RAST and skin-prick tests do not usually help to identify the asthmatic whose asthma is triggered by milk. A high index of suspicion combined with positive results in the avoidance and challenge test are the only sure ways of identifying such subjects. Milk may also play a permissive role in facilitating exercise-induced asthma.

Gastrointestinal symptoms

Milk-induced gastrointestinal problems are relatively easy to identify and treat in infancy. Although it is generally thought that symptoms clear when the child is 1 or 2 years old, this is not always the case. The childhood equivalent of the irritable bowel syndrome (IBS) – recurrent spells of abdominal pain, looseness of stools and/or constipation sometimes leading to incontinence and encopresis – may be milk or lactose induced. Milk should certainly be considered if the child was milk intolerant in infancy and is now drinking large quantities of it, or if he dislikes milk but is encouraged to drink it by well-meaning parents. There are, however, many other important causes of disturbed bowel function in children, including coeliac disease, Crohn's disease and ulcerative colitis. Although coeliac disease, Crohn's disease and ulcerative colitis may have dietary components, it is important to exclude these disorders before entertaining a diagnosis of CMA (see Chapter 41).

Irritable bowel syndrome

In the adult the IBS comprises a group of symptoms: spells of abdominal pain, flatulence, intermittent diarrhoea and sometimes constipation, with no identifiable pathology. It has been looked on as a functional disorder with a strong psychogenic component.[58] Weser and his colleagues,[70] however, found that 14 of 27 patients studied had an associated lactase deficiency and eight of these improved remarkably on milk-free and dairy-product-free diets. Bayless et al.[2] went on to demonstrate that lactase deficiencies were much more common in North American Blacks (occurring in 19 of 20 patients studied) than in American Whites (present in only two of 20 patients studied). When present, it was nearly always associated with symptoms of the IBS, with an onset at or around puberty when lactase activity tends to diminish (see Chapter 42).

The racial incidence of lactase deficiency has been mapped out by Kretchmer.[45] It is present in many African groups as well as in the Chinese and Japanese and in most races living in the Orient. If cow's milk ever becomes a staple of the Oriental diet it will almost certainly initiate an outbreak of the IBS.

Alun Jones,[43] noting that a patient with the IBS was made worse by bran, decided to look into the possibility that foods other than milk and lactose caused this syndrome. She found that 14 of 21 patients with this disorder lost their symptoms on oligoantigenic diets and that, when foods were reintroduced, wheat caused a relapse in nine, corn in five, milk and dairy products in four and coffee, tea and citrus fruits in nine others. Milk, quite apart from its lactose content, can also cause the IBS. Even Bentley,[3] who considers that psychological factors are of primary importance in the aetiology of the IBS, found that of 19 patients

studied the syndrome was precipitated by foods in three and that in two of these milk, not lactose, was the culprit. Twelve of the 14 patients studied including the three with proven food allergy, were found to have psychiatric problems, depression being the commonest. Although he thought that the psychiatric problem was primary it is possible that it accompanied rather than caused the IBS, for psychiatric problems seem to be a common accompaniment of food intolerances.[51]

Vascular: urticaria, purpura and headaches

Milk can, but does not frequently, cause urticaria[8,31] and purpura.[8] It is, however, a much more frequent cause of vascular headaches. The latter are not only common but they are commonly triggered by milk. Robert Burton[7] in The Anatomy of Melancholy, published in 1620 stated that: 'Milk and all that comes from milk are not good for those that are subject to headache.'

Headaches, whether manifestations of common or classical migraine, can be triggered by many factors, including inhalants such as perfumes and cigarette smoke, physical factors such as bright lights, noises and weather changes, but also by foods. Speer[64] in a study of 143 cases of headache, found that in approximately two-thirds foods were implicated and in half of these foods alone were to blame. The foods implicated most frequently were cow's milk and dairy products which precipitated headaches in 45 of the 143 cases. Monro[54] in her extensive review of the literature on food allergy and migraine found that cow's milk was one of the commonest foods to be implicated. Grant[32] in a series of 60 migraineurs was able to implicate cow's milk in 37% of the cases; Egger[17] in a more recent study found that 78 of 88 children with migraine were relieved of their headaches by dietary means alone. Cow's milk was the commonest single food to cause a headache (in 27 cases) and cheese caused headaches in 13 (see Chapter 37 and 38).

The urinary bladder: enuresis

There is still no consensus as to the cause of nocturnal enuresis but it is associated with a small bladder capacity.[19,65] Some enuretics have normal bladder control during the day time but not during the night time (nocturnal enuresis). Others are also caught short during the day time and wet their pants before they can reach the toilet (diurnal enuresis). A few children surprisingly are wet only during the day time, being dry at night. It is probable that all enuretic children with the exception of those presenting with polyuria due to either diabetes mellitus or insipidus have small capacity bladders.

Bray[5] was the first to suggest that enuresis might be allergic in origin and in the four cases he reported foods alone were incriminated in two, foods and inhalants in one and inhalants alone in the fourth. Milk was not one of the foods mentioned by him. Breneman,[6] who considers enuresis to be allergic in origin, found that milk was the commonest food to be incriminated. McKendry[52] compared the effectiveness of dietary management with imipramine and conditioning with a wet alarm, and found that dietary management was ineffective. Only one child in 64 became dry on dieting, whereas 23 of 43 treated with conditioning became dry. It is interesting to note that although just over half the children who were treated with dietary exclusion became dryer, a few actually became wetter. Milk was one of the foods excluded. We have found that the exclusion of milk and dairy products together with a so-called salicylate-free diet frequently leads to an increase in bladder capacity, and in approximately a third of the children to dryness.

The urinary bladder of the enuretic is partially contracted, being in spasm, and in this respect resembles the spasm of the bronchus seen in the asthmatic. The partially contracted bladder is sometimes referred to as the uninhibited bladder, for the enuretic cannot – in contrast to the normal child – relax his bladder to accommodate more urine. Spasm is relieved in some instances by dietary exclusion and in others by imipramine.[17] Because the bladder is in spasm, the child suffers frequency and urgency and cannot go through the night without emptying his bladder and wetting the bed. Urgency and frequency are often seen in the adult but in the adult they are more frequently due to beverages such as coffee and tea than to milk.

Neurological and behavioural disorders
Many authors have noted that allergic individuals have disturbances of behaviour, commonly irritability and/or fatigue, which subside with good allergy control. These individuals have been said by some to have 'allergic toxaemia' and by others[63] to have 'the tension fatigue syndrome'. Crook[13] has given details of 50 children with the syndrome, suggesting that it is relatively common. Feingold,[21] who emphasized the hyperkinetic aspects of the syndrome, has suggested that it is due to salicylates and so-called salicylate-containing foods. The children with this disorder usually have a short attention span, and the syndrome has therefore been renamed 'the attention deficit disorder'. The subject would not have been included in this chapter had not cow's milk been incriminated as a relatively common cause of the problem.

Speer,[63] who coined the term 'the tension fatigue syndrome', mentioned in his initial report the foods which precipitated symptoms in the six cases which he reported. In four cases, milk was an important offender, precipitating irritability and restlessness; when milk and dairy products together with the other foods to which they were sensitive were avoided, all the children became bright, cheerful and contented. Crook also found milk to be a common offender, the behavioural disturbances being milk-induced in 28 of the 50 patients reported by him. Rapp[59] in a smaller series of eight patients found that milk together with other foods was incriminated in six. In these six, milk caused headache in one, hyperactivity in three, spells of depression and crying in two and respiratory, not neurological, problems in one.

Interestingly, Egger,[17] studying the relationship between diet and migraine, noted that of 88 patients studied, 41 had associated behavioural disorders. In 36 patients, behaviour improved or normalized on an oligoantigenic diet. No mention was made of the foods responsible for the behavioural changes, but cow's milk was the food which most commonly caused migraine, and it is possible that it contributed to the behavioural changes seen in many of the children he studied (see Chapter 50).

Hyperactivity: attention deficit disorder
There has been much controversy over the aetiology of hyperactivity or the attention deficit disorder (ADD).[55] Feingold,[21] while emphasizing the relationship between hyperactivity and food colours and additives, unfortunately overlooked the many other foods that have been reported to cause it. The result was that double-blind studies aimed at confirming or disproving his hypothesis found little supportive evidence. Allergies are very individual, some children being sensitive to one food and others

to another. Each child must be his own control, and diets must be individualized, as in Egger's study[18] if they are to be informative.

Egger and his colleagues were the first to show that in a significant number of children foods could be, and probably are, the most important cause of ADD, with or without hyperactivity (ADHD). His own findings were confirmed by double-blind food challenges, and were later confirmed by others both in the United States[4] and in Canada.[44] They were nevertheless ignored, at least on the North American continent, by the medical profession in general, specifically by those most involved in the care of children with ADHD, namely paediatricians and psychiatrists. The putative effect of food on behaviour was even questioned in the very hospital in which Egger's studies had been undertaken, but when the studies were repeated, Egger's findings were confirmed.[9]

Food-related disturbances of behaviour also occur in infancy and in the adult. In infancy, irritability and sleeplessness[10,29] as already mentioned are probably the commonest manifestations, milk being the commonest precipitating factor. In the adult, a sense of profound exhaustion and lassitude is the characteristic component of the 'tension fatigue syndrome'. Weitkamp et al.[69] have shown that depression in the adult may have an immunological basis – the gene which carries it lies on chromosome 6, closely linked to the HLA locus. Depression, like classical allergic diseases such as asthma and hay fever, also runs in families. The concept that it too may be triggered by environmental antigens, such as milk, may therefore not be too far fetched. Schizophrenia is another relatively common psychiatric disorder which may have a dietary component for it is commoner in coeliacs than would be expected by chance and has been shown to be helped in some cases by a diet free from milk and cereals.[14,15]

Arthritis
It is well known that polyarthritis and fever can be a manifestation of serum sickness and penicillin allergy. When this is the case, the relationship between the polyarthritis and the injection of either horse serum or penicillin is self-evident. There are only a few reports of foods triggering polyarthritis.[12] This may be because when foods are taken daily and the onset of the arthritis is so gradual, the relationship to diet is not suspected. It is only when there is an unusually brisk response to a food that the relationship between the food and arthritis is obvious.[57]

Zeller[74] reported four cases of polyarthritis due to foods, two being triggered by cow's milk and a third by beef. Marshall et al.[53] in a study of rheumatoid arthritis, first fasted patients in environmental units and then gave them different foods one by one. Foods were incriminated in all instances. The commonest foods to trigger a relapse of arthritis were red meats and cereals; the best tolerated were vegetables and fruits; and milk and dairy products assumed an intermediate position. Cow's milk given orally has also been shown experimentally to be capable of inducing rheumatoid arthritis-like lesions in rabbits[11] and has also been reported as a cause of rheumatoid arthritis in man.[57] In patients with food-induced rheumatoid arthritis, challenges have been shown to lead to a fall in serotonin and to a rise in serum 5-hydroxy-indole acetic acid.[47]

ALLERGIES IN THE BREAST-FED BABY

Breast milk, in addition to containing the natural ingredients of breast milk, contains traces of foods ingested by the mother. This was first shown 80 years ago by Shannon.[62] The traces of food

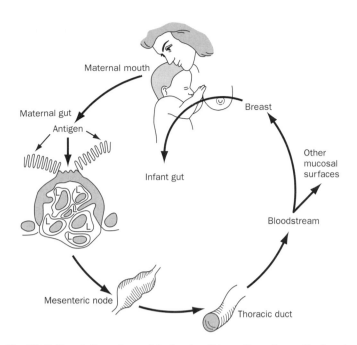

Fig. 30.5 Circulation of possible food antigens. From the mother's gut via M cells, food reaches the mesenteric nodes, thoracic duct and then the bloodstream. From there it is secreted by the breast and thus reaches the infant gut.

Presenting symptoms in 81 breast-fed babies sensitive to foods being taken by the mother	
Symptom	Percentage
Colic	40
Rhinorrhoea	23
Vomiting	21
Diarrhoea	21
Bronchitis	20
Eczema	16
Diaper (nappy) dermatitis	4
Urticaria	2

Table 30.3 Presenting symptoms in 81 breast-fed babies sensitive to foods being taken by the mother.

antigen, just like the traces of food that are absorbed by all of us, do not usually cause problems but may do so in hypersensitive babies. Paediatricians and allergists[56,66] 80 years ago were very much aware of the development of allergies in breast-fed babies to foods ingested by the mother. The problem became less apparent when formula feeding became fashionable but has become more frequent with the popularization of breast feeding (Fig. 30.5).

Symptoms

The main manifestation of allergy that concerned physicians 60 years ago was eczema and, although this was relatively uncommon, it became more common by a factor of seven when formula feeding became fashionable.[33] We are now aware that recurrent rhinorrhoea, wheezy bronchitis, vomiting and diarrhoea, and even colic[41] can be manifestations of allergy and intolerance. There has been much debate concerning the aetiology and treatment for infantile colic: the analysis of published studies on the treatment of infantile colic by Assendelft and colleagues has clearly shown that the most effective treatment is the avoidance of a cow's milk formula and its replacement by a hypoallergenic formula.

During the past 25 years, 81 breast-fed babies have been seen who developed adverse reactions to foods being ingested by the mother;[26] 35 of the cases were seen during the past 4 years. The recent increase in cases seen may be due in part to the increase in the prevalence of breast feeding – 90% of the babies leaving our hospital at the present time are on the breast – but it is also due to a greater awareness of the problem by nursing mothers and family physicians. The diagnosis was established in each case by first demonstrating relief of the baby's symptoms when the mother avoided the food or foods to which her baby was sensitive and their return when she again took the food.

The symptoms produced are listed in Table 30.3 and are similar to those seen in formula fed babies who are food sensitive. The

foods found commonly to precipitate symptoms are listed in Table 30.4. Cow's milk was by far the commonest food to be incriminated (81%), probably because mothers are encouraged to drink large quantities of milk when pregnant or when breast feeding. Egg, wheat and citrus fruits were the next most common foods to cause problems but many foods can precipitate symptoms in the baby.

Time of onset

Symptoms first develop in some 10% of the affected babies during the first week of life, suggesting that the baby may have already been sensitized *in utero*. Symptoms develop in another one-third during the next 3 weeks, in 40% during the second, third or fourth months, and in the remainder at a later date. It is possible that in some babies sensitization is triggered by the inadvertent administration of cow's milk in the nursery, but a careful enquiry in our patients suggested that this was rarely if ever the case. Once sensitization has occurred, the introduction of formula at a later date may trigger a brisk, immediate, IgE-mediated reaction. Following such an exposure, it was not unusual for the baby's symptoms to persist while still on the breast. The mother has then

Foods taken by the mother which precipitated symptoms in her baby	
Food	Percentage
Cow's milk	81
Egg	15
Wheat	11
Citrus fruits	10
Chocolate	2

Table 30.4 Foods taken by the mother which precipitated symptoms in her baby (n = 81).

had to avoid cow's milk and dairy products for the baby to be symptom-free once more.

Treatment: avoidance

As cow's milk taken by the mother is the commonest food to precipitate symptoms in the baby, it is obviously the first food which the mother of a sensitized baby should avoid. It is also, fortunately, an easy food to avoid. In children with eczema, asthma, urticaria or severe vomiting, a skin-prick test and RAST may provide additional confirmation that cow's milk and/or other foods taken by the mother are precipitating symptoms in the baby. It is much better to identify these foods and remove them from the mothers diet than to take the baby off the breast and to substitute a formula feed. If the baby is placed on a cow's milk formula he/she will probably react adversely to it and may also react adversely to other formula feeds, with final management being even more troublesome than it was when on the breast alone.

Babies who are sensitive via breast milk to foods taken by the mother are *ipso facto* highly allergic individuals. There is no easy way of distinguishing these babies from others who, although apparently equally allergic, tolerate foods taken by their mothers. When histories are taken, it is often found that the mothers of these allergic babies have consumed, while pregnant, large quantities of the food or foods to which their babies have been sensitized and this may have facilitated their sensitization.[55] However, sensitivities to foods such as peanut and egg can develop in babies whose mothers, because they disliked or were sensitive to these foods, avoided them. The complete exclusion of any one food for at least the last two trimesters of pregnancy is not easy and crossreactions between foods may nullify the attempt to prevent the sensitization of the baby. It is difficult to be sure that it is no more than coincidence if a mother who having had one baby sensitized to foods that she had eaten and who then avoided these same foods when next pregnant finds that the second baby was free from the allergies. Nevertheless, a programme of food avoidance should be recommended in such cases.

If food avoidance by the mother does not bring relief to the baby, a trial of oral cromolyn can be entertained. The starting dose for the baby is 20 mg, increasing rapidly if necessary by 20 mg increments to 100 mg dissolved in 5–10 ml hot water 20 min before each feed. Cromolyn, while not usually helpful, has occasionally relieved symptoms dramatically. In two instances, cromolyn given to the mother brought relief to the child, possibly through reducing the mother's absorption of the offending antigen.

Two forms of CMA reaction

Although symptoms produced by cow's milk in the breast- and formula-fed baby are very similar, the immunological mechanisms involved are very different.[28] The breast-fed baby is reacting to foods being taken by his mother and to trace amounts of those antigens. If he is given cow's milk as such, he will have a severe IgE-mediated reaction. He is obviously highly atopic and skin-prick tests and RAST are usually strongly positive with elevated IgE levels (Table 30.5). The symptoms in the formula-fed baby, on the other hand, although essentially the same are triggered by large amounts of antigen and are not associated with severe immediate reactions, or with positive prick and RASTs, or high levels of IgE. These two types of CMA are very clearly delineated and, as our understanding of food allergy increases, it will no doubt be

Characteristics of cow's milk allergic responses: route of administration		
Characteristic	**Via breast milk**	**Directly orally**
Quantity of allergen	Trace amounts	Large quantity
Skin-prick test	Positive	Negative
RAST	Positive	Negative
IgE	Elevated	Normal
Immediate clinical reaction	+ +	–
Delayed clinical reaction	–	+ +
'Reactivity'	Atopic	Non-atopic

Table 30.5 Characteristics of cow's milk allergic responses: route of administration and dose.

found that most allergies to foods will fall into one or other of these two categories. The brisk reaction in the breast-fed baby suggests that the hallmark of the atopic individual is his brisk response to low-dose stimulation and, although this is a handicap in modern society for it facilitates the development of atopic disease, it may have given him an advantage in primitive society when his survival was often dependent on the speed of his immunological response to parasitic infections.

CMA and intolerance

As indicated above, almost identical reactions can be triggered by trace amounts of cow's milk in breast milk. The reactions due to trace amounts are IgE mediated; this can be confirmed by RAST. By definition, the reaction is allergic. Reactions triggered by large amounts of cow's milk are said to be a manifestation of intolerance. How it triggers the intolerant reaction is not known, but it is almost certainly a biological reaction, for it is often associated with changes in the volume of the white cells, as indicated by cellular tests.[22]

From the clinical point of view, food intolerances are probably of much greater importance and frequency than classical food allergy, but many allergists avoid handling patients with food intolerances on the pretext that they do not have true allergies. Such allergists should be encouraged to broaden their outlook. But equally important is the fact that the information that those interested in food allergy have amassed is ignored by most of their specialist colleagues – paediatricians, physicians and psychiatrists alike. Children with ADHD are not placed on diets; patients with IBS are treated in every which way, but rarely with elimination diets; those with migraine headaches are offered the latest painkiller but never, or hardly ever, is an attempt made to discover the food or foods that trigger the headache; dermatologists still lean heavily on topical steroids for the treatment of eczema; and otolaryngologists, with the exception of a small group in the United States, prefer the knife and antihistamines to the sleuthing of the investigative allergist. There is a need for conventional allergists to take an interest in food intolerance, and for all allergists to educate the specialists and family physicians in the investigation and management of patients with food allergies and intolerances.

Prevention of allergies

Cow's milk, as is apparent from a perusal of this volume, is one of the commonest, if not the commonest food antigen. Breast feeding in itself is therefore to be recommended for the prevention of allergies in infancy, and this in spite of the fact that some infants develop allergies to foods ingested by the mother. What is surprising is that prolonged breast feeding, for more than 6 months, is associated with a significant reduction in the incidence of atopic disease in the child and adolescent.[61] Whether this is due to a beneficial effect of breast feeding, or to a delay in the introduction of foods, is still to be determined. But, whatever the cause, breast feeding and the delayed introduction of foods, should be encouraged for all children, and especially for those with an atopic background.

REFERENCES

1 Bahna SL, Heiner DC. *Allergies to Milk*. Grune and Stratton, New York, 1980.

2 Bayless TM, Rosensweig NS. A racial difference in incidence of lactase deficiency. *JAMA* 1966; 197: 968–72.

3 Bentley SJ, Pearson DJ, Rix KJB. Food hypersensitivity in irritable bowel syndrome. *Lancet* 1983; ii: 295–7.

4 Boris M, Mandel FS. Food and additives are common causes of the attention deficit hyperactive disorder in children. *Ann Allergy* 1994; 72: 462–7.

5 Bray GW. Enuresis of allergic origin. *Arch Dis Child* 1931; 6: 251–3.

6 Breneman JC. Nocturnal enuresis, a treatment regimen for general use. *Ann Allergy* 1965; 23: 185–91.

7 Burton R. *The Anatomy of Melancholy*. 1621. In: Dell F, Jordan-Smith P (eds) New York: Tudor, New York; 1955: 191. (Quoted by Speer F. The many facets of migraine. *Ann Allergy* 1975; 34: 273–85.)

8 Caffrey EA, Sladen GE, Isaacs PET, Clark KGA. Thrombocytopenia caused by cow's milk. *Lancet* 1981; ii: 316.

9 Carter CM, Urbanowicz M, Hemsley R *et al*. Effect of a few food diet on attention deficit disorder. *Arch Dis Child* 1993; 69: 564–8.

10 Clein NW. Cow's milk allergy in infants. *Pediatr Clin North Am* 1954; 1: 949–62.

11 Coombs RRA, Oldham G. Early rheumatoid-like joint lesions in rabbits drinking cow's milk. *Int Arch Allergy Appl Immunol* 1981; 64: 287–92.

12 Criep LH. Allergy of joints. *J Bone Joint Surg* 1946; 28: 276–9.

13 Crook WG, Harrison WW, Crawford SE, Emerson BS. Systemic manifestations due to allergy. *Pediatrics* 1961; 27: 790–9.

14 Dohan FC. Coeliac disease and schizophrenia. *Lancet* 1970; i: 897–8.

15 Dohan FC, Grasberger JC. Relapsed schizophrenia: earlier discharge from hospital after cereal-free, milk free diet. *Am J Psychiatry* 1973; 130: 685–8.

16 Durand P (ed.). *Disorders Due to Intestinal Defective Carbohydrate Digestion and Absorption*. II Pen siero Scientifico, Rome, 1964.

17 Egger J, Carter CM, Wilson J *et al*. Is migraine food allergy? *Lancet* 1983; ii: 865–9.

18 Egger J, Carter CM, Graham PJ *et al*. Controlled trial of oligoantigenic diet treatment in the hyperkinetic syndrome. *Lancet* 1985; i: 540–5.

19 Esperanca M, Gerrard JW. Nocturnal enuresis. *Can Med Assoc J* 1969; 101: 324–7.

20 Esperanca M, Gerrard JW. Nocturnal enuresis. Comparison of the effect of imipramine and dietary restriction on bladder capacity. *Can Med Assoc J* 1969; 101: 721–4.

21 Feingold BF. *Why Your Child is Hyperactive*. Random House, New York, 1975.

22 Fell PJ, Brostoff J, Pasula MJ. High correlation of the ALCAT test results with the double-blind challenge (DBC) in food sensitivity. *Ann Allergy*

23 Ford JD, Haworth JC. The fecal excretion of sugars in children. *J Pediatr* 1963; 63: 988–90.

24 Frick OL, German DF, Mills J. Development of allergy in children. I. Association with virus infections. *J Allergy Clin Immunol* 1979; 63: 228–41.

25 Gerrard JW. Familial recurrent rhinorrhea and bronchitis due to cow's milk. *JAMA* 1966; 198: 605–7.

26 Gerrard JW. Allergies in breast-fed babies to foods ingested by the mother. *Clin Rev Allergy* 1984; 2: 143–9.

27 Gerrard JW. Risk factors in developing allergic disease. *Immunology and Allergy Practice* 1984; 60: 17–24.

28 Gerrard JW, Shenassa M. Food allergy: two common types as seen in breast and formula-fed babies. *Ann Allergy* 1983; 50: 375–9.

29 Gerrard JW, Lubos MC, Hardy LW *et al*. Milk allergy: clinical picture and familial incidence. *Can Med Assoc J* 1967; 97: 780–5.

30 Gerrard JW, MacKenzie JWA, Goluboff N *et al*. Cow's milk allergy: prevalence in an unselected series of newborns. *Acta Paediatr Scand* 1973; 234 (suppl): 3–21.

31 Goldman AS, Anderson DW, Sellars WA *et al*. Milk allergy. I. Oral challenge with milk and isolated proteins in allergic children. *Pediatrics* 1963; 32: 425–43.

32 Grant ECG. Food allergies and migraine. *Lancet* 1979; i: 966–9.

33 Grulee CG, Sanford HN. The influence of breast and artificial feeding on infantile eczema. *J Pediatr* 1936; 8: 223–5.

34 Grulee CG, Sanford HN, Heron PH. Breast and artificial feeding. *JAMA* 1934; 103: 735.

35 Halpern SR, Sellars WA, Johnson RB *et al*. Development of childhood allergy in infants fed breast, soy, or cow milk. *J Allergy Clin Immunol* 1973; 51: 139–51.

36 Harrison M. Sugar malabsorption in cow's milk protein intolerance. *Lancet* 1974; i: 360–1.

37 Harrison M, Kilby A, Walker-Smith J *et al*. Cow's milk-protein intolerance: a possible association with gastroenteritis, lactose intolerance and IgA deficiency. *Br Med J* 1976; 1: 1501–4.

38 Heiner DC, Sears JW, Kniker WT. Multiple precipitins to cow's milk in chronic respiratory disease. A syndrome including poor growth, gastrointestinal symptoms, evidence of allergy, iron deficiency anemia and pulmonary hemosiderosis. *Am J Dis Child* 1962; 103: 634–54.

39a Hide W, Guyer BM. Cow's milk intolerance in Isle of Wight infants. *Br J Clin Pract* 1983; 37: 285–7.

39b Hill DJ, Hosking CS, Heine RG. Clinical spectrum of food allergy in children in Australia and South-East Asia: identification and targets for treatment. *Ann Med* 1999; 31: 272.

39c Hill DJ, Hosking CS. The cow's milk allergy complex: overlapping disease process in infancy. *Eur J Clin Nutr* 1995; 49, suppl 1:1.

40 Ingall M, Glaser J, Meltzer RS, Dreyfuss EM. Allergic rhinitis in early infancy. Review of the literature and report of a case in a newborn. *Pediatrics* 1965; 35: 105–12.

41 Jakobsson I, Lindberg T. Cow's milk as a cause of infantile colic in breast fed infants. *Lancet* 1978; ii: 437–9.

42 Jakobsson I, Lindberg T. A prospective study of cow's milk protein intolerance in Swedish infants. *Acta Paediatr Scand* 1979; 68: 853–9.

43 Alun Jones V, McLaughlan P, Shorthouse M *et al*. Food intolerance: a major factor in the pathogenesis of the irritable bowel syndrome. *Lancet* 1982; ii: 1115–17.

44a Kaplan BJ, McNichol J, Conte RA *et al*. Dietary replacement in preschool-age hyperactive boys. *Pediatrics* 1989; 83: 7–17.

44b Kjeldsen-Kagh J, Haugen M, Borchgrevink CF *et al*. Controlled trial of fasting and one-year vegetarian diet in rheumatoid arthritis. *Lancet* 338: 899.

45 Kretchmer N. Memorial lecture: lactose and lactase – a historical perspective. *Gastroenterology* 1971; 61: 805–13.

46 Lee SK, Kniker WT, Cook CD, Heiner DC. Cow's milk-induced pulmonary disease in children. *Adv Pediatr* 1978; 25: 39–57.

47 Little CH, Stewart AG, Fennessy MR. Platelet serotonin release in rheumatoid arthritis: a study in food intolerant patients. *Lancet* 1983; ii: 297–9.

48 Liu H-Y, Tsao MU, Moore B, Giday Z. Bovine milk-protein induced intestinal malabsorption of lactose and fat in infants. *Gastroenterology* 1967; 54: 27–34.

A

49a Lubos MC, Gerrard JW, Buchan DJ. Disaccharidase activities in milk sensitive and celiac patients. *J Pediatr* 1967; 70: 325–31.

49b Lucassen PLJ, Assendelft WJ, Gubbels JW, van Eijk JT, van Geldrop WJ, Neven AK. Effectiveness of treatment for infantile colic: Systematic review. *Brit Med J* 1998; 316: 1563.

50 MacFarlane PI, Miller V. Human milk in the management of protracted diarrhoea of infancy. *Arch Dis Child* 1984; 59: 260–5.

51 Mackarness R. *Not All in the Mind*. Pan, London, 1976.

52 McKendry JB, Stewart DA, Khanna F, Netley C. Primary enuresis; relative success of three methods of treatment. *Can Med Assoc J* 1975; 113: 953–5.

53 Marshall RT, Stroud RM, Kroker GF *et al.* Food challenge effects on fasted rheumatoid arthritis patients: a multicenter study. *Clin Ecol* 1984; 2: 181–90.

54 Monro J. Food allergy and migraine. *Clin Immunol Allergy* 1982; 2: 137–63.

55 National Institutes of Health Consensus Development Panel. Defined diets in childhood hyperactivity. NIH Building, No. 1, Maryland Office for Medical Applications of Research, Bethesda, 1982.

56 O'Keefe ES. The relation of food to infantile eczema. *Boston Med Surg J* 1920; 183: 569.

57 Parke AL, Hughes GRV. Rheumatoid arthritis and food: a case study. *Br Med J* 1981; 282: 2027–9.

58 Pearson DJ, Rix KJB, Bentley SJ. Food allergy: how much is in the mind? *Lancet* 1983; i: 295–7.

59 Rapp DJ. Food allergy treatment for hyperkinesis. *J Learning Disabilities* 1979; 12: 608–16.

60 Rattner B. A possible causal factor of food allergy in certain infants. *Am J Dis Child* 1936; 36: 277–88.

61 Saarinen UM, Kajosaari M. Breast feeding as prophylaxis against atopic disease: prospective follow-up study until 17 years old. *Lancet* 1995; 346: 1065–9.

62 Shannon WR. Demonstration of food proteins in human breast milk by anaphylactic experiments in guinea pigs. *Am J Dis Child* 1921; 22: 223.

63 Speer F: The allergic tension fatigue in children. *Ann Allergy* 1954; 12: 168–71.

64 Speer F. Allergy and migraine: a clinical study. *Headache* 1971; 11: 63–7.

65 Starfield B. Functional bladder capacity in enuretic and non-enuretic children. *Pediatrics* 1967; 70: 777–81.

66 Talbot FB. Eczema in childhood. *Med Clin North Am* 1918; 1: 985–96.

67 Waldmann T, Wochner RD, Laster L, Gordon RS. Allergic gastroenteropathy. *New Engl J Med* 1967; 276: 761–9.

68 Walker-Smith J, Harrison M, Kilby A *et al.* Cow's milk-sensitive enteropathy. *Arch Dis Child* 1978; 53: 375–80.

69 Weitkamp LR, Stancer HC, Persod E *et al.* Depressive disorders and HLA: a gene on chromosome 6 that can affect behavior. *New Engl J Med* 1981; 305: 1301–13.

70 Weser E, Rubin W, Ross L, Sleisenger MH. Lactase deficiency in patients with the irritable colon syndrome. *New Engl J Med* 1965; 273: 1070–5.

71 Wilson JF, Heiner DC, Lahey ME. Milk-induced gastrointestinal bleeding in infants with hypochromic microcytic anemia. *JAMA* 1964; 189: 122–6.

72 Woodbury RM. The relation between artificial feeding and infant mortality. *M J Hyg* 1922; 2: 668.

73 Wraith DG, Merrett J, Roth A *et al.* Recognition of food-allergic patients and their allergens by the RAST technique and clinical investigation. *Clin Allergy* 1979; 9: 25–36.

74 Zeller M. Rheumatoid arthritis – food allergy as a factor. *Ann Allergy* 1949; 7: 200–5.

Chapter 31

Pharmacological actions of food and drink

Timothy J. Maher

INTRODUCTION

Besides providing the nutrients required for normal growth and development, many of the foods and drinks we consume daily also contain compounds that can produce true pharmacological effects. Such dietary compounds typically mimic or antagonize endogenous neurotransmitters, neuromodulators or hormones, thereby producing effects as a result of their modification of normal biological processes; this is actually identical to the way traditional pharmacological agents (i.e. drugs) typically act. These effects can be classified as positive (i.e. therapeutic) or negative (i.e. adverse or toxic) in nature. Thus, it is not surprising to find that pharmacology and nutrition share many similarities: both disciplines are concerned with the absorption, distribution, metabolism and elimination of compounds – drugs in the case of pharmacology and foods in the case of nutrition. While dietary components that produce pharmacological effects can be classified as being either rapid in onset (e.g. minutes to hours), or being active only after chronic ingestion (e.g. months to years), in both cases the responsible dietary mediator acts similarly to a drug, and usually involves interaction with a receptor or enzyme systems.

While some of the foods and drinks consumed can provide pharmacologically active compounds, few if any drugs we use contribute to the nutritional status of the individual.[25] Occasionally, adverse symptoms experienced following consumption of such foods can be confused with the food intolerance associated with immunologically mediated food allergy, but some important differences do exist. Most significantly, true food allergy generally is independent of the amount consumed, as even a very minute amount of an allergen present in foods or drinks is typically able to produce a full, adverse response.[14] Increasing the amount of the food consumed usually has little effect on such an all-or-nothing allergic response that is produced. In contrast, following consumption of foods containing pharmacologically active compounds, the responses observed are expected to be dose-dependent. This relationship between dose and response is a characteristic generally observed with all pharmacological agents and is an important cornerstone of the discipline of pharmacology. Similarly, nutritional effects are clearly dependent on the amount of dietary exposure of a given nutrient.

METHYLXANTHINES

The methylxanthine caffeine, possibly the oldest stimulant used by humans, is typically supplied through the diet in the form of beverages and foods. Recorded history has documented the widespread use of the methylxanthines in foods and beverages for their stimulant and antisoporific effects. Decreased fatigue, elevated mood and an increase in the capacity for work have long been attributed to the ingestion of products that contain methylxanthines such as caffeine. One account in legend gives credit to the discovery of the stimulant effects of caffeine to shepherds near an Arabian convent who noticed that their sheep, following consumption of the berries from coffee plants, did not sleep, but instead were extremely active throughout the entire night. The prior of the convent hearing this report ordered that the berries be collected so that a beverage might be made to aid in their many long hours of required prayer. Today that beverage, known as coffee, is consumed by more than half of the US population.[33] Caffeine in beverages is consumed by individuals of all ages; adults enjoy tea and coffee, children and teenagers enjoy soft drinks, and even the neonate may consume caffeine through the maternal breast milk.

Caffeine

While other naturally occurring methylxanthines of importance include theobromine and theophylline, also an important synthetically derived therapeutic agent, the alkaloid caffeine is by far the most important and widely used stimulant from this chemical class. Caffeine is abundantly found in various plants throughout the world – e.g. tea, *Thea sinenis* (also contains theophylline); coffee, *Coffea arabica* (Fig. 31.1); cola, *Cola acuminata*; chocolate and cocoa, *Theobroma cacao* (also contains theobromine) – and is currently harvested and processed into many different foods and drinks. Depending upon the geographical area and local soil characteristics, the quality of the plant products, the climate during a particular growing season, the processing and manufacturing procedures, cultural differences and preparation techniques, the caffeine content of dietary products can differ greatly. Table 31.1 lists the caffeine content of a number of dietary products. Some foods, such as tea and chocolate products, contain other methylxanthines that may also exert potent pharmacological effects that are qualitatively similar to those of caffeine.

Factors influencing caffeine concentration

Factors that can significantly influence the quantity of caffeine present in coffee include the origin of the coffee bean and the brewing technique employed. Coffee prepared by the drip method tends to have greater caffeine contents than brewed or instant. Similarly, the preparation of tea can significantly influence caffeine content. For instance, increasing the brewing time from 1 min to 3 min increases the caffeine content by 75%. Colas and other soft drink beverages contain approximately 50 mg per serving (12 oz). Since even beverages such as root beer also have caffeine added, it is imperative to carefully read labels in order to determine which products contain caffeine. Some popular beverages, designed to provide extra stimulant capabilities, are advertised as having double the caffeine content of regular colas. Most

Caffeine content of various dietary products		
Product	**Serving size**	**Caffeine content (mg)**
Tea*		
brewed 1 min	5 oz	20
brewed 3 min	5 oz	35
iced	12 oz	70
Coffee		
dripped	7.5 oz	115–175
brewed	7.5 oz	80–135
instant	7.5 oz	65–100
decaffeinated	7.5 oz	3–4
Cola beverage (most brands)	12 oz	48
Cocoa†	5 oz	5
Chocolate candy bar	28 g	8

Adapted from Abbott[1] and Chou and Benowitz.[8]
* Also contains 2 mg theobromine and 1 mg theophylline (depending upon source).
† Also contains 250 mg theobromine.

Table 31.1 Caffeine content of various dietary products.

varieties of soft drinks labelled as caffeine-free contain only trace amounts or no caffeine at all. When consumed in beverages, caffeine is almost completely absorbed (99%) within the gastrointestinal tract and peak blood levels are generally observed within approximately 45 min. Caffeine is equally distributed to all tissues in the body and easily passes the blood–brain barrier. The metabolism of caffeine is extensive, as only 3% is eliminated unchanged via the kidney. The plasma half-life generally ranges from 4 to 12 hours, is age-dependent, and is significantly prolonged in individuals with impaired hepatic function or during pregnancy.

Pharmacological action of caffeine

While previously most researchers believed that caffeine produced its pharmacological actions via inhibition of phosphodiesterase, the enzyme responsible for terminating cyclic nucleotide-mediated responses, more recent work has clearly demonstrated that the pharmacological actions of caffeine involve antagonism of the adenosine receptor. Normally, the autocoid adenosine, which is constantly available in small amounts in extracellular fluid, acts to relax vascular smooth muscle in the periphery and inhibit neuronal firing in the central nervous system. Caffeine competes for binding with the endogenous adenosine and thus prevents adenosine's normal actions on purine A_1-type receptors. As there is always some adenosine interacting with receptors to produce a baseline level of cellular activity, the administration of caffeine disrupts this basal level of neuronal inhibition and leads to altered cellular firing, resulting in overt pharmacological actions. Excessive caffeine consumption can cause nervousness, agitation, and even seizures in susceptible individuals. While caffeine consumption can prolong the duration of gross motor activity tasks such as exercise, performance in tasks involving fine motor control are typically adversely affected by caffeine consumption due to muscle fasciculations and tremor.

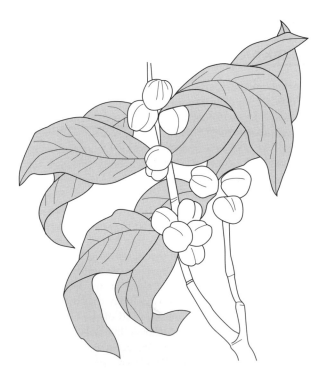

Fig. 31.1 Beans growing on a coffee plant.

Effect on the cardiovascular system

Caffeine also has prominent actions on the cardiovascular system, resulting in vasoconstriction and cardioacceleration. Together, vasoconstriction of the coronary arteries, leading to decreased coronary perfusion, and an increase in heart rate, combine to increase the oxygen demand of the heart while decreasing the oxygen supply to the heart. Such a disruption in oxygen balance can precipitate anginal attacks in susceptible individuals. Additionally, acting directly on conduction neurons in the heart, caffeine can produce premature ventricular contractions (PVCs) which can be deleterious in patients with compromised cardiovascular function. Even healthy individuals can experience palpitations and tachycardia, which certainly can be worrisome. Caffeine also produces a number of other important physiological effects when consumed (Table 31.2). However, as with most drugs, tolerance does develop to many of the effects of caffeine such that a dietary dose of caffeine delivered to a chronic caffeine consumer may have little if any effect on central nervous system and cardiovascular functions.[6,11] This same dietary dose of caffeine to a caffeine naïve individual would be expected to produce intense pharmacological effects.

SYMPATHOMIMETIC-LIKE AMINES

Tyramine, derived from the Greek word *tyros* meaning cheese, is a sympathomimetic amine that acts similarly to the noradrenaline (norepinephrine) found in the sympathetic nervous system. Like noradrenaline, tyramine can increase blood pressure and alter heart rate if given in excess. Normally the doses of tyramine found in foods and drinks we consume is small enough to be effectively degraded by the enzyme monoamine oxidase (MAO) found in the gastrointestinal tract and elsewhere in the body. Tyramine, which is formed from the amino acid L-tyrosine when foods or drinks are aged or begin to spoil, can lead to serious elevations in blood pressure, resulting in cerebrovascular accident, if the enzyme MAO is inhibited and therefore not capable of metabolizing this vasoactive amine. Under normal conditions the gastrointestinal activity of MAO is sufficient to handle even large amounts of ingested tyramine. However in patients treated with MAO inhibitors (MAOIs) for depression or other psychiatric disorders, the levels of tyramine may elevate to dangerous levels with serious consequences. The use of MAOIs that irreversibly bind the enzyme (e.g. phenelzine, tranylcypromine) have been associated with the so-called 'cheese effect' in patients who consume foods such as aged cheeses which have high tyramine content. The use of newer reversible MAOIs that less effectively inhibit the enzyme and act for a shorter period of time have not been linked to this cheese effect.[10]

Tyramine content of foods

Fermented and aged foods tend to have the highest tyramine contents. Cheeses such as Blue, Boursault, Camembert, Cheddar and Swiss usually have much higher tyramine contents than other cheeses such as American, Brie, Mozzarella, Romano and Parmesan. Sour cream and yogurt also contain some tyramine. Meats and fish that are fresh will contain less tyramine than aged meats in general. Chicken livers, Bologna, pepperoni, salami and pickled herring usually contain high amounts of tyramine and should be avoided by patients taking an irreversible MAOI. Overripe fruits and vegetables also contain high amounts of tyramine and should be avoided. Some beers and wines also need to be carefully consumed since some can precipitate a hypertensive crisis in such patients. Individuals not taking an MAOI have typically not experienced pressor responses following ingestion of even large amounts of high-tyramine containing foods.

HISTAMINE

Histamine, formed from the amino acid L-histidine via the enzyme histidine decarboxylase, is a potent endogenous autocoid that is normally found in highest concentrations in mast cells and basophils throughout the body. Metabolism is generally the result of the action of either N-methyltransferase or histaminase stored in many tissues. Histamine produces its effects via interaction with specific 7-transmembrane spanning G-protein coupled receptors, termed H_1, H_2 and H_3. H_1 receptors appear to mediate stimulation of smooth muscle activity, increased vascular permeability, pruritus and prostaglandin synthesis. H_2 receptors are mostly responsible for gastric acid and mucous secretion. Both H_1 and H_2 receptors appear to be involved in mediating the vasodilation and resultant tachycardia, flushing and headache that normally result from histamine exposure. The role of H_3 receptors is poorly understood at the present time.

The vasodilator action and increase in vascular permeability that follows histamine release significantly shifts fluid from the vascular compartment to the non-vascular space, leading to cellular oedema and congestion. Consequently, if this reallocation of vascular fluid is allowed to progress further, inadequate tissue

Physiological effects of caffeine
Central nervous system
Stimulation and decreased fatigue
Increased vigilance
Elevated mood
Cardiovascular
Increased heart rate (may initially decrease slightly)
Increased blood pressure
Premature ventricular contractions (PVCs)
Anginal symptoms
Respiratory
Increased respiratory rate
Bronchodilation
Metabolic
Increased circulating catecholamines
Increased basal metabolic rate
Increased lipolysis
Gastrointestinal
Water and sodium secretion by the small intestine
Increased secretion of gastric acid
Increased secretion of pepsin
Decreased lower oesophageal sphincter pressure
Renal
Mild diuresis

Table 31.2 Physiological effects of caffeine.

B

perfusion and circulatory collapse can result. While allergic reactions to foods, drugs and other environmental allergens may involve responses mediated by histamine released from mast cells and basophils in IgE-mediated reactions, histamine can also be released by certain agents without prior sensitization. In this situation compounds act via enhancement of intracellular Ca^{2+} and do not involve IgE. Examples include some response to morphine and other opioids, vancomycin (produces 'red-man syndrome'), and certain carbohydrate plasma expanders.[27]

Histamine can also derive directly from the diet, and if consumed in sufficient amounts can elicit typical histamine-responses including urticaria, gastrointestinal irritability, nausea and flushing. The histamine content of selected foods is listed in Table 31.3. High intakes of dietary histamine (32–250 mg) have been reported to evoke histamine-mediated responses in some individuals, while having no effect in others. When much higher amounts of histamine are consumed, as is observed in scrombroid poisoning where individuals consume badly decomposing fish such as skipjack, tuna or mackerel, histamine toxicity has been documented.[19] These food sources have been reported to contain histamine levels as high as 500 mg/100 g of fish. Patients treated for tuberculosis with isoniazid are more likely to have adverse reactions to histamine in foods as this drug is known to inhibit histaminase and prevent the clearance of histamine.[36] Some foods are also known to release.

Foods with high histamine contents	
Food	**Average amount (μg/g)**
Cheeses	
Blue	50
Monterey Jack	70
Parmesan	100–277
Meats	
Beef (sirloin)	2–3.5
Chicken liver	4–8
Chicken meat	1
Ham	0.5
Lamb	0.5–1
Salami	1
Red wines	
Burgundy	2
Bordeaux	0.02
Concord grape	0.2
Chianti	0.5–4
Lambrusco	0.05
Vegetables	
Aubergine	35
Spinach	25–60
Tomatoes	2
Yeast	
Marmite	2000

Table 31.3 Foods with high histamine contents. (Adapted from Blackwell et al.,[5] Feldman,[12] and Malone and Metcalfe.[27])

ISOFLAVONES

Certain plant-derived compounds, chemically known as isoflavones, are capable of mimicking the mammalian hormone oestrogen by virtue of their ability to act as weak agonists directly upon the oestrogen receptor. These phyto-oestrogens (plant-derived oestrogens) are chemically similar enough to oestradiol to allow for binding at the cytosolic nuclear hormone receptor; however, the interaction is weak, exhibiting only 1/1000th to 1/10 000th the potency of oestradiol.[21] Interestingly, the plasma levels of these phyto-oestrogens in individuals who regularly consume soy products in their diet, e.g. as is typically seen in many Asian cultures, average 1000 to 10 000 times those of oestradiol.[2,28,32] When present in situations where oestrogenic status is low, for instance during menopause, phyto-oestrogens act as oestrogen mimics. In contrast, when present in situations where oestrogenic status is high, for instance when hormone-dependent tumours such as breast cancer are present, phyto-oestrogens may act as oestrogen antagonists. This ability to act both as an agonist and antagonist is frequently seen in pharmacology when compounds have weak efficacy at a receptor site, and are termed partial agonists.

Soy-derived phyto-oestrogens

Soy beans (*Soya soya*) are the major source of dietary phyto-oestrogenic compounds in the human diet and chemically these can be classified as three major types that exist in four modified forms. The highest proportion of these isoflavones in soybeans exist in their glucoside form as daidzin, genestin and glycetin. These glucosides are also present as the 6″-O-acetyl and 6″-O-malonyl derivatives, but typically in much lower amounts. Additionally, these three isoflavones also exist in soy as the aglycone, where the glucoside moiety is removed, and are termed daidzein, genestein and glycetein. While the majority of isoflavone phyto-oestrogens are in the glucoside form in nature, following consumption glucosidases effectively convert these to their biologically active aglycone form.

Variation in phyto-oestrogen content

Soy products vary significantly in their phyto-oestrogen content (Table 31.4).[38] Compared to raw soybeans, non-fermented high-protein soy ingredients, such as textured vegetable protein, soy flour and roasted soybeans, contain comparable amounts of the isoflavones. Soy concentrates usually contain similarly high amounts of the isoflavones if produced with water washing. However, should alcohol washing be employed as a method to remove flatulence-producing carbohydrates such as rhaphinose, the isoflavones are also removed. Unfortunately, consumers are usually unaware of which washing procedure was utilized with a particular soy concentrate. Fermentation to produce tempeh, bean paste and miso, significantly decreases the isoflavone content and shifts the chemical form present to that of the aglycone. Second-generation soy foods such as soy hot dogs, soy bacon, tofu yogurt and soy noodles contain only 10% of the isoflavone content of an equal amount (based on weight) of soybeans. From a practical dietary stand-point, roasted soybeans and soy beverages such as soy milk provide excellent sources of phyto-oestrogens.

Effect of soy compounds in infants

Recently Setchell and colleagues[31] have determined the plasma levels of the phyto-oestrogens and a major intestinally derived

Isoflavone content of selected foods				
	Isoflavone content (mg/100 g dry weight)			
Food	Daidzein	Genistein	Glycetin	Total
Soybean (roasted)	56	87	19	162
Textured vegetable protein	47	71	20	138
Soybean (fresh)	55	73	8	136
Soyflour	23	81	9	113
Tempeh	28	32	3	63
Tofu	15	16	3	34
Tofu yogurt	6	9	1	16
Soy noodle	1	4	4	9

Table 31.4 Isoflavone content of selected foods (adapted from Wang and Murphy,[38] and Knight and Eden.[21]).

metabolite equol in infants consuming soy-based infant formulas. The results demonstrated that typical consumption of standard amounts of commercially available soy-based products in 4-month-old infants led to an exposure of 4.5–8.0 mg/kg/day total isoflavone, which yielded plasma levels in these infants 6–11 fold higher than those found in women consuming high soy diets. The contribution of isoflavones from cow's milk and breast milk was negligible. As the isoflavones have been shown to produce significant hormonal effects in women consuming soy products, a concern regarding the potential effects of infant exposure has been voiced. Much study is needed to better understand the influence of these phyto-oestrogens on health and disease in both males and females throughout the life cycle.

Anticarcinogenic effects

Epidemiological data have revealed a significantly reduced (e.g. 1/6th to 1/10th) incidence of certain cancers, including breast, endometrial, ovarian and prostate, in many Asian populations compared with those of Western societies.[29] While some studies have suggested that this difference is due to the phyto-oestrogenic content of the Asian diet, there exist significant dietary differences between these two populations which may play an even more important role in the observed reduction in the incidence of these cancers.

Besides acting at oestrogen receptors, the isoflavones are also known to influence a number of important biological processes that might help to further explain their anticarcinogenic effects. Genestein is known to be a potent inhibitor of tyrosine kinases and, thus, effectively interferes with cellular transmembrane signal transduction.[3] Additionally, genestein also inhibits topoisomerase II and angiogenesis. Genestein, soy diets, soy extracts containing a mixture of the isoflavones, but not soy extracts with the isoflavones removed, have been shown to inhibit tumour growth in a wide variety of animal models (e.g. X-ray irradiation, N-methyl-N-nitrosourea, dimethyl-benz(α)anthracene).[4,9,17,35] Epidemiological studies in humans have similarly reported a pro-

tective effect of soybean ingestion against the development of breast cancer.[7,18,22,28]

Although soy has been the focus of the majority of research on the isoflavones, these compounds are also found to a lesser degree in chickpeas, bluegrass and clover. Another chemically related class, the lignans (e.g. enterolactone and enterodiol) are found in oilseeds such as flaxseed. The pharmacological role of the various lignans is less well understood.

CARBOHYDRATES, TRYPTOPHAN AND SEROTONIN

Serotonin is an important neurotransmitter compound that is produced by enterochromaffin cells and many neurones within the central nervous system.

Tryptophan synthesis and clinical effects

Tryptophan is an essential amino acid, i.e. it cannot be readily synthesized by humans and must therefore be consumed in the diet; it is the precursor of serotonin. Serotonin-mediated functions include mood, appetite, temperature regulation, respiration, pain perception, sleep and blood pressure regulation within the central nervous system (CNS); it is also a critical haemostatic factor in the peripheral vasculature. The synthesis of serotonin occurs in two steps: initial conversion to 5-hydroxytryptophan followed by conversion to 5-hydroxytryptamine, or serotonin. The rate-limiting enzyme, tryptophan hydroxylase, is normally not saturated at normal brain concentrations of tryptophan, and thus the administration of tryptophan to animals has been shown to increase the synthesis of serotonin. Additionally, diurnal variations in the levels of tryptophan in the circulation due to consumption of foods produces predictable changes in brain serotonin.[13]

Many experiments have evaluated the ability of tryptophan administered endogenously to alter serotonergic neurotransmission. In humans, tryptophan has been shown to reduce pain, reduce food intake (especially carbohydrates), improve depression and decrease sleep latency.[16,20,37] Additionally, animals given a diet deficient in tryptophan (e.g. certain types of corn), that results in reductions in brain serotonin, experience increased pain sensitivity, a response that is reversed by tryptophan administration.[24]

Circulating levels of tryptophan are found to fluctuate depending on the composition of the food consumed.[15,26] Ingestion of a meal high in protein leads to increases in the plasma levels of the large neutral amino acids (LNAAs) valine, leucine, isoleucine, phenylalanine, tryptophan and tyrosine. Since the transport into the brain of these amino acids is competitive and via facilitated diffusion at the blood–brain barrier, the consumption of a high protein meal, which contains a small amount of tryptophan, but which also contains much more of the branched-chain amino acids (BCAAs) valine, leucine and isoleucine, actually leads to a decrease in the flux of tryptophan into the brain. Studies have indicated that in order to increase the flux of tryptophan into the brain a carbohydrate-rich meal would need to be consumed.[15] Carbohydrates elicit the release of insulin, which in addition to enhancing the uptake of glucose out of the circulation, also enhances the uptake of the BCAAs into peripheral sites such as muscle. The removal of a portion of the BCAAs from the circulation decreases the competition tryptophan is exposed to for passage across the blood–brain barrier. Thus, it is actually the ratio of the concentration of a particular amino acid in plasma to that of its competitors, the so-called 'plasma ratio', that determines the flux of that amino acid into brain.

Carbohydrate ingestion and fatigue

Following the demonstration in experimental animals that the consumption of a meal rich in carbohydrate enhances the synthesis of serotonin in the brain, studies were performed in human volunteers in an attempt to further explore the functional significance of these findings. Initial studies demonstrated that when men consumed a high-carbohydrate lunch a significant increase in feelings of fatigue were noted.[34] The high-carbohydrate meal did not have to be composed of simple sugars to trigger fatigue; a high-starch, protein-poor meal was similarly effective as long as the carbohydrate had a significant glycemic index. Others have demonstrated carbohydrate craving by obese patients and suggested that this involves a serotonergic mechanism of food self-selection.[23]

Enhancing function of serotonin

A number of studies have demonstrated the utility of various agents that act to enhance serotoninergic function (e.g. fluoxetine, dexfenfluramine) to ameliorate the mood and cognitive disturbances associated with premenstrual syndrome (PMS). Because of the relationship between macronutrient consumption in the diet and the synthesis of serotonin, the ability of a specially designed carbohydrate-rich beverage to ameliorate some of the dysphoric symptoms of PMS in women was investigated in a placebo-controlled, cross-over design study.[30] Three isocaloric beverages were designed so as to provide for different degrees of insulin release following consumption. One of the beverages containing dextrose and maltodextrin did adequately stimulate insulin release to increase significantly the ratio of tryptophan to LNAA by 29%, as compared with a placebo drink, and thus presumably enhanced serotonin neurotransmission in the CNS. Women consuming this beverage had significantly lower scores for tension, anger, depression and confusion as compared with the placebo control. Additionally, they performed better on a test of cognition. Two other drinks tested containing either protein or a carbohydrate with a greatly reduced glycaemic index were also tested but both failed to alter the tryptophan to LNAA ratio. As expected, neither of these drinks affected mood or cognition. Although it is impossible to predict what proportion of women suffering from PMS might realize symptomatic relief from such a dietary intervention, this approach appears to have associated with it essentially no significant risk of toxicity to the patient and thus should be tried in larger samples of women.

There are no dietary proteins known that have enhanced levels of tryptophan, or any other individual amino acid for that matter; there are proteins that are relatively deficient in particular amino acids, but usually more than one amino acid is deficient. Thus, dietary attempts at changing the concentration of a particular amino acid in the brain, with the exception of tryptophan, are futile. The only viable way would be to administer the isolated amino acid alone as a dietary supplement, but then this is not a food or drink and could be associated with adverse reactions.

SUMMARY AND CONCLUSIONS

The foods and drinks we consume daily contain a variety of pharmacologically active constituents that may have significant effects on the physiological systems of the body. Few would argue to the potency of caffeine as a CNS stimulant in man, and most recognize fully the dose–response characteristics of this compound. Other dietary components such as histamine and tyramine are more likely to produce adverse effects in susceptible individuals, rather than the general population. Still other compounds such as isoflavones and lignans probably require longer-term exposure to significantly affect changes in body functions. Finally, the macronutrient carbohydrate can produce short-term alterations in CNS function that may produce subtle, barely noticeable changes in behaviour, or even in some individuals overt physiological effects. Investigations into the beneficial effects of pharmacologically active compounds in red wines, green tea, antioxidant-rich fruits and vegetables, and numerous other dietary components will likely lead to improved health, although at times it may be difficult to differentiate between the nutritional contribution of a particular dietary component and its pharmacological effects, especially when chronic exposure is required to produce the desirable effect.

REFERENCES

1. Abbott PJ. Caffeine: a toxicological overview. *Med J Australia* 1986; 145: 518–21.

2. Adlercreutz H. Western diet and western diseases: some hormonal and biochemical mechanisms and associations. *Scand J Clin Lab Invest* 1990; 50(Suppl 201): 3–23.

3. Akiyama T, Ishida J, Nakagawa S *et al.* Genestein, a specific inhibitor of tyrosine-specific protein kinases. *J Biol Chem* 1987; 262: 5592–5.

4. Barnes S, Grubbs C, Setchell KDR *et al.* Soyabeans inhibit mammary tumor growth in models of breast cancer. In: Pariza MW (ed.) *Mutagens and carcinogenesis in the diet.* Wiley-Liss, New York, 1990; 239–53.

5. Blackwell B, Mabbit LA, Marley E. Histamine and tyramine content of yeast products. *J Fd Sci* 1969; 34: 47–51.

6. Casiglia E, Paleari CD, Petucco S *et al.* Haemondynamic effects of coffee and purified caffeine in normal volunteers: a placebo controlled clinical study. *J Human Hypertens* 1992; 6: 95–9.

7. Cassidy A, Bingham S, Setchell KDR. Biological effects of isoflavones present in soy in premenopausal women: implications for the prevention of breast cancer. *Am J Clin Nutr* 1994; 60: 333–40.

8. Chou TM, Benowitz NL. Caffeine and coffee: effects on health and cardiovascular disease. *Comp Biochem Physiol* 1994; 109C: 173–89.

9. Constantinous A, Kiguchi K, Huberman E. Induction of differentiation and DNA strand breakage in human HL-60 and K-562 leukemia cells by genestein. *Cancer Res* 1990; 50: 2618–24.

10. DaPrada M, Zurcher G, Wuthrich I, Haefely WE. On tyramine, food beverages and the reversible MAO inhibitor moclobemide. *J Neural Transm Suppl* 1988; 26: 31–56.

11. Denaro CP, Brown R, Jacob P, Benowitz NL. Effects of caffeine after repeated dosing. *Eur J Clin Pharmacol* 1991; 40: 273–8.

12. Feldman JM. Histaminuria from histamine-rich foods. *Arch Intern Med* 1983; 143: 2099–102.

13. Fernstrom JD, Wurtman RJ. Brain serotonin content: physiological regulation by plasma neutral amino acids. *Science* 1971; 178: 414–16.

14. Finn R, Cohen HN. Food allergy – fact or fiction. *Lancet* 1978; I: 426–8.

15. Glaeser BS, Maher TJ, Wurtman RJ. Changes in brain levels of acidic, basic, and neutral amino acids after consumption of single meals containing various proportions of protein. *J Neurochem* 1983; 41: 1016–21.

16 Hartmann E. L-Tryptophan: a rational hypnotic with clinical potential. *Am J Psychiatry* 1977; 134: 366–70.

17 Hawrylewicz EJ, Huang HH, Blair WH. Dietary soya bean isolate and methionine supplementation affect mammary tumour progression in rats. *J Nutr* 1991; 121: 1693–8.

18 Hirayama T. A large scale cohort study on cancer risks by diet – with special reference to the risk reducing effects of green-yellow vegetable consumption. In: Hayashi Y, Nagao M, Sugimura S *et al.* (eds) *Diet, Nutrition and Cancer.* VNU Sci Press, Utrecht; 1986; 41–53.

19 Hughes JM, Merson MH. Current concepts in fish and shellfish poisoning. *N Engl J Med* 1976; 295: 1117–20.

20 King RB. Pain and tryptophan. *J Neurosurg* 1980; 53: 44–52.

21 Knight DC, Eden JA. A review of the clinical effects of phytoestrogens. *Obstet Gynecol* 1996; 87: 897–904.

22 Lee HP, Gourley L, Duffy SW *et al.* Dietary effects on breast cancer risk in Singapore. *Lancet* 1991; 337: 1197–200.

23 Lieberman H, Wurtman J, Chew B. Changes in mood after carbohydrate consumption among obese individuals. *Am J Clin Nutr* 1986; 44: 772–8.

24 Lytle LD, Messing RB, Fisher L, Phebus L. Effects of long-term corn consumption on brain serotonin and the response to electric shock. *Science* 1975; 190: 692–4.

25 Maher TJ. Natural food constituents and food additives: the pharmacological connection. *J Allergy Clin Immunol* 1987; 79: 413–22.

26 Maher TJ, Glaeser BS, Wurtman RJ. Diurnal variations in plasma concentrations of basic and neutral amino acids and in red cell concentrations of aspartate and glutamate: effects of dietary protein. *Am J Clin Nutr* 1984; 39: 722–9.

27 Malone MH, Metcalfe DD. Histamine in foods: its possible role in non-allergic adverse reactions to ingestants. *NER Allergy Proc* 1986; 7: 241–5.

28 Messina MJ, Persky V, Setchell KDR *et al.* Soy intake and cancer risk: a review of the *in vitro* and *in vivo* data. *Nutr Cancer* 1994; 21: 113–31.

29 Nomura A, Henderson BE, Lee J. Breast cancer and diet among the Japanese in Hawaii. *Am J Clin Nutr* 1978; 31: 2020–5.

30 Sayegh R, Wurtman J, Spiers P, McDermott J, Wurtman R. The effect of a carbohydrate-rich beverage on mood, appetite, and cognitive function in women with premenstrual syndrome. *Obstet Gynecol* 1995; 86: 520–8.

31 Setchell KDR, Zimmer-Nechemias L, Cai J *et al.* Exposure of infants to phytoestrogens from soy-based infant formula. *Lancet* 1997; 350: 23–7.

32 Severson RK, Nomura AMY, Grove JS *et al.* A prospective study of demographics, diet, and prostate cancer among men of Japanese ancestry in Hawaii. *Cancer Res* 1989; 49: 1857–60.

33 Somani SM, Gupta P. Caffeine: a new look at an age-old drug. *Int J Clin Pharmacol Therap Toxicol* 1988; 26: 521–33.

34 Spring B. Effects of foods and nutrients on the behavior of normal individuals. In: Wurtman RJ, Wurtman JJ (eds), *Nutrition and the Brain*, Vol. 7. Raven Press, New York, 1986; 1–47.

35 Troll W, Wiesner R, Shellabarger CJ *et al.* Soybean diet lowers breast tumour incidence in irradiated rats. *Carcinogenesis* 1980; 1: 469–72.

36 Uragoda CG, Kottegoda SR. Adverse reactions to isoniazid on ingestion of fish with a high histamine content. *Tubercle* 1977; 58: 83–9.

37 VanPraag HM, Korf J. Serotonin metabolism in depression: clinical application of the probenecid test. *Int Pharmacopsychiatry* 1974; 9: 35–51.

38 Wang HJ, Murphy PA: Isoflavone content in commercial soybean foods. *J Agric Food Chem* 1994; 42: 1666–73.

B

Chapter 32

Food chemicals and their elimination

R. H. Waring

INTRODUCTION

Many different types of compound are found as food chemicals and additives, where they have a variety of uses (Table 32.1). Although they do not usually provide nutritional energy, these xenobiotics are absorbed across the wall of the gastrointestinal tract and carried *via* the portal vein to the liver where they are usually metabolized before excretion. Generally, only compounds which are relatively lipid soluble are absorbed from the gut while, since urinary excretion is the major pathway for elimination, only compounds which are fairly water-soluble can be easily removed from the body by that route. Like all living creatures, human beings rely on families of enzymes which are concentrated in the liver to transform the lipophilic food chemical into its hydrophilic metabolite. Traditionally these enzymes are divided into two major classes, Phase 1 and Phase 2 which have both endogenous and exogenous substrates (Tables 32.2, 32.3). Phase 1 reactions are often carried out *via* a haem-containing multienzyme super family, the cytochrome P450 system, which inserts or uncovers functional groups facilitating elimination (Table 32.2). One of the most important reactions is the addition of an atom of oxygen (O), taken from an oxygen molecule (O_2), into an aromatic ring

to give a phenolic derivative which is much more water-soluble than the parent compound. This reaction occurs readily, compounds such as biphenyl (E230) being hydroxylated to phenolic derivatives (Fig. 32.1). The cytochrome P450 complex exists in a number of families or isoforms which have preferred substrates; the human genome contains at least 28 P450 genes encoding individual enzymes. The nomenclature is complicated but is based on nucleotide-deduced amino acid sequences with classification into families, sub-families and individual isoenzymes (Table 32.4).

ACTIONS OF CYTOCHROME P450 ENZYMES

Induction

Many of the P450 enzymes are inducible, so that their expression can be modulated by environmental agents such as alcohol, smoking, some steroids and some drugs. The rate at which aromatic compounds can be eliminated from the body is therefore at least partially dependent on the environmental input and in some circumstances can be varied several fold. Nutrients or food additives which modify P450 activity include minerals, sulphides, isothiocyanates, thioglycosides, indoles, capsaicin, terpenes, flavones and barbecued meat so that dietary components can potentially have an important effect on metabolism.[31]

Cytochrome P450 isoforms

A further complication is that the P450 isoforms are often genetically variable, displaying 'polymorphism' in human populations. Generally, when any chemical is ingested, both the rate of elimination and the metabolite spectrum differ between individuals,

Classes of food additives

Class of compound	Examples	E-number
(a) Antioxidants	Propyl gallate	E310
	Butylated hydroxyanisole (BHA)	E320
	Butylated hydroxytoluene (BHT)	E321
(b) Colours	Tartrazine	E102
	Erythrosine BS	E127
	Sunset Yellow FCF	E110
(c) Emulsifiers/stabilizers	Sodium alginate	E402
	Fatty acid diglycerides	E471
	Sorbitan tristearate	E492
(d) Preservatives	Sodium sulphite	E221
	Benzoic acid	E210
	Ethyl 4-hydroxybenzoate	E214
(e) Sweeteners	Aspartame	—
	Mannitol	E421
	Sorbitol	E420
(f) Miscellaneous	Nicotinic acid	E375
	Magnesium sulphate	E518
	L-cysteine hydrochloride	E920

Table 32.1 Classes of food additives.

Phase 2 metabolic pathways

Substrate type	Major metabolic routes
(a) Phenols	Glucuronidation, sulphation, methylation
(b) Aromatic acids	Glucuronidation, glycine conjugation
(c) Aromatic amines, hydroxylamines	Acetylation, glucuronidation, sulphation
(d) Aliphatic amines, heterocyclic ring nitrogen	Methylation, occasionally glucuronidation
(e) Hydrazides, sulphonamides, cysteine derivatives	Acetylation
(f) Thiols	Methylation, occasionally glucuronidation
(g) Halogenated (Cl, Br) compounds, alkenes, aromatic rings, polycyclic hydrocarbons, epoxides	Glutathione conjugation

Table 32.3 Phase 2 metabolic pathways.

Phase 1 metabolic pathways

Substrate type	Major metabolic routes
(a) Aromatic (benzene) rings	Hydroxylation to phenols
(b) Aliphatic carbon chains	Hydroxylation to alcohols
(c) Aliphatic amines, heterocyclic ring nitrogens	N-oxide formation
(d) Aromatic and aliphatic sulphur	S-oxide formation
(e) O-, N- and S-alkyl compounds	Dealkylation to -OH, -NH, -SH
(f) O-, N-acetyl compounds	Deacetylation to -OH, -NH
(g) Alcohols, aldehydes	Oxidation to aldehydes, acids
(h) Amines (non-aromatic)	Oxidation to aldehydes, ketones
(i) Aldehydes, ketones	Reduction to alcohols
(j) Nitro (-NO$_2$), hydrazo (-NH-NH) azo (-N=N-)	Reduction to amines
(k) (i) Esterases, (ii) amides, (iii) epoxides	(i) Hydrolysis to acid and alcohol (ii) Acid and amine (iii) Formation of phenols or alcohols

Table 32.2 Phase 1 metabolic pathways.

Polymorphic isoforms of cytochrome P450 genes in man

Isoform	Potential substrates	Regulation
1A1	Polycyclic aromatic hydrocarbons (pah)	Cigarette smoke, pah
1A2	Aromatic amines, caffeine, cruciferous vegetables	pah, BBQ meat
2A6	Coumarin	?
2C19	Mephenytoin, diazepam, many drugs	Rifampicin, steroids
2D6	Debrisoquine, tricyclic antidepressants, many drugs	?
2E1	Nitrosamines, alcohols, carbon tetrachloride, paracetamol	Alcohol
3A3/4	Nifedipine	?
3A7	Aflatoxin	?

Table 32.4 Polymorphic isoforms of cytochrome P450 genes in man.

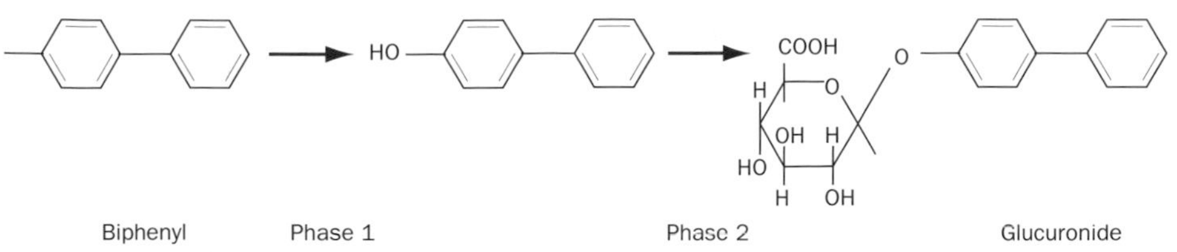

Fig. 32.1 Hydroxylation of biphenyl.

Biphenyl   Phase 1   Phase 2   Glucuronide

only identical twins giving (almost) identical results. The population distribution may appear as a Gaussian or skew Gaussian curve and is probably the summation of different variables such as absorption, metabolism and kidney function. However, in some cases, subsets of the population occur with a group having a metabolic activity which is distinct from the majority of those investigated. The population distribution may consist of overlapping Gaussian curves, with 'poor metabolizer' (PM) or 'fast metabolizer' (FM) phenotypes, reflecting differences in the gene coding for the reaction in question.

'*Pharmacological variation*' underlies many of the adverse reactions to environmental chemicals of all types. As an example, the CYP2D6 gene has been intensively studied; the gene product is a protein which catalyses the 4-hydroxylation of debrisoquine, an antihypertensive drug, and about 8% of the Caucasian population have the PM phenotype. They produce relatively little 4-hydroxy-debrisoquine, have higher blood levels of debrisoquine and are therefore more susceptible to the pharmacological effect of the parent drug since the metabolite is inactive. Many other drugs are metabolized by the same pathway and show a similarly low metabolic conversion.

Genotype variation
The PM phenotype for CYP2D6 is due to a number of mutant alleles; over 25 individual mutations are known but a base pair deletion at an intron/exon junction leading to faulty splicing of a pre-mRNA and a gene deletion are the two most important. Many of the other P450 isoforms show similar genotypic variation based on polymerase chain reaction (PCR) tests.[73,82]

Restriction fragment-length polymorphisms (RFLPs) in CYP genes have in some cases been linked to cancer risk. Cytochrome P4501A1 metabolizes polycyclic aromatic hydrocarbons while P4502E1 metabolizes N-nitrosamines and benzene; these compounds are all carcinogens and RFLPs for both P450 isoforms have been shown to be associated with lung cancer risk.[44] Similarly, expression of the enzyme catalysing the metabolic activation of benzo(a)pyrene to a 9-hydroxybenzo(a)pyrene 9-DNA adduct has a 10-fold variation in the population and RFLPs of the gene (CYP2C9) have been linked with cancer of the larynx in smokers.[5]

Phenotypic variation
Cytochrome P450 metabolism also generates free radical products and reactive oxygen species (ROS). These may initiate inflammatory disease states such as hepatitis, nephritis and scleroderma[54] and there has been speculation that ROS may also be involved in autoimmune disease and 'lupus-like' disorders.[38]

'*Idiosyncratic*' *hypersensitivity reactions* may account for up to 25% of all adverse reactions and have been suggested as being due to metabolic activation of drugs to reactive intermediates which become immunogenic through interactions with cellular macromolecules. Cytochrome P450 enzymes are thought to have key roles in this multifactorial process.[56] Autoantibodies directed against P450 2C9 and 1A2 can be induced by tienilic acid and dihydralazine, while autoimmune hepatitis type 2 is linked with autoantibodies expressed against P450 2D6.[51]

Cytochrome P450: the two-edged sword
P450 Enzymes may therefore function in an ambivalent manner, normally facilitating elimination of foreign chemicals but also giving increased formation of carcinogenic or mutagenic metabolites and toxic intermediates. Genetic differences in human P450 expression, coupled with modulation by diet and environmental factors, lead to marked inter- and intra-individual variation. Generally, for instance, low-protein and low-fat diets reduce the activity of the P450 isozymes, as does total parenteral nutrition.[32,74] The existence of susceptible subgroups in the population who may be more likely to display clinical symptoms is therefore at least partly diet-related.

Metabolism of food chemicals
Cytochrome P450 isoforms not only catalyse hydroxylation of aliphatic chains or aromatic rings but they can carry out de-alkylation reactions on nitrogen, oxygen and sulphur centres, releasing hydrophilic groups, and can also remove halogen and sulphur atoms. At low oxygen tension, especially in the gastrointestinal tract, P450s, together with nitroreductase, xanthine oxidase and cytochrome C reductase, can act to reduce nitrogen-containing compounds. Nitro groups ($-NO_2$) can be converted to amines ($-NH_2$) while azo compounds ($-N=N-$) are progressively reduced to hydrazo ($-NH-NH-$) derivatives and finally undergo reductive scission to give amines ($-NH_2 + -NH_2$) (Fig. 32.2).

Amines and food sensitivity
This reaction is particularly significant in the metabolism of food chemicals of the azo-dye type such as tartrazine (E102). As aromatic amines produced by this reaction sequence may be

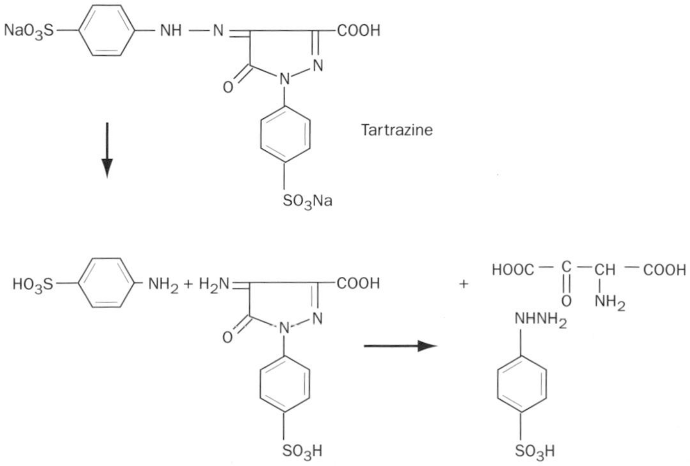

Fig. 32.2 Metabolism of tartrazime to give amines.

involved in formation of hapten–protein complexes, this could lead to sensitivity reactions. Many gut bacteria can reduce azo compounds to amines and the precise nature of the metabolites of compounds such as tartrazine probably depends on the exact species of bacteria present in the gastrointestinal tract. This can vary markedly between individuals and is also altered by diet and disease states. These factors may explain the wide variation in individual reactions; several studies have suggested that a sub-group of children may react to compounds such as tartrazine by exhibiting hyperactive behaviour[8,22,40] although other workers have not been able to confirm these effects.[29] It is possible that fluctuations in gut bacteria could underlie these inconsistencies.

PHASE I OXIDATIONS

Alcohol dehydrogenase

Other oxidations in the Phase 1 category include those carried out by alcohol and aldehyde dehydrogenases. In the simplest example, ethyl alcohol (ethanol), which may be a component of food pre-parations or coadministered, is oxidized to acetaldehyde and then to acetate, which then enters the normal endogenous pathways:

$$\underset{\substack{\text{alcohol}\\\text{dehydrogenase}}}{CH_3CH_2OH} \rightarrow \underset{\substack{\text{aldehyde}\\\text{dehydrogenase}}}{CH_3CHO} \rightarrow CH_3COO^-$$

This is the route for all primary alcohols; secondary alcohols such as propan-2-ol (isopropyl alcohol) are oxidized to ketones. The enzymes involved in these reactions have very variable activity in man, ethanol being metabolized by at least three systems – cata-lase, the microsomal oxidizing system (MEOS) and cytosolic alcohol dehydrogenase. The MEOS enzyme is inducible by alcohol and this induction is responsible for the enhanced rate of metab-olism found in regular drinkers. The reaction is catalysed by the cytochrome P450 2E1 complex which is polymorphic in man.[57] Alcohol dehydrogenase (ADH) has been more extensively studied and unusually has zero-order kinetics so that the fall in concen-tration of alcohol in the blood is linear with time. Several classes of ADH enzymes are known with variant coding alleles and interindividual and interethnic variation is high. Other substrates for the enzyme are methanol, ethylene, glycol, 1,2-propane-diol, steroids, bile acids and short-chain alcohols.[2]

Aldehyde dehydrogenase (ALDH)

This is also polymorphic in man; low ALDH activity is associated with the 'flush' reactions that can occur after drinking alcohol, due to a build-up of acetaldehyde. This phenomenon is more common in Oriental populations, especially the Japanese, but also occurs in 5–10% of Caucasians.[30]

Fish odour syndrome

Variations in oxidation of nitrogen compounds are also known. The best-studied example is that of the 'fish odour syndrome'. Normally, trimethylanine (TMA) which is present in fish and a component of choline and lecithin, is oxidized to the odourless trimethylanine-N-oxide (TMA-O) by an enzyme which is FAD (flavin adenine dinucleotide)-linked. About 5000 of the popula-tion in the UK are thought to have a defective form of this enzyme and so tend to smell 'fishy', extra fish in their diet com-pounding the problem.[45]

Sulphur oxidation

Cytochrome P450 and FAD-linked enzymes which oxidize sulphur compounds have also been described. These convert sulphur compounds to their corresponding S-oxides, which are more polar and usually less toxic than the parent molecule. FAD-linked enzymes seem to be involved in oxidation of the alkyl and dialkyl sulphides found in garlic and other members of the Allium family. These sulphur compounds give the characteristic taste and smell of onions and garlic and generally the S-oxides are less pungent although some have lacrimatory properties.[75] Allergic contact dermatitis to garlic has been reported for both man and the guinea pig and appears to be due to the presence of diallyl disulphide, allyl propyl disulphide and allyl thiol. Allicin (diallyl-sulphoxide) may act as an irritant and is possibly allergenic.[53] Intolerance to onions/garlic is relatively common in the popula-tion and probably correlates with a failure to oxidize disulphides and sulphides to their S-oxides. The enzyme system involved has not been studied but may well be polymorphic, like the FAD-linked monoamine oxidase (MAO) system.

Cysteine oxidation and autoimmune disease

Much work has been carried out on the cytosolic cysteine dioxy-genase (cdo) enzyme which catalyses the conversion of cysteine (E920) to cysteine sulphinic acid.[46] This is the initial (and rate-determining) step in the oxidative degradation of cysteine to in-organic sulphate (Fig. 32.3). The enzyme cdo is mainly present in brain, liver and kidney and is polymorphic in man, about 30% of the population having reduced and 2% having nul activity. The activity of cdo *in vivo* in man is normally assessed either by meas-uring the plasma cysteine/sulphate ratio or by giving an oral dose of S-carboxymethylcysteine (SCMC). This is a cysteine derivative and, like D-penicillamine (β,β-dimethylcysteine), a substrate for cdo, being converted to a range of S-oxide metabolites. Cysteine/sulphate plasma ratios and urinary SCMC/SCMC-S-oxide ratios correlate well,[10] showing that this is the major route of cysteine metabolism. The reduced S-oxidation phenotype appears to be linked with autoimmune disease, as about 70% of a rheumatoid arthritis (RA) population were poor S-oxidizers when challenged with SCMC.[20] An increased incidence of reduced S-oxidation has also been found in populations with primary biliary cirrhosis and systemic lupus erythematosus (SLE).[25,52] In a study of patients with chemical allergies 70% were found to be poor oxidizers of SCMC and, in agreement with these results, an investigation of patients with allergy found mean plasma sulphate levels to be about 25% of control values.[62]

It is not clear why there should be this association, but there are several possibilities. One is that cdo could metabolize a variety

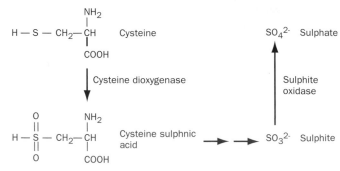

Fig. 32.3 Oxidative degradation of cysteine to inorganic sulphate.

of environmental compounds containing a free thiol group and that failure to oxidize the reactive -SH moiety leads to formation of hapten–protein complexes. It is also possible that endogenous cysteine levels are involved in some way in sensitivity responses, possibly by altering the structures of proteins. Inactivation by formation of cysteine-thiol protein dimers has been reported for C4 complement[65] and this may be involved in rheumatoid arthritis where raised cysteine levels have been shown.[76] Cysteine not only reacts with proteins, it can also combine with leukotrienes to give adducts which cause an inflammatory response.[76]

Sulphate deficit and inflammation

Another hypothesis is that inorganic sulphate levels are in some way involved in the aetiology of autoimmune disease. As well as having raised plasma cysteine levels, patients with RA and SLE have low sulphate, perhaps reflecting a fault in cdo regulation or expression.[76] There will therefore be less sulphate available for synthesis of biocomponents such as the sulphated glycosaminoglycans and mucin-type proteins which are found in synovial fluid, while any reduction in lubricant capacity in joints would be expected to worsen the disease process. A further factor in food intolerance may be the structure of mucins in the gastrointestinal tract. Several studies have shown that low sulphation of these proteins is associated with reduced tissue integrity, inflammatory responses, ulcerative colitis and Crohn's disease[48,60] and also with colonization by bacteria such as *Helicobacter pylori*.[67] As sulphate is often in short supply *in vivo* and is required for many biological processes, low levels could lead to reduced mucin sulphation and the 'leaky-gut' syndrome, with increased permeability to peptide/protein antigens. It is possible that cdo activity could be down-regulated by food components; this has not been studied but must remain an attractive hypothesis.

Sulphite oxidase

The other major enzyme in the cysteine–sulphate pathway is sulphite oxidase, found in the mitochondrial intermembrane space. This requires molybdenum (as a complex with pterins) as a cofactor and acts to convert sulphite (SO_3^{2-}) to sulphate (SO_4^{2-}). Sulphites, which are generated endogenously as part of the normal processing of sulphur-containing amino acids, occur as a consequence of fermentation and are found naturally in a number of foods. They are also added (as sulphur dioxide, sodium sulphite or calcium bisulphite) (E220, E224, E226, E227) as preservatives, controlling microbial growth and preventing browning and spoilage. Sulphite sensitivity with bronchospasm occurs most often in asthmatics, especially women, and may affect up to 0.05% of the United States population; low sulphite oxidase activity has been suggested as the trigger mechanism.[1,72]

Patients with primary biliary cirrhosis (PBC) often have circulating mitochondrial autoantigens, one of which (M4) has been identified with antigen to sulphite oxidase and is associated with a poor prognosis.[18] Patients with severe PBC often have low plasma sulphate, which may correlate with ineffective sulphite oxidase. Sulphite oxidase deficiency can exist either as an isolated enzyme defect or combined with xanthine dehydrogenase deficiency (as both enzymes have a common molybdenum cofactor) and is thought to be polymorphic in human populations.[59] A severe deficiency of the enzyme is associated with neurological symptoms, including profound mental retardation, seizures and spastic quadriparesis.[59] Patients with this syndrome excreted raised levels of sulphite, thiosulphate and S-sulphocysteine in urine.[11] This may be due to a defect in the enzyme or to low levels of the cofactor, a molybdopterin. Studies on children with both autism and food sensitivity showed that 17% had excess urinary sulphite; in about 50% of cases this was normalized when extra molybdenum was included in the diet.[34] As this cofactor appears to be bound to sulphite oxidase *via* a conserved cysteine residue, it is possible that the high plasma cysteine levels often found in autism have disrupted this process by forming disulphide bonds with the enzyme. Allergic responses to sulphite in food or in the atmosphere may reflect a mild reduction in sulphite oxidase efficiency.[39]

Esterase activity

Esterases, a family of Phase I enzymes that hydrolyse esters to their constituent acids and alcohols or phenols, can be found in both liver and plasma. There is known to be wide interindividual variation in activity in human populations. Mammals (especially the rabbit and pig) have high plasma esterase levels which may have evolved to detoxify plant alkaloids such as atropine (belladonna) or cocaine. These enzymes are relatively non-specific and can hydrolyse food-flavouring esters such as isoamyl acetate, ethyl butyrate and allyl caprate, which have been used as constituents of synthetic strawberry and pineapple flavourings. Esterase activity is readily inhibited by organophosphates, which phosphorylate serine residues at the active sites of the enzymes, often with long-lasting effects that are only reversed by degradation and resynthesis of the enzymes. As esters are more lipophilic than their constituent acids and alcohols, any reduction in esterase activity must delay their elimination.

PHASE 2 ENZYMES

The Phase 2 enzymes are equally heterogeneous and act to add a grouping which is usually large and water-soluble to either the parent compound or its derivative formed after Phase 1 metabolism, a process which in effect gives a 'handle' for further enzyme action. These Phase 2 metabolites are usually, thought not always, less toxic than the original compound and are always more readily excreted and usually more hydrophilic. The whole process is very demanding of metabolic energy, often supplied as ATP or GTP, and utilizes endogenous pathways (see Table 32.3). Because Phase 2 enzymes are involved in normal metabolism where their main substrates are biochemical intermediates and products such as steroids and bile acids, low enzyme activity can sometimes be correlated with biochemical and clinical dysfunction.

Formation of glucuronides

The most important Phase 2 enzyme system is that of the glucuronyltransferases (UGTs). These microsomal enzymes use UDPGA (uridine diphosphate glucuronic acid) to transfer a glucuronic acid residue to the substrate (Fig. 32.4). The conjugates so formed are called 'glucuronides' and usually account for 50–70% of the dose of an ingested chemical. Phenols, aromatic acids and amines all readily form glucuronides, which occur at electron-rich sites in the parent molecule.[36] Some glucuronides can interact with proteins to produce haptens, while UGTs themselves can act as hepatocellular autoantigens. The UGT enzymes are relatively easily affected by environmental conditions. They can be induced by phenobarbitone, smoking and terpenes such as menthol and borneol (the flavouring agents in peppermint oil and

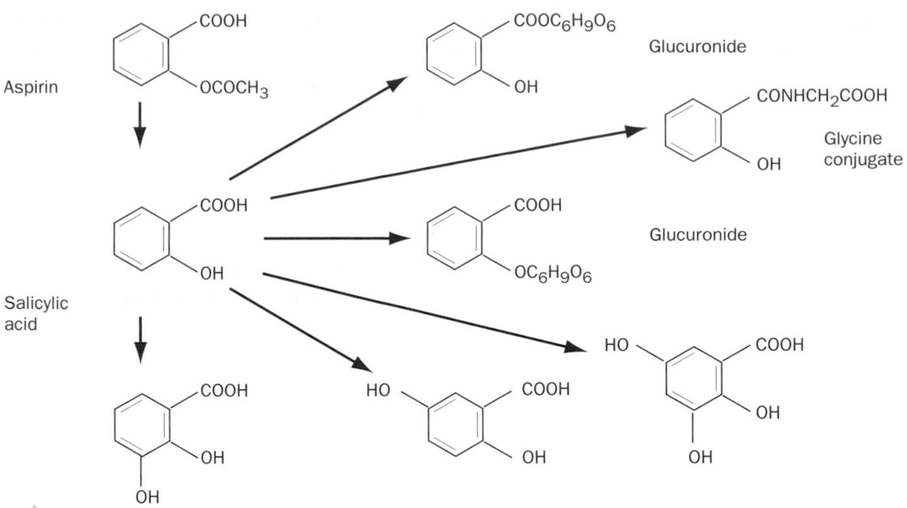

Fig. 32.4 Formation of glucunonides.

in eucalyptus).[61] They can be inhibited by viruses, especially the hepatic viruses such as hepatitis A, and even the common cold can alter metabolism and depress glucuronidation.

UGTs have relatively low activity in the neonate, adult levels only being achieved about 3 weeks after full-term gestation. Activity in old age is less predictable: some elderly individuals retain mean activity similar to that found in a student population, with others in the same age group having about a 30% decrease in mean UGT capacity. This latter group tended to be less healthy and on concurrent medication.[26]

Molecular biology of glucuronyl transferases

There are two major UGT families: the products of the UGT1 gene metabolize bilirubin and many phenols, while the UGT2 gene product accepts steroids and bile acids, both endogenous compounds, as substrates. Several isoforms of the UGT1 gene are known, each with five exons where the four exons at the 3'-end are common to all types. The exon at the 5' end has its own promoter, and mutations and deletions in this have been found. Mutations in any of the four exons at the 3' end will affect all the isoforms, since these exons are common to all UGT1 genes and will therefore affect the activity of the corresponding UGT enzymes.[12] Variants in UGT activity can have serious consequences. Patients with the Crigler–Najjar syndrome, with mutations in the UGT1 gene, are almost unable to conjugate bilirubin to its non-toxic and water-soluble glucuronide derivative and this results in severe hyperbilirubinaemia and mental retardation. Gilbert's syndrome, which is not uncommon, probably being present in about 8% of the British population, may be so mild as to be unrecognized and also involves reduced UGT1 activity. Because the same enzyme system metabolizes bilirubin and phenols, this would increase susceptibility to the action of chemicals if phenolic compounds or metabolites were involved. Aspirin (acetylsalicylic acid) is rapidly hydrolysed *in vivo* to salicylic acid (see Fig. 32.4) which can form both phenolic and acidic glucuronides. Individuals with Gilbert's syndrome would therefore be exposed to higher plasma levels of salicylic acid; this may be a factor in the reported cases of aspirin/salicylic acid sensitivity, where urticaria and rhinitis have been reported together with broncho constriction.[16]

Metabolism of polyhydroxy phenols

Polyhydroxyphenols such as gallic acid (1,2,3-trihydroxy-5-carboxy benzene) also form glucuronides as major metabolites;

they have been linked with sensitivity/allergic/intolerance responses which could be due to reduced UGT activity.[4,58] Gallate esters are widely used as food additives (E310, E311 and E312) as they act as antioxidants and scavengers of aqueous-phase free radicals while gallocatechins (green tea polyphenols) have been studied for their capacity to inhibit cancers of the gastrointestinal tract.[83] Gallic acid itself seems to have very low toxicity, though propyl gallate is slightly cytotoxic in isolated rat hepatocytes, possibly due to a greater capacity to penetrate cell membranes.[50] Reactions to gallate esters may therefore reflect a low level of esterase activity or reduced UGT detoxification.

Formation of sulphated derivatives

Sulphation is quantitatively the next most important pathway after glucuronidation (Fig. 32.5). The enzymes involved, the sulphotransferases, are usually cytosolic and catalyse the addition of a sulphate residue via PAPS (3'-phosphoadenosine-5'-phosphosulphate) to a variety of substrates including proteins, steroids and bile acids.[17] Sulphotransferases are found in most body tissues, including liver, intestine and brain and exist as a multi-gene family with many conserved sequences. The P-form of phenolsulphotransferase (PSTSULT 1A1/2) preferentially sulphates phenols while the M-form (MSTSULT 1A3) converts amines, although both enzymes can use the other substrate at higher concentrations. This is not absolute, however, MST, which sulphates endogenous neurotransmitter amines such as dopamine, also accepts the phenolic vanillin, which is often used in food flavouring. Conversely, PST sulphates the P450-hydroxylated derivatives of the heterocyclic amines which are produced when meat is grilled or barbecued. These hydroxyl amines are activated by this process and the sulphated metabolites give rise to elec-

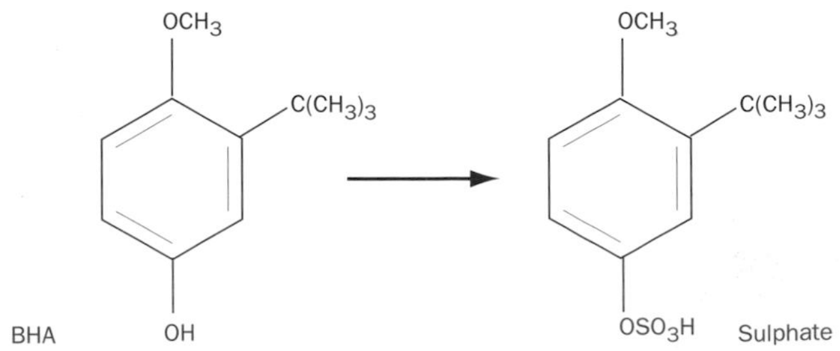

Fig. 32.5 Sulphation.

trophilic species which form adducts with DNA, thus potentially initiating the first stage in the carcinogenic process.[15] Diets with high levels of sulphotransferase inhibitors, such as the soy-bean-derived genistein, are linked with lower rates of gut cancer, suggesting that sulphated intermediates may be involved and that under some circumstances sulphation can lead to cytotoxicity rather than detoxication.[43]

Food sensitivity and migraine

The activity of PST is co-regulated in all tissues, so that measurement of PST levels in the platelet gives a good estimate of activity in the brain and gastrointestinal tract.[71] Using this approach, it has been possible to show that low PST levels correlate with clinical symptons, especially migraine. Classical food 'triggers' for migraine patients include cheese, chocolate and bananas, which contain neurotransmitter amines (tyramine, phenylethylamine and serotonin, respectively). Like the catecholamines, these are all substrates for the phenolsulphotransferases; inactivation by sulphation is a major pathway for amines in the CNS and as much as 80% of dopamine is metabolized *via* this route in man.

Sulphotransferases are inhibited by flavonoids,[23] so that citrus fruit and red wine can block sulphation of amines and then lead to a migraine headache in susceptible individuals. Although migraine is undoubtedly a multifactorial phenomcnon, the existence of food triggers implies that relatively small amounts of substrates or inhibitors can overwhelm the sulphotransferase capacity in gut and platelets, leading to an increase in neurotransmitter amines in the central nervous system. This has been shown to lead to headache.[41] The mean PST levels in migraine patients are significantly lower than those found in controls, no differences being found in cases with or without aura.[3] The mean plasma sulphate levels were not different from controls, so that the reduction in enzyme activity alone is responsible for the effects.

Both MST and PST can be inhibited *in vitro* by food components. In a study using platelet enzymes, and fruit or vegetable cytosols, spinach, oranges and pumpkin were found to be good endogenous substrates. Lettuce inhibited the M-form of the enzyme and radish, spinach, banana, beetroot, broccoli, cauliflower and leek inhibited both M- and P-forms while grapefruit, peppers and pineapple were active against the P-form of phenolsulphotransferase.[28] Ingestion of a variety of fruits and vegetables could also therefore be a factor in the onset of migraine headache, although the commonly quoted food 'triggers' are likely to be eaten in larger amounts and more frequently.

Food sensitivity and behaviour

Human liver sulphotransferases are similarly inhibited by a number of compounds that are found in food or are food additives. Vanillin gave 100% inhibition of MST and 91% inhibition of PST, while tartrazine (E102) was a strong inhibitor of the M-isoform.[6] This is of interest as tartrazine (used as a colorant in 'orange' drinks) has been linked with hyperactive behaviour in children. It is possible that inhibition of MST by tartrazine could cause increased levels of neurotransmitter amines in the CNS with subsequent effects on mood and behaviour. Vanillin, however, would be expected to cause similar symptoms if this hypothesis is true.

Hypersensitivity to food chemicals is a controversial topic, with studies showing effects in some populations but not in others. Nevertheless, many of the compounds suggested as being implicated in causing skin rashes or behaviour problems do interact with the sulphotransferase enzymes. Amines in particular readily form protein–hapten conjugates; this would be expected to happen less frequently in individuals with high sulphotransferase activity who could more easily inactivate and eliminate amines, but little work has been done in this field.

Sulphation and psychological disorders

Sulphotransferase activity has been linked with psychiatric disorders, being higher in obsessive-compulsive disorder and lower in unipolar depressive.[42] These findings probably reflect imbalances in brain amines. Similarly, about 40% of autistic children have raised serotonin levels and a general imbalance of catecholamine neurotransmitters.[7] A subset of autistic children (with parents with migraine) were shown to have low sulphotransferase levels and to be sensitive to the standard dietary 'triggers' which were linked with hyperactive or aggressive behaviour. Most autistic children (in a study of 33 patients), however, had reduced levels of plasma sulphate, the mean value (0.55 nmol/mg protein) being significantly lower than that found for control children of the same age range (4.9 nmol/mg protein).[77] With these very low levels of sulphate, even if the enzyme had normal activity the concentrations of PAPS would be inadequate to conjugate all the potential substrates. Studies in a small control population have shown that PAPS concentrations are rate-limiting, sulphation of paracetamol being saturated at ~ 650 mg when the standard dose is 1000 mg.[69] Obviously, any effects from dietary compounds which either contain amines/phenols or which inhibit their metabolism will be most marked in those individuals who have both reduced enzyme levels and low concentrations of inorganic sulphate/PAPS.

Acetylation

Genotype variation

Acetylation of aromatic amines and hydrazides occurs via the cytosolic N-acetyltransferase (NAT) enzymes with acetyl CoA as a cofactor. These have been much studied because of the pharmacogenetic variation that is seen in human populations and was, in fact, the first of its kind to be recognized. N-Acetylation is now known to be carried out by two families of enzymes: NAT1 acetylates *p*-aminobenzoic acid and *p*-aminosalicylic acid, while NAT2 acetylates a wide range of substrates including isoniazid, sulfonamides and caffeine. NAT1 shows a unimodal activity but NAT2 activity is bimodal and Caucasian populations divide into 'fast' and 'slow' acetylators with approximately 50% of the population in each category. There are striking ethnic variations, however, about 90% of Inuits are fast acetylators while about 96% of the Kung Bushmen have the slow acetylator phenotype.[55] Restriction fragment length polymorphism (RFLP) analysis has shown that there are many mutations in the gene, although three major slow acetylator alleles, each identifiable at a restriction endonuclease site, have been found in several populations.

Phenotype variation

For most practical purposes, the N-acetylation (NAT2) phenotype can be estimated by determining the individual response to caffeine. Fast acetylators are not affected by caffeine in cola or coffee drinks because the acetylated metabolite is inactive. Slow acetylators tend to require frequent infusions of caffeine and experience a mild 'lift' unlike fast acetylators. The metabolic degradation of caffeine (Fig. 32.6) involves a number of enzymes, including

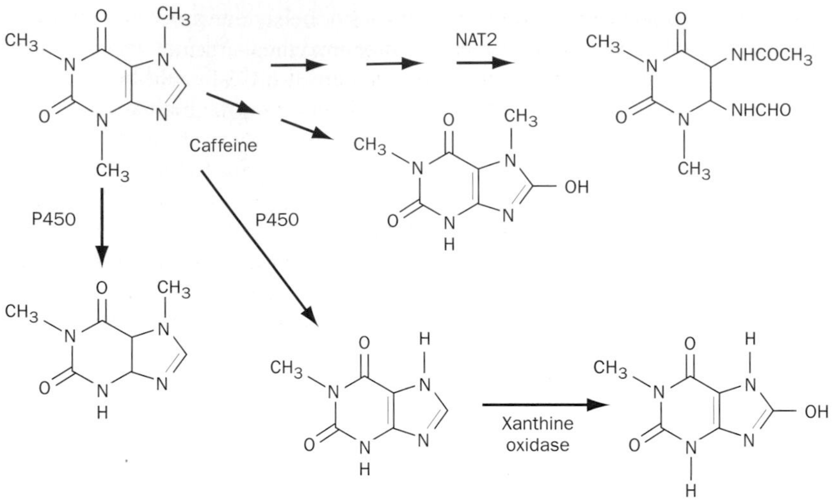

Fig. 32.6 Metabolic degradation of caffeine.

cytochrome P450 isoforms, xanthine oxidase and NAT2, but the formation of the acetylated metabolite seems to be rate-limiting pharmacologically. Other sources of substrates for the NAT enzymes come, apart from sulfonamide drugs, from carcinogenic amines generated by industrial processes and diet. The slow acetylator phenotype has been associated with bladder cancer from exposure to benzidine and β-naphthylamine.[55] Carcinogenic amines are also present in low concentrations in tobacco smoke and the urine of smokers has been found to be mutagenic, so the acetylator phenotype could be a modifying factor.[14]

Acetylation and clinical correlates

Heterocyclic amines such as 2-amino-3-methylimidazo (4,5-f) quinoline (IQ) and 2-amino-3, 8-dimethylimidazo (4,5-) quinoxaline (MeIQx) are produced when protein-rich foods are cooked at high temperatures. They are substrates for NAT2 and can also be hydroxylated by CYP1A1 and CYP1A2 and further acetylated via NAT1.[5,49] This production of N-acetoxy-N-arylamines is believed to give unstable compounds which can form carcinogenic DNA adducts. Fast acetylators might therefore be expected to be more susceptible to colorectal tumours, but a number of studies have shown that in practice there is no association between this phenotype and gastrointestinal tract cancers.[66] Japanese populations, who are generally fast acetylators (~90%), have a very low incidence of colorectal cancer. It is probable that a combination of metabolic pathways is involved here, and that NAT1/NAT2 activity cannot be taken in isolation. Industrial exposure to hydrazine can lead to SLE-like symptoms, but various studies have shown that SLE is not linked with the slow acetylator phenotype as had been proposed.[55] Naturally occurring amines and hydrazides cannot therefore be aetiological factors in the development of this disease although it is possible that again a combination of two or more metabolic routes could be involved. It would be of interest to try to correlate sensitivity to food colorants with N-acetylation status. The azo-group of dye colorants, such as tartrazine and Ponceau-4R, are reduced by gut bacteria to aromatic amines, which may form protein conjugates leading to allergic responses. As acetylation can take place in the gut, slow acetylators might be more susceptible to reactions to food colorants of this type although, since amines are also rapidly sulphated in the gastrointestinal tract by sulphotransferases, sensitivity may again depend on multifactorial input from other metabolizing enzymes.

Benzoates, diet and hyperactivity

Benzoic acid and benzoates occur naturally in small amounts in some plants and have been added to foods as preservatives. The sodium salt is more soluble but it is the undissociated acid that is active against microorganisms, particularly yeasts and bacteria. It is therefore most effective in acid solution such as fruit juices. Esters of *p*-hydroxybenzoic acid ('parabens') are also used in similar situations. Like most aromatic acids, benzoates are eliminated from the body as their glycine conjugates, which are formed via acetyl CoA (see Fig. 32.4). These metabolites are called 'hippuric' acids (the original benzoic acid–glycine conjugate was isolated from horse urine) and the formation of *p*-aminohippuric acid from *p*-aminobenzoic acid has long been used as a test of liver function (PAH test). Direct toxicity from benzoates is not common, although perioral contact urticaria has been reported from sodium benzoate.[47] This may imply a sensitive subgroup, as benzoic acid has been used in large amounts to treat non-ketotic hyperglycinaemia.[21] Pharmaceutical preparations usually contain a variety of excipients which are listed as 'inert ingredients'. A study on 102 antidiarrhoea, cough and cold, antihistamine/decongestant and analgesic/antipyretic preparations showed that sodium benzoate and methylparabens were used in 42 and 27 preparations, respectively, while dyes were common – Red Dye No. 40 and Yellow No. 6 being most found.[35] Benzoates therefore occur widely if unexpectedly. Little work seems to have been done on population studies of benzoate metabolism.

Metabolism of salicylates

Salicylic acid and salicylates (*o*-hydroxybenzoic acid and derivatives) occur naturally in many plant products, probably because salicylic acid is a plant hormone regulating many metabolic activities. Salicylic acid is usually found as the hydrolysis product of aspirin (acetylsalicylic acid) and is thought to be the active principle. Aspirin is readily hydrolysed by serum esterases and salicylic acid appears in the bloodstream about 10 min after an analgesic dose. Studies on human volunteers have shown marked variation in metabolism and all the pathways, including glycine conjugation, seem to show a wide spread in metabolite concentrations between individuals.[13] It is not clear whether any adverse effects can be attributed to any particular metabolite, but low glucuronyl transferase activity combined with low glycyltransferase would lead to increased levels of polyhydroxyphenols of the gallol and pyrogallol type, together with salicylic acid itself. The presence of high glucuronidase activity in tissues would also give raised local concentrations of phenols. These factors may underlie the aspirin-sensitive rhinosinusitis found in middle-aged patients. It may also be seen in atopic individuals who have a mixed-type rhinitis with recurrent airway infections and sensitivity to non-steroidal anti-inflammatory drugs (NSAIDs), tartrazine, food additives and alcohol. Development of nasal polyps and asthma is common.[64] These reactions may be due to a hyperactive immune system as lymphocyte and leukotriene pathway activation have been found to occur in a susceptible subset.

Glutathione conjugation

Glutathione-S-transferase activity has been much more clearly defined. The glutathione-S-transferases (GST) are a family of cytosolic enzymes which link glutathione (γ-glutamyl–cysteinyl–glycine) with electrophilic substrates. Once the substrate, usually containing an epoxide, a halogen, an alkene or aromatic ring, is linked with glutathione via the thiol group, progressive degradation takes place. A cysteinyl–glycine conjugate is first formed; this is hydrolysed to a cysteine-adduct, which is then N-acetylated to form the N-acetyl-S-substituted cysteine derivative ('mercapturic acid'). These are excreted in urine and may be further degraded in the kidney by cysteine-β-lyase enzymes to give rise to thiol-containing compounds which can be nephrotoxic (Fig. 32.7). Glutathione conjugates are notoriously difficult to find as they are chemically relatively unstable and it seems probable that GST-catalysed conjugations are more numerous than has been reported. A number of endogenous substrates are known, such as lipid hydroperoxides, prostaglandins and leukotrienes; the GST system seems to have evolved to protect the cell from electrophilic intermediary compounds which could bind to DNA or other cell constituents.[80]

Glutathione-S-transferases: isoforms

At least four classes, the α, μ, π and θ genes, have been reported and these differ markedly in size and in their intron–exon structures. GSTs are widely distributed throughout the body, although some tissues have specific isoforms. The substrate selectivities are generally described as broad and overlapping but there are some predominant findings: class α-isoenzymes usually have high peroxidase activity, while human μ-isoenzymes link polycyclic aro-

matic hydrocarbon epoxides with GSH. Products of metabolic oxidative stress, such as 9-hydroperoxylinoleic acid, 4-hydroxynon-2-enal and cholesterol-5,6-oxide are also GST substrates and the GST enzymes themselves have high antioxidant capacity.[33]

Polymorphisms: GSTM1

Polymorphisms of expression of all the genes are known. So far, five different genes expressing the μ-protein are known, GSTM1 being polymorphic with four common phenotypes resulting from homo- and heterozygotic combinations of two different alleles and a nul form. About 45% of most populations are homozygous for the deleted GSTM1*O allele, and express no μ-GST. This has been linked with Parkinson's disease and also with development of a number of cancers (adenocarcinoma, stomach and urothelial cancer), suggesting the involvement of environmental toxins which would normally be substrates for the GSTM1 gene products.[19,70]

Polymorphisms: GSTT1

The GSTT1 gene (θ-GST) is highly conserved throughout evolution and probably originated to protect against oxygen toxicity. In humans, in contrast to rats, GSTT1 is found in the erythrocytes, which may act as a detoxication sink to remove alkylating agents from the system. Two human θ-class genes are known, GSTT1 and GSTT2; GSTT1 is absent from about 25% of the British population, although marked ethnic differences occur with the nul form found in about 10% of Mexican Americans and in about 65% of Chinese populations. Subjects with a deletion of the GSTT1 gene have been shown to be more susceptible to Alzheimer's disease, again suggesting the role of environmental contaminants or ROS in neurological degeneration.[70] No correlations seem to have been made as yet between immunological dysfunction and GST genotype, although as the GST enzymes have such a wide range of substrates, there may well prove to be links in the future. GST isoforms are readily inducible by dietary flavonoids and isothiocyanates,[24,63] which therefore act as chemoprotectants.

Methyltransferases

The last of the major detoxification pathways is that of methylation, involving S-adenosyl methionine (SAM) and methyltransferase enzymes. These are usually membrane-bound and have proved resistant to isolation and characterization. O-Methyltransferases (OMTs) add methyl (CH_3) groups to phenols

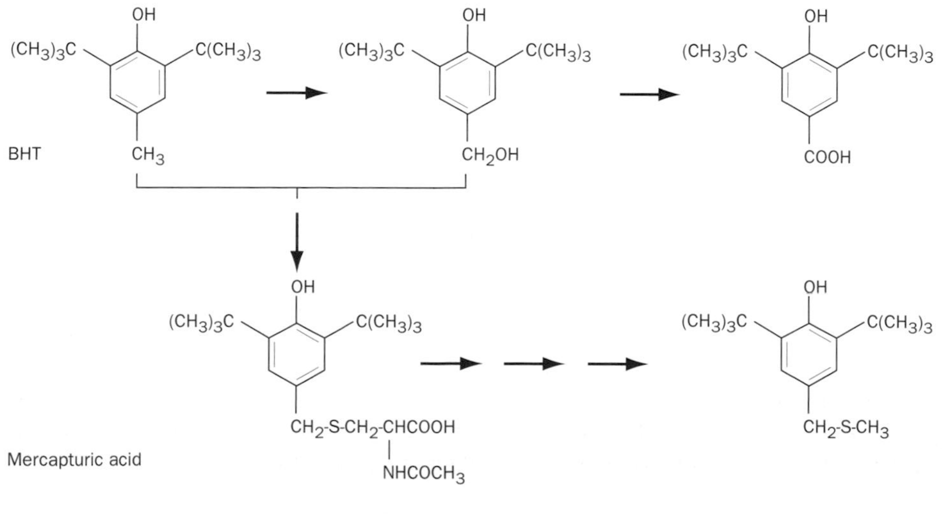

Fig. 32.7 Glutathione conjugation.

(-OH), giving the methoxy group (OCH₃). Conversion of simple phenols to these derivatives gives the corresponding anetholes, compounds which are notorious for their sickening odour, which can be detected readily at 10⁻⁹ molar concentrations. The OMT enzymes exist in liver and kidney and variants are found in anaerobic bacteria. Catechol-O-methyltransferase (COMT) enzymes also occur, and are responsible for methylation of adrenaline and noradrenaline.[79]

Polymorphisms of methylation

Erythrocyte and hepatic COMT are co-regulated in man and the enzyme shows a bimodal population distribution, which can be resolved into three overlapping peaks representing the presence of high- and low-activity alleles. Aliphatic thiolmethyltransferases (TMTs) catalyse the methylation of thiol groups and are co-regulated and may even be the same enzymes as the O-methyltransferases. TMTs have a well-recognized role in detoxication, because formation of the S-CH₃ moiety from -SH reduces any biological interactions with thiol groups on proteins and peptides. Substrates include H₂S from cleavage of cysteine (E920) and a range of aliphatic thiols, especially the propyl and allyl mercaptans produced from breakdown of S-alkyl cysteines in the Allium and Brassicae families. Hydrogen sulphide is also generated endogenously by the action of gut bacteria on either sulphur-containing amino acids from proteins or inorganic sulphate and is S-methylated to give methane thiol (CH₃SH) then dimethylsulphide (CH₃SCH₃), each time with a reduction in toxicity. Thiolmethyltransferases are ubiquitous in tissue membrane preparations, suggesting the need to protect against thiol toxicity in all organs.

Neurological disease

Reduced TMT levels have been linked with Parkinson's and Alzheimer's disease:[78] this correlates with the finding that chronic H₂S poisoning leads to damage to the basal ganglia and other parts of the brain. Individuals with low TMT would therefore be inherently more susceptible to toxicity. High TMT levels, on the other hand, are linked with motor neurone disease. The reason for this is not clear, although S-methylation in CNS tissue of the dialkylsulphides (R₁-S-R₂). that are frequently found in such vegetables as cabbages and onions would give rise to thetins, which have the R₁-S⁺-R₂(R₃) structure. Some compounds of this type have been shown to act at neuromuscular junctions, so it is possible, if speculative, that high consumption of vegetables and an endogenously high TMT level could be a factor in the disease aetiology. Low TMT activity has also been found in rheumatoid arthritis (RA); such patients would therefore be expected to be more susceptible to thiol toxicity and often show adverse reactions to the drug D-penicillamine (β,β-dimethylcysteine).[9] Patients with SLE, however, had TMT-activity distributions which were almost exactly the same as controls, showing that the two diseases are metabolically different.[76] Thiopurine methyltransferases (TPMT) also exist and methylate a number of thiopurine drugs such as 6-mercaptopurine. Two alleles, for high and low methylation, have been found and the enzyme activity is inhibited by benzoic acid derivatives and by salicylate.[79]

N-Methylation

N-Methyltransferases (NMT) methylate a number of substrates including histamine, and pyridine derivatives such as nicotine, nicotinic acid (E375) and nicotinamide, a B-vitamin. The hepatic conversion of nicotinic acid or nicotinamide to the N-methyl

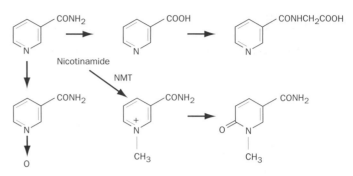

Fig. 32.8 Hepatic conversion of nicotinamide to N-methyl derivatives.

derivative gives a compound which has a charged pyridinium ring (Fig. 32.8). Pyridines and their derivatives are widely present in foods such as chocolate, tea, coffee, beer and peppermints and, being relatively lipid-soluble, are able to cross the blood–brain barrier. Methylation in the CNS would then produce charged pyridinium ions, which are highly water-soluble and so would not be able to rejoin the systemic circulation and would concentrate in brain tissue. This process could be analogous to that found with compounds such as MPTP (1-methyl-4-phenyl-2,3,5,6-tetrahydropyridine). This is converted in the CNS to the neurotoxic MPP⁺ (1-methyl-4-phenyl pyridinium ion) which can cause a Parkinsonian syndrome.[39] Generally, pyridines show low cytotoxicity but these N-methylated derivates are more damaging, at least in neuronal cell culture, probably because they mimic the structure of NAD⁺ and so block Complex 1 of the oxidative phosphorylation pathway.[27] This inhibition would reduce the supply of ATP to brain tissue, which is energetically very demanding, and the resulting energy deficit could lead to cell death.

Clinical correlaties

Reduced activity of Complex 1 and other complexes in oxidative phosphorylation has now been shown in Parkinson's disease and other neurological dysfunctions, including Alzheimer's disease.[27] A subset of patients with Parkinson's disease has been found to have increased *in vivo* N-methylation capacity, so that this may be a factor in the disease pathogenesis, especially if combined with a high intake of pyridine-containing foods.[81] Because methylation of a compound may greatly change its chemical properties, pharmacogenetic variations in methylation capacity would be expected, at least potentially, to show associations with clinical dysfunction. Current work on NMT suggests that phenotypic differences in N-methylation may be the result of mutations in the 5′-flanking region rather than in the gene itself.[68] In the long term, an understanding of genomics and proteomics will be helpful in predicting adverse reactions to food chemicals which involve any of the detoxification pathways.

SUMMARY

Elimination of food chemicals occurs *via* a number of metabolic routes which generally act to convert compounds into derivatives that are less toxic and more readily excreted. There is marked variation in individual capacity for these reactions and many of the enzyme pathways involved are polymorphic, with subsets of the population who may be inherently more susceptible to adverse reactions from environmental and dietary compounds.

REFERENCES

1 Acosta R, Granados J, Mourelle M, Perez-Alvarez V, Quezada E. Sulfite sensitivity: relationship between sulfite plasma levels and bronchospasm. *Ann Allergy* 1989; 62(5): 402–5.

2 Agarwal DP, Goedde HW. Pharmacogenetics of alcohol dehydrogenase (ADH). *Pharmacol Therap* 1990; 45: 69–83.

3 Alam Z, Coombes N, Waring RH, Williams AC, Steventon GB. Platelet sulphotransferase activity, plasma sulphate levels and sulphation capacity in patients with migraine and tension headache. *Cephalalgia* 1997; 17: 761–4.

4 Athavale NV, Srimivas CR. Contact cheilitis from propyl gallate in lipstick. *Contact Dermatitis* 1994; 30(5): 307.

5 Badawi AF, Stern SJ, Lang NP, Kadlubar FF. Cytochrome P450 and acetyltransferase expression as biomarkers of carcinogen: DNA adduct levels and human cancer susceptibility. *Progr Clin Biol Res* 1996; 395: 109–60.

6 Bamforth KJ, Jones AL, Roberts RC, Coughtrie MW. Common food additives are potent inhibitors of human liver 17-α-ethinyloestradiol and dopamine sulphotransferases. *Biochem Pharmacol* 1993; 46(10): 1713–20.

7 Barthelemy C, Bruneau N, Cottet-Eynard JM *et al*: Urinary free and conjugated catecholamines and metabolites in autistic children. *J Autism Dev Disord* 1988; 18: 583–91.

8 Boris M, Mandel FS. Food and additives are common causes of the attention deficit hyperactive disorder in children. *Ann Allergy* 1994; 72(5): 462–8.

9 Bradley H, Waring RH, Emery P. Reduced thiol methyl transferase activity in red blood cell membranes from patients with rheumatoid arthritis. *J Rheumatol* 1991; 18(12): 1787–9.

10 Bradley H, Gough A, Sokhi RS, Hassell A, Waring RH, Emery P. Sulphate metabolism is abnormal in patients with rheumatoid arthritis. *J Rheumatol* 1994; 21(7): 1192–6.

11 Brown GK, Scholem RD, Croll HB, Wraith JE, MacGill JJ. Sulfite oxidase deficiency. *Neurology* 1989; 39(2, Pt. 1): 252–7.

12 Burchell B, Coughtrie MWH. In: Kalow W (ed.) *UDP-Glucuronyl Transferases in Pharmacogenetics of Drug Metabolism*. Pergamon Press, Oxford, 1992; 195–226.

13 Caldwell JC, Hutt JA, Smith RL. The metabolism of aspirin in man: a population study. *Xenobiotica* 1986; 16: 239–49.

14 Cartwright RA, Adib R, Appleyard L *et al*. Cigarette smoking and bladder cancer: an epidemiological inquiry in West Yorkshire. *J Epidemiol Commun Health* 1983; 37: 256–63.

15 Chou HC, Lang NP, Kadlubar FF. Metabolic activation of the N-hydroxy derivative of the carcinogen 4-aminobiphenyl by human tissue sulfotransferases. *Carcinogenesis* 1995; 16(2): 413–7.

16 Corder EH, Buckley CE. Aspirin, salicylate, sulfite and tartrazine-induced bronchoconstriction. *J Clin Epidemiol* 1995; 48(10): 1269–75.

17 Coughtrie MWH. Sulphation catalysed by the human cytosolic sulphotransferases – chemical defence or molecular terrorism. *Human Exper Toxicol* 1996; 15(7): 547–55.

18 Davis PA, Leung P, Manns N *et al*. M4 and M9 antibodies in the overlap syndrome of primary biliary cirrhosis and chronic active hepatitis: epitopes or epiphenomena? *Hepatology* 1992; 16(5): 1128–36.

19 Deakin M, Elder J, Hendrickse C *et al*. Glutathione-S-transferase GSTTI genotypes and susceptibility to cancer: studies of interactions with GSTMI in lung, oral, gastric and colorectal cancers. *Carcinogenesis* 1996; 17(4): 881–4.

20 Emery P, Bradley H, Arthur V, Tunn B, Waring RH. Genetic factors influencing the outcome of early arthritis – the role of sulphoxidation status. *Brit J Rheumatol* 1992; 31: 449–51.

21 Feoli-Fonseca JC, Lambert M, Mitchell G *et al*. Chronic sodium benzoate therapy in children with inborn errors of urea synthesis. *Biochem Molec Med* 1996; 57(1): 31–6.

22 Fuglsang G, Madsen G, Halken S, Jorgenson S, Ostergaard PA, Osterballe O. Adverse reactions to food additives in children with atopic symptoms. *Allergy* 1994; 49(1): 31–7.

23 Ghazali RA, Waring RH. The effects of flavonoids on human phenolsulfotransferase. *Life Sciences* 1999; 65(16): 1625–32.

24 Ghazali R, Waring RH. Effects of flavonoids on glutathione-S-transferase in human blood platelets, rat liver, rat kidney and HT-29 colon adenocarcinoma cell-lines. *Med Sci Res* 1999; 27: 449–51.

25 Gordon C, Bradley H, Waring RH, Emery P. Abnormal sulphur-oxidation in SLE. *Lancet* 1992; 339(i): 25–6.

26 Greenblatt DJ, Sellers EM, Shader RL. Drug disposition in old age. *New Engl J Med* 1982; 306(18): 1081–8; Waring RH: unpublished observations.

27 Haas RH, Nasirian F, Nakamo K *et al*. Low platelet mitochondrial complex I and complex II/III activity in early untreated Parkinson's disease. *Ann Neurol* 1995; 37(6): 714–22.

28 Harris RM, Waring RH. Dietary modulation of human platelet phenolsulphotransferase activity. *Xenobiotica* 1996; 26(12): 1241–7.

29 Hernandez Garcia J, Garcia Selles J, Negro Alvarez JM, Pagan Aleman JA, Lopez Sanchez JD. Incidence of adverse reactions to additives. Our experience over 10 years. *Allergologia et Immunopathologia* 1994; 22(5): 233–42.

30 Higuchi S, Muramatsu T, Shigemore K *et al*. The relationship between low K_m aldehyde dehydrogenase phenotype and drinking behaviour in Japanese. *J. Stud Alcohol* 1992; 53: 170–5.

31 Ioannides C. Effect of diet and nutrition on the expression of cytochromes P450. *Xenobiotic* 1999; 29(2): 109–54.

32 Jorquera F, Culebras JM, Gonzalez-Gallego J. Influence of nutrition on liver oxidative metabolism. *Nutrition* 1996; 12(6): 442–7.

33 Ketterer B, Meyer DJ, Taylor JB, Pemble S, Coles B, Fraser G. GSTs and protection against oxidative stress. In: Hayes JD, Pickett CB, Mantle TJ (eds) *Glutathione-S-Transferases and Drug Resistance*. Taylor and Francis, London; 1990; 97–109.

34 Klovrza L, Waring RH, Williams AC. Sulphur-containing anion levels in biological fluids in neurological dysfunction. *Toxicol Lett (Suppl)* 1995; 78: 47.

35 Kumar A, Rawlings RD, Beaman DC. The mystery ingredients: sweeteners, flavourings, dyes and preservatives in preparations. *Pediatrics* 1993; 91(5): 927–33.

36 Kusper CB, Henton D: Glucuronidation. In: Jakoby WB (ed.) *Enzymatic Basis of Detoxication*, Vol. II, Academic Press, New York; 1980; 3–36.

37 Labbe P, Pelletier M, Omara FO, Girard D. Functional responses of human neutrophils to sodium sulfite (Na_2SO_3) *in vitro. Human Exper Toxicol* 1998; 17(ii): 600–5.

38 McKinnan RA, Nebert DW. Possible role of cytochromes P450 in lupus erythematosus and related disorders. *Lupus* 1994; 3(6): 473–8.

39 McNaught RS, Thull U, Carrupt PA *et al*. Nigral cell loss produced by infusion of isoquinoline derivatives structurally related to 1-methyl-4-phenyl-1,2,3,6-tetrahydropyridine. *Neurodegeneration* 1996; 5(3): 265–74.

40 Madesen C. Prevalence of food additive intolerance. *Human & Exp Toxicol* 1994; 13(6): 393–9.

41 Marazziti D, Bonucelli U, Nutt A. Platelet ^{3}H-imipramine binding and sulphotransferase activity in primary headache. *Cephalalgia* 1994; 14: 210–14.

42 Marazziti D, Palego L, Dellosso L, Balistini A, Cassano GB, Akiskal HS: Platelet sulphotransferase in different psychiatric disorders. *Psychiatry Res* 1996; 65(2): 73–8.

43 Mesina MJ, Persky V, Setchell KD, Barnes S. Soy intake and cancer risk: a review of the *in vitro* and *in vivo* data. *Nutrition and Cancer* 1994; 21(2): 113–31.

44 Minamoto T, Mai M, Ronai Z. Environmental factors as regulators and effects of multistep carcinogenesis. *Carcinogenesis* 1999; 20(4): 519–27.

45 Mitchell SC. The fish-odour syndrome. *Perspectives in Biology and Medicine* 1996; 39(4): 514–26.

46 Mitchell SC, Waring RH, Steventon GB. Variation in the S-oxidation of cysteine derivatives. In: Kalow W (ed.) *Pharmacogenetics of Drug Metabolism*. Pergamon Press, Oxford, 1992; 367–82.

47 Munoz FJ, Bellido J, Moyano JC, Alvarez M, Fonseca JL. Perioral urticaria from sodium benzoate in a toothpaste. *Contact Dermatitis* 1996; 35(1): 51.

48 Murch SH, MacDonald TT, Walker-Smith JH, Levin M, Lionetti P, Klein NJ. Disruption of sulphated glycosaminoglycans in intestinal inflammation. *Lancet* 1993; i: 711–14.

49 Nagao M, Fujita Y, Wakabayashi K, Sugimura T. Ultimate forms of mutagenic and carcinogenic heterocyclic amines produced by pyrolysis. *Biochem Biophys Res Commun* 1983; 114: 626–31.

50 Nakagawa Y, Nakajima K, Tayama S, Moldeus P. Metabolism and cytotoxicity of propyl gallate in isolated rat hepatocytes. *Molec Pharmacol* 1995; 47(5): 1021–7.

51 Obermayer-Straub P, Mannus MP. Cytochromes P450 and UDP-glucuronyl-transferases as hepatocellular autoantigens. *Bailléres Clinical Gastroenterology* 1996; 16(3): 501–32.

52 Olomu AB, Vickers CR, Waring RH *et al*. High incidence of poor sulphoxidation in patients with primary biliary cirrhosis. *New Eng J Med* 1988; 318: 1089–92.

53 Papageorgiou C, Corbet JP, Menezes-Brandao F, Pecegueiro M, Benezra C. Allergic contact dermatitis to garlic (*Allium sativum* L.). Identification of the allergens: the role of mono-di-and trisulfides present in garlic. *Arch Dermatol Res* 1983; 275: 229–34.

54 Parke DR, Sapota A. Chemical toxicity and reactive oxygen species. *Int J Occup Med Environ Health* 1996; 9(4): 331–40.

55 Price-Evans DA. *N-Acetyltransferase in Genetic Factors in Drug Therapy*. Cambridge University Press, Cambridge, 1993; 211–302.

56 Pirmohamed M, Madden S, Park BK. Idiosyncratic drug reactions. Metabolic bioactivation as a pathogenic mechanism. *Clin Pharmacokin* 1996; 31(3): 215–30.

57 Price-Evans DA. Alcohol and alcoholism. In: *Genetic Factors in Drug Therapy*. Cambridge University Press, Cambridge, 1993; 177–209.

58 Pemberton M, Yeoman CM, Clark A, Craig GT, Franklin CD, Gawkrodger DJ. Allergy to octyl gallate causing stomatitis. *Brit Dental J* 1993; 175(3): 106–8.

59 Reiss J, Christensen E, Dorche C. Molybdenum cofactor deficiency: first prenatal genetic analysis. *Prenatal Diagnosis* 1999; 19(4): 386–8.

60 Rhodes JM. Unifying hypothesis for inflammatory bowel disease: sticking the pieces together with sugar. *Lancet* 1995; i: 40–4.

61 Riley RJ, Leeder JS. *In vitro* analysis of metabolic predisposition to drug hypersensitivity reactions. *Clin Exptl Immunol* 1995; 99(1): 1–6.

62 Scadding G, Ayesh R, Brostoff J, Mitchell SC, Waring RH, Smith RL. Food sensitivity and poor S-oxidation. *Brit Med J* 1988; 297: 105–8; Waring RH, unpublished results.

63 Seow A, Shi CY, Chung FL *et al*. Urinary total isothiocyanate (ITC) in a population-based sample of middle-aged and older Chinese in Singapore: relationship with dietary total (ITC and GST011/T1/P genotypes. *Cancer Epidemiol Biomarkers and Prevention* 1998; 7(9): 775–81.

64 Schapowal AG, Simon HU, Schmitz-Schumann M. Phenomenology, pathogenesis, diagnosis and treatment of aspirin-sensitive rhinosinusitis. *Acta Oto-Rhino-Laryngologica Belgica* 1995; 49(3): 235–50.

65 Sims E. Drug-induced immune-complex disease. *Complem Inflamm* 1989; 6: 119–26.

66 Slatteny MH, Potter JD, Ma KN, Caan BJ, Leppet M, Samowitz W. Western diet, family history of colorectal cancer, NAT2 GSTT1 and risk of colon cancer. *Cancer Causes and Control* 2000; 11(i): 1–8.

67 Slomiany BL, Murty VLN, Piotrowski J, Grabska M, Slomiany A. Glycosulfatase activity of *Helicobacter pylori* toward human gastric mucosa. *Ann J Gastroenterol* 1992; 87(9): 1132–7.

68 Smith ML, Barnett D, Bennett P *et al*. A direct correlation between nicotinamide N-methyltransferase activity and protein levels using human liver cytosol. *Biochim Biophys Acta* 1998; 1422: 238–44.

69 Steventon GB, Mitchell SC, Waring RH. Human metabolism of paracetamol at different dose levels. *Drug Metab Drug Interact* 1996; 13(2): 111–18.

70 Stroombergen MCMJ, Waring RH, Bennett P, Williams AC. Determination of the GSTMI gene deletion frequency in Parkinson's disease by Allele Specific PCR. *Parkinsonism and Related Disorders* 1996; 2(3): 151–4.

71 Sundaran RS, Van Loon JA, Tucker R, Weinshilboum RM. Sulfation pharmacogenetics: correlation of human platelet and small intestinal phenolsulfotransferase. *Clin Pharm Therap* 1989; 46: 501–9.

72 Testud F, Matray D, Lambert R *et al*. Respiratory manifestations after exposure to sulfurous anhydride in wine-cellar workers. *Revue des Maladies Respiratoires* 2000; 17(1): 103–8.

73 Van Jersel MI, Verhagen H, Van Bladeren PJ. The role of biotransformation in dietary (anti) carcinogenesis. *Mutation Res* 1999; 3(1–2): 259–70.

74 Walter-Sack I, Klotz U. Influence of diet and nutritional status on drug metabolism. *Clin Pharmacokin* 1996; 31(1): 47–64.

75 Waring RH. Sulfur-sulfur compounds. In: Mitchell SC (ed) *Biological Interactions of Sulfur Compounds*. Taylor and Francis, London, 1996; 145–73.

76 Waring RH, Emery P. Genetic factors predicting persistent disease: the role of defective enzyme systems. *Baillière's Clin Rheumatol* 1992; 6(2): 337–50.

77 Waring RH, Klovrza L. Sulphur metabolism in autism. *J Nutrit Environ Med* 2000; 10: 25–32.

78 Waring RH, Sturman SG, Steventon GB, Smith MCG, Heafield MTE, Williams AC. S-Methylation in motor neurone disease and Parkinson's Disease. *Lancet* 1989; ii: 356–7.

79 Weinshilboum RM. Methyltransferase pharmacogenetics. In: Kalow W (ed.) *Pharmacogenetics of Drug Metabolism*. Pergamon Press, Oxford, 1992; 179–94.

80 Whalen R, Bayer TD. Human glutathione-S-transferases. *Seminars in Liver Disease* 1998; 18(4): 345–58.

81 Williams AC, Waring RH, Parsons RB, Ramsden DB. Idiopathic Parkinson's disease: a genetic and environmental model. *Adv Neurol* 1999; 80: 215–19.

82 Wolfe CR, Mahmood A, Henderson CJ *et al*. Modulation of the cytochrome P450 system as a mechanism of chemoprotection. *IARC Scientific Publications* 1996; 139: 165–73.

83 Yamane T, Nakatami H, Kikuoka N *et al*. Inhibitory effects and toxicity of green tea polyphenols for gastrointestinal carcinogenesis. *Cancer* 1996; 77(8 suppl): 1662–7.

Chapter 33

Exorphins and other biologically active peptides derived from diet

Michael L.G.Gardner

INTRODUCTION

The term 'exorphins' (exogenous morphine-like compounds, cp. their endogenous counterparts, the endorphins) was invented by Zioudrou et al.[165] in 1979 when they reported that digestion of wheat gluten or α-casein with pepsin *in vitro* could yield peptides with opiate-like activity. The presence of naloxone-reversible activity against a guinea pig ileum in an enzymatic digest of casein had been reported by Wajda et al.[159] As explained below, these findings have repeatedly been confirmed in other laboratories; a number of the peptides concerned have been sequenced and synthesized, and many of their physiological and potentially pathophysiological properties have been characterized. Though opioid activities have been most widely documented, the likelihood of other biological activities in peptides of dietary origin being relevant should not be ignored. It is noteworthy that Zioudrou et al. observed that pepsin hydrolysates of gluten and casein contained *many* opioid peptides, and Huebner et al.[70] corroborated this for gluten. Most of the known exorphins are opiate

agonists, but antagonists (such as the casoxins) have also been characterized.

The discoveries of the enkephalins, in 1975 by Hughes and Kosterlitz, as the natural ligands for morphine receptors,[71–73] and then of the endorphins, were rapidly recognized as key milestones in neurobiology.[1,156] However, the extent of the numerous key regulatory roles played by peptides, including these opioid peptides, was not yet fully appreciated: neuronal, endocrine and immune regulation and the integration of these mechanisms are now recognized to rely heavily on endogenous peptide signalling.[13,16,119] Now that opioid receptors have been characterized at the molecular level, structural similarities to immunoglobulins and cell-adhesion molecules are recognized.[89] The scope for interference by exogenous peptides, such as ones derived from diet, is substantial and will be discussed below. Behaviour, neural and immune function are clearly at risk. Hence, as predicted by Dohan[35,37,40] and by Zioudrou and Klee,[164] these mechanisms are now candidates to explain ill-understood effects of diet on mental health and behaviour.

B

465

AGONIST/ANTAGONIST ACTIONS OF EXORPHINS

It should be appreciated that exogenous peptides could interfere directly, e.g. by acting either as agonists or as antagonists of peptide-mediated processes, or indirectly, e.g. by inhibiting metabolism of endogenous peptides. Hence, effects of diet-derived peptides can, in theory at least, be either acute short-term or long-term effects. Since it now seems inevitable that peptides must play key roles in early neurodevelopmental processes and immunodevelopment, these particular effects are not necessarily reversible at later stages. These considerations must be borne in mind when interpreting the consequences, or lack thereof, of dietary changes and the speed at which changes may be effected.

BIOLOGICALLY ACTIVE PEPTIDES

It is clear that many proteins contain amino acid sequences corresponding to biologically active peptides: a search through an early database of protein sequences led to the conclusion that the generation of bioactive peptides during digestion was 'likely' rather than 'rare',[53] a prediction that proves now to be accurate. If these are produced during food digestion and if they are subsequently absorbed, they have the potential to modulate or interfere with cellular regulatory processes. Many peptides have a remarkably high biological potency, so that absorption of only small amounts is necessary to elicit responses. The consequences of absorption of macromolecules of botulinum toxin provide a good illustration of this principle and should dispel any preconceptions about molecular size being a barrier to absorption: the potency is such that absorption of only a few molecules (molecular weight about 10^6 daltons) is enough to cause lethal consequences.

Further, experience now shows the catalogue of activities elicited by many peptides to be so extensive, with many unsuspected activities being discovered, that it is risky to attempt to predict empirically the consequences of absorption of particular peptides or to assume that certain structures will be inactive.

PHYSIOLOGICAL SIGNALLING BY FOOD-DERIVED PEPTIDES

Although the focus here is on harmful effects of food-derived peptides, it should be recognized that some of these peptides may be normal physiological signalling molecules with roles in regulation of gastrointestinal function, satiety and hormonal response to food.[104–106,134,135] Indeed, Morley invented the term 'formones' to signify that these may be natural 'food hormones'. The two proteins most strongly implicated, gluten and casein, have of course been components of staple foods for many populations over centuries, and milk is a key substance aiding the newborn to make the transition to extra-uterine life. In the belief that milk-derived peptides may be beneficial, their commercial production as food supplements ('nutraceuticals') or as drugs has been considered.[98,99,133] Gluten, it must be noted, is also commonly added to processed foodstuffs so that its covert consumption can be significant. Although gluten and casein elimination from diet may be beneficial in some circumstances discussed below, it is conceivable that their removal without these circumstances might be disadvantageous if Morley's thesis is valid.

Previous reviews on exorphins have been provided by Zioudrou and Klee[164] and by Paroli,[114] on biologically active or regulatory peptides from milk proteins by Meisel,[100,133] and Nyberg and Brantl have edited a monograph on β-casomorphins and related peptides.[107]

A MODEL FOR GENERATION AND ACTION OF EXORPHINS

The generation of peptides from food proteins in the gastro-intestinal tract, especially the upper small intestine, is shown in Figure 33.1. Some of these peptides are active exorphins. Although the majority of the protein will be absorbed in the form of free amino acids, some partial digestion products, peptides including exorphins, are absorbed in intact form. These are subject to clearance by a variety of peptide hydrolase (peptidase) enzymes in blood and in peripheral tissues, especially liver and kidney, and they may be taken into peripheral tissues including brain, or they may act on cell-surface receptors to elicit biological or pharmacological effects: effects on the nervous and immune systems are especially relevant in the context of food intolerance. Peptides are excreted into the urine. Since many peptides are concentrated in the urine, and since urine is relatively free from peptidase activity, this fluid is particularly useful for detection and analysis of peptides. However, it is not straightforward to distinguish exogenous (food-derived) peptides from endogenous ones. These individual steps will now be considered.

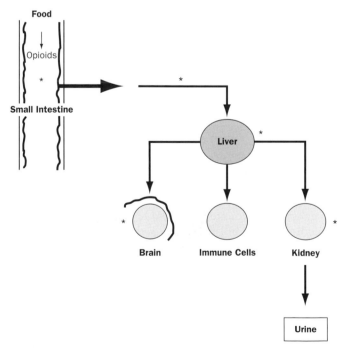

Fig. 33.1 A model for the generation of opioid peptides, exorphins, from dietary proteins and their subsequent effects on peripheral tissues, especially the nervous and immune systems. Under normal circumstances, peptides are subject to aggressive hydrolytic conditions by peptidases (denoted by *) in blood and many tissues. Urinary peptides can be measured; they originate from both exogenous sources and turnover of endogenous proteins.

GENERATION OF EXORPHINS DURING DIGESTION

Table 33.1 shows proteins that are known to yield exorphins. By far, the most information is available for those from gluten (gluten exorphins) and α- and β-caseins (casomorphins), and it is pertinent to recall that wheat and milk are also implicated in coeliac disease (gluten enteropathy) and cow's milk intolerance. Indeed, the molecular aetiology of coeliac disease is still not understood and the debate about the relative roles of enzyme- and immune-mediated mechanisms, and the relevance of gluten-induced increased intestinal permeability has much in common with current debates about a possible mechanism for gluten involvement in autism and schizophrenia.

β-casomorphin

At the same time as Zioudrou, Streaty and Klee described the production of opioid peptides (and other active peptides) during pepsin digestion of gluten and α-casein,[164,165] Brantl et al.[19] reported similar peptides – namely β-casomorphins – arising from β-casein. The β-casomorphin was sequenced and found to be a heptapeptide corresponding to residues 60–66 of β-casein; it was highly resistant to further enzymic cleavage, even by pronase or carboxypeptidase.[68] Additional work showed that the related hexa-, penta-, and tetrapeptides derived by removal of the C-terminal amino acids were all active, especially at μ-receptors, with the pentapeptide (Tyr-Pro-Phe-Pro-Gly) being the most potent.[18] In these peptides, the N-terminal tyrosine appears to be obligatory.[28,133] They also have some affinity for δ-receptors and some, but less, for κ-receptors.[79] Loukas et al. sequenced the hepta- and hexapeptides from residues 90–96 and 90–95, respectively, of α-casein and confirmed the same opioid activity in synthetic peptides.[90] Table 33.2 summarizes the sequences of some exorphins.

Gluten exorphins

Gluten exorphins were found to be of similar potency to met-enkephalin in mouse vas deferens and in a competitive binding assay in rat brain, and Zioudrou and Klee commented on the extraordinary potency of these agonists: the exorphin derived from α-casein was much less potent.[164] The peptides were resistant to trypsin and chymotrypsin activity, which would favour their survival in the gastrointestinal tract.

Proteins known to yield exorphins or related biologically active peptides on partial digestion
Albumin
α-Casein
β-Casein
κ-Casein
Cytochrome b
Gluten/glutenin
Haemoglobin
Lactalbumin
Lactoferrin
Lactoglobulin

Table 33.1 Proteins known to yield exorphins or related biologically active peptides on partial digestion.

Amino acid sequences of enkephalin and some known exorphin peptides	
Met-enkephalin	Tyr-Gly-Gly-Phe-Met
Leu-enkephalin	Tyr-Gly-Gly-Phe-Leu
Dynorphin (1–9)	Tyr-Gly-Gly-Phe-Leu-Arg-Arg-Ile-Arg
Bovine β-casomorphin-7 (β-CM7)	Tyr-Pro-Phe-Pro-Gly-Pro-Ile
Bovine β-CM6	Tyr-Pro-Phe-Pro-Gly-Pro
Bovine β-CM5	Tyr-Pro-Phe-Pro-Gly
Bovine β-CM4	Tyr-Pro-Phe-Pro
Bovine β-CM3	Tyr-Pro-Phe
Morphiceptin	Tyr-Pro-Phe-Pro-NH$_2$
Human β-casomorphin-5 (β-CM5)	Tyr-Pro-Phe-Val-Glu
Human β-CM4	Tyr-Pro-Phe-Val
α-Gliadin peptide	Tyr-Pro-Glu-Pro-Glu-Pro-Phe
Gluten B5 exorphin	Tyr-Gly-Gly-Trp-Leu
Gluten B4 exorphin	Tyr-Gly-Gly-Trp
Gluten A5 exorphin	Gly-Tyr-Tyr-Pro-Thr
Gluten A4 exorphin	Gly-Tyr-Tyr-Pro
Gluten exorphin C	Tyr-Pro-Ile-Ser-Leu
Cytochrophin-5	Tyr-Pro-Phe-Trp-Ile
Haemorphin-5	Tyr-Pro-Trp-Thr-Gln
α-Lactorphin	Tyr-Gly-Leu-Phe
β-Lactorphin	Tyr-Leu-Leu-Phe
α-Casein	Arg-Tyr-Leu-Gly-Tyr-Leu-Glu
Casoxin†	Ser-Arg-Tyr-Pro-Ser-Tyr
Casoxin A	Tyr-Pro-Ser-Tyr-Gly-Leu-Asn
Casoxin B	Tyr-Pro-Tyr-Tyr
Casoxin C	Tyr-Ile-Pro-Ile-Gln-Tyr-Val-Leu-Ser-Arg
Lactoferroxin A†	Tyr-Leu-Gly-Ser-Gly-Tyr
Lactoferroxin B	Arg-Tyr-Tyr-Gly-Tyr
Lactoferroxin C	Lys-Tyr-Leu-Gly-Pro-Gln-Tyr

† The casoxins and lactoferroxins, derived from κ-casein and lactoferrin respectively, are opiate antagonists.

Table 33.2 Amino acid sequences of enkephalin and some known exorphin peptides.

The gluten exorphins also have been sequenced,[49,50] and it is most striking that one of these sequences A5 (Gly-Tyr-Tyr-Pro-Thr) occurs 15 times in the primary structure of glutenin, a component of gluten (Fig. 33.2). This peptide was reported to be highly specific for δ-receptors. The most potent gluten exorphin, named B5 by Fukudome and Yoshikawa, was Tyr-Gly-Gly-Trp-Leu, which has the same 3 N-terminal amino acids as enkephalin, and their potencies against guinea pig ileum are closely similar.[49] A further sequence, Tyr-Pro-Ile-Ser-Leu, named exorphin C,[50] was also active in the classical guinea pig ileum and mouse vas deferens bioassays. It is thus clear that gluten is potentially a very rich source of opioid peptides.

Casoxins: opiate antagonists

Worthy of note, although much less documented, are the production of casoxins from κ-casein, which are opiate antagonists, and several immunostimulating peptides from casein.[29,30,133] Lactoferroxins are opiate antagonists obtained by peptic digestion of human lactoferrin, with lactferroxin A most active against μ-receptors and lactoferroxins B and C most active against

Food components and their reactions

```
         signal ◄─────────────────► mature
                       20                          40                                    60
MAKRLVLFVAVVVALVALTVA│EGEASEQLQCERELQELQERELKACQQVMDQQLRDISPE
                     80                       100                          120
CHPVVVSPVAGQYEQQIVVPKGGSFYPGETTPPQQLQQRIFWGIPALLKRYYPSVTSPQQ
              140                          160                          180
VSYYPGQASPQRPGQGQQPGQGQQSGQGQQ GYYPT SPQQPGQWQQPEQGQP GYYPT SPQQ
              200                          220                          240
PGQLQQPAQGQQPGQGQQGRQPGQGQP GYYPT SSQLQPGQLQQPAQGQQGQQPGQGQQGQ
              260                          280                          300
QLGQGQQ GYYPT SLQQSGQGQP GYYPT SLQQLGQGQS GYYPT SPQQPGQGQQPGQLQQPA
              320                          340                          360
QGQQPEQGQQGQQPGQGQQGQQPGQGQQPGQGQP GYYPT SPQQSGQGQP GYYPT SSQQPT
              380                          400                          420
QSQQPGQGQQGQQVGQGQQAQQPGQGQQPGQGQP GYYPT SPLQSGQGQPGYYLTSPQQSG
              440                          460                          480
QGQQPGQLQQSAQGQKGQQPGQGQQPGQGQQGQQPGQGQQGQQPGQGQP GYYPT SPQQSG
              500                          520                          540
QGQQPGQWQQPGQGQP GYYPT SPLQPGQGQPGYDPTSPQQPGQGQQPGQLQQPAQGQQGQ
              560                          580                          600
QLAQGQQGQQPAQVQQGQQPAQGQQGQQLGQGQQGQQPGQGQQPAQGQQGQQPGQGQQGQ
              620                          640                          660
QPGQGQQPGQGQPWYYPTSPQESGQGQQPGQWQQPGQWQQPGQGQPGYYLTSPLQLGQGQ
              680                          700                          720
Q GYYPT SLQQPGQGQQPGQWQQSGQGQH GYYPT SPQLSGQGQRPGQWLQPGQGQQ GYYPT
              740                          760                          780
SPQQSGQGQQLGQWLQPGQGQQ GYYPT SLQQTGQGQQSGQGQQGYYSSYHVSVEHQAASL
              800
KVAKAQQLAAQLPAMCRLEGGDEALSASQ
```

Fig. 33.2 The amino acid sequence of glutenin with gluten exorphin A5/4 shown boxed and homologous sequences of gluten exorphin A4 shown underlined. Note the very rich source of these exorphins in glutenin. (From Fukudome and Yoshikawa[49] with permission.)

κ-receptors.[149] Opioid peptides from haemoglobin have also been found in marathon runners.[62] These findings emphasize the principle that dietary proteins are an extremely rich source of potentially bioactive peptides whose actions are neither easy to predict nor to assay unless one has a preconceived activity to seek. Casomorphins or similar peptides may also be formed bacterially, e.g. during cheese production.[65]

While these studies have shown that exorphins and casomorphins can be generated under experimental conditions, especially by the action of pepsin (the major gastric protease) *in vitro*, they do not indicate whether they arise *in vivo* during assimilation of a meal. Findings on this question have been controversial and contradictory, although enough evidence has now been amassed to support the view that production of active peptides does occur in the small intestine *in vivo* under physiological conditions, and indeed these peptides can be absorbed (see below).

EXORPHIN ACTION *IN VIVO*

Fukudome and colleagues have reported that both oral and intravenous administration of the gluten exorphin A5 peptide potentiated the postprandial insulin level in rats, this effect being reversed by naloxone.[48] Hence, it is likely that the oral exorphin exerted its effect on insulin release after its absorption rather than from within the gastrointestinal lumen.

Although Teschemacher *et al.*[150] were unable to detect casomorphins in plasma of cows or calves after milk ingestion, and Petrilli *et al.*[117] believed that casomorphins were unlikely to reach significant concentrations *in vivo*, subsequent work did show the presence of casomorphins in plasma of young calves after milk ingestion.[157] Svedberg *et al.*[148] did find immunoreactive casomorphins in human small intestine during milk consumption. Similar findings, but also confirming opioid activity, have been reported for small intestinal contents of minipigs ingesting casein.[97,100] Recently, the presence of active antithrombotic peptides in duodenum and peripheral plasma of healthy adult (and infant) humans eating milk or yoghurt has been confirmed.[26,27] Singh *et al.*[139] found immunoreactive casomorphins in plasma of young dogs, but not adult dogs, suggesting that absorption might cease during intestinal maturation. Technical difficulties in preventing hydrolysis during blood collection clearly can lead to erroneous conclusions about the presence of peptides in blood samples.

GASTROINTESTINAL ABSORPTION OF INTACT PEPTIDES

The model for exorphin action shown in Fig. 33.1 depends on absorption of intact peptides in the gastrointestinal tract. The subject of protein digestion and absorption has been comprehensively reviewed by the late D M Matthews,[94] and Gardner has reviewed absorption of intact peptides.[51,52,55–57,60] A major obstacle to acceptance of dietary peptides as a source of ill-health and as a mechanism of interference with normal regulation has been the old dogma that proteins are completely digested to free amino acids before absorption. The demise of this dogma was started by the late R B Fisher in 1954,[45,46] but it was not until 1968 that proof of peptide absorption by intestinal brush-border transport systems was obtained:[93,95,96] even then, it was understood that absorbed peptides were further hydrolysed to free amino acids inside enterocytes before entry to the circulation. Subsequent work by a wide range of approaches *in vivo* and *in vitro*, in animals and in humans, has, however, shown beyond doubt that absorption of small amounts of intact peptides and even of large proteins can occur in healthy individuals – see reviews by Gardner.[52,56,59] The long-held reluctance to accept that intact peptides can be absorbed has been fuelled by the view that oral administration of peptide drugs such as insulin is unsuccessful: however, it should be stressed that nearly all investigations into insulin absorption, both in animals and in humans, have provided evidence for absorption.[56] It is the small extent of absorption together with a very large inter-subject variability that hinders the oral route of administration for insulin. The variability observed may indicate that a highly variable fate for dietary peptides may be expected, and the fate of exorphins generated during digestion seems to conform to this prediction.

The two major 'barriers' to peptide absorption are hydrolysis within the gastrointestinal tract and passage across the intestinal epithelium.[52,56,87] As outlined below, there are several routes across the epithelium that are accessible to many peptides, but factors hindering peptide hydrolysis – crucial for survival of intact peptides – are less well understood. Similar considerations apply to passage across the endothelial blood–brain barrier if peptides are to gain access to the central nervous system.

OBSERVATIONS ON PEPTIDE ABSORPTION

Although many different approaches have been applied to confirm that intact peptides can cross the gastrointestinal 'barrier', the following observations on absorption of carnosine (β-alanyl-histidine) demonstrate the process and emphasize some pitfalls in analysis of absorbed peptides, in body fluids. Healthy human subjects ingested 4 g of this dipeptide and the subsequent urinary output was measured over 5 hours.[58] Carnosine, which is present in chicken meat, simply serves as a useful model peptide which can easily be quantified. Figure 33.3 shows the urinary output for 6 subjects. It is clear that there is substantial absorption, up to 14% of the peptide being excreted in intact form, and considerable variability between subjects with excretion varying between 1.2% and 14.0%. There was no correlation between the urinary recovery of carnosine and the absorption of the intestinal permeability markers, rhamnose and lactulose, suggesting that factors other than permeability were rate-limiting for recovery. Initially,

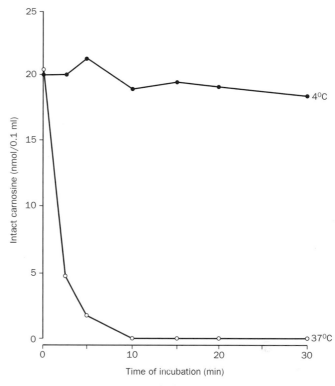

Fig. 33.4 Time course of disappearance of intact carnosine after addition to plasma *in vitro*. Samples were incubated either at 37°C (○) or on ice (•). (Reproduced from Gardner *et al*.[58] with permission.)

paradoxically, no intact carnosine could be detected in plasma even though substantial amounts were passing to urine. Then it became clear that blood possessed substantial carnosine hydrolase activity: Figure 33.4 shows the time-course of disappearance of carnosine after addition to plasma *in vitro*, conforming to a half-life of about 2 min. The variable urinary recovery of the peptide between subjects was then found to correlate significantly with the plasma carnosinase enzymic activity, confirming that post-absorptive clearance of the peptide, rather than its absorption, was limiting for its systemic fate (Fig. 33.5).

Although absorption of intact peptides is now proven beyond doubt, the amount of dietary protein that may enter the circulation in this form is still open to conjecture: it is, however, clear that the extent of this process can be augmented in a variety of pathological circumstances. As emphasized above, the potency and biological half-lives of absorbed peptides are more important than the actual amounts absorbed. Enzymic hydrolase activity, both gastrointestinal and systemic, against exorphins seems likely to be a dominating factor in determining the physiological and pathological consequences of dietary exorphins.

MECHANISMS OF PEPTIDE ABSORPTION

Peptides can probably cross the gastrointestinal 'barrier' by at least three mechanisms:

1   A transcellular route involving diffusion across the brush border membrane. This is likely to be relevant only for peptides with a high lipid solubility but, as aromatic amino acids are hydrophobic, this is no bar to absorption.

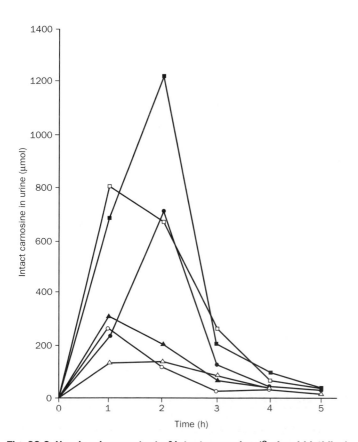

Fig. 33.3 Hourly urinary output of intact carnosine (β-alanyl-histidine) following ingestion of 4 g of this peptide by 6 healthy subjects. Each symbol represents a different subject. (Reproduced from Gardner *et al*.[58] with permission.)

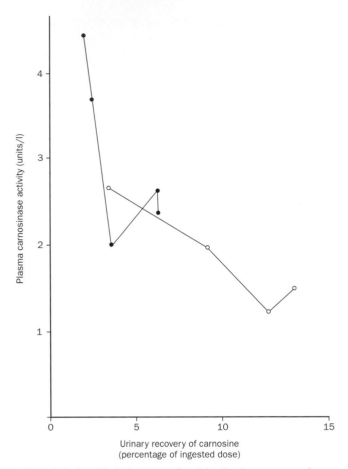

Fig. 33.5 Relationship between each subject's plasma carnosinase activity and the urinary recovery of intact carnosine during the 5 h after ingestion of 4 g of carnosine. The correlation is significant ($P = 0.004$). (•), 'exercisers'; ○, 'non-exercisers'. (Reproduced from Gardner *et al.*[58] with permission.)

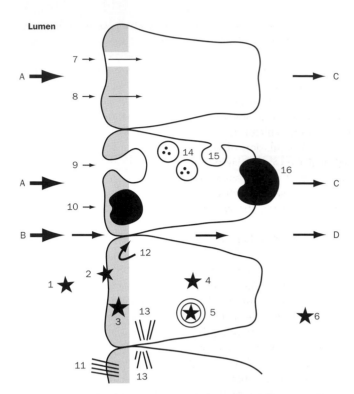

Fig. 33.6 Routes and mechanisms for absorption of intact peptides and proteins across the small intestinal epithelium. Transcellular transport is via route A to C, with hydrolysis at 3 (brush border) and 4 (cytosol), and may involve aqueous pores (7), a lipid-soluble route (8), receptor-mediated endocytosis (9) to phagolysosomes (14) and subsequent exocytosis (15), carrier-mediated transport for di-, tri-, and possibly larger, peptides (10), and a less-well characterized basolateral transport carrier (16). Paracellular transport is via route B to D through the tight junctions (12) which are subject to physiological regulation via the cytoskeletal mechanism (13). Major sites of hydrolysis are also shown (★): 1, luminal hydrolysis by pancreatic proteases and peptidases and from extruded mucosal cells, also possibly from mucosal secretions; 2, membrane-adherent enzymes; 3, brush border peptidases; 4, cytoplasmic peptidases; 5, lysosomal hydrolases; and 6, post-absorptive peptidases. (Reproduced from Gardner,[56] which provides a fuller explanation, with permission.)

2 A transcellular route involving carrier-mediated transport (carriers in the brush border membrane are well characterized; those in the basolateral membrane are identified but not fully characterized). Phagocytosis of intact proteins is a variation on this process, with binding to vesicles rather than carriers being involved, which is particularly important in the M cells (microfold cells) overlying Peyer's patches. This route may be accessible also to intact peptides.

3 A paracellular route through the inaptly named 'tight junctions', which are now believed to be under physiological control.

These routes and mechanisms are summarized in Fig. 33.6, which shows also the intestinal sites of proteolysis and peptide hydrolysis that are likely to be of critical importance to the survival of intact exorphins.

'Opening' of tight junctions

Important observations on large-scale absorption of synthetic octapeptides by rats have been made by Pappenheimer, and these focus on solvent drag drawing intact hydrolysis-resistant peptides through the tight junctions during water absorption.[111] A strong case has been made for the paracellular route being under physiological regulation, so that the tight junctions are 'opened' via cytoskeletal

filaments during absorption of a meal: luminal glucose specifically opens the junctions, decreases the transepithelial electrical impedance and permits the electron-microscopic visualization of a haem-conjugated peptide (molecular weight 40 kDa) in the intercellular space.[6,91,110,112] It is of interest that Lee has shown that a synthetic peptide (Pz-peptide: phenylazobenzyloxycarbonyl-Pro-Leu-Gly-Pro-D-Arg) can increase paracellular permeability,[88,162,163] and this raises the possibility that both glucose and peptides liberated during digestion could stimulate the opening of the paracellular pathway across the intestinal epithelium and permit the ingress of exorphins and other biologically active peptides.

PEPTIDE DIGESTIBILITY AND ABSORPTION

An early study on absorption of the N-terminal tetrapeptide sequence of the enkephalins across everted sacs of rat ileum showed no transport of Tyr-Gly-Gly-Phe, but the hydrolysis-resistant analogue L-Tyr-D-Ala-Gly-L-Phe (also opiate-active) was transported.[130] A subsequent study *in vitro* showed that absorption of the latter was enhanced by the presence of bestatin, a peptidase inhibitor, although active transport was thought not to occur.[74] These emphasize the potential importance of peptide digestibility and gastrointestinal digestive activity in determining the fate of diet-derived peptides. However, many intestinal preparations *in vitro* are now recognized to be unreliable for investigation of peptide absorption because of inadequate continuous oxygenation, which is necessary for unimpaired physiological viability and regulation of the paracellular route, and because of high leakage of cellular peptidases.[112,113,118,138] These problems, like those of post-absorptive hydrolysis during experiments *in vivo*, impose severe restrictions on interpretation of many experiments on peptide absorption.

ASSESSMENT OF INTESTINAL PERMEABILITY

Permeability has been reviewed in Chapter 15 and elsewhere.[66,103,116,152] The old concept of the gastrointestinal epithelium acting as an absolute 'barrier' to ingress of foreign materials is no longer tenable in the light of knowledge of the range of macromolecules, including intact proteins,[54,56,59] and even inert particles that can be absorbed, and since it is now recognized that intestinal permeability or 'leakiness' can be increased in many gastrointestinal diseases and in some systemic conditions. A 'leaky' gut will clearly be more liable to admit intact exorphins to the circulation, although intestinal and post-absorptive digestion will still influence the availability of peptides for passage across the gut and the subsequent fate (and half-life) of absorbed molecules, respectively. It is of particular interest that increased intestinal permeability has been reported in some patients with autism and in some schizophrenics, conditions in which hyperpeptiduria has been found and in which exorphins have been implicated (see below). Elevated intestinal permeability in coeliac disease is well documented, and hyperpeptidaemia and hyperpeptiduria in this condition have now been confirmed,[75,81,126] although the nature of the peptides still requires investigation. It is also noteworthy that André and colleagues found transient, chromoglycate-suppressible, increases in permeability in response to specific foods suspected as food allergens.[2,3] Similarly, treated coeliac patients (although not healthy control subjects) rapidly show increased intestinal permeability after a gluten challenge.[63] This may point to a mechanism where a food allergen promotes absorption of active exorphins, hence permitting a broad spectrum of systemic sequelae. However, it is unlikely that increased permeability by itself is directly causal for the mental and behavioural problems that may be exorphin-mediated, since many gastrointestinal and systemic disorders are accompanied by increased intestinal permeability without apparent psychiatric or behavioural consequences.

INTESTINAL CLOSURE

It is worth stressing that important changes in intestinal barrier function normally occur around birth. Cessation of transmission of immunoglobulins across the intestine, known as 'closure' is a complex series of events, not just a sealing of physical pores or gaps in the epithelium, involving hormonal mediation – see reviews by Baintner,[8] Brambell[17] and Walker.[160] Delays in 'closure' or incompleteness of this will permit entry to the body of abnormal amounts of some molecules whose entry would normally be restricted, and these may elicit biological activity during the critical early neurodevelopmental stages.

Perinatal absorption of exorphins

It is not known whether entry of excess exorphins in the first few weeks of life occurs, although the findings of Singh *et al.*[139] may suggest this. The possibility of effects on early development, especially of the nervous and immune systems, merits consideration. Absorption of intact α-lactalbumin (confirmed to be intact by radioimmunoassay combined with size-exclusion chromatography) has been shown to be greater in pre-term infants than in a full-term group, though it is notable that some absorption continued to occur after birth.[7,128]

Infant feeding practices

It is interesting that a reduction in childhood coeliac disease since the 1970s may be associated with changed infant feeding practices, especially the later introduction of gluten,[21] and that the onset of gluten enteropathy and increased intestinal permeability in Irish (red) setter dogs (possibly the only non-human species to be gluten-sensitive) is minimized by use of a cereal-free diet from birth.[64] Hence, early exposure during intestinal maturation to gluten may predispose to excessive intestinal permeability and/or coeliac disease in genetically susceptible individuals: the possibility of similar mechanisms influencing absorption of exorphins deserves consideration and may point to a need to exercise caution in the composition of infant feeds in families where exorphin-mediated dysfunction is suspected.

CLEARANCE OF ABSORBED EXORPHINS AND OTHER PEPTIDES FROM THE CIRCULATION

As explained above, entry to the circulation of biologically potent molecules will elicit little effect if they have a very short lifetime. Many tissues, including blood, are abundant in peptidase activity. Although numerous peptidase enzymes are known which may be active in the physiological metabolism of neuropeptides, and the view is that these enzymes act in concert rather than that specific enzymes act on each endogenous neuropeptide,[153–155] knowledge is still incomplete about their actions and relevance. The more general topic of peptide turnover seldom receives consideration.[57] Hence, it should be no surprise that information about the clearance of exorphins and other peptides of exogenous origin is scanty.

Circulating and liver peptidases may have a physiological function as scavengers of absorbed peptides – e.g. to prevent exorphins from interfering with endorphin-mediated processes – the liver being the 'first-pass' organ after gastrointestinal absorption. Hence, any defects in these enzymes may lead to dysfunction. Although only a few genetic deficiencies of peptidases have been reported,[15] this may reflect the fact that the potential significance of such defects is scarcely recognized and so they are not normally sought.

Although the peptidase(s) responsible for exorphin clearance is/are not known with certainty, Kreil *et al.*[82] concluded that an enzyme similar to dipeptidyl peptidase IV in plasma was active against casomorphins, and purified dipeptidyl peptidase IV from human lymphocytes was subsequently confirmed to be active against casomorphins.[102] Leibach and colleagues also found that rat renal dipeptidyl peptidase IV was active against these peptides. Further, they found that a Japanese strain of Fischer 344 rats specifically lacked this enzyme and that these animals excreted large amounts of prolyl and hydroxyprolyl peptides.[151] The rats also excreted large amounts of a tetrapeptide similar to casomorphin. These findings strongly implicate dipeptidyl peptidase IV in the metabolism of casomorphins, although other peptidases may also be relevant, and they draw attention to the existence of deficiencies (presumably genetic) of this enzyme.

Peptidases and β-casomorphins

Dipeptidyl peptidase IV is a serine peptidase (EC 3.4.14.5), inhibited by diisopropylfluorophosphate whose specificity allows action at Pro–X bonds. Hence, this would be expected to inactivate β-casomorphins, but not α-casomorphins or gluten exorphins. This enzyme is widely distributed in tissues: intestine, kidney and placenta are particularly rich in the enzyme. Of much interest, dipeptidyl peptidase IV is present also in lymphocytes and, classed as CD26, is regarded as an important regulator of cell growth and cytokine production.[4,5,20,47,101] Aminopeptidase P (EC 3.4.11.9) is specific for X–Pro bonds and when purified from rat brain cytosol it was found to be active against β-casomorphin.[67] It, too, is a cell-surface antigen implicated in cell signalling in the immune system.[5] Mahe *et al.*[92] observed transport of morphiceptin, which is amidated casomorphin-4 (Table 33.2), across rabbit ileum *in vitro* when the ileum had been pre-treated with diisopropylfluorophosphate, but not across untreated intestine. Though such preparations of intestine *in vitro* are liable to exude peptidases artifactually, this may implicate intestinal dipeptidylpeptidase IV in minimizing, or even preventing, passage to the circulation of intact exorphins under normal conditions. Rogers *et al.*,[130] see above, also had reported that substitution of D-Ala for Gly[2] was necessary to confer hydrolysis resistance and permit absorption of the enkephalin N-terminal tetrapeptide Tyr-Gly-Gly-Phe.

Hydrolysis and casomorphins

It is striking that Kreil *et al.*[82] observed rapid hydrolysis of immunoreactive and opioid-active β-casomorphins by rat and bovine plasma *in vitro* with a half-life of about 5 min. In view of the carnosine data reviewed above, the conclusion by these authors that casomorphins would be unlikely to survive enzymatic cleavage for long enough to reach opiate receptors is not justified. However, as with the carnosine results, these data show that failure to detect particular peptides in plasma is poor evidence about whether they have been absorbed, unless the utmost stringent precautions are taken to abolish hydrolysis during blood sampling and *ex vivo*. This error may have marred many claims that specific peptides are absent from blood.[57]

It is notable that many peptide hydrolase enzymes (although not dipeptidyl peptidase IV) are zinc-dependent,[153] and it is conceivable that deficient function of these enzymes is one of the consequences of zinc deficiency. It would be of much interest to know whether patients with hyperpeptiduria show a correlation between peptide output and body zinc content, and whether peptidase activities are compromised in these patients.

PASSAGE OF EXORPHINS AND OTHER PEPTIDES ACROSS THE BLOOD–BRAIN BARRIER AND EFFECTS ON THE BRAIN

An additional obstacle to acceptance of diet-derived peptides influencing central nervous system development and function has been scepticism that peptides can cross the blood–brain barrier. This is now unwarranted, although transport systems for peptides and endothelial cell peptidases which constitute a hydrolytic 'barrier' need consideration. Saturable transport systems for peptides have been partly characterized,[9–11] and uptake of radiolabel from labelled casomorphin into 18 brain regions has been reported with free entry to brain regions with leaky capillaries, including circumventricular organs, and restricted, but measurable, entry to other regions.[43,44] There could, of course, also be indirect mechanisms by which circulating exorphins could indirectly modulate brain function without entry to brain. Also, roles for peptides in modulating permeability of the blood–brain barrier have been postulated.[43] Additionally, maturation of the blood–brain barrier occurs around birth,[115] and defects in this process are plausible. Since, at least part of the barrier to entry is enzymic, an enzyme defect might increase the ingress of substantial amounts of intact peptide.

Effect of naloxone

Cade found that adult rats responded to intravenous human β-casomorphin-7 by expressing *Fos*-like immunoreactivity in several regions of the brain within 1 hour, the effect being blocked by systemic naloxone.[147] C-*Fos* is a neural gene whose activation is used as a marker of neural stimulation, and it was noted that the brain regions affected were ones implicated in the pathology of both schizophrenia and autism: these two conditions are discussed below as ones where exorphins may be involved. Systemic injection of β-casomorphin-5 also had an analgesic effect on young rats undergoing a heat-escape stimulus, and this was blocked by intraventricular administration of naloxone.[14] These findings strongly support a central effect of the systemic exorphin, and they imply (without proving) access to the brain of the exorphin or a signal derived from it.

In pregnant, lactating, and control women, immunoreactivity against casomorphins was found in milk, blood and cerebrospinal fluid (CSF), with a descending concentration gradient between these fluids and a significant correlation between the levels in plasma and CSF.[108] Although this suggested entry of casomorphin-like fragments across the blood–brain barrier, it was also clear that the immunoreactive material comprised fragments with several different molecular weights. This should highlight dangers inherent in assuming that immunoreactivity indicates the presence of the original antigen.

Synthetic (hydrolysis-resistant) analogues of β-casomorphins crossed cultured monolayers of cerebrovascular endothelial cells, possibly by the paracellular route,[145] though caution should be exercised in assuming that the intercellular junctions in this model behave as 'tightly' as those *in vivo*.

Brain homogenates are active in degrading β-casomorphin-4 with a half-life of 5 min (cp. <1 min in a liver homogenate), with dipeptidyl peptidase IV and other proline-specific peptidases being implicated,[144] and brain metabolism *in vivo* has also been studied.[143] Again, rapid metabolism complicates the ability to measure transport.

DIFFICULTIES IN INVESTIGATION OF PEPTIDES IN BIOLOGICAL FLUIDS

It should be stressed that much of the slow progress in understanding the roles of dietary peptides in disease is associated with a serious paucity of information on peptides in body fluids; this has arisen due to numerous methodological difficulties as well as a failure to recognize the potential pathophysiological significance of the mechanisms under discussion here.[57]

The peptide content of plasma in health is not well characterized, apart from the levels of specific hormones – indeed, the topic is not even addressed in most textbooks of biochemistry or clinical chemistry. However, about 10% of the non-protein amino-N (excluding urea) in plasma appears to be in the form of small peptides or conjugated amino acids, and the corresponding figure for urine is about 60%.[57]

IMMUNE SYSTEM AS A TARGET FOR EXORPHINS

For historical reasons, the endorphins and enkephalins tend to be regarded as neuropeptides. However, the view is clearly emerging that endogenous opioids are important regulatory signals for immune cells with already a substantial literature,[23–25,31,69,129,132,137,141,142,146] and it is extremely likely that dietary exorphins will either mimic or block their activity – hence, the inclusion of immune cells in Fig. 33.1 above. Therefore the immune, neural and endocrine systems should not be considered as discrete systems,[12,13] and Fig. 33.7 emphasizes simply the signalling cross-talk between the first two systems. T lymphocytes have receptors for enkephalins and their analogues, and both enhancing effects (probably via μ- and δ-receptors) and suppressive effects (probably via κ-receptors) occur.[22] It is also noteworthy that several aminopeptidases involved in exorphin metabolism have been identified as identical with CD (cluster differentiation) antigens in the immune system involved in signalling pathways.[5,101] Thus, as described above, dipeptidyl peptidase IV is CD26 and is likely to be involved in lymphocyte growth and cytokine production, although its role is not yet elucidated. This provides a potential set of mechanisms by which absorbed exorphins could interfere with cell-mediated immunity.

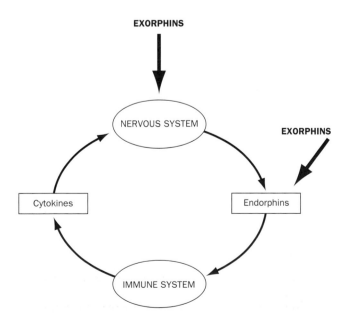

Fig. 33.7 Signalling inter-relationships between the nervous and immune systems and how exorphins would be expected to interfere profoundly.

Kurek has demonstrated histamine release from mast cells by casomorphins:[84] subsequently, a positive skin reaction was evoked in healthy children by high intradermal doses of both β- and α-casomorphins, these effects being inhibited by cetirizine, an H$_1$-antagonist.[83,85]

It is also noteworthy that endogenous opioids can cause immunosuppression (see above): if this is true also for exorphins, then this could provide a direct mechanism linking diet to susceptibility to infection.

CLINICAL SIGNIFICANCE OF EXORPHINS AND OTHER DIET-DERIVED PEPTIDES IN MENTAL AND BEHAVIOURAL ILLNESS

The original search for exorphin activity in gluten by Zioudrou et al.[165] was stimulated by the hypothesis of the late FC Dohan that wheat consumption was linked to schizophrenia.[33–35,37–42] Dohan's evidence was primarily epidemiological, considering differences between wheat-consuming and non-consuming populations and changes in incidence of mental illness during times of changed intake, e.g. times of famine. Faster improvements also had been observed in schizophrenics under treatment when gluten and casein were excluded.[40]

Following a blind challenge with gluten, Singh and Kay[140] also claimed a pathogenic involvement of gluten in schizophrenia, and it is notable that they, like Dohan,[40] had previously excluded both gluten and casein from their patients' diets. Dohan also drew attention to possible biochemical similarities between schizophrenia and coeliac disease,[36] a condition where involvement of gluten in genetically predisposed subjects is unequivocally recognized. It is interesting that the questions about the relative roles of enzyme deficiencies and immune mechanisms and active peptides in coeliac disease are remarkably similar to those now arising about gluten and mental illness. Dohan recognized a genetic component in schizophrenia, and proposed that several genetic loci combined to cause enhanced intestinal absorption of exorphins together with decreased catabolism by genetically defective enzymes,[35,37,38] a view strongly promoted by Reichelt for subsets of both schizophrenia and childhood autism.[121,122,125,127] Reichelt has reported high levels of urinary peptides, presumed to originate from diet, in schizophrenia. Initially, his methods to quantify urinary peptides were highly complex, making it difficult for other workers to reproduce his methodology or findings.[61] However, an improved method based on high-performance liquid chromatography (HPLC) is now in use and confirms hyperpeptiduria in 10 untreated schizophrenics and 57 untreated autists: casomorphin immunoreactivity, chromatographic co-elution with bovine casomorphin-8, and opioid receptor-binding were also reported in the urine.[127]

Controversy: role of gluten in schizophrenia

However, the view implicating gluten in schizophrenia has never been widely accepted, and the matter is generally regarded as highly controversial.[131] Indeed, the relevance of opioid peptides, whether deficient or in excess, in schizophrenia is disputable.[80] It seems, however, that this may well reflect the heterogeneity of the schizophrenic populations and that multiple aetiologies are involved in different subsets. Another example of a double-blind trial of gluten exclusion yielding successful remission was that by Vlissides and Jenner.[158] the small number of successful respondents (2 out of 24) should, however, probably be regarded as an indicator of the size of the subgroup with this particular aetiology (about 10% of the patient population), rather than as a failure of the dietary approach. It would have been of great interest to know whether the subgroup of responders also fell into the same subgroups if intestinal permeability and urinary peptides, especially exorphins and casomorphins, had also been measured. Failure by investigators to allow for heterogeneity of subgroups may well be responsible for a serious underestimation of the role of diet in pathogenesis.

Gut permeability in schizophrenia and autism
Dohan believed that excessive intestinal absorption of exorphins might occur, and several workers have measured intestinal permeability in schizophrenics. Although the overall conclusion has been that these patients, considered as a single group, do not have excessively 'leaky' intestines, two studies have strongly suggested the presence of subsets of patients who have abnormally high permeability.[86,161] Likewise, 8 out of 21 autistic patients studied by D'Eufemia had abnormally high permeability.[32]

Gluten and casein peptides in autism
There are also very strong evidence-based impressions that gluten- and casein-derived peptides are closely associated with the aetiology of autism although these are not widely known or accepted. The aetiology of this condition is not understood although it has some clinical similarity with schizophrenia: one proposal, advanced by Panksepp is that it arises from an opiate imbalance in the brain;[109] hence, excessive absorption of exorphins could be involved. Following his work on urinary peptides in schizophrenia, Reichelt has reported hyperpeptiduria in autism,[124,127] and the urinary peptide levels are reduced on exclusion of dietary gluten and casein concomitant with an improvement in learning as measured by quantitative behavioural tests.[76–78] The hyperpeptiduria in autism has been corroborated in another laboratory,[136] although the actual peptides have not yet been characterized: indeed, further proof of their peptide nature and rigorous quantification would be welcome. Similar findings on urinary peptides and tentative identification as casomorphins and gliadin exorphins have been obtained in both schizophrenics and autists by Cade et al.,[21a] and improvements in both peptiduria and behaviour followed exclusion of dietary gluten and casein.

Reichelt suggests that the heterogeneous peptide 'patterns' observed in patients with hyperpeptiduria reflect familial deficiencies of different peptidase enzymes, rather than one single genetic defect.[120,122,123,125,127]

It is appropriate to stress the benefit of studies where quantitative measures of learning or behaviour are made independently together with biochemical quantification of analytes such as urinary peptides and casomorphins: provided appropriate control groups are included, these studies remove the subjectivity that has often marred claims of involvement of diet with mental and behavioural health.

These findings are consistent with the model in Fig. 33.1 and, if corroborated and extended, would strongly support a major role for dietary exorphins in mental and behavioural disorders: total removal of both gluten and casein from diet would then be strongly indicated. Similar exorphin-mediated mechanisms may be operational in a broad spectrum of behavioural and mental disorders, and these should be taken seriously both for appropriate therapeutic efforts and for objective research investigations into aetiology.

CONCLUSIONS

It is clear that dietary proteins can give rise to biologically active peptides during digestion; the opioid peptides derived from gluten and casein have been the most extensively studied. It is also now clear that peptides can be absorbed in intact form, the extent of this depending on a fine balance between protein digestibility, host digestive activity and intestinal permeability. After absorption, the survival or clearance of peptides depends on peptidase enzymes in blood and other tissues, especially the liver and kidney. The consequences depend on the balance between this clearance and access to peripheral organs, especially the central nervous system and the immune system. Absorbed exorphins from the diet may cause direct effects on these systems or they may agonize or antagonize effects of endogenous neuropeptides and immune modulators. Hence, there is a sound physiological rationale for diet-derived peptides interfering with normal homeostasis and health. The newly uncovered signalling pathways providing cross-talk between the immune system, the nervous system and endocrine systems are all at risk.

An increasing body of evidence suggests that these mechanisms are implicated in at least some areas of mental, behavioural or neurodevelopmental illness for some susceptible individuals: autism, schizophrenia and Rett's syndrome are examples where peptide (or neuropeptide) metabolism appears to be abnormal. In autism and schizophrenia, some trials of dietary gluten- and casein-exclusion have provided promising results.

Now that a pathophysiological mechanism has been proven to be realistic and initial trials have been successful, fuller objective (non-anecdotal and quantitative) trials should be encouraged, although the presence of heterogeneous subgroups of patients must be amply recognized.

SUMMARY

1. Many dietary proteins contain amino acid sequences of biologically active peptides.
2. On enzymic digestion, gluten and casein yield a number of exorphins – peptides with opioid and anti-opioid activity. The sequences of these peptides are known.
3. Intact peptides, including exorphins, can be absorbed across the gastrointestinal tract.
4. Enhanced permeability of the small intestine occurs in many situations and is likely to promote absorption of intact peptides.
5. The fate and metabolic clearance of absorbed peptides varies substantially between individual subjects.
6. Peptides, including opioid peptides, are key effectors/regulators in the nervous, endocrine and immune systems and provide cross-talk signalling between these systems.
7. Absorbed exorphins are likely to be immunosuppressive.
8. Exclusion of dietary gluten and casein has been reported to be beneficial in some subsets of autistic and schizophrenic patients.
9. Absorption of active peptides, exorphins and others, from dietary gluten and casein (and possibly other proteins) provides a biochemically plausible aetiology for mental, behavioural and neurodevelopmental dysfunction.

REFERENCES

1 Akil H, Watson SJ, Young E, Lewis ME, Khachaturian H, Walker JM. Endogenous opioids: Biology and function. *Annu Rev Neurosci* 1984; 7: 223–55.

2 André C, André F, Colin L, Cavagna S. Measurement of intestinal permeability to mannitol and lactulose as a means of diagnosing food allergy and evaluating therapeutic effectiveness of disodium cromoglycate. *Ann Allergy* 1987; 59: 127–30.

3 André F, André C, Feknous M, Colin L, Cavagna S. Digestive permeability to different-sized molecules and to sodium cromoglycate in food allergy. *Allergy Proc* 1991; 12: 293–8.

4 Ansorge S, Bühling F, Kähne T *et al.* CD26/Dipeptidyl peptidase IV in lymphocyte growth regulation. In: Ansorge S, Langer J (eds) *Cellular Peptidases in Immune Functions and Diseases*. Plenum Press, New York; 1997; 127–40.

5 Ansorge S, Langner J (eds). *Cellular Peptidases in Immune Functions and Diseases*. Plenum Press, New York; 1997.

6 Atisook K, Madara JL. An oligopeptide permeates intestinal tight junctions at glucose-elicited dilatations. *Gastroenterology* 1991; 100: 719–24.

7 Axelsson I, Jakobsson I, Lindberg T, Polberger S, Benediktsson B, Raiha N. Macromolecular absorption in preterm and term infants. *Acta Paediatr Scand* 1989; 78: 532–7.

8 Baintner K. *Intestinal Absorption of Macromolecules and Immune Transmission from Mother to Young*. CRC Press, Boca Raton, Florida, 1986.

9 Banks WA, Kastin AJ. Permeability of the blood–brain barrier to neuropeptides: the case for penetration. *Psychoneuroendocrinology* 1985; 10: 385–99.

10 Banks WA, Kastin AJ. Saturable transport of peptides across the blood–brain barrier. *Life Sci* 1987; 41: 1319–38.

11 Banks WA, Kastin AJ, Fischman AJ, Coy DH, Strauss SL. Carrier-mediated transport of enkephalins and N-Tyr-MIF-1 across blood–brain barrier. *Am J Physiol* 1986; 251:E477–82.

12 Blalock JE. Shared ligands and receptors as a molecular mechanism for communication between the immune and neuroendocrine systems. *Ann NY Acad Sci* 1994; 741: 292–8.

13 Blalock JE. The syntax of immune-neuroendocrine communication. *Immunol Today* 1994; 15: 504–11.

14 Blass EM, Blom J. Beta-casomorphin causes hypoalgesia in 10-day-old rats: evidence for central mediation. *Pediatr Res* 1996; 39. 199–203.

15 Blau N, Niederwieser A, Shmerling DH. Peptiduria presumably caused by aminopeptidase-P deficiency. A new inborn error of metabolism. *J Inherited Metab Dis* 1988; 11(Suppl 2): 240–2.

16 Bloom FE. The endorphins. a growing family of pharmacologically pertinent peptides. *Annu Rev Pharmacol Toxicol* 1983; 23: 151–70.

17 Brambell FWR. *The Transmission of Passive Immunity from Mother to Young*. North-Holland, Amsterdam, 1970.

18 Brantl V, Teschemacher H, Henschen A, Lottspeich F. Novel opioid peptides derived from casein (β-casomorphins). I. Isolation from bovine casein peptone. *Z Physiol Chem* 1979; 360: 1211–16.

19 Brantl V, Teschemacher H, Henschen A, Lottspeich F. Novel opioid peptides derived from casein (β-casomorphins). I. Isolation from bovine casein peptone. *Z Physiol Chem* 1979; 360: 1211–16.

20 Bühling F, Reinhold D, Lendeckel U, Faust J, Neubert K, Ansorge S. CD26 is involved in regulation of cytokine production in natural killer cells. In: Ansorge S, Langner J (eds) *Cellular Peptidases in Immune Functions and Diseases*. Plenum Press, New York; 1997; 141–7.

21 Bullen A. Mechanisms of gluten toxicity in coeliac disease. In: Hunter JO, Alun Jones V (eds) *Food and the Gut*. Baillière-Tindall, London; 1985; 187–207.

21a Cade R, Privette M, Fregly M et al. Autism and schizophrenia. Intestinal disorders. Nutr Neuroscience 2000; 3: 57–72.

22 Caroleo MC, Arbitrio M, Melchiorri D, Nistico G. A reappraisal of the role of the various opioid receptor subtypes in cell-mediated immunity. *Neuroimmunomodulation* 1994; 1: 141–7.

23 Carr DJ. The role of endogenous opioids and their receptors in the immune system. *Proc Soc Exp Biol Med* 1991; 198: 710–20.

24 Carr DJ, Rogers TJ, Weber RJ. The relevance of opioids and opioid receptors on immunocompetence and immune homeostasis. *Proc Soc Exp Biol Med* 1996; 213: 248–57.

25 Carr DJJ, Serou M. Exogenous and endogenous opioids as biological response modifiers. *Immunopharmacology* 1995; 31: 59–71.

26 Chabance B, Jolles P, Izquierdo C et al. Characterization of an antithrombotic peptide from kappa-casein in newborn plasma after milk ingestion. *Br J Nutr* 1995; 73: 583–90.

27 Chabance B, Marteau P, Rambaud JC et al. Casein peptide release and passage to the blood in humans during digestion of milk or yoghurt. *Biochimie* 1998; 80: 155–65.

28 Chang KJ, Lillian A, Hazum E, Cuatrecasas P, Chang JK. Morphiceptin (H-Tyr-Pro-Phe-Pro-NH₂): a potent and specific agonist for morphine (μ) receptors. *Science* 1981; 212: 75–7.

29 Chiba H, Tani F, Yoshikawa M. Opioid antagonist peptides derived from kappa-casein. *J Dairy Res* 1989; 56: 363–6.

30 Coste M, Tomé D. Milk peptides with physiological activities. II. Opioid and immunostimulating peptides derived from milk proteins. *Lait* 1991; 71: 241–7.

31 Dardenne M, Savino W. Interdependence of the endocrine and immune systems. *Adv Neuroimmunol* 1996; 6: 297–307.

32 D'Eufemia P, Celli M, Finocchiaro R et al. Abnormal intestinal permeability in children with autism. *Acta Paediatr* 1996; 85: 1076–9.

33 Dohan FC. Wartime changes in hospital admissions for schizophrenia. A comparison of admission for schizophrenia and other psychoses in six countries during World War II. *Acta Psychiatr Scand* 1966; 42: 1–23.

34 Dohan FC. Schizophrenia and neuroactive peptides from food. *Lancet* 1979; 1: 1031.

35 Dohan FC. Hypothesis: genes and neuroactive peptides from food as cause of schizophrenia. In: Costa E, Trabucchi M (eds) *Neural Peptides and Neural Communication*. Raven Press, New York; 1980; 535–48.

36 Dohan FC. More on celiac disease as a model for schizophrenia. *Biol Psychiatry* 1983; 18: 561–4.

37 Dohan FC. Genetic hypothesis of idiopathic schizophrenia: its exorphin connection. *Schizophr Bull* 1988; 14: 489–94.

38 Dohan FC. Genetics and idiopathic schizophrenia. *Am J Psychiatry* 1989; 146: 1522–3.

39 Dohan FC, Grasberger JC. Relapsed schizophrenics: earlier discharge from the hospital after cereal-free, milk-free diet. *Am J Psychiatry* 1973; 130: 685–8.

40 Dohan FC, Grasberger JC, Lowell FM, Johnston HT Jr, Arbegast AW. Relapsed schizophrenics: more rapid improvement on a milk- and cereal-free diet. *Br J Psychiatry* 1969; 115: 595–6.

41 Dohan FC, Harper EH, Clark MH, Rodrigue RB, Zigas V. Is schizophrenia rare if grain is rare? *Biol Psychiatry* 1984; 19: 385–99.

42 Dohan FC, Martin L, Grasberger JC, Boehme D, Cottrell JC. Antibodies to wheat gliadin in blood of psychiatric patients: possible role of emotional factors. *Biol Psychiatry* 1972; 5: 127–37.

43 Ermisch A, Ruhle HJ, Landgraf R, Hess J. Blood–brain barrier and peptides. *J Cereb Blood Flow Metab* 1985; 5: 350–7.

44 Ermisch A, Rühle H-J, Neubert K, Hartrodt B, Landgraf R. On the blood–brain barrier to peptides: [³H]B-casomorphin-5 uptake by eighteen brain regions *in vivo. J Neurochem* 1983; 41: 1229–33.

45 Fisher RB. *Protein Metabolism*. Methuen, London; 1954.

46 Fisher RB. Absorption of proteins. *Br Med Bull* 1967; 23: 241–6.

47 Fleisher B (ed.). Dipeptidyl peptidase IV (CD26) in metabolism and the immune response. RG Landes, Austin, Texas, 1995.

48 Fukudome S, Shimatsu A, Suganuma H, Yoshikawa M: Effect of gluten exorphins A5 and B5 on the postprandial plasma insulin level in conscious rats. *Life Sci* 1995; 57: 729–34.

49 Fukudome S, Yoshikawa M. Opioid peptides derived from wheat gluten: their isolation and characterization. *FEBS Lett* 1992; 296: 107–11.

50 Fukudome S, Yoshikawa M. Gluten exorphin C. A novel opioid peptide derived from wheat gluten. *FEBS Lett* 1993; 316: 17–19.

51 Gardner MLG. Evidence for, and implications of, passage of intact peptides across the intestinal mucosa. *Biochem Soc Trans* 1983; 11: 810–13.

52 Gardner MLG. Intestinal assimilation of intact peptides and proteins from the diet – a neglected field? *Biol Rev Camb Philos Soc* 1984; 59: 289–331.

53 Gardner MLG. Production of pharmacologically active peptides from foods in the gut. In: Hunter JO, Alun Jones V (eds) *Food and the Gut*. Baillière Tindall, London; 1985; 121–34.

54 Gardner MLG. Gastrointestinal absorption of intact proteins. *Annu Rev Nutr* 1988; 8: 329–50.

55 Gardner MLG. Intestinal absorption of peptides. In: Morley JE, Sterman MB, Walsh JH (eds) *Nutritional Modulation of Neural Function*. Academic Press, San Diego; 1988; 29–38.

56 Gardner MLG. Absorption of intact proteins and peptides. In: Johnson LR (ed.) *The Physiology of the Gastrointestinal Tract*, 3 edn. Raven Press, New York; 1994; 1795–820.

57 Gardner MLG. Transmucosal passage of intact peptides. In: Grimble GK, Backwell FRC (eds) *Peptides in Mammalian Protein Metabolism: Tissue Utilization and Clinical Targeting*. Portland Press, London; 1998; 11–29.

58 Gardner MLG, Illingworth KM, Kelleher J, Wood D. Intestinal absorption of the intact peptide carnosine in Man, and comparison with intestinal permeability to lactulose. *J Physiol (Lond)* 1991; 439: 411–22.

59 Gardner MLG, Steffens K-J (eds) *Absorption of Orally Administered Enzymes*. Springer-Verlag, Berlin, 1995.

60 Gardner MLG, Wood D. Transport of peptides across the gastrointestinal tract. *Biochem Soc Trans* 1989; 17: 934–7.

61 Gilroy JJ, Ferrier IN, Crow TJ, Rowell FJ. Urinary chromatographic profiles in schizophrenia. *Biol Psychiatry* 1990; 27: 1127–32.

62 Glamsta EL, Morkrid L, Lantz I, Nyberg F. Concomitant increase in blood plasma levels of immunoreactive hemorphin-7 and beta-endorphin following long distance running. *Regul Pept* 1993; 49: 9–18.

63 Greco L, D'Adamo G, Truscelli A, Parrilli G, Mayer M, Budillon G. Intestinal permeability after single dose gluten challenge in coeliac disease. *Arch Dis Child* 1991; 66: 870–2.

64 Hall EJ, Batt RM. Dietary modulation of gluten sensitivity in a naturally occurring enteropathy of Irish Setter dogs. *Gut* 1992; 33: 198–205.

65 Hamel U, Kielwein G, Teschemacher H. Beta-casomorphin immunoreactive materials in cow's milk incubated with various bacterial species. *J Dairy Res* 1985; 52: 139–48.

66 Hamilton I. Small intestinal mucosal permeability. In: Pounder R (ed.) *Recent Advances in Gastroenterology*, Vol. 6. Churchill Livingstone, Edinburgh; 1986: 73–92.

67 Harbeck HT, Mentlein R. Aminopeptidase P from rat brain. Purification and action on bioactive peptides. *Eur J Biochem* 1991; 198: 451–8.

68 Henschen A, Lottspeich F, Brantl V, Teschemacher H. Novel opioid peptides derived from casein (beta-casomorphins). II. Structure of active components from bovine casein peptone. *Z Physiol Chem* 1979; 360: 1217–24.

69 Homo-Delarche F, Dardenne M. The neuroendocrine-immune axis. *Springer Semin Immunopathol* 1993; 14: 221–38.

70 Huebner FR, Lieberman KW, Rubino RP, Wall JS. Demonstration of high opioid-like activity in isolated peptides from wheat gluten hydrolysates. *Peptides* 1984; 5: 1139–47.

71 Hughes J, Kosterlitz HW. Opioid peptides. *Br Med Bull* 1977; 33: 157–61.

72 Hughes J, Lord JAH, Waterfield AA, Kosterlitz HW. Endogenous opioid peptides: multiple agonists and receptors. *Nature* 1977; 267: 495–9.

73 Hughes J, Smith TW, Kosterlitz HW, Fothergill LA, Morgan BA, Morris HR. Identification of two related pentapeptides from the brain with potent opiate agonist activity. *Nature* 1975; 258: 577–9.

74 Kerchner GA, Geary LE. Studies on the transport of enkephalin-like oligopeptides in rat intestinal mucosa. *J Pharmacol Exp Ther* 1983; 226: 33–8.

75 Klosse JA, Huistra DY, DeBree PK, Wardman SK, Vliegenthart JFG. An automated chromatographic system for the combined analysis of urinary peptides and amino acids. *Clin Chim Acta* 1972; 42: 409–22.

76 Knivsberg A-M. Behavioural abnormalities and childhood psychopathology: urinary peptide patterns as a potential tool in diagnosis and remediation. University of Bergen, 1997.

77 Knivsberg A-M, Reichelt KL, Nødland M, Høien T. Autistic syndromes and diet: a follow-up study. *Scand J Educ Res* 1995; 39: 223–36.

78 Knivsberg A-M, Wiig K, Lind G, Nødland M, Reichelt K-L. Dietary intervention in autistic syndromes. *Brain Dysfunct* 1990; 3: 315–27.

79 Koch G, Wiedemann K, Teschemacher H. Opioid activities of human beta-casomorphins. *Naunyn Schmiedebergs Arch Pharmacol* 1985; 331: 351–4.

80 Koob GF, Bloom FE. Behavioural effects of opioid peptides. *Br Med Bull* 1983; 39: 89–94.

81 Kowlessar OD, Warren RA, Bronstein HD. Celiac disease: enzyme defect or immune mechanism? In: Glass J (ed.) *Progress in Gastroenterology*, Vol. II. Grune and Stratton, New York; 1970; 409–29.

82 Kreil G, Umbach M, Brantl V, Teschemacher H. Studies on the enzymatic degradation of beta-casomorphins. *Life Sci* 1983; 33: 137–40.

83 Kurek M, Czerwionka-Szaflarska M, Doroszewska G. Pseudoallergic skin reactions to opiate sequences of bovine casein in healthy children. *Rocz Akad Med Bialymstoku* 1995; 40: 480–5.

84 Kurek M, Przybilla B, Hermann K, Ring J. A naturally occurring opioid peptide from cow's milk, beta-casomorphine-7, is a direct histamine releaser in man. *Int Arch Allergy Appl Immunol* 1992; 97: 115–20.

85 Kurek M, Ruëff F, Czerwionka-Szaflarska M, Doroszewska G, Przybilla B. Exorphins derived from cow's milk casein elicit pseudo-allergic wheal-and-flare reactions in healthy children. *Rev Fr Allerg* 1996; 36: 191–6.

86 Lambert MT, Bjarnason I, Connelly J *et al*. Small intestine permeability in schizophrenia. *Br J Psychiatry* 1989; 155: 619–22.

87 Lee VHL. Enzymatic barriers to peptide and protein absorption. *Crit Rev Ther Drug Carrier Syst* 1988; 5: 69–97.

88 Lee VHL. Oral route of peptide and protein drug delivery. In: Gardner MLG, Steffens K-J (eds) *Absorption of Orally Administered Enzymes*. Springer-Verlag, Berlin; 1995; 39–46.

89 Loh HH, Smith AP. Molecular characterization of opioid receptors. *Annu Rev Pharmacol Toxicol* 1990; 30: 123–47.

90 Loukas S, Varoucha D, Zioudrou C, Streaty RA, Klee WA. Opioid activities and structures of alpha-casein-derived exorphins. *Biochemistry* 1983; 22: 4567–73.

91 Madara JL, Pappenheimer JR. Structural basis for physiological regulation of paracellular pathways in intestinal epithelia. *J Membrane Biol* 1987; 100: 149–64.

92 Mahe S, Tome D, Dumontier AM, Desjeux JF. Absorption of intact morphiceptin by diisopropylfluorophosphate-treated rabbit ileum. *Peptides* 1989; 10: 45–52.

93 Matthews DM. Memorial lecture: protein absorption – then and now. *Gastroenterology* 1977; 73: 1267–79.

94 Matthews DM. *Protein Absorption: Development and Present State of the Subject*. Wiley-Liss, New York; 1991.

95 Matthews DM, Payne JW (eds) *Peptide Transport in Protein Nutrition*. North-Holland, Amsterdam; 1975.

96 Matthews DM, Payne JW. Transmembrane transport of small peptides. *Curr Top Memb Transp* 1980; 14: 331–425.

97 Meisel H. Chemical characterization and opioid activity of an exorphin isolated from *in vivo* digests of casein. *FEBS Lett* 1986; 196: 223–7.

98 Meisel H. Biochemical properties of bioactive peptides derived from milk proteins: potential nutraceuticals for food and pharmaceutical applications. *Livestock Product Sci* 1997; 50: 125–38.

99 Meisel H. Biochemical properties of regulatory peptides derived from milk proteins. *Biopolymers* 1997; 43: 119–28.

100 Meisel H, Frister H. Chemical characterization of bioactive peptides from *in vivo* digests of casein. *J Dairy Res* 1989; 56: 343–9.

101 Mentlein R, Heymann E, Scholz W, Feller AC, Flad HD. Dipeptidyl peptidase IV as a new surface marker for a subpopulation of human T-lymphocytes. *Cell Immunol* 1984; 89: 11–19.

102 Mentlein R, Rix H, Feller AC, Heymann E. Characterization of dipeptidyl peptidase IV from lymphocytes of chronic lymphocytic leukemia of T-type. *Biomed Biochim Acta* 1986; 45: 567–74.

103 Menzies IS. Transmucosal passage of inert molecules in health and disease. In: Skadhauge E, Heintze K (eds) *Intestinal Absorption and Secretion*. MTP Press, Lancaster, 1984: 527–43.

104 Morley JE. Food peptides. A new class of hormones? *JAMA* 1982; 247: 2379–80.

105 Morley JE. Neuroendocrine effects of endogenous opioid peptides in human subjects: a review. *Psychoneuroendocrinology* 1983; 8: 361–79.

106 Morley JE, Levine AS, Yamada T *et al*. Effect of exorphins on gastrointestinal function, hormonal release, and appetite. *Gastroenterology* 1983; 84: 1517–23.

107 Nyberg F, Brantl V (eds) *β-Casomorphins and Related Peptides*. Fyris-Tryck AB, Uppsala, 1990.

108 Nyberg F, Lieberman H, Lindstrom LH, Lyrenas S, Koch G, Terenius L. Immunoreactive beta-casomorphin-8 in cerebrospinal fluid from pregnant and lactating women: correlation with plasma levels. *J Clin Endocrinol Metab* 1989; 68: 283–9.

109 Panksepp J. A neurochemical theory of autism. *Trends Neurosci* 1979; 174–9.

110 Pappenheimer JR. Physiological regulation of transepithelial impedance in the intestinal mucosa of rats and hamsters. *J Membrane Biol* 1987; 100: 137–48.

111 Pappenheimer JR, Dahl CE, Karnovsky ML, Maggio JE. Intestinal absorption and excretion of octapeptides composed of D amino acids. *Proc Natl Acad Sci USA* 1994; 91: 1942–5.

112 Pappenheimer JR, Madara JL. Role of active transport in regulation of junctional permeability and paracellular absorption of nutrients by intestinal epithelia. In: Ussing HH, Fischbarg J, Sten-Knudsen O, Larsen EH, Willumsen NJ (eds) *Isotonic Transport in Leaky Epithelia* (Alfred Benzon Symposium 34). Munksgaard, Copenhagen; 1993.

113 Pappenheimer JR, Volpp K. Transmucosal impedance of small intestine: correlation with transport of sugars and amino acids. *Am J Physiol* 1992; 263:C480–93.

114 Paroli E. Opioid peptides from food (the exorphins). *World Rev Nutr Diet* 1988; 55: 58–97.

115 Pasi A, Mahler H, Lansel N, Bernasconi C, Messiha FS. Beta-Casomorphin-immunoreactivity in the brain stem of the human infant. *Res Commun Chem Pathol Pharmacol* 1993; 80: 305–22.

116 Peters TJ, Bjarnason I. Intestinal permeability. In: Hunter JO, Alun Jones V (eds) *Food and the Gut* .Baillière Tindall, London; 1985: 30–44.

117 Petrilli P, Picone D, Caporale C, Addeo F, Auricchio S, Marino G. Does casomorphin have a functional role? *FEBS Lett* 1984; 169: 53–6.

118 Plumb JA, Burston D, Baker TG, Gardner MLG. A comparison of the structural integrity of several commonly used preparations of rat small intestine *in vitro*. *Clin Sci* 1987; 73: 53–9.

119 Polak JM, Bloom SR. Peripheral regulatory peptides: a newly discovered control mechanism. In: Fink G, Whalley LJ (eds) *Neuropeptides: Basic and Clinical Aspects*. Churchill Livingstone, Edinburgh; 1982: 118–47.

120 Reichelt K-L, Scott H, Knivsberg A-M, Wiig K, Lind G, Nødland M. Childhood autism: a group of hyperpeptidergic disorders. Possible etiology and tentative treatment. In: Nyberg F, Brantl V (eds) *β-Casomorphins and Related Peptides*. Fyris-Tryck AB, Uppsala; 1990: 163–73.

121 Reichelt KL. Exorphins in schizophrenia and autism. *J Neurochem* 1994; 63 (Suppl 1):S86.

122 Reichelt KL, Hole K, Hamberger A *et al*. Biologically active peptide-containing fractions in schizophrenia and childhood autism. *Adv Biochem Psychopharmacol* 1981; 28: 627–43.

123 Reichelt KL, Knivsberg AM, Nødland M, Lind G. Nature and consequences of hyperpeptiduria and bovine casomorphins found in autistic syndromes. *Dev Brain Dysfunction* 1994; 7: 71–85.

124 Reichelt KL, Knivsberg A-M, Reichelt WH, Nødland M. Diet and autism: a four year follow up. Probable reasons and observations relevant to a dietary and genetic aetiology. In: Linfoot G, Shattock P, Finnigan R, Savery D, West S (eds) *Therapeutic Intervention in Autism: Perspectives from Research & Practice*. Autism Research Unit, Sunderland; 1996: 281–307.

125 Reichelt KL, Seim AR, Reichelt WH. Could schizophrenia be reasonably explained by Dohan's hypothesis on genetic interaction with a dietary peptide overload? *Prog Neuropsychopharmacol Biol Psychiatry* 1996; 20: 1083–114.

126 Reichelt WH, Ek J, Stensrud M, Reichelt KL. Peptide excretion in coeliac disease. *J Pediatr Gastroenterol Nutr* 1998; 26: 305–9.

127 Reichelt WH, Reichelt KL. The possible role of peptides derived from food proteins in diseases of the nervous system. In: Gobbi G (ed.) *Epilepsy and Other Neurological Disorders in Coeliac Disease*. John Libbey, London; 1997: 227–37.

128 Roberton DM, Paganelli R, Dinwiddie R, Levinsky RJ. Milk antigen absorption in the preterm and term neonate. *Arch Dis Child* 1982; 57: 369–72.

129 Roda LG, Bongiorno L, Trani E, Urbani A, Marini M. Positive and negative immunomodulation by opioid peptides. *Int J Immunopharmacol* 1996; 18: 1–16.

130 Rogers CS, Heading CE, Wilkinson S. Absorption of two tyrosine containing peptides from the ileum of the rat. *IRCS Medical Science. Biochemistry* 1980; 8: 648–9.

131 Ross-Smith P, Jenner FA. Diet (gluten) and schizophrenia. *J Hum Nutr* 1980; 34: 107–12.

132 Roy S, Loh HH. Effects of opioids on the immune system. *Neurochem Res* 1996; 21: 1375–86.

133 Schlimme E, Meisel H. Bioactive peptides derived from milk proteins. Structural, physiological and analytical aspects. *Nahrung* 1995; 39: 1–20.

134 Schusdziarra V, Henrichs I, Holland A, Klier M, Pfeiffer EF. Evidence for an effect of exorphins on plasma insulin and glucagon levels in dogs. *Diabetes* 1981; 30: 362–4.

135 Schusdziarra V, Schick A, de la Fuente A *et al*. Effect of beta-casomorphins and analogs on insulin release in dogs. *Endocrinology* 1983; 112: 885–9.

136 Shattock P, Kennedy A, Rowell F, Berney TP. Role of neuropeptides in autism and their relationships with classical neurotransmitters. *Brain Dysfunct* 1990; 3: 328–45.

137 Sibinga NE, Goldstein A. Opioid peptides and opioid receptors in cells of the immune system. *Annu Rev Immunol* 1988; 6: 219–49.

138 Silk DBA, Kim YS. Release of peptide hydrolases during incubation of intact intestinal segments *in vitro*. *J Physiol (Lond)* 1976; 258: 489–97.

139 Singh M, Rosen CL, Chang KJ, Haddad GG. Plasma beta-casomorphin-7 immunoreactive peptide increases after milk intake in newborn but not in adult dogs. *Pediatr Res* 1989; 26: 34–8.

140 Singh MM, Kay SR. Wheat gluten as a pathogenic factor in schizophrenia. *Science* 1976; 191: 401–2.

141 Singh VK. Immunoregulatory role of neuropeptides. In: Jucker E (ed.) *Progress in Drug Research*, Vol. 38. Birkhauser Verlag, Basel; 1992: 149–69.

142 Singh VK. Neuropeptides as native immune modulators. In: Jucker E (ed.) *Progress in Drug Research*, Vol. 45. Birkhauser Verlag, Basel, 1995: 9–31.

143 Stark H, Lossner B, Matthies H. Degradation of beta-casomorphin in the rat brain *in vivo*. *Biomed Biochim Acta* 1986; 45: 557–63.

144 Stark H, Lossner B, Matthies H. Metabolism of beta-casomorphin and its derivatives in rat brain and liver homogenates. *Biomed Biochim Acta* 1987; 46: 687–94.

145 Stark H, Van Bree JB, de Boer AG, Jaehde U, Breimer DD. *In vitro* penetration of des-tyrosine l-D-phenylalanine3-beta-casomorphin across the blood–brain barrier. *Peptides* 1992; 13: 47–51.

146 Stefano GB, Scharrer B, Smith EM *et al*. Opioid and opiate immunoregulatory processes. *Crit Rev Immunol* 1996; 16: 109–44.

147 Sun Z, Cade JR, Fregly MJ, Privette RM. β-Casomorphin induces *Fos*-like immunoreactivity in discrete brain regions relevant to schizophrenia and autism. *Autism* 1998; 3: 67–83.

148 Svedberg J, de Haas J, Leimenstoll G, Paul F, Teschemacher H. Demonstration of beta-casomorphin immunoreactive materials in *in vitro* digests of bovine milk and in small intestine contents after bovine milk ingestion in adult humans. *Peptides* 1985; 6: 825–30.

149 Tani F, Iio K, Chiba H, Yoshikawa M. Isolation and characterization of opioid antagonist peptides derived from human lactoferrin. *Agric Biol Chem* 1990; 54: 1803–10.

150 Teschemacher H, Ahnert G, Umbach M, Kielwein G, Lieb S. β-casomorphins – opiate-like acting peptide fragments from β-casein: determination in various milk and tissue extracts by radioimmunoassay. *Naunyn Schmiedebergs Arch Pharmacol* 1980; 311(supplement):R67.

151 Tiruppathi C, Miyamoto Y, Ganapathy V, Roesel RA, Whitford GM, Leibach FH. Hydrolysis and transport of proline-containing peptides in renal brush-border membrane vesicles from dipeptidyl peptidase IV-positive and dipeptidyl peptidase IV-negative rat strains. *J Biol Chem* 1990; 265: 1476–83.

152 Travis S, Menzies IS. Intestinal permeability: functional assessment and significance. *Clin Sci* 1992; 82: 471–88.

153 Turner AJ. Processing and metabolism of neuropeptides. *Essays Biochem* 1986; 22: 69–119.

154 Turner AJ. Neuropeptide inactivation in the central nervous system. In: Kenny AJ, Boustead CM (eds) *Cell-Surface Peptidases in Health and Disease*. BIOS Scientific Publishers, Oxford; 1997.

155 Turner AJ, Matsas R, Kenny AJ. Are there neuropeptide-specific peptidases? *Biochem Pharmacol* 1985; 34: 1347–56.

156 Udenfriend S, Kilpatrick DL. Biochemistry of the enkephalins and enkephalin-containing peptides. *Arch Biochem Biophys* 1983; 221: 309–323.

157 Umbach M, Teschemacher H, Praetorius K, Hirschhauser R, Bostedt H. Demonstration of a beta-casomorphin immunoreactive material in the plasma of newborn calves after milk intake. *Regul Pept* 1985; 12: 223–30.

158 Vlissides DN, Venulet A, Jenner FA. A double-blind gluten-free/gluten-load controlled trial in a secure ward population. *Br J Psychiatry* 1986; 148: 447–52.

159 Wajda IJ, Neidle A, Ehrenpreis S, Manigault I. Properties and distribution of morphine-like substances. In: Archer S, Collier HOJ, Goldstein A (eds) *Opiates and Endogenous Opioid Peptides*. North-Holland, Amsterdam; 1976: 129–36.

160 Walker WA. Gastrointestinal host defence: importance of gut closure in control of macromolecular transport. In: Elliott K, Whelan J (eds) *Development of Mammalian Absorptive Processes* (Ciba Foundation Symposium No 70, new series). Excerpta Medica, Amsterdam; 1979: 201–19.

161 Wood NC, Hamilton I, Axon ATR *et al*. Abnormal intestinal permeability. An aetiological factor in chronic psychiatric disorders? *Br J Psychiatry* 1987; 150: 853–6.

162 Yen WC, Lee VH. Role of Na^+ in the asymmetric paracellular transport of 4-phenylazobenzyloxycarbonyl-L-Pro-L-Leu-Gly-L-Pro-D-Arg across rabbit colonic segments and Caco-2 cell monolayers. *J Pharmacol Exp Ther* 1995; 275: 114–19.

163 Yen WCY, Lee VHL. Paracellular transport of a proteolytically labile pentapeptide across the colonic and other intestinal segments of the albino rabbit: implications for peptide drug design. *J Contr Rel* 1994; 28: 97–109.

164 Zioudrou C, Klee WA. Possible roles of peptides derived from food proteins in brain function. In: Wurtman RJ, Wurtman JJ (eds) *Nutrition and the Brain*. Raven Press, New York; 1979: 125–241.

165 Zioudrou C, Streaty RA, Klee WA. Opioid peptides derived from food proteins. The exorphins. *J Biol Chem* 1979; 254: 2446–9.

INTRODUCTION

Lectins are carbohydrate-binding proteins found in most plants. They have numerous effects on living mammalian cells and tissues, and some are toxic. Because of the ubiquity of glycoconjugates in the body (glycoproteins and glycolipids at cell surfaces and in body fluids), and because lectins are in food plants and are therefore taken regularly into the body, it is likely that they may affect our health. Allergists are familiar with the facts of food intolerance and allergy, and this chapter asks the question: 'How many adverse effects of foods are due to lectins?'.

The reason for this question is that lectins can be blocked, at least *in vitro*, by specific monosaccharides or oligosaccharides, which interfere with lectin binding in the same way as a hapten may inhibit the binding of its antibody. Our ultimate target therefore is rational therapy, should lectin-induced diseases be shown to exist (as seems likely; see below).

The development of any science is guided (perhaps distorted) by the preconceptions of its initiators, and so it has been with lectins. It was only because Stillmark, a century ago, was upset by the sufferings of the laboratory animals in his toxicology research that he turned instead to *in vitro* work on blood, and noted that certain plant extracts agglutinated the cells and coagulated the plasma.[301] It was only because lectins were originally described and defined in terms of their haemagglutinating capacity that for the next century they were thought of purely as haematology reagents,[33] and this strongly influenced the nomenclature of lectins, even though they serve totally different primary functions for the plant. So when nutrition scientists were investigating the surprisingly poor nutritional value of animal fodders based on raw beans, they were initially reluctant to believe that lectins

might be responsible.[183] It is only now that a science of clinical lectinology can be said to exist, even though much of the basic information has been available for years.

Because lectinology has grown in such a haphazard manner, there is no agreed system of nomenclature, in spite of numerous international conferences. Table 34.1 lists the names and abbreviations most frequently used; these may not be ideal but will be most easily understood by most readers.

When I reviewed the field in 1987 for the first edition of this book, much of the literature was at the stage of descriptive histochemistry. What we knew at that stage was that 'lectin x is capable of binding to tissue y' – and we were being rather daring in taking the next step of speculating that the function of tissue y might thereby be compromised. Matters have improved since then, and the evidence for true lectin-induced diseases is now very strong as I shall attempt to show. Nevertheless, our basic datum is still: 'What can bind to what?'.

This information is summarized in Table 34.2, from which it will be seen that lectins can bind virtually all cells and tissues, and that the wheat lectin (WGA) stands head and shoulders above all others; it binds to almost everything in the human body. Curious coincidence, then, that wheat is the basic daily staple for most of the Western world, and that wheat is one of the commonest foods responsible for intolerance/allergy. (But rice and maize eaters have no cause to be smug; all cereals have lectins and they are, not surprisingly, very similar.[307,352])

Note: Because the focus of this chapter is on dietary lectins, Table 34.2 does not list non-food lectins, by and large, even though they may have been studied. Note also that the mere fact of lectin binding does not tell us how avidly it binds; a tissue that binds a certain lectin well may have high affinity for that lectin or

Table 34.1 Common dietary lectins, their abbreviations and sugar specificities

Common dietary lectins, their abbreviations and sugar specificities		
Source	**Abbreviation**	**Sugar***
Wheat germ (*Triticum vulgaris*)	WGA	GNAc
Edible pea (*Pisum sativum*)	PSA	Man, Glc
Lentil (*Lens culinaris*)	LCA	Man, Glc
Peanut (*Arachis hypogaea*)	PNA	Gal
Kidney (haricot) bean (*Phaseolus vulgaris*)	PHA	Gal oligomers
Tomato (*Lycopersicon esculentum*)	LEA	LactNAc, GNAc
Potato (*Solanum tuberosum*)	STA	GNAc
Jackfruit (*Artocarpus integrifolia*)	jacalin, jac	Gal, GalNAc
Castor oil seed (*Ricinus communis*; POISON)	RCA	Gal
Soy bean (*Glycine max*)	SBA	GalNAc
Edible mushroom (*Agaricus bisporus*)	ABL	Gal
Jackbean (fodder plant; *Canavalia ensiformis*)	ConA	Man, Glc
Edible snail (*Helix pomatia*)	HPA	GalNAc

*Abbreviations for monosaccharides: GNAc = N-acetyl glucosamine. LactNAc = N-acetyl lactosamine. GalNac = N-acetyl galactosamine. Glc, Man and Gal = glucose, mannose and galactose, respectively. Others will be spelt in full.

may merely have a high density of binding sites. This can make a big difference in biological effects, but in only few cases have the necessary affinity experiments been done .

DIGESTION, COOKING AND ABSORPTION OF LECTINS

That some plants are toxic has been known since antiquity, and it was this very toxicity that started Stillmark, a century ago, on the search that led to the first description of lectins.[301] Well over 100 common foods have been shown to contain lectins,[6,97,215,261,332,352] and occasional cases of 'food poisoning' have been attributed to the lectins of undercooked beans.[106,224,239,325] One of these papers noted not only the expected diarrhoea and vomiting, but also muscle pain, rhabdomyolysis and toxic myocarditis,[325] all effects that we would expect of lectins, knowing their predilections (see below). Rolachon *et al.*[256] published a most illuminating case history in French in 1991, which I recommend to all allergists and indeed all doctors (see Box 34.1).

But acceptance of a wider role for dietary lectins in disease has been slow because lectins are proteins, and as every schoolboy knows, proteins are digested down to amino acids in the intestine. Furthermore, proteins are denatured by heat, so the cooking process surely destroys food lectins even before they are eaten.

Well, neither of these beliefs is entirely true. Many lectins are remarkably heat resistant, including those of wheat, tomato, carrot, maize, rice and peanuts[13,57,98,157,215] due to extensive disulphide crosslinking. The kidney bean lectin PHA has been most thoroughly studied, and although it is damaged by cooking, it

Box 34.1 'Diarrhèe osmotique chez un sujet vegetarien: les lectines pourraient être en cause'. 1991 report by Rolachon *et al.*[256]

A 48-year-old woman with chronic diarrhoea; 4–5 liquid stools daily. Gallbladder removed 17 years previously because of gallstones. A 20-year history of constipation, later alternating with and now supplanted by diarrhoea. Extensive upper and lower endoscopy from both ends, negative except for small prepyloric ulcer, treated with ranitidine. Diarrhoea worsened, admitted to hospital. Now 8–12 liquid motions daily. Duodenal biopsy, D-xylose test, pancreatic echogram, breath-lactulose test all normal; no evidence malabsorption or infection. Dietary history: vegetarian with high intake of vegetable fibre. Reduced intake of beans and lentils and introduced fish. Diarrhoea resolved within 48 hours.

Comment: We cannot be sure this wasn't a simple food allergy. I wish the doctor had tried feeding the patient some lactose first, which would have blocked at least some of the lectins in her diet.

retains haemagglutinating power after 4 h at 70°C and is not completely destroyed by boiling for 45 min or even by autoclaving[107,194] – that is, even though the beans are thoroughly soft and fit to eat. This is an especial problem in Third World countries, where beans are the major source of protein but fuel is scarce and expensive.[22,194] Undoubtedly, this is a factor in the vicious spiral of diarrhoea–malnutrition that kills so many in these countries.[22]

Body cells and tissues that can be bound by food lectins

Tissue	Lectins that bind to it	References
Human nasopharyngeal epithelium	WGA	56
Human labial mucosa	WGA, LCA, SBA, PNA	210
Human buccal mucosa	WGA, LCA, SBA, PNA, LEA	98, 206
Saliva, salivary gland	WGA, SBA, PNA	97, 206, 317
Human salivary IgA	WGA, PSA, PNA	99
Developing rat tooth	WGA, SBA	218
Human tonsil	WGA, SBA	90
Human stomach	WGA	220
Human parietal cells	PNA, SBA, LEA	49, 153
Human Brunner's gland	WGA, SBA	62
Human/animal intestinal, brush border	WGA, PHA, RCA, LEA, LCA, WBL, SBA	23,94,126,137,138,155, 211,217,299,336
Intestinal M cells	WGA, STA, LEA, SBA, jac	96
Human colonic mucosa	WGA, PNA, PHA, LCA, SBA	47,50,121,152,181,358
Human colonic mucus	WGA, PHA, LCA	35,50,152,181,211,336
Rat rectal mucosa	WGA	182
Human liver	WGA, PHA, PNA, SBA	214
Human gallbladder	WGA, STA, SBA, HPA, PHA, PNA	147,195
Human pancreatic duct	WGA	95
Rat pancreatic cells	WGA, PHA	141
Rodent islet cells	WGA, PNA, HPA, ABL	154,237
Human glomerulus	WGA, SBA, PNA	80,130,131,322
Human renal tubules	WGA, PHA, LCA, PSA, SBA, PNA	130,131,322
Human urothelium	WGA	221,342
Human prostate	WGA, PNA, LCA	193
Human cervix/endometrium	WGA, SBA, PNA	8,45,46,179
Human placenta	WGA	144
Human skeletal muscle	WGA, SBA, PNA, PSA, LCA	52,161
Human cardiac muscle	WGA,SBA	298
Human/animal endothelium	WGA, PNA, SBA	4,14,214,225
Human skin	WGA, LCA, PNA, SBA, HPA	29,151,270,339,343
Human sweat glands	WGA, SBA	271
Human connective tissue	WGA, PHA, LCA, jac, STA, PSA	9,274,291,316
Breast/udder; milk fat-globule membrane	WGA, PNA, SBA,	10,233,328,347
Human cartilage	WGA, SBA, PNA	78,79,105,275
Human pituitary	PNA	28
Human thyroid	WGA, SBA, PNA	201
Human thyrotropin	LCA	196
Human/animal eye tissues	WGA, PNA, PHA, SBA, PSA, ABA	34,41,166,252,255,293,306, 311,315,321
Human tears	WGA, PNA, jac, PHA	149,173
Human/animal inner ear	WGA, HPA, PSA, LCA, PHA, SBA	15,101,303,314,356
Human WBC, various	PHA	273
Human mast cells	WGA, LCA, PSA, PHA	119,162,253,286,288,362
Human platelets	WGA, STA, LCA	92,93,120,125,135
Rat nuclear pores	WGA	83,262
Human/animal axons	WGA, PSA, LCA, SBA, PHA, PNA	39,61,72,76,85,148,169,200, 216,300,318
Human myelin	WGA, PHA, LCA	134,192,248
Human amnion/chorion	WGA, LCA, PNA	168

Table 34.2 Body cells and tissues that can be bound by food lectins.

Digestion of lectins is also not straightforward. The common food lectins WGA, PHA and LEA are intrinsically resistant to proteolysis, so that up to 90% of PHA fed to animals, and most other lectins studied so far, is recoverable from the faeces unchanged or only slightly modified.[40,242] Non-digestibility of lectins in the gut is independent of their binding to the gut wall.[245] Furthermore, WGA, PHA, ConA and others profoundly interfere with enzyme function,[74,75,126,219,247,259,260,265,282,320] in most cases inhibiting their digestive functions (though occasionally enhancing).[75,143,247] Indeed, ingested lectins may damage the very architecture of the gut, as will be seen below, further undermining the body's ability to defend itself. These factors force us to the conclusion that neither cooking nor digestion will protect us very much, and should give us a sense of unease similar to the feeling of the mountain walker who, when the fog clears for a moment, discovers that for the last half-hour he has been strolling along the edge of a precipice.

Since vegetable peels and fibres are, by and large, the lectin-rich part of the plant (and also the alkaloid-rich part), I am not therefore altogether happy with the modern trend to 'whole-foods', especially the eating of raw unpeeled vegetables, and I warn my patients to be very careful when patronizing 'health food' establishments, as in my view these pose a serious hazard to the health (Box 34.2). It is a sad fact that Heaven, for its own inscrutable reasons, has seen fit to make the most nutritious plant foods also the most toxic ones.

The one 'health-food' fad that does bring a wintry smile of approval to my face is the sprouting of beans and grains, since germination usually causes the lectins to disappear over the course of a few days.[187,257,267,268] But watch out; in squash seeds (*Cucurbita ficifolia*) and possibly beans, the lectin content *increases* for the first day or two, then declines. Most sprouted seeds should be fairly safe by the end of the first week,[188,268] and some far sooner. Sprouting also causes a decline in bean trypsin inhibitors.

Armed with this information we are now ready to consider the impact of dietary lectins on the gut. Consideration of any more distant effects in the body will have to wait until we know whether lectins are absorbed into the circulation (see below).

Box 34.2 **'Healthy eating day: 1988 report from Public Health Laboratory Service**[106].

A hospital launched a 'healthy eating campaign' for staff. One of the items on the menu was a chili con carne, and there were complaints that the beans were rather hard. The first indication of something amiss was when a surgical registrar vomited in theatre about 3 hours later. Three consultants, an administrator, a works officer, an Environmental Health Officer and seven other ranks of staff suffered profuse vomiting, some with diarrhoea. All recovered within 3–4 hours (although in a similar outbreak reported in the same issue one of the victims was ill for 2 days). Food poisoning bacteria were not isolated but the beans contained 102 400 haemagglutinating units per gram. Cooked beans should not normally contain more than 200–400 units per gram by this assay, and *raw* beans not more than 70 000. These must have been particularly virulent beans.

Lesson: Don't eat hard beans.

LECTINS, THE GUT AND NUTRITION

Astonishingly, considering that the existence of these toxic proteins in foodstuffs has been known for the best part of a century, it is only within the last three decades that scientists have wondered what they do to the animals that ingest them in the food,[183,243] and as far as I know Frank Green and I were the first to note, in 1975, that we humans also eat lectins.[89] Since the pioneering work of Pusztai and colleagues about 20 years ago,[243] there has been a flurry of 'me too' research that paints a very clear picture of the effects of PHA, WGA and one or two other lectins on the animal gut. Over the last decade, feeding lectins to rats seems to have become a 'safe' research project to give to postgraduate nutrition students worldwide. Seldom in the history of biology can so many rodents have sacrificed their lives and health merely for confirmatory research, and seldom can this information have been so resolutely ignored by the health workers and administrators at whom it was aimed. But such is the fate of most research that incriminates foods as causes of illness, so blinded are we by habit and addiction.

Although we all eat lectins in our food, few humans have personally swallowed or inhaled purified lectins. Speaking at least for myself, I can confirm that we humans are not all that different from rats,[88] but as my wife banned me from more self-experimentation, most of this section will deal with non-humans.

PHA induced enteropathy

PHA fed to rats causes a syndrome very similar to human coeliac disease, with disruption of villi and microvilli, increased exfoliation and faecal mass, crypt hyperplasia and increased intestinal mass, increased gut permeability with malabsorption of nutrients and reduced mucosal enzyme function, also impaired growth, anorexia and skeletal muscle wasting. Clinically, the picture is of an emaciated and sick animal, with wasted limbs but bloated belly, and as a clinician I cannot resist the comparison with the many humans I have known with diet-related illnesses. SBA, WGA and others produce similar though not identical syndromes, and similar effects are seen in other species (Table 34.3). McPherson points out the similarity with kwashiokor; malnourished children get most of their meagre protein from legumes, which are usually undercooked because of the expense and scarcity of fuel.[22,194]

Note that Table 34.3 lists *acute* effects of lectin feeding, usually of the order of a few days or weeks. Little attention has been paid to the likely appearance of secretory antilectin antibodies after a while, and what protection they might afford, besides which the accumulation of polyamines in intestine and gut noted in Table 34.3[20,21,280] may indicate the beginnings of a repair mechanism.[346] The acute effects of PHA feeding on rats are reversible within a few days of returning the animals to their normal diet.[22,67] A couple of very long-term experiments have been done[109,122] which suggest that the body may become tolerant in the long term. However, Grant *et al.*[109] noted multiple pancreatic nodules in their rats after about 2 years (an advanced age) with splenomegaly, raising the possibility of lectin-induced neoplasia in the long term.

Lectin encourages colonization by bacteria and protozoa

A good part of the damage in lectin-fed animals is due to the fact that the lectins encourage abnormal colonization by both bacteria and protozoa. This is done both by lectin 'bridging' between mucosa and organism, and by disruption of the thin

Table 34.3 Effects on animals of lectin feeding.

Effects on animals of lectin feeding				
Species	**Lectin**	**Effect**	**Reference**
Local effects on gut			
Rat	PHA	Stomach emptying delayed	22
Rat	PHA	Stomach atrophy	22
Rat, mouse, pig, rabbit	WGA, PHA, ConA	Disruption of villi/microvilli	18,67,113,116,121, 155,174,189,243, 258,264,274,289,363
Rat	PHA, WGA	Increased intestinal weight	108,110,246,363
Rat	PHA, WGA	Raised intestinal permeability	258,289
Rat	PHA	Lumping of mucus layer with patches of naked mucosa	18
Rat	PHA	Overgrowth by abnormal microbes	18,19,247
Rat	PHA	Increased faecal weight	17,176
Rat	ConA, WGA	Reduced intestinal permeability	289
Rat	ConA, WGA	Vascularization of villi and inflammation	189,289
Rat, pig	PHA, ConA, WGA	Crypt cell hyperplasia	155,176,189,246, 296,309,363
Rat	PHA	Crypt cell polyamine accumulation	20,21,280
Rat	PHA, ConA, WGA	Increased exfoliation of mucosa	189
Rat, pig	PHA, ConA, WGA	Enzymes disrupted	155,194,219,259 189,174,2,19
Mouse, rat	PHA, PSA, LCA, SBA, RCA	Reduced nutrient uptake	69,114,129,137, 194,330,363
Effects on non-alimentary organs			
Rat	PHA, WGA	Pancreatic hypertrophy with high polyamine metabolism	22,108,110,246
Rat	PHA	Liver atrophy	2
Rat	PHA	Thymic atrophy	110,246
Rat	PHA	Splenic atrophy	110
Rat	PHA	Skeletal muscle: raised lipid mobilization, reduced protein and glycogen	24
Rat	PHA	Hypoinsulinaemia	23,109
Effects on whole animal			
Rat	PHA	Reduced food intake	174,194,258,284
Rat	PHA	Negative nitrogen balance	17,243,246
Rat	PHA, ConA, WGA	Weight loss or impaired growth	133,189,246,363, 284,176
Germ-free rat	PHA	Weight *gain*	176
Rat	PHA	Raised blood urea	110
Rat, mouse	PHA	Death	67,133,
Salmon	SBA	Poor growth	333
Mouse	taro tuber	Poor growth, slow body movements	209

layer of mucus that normally prevents microbial adherence. Bacteria and protozoa multiply and adhere in large numbers to the denuded areas of mucosa.[18] Germ-free animals suffer far milder intestinal damage than conventional ones.[18,19,139,176]

Many bacteria and viruses possess an enzyme called neuraminidase, and this is important because the carbohydrate epitopes to which lectins bind frequently terminate with N-neuraminic acid (abbrev. NANA, syn. sialic acid). This NANA reduces the ability of lectins to bind: a natural defence mechanism. But if the NANA is stripped away by microbial neuraminidase, the tissue in question becomes more susceptible to lectin binding. Thus, bacteria and viruses that possess this enzyme (e.g. pneumococci, streptococci, vibrios, influenza virus[38,338]) can promote their own binding, and the binding of lectins and other microbes, to cell and mucosal surfaces. The toxic effect of WGA on rat gut is greatly enhanced by neuraminidase pretreatment.[189] This may explain why irritable bowel syndrome and other food-intolerance states are sometimes precipitated by an enteric bacterial infection[254] or by influenza.

Stone-age diet

Allergists who use the 'Stone-Age Diet' (see Chapter 57), which eliminates most carbohydrate foods and therefore most lectins, report that this diet appears to confer a large degree of immunity to common upper respiratory infections. Many patients (and I myself) notice that they only catch colds if they were 'cheating' at the time of virus exposure, by eating bread or some other forbidden luxury. It seems plausible that this may be due to the mucus-stripping effects of dietary lectins acting at the tonsillopharyngeal mucosa, allowing viruses to gain attachment when they would otherwise have been prevented by mucus. Of course, lectins are not unique in reducing the mucus layer; acute stress in animals does the same thing;[202] I am not seeking to blame lectins for *all* ills.

PEPTIC ULCER AND COELIAC DISEASE

It is reasonably clear that peptic ulcers are caused by (i) excessive acid secretion, (ii) defective mucous protection of the mucosa and (iii) abnormal proliferation of bacteria (*Helicobacter pylori*).

Acid secretion is caused by histamine release from gastric mast cells and is amplified by anxiety and stress. Most lectins degranulate mast cells and cause histamine release,[102,119,203,284,286,288,362]and in rats the stomach (parietal cells and others) binds much more lectin (PNA) within 15 min of acute stress (surface burn), at the same time as the acute gastric mucosal lesions appear (see Figs 1, 2, 5 and 6 in Ref 164).

Lectin binding to the stomach lining is influenced by diet.[26] Commercial 'rough' rat chow, which is based on unrefined cereals to a degree that I'm surprised that 'healthfood' fanatics don't eat it more, induces more WGA and SBA binding in the gastric mucosa than a synthetic diet of cellulose and amino acids.[280] Alcohol encourages WGA binding[208] but early dietary deficiency of n_3 polyunsaturated fatty acids reduces it.[3] PNA gastric binding is enhanced in mice by a high-protein diet,[111] while sow-fed piglets have less sulphated polysaccharide in the stomach than their artificially fed counterparts, reducing lectin binding.[324] These data suggest that multiple dietary factors would affect peptic ulcers. Clinically, withdrawal of wheat products has an anecdotal reputation for healing ulcers (T H Crouch, pers comm).

The other two ulcerogenic factors – mucus disruption and abnormal bacterial infection – are also encouraged by dietary lectins, as noted above.[18] Peptic ulcer is well controlled by β₂-blockers, but allergists need to be concerned about the potential of these drugs to aggravate food intolerance, and a trial of suitable sugar lectin inhibitors in peptic ulcer would seem indicated. For WGA inhibition, adding extra yeast (a rich source of chitin, which is a GNAc polymer) would serve very well.[277]

Coelic disease

Another gut disease long overdue for a lectin inhibitor trial is coeliac disease (CD), which I reviewed for the first edition of this book.[87] The intervening period has seen a polarization and hotting-up of the lectin hypothesis debate. There is general agreement that gliadin binds in a lectin-like manner to erythrocytes, reticulin and human mucosae, especially in untreated coeliacs, and is at least partly inhibited by the WGA antagonist, GNAc;[87,170,171,295,329] on the other hand, antiWGA antibodies, which are found in high

titre in CD patients, are only partly absorbable by gluten,[295] and sugar inhibition is incomplete. In general, the binding of gliadin is not typical of lectin or immune binding and is more reminiscent of hydrophobic binding.[48,263]

Several groups have examined jejunal biopsies for lectin binding. Barresi et al.[25,26] found more WGA and SBA binding to the mucosa of coeliacs than 'normal controls' (children being investigated for short stature), and noted that the abnormality did not revert with a gluten-free diet(GFD). Vecchi et al.[337] did a very similar survey and found no difference, but his controls were patients with irritable bowel, and Barresi et al.[26] pointedly (and rightly) criticized this choice of 'control' group. A third group found only slightly raised WGA binding to CD mucosa in comparison with growth-retarded 'controls' but a big increase in SBA and PHA binding in the CD group, which *did* normalize on a GFD.[235] So the picture remains confused; CD ought to be a lectin disease but proof is tantalizingly elusive, and is likely to remain so as long as truly healthy biopsies are hard to find.

Remember that a picture indistinguishable from CD can be caused by soya intolerance,[70] and this (at least in one trial) has been reversed by administration of galactose, the SBA inhibitor.[70,87]

DO LECTINS ENTER THE SYSTEMIC CIRCULATION?

Pokeweed (*Phytolacca americana*) is a North American weed. Some children who had inadvertently eaten it were examined and reported in 1966. They showed the interesting and rare finding of transformed lymphocytes in the peripheral blood smear. Pokeweed mitogen (PWM) had been discovered, and has been beloved of cell immunologists ever since. Together with the finding of circulating antilectin antibodies after lectin ingestion in rats, this was the sum total of evidence that I was able to adduce in the first edition of this book[87] to support my contention that ingested lectins may be systemically absorbed in active form. But it did not amount to proof because one could have argued (albeit not very convincingly) that the lectin might have stimulated Peyer's patch lymphocytes without leaving the gut wall. One could have also applied that argument to the finding of activated mononuclear cells in the rat spleen a week after PHA feeding.[103]

It was already known that Peyer's patch M cells bind and endocytose dietary lectins, but that was no surprise since these cells are specialized for sampling of particles and macromolecules from the lumen[96,230] and it did not prove that the lectins get right through. It was also shown later that WGA is internalized by endocytosis into various cells in vitro,[250,349] but that also was no proof that it would get to the serosal side of the gut. Furthermore, C¹⁴-labelled PHA and ConA, when instilled *in vitro* into loops of rabbit ileum, bound strongly to the mucosal side but reached the serosal side only in low MW, non-immunoreactive form,[199] which suggested that the gut is an effective barrier. Gut mucus would be expected to bind a large proportion of any ingested lectin, and especially its SIgA, which is ideally suited to protect against lectins because of its luxuriant carbohydrate side-chains.[64,99,350,351] And even if lectins did gain access to the circulation, they would immediately be bound by plasma proteins such as Tamm–Horsfall protein[353] and IgG side-chains,[37] to say nothing of the specific antibodies that ingested lectins evoke so efficiently[65,87,312] Until 1989 my general thesis of diseases in non-alimentary organs induced by blood-borne lectins stood on uncertain foundations.

Uptake of lectin after oral feeding

In that year the clinching experiments were reported, by Pusztai and his team in Aberdeen, who compared the uptake of ^{125}I-labelled PHA with that of tomato lectin and showed TCA-precipitable, oligosaccharide-inhibitable, immunoactive PHA in venous blood, liver, kidney, pancreas and spleen after oral feeding. Tomato lectin reached the portal blood, liver and kidney in similar amounts but in much lower concentrations in systemic blood pancreas and spleen.[23,158,217,244] WGA was studied in a separate experiment in 1993; it gets from the gut lumen at least into the capillaries and lymphatics of the villi; we do not yet know about any further spread because other organs were not studied.[246] And most recently (1998) PNA was detected in human serum 1–4 hours after eating 200 g of whole peanuts.[341]

These experiments prove that of the four dietary lectins thus far studied in the whole living animal, all pass into the portal blood from the gut lumen, and at least three of the four get right through into the systemic blood and/or peripheral organs (although to be sure the concentration of active lectin diminishes a lot as it passes the 'filters' of gut, blood, liver and lungs). Lectins such as WGA which enter the *lymphatic* circulation would gain access to the general circulation without having to pass liver and lungs, although that might not avail them much as they would have to traverse lymph nodes instead.

Rapid turnover of gut enterocytes

It is interesting to note that the gut, which bears the brunt of lectin assault, has a rapid turnover of enterocytes that to a great extent is *driven by* those lectins (a fact not sufficiently acknowledged in discussions of dietary fibre). The metabolic wastefulness of that turnover is worthwhile, as it serves to keep lectins away from the deeper tissues. Since only about 0.1% of the total doses of oral PHA and LEA found their way to the kidneys, and even less to pancreas and spleen, we can understand why healthy people do not suffer the toxic effects of food lectins, and we might perhaps be forgiven for feeling complacent. After all, 99.9% or more of the dose did *not* make it that far. But that would be false reassurance since these tissues do not have a rapid turnover of cells. Once stuck into connective tissue or skeletal muscle, lectin is likely to stay, and accumulate gradually over the years. As every allergist knows, 0.1% is all you need.

And I am not sure that 'healthy' people do entirely evade lectin toxicity. I am going to argue below that areas of soft-tissue rheumatism of the type termed 'rheumatic patches' are lectin-induced, and I have found in a population survey that these patches are present in well over 60% of 'healthy' people above the age of 30, albeit not severe enough to cause much trouble. Most people consider minor aches and pains 'normal', especially with advancing age, but while it may be statistically 'normal', it is not necessarily be physiologically normal.

LECTIN–INDUCED DISEASES BEYOND THE GUT?

If one thing wears my patience thin,
  it's phytohaemagglutinin.
And I confess I'm less than keen
  on tritiated thymidine
    – anonymous wag writing in the *Lancet*, circa 1970

It is not my brief to review lectins as lymphocyte mitogens, except to note that not all lectins are mitogenic; some are anti-mitogenic[159,269,334] and some (like WGA) have both actions depending on the dose and other factors;[156,355] the same caution applies to lectin effects on granulocytes and monocytes.[81,68,117,180,198,294,345] Depending on circumstances, lectins can protect against, or enhance, infections, reviewed by Sharon in 1996[281]. The point I want to emphasize is that lectins are in general inflammatory *in vivo*, which is not surprising given their effects on every compartment of the immune system including complement.[118,124,175,249] Lectins induce rat-paw oedema and raise gut and vascular permeability,[30,136,289] an effect quite separate from the innate toxicity of many lectins.[53] Lectin-induced inflammation has been an interest of mine since the day I inhaled an aerosol of ConA and gave myself bronchopneumonia.[87]

The severity of ragweed hayfever is related to the degree to which ragweed activates that patient's complement *in vitro*,[104] and needless to say I am inclined to attribute that effect to pollen lectins (see below). Intradermal injections of PHA are used as a rough-and-ready index of lymphocyte competence in animals and humans,[32,73,340] occasionally with spectacular reactions.[273] And lastly, many lectins can stimulate non-lymphoid cells to express class II MHC antigens, either directly or via induction of IFN-γ from PBL.[82,231,240,344] The significance of that is that a non-lymphoid cell that expresses class II MHC is liable to act as a target for autoimmunity, provided that 'foreign' antigen is also attached.

Given, then, that dietary lectins are capable of (a) reaching all organs in the body and there causing (b) toxic damage, (c) inflammation and/or (d) auto-immunity, we see that they are indeed 'causes in search of diseases'.

Diabetes

There seems to be general agreement now that insulin-dependent diabetes mellitus (IDDM) is an autoimmune disease caused by cytotoxic autoantibodies that damage islet cell structure and function. For autoantobodies against islet cells to be formed, we now know, the immune cells need to find islet cells that express both surface antigen and class II MHC.

It has been known for over 20 years that WGA and many other lectins act on adipocytes and other tissue cells just like insulin in terms of anabolism, cell proliferation, lipogenesis and antilipolysis.[190,222,236,348] This is the insulinomimetic effect that I reviewed in the first edition of this book,[87] and possibly sheds new light on why wheat makes people fat. What has become known since then is that dietary lectins also bind directly to islet cells and reduce plasma insulin in rats (although blood glucose levels do not rise in the acute phase because of the simultaneous insulin-omimetic effect that substitutes for the missing insulin, at least for a while[23,154,237]). PHA and *Robinia* lectin, injected intraperitoneally, caused major up-and-down fluctuations of blood glucose over the course of a week in rodents, and although that is an artificial situation it does suggest that lectin insulinomimesis may not be a phenomenon that one could rely on long term.[16,361]

In the human, WGA binds to the same surface receptors to which islet autoantibodies bind,[165] and the dominant epitope of that receptor is Gal 1–4GNAc[327] – that is, N-acetyl lactosamine, the classic hapten for LEA and almost as inviting for WGA, STA and PNA (Table 34.1). An islet cell with bound lectins, if it also expressed HLA-DR, would be a sitting duck for autoimmune attack.

Selectivity of IDDM

But since lectin-eating is common, why do we not all get IDDM? Because the LactNAc epitope is safely hidden under a protective coat of sialic acid and not available either to antibody or lectin binding. Until, that is, some neuraminidase comes along and unmasks the epitope, allowing the lectins and autoantibodies to bind.[327]

All it will take to set the process off will be an infection by a neuraminidase-producing organism (influenza, for example) to strip the sialic acid from the beta cells just at the same time as a high level of circulating lectin (a 'binge' on chocolate biscuits, perhaps). Maybe that lends some credence to the folklore cure of fasting during a fever.

A slightly weak link in this chain of argument is the simultaneous requirement for DR expression on the target cells, as I have not yet found direct evidence in the literature for DR stimulation by lectins or IFN-γ on *beta cells*[241] (even though it has been documented for practically every other tissue[7]. All the same, the missing link is not all that speculative as the simultaneous presence of viraemia and lectinaemia, as required by my hypothesis, does sometimes occur and can result in some spectacular synergisms.[229]

Clinical studies suggest that certain foods encourage IDDM, and certainly it can be induced in genetically susceptible mice by feeding them diabetogenic foods (wheat, soya and to a lesser extent milk). Conversely, IDDM can be prevented or delayed by keeping these foodstuffs out of their diet in early life.[276] Knowledge of lectin specificities leads us to predict that all Gal and GNAc-specific lectins would be implicated, thus extending the list of diabetogens to include potato, tomato, peanut, mushroom and the other grains (Table 34.1).

Rheumatic conditions

Connective tissues of various types, from areolar tissue to cartilage, share certain characteristics. There is always a matrix or ground substance composed of carbohydrate (glycosaminoglycans and proteoglycans), whose function is to absorb water and create inflation pressure. Tensile strength is provided by long 'ropes' of collagen and/or elastin which traverse the matrix, and buried within this structure are fibroblasts and other tissue cells. It is like a balloon distended with jelly, held together by threads within.[86]

Glycosaminoglycans (GAGs): these are long-chain polymers of monosaccharides, usually of two alternating types, and are either chondroitin sulphate, keratan sulphate or dermatan sulphate. These are attached to protein backbones, like the bristles of a bottle-brush, to form proteoglycan, and the proteoglycans are linked together by enormously long-chain GAGs called hyaluronic acid. The absorption of water is largely by osmosis, brought about by the clouds of positive ions attracted by the numerous sulphate groups on the GAGs. Most of the value of connective tissues lies in their rheology: cartilage must be stiff for support and strength, and areolar tissue must be loose and wobbly to allow movement. The sheaths of muscles and tendons are of the 'stiff, strong' variety, while superficial fascia, just under the skin, is normally in the latter class.

GAGs are, however, irresistibly attractive to lectins. Hyaluronic acid binds PHA, WGA and LCA, while chondroitin sulphate A binds WGA (which also has strong affinity for heparin[274]. Keratan sulphate binds STA[316] and to complete the picture collagen, a

protein, binds WGA strongly.[291] This means that WGA binds superficial fascia and skin, especially dermis[29,151,270,291,339,343] and I propose that this forms crosslinks and alters the rheology of the tissue from flexible to stiff. This has been suggested as the cause of the abnormal stiffness of oral submucosa that allows aphthous ulcers to form[302] and it seems to me to be a likely cause for the stiffened and tender areas of skin ('trigger points', 'rheumatic patches') that cause so much misery in the form of soft-tissue rheumatism and migraine.[86] Deeper in, where these tender areas are more often (wrongly) termed 'fibrositis', we find once again that muscle and interfibrillar sheaths attract WGA and other lectins, whereas muscle tissue itself does not.[52,161]

Connective tissue cells

In terms of the *cells* of connective tissue, WGA and other lectins inhibit the motility and reproduction of fibroblasts while at the same time stimulating GAG and collagenase synthesis.[27,86,145,146,357] Furthermore, one of the key functions of fibroblasts in connective tissue is to reorganize the collagen fibrils so as to expel water and contract the gel; WGA, PHA, LCA and PSA all interfere with this function.[9] The picture that we would expect to result from these effects would be excessive fluid retention in stiffened connective tissues, or, if localized, a palisade of immobilized fibroblasts surrounding an area distended by excessive watery gel, as in fact seen in rheumatoid nodules.[86]

Arthritis

As well as other connective tissues, healthy human cartilage is strongly bound by WGA (and fibrillated cartilage binds SBA and PNA in addition to WGA).[275] When in 1985 Brauer reported a rheumatoid-like arthritis in rabbits after intra-articular lectin injections (LCA, PSA, or to a lesser extent WGA).[323] it failed to rock the rheumatology world, but now we know that lectins can get from the gut to peripheral organs that experiment comes more sharply into focus. Unlike gut and skin, joints and connective tissues are slow-turnover organs and adherent lectin is still detectable for many months.[323] It would be reasonable to anticipate inflammation, toxic damage and autoimmune attack in those areas, as noted above. But what about rheumatoid factor?

Rheumatoid factor (RF): This is an auto-antibody against altered immunoglobulin.

The normal IgG molecule has carbohydrate side-chains, as well as antigen-binding sites. In health the majority of these side-chains terminate with galactose (the 'immunodominant' sugar) and sialic acid. In Sjögren's syndrome the sialic acid is deficient,[360] and in rheumatoid disease the galactose is also missing from a high percentage of IgG molecules, exposing GNAc instead[36,54 323]which ought to be instantly bound by any circulating WGA or STA. Indeed, most of the serum GNAc in normals is in IgG[37] and lectins (albeit not edible ones) are currently used to measure blood levels of the abnormal immunoglobulin in patients.[37,54,304] It is impossible that circulating diet-derived WGA would fail to bind the abnormal IgG, although this has not yet been confirmed.[232]

Agalactosyl-IgG (G$_0$): This contributes in a major way to the circulating immune complexes found in RA;[37] these complexes cause fever and symptoms and are no mere epiphenomenon. WGA may be implicated in RA autoimmunity, particularly since wheat is one of the commonest foods to cause arthritic symptoms (see Chapter 52). A lectin causation for both RA and soft-tissue rheumatism seems tantalizingly close but we still lack the clinching evidence, and the G_0 literature is surprisingly silent on the connection, namely, that WGA must bind to G_0 IgG, that we eat wheat daily, and that wheat makes arthritis worse. WGA *must* be implicated.

Nephritis

In the 1987 edition I noted[87] that Heymann nephritis antigen (gp330 or megalin) in rats is irresistibly attractive to LCA and WGA, and that these lectins would be expected to bind tightly into the glomerular filtration apparatus, disrupting function and attracting autoimmune attack. Within 2 years, Japanese workers had induced glomerulonephritis in the isolated rat kidney by infusing first lectin and then anti-lectin antibody, with HPA and LCA,[204,278] demonstrating that it could be done.

The situation in humans is not quite so clear because there seems to be no direct counterpart for gp330,[228] but that does not prevent WGA from binding avidly to the glomerular capillary wall and tubules.[87] WGA appears to be particularly relevant to IgA nephropathy (IgAN) in humans, perhaps because IgA_1 (the major isotype deposited in IgAN) is particularly lectin-sensitive due to its O-linked oligosaccharides.[127] The evidence incriminating wheat lectin as a cause of IgAN is now impressive. The lectinic (ethanol-soluble) portion of gliadin binds to mesangial cells in both rodents and humans, and at least in rodents binds IgA, induces IgA mesangial deposits, stimulates markers of growth and differentiation and enhances TNFα and IL6 production.[5,59] Children with IgAN have high blood levels of anti-gliadin and anti-mesangium antibodies and their IgA is unusually lectin-sensitive, at least for jacalin,[128,319] favouring circulating IgA 'immune complexes' – both antibody-mediated and carbohydrate-mediated.[58,60] But is there circulating WGA in IgAN? A GNAc-specific lectin has been isolated from the blood of children with active IgAN; just like gliadin it binds to mesangial cells and stimulates IL6[184] and I would suggest that it is in fact wheat lectin from the diet. And lastly, a gluten-free diet in IgAN patients was shown to reduce proteinuria, IgA-immune complexes and IgA food antibodies.[59]

Nor is wheat the only incriminated lectin; PHA enhances rabbit immune-complex glomerulonephritis.[51] And remember the lectin-facilitating role of *infections*; PNA binding to human glomerulus is enhanced by the neuraminidase liberated during both pneumococcal and streptococcal infections,[213,338] perhaps shedding light on the nephritogenic effects of streptococci. So stick to meats and fish during acute strep infections! (The same might apply to diabetes, in which fresh PNA-binding sites become exposed on human glomerulus,[132] except that renal physicians disapprove of stone-age diets because of the high protein content. Perhaps they could be persuaded to ban peanuts, but I fear it will take a revolution to wean them from their attachment to wholemeal bread.)

Infertility and teratogenesis

Lectins and WGA in particular bind avidly to human spermatozoa, to the extent that sperm agglutination is a standard method of screening plants for lectins.[180,197,212,238,287,335] In some ways this may be beneficial; the sialic acid coat (WGA positive) may in fact serve as temporary protection for the sperm from immune attack during passage along the hostile female reproductive tract,[91] being shed just before attachment to the oocyte.[177] Human ova also bind lectins,[191] and human endometrium is likewise highly lectin-avid, changing

somewhat in step with the cycle.[8,71,292,354] In one study of women with unexplained infertility their endometrial glands were shown to have less WGA-binding than normal,[167] either because of oligosaccharide deficiency or because the WGA receptors were already saturated. The stage seems set for lectinic reproductive mischief, and several investigations have been reported.

In view of the avidity of lectins, especially WGA, for mucus, it would not be surprising if lectins interfered with sperm penetration of cervical mucus, but this has not yet been found.[290] One Russian paper reports that WGA and PHA slow the penetration of human spermatozoa through *bovine* oestrous mucus,[43] which may be of some comfort to cows during the frozen Siberian winter. On the other hand, there have been several animal experiments that I cannot afford to be flippant about.

PHA and LCA induce germinal vesicle breakdown in mice.[77] WGA infused into one horn of the guinea pig uterus completely prevented embryo implantation in that horn,[297] and WGA also interferes profoundly with mouse embryonic development.[40,66] PNA injected into anuran larvae actually changes their sex,[285] though no-one has suggested that higher animals are affected that way. Ionizing radiation increases lectin binding in mouse embryos, which may indicate a synergism in teratogenesis.[223]

Embryo effects would not be surprising in view of the fundamental changes lectins cause to membrane fluidity noted in the 1987 edition[87] and since,[63,115,186,205,226,234,305,308] and the even more disturbing effect on protein and RNA transport exerted by WGA at the rat nucleus.[83,262] Teratogenesis experiments with lectins have obviously been confined to animal embryos, but the potential for human teratogenesis is there as human placenta and other fetal organs are as sensitive as adult tissues.[168,313,331]

IgE-Type allergy

In my early twenties I developed classic perennial allergic rhinitis of the 'early-morning sneezing' variety. I would wake with the alarm clock and lie in bed waiting for the sneezing to begin, which it invariably did within about 30 seconds, irrespective of what time I woke up. For the next half-hour, while bathing and dressing, I would sneeze maybe 100 times, soaking scores of paper tissues with clear watery mucus. After about a year I mentioned it to my then chief, Dr Geoffrey Taylor, who demonstrated Dermatophagoides allergy by skin-prick testing and gave me a new treatment, still experimental: a dry spray of cromoglycate powder to sniff. Surprisingly, that cured the problem for over 30 years.

I learned to analyse the sensation. The sneezing was always preceded by an intense stinging in the nose, as though the tender mucosa was being *seized* by some multilegged creature equipped with hundreds of minute hooks. I knew about IgE and mast cells, and mused that really it was *I* who was grabbing the *allergen*, not the other way around, yet for all the world that was what it felt like. So when I first read about lectins, I instinctively put two and two together and decided that lectins in allergens must somehow be involved in allergy.

Later I bought some purified ConA powder and tried sniffing it like snuff (I used ConA because I had never consumed jackbeans and I reasoned that any response would be pure, uncoloured by any immune response). The first 2–3 doses, a few weeks apart, each gave me an unpleasant soreness of the nasopharynx after about half-an-hour, with thick mucous catarrh, sometimes blood-streaked. It was identical to the first phase of a common cold when one feels miserable but doesn't look or sound too bad. I termed this the 'mucotractive effect' and later demonstrated it in rats.[88] After a few more ConA challenges, the pattern of symptoms changed to a rapid onset of stinging, sneezing and rhinorrhoea, similar to the second phase of a cold when one sounds awful but feels a lot better, and identical to the perennial rhinitis I had had years earlier. I lacked the funds and time to develop and validate a RAST for ConA. Nevertheless, it was a piece of evidence, albeit not strong, that I had developed a Type I allergy to the lectin and that it is the *lectins* in allergens that make them divert the immune responses into IgE in susceptible people (that is, they are the elusive 'atopens' proposed over the years by numerous workers and most persuasively by Berrens.[31]) It also led me to believe that the second phase of a common cold is caused by the body's IgE-mediated attempts to sneeze out the virus – again something I have never confirmed.

The quarter-century since then have provided vindication of my hypothesis. Grass and other pollens, as well as the peritrophic membranes that encase mite faeces, do indeed contain lectins,[87,136] as do the 'toxic dusts' of grain and soya well-known to occupational health authorities.[123,227] Some of the principal allergens of banana, peanut and rubber latex (prohevein) are lectins.[1,44,55,100,172] (There has been some interest in prohevein as a possible 'natural' fungistat for food plants. It has been engineered into transgenic tomatoes where it does in fact reduce fungal attack.[178] It will probably turn up increasingly as the cause of tomato allergy.) IgE antibodies from food-allergic patients bind preferentially to the lectins of those foods, by antibody recognition and not carbohydrate binding,[24] indicating that the food lectins are important allergens. Even hen's egg, a classic food allergen but not at first sight a likely source of lectins, contains lysozyme which is a monovalent lectin that is readily transformed into a full-fledged neolectin, as or more potent than WGA.[207] The other classic

food allergen, cow's milk, contains a seasonal haemagglutinin in the early summer in the UK (from the animals' feed, perhaps), as noted independently by David Davies and I when using the tanned-cell technique to measure human anti-milk antibodies (unpublished work). And of course Bordetella pertussis, the classic IgE adjuvant, possesses a famous lectin.[87,267,326]

I suggest that ConA drives the immune system into IgE has been confirmed in rats[185] as has also a similar effect for PHA if the timing is right.[11,12] Lectin-activated human T cells induce IgE-binding receptors on lymphocytes.[160,163] And, most excitingly, WGA, LCA, PHA and PSA drive basophils to produce IL4 and IL13, the key promoters of Th$_2$ responses:[112] that is, these lectins are atopens.

Please note also the direct and indirect ways in which lectins cause mast cell degranulation, as noted in 1987[87] and amply confirmed since,[42,102,142,284,362] although in some circumstances lectins also reduce histamine release[205,359] so the system is probably quite complicated. And multiple dosing of mice with jackfruit (a human food in the tropics but also the source of the now famous lectin jacalin) does indeed induced IgE,[251] at least in mice.

Perhaps the association with 'toxic dusts' provides another clue as to why atopy goes hand in hand with industrialization.[84]

Conclusions

I consider that the evidence is now strong for a lectin causation in peptic ulcer, coeliac disease, IDDM, some arthritides and nephritides and IgE-type allergy. It would be easy to widen the scope of this theory to include diseases of the other lectin-binding organs listed in Table 34.2, but there we lack strong experimental evidence. The time is ripe for therapeutic trials of carbohydrate lectin-blockers under the conditions listed here.

REFERENCES

1 Aleinus H, Kalkkinen N, Lukka M *et al*. Prohevein from the rubber tree is a major latex allergen. *Clin Exp Allergy* 1995; 25: 659–65.

2 Aletor VA. Effect of dietary sublethal doses of lima bean lectin on relative organ weights, pancreatic and intestinal trypsin. *Nahrung* 1989; 33: 355–60.

3 Allessandri JM, Joannic JL, Delpal S, Durand G. Effect of early dietary deficiency in polyunsaturated fatty acids on two lectin binding sites in the small intestine of postweaning rats. *J Pediatr Gastroenterol* 1995; 21: 165–76.

4 Alroy J, Goyal V, Skutelsky E. Lectin histochemistry of mammalian endothelium. *Histochemistry* 1987; 86: 603–7.

5 Amore A, Cavallo F, Bocchietto E *et al*. Cytokine mRNA expression by cultured rat mesangial cells after contact with environmental lectins. *Kidney Internat Suppl* 1993; 39:S41–6.

6 Andersen MM, Ebbesen K. Screening for lectins in common foods by line-drive immunoelectrophoresis and by haemadsorption lectin test. In: van Driessche E, Bog-Hansen TC (eds) *Lectins*, Vol. V. de Gruyter, Berlin: 1986; 95–108.

7 Anonymous editorial. What triggers auto-immunity? *Lancet* 1985; ii: 78–9.

8 Aoki D, Kawakami H, Nozawa S, Udagawa Y, Iizuka R, Hirano H. Differences in lectin binding patterns of normal human endometrium between proliferative and secretory phases. *Histochemistry* 1989; 92: 177–84.

9 Asaga H, Yoshizato K. Recognition of collagen by fibroblasts through cell surface glycoproteins reactive with *Phaseolus vulgaris* agglutinin. *J Cell Sci* 1992; 101pt3: 625–33.

10 Ashorn P, Vilja P, Ashorn P, Krohn K. Lectin binding affinities of human milk fat globule membrane antigens. *Mol Immunol* 1986; 23: 221–30.

11 Astorquiza MI, Cisternas C, Leal X. Sex-dependent differences in the IgE response modulated by phytohemagglutinin. *Immunol Lett* 1987; 16: 27–30.

12 Astorquiza MI, Cisternas C. IgE suppressor factor induced by PHA. *Int Arch Allergy Appl Immunol* 1990; 92: 223–5.

13 Aub JC, Tieslau C, Lankester A. Reactions of normal and tumor-cell surfaces to enzymes I. *Proc Nat Acad Sci USA* 1963; 50: 613–9.

14 Augustin-Voss HG, Pauli BU. Migrating endothelial cells are distinctly hyperglycosylated and express specific migration-associated cell surface glycoproteins. *J Cell Biol* 1992; 119: 483–91.

15 Baird RA, Schuff NR, Bancroft J. Regional differences in lectin binding of vestibular hair cells. *Hear Res* 1991; 65: 151–63.

16 Banach M, Zaremba S, Sadowska M. Disturbances of liver and muscle glycogen level in mice following administration of lectin. *Folia Biol Krakow* 1983; 31: 177–86.

17 Banwell JG, Abramowsky CR, Weber F, Howard R, Boldt DH. Phytohemagglutinin induced diarrheal disease. *Dig Dis Sci* 1984; 29: 921–9.

18 Banwell JG, Howard R, Cooper D, Costerton JW. Intestinal microbial flora after feeding PHA lectins to rats. *Appl Environ Microbiol* 1985; 50: 68–80.

19 Banwell JG, Howard R, Kabir I, Costerton JW. Bacterial overgrowth by indigenous microflora in the PHA-fed rat. *Can J Microbiol* 1988; 34: 1009–13.

20 Bardocz S, Grant G, Brown DS, Ewen SWB, Nevison I, Pusztai A. Polyamine metabolism and uptake during *Phaseolus vulgaris* lectin induced growth in rat small intestine. *Digestion* 1990; 46(suppl)2: 360–6.

21 Bardocz S, Brown DS, Grant G, Pusztai A. Luminal and basolateral polyamine uptake by rat small intestine stimulated to grow by *Phaseolus vulgaris* lectin PHA *in vivo*. *Biochim Biophys Acta* 1990; 1034: 46–52.

22 Bardocz S, Grant G, Ewen SWB et al. Reversible effect of PHA on the growth and metabolism of rat gastrointestinal tract. Gut 1995; 37: 353–60.

23 Bardocz S, Grant G, Pusztai A, Franklin MF, Carvalho AdeFFU. The effect of PHA at different dietary concentrations on the growth, body composition and plasma insulin of the rat. Br J Nutr 1996; 76: 613–26.

24 Barnett D, Howden ME. Lectins and the radioallergosorbent test. J Allergy Clin Immunol 1987; 80: 558–61.

25 Barresi G, Tuccari G, Tedeschi A, Magazzù G. Lectin binding sites in duodeno-jejunal mucosae from coeliac children. Histochemistry 1988; 88: 105–12.

26 Barresi G, Tuccari G, Tedeschi A, Magazzu G. Lectin binding sites in the jejunal mucosa of patients with gluten-sensitive enteropathy. Gut 1990; 31: 482–3, also ibid 30: 804–10 for debate.

27 Becchetti E, Locci P, Marinucci L, Lilli C, Pezetti F, Carinci P. Age related effects of lectins on GAG metabolism in cultured chick fibroblasts. Cell Mol Biol Noisy-le-grand 1994; 40: 183–92.

28 Behncken A, Saeger W. Lectin bindings in pituitary adenomas and normal pituitaries. Pathol Res Pract 1991; 187: 629–31.

29 Bell CM, Skerrow CJ. Factors affecting the binding of lectins to normal human skin. Br J Dermatol 1984; 111: 517–26.

30 Bento CAM, Cavada BS, Oliveira JTA, Moreira RA, Barja-Fidalgo C. Rat paw edema and leukocyte immigration induced by plant lectins. Agents Actions 1993; 38: 48–54.

31 Berrens L. The chemistry of atopic allergens. Monographs in Allergy, Vol. 7, Karger, Basel, 1971.

32 Binns RM, Licence ST, Wooding FBP. PHA induces major short-term protease-sensitive lymphocyte traffic involving high endothelium venules. Eur J Immunol 1990; 20: 1067–71.

33 Bird GWG. George Bird's reminiscences. In: Bog-Hansen TC, Freed DLJ (eds) Lectins: Biology, Biochemistry, Clinical Biochemistry, Vol. 6. Sigma Publishing, St Louis; 1988: 3–5.

34 Bishop PN, Boulton M, McLeod D, Stoddart RW. Glycan localisation within the human interphotoreceptor matrix and photoreceptor inner and outer segments. Glycobiology 1993; 3: 403–12.

35 Boland CR, Roberts JA. Quantitation of lectin binding sites in human colon mucins by use of peanut and wheatgerm agglutinins. J Histochem Cytochem 1988; 36: 1305–7.

36 Bond A, Cooke A, Hay FC. Glycosylation of IgG, immune complexes and IgG subclasses in the MRL-1pr/1pr mouse model of rheumatoid arthritis. Eur J Immunol 1990; 20: 2229–33.

37 Bond A, Kerr MA, Hay FC. Distinct oligosaccharide content of rheumatoid arthritis derived immune complexes. Arthr Rheum 1995; 38: 744–9.

38 Bonn D, McGregor A. H5N1 influenza investigation eases fears of pandemic. Lancet 1998; 351: 115.

39 Borges LF, Sidman RL. Axonal transport of lectins in the peripheral nervous system. J Neurosci 1982; 2: 647–53.

40 Brady PG, Vannier AM, Banwell JG. Identification of the dietary lectin wheat germ agglutinin in human intestinal contents. Gastroenterology 1978; 75: 236–9.

41 Brandon DM, Nayak SK, Binder PS. Lectin binding patterns of the human cornea. Cornea 1988; 7: 257–66.

42 Brzezinska-Blaszczyk E, Czuwaj M, Kuna P. Histamine release from mast cells of various species induced by histamine-releasing factor from human lymphocytes. Agents Actions 1987; 21: 26–31.

43 Bulanov I, Mladenov I, Bioanovska V, Gatera I, Stanislavov R. [The effect of lectins on human spermatozoa in the capillary sperm penetration test] (Russ: English abstract). Eksp Med Morfol 1990; 29: 42–5.

44 Burks AW, Cockrell G, Connaughton C, Guin J, Allen W, Helm RM. Identification of peanut agglutinin and soybean trypsin inhibitor as minor legume allergens. Int Arch Allergy Immunol 1994; 105: 143–9.

45 Bychkov V, Toto PD. Wheat germ and peanut agglutinin binding to normal, dysplastic and neoplastic cervical epithelium. Gynecol Obstet Invest 1986; 21: 158–63.

46 Byrne P, Williams A, Rollason T. Studies of lectin binding to the human cervix uteri. Histochem J 1989; 21: 311–22.

47 Caldero J, Campo E, Ascaso C, Ramos J, Panades MJ, Rene JM. Regional distribution of glycoconjugates in normal, transitional and neo-plastic human colonic mucosa. Virchows Archiv A: Pathol Anat Histopathol 1989; 415: 347–56.

48 Calderon de la Barea AM, Yepiz-Plasciencia GM, Bog-Hansen TC. Hydrophobic interactions between gliadin and proteins and celiac disease. Life Sci 1996; 59: 1951–60.

49 Callaghan JM, Toh BH, Pettitt JM, Humphris DC, Gleeson PA. Poly-N-acetyllactosamine-specific tomato lectin interacts with gastric parietal cells. J Cell Sci 1990; 95: 563–76.

50 Campo E, Condom E, Palacin A, Quesada E, Cardesa A. Lectin binding patterns in normal and neoplastic colonic mucosa. Dis Colon Rectum 1988; 31: 892–9.

51 Camussi G, Tetta C, Bussolino F et al. Effect of leukocyte stimulation on rabbit immune complex glomerulonephritis. Kidney Internat 1990; 38: 1047–55.

52 Capaldi MJ, Dunn MJ, Sewry CA, Dubowitz V. Lectin binding in human skeletal muscle. Histochem J 1985; 17: 81–92.

53 Carlini CR, Guimaraes JA. Plant and microbial toxic proteins. Toxicon 1991; 29: 791–806.

54 Casburn-Budd R, Yoninou P, Hager H et al. Asialylated IgG in the serum and synovial fluid of patients with rheumatoid arthritis. J Rheumatol 1992; 19: 1070–4.

55 Chen Z, Posch A, Lohaus C, Raulf-Heimsoth M, Meyer HE, Baur X. Isolation and identification of hevein as a major IgE-binding polypeptide in Hevea latex. J Allergy Clin Immunol 1997; 99: 402–9.

56 Chew EC, Yuen KW, Lee JC. Lectin histochemistry of normal and neoplastic nasopharyngeal epithelium. Anticancer Res 1991; 11: 697–704.

57 Concon JM, Newburg DS, Eades SN. Lectins in wheat germ proteins. J Agric Food Chem 1983; 31: 939–41.

58 Coppo R, Amore A, Roccatello D et al. IgA antibodies to dietary antigens and lectin-binding IgA in sera from Italian, Australian and Japanese IgA nephropathy patients. Am J Kid Dis 1991; 17: 480–7.

59 Coppo R, Amore A, Roccatello D. Dietary antigens and primary IgA nephropathy. J Am Soc Nephrol 1992; 2(10suppl):S173–80.

60 Coppo R, Amore A, Gianoglio B et al. Macromolecular IgA and abnormal IgA reactivity in sera from children with IgA nephropathy. Clin Nephrol 1995; 43: 1–13.

61 Cornwall J, Phillipson OT. Afferent projections to the dorsal thalamus of the rat as shown by retrograde lectin transport. Brain Res Bull 1988; 21: 147–61.

62 Crescenzi A, Barsotti P, Anemona L, Marinozzi V. Carbohydrate histochemistry of human Brunner's glands. Histochemistry 1988; 90: 47–9.

63 Darmani H, Coakley WT, Hann AC, Brain A. Spreading of WGA-induced erythrocyte contact by formation of spatially discrete contacts. Cell Biophys 1990; 16: 105–26.

64 Davin JC, Senterre J, Mahieu PR. The high lectin-binding capacity of human SIgA protects nonspecifically mucosae against environmental antigens. Biol Neonate 1991; 59: 121–5.

65 de Aizpurua HJ, Russell-Jones GJ. Identification of classes of proteins that provoke an immune response upon oral feeding. J Exp Med 1988; 167: 440–51.

66 Dealtry GB, Sellens MH. Lectin-induced abnormalities of mouse blastocyst hatching and outgrowth in vitro. Mol Reprod Dev 1990; 26: 24–9.

67 de Oliveira AC, Vidal V deC, Sgarbieri VC. Lesions of intestinal epithelium by ingestion of bean lectins in rats. J Nutr Sci Vitaminol 1989; 35: 315–22.

68 de Oliveira PSL, Garratt RC, Mascarenhas YP et al. Crystallization and preliminary crystalographic data on a neutrophil-inducing lectin. Proteins 1997; 27: 157–9.

69 Donatucci DA, Liener IE, Gross CJ. Binding of navy bean lectin to the intestinal cells of the rat and its effect on the absorption of glucose. J Nutr 1987; 117: 2154–60.

70 Donovan K, Torres-Pinedo R. Effect of D-galactose on the fluid loss in soybean protein intolerance. Pediatr Res 1978; 12: 433.

71 Duncan DA, Mazur MT, Younger JB. Glycoconjugate distribution in normal human endometrium. Int J Gynecol Pathol 1988; 7: 236–48.

72 Edmonds BT, Koenig E. Transmembrane cytoskeletal modulation in preterminal growing axons. Cell Motil Cytoskeleton 1990; 17: 106–17.

73 Ekkel ED, Kuypers AH, Connotte GHM, Tielen MJM. The PHA skin test as an indicator of stress-induced changes in immune reactivity of pigs. *Vet Q* 1995; 17: 143–6.

74 Erickson RH, Kim YS. Interaction of purified brush-border membrane aminopeptidase N and dipeptidase N with lectin-Sepharose derivatives. *Biochim Biophys Acta* 1983; 743: 37–42.

75 Erickson RH, Kim J, Sleisinger MH, Kim YS. Effect of lectins on the activity of brush border membrane-bound enzymes of rat small intestine. *J Pediatr Gastroenterol Nutr* 1985; 4: 984–91.

76 Fabian RH, Coulter JD. Transneuronal transport of lectins. *Brain Res* 1985; 344: 41–8.

77 Fagbohun CF, Downs SM. Maturation of the mouse oocyte-cumulus cell complex: stimulation by lectins. *Biol Reprod* 1990; 42: 413–23.

78 Farnum CE. Binding of lectin-fluorescein conjugates to intracellular compartments of growth-plate chondrocytes in situ. *Am J Anat* 1985; 174: 419–35.

79 Farnum CE. In-situ localization of lectin-binding glycoconjugates in the matrix of growth-plate cartilage. *Am J Anat* 1986; 176: 65–82.

80 Farragiana T, Malchiodi F, Prado A, Churg J. Lectin-peroxidase conjugate activity in normal human kidney. *J Histochem Cytochem* 1982; 30: 451–8.

81 Felipe I, Bim S, Somensi CC. Increased clearance of C. *albicans* from the peritoneal cavity of mice pretreated with ConA or jacalin. *Braz J Med Biol Res* 1995; 28: 477–83.

82 Filipic B, Golob A, Struna T, Likar M. Porcine mitogen-induced interferon. *Acta Virol* 1994; 38: 71–5.

83 Finlay DR, Newmeyer DD, Price TM, Forbes DJ. Inhibition of *in vitro* nuclear transport by a lectin that binds to nuclear pores. *J Cell Biol* 1987; 104: 189–20.

84 Finn R. John Bostock, hay fever, and the mechanism of allergy. *Lancet* 1992; 340: 1453–5.

85 Fischer J, Csillik B. Lectin binding: a genuine marker for transganglionic regulation of human primary sensory neurons. *Neurosci Lett* 1985; 54: 263–7.

86 Fox WW, Freed DLJ. *Understanding Arthritis: the Clinical Way Forward.* Macmillan, Basingstoke, 1990.

87 Freed DLJ. Dietary lectins and disease. In: Brostoff J, Challacombe S (eds) *Food Allergy and Food Intolerance.* Bailliére Tindall, Eastbourne; 1987: 375–400.

88 Freed DLJ, Buckley CH. Mucotractive effect of lectins. *Lancet* 1978; i: 585–6.

89 Freed DLJ, Green FHY. Do dietary lectins protect against bowel cancer? *Lancet* 1975; ii: 1261.

90 Fukami K, Ohyama M. Histochemistry of glycoconjugates in tonsillar tissues. *Acta Otolaryngol Supp, Stockh* 1988; 454: 33–8.

91 Gabriel LK, Franken DR, van der Horst G, Kruger TF. FITC conjugate WGA staining of human spermatozoa and fertilisation *in vitro. Fertil Steril* 1995; 63: 894–901.

92 Ganguly P, Fossett NG. The rôle of sialic acid in the activation of platelets by wheatgerm agglutinin. *Blood* 1984; 63: 181–7.

93 Ganguly CL, Chelladurai M, Ganguly P. Protein phosphorylation and activation of platelets by wheatgerm agglutinin. *Biochem Biophys Res Comm* 1985; 132: 313–9.

94 Gelberg H, Whiteley H, Ballard G, Scott J, Kuhlenschmidt M. Temporal lectin histochemical characterization of porcine small intestine. *Am J Vet Res* 1992; 53: 1873–80.

95 Geleff S, Böck P. Pancreatic duct glands II. *Histochemistry* 1984; 80: 31–38.

96 Giannasca PJ, Giannasca KT, Falk P, Gordon JI, Neutra MR. Regional differences in glycoconjugates of intestinal M cells in mice: potential targets for mucosal vaccines. *Am J Physiol* 1994; 267:G1108–21.

97 Gibbons RJ, Dankers I. Lectin-like constituents in foods which react with components of human serum, saliva, and *Strep mutans. Appl Environ Microbiol* 1981; 41: 880–8.

98 Gibbons RJ, Dankers I. Association of food lectins with human oral epithelial cells *in vivo. Archs Oral Biol* 1983; 28: 561–6.

99 Gibbons RJ, Dankers I. Immunosorbent assay of interactions between human parotid IgA and dietary lectins. *Arch Oral Biol* 1986; 31: 477–81.

100 Gidrol X, Chrestin H, Tan HL, Kush A. Hevein, a lectin-like protein from *Hevea brasiliensis* (rubber tree) is involved in the coagulation of latex. *J Biol Chem* 1994; 269: 9278–83.

101 Gil-Loyzaga P, Brownell WE. Wheat germ agglutinin and *Helix pomatia* lectin binding in cochlear hair cells. *Hear Res* 1988; 34: 149–55.

102 Gomes JC, Ferreira RR, Cavada BS, Moreira RA, Oliveira JT. Histamine release induced by glucose (mannose)-specific lectins isolated from Brazilian beans. *Agents Actions* 1994; 41: 132–5.

103 Gómez E, Ortiz V, Ventura J, Campos R, Bourges H. Intestinal and systemic immune responses in rats to dietary lectins. *Adv Exp Med Biol* 1995; 371A: 533–6.

104 Gönczi Zs, Varga L, Hidvégi T *et al.* The severity of clinical symptoms in ragweed-allergic patients is related to the extent of ragweed-induced complement activation. *Allergy* 1997; 52: 1110–14.

105 Gotz W, Fischer G, Herken R. Lectin binding pattern in the embryonal and early fetal human vertebral column. *Anat Embryol Berlin* 1991; 184: 345–53.

106 Graham GS, Codd AA. Food poisoning from red kidney beans. Also: Gilbert RJ: Healthy eating day. *Communicable Dis Report*, 1988; 33: 3–4.

107 Grant G, More LJ, McKenzie NH, Pusztai A. The effect of heating on the haemagglutinating activity and nutritional properties of bean (*Phaseolus vulgaris*) seeds. *J Sci Food Agric* 1982; 33: 1324–6.

108 Grant G, Bardocz S, Brown DS, Watt WB, Stewart JC, Pusztai A. Involvement of polyamines in pancreatic growth induced by dietary soyabean, lectins or trypsin inhibitors. *Biochem Soc Trans* 1990; 18: 1009–10.

109 Grant G, Dorward PM, Buchan WC, Armour JC, Pusztai A. Consumption of diets containing raw soya beans, kidney beans, cowpeas or lupin seeds by rats for up to 700 days. *Br J Nutr* 1995; 73: 17–29.

110 Greer F, Brewer AC, Pusztai A. Effect of kidney bean toxin on tissue weight and composition and some metabolic functions in rats. *Br J Nutr* 1985; 54: 95–103.

111 Gupta R, Jaswal VM, Meenu-Mahmood A. Intestinal epithelial cell surface glycosylation in mice I. *Ann Nutr Metab* 1992; 36: 288–95.

112 Haas H, Falcone FH, Schramm G *et al.* Dietary lectins can induce *in vitro* release of IL-4 and IL-13 from human basophils. *Eur J Immunol* 1999; 29: 1–10.

113 Hara T, Tsukamoto I, Miyoshi M. Oral toxicity of kintoki bean lectin. *J Nutr Sci Vitaminol* 1983; 29: 589–99.

114 Hara T, Mukunoki Y, Tsukamoto I, Miyoshi M, Hasegawa K. Susceptibility of kintoki bean lectin to digestive enzymes *in vitro* and its behaviour in the digestive organs of mouse *in vivo. J Nutr Sci Vitaminol Tokyo* 1984; 30: 381–94.

115 Hare BJ, Rise F, Aubui Y, Prestegard JH. ^{13}C NMR studies of WGA interactions with GNAc at a magnetically orientated bilayer surface. *Biochemistry* 1994; 33: 10137–48.

116 Hart CA, Batt RM, Saunders JR, Getty B. Lectin-induced damage to the enterocyte brush-border. *Scand J Gastroenterol* 1988; 23: 1153–9.

117 Hartshorn KL, Daigneault DE, White MR, Tauber AI. Anomalous features of human neutrophil activation by influenza A virus. *J Leukoc Biol* 1992; 51: 230–6.

118 Hashim OH, Gendeh GS, Cheong CN, Jaafar MI. Effect of Artocarpus integer lectin on functional activity of guineapig complement. *Immunol Invest* 1994; 23: 153–60.

119 Helm RM, Froese A. Binding of the receptors of IgE by various lectins. *Int Archs Allergy Appl Immunol* 1981; 65: 81–84.

120 Helmeste DM, Chudzik J, Tang SW. Interaction of lectins with human platelet serotonin transporter. *Eur J Pharmacol* 1994; 266: 327–31.

121 Hendriks HGC, Kik MJL, Koninkx JFJ, van den Ingh TSG, Mouwen JMV. Binding of kidney bean isolectins to differentiated human colon carcinoma Caco-2 cells. *Gut* 1991; 32: 196–201.

122 Henney L, Ahmed EM, George DE, Kao KJ, Sitren HS. Tolerance to long-term feeding of isolated peanut lectin in the rat: evidence for a trophic effect on the small intestines. *J Nutri Sci Vitaminol Tokyo* 1990; 36: 599–607.

123 Hernando L, Navarro C, Marquiz M, Zapatero L, Galvan F. Asthma epidemics and soybean in Cartagena (Spain). *Lancet* 1989; i: 502.

124 Hiemstra PS, Gorter A, Stuurman ME, van Es LA, Daha MR. The IgA-binding lectin jacalin induces complement activation by inhibition of C1-inactivator function. *Scand J Immunol* 1987; 26: 111–17.

125 Higashihara N, Ozaki Y, Ohashi T, Kume S. Interaction of *Solanum tuberosum* agglutinin with human platelets. *Biochem Biophys Res Comm* 1984; 121: 27–33.

126 Higuchi M, Kawada T, Iwai K. *In vivo* binding of the winged bean basic lectin labelled with iodo [$^{2-14}$C] acetic acid to the intestinal epithelial cells of the rat. *J Nutr* 1989; 119: 490–5.

127 Hiki Y, Horii A, Iwase H *et al*. O-linked oligosaccharide on IgA$_1$ hinge region in IgA nephropathy. *Contrib Nephrol* 1995; 111: 73–84.

128 Hiki Y, Iwase H, Saitoh M *et al*. Reactivity of glomerular and serum IgA$_1$ to jacalin in IgA nephropathy. *Nephron* 1996; 72: 429–35.

129 Hisayasu S, Orimo H, Migita S *et al*. Soybean protein isolate and soybean lectin inhibit iron absorption in rats. *J Nutr* 1992; 122: 1190–6.

130 Holthöfer H. Lectin binding sites in kidney. *J Histochem Cytochem* 1983; 31: 531–7.

131 Holthöfer H, Virtanen I, Törnoth T, Miettinen A. Alterations in glomerular lectin binding sites of human kidney as detected by fluorescence microscopy. *Histochem J* 1985; 17: 905–12.

132 Holthöfer H, Pettersson E, Törnroth T. Diabetes mellitus associated changes in glomerular glycocompounds. *Histochem J* 1987; 19: 351–6.

133 Honavar PM, Shih CV, Liener IE. Inhibition of the growth of rats by purified hemagglutinin fractions isolated from *Phaseolus vulgaris*. *J Nutr* 1962; 77: 109–114.

134 Hukkanen V. Lectin-reactive components in white matter membranes from normal and multiple sclerosis brains. *J Neurochem* 1982; 38: 1537–41.

135 Hwang S-B, Wang S. Wheatgerm agglutinin potentiates specific binding of platelet-activating factor to human platelet membranes. *Mol Pharmacol* 1991; 39: 788–97.

136 Imamura T, Di Virgilio S, Bagarozzi DA, Matheson N, Travis J. Induction of histamine release from non-immunized guineapigs. *Int Arch Allergy Immunol* 1996; 111: 161–5.

137 Ishiguro M, Matori Y, Tanabe S, Kawase Y, Sekine I, Sakakibara R. Biochemical studies on oral toxicity of ricin V. The rôle of lectin activity. *Chem Pharm Bull Tokyo* 1992; 40: 1216–20.

138 Jaeger LA, Lamar CH, Turek JJ. Lectin binding to small intestinal goblet cells of newborn, suckling and weaned pigs. *Am J Vet Res* 1989; 50: 1984–7.

139 Jayne-Williams DJ. Influence of dietary jackbeans and of Con A on the growth of conventional and gnotobiotic Japanese quail (*Coturnix coturnix japonica*). *Nature New Biol* 1973; 243: 150–51.

140 Johnson LV. WGA induces compaction- and cavitation-like events in two-cell mouse embryos. *Dev Biol* 1986; 113: 1–9.

141 Jonas L, Putzke HP. Light and electron microscopic studies of lectin binding to the glycocalyx of rat pancreatic cells. *Acta Histochem* 1992; 93: 388–96.

142 Jones CJ, Kirkpatrick CJ, Stoddart RW. An ultrastructural study of the morphology and lectin-binding properties of human mast cell granules. *Histochem J* 1988; 20: 433–42.

143 Jordinson M, Deprez PH, Playford RJ, Heal S, Freeman TC, Alison M, Calam J. Soybean lectin stimulates pancreatic exocrine secretion via CCK-A receptors in rats. *Am J Physiol* 1996; 270(4pt1):G653–9.

144 Juan FT, Hoshima M, Manalo AM, Mochizuki M. Lectin binding in tissues from hydatidiform mole, invasive mole and choriocarcinoma to ConA, WGA and PNA. *Asia Oceania J Obstet Gynaecol* 1989; 15: 383–93.

145 Kaplowitz PB. WGA and ConA inhibit the response of human fibroblasts to peptide growth factors by a post-receptor mechanism. *J Cell Physiol* 1985; 124: 474–80.

146 Kaplowitz PB, Haar JL. Antimitogenic actions of lectins in cultured human fibroblasts. *J Cell Physiol* 1988; 136: 13–22.

147 Karayannopoulon G, Damjanov I. Lectin binding sites in the human gallbladder and cystic duct. *Histochemistry* 1987; 88: 75–83.

148 Katz DM, White ME, Hall AK. Lectin binding distinguishes between neuroendocrine and neuronal derivatives of the sympathoadrenal neural crest. *J Neurobiol* 1995; 26: 241–52.

149 Kawano K, Uehara F, Ohba N. Lectin-cytochemical study on epithelial mucus glycoprotein of conjunctiva and pterygium. *Exp Eye Res* 1988; 47: 43–51.

150 Kean EL, Sharon N. Inhibition of yeast binding to mouse peritoneal macrophages by wheat germ agglutinin. *Biochem Biophys Res Comm* 1987; 148: 1202–7.

151 Keeble S, Watt FM. Characterisation of the peanut lectin-binding glycoproteins of human epidermal keratinocytes. *Differentiation* 1990; 43: 139–45.

152 Kellokumpu I, Karhi K, Andersson LC. Lectin-binding sites in normal, hyperplastic, adenomatous and carcinomatous human colorectal mucosa. *Acta Pathol Microbiol Immunol Scand [A]* 1986; 94: 271–80.

153 Kessimian N, Langner BJ, McMillan PN, Jauregui HO. Lectin binding to parietal cells of human gastric mucosa. *J Histochem Cytochem* 1986; 34: 237–43.

154 Khalid P, Ahmad F, Khan MM, Rastogi AK, Kidwai JR. Effect of age on the binding of lectin ^{125}I-PHA-B to pancreatic islets of rat *in vitro* and stimulation of some cellular events. *Acta Diabetol Lat* 1989; 26: 171–80.

155 Kik MJ, Koninkx JF, van-den-Muysenberg A, Hendriksen F. Pathological effects of *Phaseolus vulgaris* isolectins on pig jejunal mucosa in organ culture. *Gut* 1991; 32: 886–92.

156 Kilpatrick DC, McCurrach PM. Wheat germ agglutinin is mitogenic, nonmitogenic and anti-mitogenic for human lymphocytes. *Scand J Immunol* 1987; 25: 343–8.

157 Kilpatrick DC, Graham C, Urbaniak SJ. The immunosuppressive nature of tomato lectin and its possible clinical relevance. In: Breborowicz J, Bog-Hansen TC (eds) *Lectins: Biology, Biochemistry, Clinical Biochemistry*, Vol. IV, de Gruyter, Berlin; 1985; 3–13.

158 Kilpatrick DC, Pusztai A, Grant G, Graham C, Ewen SWB. Tomato lectin resists digestion in the mammalian alimentary canal and binds to intestinal villi without deleterious effects. *FEBS Lett* 1985; 185: 299–305.

159 Kilpatrick DC, Graham C, Urbaniak SJ. Inhibition of human lymphocyte transformation by tomato lectin. *Scand J Immunol* 1986; 24: 11–19.

160 Kim KM, Tanaka M, Yoshimura T, Katanura K, Mayumi M, Mikawa H. Regulation of IgE receptor expression of human PBL by lymphocytosis-promoting factor, lectins and dexamethasone. *Clin Exp Immunol* 1987; 68: 418–26.

161 Kirkeby S. Glycosylation pattern and enzyme activities in atrophic, angulated skeletal muscle fibres from ageing rats. *Virchs Arch* 1994; 424: 279–85.

162 Kirkpatrick CJ, Jones CJP, Stoddart RW. Lectin histochemistry of the mast cell. *Histochem J* 1988; 20: 139–46.

163 Kisaki T, Huff TF, Conrad DH, Yodoi J, Ishizaka K. Monoclonal antibody specific for T-cell-derived human IgE binding factors. *J Immunol* 1987; 138: 3345–51.

164 Kitajima M, Mogi M, Kiuchi T *et al*. Alternation of gastric mucosal glycoprotein (lectin-binding pattern) in gastric mucosa in stress. *J Clin Gastroenterol* 1990; 12suppl: S1–S7.

165 Kitano N, Taminato T, Ida T *et al*. Detection of antibodies against WGA-bound glycoproteins on the islet-cell membrane. *Diabet Med* 1988; 5: 139–44.

166 Kivela T. Characterization of galactose-containing glycoconjugates in the human retina. *Curr Eye Res* 1990; 9: 1195–209.

167 Klentzeris LD, Bulmer JN, Morrison L, Warren A, Cooke LD. Lectin binding of endometrium in women with unexplained infertility. *Fertil Steril* 1991; 56: 660–7.

168 Klima G, Zerlanth B, Wolf H, Schellnast R. A study of lectin bindings to the fetal membranes. *Anat Anz* 1991; 173: 87–91.

169 Ko CP. A lectin, PNA, as a probe for the extracellular matrix in living neuromuscular junctions. *J Neurocytol* 1987; 16: 567–76.

170 Kolberg J, Sollid L. Lectin activity of gluten identified as wheat germ agglutinin. *Biochem Biophys Res Comm* 1985; 130: 867–72.

171 Kolberg J, Wedege E, Sollid L. Immunoblotting detection of lectins in gluten and white rice flour. *Biochem Biophys Res Comm* 1987; 142: 717–23.

172 Koshte VL, Aalbers M, Calkhoven PG, Aalberse RC. The potent IgG$_4$-inducing antigen in banana is a mannose-binding lectin. *Int Arch Allergy Immunol* 1992; 97: 17–24.

173 Kuizenga A, van Haeringen NJ, Kijlstra A. Identification of lectin binding proteins in human tears. *Invest Ophthalmol Vis Sci* 1991; 32: 3277–84.

174 Lafont J, Rouanet J-M, Gabrion J, Assouad JL, Zambonino-Infante JL, Besancon P. Duodenal toxicity of dietary *Phaseolus vulgaris* lectins in the rat: an integrative assay. *Digestion* 1988; 41: 83–93.

175 Langone JJ, Boyle MDP, Borsos T. Effect of ConA on the classical complement pathway. *J Immunol* 1977; 118: 1622.

176 Larson G, Falk P, Howard R, Banwell JG. Intestinal sphingolipid excretion associated with lectin feeding. *Glycoconj J* 1989; 6: 539–50.

177 Lassalle B, Testart J. Are sperm WGA receptors involved in fertilization? *Fertil Steril* 1996; 65: 448–50.

178 Lee HI, Raikhel NV. Prohevein is poorly processed but shows enhanced resistance to a chitin-binding fungus in transgenic tomato plants. *Braz J Med Biol Res* 1995; 28: 743–50.

179 Lee M-C, Damjanov I. Pregnancy-related changes in the human endometrium revealed by lectin histochemistry. *Histochemistry* 1985; 82: 275–80.

180 Lee M-C, Damjanov I. Lectin binding sites on human sperm and spermatogenic cells. *Anat Rec* 1985; 212: 282–7.

181 Lee YS. Lectin reactivity in human large bowel. *Pathology* 1987; 19: 397–401.

182 Lee YS. Lectin expression in neoplastic and non-neoplastic lesions of the rectum. *Pathology* 1988; 20: 157–65.

183 Leiner IE. Nutritional significance of lectins in the diet. In: Liener IE, Sharon N, Goldstein IJ (eds) *The Lectins*. Academic Press, London; 1986; 527–52.

184 Libetta C, Rampino T, Palumbo G, Esposito C, dal Canton A. Circulating serum lectins of patients with IgA nephropathy stimulate IL-6 release from mesangial cells. *J Am Soc Nephrol* 1997; 8: 208–13.

185 Lim BO, Yamada K, Sugano M. Effects of bile acids and lectins on immunoglobulin production in rat mesenteric lymphnode lymphocytes. *In Vitro Cell Dev Biol Anim* 1994; 30A: 407–13.

186 Lin S, Huestis WH. WGA stabilization of erythrocyte shape. *Biochim Biophys Acta* 1995; 1233: 47–56.

187 Lis H, Sharon N. Lectins in higher plants. In: Marcus A (ed) *The Biochemistry of Plants, Vol. VI: Proteins and Nucleic Acids*. Academic Press, New York; 1981.

188 Lorenc-Kubis J, Klimczak A, Morawiecka B. Lectins from squash seedlings. *Acta Biochim Pol* 1993; 40: 103–5.

189 Lorenz-Meyer H, Roth H, Elsässer P, Hahn U. Cytotoxicity of lectins on rat intestinal mucosa enhanced by neuraminidase. *Eur J Clin Invest* 1985; 15: 227–34.

190 Lotan RM, Barzilai D. Effect of WGA and ConA on insulin binding and response by Madin-Darby canine kidney cells. *Isr J Med Sci* 1990; 26: 5–11.

191 Lucas H, Bercegeay S, LePendu J, Jean M, Mirallie S, Barriere P. A fucose-containing epitope potentially involved in gamete interaction on the human zona pellucida. *Hum Reprod* 1994; 9: 1532–8.

192 McIntyre LJ, Quarles RH, Brady RO. Lectin-binding proteins in CNS myelin. *Biochem J* 1979; 183: 205–12.

193 McNeal JE, Leav I, Alroy J, Skutelsky E. Differential lectin staining of central and peripheral zones of the prostate. *Am J Clin Pathol* 1988; 89: 41–8.

194 McPherson L. Lectins in the etiology of protein-energy malnutrition. *J Roy Soc Health* 1989; 109: 66–8.

195 Madrid JF, Ballesta J, Galera T, Castells MT, Perez-Tomas R. Histochemistry of glycoconjugates in the gallbladder epithelium of ten animal species. *Histochemistry* 1989; 91: 437–43.

196 Magner JA, Kane J. Binding of thyrotropin to lentil lectin is unchanged by thyrotropin-releasing hormone. *Endocr Res* 1992; 18: 163–73.

197 Malmi R, Kallajoki M, Suominen J: Distribution of glycoconjugates in human testis. *Andrologia* 1987; 19: 322–32.

198 Mangnisson KE, Dahlgren C, Sjolander A. Distinct patterns of granulocyte luminol dependent chemoluminescence response to lectins. *Inflammation* 1988; 12: 17–24.

199 Marcon-Genty D, Krempf M, Tome D. Transmucosal transport of PHA, Con A and alpha-lactalbumin across rabbit ileum in vitro. *Gastroenterol Clin Biol* 1991; 15: 10–15.

200 Mares V, Borges LF, Sidman RL. Uptake and transport of lectins from the cerebrospinal fluid by cells of the immature mouse brain. *Acta Histochem* 1984; 74: 11–19.

201 Martin-Lacane I, Mora-Marin J, Montero-Linares C, Galera-Davidson H. Lectin histochemistry of the thyroid gland. *Cancer* 1988; 62: 2354–62.

202 Mason CM, Azizi SQ, Dal-Nogare AR. Respiratory epithelial carbohydrate levels of rats with gram negative bacillary colonization. *J Lab Clin Med* 1992; 120: 740–5.

203 Matsuda K, Aoki J, Uchida MK, Suzuki-Nishimura T. Datura stramonium agglutinin released histamine from rat peritoneal mast cells. *Jpn J Pharmacol* 1994; 66: 195–204.

204 Matsuo S, Yoshida F, Yuzawa Y et al. Experimental glomerulonephritis induced in rats by a lectin and its antibodies. *Kidney Internat* 1989; 36: 1101–21.

205 Matsuya Y, Yamane T. Cell hybridization and cell agglutination. I: Enhancement of cell hybridization by lectins. *J Cell Sci* 1985; 78: 263–71.

206 May DP, Sloan P. Lectin binding to normal mucosa, leukoplakia and squamous cell carcinoma. *Med Lab Sci* 1991; 48: 6–18.

207 Mega T, Hase S. Conversion of egg-white lysozyme to a lectin-like protein with agglutinating activity analogous to WGA. *Biochim Biophys Acta* 1994; 1200: 331–3.

208 Mitchell PA, Miller TA, Schmidt KL. Effects of alcohol on lectin binding affinity in rat gastric mucosa. *Dig Dis Sci* 1990; 35: 865–72.

209 Miyoshi M. The effect of lectin from Taro tuber (*Colocasia antiquorum*) given by force-feeding on the growth of mice. *J Nutri Sci Vitaminol Tokyo* 1990; 36: 277–85.

210 Mizukawa Y, Takata K, Ookusa Y, Nagashima M, Hirano H. Lectin binding pattern in normal human labial mucosa. *Histochem J* 1994; 26: 863–9.

211 Moré J, Fioramonti J, Bénazet F, Buéno L. Histochemical characterization of glycoproteins present in jejunal and colonic goblet cells of pigs on different diets. *Histochemistry* 1987; 87: 189–94.

212 Mortimer D, Curtis EF, Camenzind AR. Combined use of fluorescent PNA and Hoechst 33258 to monitor acrosomal status and vitality of human spermatozoa. *Human Reprod* 1990; 5: 99–103.

213 Mosquera JA, Rodríguez-Iturbe B. Glomerular binding sites for peanut agglutinin in acute poststreptococcal glomerulonephritis. *Clin Nephrol* 1986; 26: 227–34.

214 Murakami I, Sarker AB, Hayashi K, Akagi T. Lectin binding patterns in normal liver. *Acta Pathol Jpn* 1992; 42: 566–72.

215 Nachbar MS, Oppenheim JD. Lectins in the US diet. *Am J Clin Nutr* 1980; 33: 2338–45.

216 Nagao M, Kamo H, Akiguchi I, Kimura J. SBA binds commonly to a subpopulation of small diameter neurons. *Neurosci Lett* 1992; 142: 131–4.

217 Naisbett B, Woodley J. Binding of tomato lectin to the intestinal mucosa and its potential for oral drug delivery. *Biochem Soc Trans* 1990; 18: 879–80.

218 Nakai M, Tatemoto Y, Mori H, Mori M. Lectin-binding patterns in the developing tooth. *Histochemistry* 1985; 83: 455–63.

219 Nakata S, Kimura T. Effect of ingested toxic bean lectins on the gastrointestinal tract in the rat. *J Nutri* 1985; 115: 1621–9.

220 Narita T, Numao H. Lectin binding patterns in normal metaplastic and neoplastic gastric mucosa. *J Histochem Cytochem* 1992; 40: 681–7.

221 Neal DE, Charlton RG, Bennett MK. Histochemical study of lectin binding in neoplastic and non-neoplastic urothelium. *Br J Urol* 1987; 60: 399–404.

222 Ng TB, Li WW, Yeung HW. Effects of lectins with various carbohydrate binding specificities on lipid metabolism in isolated rat and hamster adipocytes. *Int J Biochem* 1989; 21: 149–55.

223 Nievergelt-Egido MC, Michel C, Schmahl W. Histochemical investigations on lectin binding in normal and irradiated mouse embryos. *Radiat Environ Biophysics* 1993; 32: 119–28.

224 Noah ND, Bender AE, Reaidi GB, Gilbert RJ. Food poisoning from raw red kidney beans. *Br Med J* 1980; ii: 236–7.

225 Northover AM, Northover BJ. Lectin-induced increase in microvascular permeability to colloidal carbon *in vitro* may involve protein kinase C activation. *Agents Actions* 1994; 41: 136–9.

226 Ohtoyo T, Shimagaki M, Otoda K, Kimura S, Imanishi Y. Change in membrane fluidity induced by lectin. *Biochem* 1988; 27: 6458–63.

227 Olenchock SA, Lewis DM, Mull JC. Composition of extracts of airborne grain dusts: lectins and lymphocyte mitogens. *Environ Health Perspect* 1986; 66: 119–23.

228 Oliveira DBG. Membranous nephropathy: an IgG$_4$-mediated disease. *Lancet* 1998; 351: 670–1.

229 Osunkoya BO, Ajayi O, Akinyemi AA, Ukaejiofo EO. Blood lymphocytes and measles viraemia. *Afr J Med Med Sci* 1987; 16: 181–6.

230 Owen RL, Bhalla DK. Cytochemical analysis of alkaline phosphatase and esterase activities and of lectin-binding and anionic sites in rat and mouse Peyer's patch M cells. *Am J Anat* 1983; 168: 199–212.

231 Papiha SS, Boddy J, Roberts DF, Bates D. PHA-induced interferon in multiple sclerosis. *Acta Neurol Scand* 1989; 80: 145–50.

232 Parkkinen J. Aberrant lectin-binding activity of IgG in serum from RA patients. *Clin Chem* 1989; 35: 1638–43.

233 Patton S, Huston GE, Jenness R, Vaucher Y. Differences between individuals in high molecular weight glycoproteins from mammary epithelia of several species. *Biochim Biophys Acta* 1989; 980: 333–8.

234 Peters MW, Grant CWM. Freeze-etch study of an unmodified lectin interacting with its receptors in model membranes. *Biochim Biophys Acta* 1984; 775: 273–82.

235 Pittschieler K, Ladinser B, Petell JK. Reactivity of gliadin and lectins with celiac intestinal mucosa. *Pediatr Res* 1994; 36: 635–41.

236 Ponzio G, Debant A, Contreres J-O, Rossi B. WGA mimics metabolic effects of insulin without increasing receptor autophosphorylation. *Cell Signal* 1990; 2: 377–86.

237 Pour P, Burnett D, Uchida E. Lectin binding affinities of induced pancreatic lesions in the hamster model. *Carcinogenesis* 1985; 6: 1775–80.

238 Promplook P, Chulavatnatol M. Three sperm-agglutinating isoagglutinins from tubers of Taro. In: van Driessche E, Bog-Hansen TC (eds) *Lectins: Chemistry, Biochemistry, Clinical Biochemistry*, vol 5. de Gruyter, Berlin, 1986.

239 Public Health Laboratory Service. Unusual outbreak of food poisoning. *Br Med J* 1976; ii: 1268.

240 Pujol-Borrell R, Hanafusa T, Chiovato L, Bottazzo GF. Lectin-induced expression of DR antigen on human cultured follicular thyroid cells. *Nature* 1983; 304: 71–73.

241 Pujol-Borrell R, Todd I, Doshi M, Gray D, Feldmann M, Bottazzo GF. Differential expression and regulation of MHC products in the endocrine and exocrine pancreas. *Clin Exp Immunol* 1986; 65: 128–39.

242 Pusztai A. Transport of proteins through the membranes of the adult gastro-intestinal tract – a potential for drug delivery? *Adv Drug Delivery Rev* 1989; 3: 215–228.

243 Pusztai A, King TP, Clarke EMW. Recent advances in the study of the nutritional toxicity of kidney bean lectins in rats. *Toxicon* 1982; 20: 195–7.

244 Pusztai A, Greer F, Grant G. Specific uptake of dietary lectins into the systemic circulation of rats. *Biochem Soc Trans* 1989; 17: 481–2.

245 Pusztai A, Ewen SW, Grant G et al. Relationship between survival and binding of plant lectins during small intestinal passage and their effectiveness as growth factors. *Digestion* 1990; 46 (suppl 2): 308–16.

246 Pusztai A, Ewen SW, Grant G et al. Antinutritive effects of wheat-germ agglutinin and other GNAc-specific lectins. *Br J Nutr* 1993; 70: 313–21.

247 Pusztai A, Ewen SWB, Grant G, Peumans WJ, van Damme EJM, Coates ME, Bardocz S. Lectins and also bacteria modify the glycosylation of gut surface receptors in the rat. *Glycoconj J* 1995; 12: 22–35.

248 Quarles RH, McIntyre LJ, Pasnak CF. Lectin-binding proteins in CNS myelin II. *Biochem J* 1979; 183: 213–21.

249 Ramos OF, Sarmay G, Eggersten G, Nilsson B, Klein E, Gergely J. Alternative pathway of complement activation by stimulated T lymphocytes. *Eur J Immunol* 1987; 17: 975–9 and 969–74.

250 Raub TJ, Koroly MJ, Roberts RM. Endocytosis of WGA binding sites from the cell surface into a tubular endosomal network. *J Cell Physiol* 1990; 143: 1–12.

251 Restum-Miguel N, Provost-Danon A. Effects of multiple oral dosing on IgE synthesis in mice. *Immunology* 1985; 54: 497–504.

252 Rittig M, Brigel C, Lutjen-Drecoll E. Lectin binding sites in the anterior segment of the human eye. *Graefes Arch Clin Exp Ophthalmol* 1990; 228: 528–32.

253 Roberts ISD, Jones CJP, Stoddart RW. Lectin histochemistry of the mast cell. *Histochem J* 1990; 22: 73–80.

254 Rodríguez LAG, Ruigómez A. Increased risk of irritable bowel syndrome after bacterial gastroenteritis: cohort study. *Br Med J* 1999; 318: 565–6.

255 Rohlich P, Szel A, Johnson LV, Hageman GS. Carbohydrate components recognized by the cone-specific monoclonal antibody CSA-1 and by peanut agglutinin are associated with red and green-sensitive cone photoreceptors. *J Comp Neurol* 1989; 289: 395–400.

256 Rolachon A, Groslambert P, Paillet D, Hostein J. Diarrhèe osmotique chez un sujet vegetarien: les lectines pourraient être en cause. *Gastroenterol Clin Biol* 1991; 15: 267–8.

257 Roozen JP, de Groot J. Analysis of trypsin inhibitors and lectins in white kidney beans, in a combined method. *J Assoc Off Anal Chem* 1991; 74: 940–3.

258 Rossi MA, Filho JM, Lajolo FM. Jejunal ultrastructural changes induced by kidney bean lectins in rats. *Br J Exp Pathol* 1984; 65: 117–23.

259 Rouanet J-M, Besancon P, Lafont J. Effect of lectin from leguminous seeds on rat duodenal enterokinase activity. *Experientia* 1983; 39: 1356–58.

260 Rouanet JM, Lafont J, Zambonino-Infante JL, Besancon P. Selective effects of PHA on rat brush border hydrolases along the crypt-villus axis. *Experientia* 1988; 44: 340–1.

261 Roy S, Bhalla V. Haemagglutinins and lysins in plants. *Aust J Exp Biol Med Sci* 1981; 59: 195–201.

262 Rutherford SA, Goldberg MW, Allen TD. Three-dimensional visualisation of the route of protein import: the role of nuclear pore complex substructures. *Exp Cell Res* 1997; 232: 146–60.

263 Rühlmann J, Sinha P, Hansen G, Tauber R, Köttgen E. Studies on the aetiology of coeliac disease: no evidence for lectin-like components in wheat gluten. *Biochim Biophys Acta* 1993; 1181: 249–56.

264 Saccia M, Rutigliano V, Rigillo N, Bosco L, Rizzo G, e Fini M. [Modificazioni indotte sulla mucosa intestinale di ratto dopo] (English abstract). *Boll Soc Ital Biol Sper* 1987; 63: 209–16.

265 Sandholm M, Scott ML. Binding of lipase, amylase and protease to intestinal epithelium as affected by carbohydrate and lectin *in vitro*. *Acta Vet Scand* 1979; 20: 329–42.

266 Sandros J, Rozdzinski E, Zheng J, Cowburn D, Tuomanen E. Lectin domains in the toxin of Bordetella pertussis: selectin mimicry linked to microbial pathogenesis. *Glycoconj J* 1994; 11: 501–6.

267 Savelkoul PH, van der Poel AF, Tamminga S. The presence and inactivation of trypsin inhibitors, tannins, lectins and amylase inhibitors in legume seeds during germination. *Plant Foods Hum Nutr* 1992; 42: 71–85.

268 Savelkoul PH, Tamminga S, Leenaars PP, Schering J, Ter-Maat DW. The degradation of lectins, phaseolin and trypsin inhibitors during germination of white kidney beans. *Plant Foods Hum Nutr* 1994; 45: 213–22.

269 Saxon A, Tsui F, Martinez-Mazo O. Jacalin, an IgA-binding lectin, inhibits differentiation of human B cells. *Cell Immunol* 1987; 104: 134–41.

270 Schaumberg-Lever G. Ultrastructural localization of lectin-binding sites in normal skin. *J Invest Dermatol* 1990; 94: 465–70.

271 Schaumberg-Lever G, Metzler G, Trounier M. Ultrastructural localization of lectin-binding sites in normal human eccrine and apocrine glands. *J Dermatol Sci* 1991; 2: 55–61.

272 Schiavino D, Nucera E, Murzilli F et al. Anaphylactic shock after skin test with PHA. *Allergy* 1992; 47/2pt2: 121–2.

273 Schumacher U, Horny HP, Welsch U. The lectin leucoagglutinin binds specifically to human granulocytes, monocytes and tissue mast cells. *Br J Haematol* 1987; 66: 405–6.

274 Schumacher U, Thielke E, Adam E. A dot blot technique for the analysis of interactions of lectins with glycosaminoglycans. *Histochem J* 1992; 24: 453–5.

275 Schunke M, Schumacher U, Tillmann B. Lectin binding in normal and fibrillated cartilage of human patellae. *Virchows Archiv A* 1985; 407: 221–31.

276 Scott FW, Kolb H. Cows' milk and insulin-dependent diabetes mellitus. *Lancet* 1996; 348: 613.

277 Segal E. Inhibitors of C. *albicans* adhesion to prevent candidiasis. *Adv Exp Med Biol* 1996; 408: 197–206.

278 Sekiyama S, Yoshida F, Yuzawa Y *et al*. Mesangial proliferative glomeru-lonephritis induced in rats by a lentil lectin and its antibodies. *J Lab Clin Med* 1993; 121: 71–82.

279 Sessa A, Tunici P, Rabellotti E *et al*. Response of intestinal transgluta-minase activity to dietary PHA. *Biochim Biophys Acta* 1996; 1314: 66–70.

280 Sharma R, Schumacher U. The influence of diets and gut microflora on lectin binding patterns of intestinal mucins in rats. *Lab Invest* 1995; 73: 558–64.

281 Sharon N. Carbohydrate-lectin interactions in infectious disease. *Adv Exp Med Biol* 1996; 408: 1–8.

282 Shaw LM, Peterson-Archer L. Interaction of gamma-glutamyltrans-ferase from human tissues with insolubilized lectins. *Clin Biochem* 1979; 12: 256–260.

283 Shet MS, Madaiah M, Ahamed RN. Effect of raw winged bean (*Psophocarpus tetragonolobus*) tuber lectin on gastrointestinal tract of growing rats. *Indian J Exp Biol* 1989; 27: 58–61.

284 Shibasaki M, Sumuzaki R, Isoyama S, Takita H. Interaction of lectins with human IgE. *Int Archs Allergy Immunol* 1992; 98: 18–25.

285 Shirane T. Role of peanut-lectin-affinity molecules (PLAM) on pri-mordial germ cells in the initial determination of sex in Anura. *J Exp Zool* 1987; 243: 495–502.

286 Silva Lima M, Oliveira MC, Moriera RA, Prouvost-Danon RA. Metabolic energy dependent exocytosis of mouse mast cells by lectin of *Dioclea grandiflora*. *Biochem Pharmacol* 1985; 34: 4169–70.

287 Singer R, Sagiv M, Allalouf D *et al*. Separation of normozoospermic human spermatozoa into subpopulations by selective agglutination with PNA. *Andrologia* 1986; 18: 17–24.

288 Siraganian RP, Siraganian PA. Mechanism of action of concanavalin A on human basophils. *J Immunol* 1975; 114: 886–893.

289 Sjölander A, Magnusson K-E, Latkovic S. The effect of ConA and WGA on the ultrastructure and permeability of rat intestine: a possible model for an intestinal allergic reaction. *Int Arch Allergy Appl Immunol* 1984; 75: 230–6.

290 Snyder MC, Zaneveld LJD. Treatment of cervical mucus with lectins: effect on sperm migration. *Fertil Steril* 1985; 44: 633–7.

291 Söderström KO. Lectin binding to collagen strands in histologic tissue sections. *Histochemistry* 1987; 87: 557–60.

292 Soderstrom KO. Lectin binding to formalin-fixed paraffin sections of human endometrium. *Int J Gynecol Pathol* 1987; 6: 55–65.

293 Söderstrom KO. Lectin binding to the human retina. *Anat Rec* 1988; 220: 219–23.

294 Sokal I, Kulacz A, Gorczyca W, Janusz M, Lisowski J. Guineapig peri-toneal macrophages: Differential effects of lectins. *Cell Biochem Funct* 1995; 13: 25–30.

295 Sollid LM, Kolberg J, Scott H, Ek J, Fausa O, Brantzaeg P. Antibodies to wheatgerm agglutinin in coeliac disease. *Clin Exp Immunol* 1986; 63: 95–100.

296 Speekenbrink AB, Parrott DM. Modulation of *in vitro* thymidine incor-poration into crypt cells from the murine small intestine. *Cell Tissue Kinet* 1987; 20: 135–44.

297 Sretarugsa P, Sobhon P, Bubpaniroj P, Yodyingynad V. Inhibition of implantation of hamster embryos by lectins. *Contraception* 1987; 35: 507–15.

298 Stegemann M, Meyer R, Haas HG, Robert-Nicoud M. The cell surface of isolated cardiomyocytes. *J Mol Cell Cardiol* 1990; 22: 787–803.

299 Stern M, Knauss M, Stallmach A. Crypt-villus differentiation reflected by lectin and protein binding to rat small intestinal brush border mem-branes. *Dig Dis Sci* 1995; 40: 2438–45.

300 Stieber A, Erulkar SD, Gonatas NK. A hypothesis for the superior sen-sitivity of WGA as a neuroanatomical probe. *Brain Res* 1989; 495: 131–9.

301 Stillmark H. Ueber ricin, ein giftiges ferment. Doctoral Thesis, University of Dorpat, 1888.

302 Stone OJ. Aphthous stomatitis (canker sores): a consequence of high oral submucosal viscosity (the rôle of extracellular matrix and the pos-sible rôle of lectins). *Med Hypoth* 1991; 36: 341–4.

303 Sugiyama S, Spicer SS, Munyer PD, Schulte BA. Distribution of gly-coconjugates in ion transport cells of gerbil inner ear. *J Histochem Cytochem* 1991; 39: 425–34.

304 Sumar N, Bodman KB, Rademacher TW *et al*. Analysis of glycosylation changes in IgG using lectins. *J Immunol Methods* 1990; 131: 127–36.

305 Sung LA, Kabat EA. Agglutination-induced erythrocyte deformation. *Biorheology* 1994; 31: 353–64.

306 Suzuki T. [Lectin binding pattern of the normal rat lens] (Engl abstr) *Nippon Ganka Gakkai Zasshi* 1989; 93: 307–14.

307 Tabary F, Font J, Bourillon R. Isolation, molecular and biological prop-erties of a lectin from rice embryo. *Arch Biochem Biophys* 1987; 259: 79–88.

308 Tajima M, Araiso T, Koyama T, Fujinaga T, Otomo K, Koike T. Membrane viscosity of lymphocytes and influence of PHA. *Biorheology* 1989; 26: 454.

309 Tajiri H, Klein RM, Lebenthal E, Lee P-C. Oral feeding of isolated lectins from red kidney bean stimulates rat small intestinal mucosal DNA synthesis and crypt cell division. *Dig Dis Sci* 1988; 33: 1364–9.

310 Takai Y, Noda Y, Sumitomo S-I, Sagara S, Mori M. Different bindings to lectin in human submandibular gland after enzymatic digestion. *Acta Histochem* 1986; 78: 111–21.

311 Takumi K, Uehara F. *In vivo* lectin-binding of photoreceptors and inter-photoreceptor matrix in rat. *Jpn J Ophthalmol* 1991; 35: 16–22.

312 Tchernychev B, Wilchek M. Natural human antibodies to dietary lectins. *FEBS Lett* 1996; 397: 139–42.

313 Thrower S, Bulmer JN, Griffin NR, Wells M. Further studies of lectin binding by villous and extravillous trophoblast in normal and patholog-ical pregnancy. *Int J Gynecol Pathol* 1991; 10: 238–51.

314 Tian Q, Rask-Andersen H, Linthicum FH Jr. The identification of sub-stances in the endolymphatic sac. *Acta Otolaryngol Stockh* 1994; 114: 632–6.

315 Tien L, Rayborn ME, Hollyfield JG. Characterization of the interpho-toreceptor matrix surrounding rod photoreceptors in the human retina. *Exp Eye Res* 1992; 55: 297–306.

316 Toda N, Doi A, Jimbo A, Matsumoto I, Seno N. Interaction of sul-phated glycosaminoglycans with lectins. *J Biol Chem* 1981; 256: 5345–9.

317 Tolson ND, Daley TD, Wysocki GP. Lectin probes of glycoconjugates in human salivary glands. *J Oral Pathol* 1985; 14: 523–30.

318 Tomimoto H, Kamo H, Araki M, Kimura H. An economic anterograde axonal tracing method using PHA P-form. *J Neurosci Methods* 1987; 22: 1–8.

319 Tomino Y, Ohmuro H, Takahashi Y *et al*. Binding capacity of serum IgA to jacalin in patients with IgA nephropathy. *Nephron* 1995; 70: 329–33.

320 Triadou N, Audran E. Interaction of brush-border hydrolases of the human small intestine with lectins. *Digestion* 1983; 27: 1–7.

321 Tripathi BJ, Marcus CH, Tripathi RC, Millard CB, Gulcher J, Stefansson K. Monoclonal antibodies and lectins as probes for investigation of the cell biology of the human trabecular meshwork. *Ophthalmol Res* 1989; 21: 27–32.

322 Truong LD, Phung VT, Yoshikawa Y, Mattioli CA. Glycoconjugates in normal human kidney. *Histochemistry* 1988; 90: 51–60.

323 Tsuchiya N, Endo T, Shiota M, Kochibe N, Ito K, Kobata A. Distribution of glycosylation abnormality among serum IgG subclasses from patients with rheumatoid arthritis. *Clin Immunol Immunopathol* 1994; 70: 47–50.

324 Turck D, Feste AS, Lifschitz CH. Age and diet affect the composition of porcine colonic mucins. *Pediatr Res* 1993; 33: 564–7.

325 Tuxen MK, Nielsen HV, Birgens H. [Forgiftning med kidneybonner] (Danish: English abstract) *Ugeskr Laeger* 1991; 153: 3628–9.

326 Tyrrell GJ, Peppler MS, Bonnah RA, Clark CG, Chong P, Armstrong GD. Lectin-like properties of pertussis toxin. *Infect Immunol* 1989; 57: 1854–7.

327 Uchigata Y, Spitalnik SL, Tachiwaki O, Salata KF, Notkins AL. Pancreatic islet cell surface glycoproteins containing Gal 1-4GNAc-R identified by a cytotoxic monoclonal autoantibody. *J Exp Med* 1987; 165: 124–139.

328 Ujita M, Furukawa K, Aoki N *et al*. A change in soybean agglutinin binding patterns of bovine milk fat globule membrane glycoproteins during early lactation. *FEBS Lett* 1993; 332: 119–22.

329 Unsworth DJ, Leonard JN, Hobday CM *et al*. Gliadins bind to retic-ulin in a lectin-like manner. *Arch Dermatol Res* 1987; 279: 232–5.

330 Utal AK, Verma K, Soni GL, Singh R. Effect of pea and lentil lectins on in vitro absorption of nutrients. *Indian J Exp Biol* 1990; 28: 93–5.

331 Valette A, Rouge P, Coulais E, Potonnier G, Cros J, Simon EJ. Interaction with lectin of kappa opioid binding sites solubilized from human placenta. *Life Sci* 1987; 40: 535–40.

332 van Damme EJ, Grossens K, Smeets K, van-Leuven F, Verhaert P, Peumans WJ. The major tuber storage protein of araceae species is a lectin. *Plant Physiol* 1995; 107: 1147–58.

333 van den Ingh TS, Krogdahl A. [Negatieve effecten van antinutritionele factoren in soyabonen bij salmoniden] (Dutch, Eng abstr). *Tijdschr-Diergeneeskd* 1990; 115: 935–8.

334 Vargas-Albores F, Hernández J, Córdoba F, Zenteno E. Isolation of an immunosuppressive lectin from *Phaseolus vulgaris*. *Prep Biochem* 1993; 23: 473–83.

335 Vasquez JM, Magargee SF, Kunze E, Hammerstedt RH. Lectins and heparin-binding features of human spermatozoa as analysed by flow cytometry. *Am J Obstet Gynecol* 1990; 163(6pt1): 2006–12.

336 Vecchi M, Torqano G, Monti M *et al.* Evaluation of structural and secretory glycoconjugates in normal human duodenum. *Histochemistry* 1987; 86: 359–64.

337 Vecchi M, Torgano G, de Franchis R, Tronconi S, Agape D, Ronchi G. Evidence of altered structural and secretory glycoconjugates in the jejunal mucosa of patients with gluten-sensitive enteropathy and subtotal villous atrophy. *Gut* 1989; 30: 804–10, see also *ibid* 31: 482–3 for debate.

338 Vierbuchen M, Klein PJ. Histochemical demonstration of neuraminidase effects in pneumococcal meningitis. *Lab Invest* 1983; 48: 181–6.

339 Virtanen I, Kareniemi I, Holthöfer H, Lehto V-P. Fluorochrome-coupled lectins reveal distinct cellular domains in human epidermis. *J Histochem Cytochem* 1986; 34: 307–15.

340 Visser JJ, Meyer S, de Jong D. PHA skin testing in critically ill surgical patients. *Acute Care* 1986; 12: 52–7.

341 Wang Q, Yu L-G, Campbell BJ, Milton J, Rhodes JM. Identification of intact peanut lectin in peripheral venous blood. *Lancet* 1998; 352: 1831–2.

342 Ward GK, Stewart SS, Price GB, Mackillop WJ. Cellular heterogeneity in normal human urothelium. *Histochem J* 1987; 19: 337–44.

343 Watt FM, Jones PH. Changes in cell surface carbohydrate during terminal differentiation of human epidermal keratinocytes. *Biochem Soc Trans* 1992; 20: 235–8.

344 Weetman AP, Volkman DJ, Burman KD, Gerrard TL, Fauci AS. The *in vitro* regulation of human thyrocyte HLA-DR antigen expression. *J Clin Endocrinol Metab* 1985; 61: 817–24.

345 Wei WZ, Lindquist RR. WGA initiates monocytoid cell killing of non-antibody-coated erythrocytes. *Immunology* 1983; 25: 617.

346 Weinman MD, Allan CH, Trier JS, Hagen SJ. Repair of microvilli in the rat small intestine after damage with lectins contained in the red kidney bean. *Gastroenterology* 1989; 97: 1193–204.

347 Welsch U, Schumacher U, Buchheim W, Schinko I, Jenness P, Patton S. Histochemical and biochemical observations on milk fat-globule membranes from several mammalian species. *Acta Histochem* suppl 1990; 40: 59–64.

348 Wilden PA, Morrison BD, Pessin JE. Wheat germ agglutinin stimulation of heterodimeric insulin receptor. *Endocrinol* 1989; 124: 971–9.

349 Wirth C, Schwuchow J, Jonas L. Internalization of WGA by rat pancreatic cells *in vivo* and *in vitro*. *Acta Histochem* 1996; 98: 165–72.

350 Wold AE, Mestecky J, Tomana M *et al.* Secretory IgA carries oligosaccharide receptors for *E. coli* type 1 fimbrial lectin. *Infect Immun* 1990; 58: 3073–7.

351 Wold AE, Motas C, Svanborg C, Hanson LA, Mestecky J. Characterization of IgA$_1$, IgA$_2$ and secretory IgA carbohydrate chains using plant lectins. *Adv Exp Med Biol* 1995; 371A: 585–9.

352 Wright HT, Sandrasageram G, Wright CS. Evolution of a family of GNac-binding proteins containing the disulphide-rich domain of wheat germ agglutinin. *J Mol Evol* 1991; 33: 283–94.

353 Wu AM, Watkins WM, Chen C-P, Song SC, Chow L-P, Lin J-Y. Native and/or asialo-Tamm-Horsfall glycoproteins Sd(a+) are important receptors for WGA and three toxic lectins. *FEBS Lett* 1995; 371: 32–4.

354 Wu TCJ, Lee SM, Jih MH, Liu JT, Wan YJY. Differential distribution of glycoconjugates in human reproductive tract. *Fertil Steril* 1993; 59: 60–4.

355 Yachie A, Hernandez D, Blaese RM. T3-T cell receptor (Ti) complex-independent activation of T cells by wheat germ agglutinin. *J Immunol* 1987; 138: 2843–7.

356 Yamashita H, Bagger-Sjoback D, Wersall J, Sekitani T. Glycoconjugates in the human fetal endolymphatic sac as detected by lectins. *J Laryngol Otol* 1991; 105: 711–5.

357 Yan WQ, Nakashima K, Iwamoto M, Kato Y. Stimulation by ConA of cartilage matrix proteoglycan synthesis in chondrocyte cultures. *J Biol Chem* 1990; 265: 10125–31.

358 Yang K, Cohen L, Lipkin M. Lectin soybean agglutinin: measurements in colonic epithelial cells of human subjects following supplementary dietary calcium. *Cancer Lett* 1991; 56: 65–9.

359 Yoshino Y, Nagaya K, Sekino H, Uchida MK, Suzuki-Nishimura T. Comparison of histamine release induced by synthetic polycations with that by compound 48/80 from rat mast cells. *Jpn J Pharmacol* 1990; 52: 387–95.

360 Youinou P, Pennec YL, Casburn-Budd R, Dueymes M, Letoux G, Lamour A. Galactose terminating oligosaccharides of IgG in patients with primary Sjögren's syndrome. *J Autoimmun* 1992; 5: 393–400.

361 Zaremba S, Gwozdz H, Banach M. Effect of lectin from *Phaseolus vulgaris* on the glucose content in the blood and the content of glycogen in the mouse liver and muscles. *Folia Biol Krakow* 1987; 35: 3–12.

362 Zavázal V, Krauz V. Lectin-binding ability of immunoglobulin E and its participation in triggering of mast cells. *Folia Microbiol (Praha)* 1985; 30: 237–46.

363 Zucoloto S, Scaramello AC, Lajolo FM, Muccillo G. Effect of oral PHA intake on cell adaptation in the epithelium of the small intestine of the rat. *Int J Exp Pathol* 1991; 72: 41–5.

Chapter 35
Rhinitis, secretory otitis media and sinus disease caused by food allergy

Zdenek Pelikan

INTRODUCTION

The role of food allergy and intolerance in subjects with allergic disorders, especially in those suffering from rhinitis, otitis media, sinusitis and bronchial asthma, is still underestimated by clinicians[5]. This is for three reasons: 1) these allergic disorders have in the past been attributed only to the immediate (Type I) hypersensitivity mech-anisms and the suspected allergens have been those acquired by the inhalation route; 2) there may exist different mechanisms by which foods can cause clinical disorders in patients, of which the hypersensitivity mechanism is only one; 3) the diagnosis of food allergy and its confirmation in the symptomatology of patients is not always easy and requires both experience and a clear diagnostic system, as well as patience from both the clinician and the patient.[1,5,6,57,58,70,80,83]

Definition

Food allergy or hypersensitivity may be defined as the clinical manifestation of an immunological process in which foods or their parts are able first to act as antigens or haptens to stimulate the production of specific antibodies or to sensitize the particular T cell population (subset). Second, they are capable of interacting with these antibodies or cells, a process resulting in an allergic (hypersensitivity) reaction. The foods may then be responsible for the immunological injury by any of the classical types of hypersensitivity reactions[1,5,70,80,82,83].

Differential diagnosis

A distinction must be made between genuine food allergy which is caused by an immunological process and disorders which can also be caused by foods, their ingredients or factors related to them, which can produce similar symptoms, but which are due to completely different mechanisms (Table 35.1).[6,8,48,57,59,64,70,74,79,80,83,95,96,97]

Forms of food allergy

There are two basic forms of food allergy.[70,78,79,80,83]

The first is the *primary form*, where the food alone causes the defined clinical symptoms by an immunological process. In such a case, the food is the primary and sole cause of activation of the hypersensitivity mechanism and the resulting symptoms.

The *secondary form* is where one or more foods potentiate the already existing hypersensitivity mechanism(s) caused by different antigens (e.g. inhalant antigens, etc.). The foods may act by different pathways in potentiating the particular responses. Here, the food allergy is a complementary process to another hypersensitivity state which is the primary and basic event. This secondary form of food allergy occurs more frequently than the primary form and is regularly overlooked in practice.[79,82,83]

IMMUNOLOGICAL CHARACTERISTICS OF FOOD ALLERGY

Food usually enters the body via the digestive tract, i.e. by ingestion. Food can also cause hypersensitivity reactions by contact with the skin, gingiva, lips or tongue, and also through inhalation on and in the nasal or bronchial mucosa.[45,48,70,80,110]

The antibodies involved in food allergy have classically been understood to be of the IgE class. However, antibodies of other classes, for example IgG and IgM, as well as IgA and immune complexes, may also be involved.[8,23,68] There is evidence that T lymphocytes may also be involved in those mechanisms caused by foods. [2,8,14,29,30,33,47,48,61,62,104,106]

All four basic types of hypersensitivity, i.e. Types I–IV, may be involved in food allergy and can lead to the appearance of clinical symptoms. However, the immediate (Type I) and the late type (Type III) reactions have been most investigated and documented. Recently, the delayed type of response (Type IV) caused by foods has been demonstrated in subjects with rhinitis, bronchial asthma, atopic eczema, urticaria, migraine and other disorders (Fig. 35.1).[8,22,33,69a,70,70a,71a,72a,73a,74,74a,79,80,82,83,97,108]

The terms 'food allergy' or 'food hypersensitivity' imply an immunological mechanism but in many instances the exact immunopathological mechanism producing particular symptoms remains unknown. It would therefore be more appropriate to use the term 'adverse reactions to foods', where genuine food hypersensitivity represents one of the suspected mechanisms.[5,58,82,83]

Food additives

Chemical additives in food represent a special problem, not only with respect to their frequent occurrence in manufactured foods and their heterogeneity of presentation, but also because of the lack of the understanding concerning their mode of action and the

Survey of the disorders caused by foods
1. Idiosyncrasy
2. Intolerance (e.g. enzymatic)
3. Non-specific hyperreactivity (e.g. histamine or other mediator liberators, food additives)
4. Toxicity caused by (a) non-controlled chemical compounds (e.g. insecticides, contaminants) (b) microorganisms (c) products of microorganisms, e.g. bacterial toxins or mycotoxins (d) controlled chemical compounds exceeding their permitted threshold or individual subjects having increased susceptibility to these compounds (e.g. disinfectants) caused by other metabolic disorders
5. Adverse non-immunological reaction to additives (controlled chemical compounds) (a) preservation and conservation compounds (b) colouring compounds (c) flavouring compounds (d) consistency correcting compounds (emulsifiers and stabilizers) (e) antioxidants (f) adjuvants
6. Psychological disorders

Table 35.1 Survey of the disorders caused by foods, their ingredients or factors relating to them, which can lead to symptoms similar to those due to the food allergy mechanism.

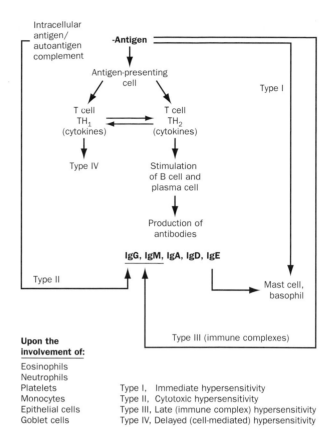

Fig. 35.1 Basic types of hypersensitivity (allergy) reactions.

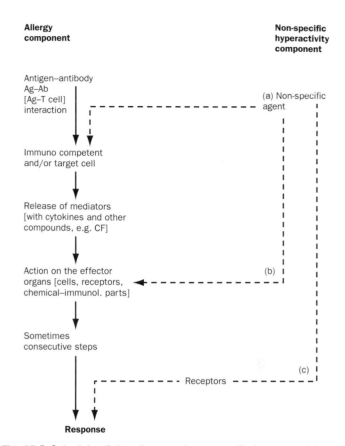

Fig. 35.2 Schedule of the allergy and non-specific hyperreactivity pathways.

mechanisms through which additives may produce clinical symptoms. There is clear evidence that additives may cause clinical symptoms in various organs, as has been demonstrated by clinical oral challenge studies.[52,95–97] Although clinical manifestations are associated with the ingestion of additives, specific antibodies of IgE or other classes or, indeed, sensitized T lymphocytes have not yet been unequivocally demonstrated in affected patients.[5,11,51,64]

Oral disodium cromoglycate is very effective in preventing the clinical symptoms which follow ingestion challenge with foods. However, there is little evidence for a comparable protective effect of this drug in preventing symptoms after oral challenge with additives. This suggests that additives may produce clinical symptoms through non-immunological and non-specific mechanisms. These may include non-specific hyperreactivity, non-specific direct release of mediators and other factors without any preceding antigen–antibody interaction and other direct effects on various effector organs, for example, pharmacological or subtoxic effects.[10,28,59,82,83,113–15]

Isolated adverse reactions to additives are diagnosed rarely and only in a very small number of patients reporting suspicion of adverse reactions to foods. In the majority of these patients either food hypersensitivity appears alone, or it is supplemented by adverse reactions to food additives. Diagnostic confirmation of the causal role of additives in precipitating the patient's symptoms is often difficult to obtain.

RHINITIS

Basic facts

Allergic rhinitis is a non-infectious disorder characterized by nasal obstruction caused by the swelling of the nasal mucosa, hyper-

secretion, sneezing and mucosal itching. Nasal symptoms may be caused by two different mechanisms – an allergic and a non-specific hyperreactivity component. Both of these components may play a role in the same patient to various degrees (Fig. 35.2).[79,80,82,83]

The allergic component

The allergic component is due to the antigen–antibody or antigen–T cell interactions influencing the immunocompetent or target cell(s), a process which leads to the release of mediators which act either directly on the various effector organs (e.g. smooth muscle, mucosal glands, goblet cells, capillary network, neurosynapses, receptors, etc.) or indirectly through effects on other cell types. The combined response of the effector organs results in a variety of clinical symptoms representing the particular allergic disorder. The allergic component may be of a seasonal or non-seasonal (perennial) character, depending on the kind of allergens involved.

Of the four basic types of hypersensitivity reaction, three (Type I, immediate; Type III, late; and Type IV, delayed) can be involved in the production of symptoms in the patient with rhinitis. However, immediate hypersensitivity (Type I) is most commonly involved in these patients, causing an *immediate nasal response* (INR). This occurs within 120 min after alltergen exposure (food ingestion). In addition to the immediate nasal response, non-immediate nasal responses may also occur. The *late nasal response* (LYNR), appearing 4–24 h after allergen exposure, may be caused by late (Type III) hypersensitivity, whereas the *delayed nasal response* (DYNR), occurring 30–56 h after allergen exposure, may suggest possible involvement of delayed type hypersensitivity (Type IV).

The particular types of nasal response can be demonstrated by nasal provocation tests with allergens or by ingestion challenge with the appropriate food, in combination with rhinomanometry, otitis media, simuhoponia.[29,39,75,79,80,83]

The non-specific hyperreactivity component

Non-specific hyperreactivity may lead to a similar spectrum of nasal symptoms as that caused by an immunological mechanism (Type 1=immediate hypersensivity), however without any initial antigen-antibody interaction. These non-specific agents may be small molecular chemical compounds, physical factors such as temperature differences, vapours and smoke, or mechanical factors such as non-organic dusts. Such agents may act in a variety of different ways.

1. They may influence the immunocompetent or target cell directly, causing a non-specific release of mediators, or they may do so indirectly, through the stimulation of the nasal mucosal sensory nerves and/or a variety of mucosal receptors. This then causes activation and release of various neuropeptides, which affect the immunocompetent cells.[82]
2. They may act by the stimulation of mediator precursors, leading first to the stimulation of mediator production (which then acts directly on the effector organs) and, secondly, to the feedback inhibition of these mediators or the immunocompetent cells.
3. They may exert their influence directly on the effector organs and their receptors to cause clinical effects (Fig. 35.2).[79,82,83]

The involvement of non-specific hyperreactivity in patients with rhinitis may be confirmed by nasal challenge with histamine and/or one of the methacholines. Decreased thresholds of these chemicals are regularly seen in the nose.[75]

In approximately 60% of patients with rhinitis, an allergy component and a non-specific hyperreactivity component may be combined to various degrees in precipitating the patient's complaints. In the remaining patients only one of these components may be found. Such cases of rhinitis in which nasal complaints are solely due to the non-specific hyperreactivity component can be called vasomotor rhinitis. In the past, the role of foods in producing symptoms in patients with allergic rhinitis has been the subject of considerable controversy in the literature. More recently, the role of foods has been recognized and confirmed by clinical experiments and food ingestion challenges.[8,13,39,53,55,101,104,112] This does not imply that all clinical responses to food involve immunological hypersensitivity mechanisms, but this is probably the case with most.

Diagnostic procedures in vivo
Disease history and physical examination
In all patients with rhinitis, otitis media, sinusitis, bronchial asthma, urticaria, atopic eczema and other disorders with a possible allergic component, the case history should be taken with special emphasis on dietary habit. In our clinical experience approximately 38% of patients with rhinitis, 27% with otitis media, 20% with sinusitis, 19% with bronchial asthma, 73% with atopic eczema, 69% with urticaria 82% with chronic Colotis, 39% with aphthae, 33% with rheumatoid arthritis, and 93% with migraine give a history which suggests the possibility of adverse reaction to foods.[79,82,83] The food-positive history in the patients with rhinitis reported by Wilson (16%)[110] and Eriksson (24%)[36] is roughly in accordance with the author's findings. In practice, insufficient attention is paid to dietary history in the routine assessment of these patients.[82,89]

Moreover, the presence in an allergic rhinitis sufferer of a concomitant disorder in which food hypersensitivity may be implicated (such as urticaria, atopic eczema or irritable bowel syndrome) increases the possibility of food-related causation.[69a,70,70a,74,76a,78a,79,82,83]

Laboratory and X-ray examination
Basic laboratory screening and X-ray or echography of the paranasal sinuses are important in these patients from the point of view of differential diagnosis. Slight abnormality of blood sedimentation rate, leukocytosis and eosinophilia, together with a mild mucosal oedema in the maxillary sinuses, are frequently present.

Skin tests
Skin prick or scratch (dermal) tests followed by intradermal (intracutaneous) tests are usually used. However, there are some problems concerning skin tests with food extracts.

1. The standardization of food extracts.
2. The technology and purification of food allergens.
3. The method of testing.
4. Correlation of results of skin tests with other *in vivo* and *in vitro* tests.
5. Correlation with the clinical disorder.

The reported correlation between the results of skin tests and clinical symptoms or disorders varies widely in the literature. In patients with rhinitis where food allergy is suspected, skin testing with food extracts has been found to be a useful diagnostic test by some investigators,[5,6,57] but it has not been confirmed by other authors.[4,6,13,112]

In the author's department, skin tests with food extracts in patients with allergic rhinitis caused by food allergy correlated with other diagnostic parameters in only 60%, which is unsatisfactory. The immediate skin response was positive in 55% of patients demonstrating the immediate nasal response. The late skin response was positive in 48% of patients developing the late nasal response. The delayed skin response was positive in only 32% of those demonstrating the delayed nasal response (Table 35.2).[74,80,82,83]

Schedule for skin testing
The schedule for skin tests in this department is as follows. Skin prick or scratch tests are performed and evaluated after 20 min. If they are negative (as is the case in approximately 95% of patients), then intracutaneous tests are carried out and evaluated after 20 min for the immediate skin response (Fig. 35.3a). They are then evaluated every 4 h for up to 12 h to detect late skin response (Fig. 35.3b) and after 24, 28, 32, 36, 40, 48, 56, 60 and 72 h for the delayed skin response (Fig. 35.3c). If necessary, skin tests are examined for a longer period of time up to the full disappearance of the wheal and/or induration. It should be emphasized, as has been mentioned above, that skin tests alone are not a sufficient parameter for the diagnosis of food allergy. They should be followed by food ingestion challenge.[8,65,67,108,112]

Provocation tests with foods
Ingestion challenge with appropriate foods should be considered to be the cornerstone of diagnostic confirmation of the role of food allergy in patients with rhinitis. Provocation tests should demonstrate the appearance of nasal symptoms after ingestion of the suspected food.[66,79,82] The food ingestion challenge should be regarded as a model investigation and as a simulated reproduction of the patient's complaints after exposure to the particular allergen.

Association of various types of nasal response to food ingestion challenge with other diagnostic parameters				
	Nasal mucosa response to ingested food			
	Immediate (*n* = 267)	Late (*n* = 203)	Delayed (*n* = 164)	Negative (*n* = 309)
Positive skin response				
Immediate	146 (55)			48 (16)
Late		98 (48)		11 (4)
Delayed			69 (42)	3 (1)
Increase in total serum IgE (PRIST)	11 (4)	1 (0.5)	0	3 (1)
Increase in specific serum IgE (RAST)	38 (14)	3 (1.5)	1 (0.6)	4 (1)
Increase in blood eosinophils	14 (5)	17 (8)	2 (1)	2 (0.6)
Increase in blood leukocytes	10 (4)	18 (9)	11 (7)	3 (1)
Aspects of the nasal mucosa				
Hyperaemia	197 (74)	48 (24)	1 (0.6)	5 (2)
Violaceous aspect	70 (26)	155 (76)	163 (99)	0
Nasal mucosa haemorrhages	0	42 (21)	72 (44)	0
Nasal secretions				
Changes in count				
Eosinophils	201 (75)	128 (63)	53 (32)	21 (7)
Mast cells/basophils	53 (20)	30 (15)	6 (4)	0
Neutrophils	108 (40)	142 (70)	151 (92)	15 (5)
Goblet cells	39 (15)	103 (51)	114 (70)	2 (0.6)
Lymphocytes	9 (3)	5 (2)	146 (89)	0
Epithelial cells	17 (6)	93 (46)	158 (96)	3 (1)
Monocytes	2 (0.7)	3 (1.5)	0	1 (0.3)
Plasma cells	0	1 (0.5)	0	1 (0.3)

Values in parentheses are percentages. PRIST, RAST, radioallergosorbent test.

Table 35.2 Association of various types of nasal response to food ingestion challenge with other diagnostic parameters.

There are two main aspects concerning provocation tests. First, the qualitative aspect; the test should demonstrate that the particular organ does indeed react to the suspected food allergen by the occurrence of typical complaints and the development of a certain type of organ response. Second, the quantitative aspect; the test should confirm that the suspected food allergen, in a particular dose and during a particular time of exposure, may cause a specific organ response which can be quantified and recorded. This is the time–and dose–response principle.

A most important aspect of the provocation test is the comparison of objective parameters and simultaneous subjective complaints before and repeatedly after challenge with the allergen, in this case before and after food ingestion challenge. Various modifications of provocation tests with foods have been described in the literature. Ingestion challenge with foods in their natural form, so-called open oral challenge, is frequently used in this department as well as by the other investigators.[5,53,55,87]

The challenge can be combined with recording of various *in vivo* and *in vitro* diagnostic parameters, such as clinical symptoms,[45] pulse rate,[5,87] nasal resistance and/or lung function and other parameters.[7,69,70,74,75,80,112] Other authors may prefer single blind challenge,[5] open challenge with disguised foods,[24,87] double blind challenge with foods processed in capsules,[53,57,92,93] or so-called sublingual testing, where the foods in their natural form or their extracts in dilutions are placed under the tongue.[41,43,87]

Elimination and rotation diets[5,87], where the appropriate food is reintroduced a specific time after elimination, can also be used for diagnostic purposes (see Chapter 52).

There are few published data concerning the role of foods and food allergy in patients with allergic rhinitis, secretory otitis media and sinusopathy. Particularly rare are reports of nasal, conjunctival, paranasal sinuses, middle ear and bronchial tree responses after food ingestion challenge combined with quantitative recording of objective parameters.[74,75,80,111,112]

Precautions for oral challenge

The following requirements should be met before oral provocation tests with foods are performed.

1. The tests should be safe, reproducible, free of artifacts, reliable and sufficiently sensitive to show genuine results. The patient should not be able to influence the results with knowledge of the challenging agent.
2. A careful system for the evaluation of indications and contraindications for the individual patient is necessary. This

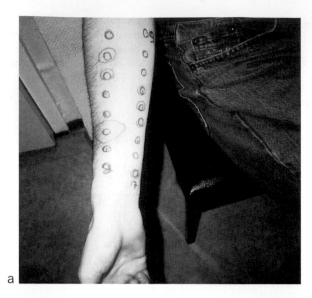

a

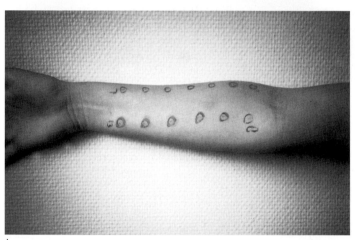

b

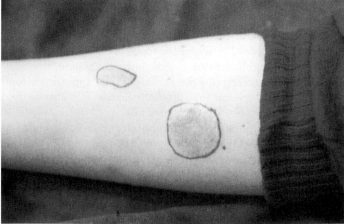

c

Fig. 35.3 Particular types of skin response after intracutaneous injections with various food extracts. (**a**) Immediate skin responses (20 min after injection) to cheese (no. 3), cow's milk (no. 16), cocoa powder (no. 12), kiwi (no. 13), tomato (no. 14), shrimps (no. 17). (**b**) Late skin responses (after 8 h) to cow's milk (no. 9), almond (no. 10), spinach (no. 11), cucumber (no. 12), mushrooms (no. 13).

(**c**) Delayed skin responses (after 56 h) to peanuts (the larger response) and hazel nuts (the smaller response).

involves a detailed disease history, general physical examination, laboratory screening and basic skin tests before the oral challenge is performed.

3. An absolute contraindication for this test is any suspicion or presumption of an anaphylactic reaction or any life-threatening event which might conceivably be associated with the specific food in the particular patient. Pregnancy and any state or disorder which might be irreversibly affected by food ingestion challenge should also be regarded as contraindications.

4. Any medication which can mask or influence the results of the challenge is contraindicated. The patient should be tested while they are receiving no restricted treatments and have no intercurrent illness or other relevant allergic symptoms.

5. Where the clinical response is not expected to be dangerous or severe (e.g. mild diarrhoea), oral food challenge can be performed as an outpatient. Other oral challenges where some severe response, such as acute dyspnoea caused by bronchospasm, oedema of epiglottis, paroxysmal hypertension attack, severe migraine attack, or severe gastrointestinal upset may occur or where a late-phase reaction is expected, should be performed as an inpatient with adequate facilities for resuscitation and the management of any emergency or unexpected complication. Such oral challenges should be carried out under the direct supervision of experienced medical staff in standard conditioning.

6. Foods or additives suspected of causing adverse reactions, together with possible crossreacting foods, should be excluded from the diet for a sufficient period of time before ingestion challenge. Opinions concerning this exclusion period vary. Some authors have recommended 1–2 weeks as a suitable elimination period.[58,59,113,114] However, clinical experience in this department suggests that, if a large number of foods need to be excluded, a 3-day avoidance before ingestion challenge may be sufficient.[80]

Techniques for oral provocation with foods

Two basic techniques for oral provocation tests with foods are usually used, double blind and open challenge with natural foods. Both of these techniques have advantages and disadvantages.[13,20,60,92,101]

In many cases we prefer open challenge with foods, our results being comparable with those obtained by the double blind technique. Open challenge is satisfactory where objective measurements of the responses to the ingested food can be made, such as bronchial function, nasal resistance, skin appearance X-ray or echography of paranasal stimulus or middle ear pressure. Double blind or crossover challenge is important in instances where pharmacological intervention is being investigated or when objective parameters cannot be quantified and recorded, such as in arthralgia or pruritus cutis or where there may be a psychosomatic component.

Double blind oral challenge with foods

Outweighing its obvious advantages, double blind challenge, performed usually with lyophilized (and/or freeze-dried) food in capsules, has a number of disadvantages.[53]

1. The maximum content of the capsules is 500 mg, which is considerably less than the quantity of the food usually being consumed. If the quantity of freeze-dried food in the capsules is to be comparable with the normal portion (e.g. 100 g of meat), then more than 200 capsules would be necessary.

2. Ideally, the food should be colourless, odourless and tasteless. Processing foods to make them suitable for such administra-

tion will inevitably lead to changes in their physical properties, and in some cases to changes in their chemical structure.

3. By administering the foods in capsules, direct contact with the buccal mucosa, tongue, oesophagus and parts of the stomach is mostly excluded.

4. By administering the food in capsules, direct the digestive process, which begins in the mouth, may be prolonged and the expected response may be delayed.

5. Providing a suitable placebo that matches the offending food in quantity, consistency, colour and taste is not always possible.[58]

6. Double blind challenge with foods and placebo hidden in capsules may be preferable for research purposes, but this technique is impractical for routine clinical use because of the expense, difficulties with patient compliance, and the problem of choosing a truly inert placebo.

7. The long dietary restriction for 1 to 2 or more weeks, as suggested by some authors,[57] can sometimes cause other problems.

Open challenge

The following schedule of food ingestion challenge is used in this department (Fig. 35.4). After a 72-h avoidance of the appropriate and related foods, food ingestion challenge is performed with the food in its natural form. The challenge may be combined with rhinomanometry (nasal airway resistance and/or nasal air flow pressure differences) typanometry, x-ray and/or echography of paranasal sinuse, lung functions and, if necessary, other diagnostic parameters. After the one-hour waiting interval, the actual post-challenge parameters are recorded for up to 36 or 56 h, and, if necessary, for a longer period of time. For control challenges (placebo) we use cooked rice, glucose or cooked potatoes, depending on the patient's symptoms and diet history.[69,70]

The amounts of particular foods used for the ingestion challenge are shown in Table 35.3. In general, for ingestion challenges we prefer quantities of foods that correspond to the usual consumption of those foods in daily life.

Nasal challenge

The food ingestion challenge can sometimes be replaced by a nasal challenge with corresponding food extract(s), especially in patients with a risk of anaphylactic reaction, severe circulatory, respiratory or metabolic disorders, or laryngeal oedema. Pregnancy is also a contraindication for the food ingestion challenge. We have shown satisfactory correlation between the results generated by food ingestion challenge and results generated by nasal challenge.[78]

Diagnostic procedures *in vitro*
Serum immunoglobulins
Total IgE

The level of total IgE as measured by the paper radioimmunosolvent test(PRIST) has not been found to be significantly related to rhinitis, sinus disease or secretory otitis media where food allergy is involved (Table 35.4).[40]

Specific IgE

The radioallergosorbent test (RAST) is the most frequently used technique,[26,49,82,91] but also one of the most controversial. This is so because of its unsatisfactory correlation with the clinical state and other *in vivo* diagnostic parameters[1] and there are also questions about interpretation and methodology.[3,4,6,32,37,40,91]

The author has studied the correlation of RAST and other diagnostic parameters with food ingestion challenge in patients with rhinitis caused by food allergy. A positive RAST was found in only 14% of patients who showed immediate nasal response to food ingestion challenge (Table 35.2). There was a better correlation between a negative ingestion challenge and a negative RAST (Fig. 35.5). Total IgE was found to be unchanged in most patients with an immediate nasal response to food ingestion challenge (Table 35.2 and 35.4). We conclude that RAST has little value in the diagnosis of food-related rhinitis. This conclusion is in accordance with the findings and experience of other investigators.[26,91,92]

Other immunoglobulins

There is partial evidence that antibodies of other classes, e.g. IgG, IgA and IgM, may be involved in the nasal response to foods. These immunoglobulins seem to be especially relevant to the late nasal response after food ingestion challenge.[8,30,47,108] There is also evidence for other, non-immediate types of hypersensitivity (Type III or Type IV) in food-induced reactions.

Nasal secretions

The study of nasal secretions is a useful supplement to rhinomanometry after oral provocation. The patient blows his nose onto a polyethylene sheet before and after food challenge and the specimens are processed by various methods: the air-dried specimens, fixed by polyethylene glycol, are stained by a modified Hansel's technique; the air-dried specimens are stained by the May–Grünwald–Giemsa technique; the methanol-fixed specimens are stained by toluidine blue. Changes in the numbers of particular cell types, accompanying the particular types of nasal response to the ingested food suggest their involvement in these responses (Fig. 35.6a–g and Tables 35.2, 35.5–8).[74,79,80,82,83,101]

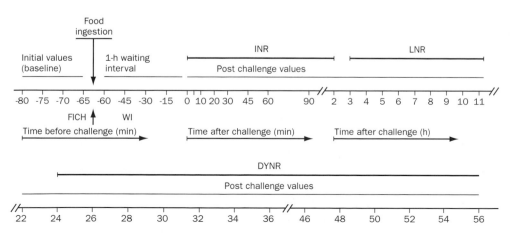

Fig. 35.4 Schedule of food ingestion challenge. INR, immediate nasal response; LNR, late nasal response; DYNR, delayed nasal response; FICH, food ingestion challenge; WI

Survey of food quantities used for ingestion challenge

Food	Quantity used for ingestion challenge
1. *Basic foods of solid consistency consumed in various quantities, usually more than 100 g at one time:* cheese, chocolate, cocoa powder, peanuts, walnuts, almonds, hazelnuts, soya, fruits, vegetables crustaceans and molluscs, meats, honey, grain and flour (barley, wheat, buck wheat, corn, maize, oat, rye)	Up to 100 g of each
2. *Basic foods of fluid consistency consumed in various quantities, usually more than 100 g at one time:* milk, yoghurt, non-alcoholic beverages (Coca-cola, 7-up, Fanta, etc.), fruit juices, coffee, tea, hot chocolate and other non-alcoholic beverages	100 ml of each
3. *Egg:* white, yellow	Amount contained in one egg (weighed)
4. *Foods, parts of foods or foodstuffs, usually with a well defined flavour or taste, only added to the basic foods in very small quantities:* spices and herbs, vegetables (garlic, onion, paprika, chilli, horseradish, sunflower, etc.), miscellaneous (casein, lactose, glucose, sucrose, olive oil, butter, margarine, vinegar, etc.)	5 g of each on brown bread with butter
5. *Alcoholic beverages:* Soft: beer, wine, sherry, port, shandy, etc. Liquor: whisky/scotch, gin, cognac, brandy, vodka, liqueurs, etc.	100 ml of each 5 ml of each
6. Additives are used in quantities corresponding with those occurring in 100 g or 100 ml of the basic foods or in 5 g or 5 ml of the 'flavouring' foods and appetizer (e.g. vinegar, ketchup, dressings, mayonnaise, mustard, etc.)	Usually 1–10 mg, sometimes more

Table 35.3 Survey of food quantities used for ingestion challenge.

Survey of total serum IgE antibodies in patients with positive immediate nasal responses to ingestion challenge with foods

	IgE (IU/ml)				
	0–50	50–100	100–500	500–1000	>1000
Subjects (*n* = 134)	84 (63)	39 (29)	7 (5)	2 (1.5)	2 (1.5)

Values in parentheses are percentages.

Table 35.4 Survey of total serum IgE antibodies (PRIST) in patients with positive immediate nasal responses to ingestion challenge with foods.

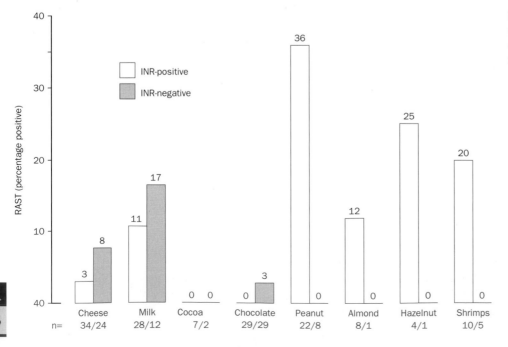

Fig. 35.5 Specific IgE antibodies in serum of patients with immediate nasal response (INR) after food ingestion challenge. RAST, radioallergosorbent test.

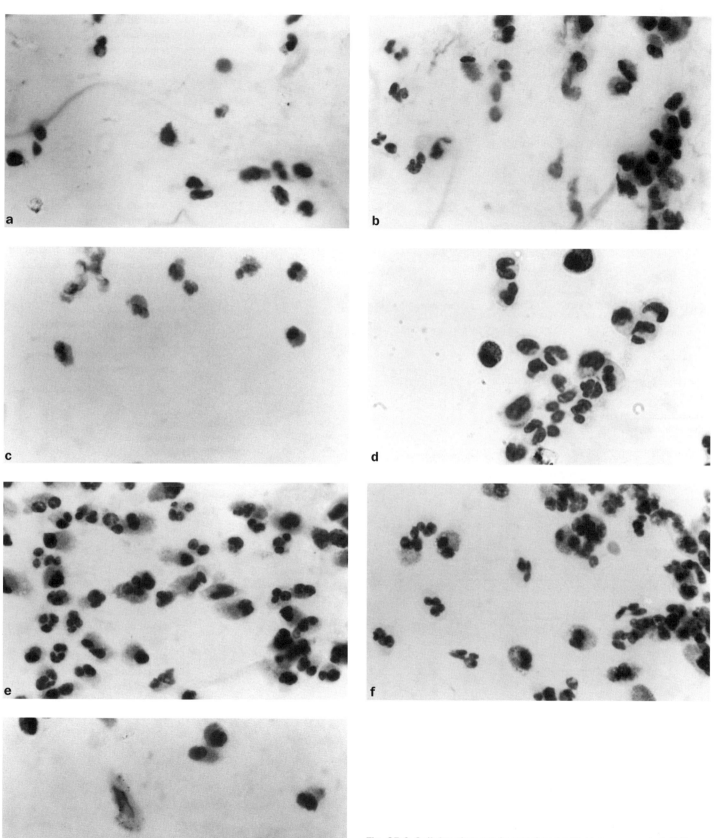

Fig. 35.6 Cellular changes in nasal secretions accompanying: (i) the immediate nasal response to food ingestion challenge with milk (a) before challenge; (b) 120 min after challenge; (c) 180 min after challenge; and (ii) the late nasal response to challenge with peanuts (d) before challenge; (e) at the fifth hour, i.e. just before the onset of the late response; (f) at the eight hour, i.e. at the maximal peak of the late response; (g) at the twelfth hour, i.e. 1 h after the late nasal response has resolved.

Time course of individual clinical types of nasal response to food ingestion challenge

	Onset	Maximum	Resolving
Immediate	10–20 min	30–45 min	90–120 min
Late	4–6 h	6–10 h	10–12 h
Delayed	24–28 h	30–36 h	42–52 h

The time is expressed in minutes or hours after a 60-min waiting interval after food ingestion.

Table 35.5 Time course of individual clinical types of nasal response to food ingestion challenge.

Presence of particular cell types in nasal secretions and changes in cell count during the non-pretreated and pretreated immediate nasal response to food ingestion challenge

	Non-pretreated		Pretreated			
			DSCG		Placebo	
Cells	Presence	Changes	Presence	Changes	Presence	Changes
Eosinophils	80	73*	20*	0*	73	67
Neutrophils	67	52*	13*	6*	67	60
Basophils	20	20*	0*	0*	13	13
Mast cells	6	0	0	0	0	0
Epithelial cells	73	20+	6*	0*	73	26
Goblet cells	13	0	0+	0	20	6
Monocytes	6	0	6	0	0	0
Plasma cells	0	0	0	0	6	0
Lymphocytes	26	0	20	6	20	0

$*P < 0.05$, statistically significant; $+P = 0.05$, statistically borderline.

Table 35.6 Presence of particular cell types in nasal secretions and changes in cell count during the non-pretreated immediate nasal response to food ingestion challenge and in those pretreated with oral Cromolyn (disodium cromoglycate; DSCG) and placebo, with respect to the prechallenge count (in percentage of cases).

Presence of particular cell types in nasal secretions and changes in cell count during the non-pretreated and pretreated late nasal response to food ingestion challenge

	Non-pretreated		Pretreated			
			DSCG		Placebo	
Cells	Presence	Changes	Presence	Changes	Presence	Changes
Eosinophils	83	72*	28*	6*	77	72
Neutrophils	100	88*	33*	11*	100	94
Basophils	28	28*	17*	0*	22	17
Mast cells	0	0	0	0	0	0
Epithelial cells	77	56*	33*	6*	72	44
Goblet cells	39	28+	6*	0+	33	22
Monocytes	17	0	11	0	11	0
Plasma cells	6	0	0	0	0	0
Lymphocytes	17	0	6+	0	22	0

$*P < 0.05$, statistically significant; $+P = 0.05$, statistically borderline.

Table 35.7 Presence of particular cell types in nasal secretions and changes in cell count during the non-pretreated late nasal response to food ingestion challenge and in those pretreated with oral Cromolyn (disodium cromoglycate, DSCG) and placebo, with respect to the prechallenge count (in percentage of cases).

Presence of particular cell types in nasal secretions and changes in cell count during the non-pretreated and pretreated delayed nasal response to food ingestion challenge						
	Non-pretreated		**Pretreated**			
			DSCG		**Placebo**	
Cells	**Presence**	**Changes**	**Presence**	**Changes**	**Presence**	**Changes**
Eosinophils	40	40*	10*	0*	30	30
Neutrophils	70	60*	20*	10*	70	70
Basophils	10	0	0	0	10	10
Mast cells	0	0	0	0	0	0
Epithelial cells	80	70+	20*	20*	90	60
Goblet cells	20	20+	10+	0+	20	20
Monocytes	30	20	30	0+	30	10
Plasma cells	0	0	0	0	0	0
Lymphocytes	100	80+	60*	50+	100	90

*$P < 0.05$, statistically significant; +$P = 0.05$, statistically borderline.

Table 35.8 Presence of particular cell types in nasal secretions and changes in cell count during the non-pretreated delayed nasal response to food ingestion challenge and in those pretreated with oral Cromolyn (disodium cromoglycate, DSCG) and placebo, with respect to the prechallenge count (in percentage of cases).

Author's clinical studies

We have studied the role of food allergy in rhinitis, sinusitis, headache, conjunctivitis and otitis media.[69,74,80,83] In 60% of patients with allergic rhinitis, food allergy participated in producing the nasal complaints. In most of these patients the nasal symptoms were caused primarily by various inhalant allergens and the foods were involved secondarily. However, in 19% food allergy was found to be the sole cause of the rhinitis.

Basic types of nasal response to foods

Three types of nasal response were recorded after food ingestion challenge (Table 35.5).

1. An immediate response occurring within 70 min of the food ingestion challenge, peaking at 100–120 min and resolving within 180 min (Fig. 35.7).
2. A late response starting 7 h after the food ingestion challenge, peaking at 9–11 h and resolving within 12–24 h (Fig. 35.7).
3. The delayed response appearing at 24–28 h, achieving its maximum at 34–38 h and resolving within 52–56 h (Fig. 35.8).

The late and delayed responses could be observed either in an isolated form or in a simultaneous combination with the immediate type, so-called dual late or dual delayed responses (Figs 35.7 and 35.8). A waiting interval of 1 h after the ingestion challenge with

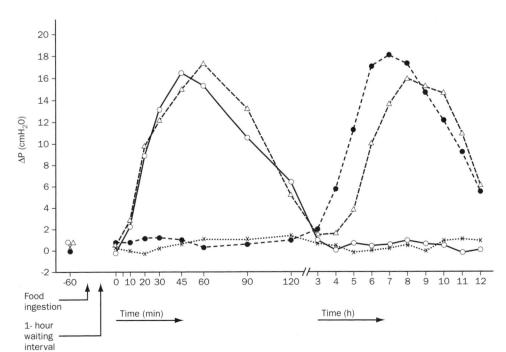

Fig. 35.7 Immediate, late and dual late nasal response to food ingestion challenge. Mean nasopharynx–nostril pressure gradient values recorded after the challenge were calculated from all patients developing the same type of nasal response. O———O, isolated immediate response ($n = 10$); ●– – – –●, isolated late response ($n = 15$); △———△, dual late response ($n = 6$); ×······×, control food challenge ($n = 28$).

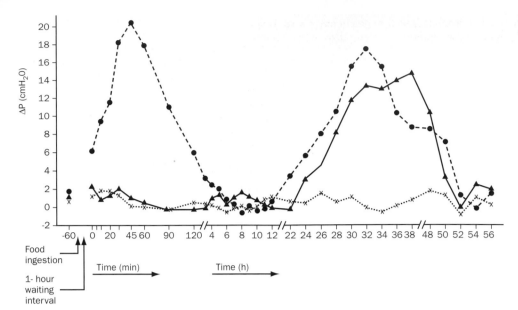

Fig. 35.8 Delayed nasal response to food ingestion challenge. Mean nasopharynx–nostril pressure gradient values recorded after food ingestion challenge were calculated from all patients developing the same type of nasal response.
▲———▲, isolated delayed response (*n* = 18); ●– – – –●, dual delayed response (*n* = 15); ×·······×, control food challenge (*n* = 35).

a particular food has already been included in the above described time courses of the particular response types.

The frequency of occurrence of the particular types of nasal responses to food ingestion has been found to be as follows: the isolated immediate type 20%; the isolated late type 35%; the dual late type 30%; the isolated delayed type 10%; and the dual delayed type less than 5% of all cases.[74,80,83] The combined data are shown in Table 35.2.

The frequency with which particular foods may cause nasal, middle ear or paranasal sinus symptoms after ingestion challenge varies, but the most common foods implicated are dairy products (milk, cheese), mayonnaise, ice-cream, chocolate, peanuts, hazelnuts, apple, green peas, cauliflower, celery, almonds, walnuts, soya, onion, garlic, mushrooms, cabbage, tomato, spinach, beans, lettuce, lobster, shrimps, mussels, oysters, crab, various fish (salmon, herring, tuna), cucumber, strawberries, kiwi, mango, flour (wheat, barley, corn, maize, oat, rye, buck-wheat) sweets, banana, eggs, spices (paprika powder, mustard, nutmeg, sambal, horse-radish, coriander, ketjap, ketchup, vanilla, ginger etc) beer, wine, sherry, port and non-alcoholic beverages(coca-cola, 7-up, fanta), and miscellaneous such as casein, glucose, sucrose, olive oil, butter, margarine, vinegars, honey etc.[70,74,79,80,82,83]

Coexistence of food-induced rhinitis and other allergic disorders

Nasal responses caused by food allergy can occur simultaneously with other clinical disorders and with other organ responses (Table 35.9).[16,24,74,79,80,109] There appear to be two basic forms of such coexistence, a primary (independent or non-associated) form and a secondary (dependent or associated) form.

In the primary form, the food, acting through a food hypersensitivity mechanism, causes not only the nasal response, but simultaneous and independent response(s) elsewhere.

For example, symptoms may occur relating to hypersensitivity responses in the oral mucosa (aphthae, stomatitis), conjunctiva, eyelids, middle ear, bronchial tree bronchospasm, skin (acute excerbation of atopic eczema, urticaria or angio-oedema, joints (arthralgia), central nervous system (headache, migraine) or gastrointestinal system (vomiting, diarrhoea, intestinal spasm, colitis, gastroenteritis), interstitial cystitis, circulatory tract hypo or hyper-tension, tachy-or brachycardio lymphoden opathia, general malaise.

In the secondary form, food ingestion leads primarily to a nasal response, which then induces a secondary response in another organ.

Such secondary responses may occur in the paranasal sinuses, middle ear, eye, tongue or bronchial tree.[74,79,80,83] Migraine and headaches may also occur as a secondary and dependent manifestation of food-induced rhinitis (Table 35.9 and Fig. 35.9).

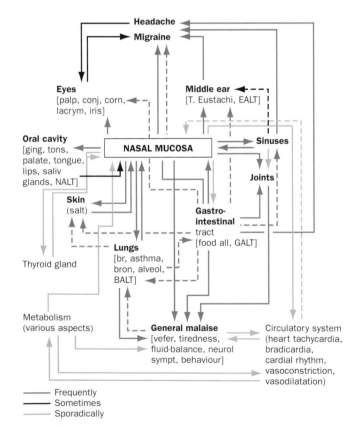

Fig. 35.9 Possible relationships between the nasal mucosa (allergy, response) and other organs. BALT, bronchi-associated lymphoid tissue; EALT, ear-associated lymphoid tissue; GALT, gut-associated lymphoid tissue; NALT, nasal-associated lymphoid tissue; SALT, skin-associated lymphoid tissue.

Review of nasal complaints and those in other organs accompanying the various types of nasal response to food ingestion challenge				
	Nasal mucosa response to ingested food			
	Immediate (n = 267)	Late (n = 203)	Delayed (n = 164)	Negative (n = 309)
Nasal complaints				
Obstruction	267 (100)	203 (100)	164 (100)	0
Sneezing	19 (7)	1 (0.5)	0	1 (0.3)
Hypersecretion	193 (72)	166 (82)	39 (24)	16 (5)
Itching	181 (68)	75 (37)	145 (88)	13 (4)
General malaise complaints	22 (8)	54 (27)	49 (30)	1 (0.3)
Conjunctival injection	35 (13)	18 (9)	6 (4)	0
Middle ear response (otalgia, decrease in hearing, change of middle ear pressure)	31 (12)	19 (9)	13 (8)	10 (3)
Pressure in the sinuses (maxillary and frontal, acute oedema of the sinus mucosa)	45 (17)	32 (16)	33 (20)	7 (2)
Cephalgia	56 (21)	91 (45)	125 (76)	42 (14)
Urticaria	4 (1.5)	7 (3)	8 (5)	5 (1.6)
Angioneurotic oedema (labial, palpebral or elsewhere)	9 (3)	6 (3)	3 (2)	3 (1)
Increase in body temperature	4 (1.5)	21 (10)	1 (0.6)	0
Bronchial complaints (mostly secondary bronchospasm, sometimes also wheezing and/or cough)	13 (5)	15 (7)	12 (7)	8 (3)
Other complaints	2 (0.7)	1 (0.5)	2 (1)	0

Values in parentheses are percentages.

Table 35.9 Review of nasal complaints and those in other organs accompanying the various types of nasal response to food ingestion challenge.

Management and treatment

The management of the patient with allergic rhinitis because of food allergy has two main issues: the avoidance of the incriminating foods and the pharmacological approach.

Elimination diet

The avoidance of the offending food is the most important part of the management of food allergy, especially in cases in which only a small number of foods are involved. Two precautions are important: first, the diagnostic procedures must have confirmed the involvement of these foodgroups in the patient's complaints; and second, it must be possible for the incriminated food or food groups to be completely avoided by the patient.

Various schedules and modifications of the elimination diet have been reported in the literature.

Pharmacological treatment

Oral disodium cromoglycate

Disodium cromoglycate (DSCG) administered orally in a dose of 100–200 mg four times daily has been found to be effective in patients suffering from rhinitis, sinus disease, secretory otitis media and conjunctivitis, and even in patients with bronchial asthma, colitis, migraine, atopic eczema, urticaria and angio-oedema, aphthoe and interstitial cystitis in which food allergy has been involved (Figs 35.10a–e).[10,25,28,31,68,74,107,111,115] Data showed that oral DSCG significantly prevented both the immediate (83%; $P < 0.001$) and late (79%; $P < 0.01$) nasal responses to food ingestion challenge and partly also the delayed nasal response (51%; $P < 0.05$) (Figs 35.10–13).[74,79,83,111]

Topical treatment

Disodium cromoglycate

DSCG has been found to be effective in the topical treatment of nasal allergy, especially in cases where the immediate and/or late nasal response may dominate the clinical picture.[76,77,79,82,83]

Glucocorticosteroids

Glucocorticosteroids such as beclomethasone dipropionate, budesonide, or fluticasones have demonstrated significant protective effects on the late and especially the delayed nasal response to inhalant allergen challenge.[79,82,83]

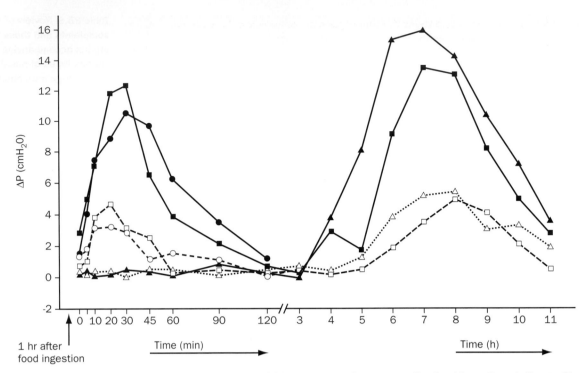

Fig. 35.10a Protective effects of oral disodium cromoglycate (DSCG) on the nasal response after food ingestion challenge. The mean nasopharynx–nostril pressure gradient values after non-pretreated and pretreated nasal mucosa responses because of the ingestion challenge, with respect to the appropriate 'Coca's solution' values, were always calculated from patients developing the same type of nasal response. Isolated immediate response (m=11) ●———● = non pretreated; ○– – –○ = pretreated with DSCG. Isolated late response (m=12) ▲———▲ = non pretreated; △– – –△ = pretreated with DSCG. Dual response (immediate+late) (m=22) ■———■ = non pretreated; □– – –□ = pretreated with DSCG

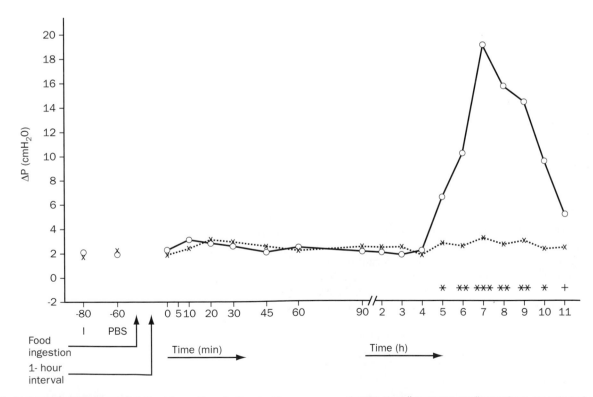

Fig. 35.10b Late nasal response after food ingestion challenge. The mean nasopharynx–nostril pressure gradient values, recorded after the non-pretreated food ingestion challenge and the control ingestion challenge with indifferent food, were calculated from 14 patients. I, initial value (mean); PBS, control challenge with phosphate-buffered saline (mean). $^{+}P \leq 0.05$; $^{*}P < 0.05$; $^{**}P < 0.01$; $^{***}P < 0.001$. ○———○, Non-pretreated late nasal response ($n = 14$); ×------×, control ingestion challenge ($n = 14$).

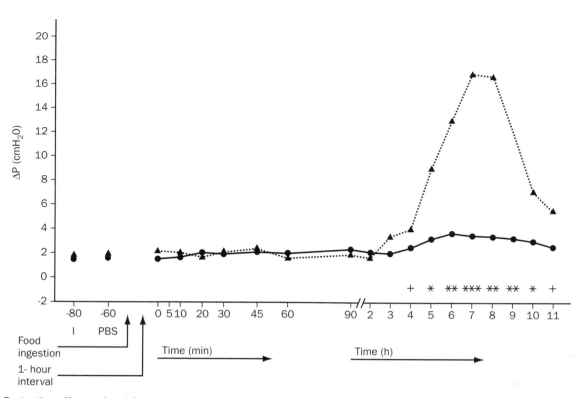

Fig 35.10c Protective effects of oral Cromolyn (Disodium chromoglycate, DSCG)on the late nasal response after food ingestion challenge. The mean nasopharynx–nostril pressure gradient values, recorded after the food ingestion challenges pretreated with oral disodium cromoglycate (Cromolyn, DSCG) and with placebo, were calculated from 14 patients. I, initial value (mean); PBS, phosphate-buffered saline (mean). Protective effects of DSCG with respect to the placebo: $^+P - 0.05$; $^*P < 0.05$; $^{**}P < 0.01$; $^{***}P < 0.001$. ●———●, late nasal response pretreated with oral DSCG ($n = 14$); ▲– – – –▲, late nasal response pretreated with oral placebo ($n = 14$).

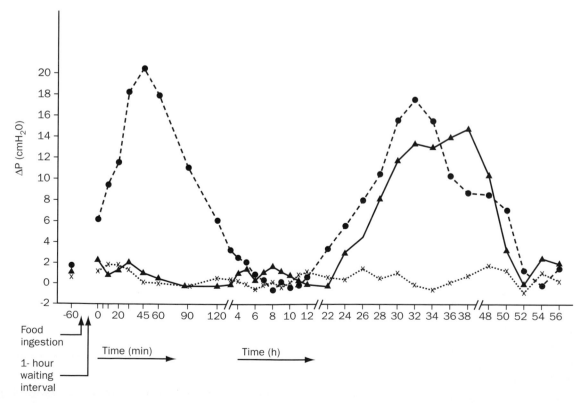

Fig. 35.10d Delayed nasal response to food ingestion challenge. Mean nasopharynx–nostril pressure gradient values recorded after food ingestion challenge were calculated from all patients developing the same type of nasal response. ▲———▲, isolated delayed response ($n = 18$); ●– – – –●, dual delayed response ($n = 15$); ×·······×, control food challenge ($n = 33$).

End-organ effect

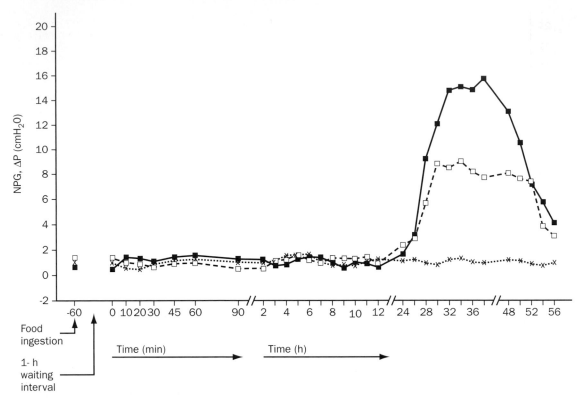

Fig. 35.10e Protective effects of oral disodium cromoglycate (DSCG) on the delayed nasal response after food ingestion challenge. The mean nasopharynx–nostril pressure gradient values after non-pretreated and pretreated nasal mucosa responses due to the food ingestion challenge, with respect to the appropriate control nasopharynx–nostril pressure gradient values, were calculated from all patients, developing the some type of nasal response. ■———■, non-pretreated delayed response(m=6); □– – – –□, pretreated with DSCG(m=6); ×------×, controls (n = 6).

H₁-receptor antagonists
These are also available for topical use, e.g. azelastine or levocabastine.

Nedocromil sodium
This has been shown to prevent significantly the immediate, the late and also partly the delayed nasal responses to nasal challenge with inhalant allergens.[82]

H₁-receptor antagonists
These can be used for oral (systemic) use, especially those of the third generation such as cetirizine or loratadine.

These drugs should be considered when oral DSCG is not able to prevent fully the nasal symptoms caused by the ingested food, when nasal allergy due to inhalant allergens is also present, or when late or delayed nasal responses predominate.[71,73,76,77,81]

Supplementary treatment
In some patients with allergic rhinitis, non-specific hyperreactivity participates in the precipitation of nasal symptoms. In this case, supplementary treatment may be needed to achieve optimal symptom control. This may include anticholinergic drugs (ipratropium bromide or oxyphenonium), additional H₁-receptor antagonists (acrivastine hydroxyzine), or H₂-receptor antagonists (cimetidine and ranitidine).

Controversial and unproven procedures
The basic requirement for every diagnostic and therapeutic procedure is a scientific basis, reasonable effectiveness and minimal risk for the patient. It must be added that some tests are routinely performed when there is neither a clear scientific basis nor are the clinical responses that result from the application of such tests supported by an existing consensus. Such tests are not listed or discussed in this section.

Conclusion
It can be concluded that the involvement of foods in allergic rhimitis is more frequent than is usually expected. The definite confirmation of the role of a certain food in these patients should be provided by the food ingestion challenge demonstrating one of the clinical types of masal response. The management of the patient with allergic rhimitis due to the food allergy has two main issues:(a) the avoidance of imeriminating foods(=e.g. elimination diet) and (b) the pharmacological approach. The pharmacological treatment consists of: oral disodium cromoglycate (Cromolyn, DSCG, Nalcrom^R, 4x100-200mg daily), accompanied by one of the third generation of the oral H₁-receptors antagonists(e.g. cetirizime, loratadine, ebastine) and eventually complemented by topical(=intranasal) DSCG, glucocorticosteroids, anticholiuespics, H₁-and H₂-receptor antagonists.

SECRETORY OTITIS MEDIA

Basic facts
Secretory otitis media (SOM), or otitis media with effusion, is an especially common disorder in children and adolescents but can occur also in adults.[35] It can be divided with respect to the appearance into an acute and a chronic form. It can also be classified

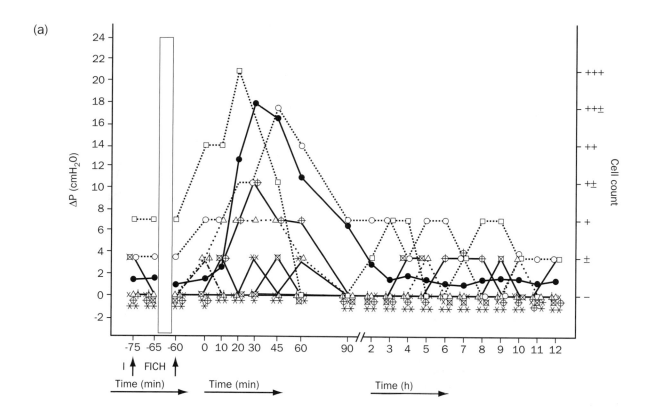

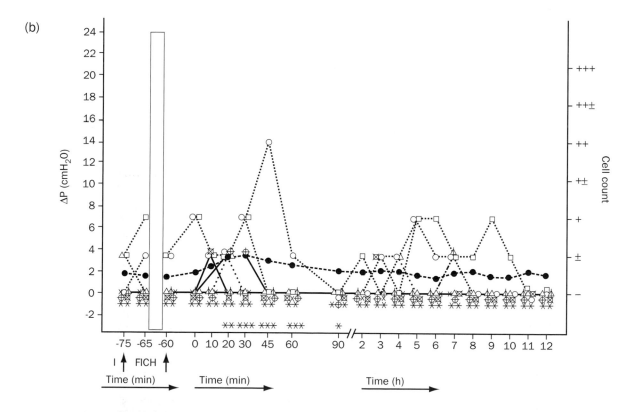

Fig. 35.11 Immediate nasal response (INR) to food ingestion challenge (FICH) and the accompanying cytological changes in the nasal secretions: (a) without pretreatment; (b) after pretreatment with oral disodium cromoglycate (DSCG). The mean changes in the individual cell counts in the nasal secretions were calculated of all patients (m=15). I, initial values. Protective effects of DSCG: $^{+}P = 0.05$; $^{*}P < 0.05$; $^{**}P < 0.01$; $^{***}P < 0.001$.
●———●, Non-pretreated immediate nasal response ($n = 15$); ●- - - - -●, immediate nasal response [INR] pretreated otith oral DSCG ($n = 15$); □- - - - -□, eosinophils; △- - - - - -△, basophils; ▲—·—·—▲, mast cells; ○- - - - - -○, neutrophils; ×———×, goblet cells; ⊠———⊠, lymphocytes; ⊕———⊕, epithelial cells; *———*, plasma cells; *—·—·—*, monocytes.

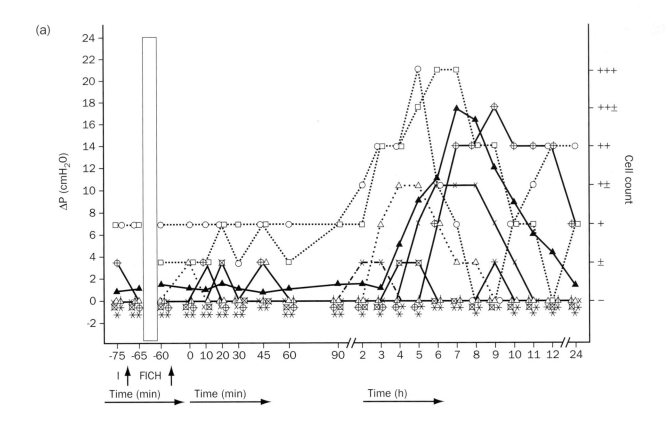

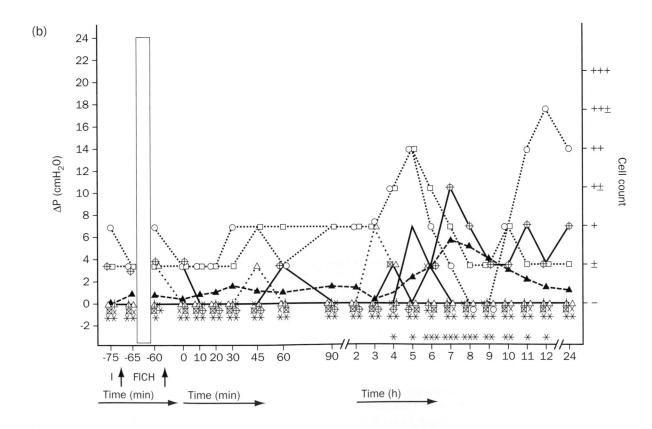

Fig. 35.12 Late nasal response to(LNR) food ingestion challenge (FICH) in 18 patients and the accompanying cytological changes in the nasal secretions: (a) without pretreatment; (b)after pretreatment with oral disodium cromoglycate (DSCG). See Fig. 35.11 for full key details.
▲- - - - -▲, late nasal response(LNR) pretreated with DSCG (*n* = 18). ▲——▲, non-pretreated late nasal response (LNR) (m=18).

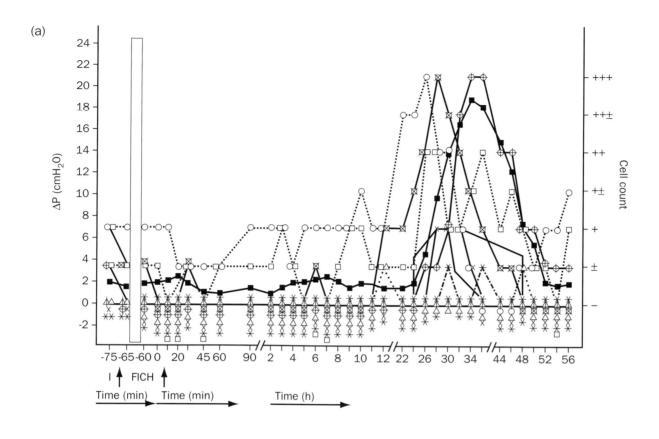

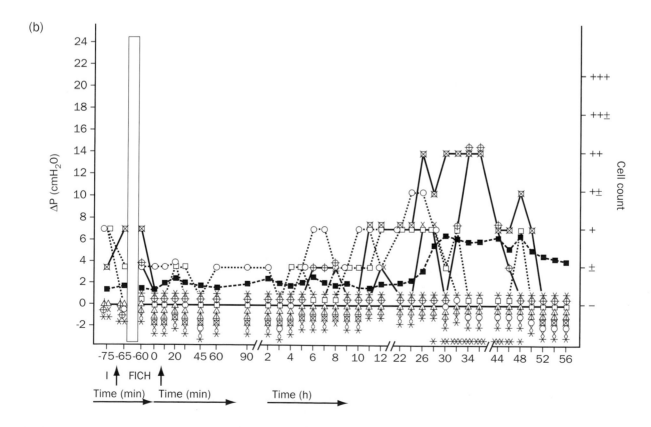

Fig. 35.13 Delayed nasal response to (DYNR) food ingestion challenge (FICH) in 10 patients and the accompanying cytological changes in the nasal secretions: (a) without pretreatment; (b) after pretreatment with oral disodium cromoglycate (DSCG). See Fig. 35.11 for full key details. ■———■, Non-pretreated delayed nasal response(DYNR) (*n* = 10) ■-------■,delayed nasal response(DYNR) pretreated with oral DSCG (m=10).

according to the middle ear fluid production, either as serous, mucoid or purulent (so-called 'glue ear').[16–19] The purulent form of acute, as well as of chronic, otitis media is generally caused by bacterial agents (e.g. *Streptococcus pneumoniae*, 40%; *Haemophilus influenzae*, 20%; *Streptococcus pyogenes*, 5%). In approximately 25% of these cases no bacteria can be identified in the middle ear effusions.[19] The most common cause of acute serous secretory otitis media is presumed to be bacterial infection whereas, in contrast, hypersensitivity mechanisms and in particular allergy, are presumed to be the most important and frequent cause of chronic SOM.[12,16,18,19]

Epidemiology of secretory otitis media

The estimates reported in the literature concerning the incidence of SOM vary widely, from 15% to 64% of children.[16,18,19,35,44,50,98] SOM occurs mainly unilaterally, and the bilateral form is rare.[16,19,89] Epidemiological data concerning SOM in adults are difficult to find. The condition is more frequent during the first 2 years of life and decreases slowly in incidence towards the teenage years. There is no gender difference, but there is a greater frequency of SOM during the winter and early spring than in summer[16,17].

Pathophysiology and aetiology of secretory otitis media

SOM is an accumulation of serous or sometimes mucoid fluid in the middle ear. It is associated with changes in middle ear pressure and with dysfunction of the middle ear structures.[16,17,19] SOM has multiple aetiologies, which are discussed later in this section.

The Eustachian tube

The pathogenesis of SOM appears to be related to abnormal function of the Eustachian tube[15].

The Eustachian tube executes three basic functions: first, protection of the middle ear from the nasopharyngeal secretions; second, ventilation of the middle ear to equilibrate the air pressure in the middle ear with the atmospheric pressure; and third, drainage of the secretions from the middle ear into the nasopharynx.

The major types of abnormal function of the Eustachian tube that may cause SOM are obstruction, abnormal patency or a combination of both.

Obstruction

Obstruction of the Eustachian tube can be caused by various factors.

For example, mechanical obstruction owing to extrinsic causes, such as adenoid hypertrophy, or intrinsic causes such as infection or allergy.

Functional obstruction can be caused by an increased compliance by the abnormally active opening mechanism or by the nasal obstruction(so-called Toynbee phenomenon). In this form, the allergy may usually be involved. The persistent high negative middle ear pressure is associated with a collapse or retraction of the tympanic membrane (atelectasis).

1. Ventilation of the Eustachian tube may occur, and because of the high negative middle ear pressure, the nasopharyngeal secretions become aspirated into the middle ear, which results in an acute otitis media with effusion.
2. Alternatively, ventilation of the Eustachian tube may not occur and persistent obstruction of the tube results in an otitis media with effusion, because there is insufficient drainage of the middle ear. In this case, the occurance of the

SOM may be dependent on the degree and the duration of the negative pressure as well as the middle ear hypoxia or hypercapnia, which can lead to the stimulation of the secretion and local exudation.[15,16,17,,18,19,38]

Relationship between the middle ear and nose

Nasal obstruction

Nasal obstruction may also be involved in the pathogenesis of SOM. This can lead either to an oedematous obstruction of the Eustachian tube or to an increase in the negative pressure in the nasopharynx resulting in an obstruction of the Eustachian tube and an increase in negative pressure in the middle ear. The corollary is that nasal obstruction can lead to an increase in the positive nasopharyngeal pressure, causing aspiration of nasopharyngeal secretions into the middle ear.

The relationship of SOM with other allergic disorders, especially those of the nose, has already long been recognized. Allergy is presumed to be one of the most important aetiological factors in SOM, because it occurs so frequently in subjects with other allergic disorders.[84,109] Moreover, reliable management of the other allergic disorder regularly leads to a distinct improvement in the SOM. The majority of patients with this condition also suffer from nasal allergy, either because of inhalant allergens or to food, or to both.[109] In these patients treatment and management which is focused on the food allergy component may be extremely successful.[18,27,83,90]

Involvement of allergy in secretory otitis media

In spite of evidence of the involvement of allergy in SOM, the exact mechanism of this involvement is not yet fully understood. Mogi[63] has found IgE levels in SOM effusions to be lower than IgE levels in the serum. From this finding he has concluded that allergy is probably not a major cause of SOM. In contrast, Phillips *et al.*[84] and Lim *et al.*[56] have found distinctly higher levels of IgE in middle ear effusions than in serum and they therefore concluded that Type I allergy (immediate hypersensitivity) may be the major cause of SOM, a view endorsed by Dockhorn.[34] However, the findings of high concentrations of IgG and IgA antibodies in middle ear effusions may suggest that other hypersensitivity mechanisms might also be involved. Hall *et al.*[44] have suggested that allergy is not the primary aetiological factor in chronic SOM, but only a contributing factor. Ruokonen *et al.*[89,90] and Clemis[27] have concluded that foods and food allergy are regularly involved in SOM. Moreover, Clemis[27] believes that food allergens are of greater importance than inhalant allergens in the allergic diseases of the upper airway.

Author's clinical studies

From our own studies it would appear that in approximately 80% of patients with SOM, an allergic rhinitis has also been found. The corollary is that in approximately 8% of patients with allergic rhinitis, coexistent SOM has been confirmed. In some patients with allergic rhinitis an increase in negative middle ear pressure has been recorded after nasal challenge with inhalant allergens and also after ingestion challenge with foods. An increased negative pressure in the middle ear after intranasal allergen challenge can also be found in patients with a clinically negative nasal response (Tables 35.10–12).

We have also found that some patients with both positive and negative nasal provocation tests have reported a sharp pain in the middle ear (otalgia) or a sudden decrease in hearing after allergen

Survey of patients with secretory otitis media					
History of nasal allergy	No.	Skin test		RAST	
		+	–	+	–
Suggestive	23	19	4	5	18
Unknown	15	12	3	1	14

RAST, radioallergasorbent test.

Table 35.10 Survey of patients with secretory otitis media (*n* = 38).

Middle ear response to nasal allergen challenge in patients with secretory otitis media			
Nasal response	Ear response		
	Positive	Negative	Total
In 31 patients			
Positive	65	11	76
Negative	6	15	21
In 7 patients			
Negative	8*	4+	12

* Responses in five patients; +responses in two patients. In 38 control challenges with phosphate-buffered saline there was neither nasal nor ear response.

Table 35.11 Middle ear response to nasal allergen challenge in 38 patients with secretory otitis media. Survey of nasal (rhinomanometry) and ear (tympanometry) responses after nasal challenge with allergens.

Middle ear response to nasal allergen challenge in 38 patients with secretory otitis media. Survey of the otological complaints during particular types of nasal response					
Nasal response	No.	Changes in MEP* accompanied by			
		Otalgia	Decrease in hearing	Secretions†	Otalgia only
Positive (76)	61	56	35	13	4
Isolated immediate (21)	19	18	6	4	2
Isolated late (24)	17	17	13	5	1
Dual late (15)	12	10	9	1	0
Isolated delayed (11)	9	9	4	2	0
Dual delayed (5)	4	2	3	1	1
Negative (33)	13	6	2	1	1

* MEP, middle ear pressure recorded by tympanometry; †secretions, rapid increase in the middle ear effusions through the monolateral or bilateral ventilation tube(s).

Table 35.12 Middle ear response to nasal allergen challenge in 38 patients with secretory otitis media. Survey of the otological complaints during particular types of nasal response.

Survey of total IgE antibodies in the serum of 29 patients with positive immediate middle ear response to food ingestion challenge					
	IgE (IU/ml)				
	0–50	50–100	100–500	500–1000	>1000
Subjects (*n* = 29)	16 (55)	9 (31)	1 (3.5)	2 (7)	1 (3.5)

Values in parentheses are percentages.

Table 35.13 Survey of total IgE antibodies in the serum of 29 patients with positive immediate middle ear response to food ingestion challenge.

challenge, whereas the middle ear pressure (as measured by tympanometry) remained unchanged (Table 35.12).

Forms of secretory otitis media and types of response

Observations implicate two possible mechanisms of involvement of food allergy in SOM.[80] The middle ear response may either be primary (non-associated), caused by a direct effect via the bloodstream or secondary (associated), as a consequence of nasal mucosa response, the nasal mucosa being the primary site of the hyper-

sensitivity reaction and thus the primary effector organ. In this secondary form, the nasal mucosa response (oedema, hypersecretion and other changes) leads to swelling of the peritubal and lymphatic tissue of the pharyngeal orifice of the Eustachian tube, causing its partial or full obstruction and resulting in the secondary SOM (Tables 35.11 and 35.12).[80]

Three basic types of middle ear response to food allergy, whether of the primary or secondary form, have been observed and repeatedly demonstrated. The first is the early middle ear response, with

Survey of nasal and middle ear responses after food ingestion challenge			
	Ear response		
Nasal response	Positive	Negative	Total
In 21 patients			
Positive	19	6	25
Negative	4	2	6
In 7 patients			
Negative	9*	5†	14

* Responses in five patients; † responses in two patients. In 28 control challenges there was neither nasal nor ear response.

Table 35.14 Survey of nasal and middle ear responses after food ingestion challenge in 28 patients.

onset within 80 min, maximum within 125–150 min and resolving within 3 h after the food ingestion challenge. The second is the late middle ear response, with onset within 5–6 h, maximum within 7–10 h and resolving within 12–24 h after the food ingestion. Third is the delayed middle ear response, with onset within 26–30 h, maximum within 31–37 h and resolving within 48–52 h after the food ingestion challenge.[79,80,82,83] In some patients, early, late and delayed middle ear responses may present concurrently (Tables 35.14 and 35.15, Figs 35.14 and 35.15).

Diagnostic procedures

The diagnostic procedures should include: general examination; ear, nose, throat and paranasal sinuses examination; and allergo-logical–immunological examination.

1. General examination should consist of: a detailed case history; a physical examination; laboratory screening tests; X-ray

Middle ear and nasal responses after food ingestion challenge in 28 patients with secretory otitis media. Survey of the tympanometric and otological parameters						
		Changes in MEP* accompanied by				
Nasal response	No.	Otalgia	Decrease in hearing	Paracusia/ ruslting	†Secretions	Otalgia only
Positive (25)	19	18	6	3	7	0
Isolated immediate (7)	6	6	1	0	2	0
Isolated late (10)	9	9	4	2	3	0
Dual late (4)	2	1	0	0	0	0
Isolated delayed (3)	1	1	1	1	1	0
Dual delayed (1)	1	1	0	0	1	0
Negative (20)	13	11	4	1	1	1

* MEP, middle ear pressure recorded by tympanometry (increase in the pressure negativity); †secretions, rapid increase in the middle ear effusions through the monolateral or bilateral ventilation tube(s).

Table 35.15 Middle ear and nasal responses after food ingestion challenge in 28 patients with secretory otitis media. Survey of the tympanometric and otological parameters.

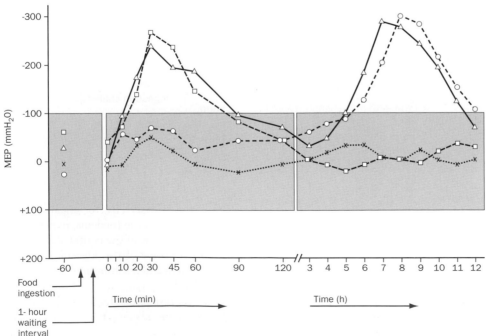

Fig. 35.14 Middle ear response to food ingestion challenges in 35 patients with SOM. The tympanometric values (MEP, middle ear pressure) were calculated from all patients with the same type of middle ear response. The spotted area represents the normal value range of MEP. □– – –□, isolated immediate ear response (n = 17); △——△, dual late response (n = 10); ○– – –○, isolated late response (n = 8); ×·······×, control food challenge (n = 35).

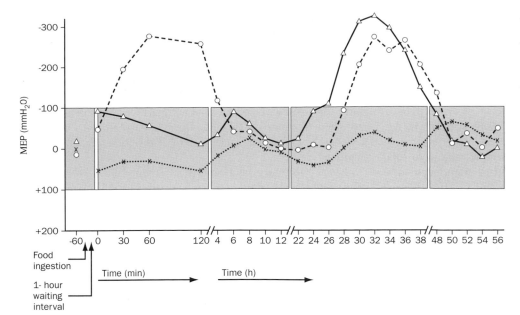

Fig. 35.15 Middle ear response to food ingestion challenge in patients with SOM. The tympanometric values (MEP, middle ear pressure) were calculated from all patients with the same type of middle ear response. The spotted area indicates the normal value range of MEP. $\triangle$————$\triangle$, isolated delayed ear response ($n = 21$); $\bigcirc$-----$\bigcirc$, dual delayed response ($n = 13$); $\times$------$\times$, control food challenge ($n = 34$).

examination, for example, of the middle ear and/of paranasal sinuses.

2. An ear, nose and throat examination should consist of: an otolaryngological physical examination, including rhinoscopy and otoscopy; tympanometry; pneumatoscopy and audiometry; echography of the paranasal sinuses; and, if necessary, a diagnostic aspiration of the middle ear effusions should be performed for cytological, immunological and bacteriological purposes.

3. Allergological–immunological examination may include: skin testing with basic inhalant and food allergen extracts; nasal provocation tests with inhalant allergens and food ingestion challenges, or both of them in combination with rhinomanometry and tympanometry; and the determination of immunoglobulins of various classes, such as total IgE, specific IgE, total IgG, subclasses of IgG, total IgM and IgA in the blood, nasal secretions and/or middle ear effusions.

In some cases, the determination of various other immunological factors and parameters, such as mediators, chemotactic factors, cytokines, etc. should be performed. The determination of total serum IgE did not demonstrate any diagnostic value for SOM (Table 35.13), whereas the determination of the allergen-specific IgE may sometimes be of value.

Management and treatment
Otitis media caused by infection
Acute otitis media
Antibiotics, analgesics and nasal decongestants, if indicated, may be used. If fever and pain persist for longer than 24–48 h, myringotomy may be then indicated. In the case of recurrent otitis media, the insertion of ventilation tubes, at least temporarily, may be helpful.[12,16,18,19]

Chronic otitis media
Prophylactic antimicrobial therapy, nasal decongestants and myringotomy with insertion of ventilation tubes may be used in treatment. Occasionally, inflation of the middle ear

(Politzer's manoeuvre) may be helpful and may prevent further complications.[12,16,18,19]

Secretory otitis media with an allergic component
Acute secretory otitis media
In the isolated(non-associated)form of acute SOM, confirmation of allergy involvement is usually difficult. Treatment consists of nasal decongestants, antihistamines (H_1-receptor antagonists) and the elimination of the presumed allergen(s).In the associated-form of SOM, which is induced by the allergic reaction occuring primarily in the nasal mucosa, the treatment should include the topical (intranasal)DSCG, H_1- receptor ontagonists, nasal decongestans(temporarily), and if necessary topical corticosteroids.[82]

Chronic SOM
In the case of primary(non-associated) SOM ,H_1-receptor antagonists (antihistamines) and, if necessary, myringotomy may be indicated. Every effort should be made to avoid the allergens involved.

The treatment of secondary (associated) SOM allergy consists of long-term intranasal administration of DSCG, supplemented by H_1-receptor antagonists and sometimes by immunotherapy. In the case of non-immediate nasal responses to the allergen, topical glucocorticosteroids in the form of nasal sprays should also be considered. Every effort should again be made to avoid the allergens involved. If middle ear effusions occur, myringotomy followed by possible insertion of ventilation tubes should be considered.[12,15,16,18,19,98]

Involvement of food allergy in SOM
The avoidance of the incriminating foods should be the first step in the management of this disorder.[90]

Secretary otitis media induced by the nasal mucosa response due to the food allergy
In cases where SOM is induced by nasal mucosal response to food allergy, elimination of the offending foods combined with topical intranasal DSCG and supplemented by H_1-receptor antagonists is effective in a large number of patients. In patients in

whom a late or delayed type of nasal response to foods has also been demonstrated, topical intranasal corticosteroids should also be used. If the topical intranasal DSCG is not sufficiently effective, then treatment with oral DSCG preparation (100–200 mg four times daily) is indicated. The treatment should be supplemented by rinsing of the nose with sterile saline.

Secrotary otitis media due directly to the food allergy without any involvement of the nasal mucosa

In cases where SOM is thought to be directly related to food allergy, the elimination of the presumed and/or offending food(s) and the prophylactic treatment with oral DSCG (100–200 mg four times daily) is the treatment of first choice.[74,82,83]

Conclusion

The involvement of food and inhalant allergens in the pathogenesis of secretory middle ear disease is becoming more widely recognized. A diligent search for extrinsic causes should be pursued in all cases of SOM, because the removal of such aetiological agents results in the resolution of the disease. Other therapeutic manoeuvres are obviously necessary when the invoking agents are not discovered or when their elimination is not fully possible.

SINUS DISEASE

Basic facts

Acute sinusitis may be caused almost exclusively by bacterial or viral infections, with allergy only rarely playing a causal role in this form of sinus disease. Acute sinusitis is a common disorder, both in children and in adults.[75,102]

Chronic sinusitis, especially chronic maxillary sinusitis, is a common disorder in adults and sometimes in older children. The association of sinusitis with rhinitis is well known.[75,102]

The role of allergy and the involvement of hypersensitivity mechanisms in some forms of sinus disease has been discussed in the literature.[38,42,62,75,85,94,103,105] The use of the term 'sinusitis' for a disorder caused by an immunological process does not appear to be fully suitable. This disorder would be better designated as allergic sinus disease.[75]

With respect to the localization of particular kinds of paranasal sinuses, such as maxillary, frontal, sphenoid and ethmoidal (anterior and posterior), sinus disease related to allergy may appear most commonly in the maxillary sinuses, sporadically in the frontal sinuses, and has not been reported in the sphenoid or ethmoidal sinuses.[69,75,82,83] Some investigators have postulated that disease of the maxillary and frontal sinuses, especially of bacterial and viral aetiology, is almost always accompanied, if not preceded, by disease of the ipsilateral anterior ethmoidal region, since all three sinus types communicate at the middle meatus, the region known as the ostiomeatal complex.

Basic forms of sinus disease caused by hypersensitivity

Our observations implicate two basic mechanisms of involvement of hypersensitivity in sinus disease.

In the primary (non-associated) form of allergic sinus disease, the antigen–antibody interaction takes place in the mucosal membrane of the sinuses. This primary form of sinus disease can be elicited by inhalant allergens passing the nasal mucosal barrier and the mucosal filter without initiating any hypersensitivity reaction in the nasal mucosa. The allergen may then be directly trapped into the appropriate sinus and an antigen–antibody or sensitised T-lymphocyre reaction takes place, resulting in a primary sinus response without any accompanying nasal response. The opening of the sinus into the nasal cavity e.g. ostium, is the most probable site of the trapping. Such a mechanism has previously been proposed by Slavin and colleagues.[102,103] The primary form can also be caused by food antigens which, after digestion, are then transported through the bloodstream into the sinus mucosa, where they interact with local antibodies or sensitized T lymphocytes.

In the secondary (associated) form, inhalant allergens penetrating into the nasal mucosa from outside or food antigens which have been delivered to the nasal mucosa from the gut by the bloodstream, interact with the antibody or sensitized T lymphocytes, primarily in the nasal mucosa. This primary antigen–antibody interaction in the nasal mucosa leads to the development of the primary nasal mucosa response, which then induces the secondary response of the particular sinuses and/or sinus mucosa.[75] The secondary form of the sinus response due to allergy occurs much more frequently than the primary form.[75]

Pathological aspects of sinus disease due to allergy

Allergic mechanisms occurring in the nasal mucosa may lead to various symptoms. Nasal obstruction caused by swelling of the nasal mucosa is the most important of these symptoms. Oedema of the nasal mucosa leads to obstruction of the paranasal sinus orifice, in the case of the maxillary sinuses the nasal ostia, and to the decreased ciliary action and increased mucus production in the paranasal sinuses. The whole process results in accumulation of mucus and gas in the sinuses, with the subsequent thickening of the mucosal membrane in the sinuses due to oedema. Topical infiltration of the sinus mucosa, a decrease in aeration and an increase in opacification may also occur sometimes associated with the formation of a fluid level and soft tissue mass in the maxillary sinuses.[21,85,94,102,103,105]

Basic types of sinus response

Sinus disease in which hypersensitivity mechanisms play the causal role is almost exclusively chronic sinus disease. When challenged intranasally by an allergen or exceptionally by a nonspecific hyperreactivity agent, patients with chronic sinus disease may develop different types of paranasal sinus response.[69,75,82,83]

Primary(non-associated) paranasal sinus response

This type of paranasal sinus response, without any preceding or accompanying nasal response, occurs in less than 5% of all positive paranasal sinus responses, and may be observed only in maxillary sinuses.[69,75,82,83] The primary form appears to be induced only by intranasal challenge with an allergen but not with a nonspecific hyperreactivity agent.

Three types of the primary form of maxillary sinus response may be observed: an early response in approximately 3.5%, a late response in approximately 1% of cases, and a delayed response in less than 1%.

Secondary (associated)paranasal sinus response

This type of paranasal sinus response is induced secondarily by hypersensitivity mechanism(s) appearing primarily in the nasal mucosa. The nasal response because of the hypersensitivity mechanism acts as a preceding and as an accompanying causal factor that then induces the secondary sinus response. The secondary form of the paranasal sinus response is a very common disorder in both adults and children, and may be observed in 95% of subjects suffering from allergic chronic sinus disorders. The secondary form of the paranasal response is not limited to the maxillary sinuses only, but may also regularly be observed in the frontal sinuses. This form of response, induced by the primary nasal response both in the maxillary and frontal sinuses, occurs bilaterally in the majority of cases (70–80%) and on one side only in a minority of cases (20–30%).[75]

Three types of the secondary or associated form of sinus response have been recorded: early, late and delayed types. All three types are associated with the preceding and inducing nasal response of the appropriate type. However, the clinical course of the particular sinus response, especially its onset, is usually shifted in time and the sinus response appears 10–30 min later than the corresponding and inducing nasal response type.[69,75,79,82]

In most subjects suffering from immunologically mediated chronic sinus disease (besides allergic rhinitis), an additional allergic (disorder because of the participation of the hypersensitivity mechanisms), such as bronchial asthma in approximately 12%, allergic conjunctivitis in 7% and otitis media (secretory) in 6%, may be observed.[69,75,79,82]

Paranasal sinus response to foods

Primary (non-associated) form

The primary form of sinus response to ingested foods has been recorded more frequently than any response to inhalant allergens, and occurs in approximately 12% of all cases of sinus response to foods. The appearance of particular types of primary sinus responses to foods has been found as follows: (a) an *early sinus response* in 4%; (b) a *late sinus response* in 7%; and (c) a *delayed sinus response* in 1% of cases. In contrast to the primary sinus responses to inhalant allergens where responses appear to be confined to the maxillary sinuses, primary sinus responses to foods have appeared simultaneously in the maxillary and frontal sinuses.

The clinical course of the primary sinus response to foods, recorded by echography in combination with radiography, has demonstrated some differences from the clinical course of the primary sinus response to inhalant allergens (the figures for inhalant allergen responses are given in brackets): (a) early sinus response: onset within 2–3 h (1 h), maximum within 3–4 h (1–2 h) and resolving within 8–10 h (6h); late sinus response: onset within 6–8 h(4–6h), maximum within 10–12(8–10h) hours and resolving within 12–24 h(8–12h); delayed sinus response: onset within 28–30 h (24–28 h) maximum within 40 h (30–40 h) and resolving within 56–60 h (50–56 h) after the food ingestion challenge.[69,79,82]

The other *in vivo* and *in vitro* diagnostic parameters recorded during the particular types of the 'non-associated' form of sinus response to the food ingestion challenge did not differ substantially from those having been recorded during the particular types of the non-associated form of the sinus response to the inhalant allergen. However, one exception has been observed, and the positive or suspect history for a sinus response to foods has been found to a significantly lower degree, in 21% of cases only.[69,75,79,82,83]

Secondary form

The secondary (associated) form of sinus response to ingested foods has been observed in approximately 88% of all cases of sinus response to foods. As with the primary form of sinus response to food, the secondary form is not limited to the maxillary sinuses, but includes also the frontal sinuses. In the majority of the cases($\pm$75%), there is bilateral involvement.

The appearance of particular types of secondary sinus response to foods has been found to be as follows: (a) an early sinus response in approximately 48%; (b) a late sinus response in 44%; and (c) a delayed sinus response in 58% of cases (Fig. 35.19)[75].

The clinical course of particular types of the secondary form of sinus responses to foods is similar to that of the primary forms of sinus response (see above).

Diagnostic procedures

The general examination, allergological and immunological examinations have already been described in the section on Rhinitis earlier in this chapter. Nevertheless, there are additional diagnostic procedures which may be helpful for the confirmation of the causal role of foods in the paranasal sinus response.

Ingestion challenge with food(s) may be combined with monitoring of nasal resistance (rhinomanometry) combined with one or more imaging techniques of the paranasal sinuses, echography and/or radiography (X-ray) (Fig. 35.19).[75]

Ingestion challenge with food(s) may be combined with endoscopic examination of the paranasal sinuses, in most cases the maxillary sinuses, combined with lavage of the sinuse for histological, cytological, immunological and bacteriological examination.[38,46,62,86,100]

Monitoring of the paranasal sinus response

The response of the paranasal sinuses can be recorded by means of the imaging techniques.[9,54,88,99,117,118] There are several techniques for imaging the sinuses, the diagnostic values of which depend not only on the application, but also on the investigator's experience and resources. In the investigation of the role of an allergic reaction in sinus disease, repeated examinations before and after allergen exposure or challenge is the basic rule.[9,13,69,75,88]

Diagnostic imaging of the paranasal sinuses may include the following techniques.

1. Transillumination.
2. Radiography (Table 35.16. Fig. 35.16).
3. Plain tomography.
4. Computed tomography (CT).
5. Echography (Table 35.16, Fig. 35.16).
6. Magnetic resonance imaging (MRI).
7. Single photon emission computerized tomography (SPECT).

Further description of the particular imaging techniques, their practical performance and application in detail would exceed the scope of this chapter and is exhaustingly reviewed in the literature.[9,21,62,86,88,99,102,103,117,118]

Therapeutic approach

The treatment of sinus disease caused by allergy should be considered a logical consequence of the reliable identification of specific allergens. Treatment should be as comprehensive as possible and should be based on an understanding of the various primary and secondary mechanisms involved.

Therapeutic possibilities for controlling the primary form of sinus response to foods may include: the avoidance of those food(s) as far as possible; oral H_1-receptor antagonist(s); or oral DSCG 100–200 mg four times daily, either in the form of powder

Survey of radiographic and echographic changes in the maxillary sinuses		
	Changes	
Nasal response	**Radiographs**	**Echographs**
Isolated immediate	9	7	9
Isolated late	12	11	8
Dual late	4	3	3
Isolated delayed	5	5	4
Dual delayed	3	1	2
Negative	9	4	2

Statistical correlation between the radiographs and the echographs was significant (*P* < 0.05)

Table 35.16 Survey of radiographic and echographic changes in the maxillary sinuses (increase in thickening of the mucosal membrane, increased opacification and/or decreased aeration) in 28 patients suffering from chronic maxillary sinusopathy and rhinitis after 42 food ingestion challenges.

in capsules (one capsule contains 100 mg DSCG powder) or in the form of solution (1 ampule contains 100 or 200 mg DSCG).

Treatment of the secondary form of sinus response may include not only the measures mentioned above, but also therapeutic measures directed to the primary food-triggered hypersensitivity event in the nasal mucosa. These additional measures have already been described in the section on Rhinitis above.

Conclusion

Foods, acting through as yet ill-defined hypersensitivity mechanioms, are regularly involved in paranasal sinus responses. These responses can exist in two basic forms, either as a primary (or non-associated) event or as a secondary (or associated) event. In the latter case the primary response to foods takes place in the nasal mucosa, and then induces the sinus response. Three basic types of sinus response to ingested foods have been demonstrated: early, late and delayed. All three types can occur either as a primary or as a secondary event. Food ingestion challenge performed whilst monitoring nasal resistance (rhinomano-metry) and in combination with one of the paranasal sinus imaging techniques (e.g. echography, radiography) may add weight to the evidence for the role of food(s) in sinus disease. This disorder can then be approached by various therapeutic measures.

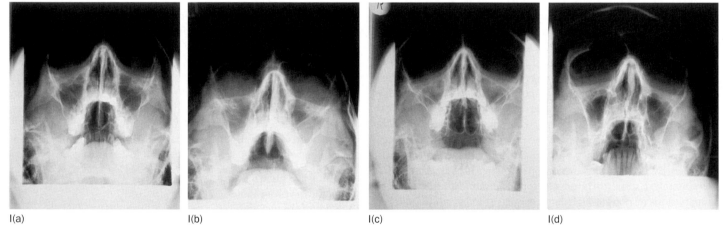

I(a)   I(b)   I(c)   I(d)

Figure 35.16(I) Radiographs of the paranasal sinuses of a patient developing the associated form of the late sinus response (LSR-MS), induced by the late nasal response (LNR) to ingestion challenge with cow's milk.

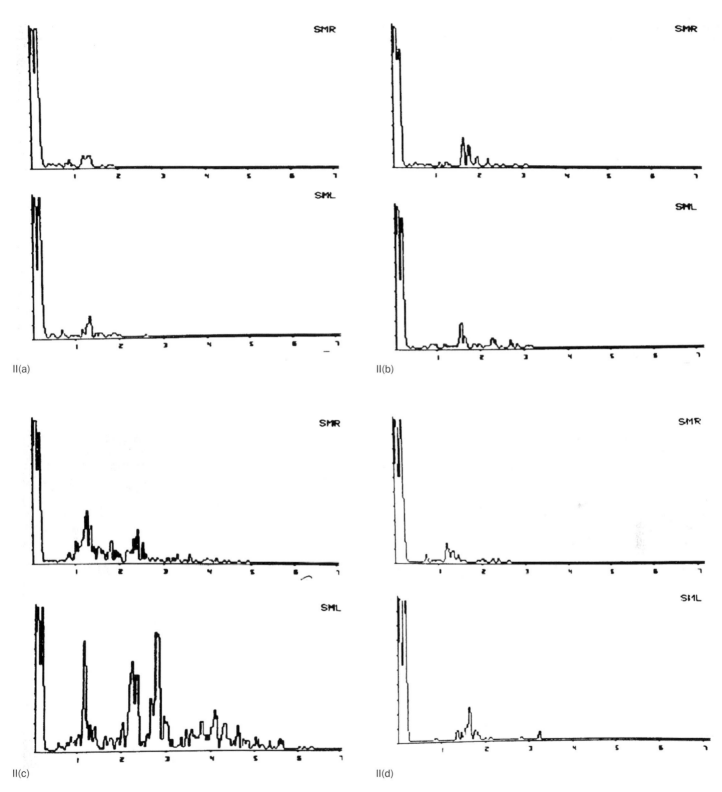

II(a)   II(b)   II(c)   II(d)

Figure 35.16(II) Echographs of the paranasal sinuses of a patient developing the associated form of the late late sinus response (LSR-MS), induced by the late nasal response (LNR) to ingestion challenge with cow's milk.

REFERENCES

1 Aas K. The critical approach to food allergy. *Ann Allergy* 1983; 51: 256–9.

2 Abernathy Carver KJ, Sampson HA, Picker LJ, Leung DY. Milk-induced eczema is associated with the expansion of T cells expressing cutaneous lymphocyte antigen. *J Clin Invest* 1995; 95: 913–18.

3 Adkinson NF. The radioallergosorbent test. *J Allergy Clin Immunol* 1980; 66: 174–5.

4 Adkinson NF. The radioallergosorbent test: uses and abuses. *J Allergy Clin Immunol* 1980; 65: 1–4.

5 Anderson JA, Sogn DD. Committee on adverse reactions to foods of the American Academy of Allergy and Immunology and National Institute of Allergy and Infectious Disease. In: *Adverse Reactions to Foods*, Washington: US Department of Health and Human Services, 1984; NIH Publication No. 84-2442.

6 Atkins FM, Steinberg SS, Metcalfe DD. Evaluation of immediate adverse reactions to foods in adult patients. Parts I and II. *J Allergy Clin Immunol* 1985; 75: 348–55 and 356–63.

7 Bahna SL, Ghandi MD. Milk hypersensitivity. II. Practical aspects of diagnosis, treatment and prevention. *Ann Allergy* 1983; 50: 295–301.

8 Barrett KE, Metcalfe DD. Immunologic mechanisms in food allergy. In: *Food Allergy, a Practical Approach to Diagnosis and Management*, (Chiaramonte LT, Scneider AT, Lifshitz F, eds). Marcel Dekker Inc, New York, Basel, 1988: 23–43.

9 Benson ML, Oliverio PJ, Zinreich SJ. Imaging techniques: conventional radiography, computed tomography, magnetic resonance, and ultra-sonography of the paranasal sinuses. In: *Disease of the sinuses*, (Gershwin ME, Incaudo GA, eds). Humana Press Inc, Totowa (NJ), 1996: 63–83.

10 Berman BA. Cromolyn: past, present and future. *Pediatr Clin North Am* 1983; 30 (5): 915–30.

11 Bernstein IL, Johnson CL, Gallagher JS, Archer D, Johnson H. Are tar-trazine reactions mediated by IgE? *J Allergy Clin Immunol* 1978; 61: 191 (Abstract).

12 Bernstein JM. Recent advances in immunologic reactivity in otitis media. *J Allergy Clin Immunol* 1988; 81: 1004–9.

13 Bernstein M, Day JM, Welsh A. Double blind food challenge in the diagnosis of food sensitivity in the adult. *J Allergy Clin Immunol* 1982; 70: 205–10.

14 Bindslev-Jensen, Poulsen LK. In vitro diagnostic methods in the eval-uation of food hypersensitivity. In: *Food Allergy: Adverse Reactions to Foods and Food Additives*, 2nd edn, Metcalfe DD, Sampson HA, Simon RA, (eds). Blackwell Sci Ltd, Oxford, 1997: 137–50.

15 Bluestone CD. Anatomy and physiology of eustachian tube and middle ear related to otitis media. *J Allergy Clin Immunol* 1988; 81: 997–1003.

16 Bluestone ChD, Douglas DS, Bernstein JM. Otitis media. In: *Allergy, Principles and Practice*, 1st edn (Middleton E, Reed ChE, Ellis EF, eds). CV Mosby, St Louis 1978: 1023–38.

17 Bluestone ChD, Klein JD. *Otitis Media in Infants and Children*. WB Saunders, Philadelphia, 1988: 15–29.

18 Bluestone ChD. Eustachian tube function and allergy in otitis media. *Pediatrics* 1978; 61: 753–60.

19 Bluestone ChD. Recent advances in the pathogenesis, diagnosis and management of otitis media. *Pediatr Clin North Am* 1981; 28: 727–55.

20 Bock SA. In vivo diagnosis: skin testing and oral challenge procedures. In: *Food Allergy: Adverse Reactions to Foods and Food Additives*, 2nd Edn. (Metcalfe DD, Sampson HA, Simon RA, eds). Oxford, Blackwell Sci Ltd, 1997: 151–66.

21 Bolger WE, Butzin CA, Parsons DS. Paranasal sinus bony anatomic variations and mucosal abnormalities: CT analysis for endoscopic sinus surgery. *Laryngoscope* 1991; 101: 56–64.

22 Bousquet J, Chañez P, Michel F-B. The respiratory tract and food hypersensitivity. In: *Food Allergy: Adverse Reactions to Foods and Food Additives*; 2nd Edn. (Metcalfe DD, Sampson HA, Simon RA, eds). Oxford, Blackwell Sci Ltd, 1997: 235–44.

23 Brostoff J, Canini C, Wraith DG, Paganelli R, Levinsky RJ. Immune-complex in atopy. In *The Mast Cell – Its Role in Health and Disease*, (Pepys J, Edwards AM, eds). Pitman Medical, Tunbridge Wells, 1979: 380–93.

24 Buisseret PD. Common manifestations of cow's milk allergy in children. *Lancet* 1978; i: 304–5.

25 Businco L, Cantani A, Benincori N *et al*. Effectiveness of oral sodium cromoglycate (SCG) in preventing food allergy in children. *Ann Allergy* 1983; 51: 47–50.

26 Chua YY, Bremner K, Lakdawalla N, Llobet JL, Kokubu HL, Orange RP, Collins-Williams C. In vivo and in vitro correlates of food allergy. *J Allergy Clin Immunol* 1976; 58: 299–307.

27 Clemis JD. Identification of allergic factors in middle ear effusions. *Ann Otol Rhinol Laryngol* 1976; 23: 234–7.

28 Collins-Williams C. The role of pharmacologic agents in the prevention or treatment of allergic food disorders. *Ann Allergy* 1986; 57: 53–60.

29 Coombs RRA. Pathogenesis and mechanisms. In: *Proceedings of the First Food Allergy Workshop*, (Coombs RRA, ed.). Medical Education Services, Oxford, 1980; 7–8: 13–27.

30 Cunningham-Rundles C, Brandeis WE, Good RA, Day NK. Milk pre-cipitants, circulating immune complexes and IgA deficiency. *Proc Natl Acad Sci USA* 1978; 75: 3387–9.

31 Dahl R, Zetterstrom O. The effect of orally administered sodium cro-moglycate on allergic reactions caused by food allergens. *Clin Allergy* 1978; 8: 419–422.

32 Dannaeus A. Management of food allergy in infancy. *Ann Allergy* 1983; 51: 303–6.

33 Delire M. Detection of circulating immune-complexes in infants fed on cow's milk. In: *The mast cell – Its role in health and disease*. Pepys J, Edwards AM, (eds). Tunbridge Wells Pitman Medical, 1979: 375–9.

34 Dockhorn RJ. Otolaryngologic allergy in children. *Otolaryngol Clin North Am* 1977; 10: 103–12.

35 Draper WL. Secretory otitis media in children: a study of 540 children. *Laryngoscope* 1967; 77: 636–56.

36 Eriksson NS. Food sensitivity reported by patients with asthma and hay fever. *Allergy* 1978; 33: 189–96.

37 Evans R III. Variability in the measurement of specific immunoglobu-lin E antibody by the RAST procedure. *J Allergy Clin Immunol* 1982; 69: 245–52.

38 Fireman P. Diagnosis of sinuses in children: emphasis on the history and physical examination. *J Allergy Clin Immunol* 1992; 90: 433–6.

39 Fireman P. Nasal provocation testing: an objective assessment for nasal and eustachian tube obstruction. *J Allergy Clin Immunol* 1988; 81: 953–60.

40 Freed DLJ. Laboratory diagnosis of food intolerance. In: *Clinics in Immunology and Allergy – Food Allergy*, (Brostoff J, Challacombe SJ, eds). WB Saunders, Philadelphia; 1982: 181–203.

41 Gerrard JW. The diagnosis of the food-allergic patient. In: *The mast cell – Its role in health and disease*. (Pepys J, Edwards AM, eds).Tunbridge Wells, Pitman Medical, 1979: 416–21.

42 Goodman GM, Slavin RG. Medical management of sinusitis in adults. *Immunol Allergy Clin N Amer* 1994; 14(1): 69–87.

43 Green M. Sublingual provocative testing for food and FD and C dyes. *Ann Allergy* 1974; 33: 274–81.

44 Hall LJ, Asuncion J, Lukat M. Allergy skin testing under general anes-thesia with treatment response in ninety-two patients with chronic serous otitis media. *Am J Otol* 1980; 2: 150–7.

45 Halpern GM. Alimentary allergy. *J Asthma* 1983; 20(4): 251–84.

46 Harlin SL, Ansel DG, Lane SR, Myers J, Kephart GM, Gleich GJ. A clinical and pathologic study of chronic sinusitis: the role of the eosinophil. *J Allergy Clin Immunol* 1988; 81: 867–75.

47 Heiner DC, Sears JW, Kniker WT. Multiple precipitins to cow's milk in chronic respiratory disease. *Am J Dis Child* 1962; 103: 634–54.

48 Heiner DC. Food allergy and respiratory disease. *Ann Allergy* 1983; 51: 273–4.

49 Hoffman DR, Haddad ZH. Diagnosis of IgE-mediated reactions to food antigens by radioimmunoassay. *J Allergy Clin Immunol* 1974; 54: 165–73.

50 Ingvarsson L, Lundgren K, Olofsson B, Wall S. Epidemiology of acute otitis media in children. *Acta Oto-Laryngol* (Stockh) 1982; Suppl 388: 1–52.

51 Juhlin L, Michaelsson G, Zetterstrom O. Urticaria and asthma induced by food- and drug-additives in patients with aspirin hypersensitivity. *J Allergy Clin Immunol* 1972; 50: 92–8.

52 Juhlin L. Incidence of intolerance to food additives. *Int J Dermatol* 1980; 19: 548–51.

53 Kettelhut BV, Metcalfe DD. Provocation tests in the diagnosis of suspected adverse reactions to food and food additives. *J Allergy Clin Immunol* 1986. Proceedings of the XIIth International Congress Allergol Clin Immunol, Washington (DC), Oct 20–25, 1985. Reed Ch E (ed). CV Mosby, St Louis (MO), 1986: 475–80.

54 Landman MD. Ultrasound screening for sinus diseases. *Otolaryngol Head Neck Surg* 1986; 94: 157–64.

55 Lee CH, Williams RI, Binkley EL. Provocative testing and treatment for foods. *Arch Otolaryngol* 1969; 90: 87–94.

56 Lim DJ, Liu YS, Schram J, Birck HG. Immunoglobulin E in chronic middle ear effusions. *Ann Otol Rhinol Laryngol* 1976; 85 (Suppl. 25): 117–23.

57 May CD, Bock SA. A modern clinical approach to food hypersensitivity. *Allergy* 1978; 33: 166–88.

58 May CD, Bock SA. Adverse reactions to foods due to hypersensitivity. In: *Allergy, Principles and Practice*, 1st edn, (Middleton E Jr, Reed CE, Ellis EF, eds). CV Mosby, St Louis, 1978: 1159–71.

59 May CD. Immunologic versus toxic adverse reactions to foodstuffs. *Ann Allergy* 1983; 51: 267–8.

60 Metcalfe DD. Food allergy in adults. In: *Food Allergy: Adverse Reactions to Foods and Food Additives*; 2nd Edn., (Metcalfe DD, Sampson HA, Simon RA, eds). Oxford, Blackwell Sci Ltd, 1997: 183–91.

61 Minor JD, Tolber SG, Frick OL. Leukocyte inhibition factor in delayed-onset food allergy. *J Allergy Clin Immunol* 1980; 66: 314–21.

62 Minotti DA. Allergic rhinitis and sinusitis. *Immunol Allergy Clin N Am* 1994; 14(1): 113–27.

63 Mogi G. Secretory IgA and antibody activities in middle ear effusion. *Ann Otol Rhinol Laryngol* 1976; 85(25): 97–102.

64 Moneret-Vautrin DA. Non specific reactions to foodstuffs: false food allergies. In: *Proceedings of the XIth International Congress of Allergology and Clinical Immunology*, London, Oct 17–22, 1982, (Kerr JW, Ganderton MA, eds). Macmillan, London and Basingstoke, 1982: 175–9.

65 Novembre E, Martino de M, Vierucci A. Foods and respiratory allergy. *J Allergy Clin Immunol* 1988; 81: 1059–65.

66 Ogle KA, Bullock JD. Children with allergic rhinitis and/or bronchial asthma treated with elimination diet. *Ann Allergy* 1977; 39: 8–11.

67 Ogle KA, Bullock JD. Children with allergic rhinitis and/or bronchial asthma treated with elimination diet: a five-year follow-up. *Ann Allergy* 1980; 44: 273–8.

68 Paganelli R, Levinsky RJ, Brostoff J, Wraith DG. Immune complexes containing food proteins in normal and atopic subjects after oral challenge and effect of sodium cromoglycate on antigen absorption. *Lancet* 1979; i: 1270–2.

69 Pelikan Z, Pelikan-Filipek M, Ossekoppele R. Chronic sinusitis maxillaris (CSM) – the role of nasal allergy and the diagnostic value of echography and radiographs. *Allergy Clin Immunol News* 1994; Suppl No 2: 415.

70 Pelikan Z, Pelikan-Filipek M. Bronchial response to the food ingestion challenge. *Ann Allergy* 1987; 58: 164–72.

71 Pelikan Z, Pelikan-Filipek M. Cytologic changes in nasal secretions during the immediate nasal response. *J Allergy Clin Immunol* 1988; 82: 1103–12.

72 Pelikan Z, Pelikan-Filipek M. Cytologic changes in nasal secretions (NS) during the late nasal response (LNR) pretreated with disodium cromoglycate (DSCG) and beclomethasone dipropionate (BDA) or budesonide (BSA). *J Allergy Clin Immunol* 1991; 87: 28.

73 Pelikan Z, Pelikan-Filipek M. Cytologic changes in the nasal secretions during the late nasal response. *J Allergy Clin Immunol* 1989; 83: 1068–79.

74 Pelikan Z, Pelikan-Filipek M. Effects of oral cromolyn on the nasal response due to foods. *Arch Otolaryngol Head Neck Surg* 1989; 115: 1238–43.

75 Pelikan Z, Pelikan-Filipek M. Role of nasal allergy in chronic maxillary sinusitis – diagnostic value of nasal challenge with allergen. *J Allergy Clin Immunol* 1990; 86: 484–91.

76 Pelikan Z, Pelikan-Filipek M. The effects of disodium cromoglycate and beclomethasone dipropionate on the immediate response of the nasal mucosa to allergen challenge. *Ann Allergy* 1982; 49: 283–92.

77 Pelikan Z, Pelikan-Filipek M. The effects of disodium cromoglycate and beclomethasone dipropionate on the late nasal mucosa response to allergen challenge. *Ann Allergy* 1982; 49: 200–12.

78 Pelikan Z. Food ingestion challenge (FICH) and nasal challenge with food extracts in patients with nasal complaints due to the foods. *Allergy* 1992; 47 (Suppl.): 304.

79 Pelikan Z. Late nasal response – its clinical characteristics, features, and possible mechanisms. In: *Late Phase Allergic Reactions*, (Dorsch W, ed.). CRC Press, Boca Raton , 1990: 111–55.

80 Pelikan Z. Nasal response to food ingestion challenge. *Arch Otolaryngol Head Neck Surgery* 1988; 114: 525–30.

81 Pelikan Z. The effects of disodium cromoglycate and beclomethasone dipropionate on the delayed nasal mucosa response to allergen challenge. *Ann Allergy* 1984; 52: 111–24.

82 Pelikan Z. *The late nasal response*. Thesis. Free University Amsterdam, The Netherlands, 1996.

83 Pelikan Z. The role of allergy in sinus disease. In: *Diseases of the Sinuses*, (Gershwin ME, Incaudo GA, eds). Humana Press, Totowa (NJ), 1996: 97–165.

84 Phillips MJ, Knight NJ, Manning H, Abbott AL, Tripp WG. IgE and secretory otitis media. *Lancet* 1974; ii: 1176–8.

85 Pinczower EF, Weymuller EA. Nasal obstruction. *Immunol Allergy Clin N Am* 1994; 14(1): 129–42.

86 Rachelefsky GS, Goldberg M, Katz RM *et al*. Sinus disease in children with respiratory allergy. *J Allergy Clin Immunol* 1978; 61: 310–14.

87 Radcliffe MJ. Clinical methods for diagnosis. In: *Clinics in Immunology and Allergy – Food Allergy*, (Brostoff J, Challacombe SJ, eds). WB Saunders, London, 1982; 205–20.

88 Revonta M. Ultrasound in the diagnosis of maxillary and frontal sinusitis. *Acta Otolaryngol* 1980; 370 (Suppl.): 1–54.

89 Ruokonen J, Holopainen E, Palva T, Backman A. Secretory otitis media and allergy. *Allergy* 1981; 36: 59–68.

90 Ruokonen J, Paganus A, Lehti H. Elimination diets in the treatment of secretory otitis media. *Int J Pediatr Otorhinolaryngol* 1982; 4: 39–46.

91 Sachs MI. Value of food antigen specific IgE-RAST and immediate reaction skin test. *Ann Allergy* 1983; 51: 264–6.

92 Sampson HA, Albergo R. Comparison of results of skin tests, RAST and double-blind, placebo controlled food challenges in children with atopic dermatitis. *J Allergy Clin Immunol* 1984; 74: 26–33.

93 Sampson HA. Role of immediate food hypersensitivity in the pathogenesis of atopic dermatitis. *J Allergy Clin Immunol* 1983; 71: 473–80.

94 Savolainen S. Allergy in patients with acute maxillary sinusitis. *Allergy* 1989; 44: 116–22.

95 Schlumberger HD. Pseudo-allergic reactions to drugs and chemicals. *Ann Allergy* 1983; 51: 317–24.

96 Schwartz HJ. Sensitivity to ingested metabisulfite: variation in clinical presentation. *J Allergy Clin Immunol* 1983; 71: 487–9.

97 Settipane GA, Chafee FH, Postman IM *et al*. Significance of tartrazine sensitivity in chronic urticaria of unknown etiology. *J Allergy Clin Immunol* 1976; 57: 541–6.

98 Shanon E, Englender M, Beizer M. A clinical pilot study of disodium cromoglycate in the treatment of secretory otitis media. In: *The Mast Cell – Its Role in Health and Disease*, (Pepys J, Edwards AM, eds). Pitman Medical, Tunbridge Wells, 1979: 791–4.

99 Shapiro GG, Furukawa CT, Pierson WE, Gilbertson E, Bierman CW. Blinded comparison of maxillary sinus radiography and ultrasound for diagnosis of sinusitis. *J Allergy Clin Immunol* 1986; 77: 59–64.

100 Shapiro GG. Sinusitis in children. *J Allergy Clin Immunol* 1988: 1025–7.

101 Shioda H, Mishima T, Yamada S, Shioda S, Nakai Y. Nasal smears in the diagnosis of food allergy. In: *The Mast Cell – Its Role in Health and Disease*, (Pepys J, Edwards AM, eds). Pitman Medical, Tunbridge Wells, 1979: 422–30.

102 Slavin RG. Nasal polyps and sinusitis. In: *Allergy, Principles and Practice*, 4th edn, (Middleton E, Reed ChE, Ellis EF *et al.*, eds). Mosby Year Book, St Louis (MO), 1993: 1455–70.

103 Slavin RG. Sinusitis in adults. *J Allergy Clin Immunol* 1988; 81: 1028–32.

104 Soothill J. Food allergy. In: *The Mast Cell – Its Role in Health and Disease*, (Pepys J, Edwards AN, eds). Pitman Medical, Tunbridge Wells, 1979: 367–70.

105 Spector SL. The role of allergy in sinus in adults. *J Allergy Clin Immunol* 1992; 90: 518–20.

106 Strobel S. Oral tolerance: immune response to food antigens. In: *Food Allergy: Adverse Reactions to Foods and Food Additives;* 2nd Edn. (Metcalfe DD, Sampson HA, Simon RA, eds). Oxford, Blackwell Sci Ltd, 1997: 107–35.

107 Syme J. Investigation and treatment of multiple intestinal food allergy in childhood. In: *The Mast Cell – Its Role in Health and Disease*, (Pepys J, Edwards AM, eds). Pitman Medical, Tunbridge Wells, 1979: 438–42.

108 Wershil BK, Walker WA. Milk allergies and other food allergies in children. *Immunology Allergy Clinics N Am* 1988; 8: 485–504.

109 Whitcomb NJ. Allergy therapy in serous otitis media associated with allergic rhinitis. *Ann Allergy* 1965; 23: 232–6.

110 Wilson CMW. Food sensitivities, taste changes, aphthous ulcers and atopic symptoms in allergic disease. *Ann Allergy* 1980; 44: 302–7.

111 Wraith DG, Young GVM, Lee TH. The management of food allergy with diet and Nalcrom. In: *The Mast Cell – Its Role in Health and Disease*. Pepys J, Edwards AM, eds). Pitman Medical, Tunbridge Wells, 1979; 443–6.

112 Wraith DG. Asthma and rhinitis: In: *Clinics in Immunology and Allergy – Food Allergy*, (Brostoff J, Challacombe SJ, eds). WB Saunders, Philadelphia, 1982: 101–12.

113 Yalamanchili AK Rao, Bahna SL. Dietary management of food allergies. In: *Food Allergy*, (Chiaramonte LT, Schneider AT, Lifshitz F, eds). Marcel Dekker Inc, New York, Basel, 1988: 351–64.

114 Zanussi C, Ortolani C, Pastorello E. Dietary and pharmacologic management of food intolerance in adults. *Ann Allergy* 1983; 51: 307–10.

115 Zanussi C. Food allergy treatment. *Clinics Immunol Allergy*, 1982; 2: 221–40.

116 Zanussi C. Food allergy treatment. In: *Clinics in Immunology and Allergy – Food Allergy*, (Brostoff J, Challacombe SJ, eds). WB Saunders, Philadelphia, 1982; 221–40.

117 Zinreich J. Imaging of inflammatory sinus disease. *Immunol Allergy Clin N Am* 1994; 14(1): 17–29.

118 Zizmor J, Noyek AM. Radiology of the nose and paranasal sinuses. In: *Otolaryngology*, Vol 1, (Paparella MM, Shumrick DA, eds). WB Saunders, Philadelphia, 1983: 1043–95.

Chapter 36

Food-induced asthma

J. G. Ayres and J. C. Baker

INTRODUCTION

Asthma is a very common condition worldwide, with significant morbidity and measurable mortality rates. It is a condition which has a number of identifiable causes, notably inhaled allergens both in the outdoor environment and indoors (domestic and occupational). While the role of food intolerance in asthma is well recognized it has been poorly quantified in the asthmatic population to date. There are considerable difficulties in recognizing food intolerance and the logistics of so doing has dissuaded many clinicians from trying. In addition, the relatively poor understanding of the mechanisms involved in food intolerance has meant that its very existence has been doubted. However, where a food intolerance is recognized and food avoidance measures instituted, considerable improvement in asthma symptoms and reduction in drug therapy can result in some, but not all, patients. These benefits may have greater impact in those patients with greater symptoms. However, the promise of such benefits should not result in an approach which ignores inhaled drug therapy or in a dietary regime which is inappropriate in the face of mild symptoms.

This chapter will briefly cover asthma as a condition in clinical, epidemiological and mechanistic terms. The problems of definition and the difficulties in interpreting the epidemiology are addressed, as are the diagnosis and management of food intolerance.

ASTHMA

Definition

Asthma is a condition which has been defined in a number of ways (clinically, physiologically and pathologically), an all-encompassing definition being elusive because of the differing clinical phenotypes met in practice. A physiological definition was established at the CIBA symposium of 1956, but this has been superseded to an extent by a pathophysiological definition incorporating airway inflammation as the critical factor. Such definitions are to an extent unhelpful in the clinical setting, although they become crucial when considering epidemiological studies where comparison of findings between different geographical areas requires a uniform definition.

Pathogenesis

Nevertheless, asthma is an inflammatory condition resulting in increased bronchial responsiveness and consequently airway narrowing in response to inhaled and ingested triggers. These inflammatory processes are characterized by mucosal oedema, mucus hypersecretion and bronchial smooth muscle hypertrophy and constriction, all of which reduce the airway lumen. There are a number of inflammatory pathways that are important in the genesis of asthmatic inflammation (e.g. leukotrienes, prostaglandins), but IgE production, with mast cell and eosinophil

A

activation after exposure to relevant inhaled or ingested allergens, is the major route of inflammation. The consequent airway narrowing results in the characteristic symptoms of breathlessness, wheeze, chest tightness and cough.

Epidemiology

It is generally believed that the prevalence of asthma has increased, in particular over the past 30 years, in the Western world. The reasons for this are likely to be multifactorial, but sensitization to allergens does seem to be an important factor. In the UK, asthma is present in about 1 in 15 school children up to the age of 10 years and in 5–6% of adults, with a slight predominance in women over men, although there is wide variation in prevalence worldwide.[24] In general, the highest rates are found in conditions of temperature and humidity which encourage the house dust mite (*Dermatophagoides pteronyssinus* or *D. farinae*). Sensitization to the proteases in the faecal pellets of these mites is a major cause of the development of asthma throughout the world. In areas where the mite is less likely to thrive, low rates of asthma are found, for example in rural black African populations and in Inuits.

An acute asthma attack can result in death. The rise and subsequent fall in asthma deaths in the 1960s in the UK and in other countries was attributed at the time to the use of isoprenaline inhalers, although this interpretation remains hotly debated and the role of inhaled aeroallergens has not been excluded. Since the early 1970s, mortality rates from asthma have increased gradually in the UK, peaking in the early 1990s at around 2000 deaths per year. Subsequently, asthma deaths have fallen, by 1996 reaching around 1400. In a number of cases these deaths were because of anaphylaxis from ingestion of foods which can trigger such events, but in the majority of cases such a clearcut trigger cannot be identified. Apart from death, morbidity rates from repeated hospital admissions are high in patients with severe asthma and it has been estimated that 60% of the total costs for asthma to the National Health Service are consumed by the most severe 10% of the asthmatic population.[61]

Causal factors

While the true reasons for the increase in asthma witnessed during the 1970s and 1980s are not clearly understood, there is little doubt that allergen exposure represents an important factor, perhaps particularly in early life. Inhaled allergens are reckoned to be the most important in this regard, particularly house dust mite allergens (Der P1) and pet allergens, notably cat dander (Fel D1).[58] Occupational exposure to allergenic and non-allergenic sensitizers is more common than is recognized, and is said to be responsible for 1 out of every 20 new cases of asthma occurring during adult life in the working population in the UK.[62] A number of these occupational causes are associated with food-related antigens (e.g. flour), but the role of chronic ingestion of food allergens as a cause for initiation of asthma is not known. Consequently, this chapter will deal with exacerbations of asthma and the role that food allergens may play in maintaining airway inflammation once it has been established.

Severity

The great majority of patients with asthma have mild symptoms that are easily controlled. The treatment of asthma is relatively straightforward in these patients, inhaled therapy being simple and safe. Where obvious simple allergen avoidance steps can be undertaken these may help some patients, although in many cases neither the patient nor the physician are overenthusiastic in undertaking what are often difficult and time-consuming steps when the symptoms are few.

At higher levels of severity, management becomes more difficult, and identification and treatment of recognized causes becomes more relevant as far as many physicians and patients are concerned. Severity can be classified by the amount of inhaled corticosteroids used, the degree of loss of lung function or the level of symptoms. Some severe groups can be recognized by their pattern of symptoms, e.g. nocturnal asthma, aspirin-sensitive asthma. Brittle asthma is one such group. This has been classified into two types, both susceptible to severe repeated attacks, either on a background of poor asthma control (type I) or apparently good asthma control (type II).[9] Food sensitivity appears to be important in both but in particular in the type I patient.

FOOD-INDUCED ASTHMA

Definitions

It is important to clarify terminology and establish working definitions in this area. Different schemes have been suggested but the one now generally accepted in the UK is that proposed by the Royal College of Physicians.[1] This identifies adverse reactions to foods as being because of either food intolerance or food aversion (Table 36.1).

The differentiating factor between these two is the repeatability of the reaction if the food is given in a disguised form, with the reaction being repeatable in food intolerance. There are different mechanisms known to underlie these reactions (e.g. enzyme defects, toxic effects, pharmacological effects), which are covered in Chapter X. Food allergy is a form of food intolerance in which there is evidence of an abnormal immunological reaction to the food.

Epidemiology

Most studies of the prevalence of food intolerance are questionnaire-based, relying on self-reported perceived adverse responses to food. The European Community Respiratory Health Survey (ECRHS) employed a validated questionnaire[23] which has been used in epidemiological studies.[38,39] There are scant data on the reproducibility of different questionnaires used in other studies. Objective measures of food intolerance give a better idea of the true prevalence but this involves challenge of each patient with a range of foodstuffs. The double blind placebo-controlled food

Food aversion and intolerance	
Food aversion	**Food intolerance**
Psychological food intolerance	Enzyme defects
Food avoidance	Pharmacological
	Irritant and toxic
	Allergic
	Fermentation of food residues
	Other

Table 36.1 Food aversion and intolerance.

challenge (DBPCFC: see below) is considered to be the 'gold standard'[59] procedure to confirm or refute a diagnosis of food allergy, but the logistics of this are substantial and it cannot be used as an epidemiological tool. It should also be recognized that, even in an individual with proven food intolerance, their response to ingestion of a particular food may vary over time. Because of this problem, estimates of the prevalence of adverse reactions to food in either general or asthmatic populations should be regarded with caution unless they are supported by an objective measure.

Food allergy and intolerance in general populations

There are few estimates of the prevalence of food allergy and intolerance in general populations before 1990. In the UK, a study from 1970[14] stated that rates ranged from 1% to 4%, and considered that true food allergy occurred in less than 0.5% of a general population. However, amongst university teaching staff, a later study[11] found a history of adverse reactions to food in 33% of subjects, although this was in a highly selected population. A study from a small town in South Wales in 1983[19] found that 14% of men and 18% of women reported adverse effects to some foods. However, in none of these studies was confirmation obtained by blinded food challenge testing. Of the more recent studies reported in the 1990s (Table 36.2), two included food challenge testing, revealing much lower objective rates and confirming the difference between subjective and objective measures of food intolerance.

Food allergy and mild–moderate asthma

A number of studies have been conducted in a range of countries over the past 20 years in subjects with mild–moderate asthma. The populations have been a mix of general populations and selected groups, and it is difficult to determine any clear pattern from the figures. In general, rates of self-reported food intolerance in asthma are found to be similar to those in the general population whether considering self-reported or objectively confirmed adverse reactions (Table 36.3).

The discrepancy between perception and objective evidence of an adverse reaction to food is again clear, the lowest figures for prevalence being in studies where food challenges have been conducted. The major difficulty in determining an adverse reaction to a food, either by the doctor or patient, is the ill-defined time relationship between ingestion and the appearance of symptoms. The patient is unlikely to appreciate a reaction to a food if the time delay is long and if the food is eaten frequently. While recognizing the substantial logistical difficulties of the DBPCFC, unless it is used as a standard test or until a logistically simpler test of equivalent sensitivity and specificity is found,[28] it will be difficult to determine the true prevalence of food intolerance in asthma.

Food allergy and severe asthma

Even less information is available for patients with more severe asthma. In our clinic population of patients with brittle asthma, 65% (19 of 29) reported at least one food which could exacerbate their asthma, the main identified foods being wheat and milk or milk products. In a selected proportion (around 60% of the total clinic population) of these patients (selected on the basis of at least one reported food intolerance or one positive skin test to a food stuff), food challenge studies were performed. A protocol of dietary exclusion followed by open food challenges (OFCs) showed that 52% of this subgroup reacted to at least one food (Table 36.4). A protocol of dietary exclusion followed by DBPCFCs twice daily was subsequently altered to DBPCFCs once daily to avoid missing late responses.[10] This supported the questionnaire findings of a high prevalence of food allergy in this population. The figures cannot be extrapolated to all asthma at the severe end of the spectrum, but the findings would support the hypothesis that the more severe the bronchial hyperresponsiveness the more likely it is that a positive response to food may be demonstrated.

Mechanisms

The mechanisms for food intolerance and allergy are covered in Chapter X. There are no mechanisms that are recognized to relate specifically to food-induced asthma compared to food intolerance involving other systems, although the role of immune complexes containing IgE and allergen cannot be discounted.

Prevalence of food allergy in general populations					
Country	Date	Sample size	% Self-reported food intolerance	Confirmation by food challenge	% Population prevalence
China[66]	1990	10 144	4.9	No	n/k
Germany[33]	1994	n/k	n/k	n/k	1.0
UK[71]	1994	20 000	20.4	Yes	1.4–1.8
Holland[37]	1994	1483	12.4	Yes	2.0–4.0
Sweden[13]	1996	1379	25.0	No	n/k
Spain[22]	1996	7698	1.8	No	n/k
Australia[68]	1998	669	17.0	No	n/k
n/k, Not known.					

Table 36.2 Prevalence of food allergy in general populations.

Prevalence of food allergy in mild–moderate asthma							
Country	Date	Sample size and population			% Self-reported		Confirmation by food challenge
		General	Asthma	Food intolerance	Food intolerance	Asthma	
Sweden[49]	1978	n/a	1129	n/a	24.0	n/a	No
Switzerland[18]	1983–5	n/a	n/a	229	n/a	24.1	No
Wales[54]	1986	n/a	72	n/a	4.0	n/a	Yes
France[47]	1987	n/a	300	n/a	2.0	n/a	Yes
France[55]	1987	n/a	67	n/a	5.8	n/a	Yes
China[66]	1990	10 144	n/a	n/a	4.9	3.8	No
Italy[69]	1992	n/a	n/a	1339	n/a	2.6	Yes
Australia[40]	1996	n/a	914	n/a	45.3	n/a	No
Turkey[40]	1996	1884	584	n/a	4.5	13.5	No

Studies of general populations and mixed groups make it difficult to determine any clear pattern but, in general, rates of self-reported food intolerance in asthma are found to be similar to those in a general population. n/a, Not applicable.

Table 36.3 Prevalence of food allergy in mild–moderate asthma.

Prevalence of food allergy in brittle asthma			
	OFC	DBPCFC Twice daily	DBPCFC Once daily
No. of subjects	29	22	18
No. of subjects reacting to at least one food	15 (52)	12 (55)	12 (66)
No. of subjects by no. of foods causing reaction			
1	0 (0)	3 (25)	1 (8)
2	6 (40)	3 (25)	2 (15)
3	4 (27)	2 (17)	2 (15)
4	5 (33)	1 (8)	2 (15)
5	0 (0)	2 (17)	3 (23)
6	n/a	1 (8)	0 (0)
7	n/a	0 (0)	2 (15)

The various protocols used in the diagnosis of food intolerance in patients with brittle asthma all demonstrate a higher prevalence of food intolerance in these patients than in those with mild–moderate asthma. OFC, open food challenges; DBPCFC, double blind placebo-controlled food challenges; n/a, not applicable. Values in parentheses are percentages.

Table 36.4 Prevalence of food allergy in brittle asthma.

Psychology

Asthma is well recognized to be associated with psychological triggers, both in the long term and when asthma deteriorates.[32] Some individuals can develop an attack of asthma by suggestion,[50] which immediately raises a problem as far as food-induced asthma is concerned. Subjects who believe that they will always develop an attack in response to a specific food may thus be almost certain to do so, but the mechanism will not be an immunological response to a food allergen (it may be a conditioned response but in an allergic subject). This may explain, at least in part, the difference in reported compared to true rates of food intolerance, although this can also be because of the risk of underestimation of food intolerance when using DBPCFCs. (The drawbacks of DBPCFC are addressed below.) The problems of psychology are a particular feature in brittle asthma which, albeit a very rare form of asthma, presents problems because of the psychosocial aspects of the condition. Some of our patients have persistently shown a bronchoconstrictor response to hypoallergenic foods

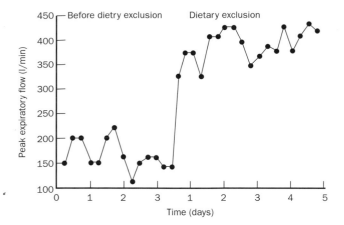

Fig. 36.1 Dietary exclusion in a patient with brittle asthma. In the week before dietary exclusion daily mean, maximum and minimum peak expiratory flows (PEF) were 160 l/min, 200 l/min and 130 l/min, respectively. After 5 days' dietary exclusion daily mean PEF had increased from 230 l/min on day 1 to 420 l/min (+81%) on day 5.

(even to warm water) when given blind, which makes assessment of true food allergy impossible. In addition, some with a severe psychological disturbance may even use knowledge of their true food allergies to induce asthma attacks. These factors need to be carefully considered before attributing difficult asthma to food and whether apparent avoidance of foods has or has not resulted in benefit to the individual.

Diagnosis

While some take the view that detection of food intolerance in asthmatic subjects is of limited value,[67] some patients in whom specific foods are identified as being causally related to their asthma benefit substantially from excluding them from their diet.[17,54,]

History

Although a positive history of an adverse reaction to a food is helpful in deciding whether an individual patient may have a food intolerance, most subjects with proven food intolerance on challenge give no such history. The main reason for this is that the unrecognized foods are those which are staple foods (e.g. wheat, milk or milk products) which are consumed every day and presumably act as chronic potentiators of airway inflammation. Where a history is positive, the pattern of symptoms is similar to any other exacerbation of asthma, although there may be associated symptoms in other systems such as headache, abdominal pain and bloating, nasal symptoms and, occasionally, skin rash. More credence can be given to such a history where the response is repeatable and involves more than one system.

Skin prick tests

Burrows *et al.*[20] stated that the use of skin prick tests in respiratory allergic disease should be 'used as an indicator of a subject's atopic predisposition rather than as a guide to the specific cause of his complaints'. This cautious approach was supported by later work[59] which showed them to have poor positive predictability (25–75%) for food-induced asthma. In brittle asthma, skin prick tests have

a 71% sensitivity and a 77% specificity in predicting a positive DBPCFC.[10] They are now acknowledged not to be diagnostic for the triggering of asthma by foods.[43]

Radioallergosorbent tests

Radioallergosorbent tests (RAST) have also been shown to have poor positive predictability (0–57%)[59] and are considered to help in the diagnosis of food allergy but, again, not to be diagnostic in themselves.[43] In patients with brittle asthma, RAST were shown to have a sensitivity of 40% and specificity of 74% in predicting a positive DBPCFC.[10]

It is thus inappropriate, on the basis of skin prick tests and RAST alone, to recommend restrictive diets.[42]

Total serum IgE

Levels of total serum IgE have not been shown to be consistently related to the presence of a positive food challenge.

Histamine release test

The diagnostic value of the histamine release test in whole blood of patients with food allergy has been suggested as a diagnostic test for food allergy in asthma[52,53] but has yet to be tested against DBPCFC.

TOP-CAST/CAST ELISA

The cellular antigen stimulation test (CAST) is an enzyme-labelled immunosorbent assay (ELISA) which measures sulphidoleukotriene generation by leukocytes on specific allergen challenge. In one study[45] which aimed to establish the usefulness of the test in differentiating between allergic and non-allergic status, the test yielded a 100% sensitivity and did not produce any false-positives. However, it was unable to distinguish between health and disease states, and its role in food allergy in relation to asthma remains to be determined.

Methacholine responsiveness

Bronchial hyperresponsiveness to methacholine is well recognized as a marker of asthma and has been shown to increase in response to antigen challenge both in the laboratory and occupational setting. In the setting of response to food challenge the picture is less clearcut. In one study, methacholine response before and 24 h after DBPCFCs in 11 subjects with asthma and a history of food-induced asthma and positive skin prick tests to the suspect food[73] revealed no difference in response after food challenge compared to placebo challenge. In another study, airway hyperresponsiveness was measured by methacholine challenge performed before and 4 h after DBPCFC in 26 food-allergic asthmatic patients. The results indicated that food-induced allergic reactions can increase airway responsiveness and may do so without inducing acute asthma.[36]

Dietary manipulation

As no single laboratory test has yet been devised to identify food intolerance or even provide a broad screening test, dietary manipulation is considered to be the cornerstone of diagnosis and treatment. Various procedures for dietary manipulation (see Chapter X) may be used. The method of choice for investigators is usually that outlined by Bock *et al.*[15] which comprises three main components.

A period of dietary exclusion before food challenge[34]

The length of time for such exclusion varies. Up to 14 days[44] may be necessary to stabilize a patient's symptoms before food challenge.

Changes in aeroallergen exposure and other environmental factors do not produce the degree of improvement in lung function (except occasionally but only over a longer period of time) in this group of patients when they are routinely admitted to hospital for exacerbations of asthma as are seen during investigations for food intolerance.

'Few Foods' diets[60] (providing the patients with a minimal number of hypoallergenic foods to provide optimal nutrition) are usually used during the period of dietary exclusion. In this group of patients, some have adversely reacted to the foods normally used in these diets. Whilst a Few Foods diet can be adapted to the needs of each individual, a standardized methodology using a hypoallergenic formula drink (Elemental 028 Extra Liquid, Scientific Hospital Supplies Ltd, UK) for every patient is preferable. If a patient does show an airways response to E028 or finds the drink unpalatable then unflavoured crystalline E028 can be reconstituted and administered orally or via a nasogastric tube.

A DBPCFC methodology[65]

Food challenges are usually given as lyophilized foods in opaque, dye-free capsules. In preparing antigens for hiding in capsules, freeze drying and purification have been shown to decrease or even destroy the allergenic activity of the agent.[15] While this is considered the most convenient method,[34] it does not facilitate food being given in the 'natural form' and problems may also arise concerning the quantity of dried foods needed to elicit symptoms, the number of capsules required and time taken for dissolution of the capsule. Less frequently, because of difficulty in devising recipes, masked foods are used for challenges.[15,44] This method does, however, enable challenge foods to be given in portion-sized doses and in the 'natural form', i.e. how it was eaten when the reaction occurred. The challenge of the methodology, if there is to be standardization, is to devise a masking agent suitable for all the foods in the challenge panel to be masked for every subject in a study. When masked in food, the suspected agent must be undetectable by taste, smell, colour and texture.

In our method the portion-sized doses are sufficient to elicit a response in sensitized patients, while not resulting in anaphylaxis. However, the degree of response suggests that in some less sensitive individuals smaller doses could be employed, although this runs the risk of missing lesser degrees of response. We choose to challenge with those foods that are most likely to produce a response in hospital. These are undertaken in supervised, controlled conditions with full resuscitation facilities on hand. Compliance with the methodology is good; in our clinic 14 of 18 (78%) patients studied in this way completed the DBPCFC programme.

Responses to food allergens can be limited to an immediate response (Fig. 36.2), a late response or a dual response. It has been reported that isolated late responses are rare, but we have found a significant number in our patients with severe asthma (Fig. 36.3).

A subsequent diet which is nutritionally adequate

This is based on the evidence of a positive food challenge,[65] is acceptable to the patient and is not more troublesome than any of the symptoms it has alleviated.

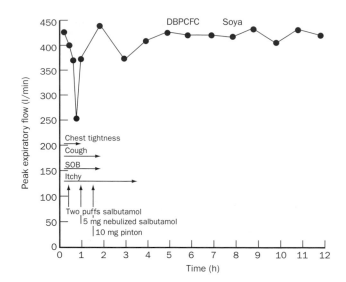

Fig. 36.2 Immediate positive response to DBPCFC in a patient with brittle asthma. SOB=Shortness of Breath

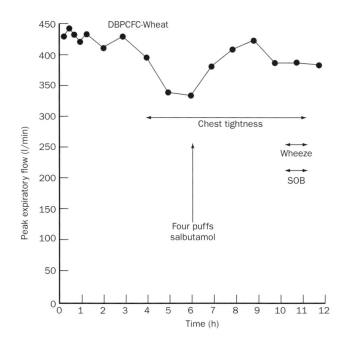

Fig. 36.3 Late positive response to DBPCFC in a patient with brittle asthma. SOB=Shortness of Breath

There have been a number of variations on this design; these are addressed in Chapter X. From the asthma point of view, Appendix 36.1 describes the DBPCFC protocol that was developed in this department for the diagnosis of food allergy in patients with brittle asthma. There are a number of aspects in which our method differs from existing methodology, although many areas of importance are the same. It is possible that the precautions we have taken for brittle asthma may not need to be quite as stringent for asthma of lesser severity, although there is no doubt that some reactions can be severe, even in patients whose asthma would not appear to be quite as chaotic as that of a patient with brittle asthma. The severity of the asthma and the potential severity of the impact of the food challenges makes it essential to admit these patients to hospital. We have found that 5 days' dietary exclusion is, in most cases, sufficient time for both objective (20% improvement in peak expiratory flow (PEF) and/or forced expiratory volume in 1 s (FEV$_1$)) and subjective changes (symptom improvement) to occur. This allows assessment of the appropriateness of going on to food challenge, although we accept that we may have missed some real potential responders by limiting ourselves to just 5 days. If doubt exists as to whether the improvement is real or not, 1 or 2 further days of exclusion is employed. If such an improvement is not seen, challenges do not take place.

TREATMENT OF ESTABLISHED FOOD ALLERGY IN ASTHMA

Dietary avoidance

There is conflicting evidence as to whether oral challenge with food causes a direct asthmatic response, or may lead to an alteration in bronchial hyperresponsiveness thus priming the bronchi for a subsequent provocation.[35] Nevertheless, the purpose of any dietary avoidance is to have a direct impact on symptoms, and food allergy is primarily treated by dietary avoidance of the offending foods.[4] The most important factor influencing the effective control of symptoms is complete avoidance. Detail concerning dietary avoidance is provided in Chapter X.

Drug therapy

In the 1970s inhaled sodium cromoglycate was developed as a therapy for patients with asthma, particularly those with an allergic component.[3] Subsequently, its use was assessed in asthma and urticaria due to foods. Oral sodium cromoglycate in a dosage of 800 mg/day for 1 week or a single dose of 1.0 g did not block any of the asthmatic reactions, but by inhalation it blocked the airway responses after food challenge (Fig. 36.4).[16] In a study of fish-induced asthma, oral sodium cromoglycate blocked the fall in FEV$_1$ either completely or significantly in 16 of 20 patients.[16] The cromone-like drug ketotifen has been considered to offer help in food allergy.[56] In a study[51] of 24 patients it was found to afford protection against the bronchial response to food challenge in asthmatic subjects. The mean reduction in PEF response to repeated oral provocation tests was smaller than the reduction induced by the initial challenge.

Inhaled bronchodilators offer the best treatment for an acute episode when induced by food but when the attacks are severe and rapid, and are similar in speed of onset to an anaphylactic reaction, we have found self-injected adrenaline (EpiPen, AnaPen) to be very effective in some patients.

Vitamin therapy

Vitamin C is considered by some to have a protective role in asthma and other allergic diseases but this is not well defined. The current literature[31] does not support a definite indication for the use of vitamin C in asthma and allergy, and further studies are needed to define its role and indications to support its continuing use.

FOODS IMPLICATED IN ASTHMA

Diet

Diet has been implicated in asthma in many ways, some of which do not concern us here and some remain contentious. For

Reactions to specific foods		
	OFC	DBPCFC
No. of subjects	29	18
No. of reactions to specific foods		
Egg	6 (40)	10 (77)
Milk	7 (47)	8 (62)
Wheat	5 (33)	8 (62)
Fish	6 (40)	6 (46)
Orange	3 (20)	4 (31)
Peanut	nc	7 (54)
Soya	nc	5 (38)

OFC, open food challenge; DBPCFC, double blind placebo-controlled food challenge; nc, no challenge. Values in parentheses are percentages.

Table 36.5 Reactions to specific foods.

instance, a review of the studies relating to dietary salt intake and asthma concluded that a relationship had not been proved definitively between bronchial responsiveness and dietary sodium.[27]

In food allergy, adverse responses have been documented to most foods, but those found to be the most allergenic are egg, milk, wheat, fish, citrus fruits, peanuts and soya.[46] These foods are either staple dietary constituents and/or are nutritionally significant. The respiratory, as well as gastrointestinal and dermatological systems, are all documented as being affected by these adverse responses.

In patients with brittle asthma a very similar pattern of food responses is seen, suggesting that it is the allergenic moieties which are of importance, rather than the end-organ sensitivity, in determining which foods are important in asthma.

Using our protocol (see Appendix 36.1), two-thirds of subjects had positive respiratory reactions with 55% of challenges being positive. A total of 46% of the positive challenges resulted in an immediate-only response, 12% in a late-only response, and 42% a dual response. Egg, orange, peanut and soya were the foods causing an immediate-only response, with milk, wheat and fish the foods causing a late-only response (Table 36.6).

Food additives

Food additives have perhaps been more frequently cited as a group of foodstuffs causing problems in asthma. Some patients with asthma report adverse responses to monosodium glutamate (MSG), particularly if high doses are consumed.[30] A more recent study[12] concluded that oral challenge with MSG reproduced symptoms in some subjects but that the mechanism was unknown, although the symptom characteristics did not support an IgE-mediated mechanism. The same study recommended that the symptoms originally called the 'Chinese Restaurant' syndrome would be better referred to as the MSG symptom complex.

A review of tartrazine sensitivity[72] found that this is most frequently manifested by urticaria and asthma but that the mechanism is obscure and pseudoallergic.

There is conflicting evidence concerning sulphited foods and asthma. It has been reported that about one in nine people with asthma gives a history of asthma worsened by drinking 'soft

Numbers of immediate and late responses				
Challenge food	Positive challenge	Immediate response	Late response	Dual response
Egg	9	5	0	4
Milk	6	3	2	1
Wheat	7	1	2	4
Fish	6	1	1	4
Orange	4	1	0	3
Peanut	6	6	0	0
Soya	3	2	0	1
Totals	41 (55)	19 (46)	5 (12)	17 (42)

Values in parentheses are percentages.

Table 36.6 Numbers of immediate and late responses.

drinks' containing sulphur dioxide,[16] although sulphite-sensitive individuals may not necessarily react after each ingestion of sulphited food.[48]

Salicylates

Some patients with asthma are known to be sensitized to aspirin and aspirin-induced asthma is well recognized. Salicylate-free diets are prescribed by some to improve the asthma symptoms of these individuals. There are no published studies demonstrating the efficacy of this treatment, but anecdotal evidence suggests that it is helpful in some patients.

Alcohol-induced asthma

Although alcohol itself is a modest bronchodilator,[70] many patients with asthma report worsening of their symptoms with ingestion of alcohol. In one series, 25% of a hospital outpatient population reported that at least one alcoholic drink made their asthma worse (Ayres questionnaire).[26] Rarely, an individual is unable to tolerate any form of alcohol, but this may be a pharmacological response to ethyl alcohol mediated through vascular permeability and subsequent airway oedema. The main drinks implicated are red wine, white wine, fortified wines, beers and whisky.[26]

The mechanisms of alcohol-induced asthma are multiple, one candidate being an adverse reaction to chemicals in the drinks, notably preservatives. Sulphur dioxide, a potent bronchoconstrictor in patients with asthma, is found in some alcoholic beverages, notably red wine[29] and, often in high levels, in 'home brew' beers and wines. Alcoholic beverages also contain allergens of vegetable origin such as yeasts and hop residues, allergy to which can initiate worsening asthma. Adverse reactions to alcohol may be worse in asthmatic patients who are also taking the oral hypoglycaemic agent, chlorpropamide,[63] the mechanism for which is unclear but may involve the production of endorphins.[6]

Other foods

Foods of minor significance nutritionally, but nevertheless cited recently as the cause of severe asthmatic responses, are shellfish,[8] royal jelly[5] and fenugreek,[25] and are probably IgE-mediated responses.

CONCLUSION

Food-allergic responses in asthma are now sufficiently well documented to be regarded as real, and recognition of these can result in significant improvement at an individual level. However, there are many gaps in our knowledge and the true overall importance of adverse responses in asthma is unknown. We have no clear idea of the true prevalence of adverse responses to foods in asthmatic populations, and it is unlikely that good estimates will be available until an easy objective assessment is found. For the time being it is reasonable to assume that, overall, the prevalence of food responses in asthma is much less than 10%, although this does seem to increase with increasing severity. We also know that relying on skin prick tests to determine food allergy is inaccurate and unwise. Consequently, the widespread use of food avoidance measures, sometimes extreme, in individuals with modest asthma is to be deplored.

Some foods, such as peanuts and shellfish, can easily be recognized as causes of acute severe responses. While potentially causing life-threatening attacks, these are unlikely to be the cause of long-term destabilization of asthma. Conversely, where recognized, allergy to staple foods such as milk and milk products and wheat is much more important as this means that a major change in dietary habits is required, which is often difficult to undertake consistently. This can be reinforced by the observation that some patients, known to be allergic to a specific food stuff, can 'get away with' eating the forbidden food if their asthma is going through a good period, whereas they daren't try the food if their asthma is at the time poorly controlled. Whether such occasional doses of allergen maintain the adverse immune response in these patients or whether it is of no import in the long run is not known. It does suggest, however, the need to balance the other needs of the patient who may have been advised to avoid a food which is a great favourite and may feel that an occasional treat is well worth the potential risk.

KEY FACTS

1. Food-allergic responses in asthma are well documented and recognized as real.

2. The true prevalence and importance of these responses is not known.

3. Identification and avoidance of the food causing the allergic response can lead to significant improvement in the asthma of some individuals.

4. There appears to be a higher prevalence of food allergy amongst individuals with brittle asthma than those with less severe asthma.

5. There is no simple diagnostic tool for food-allergic asthma – dietary exclusion followed by food challenge is the most reliable method and DBPCFC is the 'gold standard'.

6. Seven foods are most commonly implicated: egg, milk/milk products, wheat, fish, citrus fruits, peanut and soya.

7. Dietary avoidance of the offending food allergen is the only treatment.

8. For a dietary regime to be useful it must be more acceptable to the patient than the symptoms it has alleviated.

REFERENCES

1 A joint report of the Royal College of Physicians and the British Nutrition Foundation. Food intolerance and food aversion. *J R Coll Phys* 1984; 18: 2.

2 Anonymous. An epidemiologic study of severe anaphylactic and anaphylactoid reactions among hospital patients: methods and overall risks. The International Collaborative Study of Severe Anaphylaxis. *Epidemiology* 1998; 9: 141–6.

3 Atkins FM, Steinberg SS, Metcalfe MD. Evaluation of immediate adverse reactions to foods in adult patients. *J Allergy Clin Immunol* 1985; 75: 348–55.

4 Atkins FM. A critical evaluation of clinical trials in adverse reactions to foods in adults. *J Allergy Clin Immunol* 1986; 78: 174–82.

5 Ayres JG, Clarke TJH. Alcoholic drinks and asthma: a survey. *Br J Dis Chest* 1983; 77: 370–5.

6 Ayres JG, Ancic P, Clark TJH. Airway responses to oral ethanol in normal subjects and in patients with asthma. *J R Soc Med* 1982; 75: 699–704.

7 Ayres JG, Clark TJH. Alcohol in asthma and the bronchoconstrictor effect of chlorpropamide. *Br J Dis Chest* 1982; 76: 79–87.

8 Ayres JG, Clark TJH. Intravenous ethanol can provide bronchodilatation in asthma. *Clin Sci* 1983; 74: 555–7.

9 Ayres JG, Miles JF, Barnes PJ. Brittle asthma. *Thorax* 1998; 53: 315–21.

10 Baker JC, Tunnicliffe WS, Duncanson RC, Ayres JG. Double-blind placebo controlled food challenge in Type 1 and Type 2 brittle asthma. *Thorax* 1996; 51 (Suppl. 3): A2.

11 Bender AE, Matthews DR. Adverse reactions to foods. *Br J Nutr* 1981; 46: 403–7.

12 Bielory L, Gandhi R. Asthma and vitamin C. *Ann Allergy* 1994; 73: 89–96.

13 Bjornsson E, Janson C, Plasschke P *et al*. Prevalence of sensitisation to food allergens in adult Swedes. *Ann Allergy Asthma Immunol* 1996; 77: 327–32.

14 Bleumink E. Food allergy: the chemical nature of the substances eliciting symptoms. *World Rev Nutr Diet* 1970; 12: 505–70.

15 Bock SA, Sampson HA, Atkins FM *et al*. Double-blind placebo controlled food challenge (DBPCFC) as an office procedure: a manual. *J Allergy Clin Immunol* 1988; 82: 986–97.

16 Bock SA. Oral challenge procedures. In: *Food Allergy: Adverse Reactions to Food and Food Additives*, (Metcalfe DD, Sampson HA, Simon RA, eds). Blackwell Scientific Publications, Boston, 1991: 83.

17 Bousquet J, Michel FB. Food allergy and asthma. *Ann Allergy* 1988; 61: 70–3.

18 Burr ML, Fehily AM, Stott NCH *et al*. Food-allergic asthma in general practice. *Hum Nutr Appl Nutr* 1985; 39A: 349–55.

19 Burr ML, Merrett TG. Food intolerance: a community survey. *Br J Nutr* 1983; 49: 217–19.

20 Burrows B, Lebowitz MD, Barbee RA. Respiratory disorders and allergy skin test reactions. *Ann Intern Med* 1976; 84: 134–9.

21 Castillo R, Carrilo T, Blanco C *et al*. Shellfish hypersensitivity: chemical and immunological characteristics. *Allergol Immunopathol* 1994; 22: 83–7.

22 Castillo R, Delgado J, Quiratte J *et al*. Food hypersensitivity among adult patients: epidemiological and clinical aspects. *Allergol Immunopathol* 1996; 24: 943–97.

23 Chinn S, Zanolin E, Lai E *et al*. Adjustment of reported prevalence of respiratory symptoms for non-response in a multi-centre health survey. *Int J Epidemiol* 1995; 24: 603–11.

24 Committee on the Medical Effects of Air Pollution. *Asthma and Outdoor Air Pollution*. HMSO, London, 1995; 85–130.

25 Dahl R, Henriksen JM, Harving H. Red wine asthma: a controlled challenge study. *J Allergy Clin Immunol* 1986; 78: 1126–9.

26 Dipalma JR. Tartrazine sensitivity. *Am Fam Phys* 1990; 42: 1347–50.

27 Ellul-Micallef R. Effect of oral sodium cromoglycate and ketotifen in fish-induced bronchial asthma. *Thorax* 1983; 38: 527–30.

28 Eriksson NE. Food sensitivity reported by patients with asthma and hay fever. *Allergy* 1978; 33: 189–96.

29 Freedman BJ. Sulphur dioxide in foods and beverages its use as a preservative and its effect on asthma. *Br J Dis Chest* 1980; 74: 128–34.

30 Furlan J, Suskovic S, Rus A. The effect of food on the bronchial response in adult asthmatic patients and the protective role of ketotifen. *Allergol Immunopathol Madr* 1987; 15: 73–81.

31 Harries MG, O'Brien IM, Burge PS *et al*. Effects of orally administered sodium cromoglycate in asthma and urticaria due to foods. *Clin Allergy* 1978; 8: 423–7.

32 Harrison BDW. Psychosocial aspects of asthma in adults. *Thorax* 1998; 53: 519–25.

33 Hebling A. Food allergy (review). *Therapeutische Umschau* 1994; 51: 31–7.

34 Hodge L, Yan KY, Loblay RL. Assessment of food chemical intolerance in adult asthmatic subjects. *Thorax* 1996; 51: 805–9.

35 Huijbers GB, Colen AAM, Niestijl JJ *et al*. Masking foods for challenge: practical aspects of masking foods for a double-blind placebo-controlled food challenge. *J Am Diet Assoc* 1994; 94: 644–9.

36 James JM, Eigenmann PA, Peyton A *et al*. Airway reactivity changes in asthmatic patients undergoing blinded food challenges. *Am J Respir Crit Care Med* 1996; 150: 597–603.

37 Jansen JJ, Kardinaal AFM, Huijbers G *et al*. Prevalence of food allergy in the adult Dutch population. *J Allergy Clin Immunol* 1994; 93: 446–56.

38 Janson C, Chinn S, Jarvis D, Burney P. Physician diagnosed asthma and drug utilisation in the European Community Respiratory Health Survey. *Eur Respir J* 1997; 10: 1795–802.

39 Jarvis D, Chinn S, Luczynska C, Burney P. The association of respiratory symptoms and lung function with the use of gas for cooking. European Community Respiratory Health Survey. *Eur Respir J* 1998; 11: 651–8.

40 Kalyoncu AF, Karakoca Y, Demir AU *et al*. Prevalence of asthma and allergic disease in Turkish university students in Ankara. *Allergol Immunopathol* 1996; 24: 152–7.

41 Lawrence T, Chiaramonte MD. Food sensitivity in asthma: perception and reality. *J Asthma* 1991; 28: 5–9.

42 Leinhas J, McCaskill CC, Sampson HA. Food allergy challenges: guidelines and implications. *J Am Diet Assoc* 1987; 87: 604–8.

43 Lessof MH. *Food Intolerance*. Chapman Hall, London, 1992; 122.

44 Lessof MH. *Food Intolerance*. Chapman and Hall, London, 1992: 109.

45 Medrala W, Wolariczyk-Medrala A, Malplepszy J *et al*. Comparative study between SPTs and TOP-CAST allergen leukocyte stimulation in diagnosis of allergic status. *J Invest Allergol Clin Immunol* 1997; 7(2)115–18.

46 Molkhon P, Dupont C. Ketotifen in prevention and therapy of food allergy. *Ann Allergy* 1987; 59: 187–93.

A

47 Moneret-Vautrin DA, Mohr N, Gerard H *et al*. Occurrence of IgE-dependent food allergy in asthmatic disease. *Allergie Immunologie* 1987; 19: 410–14.

48 Moneret-Vautrin DA. Monosodium glutamate-induced asthma: a study of the potential risk of 30 asthmatics and review of the literature. *Allergie Immunologie* 1987; 19: 29–35.

49 Muhlemann RJ, Wuthrich B. Food allergies 1983–1987. *J Suisse Med* 1991; 121: 1679–700.

50 Neild JE, Cameron IR. Bronchoconstriction in response to suggestion: its prevention by an inhaled anticholinergic agent. *BMJ* 1985; 290: 674.

51 Nizani RM, Lewin PK, Baboo MT. Oral cromolyn therapy in patients with food allergy: a preliminary report. *Ann Allergy* 1977; 39: 102–5.

52 Oehling A, Garcia B, Santo F *et al*. Food allergy as a cause of rhinitis and/or asthma. *J Inv Allergol Clin Immunol* 1992; 2: 78–83.

53 Oehling A, Ona J, Trento H *et al*. The diagnostic value of the histamine release test in food allergy. *Allergol Immunopathol* 1984; 12: 439–48.

54 Onorato J, Merland L, Terral C *et al*. Placebo-controlled double-blind food challenge in asthma. *J Allergy Clin Immunol* 1986; 78: 1139–46.

55 Pacor MZ, Mardi G, Cortina P *et al*. Food allergy and asthma. *Rec Progr Med* 1991; 83: 64–6.

56 Pastorello EA, Stocchi L, Pravettoni V *et al*. Role of the elimination diet in adults with food allergy. *J Allergy Clin Immunol* 1989; 84: 475–83.

57 Patil SP, Niphadkar PV, Bapat MM. Allergy to fenugreek (*Trigonella foenum graecum*). *Ann Allergy Asth Immunol* 1997; 78: 329–30.

58 Pirhonen I, Nevalainen A, Husman T, Pekkanen J. Home dampness, moulds and their influence on respiratory infections and symptoms in adults in Finland. *Eur Resp J* 1996; 9: 2618–22.

59 Sampson HA, Albergo R. Comparison of results of skin tests, RAST, and double-blind, placebo-controlled food challenges in children with atopic dermatitis. *J Allergy Clin Immunol* 1984; 74: 26–33.

60 Sampson HA. Immunologically mediated food allergy: the importance of food challenge procedures. *Ann Allergy* 1988; 60: 262–9.

61 Sullivan SD. Economics of asthma and asthma treatments. *Eur Resp Rev* 1998; 8: 59: 351–5.

62 SWORD '96 (Ross DJ, Keynes HL, McDonald JC). Surveillance of work-related and occupational respiratory disease in the UK. *Occup Med* 1997; 47: 377–81.

63 Taylor SL, Bush RK, Selner JC *et al*. Sensitivity to sulphited foods among sulphite-sensitive subjects with asthma. *J Allergy Clin Immunol* 1988; 81: 1159–67.

64 Thien FC, Leung R, Baldo BA *et al*. Asthma and anaphylaxis induced by royal jelly. *Clin Exp Allergy* 1996; 26: 216–22.

65 Thomas B (ed.). *Manual of Dietetic Practice*. Blackwell Scientific Publications, 1988.

66 Wang Z. An allergy prevalence study in a population of 10,144 people. *Chinese J Epidemiol* 1990; 11: 100–2.

67 Warner JO. Food intolerance and asthma. *Clin Exp Allergy* 1995; 25 (Suppl. 1): 29–30.

68 Woods RK, Abramson M, Raven JM *et al*. Reported food intolerance and respiratory symptoms in young adults. *Eur Respir J* 1998; 11: 151–5.

69 Woods RK, Weiner J, Abramson M *et al*. Patients' perceptions of food-induced asthma. *Aust NZ J Med* 1996; 26: 504–12.

70 Yang WH, Drouin MA, Herbert M *et al*. The MSG symptom complex: assessment in a double-blind, placebo-controlled randomised study. *J Allergy Clin Immunol* 1997; 99: 757–62.

71 Young E, Stoneham MD, Petruschevitch A *et al*. A population study of food intolerance. *Lancet* 1994; 343: 1127–30.

72 Zoia MC, Fanfulla F, Bruschi C *et al*. Chronic respiratory symptoms, bronchial responsiveness and dietary sodium and potassium: a population-based study. *Monaldi Arch Chest Dis* 1995; 50: 104–8.

73 Zwetchkenbaum JF, Skufea R, Nelson HS. An examination of increased bronchial responsiveness to inhaled methacholine. *J Allergy Clin Immunol* 1991; 88: 360–4.

APPENDIX 36.1 PROTOCOL FOR DIETARY EXCLUSION AND DBPCFCS

STAGE 1

- For 3 days before admission the patient keeps a record of their normal food and drink intake and peak expiratory flow (PEF) (best of three values, three times daily) in a diary.

STAGE 2

- Patient is admitted to a dedicated respiratory ward for 10 days.
- During days 1–5 they undergo dietary exclusion, drinking only 'still' bottled water. Their nutritional needs are met by drinking a hypoallergenic elemental formula (Elemental 028 Extra Liquid).
- On day 1 their medication is assessed for any potential food allergens contained as excipients (e.g. cornstarch) and alternative preparations given if necessary.
- PEF (best of three on each occasion) and FEV_1 is measured four times a day throughout the 5 days using a handheld, portable electronic spirometer (Micromed, UK) for the supervised measurement and recording of PEF and FEV_1.
- Skin prick tests are undertaken to ingested allergens (egg, milk, wheat, fish, orange, peanut and soya) and to inhaled allergens. The maximum diameter (excluding pseudopodia) is measured with the diameter at right angles to it, the mean value of the two being recorded. A positive response is taken as a wheal at least 3 mm greater than a saline control.[68] Total serum IgE is measured.
- A detailed dietary history is obtained concerning foods previously excluded from the patient's diet because they were perceived as allergens and/or were known to cause anaphylaxis. Any food known to cause anaphylaxis in a particular patient is not administered to that individual in any subsequent series of challenges.

STAGE 3

- At the end of day 5, if there is an improvement in mean daily PEF and/or FEV_1 of more than or equal to 20%, the programme of DBPCFCs to egg, milk, wheat, fish, orange, peanut, soya and placebo (see soup recipe below) is started.
- Foods other than the standard panel which are suspected as allergens for any patient are included in the challenge programme for that individual.
- It is advised that the patient's medication is assessed before DBPCFCs and that the following drugs be discontinued before the challenge procedure: antihistamines (72–96 h), β-agonists (12 h), theophylline (12 h), cromolyn (12 h) and probably tricyclic antidepressants (96 h or possibly longer).[28] It is medically inappropriate to remove these drugs from the treatment of patients with brittle asthma and the DBPCFCs are conducted under these conditions. However, the dosage of drug for each patient remains the same throughout the challenge period.

SOUP RECIPE

- A soup recipe is given as the placebo and used as the vehicle for each challenge food (Table A36.1).
- The soup is cooked, either plain or with the challenge food added, and then liquidized to mask for texture. It is given to the patient to drink in a covered, opaque beaker with a built-in straw to mask sight and smell. The patient drinks the soup wearing nose clips and takes a glass of mineral water after drinking the soup and before removing the nose clips, to mask smell and taste.
- On the first day of this stage the patient is given one dose of the placebo.
- If this produces a negative response, on subsequent days patients are given one of the challenge foods masked in the soup (Table A36.2).
- The order of the challenges is randomized and double blind.
- The soup is also served to any patient who desires a palatable alternative and complementary source of food and nutrition to the E028.
- A specialist dietitian, specialist nurse and physician oversee each challenge.
- Outcomes are recorded as symptoms and changes in PEF and FEV_1 at 15, 30 and 60 min and then at hourly intervals for 12h.
- A positive reaction is defined as a fall in PEF and/or FEV_1 of more than or equal to 15% with symptoms, or a fall in PEF and/or FEV_1 of more than or equal to 20% plus or minus symptoms.

CONTINUATION STAGE

- At the end of challenge with the seven standard foods and placebo, the codes are broken.
- The patient is advised of any positive results and how to exclude the offending food(s) from their diet while maintaining a nutritionally balanced dietary intake.
- The E028 and mineral water are discontinued, a vitamin and mineral supplement prescribed and the patient is discharged to continue introducing one new food daily at home until they have reintroduced into their diet all the foods they normally eat.

Placebo soup recipe	
Ingredients	300 ml tap water, 30 g dried lentils, 30 g carrot, 30 g onion, salt and pepper
Method	Place all ingredients in a pan, bring to boil, simmer for 20 min, liquidize
Protein	9.1 g
Energy	138 kcal
Fat	0.64 g

Table A36.1 Placebo soup recipe.

Food challenge recipes			
Challenge	**Quantity**	**Add to soup recipe**	**Cooking instructions**
Egg	50 g, fresh	One whole egg, raw	Beat, add to raw ingredients, cook, etc.
Milk	300 ml	Whole, pasteurized	Use in place of water
Wheat	60 g	Wholemeal flour	Mix to a paste, add to raw ingredients, cook, etc.
Fish	60 g	Cod, raw	Add to raw ingredients, cook, etc.
Orange	60 g	Flesh of one orange	Add to soup after cooking, liquidize
Peanut	10 g	Approximately 10 peanuts	Add to soup after cooking, liquidize
Soya	300 ml	Soya milk, UHT	Use in place of water

Table A36.2 Food challenge recipes.

- The patient continues to record symptoms and PEF, as in hospital, in the diary booklet.
- Contact telephone numbers are provided.

- Regular outpatient attendance ensures that the ultimate dietary regime is assessed for nutritional adequacy and is not more troublesome to the patient than any symptoms it has alleviated.

INTRODUCTION

An earlier book edited by Brostoff and Challacombe concerning food allergy included contributions from 19 authors, four countries and both sides of the Atlantic.[14] It was published in 1982 and was followed in 1984 by the report on food intolerance and food aversion by the joint committee of the Royal College of Physicians and the British Nutrition Foundation.[35] Both publications provided testimony to the increasing awareness and respect that the subject of food allergy had commanded over the preceding decade, a decade that began with the very existence of food allergy being described in editorial comment as 'beyond the fringe of credibility'.[43] Neither publication, however, acknowledged even the possibility that food allergy could produce a direct effect in the gas exchanging tissues of the lung. Our task in the first edition of *Food Allergy and Intolerance* was therefore a limited one – to consider whether alveolitis (i.e. pneumonitis) attributable to food allergy or intolerance lay within the fringe of credibility. We concluded that it did, but only just.

For this second edition the experience of a further decade has become available, and this has produced important examples in both man and other animals where food (or food contaminants)

has led to serious disruption of parenchymal lung function. The precise mechanisms are not all fully clear. Although the immune system is undoubtedly critical in pathogenesis, the initiating events may owe more to toxic mechanisms and 'intolerance' than to allergy. Because few parenchymal diseases of the lung affect the alveoli in isolation, we shall interpret our 'alveolitis' brief quite widely and consider the lung parenchyma together with the bronchioles, in addition to the alveoli themselves.

CLINICAL CONSIDERATIONS

Could food allergy cause alveolitis?

There are excellent theoretical reasons for supposing that food allergy could cause alveolitis (and its end stage, diffuse pulmonary fibrosis), a good deal of which is currently considered to be idiopathic or 'cryptogenic' in origin. The most important aetiological agents in conventional types of extrinsic allergic alveolitis (EAA), which is also widely known as hypersensitivity pneumonitis, are derived from vegetable (and microbial) dusts and from birds. With both, relevant antigens (or toxins) are likely to find their way into food products. Food processing and cooking will, in many instances, destroy or modify much of the antigenic specificity, and that which survives will be further degraded by digestive processes within the alimentary tract. On the other hand, the magnitude of an ingested antigenic challenge may be substantially larger than that which is experienced in the alveoli directly following airborne exposure, and toxic constituents may be less readily degraded. Furthermore, not all antigenic food is fully denatured by cooking or digestion, and it is now well recognized that many macromolecules cross the intestinal mucosa antigenically intact.[37,62] These can be identified in the milk of nursing mothers whose infants may occasionally suffer allergic symptoms as a consequence.[2,34,59] The fact that food allergy may present in almost any organ beyond the gut is itself supportive evidence that food components may be absorbed with preserved antigenicity and distributed systemically. That this distribution can be of clinical significance to the lungs is shown by numerous reports of asthma following the ingestion of foods or food additives.

Food additives

With food additives (such as the colouring agent tartrazine, benzoate preservatives and salicylates), the chances of heat or enzymic denaturation are much less than with antigens of food itself, and these additives are, perhaps, a more important cause of asthma provoked by foodstuffs. With agents of this type there is little evidence that specific immunological mechanisms are responsible and, with salicylates (which occur naturally in certain fruits and vegetables, and are added to flavour a variety of food products), the major mechanism probably involves inhibition of prostaglandin synthesis and the direct release of mast cell mediators.

Antibiotics

Antibiotics may contaminate food and with penicillins there is interesting confirmation that, once the airways are sensitized by the inhalation route, further asthmatic reactions can be produced when the provoking agent is ingested.[18] The subjects concerned were employed in the manufacture of ampicillin from benzylpenicillin and developed occupational asthma as a result of continual exposure to fine airborne dust containing these antibiotics. Inhalation provocation tests lasting 30 min using an airborne dust from a mixture of 250 g lactose containing 1–10 g of antibiotic powder led to typical and reproducible late asthmatic responses which were duplicated when 500 mg of each drug were ingested (Fig. 37.1). It is interesting that the ingested challenges provoked, in addition, late reactions in the gastrointestinal tract (diarrhoea) and skin (urticaria). It is difficult to estimate the actual dose deposited in the lungs and absorbed systemically after the airborne challenges, but this must have been substantially less than that responsible for the orally provoked responses.

Relevance to alveolitis

The possible relevance of these observations to food-induced alveolitis is twofold. Firstly, many airborne dusts which induce EAA (and which induce asthma also) are likely to contribute to the allergenicity of food or share relevant antigens with components or contaminants of foodstuffs. Flour and grain dust with bread; avian bloom, urine and faeces with egg; yeasts and other fungi with various food 'extracts' and alcoholic beverages, are examples. In each case ingestion of the end product is known to provoke asthma in some individuals, not necessarily those

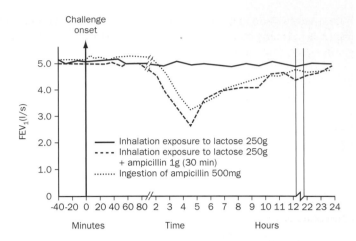

Fig. 37.1 Inhalation and ingestion provocation tests with ampicillin in a 26-year-old production worker. From: Occupational lung disease. In: Simmons DH, ed. *Current Pulmonology*, vol. 3, John Wiley, New York, 1981, with permission.

sensitized initially by the inhalation route. Secondly, a number of drugs, including a further antibiotic – nitrofurantoin – may cause alveolitis when ingested.[13,55] This occurs in the absence of apparent prior sensitization by the respiratory route, a point of potential importance. The relevant drugs and the doses involved are not, however, likely to be encountered in everyday foods. Most are cytotoxic agents and some, such as bleomycin, exert their effects largely through toxic mechanisms. Individual susceptibility (i.e. intolerance) does, however, play a major role. With other cytotoxic agents, such as methotrexate, hypersensitivity mechanisms appear more probable, although the definite participation of immunological processes has not yet been confirmed. Nevertheless, the clinical picture of the alveolitic response to many of these agents is identical to that observed in classical types of EAA.

IMMUNOLOGICAL CONSIDERATIONS

Before considering further the clinical evidence that immunological reactions against food antigens (or food additives or food contaminants) might induce alveolitis, it is important to consider the immunological responses which may be relevant. Earlier chapters which have dealt with immunological mechanisms have stressed the preoccupation of bowel mucosal immunity with local defence. Thus, local antigen challenge, whether with microbial, chemical (haptenic) or environmental antigens such as foods, generally induces local immunity only. Systemic immunization does not normally occur even if the antigens traverse the bowel mucosa, as occurs frequently in the case of food antigens. This failure of systemic priming applies to both systemic humoral (mainly IgG) and cellular (principally T lymphocyte) limbs of the immune response system and a principal mechanism is active suppression by T lymphocytes.[58]

Route of antigen presentation

The route of initial antigenic presentation to the specialized cells of the monocyte/macrophage series, now referred to as antigen-presenting cells, appears crucial to the outcome of mucosal compared to systemic antigen challenge. For systemic immunization to follow antigen penetration of the bowel mucosa, the antigen must not only evade local mechanisms for generating suppression but must also run the gauntlet of the liver reticuloendothelial system. The latter is also responsible for induction of specific systemic suppression after immunization with certain soluble antigens and haptens by the hepatic portal vein route.[15] Consideration of these observations is of particular relevance to alveolitis. For such distant disease to occur as a result of food absorption, either the mechanisms for systemic suppression must have been bypassed, or prior sensitization of the systemic immune system by another route of presentation must have occurred.

Abrogation of systemic suppression

Possible ways in which the first criterion might be met include failure of local immune mechanisms (e.g. IgA deficiency), inflammatory bowel disease permitting a generalized increase in mucosal permeability, local immunological disorders of the bowel (e.g. coeliac disease), or generalized immunological disorders associated with abnormal immune responses.

Primary sensitization via airways

In the context of parenchymal lung disease, the most likely route for primary systemic sensitization would be via the airway mucosa itself. There is sparse information available about local and systemic immune responses generated as a result of bronchial antigenic challenge. The bronchial tree possesses a secretory mucosal immune system similar to that of the gastrointestinal tract, but from the limited experimental data available it appears unlikely that antigen presentation via this route is geared to the induction of systemic immune suppression to quite the same degree. This probably reflects the nature of the antigenic challenge to which the respiratory mucosa is normally exposed; inhaled pathogenic microorganisms rather than non-pathogenic food. Clinical evidence supports this view. IgG antibodies directed against vegetable and animal antigens associated with EAA are found in serum and alveolar fluid in both asymptomatic and clinically affected individuals exposed to the relevant antigens. The levels are generally greater in those who are clinically affected, however.

It therefore appears that airway exposure to food antigens would provide a more immunogenic form of antigen presentation than would their absorption through healthy bowel. These considerations do not apply if the bowel is diseased and there is increased absorption of food antigens (Table 37.1).

Factors increasing gut absorption of food antigens
Immature gut
IgA deficiency
Inflammatory bowel disease
Local immunological disorders of the bowel, e.g. coeliac disease
Post diarrhoea states

Table 37.1 Factors increasing gut absorption of food antigens.

Neonatal antigen challenge

Antigenic challenge in the neonate is worthy of special consideration. IgA production increases after a variable period following birth, and in the immediate postnatal period a number of immunological responses remain immature. In particular, food antigen penetration of the bowel is liable to occur to a greater degree at this age. This immaturity of mucosal immune exclusion in the neonate is compounded by an inherent increased permeability of the neonatal gut, which may represent the residuum of a primitive absorption mechanism.[63] A third relevant consideration is that in early infancy aspiration of food is frequent, creating the possibility of an alternative route of sensitization prior to the development of specific tolerance. These three factors probably combine to induce the high levels of precipitating (IgG) antibodies directed against food antigens which are invariably found in *normal* infants. Such antibodies generally persist in readily detectable quantities for about 3 years, after which their concentration and prevalence drop sharply.[25]

IgE-mediated mechanisms

This discussion of gastrointestinal and respiratory immune responses to food antigens and their interrelationships has to this point excluded IgE. This class of antibody is not thought to be of major importance in the initiation or perpetuation of parenchymal lung disease. Nevertheless, IgE antibodies against food antigens will, in some cases, form part of the humoral immune response generated at gastrointestinal mucosal surfaces, particularly in atopic subjects. This antibody, although synthesized locally in the gut mucosa and mesenteric lymph nodes, will disseminate systemically, thereby sensitizing mast cells in other mucosal and epithelial surfaces. It could then be responsible for distant immediate reactions after food ingestion. IgE antibody production is under separate class-specific regulatory control, and is very dependent upon the concentration of sensitizing antigen. Therefore, in genetically predisposed subjects exposed to antigen under appropriate conditions, specific IgE responses may occur with resulting distant consequences, even though the other major limbs of the immune response outside the gut mucosa are not primed to the same antigen.

MECHANISMS RESPONSIBLE FOR THE INDUCTION OF EXTRINSIC ALLERGIC ALVEOLITIS

Conflicting evidence for Type III hypersensitivity

The possible pathogenic immunological mechanisms responsible for the induction of EAA are of interest and importance. The similar time course of response to exposure to that of the experimental Arthus reaction, and the almost invariable finding of precipitating antibodies to provocation antigens in the serum of affected subjects, initially encouraged the belief that the disease was the result of immune complex formation at sites of antigen deposition. To accommodate the view that IgG-class antibody and complement were largely responsible for the associated parenchymal lung damage, certain conflicting pieces of evidence were overlooked. In particular, evidence of local vasculitis, a cardinal feature of the experimental Arthus reaction, is lacking in most cases of EAA, while evidence of immune complex and complement deposition in affected tissue is unconvincing. The histological findings in EAA of granulomatous lesions associated with mononuclear infiltration of alveoli and interstitial tissue are also atypical of immune complex-induced disease but are more consistent with T cell-mediated hypersensitivity. Finally, precipitating antibodies cannot always be demonstrated in the serum of affected subjects, although they may be found in similarly exposed individuals who have no symptoms.

T cell-mediated hypersensitivity

The preoccupation with antibody-mediated mechanisms has undoubtedly resulted from the ease with which these specific immunoglobulins can be detected when contrasted with the difficulty, until recently, of studying specific T lymphocytic responses in humans. Animal models of disease are now increasing our understanding. They have confirmed that, while acute necrotizing lesions associated with polymorph infiltration can be readily induced experimentally by humoral immunization or serum transfer into immunologically naïve, antigenically challenged animals, T lymphocyte responses induced by adjuvant sensitization are essential to produce the clinical and histological features of chronic hypersensitivity alveolitis. In animal models, alveolitis can be passively transferred to naïve recipient exposed animals by CD4+ T (helper) lymphocytes.[56] Gamma-interferon (IFNγ) gene knock-out mice fail to generate pulmonary inflammatory disease when exposed to thermophilic bacteria, but granulomatous inflammation can be restored to these animals by the exogenous administration of IFNγ.[24]

These two pieces of experimental evidence suggest that a CD4 helper T cell-mediated immune reaction with the characteristics of a TH1 cytokine-producing cell population is responsible for experimental hypersensitivity alveolitis. In chronic human alveolitis the CD8 T cell is the predominant cell type found in bronchoalveolar lavage,[57] again indicating the probable importance of T cell mechanisms in disease production. Since the T cell epitopes on antigens are linear peptide sequences bound by and presented with histocompatibility molecules on antigen-presenting cells, it is simple to envisage triggering T cell antigens being relatively preserved during intestinal digestion when compared to the three-dimensional folded protein antigens bound by antibodies and B lymphocytes.

Summary

Systemic sensitization to ingested food antigens is unlikely to occur in the presence of mature local and systemic immune systems and normal gastrointestinal mucosal permeability. Nevertheless, food allergy (or food intolerance attributable to toxic mechanisms) could account for a proportion of the alveolitic disorders whose aetiology is currently unknown. To explore this possibility further, we shall turn to six illustrative topics: (1) an alveolar disorder of children resembling pulmonary haemosiderosis which has been attributed to milk and buckwheat allergy; (2) the alleged association between alveolitis and coeliac disease; (3) the speculative suggestion that bird fancier's lung could be exacerbated or even initiated by egg allergy; (4) an apparently toxic pneumonitis from ingesting a contaminated cooking oil; (5) the development of an obstructive bronchiolitis/alveolitis after ingestion of leaf extracts from the Asian shrub, *Sauropus androgynus*; and (6) alveolar/bronchiolar disorders of other mammalian species which are thought to result from food ingestion.

PULMONARY HAEMOSIDEROSIS AND MILK ALLERGY

Pulmonary haemosiderosis is a rare disorder characterized by pulmonary haemorrhage at alveolar level. Its major clinical features are haemoptysis and iron-deficient anaemia. These features may also be prominent in systemic lupus erythematosus (SLE) and Goodpasture's syndrome, diseases which are known to be mediated by circulatory or cell bound immune complexes. In SLE, circulating complexes are selectively deposited in pulmonary capillaries by a mechanism which remains unclear. Deposition in other sites leads to the multisystem dysfunction typical of this disease. In Goodpasture's syndrome the immune complexes are formed *in situ* by the complexing of a specific circulating IgG with basement membranes of capillaries in both alveoli and renal glomeruli. When pulmonary alveolar haemorrhage occurs in isolation, these immunological abnormalities are found (or sought) less often, and the disorder is conventionally labelled idiopathic pulmonary haemosiderosis (IPH).

In 1962, Heiner and colleagues[26] reported the curious case of an 8-month-old North American infant who had a severe and persistent cough, recurrent diarrhoea and failure to thrive. Investigation revealed recurrent pulmonary infiltrates on chest radiographs and a persistent iron-deficiency anaemia. No infecting microorganisms were discovered and cystic fibrosis was excluded. Although skin tests for tuberculosis, histoplasmosis, blastomycosis and coccidioidomycosis proved to be negative, the child's serum gave a strong precipitin reaction with a culture filtrate of a virulent strain of *Mycobacterium tuberculosis*. With culture filtrates from five other virulent strains of *M. tuberculosis* no immunological reactions were observed. It transpired that the filtrate giving the positive reaction had been cultured from a medium containing bovine serum, the latter sharing antigens with raw cow's milk. An appropriate cow's milk exclusion diet was recommended and the child improved dramatically.

As a result of this experience, these investigators studied sera from 65 further children with respiratory diseases of uncertain aetiology (cases), and an additional 1980 subjects who were either well or had diseases of established cause (controls). Seven of the cases gave precipitin responses to cow's milk that closely resembled those from the index case. That is, strong precipitin lines were seen to at least five components of cow's milk. A further 18 sera gave precipitin reactions to one to three components of cow's milk only. One child with a strong precipitin response could not be evaluated fully but the other six, together with the index case, were found to exhibit a remarkable constellation of similar clinical features. Those with less strong responses did not.

Clinical features

The seven affected subjects were infants aged 13 days to 6 months when they became ill. They were troubled by chronic cough and rhinitis, persistent tachypnoea and recurrent fever. In six, poor weight gain and pallor, together with recurrent diarrhoea and otitis media, were associated features. In addition, five experienced recurrent vomiting and four recurrent haemoptysis. Investigation confirmed the presence of recurrent pulmonary infiltrates in all the children. Six had hypochromic anaemias and six had weights below the tenth percentile. Eosinophilia was seen in six. All seven underwent diagnostic aspiration of gastric or bronchial secretions which, on examination, revealed an excess of iron-laden macrophages in four. A similar excess was noted following needle aspiration of the lung in one. These findings led the authors to suggest that the iron-deficient anaemias were due to bleeding from the gut and lungs. The pulmonary component of the syndrome therefore resembled pulmonary haemosiderosis.

In six of these infants major changes in diet were introduced. Five received evaporated or boiled milk but no raw cow's milk, and two became symptom-free within 2 days. The four who remained symptomatic were then given soybean substitute feeds and cow's milk was withdrawn altogether. All recovered fully. After 3–6 months, cow's milk was reinstituted in the diet of each infant. Two developed a recurrence of all former symptoms but four appeared to have become partially tolerant. The authors believed the syndrome described was caused by allergy to ingested cow's milk. It is interesting that as many as six of the seven infants were breast fed initially, which did not therefore confer protection.

Precipitins to cow's milk and other food allergens

Heiner and colleagues[26] remarked that precipitins to cow's milk are also commonly observed in children with coeliac disease, but the absence of precipitins to wheat made coeliac disease unlikely in their particular cases. Like a small number of other investigators, they did, however, refer to a further case in which pulmonary haemosiderosis (proved at autopsy) and coeliac disease appeared to have coexisted. Precipitins were detected to both cow's milk and gliadin. They also remarked that precipitins to cow's milk are not always found with pulmonary haemosiderosis, implying that milk allergy is simply one possible cause of this disorder in childhood. Finally, this landmark publication briefly reported the outcome of a further survey of 1284 sera obtained from subjects with some clinical suspicion of this interesting syndrome. Strong precipitin responses to cow's milk were noted in 26. With 10 there was iron deficiency anaemia but no evidence of pulmonary disease. With eight, both gastrointestinal and pulmonary disorders were evident, and these improved with cow's milk avoidance.

The evidence presented by these investigators is very persuasive and other authors have subsequently reported similar cases. It is possible that sensitization could have resulted primarily from regurgitation and aspiration of ingested milk into the lungs, and subsequent experience suggests that this may indeed occur in infants with this syndrome. It does not appear to be a uniform finding, however. Until recently, the syndrome had not been related to foods other than cow's milk. Its description in 1997 in a Japanese child following the ingestion of buckwheat is therefore of considerable interest since it demonstrates that, although cow's milk undoubtedly has unusual potency, it does not possess a unique property in inducing this curious disorder.[1]

Mechanism of pulmonary damage

The mechanism of pulmonary damage in this syndrome has not been investigated by immunopathological techniques, but the evidence that circulating immune complexes can initiate similar effects in a small proportion of patients with SLE suggests the possibility that circulating food-containing immune complexes could be responsible. The low incidence of this complication in milk-allergic infants in general would then illustrate the recognized variability between individuals in sites of immune complex deposition or in susceptibility.

In adults with IPH there is no direct evidence suggesting an association with food hypersensitivity, although occasional case reports have suggested a link with malabsorption.[7,11,41] In a study designed to investigate this possible association in more detail, jejunal biopsies were obtained in six patients with IPH.[65] Abnormal morphological appearances were revealed in two. IPH is an uncommon disease, however, and further studies are needed before its possible association with coeliac disease can be verified and quantified.

ALVEOLITIS AND COELIAC DISEASE

Interest in a possible association between a true diffuse alveolitis and coeliac disease (and hence food allergy) was first kindled in the early 1970s. The report by Hood and Mason[33] described two patients with both disorders but gave no indication of the size of the population from which they had emerged. Whether the association could have been one of chance alone could not consequently be assessed. Lancaster-Smith and colleagues[39] reported alveolitis in three of a selected group of 24 patients with coeliac disease, but when the group was increased to 57 no further cases of diffuse lung disease were noted.[40] Following the suggestion of Berrill and colleagues[9,10] that coeliac disease was associated specifically with bird fancier's lung (BFL), case reports have emerged linking coeliac disease with farmer's lung,[53,54] and there is now much speculation that this intestinal food allergy may be associated with both cryptogenic fibrosing alveolitis and EAA.[3,4,16]

Clinical significance of precipitins to bird serum

Sera from the initial 24 patients reported by Lancaster-Smith et al. were examined for a number of antibodies to both autoantigens and extrinsic antigens. Faux (personal communication, 1978) found a high proportion (seven of 28) to have precipitins directed against the sera of many species of bird, but these did not cross-react with the appropriate droppings extracts, indicating that there was no common allergen. This response pattern is not characteristic of BFL.[22] Furthermore, none of the patients concerned appeared to be exposed to birds at the time, and when avian inhalation provocation tests were performed on two of the three with alveolitis, no reactions were produced.[8] It was concluded that these precipitins to bird serum were 'non-specific'. Similar observations were reported independently by Morris and colleagues at about the same time.[47]

The presence of precipitins to bird serum was an important diagnostic feature in the study of Berrill et al.,[9] although their 'specificity' was unknown. These investigators reported a high prevalence of villous atrophy in small bowel biopsies taken from patients with presumed BFL. Of 18 patients thought to have BFL, nine underwent jejunal biopsy and villous atrophy was demonstrated in five. No inhalation provocation tests were performed with avian antigens, and only one of the five subsequently achieved an adequate and persisting pulmonary response from bird avoidance alone. The specific diagnosis of BFL could therefore be questioned, as could the strength of the suggested association with coeliac disease. That villous atrophy should have been found so commonly in patients with diffuse pulmonary disease of whatever cause is, however, surprising and it is possible that selection bias may have exerted an influence.

The clinical significance of the 'non-specific' precipitin response to bird sera has now been clarified by Faux and her colleagues.[22,29] Precipitin responses to bird serum, droppings and eggs from a number of species were examined in current and former bird fanciers, patients with BFL proved by inhalation provocation tests, control subjects unexposed to birds, and patients with biopsy-proved coeliac disease. Two patterns of response were distinguished.

Bird fancier's lung-associated precipitins

The response illustrated in Fig. 37.2 shows reactions of identity (or partial identity) between the bird serum and droppings of exposure. Although there is some crossreactivity with other species, the responses are most marked to the species of exposure. Their strength is also dependent on the degree of current exposure (i.e. number of birds). This pattern proved to be significantly related not only to current bird exposure but to BFL itself.

The immunologically identical antigens of the birds' blood and excreta which are responsible were consequently termed 'BFL-associated' and the corresponding antibodies 'BFL-associated precipitins'. A number of different antigens may be involved, some of which may be found in egg.

Coeliac disease-associated precipitins

Fig. 37.3 shows the second pattern of response which involves a single reaction and presumably a single antigen. The common reaction observed indicates that the single antigen is present equally in the sera of a number of avian species and in chicken egg yolk, but not in droppings. This pattern was not related to BFL or even bird exposure, but it was closely related to coeliac disease. The precipitins were therefore termed 'coeliac disease-associated'.

It was assumed that this antibody response to the coeliac disease-associated antigen was provoked by dietary egg, and a relationship was sought between its presence and the degree of

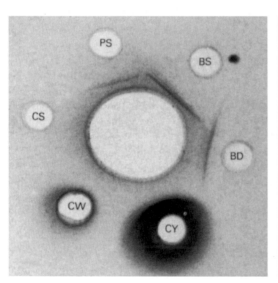 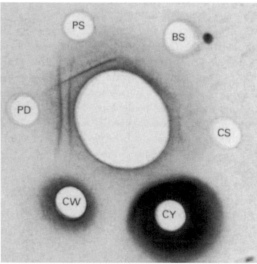

Fig. 37.2 Bird fancier's lung-associated precipitins from a budgerigar fancier (single bird) and pigeon breeder, respectively. BD, budgerigar droppings; BS, budgerigar serum; CS, chicken serum; CW, chicken egg white; CY, chicken egg yolk; PD, pigeon droppings; PS, pigeon serum.

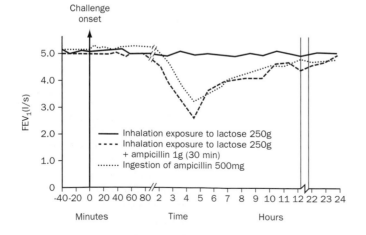

Fig. 37.3 Coeliac disease-associated precipitins. For abbreviations, see legend to Fig. 37.2. G, gluten.

derangement of the small bowel mucosa.[29] Precipitin tests were carried out on the sera of 25 patients with coeliac disease who had undergone initial or follow up small bowel biopsies within the preceding 3 years. Each biopsy was paired with the temporally most closely related precipitin test, and a 0–9 point scoring system was devised to quantify the mucosal abnormalities. The villi, crypts and lamina propria were scored independently 0–3 by a pathologist with special interest in coeliac disease. He had no prior knowledge of the source of each biopsy. The coeliac disease-associated precipitins were indeed found chiefly among the patients with the greater degrees of mucosal derangement (Fig. 37.4), and the mean scores of the precipitin-positive patients proved to be significantly greater than those who were precipitin-negative (Table 37.2).

Patients with active coeliac disease are consequently likely to show positive precipitin test results to bird serum irrespective of bird exposure or lung disease, and special care should be taken in interpreting the results when BFL is suspected in such patients.

Effect of smoking
The results of precipitin tests may also be seriously confounded by cigarette smoking. A number of investigators have now shown that precipitin responses to aetiological agents of EAA are diminished in smokers.[12,45,46,64] Some suggest that EAA is itself less common in smokers, but this is not easily confirmed or excluded in the absence of a precipitin response unless inhalation provo-

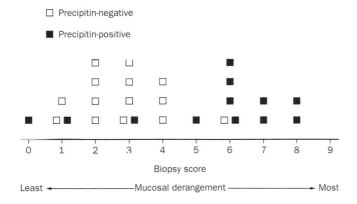

Fig. 37.4 Distribution of small bowel biopsy scores in subjects with and without coeliac disease-associated precipitins.

cation tests are performed. Definitive tests of this type were widely used by Faux and colleagues irrespective of the results of precipitin tests. Although precipitin responses were indeed less common in the smokers, it was less clear that BFL itself was associated with not smoking (Table 37.3).

Bird fancier's lung and coeliac disease
Inhalation provocation tests have been used to re-examine the suggested association between BFL and coeliac disease.[29] Thirteen consecutive patients proved to have BFL by these tests were invited to undergo small bowel biopsy, and 12 obliged. No biopsy was suggestive of coeliac disease. The mean biopsy score was 0.4 (compared with a maximum possible of 9.0), the range being 0–2. In a parallel study of 81 patients with biopsy-established coeliac disease, seven were found to be currently exposed to birds.[29] Three of these reported the onset of undue breathlessness during the period of bird exposure, and all three underwent inhalation provocation tests with appropriate avian antigens. One patient with several clinical features of EAA gave reproducible positive results. She was one of four currently exposed to budgerigars, a proportion which may be compared to a prevalence of BFL predicted among current budgerigar fanciers[28] in general of 0.5–7.5%.

Little significance can be attached to this single case in a statistical sense, and the investigators concluded that an association between these interesting disorders must be a weak one if it exists at all. They have since reported a second patient with both disorders.[48] Tarlo and colleagues[60] have, however, failed to find any evidence of an excess of diffuse alveolitis (of any cause) in a sample of 18 (of 28) patients with coeliac disease compared with 18 control subjects, while Berrill and colleagues[20] have reported villous atrophy in three of 28 further patients presumed to have BFL.

More recently, the British Thoracic Society has published its findings from a multicentre national survey of BFL.[52] Jejunal villous atrophy was demonstrated in five of 143 subjects thought to have BFL, a mild but significant excess over the expected prevalence in a normal population. The diagnostic criteria for BFL were not strict, however, and collaborating physicians were alerted to possible markers of coeliac disease at the time they entered patients into the study. This could have introduced a mild but important selection bias. The strength (or validity) of the suggested association between coeliac disease and alveolitis therefore remains controversial, and it may be that chance alone accounts for many of the reported cases where these two disorders coexist.

Mean small bowel biopsy scores of subjects with and without coeliac disease-associated precipitins		
Precipitins	**Biopsy scores**	
	Precipitin & biopsy intervals (mean)	
	<36 months (6.0) 26 paired results*	**<3 months (1.1) 11 paired results**
Present	5.3	6.2
Absent	2.9	3.0
P <	0.05	0.05

*One subject contributed two pairs.

Table 37.2 Mean small bowel biopsy scores of subjects with and without coeliac disease-associated precipitins.

Relation of smoking to bird fancier's lung (BFL) in 24 current bird fanciers (BF) undergoing diagnostic inhalation provocation tests with avian antigens		
	BF (n = 24)	**BFL confirmed (n = 15)**
Current smokers	7	4 (57%)
Current non-smokers	17	11 (65%)
P, n.s.		

Table 37.3 Relation of smoking to bird fancier's lung (BFL) in 24 current bird fanciers (BF) undergoing diagnostic inhalation provocation tests with avian antigens.

BIRD FANCIER'S LUNG AND EGG ALLERGY

There is the theoretical possibility that ingested egg could exacerbate or even initiate BFL. BFL-associated antigens can be demonstrated in chicken egg, and ingested chicken egg (and inhaled avian dust) can provoke asthmatic reactions in the lungs of sensitized individuals.[32] In most cases asthmatic sensitization probably results from gastrointestinal challenge, though occupational asthma attributable to allergy to inhaled egg has been described.[21] The affected workers used a spray system to coat meat rolls with egg solution. One also reported intolerance of ingested egg, but this was noted by a proportion of the unaffected workers.

Allergy to ingested egg appears to be the chief, if not sole, cause of adverse reactions to systemically administered vaccines that are raised in egg and contaminated by it.[17,51] Since they include skin rashes, asthma, angio-oedema, alveolitis and even fatal anaphylaxis, it seems undeniable that ingested egg, like cow's milk, can occasionally lead to a systemic hypersensitivity state. That BFL could become a consequence of childhood egg allergy in subjects who later become exposed to birds is thus an intriguing idea, but it is an idea that currently lacks any published confirmatory evidence. Similarly, the suggestion of a number of authors that ingested egg could adversely affect lungs that have become sensitized to inhaled avian dust (the so-called 'bird–egg syndrome'[42]) is supported chiefly by anecdotal experience. This stimulated us to review our data concerning possible egg intolerance among our own patients investigated for BFL.[29]

Like or dislike of chicken egg was compared in three groups of patients: the 15 in whom BFL was confirmed by inhalation provocation tests, the 12 in whom BFL was excluded using these tests, and 20 control patients who were selected at random from a respiratory ward. The results are given in Table 37.4. They show that a dislike of egg was significantly associated with BFL. Not all those disliking eggs admitted to definite adverse reactions, whereas two subjects who did describe adverse reactions claimed to enjoy eating eggs. Overall, six of the BFL group (40%) claimed adverse reactions compared with three (9%) from the other two groups. Most reported abdominal discomfort or diarrhoea, but some complained of nausea, an unpleasant taste, malaise or even (in two cases) increased breathlessness on exertion. It is interesting that some strongly related the onset of their intolerance to egg to the onset of their respiratory diseases, while others claimed the intolerance to be lifelong.

TOXIC (COOKING) OIL SYNDROME

In early 1981 an illegal unlabelled denatured rapeseed 'cooking' oil was sold widely to economically poorly privileged homes in the Madrid region of Spain, largely by door-to-door salesmen. The oil was cheap, had been denatured with aniline to ensure that it was used only in industry, and was 'diluted' with other oils of both vegetable and animal origin. However, it was subsequently refined in the hope that the aniline would be removed and the oil would be fit for human consumption. Over the following 12 months, some 20 000 consumers experienced a wide variety of serious adverse effects in many organs, and over 350 died.[5,6,36,61] Fortunately, the cause was quickly established, and with prompt government and news media action, the epidemic was quickly controlled. A pneumonic picture (with or without pleural effusion) with fever and flu-like symptoms dominated the earliest phase of the illness of those who became most intoxicated, and many of the deaths were a consequence of respiratory failure. In the survivors, a number of other effects were seen over the following months, and three distinct phases to the illness eventually became evident.

The first phase (week 1) was characterized principally by flu-like symptoms, cough, breathlessness, pulmonary infiltrates, pleural effusions, encephalitis, generalized lymphadenopathy and pruritic skin rashes. The intermediate phase, over the following 8 weeks, was dominated by gastrointestinal problems of abdominal pain, dysphagia, nausea and diarrhoea, and by eosinophilic leukocytosis. Finally, during the ensuing months of the third phase, some patients developed a prominent paralytic neuromuscular disorder, 'rheumatological' abnormalities such as arthritis and dry mouth, thromboembolic disorders or a scleroderma-like picture. Although the great majority of affected subjects survived, many were left with persisting disablement.

The more severely affected subjects tended to produce antinuclear autoantibodies (often in low titres) together with eosinophilia with raised IgE levels, and so immunological mechanisms have been postulated in addition to those which are more obviously toxic in nature. A widespread vasculitic picture became evident also from biopsy and autopsy material. Anilide derivatives of aniline, particularly oleoanilide, were subsequently reported to be the probable aetiological agents, but the precise mechanism of action has not been established.

For most diseases caused by environmental agents there is a wide spectrum of individual susceptibility and hence intolerance, and for some both toxic and hypersensitivity mechanisms are relevant. In the example of toxic cooking oil syndrome, toxic mechanisms clearly dominated, and potency was so great that the relevance of the food product was quickly recognized. Toxic agents of lesser potency would be recognized less readily, particularly if they are consumed irregularly, by smaller proportions of the population, or if only a proportion of the population was susceptible to hypersensitivity. This tragic example of 'food intolerance' in its widest sense provides an important stimulus to consideration of the possibility that ingested foods (and/or additives or contaminants) may indeed be relevant to some forms of parenchymal lung disease which are currently considered 'cryptogenic' in origin. The following sections provide additional stimuli.

BRONCHIOLITIS OBLITERANS AFTER INGESTION OF SAUROPUS ANDROGYNUS

Sauropus androgynus is an Asian shrub of the Euphoriaceae family, the leaves of which are thought (by some Asian people) to have

Dislike of egg in patients with bird fancier's lung (BFL)	
Subject group	Prevalence (%)
Confirmed BFL ($n = 15$)	47
Disproved BFL ($n = 12$)	8
Respiratory controls ($n = 20$)	10
$P = 0.01$.	

Table 37.4 Dislike of egg in patients with bird fancier's lung (BFL).

the property of controlling weight. The effect is not proven. In 1996 a more convincing property came to light, one which was most unexpected. In a remarkable period of less than 6 months, more than 60 patients who had ingested juice containing uncooked leaf extract of *Sauropus androgynus* presented to hospital in Taiwan with progressive undue breathlessness. In a study population of 23 of these patients breathlessness was severe and they were admitted to hospital, but the size of the population ingesting the extract from which the initial 60 were drawn (the denominator) is not known. The epidemiological significance of the outbreak (described by Lai and colleagues[38]) is consequently unclear, particularly as news media interest stimulated many of the initial presentations.

Clinical features

All 23 patients had progressive undue breathlessness, and 21 had cough which was usually non-productive. There was generally tachypnoea with impaired breath sounds, and there were crackles in 17 and wheezes in three. The mean forced expiratory volume in 1 second (FEV_1) was only 26% of predicted and the forced vital capacity (FVC) 51%, and there was no significant response to a bronchodilator. An elevated mean residual volume but not total lung capacity indicated air trapping, but the corrected gas transfer factor for carbon monoxide was said to be normal in 17. The diagnosis rested essentially on the appearances from high resolution computed tomography (CT) which showed patchy low attenuation of the lung parenchyma with a mosaic perfusion pattern in the expiratory images of all patients and in the inspiratory images of 11, abnormalities which are now recognized to be characteristic of obstructive bronchiolitis. All scans additionally showed bronchiectasis in the segmental and subsegmental bronchi. The plain radiographs were essentially normal.

Four patients underwent open lung biopsy, which revealed the characteristic appearance of obstructive bronchiolitis with a predominance of T lymphocytes. There was no histological or serological evidence of infection, and material from two biopsies gave negative results when cultured for viruses. The authors speculated that the disease was immunologically mediated.

Neither bronchodilator nor corticosteroid medication had any discernible beneficial effect, and there was no spontaneous resolution once ingestion of the leaf extract was discontinued. Severe respiratory impairment was, however, already established before the diagnosis was confirmed in any subject. The authors did not report whether there was continued progression after ingestion ceased.

Heat degradation and the role of cooking

The 23 patients were all women and non-smokers, and all had been well previously. Five had bought the leaf extract as a juice from local stores, and 18 had used home-made preparations. The authors remarked that the extract was commonly uncooked when consumed, although it is more generally used in Taiwan after cooking. Cooking might therefore 'detoxify' the relevant inducer of the bronchiolar disease. Significant heat denaturation would, however, reduce the possibility that the pulmonary reaction was the consequence of papaverine within the fresh leaves (about 580 mg/100 g), since this is resistant to such levels of heat. The leaf extract was apparently consumed in considerable quantities by each of the affected women (estimated range 2–21 kg over 10 weeks, mean 8 kg), and so other components will merit consideration as the primary inducing agent.

Comment

Although bronchiolitis obliterans is not commonly recognized in adults it is frequently diagnosed in childhood after adenovirus infection. Other established causes include autoimmune disease such as rheumatoid disease, and the inhalation of a number of toxic chemicals such as ammonia, chlorine and nitrogen dioxide. The disorder has gained particular prominence over recent years because of its occurrence complicating heart and lung transplantation, and this has identified the benefit (for this particular cause) of prompt immunosuppressive therapy. It is clear, therefore, that both toxic and immunological processes may be involved in pathogenesis.

Bronchiolitis obliterans is characterized by persistent inflammation of the bronchioli and proliferative occlusion of the lumina with fibroblasts and smooth muscle cells. Inflammatory cells, usually lymphocytes, are seen in the earlier stages. Once there is advanced fibrotic obliteration, little can be offered in terms of treatment, and so there has been a quest for methods of earlier diagnosis. In many cases the bronchiolar disease extends centrally to involve bronchi, which causes bronchiectasis. If it extends more distally to involve the alveoli there may be evidence of an organizing pneumonia, and a further disorder of unknown aetiology may be simulated – bronchiolitis obliterans and organizing pneumonia (BOOP).[23]

While pulmonary toxicity from a variety of oral medications is well recognized (for example, pulmonary hypertension from certain pharmacological appetite suppressants, and pulmonary fibrosis from certain cytotoxic agents) and regulatory mechanisms now greatly limit the chances of important adverse effects in epidemiological terms, the ingestion of unlicensed medications or 'fad' foods carries unknown risks and adverse effects are not readily identified. The novel discovery that bronchiolitis obliterans may occur, perhaps commonly, in populations ingesting the natural products of certain plants usefully illustrates that the lungs can be readily damaged by toxic or allergenic agents whose portal of entry is the gastrointestinal tract rather than the airways, and that serendipity is often necessary before such a problem is recognized.

FOOD-INDUCED ALVEOLAR/BRONCHIOLAR DISORDERS IN OTHER SPECIES

Fog fever

A naturally occurring febrile pneumonic disease of cattle follows their return from poor summer grazing in high moorland pasture to lush valley meadows recovering unmolested from earlier hay harvests. It is generally known in Britain as 'fog fever', fog being a northern term for autumn or the fall.[44] It is characterized by pulmonary consolidation and emphysema. Its precise cause is uncertain, though it is presumably related to a noxious constituent or metabolite of grass (perhaps D,L-tryptophan) or a contaminant (perhaps mould) which is particularly prevalent in autumn and to which the cattle lose tolerance during their summer months in different pastures. Toxic mechanisms appear more likely than those of hypersensitivity, and it should be noted that fog fever is not 'farmer's lung (i.e. EAA attributable to mouldy hay) in cattle'.

Sweet potatoes and *Fusarium* contamination

An apparently similar disease associated with feeding cattle mouldy sweet potatoes has been recognized for 50 years in North

America,[50] and more recently in Australia.[31] It too is characterized by pneumonic infiltration and emphysema, and it is more clearly related to mould contamination. In one outbreak in Texas as many as 69 from a herd of 275 cows died of the disorder.[50] Respiratory distress, rapid breathing, cough and a frothy exudate around the mouth shortly before death are common clinical features, and autopsy examinations have demonstrated the presence of marked oedema, inflammatory cell infiltration (including eosinophils), alveolar wall proliferation, hyaline membranes, haemorrhagic foci, bronchiolitis obliterans and emphysema in the absence of any microorganisms. After the Texas incident, the sweet potatoes were examined for mould contamination and many species were discovered, possibly because the potatoes had been stored for some weeks in conditions of moisture and temperature which particularly favoured mould growth. When oven-dried samples of the mouldy sweet potatoes were fed experimentally to chicks there was a consistent pattern of death which provided useful supportive evidence that the contaminated sweet potatoes were indeed responsible for the cattle deaths, although other members of the herd and a hog appeared unaffected.

Aetiological suspicion fell on a number of species of *Fusarium*. An isolate of *F. solani* was used to infest other (viable) sweet potatoes experimentally and when these were fed to 16 cattle an apparently identical respiratory disease caused death in three. Furthermore, there was a parallel mortality rate when chicks were fed with corn on which the same isolate had been grown.

The explanation for this dramatic food-induced 'alveolar' disease has proved to be complex and fascinating, and cattle have proved to be particularly susceptible. When stressed (for example by mechanical injury, insect invasion or microbial infection), the sweet potato may produce phytoalexin metabolites. These may in turn be catabolized by certain species of *Fusarium* to produce a number of toxic furanoterpenoid compounds. One of these, 4-ipomeanol, has been produced synthetically and has been shown to reproduce 'mouldy sweet potato respiratory disease' in both cattle and laboratory mice after oral administration.[19] It is difficult to imagine such complexity being uncovered from the study of human respiratory disease. Individual members of human population groups rarely consume identical diets, and very rarely consume these consistently from day to day in large quantities; hence, the epidemiological conditions under which this disease has been recognized in cattle are not likely to arise in humans. This is not to say that similar mechanisms do not operate sporadically in humans with cryptogenic forms of parenchymal lung disease.

Crotalaria juncea seed

A further reported example of a pulmonary toxin ingested as a foodstuff in a mammal is the *Crotalaria juncea* seed.[49] The genus *Crotalaria* is a legume which valuably contributes humus and nitrogen to the soil for horticulture. Its seeds are used as a fertilizer but, because of their high protein content and their ready availability on a farm in Brazil, they were fed with maize (40:60) to 20 adult horses and a number of cattle. Within 30 days all the horses, but none of the cattle, died of a similar disease which was characterized by a diffuse fibrosing alveolitis with inflammatory infiltration and interstitial oedema. In addition, there was congestion of the liver, but the pulmonary abnormalities dominated and were considered to be the primary cause of death. The cattle appeared unaffected. *Crotalaria* species are known to produce toxic pyrrolizidine alkaloids, and these are recognized to pose a risk of hepatotoxicity to a number of domesticated animals if ingested. Metabolism within the host liver is generally necessary to produce the metabolites of greatest toxicity, and so different susceptibilities between species is to be expected. Pulmonary toxicity had not previously been reported, but the seeds appear not to have been used previously as a major foodstuff for horses.

CONCLUSIONS

While evidence linking ingested foods (or food additives/contaminants) with, specifically, alveolitis remains limited in humans, there is increasing recognition that the gastrointestinal tract may provide a portal of entry for agents which cause disease of the lung parenchyma in a number of species. Some involve the alveoli, lung interstitium, and/or adjacent bronchioli, and both hypersensitivity and toxic mechanisms may be involved. Alveolitis attributable to food allergy or intolerance consequently lies well within the fringe of credibility, and may eventually provide the explanation for a number of parenchymal disorders of the lung which are currently considered 'cryptogenic' in origin.

ACKNOWLEDGEMENTS

We are grateful to Dr J A Faux for Figs 37.2 and 37.3 and for her collaboration in much of the work we have quoted concerning bird fancier's lung and coeliac disease. We are also grateful to Prof T Higenbottam who allowed us to use text (partly modified) from an article he wrote with DJH concerning *Sauropus androgynus*.[30]

REFERENCES

1 Agata H, Kondo N, Fukutomi O *et al*. Pulmonary hemosiderosis with hypersensitivity to buckwheat. *Ann Allergy Asthma Immunol* 1997; 78: 233–7.

2 Anonymous. Antigen absorption by the gut [Editorial]. *Lancet* 1978; ii: 715.

3 Anonymous. Bird fancier's lung and jejunal villous atrophy [Editorial]. *Med J Aust* 1976; 1: 813.

4 Anonymous. Coeliac lung disease [Editorial]. *Lancet* 1978; i: 917.

5 Anonymous. Toxic epidemic syndrome, Spain, 1981. *Lancet* 1982; ii: 696–702.

6 Anonymous. Toxic oil syndrome [Editorial]. *Lancet* 1983; i: 1257–8.

7 Bailey P, Groden BM. Idiopathic pulmonary haemo-siderosis: report of two cases and review of the literature. *Postgrad Med J* 1979; 55: 266–72.

8 Benson MK, Lancaster-Smith MJ, Perrin J *et al*. Serum immunoglobulins, autoantibodies and avian precipitins in adult coeliac disease, and avian antigen inhalation provocation tests in patients with adult coeliac disease and diffuse interstitial lung disease. *Arch Fr Mal App Digestift* 1972; 61: 398.

9 Berrill WT, Eade OE, Fitzpatrick PF *et al*. Bird fancier's lung and jejunal villous atrophy. *Lancet* 1975; ii: 1006.

10 Berrill WT, Eade OE, Macleod WM *et al*. Proceedings: bird fancier's lung and coeliac disease. *Gut* 1975; 16: 825–6.

11 Bouros D, Panagou P, Rokkas T, Siafakas NM. Bronchoalveolar lavage findings in a young adult with idiopathic pulmonary haemosiderosis and coeliac disease. *Eur Respir J* 1994; 7: 1009–12.

12 Boyd G, Madkour M, Middleton S, Lynch P. Effect of smoking on circulating antibody levels to avian protein in pigeon breeder's disease. *Thorax* 1977; 32: 651.

13 Brettner A, Heitzman ER, Woodin WG. Pulmonary complications of drug therapy. *Radiology* 1970; 96: 31.

14 Brostoff J, Challacombe SJ (eds). *Food allergy. Clinics in Immunology and Allergy*. WB Saunders, London, 1982.

15 Cantor HM, Dumont AE. Hepatic suppression of sensitization to antigen absorbed into the portal system. *Nature* 1967; 215: 744–5.

16 Cummiskey J, Keelan P, Weir DG. Coeliac disease and diffuse pulmonary disease (corresp). *BMJ* 1976; i: 1401.

17 Davies RJ, Pepys J. Egg allergy, influenza vaccine and immunoglobulin E antibody. *J Allergy Clin Immunol* 1976; 57: 373.

18 Davies RJ, Hendrick DJ, Pepys J. Asthma due to inhaled chemical agents: ampicillin, benzyl penicillin, 6 amino penicillanic acid and related substances. *Clin Allergy* 1974; 4: 227.

19 Doster AR, Mitchell FE, Farrell RL, Wilson BJ. Effects of 4-ipomeanol, a product from mould-damaged sweet potatoes, on the bovine lung. *Vet Pathol* 1978; 15: 367–75.

20 Eade OE, Hodges JR, Berrill WT *et al*. Immunofluorescent antibodies in patients with bird fancier's lung. *Clin Exp Immunol* 1978; 132: 263.

21 Edwards JH, McConnachie K, Trotman DM *et al*. Allergy to inhaled egg material. *Clin Allergy* 1983; 13: 427–32.

22 Faux JA, Hendrick DJ, Anand BS. Precipitins to different avian serum antigens in bird fancier's lung and coeliac disease. *Clin Allergy* 1977; 8: 101.

23 Geddes DM, Corrin B, Brewerton D, David RJ, Turner-Warwick M. Progressive airway obliteration in adults and its association with rheumatoid disease. *Q J Med* 1977; 46: 427–44.

24 Gudmundsson G, Hunninghake GW. Interferon γ is necessary for the expression of hypersensitivity pneumonitis. *J Clin Invest* 1997; 99: 2386 90.

25 Gunther M, Aschaffenberg R, Matthews RH *et al*. The level of antibodies to proteins of cow's milk in the serum of normal infants. *Immunology* 1960; 3: 296–306.

26 Heiner DC, Sears JW, Kniker WT. Multiple precipitins to cow's milk in chronic respiratory disease. *Am J Dis Child* 1962; 103: 634.

27 Hendrick DJ. *Bird Fancier's Lung – Clinical, epidemiological and laboratory features*. MD Thesis, University of London, 1979.

28 Hendrick DJ, Faux JA, Marshall R. Budgerigar fancier's lung: the commonest variety of allergic alveolitis in Britain. *BMJ* 1978; ii: 81.

29 Hendrick DJ, Faux JA, Anand B *et al*. Is bird fancier's lung associated with coeliac disease? *Thorax* 1978; 33: 425.

30 Higenbottam T W. Bronchiolitis obliterms following the ingestion of an Asian shrub leaf. *Thorax* 1997; 52(suppl 3): S68–72.

31 Hill BD, Wright HF. Acute interstitial pneumonia in cattle associated with consumption of mould-damaged sweet potatoes (*Ipomoea batatas*). *Aust Vet J* 1992; 69: 36–7.

32 Hoigne R, Scherrer M. An attack of bronchial asthma produced by egg-white and studied by means of lung function tests. *Int Arch Allergy* 1960; 17: 152.

33 Hood J, Mason AMS. Diffuse pulmonary disease with transfer defect occurring with coeliac disease. *Lancet* 1970; i: 445.

34 Jakobsson I, Linberg T. Cow's milk as a cause of infantile colic in breast-fed infants. *Lancet* 1978; ii: 437.

35 Joint Report of the Royal College of Physicians and the British Nutrition Foundation. Food intolerance and food aversion. *R Coll Physicians Lond J* 1984; 18: 83–123.

36 Kilbourne EM, Rigau-Perez JG, Heath CW *et al*. Clinical epidemiology of toxic oil syndrome. *N Engl J Med* 1983; 309: 1408–14.

37 Kuroume T, Oguri M, Matsumura T *et al*. Milk sensitivity and soybean sensitivity in the production of eczematous manifestations in breast-fed infants with particular reference to intrauterine sensitization. *Ann Allergy* 1976; 37: 41.

38 Lai R-S, Chiang AA, Wu M-T *et al*. Outbreak of bronchiolitis obliterans associated with consumption of *Sauropus androgynus*. *Lancet* 1996; 348: 83–5.

39 Lancaster-Smith MJ, Benson MK, Strickland ID. Coeliac disease and diffuse interstitial lung disease. *Lancet* 1971; i: 473.

40 Lancaster-Smith MJ, Swarbrick ET, Perrin J, Wright JT. Coeliac disease and autoimmunity. *Postgrad Med* 1974; 50: 45.

41 Lane DJ, Hamilton WS. Idiopathic steatorrhoea and idiopathic pulmonary haemosiderosis. *BMJ* 1971; ii: 89–90.

42 Mandallaz MM, Dahinden CA, de Weck AL. Bird-egg syndrome. *Int Arch Allergy Appl Immunol* 1988; 87: 143–50.

43 May CD. Food allergy – a commentary. *Pediatr Clin North Am* 1975; 122: 217.

44 MacKenzie A. Fog fever in cattle. *Proc R Soc Med* 1966; 59: 1008.

45 Morgan DC, Smyth JT, Lister RW, Pethybridge RJ. Chest symptoms and farmer's lung: a community survey. *Br J Ind Med* 1973; 30: 1259–65.

46 Morgan DC, Smyth JT, Lister RW *et al*. Chest symptoms in farming communities with special reference to farmer's lung. *Br J Ind Med* 1975; 132: 228–34.

47 Morris JS, Read AE, Jones B *et al*. Coeliac disease and lung disease. *Lancet* 1971; i: 754.

48 Muers MF, Faux JA, Ting A, Morris PJ. HLA A, B, C, and HLA-DR antigens in extrinsic allergic alveolitis (budgerigar fancier's lung disease). *Clin Allergy* 1982; 12: 47–57.

49 Nobre D, Dagli MLZ, Haraguchi M. *Crotalaria juncea* intoxication in horses. *Vet Human Toxicol* 1994; 36: 445–8.

50 Peckham JC, Mitchell FE, Jones OH, Doupnik B. Atypical interstitial pneumonia in cattle fed mouldy sweet potatoes. *J Am Vet Med Assoc* 1972; 160: 169–72.

51 Ratner B, Untracht S. Allergy to virus and rickettsial vaccines. 1. Allergy to influenza A and B vaccine in children. *JAMA* 1946; 132: 899.

52 Report to the Research Committee of the British Thoracic Society. A national survey of bird fancier's lung: including its possible association with jejunal villous atrophy. *Br J Dis Chest* 1984; 178: 75–88.

53 Robinson TJ. Coeliac disease with farmer's lung. *BMJ* 1976; ii: 745.

54 Robinson TJ. Coeliac disease with farmer's lung (corresp). *BMJ* 1976; ii: 593.

55 Rosenow EC. The spectrum of drug-induced pulmonary disease. *Ann Intern Med* 1972; 77: 977.

56 Schuyler M, Gott K, Edwards B. Experimental hypersensitivity pneumonitis: cellular requirements. *Clin Exp Immunol* 1996; 105: 169–75.

57 Semenzato G, Zambello R, Trentin L, Agostini C. Cellular immunity in sarcoidosis and hypersensitivity pneumonitis: recent advances. *Chest* 1993; 103: 1395.

58 Strobel S, Mowat AM, Drummond HE *et al*. Immunological responses to fed protein antigens in mice. 2. Oral tolerance for CM 1 is due to activation of cyclophosphamide sensitive cells by gut processed antigen. *Immunology* 1983; 149: 457–66.

59 Stuart CA, Twiselton R, Nicholas MK, Wilde DW. Passage of cow's milk protein in breast milk. *Clin Allergy* 1984; 14: 573–5.

60 Tarlo SM, Brodes I, Prokipchuk EJ *et al*. Association between coeliac disease and lung disease. *Chest* 1981; 80: 715–18.

61 Tabuenca JM. Toxic-allergic syndrome caused by ingestion of rapeseed oil denatured with aniline. *Lancet* 1981; ii: 567–8.

62 Walker WA. Antigen absorption from the small intestine and gastrointestinal disease. *Pediatr Clin N Am* 1975; 22: 731.

63 Walker WA. Antigenic uptake in the gut: immunological implications. *Immunol Today* 1981; 2: 30–4.

64 Warren CPW. Extrinsic allergic alveolitis: a disease commoner in non-smokers. *Thorax* 1977; 32: 567–9.

65 Wright PH, Menzies IS, Pounder RE, Keeling PIWN. Adult idiopathic pulmonary haemosiderosis and coeliac disease. *Q J Med* 1981; 50: 95–102.

66 Hendrick DJ, Marshall R, Faux JA, Krall JM. Positive 'alveolar' response to antigen inhalation provocation tests: their validity and recognition. *Thorax* 1980; 35: 415–27.

A

Chapter 38

Intestinal manifestations of food allergy and intolerance

Stephan C. Bischoff and Julika H. Mayer

INTRODUCTION

There have frequently been doubts as to the clinical relevance of food allergy, in particular as far as the involvement of the intestinal tract is concerned. Whereas the importance of food allergic reactions as a cause of intestinal disorders in children is well accepted, the significance of gastrointestinal (GI) allergy in adults is still questioned. However, there is substantial evidence in the literature as well as from our own experience that allergic reactions exist in the GI tract, and that this food allergic enteropathy is of relevance not only in children, but in certain adult patients as well.[10,22,45]

The doubts confronting GI allergy are mainly because of the fact that these manifestations can hardly be visualized, as is possible in skin reactions, or measured, as by bronchial obstruction or hyperresponsiveness in allergic asthma. Because of both a lack of standardized diagnostic procedures and inaccessibility of the target organ, current knowledge of epidemiology, clinical manifestations, involved pathomechanisms and specific therapy is poor. The role of GI hypersensitivity reactions in the natural history of disorders such as inflammatory bowel disease (e.g. Crohn's disease and ulcerative colitis) and irritable bowel syndrome remains controversial.[3,28,50]

EPIDEMIOLOGY

Probably the most reliable data concerning the epidemiology of food allergy in adults are presented in a population study by Young et al.[49] This survey used double blind placebo-controlled food challenges to confirm reported reactions to food on an objective basis. The results of this investigation suggest that the prevalence of food allergy in adults is about 1.4%. In this study, 28% of the individuals with diagnosed food allergy had intestinal symptoms.

Compared to adults, a higher prevalence of food allergy is found in children under 3 years of age. According to the literature, 2–8% of children are afflicted.[15,29] The most relevant allergen in childhood seems to be cow's milk, with 2.2% of children having been described to suffer from cow's milk allergy.[15,26] Most children tend to outgrow their allergy by the third[26] or, at the latest, sixth[14] year of age.

CLINICAL MANIFESTATIONS

Allergic reactions of the GI tract may occur within minutes to several hours after ingestion of the offending food allergen and present as a variety of clinical findings. They include nausea, vomiting, abdominal pain, cramps and distension, flatulence, constipation, or diarrhoea.[10,13,16,22] Occult faecal blood loss and malabsorption have also been reported in association with GI tract allergic response. Unfortunately, these features also typify other GI disorders such as Crohn's disease, ulcerative colitis,[37,38] or irritable bowel syndrome, so a differential diagnosis often proves to be difficult. At present, it is unclear whether there exists (beside the immediate type reactions following allergen contact) a delayed-type or chronic form of allergic enteropathy with persistent inflammatory alterations of the intestinal mucosa.

In the experience of this department, the most relevant allergens for intestinal food allergy are milk proteins, hazelnut, wheat, apple, pork and egg.[12] Important clinical aspects of intestinal allergic reactions are summarized in Table 38.1.

Eosinophilic gastroenteritis

In the context of intestinal allergy, eosinophilic gastroenteritis must also be mentioned. It is a rare disease of unknown aetiology characterized by pronounced eosinophil accumulation and activation in

Clinical aspects of gastrointestinal allergic reactions in adults

Clinical syptoms	Relevant allergens	Differential diagnosis
Nausea	Milk	Crohn's disease
Vomiting	Hazelnut	Ulcerative colitis
Abdominal pains	Wheat	Eosinophilic gastroenteritis
Cramping	Apple	Coeliac disease
Distension	Pork	Lactase deficiency
Flatulence	Egg	Infectious diseases
Constipation	Celery	Tumour diseases
Diarrhoea	Carrots	Irritable bowel syndrome
Intestinal oedema	Inhalation?	Pseudoallergic reactions

Table 38.1 Clinical aspects of gastrointestinal allergic reactions in adults.

the GI tract. Eosinophil infiltration can involve all parts of the GI tract, from the oesophagus to the rectum. In most cases, infiltration is limited to the mucosa, but sometimes the muscle layer or the subserosa are predominantly affected. This disease presents clinically with abdominal pain, cramps, nausea, diarrhoea, malabsorption and, if the subserosa is infiltrated, eosinophilic ascites. It is interesting that 25–50% of patients are reported to have a food allergy.[34,48]

PATHOGENESIS

Whereas allergic reactions have been studied extensively in human skin and respiratory mucosa, little is known about the pathophysiology of intestinal hypersensitivity reactions, and most available information comes from animal studies.[18]

Mast cells, the well recognized key cells of type I hypersensitivity reactions, are found at multiple body sites, including the GI tract. The mast cell density in the intestinal mucosa is even higher than in the skin, for example 2–3% of the lamina propria cells in the gut are mast cells and are located in the neighbourhood of blood vessels, nerves and lymphatic tissue. Mast cells have been known for 20 years to be involved in the pathomechanisms of intestinal disorders such as Crohn's disease, ulcerative colitis and coeliac disease. For example, degranulating mast cells have been found in the gut mucosa of patients with Crohn's disease,[21] and elevated mast cell numbers in jejunal mucosa were detected in patients with coeliac disease.[47]

Mast cell activation also seems to be of importance in GI food allergy. Research has shown that intestinal mucosal mast cells degranulate and release histamine upon allergen stimulation in rats that are sensitized against cow's milk or egg albumin.[36] Some human studies have demonstrated the involvement of mast cells in hypersensitivity reactions of the GI tract. In endoscopic intragastral provocation tests performed by Reimann and Lewin[42] and Bagnato et al.,[2] mast cell and histamine changes in the mucosa were reported. Consistent with these findings, this unit also found mast

cell activation in caecal biopsies after colonoscopic allergen provocation (Fig. 38.1).[13] Mast cell stimulation results in the release of various mediators and proteases (e.g. histamine, tryptase, chymase, leukotrienes). By virtue of these biologically active substances, mast cells have a significant potential to modulate gut function. Crosslinking of immunoglobulin (Ig)E receptors has been shown to stimulate epithelial ion transport, increase vascular permeability, diminish barrier integrity, cause mucosal oedema and contraction of intestinal smooth muscle.[20,36] These alterations may account for the clinical findings associated with food-allergic enteropathy.

Several recent studies and reviews have focused on the function of eosinophilic granulocytes in GI disease.[23,32] There is increasing evidence that activation of eosinophils plays a role in the pathogenesis of non-infectious inflammatory bowel diseases such as Crohn's disease, ulcerative colitis and coeliac disease.[9,33,39] Less is known about the role of eosinophils in the pathophysiology of GI hypersensitivity reactions, although the importance of eosinophils in allergic conditions of other organs is well established.[43] In recent years, however, some findings have been reported that imply an involvement of eosinophils in food-allergic reactions of the gut. For example, the present authors and others

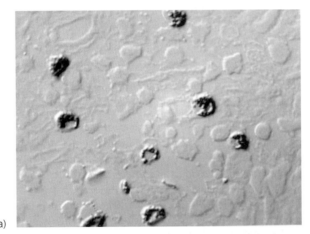

(a)

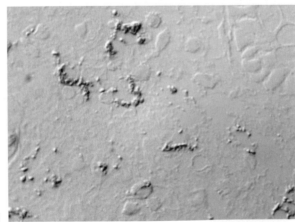

(b)

Fig. 38.1 Mast cell degranulation after colonoscopic allergen provocation. The figure demonstrates mast cells in the lamina propria of caecal mucosa in an individual having food allergy. Mast cells were stained by immunohistochemistry using an anti-histamine antibody. (a) In endoscopically normal, unstimulated mucosa, mast cells are densely filled with granula. (b) Intramucosal provocation with apple allergen in the COLAP test led to a clear macroscopic weal and flare reaction. In biopsies of this area, significant mast cell degranulation is found.

have found that the levels of eosinophil granule proteins such as eosinophil cationic protein (ECP) or eosinophil protein X (EPX) in faeces are elevated in patients with intestinal food allergy.[9,31] Local stimulation of the gut mucosa of food-allergic patients with the relevant antigens led to an activation of mucosal eosinophils which was detected by electron microscopy[13] and immunohistochemistry (Bischoff and Mayer, unpublished data), as well as to an intestinal secretion of ECP.[5] In both studies, eosinophil activation took place within 20 min of allergen challenge of the mucosa, whereas, to date, eosinophil activation has been associated particularly with allergic late phase reactions occurring 2–4 h after allergen challenge in some individuals, mainly in the respiratory system and skin.[43] The mechanism of the observed rapid eosinophil activation is unclear. Both a directly stimulating effect of the allergen on eosinophils by crosslinking surface-bound IgE[17] and IgA, or an indirect effect, e.g. via mast cell mediators, which may induce eosinophil degranulation,[40] may be anticipated. These data suggest that eosinophils may be involved in the immediate phase of food-allergic enteropathy. Figure 38.2 illustrates the pathogenesis of GI allergic reactions.

DIAGNOSTIC PROCEDURES

The methods available to confirm the diagnosis of GI allergy are insufficient at present, and therefore it remains difficult to identify afflicted patients on an objective basis. The classical allergologic tests (skin test, radioallergosorbent test; RAST) often fail to deliver reliable results in cases in which the GI tract is involved exclusively. Thus, new laboratory methods have been established to measure IgE or eosinophil-derived mediators in stool samples.[9,30,39] In addition, some attempts have been made to develop local provocation tests. Most have to date, however, not exceeded experimental status.

A selection of diagnostic procedures for intestinal allergy is discussed below. Nevertheless, in addition to the allergologic tests, it is important to perform careful *gastroenterological work-up*. Since the symptoms of intestinal allergy are non-specific and variable, the diagnosis is, to a large degree, made by exclusion. Lactose tolerance and malabsorption tests, microbiological examinations, ultrasound and endoscopy can serve to exclude non-allergic causes of GI disorders.[16]

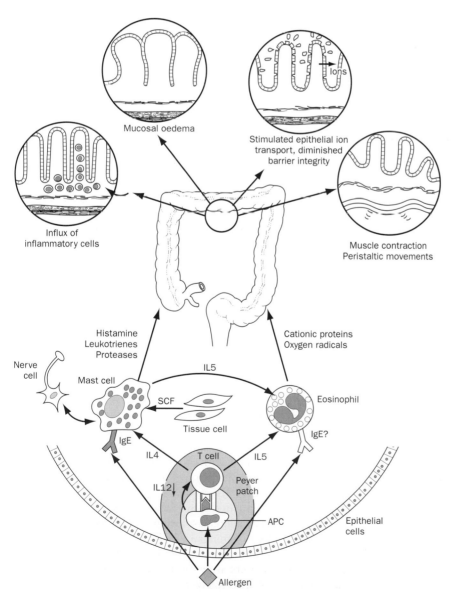

Fig. 38.2 Pathogenesis of gastrointestinal allergic reactions. APC, antigen-presenting cell; SCF, stem cell factor.

In vitro tests

Radioallergosorbent test

The RAST, or other appropriate enzymatic tests, allow the quantification of allergen-specific IgE in serum. Elevated total IgE or high levels of IgE antibodies to specific foods may argue for the presence of an IgE-mediated allergic disorder. They cannot, however, establish the diagnosis of a clinical food allergy, particularly as sensitivity is low compared to oral food challenge tests and normal values of such parameters do not exclude intestinal allergy.[5,12,44] A possible explanation of this discrepancy may be that hypersensitivity reactions of the gut are mediated by *local* IgE that is not necessarily reflected by serum levels. Older studies have shown that IgE concentration in faeces and intestinal juice does not correlate with IgE concentration in the blood.[4,30] Huggins and Brostoff[27] described a group of patients with dust mite allergic rhinitis who had a negative RAST and skin test, whereas in nasal fluid, specific IgE was detected that did not correlate with serum levels. A similar phenomenon might be present in the GI mucosa.

Measurement of parameters in faeces

In patients with allergic enteropathy, elevated levels of eosinophilic granule proteins, e.g. ECP and EPX can be measured in faeces,[9,31] suggesting eosinophil activation in the gut mucosa. However, increased faecal concentrations of ECP and EPX are also found in patients with Crohn's disease and ulcerative colitis.[7,9,11,39] Single attempts have also been made to measure IgE levels in faeces from allergic individuals.[1,30]

'Ex vivo' stimulation tests

Basophil histamine release test

It can be shown that isolated peripheral blood-derived basophils from patients with food allergy have an increased rate of spontaneous histamine release compared to controls.[46] Dispersed mast cells and basophils from jejunal mucosa of patients with food allergy were found to release histamine when stimulated with the relevant food extracts.[35] These test procedures, however, are of experimental character and are not yet established for routine diagnosis.

Cellular allergen stimulation test

The cellular allergen stimulation test is an alternative *in vitro* approach similar to the basophil histamine release test.[19] There is limited experience with this test procedure to date, but sensitivity and specificity seem to be at least comparable to those of the RAST.

Tissue oxygenation provocation

Intestinal biopsies taken endoscopically undergo oxygenation in a so-called 'Tabbox' system and are incubated with food antigens. Relevant allergens lead to significantly increased rates of mediator secretion (tryptase, ECP, tumour necrosis factor; TNF) from intestinal tissue. These functional release experiments are used for allergen identification. The results of mucosa oxygenation and mediator determination have been found to predict the outcome of oral food challenge tests[41] with a sensitivity of 78% and a specificity of 100%. An appreciable advantage of this method is the ability to challenge the involved organ in an 'ex vivo' manner without the risk of inducing an anaphylactic reaction in the patient. However, controlled studies to validate these preliminary data are still awaited.

In vivo provocation tests

Skin prick test

Similar to the RAST, the skin prick test (SPT) indicates the presence of systemic allergen-specific IgE, and thus, it has similar drawbacks to the RAST. A patient who experiences hypersensitivity reactions in the GI tract does not necessarily have positive skin reactions after prick test provocation, possibly because of local intestinal IgE production. Accordingly, the use of this test in the diagnosis of intestinal hypersensitivity has serious limitations.[13,44]

Elimination and re-challenge diet

Elimination diet and re-challenge can be a valid, objective method for confirming a diagnosis of food-allergic enteropathy[22] but, in practice, this approach has limitations because of difficulties in eliminating the suspected food allergens. This method depends on the correct choice of food to be avoided, patient compliance, and the type of food. In addition, a properly carried out elimination and re-introduction diet is a protracted procedure, taking days or even weeks. To avoid fatal reactions, patients must be carefully selected, and challenges should be performed in hospital settings.

Double blind placebo-controlled food challenge

Oral challenge procedures with food substances are acknowledged as the gold standard for the confirmation of intestinal food allergy.[16,44] In this method, food antigen as well as placebo is given in blinded form (e.g. in capsules), and the patients' symptoms after ingestion are registered. At present, a positive double blind placebo-controlled food challenge (DBPCFC) is considered the only conclusive evidence of food allergy provided it is performed properly.[16] However, there are several practical problems connected with the DBPCFC. One of these problems is the read-out system. The test procedure was originally developed for patients with food-induced urticaria or atopic dermatitis. In these patients, symptoms after ingestion of a food can easily be demonstrated and registered. The most important drawback of the DBPCFC in GI allergy, however, is that most patients present only subjective symptoms which cannot be objectively verified (e.g. abdominal pain, cramps, nausea), so the interpretation of test results is often unsatisfactory.[16] In most cases of intestinal allergy, the read-out systems depend on the patients' subjective reports of their experienced symptoms, although the test procedure itself is performed in an objective, placebo-controlled manner. An additional disadvantage is the variable time interval between ingestion and onset of symptoms, which may occur hours or days after ingestion if, for example, the colonic mucosa is the target organ. Finally, the DBPCFC does not discriminate between food allergy and food intolerance. The experiences in this department with the DBPCFC in patients with allergic enteropathy have been largely disappointing.[13]

Jejunal perfusion

An alternative approach with a more objective read-out system has been proposed by Bengtsson *et al.*[6] During endoscopy of the upper intestinal tract, a 10-cm long segment in the proximal part of the jejunum was isolated using a two-balloon six-channel tube and perfused with an allergen solution. Samples of the perfusate were collected after 20 min, and ECP and histamine levels were measured. The authors found increased mediator concentrations in food-allergic patients after allergen challenge. This methodology has been performed solely in patients with cow's milk allergy to date. The rather large amount of allergen solution required for the challenge (10 ml cow's milk) increases the risk of anaphylactic reaction. A minor disadvantage of this technically complicated procedure is that the changes in the mucosa are not visible, and biopsies cannot be taken. So far, this technique is reserved to research settings.

Gastroscopic provocation tests

In previous studies, attempts have been made to challenge gastric mucosa with food allergens during gastroscopy. Mucosal changes with oedema, reddening and bleeding of the stimulated area were reported in cases of challenges with a food allergen. However, these tests could not be established for clinical practice.[2,42]

Colonoscopic allergen provocation test

The idea of local challenge in the GI tract was used to develop the colonoscopic allergen provocation (COLAP) test.[12,13] During colonoscopy, liquid (food) antigen extracts, a buffer control and a positive control containing histamine are injected into the mucosa of the caecum with a fine needle. The antigen extracts are selected according to patient's history and/or RAST results. Three to four different antigens are tested in each patient. After 20 min, the weal and flare reaction of the provoked mucosa is registered semiquantitatively using a score from 0 to 4, and biopsies are taken from the provocation areas as well as from unprovoked caecal mucosa (Fig. 38.3). To date, more than 100 patients with suspected GI food allergy and 10 healthy volunteers have undergone the COLAP test. There has been no systemic anaphylactic reaction in response to intestinal challenge, except in one patient who had generalized urticaria. When there was a positive reaction, weal and flare began approximately 2 min after antigen challenge and was at its maximum after 10–15 min. Whereas there was no positive mucosal reaction to antigen challenge in the control group, about 50% of all antigens tested positive in the patient group. Histamine injection led to a mucosal weal and flare reaction in 70% of the patients and 80% of the control individuals, and buffer injection was always negative. Antigen-induced weal and flare reactions were correlated with patients' history of adverse reactions to food, but not with serum levels of total or specific IgE or skin test results (Table 38.2).

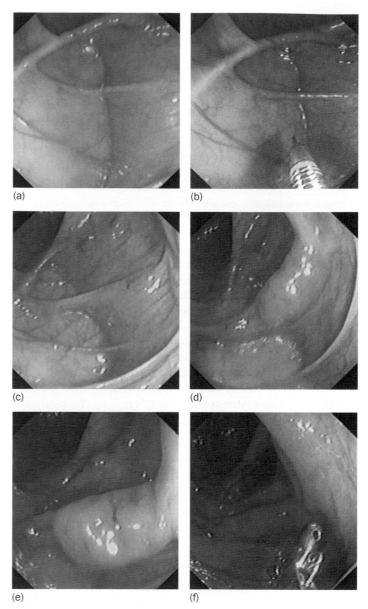

(a)   (b)
(c)   (d)
(e)   (f)

Fig. 38.3 Colonoscopic allergen provocation. During colonoscopy of a suspected food-allergic patient, wheat allergen extract is injected into the mucosa of the caecum using a fine needle (**a–c**). After 15 min, a significant weal and flare reaction develops in the provoked area (**d,e**). After 20 min, biopsies are taken (**f**).

Correlation of different clinical test results in patients with food allergy			
Clinical test			**P**
Clinical history	versus	RAST	n.s.
Clinical history	versus	Skin prick test	n.s.
Skin prick test	versus	RAST	<0.01
COLAP	versus	Skin prick test	n.s.
COLAP	versus	RAST	n.s./<0.03*
COLAP	versus	Clinical history	<0.02

COLAP, colonoscopic allergen provocation test; RAST, radioallergosorbent test. *Interestingly, there was a correlation between COLAP test results and RAST in case already CAP class ≥ 1 was considered positive (P<0.03), whereas no correlation was found in case CAP class ≥ 2 – as usual – was considered positive. This finding suggests that minor specific IgE levels in serum may be of clinical relevance in intestinal allergy (Statistical test, Pearson's χ^2; n = 70.)

Table 38.2 Correlation of different clinical test results in patients with food allergy.

The clinical relevance of the COLAP test results has yet to be evaluated. A preliminary follow up showed that an individual diet with strict elimination of each food that tested positive in the COLAP, in a few cases combined with additional antiallergic medication, seems to achieve an improvement of symptoms in the majority of patients.[13]

A disadvantage of this technique is that late-phase reactions escape diagnosis unless a second colonoscopy with re-evaluation of the provoked areas is performed the next day. Table 38.3 shows a synopsis of the different diagnostic methods.

THERAPY

In cases in which a relevant food allergen can be identified as a cause of GI complaints, a diet with elimination of the responsible

Diagnostic procedures to confirm the diagnosis of gastrointestinal food allergy		
In vitro	**Ex vivo**	**In vivo**
Total IgE in stool and serum	Basophil histamine release test	Skin prick test
Specific IgE in serum (RAST)	Cellular allergen stimulation test	Elimination and re-challenge diet
ECP, EPX in stool and serum	Tissue oxygenation provocation	Oral food challenge (DBPCFC)
		Endoscopic challenge (gastric challenge, COLAP, jejunal perfusion)
COLAP, colonoscopic allergen provocation test; DBPCFC, double blind placebo-controlled food challenge; ECP, eosinophil cationic protein; EPX, eosinophil protein X; RAST, radioallergosorbent test.		

Table 38.3 Diagnostic procedures to confirm the diagnosis of gastrointestinal food allergy.

food is a causal therapy. The practicability of such an elimination diet is, however, limited by the number of allergens and quite often also by the frequency of the allergen within normal nutrition. Food (extracts) that serve as ingredients for common products, e.g. egg, wheat, soy, spice, can hardly be eliminated.

If an elimination diet cannot be performed properly because of the reasons listed above or because the responsible foods cannot be identified, antiallergic medication is required. A preparation of disodium chromoglycate that is effective locally in the GI tract is available. Because there are few side effects, oral chromoglycate can be used in children as well. In more severe cases, therapy with steroids might be inevitable. How helpful locally effective steroids, e.g. budesonide, are in GI food allergy has not yet been studied. In conclusion, therapeutic options for hypersensitivity reactions in the gut are as yet poorly evaluated. It is unclear whether innovative antiallergic drugs under development at present, e.g. tolerogenic peptides, anti-CD4, anti-IgE or anti-IL4 strategies, will be effective in the GI tract.

FUTURE DIRECTIONS

Many questions remain to be answered in the field of GI food allergy, including the most appropriate means of diagnosis and the basic pathomechanisms involved in intestinal allergic reactions. Clinical manifestations of GI allergy are variable and unspecific, including symptoms such as abdominal pain, cramping and diarrhoea.

A crucial aspect to focus on is the relationship between GI hypersensitivity reactions and other GI disorders. There are, for instance, few studies suggesting a relation between food allergy and the irritable bowel syndrome.[50] Furthermore, the relationship between food-allergic enteropathy and inflammatory bowel diseases (Crohn's disease and ulcerative colitis) remains to be elucidated. Although there are hints in the literature that there might be a relationship between these disorders,[3,10,28] a distinct causality has not been proven so far, and clear epidemiological data do not exist at present. The same applies to coeliac disease, where the responsible agent (wheat protein gliadin) is well known; the mechanism, however, by which the disease is caused is not yet understood.[25]

Oral challenge procedures with blinded food antigens are currently accepted as the gold standard in diagnosing food allergy, although these tests have several practical problems, especially in patients with intestinal manifestations of food hypersensitivity. However, new test systems have been developed, such as measurement of IgE and eosinophil parameters in stool samples and endoscopic provocation tests performed locally in the intestinal mucosa. These tests may improve the identification of patients with food-allergic enteropathy and, in addition, they can provide new insights into the pathophysiology of intestinal hypersensitivity reactions. There is increasing evidence that, consistent with findings in skin and the respiratory system, mast cells and eosinophils play a critical role in mediating intestinal allergic reactions. However, the basic mechanisms of allergic enteropathy still remain largely unclear. Further investigations are necessary to understand the pathophysiology of GI allergy, because such knowledge is important for the development of reliable diagnostic tests and pharmacological agents for treatment of this disease.

REFERENCES

1 Andre F, Andre C, Colin L, Cavagna S. IgE in stools as indicator of food sensitization. *Allergy* 1995; 50: 328–33.

2 Bagnato GF, Di Cesare E, Caruso RA *et al.* Gastric mucosal mast cells in atopic subjects. *Allergy* 1995; 50: 322–7.

3 Ballegaard M, Bjergstrom A, Bronndum S, Hylander E, Jensen L. Self-reported food intolerance in chronic inflammatory bowel disease. *Scand J Gastroenterol* 1997; 32: 569–71.

4 Belut D, Moneret-Vautrin DA, Nicolas JP, Grilliat JP. IgE levels in intestinal juice. *Dig Dis Sci* 1980; 25: 323–32.

5 Bengtsson U, Nilsson-Balnäs U, Hanson LÅ, Ahlstedt S. Double blind, placebo controlled food reactions do not correlate to IgE allergy in the diagnosis of staple food related gastrointestinal symptoms. *Gut* 1996; 39: 130–5.

6 Bengtsson U, Knutson TW, Knutson L, Dannaeus A, Hällgren R, Ahlstedt S. Eosinophil cationic protein and histamine after intestinal challenge in patients with cow's milk intolerance. *J Allergy Clin Immunol* 1997; 100: 216–21.

7 Berstad A, Borkje B, Riedel B, Elsayed S, Berstad A. Increased fecal eosinophil cationic protein in inflammatory bowel disease. *Hepatogastroenterol* 1993; 40: 276–8.

8 Bischoff SC. Mucosal allergy: role of mast cells and eosinophil granulocytes in the gut. In: *Liver and Gastrointestinal Immunology* (Manns MP, ed.). Baillière's Clinical Gastroenterology 1996; 10: 443–59.

9 Bischoff SC, Grabowsky J, Manns MP. Quantification of inflammatory mediators in stool samples of patients with inflammatory bowel disorders and controls. *Dig Dis Sci* 1997; 42: 394–403.

10 Bischoff SC, Herrmann A, Manns MP. Prevalence of adverse reactions to food in patients with gastrointestinal disease. *Allergy* 1996; 51: 811–18.

11 Bischoff SC, Mayer JH, Nguyen Q-T, Stolte M, Manns MP. Immunohistological assessment of intestinal eosinophil activation in patients with eosinophilic gastroenteritis and inflammatory bowel disease. *Am J Gastroenterol* 1999; 93: 3521–9.

12 Bischoff SC, Mayer J, Meier PN, Zeck-Kapp G, Manns MP . Clinical significance of the colonoscopic allergen provocation test. *Int Arch Allergy Immunol* 1997; 113: 348–51.

13 Bischoff SC, Mayer J, Wedemeyer J *et al.* Colonoscopic allergen provocation (COLAP): a new diagnostic approach for gastrointestinal food allergy. *Gut* 1997; 40: 745–53.

14 Bishop JM, Hill DJ, Hosking CS. Natural history of cow milk allergy: clinical outcome. *J Pediatr* 1990; 116: 862–7.

15 Bock SA. Prospective appraisal of complaints of adverse reactions to foods in children during the first 3 years of life. *Pediatrics* 1987; 79: 683–8.

16 Bruijnzeel-Koomen C, Ortolani C, Aas K *et al.* Adverse reactions to food. *Allergy* 1995; 50: 623–35.

17 Capron M, Gounni SA, Morita M *et al.* Eosinophils: from low- to high-affinity immunoglobulin E receptors. *Allergy* 1995; 50(Suppl. 25): 20–3.

18 Crowe SE, Perdue MH. Gastrointestinal food hypersensitivity: basic mechanisms of pathophysiology. *Gastroenterology* 1992; 103: 1075–95.

19 De Weck AL, Stadler BM, Urwyler A, Wehner HU, Bühlmann RP. Cellular allergen stimulation test (CAST) – a new dimension in allergy diagnostics. *ACI News* 1993; 5: 9–14.

20 D'Inca R, Ramage JK, Hunt RH, Perdue MH. Antigen-induced mucosal damage and restitution in the small intestine of the immunized rat. *Int Arch Allergy Appl Immunol* 1990; 91: 270–7.

21 Dvorak AM, Monahan RA, Osage JE, Dickersin GR. Mast cell degranulation in Crohn's disease. *Lancet* 1978; i: 498.

22 Finn R. Food allergy – fact or fiction: a review. *J Roy Soc Med* 1992; 85: 560–4.

23 Furuta GT, Ackerman SJ, Wershil BK. The role of the eosinophil in gastrointestinal diseases. *Curr Opin Gastroenterol* 1995; 11: 541–7.

24 Hällgren R, Colombel JF, Dahl R *et al.* Neutrophil and eosinophil involvement of the small bowel in patients with celiac disease and Crohn's disease: studies on the secretion rate and immunohistochemical localization of granulocyte granule constituents. *Am J Med* 1989; 86: 56–64.

25 Hed J. Coeliac disease: a food allergy? *Monogr Allergy* 1996; 32: 204–10.

26 Host A, Halken S. A prospective study of cow milk allergy in Danish infants during the first 3 years of life. Clinical course in relation to clinical and immunological type of hypersensitivity reaction. *Allergy* 1990; 45: 587–96.

27 Huggins KG, Brostoff J. Local production of specific IgE antibodies in allergic-rhinitis patients with negative skin tests. *Lancet* 1975; ii: 148–50.

28 Jones VA, Dickinson RJ, Workman E, Wilson AJ, Freeman AH, Hunter JO. Crohn's disease: maintainance of remission by diet. *Lancet* 1985; ii: 177–80.

29 Kristjansson I, Ardal B, Jonsson JS, Sirudsson JA, Foldevi M, Bjorksten B. Adverse reaction to food and food allergy in young children in Iceland and Sweden. *Scand J Prim Health Care* 1999; 17: 30–4.

30 Kolmannskog S, Haneberg B. Immunoglobin E in feces from children with allergy. *Int Arch Allergy Appl Immunol* 1985; 76: 133–7.

31 Kosa L, Kereki E, Borzsonyl L. Copro-eosinophil cationic protein (ECP) in food allergy. *Allergy* 1996; 51: 964–6.

32 Levy AM, Kita K. The eosinophil in gut inflammation: effector or director? *Gastroenterology* 1996; 110: 952–4.

33 Levy AM, Gleich GJ, Sandborn WJ, Tremaine WJ, Steiner ML, Phillips SF. Increased eosinophil granule proteins in gut lavage fluid from patients with inflammatory bowel disease. *Mayo Clin Proc* 1997; 72: 117–23.

34 Naylor AR. Eosinophilic gastroenteritis. *Scot Med J* 1990; 35: 163–5.

35 Nolte H, Stahl-Skov P, Kruse A, Schiotz PO. Histamine release from dispersed human intestinal mast cells. A method using biopsies from children and adults. *Allergy* 1989; 44: 543–53.

36 Patrick MK, Dunn IJ, Buret A *et al.* Mast cell protease release and mucosal ultrastructure during intestinal anaphylaxis in the rat. *Gastroenterology* 1988; 94: 1–9.

37 Podolsky D. Inflammatory bowel disease. Second of two parts. *N Engl J Med* 1991; 325: 1008–18.

38 Podolsky D. Inflammatory bowel disease. First of two parts. *N Engl J Medicine* 1991; 325: 928–37.

39 Raab Y, Fredens K, Gerdin B, Hällgren R. Eosinophil activation in ulcerative colitis. *Dig Dis Sci* 1998; 43: 1061–70.

40 Raible DG, Schulman ES, DiMuzio J, Cardillo R, Post TJ. Mast cell mediators prostaglandin-D$_2$ and histamine activate human eosinophils. *J Immunol* 1992; 148: 3536–42.

41 Raithel M, Matek M, Baenkler HW, Jorde W, Hahn EG. Mucosal histamine content and histamine secretion in Crohn's disease, ulcerative colitis and allergic enteropathy. *Int Arch Allergy Immunol* 1995; 108: 127–33.

42 Reimann HJ, Lewin J. Gastric mucosal reactions in patients with food allergy. *Am J Gastroenterol* 1988; 11: 1212–19.

43 Rothenberg ME. Eosinophilia. *N Engl J Med* 1998; 338: 1592–600.

44 Sampson HA. Food allergy. Part 2: diagnosis and management. *J Allergy Clin Immunol* 1999; 103: 981–9.

45 Sampson HA. Food allergy. Part 1: Immunopathogenesis and clinical disorders. *J Allergy Clin Immunol* 1999; 103: 717–28.

46 Sampson HA, Broadbent KR, Bernhisel-Broadbent J. Spontaneous release of histamine from basophils and histamine-releasing factor in patients with atopic dermatitis and food hypersensitivity. *N Engl J Med* 1989; 321: 228–32.

47 Strobel S, Busuttil A, Ferguson A. Human intestinal mast cells: expanded population in untreated coelic disease. *Gut* 1983; 24: 222–7.

48 Talley NJ, Shorter RG, Phillips SF, Zinsmeister AR. Eosinophilic gastroenteritis: a clinicopathological study of patients with disease of the mucosa, muscle layer, and subserosal tissues. *Gut* 1990; 31: 54–8.

49 Young E, Stoneham MD, Petruckevitch A, Barton J, Rona R. A population study of food intolerance. *Lancet* 1994; 343: 1127–30.

50 Zwetschenbaum JF, Burakoff R. Food allergy and the irritable bowel syndrome. *Am J Gastroenterol* 1988; 83: 901–4.

Chapter 39

Oral manifestations of food allergy and intolerance

David. Wray

INTRODUCTION

As the portal of entry to the gastrointestinal tract, the mouth is exposed to a wide spectrum of external antigenic agents, including foodstuffs, drugs, cosmetics, eating utensils, dental materials (including heavy metals), and bacteria, both commensal and pathogenic. It would be surprising, therefore, if oral mucosal reactions to external antigens did not occur, and indeed examples of adverse reactions to all of the above are apparent.

Food allergy or hypersensitivity *per se* is not, however, widely regarded as an important cause of oral disease. This is in part because of incomplete understanding of the aetiopathogenesis of many mucosal diseases and to difficulties in objectively assessing mucosal allergy, rather than an absence of a role for foodstuffs in many mucosal disease processes. It is now increasingly clear that food allergy or sensitivity has a direct aetiological effect in some oral diseases and is an important factor in the pathogenesis of several others.

The immune mechanisms clearly vary from one disease to another, and examples of each type of immune sensitivity can be shown (see later), although a detailed discussion of immune mechanisms is not included within this chapter.

Oral lesions may result from immune responses to foods in direct contact with the oral mucosa, as can occur in recurrent aphthous stomatitis (RAS), or they may arise as an oral manifestation of a more systemic adverse reaction to foods, such as in anaphylaxis.

INVESTIGATION OF ORAL FOOD ALLERGY

As discussed elsewhere in this text, the gastrointestinal immune responses differ significantly from cutaneous responses, and may even be reciprocal. Thus, *in vitro* or cutaneous *in vivo* testing for allergy may not be relevant to oral disease, while oral food challenge may not be objective. The evidence supporting a role for food allergy in oral disease must therefore be seen in the context of the available methods of investigating food sensitivity relevant to oral disease.

In vitro assays

A number of *in vitro* tests have been used to investigate the pathogenesis of oral disease. Early studies included the measurement of serum antibodies to foods[79,80] although whether the presence of such antibodies was of aetiological significance or secondary to mucosal disease could not be determined. More recent studies, for example, on the significance of α-gliadin antibodies in patients with recurrent oral ulceration, suggest a specific use for these assays.[50]

Radioallergosorbent tests (RAST) provide a simple method of assessing specific immunoglobulin (lg)E-mediated food allergies, although the scope of allergens which can be tested commercially limits their usefulness. RAST assays for latex are widely available, latex allergy is of increasing importance, particularly among healthcare workers.[61] The frequency of crossreacting IgE antibodies between latex and some fruits (including avocado, papaya, kiwi, pineapple, banana, peach, chestnuts, etc.) makes the 'latex–fruit syndrome' of real concern.[10,49]

Basophil histamine release can also be used to study human allergy,[73] and this has been applied to the assessment of the role of allergy in RAS.[102] Lymphocyte proliferation assays have recently become commercially available, especially for putative sensitivity to heavy metals, although evidence for their value in routine assessment of oral allergy is lacking.

In vivo testing

The mainstay of *in vivo* testing is conventional epicutaneous patch testing. This is usually used for contact sensitivity,[1,75] but also includes foodstuffs.[48,100] Clinical improvement on antigen withdrawal suggests a relevance for positive reactions.[48,100] Elimination diets[69] or dietary elimination[102] have also been shown to be effective.

Early studies of buccal or labial food challenges, especially with weak organic acids, showed a sensitivity among patients with recurrent oral ulceration,[82–84] and subsequently Amlot *et al.*,[4] showed a good correlation between buccal challenge and symptoms, although they found skin more sensitive than mucosa. More recently, Rance and Dutau[55] found that positive labial food challenge indicated the presence of food allergy, but negative responses required further investigation.

LOCALIZED DISEASE

A variety of oral conditions are associated with food allergy and those discussed in this chapter are shown in Table 39.1.

The clinical features of each condition will be detailed, together with the evidence for, and the relevance of, associated food allergies.

Recurrent aphthous stomatitis

RAS is characterized by recurrent, self-healing oral ulcers affecting exclusively the non-keratinized oral mucosa[95] (Fig. 39.1). Clinically, the lesions can be distinguished into the following:

1. Minor, characterized by crops of 1–10 ulcers, usually 2–4 mm in diameter which heal within 10–14 days without scarring.
2. Major, which are larger (usually more than 1 cm), more intransigent (lasting 6 weeks to 6 months) and heal by scarring.
3. Herpetiform ulcers, so called because of their resemblance to herpetic ulceration although they are not viral in nature. They are characterized by crops of 10–100 ulcers which are 1–2 mm in size and which heal spontaneously after 10–14 days without scarring.

Behçet's syndrome is a multisystem disorder characterized by RAS and other systemic involvement, including genital ulceration, eye involvement, arthritis and neurological or gastrointestinal manifestations. It is thought to have an immune complex component and patients show enhanced polymorph chemotaxis. There appears to be a clear immunogenetic basis.

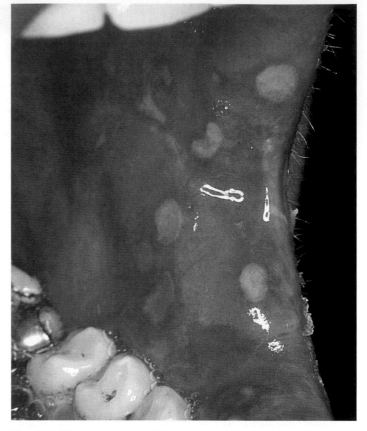

Fig. 39.1 Minor recurrent aphthous stomatitis affecting the non-keratinized buccal mucosa.

RAS arises as a result of immunologically mediated epithelial damage which is influenced by a number of host and environmental factors (Table 39.2). Host factors appear to alter the patient's disease susceptibility and include genetic, nutritional and endocrine factors as well as systemic diseases. A positive family history exists in the majority of patients despite a population prevalence[72] of only 20%, and there is a high concordance (90%) in identical twins.[47] There is also a weak HLA association.[12,101]

Nutritional deficiencies of iron, folic acid or vitamin B12 can be shown to be present in 20% of patients who present with RAS, and ulceration improves or remits with replacement therapy.[11,30,98] Endocrine factors are implicated since 80% of women have remission of ulcers during pregnancy[93] and ulceration can be suppressed

Oral conditions associated with food allergy
Recurrent aphthous stomatitis
Orofacial granulomatosis
Lichen planus
Erythema multiforme
Angio-oedema
Allergic stomatitis
Pruritus and burning mouth
Cheilitis and contact dermatitis
Miscellaneous conditions

Table 39.1 Oral conditions associated with food allergy.

Associated factors in the aetiopathogenesis of recurrent aphthous stomatitis	
Host	**Environmental**
Genetic	Trauma
Nutritional	Allergy
Endocrine	
Systemic disease	

Table 39.2 Associated factors in the aetiopathogenesis of recurrent aphthous stomatitis.

by sex hormones,[9] especially in those with a premenstrual accentuation of their ulceration.[22]

RAS type ulceration can be associated with a number of systemic diseases,[98] especially coeliac disease (see later),[23,24] and may be associated with a number of other overt or occult gastrointestinal diseases, including Crohn's disease and ulcerative colitis.[98] It should be stressed that there are many forms of oral ulceration in addition to RAS.

Environmental factors are associated with the initiation of individual episodes of ulceration, and include trauma and allergy.

Although ulceration may arise in anyone whose mucosa is traumatized by broken teeth or ill-fitting dentures, those with RAS may develop ulceration in response to mild trauma arising from sharp foods, toothbrushing, etc., presumably because of the release of inflammatory mediators such as histamine.[100]

Evidence for food allergy in recurrent aphthous stomatitis

The evidence supporting a role for food allergy in the pathogenesis of RAS is extensive. Since Alvarez[3] originally described an association between food ingestion and RAS in 1937, several authors have shown that foodstuffs were of aetiological significance.[62,64,82–84] Also, a positive correlation between a history of atopic disease and RAS has been reported on several occasions.[77,82,91] In 1960, Ship[70] claimed complete remission in seven patients with RAS when placed on an elemental diet, but failed to confirm this in a further series of six patients.[71] The involvement of components of food in the causation of RAS was tested in 17 selected patients by Hay and Reede.[27] These patients, with RAS which had been resistant to other forms of treatment, were studied with the aid of a strict elimination diet. Five patients abandoned the diet and five patients had a remission of ulcers while on the diet. In four of these five patients a particular food was identified which, when eliminated from the subsequent normal diet, led to either marked improvement or resolution. The elimination diet had been maintained for approximately 8 weeks in the patients who were not free of ulcers for more than a few days. The results of this study indicate that, in a small proportion of cases of RAS, reactions to food components may participate in the aetiology of the oral ulceration.

Several authors have claimed that foodstuffs were of aetiological significance in RAS: Tuff et al.[82–84] reported a sensitivity to weak organic acids, citric and acetic. Kutscher et al.,[36] however, did not show sensitivity to these acids in their study. Rowe and Thomas[64] and Rosenbaum[62] claimed an association with a variety of foods but this could not be confirmed by Sircus et al.[74]

Wray et al.[102] studied the basophil histamine release in response to food antigens in patients with RAS. Of 60 patients tested, 23 showed significant histamine release to food antigens. Only five of these subjects had given a history of allergy to food antigens, while three subjects who gave a history did not show significant histamine release. Overall, the ability of patients to correlate clinical food allergy to the histamine assay was less specific than for respiratory allergies.

An interesting finding was that a higher proportion of non-atopic patients showed histamine release from leukocytes in response to food antigens compared with non-atopic controls. Atopic patients and atopic controls both showed a higher prevalence of histamine release to foods and were not significantly different statistically. Overall, no difference was found between patients and controls.

This study[103] was extended to the elimination of specific foods in those patients who had histamine release to foods in an attempt to correlate in vitro histamine release to the development of oral ulcers. Of the patients, 30% had a decreased incidence of ulcers after eliminating foods which had induced in vitro histamine release. On re-challenge in a double blind manner, 30% of foods which caused histamine release also correlated with an increased incidence of oral lesions (though 70% did not) and, in eight patients, ingestion of specific foods was correlated with oral ulceration by food challenge and then elimination on an open trial basis.

These results suggest that sensitivity to food may play a minor role in the development of some cases of RAS, although it should be noted that dietary manipulation did not eliminate the ulceration in any of the patients.

Association of recurrent aphthous stomatitis with nuts

Exacerbations of Behçet's syndrome and RAS have been reported to occur after the ingestion of English and black walnuts in some patients.[45] The meat of these nuts appears to be mitogenic to lymphocytes and chemotactic for mononuclear leukocytes in vitro in both patients and controls.[52] Basophils from all patients with clinically symptomatic unrelated allergies released a significant proportion of their histamine when exposed to mitogen-containing extracts of black walnut meat. In contrast, non-allergenic subjects released little or none.[52] The pellicle from these walnuts is rich in heat-labile tannins, which significantly depress lymphocyte transformation.[52]

When walnuts are ingested they cause a 50% reduction in lymphocytes proliferating in vitro to all stimulants in both patients and controls within 48 h.[45] It is therefore suggested that a temporary depression of functional T cell populations by walnuts may indirectly allow B cells to produce more immunoglobulin and cause an exacerbation of the disease.[45] Eversole et al.,[21] however, found no significant increase in walnut sensitivity on challenging 58 patients with RAS compared to controls.

IgE-bearing lymphocytes are significantly increased in aphthous lesions,[8] and mast cells are increased in tissue sections from the prodromal stage of recurrent ulcers.[37] These mast cells degranulate within 48 h of new ulcer formation,[13] and disodium cromoglycate is partially effective in the treatment of RAS.[14,25,35,86]

In addition, patients with RAS have been shown to display increased serum antibodies to cows' milk proteins and other food antigens compared to normal but not when compared to patients with other ulcerative conditions.[79,80] This suggests that ulceration of any type allows increased antigen access to the immune system.

More recently, Nolan et al.[48] showed improvement in 18 of 20 patients with RAS who were patch test-positive to foodstuffs and underwent dietary manipulation. Wray et al.[100] studied 352 patients with RAS and 100 disease-free controls who underwent percutaneous patch testing and contact urticaria testing (Table 39.3). Of those tested, 289 (82%) were patch test-positive for one or more groups of allergens (European Standard Series, food additives, perfumes and flavourings, and chocolate). A total of 169 (48%) reacted positively to food additives, especially benzoic acid ($n = 158$; 45%) compared to 33% of controls (benzoic acid 23%; $P < 0.02$). There was reaction in 129 (37%) to perfumes and flavourings (cinnamaldehyde 32%) compared with 7% of controls (cinnamaldehyde 7%; $P < 0.01$) and 15 (4%) reacted to chocolate compared to 1% of controls (P, n.s.).

Patch and contact urticaria testing in patients with oral diseases (percentage positive reactions)					
	Food additives	Benzoic acid	Perfumes and flavourings	Cinnamon	Chocolate
Controls (n = 100)	33	23	7	7	1
RAS (n = 352)	48*	45*	37†	32†	4
OFG (n = 240)	48*	45*	36†	34†	9*
Lichen planus (n = 228)	31	27	23*	18*	2
Angio-oedema (n = 31)	35	26	32†	19*	0
Erythema multiforme (n = 22)	45	41	32†	23*	5

RAS, recurrent aphthous stomatitis; OFG, orofacial granulomatosis. *P < 0.05, †P < 0.01.

Table 39.3 Patch and contact urticaria testing in patients with oral diseases (percentage positive reactions).

The majority of patients reported clinical improvement after self-assessed compliance with dietary avoidance.

Food allergy appears, in the same way as trauma, to stimulate the release of acute inflammatory mediators such as histamine. This has an immunomodulating effect on the mucosal immunocyte population, thus initiating RAS. Allergy is not the sole aetiological agent and even successful dietary avoidance will not lead to complete cure. Dietary manipulation in response to percutaneous patch test investigation and empirical avoidance of suspect foods in the absence of formal patch testing seems justified in patients with troublesome RAS.

Orofacial granulomatosis

Wiesenfeld et al.[89] introduced the term orofacial granulomatosis (OFG) to describe the clinical features of individuals with signs and symptoms resembling oral Crohn's disease but who did not have gastrointestinal involvement. The term is currently an umbrella term, encompassing patients with orofacial Crohn's disease, orofacial sarcoidosis, Melkersson–Rosenthal syndrome and clinical orofacial lymphoedema.[90] The condition is increasing in prevalence: oral Crohn's disease was first described in 1969[17] and recently clinical aspects have been reported in a series of 264 patients with OFG in the west of Scotland.[26]

Clinical features include lip and facial swelling with associated mucosal oedema and ulceration, angular cheilitis and gingivitis[90] (Figs 39.2 and 39.3).

The aetiology of Crohn's disease and OFG is unknown. It has been suggested that Crohn's disease may be caused by infection with *Mycobacterium paratuberculosis*,[66] although this could not be confirmed in patients with OFG.[58]

Evidence for food allergy in orofacial granulomatosis

Extensive evidence suggests a role for food allergy in the pathogenesis of OFG: allergic causes have been proposed[31,53] and elimination diets have been used with some success,[29,53] although these studies were not controlled. James et al.[31] established an association between OFG and atopy when 60% of a group of 75 patients with OFG were found to be atopic compared with 15% of 200 controls. In 1985, Patton et al.[54] suggested an association

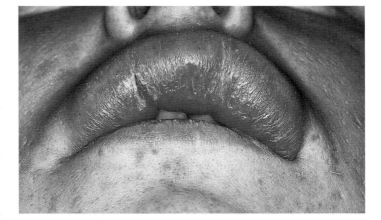

Fig. 39.2 Chronic lip swelling in a patient with orofacial granulomatosis showing associated vertical fissuring.

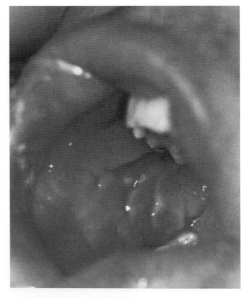

Fig. 39.3 Buccal cobblestoning because of lymphoedema with associated mucosal tags in a patient with orofacial granulomatosis.

between OFG and allergy to foodstuffs with 14 of 80 patients with OFG reporting intolerance to foods or flavourings. Subsequently, in 1986 Sweatman *et al.*[78] reported relapse in a single patient with atopy and OFG on exposure to food additives in a double blind diet provocation test. Other anecdotal reports suggest clinical exacerbations on exposure to food allergens.[51,56,65] More recently, Armstrong *et al.*[6] investigated 48 patients by percutaneous patch testing and showed 10 with positive responses to food stuffs, of whom seven improved on dietary elimination.

Wray *et al.*[100] studied 240 patients with OFG and 100 controls by percutaneous patch testing and contact urticaria testing (Table 39.3). Of those tested, 181 (75%) were patch test-positive for one or more groups of allergens (European Standard Series, food additives, perfumes and flavourings, and chocolate). In all, 115 (48%) reacted to food additives, especially benzoic acid ($n = 108$; 45%) compared to 33% of controls (benzoic acid 23%; $P < 0.05$). Eighty-seven (36%) reacted to perfumes and flavourings (cinnam aldehyde 34%) compared to 7% of controls (cinnam aldehyde 7%) and 21 (9%) reacted to chocolate compared to 1% of controls.

In a separate study in the same centre, Gibson *et al.*[26] studied 264 patients for OFG who underwent patch testing and were subsequently analysed with respect to outcome for dietary elimination. Of these, there were 234 patients who gave positive reactions on patch testing. Symptoms and signs scores were assessed during dietary elimination, indicating an improvement in symptoms and signs of more than 50% among those with intestinal Crohn's disease ($n = 30$), and more than 70% in those with localized OFG ($n = 201$).

Patients with OFG can develop rapid lip and face swelling within hours of exposure to dietary allergens, but chronic lip swelling is the most common clinical manifestation. Histology of the lesions reveals non-caseating granulomas in the majority of cases.[89] These granulomas may arise directly as a result of chronic exposure with hypersensitivity to exogenous food allergens, or they could arise as a result of infection with, for example, *M. paratuberculosis*.[58] Superimposed food allergy may then exacerbate the clinical lymphoedema and render it clinically manifest. Regardless, dietary manipulation after patch testing causes significant clinical improvement in the majority of cases.

Lichen planus and lichenoid reactions

Lichen planus is a relatively common mucocutaneous disorder. Oral lesions of lichen planus may be reticular (Fig. 39.4), plaque-like, papular, atrophic or erosive. Oral lichen planus affects up to 4% of adults.[67] The condition has a complex aetiology and most data suggest cellular immune mechanisms are fundamental to the pathogenesis. In a proportion of patients, exogenous antigenic agents such as drugs can be shown to be of aetiological significance and the term lichenoid reaction is used. The main antigenic culprit is reported to be mercury. In 1994, Skoglund and Egelrud[75] showed a patch test positivity in 19 of 48 patients with oral lichenoid reactions to mercury. Eighteen of those who were patch test-positive showed regression of their lesions on removal of their amalgams, but even among those with negative responses, 83% improved on removal of amalgam restorations. Previously, a minority of patients with lichenoid reactions have shown reactions to certain foods[19] and some to food additives, especially cinnam aldehyde.[2,40]

Wray *et al.*[100] reported on the percutaneous patch testing and contact urticaria testing of 228 patients with lichen planus or lichenoid reactions and compared these to 100 controls (Table

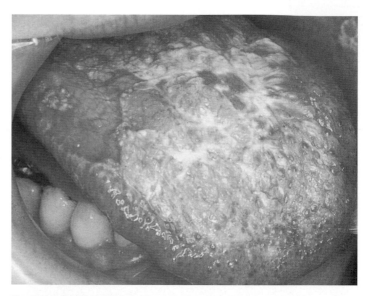

Fig. 39.4 Reticular lichen planus affecting the dorsum of the tongue in a 46-year-old male.

39.3). In all, 184 (81%) were patch test-positive to one or more groups of allergens (European Standards Series, food additives, perfumes and flavourings, and chocolate). Seventy-one (31%) reacted positively to food additives, especially benzoic acid ($n = 62$; 27%), which was not significantly different from the 33% of controls (benzoic acid 23%). However, 52 (23%) reacted to perfumes and flavourings (cinnam aldehyde 18%) compared with 7% of controls ($P < 0.01$), and five (2%) reacted to chocolate compared to 1% of controls (n. s.).

Lichenoid reactions occur to many drugs, especially non-steroidal anti-inflammatories (NSAIDs) and antihypertensives.[59] Also, amalgam restorations seem to be of pathogenic significance in a proportion of individuals. The above data suggest a similar role for food allergens in some patients, and patch testing is warranted in intransigent or symptomatic disease.

Erythema multiforme

Erythema multiforme is a mucocutaneous disorder characterized by circulating immune complexes that localize to vascular walls and are associated with complement fixation. Erythema multiforme may present as cutaneous target lesions, crusting of the lips or stomatitis (Fig. 39.5). Various drugs, particularly sulpha drugs and infectious agents, primarily Herpes simplex virus, have been implicated.[20]

Wray *et al.*[100] performed percutaneous patch testing and contact urticaria testing on 22 patients with erythema multiforme compared to 100 controls (Table 39.3). Of the 22 patients with erythema multiforme tested, 18 (82%) were positive to one or more groups of allergens (European Standard Series, food additives, perfumes and flavourings, and chocolate). Of those, 10 (45%) reacted to food additives, especially benzoic acid ($n = 9$; 41%), compared with 33% of controls (benzoic acid 23%; n.s.). Seven patients (32%) reacted to perfumes and flavourings (cinnam aldehyde 23%) compared to 7% of controls (cinnam aldehyde 7%; $P < 0.01$) and one (5%) reacted to chocolate compared to 1% of controls (n.s.).

Erythema multiforme can be a severe condition, with 5–15% mortality rates in severe cases.[18] In the absence of drug-associated causes and a negative response to antiviral prophylaxis, percuta-

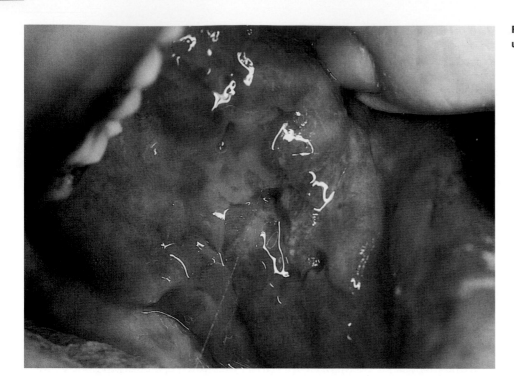

Fig. 39.5 Erythema multiforme causing ulcerative stomatitis.

neous patch testing is warranted since a proportion of patients may benefit from dietary avoidance.

Angio-oedema

Angio-oedema may be hereditary or acquired. Acquired angio-oedema may arise because of deficiency of C1 esterase inhibitor secondary to autoimmunity or an associated lymphoproliferative disorder, or it may be induced by allergy.[57] Allergy to ACE inhibitors is most common,[76] but other substances include NSAIDs[68] and allergic reactions to food additives[41] and latex.[61]

Wray *et al.*[100] performed percutaneous patch testing and contact urticaria testing on 31 patients with angio-oedema and compared the results to those of 100 control subjects (Table 39.3). Of the 31 patients tested, 22 (71%) were positive to one or more groups of allergens (European Standard Series, food additives, perfumes and flavourings, and chocolate). Of those who were positive, 11 (35%) reacted to food additives, especially benzoic acid (*n* = 8; 26%) which was similar to the 33% of controls (benzoic acid 23%; n.s.). Ten (32%) reacted to perfumes and flavourings (cinnam aldehyde 19%) compared to 7% of controls (cinnam aldehyde 7%; *P* < 0.01).

Clearly, there is a less obvious trend in allergy to foodstuffs assessed by percutaneous patch testing than the aforementioned disorders, but some patients reacted and had a positive response to dietary elimination. It is important that all patients with allergic type reactions are fully investigated since these reactions are potentially life-threatening. Patch testing is therefore indicated where appropriate to identify potential allergens.

Allergic stomatitis

Contact stomatitis is analogous to contact dermatitis.[15] The mucosa is less readily sensitized than the skin, probably because of shorter contact times, the cleansing effect of saliva, and the rapid absorption and dispersion of allergens because of the high mucosal vascularity.[32] Contact stomatitis is rare, however, even to dental prostheses, although a number of reactions to foodstuffs and flavourings have been reported, particularly menthol, eugenol, cinnamon and orange.[33,34,39,46,74]

Pruritus and burning mouth

Pruritus is an uncommon intraoral complaint, although itching of the soft palate is often associated with allergic rhinitis.

Burning mouth is a clinical symptom which has various causes, including vitamin deficiencies, diabetes, dental problems, denture problems, candidosis and allergy.[96] Very few reports have implicated food allergies such as peanut sensitivity[88] in the aetiology, although responses to dental materials are more common.[1]

Oral allergy syndrome

Oral allergy syndrome is regarded as a distinct entity by allergists and results from direct contact between the food allergen and the oral mucosa. Patients are allergic to pollens, particularly birch pollen,[103] and 20% may also be allergic to apples, peaches, kiwi fruit and rarely chestnut[5] or salami.[38] It seems that, like latex, which shares common allergens with some foods (see above), a specific allergen, Bet v 1, appears to be specific to birch and apples.[63] Affected patients may have intraoral swelling associated with periorbital and pharyngeal swelling.

Cheilitis and contact dermatitis

Allergic contact stomatitis is often associated with cheilitis which manifests as dryness, scaling and fissuring of the lips. In severe reactions perioral skin may be involved. The vermilion border is more likely, however, to develop reactions than intraoral sites, and angular cheilitis may be the only manifestation of allergy. Angular cheilitis may also present as part of OFG (see above). Allergic cheilitis may arise because of food allergy although there is no evidence in the literature to support the notion that this is a significant cause.

Miscellaneous conditions

Several miscellaneous diseases affecting the oral cavity have an allergic basis. Although geographic tongue is associated with an increased prevalence of atopy[43,44,85], there is no convincing evidence for a role for foodstuffs in the aetiology of this complaint. Similarly, desquamative gingivitis is often allergic in nature, although this is usually due to the ingredients of toothpastes rather than foods. Also, candidal infections can be aggravated by concurrent allergy which makes clinical resolution more difficult. There is no evidence in the literature, however, to support these observations, although patch testing may have a role in patients who present with management problems.

ORAL MANIFESTATION OF DISTANT ALLERGIC REACTIONS

In addition to the direct effects of exogenous antigens on the oral and paraoral tissues causing specific oral disease as discussed above, oral manifestations may arise as part of a generalized allergic disorder such as anaphylaxis (discussed elsewhere). In these circumstances, local oral pathology is overshadowed by the severe systemic consequences of the acute allergic response.

Oral disease may also arise as a consequence of allergic disorders elsewhere in the body. This may be seen as a non-specific oral response to cutaneous contact sensitivity. Indeed, it is well recognized that cheilitis or stomatitis may be exacerbated in response to contact with an allergen at a distant site in the body.

More specifically, however, oral disease may be a manifestation of some gastrointestinal disorders, such as coeliac disease or inflammatory bowel disease, which have an allergic basis. The relationship of these disorders to food sensitivity is discussed elsewhere, hence only their relationship to oral disease will be considered here.

Coeliac disease

Before the discovery of the relationship between wheat ingestion and coeliac disease the condition was often referred to as idiopathic steatorrhoea or sprue. The term sprue is derived from the Dutch word 'spruw' which means aphthous disease[16] and, indeed, in 1930 Manson-Bahr and Willoughby[42] classified sprue on the basis of the presence or absence of aphthous stomatitis since 22% of their cases suffered from this condition, and occasionally aphthae dominated the clinical picture.

Subsequently, Wray et al.[97] showed an increased prevalence of coeliac disease in patients with RAS, and later Ferguson et al.[24] claimed that 33% of patients with RAS had gluten-sensitive enteropathy. Others have, however, been unable to confirm the high prevalence seen in the latter study.[23,60] In the original series by Wray et al.,[98] 5.3% of patients had malabsorption and gluten-sensitive enteropathy. Indeed, all patients with folate deficiency were identified as having villous atrophy. One patient had an incomplete response to folate replacement and only became free of ulcers on withdrawal of gluten.[98] The others all became ulcer-free with folate replacement alone. Subsequently, Ferguson et al.[23] demonstrated villous atrophy in only two of 50 patients with RAS and both of those with coeliac disease were deficient in folate. More recently, Walker et al.[87] showed a favourable response to gluten withdrawal in a small series of patients with RAS without enteropathy. In 1981, Wray[92] placed 20 patients with RAS who had normal jejunal morphology on a gluten-free diet. Five patients showed a favourable response to gluten withdrawal and a positive gluten challenge. This was extended to a further 18 patients with normal jejunal morphology, 14 of whom were deficient in folate.[93]

Five of the 18 patients (28%) showed a reduction in ulcers in response to gluten withdrawal. Three of these without folic acid deficiency were found to release histamine in vitro by their basophils on incubation with wheat and cereals. The fourth patient with folate deficiency also released histamine in vitro on incubation with wheat and cereals, but showed no haematological improvement during the period of gluten withdrawal. The fifth patient, a 33-year-old woman with folate deficiency, did not show histamine release in vitro to any foods tested.[93]

These studies suggest that coeliac disease may cause oral disease indirectly by causing folate deficiency. The data also suggest an additional direct effect of gluten on the oral cavity in some patients with coeliac disease.

Crohn's disease

The relationship between oral manifestations and intestinal Crohn's disease has been discussed above.

The prevalence of oral lesions in patients with intestinal Crohn's disease[7,90] is between 6 and 20%. Whether the oral and intestinal lesions share a common aetiology and whether food sensitivity is concurrent to both oral and intestinal lesions is speculative.

Another extraintestinal manifestation of inflammatory bowel disease, including Crohn's disease, is pyostomatitis vegetans which is considered below with ulcerative colitis.

Ulcerative colitis

Ulcerative colitis may cause oral disease as a result of haematinic deficiency resulting from either malabsorption or blood loss.[98] However, activity of oral lesions seems to parallel bowel activity. A specific oral manifestation of inflammatory bowel disease is pyostomatitis vegetans and this may arise in association with either Crohn's disease or ulcerative colitis[28,81,94] and may persist even after colectomy.[94] The aetiological relationship between pyostomatitis and inflammatory bowel disease has not been investigated.

CONCLUSIONS

It is clear that several oral diseases may arise in association with food allergy or intolerance and that these may result from a number of diverse mechanisms, as shown in Fig. 39.6.

It seems clear that angio-oedema may arise as a result of IgE-mediated hypersensitivity (type I), causing immunologically mediated oral effects. Type I hypersensitivity may also be of pathogenic significance in RAS, when food allergy may stimulate the release of inflammatory mediators which will have an immunomodulating effect on the process of mucosal destruction. Similarly, food allergy can clearly exacerbate OFG. Whether this is a result of causing superadded lymphoedema because of type I hypersensitivity on a pre-existing type IV reaction to, for example, M. paratuberculosis or whether foodstuffs can directly cause granulomatous inflammation is unclear. Erythema multiforme, in contrast, is an immune complex-related disorder and foodstuffs may induce a type III reaction. Lichen planus probably arises from a cell-mediated reaction to external stimulae (type IV), whether they be foodstuffs, drugs or dental materials.

The mechanisms involved in the implication of foodstuffs in the aetiopathogenesis of mucosal disease are complex. Regardless, identifying putative food reactions is of increasing importance in the appropriate management of those with oral disease.

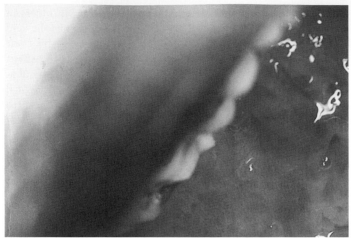

Fig. 39.6 Potential mechanisms for hypersensitivity reactions causing immune modulation leading to mucosal disease. LP, lichen planus; OFG, orofacial granulomatosis; RAS, recurrent aphthous stomatitis; GVH, graft *versus* host disease; AE, angio-oedema; EM, erythema multiforme. Type of immune hypersensitivity shown in parentheses.

KEY FACTS

1. Oral lesions may result directly or indirectly from sensitivity to foodstuffs.
2. Important oral disorders which have a significant association with food sensitivity include recurrent aphthous stomatitis, orofacial granulomatosis, lichen planus, erythema multiforme and angio-oedema.
3. Patch testing is a useful tool in the management of patients with oral mucosal disease.
4. Allergy to food additives and flavourings, especially benzoic acid and cinnam aldehyde, can be demonstrated in a significant proportion of patients with RAS and OFG.
5. Allergy to food additives and flavourings can be demonstrated in a proportion of patients with lichen planus, erythema multiforme and angio-oedema.
6. Oral mucosal disease is more prevalent among those with gastrointestinal diseases, including coeliac disease and inflammatory bowel diseases.
7. Foodstuffs associated with oral mucosal disease may mediate their effects by a variety of immune mechanisms.

REFERENCES

1 Alanko K, Kanerva L, Jolanki R, Kannas L, Estlander T. Oral mucosal diseases investigated by patch testing with a dental screening series. *Contact Dermatitis* 1996; 34: 263–7.

2 Allen CM, Bloziz GG. Oral mucosal reactions to cinnamon-flavoured chewing gum. *J Am Dent Assoc* 1988; 116: 664–7.

3 Alvarez WC. Canker sores. *Minn Med* 1937; 20: 602.

4 Amlot PL, Urbanek R, Youlten LJ. Allergy to egg and milk proteins: comparison of skin prick tests with nasal buccal and gastric provocation tests. *Allergy Appl Immunol* 1985; 77: 171–3.

5 Antico A. Oral allergy syndrome induced by chestnut (*Castanea sativa*). *Annals of Allergy Asthma and Immunology* 1996; 76: 37–40.

6 Armstrong DKB, Biagioni P, Lamey PJ, Burrows D. Contact hypersensitivity in patients with orofacial granulomatosis. *Am J Contact Dermatol* 1997; 8: 35–8.

7 Basu MK, Asquith P. Oral manifestations of inflammatory bowel disease. *Clin Gastroenterol* 1980; 9: 307–21.

8 Bays RA, Hamerlinck F, Cormane RH. Immunoglobulin-bearing lymphocytes and polymorphonuclear leukocytes in recurrent aphthous ulcers in man. *Arch Oral Biol* 1977; 22: 147–53.

9 Bishop PMF, Harris PWR, Trafford JAP. Oestrogen treatment of recurrent aphthous mouth ulcers. *Lancet* 1967; i: 1345–7.

10 Brehler R, Theissen U, Mohr C, Luger T. 'Latex-fruit syndrome': frequency of cross-reacting IgE antibodies. *Allergy* 1997; 52: 404–10.

11 Challacombe SJ, Barkhan P, Lehner T. Haematological features and differentiation of recurrent oral ulceration. *Oral Surgery* 1977; 15: 37–48.

12 Challacombe SJ, Batchelor JR, Kennedy LA, Lehner T. HLA antigens in recurrent oral ulceration. *Dermatologica* 1977; 113: 1717–19.

13 Dolby AE, Allison RT. Quantitative changes in the mast cell population in Mikulicez's recurrent oral aphthae. *J Dent Res* 1969; 48: 901–3.

14 Dolby AE, Walker DM. A trial of cromoglycic acid in recurrent aphthous ulceration. *Br J Oral Surg* 1975; 12: 292–5.

15 Dower FH, Stevenson CJ. Contact dermatitis from topical drugs. *Adverse Drug React Bull* 1998; 42: 136–9.

16 Dubois A, Van den Berghe L . *Diseases of the Warm Climates.* Grune & Stratton, New York, 1948: 390 pp.

17 Dudeney TP, Todd IP. Crohn's disease of the mouth. *Proc R Soc Med* 1969; 62: 1237.

18 Ebersole R, Millard D, Mason DK (eds) Perspectives on 1993 World Workshop on Oral Medicine, *Oral Mucosal Diseases.* Mosby Year Book Inc, Chicago, 1995; 108–59.

19 Eisen D. The therapy of oral lichen planus. *Crit Rev Oral Biol Med* 1998; 4: 141–58.

20 Eversole LR. Millard HD, Mason DK (eds). Perspectives on 1988 World Workshop on Oral Medicine, *Diseases of Oral Mucosa.* Year Book Medical Publishers, Chicago, 1989; 54–121.

21 Eversole LR, Shopper TP, Chambers DW. Effects of suspected foodstuff challenging agents in the aetiology of recurrent aphthous stomatitis. *Oral Surgery* 1982; 54: 33–8.

22 Ferguson MM, Hart D, Lindsay R, Stephen KW. Progesterone therapy for menstrually related aphthae. *Int J Oral Surg* 1978; 54: 33–8.

23 Ferguson MM, Wray D, Carmichael HA, Russell RI, Lee FD. Coeliac disease associated with recurrent aphthae. *Gut* 1980; 21: 223–6.

24 Ferguson R, Basu MK, Asquith P, Cooke WT. Jejunal abnormalities in patients with recurrent aphthous ulceration. *BMJ* 1976; i: 11–13.

25 Frost M. Cromoglycate in aphthous stomatitis. *Lancet* 1973; ii: 389.

26 Gibson J, Wray A, Neilly B *et al.* Technetium-99m-HMPAO leucocyte labelling in OFG and intestinal Crohn's disease. *J Dent Res* 1998; 77: 895 (Abstract).

27 Hay KD, Reade PC. The use of an elimination diet in the treatment of recurrent aphthous ulceration of the oral cavity. *Oral Surgery* 1985; 57: 504–7.

28 Healy CM, Farthing PM, Williams DM, Thornhill MH. Pyostomatitis vegetans and associated systemic disease – a review and 2 case reports. *Oral Surg Oral Med Oral Pathol Oral Radiol Endodontics* 1994; 78: 323–8.

29 Hernandez G, Hernandez F, Lucas M. Miescher's granulomatous cheilitis: literature review and report of a case. *J Oral Maxillofac Surg* 1986; 44: 474–8.

30 Hutcheon AW, Wray D, Ferguson MM, Dagg JH, Mason DK, Lucie NP. Clinical and haematological screening in recurrent aphthae. *Postgrad Med J* 1978; 54: 779–83.

31 James J, Patton DW, Lewis CJ, Kirkwood EM, Ferguson MM. Oro-facial granulomatosis and clinical atopy. *J Oral Med* 1986; 41: 29–30.

32 Jones DH, Beltrani VS. Oral mucous membrane contact dermatitis. *Immunol Allergy Clin N Am* 1997; 17: 471–87.

33 Kirton V, Wilkinson DS. Contact sensitivity to toothpaste. *BMJ* 1973; ii: 115–16.

34 Kowitz GM, Lucatorto FM, Bennett W. Effects of dentifrices on soft tissues of the oral cavity. *J Oral Med* 1973; 22: 105–9.

35   Kowolik MJ, Muir KF, MacPhee IT. Di-sodium cromoglycate in the treatment of recurrent aphthous ulceration. *Br Dent J* 1974; 136: 452–4.

36   Kutscher AH, Barbash R, Zegarelli EV, Amphlett J. Citric acid sensitivity in recurrent ulcerative (aphthous) stomatitis. *J Allergy* 1958; 29: 438–41.

37   Lehner T. Pathology of recurrent oral ulceration and oral ulceration in Behcet's syndrome: light, electron and fluorescence microscopy. *J Pathol* 1969; 97: 481–94.

38   Liccardi G, D'Amato M, D'Amato G. Oral allergy syndrome after ingestion of salami in a subject with monosensitization to mite allergens. *J Allergy Clin Immunol* 1996; 98: 850–2.

39   Lysell L. Contact allergy to rosin in a periodontal dressing. *J Oral Med* 1976; 31: 24–5.

40   Maibach HI. Cheilitis: occult allergy to cinnamic aldehyde. *Contact Dermatitis* 1986; 15: 106–7.

41   Malanin G, Kalimo K. The results of skin testing with food additives and the effect of an elimination diet in chronic and recurrent urticaria and recurrent angioedema. *Clin Exp Allergy* 1989; 19: 539–43.

42   Manson-Bahr P, Willoughby H. Studies on sprue with special reference to treatment. *Quart J Med* 1930; 23: 411–42.

43   Marks R, Czarny D. Geographic tongue: sensitivity to the environment. *Oral Surg Oral Med Oral Pathol* 1984; 58: 156–9.

44   Marks R, Radden BG. Geographic tongue: a clinicopathological review. *Aust J Dermatol* 1981; 22: 72–9.

45   Marquardt JL, Synderman R, Oppenheim JJ. Depression of lymphocyte transformation and exacerbation of Behcet's syndrome by ingestion of English walnuts. *Cell Immunol* 1973; 9: 263–72.

46   Millard LG. Contact sensitivity to toothpaste. *BMJ* 1973; i: 676.

47   Miller MF, Garfunkel AA, Ram CC, Ship II. Inheritance patterns in recurrent aphthous ulcers: twin and pedigree data. *Oral Surgery* 1977; 43: 487–93.

48   Nolan A, Lamey PJ, Milligan KA, Forsyth A. Recurrent aphthous ulceration and food sensitivity. *J Oral Pathol Med* 1991; 20: 473–5.

49   Novembre E, Bernardini R, Brizzi I *et al*. The prevalence of latex allergy in children seen in a university hospital allergy clinic. *Allergy* 1997; 52: 101–5.

50   OFarrelly C, Omahony C, GraemeCook F, Feighery C, McCartan BE, Weir DG. Gliadin antibodies identify gluten-sensitive oral ulceration in the absence of villous atrophy. *J Oral Pathol Med* 1991; 20: 476–8.

51   Oliver AJ, Reade PC, Varigos GA, Radden BG. Monosodium glutamate-related orofacial granulomatosis. *Oral Surg Oral Med Oral Pathol* 1991; 71: 560–4.

52   Oppenheim JJ, Sandberg AL, Altman LC, Hook WA, Dougherty SF. Relationship of mitogen and tannins in walnuts to suppression of lymphocyte transformation after ingestion of walnuts. *Proceedings of the Eighth Leucocyte Conference* 1973; 79–84.

53   Pachor ML, Urbani G, Cortina P. Is the Melkersson–Rosenthal syndrome related to the exposure of food additives? *Oral Surg Oral Med Oral Pathol* 1989; 67: 393–6.

54   Patton DW, Ferguson MM, Forsyth A, James J. Oro-facial granulomatosis: a possible allergic basis. *Br J Oral maxillofac Surg* 1985; 23: 235–42.

55   Rance F, Dutau G. Labial food challenge in children with food allergy. *Paediatric Allergy and Immunology* 1997; 8: 41–4.

56   Reed BE, Barrett AP, Katelaris C, Bilous M. Orofacial sensitivity reactions and the role of dietary components. Case reports. *Aust Dent J* 1993; 38: 287–91.

57   Rees SR, Gibson J. Angioedema and swellings of the orofacial region. *Oral Diseases* 1997; 3: 39–42.

58   Riggio MP, Gibson J, Lennon A, Wray D, MacDonald DG. Search for *Mycobacterium paratuberculosis* DNA in orofacial granulomatosis and oral Crohn's disease tissue by polymerase chain reaction. *Gut* 1997; 41: 646–50.

59   Robertson WD, Wray D. Immunohistochemical study of oral keratoses including lichen planus. *J Oral Pathol Med* 1993; 22: 180–2.

60   Rose JDR, Smith DM, Allan FG, Sircus W. Recurrent aphthous ulceration and jejunal biopsy. *BMJ* 1978; i: 1145.

61   Rosen A, Isaacson D, Brady M. Hypersensitivity to latex in health care workers: report on five cases. *Otolaryngol Head Neck Surg* 1993; 109: 731–4.

62   Rosenbaum JG. Aphthous stomatitis. *J Am Med Assn* 1960; 174: 1360.

63   Rossi RE, Monasterolo G, Operti D, Corsi M. Evaluation of recombinant allergens Bet v 1 and Bet v 2 (profilin) by Pharmacia CAP system in patients with pollen-related allergy to birch and apple. *Allergy* 1996; 51: 940–5.

64   Rowe AH, (ed.). *Food Allergy: Its Manifestations and Control and the Elimination Diets.*, C.C. Thomas, Springfield, Ill, 1972; 101–10.

65   Sakuntabhai A, Macleod RI, Lawrence CM. Intralesional steroid injection after nerve block anaesthesia in the treatment of orofacial granulomatosis. *Arch Dermatol* 1993; 129: 477–80.

66   Sanderson JD, Moss MT, Tizard MLV, Hermon-Taylor J. *Mycobacterium paratuberculosis* DNA in Crohn's disease tissue. *Gut* 1992; 33: 890–6.

67   Scully C, Beyli M, Ferreiro MC *et al*. Update on oral lichen planus: etiopathogenesis and management. *Crit Rev Oral Biol Med* 1998; 9: 86–122.

68   Shapiro N. Acute angioedema after ketorolac ingestion. *J Oral Maxillofac Surg* 1994; 52: 626–7.

69   Ship II. The etiology of recurrent aphthous stomatitis: the effect of a non-allergenic regime in hospitalized patients. *J Dent Res* 1960; 39: 748.

70   Ship II. The etiology of recurrent aphthous stomatitis: the effect of a non-allergenic regime in hospitalized patients. *J Dent Res* 1960; 39: 748.

71   Ship II. Recurrent aphthous ulcers. *J Am Med Assn* 1962; 32: 32–43.

72   Ship II. Inheritance of aphthous ulcers in the mouth. *J Dent Res* 1965; 44: 837–44.

73   Siraganian RP, Hook WA, Rose NR, Friedman H (eds). Histamine Release and Assay methods for the Study of Human allergy, Manual of Clinical Immunology. American Society of Microbiology, Washington DC, 1980; 808–21.

74   Sircus W, Church R, Kelleher J. Recurrent aphthous ulceration of the mouth: a study of the natural history aetiology and treatment. *Quart J Med* 1957; 26: 235–49.

75   Skoglund A, Egelrud T. Hypersensitivity reactions to dental materials in patients with lichenoid oral mucosal lesions and in patients with burning mouth syndrome. *Scand J Dental Res* 1991; 99: 320–8.

76   Slater EE, Merrill DD, Guess HA. Clinical profile of angioedema associated with angiotensin-converting-enzyme inhibition. *J Am Med Assn* 1988; 260: 967–70.

77   Spouge JD, Diamond HF. Hypersensitivity reactions in mucous membranes. The statistical relationship between hypersensitivity disease and recurrent oral ulcerations. *Oral Surg* 1963; 16: 412–21.

78   Sweatman MC, Tasker R, Warner JO, Ferguson MM, Mitchell DN. Oro-facial granulomatosis. Response to elemental diet and provocation by food additives. *Clinical Allergy* 1986; 16: 331–8.

79   Taylor KB, Truelove SC, Wright R. Serological reaction to gluten and cow's milk proteins in gastrointestinal disease. *Gastroenterology* 1964; 46: 99–109.

80   Thomas HC, Ferguson A, McLennan JG, Mason DK. Food antibodies in oral disease: a study of serum antibodies to food proteins in aphthous ulceration and other oral diseases. *Clin Pathol* 1973; 26: 371–4.

81   Thornhill MH, Zakrzewska JM, Gilkes JJH. Pyostomatitis vegetans – report of 3 cases and review of the literature. *J Oral Pathol Med* 1992; 21: 128–33.

82   Tuft L, Ettelson LN. Canker sores from allergy to weak organic acids (citric and acetic). *Allergy* 1956; 27: 536–43.

83   Tuft L, Girsh LS. Buccal mucosal tests in patients with canker sores (aphthous stomatitis). *Allergy* 1958; 29: 502–10.

84   Tuft L, Girsh LS, Ettelson LN. Canker sores. *J Am Med Assn* 1961; 175: 924.

85   Ullmann W. Korrelationen zwischen exfolation linguae areata und atopie. *Hautzard* 1981; 32: 629–31.

86   Walker DM, Dolby AE. Aphthous ulceration cromoglycic acid and cellular immune response. *Lancet* 1975; i: 1390.

87   Walker DM, Rhodes J, Llewelyn J, Mead J, Dolby AE. Gluten hypersensitivity in recurrent aphthous ulceration. *J Dent Res* 1979; 58: 1271.

88   Whitley BD, Holmes AR, Shepherd MG, Ferguson MM. Peanut sensitivity as a cause of burning mouth. *Oral Surg Oral Med Oral Pathol Oral Radiol Endodontics* 1991; 72: 671–4.

89 Wiesenfeld D, Ferguson MM, Mitchell DN. Oro-facial granulomatosis – a clinical and pathological analysis. *Quart J Med* 1985; 213: 101–13.

90 Williams AJK, Wray D, Ferguson A. The clinical entity of orofacial Crohn's disease. *Quart J Med* 1991; 289: 451–8.

91 Wilson CWM. Food sensitivities, taste changes, aphthous ulcers and atopic symptoms in allergic disease. *Ann Allergy* 1980; 44: 301–7.

92 Wray D. Gluten-sensitive recurrent aphthous stomatitis. *Dig Dis Sci* 1981; 26: 737.

93 Wray D. Recurrent aphthous stomatitis: clinical and immunological studies. MD Thesis 1982; University of Glasgow.

94 Wray D. Pyostomatitis vegetans. *Br Dent J* 1984; 157: 316–18.

95 Wray D. Recurrent aphthous stomatitis. *J R Soc Med* 1984; 77: 1–3.

96 Wray D. The clinical presentation of functional facial pain syndromes. *Proc R Coll Physicians Edinb* 1996; 26: 14–19.

97 Wray D, Ferguson MM, Hutcheon AW, Dagg JH. Nutritional deficiencies in recurrent aphthae. *J Oral Pathol* 1978; 7: 418–23.

98 Wray D, Ferguson MM, Mason DK, Hutcheon AW, Dagg JH. Recurrent aphthae: treatment with vitamin B12, folic acid and iron. *BMJ* 1975; ii: 490–3.

99 Wray D, Graykowski EA, Notkins AL. Role of mucosal injury in initiating recurrent aphthous stomatitis. *BMJ* 1981; ii: 1569–70.

100 Wray D, Rees SR, Gibson J, Forsyth A. The role of allergy in oral mucosal diseases. *Quart J Med* 2000; 93: 507–11.

101 Wray D, Rubinstein P, Walker M. Inheritance and HLA markers in recurrent aphthous stomatitis (RAS). *J Dent Res* 1981; 60: 378 (Abstract).

102 Wray D, Vlagopolous T, Siraganian RP. The role of food allergens and basophil histamine release in recurrent aphthous stomatitis. *Oral Surgery* 1982; 54: 388–95.

103 Yamamoto T, Kukuminato Y, Nui I *et al*. Relationship between birch pollen allergy and oral and pharyngeal hypersensitivity to fruit. *Journal of the Oto-Rhino-Laryngological Society of Japan* 1995; 98: 1086–91.

Chapter 40

Gluten toxicity in coeliac disease

Paul J. Ciclitira and H. Julia Ellis

INTRODUCTION

Coeliac disease was first reported in the 2nd century but has been recognized as a gluten-sensitive enteropathy only since World War II. The general prevalence is 1 in 1000, although it may be as high as 1 in 300 in certain population groups. A characteristic histology is now established and changes appear within hours of a gluten challenge. Dermatitis herpetiformis is associated with a patchy form of coeliac disease. Toxic peptides from the α-gliadin subfraction have been identified and established to be active both *in vitro* and *in vivo*. These studies suggest that coeliac disease is an abnormal primary immune response of the small intestinal mucosa to gluten which results in allergic phenomena. There is a strong HLA association with the DQA1*0501 and DQB1*0201 genes. The main management of coeliac disease is by avoidance and thus a gluten-free diet.

DEFINITION

Coeliac disease is defined as a condition in which there is an abnormal small intestinal mucosa which improves morphologically when the patient is treated with a gluten-free diet and relapses when gluten is reintroduced. The condition, sometimes known as coeliac sprue or gluten-sensitive enteropathy, was previously called non-tropical sprue, coeliac syndrome, idiopathic steatorrhoea or primary malabsorption. Dermatitis herpetiformis is a related condition in which there is an itchy blistering skin eruption, which frequently affects the knees, elbows, buttocks and back, with deposition of granular IgA at the dermoepidermal junction, including uninvolved skin. The majority of patients with dermatitis herpetiformis have a small intestinal enteropathy which improves on gluten withdrawal.

HISTORICAL ASPECTS

Coeliac disease was reported by Aretaeus the Cappadocian in the 2nd century AD.[1] 'Diarrhoea does not proceed from a slight cause of only one or two days' duration and if, in addition, the patient's general symptoms be debilitated by atrophy of the body, the coeliac disease of a chronic nature is formed'. Aretaeus thought that the condition only affected adults.

Samuel Gee drew attention to the condition in his report in 1887.[33] He noted that the disease affected all ages and thought that to 'regulate the food was the main part of treatment'. In his article he described a child who was fed on a quart of the best Dutch mussels daily, throve wonderfully, but relapsed when the season for mussels was over. The following season the child could not be prevailed upon to take the diet once again. It is of interest that Samuel Gee states in his article that 'if the patient can be cured at all, it must be by means of the diet'. In 1918 Still[79] commented that 'the most striking feature is the surprising inconsistency of the child's size with its age. What appears to be an infant little more than twelve months old, startles one by unexpectedly talking and so reveals the fact it is at least a year or two older, possibly even three or four, than its appearance would suggest.[79] In 1924, Haas described his treatment of coeliac disease.[36] Following the successful treatment of a patient with anorexia nervosa he thought it logical to try a banana diet in children with coeliac disease and anorexia. Haas's treatment was purely dietary, excluding bread, crackers, potatoes and cereals. Bananas were gradually added to the diet, usually from the fourth to the eighth day. This treatment was continued for an indefinite period. He believed that, ultimately, all children would tolerate most food.[37]

Treatment of coeliac disease with a banana diet continued well into the 1950s. During World War II children with coeliac disease in the UK were treated as a special case, being allowed extra bananas at a time of shortage. During the same period in the Netherlands there was a scarcity of cereals, and bread in particular. Dicke, a Dutch paediatrician, observed that coeliac sprue diminished remarkably during this period of shortage.[19] After Swedish planes dropped bread into the fields in Holland it was observed that children with coeliac disease quickly relapsed. It was this that helped to convince Dicke of the toxicity of wheat to individuals with coeliac disease. Dicke and coworkers went on to prove that wheat flour was the offending substance and that the toxicity resided in the gluten fraction.[19,86]

Early diagnosis was made on clinical grounds.[69] The relatively late description of the characteristic histology was because of the presumption that the abnormal changes previously noted at autopsy were post-mortem artifacts.[82] In 1957, Paulley[58,59] reported on the histology of coeliac jejunal mucosa obtained operatively. Shiner[73,74] independently developed methods for biopsy of the duodenum, followed by Crosby and Kugler,[18] who recognized the need for a more flexible instrument.

EPIDEMIOLOGY

The prevalence throughout Europe was previously thought to be about 1:1000 with only 1:6000 affected in North America.[39,64,67] However serological test's on blood donors indicate that the actual number both in Europe and in America may be closer to 1:250. The condition may be even more common in Celtic populations. A report from Ireland suggests a prevelance of 1:120.[57]

Coeliac disease occurs in non-caucasians, although the incidence is probably lower. It has been reported from the wheat-eating areas of Bengal and the Punjab rather than the predominantly rice-eating area of southern India. The condition has been reported in Arabs, Hispanics, Israeli Jews and Sudanese of mixed Arab–Negro stock. The condition rarely, if ever, affects people from a purely Afro–Caribbean or Chinese background. However coeliac disease should be considered a possibility in individuals of any racial background.[16]

Suggestions that coeliac disease was disappearing have now been shown to be incorrect. It appears that changes in infant feeding practices may have altered the age and mode of presentation, but the condition is more rather than less prevelant than previously suspected.

Sex incidence
A number of papers suggest that the female:male ratio is 2:1, but in other series the sexes are more equally affected.[16]

Twin studies
Concordance in identical or apparently identical twins is well documented. Discordance was recorded in infancy with normal biopsy findings in an 11-month-old twin who was ahead of his monozygotic twin in developmental age.[89] However, gluten loading had not been undertaken and it should not be forgotten that prolonged follow up of discordance of monozygotic twins results in the unaffected twin subsequently developing the condition.

Mortality rates
The outlook for individuals with coeliac disease before the introduction of a gluten-free diet was poor, with published mortality rates varying between 10 and 30%, probably lying closer to 20%. The introduction of a gluten-free diet allowed this mortality rate[70] to fall to 0.4%. However patients diagnosed in childhood and well treated with a strict gluten-free diet may have a life expectancy very similar to the general population.[41]

PATHOLOGY

Coeliac disease affects the mucosa of the proximal small intestine, with damage gradually decreasing in severity towards the distal ileum, although in severe cases changes are seen well into the ileal mucosa.[65] Abnormalities of the rectal mucosa have also been observed in severe cases.[50]

Examination of the small intestinal mucosa with a dissecting microscope is valuable. The observer may distinguish between normal and flat biopsies with degrees of abnormality falling between these two categories.[65] The normal mucosa exhibits digitate villi, leaf forms and ridges. They may vary in size, shape and height but are usually three times longer in height than width. There are differences in appearances of the jejunum in apparently normal subjects, depending on whether they reside in temperate or tropical climates. Fully convoluted appearances occur in more than 5% of normal subjects in tropical areas. Convolutions are long ridges, which may be regarded as villi having fused and buckled. Infants exhibit broad leaves and villi, with finger-shaped villi rarely present.[88] The jejunal mucosa in coeliac disease may be flat and featureless but it exhibits a mosaic pattern caused by intersection of deep depressions leaving elevated mounds. Each mound has 8–40 crypt openings.[61] Examination of a biopsy by dissecting microscopy is of value in assessing the whole specimen for patchiness of mucosal abnormality. This is particularly important in dermatitis herpetiformis, where a characteristic patchy lesion is more common.

Characteristic histology
The characteristic histological appearances of the jejunal mucosa in normal individuals are shown in Fig. 40.1, compared to the appearance of a jejunal mucosa from a patient with untreated coeliac disease in Fig. 40.2. The classic flat mucosa exhibits no villi, a loss of the villous architecture and a reduction in the normal height:crypt depth ratio[72] of between 5:1 and 3:1. There is a general flattening of the mucosa which can vary from mild to partial villous atrophy to a total absence of villi. The total thickness of the mucosa may be increased because of crypt hyperplasia and infiltration of the lamina propria by plasma cells and lymphocytes. The surface epithelial cells become pseudostratified compared to their normal tall columnar shape. Enterocyte surface cell height is reduced. Crypt mitotic activity is normally confined to the lower third of the crypt, but in coeliac disease this may be increased and continue to the crypt surface, although the histological appearance of the crypt appears normal.

The time taken for cells to migrate from the crypt to the surface is reduced from the normal 3–5 days to between 1 and 2

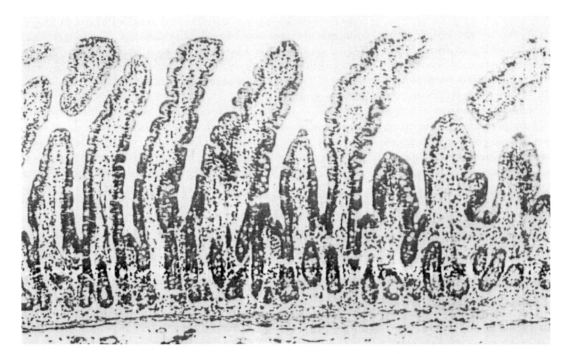

Fig 40.1 Histological appearance of a normal small intestinal biopsy.

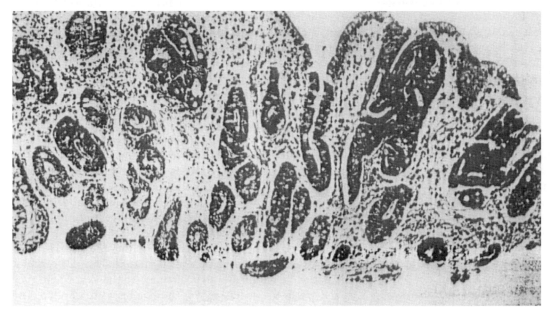

Fig 40.2 Histological appearance of a small intestinal biopsy from a patient with untreated coeliac disease. Showing a classic flat mucosa. There is a loss of villi and a reduction in the normal height: crypt depth ratio which is normally between 5:1 and 3:1

days. The number of intraepithelial lymphocytes in relation to the number of surface cell enterocytes is increased in patients with active disease. Crypt abscesses have been described and small ulcers may be encountered. These ulcers may become problematical, developing into the small intestinal T cell lymphoma that may complicate 10% of cases of untreated coeliac disease.

Goblet cells are apparent throughout the crypts along the surface of the epithelium. Paneth cells in coeliac disease may more readily discharge their contents into the crypt lumen, making recognition difficult and resulting in an apparent reduction in their numbers. There have been reports of both increased and decreased numbers of endocrine-secreting cells in the small intestine of patients with untreated coeliac disease. The basement membrane may be thickened, changes often being patchy and having the staining characteristics of collagen rather than reticulin. Previous controversy has occurred regarding the specific

diagnosis of collagenous sprue as opposed to coeliac disease. This has now been resolved through the appreciation that the condition represents a variation of the histological appearance of coeliac disease. The presence of a thickened basement membrane was suggested to imply a slow response to a gluten-free diet.[6]

Chronic inflammatory cells are found infiltrating the small intestinal mucosa in patients with untreated coeliac disease. Increased numbers of plasma cells are found in the lamina propria[53] and lymphocytes in the surface epithelium. The majority of intraepithelial lymphocytes express the common lymphocyte antigen CD3, 70% express the suppressor/cytotoxic phenotypic CD8, 5% express the helper/inducer CD4 phenotype and 20% of the cells, while they are CD3[+], are CD4[-] and CD8[-], the majority of which express the γ and δ T cell receptor.[29,46,77,78]

Electron microscopy

Scanning electron microscopy reveals the surface of villi from normal subjects to be traversed by a series of furrows. In untreated coeliac disease shallow depressions can be seen on the surface of the mucosa into which two to four crypts open. Higher magnification shows that the microvilli are thicker than normal and appear to bear rounded projections. Transmission electron microscopic studies of normal enterocytes show that the brush border is composed of tall, regular microvilli covered by a glycocalyx. Below this is found the terminal web where the cells appear tightly bound together by an apparent fusion of the lateral cell membranes. The epithelium in untreated coeliac disease reveals stratified cells;[55] the microvilli show varying degrees of abnormality from shortening to gross disorganization and disappearance. Abnormalities within the enterocytes include an increase in the number of lysosome-like bodies, swelling into the mitochondria, increased vacuolation and evidence of cellular degeneration.

DERMATITIS HERPETIFORMIS

Skin disorders in coeliac disease are common, and include psoriasis, eczema and pustular dermatitis.[17] Atopic eczema in coeliac patients may respond to a gluten-free diet. There are rare skin disorders which have been reported in association with gluten-sensitive enteropathy, including cutaneous amyloid, cutaneous vasculitis, nodular prurigo, acquired ichthyosis, epidermal necrolysis, pityriasis rubra pilaris and mycosis fungoides (Table 40.1). The most important skin disorder associated with coeliac disease remains dermatitis herpetiformis. It would appear that small intestinal mucosal damage in this condition is very similar to that seen in coeliac disease, but less severe.

Dermatitis herpetiformis (see Chapter 46) is characterized by itchy vesicular eruption, usually located symmetrically on the elbows, knees, buttocks, sacrum, face, neck, trunk and, occasionally, in the mouth.[22] Common symptoms include itching and burning which may be so severe as to cause pain, with bursting of the blisters leading to rapid relief of the symptomatic irritation. The earliest abnormality of the rash consists of a small erythematous macule 2–3 mm in diameter which rapidly develops into a papule. Small vesicles then appear, which coalesce. Scratching causes them to rupture, dry out and quickly leave an area of pigmentation and scarring. The vesicles appear tense and shiny, containing a clear fluid which clouds as the lesion progresses, and which may be tinged with blood in rapidly growing blisters.

Solitary vesicles may occur. Lesions tend to occur in crops, although all stages may be evident at one time. The blisters take 7–10 days to evolve. The tendency to suffer from attacks continues throughout life, although complete remission has been reported. The disorder is uncommon in childhood and usually presents in adults.

Common symptoms experienced by patients with dermatitis herpetiformis are the same as those in coeliac disease, although they may be milder. These include lassitude, diarrhoea, abdominal pain and distension. The degree of malabsorption in patients with dermatitis herpetiformis is frequently less than that in coeliac disease, with only 10% of these patients having symptoms directly attributable to malabsorption. The increased risk of gastrointestinal lymphoma and other gastroenterological neoplasias in patients with coeliac disease also matches those with dermatitis herpetiformis.[30]

In patients with dermatitis herpetiformis the serological changes found are similar to those that occur in coeliac disease, frequently with lowered IgM and IgA and variable changes in IgG antibodies. There are elevated titres of both IgG and IgA class antibodies to gliadin, reticulin and also endomysium.

The diagnosis of dermatitis herpetiformis depends on the finding of granular IgA in a skin biopsy. Deposition, which should be sought in an area of skin not affected by the blistering, is granular and occurs at the dermoepidermal junction.[32] This allows diagnostic separation from linear IgA disease which is not associated with gluten-sensitive enteropathy (see Chapter 46).[12]

Patients with dermatitis herpetiformis have an abnormal small intestinal mucosa, with abnormalities occurring in nearly 90% of patients if several biopsies are assessed, suggesting that the lesion may be patchy.[68] While some patients have an apparently normal jejunal mucosa on initial inspection there are usually increased numbers of lymphocytes in the epithelium which decrease in number when a gluten-free diet is introduced. It should not be forgotten that the degree of mucosal abnormality may depend on the amount of gluten ingested as well as individual sensitivity. The precise relationship of gluten-sensitive enteropathy in patients with dermatitis herpetiformis and coeliac disease remains unclear. It has been suggested that the pathogenesis of dermatitis herpetiformis is that antibodies form in the gut as a result of stimulation by gluten and then circulate to the skin where they fix and create the conditions for the skin lesion to develop. The treatment of dermatitis herpetiformis is dapsone 50–100 mg/day. Patients should also be advised to take a gluten-free diet as this results in a significant improvement after some months (usually six), frequently permitting the dosage of dapsone to be reduced or removed totally.[32] Months or years are usually necessary for the full benefit of a gluten-free diet to be obtained; many patients are unwilling to cooperate for this long.

TOXIC CEREAL PEPTIDES IN COELIAC DISEASE

Although it is known that wheat, rye, barley and possibly oats can all exacerbate the condition, the cereal fraction of wheat has been characterized in view of its nutritional importance. Wheat grains can be divided into three fractions: the outer husk or bran; the germ from which the plants grow; and the flour or endosperm which normally represents 72% of the grain by weight.

In early feeding studies in which these three components were mixed separately in water and fed to an 8-year-old child, the

Skin disorders associated with coeliac disease	
Common	Dermatitis herpetiformis
	Psoriasis
	Pustular dermatitis
Rare	Cutaneous amyloid
	Cutaneous vasculitis
	Nodular prurigo
	Acquired Ichthyosis
	Epidermal necrosis
	Pityriasis rubra pilaris
	Mycosis fungoides

Table 40.1 Skin disorders associated with coeliac disease.

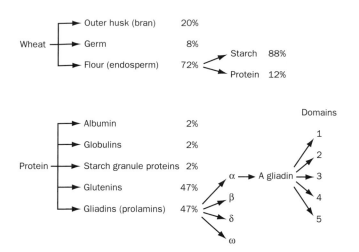

Fig 40.3 Characterization of wheat proteins.

major toxic fraction was demonstrated to be in the endosperm or flour. The child suffered from vomiting, diarrhoea and collapse with this fraction.[19] The investigators extended their study by fractionating wheat flour, which comprises water-soluble starch and protein. The protein fraction comprises 8–14% of the flour by weight, depending on whether it is a weak/soft or hard/strong flour, as used for bread-making.

The protein fraction can be subdivided into further groups (Fig. 40.3). These comprise the albumin and globulins and starch granule proteins which represent only a minor fraction of the whole, and the glutenins and gliadins, each of which correspond to approximately 50% of the protein in wheat flour. The glutenins are proteins of between 60 kDa and several million daltons which provide wheat flour with its characteristic baking qualities by entrapping carbon dioxide, allowing dough to prove.

Early feeding studies revealed that the major coeliac toxic fraction was the gliadin fraction. Gliadins are alcohol-soluble proteins otherwise known as prolamins. The proteins can be divided into α, β, γ and ω subfractions according to their relative electrophoretic mobility by either starch or polyacrylamide gel electrophoresis. An alternative classification is based on N-terminal amino acid sequences of the gliadins, and on this basis the groups are the α-type, γ-type and ω-type gliadin.[2] Gliadins are unusual in that they are comprised of 10–15% proline and 35% glutamine. We, and others, have used coeliac jejeunal biopsy organ culture to investigate the coeliac toxicity of the α, β, γ and ω protein fractions. The main principle of the assay is that, in the absence of gluten, cultured biopsies from untreated coeliac patients show an improvement in the enterocyte cell surface height. However, in the presence of gluten, biopsies from untreated patients showed no improvement, or in some cases, a further reduction in enterocyte cell surface height. Using this system, in vitro toxicity of not only α, but also β, γ and ω fractions of wheat gliadin has been shown.[43]

Structure and pathogenicity of gliadin subfractions
The antigenicity of these subfractions was further investigated by raising a set of polyclonal antisera. They were assessed initially in Ouchterlony double diffusion assays which demonstrated that the complex antigenicity of these proteins[11] was shared with similar proteins from rye, termed secalins, and hordeins from barley.

It subsequently proved possible to sequence individual gliadin proteins including A or aggregable gliadin, an individual protein within the wheat α-gliadin fraction. The structure of this protein could be divided into five domains.[49] Kagnoff et al.[47] went on to report a sequence homology of eight amino acids within the C-terminal region of A-gliadin amino acids 206–216 and the E1b coat protein of human adenovirus 12. Wieser et al.[93,94] produced a series of N-terminal peptides of A-gliadin that were tested by coeliac jejunal biopsy in in vitro organ culture. The result of these studies implied that the N-terminal region of A-gliadin was toxic to patients with coeliac disease.

Sollid and colleagues have cloned gluten-sensitive T cells from both the peripheral blood and small intestinal biopsies of patients with coeliac disease.[34] A peripheral blood clone recognized a peptide from A-gliadin corresponding to amino acids 31–49. In addition, we have made monoclonal antibodies to peptides from the N-terminal region of A-gliadin and showed that a monoclonal antibody which bound in the region of amino acid 36 crossreacted with coeliac toxic cereals but not non-toxic cereals.[24]

Gliadin peptides
Based on the above findings three gliadin peptides were synthesized. Peptide A corresponded to amino acids 31–49 of A-gliadin, peptide B to amino acids 202–220 and peptide C corresponded to amino acids 3–21. In vitro organ culture system was then used to assess these peptides. Using a peptic tryptic digest of gluten, which served as a positive control, there was a fall in enterocyte surface cell height in jejunal biopsies from treated as well as untreated coeliac patients. This also occurred with peptide A but not with peptides B or C or ovalbumin, the latter of which served as a negative control.[71]

These findings were then extended in vivo using treated patient volunteers. A Quinton multiple jejunal biopsy capsule was placed, under X-ray control, into the proximal jejunum. To this was taped an infusion catheter which allowed test fractions to be infused into the duodenum. Unfractionated gliadin was initially used as a positive control. Jejunal biopsies were taken hourly, for 6 h, since it had previously been shown that in most of the subjects assessed, initial damage to the mucosa is seen 2 h after commencing the infusion of gliadin, but that the most marked changes were observed between 4 and 6 h, after which the mucosa gradually improves (Table 40.2).[13]

To assess the potential coeliac toxicity of amino sequenced A-gliadin peptides, the histology of biopsies taken at time 0 was compared with those taken at 6 h after commencing the challenge. In the four patients studied an initial 1 g gliadin challenge was given. Then, with at least 1 week between challenges, the three peptide fractions were tested in the four subjects.

Changes in intestinal epithelium after gluten challenge
Change in dissecting microscopic appearance
Fall in villous height:crypt depth ratio
Fall in enterocyte surface cell height
Increase in intraepithelial lymphocyte count[13]
Increased expression of ICAM in the subepithelial lamina propria[81]
Increased expression of HLA Class II antigen by crypt enterocytes[14]

Table 40.2 Changes in intestinal epithelium after gluten challenge.

There was damage to the villous morphology in the four patients challenged with peptide A. In one patient there were some minimal mucosal changes with peptide B (amino acids 202–220 of A-gliadin). Peptide C, corresponding to amino acids 3–21 of A-gliadin, caused no change in any of the morphometric parameters measured.[80] In subsequent experiments, coeliac biopsies taken at time 0 were compared with those taken 2–4 h after the infusion of the three peptides A, B and C for expression of mRNA encoding proinflammatory cytokines. There was evidence of mRNA for the proinflammatory cytokines interferon-γ and IL2 within 2 h of challenge with both unfractionated gliadin and also peptide A,[51] but not with peptide C. A minimal increase of proinflammatory cytokines was observed 2 h after the infusion of peptide B in the patient who had shown minimal mucosal changes. Thus we believe that these experiments show that a peptide corresponding to amino acid residues 31–49 of A-gliadin exacerbates coeliac disease, whilst a peptide corresponding to amino acids 3–21 does not and another corresponding to 202–220 may produce minimal changes in some patients.

Since this time a number of T cell clones have been isolated from the small bowel of patients with CD. Two DQ2-restricted α-gliadin epitopes are of particular interest in that they comprise overlapping sequences, and when tested with a panel of clones from DQ2-positive Norwegian patients between them caused stimulation of all clones. A very similar peptide was found to stimulate γ-interferon production from peripheral blood T cells of coeliac patients following gluten challenge. It has been suggested that these peptides may represent the immunodominant epitopes in coeliac disease, however this awaits confirmation.

HYPOTHESIS FOR PATHOGENESIS

The three main hypotheses for the pathogenesis of coeliac disease are: a small intestinal enzyme deficiency; an enterocyte membrane defect, allowing lectin-like binding of gliadin to the small intestine enterocytes; and a primary abnormal immune response to specific cereal peptides.

Enzyme deficiency hypothesis

It is postulated that there is an absence of a specific peptidase from the jejunal mucosa of coeliac patients, resulting in an inability to digest gluten which, in turn, damages the intestinal mucosa. This hypothesis followed the report that gluten, subjected to complete acid hydrolysis, deamination by acid and treatment with papain,[48] resulted in the loss of its deleterious properties. However, peptic tryptic digestion of gluten does not significantly reduce its toxicity.[28] Batt et al.[3] suggested that the primary abnormality is late development during infancy of the ability to produce small intestinal N-peptidase.[3] This abnormality then permits peptides to be absorbed into the circulation and establish a hypersensitivity to specific cereal peptides.

Lectin-binding hypothesis

This hypothesis suggests a defect in the cell surface of small intestinal enterocytes, either an abnormal glycoprotein or glycolipid structured element, or reduced biosynthesis of one of these cell wall components.[66,92] Immunohistochemical studies suggested that gliadin bound only to coeliac and not to normal small intestinal enterocytes, but these findings have not been confirmed, either by similar techniques or by radioimmunoassay binding studies.[9,15] This hypothesis has fallen into disrepute.

HYPOTHESIS FOR AETIOLOGY

Primary immune hypothesis

This hypothesis suggests there is an abnormal primary immune response of the small intestinal mucosa to gluten that results in allergic phenomena. There is considerable evidence to support this. The rare occurrence of 'gluten shock' (vomiting, diarrhoea, tachycardia and cardiovascular collapse)[87] in a small number of treated coeliac patients after gluten challenge implies an immune aetiology.

There is dense infiltration of the lamina propria of small intestinal mucosa with untreated coeliac disease by lymphocytes and plasma cells. There is a significant increase in the ratio of intraepithelial lymphocytes to surface cell enterocytes,[27] the majority of which express the suppressor/cytotoxic phenotype[78] and which have the appearance of immunoblasts.[54] Freedman et al.[29] showed that, in the majority of treated coeliac patients subject to gluten challenge, there is a deterioration in villous morphology concomitant with an increase in the ratio of T lymphocytes to surface small intestinal enterocytes 1–2 h after challenge. The reversal of both the symptoms and histological abnormalities of the small intestine in coeliac patients when treated with a gluten-free diet or systemic steroids implies an immune-mediated aetiology. Splenic atrophy, which occurs in coeliac patients,[5] and the strong association with the histocompatibility antigens HLA DQ2 and DQ8, often associated with autoimmune disorders, further support this hypothesis.[84]

The presence of circulating antibodies to gluten after ingestion by coeliac patients[10] also points to an immune mechanism. The presence of antibodies to a variety of food antigens in these patients implies that these antibodies could be secondary to small intestinal damage, allowing non-specific absorption of food antigen.

We now believe that coeliac disease can be considered to be an aberrant immune response to gliadin which triggers a cascade of events that results in a chronic enteropathy. The demonstration of gliadin-specific T cell HLA DQ2 in the small intestine of patients with coeliac disease strongly supports a role of the immune system in the pathogenesis of this condition. The isolation of gliadin-specific T cells that are HLA DR, DP or DQ restricted from the peripheral blood of not only coeliac disease patients but also of healthy controls, suggests that the triggering of the immune system in coeliac disease may be a consequence of the primary pathogenic event rather than being the primary pathogenic event itself.

Role of enterocytes in antigen presentation

We believe that antigen-presenting cells are involved in the processing and presentation of gliadin to the immune system. In vitro evidence suggests that enterocytes may act as antigen-presenting cells. Zimmer et al.[96] suggested that enterocytes might have a role in the induction of the immune response in coeliac disease. In particular, they have shown that gliadin is translocated into vacuoles positive for MHC Class II antigens in enterocytes of untreated coeliac patients but not of healthy controls.[96]

Friis et al.,[31] using an immunofluorescent method with gliadin polyclonal antibodies, have shown that the enterocytes of healthy controls and coeliac patients have different staining patterns just 20 min after the start of an infusion of gliadin. The enterocytes of healthy controls are characterized by a diffuse, homogeneous staining pattern, whereas those of coeliac patients exhibit a more intense granular staining pattern in the apical region, and a conspicuous fluorescence in the intercellular space.

The difference in staining patterns might imply a different distribution of the gliadin in the enterocytes of healthy controls and coeliac patients. Thus in healthy controls gliadin appears to be in the cytoplasm of the enterocytes in a diffuse pattern, but in coeliac patients it appears to be in an endocytic compartment in a granular pattern that resembles the MHC Class II positive vacuoles containing gliadin as described by Zimmer *et al.*[96]

It is generally accepted that the factor that determines whether a peptide is processed in the MHC Class I endogenous pathway or in the MHC Class II pathway is its site within the cell.[52] In coeliac disease the enterocytes might metabolize gliadin through a MHC Class II immunogenic pathway. This would result in an abnormal presentation to the immune system, which, mistaking gliadin for a pathogen, triggers an immune response that results in enteropathy.[4]

Tissue transglutaminase

Tissue transglutaminase (tTG), a cytoplasmic enzyme for which gliadin is an excellent substrate, has recently been shown to be the antigen for endomysial antibodies.[20] Endomysial antibodies are unlikely to be essential for the development of the disorder, since patients with hypogammaglobulinaemia can develop the condition.[91] However, it has been suggested that tTG forms complexes with gliadin and that the neoepitopes trigger the immune response that causes coeliac disease.[88] Recently, it has been suggested that gliadin-specific T cells could provide help for tTG B cells.[75] Perhaps the abnormal compartmentalization of gliadin in enterocytes might be the predisposing factor for binding to tTG. Thus tTG might also be presented to the immune system in an abnormal way, which would produce antibodies against it. The withdrawal of gliadin from the diet would eliminate the abnormal presentation of tTG by either of the above routes to the immune system. This could explain the very high sensitivity of endomysial antibodies for coeliac disease.

We believe it is therefore critical to explore this hypothesis in the study of absorption of gliadin and other dietary peptides in coeliac disease and also provide a further understanding of the role of increased epithelial lymphocytes in coeliac disease and their putative suppressor functions.

GENETICS

The precise inheritance of coeliac disease and dermatitis herpetiformis is unknown, although 10% of first degree relatives of coeliac patients are affected by the condition. Efforts to understand the mechanisms and genetics of polygenic human disease have focused on the identification of DNA and protein markers that segregate with diseases in populations and families. The most significant observation is the increased frequency of specific serologically defined lymphoid cell surface proteins encoded in the HLA D region of the MHC and referred to as HLA Class II antigens. These consist of α- and β-chain transmembrane glycosylated heterodimers. The genes for these are organized into three subregions termed DR, DP and DQ.[85]

Recently, a DQ-A gene[7] and an HLA DP locus association, although weaker, have also been demonstrated.[8,44,62,63] The genes are encoded within the HLA Class II region of the MHC on the short arm of chromosome 6. The association of particular HLA DR and DQ types with both coeliac disease and dermatitis herpetiformis is well established.[38,76] Associations with the HLA DP region and the TNFα genes have been reported but are thought to be secondary to linkage disequilibrium with HLA DR and DQ haplotypes. The genes most strongly associated with coeliac disease are DQA1*0501 and DQB1*0201; 98% of northern European individuals with coeliac disease have these alleles in *cis* (DQ2), whereas in southern Europe a third of the disease population express the same Class II molecule from these alleles in *trans* (DR5,7).[76] Italian and Argentinian populations of patients with coeliac disease are also reported to have an increased frequency of the DR5,7 genotype.[40] In Israel an association has been found between possession of the HLA DR4 DQ8 genotype and coeliac disease. This genotype encodes for a Class II molecule with considerable similarities in the peptide binding groove configuration to that produced by the DQ2 genes, supporting a central role for the Class II molecule in an immune-mediated model of coeliac disease.[83]

It is estimated that the HLA associations account for only 30% of the genetic susceptibility to coeliac disease, as evidenced by the prevalence of the susceptible DR3 DQ2 haplotype of up to 25% in the general UK and US populations. Segregation analyses propose an oligogenic model involving both the HLA DQ alleles and one or more genes located elsewhere in the genome.[35,60] Genomewide screening to identify these remaining susceptibility alleles is being undertaken in a number of centres using either sibling pair analysis or multigeneration multiply affected families. The first reports of possible linkage from a sibling pair analysis[95] have yet to be confirmed.

TREATMENT

Coeliac disease is treated with a gluten-free diet, avoiding products containing wheat, rye, barley and oats.[19] There is disagreement concerning the toxicity of oats,[21] and some physicians permit oats to be taken in the diet. Recent studies have suggested that moderate quantities of oats may not be harmful to most patients.[45] Holmes *et al.*[42] recently showed that a gluten-free diet decreased the incidence of small intestinal T cell lymphomas in coeliac patients.[42] We therefore believe that, to protect against long-term complications, coeliac patients with relatively few symptoms should be advised to take a strict gluten-free diet. Some patients improve well on a partially gluten-free diet, symptomatic sensitivity to gluten varying widely. A few patients with untreated coeliac disease can become very ill and require treatment with a short course of oral or parenteral steroids.

Oral steroids can be given as prednisolone 20 mg/day or, if the patient is severely ill, hydrocortisone 100 mg iv 6-hourly. A gluten-free diet is very low in fibre and therefore may induce troublesome constipation. This usually responds to the addition of regular dietary rice bran or ispaghula husk. Patients may supplement their diet with commercial gluten-free products which are available on prescription in many European countries. Specific dietary deficiencies which occur should be corrected. These include iron, folic acid, calcium and, very rarely, vitamin B12 deficiency.

After 3–4 months of treatment with a gluten-free diet, a repeat small intestinal biopsy should be taken to demonstrate improvement in the appearance of the jejunal biopsy morphology. If this has not occurred, other possible causes of small intestinal villous atrophy, such as giardiasis or cow's milk protein allergy, should be excluded. Even if improvement in small bowel morphology is not seen, if symptomatic improvement has occurred the diet should be continued and jejunal biopsy should then be repeated after a further 6–9 months.

Should an improvement in jejunal biopsy morphology and symptoms have occurred, we advocate further confirmation of the diagnosis of deterioration of small intestinal morphology by a repeat small intestinal biopsy after gluten challenge. This is particularly important in children, in whom conditions such as infectious diarrhoea and cow's milk intolerance may produce similar abnormalities in small intestinal morphology. The most convenient way to give a gluten challenge is to ask the patient to ingest at least 10 g of gluten or four slices of normal bread per day for 4–6 weeks. If this causes severe symptoms then the next biopsy date should be brought forward. The European Society of Paediatric Gastroenterology and Nutrition (ESPGAN) have suggested that it is not mandatory to undertake a repeat jejunal biopsy after a gluten challenge if a gluten-free diet has produced a good improvement in symptoms and the morphology of small intestinal biopsy.[90] Many physicians therefore do not practise gluten challenge as confirmation of the diagnosis.

The biopsy after gluten challenge should exhibit relapse in small intestinal morphology compared to the previous biopsy taken after at least 3 months of treatment with a gluten-free diet. If the patient's symptoms persist or the jejunal biopsy morphology remains grossly abnormal while continuing on gluten-free diet, commercial gluten-free products based on wheat starch should be discontinued and the initial diagnosis be questioned. It should not be forgotten that the commonest reason for the lack of response to a gluten-free diet is lack of patient compliance with dietary therapy.

Failure to respond to a gluten-free diet

Patients who fail to adhere strictly to a gluten-free diet frequently continue with ill health and recurring symptoms which can usually be traced to dietary lapses, either deliberate or accidental. Difficulty may arise when a food is taken which is thought to be gluten-free but which contains gluten. Misconceptions have arisen over the years as to the suitability of foods containing malted barley and its derivatives such as malt extract. There is no evidence that hydrolysis with enzymes during malting abolishes the coeliac toxicity of barley. All beers and lagers and all forms of malt and malt extract should be avoided by patients with coeliac disease.[23,25,26] A rare failure to respond to a true gluten-free diet is the development of small intestinal lymphoma or jejunal ulceration or unmasking of another condition such as chronic pancreatitis. Rarely, a patient on treatment may deteriorate and die unaccountably.

It was previously reported that 70% of coeliac patients on a gluten-free diet quickly return to normal health, with improvement within 2 weeks. The remaining 30% can be divided into three groups. Patients in the first group experienced progressive deterioration which was halted in some cases by corticosteroids but which continued to death in others. Patients in the second group often have an associated pancreatic lesion; those in the third group were found not to adhere strictly to the diet, but even when this was corrected minor abdominal symptoms and diarrhoea persisted.

Treatment of complications

Many patients with coeliac disease have lactose or sucrose intolerance at the time of diagnosis. A small percentage of treated coeliac patients continue to be troubled with disaccharidase deficiencies. Such patients develop diarrhoea and abdominal pain with lactose in the case of alactasia, and with sucrose in the case of asucrasia. These conditions may be diagnosed either by enzyme assays of the mucosa from part of a repeat small intestinal biopsy or the appropriate sugar peroral permeability study.[56] Should concomitant disaccharidase deficiency be diagnosed, then the appropriate disaccharide should be excluded from the gluten-free diet.

A small number of treated coeliac patients suffer from small intestinal bacterial overgrowth. This is diagnosed from abnormal breath hydrogen or bile acid breath tests, or an abnormally high small intestine aspirate bacteriological count. If small intestinal bacterial overgrowth is a persistent problem, patients may be treated with antibiotics such as oxytetracycline 250 mg four times a day, which may be rotated with another agent such as cotrimaxozole one tablet twice a day. A short 10-day course of metronidazole 200 mg three times a day is frequently helpful if small bowel bacterial overgrowth is a problem, although this agent cannot be continued in the long term because of neurological problems.

CONCLUSIONS

It has been proposed that coeliac disease is a condition in which susceptible individuals have an abnormal response to the ingestion of certain cereal peptides. The result of immunogenetic studies suggests that particular HLA DQ2 or DQ8 molecules are required to present certain cereal epitopes to a clone of wheat gliadin antigen-sensitive T helper cells. The increased incidence of gastrointestinal lymphoma in coeliac disease implies that chronic stimulation of a clone of T cells occasionally proceeds to a neoplastic state, allowing a lymphoma to develop. This is further supported by recent evidence showing a reduction in the incidence of lymphoma complicating coeliac disease in those patients who have been treated with a strict gluten-free diet.[42]

ACKNOWLEDGEMENTS

H.J. Ellis wishes to acknowledge financial support from the St Thomas' Hospital Research (Endowments) Committee and P.J. Ciclitira is in receipt of a grant from the National Institutes of Health, Bethesda, MD, USA (RO1 DK47716).

REFERENCES

1 Adams F. The extant works of Aretaeus the Cappadocian. *London Sydenham Society* 1856; 297: 350.

2 Autran JC, Ellen J, Law L, Nimmo CC, Kasarda DD. N-terminal amino acid sequencing of prolamins of wheat and related species. *Nature* 1979; 282: 527–9.

3 Batt RM, Carter MW, McLean L. Developmental brush border defect associated with cereal sensitivity in the Irish setter dog. *Clin Sci* 1984; 66: 38.

4 Biagi F, Zimmer KP, Thomas PD, Ellis HJ, Ciclitira PJ. Coeliac disease as a case of 'immunological friendly fire': a new pathogenic hypothesis. *Lancet* 1998;38: 42.

5 Blumgart HL. Three fatal cases of malabsorption of fat with emaciation and anaemia and in two acidosis and tetany. *Arch Int Med* 1923; 32: 113–28.

6 Bossart R, Henry K, Booth CC, Doe WF. Subepithelial collagen in intestinal malabsorption. *Gut* 1975; 16: 18–22.

7 Bugawan TL, Angelini G, Larrick J, Aurrichio S, Ferrara GB, Erlich HA. A combination of a particular HLA-DPβ allele and an HLA-DQ heterodimer confers susceptibility to coeliac disease. *Nature* 1989; 339: 470–3.

8 Bugawan TL, Horn GT, Long CM *et al.* Analysis of HLA-DP allelic sequence polymorphism using *in vitro* enzymatic DNA amplification of DP-α and DP-β loci. *J Immunol* 1988; 141: 4024–30.

9 Ciclitira PJ, Nelufer JM. Immunohistochemical investigation of pathogenetic mechanisms in coeliac disease. *Clin Sci* 1985; 68(11): 64P.

10 Ciclitira PJ, Ellis HJ, Evans DJ. A solid-phase radioimmunoassay for measurement of circulating antibody titres to wheat gliadin and its subfractions in patients with adult coeliac disease. *J Immunol Meth* 1983; 62: 231–9.

11 Ciclitira PJ, Ellis HJ, Evans DJ, Lennox ES. Relationship of antigenic structure of cereal proteins to their toxicity in coeliac patients. *Br J Nutr* 1985; 53: 39–45.

12 Ciclitira PJ, Ellis HJ, Venning VA *et al.* Circulating antibodies to gliadin subfractions in dermatitis herpetiformis and linear IgA dermatosis of adults and children. *Clin Exp Dermatol* 1986; 11: 502–9.

13 Ciclitira PJ, Evans DJ, Fagg NLK, Lennox ES, Dowling RH. Clinical testing of gliadin fractions in coeliac patients. *Clin Sci* 1984; 66: 357–64.

14 Ciclitira PJ, Nelufer JM, Ellis HJ, Evans DJ. The effect of gluten on HLA-DR in the small intestinal epithelium of patients with coeliac disease. *Clin Exp Immunol* 1986; 63: 101–4.

15 Colyer J, Farthing MJG, Kumar PJ, Clark ML, Obannesian AD, Waldron NM. Reappraisal of the lectin hypothesis in the aetiopathogenesis of coeliac disease. *Clin Sci* 1986; 71, 105–10.

16 Cooke WT, Holmes GKT. Coeliac disease definition and epidemiology. In: *Coeliac Disease* (Cooke WT, Holmes GKT, eds). Churchill Livingstone, London, 1983: 2–22.

17 Cooke WT, Holmes GKT. Skin manifestation and dermatitis herpetiformis. In: *Coeliac Disease* (Cooke WT, Holmes GKT, eds). Churchill Livingstone, London, 1984: 204–24.

18 Crosby WH, Kugler HW. Intraluminal biopsy of the small intestine. *Am J Dig Dis* 1957; 2: 236–41.

19 Dicke WK, Weijers NA, Van Der Kamer JH. Coeliac disease. The presence in wheat of a factor having a deleterious effect in cases of coeliac disease. *Acta Paed* 1953; 42: 34–42.

20 Dieterich W, Ehnis T, Bauer M *et al.* Identification of tissue transglutaminase as the autoantigen of coeliac disease. *Nature Medicine* 1997; 3(7): 797–801.

21 Dissanayake AJ, Truelove SC, Whitehead R. Lack of harmful effect of oats on small intestinal mucosa in coeliac disease. *BMJ* 1974; i: 189–91.

22 Duhring LA. Dermatitis herptiformis. *JAMA* 1884; 3, 225–29.

23 Ellis HJ, Doyle AP, Day P, Wieser H, Ciclitira PJ. Demonstration of the presence of coeliac-activating gliadin-like epitopes in malted barley. *Int Arch Allergy Immunol* 1994; 104: 308–10.

24 Ellis HJ, Doyle AP, Wieser H, Sturgess RP, Ciclitira PJ. Specificities of monoclonal antibodies to domain 1 of α-gliadins. *Scand J Gastroenterol* 1993; 28: 212–16.

25 Ellis HJ, Freedman AR, Ciclitira PJ. Detection and estimation of the barley prolamin content of beer and malt to assess their suitability for patients with coeliac disease. *Clin Chim Acta* 1990; 189: 123–30.

26 Ellis HJ, Parnell NDJ, Ciclitira PJ. Cornflakes and coeliac disease. *Gut* 1998; 42(1): A35.

27 Ferguson A, Murray D. Quantitation of intraepithelial lymphocytes in human jejunum. *Gut* 1971; 12: 988–94.

28 Frazer AC, Fletcher RF, Ross CAC, Shaw B, Sammons HG, Schneider R. Gluten-induced enteropathy. The effect of partially digested gluten. *Lancet* 1959; ii: 252–5.

29 Freedman AR, Macartney JC, Nelufer JM, Ciclitira PJ. Timing of infiltration of T-lymphocytes induced by gluten into the small intestine in coeliac disease. *J Clin Pathol* 1987; 40: 741–5.

30 Freeman HJ, Weinstein WM, Shintka TK, Piercy JRA, Wensel RH. Primary abdominal lymphoma. Presenting manifestation of coeliac sprue at complicating dermatitis herpetiformis. *Am J Med* 1977; 63: 585–94.

31 Friis S, Dabelsteen E, Sjöström H, Norén O, Jarnum S. Gliadin uptake in human enterocytes. Differences between coeliac patients in remission and control individuals. *Gut* 1992; 33: 1487–92.

32 Fry L, Seah PP, Riches DJ, Hoffbrand AV. Clearance of skin lesions in dermatitis herpetiformis after gluten withdrawal. *Lancet* 1973; i: 288–91.

33 Gee S. On the coeliac affection. *St Bartholomew's Hospital Report* 1888; 24: 17–20.

34 Gjertsen HA, Lundin K, Sollid LM, Eriksen J, Thorsby E. T-cells recognise a peptide derived from A-gliadin presented by the coeliac disease associated HLA-DQ (α1*0501/β1*0201) heterodimer. *Human Immunol* 1994; 39: 243–52.

35 Greenberg DA, Lange KL. A maximum likelihood test of the two locus model for coeliac disease. *Am J Med Gen* 1982; 12: 75–82.

36 Haas SV. Value of bananas in the treatment of coeliac disease. *Am J Dis Child* 1924; 38: 42.

37 Hass SV. Coeliac disease: its specific treatment and care without nutritional relapse. *JAMA* 1932; 99: 488.

38 Hall MA, Lanchbury JSS, Bolsover WJ, Welsh MI, Ciclitira PJ. Coeliac disease is associated with an extended HLA-DR3 haplotype which includes HLA-DPw1. *Human Immunol* 1990; 27: 220–8.

39 Hallart C, Gotthard R, Norby K, Wallace A. On the prevalence of adult coeliac disease in Sweden. *Scand J Gastroenterol* 1981; 16: 257–61.

40 Herrera M, Chertkoff L, Palavecino E. Restriction fragment length polymorphism in HLA-class II genes of Latin American caucasian coeliac disease patients. *Human Immunol* 1989; 26: 272–80.

41 Holmes GKT, Stokes PL, Sorahan TM, Prior P, Waterhouse JAH, Cooke WT. Coeliac disease, gluten-free diet and malignancy. *Gut* 1976; 17: 612–19.

42 Holmes GKT, Prior P, Lane MR, Poke D, Allan RN. Malignancy in coeliac disease – effect of a gluten-free diet. *Gut* 1989; 30: 333–8.

43 Howdle PD, Ciclitira PJ, Simpson FG, Losowsky MS. Are all gliadins toxic in coeliac disease? An *in vitro* study of α, β, γ, ω-gliadins. *Scand J Gastroenterol* 1984; 19: 41–7.

44 Howell MD, Smith JR, Austin RK *et al.* An extended HLA-D region haplotype associated with coeliac disease. *Proc Natl Acad Sci USA* 1988; 85: 222–6.

45 Janatuinen EK, Pikkarainen PH, Kemppainen TA *et al.* A comparison of diets with and without oats in adults with coeliac disease. *N Engl J Med* 1995; 333: 1033–7.

46 Jenkins D, Goodall A, Scott BB. T-lymphocyte populations in normal and coeliac small intestinal mucosa defined by monoclonal antibodies. *Gut* 1986; 27: 1330–7.

47 Kagnoff MF, Raleigh KA, Hubert JJ, Bernardin JE, Kasarda DD. Possible role for a human adenovirus in the pathogenesis of coeliac disease. *J Exp Med* 1984; 160: 1544–1557.

48 Kantor JL. The roentgen diagnosis of dispathic steatorrhoea and allied conditions. Practical value of the 'moulage' sign. *Am J Roentgenol* 1939; 41: 738–78.

49 Kasarda DD, Okita TW, Bernardin JE *et al.* Nucleic acid (cDNA) and amino acid sequences of α-type gliadins from wheat (*Triticum aestivum*). *Proc Natl Acad Sci USA* 1984; 87: 4712–16.

50 Kiln G, Holmes GKT, Cooper BT, Thompson H, Allan RN. Association of coeliac disease and inflammatory bowel disease. *Gut* 1980; 21: 636–41.

51 Kontakou M, Przemioslo RT, Sturgess RP *et al.* Cytokine mRNA expression in the mucosa of treated coeliac patients after wheat peptide challenge. *Gut* 1995; 37: 52–7.

52 Kuby J. *Immunology*, 3rd edn. WH Freeman and Company, New York, 1997.

53 Lancaster-Smith MJ, Kumar P, Marks R, Clark ML, Dawson AM. Jejunal mucosa immunoglobulin containing cells and jejunal fluid immunoglobulins in adult coeliac disease and dermatitis herpetiformis. *Gut* 1974; 15: 371–6.

54 Marsh MN. Immunocytes, enterocytes and the lamina propria: an immunopathological framework of coeliac disease. *J R Coll Phys Lond* 1983; 17: 205–12.

55 Marsh MN, Brown AC, Swift JA. The surface ultra-structure of the small intestinal mucosa of normal control human subjects and of patients with untreated and treated coeliac disease using the scanning electron microscope. In: *Coeliac Disease* (Booth CC, Dowling RH, eds). Churchill Livingstone, Edinburgh, 1979; 26–44.

56 Menzies IS. Transmucosal passage of inert molecules in health and disease. In: *Intestinal Absorption and Secretion*, (Heintze K, Sradhauge E, eds). MTP Press, Lancaster, 1984; 39: 243–52.

57 Mylotte M, Egan-Mitchell B, McCarthy CF, McNicholl N. Incidence of coeliac disease in Western Ireland. *BMJ* 1973; i: 703–5.

58 Paulley JW. Personal communications. *Proc R Soc Med* 1949; 42: 241.

59 Paulley JW, Fairweather FA, Leemin A. Postgastrectomy steatorrhea and patchy jejunal atrophy. *Lancet* 1957; i: 406–7.

60 Pena AS, Mann DL, Hague NE *et al.* Genetic basis of gluten-sensitive enteropathy. *Gastroenterology* 1978; 75: 230–5.

61 Ray-Choudhury DC, Cooke WT, Tan DT, Banwell JG, Smits BJ. Jejunal biopsy: criteria and significance. *Scand J Gastroenterol* 1966; i: 57–74.

62 Roep BO, Bontrop RE, Pena AS, Van Eggermond MCJA, Van Rood JJ, Giphart MJ. An HLA-DQα allele identified at DNA and protein level is strongly associated with coeliac disease. *Human Immunol* 1988; 23: 271–9.

63 Rosenberg WMC, Wordsworth BP, Jewell DP, Bell JI. A locus telomeric to HLA-DPB encodes suscepibility to coeliac disease. *Immunogenetics* 1989; 30: 307–10.

64 Rossipal E. Incidence of coeliac disease in children in Austria. *Zeitschr Kinderheilkunde* 1975; 119: 143–9.

65 Rubin CF, Brandborg LL, Flick AL *et al.* Biopsy studies on the pathogenesis of coeliac sprue. In: *Intestinal Biopsy*, (Wolstenholme GEW, Cameron MP, eds). Ciba Foundation Study Group 14, London, 1962; 67–83.

66 Rubin CF, Cauci AS, Sleisenger MH, Jeffries GH, Margolis S. Immunofluorescent studies in adult coeliac disease. *J Clin Invest* 1965; 44: 475–85.

67 Schmerling DH, Leisinger P, Prader A. On the familial occurrence of coeliac disease. *Acta Paed Scand* 1972; 61: 501.

68 Scott BB, Losowsky MS. Patchiness and duodenal-jejunal variation of the mucosal abnormalities in coeliac disease and dermatitis herpetiformis. *Gut* 1976; 17: 984–92.

69 Sheehy TW. Intestinal biopsy. *Lancet* 1964; i: 959–62.

70 Sheldon W. Prognosis in early adult life of coeliac children treated with a gluten-free diet. *BMJ* 1969; ii: 401–4.

71 Shidrawi RG, Day P, Przemioslo RT, Ellis HJ, Nelufer JM, Ciclitira PJ. *In vitro* toxicity of gluten peptides in coeliac disease assessed by organ culture. *Scand J Gastroenterol* 1995; 30(5): 758–63.

72 Shiner M, Doniach I. Histopathological studies in steatorrhea. *Gastroenterology* 1960; 38: 419–40.

73 Shiner M. Duodenal biopsy. *Lancet* 1956; i: 17–19.

74 Shiner M. Jejunal biopsy tube. *Lancet* 1956; i: 85.

75 Sollid L, Molberg O, McAdam S, Lundin KEA. Autoantibodies in coeliac disease: tissue transglutaminase – guilt by association? *Gut* 1997; 41: 851–2.

76 Sollid LM, Markussen G, Ek J, Gjerde H, Vartdal F, Thorsby E. Evidence for a primary association of coeliac disease to a particular HLA-DQ α/β heterodimer. *J Exp Med* 1989; 169: 345–50.

77 Spencer J, Isaacson PG, Diss TC, MacDonald TT. Expression of disulphide-linked and non-disulphide-linked forms of the T-cell receptor γ/δ heterodimer in human intra-epithelial lymphocytes. *Eur J Immunol* 1989; 19: 1331–8.

78 Spencer J, MacDonald TT, Diss TC, Walker-Smith JA, Ciclitira PJ, Isaacson PG. Changes in intra-epithelial lymphocyte subpopulations in coeliac disease and enteropathy associated T-cell lymphoma (malignant histocytosis of the intestine). *Gut* 1989; 30: 339–46.

79 Still CF. Lumelieu lectures on coeliac disease. *Lancet* 1918; ii: 163–6, 193–7, 227–9.

80 Sturgess RP, Day P, Ellis HJ *et al.* Wheat peptide challenge in coeliac disease. *Lancet* 1994; 343: 758–61.

81 Sturgess RP, Macartney C, Makgoba MW, Hung C-H, Haskard DO, Ciclitira PJ. Differential upregulation of intercellular adhesion molecule-1 in coeliac disease. *Clin Exp Immunol* 1990; 82: 489–92.

82 Thaysen IEH. *Non-tropical sprue.* Levin & Munksgaard, Copenhagen; Humphrey Milford, London, 1932.

83 Tighe MR, Hall MA, Ashkenazi A, Siegler E, Lanchbury JSS, Ciclitira PJ. Coeliac disease among Ashkenazi Jews from Israel: a study of the HLA-class II alleles and their association with disease susceptibility. *Human Immunol* 1993; 38: 270–6.

84 Tosi R, Vismara D, Tanigaki N. Evidence that coeliac disease is intimately associated with a DC locus allelic specificity. *Clin Immunol Immunopathol* 1983; 28: 395–404.

85 Trowsdale J, Campbell RD. Physical map of the human HLA region. *Immunol Today* 1988; 9: 2–34.

86 van de Kamer JH, Weijers HA, Dicke WK. Coeliac disease IV. An investigation into the injurious constituents of wheat in connection with their action on patients with coeliac disease. *Acta Paed* 1953; 42: 223–31.

87 von Krainick HG, Debatin F, Gautier E, Tobler R, Velasco JA. Additional research on the injurious effect of wheat flour in coeliac disease I. Acute gliadin reactions (gliadin shock). *Helv Paed Acta* 1958; 13: 432–54.

88 Walker-Smith JA. Small bowel morphology in childhood. *Med J Aust* 1969; i: 382–7.

89 Walker-Smith JA. Discordance for childhood coeliac disease. *Gut* 1973; 14: 374–5.

90 Walker-Smith JA, Guandalini S, Schmitz J, Schmerling DM, Visakorpi JK. Revised criteria for diagnosis of coeliac disease. *Arch Dis Child* 1990; 65: 909–11.

91 Webster ADB, Slavil G, Shiver M, Platts-Mills TAE, Ashersan G. Coeliac disease with severe hypogammaglobulinaemia. *Gut* 1981; 22: 153–7.

92 Weiser MM, Douglas AP. An alternative mechanism for gluten toxicity in coeliac disease. *Lancet* 1976; i: 567–9.

93 Wieser H, Belitz H-D, Ashkenazi A. Amino acid sequence of the coeliac active peptide B3142. *Z Lebensum Unters Forsch* 1984; 179: 371–6.

94 Wieser H, Belitz H-D, Idar D, Ashkenazi A. Coeliac activity of gliadin peptides CT-1 and CT-2. *Z Lebens Unters Forsch* 1986; 182: 115–7.

95 Zhong F, McCombs CC, Olson JM *et al.* An autosomal screen for genes that predispose to coeliac disease in the western counties of Ireland. *Nature Genetics* 1996; 14: 229–333.

96 Zimmer KP, Poremba C, Weber P, Ciclitira PJ, Harms E. Translocation of gliadin into HLA-DR antigen containing lysosomes in coeliac disease enterocytes. *Gut* 1995; 36(5): 703–9.

Chapter 41

Irritable bowel syndrome, Crohn's disease and ulcerative colitis

K. L. E. Dear and J. O. Hunter

INTRODUCTION

The concept of food intolerance as an aetiological factor in gastrointestinal disease has attracted a great deal of attention in recent years. However, as early as 1771 the King's Physician, Sir George Bates, presented to the Royal College of Physicians, a patient whose abdominal symptoms improved on a diet of 'sea biscuits and salt meat'.[32] Reports early in the 20th century described patients with abdominal pain, vomiting and diarrhoea provoked by ingestion of a variety of foods such as honey, eggs and beef. Relief of symptoms occurred only on avoidance of such foods and returned with a repeat challenge.[33] It was only subsequent to such observations that W. K. Dicke[117] discovered the causal link between gluten and coeliac disease, allowing a simple dietary change to relieve what was frequently previously a dangerous disease. Food, and an intolerance to it, has subsequently been shown to play an important role in other gastrointestinal disorders such as irritable bowel syndrome (IBS), Crohn's disease and, to a lesser extent, ulcerative colitis.

IRRITABLE BOWEL SYNDROME (IBS)

Epidemiology

IBS is a condition of unknown aetiology diagnosed by the fulfilment of specific criteria in the absence of any other bowel pathology.[112] Patients have at least a 3-month history of abdominal pain, commonly situated over the sigmoid colon, relieved by defaecation or associated with a change in stool frequency or form or alteration in the passage of stool. Associated features include abdominal bloating and the passage of mucus per rectum. The condition is frequently a chronic relapsing disorder, with periods of wellbeing interrupted by attacks of symptoms. It has been estimated that between 14 and 22% of the general population suffer with such symptoms at some time in their life.[59, 113] The condition is commoner in young women, who are affected twice as frequently as men. The onset of symptoms occurs before the age of 35 years in 50% of patients.

Aetiology

Despite the frequency of the condition, the aetiology of IBS is uncertain but many hypotheses exist. Abnormalities in small bowel motility have been shown, e.g. shorter duration of postprandial electrical activity with longer episodes of postprandial motor quiescence together with clusters of contractions associated with abdominal pain.[1] Abnormalities seen in colonic motility include colonic hypermotility with high pressure waves which is associated with pain-predominant IBS.[17] Many patients have also been shown to have visceral hyperalgesia, with abdominal pain experienced at lower volumes of rectal balloon distension than controls.[63] Psychological factors have also been suggested to be important, with patients scoring higher on standard anxiety and depression scores than controls.[119] The similarity of symptoms to patients with hypolactasia has led us and others to show that many patients improve with dietary restrictions of foods to which they seem intolerant. Such varying hypotheses have led many to consider that the syndrome is probably multifactorial (see Chapter 23).

Food intolerance in irritable bowel syndrome

There have been several trials to determine the effect of dietary restriction in IBS. The results of the major trials are shown in Table 41.1. The protocols for all the studies are similar. Patients follow a bland diet for between 1 and 3 weeks. This enables any intolerant foods to be cleared from the body before the process of food testing. The composition of these diets has varied. Initially, a diet composed solely of lamb, rice and pears was used. Such a strict diet may be the reason that initial studies produced better results than subsequent ones where diets were less strict. Indeed, Farah et al.[39] included citrus fruits and corn in their initial diet, foods of which many patients are intolerant. Since these diets are very restrictive, compliance may be poor. This led us to develop a less restricted exclusion diet which avoided only those foods which upset 20% or more patients. The results reported by Parker et al.[88] showed that 200 of the original 253 patients were able to complete the diet, the compliance being no better than that reported by Alun Jones et al.[3] of 21 of 25 on a very restricted diet.

Patients then introduced one food at a time into their diet every 24–48 h. A food to which they are intolerant will reproduce their symptoms and the patient is instructed to avoid that food. Patients are usually asked to repeat the challenge two or three times to confirm the intolerance over a period of weeks. Such open food challenges are open to subjective bias, patients often having preconceived ideas about which foods they tolerate. Confirmation by double blind placebo-controlled food challenges is the gold standard, the food being either coated in capsular form or given via a nasogastric tube, thereby eliminating taste. However, such studies are difficult to design and tedious to perform. All studies to date have performed double blind challenges on only a selected few patients, with varying confirmatory results. It is difficult to define patients who will respond to such a regime. Nanda et al.[84] showed that women under 30 years of age with a history of food intolerance were more likely to respond, together with patients over 50 years with flatus as a predominant symptom. Our experience has been that the age and sex of patients are immaterial, and many patients with no suspicion of food intolerance do very well. The symptoms most likely to respond to an exclusion diet are listed in Table 41.2.

Long-term follow up of IBS patients treated by dietary manipulation is limited, but those who remain on their diets do well. Nanda et al.[84] reviewed their 91 responders to diet after 18 months, finding that 73 of these were still following their safe diet and all but one were free of symptoms. Our own follow up data over 22–39 months showed continuing remission in 53 of 61 patients who were still following a diet.[54]

Implicated foods

The foods which have been commonly implicated in IBS vary between studies (Table 41.3).

Most studies have shown that cereals, especially wheat, and dairy products, are the foods most commonly to blame. Many patients have multiple food intolerances. We have found that only 5% have a single intolerance, 28% have between two and five, 35% have between six and ten, and 32% have more than ten intolerances, with half of these having over 20.[54] Such multiple intolerances are difficult to manage by diet alone since such restricted diets may often be nutritionally inadequate.

Immunological abnormalities
True food allergies

Food intolerance is reported by a large proportion of the adult population,[76] but this does not represent true food allergy. By definition, food allergy constitutes an immune-mediated reaction. Most true food allergies appear to be IgE-mediated,[47] causing a type 1 hypersensitivity reaction with presensitized IgE antibodies on the surface of mast cells. The food allergen is bound,

Frequency of food intolerances in patients with irritable bowel syndrome as shown in the major trials to date					
Authors	Year	Reference	No. of patients	Responders	Positive double blind challenges
Alun Jones et al.	1982	3	25	14	5 of 6
Bentley et al.	1983	12	27	10	3 of 10
Farah et al.	1985	39	49	13	3 of 8
Nanda et al.	1989	84	200	91	—
Parker et al.	1995	88	253	100	—

Table 41.1 Frequency of food intolerances in patients with irritable bowel syndrome as shown in the major trials to date.

Analysis of presenting symptoms suffered by 122 patients subsequently found to be food intolerant	
Symptom	**%**
Abdominal pain	73
Diarrhoea	60
Tiredness	42
Headaches	38
Constipation	22.5
Abdominal distension	21.5
Related conditions	
Migraine	11
Atopy	10

From Hunter et al.,[54] with kind permission from the authors and publisher, Blackwell Scientific.

Table 41.2 Analysis of presenting symptoms suffered by 122 patients subsequently found to be food intolerant. In addition to the abdominal symptoms a significant proportion of 188 patients also complain of lethergy and headache

Common food intolerances as shown in the major studies to date. Values are percentages			
Food	**Hunter et al.[54]**	**Lessof et al.[65]**	**Nanda et al.[84]**
Milk	44	46	31.9
Egg	26	40	23.3
Nuts	22	22	18
Fish/shellfish	10	22	2.2
Wheat	60	9	29.7
Chocolate	22	9	27.5
Colourings	—	7	2.2
Pork	14	7	2.2
Chicken	13	6	—
Tomatoes	11	6	5.5
Onions	22	6	35.2
Soft fruits	8	6	7.7
Cheese	39	5	35.2
Yeast	20	3	5.5
Coffee	33	—	24.2
Tea	25	—	17.6

Table 41.3 Common food intolerances as shown in the major studies to date. Values are percentages.

resulting in mast cell degranulation, with the release of proinflammatory mediators such as histamine, proteases, heparin, proteoglycans and chemotactic factors. This leads to increased bowel wall permeability, increased mucus production, inflammatory cell infiltration and stimulation of pain fibres. This results in symptoms of pain, diarrhoea, nausea and vomiting. Such reactions often also cause non-gastrointestinal symptoms such as asthma, rhinorrhoea, urticaria and even angio-oedema.

Tests for specific IgE

A diagnosis of food allergy demands that symptoms follow food exposure and that there is evidence of an immunological cause. Commonly employed immunological tests include the radio-allergosorbent test (RAST), enzyme-linked immunosorbent assay (ELISA) and leukocyte histamine release. The RAST involves the incubation of patient's serum with food antigen on a paper disc.[76] Non-specific antibody is washed off and any resulting immune complex is demonstrated by radiolabelled anti-IgE antibody. The ELISA follows the same principle but the resulting immune complex is demonstrated by an enzyme marker. Leukocyte histamine release measures the amount of histamine released by patient's leukocytes after exposure to dilute suspensions of food antigens. The other commonly carried out tests are skin prick tests,[47] where solutions of food antigens are applied to the skin and the skin pricked with a sterile lancet. A positive result produces a wheal when read 15 min later. Such tests seem no less sensitive nor specific than other immunological tests.[121] However, a positive immunological test does not prove food allergy unless the patient gives a history of intolerance to that food. Therefore, immunological tests should be limited to those foods identified from the history as causing symptoms. Ideally, such a food allergy should then be confirmed by a double blind food challenge.

Incidence of true food allergy in irritable bowel syndrome

There have been few trials assessing the frequency of true food allergy in IBS. Petitpierre et al.[92] studied 24 patients, of whom 12 were considered to be atopic according to the classical criteria (personal and family history, atopic symptoms, positive immediate skin tests and RAST). Such a high percentage of atopy is unusual in the general population of IBS patients. All patients underwent skin testing for 20 foods, IgE, RAST, and total IgE. Fourteen patients had symptoms with one or more foods and nine of these had positive immunological tests, all nine being atopic. The high positive rate was a reflection of the abnormally high percentage of atopics.

Bentley et al.[12] studied 27 patients, all of whom underwent skin testing. Food allergy was confirmed in only three of the 27 patients, all of whom, again, had a history of atopy. Zwetchenbaum et al.[129] studied 10 non-atopic patients who were assessed by skin tests and IgE RAST panel to common foods. Six patients had positive skin tests, only one also having an elevated IgE RAST. However, no patients responded to a food rechallenge.

Alun Jones et al.[3] studied six patients with IBS who had previously responded to an exclusion diet. Histamine concentrations, immune complexes and total IgE levels were measured after blind food challenges which confirmed a clinical reaction to the food. No positive immunological responses were detected in any of the above.

Delayed allergic response

Such studies suggest that an explanation other than IgE-mediated immunity must account for the majority of cases of food intolerance in patients with IBS. A delayed allergic response has been suggested[60] which may occur between 1 and several days after ingestion of the offending food. Such reactions are difficult to detect by history or double blind food challenges. Some of these delayed food reactions have been attributed to IgE antibodies,[8,60] but most appear not to be.[70] It is currently believed that such delayed reactions, when a true immunological reaction has been demonstrated, are associated with IgG, in particular IgG4.[48,107] Furthermore, allergen-specific IgG4 is found at higher levels in allergic subjects compared to controls and can be found in allergic subjects with low IgE and negative RAST and skin prick tests. IgG receptors have also been found on mast cells and basophils.[83] Further evidence that mast cells are important in cases of food intolerance in IBS comes from studies using the mast cell stabilizing agent sodium cromoglycate. Lunardi et al.[66] studied 20 patients with IBS and positive double blind food challenges to various foods. Only two patients had positive IgE RAST and skin prick tests. Patients were randomized to 8 weeks of treatment with sodium cromoglycate and placebo in a crossover study with a washout interval of 4 weeks between treatments. Compared to controls, 17 improved significantly on sodium cromoglycate when challenged with intolerant foods. Similar encouraging results have been achieved by others.[25,28] Sodium cromoglycate has been shown to inhibit the passage of macromolecules across the intestinal mucosa, preventing the formation of immune complexes[6] thereby providing a further protective mechanism in food intolerance.

Prostaglandins in food intolerance

Prostaglandins have been implicated in the pathogenesis of food intolerance. Administration of PGE_2 and $PGF_{2\alpha}$ produce gastrointestinal symptoms such as nausea, vomiting, colicky abdominal pain and bloating, symptoms typical of IBS.[79] Rises in PGE_2 and $PGF_{2\alpha}$ have been shown to occur in plasma and stool after challenge with intolerant foods.[24] Rises in PGF_2 have also been found in the rectal mucosa after a positive food challenge.[3] These correlated with faecal weight and, hence, with diarrhoea. Symptoms have been shown to improve with the use of non-selective prostaglandin inhibitors accompanied by a decrease in prostaglandin levels.[23]

Other possible mechanisms of food intolerance

Enzyme deficiencies

Non-immune mechanisms of food intolerance include intestinal enzyme deficiencies such as lactase deficiency. This has been demonstrated to occur in up to 25% of all patients presenting with IBS-like symptoms to this department.[89] Occasionally, other disaccharide deficiencies occur, such as trehalase deficiency (found in 8% of people living in Greenland but in 0 of 402 patients in Nottingham),[89] and isomaltase–sucrase deficiency, but the infrequency of such deficiencies makes them unlikely to be important in IBS. Foods themselves may contain toxic constituents, e.g. vasoactive amines in cheese, wine, avocados and bananas, oxalates in rhubarb and alkaloids in mushrooms. Food additives such as monosodium glutamate or preservatives such as sodium benzoate, nitrites and colouring agents may all have direct toxic effects.

Colonic flora

The effect of food on the colonic flora has also been proposed as a possible mechanism for food intolerance in IBS (see Chapter XX). In a healthy individual the composition of the gut flora is affected by complex regulatory forces such as the microbial community and the host's physiological and immunological status.[102]

Although the rank order of species in the flora is usually stable, the characteristics of the population may change with diet.[128] Balsari et al.[10] found that six of 20 patients with IBS had facultative species (Pseudomonas and Enterobacter) which were not present in controls. Patients also had lower numbers of Escherichia coli and Bifidobacter species. Bayliss et al.[11] showed that patients with food intolerances had higher numbers of aerobes in a faecal sample compared to controls. Food challenges produced noticeable changes in the predominant aerobic flora of four of six patients and in the anaerobic flora of three of six patients.

Bradley et al.[21] showed an increase in Gram-negative facultative bacteria in food-intolerant individuals. Thus, from the limited studies to date, there does appear to be a change in the intestinal bacteria, but changes do not appear to be consistent.

Psychological disorders

Finally, psychological studies of patients referred with suspected food allergies have revealed a high prevalence of psychiatric disorders.[90] Psychological disorders such as anxiety and depression may have a direct effect upon the gut mediated via neurohormond agents and there is no evidence as yet to suggest a psychopathological role in food intolerance. Indeed amongst IBS patients, a higher prevalence of psychological disorder appears to be restricted to the few who seek medical intervertion, representing a determinant of health-seeking behaviour, rather than being a risk factor for IBS.

Conclusion

IBS is a common disorder of unknown aetiology. Food intolerance is seen in approximately 50% who respond well to an exclusion diet. Those who respond initially are likely to enjoy long-term improvement if they avoid the relevant foods. No consistent immunological abnormality has been documented in the majority of patients with food intolerance. Other possible aetiologies for food intolerance in IBS may include direct toxic effects of some foods or preservatives and changes in the bacterial flora.

FOOD INTOLERANCE IN CROHN'S DISEASE

Introduction

Crohn's disease is a chronic inflammatory disease of unknown aetiology that can involve any part of the gastrointestinal system from the mouth to the anus. It is characterized by episodes of relapse and remission. Pathologically active disease is seen as areas of transmural inflammation with granulomas present in approximately 50% of cases. The sites of inflammation are often discontinuous, with areas of normal mucosa between. The first series of patients was described by Dalziel in 1913, followed by Crohn[27] in 1932. The disease affects the small bowel alone in 30–40%, small and large bowel in 40–50% and the large bowel alone in 15–25%. Of the 75% or so with small bowel disease, the terminal ileum is involved in 90%.

The prevalence of Crohn's disease varies throughout the world, with the highest prevalence being in industrialized north-west Europe, North America, Australia and South Africa. The incidence of Crohn's disease has steadily risen since its initial description by Crohn, but may now have reached a plateau.[35] Such epidemiological evidence has led some to believe that the evolution of a highly processed Western diet is important in the aetiology of this condition.[104]

Foods implicated in the pathogenesis

Refined sugar

Several authors have reported an increased incidence of Crohn's disease in individuals who consume higher quantities of refined sugar before the onset of their disease as compared to healthy controls.[69,106] Others failed to show such a relationship,[43,94] and this has subsequently been confirmed by a recent review by Riordan et al.[97] of all such studies. Several studies have also shown that patients with Crohn's disease consume more refined sugar than controls, both adding more sugar to food[72] and eating more sweet food and confectionery.[71] It seems likely that increased sugar intake may simply be a convenient way of meeting energy demand although this was disputed by Thornton et al.,[114] who found no difference in the intake of refined sugar between patients with recent onset and longstanding symptoms. However, controlled trials of high fibre, low sugar diets have shown no benefit in Crohn's disease.[98]

Fibre

Several researchers have shown that patients with Crohn's disease have a decreased consumption of fruit and fibre.[14,114] However, such studies are difficult to interpret since patients with Crohn's tend to avoid high fibre foods since they often provoke symptoms and because they may be instructed so to do by their physicians. Breakfast cereals and bread have been reported by others to be consumed in larger quantities in patients with Crohn's disease.[55,91] The authors suggested that consumption of such foods on an empty stomach for breakfast would more likely allow them to reach affected parts of the bowel.

The low fibre, high refined sugar diets are typical of Western cultures and have become increasingly popular since World War II, which reflects the epidemiology of Crohn's. Another Western food habit, that of fast, highly processed foods, has also been implicated. Persson et al.[91] showed that consumption of such foods at least twice a week was associated with a three to fourfold increased risk of developing Crohn's, but this may just reflect increased consumption of the low fibre, high refined sugar content of such foods.

Induction of remission

Conventionally, this has been achieved by the use of corticosteroids ever since the studies of Truelove and Witt.[116] Such treatment induces remission in 80–90% of cases. However, such treatment is not without side effects, which has led towards the development of other treatments.

Total parenteral nutrition

Total parenteral nutrition (TPN) was initially used before surgery to improve the nutrition of patients, and to minimize problems after surgery such as poor wound healing and infection. However, it has been shown to have a therapeutic effect independent of improved nutrition.[29,40,95] The mechanism was thought to be through resting the bowel and removing food antigens from the gut lumen. Ostro et al.[87] reported a remission rate of 77 of 100 patients with acute Crohn's disease. The number still in remission after 3 months and 12 months was 75% and 58%, respectively. They found a similar efficacy in small and large bowel disease. Patients with subacute obstruction or an inflammatory mass did well; those with fistulous disease did less well. Others report a lower success rate of around 40% induction of remission, although

these earlier studies involved a mixture of patients with Crohn's and ulcerative colitis. Hanauer et al.[49] looked solely at patients with ulcerative colitis, finding that only 19 of 40 responded to TPN, of whom four relapsed in the following 2 years.

The mechanism of action does not seem to be solely bowel rest. Greenberg et al.[45] found no significant difference in remission or relapse rates between patients receiving parenteral nutrition alone, parenteral nutrition and unrestricted diet or enteral polymeric diet.

TPN is costly and not without complications. Mullen et al.[80] reported a complication rate of 10%, with 4% having a pneumothorax, 4% catheter-related sepsis and 2% metabolic complications. Thus, since bowel rest did not seem essential for the beneficial effects of TPN, enteral preparations were developed as treatments to avoid the cost and complications of TPN.

Elemental diet

Elemental diets are synthetic liquid diets which have been proven to be nutritionally adequate.[124] Protein is supplied as amino acids, carbohydrate as maltodextrins and sugar, fat as small quantities of defined oils with the addition of vitamins and minerals. They were initially used as an alternative to TPN to provide preoperative nutritional support, but patients fed such diets while awaiting surgery experienced clinical improvements of their disease as well as improved nutrition.[118] Several subsequent reports compared their efficacy with that of corticosteroids.[42,53,103] O'Morain et al.[86] showed a remission rate of 82% for elemental diet as compared to 80% for steroids. Alun Jones[5] showed elemental diet to be as effective and rapid in response for the control of inflammation and correction of malnutrition as TPN. Initially, it was thought that these feeds worked by the avoidance of antigenic whole proteins which were replaced by the constitutive amino acids.[5] However, many have subsequently shown that feeds containing oligopeptides and even whole proteins are as effective in inducing remission.[68,77,100]

Other mechanisms of action have thus been considered, including the role of other constituents. Enteral feeds differ widely in their source and content of fat. Elemental feeds have minimal fat content, with less than 2% of the total energy of these feeds being derived from fat, compared to some peptide and polymeric diets in which fat supplies as much as 30% of the total energy. Gassull et al.[41] showed that diets with intermediate or high levels of fat were inferior to those of low fat content. One possible mechanism of action of low fat diets is that such diets reduce the triglycerides that can be subsequently converted to pro-inflammatory eicosanoids. Middleton et al.,[78] however, showed that it may not be the overall level of fat that is important but the quantity of long chain triglycerides (Table 41.4), since a greater number of patients achieved remission with use of enteral feeds containing a low percentage of long chain triglycerides (Table 41.5).

Elemental diets are absorbed in the small bowel, therefore the only materials reaching the colon are enterocytes and mucus shed from the intestinal wall. It is therefore not surprising that there is a profound reduction in faecal wet and dry weight on enteral feeds and a reduction in colonic bacterial mass.[81] This would lead to reduction in bacterial antigens which could be a further possible mechanism of action. Winitz et al.[123] showed a reduction in all types of bacteria while an elemental diet was taken, but such findings have not been reproduced by others.[9,20]

Nomenclature of fatty acids commonly found in foods				
Carbon: double bonds	Class	*Name	Structure	Common natural sources
4:0	Short chain/saturated	Butyric (tetranoic)	$CH_3(CH_2)_2CO_2H$	
6:0	Short chain/saturated	Caproic (hexanoic)	$CH_3(CH_2)_3CO_2H$	
8:0	Short chain/saturated	Caprylic (octanoic)	$CH_3(CH_2)_4CO_2H$	Coconut oil and dairy products
10:0	Medium chain/saturated	Capric (decanoic)	$CH_3(CH_2)_5CO_2H$	
12:0	Medium chain/saturated	Lauric (dodecanoic)	$CH_3(CH_2)_6CO_2H$	
14:0	Long chain/saturated	Myristic (tetradecanoic)	$CH_3(CH_2)_7CO_2H$	
16:0	Long chain/saturated	Palmitic (hexadecanoic)	$CH_3(CH_2)_8CO_2H$	Palm oil, butter, meat
18:0	Long chain/saturated	Stearic (octadecanoic)	$CH_3(CH_2)_9CO_2H$	Meat, butter and chocolate
20:0	Long chain/saturated	Arachidic (eicosanoic)	$CH_3(CH_2)_{10}CO_2H$	Nut and seed oils
22:0	Long chain/saturated	Behanic (docosanoic)	$CH_3(CH_2)_{11}CO_2H$	Peanut oil, peanuts
16:1n7	Long chain/ monounsaturated	Palmitoleic (9 cis-hexadecenoic)	$CH_3(CH_2)_5CH=CH(CH_2)_7CO_2H$	Cod liver oil, meat fat, fish
18:1n9	Long chain/ monounsaturated	Oleic (9 cis-octadecanoic)	$CH_3(CH_2)_7CH=CH(CH_2)_7CO_2H$	Olive oil, nut and seed oils, eggs, butter
22:1n9	Long chain/ monounsaturated	Eruic (13 cis-docosaenoic)	$CH_3(CH_2)_7CH=CH(CH_2)_{11}CO_2H$	Rapeseed (if not a low eruic variety)
18:2n6	Long chain/ polyunsaturated	Linoleic (9,12 cis-octadecadienoic)	$CH_3(CH_2)_4(CH=CHCH_2)_2(CH_2)_6CO_2H$	Vegetable oils, nuts, lean meat and eggs
18:3n3	Long chain/ polyunsaturated	Alpha-linolenic (9,12,15 all cis-octadecatrienoic)	$CH_3CH_2(CH=CHCH_2)_3(CH_2)_6CO_2H$	Soyabean and rapeseed oils
20:4n6	Long chain/ polyunsaturated	Arachidonic (5,8,11,14, all cis-eicosatetraenoic)	$CH_3(CH_2)_4(CH=CHCH_2)_3(CH_2)_3CO_2H$	Offal, game, lean meat, egg

* Systematic name in brackets.

Table 41.4 Nomenclature of fatty acids commonly found in foods.

Maintenance of remission

Although elemental diets and TPN are effective at inducing remission, patients cannot stay on such treatments indefinitely and it is usual to restart regular food after a period of 2–4 weeks. This results in relapse in many patients. Teahon et al.[111] reported a relapse rate of 22% in the first 6 months after induction of remission with elemental diet. There was a subsequent annual relapse rate of 8–10%, with a probability of maintaining remission of 38% at 3 years. Those continuing on steroids relapsed at the same rate, with the ineffectiveness of steroids in maintaining remission also being shown by two large multicentre trials in Crohn's disease.[67,109]

Use of an exclusion diet

Alun Jones et al.[4] showed that the use of an exclusion diet to identify intolerant foods after induction of remission by either TPN or elemental diet, maintained remission in seven of 10 patients as compared to none of 10 patients fed on a diet containing substantial amounts of unrefined carbohydrate. Subsequent follow up of 77 patients treated by exclusion diets showed 51 patients still in remission on such a diet over a period of follow up of up to 51 months. The East Anglian Multicentre trial[96] compared maintenance to a slowly reducing regime of prednisolone over 12 weeks to an exclusion diet after induction of remission with elemental diet. Median length of remission

Composition of some of the enteral feeds produced by SHS International Limited as used by Middleton et al.[78]				
Enteral feed	Peptide 2+	EO28	E028 LCT	E028 MCT
Feed type	Semi-elemental	Elemental	Elemental	Elemental
Energy (kcal)	469	382	443	500
Protein/100 g dry weight (% energy)	13.8 (11.8)	10 (10.5)	12.2 (11.2)	12.5 (10)
Source	Meat and soya	Synthetic	Synthetic	Synthetic
Carbohydrate/100 g dry weight (% energy)	64.5 (55.0)	70.5 (73.8)	59 (53.3)	73 (58.4)
Source	Maltodextrins	Maltodextrin and sugar	Maltodextrin and sugar	Maltodextrin and sugar
Total fat/100 g dry weight (% energy)	17.3 (33.2)	6.6 (15.6)	17.5 (35.6)	17.5 (31.6)
Total LCT/100 g dry weight (% energy)	11.2 (21.6)	6.6 (15.6)	17.5 (35.6)	11.4 (20.5)
LCT source	Maize oil	†Arachis oil	Safflower and *canola	Safflower and *canola
Total MCT/100 g dry weight (% energy)	6.1 (11.6)	0 (0)	0 (0)	6.1 (11.1)
MCT source	Coconut oil	None	None	Coconut oil
Saturated fat (% total fat)	65.4	17.1	11.1	44
Monounsaturated fat (% total fat)	11.7	56.9	67.2	42
Polyunsaturated fat (% total)	22.9	26	21.7	14

Dietary data calculated for ready flavoured feeds or with orange flavouring added (Peptide 2+). *Canola also known as rapeseed, †Arachis oil also known as peanut oil. LCT, long chain triglycerides; MCT, medium chain triglycerides.

Table 41.5 Composition of some of the enteral feeds produced by SHS International Limited as used by Middleton et al.[78]

was 3.8 months for the steroid group compared to 7.5 months for the diet group ($P<0.05$) (Fig. 41.1). Although these figures

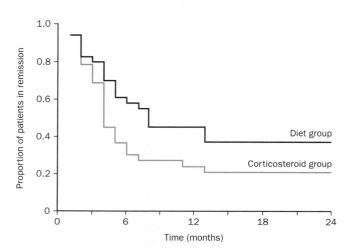

Fig. 41.1 Proportion of patients remaining in clinical remission on an exclusion diet in comparison to steroid reduction over time. From the East Anglian Multicentre controlled trial (Riordan et al.[96]).

are disappointing compared to some, it clearly shows exclusion diets do prolong remission (Fig. 41.2).

Commonly implicated foods

It has been found that the foods commonly implicated in food intolerance are similar to those in IBS, with wheat and dairy products being very important (see Table 41.3). Multiple food intolerances occur frequently, but not quite to the same degree as in irritable bowel syndrome. Alun Jones et al.[4] reported that 35 of 59 patients had less than five intolerances, and 54 of 59 had less than 10.

Current practice in this department is to introduce a new food daily once remission has been achieved. Each food needs to be consumed in large quantities on two or three occasions on the test day. If the food is tolerated without symptoms, it is presumed safe and introduced into the regular diet. If a person reacts to a food, this is then excluded from the diet temporarily, to be retested later to confirm an intolerance. If there is doubt regarding a food, it is avoided initially and rechallenged at a later date for a longer period of 4 days. All foods which provoke a reaction should ideally be confirmed by double blind challenge.

After every 7 days of food testing, a patient is allowed 2 rest days on which no new foods are tested, to help identify delayed

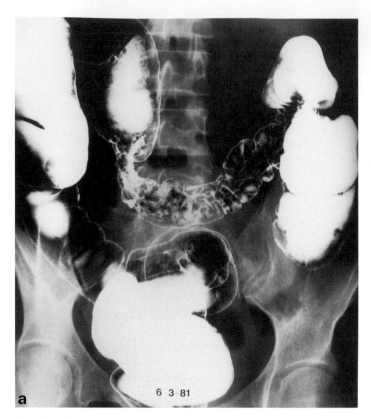
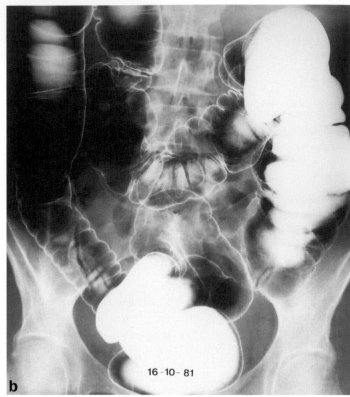

Fig. 41.2 Barium enema. (a) March 6, 1981, showing transverse colon affected by narrowing, ulceration, obliteration of the haustra and skip lesions; (b) October 16, 1981 showing no ulceration and a normally distensible colon, with puckering and pseudodiverticulum formation because of fibrosis from burnt-out Crohn's disease. From Alun Jones *et al.*,[4] with permission.

food reactions. Foods are only tested when a patient is asymptomatic. Severe reactions can take several days to settle, often requiring a patient to go back to elemental feeding for a few days. Foods least likely to cause a reaction are tested first to help build up confidence and to allow the patient off the elemental diet. The elemental diet is gradually reduced until enough foods have been introduced to provide adequate nutrition. The final diet is assessed by a dietitian to ensure it is nutritionally adequate.

LOFFLEX diet

Food reintroduction in patients with Crohn's disease is a slow process, often taking up to 3 months. In addition, patients have to continue an elemental diet for several weeks while food testing continues. Patients require great discipline and many are unwilling to follow such a regime. This is reflected in the East Anglian Multicentre trial where 31% of patients failed to tolerate such a diet.

From our experience with exclusion diets, we have found the foods which commonly elicit symptoms in patients with Crohn's; these are represented in Table 41.6. Using this knowledge, a diet was devised which avoided those foods which provoked symptoms in more than 5% of patients, along with high fibre and high fat foods, which also often produce symptoms. These were replaced with suitable alternatives of a similar nutritional content. This led to the low fibre, fat limited exclusion diet (LOFFLEX). Remission is induced in the usual way with an elemental diet. The patient is then put on the LOFFLEX diet and, since this is nutritionally complete, patients can stop elemental diet. As the patient

Foods reported by over 5% of patients with Crohn's disease as causing symptoms when reintroduced after enteral feeding			
Food	**Patients (%)**	**Food**	**Patients %**
Wheat products	25	Yeast	11
Onion	19	Eggs	11
Coffee	19	Apple	10
Corn	17.5	Tea	10
Oats	17.5	Chocolate	10
Milk	16	Nuts	10
Dairy products	16	Pork	9
Citrus fruits	16	Pulses	9
High fibre	15	High fat	7.5
Rye	15	Alcoholic drinks	7.5
Tomato	12.5	Bananas	6

Table 41.6 Foods reported by over 5% of patients with Crohn's disease as causing symptoms when reintroduced after enteral feeding. (From a review of 80 patients, 1994, data not published.)

is allowed to consume a relatively wide range of foods, they are more likely to be compliant and complete the diet. Since fewer foods are excluded, the process of food testing is faster, allowing more time between testing individual foods, usually 4 days, which allows improved detection of delayed food reactions.

Woolner et al.[125] described the application of this diet. Remission was induced by means of elemental diet and then subjects were offered a conventional diet or the LOFFLEX diet. Four of 28 patients(14%) did not comply with the exclusion diet compared to four of 48(8%) on the LOFFLEX diet. Of the 28 patients on the exclusion diet 21(75%) maintained remission , compared to 38 of 48(79%) on a LOFFLEX diet. Such a diet seems as effective, if not more so, than a conventional exclusion diet and is certainly better tolerated.

Immunological abnormalities
Luminal antigens
The intestine is constantly bombarded with luminal antigens, primarily from food and the endogenous microflora. Evidence that such luminal contents are essential for the development of Crohn's disease comes from postoperative studies. Recurrent disease invariably occurs at the anastomotic site with time. However, if the anastomosis is protected by a proximal ileostomy, recurrent anastomotic disease does not occur. Ulceration promptly recurs within 6 months of closure of the proximal stoma.[101] The fact that we do not all develop inflammation in response to such an antigenic load is because of the presence of immunological protective mechanisms involving the humoral and cellular immune systems.

Protective humoral mechanisms are based on secretory IgA. Produced in response to such antigens as food, it forms an immune complex, the size of which prevents absorption of the antigen across the mucosa. Secretory IgA complexes lack the ability to fix complement and therefore fail to induce a local inflammatory response.[15] IgA-specific immune responses have also been linked to the induction of tolerance to the inducing antigen.[26] Therefore, to precipitate inflammation, food may induce alternative immune mechanisms to IgA in IBD. Alternatively, IgA deficiency may lead to a reduction of the usual IgA-mediated tolerance to food antigens.

IgE antibodies and mast cells
Other humoral responses may well involve IgE, as seen in classical food allergy. Heatley et al.[50] showed an abundance of IgE in rectal mucosal biopsies in patients with active proctitis, but few in quiescent disease. O'Donoghue and Kumar[85] confirmed such findings in active disease but also found raised levels in quiescent disease. Raised levels of mast cells have also been demonstrated in areas of active disease, occupying the submucosal and muscular layers.[34,93] Such cells are often seen in a degranulated state, suggesting that they are not merely inactive bystanders. Further evidence that mast cells may be important in this disorder is that the mast cell stabilizing agent, sodium cromoglycate, was reported to have a beneficial effect in this disorder. Heatley et al.[51] showed a symptomatic improvement in 14 of 26 patients with proctitis using this agent but this was not confirmed by later studies.[73] Such evidence suggests that IgE-mediated responses may have a role in Crohn's disease, but the relation of such responses to food intolerance is less clear. Jewell and Truelove[58] looked at immunological reactions to milk proteins. They demonstrated that the percentage of positive reactions was similar in Crohn's disease

and ulcerative colitis as in controls. No circulating IgE antibodies were found and IgA and IgG antibodies found showed no correlation to the skin prick results.

Crossreacting antigens
These have been found between bacteria commonly resident in the healthy bowel and colonic epithelial cells.[105] Such crossreactions may similarly occur with food antigens. Antibodies to bovine protein have been detected in IBD,[38] but have also been found in other gastrointestinal disorders such as coeliac disease and even in normal individuals.

IgA deficiency
The importance of IgA deficiency in allergic disease was suggested by Taylor et al.,[110] who showed atopy was more common in children with transient IgA deficiency. However, no such deficiency has been observed in IBD. Indeed, to the contrary, Hodgson and Jewell[52] showed IgA levels were raised significantly in ulcerative colitis, with a similar trend in Crohn's disease as compared to healthy controls. However, Kett et al.[64] subsequently showed that both IgA1 and IgA2 immunoglobulin subclasses in IBD produced less J chain peptide necessary for the production of the secretory form than healthy controls. In addition, IgA1 was the predominant subclass compared to controls, where IgA2 was the dominant subclass. They showed IgA2 lymphocytes produced more J peptide than IgA1 lymphocytes, thus leading to further lowering of J peptide production. Thus, although there is an overall increase in IgA production in IBD, there is a reduction in secretory IgA. In addition, the IgA1 subclass which dominates in IBD is more susceptible to microbial proteases.

Cellular mechanisms
Such mechanisms protect against immunological reactions to all mucosal antigens and include induction of T cell subsets mediating suppression and, probably less importantly in the gastrointestinal system, the induction of clonal anergy. T cells which suppress responses via TGFβ seem to be particularly prominent in the Peyer's patches. Strober and Kelsall,[108] in a recent review of the mucosal cellular immune system, stressed the importance of the balance between proinflammatory helper T cell response, characterized by the production of IFNγ and TNFα, and the anti-inflammatory T cell down-regulatory response, characterized by the production of TGFβ. In health, most encounters between mucosal antigens and the mucosal cellular immune system result in a predominant TGFβ producing a T cell response resulting in tolerance to luminal antigen. However, in disease states such as IBD it is believed that the normal mechanisms of tolerance are bypassed in some manner, resulting in an excessive proinflammatory T cell response, dominated by T1 helper cells and the production of large amounts of TNFα and INFγ.

Suppressor responses
The importance of suppressor responses in colitis is elegantly illustrated by the trinitrobenzene sulphonic acid (TNBS) model of murine colitis (Fig. 41.3). This is characterized by a massive transmural infiltration of TH1 helper cells, together with IFNγ and TNFα. If, however, proteins haptenized by TNBS are given orally at the same time as TNBS given rectally, colitis does not develop.[61] It is presumed that the oral administration of this agent stimulates the TGFβ cells of the Peyer's patches to produce TGFβ which

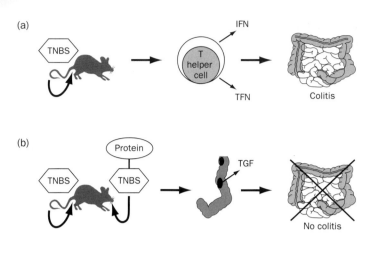

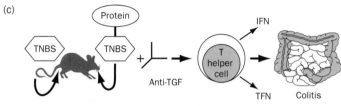

Fig. 41.3 Oral *versus* systemic challenge in the murine trinitrobenzene sulphonic acid (TNBS) model of colitis. (a) Rectally administered TNBS induces colitis in mice by causing massive transmural infiltration of T_1 helper cells into the colon. (b) Coadministration of oral proteins haptenized by TNBS together with rectally administered TNBS fails to induce colitis, by stimulation of TGF from the Peyer's patches. TGF suppresses the T helper-driven inflammatory response. (c) Coadministration of oral proteins haptenized by TNBS together with rectally administered TNBS will once again induce colitis after blockade of TGF production with specific antibodies.

suppresses the T helper-driven inflammatory response, inducing tolerance to the proteins. That this is the case is shown by the administration of anti-TGFβ at the same time mice are fed TNBS protein and given rectal TNBS. This results, once again, in colitis.

Thus, to precipitate food intolerance, food antigens may stimulate an unregulated T helper response either by somehow bypassing normal mucosal immunoregulation, or by stimulating a response in a genetically susceptible individual with deficient mucosal immunoregulation.

Conclusion

Crohn's disease is a condition that has been studied only since the 1930s and has risen in incidence with the development of Western culture and the consmption of highly processed diets . It is still rare in underdeveloped countries. Food intolerances occur frequently in this condition and prolonged remission can be achieved by the use of exclusion diets. Similar immunological abnormalities involving IgE immune responses have been seen in this condition as with some cases of IBS and true food allergy, but their relationship to food intolerances other than milk remains uncertain.

FOOD INTOLERANCE IN ULCERATIVE COLITIS

Introduction

Ulcerative colitis is a chronic inflammatory disorder of the colon of unknown aetiology. Clinically it is characterized by exacerba-

tions of bloody diarrhoea and abdominal pain interspersed with periods of relative wellbeing. Histologically, there is inflammation, usually confined to the colonic mucosa. In approximately 40–50% of patients the disease is confined to the rectum and rectosigmoid areas, whereas 20% have a total colitis. The remaining 30–40% have disease proximal to the sigmoid colon but not involving the entire colon. The disease was first identified as a distinct entity from bacillary dysentery by Samuel Wilks, with the first complete descriptions of the disease being provided by Sir Arthur Hurst at the beginning of the century. Ulcerative colitis is a worldwide disorder. Areas of high incidence include the UK, northern Europe, USA and Australia. Amongst the Caucasian population the incidence ranges from 3 to 15/100 000, with a prevalence of 50/100 000. The incidence of this condition has remained constant from the 1950s onwards, in contrast to the rising incidence of Crohn's disease. The incidence is substantially lower in southern and eastern Europe, Asia, Japan and South America.[75]

Foods implicated in the pathogenesis

Fibre

As in Crohn's disease, some have reported that a decreased consumption of fruit and vegetables in patients with colitis is associated with an increased incidence of the disease.[14,22] As mentioned previously, such studies are difficult to interpret since those with colonic symptoms often avoid high fibre foods because they frequently exacerbate their symptoms. However, others have shown an increased consumption of cereal and bread for breakfast is associated with a slight increase of colitis, suggesting that consumption of such foods on an empty stomach allows them to reach inflamed areas.[69]

Fatty foods

Long chain fatty acids are the precursors of eicosanoids. Some of the arachidonic acid-derived eicosanoids (PGE_2, leukotriene B_4 and thromboxane A_2) have been implicated in the pathogenesis of IBD, since increased concentrations of such compounds are found in the inflamed intestinal mucosa. Katschinski and Goebell[62] showed that individuals ingesting diets high in n-3 fatty acids before the onset of symptoms had an increased risk of developing colitis. Others have shown increased levels of n-3 fatty acids in the plasma of patients with colitis with both active[37] and quiescent[36] disease, suggesting the importance of ingestion of polyunsaturated fatty acids. Others have looked at the beneficial effects of the essential fatty acid gamma-linolenic acid,[46] which is rapidly converted *in vivo* to dihomogamma-linolenic acid. This compound competes with arachidonic acid for the cyclo-oxygenase enzyme in cell membranes, suppressing production of the series two prostaglandins in favour of PGE_1, which inhibits phospholipase, further limiting the production of the proinflammatory series two eicosanoids. However, this was not found to have a significant therapeutic effect in active colitis.

Breast feeding

Early artificial feeding may predispose to the future development of ulcerative colitis. Acheson and Truelove[2] reported that 30.3% of patients with colitis were not breast fed in comparison with 14.7% of controls. Such a difference was not significantly different after 1 month of life. It was concluded that early artificial feeding increases the chance of subsequently developing ulcerative colitis. Possible mechanisms may be early sensitization to cow's milk, increased intestinal permeability, or perhaps because of alterations in the bacterial flora at a time when sensitization to bacterial antigens may occur. Similar results were reported by Whorwell et al.,[120] who also suggested that breast milk may be protective against gastroenteritis in infancy, which could provide the triggering antigens for the subsequent development of colitis. However, although there was an increase in the number of cases of gastroenteritis in those with colitis compared to controls, this increase was not significant.

Cow's milk protein sensitivity during infancy

It has been suggested that infants with cow's milk protein sensitivity have an increased risk of subsequently developing ulcerative colitis. Glassman et al.[44] showed, in a retrospective questionnaire study of children and adolescents, that the frequency of a history compatible with infantile cow's milk sensitivity was 2.8% in controls (one of 36) compared to a frequency of 20.9% in patients with ulcerative colitis (nine of 43), with no significant difference being seen in Crohn's disease. They also showed that colitis began, on average, 4 years earlier in those with a history of cow's milk protein sensitivity in infancy. They hypothesized that, in patients with colitis with such a history, colonic antigens released by the inflamed mucosa could initiate the immunological reactions seen in the condition, possibly by the induction of autoantibodies. Berezin et al.[13] demonstrated an intense inflammatory reaction in the colon of infants with cow's milk sensitivity that was indistinguishable from the appearance in IBD.

Milk intolerance

As long ago as 1942, Andreson[7] suggested that ulcerative colitis might be caused by an allergy to milk, claiming that two-thirds of his patients had a food allergy, of whom 84% were sensitive to milk. Truelove[115] reintroduced milk into the diets of patients with ulcerative colitis who had previously responded to a milk-free diet and found that they relapsed. A subsequent controlled trial[126] of a milk-free diet showed that 10 of 26 patients on a milk-free diet, compared to five of 24 on a normal diet, remained asymptomatic for 1 year. They concluded that about 20% of patients improve on a milk-free diet. Raised antibodies have been found against milk, although none of the IgE class, and no correlation has been shown between the height of the antibody titre and severity or extent of disease.[57]

Diet as primary therapy

Unfortunately, unlike Crohn's disease, ulcerative colitis does not respond to dietary manipulation apart from those responding to a dairy-free diet as mentioned above. McIntyre et al.[74] showed that the outcome of a severe attack of colitis was not influenced by whether a patient was fed orally or intravenously to allow bowel rest and removal of food antigens from the gut lumen. Patients were given either TPN or hospital diets, supplemented if necessary to ensure adequate nitrogen and calorie intake, with no difference in the outcome of these groups of patients. Such lack of response has been confirmed by others.[29]

Immunological abnormalities

As in Crohn's disease, several groups have looked for abnormalities in IgE-mediated immunity in this condition. Increased numbers of mast cells have been found in the submucosa and lamina propria of the colon and rectum,[73] along with an increased histamine content in rectal biopsies.[16] Wright and Truelove[127] found increased numbers of circulating and tissue eosinophils in patients who had a relapse of their colitis (54 of 155) compared to those in remission (67 of 442). They subsequently showed that treatment with steroids caused levels to fall and concluded that eosinophils are associated with disease activity. Rosekrans et al.[99] suggested that there was a specific group of patients with proctitis with increased IgE-containing cells in the lamina propria of the rectal mucosa. He showed that eight of 12 patients in this subgroup responded to treatment with the mast cell stabilizing agent sodium cromoglycate. This agent has shown promise in other trials, with many showing both clinical and histological improvement with this agent in acute attacks. Others, however, have shown it to be inferior to sulfasalazine in maintenance of remission.[31, 122] As in Crohn's disease, there is an increased incidence of atopy in patients with colitis, with Jewell reporting an incidence of 15.2% in colitis compared to 1.2% in normal controls. However, as in Crohn's disease, no clear abnormalities of IgE immunity have been shown to correspond to food sensitivity in colitis.

Infantile colitis

Despite lack of evidence of food intolerance in adults with ulcerative colitis, food allergy may play a major role in infantile colitis. Jenkins et al.[56] reported on 46 children with colitis, showing that all eight infants under the age of 2 years had a food-allergic colitis, which histologically appeared different to ulcerative colitis, with normal crypt architecture and goblet cell preservation, and a predominance of eosinophils and IgE mononuclear cells in the lamina propria. Most of these patients became symptomatic after the introduction of foods other than breast milk. Commonly, cow's milk was implicated, but also soya and beef. Patients had a raised serum eosinophil and IgE level, four had positive skin prick tests and a family history of atopy was common. All responded to exclusion of the appropriate foods. Rechallenging the patients over the following 9 months reproduced symptoms.

Conclusion

Unlike Crohn's disease, most cases of ulcerative colitis do not respond to dietary intervention. The possible exceptions to this are infants under 2 years who often seem to respond to diet, although this disease may be a separate entity to ulcerative colitis. Although it is clinically similar, many of the classical histological findings are absent. Patients with a history of milk intolerance may also improve on a milk-free diet. Despite the lack of response to dietary manipulation, many of the immunological abnormalities are similar to those in Crohn's disease, with evidence of involvement of IgE immune responses typically seen in food allergy and other atopic disorders.

REFERENCES

1 Accarino AM, Azpiroz F, Malagelada JR. Selective dysfunction of mechanosensitive intestinal afferents in irritable bowel syndrome. *Gastroenterology* 1995; 108: 636–43.

2 Acheson ED, Truelove SC. Early weaning in the aetiology of ulcerative colitis. *BMJ* 1961; ii: 929–33.

3 Alun Jones V, Shorthouse M, McLaughlan P, Workman E, Hunter JO. Food intolerance: a major factor in the pathogenesis of irritable bowel disease. *Lancet* 1982; ii: 1115–1.

4 Alun Jones V, Workman E, Dickinson RJ, Wilson AJ, Freeman AH, Hunter JO. Crohn's disease: maintenance of remission by diet. *Lancet* 1985; ii: 177–80.

5 Alun Jones V. Comparison of total parenteral nutrition and elemental diet in induction of remission of Crohn's disease. Long-term maintenance of remission by personalised food exclusion diets. *Dig Dis Sci* 1987; 32: 100–7S.

6 Andre C, Andre F, Colin L. Effect of allergen ingestion challenge with and without cromoglycate cover, on intestinal permeability in atopic dermatitis, urticaria and other symptoms of food allergy. *Allergy* 1989; 4(Suppl. 9): 47–51.

7 Andreson AFR. Ulcerative colitis – an allergic phenomenon. *Am J Dig Dis* 1942; 9: 91.

8 Atkins CA, Zweiman B. IgE-mediated late phase skin response: unraveling the enigma. *J Allergy Clin Immunol* 1987; 79: 12–15.

9 Axelsson CK, Justessen T. Studies of the duodenal and faecal flora in gastrointestinal disorders during treatment with an elemental diet. *Gastroenterology* 1977; 72: 397–401.

10 Balsari A, Ceccarelli A, Dubin F, Fosce E, Poli G. The faecal microbial population in the irritable bowel syndrome. *Microbiologica* 1982; 5: 185–94.

11 Bayliss CE, Houston AP, Alun Jones V, Hishon S, Hunter JO. Microbiological studies on food intolerance. *Proc Nutr Soc* 1984; 43: 16A.

12 Bentley SJ, Pearson DJ, Rix KJB. Food hypersensitivity in irritable bowel syndrome. *Lancet* 1983; ii: 295–7.

13 Berezin S, Schwartz SM, Glassman MS *et al.* Gastrointestinal milk intolerance of infancy. *Am J Dis Child* 1989; 143: 361–2.

14 Bianchi Porro G, Panza E. Smoking, sugar and inflammatory bowel disease. *BMJ* 1985; 291: 971–2.

15 Bienstock J, Befus AD. Mucosal immunology. *Immunology* 1981; 41: 249–63.

16 Binder V, Hviderg E. Histamine content of rectal mucosa in ulcerative colitis. *Gut* 1967; 8: 24–8.

17 Blanchard EB, Scharff L, Schwartz SP, Sulus JM, Barlow DH. The role of anxiety and depression in the irritable bowel syndrome. *Behav Res Ther* 1990; 28: 401–5.

18 Bock SA, Buckley J, Holt A *et al.* Proper use of skin tests with food extracts in the diagnosis of hypersensitivity to food in children. *Clin Exp Allergy* 1977; 7: 375–83.

19 Bock SA, Sampson HA, Atkins FM *et al.* Double-blind placebo controlled food challenge as an office procedure: a manual. *J Allergy Clin Immunol* 1988; 82: 986–97.

20 Bounous G, Devreede GJ. Effects of an elemental diet on human faecal flora. *Gastroenterology* 1974; 66: 210–14.

21 Bradley HK, Bayliss CE, Wyatt GM, Smyth AF, Alun Jones V, Hunter JO. Food intolerance and microbial populations in the human colon. In: *Recent Advances in Anaerobic Bacteriology*, Martinus Nijhoff, Dordrecht, 1985.

22 Brandes JW, Stenner A, Martini GA. Ernährungsgewohnheiten der patienten mit colitis ulcerosa. *Zeitschrift für Gastroenterologie* 1979; 17: 834–42.

23 Buhave K, Rask-Masden J. An approach to evaluation of local intestinal prostaglandin production and clinical assessment of its inhibition by indomethacin in chronic diarrhoea. *Adv Prostaglandin Thromboxane Res* 1980; 8: 1627–31.

24 Buisseret PD, Heinzelman DI, Youlton LJF, Lessoff MH. Prostaglandin synthesis inhibitors in prophylaxis of food intolerance. *Lancet* 1978; i: 906–8.

25 Canoica GW, Ciprandi G, Bagnasco M, Scordamaglia A. Oral cromolyn in food allergy: in vivo and in vitro effects. *Clin Immunol Immunopathol* 1986; 41: 154–8.

26 Chase MW. Inhibition of experimental drug allergy by prior feeding of the sensitising agent. *Proc Soc Exp Biol Med* 1946; 61: 257–9.

27 Crohn BB, Gilzberg L, Oppenheimer GD. Regional enteritis: a pathological and clinical entity. *JAMA* 1932; 99: 1323.

28 Dahl R. Oral and inhaled sodium cromoglycate in challenge test with food allergens or acetylsalicylic acid. *Allergy* 1981; 36: 161–5.

29 Dickinson RJ, Ashton MG, Axon ATR *et al.* Controlled trial of intravenous hyperalimentation and total bowel rest as an adjunct to the routine therapy of acute colitis. *Gastroenterology* 1980; 79: 1199–204.

30 Dickinson RJ, Ashton MG, Axon ATR, Smith RC, Yeung CH, Hill GL. Controlled trial of intravenous hyperalimentation and total bowel rest as an adjunct to the routine therapy of active ulcerative colitis. *Gastroenterology* 1980; 79: 1199–204.

31 Dronfield MW, Langman MJS. Controlled comparison of sodium cromoglycate and sulphasalazine in the maintenance of remission in ulcerative colitis. *Gut* 1977; 18: A473.

32 Drummond JC, Wilbraham A. *The Englishman's Food.* Johnathan Cope, London, 1954: 254 pp.

33 Duke WW. Food allergy as a cause of abdominal pain. *Arch Int Med* 1921; 28: 151–65.

34 Dvorak AM, Monahan RA, Osage JE, Dickerson R. Crohn's disease; transmission electron microscopic studies. II. Immunologic inflammatory response. Alterations of mast cells, basophils, eosinophils and the microvasculature. *Human Path* 1980; 11: 606–19.

35 Ekbom A, Helmich C, Zak M, Admani HO. The epidemiology of inflammatory bowel disease: a large population-based study in Sweden. *Gastroenterology* 1991; 100: 350–8.

36 Esteve-Comas M, Núñez MC, Fernández-Bañares F *et al.* Abnormal plasma polyunsaturated fatty acid pattern in non active inflammatory bowel disease. *Gut* 1993; 34: 1370–3.

37 Esteve-Comas M, Ramíroe M, Fernández-Bañares F *et al.* Plasma polyunsaturated fatty acid pattern in active inflammatory bowel disease. *Gut* 1992; 33: 1365–9.

38 Falchuck KR, Isselbacher KJ. Circulating antibodies to bovine albumin in ulcerative colitis and Crohn's disease. *Gastroenterology* 1976; 70: 5–8.

39 Farah DA, Calder I, Benson L, Mackenzie JF. Specific food intolerance: its place as a cause of gastrointestinal symptoms. *Gut* 1985; 26: 164–8.

40 Fischer JE, Foster GS, Abel RM, Abbott WM, Ryan JA. Hyperalimentation as primary therapy for inflammatory bowel disease. *Am J Surg* 1973; 125: 165–75.

41 Gassall MA, Fernandez-Banares F, Esteve Comas M. *Nutrition in Inflammatory Bowel Disease. Artificial Nutritional Support in Clinical Practice.* London: Edward Arnold, 1995.

42 Gerrard DA, Hunt JB, Payne-James JJ *et al.* Initial response and subsequent course of Crohn's disease treated with elemental diet or prednisolone. *Gut* 1993; 34: 1198–202.

43 Gilat T, Wacoben D, Lilos P, Langman MJS. Childhood factors in ulcerative colitis and Crohn's disease. An international co-operative study. *Scand J Gastroenterol* 1987; 22: 1009–29.

44 Glassman MS, Newman LJ, Berezin S, Gryboski J. Cow's milk protein sensitivity during infancy in patients with inflammatory bowel disease. *Am J Gastroenterol* 1990; 85: 838–40.

45 Greenberg GR, Fleming CR, Jeejeebhoy KN *et al.* Controlled trial of bowel rest and nutritional support in the management of Crohn's disease. *Gut* 1988; 29: 1309–15.

46 Greenfield SM, Green AT, Teare JP *et al.* A randomised controlled study of evening primrose oil and fish oil in ulcerative colitis. *Alim Pharmacol Ther* 1993; 7: 159–66.

47 Haddard ZH. Clinical and immunological aspects of food hypersensitivity. *Ann Allergy* 1982; 49: 29–36.

48 Halpern GM, Scott JR. Non-IgE antibody mediated mechanisms in food allergy. *Ann Allergy* 1987; 58: 14–27.

49 Hanauer SB, Sitrin MD, Bengoa JM, Neurcomb SA, Kirsner JB. Long-term follow up of patients with Crohn's disease treated by supportive total parenteral nutrition. *Gastroenterology* 1984; 86: 1106.

50 Heatley RV, Rhodes J, Calcraft BJ *et al.* Immunoglobulins in rectal mucosa of patients with proctitis. *Lancet* 1975; ii: 1010–12.

51 Heatley RV, Calcraft BJ, Rhodes J *et al.* Disodium cromoglycate in the treatment of chronic proctitis. *Gut* 1975; 16: 559–63.

52 Hodgson HJF, Jewell DP. The humoral immune system in inflammatory bowel disease. II. Immunoglobulin levels. *Am J Dig Dis* 1978; 23: 123–8.

53 Hunt JB, Payne-James JJ, Palmer KR *et al.* A randomised controlled trial of elemental diet and prednisolone as primary therapy in acute exacerbations of Crohn's disease. *Gastroenterology* 1989; 96: A224.

54 Hunter JO, Workman E, Alun Jones V. Dietary studies. *Topics in Gastroenterology*, 12. Blackwell Scientific Publications, 1985; 305–13.

55 James AH. Breakfast and Crohn's disease. *BMJ* 1977; i: 943–5.

56 Jenkins HR, Pincott JF, Soothill JF, Milla PJ, Harries JT. Food allergy: the major cause of infantile colitis. *Arch Dis Child* 1984; 59: 326–9.

57 Jewell DP, Truelove SC. Circulating antibodies to cow's milk proteins in ulcerative colitis. *Gut* 1972; 13: 796–801.

58 Jewell DP, Truelove SC. Reagenic hypersensitivity in ulcerative colitis. *Gut* 1972; 13: 903–6.

59 Jones R, Lydeard S. Irritable bowel syndrome in the general population. *BMJ* 1992; 304: 87–90.

60 Kaliner M. Hypothesis on the contribution of late-phase allergic responses to the understanding and treatment of allergic diseases. *J Allergy Clin Immunol* 1984; 73: 311–15.

61 Kapikaan AZ, Chanock RM. In: *Fields' Virology*, 3rd ed, (Fields BN ed). Lippincott-Raven, Philadelphia, 1996.

62 Katschinski B, Goebell H. Dietary essential fatty acids and the risk of ulcerative colitis. *Gastroenterology* 1991; 100: A9.

63 Kellow JE, Gill RC, Wingate DL. Prolonged ambulant recordings of small bowel motility demonstrate abnormalities in the irritable bowel syndrome. *Gastroenterology* 1990; 98: 1208–18.

64 Kett K, Brantzaeg P, Fausa O. J-chain expression is more prominent in immunoglobulin A2 than in immunoglobulin A1 colonic immunocytes and is decreased in both subclasses associated with inflammatory bowel disease. *Gastroenterology* 1988; 94: 1419–25.

65 Lessof MH, Wraith DG, Merrett TG, Merrett J, Buisseret PD. Food allergy and intolerance in 100 patients – local and systemic effects. *Q J Med* 1980; 49: 259–71.

66 Lunardi C, Bambara LM, Biasi D *et al.* Double-blind cross-over trial of oral sodium cromoglycate in patients with irritable bowel syndrome due to food intolerance. *Clin Exp Allergy* 1991; 21: 569–72.

67 Malchow H, Ewe K, Brandes JW *et al.* European co-operative Crohn's disease study: results of drug treatment. *Gastroenterology* 1984; 86: 249–66.

68 Mansfield JC, Giaffer MH, Holdsworth CD. Controlled trial of oligopeptide versus amino acid diet in the treatment of active Crohn's disease. *Gut* 1995; 36: 60–6.

69 Martini GA, Brandes JW. Increased consumption of refined carbohydrates in patients with Crohn's disease. *Klin Wochensch* 1976; 54: 367–71.

70 May CD, Bock SA. A modern clinical approach to food hypersensitivity. *Allergy* 1978; 33: 166–88.

71 Maybery JF, Rhodes J, Allan R *et al.* Diet in Crohn's disease. Two studies of current and previous habits in newly diagnosed patients. *Dig Dis Sci* 1981; 26: 444–8.

72 Maybery JF, Rhodes J, Newcombe RG. Increased sugar consumption in Crohn's disease. *BMJ* 1980; ii: 1401.

73 McAuley RC, Sheldon C, Sommes SC. Mast cells in non specific ulcerative colitis. *Am J Dig Dis* 1961; 6: 233–6.

74 McIntyre PB, Powell-Truck J, Wood SR *et al.* Controlled trial of bowel rest in the treatment of severe acute colitis. *Gut* 1986; 27: 481–5.

75 Mendeloff AI, Calcins BM. Epidemiology of idiopathic inflammatory bowel disease. In: *Inflammatory Bowel Disease*, 3rd edn. (Kirsner JB, Shorter RG, eds). Lea & Febiger, Philadelphia, 1988: 3.

76 Metcalfe DD, Kaliner MA. 'What food is to one …' *N Eng J Med* 1984; 311: 399–400.

77 Middleton SJ, Riordan AM, Hunter JO. Comparison of elemental and peptide based diets in the treatment of acute Crohn's disease. *Ital J Gastroenterol* 1991; 23: 609.

78 Middleton SJ, Rucker JT, Kirby GA, Riordan AM, Hunter JO. Long-chain triglycerides reduce the efficacy of enteral feeds in patients with active Crohn's disease. *Clin Nutr* 1995; 14: 229–36.

79 Misiewitz JJ, Waller SL, Kiley N, Horton EW. Effect of oral prostaglandin E on intestinal transit in man. *Lancet* 1969; i: 648–51.

80 Mullen JL, Clark Hargrove W, Dudrick SJ, Fitts WT, Rosato EF. Ten years experience with hyperalimentation and inflammatory bowel disease. *Ann Surg* 1978; 187: 523–9.

81 Murphy JL, Wootton SA, Rucker JT, Kirby GA, Hunter JO. The effect of an elemental diet on stool output in irritable bowel syndrome. *Proc Nutr Soc* 1994; 53: 223A.

82 Murray IA, Smith JA, Coupland K, Long RG. Intestinal trehalase activity: establishing a normal range and the effect of disease. *Gut* 1998; 42: A35.

83 Nakagawa T, DeWeck AL. Membrane receptors for the IgG4 subclass of human basophils and mast cells. *Clin Rev Allergy* 1983; 1: 197–206.

84 Nanda R, James R, Smith H, Dudley CRK, Jewell DP. Food intolerance and the irritable bowel syndrome. *Gut* 1989; 30: 1099–104.

85 O'Donoghue DP, Kumar P. Rectal IgE cells in inflammatory bowel disease. *Gut* 1979; 20: 149–53.

86 O'Morain C, Segal AW, Levi AJ. Elemental diet as primary therapy of acute Crohn's disease: a controlled trial. *BMJ* 1984; 288: 1859–62.

87 Ostro MJ, Greenberg GR, Jeejeebhoy KN. Total parenteral nutrition and complete bowel rest in the management of Crohn's disease. *Gastroenterology* 1984; 86: 1203A.

88 Parker TJ, Naylor SJ, Riordan AM, Hunter JO. Management of patients with food intolerance in irritable bowel syndrome: the development and use of an exclusion diet. *J Hum Nutr Dietetics* 1995; 8: 159–66.

89 Parker TJ, Woolner JT, Tuffnell Q, Shorthouse M, Hunter JO. The importance of hypolactasia in irritable bowel syndrome. *Gut* 1997; 41(Suppl. 3): A219.

90 Pearson DJ, Rix KJB, Bently SJ. Food allergy: how much in the mind? A clinical and psychiatric study of suspected food hypersensitivity. *Lancet* 1983; i: 1259–61.

91 Persson PG, Ahlbom A, Hellers G. Diet and inflammatory bowel disease: a case control study. *Epidemiology* 1992; 3: 47–52.

92 Petitpierre M, Gumowski P, Girard JP. Irritable bowel syndrome and hypersensitivity to food. *Ann Allergy* 1985; 54: 538–40.

93 Rao SN. Mast cells as a component of the granuloma in Crohn's disease. *J Path* 1973; 109: 79–82.

94 Rawcliffe PM, Truelove SC. Breakfast and Crohn's disease. *BMJ* 1978; ii: 971–2.

95 Reilly J, Ryan JA, Strole W, Fischer JE. Hyperalimentation in inflammatory bowel disease. *Am J Surg* 1976; 131: 192–200.

96 Riordan AM, Hunter JO, Cowan RE *et al.* Treatment of active Crohn's disease by exclusion diet: East Anglian multi-centre controlled trial. *Lancet* 1993; 342: 1131–4.

97 Riordan AM, Ruxton CHS, Hunter JO. A review of association between Crohn's disease and consumption of sugars. *Eur J Clin Nutr* 1998; 52: 229–38.

98 Ritchie JK, Wadsworth J, Lennard-Jones JL, Rogerson G. Controlled multicentre therapeutic trial of an unrefined carbohydrate, fibre rich diet in Crohn's disease. *Br Med J Clin Res* 1987; 295: 517–20.

99 Rosekrans PCM, Meijer CJLM, Van Der Wal AM *et al.* Allergic proctitis, a clinical and immunological entity. *Gut* 1980; 21: 1017.

100 Royall D, Jeejeebhoy KN, Baker JP *et al.* Comparison of amino acid versus peptide based enteral diets in active Crohn's disease: clinical and nutritional outcome. *Gut* 1994; 35: 783–7.

101 Rutgeerts P, Goboes K, Peeters M *et al.* Effect of faecal stream diversion on recurrence of Crohn's disease in the neoterminal ileum. *Lancet* 1991; 338: 771–4.

102 Savage DC. *Effect of food and fibre on the intestinal luminal environment. Fibre in human and animal nutrition.* Royal Society of New Zealand, Wellington; 1983: 125–9.

103 Seidman EG, Lohoues MJ, Turgeon J, Bouthillier L, Morin CL. Elemental diet versus prednisolone as initial therapy in Crohn's

disease. Early and long-term results. *Gastroenterology* 1991; 100: A250.

104 Shoda R, Matsueda K, Yamato S, Umeda N. Epidemiologic analysis of Crohn's disease in Japan: increased dietary intake of N-6 polyunsaturated fatty acids and animal proteins relates to the increased incidence of Crohn's disease in Japan. *Am J Clin Nutr* 1996; 63: 741–5.

105 Shorter RC, Cordoza M, Spender RJ, Huizenga KA. Further studies of in vitro cytotoxicity of lymphocytes from patients with ulcerative colitis and granulomatous colitis for allergenic colonic epithelial cells, including the effects of colectomy. *Gastroenterology* 1969; 56: 304–9.

106 Silkoff K, Wallak A, Vegena L *et al.* Consumption of refined carbohydrate by patients with Crohn's disease in Tel Aviv. *Yago Postgrad Med J* 1980; 56(662): 842–6.

107 Stanworth DR. Immunochemical aspects of human IgG4. *Clin Rev Allergy* 1983; 1: 183–95.

108 Strober W, Kelsall B. To be responsive or not to be responsive, that is the mucosal question. *Gastroenterology* 1998; 114: 214–17.

109 Summers RW, Switz DM, Sessions JT *et al.* The national co-operative Crohn's disease study. *Gastroenterology* 1979; 77: 847–69.

110 Taylor B, Norman AP, Orgel HA, Stokes CR, Turner MW, Soothill JF. Transient IgA deficiency and pathogenesis of atopy. *Lancet* 1973; ii: 111–13.

111 Teahon K, Bjarnason I, Pearson M, Levi AJ. Ten years' experience with an elemental diet in the management of Crohn's disease. *Gut* 1990; 31: 1133–7.

112 Thompson WG, Creed F, Drossman DA, Heaton KW, Muzzacca G. Functional bowel disease and functional abdominal pain. *Gastroenterol Int* 1992; 5: 75–91.

113 Thompson WG, Heaton KW. Functional bowel disorders in apparently healthy people. *Gastroenterology* 1980; 79: 283–8.

114 Thornton JR, Emmett PM, Heaton KW. Diet and Crohn's disease, characterisation of the pre-illness diet. *BMJ* 1974; ii: 760–5.

115 Truelove SC. Ulcerative colitis provoked by milk. *BMJ* 1961; i: 154.

116 Truelove SC, Witts LJ. Cortisone in ulcerative colitis: final report on a therapeutic trial. *BMJ* 1955; ii: 1041–8.

117 Van der Kamer JH, Weijers HA, Dicke WK. Coeliac disease. An investigation into the injurious constituents of wheat in connection with their action on patients with coeliac disease. *Acta Paediatr* 1953; 42: 223.

118 Voitk AJ, Echave V, Feller JH, Brown RA, Gurd FN, Ottawa MD. Experience with elemental diet in the treatment of inflammatory bowel disease: is this primary therapy? *Arch Surg* 1973; 107: 329–37.

119 Wangel AG, Deller DJ. Intestinal motility in man; mechanisms of constipation and diarrhoea with particular reference to the irritable colon syndrome. *Gastroenterology* 1965; 48: 69–84.

120 Whorwell PJ, Holdstock G, Whorwell GM, Wright R. Bottle feeding, early gastroenteritis and inflammatory bowel disease. *BMJ* 1979; i: 382.

121 Wide L, Bennich L, Johansson SGO. Diagnosis of allergy by an in vitro test for allergen antibodies. *Lancet* 1967; ii: 1105–7.

122 Willoughby CP, Piris J, Heyworth MF, Truelove SC. Comparison of disodium cromoglycate and sulphasalazine as maintainance therapy for ulcerative colitis. *Lancet* 1979; i: 119–22.

123 Winitz M, Adams RF, Seedman DA *et al.* Studies in metabolic nutrition employing chemically defined diets: effect on gut microflora populations. *Am J Clin Nutr* 1970; 23: 546–54.

124 Winitz M, Seedman DA, Graff J. Studies in metabolic nutrition employing chemically defined diets. Extended feeding of normal adult males. *Am J Clin Nutr* 1970; 23: 525–45.

125 Woolner JT, Parker TJ, Kirby GA, Hunter JO. The development and evaluation of a diet for maintaining remission in Crohn's disease. *J Hum Nutr Dietetics* 1998; 11: 1–11.

126 Wright R, Truelove SC. A controlled therapeutic trial of various diets in ulcerative colitis. *BMJ* 1965; ii: 138.

127 Wright R, Truelove SC. Circulating and tissue eosinophils in ulcerative colitis. *Am J Dig Dis* 1966; 11: 831–46.

128 Wyatt GM, Bayliss CE, Holcroft JD. A change in human faecal flora in response to inclusion of gum arabic in the diet. *Br J Nutrition* 1986; 55: 261–6.

129 Zwetchenbaum JF, Burakoff R. The irritable bowel syndrome and food hypersensitivity. *Ann Allergy* 1988; 61: 47–9.

Section B Gastrointestinal Tract

Chapter 42

Paediatric gastrointestinal food-allergic disease

R.P.K. Ford and John Walker-Smith

INTRODUCTION

Gastrointestinal food-allergic diseases may be defined as those clinical syndromes characterized by the onset of gastrointestinal symptoms following food ingestion, in which the underlying mechanism is an immunologically mediated reaction within the gastrointestinal tract. These symptoms may be accompanied by other manifestations outside the alimentary tract, such as in the skin or respiratory tract.

PATTERNS OF ILLNESS

The number of adverse reactions to foods claimed to affect the gastrointestinal tract is vast. They range from an acute anaphylactic reaction, even leading to death, to relatively minor symptoms which are difficult to distinguish from other disorders such as toddler's diarrhoea or psychological disorders with gastrointestinal symptoms.

More than one system is frequently involved in an adverse reaction to a food and the observed patterns of system involvement vary considerably between authors. The overall clinical pat-

terns of system involvement for milk sensitivity are shown in Table 42.1. Gastrointestinal manifestations have been reported in the majority of children in most studies and often gastrointestinal symptoms are seen alone. The large variations between observations can probably be explained by the differences in criteria used to establish the diagnosis, the preselection bias of the investigators, the age of the patients and perhaps the pattern of infant feeding in a particular community.

In infancy and early childhood the proteins of cow's milk and soya have been highlighted as the major causes of food-allergic syndromes, although wheat (in individuals in whom coeliac disease has been excluded), egg, rice, fish, chicken meat and corn, as well as tomatoes, oranges, bananas and chocolate, have been reported to produce gastrointestinal symptoms in some individuals. The adverse responses to some of these foods have been much better documented than others as causes of gastrointestinal allergic disease. There is not always a consistent association between an individual food and a particular symptom or symptom complex. While in some individuals a single food may cause an adverse response, in others there may be clinical intolerance to multiple foods. A clear example of this is the varied gastrointestinal

Patterns of system involvement in cow's milk hypersensitivity						
Author(s)	No. of patients	Age (years)	System involved (%)			
			Cutaneous	Respiratory	Gastrointestinal	Gastrointestinal symptoms only
Clein[8]	140	0–1	43	10	51	17
Goldman et al.[28]	89	0–11	45	46	65	17
Gerrard et al.[27]	59	0–2	46	44	61	15
Buisseret[6]	79	1–16	82	93	84	0
Stintzing and Zetterstrom[77]	25	not stated	40	16	84	50
Hill et al.[40]	17	0–5	41	12	59	47

Table 42.1 Patterns of system involvement in cow's milk hypersensitivity.

responses that may be provoked by the ingestion of cow's milk protein, as shown in Table 42.2. Furthermore, in the case of cow's milk protein intolerance the symptoms may change with increasing age in one individual. For example, a child who developed diarrhoea and lethargy in infancy might later develop abdominal pain and irritability, although eventually becoming completely tolerant to cow's milk.

AGE OF ONSET AND DURATION

The incidence of gastrointestinal food-allergic diseases is greatest in the first months and years of life and decreases with age. The natural history of gastrointestinal food-allergic disease is best documented for reactions to cow's milk, with most such children developing their adverse symptoms to milk within the first 3 months of life (Table 42.3).

The reported ranges of age of onset extend from 1 day to 15 months' old. The age at which these children were first exposed to milk will, of course, influence this to some extent. Adverse symptoms become less severe with increasing age,[11] and most children have become fully tolerant of milk by 2 years of age. Adequate catch-up growth has usually occurred by this time if there has been a period of growth failure. Verkasalo et al.[80] found that, after clinical tolerance to cow's milk had developed, one-third of their patients had persistent minor symptoms that did not

Range of gastrointestinal manifestations seen in cow's milk hypersensitivity
Common well documented manifestations
Anaphylaxis
Vomiting
Diarrhoea, malabsorption, failure to thrive
Colic, abdominal pain, nausea
Less common, well documented manifestations
Occult intestinal haemorrhage
Protein-losing enteropathy
Milk-induced colitis
Functional intestinal obstruction
Other manifestations
Intussusception
Constipation

Table 42.2 Range of gastrointestinal manifestations seen in cow's milk hypersensitivity.

Age of onset and resolution of cow's milk hypersensitivity			
Author(s)	No. of patients	Age of onset (range)	Age of resolution (range)
Gybroski[32]	21	'Most' by 6 weeks (2 days to 4 months)	'Most' by 2 years (8 months to 5 years)
Visakorpi and Immonen[81]	12	Not stated	90% by 1 year, 100% by 2 years
Kuitunen et al.[54, 55]	54	Mean 9 weeks (1 day to 22 weeks)	Mean 13 months (7 months to 2 years)
Harrison et al.[37]	25	Mean 10 weeks (1 week to 15 months)	Mean 18.4 months (7 months to 4 years)
Walker-Smith et al.[88]	5	Mean 2 weeks (1 week to 3 weeks)	100% by 2 years
Verkasalo et al.[80]	65	Mean 9 weeks	97% by 2 years, 100% by 3 years

Table 42.3 Age of onset and resolution of cow's milk hypersensitivity.

seem to be associated with drinking milk. These symptoms included occasional abdominal pains, a tendency to have loose stools or constipation, eczema and recurrent respiratory infections, particularly otitis media. It is not known whether these symptoms are related to an underlying gastrointestinal food allergy.

CLINICAL SYNDROMES

The major adverse gastrointestinal reactions to cow's milk are vomiting, diarrhoea and abdominal pain. These symptoms are also frequently seen in many childhood illnesses such as generalized infections, gastroenteritis, parasitic infestation, sugar malabsorption and stress-related psychosomatic illnesses. Symptoms must therefore be accurately assessed in relation to milk ingestion, and careful guidelines used for the diagnostic differentiation of gastrointestinal food-allergic disease from other conditions.

Time of onset of symptoms
Broadly, gastrointestinal reactions to food may be divided into those which manifest quickly, within minutes to an hour after taking the food, and those in which the onset is slower, taking several hours and even days to become manifest.[22,64] The former syndromes are usually easy to diagnose on historical grounds, and levels of food-specific immunoglobulin (Ig)E antibodies are usually raised. By contrast, the slow onset reactions are often difficult to diagnose clinically and the currently available diagnostic investigations may be impractical for general use.

An outline of the manifestations and clinical syndromes of gastrointestinal food-allergic disease is shown in Table 42.4.

Quick onset reactions
Anaphylaxis
Acute anaphylaxis is the most serious of the quick onset gastrointestinal food reactions. Anaphylaxis results from a generalized immediate IgE-mediated reaction following the introduction of a sufficient amount of antigen into a previously sensitized individual which releases histamine and other biologically active mediators from sensitized mast cells. This phenomenon of an acute anaphylactic reaction to an ingested food represents the most severe extreme of the clinical spectrum of gastrointestinal food-allergic disease[12,28] and may even result in death.[19] (Anaphylaxis is discussed in Chapter 28.)

Vomiting, diarrhoea and abdominal pain
Acute vomiting, with or without diarrhoea and frequently accompanied by other system involvement, is commonly the presenting feature of quick onset gastrointestinal reactions. These reactions occur within minutes to an hour of the food being ingested with often only small amounts of food needed to precipitate such a reaction. Such a reaction may occur at the first exposure to the food, the child having been previously sensitized via the breast milk[5] or even *in utero*.[59] Many foods may produce such reactions.

Breast feeding and cow's milk allergy
Some entirely breast fed infants are exquisitely sensitive to cow's milk. Small amounts of cow's milk given as a complement feed or in solids may lead to a rapid onset of vomiting which will cease when cow's milk is completely withdrawn from the diet. Often such vomiting may be accompanied by the onset of eczema. In some infants the lips and tongue may swell immediately upon contact with cow's milk and this oedema is sometimes associated with urticaria and angio-oedema which may in fact be the major presenting clinical problem. Characteristically, these children have increased levels of total serum IgE and elevated milk-specific IgE antibodies[22] which can be demonstrated by skin prick test and radioallergosorbent test (RAST) responses. They also tend to have lower titres of IgG, IgA and IgM milk antibodies than do infants who develop cow's milk protein intolerance some months after they have been fed with cow's milk.[70]

Egg hypersensitivity
Vomiting within a few minutes to an hour of egg ingestion is seen in about a quarter of children with egg hypersensitivity[57] (Chapter 21). Diarrhoea, abdominal pain and nausea may also occur.[21] However, skin and respiratory manifestations also frequently occur and are usually a more important part of the clinical presentation than gastrointestinal symptoms. Again, skin prick test and RAST responses to egg are usually positive.

Acute abdominal pain
Acute abdominal pain seems to be a particular feature of fish hypersensitivity,[67] while peanuts often produce immediate reactions of the oral mucosa[97] as well as abdominal pain.

Multiple food sensitivities
Some individuals have gastrointestinal and other symptoms related to a wide variety of foods. Such patients characteristically have a number of quick onset symptoms such as vomiting, urticaria or wheezing upon exposure to multiple foods. They often have an individual and family history of atopy, peripheral eosinophilia, elevated total serum IgE and positive RAST and skin tests to specific foods. Diets involving the elimination of a number of foods may be impractical or ineffective on their own. However, treatment with sodium cromoglycate may be highly

Manifestations and clinical syndromes seen in gastrointestinal food-allergic disease in children
Quick onset reactions
Anaphylaxis
Vomiting, diarrhoea and abdominal pain
Slow onset reactions
Vomiting, pallor and irritability
Food-sensitive enteropathies
Transient gluten intolerance
Other gastrointestinal reactions
Milk-induced colitis
Infantile colic
Occult intestinal haemorrhage
Protein-losing enteropathy
Functional intestinal obstruction
Oesophagitis
Allergic gastroenteropathy
Eosinophilic gastroenteritis

Table 42.4 Manifestations and clinical syndromes seen in gastrointestinal food-allergic disease in children.

effective, as has been shown in the group of children described by Syme,[78] and also in older patients reported by Wraith et al.,[97] but the therapeutic dose is empirical at present.[53] Curiously, if oral sodium cromoglycate alleviates the symptoms then these may not relapse when the drug is subsequently discontinued. These patients need to be distinguished from those with eosinophilic gastroenteritis.

Slow onset reactions

Slow onset reactions are much more difficult to diagnose because of the difficulty of associating symptoms with a food taken hours or even days before. However, in general the pathology is more site-specific. The problem is usually one of establishing whether or not the observed gastrointestinal pathology is in fact caused by an adverse immunological reaction to a food. Here, elimination of the suspected food or foods and their subsequent reintroduction into the diet as food challenge is at the heart of the diagnostic approach.

Food-sensitive small intestinal enteropathies

Changes in the structure of the small intestinal mucosa in response to the ingestion of particular foods provide clear objective evidence of food-sensitive disorders involving the small intestinal mucosa. The approach of using serial small intestinal mucosal biopsies combined with dietary elimination and challenge has been adapted from the Interlaken Criteria used to diagnose coeliac disease.[62] However, the time scale is compressed in these disorders which, unlike coeliac disease, are transient conditions. Using this approach, a number of foods have now been shown to produce food sensitive enteropathy (Table 42.5).

Mechanisms

From the studies reported by Ferguson[18] in experimental animals, it seems likely that enteropathy may be caused by a Type IV or T cell - mediated reaction.[26] A Type I reaction in the gut is associated with only minimal changes of mast cell degranulation and some oedema, while Type III reactions are associated with polymorph infiltration and do not cause crypt hyperplasia. Of course, more than one type of allergic response may coexist within the mucosa at any one time. In further experimental studies of human fetal small intestinal lamina propria, in vitro features of small intestinal enteropathy, i.e. villous atrophy, crypt cell proliferation and raised levels of intraepithelial lymphocytes have been described.[61] Some degree of morphological features are characteristic of cow's milk-sensitive enteropathy.

Food-sensitive enteropathies described to date
Cow's milk
Wheat
Soya
Chicken
Egg
Fish
Rice

Table 42.5 Food-sensitive enteropathies described to date.

Gastroenteritis

It sometimes appears that acute gastroenteritis may precede the development of food sensitivity enteropathy. However, although there is an association between post-enteritis enteropathy and food-sensitive enteropathy in early infancy,[82,86] which condition came first is often impossible to establish. Acute gastroenteritis causes damage to the small bowel mucosal epithelium,[2] which may permit the entry of excess food antigen into the body with subsequent food protein sensitization. There is firm evidence from animal models that there is increased absorption of macromolecules in gastrointestinal infection.[39,89] It is therefore possible that gastroenteritis may predispose to the development of food hypersensitivity. Clinical support for this concept has been given by two groups[33,37] who have both implicated an IgA deficiency as an underlying factor. However, the relationship between gastroenteritis and milk hypersensitivity has not been found by others.[35] It is possible that gastrointestinal infection may merely unmask pre-existing cow's milk-sensitive enteropathy.[92]

IgA deficiency

There is evidence that IgA deficiency is associated with the development of gastrointestinal food hypersensitivity. This may be because of inadequate immune exclusion in the early months of life, allowing sensitization to inhaled and ingested antigens.[76] IgA in colostrum and breast milk may give passive mucosal protection in this vulnerable period.[30] IgA deficiency has been found associated with milk hypersensitivity,[33,37,65]. A defect in the quality of the IgA produced is also possible[60] but transforming growth factor-β (TGF-β) may play a key role. Using the ELISPOT technique, it has been shown that levels of circulating IgA secretory cells are low at diagnosis of cow's milk allergy but rise to control levels when tolerance to cow's milk is achieved.[42]

Food antigen absorption

Food antigens can be absorbed unaltered through the intestinal mucosa.[73,84] These antigenically active proteins are not absorbed in sufficient quantity to be of nutritional importance, but enough can be absorbed to stimulate antibody production.[7] The vast majority of individuals show no ill effects from this limited intestinal permeability to large molecules, so it seems likely that other factors must be involved before clinical food protein hypersensitivity occurs.

Premature and newborn infants have been shown to have increased gastrointestinal permeability to β-lactoglobulin compared to older children or adults,[70] which seems to be related to gut immaturity. A similar pattern of intestinal permeability has been found using small inert sugars as permeability probes.[3]

Increased levels of food antigen are found in patients with diseases that damage the gastrointestinal tract, such as gastroenteritis,[31] inflammatory bowel disease[75] and coeliac disease. Also, increased gastrointestinal permeability to polyethylene glycol (PEG) has been found in children with eczema, whether or not they had any food protein hypersensitivity.[47] In addition, studies with horseradish peroxidase have established that there is increased antigen entry via damaged enterocytes in cases of post-enteritis enteropathy.[46] However, to date no clear relationship has been found between food protein hypersensitivity and altered gastrointestinal transport of macromolecules. A hypothesis incorporating these interrelationships is illustrated in Fig. 42.1. Sugar permeability in gastroenteritis is shown in Fig. 42.2.

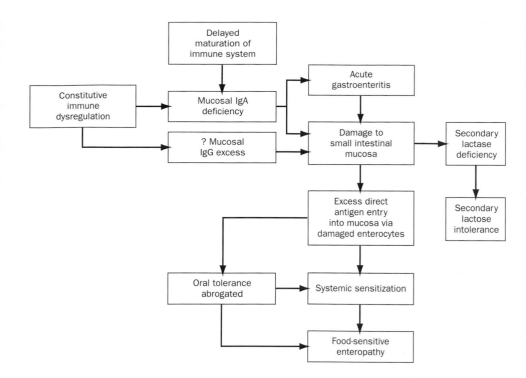

Fig. 42.1 Proposed interrelationship between gastroenteritis, immune deficiency and food-sensitive enteropathy (Walker-Smith and Murch, 1997 unpublished).

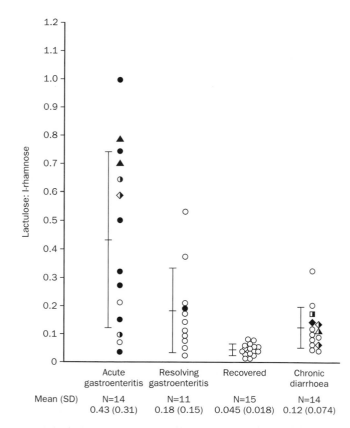

Fig. 42.2 Lactulose:L-rhamnose urinary excretion ratios expressed as percentage of the oral load, and pathogens detected in each clinical group. The dashed line represents the upper limit of normal. Horizontal bars with vertical lines denote mean and standard deviation of each group. Symbols: ○, none detected or no sample; ●, rotavirus; ▲, adenovirus; ◆, cornavirus; ◑, *Campylobacter*; ◇, *Cryptosporidia*; ◨, *Escherichia coli*; ▲, *Salmonella* □, *Giardia*. From Ford RPK *et al*. Intestinal sugar permeability: relationship to diarrhoeal disease and small bowel morphology. *J Pediatr Gastroenterol Nutr* 1985; 4: 568–74.

MAJOR FOOD-SENSITIVE ENTEROPATHIES

Cow's milk-sensitive enteropathy

Cow's milk-sensitive enteropathy is a condition usually characterized by combinations of diarrhoea, vomiting, abdominal pain and failure to thrive following the ingestion of cow's milk protein in infancy. This reaction to milk is usually slow in onset, and is not associated with atopic illness or positive specific IgE responses to milk.[22] Various tests to assess the integrity of the small bowel mucosa have been used to investigate this condition but often with conflicting reports of their diagnostic value.

Initially, the use of small bowel biopsy convincingly demonstrated that cow's milk protein could cause severe small bowel mucosal damage in young infants who had diarrhoea and were failing to thrive.[54] Once this relationship between cow's milk protein and mucosal damage had been established, further studies performed before and after milk challenge documented mucosal changes after milk provocation.[55] Iyngkaran *et al*.[44] subsequently suggested that evidence of mucosal damage should be necessary for the firm diagnosis of gastrointestinal milk hypersensitivity. However, not all children with gastrointestinal symptoms provoked by cow's milk protein have this recognizable mucosal damage[25,40] and, conversely, histological damage has been observed in children who have developed no clinical symptoms with milk.[72,74] Thus, unlike coeliac disease, this enteropathy is not necessarily an invariable finding on a single proximal biopsy from all such children. Nevertheless, when present, the enteropathy can be shown to be cow's milk-sensitive by serial biopsies related to withdrawal and challenge with cow's milk (Fig. 42.3).

Pathology

Unlike the gluten-sensitive enteropathy of untreated coeliac disease, cow's milk-sensitive enteropathy is of variable severity on proximal mucosal biopsy, and patchy in its distribution. There is typically a thin mucosa,[58] although a flat mucosa indistinguishable

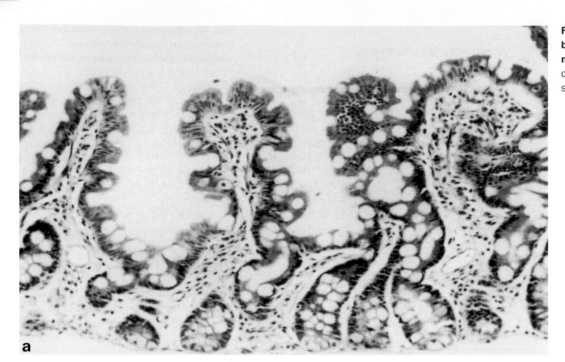

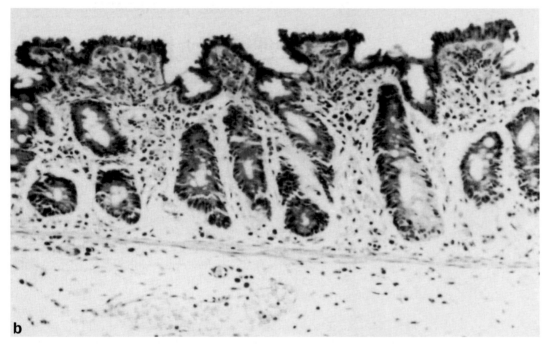

Fig. 42.3 Serial small intestinal biopsy before and after cow's milk challenge. (a) Cow's milk-free diet; (b) after cow's milk challenge, showing a flattening of the mucosa.

from the mucosal appearances found in coeliac disease may also occur. More often lesser degrees of mucosal abnormality are found. After a positive milk challenge, alteration in microvilli of the enterocyte may be seen in parallel with a fall in disaccharidase activity. In untreated cow's milk-sensitive enteropathy, intra-epithelial lymphocyte numbers are high, although not as high as that found in coeliac disease. Subsequently, these fall to a level below normal on a milk-free diet. Although the numbers of intraepithelial lymphocytes may rise again after a positive milk challenge, the level reached is usually within the normal range.[69]

Clinical features

Most children with gastrointestinal symptoms because of cow's milk protein intolerance develop their sensitivity to milk within the first 6 months of life. In most of these children there is no family history of atopy or cow's milk protein intolerance. Symptoms may either present acutely or with the gradual onset of chronic diarrhoea.

Those with an acute presentation usually have sudden vomiting, with or without diarrhoea, occurring within 1–4 h of drinking milk. This often follows their first known drink of milk. The vomiting may be stained with bile. It is frequently associated with pallor, lethargy, limpness and tachypnoea. The vomiting is usually short-lived but can be protracted for several hours. If no further milk is given, the child will recover completely within 4–6h. This type of reaction is not usually associated with skin eruptions, although in a child with eczema existing lesions may transiently become red and itchy. If cow's milk continues to be given, the symptoms will persist but often with less intensity.

Differential diagnosis

It may at first be impossible to distinguish such symptoms from an acute episode of gastroenteritis, especially as it is not possible to detect a stool pathogen in most cases of acute gastroenteritis unless stool electron microscopy can be used to identify viral particles. Furthermore, cow's milk protein intolerance may itself be a sequel to gastroenteritis. Such infants may have been tolerating cow's milk for several months up until this time. It is also important to recognize post-enteritis lactose intolerance, but the two disorders may overlap.[86]

Chronic symptomatology

The chronic presentation of cow's milk-sensitive enteropathy usually manifests as chronic diarrhoea with failure to thrive. The clinical features are suggestive of coeliac disease except that the child may not be taking gluten. These children have usually been bottle fed from birth, with their symptoms developing within the first 6 months of life. They often have a history of irritability and colic.

Soya-sensitive enteropathy

Ament and Rubin[1] have described damage of the small intestinal mucosa which improved with withdrawal of soya protein from the diet. The prevalence of soya-induced enteropathy is not known, but is likely to increase if soya-based formulae are chosen more frequently as the feeding formulae for normal infants.

The events of soya enteropathy have been assumed to mirror those of cow's milk-sensitive enteropathy. The close morphological similarity between cow's milk-sensitive and soya-sensitive enteropathy has now been demonstrated in a thorough histological and immunological study by Perkkio et al.[68] Soya-sensitive enteropathy may occur on its own or as a sequel to cow's milk-sensitive enteropathy.

Transient gluten intolerance

Transient gluten intolerance may be defined as the syndrome seen when a child with gastrointestinal symptoms and an abnormal small intestinal mucosa responds clinically and histopathologically to a gluten-free diet, but who subsequently thrives on a normal gluten-containing diet with the small intestinal mucosa remaining normal. Dicke in Holland, in 1952, described a transient wheat sensitivity in preschool children after enteritis.[13,14] Later, a similar state of transient gluten intolerance was described in 28 children, which in some cases was associated with cow's milk protein intolerance.[81] However, these reports did not include serial small intestinal biopsies. Children with transient gluten intolerance investigated by serial biopsies have subsequently been described.[85,87]

Pathology

The small intestinal mucosa is by definition abnormal, with partial or total villus atrophy. Only long-term follow up with serial small bowel biopsies can allow this retrospective diagnosis to be made in a child with a flat mucosa who earlier responded clinically to gluten withdrawal, but who subsequently has thrived on a gluten-containing diet.

Clinical features

In infants less than 1 year of age, transient gluten intolerance should be considered as part of the differential diagnosis of an infant who develops gastrointestinal symptoms when he first encounters wheat protein, especially when intolerances to other food proteins such as milk and egg are present. This diagnosis should also be considered as a possibility in a child whose diet includes gluten and who fails to thrive following gastroenteritis in the presence of an abnormal small intestinal mucosa.

Genetic differences in HLAYDR phenotypes between children with transient gluten intolerance and coeliac disease have been described.[63] As children diagnosed with transient gluten intolerance could theoretically relapse even after many years, it is very difficult, at least at present, ever to make a final diagnosis of transient gluten intolerance.[93]

Other food-sensitive enteropathies

Infants have also been described with food-sensitive enteropathies to fish, rice, chicken[82] and egg[43] diagnosed by serial small bowel biopsies in conjunction with dietary elimination and challenge. In all cases intolerance to these foods was preceded by cow's milk protein intolerance and was temporary. Thus, present evidence indicates that a number of transient food-sensitive enteropathies do exist in infancy.

OTHER GASTROINTESTINAL REACTIONS

The following types of gastrointestinal reaction are for the most part probably related to the slow onset type pattern, and so are generally not associated with the presence of food-specific IgE antibodies.

Food-sensitive colitis

In 1940, Rubin described rectal loss of fresh blood which responded to cow's milk withdrawal.[71] In 1967, Gryboski described eight children with cow's milk colitis established by elimination and challenge.[32] The main clinical features were explosive bloody diarrhoea, shock, pallor and colitis. This diagnosis was based upon evaluation of sigmoidoscopic appearances. No pathogens were isolated. The advent of safe colonoscopy and multiple mucosal biopsy even in early infancy has clearly established eosinophilic or allergic colitis as an important cause of chronic bloody diarrhoea in infancy.[10,50] On colonoscopy there is erythema of the mucosa, with aphthoid ulceration. Histopathologically, infiltration with eosinophils has been reported, although Gryboski and Walker[34] describe a histopathological appearance not dissimilar to ulcerative colitis. Even breast fed infants whose mothers drink much cow's milk may develop cow's milk colitis.[56] β-Lactoglobulin has been demonstrated in the breast milk of lactating mothers, although the amounts are very small .

Differential diagnosis

This disorder should be distinguished from ulcerative colitis and Crohn's colitis. Ulcerative colitis has been observed to remit in a group of five children when on a milk-free diet, all having both symptomatic and histological relapse after milk was reintroduced.[79] It is possible that this was a secondary effect of increased antigen absorption through a diseased bowel mucosa with subsequent immune complex deposition causing symptoms. Milk-specific antibodies were not measured in these children, although a later study[98] showed that children with high levels of specific antibodies to whole cow's milk relapsed more frequently than those with lower levels. These relapses were not necessarily caused by milk ingestion. It has also been suggested that proctitis may at times be caused by local IgE-mediated reaction to cow's milk protein.[38]

Thus a response to cow's milk elimination may not accurately discriminate between these disorders, and the diagnosis rests upon the histopathology demonstrated by mucosal biopsy and the subsequent clinical course. In food-sensitive colitis there is usually a dense infiltration of eosinophils in the mucosa with the lesion resolving on food elimination.

Occult intestinal haemorrhage

Occult gastrointestinal blood loss has been described in association with cow's milk ingestion. The first report[95] concerned 13 infants seen in a Well Baby Clinic aged 7–84 months, who had iron deficiency anaemia. Nine of these children had been fed with homogenized milk, of whom seven (78%) had precipitins to whole cow's milk compared to only two (17%) of 12 controls. These findings were later confirmed[96] with another 17 children who had occult gastrointestinal blood loss induced by whole cow's milk. In some children it was associated with hypoproteinaemia and oedema. Heat-labile cow's milk proteins, possibly bovine serum protein, were incriminated as aetiological agents. Occult blood loss was also observed after the ingestion of fresh goat's milk in some children, but was not seen with boiled cow's milk, proprietary heat-modified cow's milk formulae or soya-based formulae. When iron supplements were given while cow's milk ingestion was continued, the iron deficiency anaemia improved in only 20% of the children, but improvement was seen in all children as soon as milk was withdrawn from the diet.

Others[66] have suggested that the increased milk precipitins and hypoproteinaemia may have resulted from altered gut permeability caused by iron deficiency rather than a primary hypersensitivity to milk. Holland et al.[41] also observed an association between the presence of serum precipitins to cow's milk and the incidence of recurrent respiratory tract disease, iron deficiency anaemia and failure to thrive. Precipitins to bovine serum albumin and bovine γ-globulin were the most common. However, 17% of these children with increased precipitins to milk had no ill health despite continued milk ingestion.

Gastritis

Gastritis may also be a cause of gastrointestinal blood loss caused by cow's milk hypersensitivity. Four infants have been described[9] who had erosive gastritis or gastroduodenitis diagnosed by endoscopy. Vomiting, poor growth and iron deficiency anaemia were the prominent clinical features associated with occult blood loss. One child had chronic diarrhoea. All children became asymptomatic on a milk-free diet, with adequate weight gain and the endoscopic appearances of the upper gastrointestinal tract returned to normal. With later milk provocation, all children developed slow onset reactions.

Protein-losing enteropathy

Waldmann et al.[83] described six children presenting with peripheral oedema. This was associated with intermittent diarrhoea and vomiting, anaemia, hypoalbuminaemia, hypogammaglobulinaemia, eosinophilia and growth retardation. Loss of plasma proteins into the gastrointestinal tract was demonstrated in all patients. All of these children developed diarrhoea and vomiting after drinking milk. Three children had detailed studies with milk

elimination and challenge, which confirmed that the abnormal gastrointestinal protein loss was linked to the drinking of cow's milk.

Functional intestinal obstruction

Three children have been described who repeatedly developed functional intestinal obstruction with symptoms of vomiting and abdominal distension after milk ingestion.[24] No physical obstruction could be demonstrated by X-ray studies, and when milk was eliminated from the diet the symptoms disappeared and there was an improvement in weight gain, appetite and mood.

Intussusception

Two children have been described who developed ileocolic intussusceptions during a period of milk ingestion.[32] They had been diagnosed as being hypersensitive to milk by fulfilling the criteria of Goldman et al.[28] At surgery they had enlarged mesenteric lymph nodes. There was good evidence to implicate milk as the aetiological agent.

Constipation

In one study[8] chronic constipation was found in 5% of infants and children thought to have milk hypersensitivity. They developed normal stools when milk was removed from the diet. Another study[6] mentions constipation as a symptom of milk hypersensitivity, but its frequency and severity were not mentioned. Weaning on to cow's milk is frequently associated with the faeces becoming firmer and less frequent.

Aphthous ulcers

Mouth, oesophageal and stomach aphthous ulcers have been reported in up to 20% of the population.[29] They may occur in association with coeliac disease and Crohn's disease. Dolby and Walker[15] have reported the successful use of sodium cromoglycate in a proportion of such ulcers, but whether they are truly food-allergic in nature is uncertain. Forget et al.[23] have described eosinophilic infiltration of the oesophagus which may be food-related. Katz et al.[52] have described eosinophilic infiltration of the stomach associated with a history of food intolerance, response to food avoidance and laboratory evidence of reaginic allergy (Chapter 31).

Eosinophilic gastroenteritis

Eosinophilic gastroenteritis is characterized by protein losing enteropathy, peripheral eosinophilia and iron deficiency anaemia secondary to gastrointestinal blood loss. This condition must be distinguished from cow's milk-sensitive enteropathy, although it merges with other disorders such as the 'allergic gastroenteropathy' described by Waldmann et al.[83] The pathological classification is confused,[51] and not all reports clearly indicate that this is a definite food-allergic disorder. Some patients appear resistant to elimination diets and require treatment with corticosteroids, thus suggesting a different pathogenesis.

Infantile colic

'Colic' is a ubiquitous part of infant behaviour in westernized societies. It usually refers to a picture of episodes of restlessness or crying because of presumed abdominal discomfort with eructation and flatulence. Many causes, such as maternal anxiety or aerophagy distending the gut, have been put forward. This behaviour pattern is so common that it is likely that many causes exist, but several studies have suggested that colic is frequently associated with milk ingestion.[27,28] Although older children may perhaps also have abdominal pain or nausea, available data refer only to infants.

Increased numbers of IgE-producing plasma cells have been found in the duodenal biopsy tissue of infants with colic after 7 days of cow's milk feeding, suggesting that colic may be an IgE-mediated response to cow's milk protein.[36] However, most such children have negative skin prick responses to milk.

Relief from colic has been observed in breast fed infants whose mothers have been put on a diet free of cow's milk and dairy products, the colic returning when maternal milk ingestion was recommended.[48] On the other hand, a similar study[17] found no such association between milk ingestion by the mother and colic in the infant. Colic was not significantly more common on days when mothers drank cow's milk, but increased with increasing diversity of maternal diet. These studies also showed that cow's milk antigen was found in mother's milk equally often in infants with or without colic.

A prospective study by Jacobsson and Lindberg[49] in Sweden diagnosed, with two clinically positive challenges, 20 of nearly 1000 infants as having cow's milk intolerance; all 20 had colic and seven had gastrointestinal symptoms only. Four of these infants were breast fed and suffered colic unless their mothers avoided cow's milk in their diet.

It seems that, without a clear clinical picture of relapse on challenge or evidence of major atopy, cow's milk avoidance as a treatment for so common a disorder as infantile colic may have little other than a placebo effect in the majority of babies for whom it might be considered. Thus, although children with cow's milk protein intolerance frequently have colic, children with colic do not necessarily have cow's milk protein intolerance.

Migraine-related gastrointestinal symptoms

Egger et al.[16] reported a study investigating the effect of an oligoantigenic diet on 88 children with severe migraine. Two-thirds of these children had accompanying symptoms of abdominal pain, diarrhoea and flatulence. When treated for their migraine with the oligoantigenic diet, the majority (86%) also had alleviation of their gastrointestinal symptoms. The mechanism of these reactions was presumed to be of an allergic nature. That it was food causing these symptoms was confirmed by double blind food provocation.

CONCLUSIONS

The range of gastrointestinal manifestations caused by allergic food disease is vast. These can be broadly clinically categorized into quick and slow onset reactions. The quick onset reactions, which occur within minutes to an hour of taking the food, are usually associated with elevated specific food IgE antibodies, positive skin prick tests and atopy. Only small amounts of the foods are usually required to provoke such reactions. The slow onset reactions usually occur between 1 and 4 h after food ingestion, but may take days to manifest. These reactions are not associated with increased IgE-specific antibodies and often more of the food is required to produce any symptoms.

REFERENCES

1 Ament ME, Rubin CE. Soy protein – another cause of the flat intestinal lesion. *Gastroenterology* 1972; 62: 227–34.

2 Barnes GL, Townley RRW. Duodenal mucosal damage in 31 infants with gastroenteritis. *Arch Dis Child* 1973; 48: 343–9.

3 Beach RC, Menzies IS, Clayden GS, Scopes JW. Gastrointestinal permeability changes in the preterm neonate. *Arch Dis Child* 1982; 57: 141–5.

4 Bleumink E. Allergies and toxic protein in food. In: *Coeliac Disease* (Hekkens WTJM, Pena AS, eds), Kroese, Leyden, 1975: 46–55.

5 Bjorksten F, Saarinen UM. IgE antibodies to cow's milk in infants fed breast milk and milk formulae. *Lancet* 1978; ii: 624–5.

6 Buisseret PD. Common manifestations of cow's milk allergy in children. *Lancet* 1978; i: 304–5.

7 Carswell F, Ferguson A. Food antibodies in serum – a screening test for coeliac disease. *Arch Dis Child* 1972; 47: 594–6.

8 Clein NW. Cow's milk allergy in infants. *Ann Allergy* 1951; 9: 195–204.

9 Coello-Ramirez P, Larraso-Haro A. Gastrointestinal occult hemorrhage and gastroduodenitis in cow's milk protein intolerance. *J Pediatr Gastroenterol Nutr* 1984; 3: 215–18.

10 Cucchiara S, Guandalini S, Staiano A *et al.* Sigmoidoscopy, colonoscopy and radiology in the evaluation of children with rectal bleeding. *J Pediatr Gastroenterol Nutr* 1983; 2: 667–71.

11 Dannaeus A, Johansson SGO. A follow-up of infants with adverse reactions to cow's milk. *Acta Paediatr Scand* 1979; 68: 377–82.

12 de Peyer E, Walker-Smith JA. Cow's milk intolerance presenting as necrotizing enterotizing enterocolitis. *Helv Paediatr Acta* 1977; 32: 509.

13 Dicke WK. De subacute, chronische en reciverende darmstoornis van de kleuter. *Ned Tijdschr Geneesk* 1952; 96: 860.

14 Dicke WK, Weijers HA, van de Kamer JH. Coeliac disease presence in wheat of a factor having a deleterious effect in coeliac disease. *Acta Paediatr Scand* 1953; 42: 34–42.

15 Dolby AE, Walker DMA. Trial of cromoglycic acid in recurrent aphthous ulceration. *Br J Oral Surg* 1975; 12: 292–5.

16 Egger J, Carter C, Wilson J *et al*. Is migraine food allergy? *Lancet* 1983; ii: 865–8.

17 Evans RW, Fergusson DM, Allardyce RA, Taylor B. Maternal diet and infantile colic in breast fed infants. *Lancet* 1981; i: 1340–2.

18 Ferguson A. Pathogenesis and mechanisms in the gastrointestinal tract. In: *Proceedings of the First Fisons Food Allergy Workshop*, Medicine Publishing Foundation, Oxford; 1980: 28–38.

19 Finkelstein H. Kuhmilch als ursache akuter ernathrungstorungen bei sauglingen. *Monatsschr Kinderheilkd* 1905; 4: 65–72.

20 Firer MA, Hosking CS, Hill DJ. Effect of antigen load on development of milk antibodies in infants allergic to milk. *BMJ* 1981; 283: 693–6.

21 Ford RPK, Taylor B. Natural history of egg hypersensitivity in childhood. *Arch Dis Child* 1982; 57: 649–52.

22 Ford RPK, Hill DJ, Hosking CS. Cows milk hypersensitivity: immediate and delayed onset clinical patterns. *Arch Dis Child* 1983; 58: 856–62.

23 Forget P, Eggermont E, Marchall G *et al*. Eosinophilic infiltration of the oesophagus in the infant. *Acta Paediatr Belg* 1978; 31: 91–3.

24 Freier S. Paediatric gastrointestinal allergy. *Clin Allergy* 1973; 3 (Suppl.): 597–618.

25 Freier S, Kletter N, Gery I *et al*. Intolerance to milk protein. *J Pediatr* 1969; 75: 623–31.

26 Gell PGH, Coombs RRA. Classification of allergic reactions. In: *Clinical Aspects of Immunology* (Gell RGH, Coombs RRA, eds) Blackwell Scientific Publications, Oxford,

27 Gerrard JW, MacKenzie JW, Golubuff N *et al*. Cow's milk allergy: prevalence and manifestations in an unselected series of newborns. *Acta Paediatr Scand* 1973; 234 (Suppl.): 1–21.

28 Goldman AS, Anderson DW, Sellers WA *et al*. Milk allergy. *Pediatrics* 1963; 32: 425–43.

29 Graysowski EA, Barile MF, Lee WB, Stanley HR. Recurrent aphthous stomatitis; clinical, therapeutic, histopathologic, and hypersensitivity aspects. *JAMA* 1966; 196: 637–44.

30 Gross SJ, Buckiey RH, Wakil SS *et al*. Elevated IgA concentration in milk produced by mothers delivered of preterm infants. *J Pediatr* 1981; 99: 389–93.

31 Gruskay FL, Cooke RE. The gastrointestinal absorption of unaltered protein in normal infants and in infants recovering from diarrhoea. *Pediatrics* 1965; 16: 763–7.

32 Gryboski JD. Gastrointestinal milk allergy in infants. *Pediatrics* 1967; 40: 354–62.

33 Gryboski JD, Kochoshis S. Immunoglobulin deficiency in gastrointestinal allergies. *J Clin Gastroenterol* 1980; 2: 71–6.

34 Gryboski JD, Walker WA. The colon, rectum and anus. In: *Gastrointestinal Problems in the Infant*, (Gryboski JD, Walker WA, eds) 2nd ed; WB Saunders, Philadelphia, 1983: 524.

35 Halliday K, Edmeades R, Shepherd R. Persistent post-enteritis diarrhoea in childhood. A prospective analysis of clinical features, predisposing factors and sequelae. *Med J Aust* 1982; 18: 2.

36 Harris M, Petts V, Penny P. Cow's milk allergy as a cause of infantile colic: immunofluorescent studies on jejunal mucosa. *Aust Paediatr J* 1977; 13: 276–81.

37 Harrison M, Kilby A, Walker-Smith JA *et al*. Cow's milk protein intolerance: a possible association with gastroenteritis, lactose intolerance, and IgA deficiency. *BMJ* 1976; i: 1501–4.

38 Heatley RV, Calcraft BJ, Fifield R. Immunoglobulins in rectal mucosa of patients with proctitis. *Lancet* 1975; ii: 1010–12.

39 Heyman M, Corthier G, Lucas F, Meslin JC, Desjeux JF. Evolution of the caecal epithelial barrier during *Clostridium difficile* infection in the mouse. *Gut* 1989; 30: 8: 1087–93.

40 Hill DJ, Davidson GP, Cameron DJS, Barnes GL. The spectrum of cow's milk allergy in childhood. *Acta Paediatr Scand* 1979; 68: 847–52.

41 Holland NH, Hong R, Davis NC, West CD. Significance of precipitating antibodies to milk proteins in the serum of infants and children. *J Pediatr* 1962; 61: 181–95.

42 Isolauri E, Suomalainen H, Kaila M *et al*. Local immune response in patients with cow's milk allergy: follow-up of patients retaining allergy or becoming tolerant. *J Paediatr* 1992; 120: 9–15.

43 Iyngkaran N, Abidain Z, Meng LL, Yadav M. Egg-protein-induced villous atrophy. *J Pediatr Gastroenterol Nutr* 1982; 1: 29–35.

44 Iyngkaran N, Robinson MJ, Prathap K *et al*. Cow's milk protein sensitive enteropathy: combined clinical and histological criteria for diagnosis. *Arch Dis Child* 1978; 53: 20.

45 Iyngkaran N, Robinson NJ, Sumithran E *et al*. Cow's milk protein-sensitive enteropathy. An important factor in prolonging diarrhoea in acute infective enteritis in early infancy. *Arch Dis Child* 1978; 53: 150–3.

46 Jackson D, Walker-Smith JA, Phillips AD. Macromolecular absorption by histologically normal and abnormal small intestinal mucosa in childhood: an in vitro study using organ culture. *J Pediatr Gastroenterol Nutr* 1983; 2: 235–48.

47 Jackson PG, Lessof MH, Baker RWR *et al*. Intestinal permeability in patients with eczema and food allergy. *Lancet* 1981; i: 1285–6.

48 Jacobsson I, Lindberg T. Cow's milk as a cause of infantile colic in breast fed infants. *Lancet* 1978; i: 437–9.

49 Jacobsson T, Lindberg T. Prospective study of cow's milk protein intolerance in Swedish infants. *Acta Paediatr Scand* 1979; 68: 853–9.

50 Jenkins HR, Milla PJ, Pincott TR *et al*. Food allergy: the major cause of infantile colitis. *Pediatr Res* 1983; 431 (Abstract).

51 Johnstone JM, Morson BC. Eosinophilic gastroenteritis. *Histopathology* 1978; 2: 335–48.

52 Katz AJ, Goldman H, Grand RJ. Gastric mucosal biopsy in eosinophilic (allergic) gastroenteritis. *Gastroenterology* 1977; 73: 705–9.

53 Kochoshis S, Gryboski JD. Use of cromolyn in combined gastrointestinal allergy. *JAMA* 1979; 242: 1169–73.

54 Kuitunen P, Visakorpi JK, Hallman N. Histopathology of duodenal mucosa in malabsorption syndrome induced by cow's milk. *Ann Paediatr* 1965; 205: 54–63.

55 Kuitunen P, Rapola J, Savilahti E, Visakorpi JK. Light and electron microscopic changes in the small intestinal mucosa in patients with cow's milk induced malabsorption syndrome. *Acta Paediatr Scand* 1972; 61: 237.

56 Lake AM, Whitington PF, Hamilton SR. Dietary protein-induced colitis in breast fed infants. *J Pediatr* 1982; 101: 906–10.

57 Langeland T. A clinical and immunological study of allergy to hen's egg white. *Clin Allergy* 1983; 13: 371–82.

58 Maluenda C, Phillips AD, Briddon A, Walker-Smith JA. Quantitative analysis of small intestinal mucosa in cow's milk sensitive enteropathy. *J Pediatr Gastroenterol Nutr* 1984; 3: 349–56.

59 Matsumura T, Kuroume T, Oguri M *et al*. Egg sensitivity and eczematous manifestations in breast-fed newborns with particular reference to intrauterine sensitization. *Ann Allergy* 1975; 35: 221–9.

60 MacDonald D, Habeshaw J, Malpas JS *et al*. Case report of an unusual immune deficiency syndrome. *Paediatric Research Society of Australia, Annual Meeting*; 1983.

61 MacDonald TT, Spencer J. Evidence that activated mucosal T cells play a role in the pathogenesis of enteropathy in human small intestine. *J Exp Med* 1988; 167: 1341–9.

62 Meeuwisse G: Diagnostic criteria in coeliac disease. *Acta Paediatr Scand* 1970; 59: 461–3.

63 Meuli R, Pichler WJ, Gaze H, Lentze MJ. Genetic difference in HLA-DR phenotypes between coeliac disease and transitory gluten intolerance. *Arch Dis Child* 1995; 72: 29–32.

64 Minford AMB, MacDonald A, Littlewood JM. Food intolerance and food allergy in children: a review of 68 cases. *Arch Dis Child* 1982; 57: 742–7.

65 Minor JD, Tolber SG, Frick OL. Leukocyte inhibition factors in delayed-onset food allergy. *J Pediatr* 1980; 66: 314–21.

66 Naiman JL, Oski EA, Diamond LK *et al*. The gastrointestinal effects of iron-deficiency anemia. *Pediatrics* 1964; 33: 83–99.

67 Nizami RM, Lewin PK, Baloo MT. Oral cromolyn therapy in patients with food allergy: a preliminary report. *Ann Allergy* 1977; 39: 102–5.

68 Perkkio M, Savilahti E, Kuitunen P. Morphometric and immunochemical study of jejunal biopsies from children with intestinal soy allergy. *Eur J Pediatr* 1981; 137: 63–9.

69 Phillips AD, Rice SJ, France NE, Walker-Smith JA. Small intestinal lymphocyte levels in cow's milk protein intolerance. *Gut* 1979; 20: 509–12.

70 Roberton DM, Paganelli R, Dinwiddie R, Levensky RJ. Milk antigen absorption in the preterm and term neonate. *Arch Dis Child* 1982; 57: 369–72.

71 Rubin MI. Allergic intestinal bleeding in the newborn – a clinical syndrome. *Am J Med Sci* 1940; 200: 385–90.

72 Savilanti E. Immunochemical study of the malabsorption syndrome with cow's milk intolerance. *Gut* 1973; 14: 491–501.

73 Schloss OM, Warthen TW. The permeability of the gastroenteric tract of infants to undigested protein. *Am J Dis Child* 1916; 11: 342–62.

74 Shiner M, Ballard J, Brook CGD, Herman S. Intestinal biopsy in the diagnosis of cow's milk protein intolerance without acute symptoms. *Lancet* 1975; ii: 1060–3.

75 Shorter RG, Huizenga KA, Spencer RJ. A working hypothesis of the etiology and pathogenesis of nonspecific inflammatory bowel disease. *Am J Digest Dis* 1972; 17: 1024–32.

76 Soothill JF, Stokes CR, Turner MW *et al*. Predisposing factors and the development of reaginic allergy in infancy. *Clin Allergy* 1976; 6: 305–19.

77 Stintzing G, Zetterstrom R. Cow's milk allergy, incidence and pathogenic role of early exposure to cow's milk formula. *Acta Paediatr Scand* 1979; 68: 383–7.

78 Syme J. Investigation and treatment of multiple intestinal food allergy in childhood. In: *The Mast Cell: its Role in Health and Disease* (Pepys J, Edwards AM, eds), Pitman Medical, Tunbridge Wells, 1979: 438–42.

79 Truelove SC. Ulcerative colitis provoked by milk. *BMJ* 1961; i: 154–60.

80 Verkasalo M, Kuitunen P, Savilahti E, Tiilikainen A. Changing pattern of cow's milk intolerance. *Acta Paediatr Scand* 1981; 702: 289–295.

81 Visakorpi JK, Immonen P. Intolerance to cow's milk and wheat gluten in the primary malabsorption syndrome in infancy. *Acta Paediatr Scand* 1967; 56: 49–56.

82 Vitoria JC, Camarero C, Sojo A *et al*. Enteropathy related to fish, rice and chicken. *Arch Dis Child* 1982; 57: 44–8.

83 Waldmann TA, Wochner RD, Laster L, Gordon RS Jr. Allergic gastroen-teropathy. A cause of excessive gastrointestinal protein loss. *N Engl J Med* 1967; 276: 761–9.

84 Walker WA, Isselbacher KJ. Progress in gastroenterology uptake and transport of macromolecules by the intestine. Possible role in clinical disorders. *Gastroenterology* 1974; 67: 531–50.

85 Walker-Smith JA. Transient gluten intolerance. *Arch Dis Child* 1970; 45: 523–6.

86 Walker-Smith JA. Cow's milk intolerance as a cause of post-enteritis diarrhoea. *J Pediatr Gastroenterol Nutr* 1982; 1: 163–75.

87 Walker-Smith JA, Phillips AD. The pathology of gastrointestinal allergy. In: *The Mast Cell: its Role in Health and Disease* (Pepys J, Edwards AM, eds), Pitman Medical, Tunbridge Wells, 1979: 31–9.

88 Walker-Smith JA, Harrison M, Kilby A *et al.* Cow's milk sensitive enteropathy. *Arch Dis Child* 1978; 53: 375–80.

89 Walker-Smith JA. Gastrointestinal food allergy in childhood: current problems. *Nutrition Research* 1992; 12: 123–35.

90 Walker-Smith JA. Objective assessment of allergenicity of infant feeding formulae. *Clin Exp Allergy* 1992; 22: 595–6.

91 Walker-Smith JA. Cow's milk sensitive enteropathy: predisposing factors and treatment. *J Paed* 1992; 121 (5pt2)Suppl. 111–15.

92 Walker-Smith JA. Food sensitive enteropathy: overview and update. *Acta Paed Jap* 1994; 36: 545–50.

93 Walker-Smith JA. Transient gluten intolerance. *Arch Dis Child* 1996; 74: 183–4.

94 Walker-Smith JA, Murch SH. *Diseases of the small intestine in childhood*. Fourth edition, 1999.

95 Wilson JF, Heiner DC, Lahey ME. Studies on iron metabolism: I. Evidence of gastrointestinal dysfunction in infants with iron deficiency anaemia; a preliminary report. *J Pediatr* 1962; 60: 787–800.

96 Wilson JF, Lahey ME, Heiner DC. Studies on iron metabolism. V. Further observations on cow's milk-induced gastrointestinal bleeding in infants with iron-deficiency anaemia. *J Pediatr* 1974; 84: 335–44.

97 Wraith DG, Young GVW, Lee TH. The management of food allergy with diet and Nalcrom. In: *The Mast Cell: its Role in Health and Disease* (Pepys J, Edwards AM, eds), Pitman Medical, Tunbridge Wells, 1979: 443–6.

98 Wright R, Truelove SC. Circulating antibodies to dietary proteins in ulcerative colitis. *BMJ* 1965; ii: 142–4.

INCIDENCE

The incidence of atopic dermatitis (AD) has been increasing for 40 years and is now estimated to affect between 10 and 20% of the paediatric population.[36] A more recent study of 270 adults with AD found that 60% of their children were also affected. The prevalence in children when both parents had the condition was 81%, 59% when one parent had AD or respiratory atopy, and 56% when one parent had neither AD nor respiratory atopy.[127] The current high population prevalence of atopy[18] of 40–50%, should result in 16–25% of all marriages being between atopics.[81]

GENETIC AND EXOGENOUS FACTORS

The cause of AD is unknown, but it is clear that hereditary predisposition is one of the most important factors in this chronically recurring skin disease.[66] Twin studies support the role of genetics in atopic disorders, with concordance rates for AD of 77% and 15% in monozygotic and dizygotic twins, respectively.[66] This is remarkably similar to the concordance with atopic respiratory disease, where 65% monozygotic and 25% dizygotic twin concordance has been shown.[29] Therefore, twin studies indicate that, while genetic factors play a definite part in the predisposition to atopic disorders and regulation of total serum immunoglobulin (Ig)E levels, environmental factors have considerable influence in determining specific antigen sensitivities and manifestation of the atopic disease.[20]

Non-genetic factors known to influence the expression of atopic disease include season of birth (with a peak incidence in April and a trough in late October),[62] animal exposure during the first few months of life,[130] birth order and exposure to viral infections.[76,137] The possible protective effect of breast feeding against the development of AD is controversial.[64]

The hygiene hypothesis

Children from large families are at a reduced risk of developing hay fever, eczema and allergic sensitization to common allergens. This observation led Strachan in 1989 to propose the 'hygiene' hypothesis, so challenging the immunological opinion of the time.[116,117] Children are likely to experience more severe infections at an earlier age with a greater number of older siblings. Thus, it was suggested that infections in early childhood might protect against atopy and that successive cohorts of children have progressively lost their protection. Since then, however, our understanding of T lymphocyte differentiation has suggested a possible mechanism for a protective effect.[48,93] The 'natural' immune response to infections occurring in early life, perhaps specifically at the time of first exposure to the relevant allergen, may inhibit the proliferation of Th2 cell clones through the preferential induction of Th1 type cytokines, and thereby prevent allergy.[75] These effects may, however, depend more on infective dose than on age at infection. More recently, Jarvis et al.[54] found slightly stronger associations of hay fever and specific IgE with sibship size than with birth order, suggesting that family size is of greater importance than position within the household. More direct evidence that childhood infection might prevent atopy comes from a recent historical cohort study in Guinea-Bissau, West Africa.[108] It was found that young adults who had experienced measles in childhood during a severe epidemic were significantly less likely to be atopic than those who had been vaccinated and not had measles. At present it is not known if this protection applies to other respiratory viruses since these are more difficult to examine in population-based studies. Measles may, however, be a special case in that it can cause severe damage to the thymus[139] and has been associated with reductions in cell-mediated immunity 3 years after infection.[109] However, a recent study in young Italian adults has also confirmed an inverse relationship between previous viral infection (in particular, hepatitis A) and the incidence of atopy.[76]

Regulation of immune response to antigens

Two major mechanisms, non-antigen-specific (total IgE levels) and antigen-specific (specific IgE antibodies and skin tests), have been proposed to regulate the immune response to allergens in humans. Firstly, gene(s) independent of the HLA system which are involved in the regulation of total IgE levels, and secondly, specific immune response gene(s) associated with MHC Class II genes which are involved in antigen-specific mechanisms.[8] Candidate genes have been proposed for both mechanisms. Thus,

genes linked to IgE and environmental influences appear to be important in determining the overall risk of allergy. Both genetic and non-genetic maternal effects may also play a part, and substantial evidence supports[19] the maternal inheritance of atopy underlying atopic respiratory disease by a gene or genes localized to 11q13. More recently, two candidate genes for atopy were identified in the region of 11q13; CD20, a molecule involved in B cell differentiation, and Fcε-RI β, the β subunit of the high affinity IgE receptor. Studies of variations in the inheritance of alleles of these genes found only Fcε-RI β to be maternally linked to atopy.[103]

Other factors, such as inheritance of genes for IL4 and mast cell tryptase, have also been suggested to have a direct effect on atopy,[50] but the critical timing and route of exposure remain unknown. A group in Finland[120] found that increased numbers of tryptase-positive mast cells contribute to promotion of inflammation, whereas chymase partially lacked the capability to suppress inflammation. This dysregulation of proteinases may explain why some people are more prone to inflammatory changes than others.[38]

Concentration of environmental antigens

Environmental antigens may initiate the atopic phenotype and contribute to its persistence and, postnatally, dietary antigens predominate.[6] High levels of antigen exposure during the first few months of life may predispose children to allergic sensitization.[2] More recently, the influences which exert their effect(s) prenatally, perhaps even affecting the very development of immune function before the fetus has been exposed (in the classical sense) to direct immune challenges from the extrauterine environment, have been investigated. In particular, Szepfalusi et al.[120] have provided evidence of prenatal priming of T cells. They documented proliferative responses of cord blood mononuclear cells to cow's milk proteins α-lactalbumin, β-lactoglobulin and α-casein, which were specific and required the presence of antigen-presenting cells. These responses were seen in nearly all of the 39 infants tested. The relevance of these responses to the later development of asthma and/or atopy is unclear, as this and other reports of such responses do not consistently show a relationship to either parental history of atopic disease or subsequent development of such disorders in the infant.[120] This work did not assess whether maternal T cells reacted to the same antigens. An association between maternal history of allergy and detectable cord blood IgE, and the subsequent development of eczema and asthma during infancy has already been demonstrated; an association with paternal history of allergy has not been shown.[38]

The previous finding that cutaneous lymphocyte antigen-positive mononuclear cells from children with milk-inducible AD can be expanded in vitro with casein, points to a possible significance of food-specific T cell responses in the pathogenesis of AD in these patients. This is echoed by the fact that double blind placebo-controlled food challenge abolishes antigen-specific interferon γ production in the peripheral blood of children with AD and cow's milk allergy.

Intestinal mucosa as organ of defence

The intestinal mucosa has two opposing functions: first, to provide a barrier that excludes numerous harmful antigens derived from microorganisms and food; and, second, to transfer antigens essential for evoking specific immune responses. Most macromolecules, including dietary antigens, are excluded by the intestine's mucosal barrier.[135] In health, antigen transfer is well controlled and aberrant antigen absorption does not occur. During mucosal dysfunction caused by immaturity, infection or hypersensitivity reactions, the normal pattern of antigen handling is impaired and this may evoke aberrant immune responses and lead to sensitization.[30] In 1996, Majamaa et al[78] found an increased protein absorption and permeability in children with AD, therefore implying impaired gut mucosal barrier function to low molecular weight proteins. The authors suggest that this may reflect a primarily altered antigen transfer in those who have AD. Aberrant antigen absorption could partly explain why patients with the condition frequently show prompt immune responses to common environmental antigens, including dietary antigens.[112] Work on immunohistology of gut in patients with AD is unfortunately lacking, but jejunal aspirate and radioallergosorbent test (RAST) results would be in keeping with this theory.[112]

IMMUNOPATHOGENESIS OF ATOPIC DERMATITIS

In both acute and chronic eczematous lesions a prominent dermal lymphocytic infiltrate is seen. Immunohistochemical staining has demonstrated that the infiltrate is comprised predominantly of activated T cells, bearing CD3, CD4 and CD45 Ro antigens,[10,67] and that the CD4+, CD25+ and CD45 Ro+ cells have TH2 cytokine characteristics. The majority of T lymphocytes migrating into the skin bear the cutaneous lymphocyte antigen (CLA) which functions as a skin homing receptor for T cells.[88] Vascular endothelial cells in AD lesions express elevated levels of the receptor, VCAM 1[131] which plays an important role in targeting the homing of CLA+ T cells to sites of skin inflammation.[95] Increased numbers of Langerhans cells are found in chronic AD lesions and have been shown to have increased expression of high (FCϵ-RI) and low affinity FCϵ-RII IgE receptors and surface-bound IgE.[12] Mast cell numbers are also elevated in chronic AD lesions. Despite the large number of CLA+ T cells in the skin these are only a small percentage of aeroallergen-specific T cells in the skin of patients with positive skin prick tests to these aeroallergens and at present it is not known whether any of these are dietary allergen-specific.

HYPOTHESES FOR THE ROLE OF FOOD IN THE PATHOGENESIS OF ATOPIC ECZEMA

A metabolic effect?

There is overwhelming evidence that there is an immunological basis to AD, but could this be linked to an underlying nutritional disturbance? It was suggested many years ago that these patients had a relative deficiency of unsaturated fatty acids[41] and sources rich in essential fatty acids (EFA) have been reported to be beneficial.[41,141] Wright and Burton[141] suggested that a deficiency of the enzyme Δ6-desaturase might be present in patients with AD and support for this hypothesis is provided by plasma EFA profiles.[74] Δ6-desaturase is responsible for the conversion of linoleic to γ-linolenic acid and the supplementation of γ-linolenic acid in evening primrose seed oil is thought to overcome this deficiency.[141] Horrobin et al.[49] have reported that prostaglandin E1, a metabolite of γ-linolenic acid, is an important factor in controlling T lymphocyte function and that defective EFA metab-

olism contributes to the T lymphocyte abnormalities in patients with AD.[15]

An abnormality of food antigen handling?
Absorption of antigen from the gut

The absorption of intact antigens is a feature of normal gastrointestinal function.[134] The amounts which enter the circulation are nutritionally insignificant but are undoubtedly sufficient to immunize since antibodies to intact food proteins can be demonstrated in most healthy individuals.[87] It is assumed that the function of these antibodies is the safe elimination of those food antigens that succeed in gaining access to the circulation. It is likely that the complexes formed by the combination of antibody and food antigen are removed from the blood by phagocytic cells and that this occurs asymptomatically after each meal. It is possible that this system has broken down in the individual with food-responsive AD, and that the eczema arises as a direct consequence of defective handling of normally harmless antigens which have entered the circulation by the gastrointestinal route (see Fig. 43.5).

Antigen elimination: role of mucosal immunity

Under normal circumstances, the safe elimination of circulating antigenic proteins derived from food and airborne particulate matter is probably mediated by serum IgA.[37] In a child with AD, some food antigen will enter the circulation after a meal, as in normal children. Preliminary evidence indicates the possibility that the entry of such antigens may be greater in at least some atopics.[23,85]

Mucosal hypersensitivity and antigen absorption

Rats which have been reaginically sensitized against food antigens demonstrate enhanced gastrointestinal permeability to the same antigens subsequently given by mouth.[14] The increased permeability appears to be the consequence of an IgE-mediated hypersensitivity reaction and, in these rat experiments, could be blocked by parenteral cyproheptadine or by oral sodium cromoglycate. Bloch et al.[7] demonstrated enhanced uptake of orally administered bovine serum albumin into the circulation of rats subjected to a mild degree of systemic anaphylaxis. Anaphylaxis was induced by intravenously injecting rats infected by the nematode Nippostrongylus brasiliensis with an extract of the same parasite. This result implies that antigen entry enhanced by this mechanism is enhanced in an antigen non-specific way. Support for this concept has also been provided by interesting findings from experiments in preruminant calves made allergic to soya flour, in which simultaneous administration of soya enhanced the absorption of β-lactoglobulin.[61]

Abnormal gastrointestinal mucosa

Minor morphological abnormalities of the small intestinal mucosa have been demonstrated in a proportion of children with AD,[63,70,111] which might reflect the long-term impact of this type of allergic reaction. Occasionally AD is complicated by full-blown protein-losing enteropathy which, likewise, is assumed to have an allergic cause.[56,132]

Indirect evidence of more subtle mucosal damage is provided by reports of increased gastrointestinal permeability to inert molecules which are not normally subject to significant absorption from the gut lumen, such as polyethylene glycol[52] of mean molecular weight 4000 and lactulose.[86,89,128]

Taken together, these findings suggest that the absorption of macromolecular antigens from the gastrointestinal tract is increased in at least some patients with atopic eczema. These phenomenon are often associated with a mild degree of mucosal damage and the mechanism in both cases may be an IgE-mediated hypersensitivity reaction in the gut wall. Although the initial hypersensitivity reaction is clearly antigen-specific, the resulting enhancement of permeability is likely not to be.

Fate of absorbed food antigens

Most food antigens which gain access to the systemic circulation will become bound shortly afterwards by antibodies. Their subsequent fate probably depends largely upon the properties of the antigen–antibody complexes thus formed (see Fig. 43.5). The appearance of circulating antigen–antibody complexes after food challenge has been demonstrated in normal subjects.[11,84] The antibodies in these complexes appear to be predominantly of IgA class[11] and the formation of such complexes is not associated with the development of symptoms. The harmless nature of these complexes is almost certainly related to the relative biological inertness of IgA, which does not activate complement by the classical pathway.[21] Under the same conditions, it has been found that many patients with AD form not only IgA-containing complexes, but also complexes containing IgG and IgE, and complexes which bind to Clq.[11] These complexes can be shown to contain food antigens.[84] Their fate is unknown, but it does not seem impossible that AD could result from the deposition of such complexes in the skin.

FOOD ALLERGY AND ATOPIC ECZEMA

Clinical presentation

AD is a chronically relapsing skin disease characterized by pruritic, erythematous, papulovesicular lesions which may become crusted and lichenified.[22] Onset is usually early in infancy (occasionally appearing for the first time in adult life), with 50% of cases developing the disease by 6 months of age and 75% by 12 months.

Pruritic lesions generally appear first on the convexities of the face and then spread to the limbs. Subsequently the face clears and the disease tends to settle in the limb flexures, though in the more severely affected it can become widespread (Fig. 43.1). The disease characteristically fluctuates in severity, with a trend to spontaneous resolution. Remission occurs within 5 years of onset in 90% of children and in only about 5% of cases does the disease persist into adult life. It also appears generally true that the later the onset, the worse the prognosis for long-term recovery.

Introduction

Whether food allergy is pathogenic in AD has been disputed for nearly a century.[104] Several lines of evidence support a pathogenic role for food hypersensitivity in AD:

1. Studies of food allergen avoidance indicate that AD can be prevented in some infants.
2. Food challenge studies provoke immunological changes that have been associated with the development of eczematous lesions.
3. Identification and elimination of food allergens leads to clinical improvement and return of abnormal immunological parameters to normal.

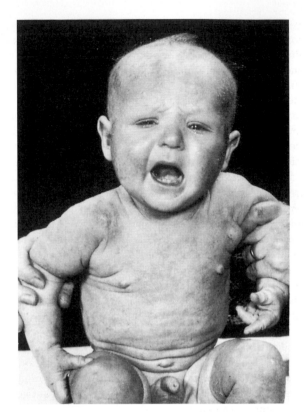

Fig. 43.1 Generalized atopic eczema in a severely affected 10-month-old boy.

A study from the USA reported that approximately one-third of children seen in a university combined dermatology and allergy clinic had food hypersensitivity contributing to their skin symptoms,[13] and a second study from France demonstrated that the more severe the AD, the more likely that food allergy was pathogenic.[33]

Avoidance

Hide *et al.*[45] confirmed benefits of maternal and infant allergen avoidance in a study of infants at high risk for atopy (atopy in both parents, one parent and a sibling, or two siblings; or atopy in one first-degree relative and elevated cord IgE level). Infants in the prophylactic group were either breast fed by mothers on a hypoallergenic diet or fed soy-based protein hydrolysate, with dairy products, eggs, wheat, oranges, fish, nuts and unhydrolysed soy excluded from the diet until 9 months of age. In addition, the homes of infants in the prophylactic group were treated to minimize contact with house dust mites. Control group infants had no dietary or environmental restrictions. Infants in the control group had a significantly greater risk for asthma and AD at 1 year of age and for AD but not asthma at 2 years of age.

Sigurs *et al.*[110] determined that the cumulative incidence and current prevalance of AD were reduced in high-risk children at 4 years of age whose mothers had avoided eating eggs, cow's milk and fish during lactation.

Cow's milk allergy

This frequently comprises the first major allergy in infants, probably because cow's milk is the first important source of antigenic protein consumed in large quantities. Allergy to cow's milk is most prevalent at the age of 1 year, and it coincides with the peak prevalence of AD. Cow's milk allergy has been reported in 2.5% of the general population.[105] In infants with AD, studies with double blind placebo-controlled oral challenge showed the incidence[51] of cow's milk allergy to be 50–60%. It follows, therefore, that infants wholly breast fed by mothers on cow's milk-free diet should have less eczema.[17,32,69,77,96] Nevertheless, conclusive proof is lacking and several studies have failed to demonstrate this effect.[39,44,69] A number of problems are encountered in the design and execution of such studies which help to explain these inconsistencies. One problem is that it is very difficult to be certain that breast feeding has been truly exclusive. Also, it would clearly be unethical to allocate a feeding method against maternal preference. A belief that breast feeding may prevent allergic disease is now widespread in the community, so that mothers who themselves have allergic diseases, or whose husbands or children have them, will tend to elect to breast feed more frequently than other mothers.[44] Furthermore, this trend is likely to be particularly pronounced in mothers of higher socioeconomic class. Since a positive family history and high socioeconomic class are both associated with an increased risk of AD,[122] this might easily introduce a bias towards more eczema in the breast fed infants, which would in its turn tend to obscure any real protective effect.

Maternal and infant food allergen avoidance

A prospective, randomized allergy prevention trial recently compared the benefits of maternal and infant food allergen avoidance in the prevention of allergic disease in infants at high risk for AD.[144-147] Breast feeding was encouraged in both prophylactic and control groups. In the prophylactic group, both the diets of lactating mothers and infants were restricted of eggs, cow's milk and peanuts. The control infants received cow's milk formula for supplementation. The period prevalences of food allergy, cow's milk sensitization and AD in the prophylactic group were reduced significantly during the first 2 years compared to the control group, but were no longer significantly different beyond 2 years. The cumulative prevalence of food allergy remained lower in the prophylactic group at 4 and 7 years' follow up, suggesting that the benefits of food allergy preventive measures are of limited duration, primarily because of the frequent remission of food allergy in early childhood. Overall, it appears that food allergen avoidance diets for genetically predisposed infants have their greatest effect on the development of AD, but that this effect may be limited to those with milder disease who are likely to 'outgrow' it after the first few years.[147]

Food challenge studies

Patients with AD differ from those with asthma and hay fever in having a much higher frequency of positive immediate skin tests to foods[5] and much greater levels of circulating food-specific IgE as measured by RAST.[126] They are particularly liable to immediate contact hypersensitivity to foods or food-induced contact urticaria syndrome in which urticaria develops within a few minutes at the site of contact with food (Fig. 43.2). This may be followed by eczematous reactions.[83] Immediate contact hypersensitivity to food is comparable to protein contact dermatitis which is characterized by dermatitis with episodic acute flares within minutes of contact with an allergen. Protein contact dermatitis is an important cause of occupational skin disease in food handlers, bakers, butchers and veterinarians. Atopic skin is particularly prone to this type of dermatitis because of its increased

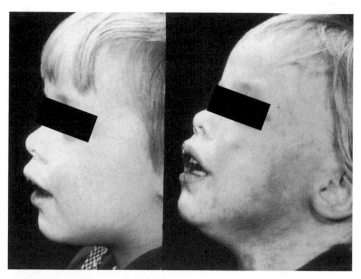

Fig. 43.2 Contact urticaria to egg. This 3-year-old boy with atopic eczema was photographed before, and 15 min after, the application of raw egg-white to his cheek.

susceptibility to irritants, impaired skin barrier function and the presence of increased amounts of inflammatory mediators.[53]

Several workers have reported results of studies in which specific foods were administered to eczematous atopic subjects as a challenge in an attempt to elucidate the aetiological role of foods (Table 43.1). Studies in which patients have been re-challenged 1–2 years after completely eliminating the response food allergen from their diets show that approximately one-third of symptomatic food allergies had resolved.[100] The likelihood of developing clinical tolerance was dependent upon the food to which the child was reactive; e.g. the development of tolerance to soy was common whereas development of tolerance to peanut was extremely rare. Results of skin prick tests were of little value in predicting loss of clinical reactivity since most remained virtually unchanged for years after the child could tolerate a specific food.

Any attempt to draw conclusions from the double blind placebo-controlled food challenge studies performed so far is extremely difficult as there is a lack of standardization. The dose of food, frequency of challenge, delay between challenges and the exact definition of a positive reaction are variable. Also, the preparation of the patients varies, some having been treated previously, while others have not, some have had a washout period from treatment, and all have had variable time without the suspected food. However, Sampson's group[102] have found that five foods account for nearly 90% of the food-induced reactions seen: egg, milk, peanut, soy and wheat. Egg allergy was most prevalent, affecting nearly two-thirds of the children with food hypersensitivity.

Elimination studies
Treatment by excluding egg and milk

Successful treatment of AD by exclusion of particular foods from the diet has been reported by numerous authors.[35,40,58,60,68,94,107,118,121,129] These reports describe the open evaluation of simple empirical elimination diets in fairly large numbers of children with AD. The first controlled study was that of milk and egg exclusion in childhood eczema, by Atherton et al.[4] In this study, a diet excluding milk and eggs was selected for trial. This was on an entirely empirical basis because these were the

Food challenge studies in atopic eczema										
Author(s)	No. of subjects	Food	Skin tests or RAST		History of provocation		Response to dietary elimination	Skin lesions on challenge		
			Positive	Negative	Positive	Negative		Eczema	Urticaria	All
Meara[65]	112	Egg	29(26)		–	–	11 of 29(38)	2(7)	8(28)	8(28)
				83(74)	–	–	–	–	–	–
Freedman[24]	48	Milk	14(29)	34(71)	12(25)	36(75)	1(2)	0	0	0
Goldman et al.[25]	37	Milk	–	–	37(100)	0	–	31(84)	–	–
Stifler[89]	40	Various	27(68)	–	–	–	10/27(37)	10(25)	–	–
				13(32)	–	–	–	–	–	–
Sedis[85]	38	Egg	27(71)	–	–	–	5 of 27(19)	16 of 27(59)	17 of 27(63)	
				11(29)	–	–	–	2 of 11(18)	4 of 11(36)	4 of 11(36)
Hammar[33]	81	Milk	–	–	7(9)	–	6 of 7(86)	–	–	–
						74(91)	–	8 of 74(11)	–	–
Bonifazi et al.[9]	134	Egg	37(28)	–	24(18)		–	3 of 24(13)	–	–
		Milk	28(21)			110(82)	–	–	–	–
Bonifazi et al.[10]	541	Various	–	–	42(8)	500(92)	–	13 of 42(31)	–	–
Juto et al.[47]	20	Milk	–	–	–	–	7 of 20(35)	12 of 19(63)	–	–
Bock et al.[8]	7	Various	7(100)	0	7(100)	0	–	4(57)	3(43)	5(71)

Values in parentheses are percentages.

Table 43.1 Food challenge studies in atopic eczema.

foods most frequently implicated by other authors. The problem of a control diet was overcome by the use of a soya substitute, with the patients being unaware of the constituents of either diet (it should be remembered that soya preparations were not in current use at that time). A double blind crossover design was used in which both diets were taken by every patient, each for a period of 4 weeks in random order, with an intervening washout period. Neither of the two dermatologists making the clinical evaluations had previously employed dietary therapy, and both were impressed and somewhat surprised by the unequivocal nature of the results of this study despite the relatively small number of patients taking part. Over half of the children showed clear preference for, and worthwhile benefit from, the regime avoiding egg and milk. Poor predictive value of an appropriate history, skin tests and RASTs made the findings of the above study more important. Of note is the point that many of the children benefited from egg and milk avoidance in the absence of any previous suspicion that these foods had aggravated their eczema. Also of interest was the lack of any association between response to diet and the presence or absence of positive immediate skin tests or raised serum levels of IgE antibodies to milk and egg antigens.[3] Therefore, neither these tests nor a careful history would

have allowed reliable identification of individuals likely to benefit from dietary therapy.

Commonly implicated foods

In 1992, Guillet and Guillet[33] published results confirming the relationship between food allergy and atopic disease in 250 children with AD. Of those with severe AD, 96% had food sensitivity, verified by alleviation of their condition with elimination of the allergenic food. The most commonly implicated foods were egg, milk, shellfish, corn starch, peanuts, fish and soy beans. Food sensitivity persisted in 67% of children (7–16 years old) with severe AD and was always associated with aeroallergen sensitivity in this age group.

In a prospective follow up study of 34 patients with AD, 17 children with food allergy (group 1) were appropriately diagnosed and placed on an allergen elimination diet. They experienced a marked and significantly greater improvement in their eczematous rash after 1–2 years and 3–4 years of follow up rather than 12 similar patients who did not have food allergy (group 2) and five children who were food-allergic but did not adhere to the elimination diet (group 3).[100] Only children in group I had a significant fall in their serum IgE concentrations over the 3–4-year follow up (serum IgE concentration correlates roughly with disease severity).[97–101]

Challenge studies

Juto et al.[58] challenged 19 children under 2 years of age with AD by repeated administration of cow's milk after a period of elimination. Eczematous reactions were reported in 12 of the 19. Bock et al.[9] used a double blind challenge technique to study children with histories of a variety of reactions to foods. Among these were seven children with eczema whose parents had implicated specific foods, particularly peanuts, eggs and milk. The authors were able to demonstrate exacerbation of eczema on appropriate challenge in four of these seven children.

Change in gut permeability

Changes associated with the elimination of allergens from the diet are not confined to skin in food-allergic patients. Lactulose absorption studies (a measure of gastrointestinal permeability) were abnormal in food-allergic children with AD when ingesting food allergens, but subsequently became normal when the responsible food allergens were eliminated from the diet.[31] The authors concluded that the presence of food allergy is indicative of a prognosis of severe AD and of associated respiratory atopy.

As food allergy can be overestimated by patients or their parents, it is important to verify allergy objectively in patients with AD to prevent potentially unsafe food avoidance practices.[92] Thus double blind placebo-controlled food challenges have been performed and these all show discrepancy between the perception of food allergy and objective measures.[82,142]

Placebo-controlled food challenge

Sampson's group[101] has demonstrated positive challenges to food in a series of double blind placebo-controlled challenges in children with chronic AD by using up to 10 g of dehydrated food or placebo disguised in opaque capsules or juice. Positive challenges are manifested by immediate skin symptoms consisting of an erythematous macular rash, sometimes followed by a macular rash 6–8 h later. Positive tests were associated with an increase in plasma histamine levels. In a series of 514 double blind placebo-controlled food challenges in 160 patients of mean age 5.3 years (range 3 months–24 years), there were 180 positive tests and 334 negative tests. Positive challenge tests were more common in children under 2 years old.

Conclusions

Taking the data available from the literature as a whole, a strong case can be made for a link between AD and foods in at least a proportion of affected individuals. The precise nature of this link and the proportion of patients affected remain unclear, nor, as yet, have any in vivo or in vitro characteristics been described that reliably identify these patients. If future studies are to help answer these questions, a number of guidelines need to be established.

1. Identification of patients

Patients considered for dietary treatment with food exclusion and challenge should not be identified solely on the basis of history or IgE-based investigations such as skin prick tests and RAST. Apart from doubts about the role of IgE antibodies in pathogenesis, the general relevance of currently available tests for such antibodies in food allergy is questionable for a number of reasons.

For example, important unrecognized antigens could be inactivated during the preparation of extracts for prick testing or RAST. Maibach[73] described a patient in whom immediate wealing reactions followed application of fresh foods to the skin, whereas prick tests to the same foods using commercially prepared extracts were negative.

It is also quite possible that some important antigens appear only during digestive degradation in the gastrointestinal tract. Spies et al.[114,115] demonstrated the production of potent new antigens by pepsin hydrolysis of a milk protein, β-lactoglobulin. Haddad et al.[34] have published preliminary data suggesting that some patients have IgE antibodies to digestion products of this protein in the absence of antibodies to the intact parent protein. More recently, however, Schwartz et al.[106] studied patients with various symptoms apparently caused by allergy to cow's milk, and found crossreactivity in the RAST in patients who were positive to the parent protein and new antigens produced by pepsin hydrolysis. However, little crossreactivity was observed when food allergens were actually ingested.

2. Avoidance of food antigens

All relevant food antigens must be avoided for an adequate period of time to allow improvement to occur. As reported by Hathaway and Warner,[42] this may mean excluding a large number of foods for several weeks. Clearly, food challenge studies are only relevant once adequate food elimination has produced an improvement. Diagnostic challenges undertaken in an individual whose eczema is constantly being exacerbated by the foods which continue to be eaten are clearly unlikely to produce identifiable changes in the condition.

3. Diagnostic challenges: double blind

Diagnostic challenges should be given double blind, though obviously this can be exceedingly difficult. A particular problem in AD is that the quantity of food generally required to induce a reaction may be relatively large, so that concealment in a capsule is unlikely to be adequate. However, it is possible to conceal reasonable amounts of such foods as tomato, pork, beef and chicken in a fairly strongly flavoured savoury base comprising rice flour, carrots, sage, onion and some caramel to provide additional colour. The base alone can be used as the control material provided the patient has been shown not to react to any of its constituents. Other foods, such as cow's milk, egg and wheat, can more easily be concealed in a sweet base containing banana, sugar, rice flour and citric acid. All these challenges are prepared in tins, giving a prolonged shelf life. (These products have been supplied in the past by H.J. Heinz Co. Ltd on special request.)

4. Single challenges

Single diagnostic challenges are almost certainly inadequate. The evidence for this statement is largely anecdotal but it has been our own experience that, while single challenges frequently fail to elicit an exacerbation of eczema, repeated challenges on successive days may succeed in doing so. Such challenges may need to be given for as many as 7 consecutive days before one can conclude that no reaction has occurred.

5. Time of reactions

Patients should be monitored for urticarial and eczematous reactions for at least 48 h after the last challenge dose, especially if few test doses were given. Eczematous reactions are often slow to develop,[40] and their onset may be delayed for as long as 72 h after challenge.

6. Location of challenge

Ideally, diagnostic challenges should be undertaken in the patient's home; however, this poses a problem of monitoring. The studies mentioned above have largely been conducted in hospital, where the additional benefit of house dust mite avoidance could have contributed to the results.[90]

THERAPEUTIC IMPLICATIONS

'Simple' empirical diets

All dietary manipulations are difficult if performed properly, and it is therefore our view that dietary treatment of AD should only be proposed when other less uncomfortable measures such as emollients, mild topical corticosteroids and oral antihistamines have themselves failed to secure adequate improvement. If this is the case, and the patient and family (in the case of children) are suitable, then it is our practice in the first instance to recommend the empirical elimination from the diet of eggs, chicken (as this shares antigens with egg[65]), cow's milk, and artificial colourings and preservatives. If there is a good history of adverse reactions of any kind to other foods, it is clearly wise to ensure that these are also eliminated. It is important that the relevant foods are excluded totally, which implies the careful identification and avoidance of manufactured foods containing these products.

Duration of diet

An elimination diet should be maintained for a minimum of 4 weeks as benefit may not be apparent if it is any shorter than this. Then, if improvement has occurred, each of the excluded items should be reintroduced separately, allocating 7 days for each item and starting with small quantities on the first day of each introduction (see note on anaphylaxis, below). From the second day, each food should be given in at least one normal serving for every day of the introductory week. A period in which the child's eczema is fairly stable should be selected for food introductions, and any deterioration during the course of the week of reintroduction should signal the need to renew avoidance of the relevant food for a further period. Where there is suspicion that deterioration may have occurred for other reasons, reintroduction should be attempted again fairly soon afterwards.

Oligoantigenic (oligoallergenic and hypoallergenic) diets

In individuals with troublesome eczema despite adequate topical therapy and a thorough empirical diet, the possibility of a provocative role for other foods must be considered. However, the response rate to more complex diets has been of the order of 25% where an empirical diet has already failed. Therefore, given the considerable difficulties involved, such manoeuvres should be reserved for carefully selected individuals and families in a setting of experienced medical and dietetic support.

The use of hypoallergenic or oligoantigenic diets, such as those in Table 43.2, represents a compromise between the theoretical ideal and generally unacceptable option of an elemental diet. The individual is restricted for a period of 3 or 4 weeks to a limited diet comprising foods which appear to be infrequently involved in provoking eczema.

Outline of two examples of oligoallergenic diets	
Diet 1	**Diet 2**
Duck	Rabbit
Potato and potato floor	Rice and rice flour
Carrots, parsnips and swedes	Brassica vegetables
Olive oil	Sunflower oil
Grapes and grape juice	Rhubarb and rhubarb juice
Calcium and vitamin supplement	Calcium and vitamin supplement

Table 43.2 Outline of two examples of oligoallergenic diets.

Principles for reintroduction of foods

If the patient shows an unequivocal clinical improvement during the period, then consecutive diagnostic reintroduction of all the excluded items can be undertaken. The principles of dietary exclusion are the same as those outlined above in relation to empirical elimination diets. The child and parents carefully identify those foods that appear to exacerbate the eczema during individual reintroduction over 7 successive days. If no adverse reaction is noted, each food tested in this way can be added to the basic diet and subsequently eaten freely. If any reaction is noted, particularly a cutaneous reaction, the parents note the details in a special diary, and the food is not given again.

There are, of course, special problems with those foods containing several constituents, such as bread, in which the ingredients may include wheat, soya, yeast and often also milk and pork fat. With such foods, particular recipes or commercial brands with well specified contents should be used and, if a reaction occurs, the constituents should subsequently be introduced individually. Similarly, with a number of infrequently implicated foods it may be reasonable to introduce two foods concurrently, with the proviso that both will need to be excluded and introduced individually should the eczema deteriorate.

If the child fails to improve during the initial phase, one may surmise either that foods are not the main aetiological factor in that child's case, or that the child is reacting to one or more of those foods which remain in the oligoantigenic regimen. The latter possibility might be overcome by utilizing a second diet, which comprises entirely different foods, as illustrated in Table 43.2.

Fluctuation of eczema

The identification of provoking foods may be hampered by unrelated fluctuations in the eczema and, if there is any doubt, a food should be excluded and tried a second time at a later date. At the end of several months, the patient will have identified a list of foods for which a provocative role is suspected.

PROBLEMS ASSOCIATED WITH DIETARY TREATMENT

Nutritional hazards

A recent report highlighted the risk of nutritional deficiencies, particularly of calcium, developing in children on exclusion diets for eczema.[25] This is a hazard of even the simplest dietary manipulation and is a special problem in young children in whom a few individual foods may play an essential nutritional role. For example, cow's milk contributes an increasingly large proportion of dietary protein and calcium the younger the child; 500 ml of cow's milk would supply a 2 year old with almost 100% of his daily calcium and riboflavin requirements, with about 50% of his protein and 25% of his calorie intake. Hence, if cow's milk is excluded for any length of time, an alternative source of these nutrients must be found. Furthermore, this milk substitute must be of an appropriate constitution and osmolarity for the child's age, palatable and neither strongly sensitizing in its own right nor antigenically crossreactive with cow's milk.

Milk substitutes: soya and casein hydrolysate formulae

Appropriately modified soya milk products such as Cow & Gate Formula S, Prosobee (Mead Johnson) and Wysoy (Wyeth) provide a nutritionally adequate alternative to cow's milk for all age groups. Although allergic sensitization to soya may occur, this seems to be less of a problem than in gastrointestinal disease. The casein hydrolysate formula Pregestimil (Mead Johnson) is nutritionally suitable for all ages and Nutramigen (Mead Johnson) is appropriate for those over 4 months old. Studies by McLaughlan et al.[71] on Pregestimil suggest that such casein hydrolysate-based formulae are both non-antigenic in themselves and only minimally crossreactive with cow's milk.

Both soya formulae and casein hydrolysate-based formulae may be refused as unpalatable, particularly by older children. The use of a trainer beaker or a straw rather than an open cup may help by minimizing the unpleasant aroma of these feeds.

Milk substitutes: goat's milk

Goat's milk provides a more palatable option but is associated with a number of other drawbacks which warrant consideration. Liquid goat's milk is now widely available but it is almost invariably unpasteurized. The conditions under which goats are kept and milked are not subject to the controls mandatory in the dairy industry. Hence, goat's milk frequently contains potentially pathogenic bacteria, including *Salmonella* spp., *Staphylococcus aureus*, *Escherichia coli*, *Klebsiella* spp. and *Campylobacter jejuni*, derived from clinical and subclinical mastitis in goats, and from faecal contamination from both goats and herdsmen. Although reports of tuberculosis and brucellosis are very rare among British goats, the risk of contracting these infections from goat's milk remains a real one. For these reasons, goat's milk should be heat-treated to destroy such organisms before it is drunk, particularly when it is to be given to young children. Since pasteurization is not a practical proposition in the home, this will mean boiling the milk. Unfortunately, this process reduces the nutritional value of the milk by decreasing the content of heat-labile vitamins, particularly folic acid.[123] Supplementary vitamins A, D, C, B12 and folic acid may be required.

A further problem relates to the considerable antigenic crossreactivity demonstrable between goat's and cow's milk. In guinea pigs anaphylactically sensitized to cow's milk, an intravenous challenge with raw goat's milk produced anaphylaxis in 70% of animals challenged.[72] However, the authors showed that boiling considerably reduced the antigenicity of both cow's and goat's milk, and this was particularly marked in the case of goat's milk. Thus boiling has two benefits, the one immunological and the

other microbiological. Nevertheless, some crossreactivity remains after boiling, and this reduces the value of goat's milk as a substitute for cow's milk in these diets. New substitutes on the market try to address these drawbacks. 'Nanny' goats' milk, for example, has been pasteurized and appropriately supplemented with minerals and vitamins; even the aroma has been adjusted to make it more palatable.

In the school-aged child in whom none of these alternatives are acceptable for one reason or another, the option is to provide no milk substitute but to give supplementary calcium in tablet form. In any child on an elimination diet, a close watch will need to be kept on the nutritional value of what is eaten in relation to protein, calories, vitamins and calcium.

SOCIAL AND EMOTIONAL PROBLEMS OF ELIMINATION DIETS

The ubiquity of substances such as cow's milk, egg and artificial colours and preservatives in processed foods means that even the simplest elimination diet requires careful dietetic advice and will involve the family in extra time and expense when shopping or preparing food. The emotional consequences to the child must also be borne in mind. Not only is there a daily preoccupation with what he can and cannot eat, but he also may not be able to partake fully in social and festive occasions.

On a more disturbing note, Warner and Hathaway[136] have illustrated the susceptibility of the concept of food-allergic disease to abuse by disturbed parents who may fabricate 'allergic' symptoms for their child, resulting in unnecessary investigation and dietary restriction (Meadow's syndrome or 'Munchausen syndrome by proxy').

ANAPHYLAXIS

As has been discussed above, immediate IgE-mediated reactions to foods are relatively common in children with AD. The vast majority of these are not serious but in 1984 David[24] drew attention to the small but worrying risk of anaphylaxis when previously eliminated foods are reintroduced, whether intentionally or inadvertently, to atopic children. In his series, this occurred in four of 1862 food introductions in 80 patients. Particularly disturbing was the apparent inability to predict these reactions in individuals, though the possible value of skin prick test responses or the IgE RAST was not discussed. It is, however, worth noting that in two patients there was evidence of contact urticaria to the relevant food or to a closely related one. Another worrying finding was the development in one patient of the anaphylactic reaction as long as 10 h after the food was first eaten.

'Test' doses

It therefore seems more prudent to reintroduce any food with a very small 'test' dose. This should minimize the risk of serious reaction and special precautions should be taken with foods which have previously caused immediate-type reactions such as angiooedema, contact urticaria and vomiting, and with any food associated with a strongly positive skin prick test response or a very high level of circulating IgE antibody. In such cases, a little of the relevant food should first be rubbed on to the lips. If the lips become swollen, the reintroduction is abandoned. After 90 min, if no swelling occurs, a minute test dose is given by mouth, 1 ml

C

in the case of milk (diluted with a little water) and equivalent amounts in the case of other foods. If 1 ml is taken without ill effect, 10 ml may be taken 90 min later, then 100 ml. However, as David points out, these measures may not obviate the very occasional severe reaction with a later onset.

NON-FOOD ALLERGENS AND THEIR ROUTE OF ENTRY

Although publications concerned with the role of food allergy in AD are numerous, relatively little attention has been paid to the possible relevance of common environmental non-food allergens. A number of cases have been reported in the literature in which AD appears to have been provoked by such allergens.[16,43,57,94,125,133] The most common in the UK is the house dust mite, and evidence exists that at least some patients will benefit from house dust mite elimination procedures.[1,124] Some may also benefit from specific hyposensitization using non-food allergens.[27,28,59,143]

Airborne allergens

If an allergen entering the circulation can provoke AD, it seems unlikely that the route by which it does so would be of particular importance. Those who have treated patients by specific parenteral hyposensitization regularly comment on the marked provocation of eczema that may follow antigen injection.[26,28] From the point of view of aeroallergen absorption, the gastrointestinal tract is likely to be more relevant than the lower respiratory tract. It should be remembered that airborne particulate matter is largely deposited in the oropharynx, from where it passes to the gastrointestinal tract, with only a very small proportion entering the lower airways.[140] However, it seems possible that the nasal mucosa could be an important site of aeroallergen absorption, perhaps more important than the gastrointestinal tract by virtue

of the absence of either intraluminal digestion or hepatic clearance of antigen.

Skin contact with allergens

There is, in addition, evidence that eczema can be aggravated by direct cutaneous contact with both food and non-food antigens to which immediate skin test reactivity is present.[16,46,73,80,119] This may be the cause of much eczema that is localized to the perioral area and/or the hands. Epicutaneous application of aeroallergens can induce eczematous lesions[13] and the distribution of AD can often be localized to the exposed sites on these patients. What is not known is whether other routes of entry for the aeroallergen may also cause activation of the disease.

ECZEMA AND URTICARIA: DIFFERENT MANIFESTATIONS OF A SIMILAR PATHOLOGICAL PROCESS?

Eczema and urticaria may be reflections of similar degrees of cutaneous microvascular damage affecting vessels at somewhat different levels in the skin. Is 'eczema' simply 'urticaria' occurring very superficially in the dermis? In urticaria, perivascular inflammation is typically seen at the level of the mid-dermis, sparing the fingerlike dermal papillae which project up into the epidermis. On the other hand, in eczema the perivascular inflammation predominantly affects the upper dermis, and the dermal papillae in particular. The resulting oedema and inflammatory cell infiltrate would be unable to escape in any direction other than into the epidermis, which effectively surrounds these dermal papillae (Fig. 43.3). Although it might initially be contained by the structures comprising the basement membrane at the dermoepidermal junction, when the inflammation is intense, it would probably eventually 'burst' through into the epidermis (Fig. 43.4). Indeed,

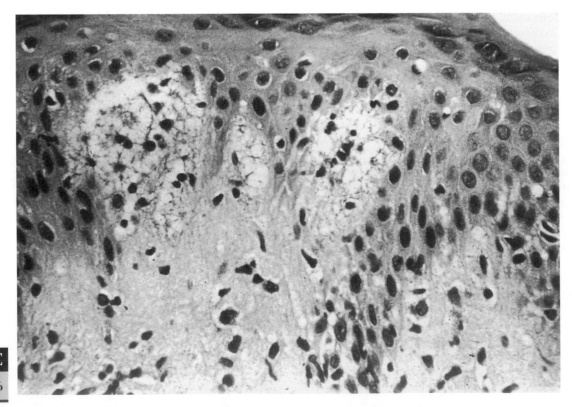

Fig. 43.3 Atopic eczema showing intense oedema of the dermal papillae.

the existence of individual elements of this sequence, much of what we have suggested is unconfirmed and, as a whole, it must be regarded as entirely hypothetical. Nevertheless, it would seem important to have a working hypothesis to test experimentally.

Finally, mention should be made of the reports that immunoglobulin deposition can be demonstrated by direct immunofluorescence in the basement membrane zone at the dermoepidermal junction.[47,91] Similar immunoglobulin deposition is also a feature of both systemic lupus erythematosus and allergic vasculitis, and it seems possible that the basement membrane zone in all these disorders is simply acting as a non-specific trap for antigen–antibody complexes that have escaped from vessels in the upper dermis.

CONCLUSIONS

In this chapter, the relationship between foods and AD has been considered by posing three principal questions.

1. What is the evidence that food allergy is an important aetiological factor in AD? While a substantial amount has been written on this subject, it remains impossible to arrive at firm conclusions. Much of the available data are open to scientific criticism, but it is our view that, overall, a reasonable case has been made for a role for foods in the aetiology of AD in many patients, particularly children. The relative importance of foods *vis à vis* other aetiological factors is unclear, and in this context the possible contribution of non-food environmental allergens should perhaps not be underestimated. It is uncommon for foods alone to be responsible for an individual's AD.

2. What are the therapeutic implications of what we know about food allergy in AD? In our opinion, a case for a dietary approach to treatment has been made, though the best method is still to be established.

3. What is the sequence of pathological events by which foods induce eczema? It is important to be aware that we are so far from answering this question that, for the present, we can only assume that the mechanisms are principally immunological rather than nutritional. However, that the two are not mutually exclusive is illustrated by the proposed link between essential fatty acid metabolism and T lymphocyte function.

We have postulated a hypothetical sequence of pathological events initiated by the absorption of intact food antigens from the alimentary tract (Fig. 43.5). Gastrointestinal absorption of food antigens is possibly increased in AD, and their handling subsequent to absorption may be abnormal. It has been speculated that, while in normal subjects they become complexed predominantly with IgA, these IgA complexes being rapidly and safely cleared, possibly by the liver, in AD they may be complexed to a significant degree with antibodies of the IgG or IgE class, and a chain of events initiated that results in damage to the superficial dermal microvasculature, leading in its turn to oedema and infiltration of the dermal papillae by inflammatory cells. The presence of oedema and inflammatory cells into the epidermis is the final event and the hallmark of eczema.

Tolerance is also thought to be important in AD. Oral tolerance describes the observation that a state of hyporesponsiveness follows immunization with a previously fed protein. Immunological tolerance is a fundamental property of the immune system in that it

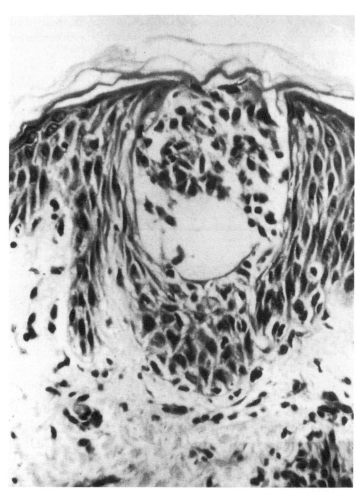

Fig. 43.4 Atopic eczema showing intense epidermal intercellular oedema ('spongiosis') with an intraepidermal vesicle.

the presence of oedema ('spongiosis') and inflammatory cells (principally lymphocytes and monocyte macrophages) within the epidermis are the histological hallmarks of acute eczema, the clinical counterparts being vesiculation and exudation.

Some support for such a hypothetical sequence is provided by the observation by many parents that exacerbation of their children's eczema by foods is regularly preceded by widespread erythema, or even by frank urticaria. This pattern has been reported experimentally by Stifler[118] and by Sedlis.[107]

Histological features of atopic eczema
The histological features observed in AD are perfectly consistent with such a sequence of events. Mihm *et al.*[79] reported prominent changes in the vessel walls of the superficial dermal venular plexus that included endothelial cell hypertrophy, and thickening and reduplication of the vascular basement membrane. These changes are entirely compatible with deposition of antigen–antibody complexes. As one would anticipate, these changes were also observed, albeit to a milder degree, in skin that appeared clinically uninvolved.

Proposed sequence of events
The sequence of events proposed is a complex one, which may involve hypersensitivity reactions of types I, III and possibly also IV at different stages. Although there is some evidence to support

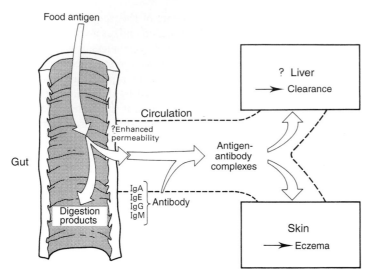

Fig. 43.5 A hypothetical pathway for the pathogenesis of atopic eczema. In normal individuals, food antigen–antibody complexes are formed in the circulation in small quantities after meals, and these appear to be rapidly cleared by the reticuloendothelial system. The evidence suggests that, in individuals with atopic eczema, such complexes may be formed in greater quantity and that they have different properties. It seems possible that eczema results from their deposition in the cutaneous microvasculature. Reprinted from Atherton DJ. Atopic eczema. *Clin Immunol Allergy* 1982; 2: 77–100, with permission.

provides a mechanism for self–non-self discrimination. Thus, the immune system can protect the host from external pathogens without eliciting autoimmune disease.[138] The induction of oral tolerance by oral immunization has been well recognized, and oral administration of certain allergens can prevent and reduce AD.[113] A double blind placebo-controlled trial looking at children with cow's milk allergy was published in 1992.[55] These authors challenged a small number of patients annually and showed loss of clinical reactivity in 38% of their patients. These patients were also noted to have lower IgE-specific antibody concentrations and IgE:IgG-specific ratios for casein-specific and beta-lactoglobulin-specific IgE. These concentrations also decreased significantly with time in comparison with those in the group who retained clinical sensitivity. Thus it was concluded that cow's milk-specific antibody responses correlated with the development of clinical tolerance. Many mechanisms have been postulated for oral tolerance and

it has been noted that tolerance is slow to develop postnatally and therefore provides a possible basis for the increased risk of allergic sensitization recognized in infancy.

We are often asked by sceptical colleagues, 'Do you really believe all this "food business"?' It remains one of the sadder aspects of mainstream medicine that we should see such an important problem as a question of 'belief' or 'non-belief'. What is actually needed is an open, enquiring attitude and careful, critical investigation. By failing to study the relationship between foods and AD scientifically we might deny ourselves the opportunity of understanding and thus eventually overcoming this common and distressing disease.

KEY FACTS

Although the role of food allergy and intolerance in AD is controversial, general conclusions have been drawn:

1. Breast feeding, especially in conjunction with maternal hypoallergenic diets, appears to decrease the prevalence of AD in high-risk infants.
2. Food allergy may trigger AD or urticaria in a small subgroup of patients and is more commonly a trigger in children than in adults.
3. It is appropriate to consider food allergy in the management of AD when there is a history of provocation with food or when conventional treatment measures are ineffective, or both.
4. Positive skin tests to egg, milk, peanuts, nuts, fish, soy, wheat, shellfish or any food implicated by history should be followed by an elimination diet (if nutrition is not compromised); if there is improvement with elimination and only one or two foods are involved, continued avoidance is appropriate; if several foods are involved, double blind placebo-controlled food challenges can be performed to attempt to return foods to the diet.
5. Sensitivity to food in children, with the exception of peanut, tends to wane with time; after 1 year, consideration can be given to returning eliminated foods to the diet.

Endnote

Copies of diet sheets for the 'simple' empirical diets (excluding egg, cow's milk, etc.) used at The Hospital for Sick Children, London may be obtained from The Allergy Dietitian, The Hospital for Sick Children, Great Ormond Street, London WC1 3JH, UK.

REFERENCES

1 Alani M, Hjorth N. Sensitivity to house-dust mites in atopic dermatitis. *Acta Allergol* 1970; 25: 41–7.
2 Arshad SH, Twiselton R, Smith J, Hide DW. Influence of genetic and environmental factors on the level of IgE at birth. *Pediatr Allergy Immunol* 1992; 3: 79–83.
3 Atherton DJ. Dietary antigen avoidance in the treatment of atopic eczema. *Acta Derm Venereol (Stockh)* 1980; Suppl. 92: 99–102.
4 Atherton DJ, Sewell M, Soothill JF *et al.* A double-blind controlled crossover trial of an antigen avoidance diet in atopic eczema. *Lancet* 1978; i: 401–3.
5 Barnetson RSTC. Hyperimmunoglobulinaemia B in atopic eczema (atopic dermatitis) is associated with 'food allergy'. *Acta Derm Venereol (Stockh)* 1980; Suppl. 92: 94–6.

6 Björkstén B. Risk factors in early childhood for the development of atopic diseases. *J Allergy Clin Immunol* 1980; 65: 403–5.
7 Bloch KJ, Bloch DB, Stearns M, Walker WA. Intestinal uptake of macromolecules. VI. Uptake of protein antigen in vivo in normal rats and in rats infected with *Nippostrongylus brasiliensis* or subjected to mild systemic anaphylaxis. *Gastroenterology* 1979; 77: 1039–44.
8 Blumenthal MN, Mendell N, Yunis E. Immunogenetics of atopic diseases. *J Allergy Clin Immunol* 1980; 65: 403–5.
9 Bock SA, Lee W-Y, Remigio LK, May CD. Studies of hypersensitivity reactions to foods in infants and children. *J Allergy Clin Immunol* 1978; 62: 327–34.
10 Boss JD, Hagenara C, Das PK *et al.* Predominance of 'memory' T cells (CD4+, CD29+) over 'naïve' T cells (CD4+, CD45R+) in both normal and diseased human skin. *Arch Dermatol Res* 1989; 81: 24–30.

11 Brostoff J, Carini C, Wraith DG *et al.* Immune complexes in atopy. In: *The Mast Cell: its Role in Health and Disease* (Pepys J, Edwards AM, eds), Pitman, London; 1979; 380–93.

12 Bruynzeel-Koomen C, Van Wicken DF, Toonstra J *et al.* The presence of Ig E molecules on epidermal Langerhans cells in patients with atopic dermatitis. *Arch Derm Res* 1989; 287: 199–205.

13 Burks AW, Mallory SB, Williams LW, Shirrell MA. Atopic dermatitis: clinical relevance of food hypersensitivity reactions. *J Pediatr* 1988; 113: 447–51.

14 Byars NE, Ferraresi RW. Intestinal anaphylaxis in the rat as a model of food allergy. *Clin Exp Immunol* 1976; 24: 352–6.

15 Byrom NA, Timlin DM. Immune status in atopic eczema: a survey. *Br J Dermatol* 1979; 100: 491–8.

16 Champion RH. Atopic sensitivity to algae and lichens. *Br J Dermatol* 1971; 85: 551–7.

17 Chandra RK. Prospective studies of the effect of breast feeding on the incidence of infection and allergy. *Acta Paediatr Scand* 1979; 68: 691–4.

18 Cline MG, Burrows B. Distribution of allergy in a population sample residing in Tuscon, Arizona. *Thorax* 1989; 44: 425–31.

19 Coleman R, Trembath RC, Harper JI. Chromosome 11q13 and atopy underlying atopic eczema. *Lancet* 1993; 341(8853): 1121–2.

20 Coleman R, Trembath RC, Harper JI. Genetic studies of atopy and atopic dermatitis. *Br J Dermatol* 1997; 136: 1–5.

21 Colten HR, Bienenstock J. Lack of C3 activation through classical or alternate pathways by human secretory IgA antiblood group A antibody. *Adv Exp Med Biol* 1974; 45: 305–13.

22 Consensus Report of the European Task Force on atopic dermatitis. Severity scoring of atopic dermatitis: the SCORAD index. *Dermatology* 1993; 186: 23–31.

23 Dannaeus A, Inganaes M, Johansson SGO, Foucard T. Intestinal uptake of ovalbumin in malabsorption and food allergy in relation to serum IgG antibody and orally administered sodium cromoglycate. *Clin Allergy* 1979; 9: 263–70.

24 David TJ. Anaphylactic shock during elimination diets for severe atopic eczema. *Arch Dis Child* 1984; 59: 983–6.

25 David TJ, Waddington E, Stanton RHJ. Nutritional hazards of elimination diet, in children with atopic eczema. *Arch Dis Child* 1984; 59: 323–5.

26 Derbes VJ, Caro MR. Localised eczema induced by house dust extract injections. *Areb Dermatol* 1957; 74: 804–5.

27 Diamond HE. Atopic dermatitis caused by inhalant antigens and its immunologic therapy. *Ann Allergy* 1953; 11: 146–56.

28 Di Prisco de Fuenmayor MC, Champion RM. Specific hyposensitization in atopic dermatitis. *Br J Dermatol* 1979; 101: 697–700.

29 Duffy DL, Martin NG, Battistutta D *et al.* Genetics of asthma and hayfever in Australian twins. *Am Rev Respir Dis* 1990; 142: 1351–8.

30 Fargeas MJ, Theodoran V, More J *et al.* Boosted systemic immune and local responsiveness after intestinal inflammation in orally sensitized guineapigs. *Gastroenterology* 1995; 109: 53–62.

31 Flick J, Sampson HA, Perman J. Intestinal permeability to carbohydrates in children with atopic dermatitis and food hypersensitivity. *Pediatr Res* 1988; 23: 303A.

32 Grulee CG, Sanford HN. The influence of breast and artificial feeding on infantile eczema. *J Pediatr* 1936; 9: 223–5.

33 Guillet G, Guillet MH. Natural history of sensitizations in atopic dermatitis: a 3-year follow-up in 250 children. *Arch Dermatol* 1992; 128: 187–92.

34 Haddad ZH, Verma S, Kalra V. IgE antibodies to peptic and peptic-tryptic digests of beta-lactoglobulin: significance in food hypersensitivity. *J Allergy Clin Immunol* 1979; 63: 198.

35 Hagerman G. The importance of food factors in atopic dermatitis. *Acta Derm Venereol (Stockh)* 1966; 81–6.

36 Hanifin JM. Epidermology of atopic dermatitis. *Monogr Allergy* 1987; 21: 116–31.

37 Hall JG, Andrew E. Biliglobulin: a new look at IgA. *Immunol Today* 1980; 1(5): 100–4.

38 Halonen M, Stern D, Tanssig LM *et al.* The predictive relationship between serum IgE levels at birth and subsequent incidences of lower respiratory illnesses and eczema in infants. *Am Rev Respir Dis* 1992; 146: 866–70.

39 Halpern SR, Sellars WA, Johnson RB *et al.* Development of childhood allergy in infants fed breast, soy or cow milk. *J Allergy Clin Immunol* 1973; 51: 139–51.

40 Hammar H. Provocation with cow's milk and cereals in atopic dermatitis. *Acta Derm Venereol (Stockh)* 1977; 57: 159–63.

41 Hansen AE, Knott EM, Wiese HF *et al.* Eczema and essential fatty acids. *Am J Dis Child* 1947; 73: 1–16.

42 Hathaway MJ, Warner JO. Compliance problems in the dietary management of eczema. *Arch Dis Child* 1983; 58: 463–4.

43 Hewitt M, Barrow GI, Miller DL *et al.* Mites in the personal environment and their role in skin disorders. *Br J Dermatol* 1973; 89: 401–9.

44 Hide DW, Guyer BM. Clinical manifestations of allergy related to breast and cow's milk feeding. *Arch Dis Child* 1981; 56: 172–5.

45 Hide DW, Matthews S, Matthews L *et al.* Effect of allergen avoidance in infancy on allergic manifestations at age two years. *J Allergy Clin Immunol* 1994; 93: 842–6.

46 Hjorth N, Roed-Petersen J. Occupational protein contact dermatitis in food handlers. *Contact Dermatitis* 1976; 2: 28–42.

47 Hodgkinson GI, Everall JD, Smith HV. Immunofluorescent patterns in the skin of Besnier's prurigo. *Br J Dermatol* 1977; 96: 357–66.

48 Holt PG. A potential vaccine strategy for asthma and allied atopic diseases during early childhood. *Lancet* 1994; 344: 456–8.

49 Horrobin DF, Manku MS, Oka M. The nutritional regulation of T-lymphocyte function. *Med Hypotheses* 1979; 5: 969–85.

50 Irani AM, Sampson HA, Schwartz LB. Mast cells in atopic dermatitis. *Allergy* 1989; 44(Suppl. 9): 31–4.

51 Isolauri E, Turjanmaa K. Combined skin prick and patch testing enhances identification of food allergy in infants with atopic dermatitis. *J Allergy Clin Immunol* 1996; 97: 640–4.

52 Jackson PG, Lessof MH, Baker RWR *et al.* Intestinal permeability in patients with eczema and food allergy. *Lancet* 1981; i: 1285–6.

53 Janssens V, Morren M, Dooms-Goossens A *et al.* Protein contact dermatitis: myth or reality? *Br J Dermatol* 1995; 132: 1–6.

54 Jarvis D, Chinn S, Luczynska C, Burney P. The association of family size with atopy and atopic disease. *Clin Exp Allergy* 1997; 27: 240–5.

55 James JM, Sampson HA. Immunologic changes associated with the development of tolerance in children with cow milk allergy. *J Pediatr* 1992; 121: 371–7.

56 Jenkins HR, Walker-Smith JA, Atherton DJ. Protein-losing enteropathy in atopic dermatitis. *Pediatr Dermatol* 1986; 3:125–9.

57 Jillson OF, Adami M. Allergic dermatitis produced by inhalant moulds. *Areb Dermatol* 1955; 72: 411–19.

58 Juto P, Engberg S, Winberg J. Treatment of infantile atopic eczema with a strict elimination diet. *Clin Allergy* 1978; 8: 493–500.

59 Kaufman H, Roth HL. Hyposensitization with alum precipitated extracts in atopic dermatitis: a placebo controlled study. *Ann Allergy* 1974; 32: 321–30.

60 Kesten BM. Allergic eczema. *NY State J Med* 1954; 54: 2441–8.

61 Kilshaw PJ, Slade H. Passage of ingested protein into the blood during gastrointestinal hypersensitivity reactions: experiments in the preruminant calf. *Clin Exp Immunol* 1980; 41: 575–82.

62 Kimpen J, Callaert H, Embrechts P, Bosmans E. Cord blood Ig E and month of birth. *Arch Dis Child* 1987; 62: 478–82.

63 Kokkonen J, Simila S, Herva R. Gastrointestinal findings in atopic children. *Eur J Paediatr* 1980; 134: 249–54.

64 Kramer DS. Does breast feeding help protect against atopic disease? Biology, methodology, and a golden jubilee of controversy. *J Pediatr* 1988; 112: 181–90.

65 Langeland T. A clinical and immunological study of allergy to hen's egg white. VI. Occurrence of proteins crossreacting with allergens in hen's egg white as studied in egg white from turkey, duck, goose, seagull and hen's egg yolk, and hen's and chicken's sera and flesh. *Allergy* 1983; 38: 399–412.

66 Larsen FS, Holm NV, Henning K. Atopic dermatitis: a genetic-epidemiologic study in a population-based twin sample. *J Am Acad Dermatol* 1993; 28: 719–23.

67 Leung DYM, Bhan AK, Schneeberger EE *et al.* Characterisation of mononuclear cell infiltrate in atopic dermatitis using monoclonal antibodies. *J Allergy Clin Immunol* 1983; 71: 47–56.

68 Longo G, Poli F. Trattamento dell'eczema atopico infantile con dicta de eliminazione. *Rev Ital Pediatr* 1980; 6: 41–9.

69 Lucas A, Brooke O, Morley R, Cole T, Bamford M. Early diet of preterm infants and development of allergic or atopic disease: randomised prospective study. *BMJ* 1990; 300: 837–40.

70 McCalla R, Savilahti E, Perkkio M *et al.* Morphology of the jejunum in children with eczema due to food allergy. *Allergy* 1980; 35: 563–71.

71 McLaughlan P, Anderson KJ, Coombs RRA. An oral screening procedure to determine the sensitizing capacity of infant feeding formulae. *Clin Allergy* 1981; 11: 311–18.

72 McLaughlan P, Anderson KJ, Widdowson EM, Coombs RRA. Effect of heat on the anaphylactic sensitizing capacity of cow's milk, goat's milk and various infant formulae fed to guineapigs. *Arch Dis Child* 1981; 56: 165–71.

73 Maibach H. Immediate hypersensitivity in hand dermatitis. *Arch Dermatol* 1976; 112: 1289–91.

74 Manku MS, Horrobin DF, Morse NL *et al.* Essential fatty acids in the plasma phospholipids of patients with atopic eczema. *Br J Dermatol* 1984; 110: 643–8.

75 Martinez FD. Role of viral infections in the inception of asthma and allergies during childhood: could they be protective? *Thorax* 1994; 49: 1189–91.

76 Matricardi PM, Rosmini F, Ferrigno L *et al.* Cross sectional retrospective study of prevalance of atopy among Italian military students with antibodies against hepatitis A virus. *BMJ* 1997; 314: 999–1003.

77 Matthew DJ, Taylor B, Norman AP *et al.* Prevention of eczema. *Lancet* 1977; i: 321–4.

78 Majamaa H, Isolauri E. Evaluation of gut mucosal barrier: evidence for increased antigen transfer in children with atopic eczema. *J Allergy Clin Immunol* 1996; 97: 985–90.

79 Mihm MC, Soter NA, Dvorak HF, Austen KF. The structure of normal skin and the morphology of atopic eczema. *J Invest Dermatol* 1976; 67: 305–12.

80 Mitchell EB, Chapman MD, Pope FM *et al.* Basophils in allergen-induced patch test sites in atopic dermatitis. *Lancet* 1982; i: 127–30.

81 Moffat MF, Sharp PA, Faux JA *et al.* Factors confounding genetic linkage between atopic and chromosome 11q. *Clin Exp Allergy* 1992; 22: 1042–51.

82 Niestijl Jansen JJ, Kardinaal AFM, Huijbers G *et al.* Prevalence of food allergy and intolerance in the adult Dutch population. *J Allergy Clin Immunol* 1994; 93: 446–56.

83 Oranje AP, Aarsen RSR, Mulder PGH *et al.* Food immediate-contact hypersensitivity (FICH) and elimination diet in young children with atopic dermatitis: preliminary results in 107 children. *Acta Derm Venereol Suppl (Stockh)* 1992; 176: 41–4.

84 Paganelli R, Levinsky RJ, Atherton DJ. Detection of specific antigen within circulating immune complexes. Validation of the assay and its application to food antigen–antibody complexes found in healthy and food allergic subjects. *Clin Exp Immunol* 1981; 46: 44–53.

85 Paganelli R, Levinsky RJ, Brostoff J, Wraith DG. Immune complexes containing food proteins in normal and atopic subjects after oral challenge, and effect of sodium cromoglycate on antigen absorption. *Lancet* 1979; i: 1270–2.

86 Parrilli G, Ayala F, Lembo G *et al.* Abnormal intestinal permeability to lactulose in patients with atopic dermatitis. In: *Immunodermatology* (MacDonald DM, ed.), Butterworths, London, 1984; 21–2.

87 Peterson RDA, Good RA. Antibodies to cow's milk proteins – their presence and significance. *Pediatrics* 1963; 31: 209–21.

88 Picker LJ, Martin RJ, Trumble A *et al.* Differential expression of lymphocyte homing receptors by human memory/effector T cells in pulmonary versus cutaneous immune effector sites. *Eur J Immunol* 1994; 24: 1269–77.

89 Pike M, Heddle RJ, Boulton P *et al.* Increased intestinal permeability in atopic eczema. *J Invest Dermatol* 1986; 86: 101–4.

90 Platts-Mills TA, Mitchell EB, Rowntree S, Chapman MD, Wilkins SR. The role of dust mite allergen in atopic dermatitis. *Clin Exp Derm* 1983; 8: 233–47.

91 Ring J, Senter T, Cornell RC *et al.* Complement and immunoglobulin deposits in the skin of patients with atopic dermatitis. *Br J Dermatol* 1978; 99: 495–501.

92 Rothe MJ, Grant-Kels JM. Atopic dermatitis: an update. *J Am Acad Dermatol* 1996; 35: 1–13.

93 Romagnani S. Induction of Th1 and Th2 responses: a key role for the 'natural' immune response? *Immunol Today* 1992; 13: 379–81.

94 Rowe A, Rowe AH. Atopic dermatitis in infants and children. *J Pediatr* 1951; 39: 80–6.

95 Rossiter H, Van Reijsen F, Mudde G. Skin disease-related T cells bind to endothelial selectins: expression of cutaneous lymphocyte antigen (CLA) predicts E-selectin but not P-selectin binding. *Eur J Immunol* 1994; 24: 205–10.

96 Saarinen UM, Kajossari M, Backman A, Siimes MA. Prolonged breast feeding as prophylaxis for atopic disease. *Lancet* 1979; ii: 163–6.

97 Sampson HA. Role of immediate food hypersensitivity in the pathogenesis of atopic dermatitis. *J Allergy Clin Immunol* 1983; 71: 473.

98 Sampson HA, Jolie PA. Increased plasma histamine concentration after food challenges in children with atopic dermatitis. *New Engl J Med* 1984; 311: 372.

99 Sampson HA, McCaskill CM. Food hypersensitivity in atopic dermatitis: evaluation of 113 patients. *J Paediatrics* 1985; 107: 669.

100 Sampson HA, Scanlon SM. Natural history of food hypersensitivity in children with atopic dermatitis. *J Pediatr* 1989; 115: 23–7.

101 Sampson HA. Food hypersensitivity and dietary management in atopic dermatitis. *Pediatr Dermatol* 1992; 9: 376–9.

102 Sampson HA. Food sensitivity and the pathogenesis of atopic dermatitis. *J R Soc Med* 1997; 90(Suppl. 30): 2–8.

103 Sandford AJ, Shirakawa T, Moffatt MF *et al.* Localisation of atopy and β subunit of high affinity Ig E receptor (FcεR I) on chromosome 11q. *Lancet* 1993; 341: 332–4.

104 Schloss OM. Allergy to common foods. *Trans Am Pediatr* 1988; 113: 447–51.

105 Schrander JP, Van den Bogart JPH, Forget PP, Schrander-stumpel CTRM, Kuijten RH, Kester ADM. Cow's milk protein intolerance in infants under 1 year of age: a prospective epidemiological study. *Eur J Pediatr* 1993; 152: 640–4.

106 Schwartz HR, Nerurka LS, Spies JR *et al.* Milk hypersensitivity: RAST studies using new antigens generated by pepsin hydrolysis of beta-lactoglobulin. *Ann Allergy* 1980; 45: 242.

107 Sedlis E. Conference on infantile atopic eczema: some challenge studies with foods. *J Pediatr* 1965; 66 (Suppl.): 235–41.

108 Shaheen SO, Aaby P, Hall AJ *et al.* Measles and atopy in Guinea-Bissau. *Lancet* 1996; 347: 1792–6.

109 Shaheen SO, Aaby P, Hall AJ *et al.* Cell-mediated immunity after measles infection in Guinea-Bissau: historical cohort study. *BMJ* 1996; 313: 969–74.

110 Sigurs N, Hatterig G, Kjellman B. Maternal avoidance of eggs, cows milk and fish during lactation: effect on allergic manifestations, skin-prick tests and specific Ig E antibodies in children at age 4 years. *Pediatrics* 1992; 89: 735–9.

111 Sloper KS, Brook CGD, Kingston D *et al.* Eczema and atopy in early childhood; low IgA plasma cell counts in the jejunal mucosa. *Arch Dis Child* 1981; 56: 939–42.

112 Sloper KS, Wadsworth J, Brostoff J. Children with atopic eczema: clinical response to food elimination and subsequent double-blind food challenge. *Quart J Med* 1991; 292: 677–93 and 695–705.

113 Sosroseno W. A review of the mechanisms of oral tolerance and immunotherapy. *J R Soc Med* 1995; 88: 14–17.

114 Spies JR, Stevan MA, Stein WJ. A method for estimation of the relative antigenic potencies of preparations containing common new antigens derived from a precursor protein (β-lactoglobulin). *J Immunol Methods* 1972; 2: 35–43.

115 Spies JR, Stevan MA, Stein WJ. The chemistry of allergens. XXI. Eight new antigens generated by successive pepsin hydrolysis of bovine β-lactoglobulin. *J Allergy Clin Immunol* 1972; 50: 82–91.

116 Strachan DP, Taylor EM, Carpenter RG. Family size, neonatal infection and hay fever in adolescence. *Arch Dis Child* 1996; 74: 422–6.

117 Strachan DP. Allergy and family size: a riddle worth solving. *Clin Exp Allergy* 1997; 27: 235–6.

118 Stifler WC. Conference on infantile atopic eczema: some challenge studies with foods. *J Pediatr* 1965; 66 (Suppl): 235–41.

119 Strauss JS, Kligman AM. The relationship of atopic allergy and dermatitis. *Arch Dermatol* 1957; 75: 806–11.

120 Van Daran-schmidt K, Pichler J, Ebner C, Szepfalusi Z *et al.* Prenatal allergen contact with milk proteins. *Clin Exp Allergy* 1997; 27: 28–35.

121 Talbot FB. Eczema in childhood. *Med Clin North Am* 1918; 1: 985–96.

122 Taylor B, Wadsworth J, Wadsworth M, Peckham C. Changes in the reported prevalence of childhood eczema since the 1939–45 war. *Lancet* 1984; ii: 1255–7.

123 Tripp JH, Francis DEM, Knight JA, Harries JT. Infant feeding practices: a cause for concern. *BMJ* 1979; ii: 707–9.

124 Tuft LA. The importance of inhalant allergens in atopic dermatitis. *J Invest Dermatol* 1949; 12: 211–19.

125 Tuft L, Tuft HS, Heck VM. Atopic dermatitis. I. An experimental clinical study of the role of inhalant allergens. *J Allergy* 1950; 21: 181–6.

126 Turner MW, Brostoff I, Mowbray JF, Skelton A. The atopic syndrome: in vitro immunological characteristics of clinically defined subgroups of atopic subjects. *Clin Allergy* 1980; 10: 575–84.

127 Uehara M, Kimura C. Descendant family history of atopic dermatitis. *Acta Derm Venereol (Stockh)* 1993; 73: 62–3.

128 Ukabam SO, Mann RJ, Cooper BT. Small intestinal permeability to sugars in patients with atopic eczema. *Br J Dermatol* 1984; 110: 649–52.

129 Van Asperen PP, Lewis M, Rogers M *et al.* Experience with an elimination diet in children with atopic dermatitis. *Clin Allergy* 1983; 13: 479–85.

130 Vanto T, Kovikko A. Dog hypersensitivity in asthmatic children. *Acta Paediatr Scand* 1983; 72: 571–5.

131 Wakita H, Sakamoto T, Tokura Y, Takigawa M. E-Selectin and vascular cell adhesion molecule-1 as critical adhesion molecules for infiltration of T lymphocytes and eosinophils in atopic dermatitis. *J Cutan Pathol* 1994; 21: 33–9.

132 Waldmann TA, Wochner RD, Laster L, Gordon RS. Allergic gastroenteropathy. *N Engl J Med* 1967; 276: 761–7.

133 Walker C. Causation of eczema, urticaria and angioneurotic oedema by proteins other than those derived from food. *JAMA* 1918; 70: 897–900.

134 Walker WA, Isselbacher KJ. Uptake and transport of macromolecules by the intestine. *Gastroenterology* 1974; 67: 531–50.

135 Walker WA. Transmural passage of antigen. In *Food Allergy* (Schmidt E, ed.), Vevey/Raven Press, New York, 1988: 15–32.

136 Warner JO, Hathaway MJ. Allergic form of Meadow's syndrome (Munchausen by proxy). *Arch Dis Child* 1984; 59: 151–6.

137 Welliver RC, Sun M, Rinaldo D, Ogra PL. Predictive value of respiratory syncitial virus-specific IgE responses for recurrent wheezing following bronchiolitis. *J Pediatr* 1986; 109: 776–80.

138 Weiner HL. Oral tolerance: immune mechanisms and treatment of autoimmune diseases. *Immunol Today* 1997; 18: 335–43.

139 White RG, Boyd JE. The effect of measles on the thymus and other lymphoid tissues. *Clin Exp Immunol* 1973; 13: 343–57.

140 Wilson AF, Novey HS, Berke BA, Surprenant EL. Deposition of inhaled pollen and pollen extract in human airways. *N Engl J Med* 1973; 288: 1056–8.

141 Wright S, Burton JL. Oral evening primrose seed oil improves atopic eczema. *Lancet* 1982; ii: 1120–2.

142 Young E, Stoneham MD, Petruckevitch A *et al.* A population study of food intolerance. *Lancet* 1994; 343: 1127–30.

143 Zachariae H, Thestrup-Pedersen K, Thulin H *et al.* Experimental treatment in atopic dermatitis: immunological background and preliminary results. *Acta Derm Venereol (Stockh)* 1980; (Suppl. 92): 121–7.

144 Zeiger R, Heller S, Mellon M, Forsythe A, O'Connor R, Hamburger R. Effect of combined maternal and infant food-allergen avoidance on development of atopy in early infancy: a randomized study. *J Allergy Clin Immunol* 1989; 84: 72–89.

145 Zeiger R. Prevention of food allergy in infancy. *Ann Allergy* 1990; 65: 430–41.

146 Zeiger R, Heller S, Mellon M, Halsey J, Hamburger R, Sampson H. Genetic and environmental factors affecting the development of atopy through age 4 in children of atopic parents: a prospective randomised study of food allergen avoidance. *Pediatr Allergy Immunol* 1992; 3: 110–27.

147 Zeiger R, Heller S. The development and prediction of atopy in high-risk children: follow-up at seven years in a prospective randomised study of combined maternal and infant food allergen avoidance. *J Allergy Clin Immunol* 1995; 95: 1179–90.

Chapter 44

Food intolerance in urticaria and angio-oedema and urticarial vasculitis

Malcolm Greaves

INTRODUCTION

Most patients with urticaria and angio-oedema believe, at least initially, that adverse reactivity to one or more foods underlies their urticaria. This belief is shared in many cases by their doctors. Food allergy or intolerance is undoubtedly the cause of many cases of acute urticaria although this causal relationship can less often be established in chronic urticaria and angio-oedema or urticarial vasculitis. It is the purpose of this account to discuss critically the evidence for and against adverse reactions to food as a cause of these different forms of urticaria.

ACUTE URTICARIA

Acute urticaria is arbitrarily defined as a single bout of urticaria continuing for no more than 6 weeks. However, it can pursue an intermittent course with repeated bouts over a prolonged period. Acute urticaria is common; probably at least 10–15% of the population experience it at some time in their lives.[55] However, up to date figures for its epidemiology are lacking.

Pathology

Acute urticaria is an archetypal type 1 hyperactivity reaction involving activation and degranulation of cutaneous mast cells, and release of histamine and other preformed mediators. Mast cell activation may occur via crosslinking of the high affinity IgE receptor (Fcε-RI) (e.g. by specific antigen) or independently of Fcε-RI (e.g. acute urticaria and angio-oedema due to aspirin).

Clinical features

Acute onset of widespread urticarial wheals with itching, with or without angio-oedema, is the rule. The urticarial weals, which vary from a few millimetres to several centimetres in diameter, may show pseudopodia and are usually surrounded by a bright red flare. Angio-oedema, which may affect mucous membranes as well as skin is pale, usually non-irritant, and is subcutaneous or submucosal. Urticarial weals which untreated last less than 24 h, but more than 8–12 h, fade without scaling or staining unless they have been scratched.

Acute urticaria, with or without angio-oedema, is often associated with systemic symptoms including wheezing, headache, palpitations, nausea and vomiting, and faintness or syncope, sometimes amounting to full anaphylactic episodes.

Aetiology

The cause of acute urticaria is often apparent to patient and physician alike. For this reason many patients never come to the attention of the specialist allergologist or dermatologist. Figures for the relative prevalences of food allergies, infections and 'pseudoallergies' (idiosyncratic reactions to specific agents which mimic true allergic reactions clinically and pathologically, but which do not depend on an identifiable immunological mechanism) vary greatly depending on the source. Acute urticaria is common in children as well as adults and shows little or no predilection for atopic subjects.[11,59] Although recent studies have cast doubt on the frequency with which an identifiable culprit allergen can be identified,[2,59] this may be attributable to the hospital outpatient referral database used. Patients who recognize a food or drug allergen as the culprit may see little purpose in attending a hospital clinic to have a self-evident cause confirmed. Aoki *et al.*[2] found that most of 50 patients studied had a history suggestive of a preceding infection. Most cleared up within 2 weeks. Pseudoallergic reactions[59] to analgesics and aspirin were identified as a cause in only 9%. In the general community, however, food allergens (nuts, seafood, egg) are common allergens. In infants, dairy products are recognized causes. In these food-provoked cases of acute urticaria it is presumed that an IgE-dependent mechanism is involved.

Diagnosis

A careful history is often sufficient to incriminate one or more items of food as a cause. Oral provocation testing is obviously hazardous in patients with a history of acute urticaria or angio-oedema and can rarely, if ever, be safely undertaken. Skin prick testing may be undertaken in patients in whom there is a degree of uncertainty. It should only be carried out where facilities for resuscitation are available because of the significant, albeit remote, risk of an anaphylactic response. Radioallergosorbent tests can identify circulating serum levels of specific IgE to penicillin and certain foods. This is helpful but does not confirm IgE-mediated allergy since there is a poor correlation between the levels of circulating specific IgE and clinical reactivity.

Management

Apart from avoidance of the offending culprit, H1-antihistamines remain the mainstay of treatment. For acute urticaria and angio-oedema patients may find an adrenaline aerosol spray (two or three puffs as required) useful for swellings in and around the oropharynx. One per cent menthol in aqueous cream is useful as a soothing balm for patients with highly irritant urticaria. Desensitization regimens for food allergens have not been found successful and are not an option in recurrent cases.

PHYSICAL URTICARIAS

Physical urticarias are chronic urticarias in which external physical stimuli (local pressure, stroking, cold, heat, sunlight, water) cause a local urticarial reaction at the site of application of the stimulus. It is important to identify patients in whom physical urticaria is the sole or predominant problem. This is because food or drug intolerance is not a significant cause in these cases. Cholinergic urticaria (urticaria induced by exercise, heat and emotional stimuli) is also included in this group for convenience.

Delayed pressure urticaria

This type of physical urticaria occurs at sites of local pressure, including the skin under the waist band, the soles of the feet and palms of the hands, and the skin underlying the strap of a heavy bag or basket. The swellings, which may be itchy or painful, occur several hours after application of pressure and may last for 24 h or more. Chronic 'idiopathic' urticaria is associated with delayed pressure urticaria in 37% of patients. The diagnosis is made by challenge testing, with local pressure applied in a graded fashion at right angles to the skin.[4,14] This causes whealing after a latent period of 2–4 h, lasting 24 h or more. There is no evidence that food intolerance plays any part in delayed pressure urticaria, the aetiology of which is unknown.

Symptomatic dermographism (*syn* factitious urticaria)

Whealing associated with intense itching occurs immediately after gentle stroking of clinically normal looking skin. Subsequently it is possible to 'write' on the skin – hence this physical urticaria's name. Caused by histamine release from skin mast cells,[23] the whealing lasts for 10–20 min before fading. A similar reaction occurs in the involved skin of patients with urticaria pigmentosa (cutaneous mastocytosis). In the latter there is a great increase in the population density of mast cells, whereas in symptomatic dermographism the mast cell population is within normal limits. The diagnosis is made by gentle stroking of the skin with a spring-loaded dermographometer,[39] which causes immediate local whealing.

The cause of symptomatic dermographism is unclear, although in some patients the capacity to confer skin reactivity is passively transferable by serum.[44] There is no suggestion in the literature of any involvement of food intolerance in the aetiology.

Cholinergic urticaria

Unlike physical urticarias, in which there is no predilection for atopic subjects, cholinergic urticaria occurs more frequently in patients with a history of eczema, asthma and hay fever. It is common, occurring at least in a mild form in 5–10% of the population. It is frequent in young adults who complain of episodes of a symmetrical monomorphic punctate eruption with a burning itch occurring on the face, neck, upper trunk and upper limbs. The rash may be much more widespread, including the scalp and lower limbs. Occasionally wheals are larger, becoming confluent and leading to large areas of brawny oedema. Systemic symptoms (wheezing, palpitations, flushing and faintness) may occur. Attacks occur within minutes of physical exertion, hot baths, emotional stress, ingestion of spicy foods and indeed any activity which leads to sweating. Exercise-induced anaphylaxis is probably a variant of this condition.[33] As its name suggests, the lesions are mediated by acetylcholine released from the sympathetic cholinergic innervation of eccrine sweat glands, since atropinization of the skin blocks the rash. Subsequent molecular events involve release of histamine from cutaneous mast cells.[28] A circulating factor is also involved since the disease can be passively transferred by serum in some patients.[45] The diagnosis is confirmed by challenge testing by exercise or a hot bath or shower.[12] Clinical variants of cholinergic urticaria include persistent cholinergic erythema[43] and cholinergic urticaria with angio-oedema.[37] The natural history is for gradual improvement and the condition is rare in the elderly. H1-antihistamines form the routine treatment, but anabolic steroids have been shown to be effective in more severely disabled patients.[57] The clinical features, pathophysiology and management have been fully reviewed.[30,31]

Food–exercise-induced cholinergic urticaria

That food factors are involved in a small minority of patients with cholinergic urticaria is suggested by a number of reports. In these patients, food ingestion is necessary but not sufficient for development of the rash of cholinergic urticaria. Ingestion of specific items of food (e.g. gliadin or celery), followed by exercise, leads to an outbreak of exercise-induced urticaria.[35,56] In others, the act of eating any food rather than any specific food item followed by exercise is a prerequisite for development of the rash.[35] In those cases involving a specific food allergen, intracutaneous testing is positive. In the non-specific food ingestion–exercise-provoked patients, exercise within 2 h of food intake causes an attack. Exercise occurring without recent food ingestion has no effect and neither does food intake alone. It seems conceivable that in either type of food–exercise-induced cholinergic urticaria, 'priming' of the mast cells (by neurogenic mediators released non-specifically after eating or by an IgE-dependent process in the case of food allergen-specific provocation) has a permissive action on exercise-evoked mast cell degranulation.

Other physical urticarias

These rare physical urticarias include cold urticaria, solar urticaria, aquagenic urticaria and vibration urticaria. Their diagnosis has been the subject of a recent consensus conference.[10] None of these is known to be provoked by food intolerance.

CHRONIC 'IDIOPATHIC' URTICARIA

Chronic urticaria is defined as the occurrence of daily (or almost daily) urticaria for at least 6 weeks. It is associated with angio-oedema in 50% of patients and with delayed pressure urticaria[20] in about 37%.

Pathology

Unlike urticarial vasculitis (see below) there is no evidence of vascular damage. When a skin biopsy is examined histologically, the predominant cell types are lymphocytes of the T helper phenotype arranged in a perivascular distribution, with a preponderance of CD4+ over CD8+ cells.[6] Immunocytochemical studies show increased expression of ICAM-1 on vascular endothelium and VCAM-1 on perivascular cells.[5] Mast cell numbers have been reported to be increased[46] or normal.[6]

Immunopathology

Perivascular deposition of immunoreactants, including complement C'3, IgG and IgM, is occasionally found, but this finding is not associated with other evidence of vasculitis (endothelial cell damage, leukocytoclasis). A few eosinophils are often found within the inflammatory infiltrate.

Pathophysiology

That the wheals and itching of chronic urticaria are at least partly caused by release of histamine from cutaneous mast cells has been confirmed by direct measurements using a suction bulla technique.[32] However, since the duration of the wheals (8–12 h in most patients) is considerably longer than that of a straight-forward histamine-induced wheal, it is clear that other factors are involved in its pathogenesis. These include fibrin deposition and mast cell or other mononuclear cell-derived mediators, including eicosanoids and cytokines. Histamine also evokes tachyphylaxis with regard to increased vascular permeability which rules it out as a mediator of all but the most short-lived wheals.[22] The possibility that activated basophil leukocytes may also be involved in the pathogenesis of chronic urticaria needs to be considered (see below).

Clinical features

The wheals in chronic urticaria are smooth, raised pink or red, and are surrounded by a bright red flare. They may occur anywhere on the body, including the scalp, palms of hands and soles of feet. In shape they may be annular, papular, circinate or in the form of larger plaques. The centre of the wheal is often paler than the periphery because of the compressive effect of dermal oedema on the postcapillary venous plexus. The wheals are almost invariably itchy but, unless vigorously rubbed, they fade without leaving any mark or scaling in the skin. The wheals last less than 24 h. Residual purpura or staining suggests urticarial vasculitis rather than chronic idiopathic urticaria.

Delayed pressure urticaria occurs in 37% and angio-oedema in 50% of patients with chronic idiopathic urticaria. The swellings of angio-oedema affect skin or mucous membranes and frequently involve the face, lips, eyelids and genitalia. Cutaneous angio-oedema is skin-coloured and is caused by oedema of the deep dermis and subcutis or submucosa. The tongue, palate, throat and oesophagus are affected in some patients, causing considerable distress although the angio-oedema associated with chronic urticaria is rarely, if ever, life threatening. Itching is usually burning or pricking in quality, is worse when the patient is warm and at night time, and induces rubbing rather than scratching.

Systemic symptoms are variable, usually mild, and include dyspnoea, palpitations, dysphasia, vomiting, diarrhoea and tiredness. When present, joint pain favours a diagnosis of urticarial vasculitis. Laboratory evidence of systemic involvement is rare, although the erythrocyte sendimentation rate (ESR) may be raised and acute phase proteins may also be elevated in the blood. The serum IgE is within normal limits in chronic urticaria.[24]

Aetiology

Most patients with chronic urticaria (and frequently their medical carers) believe, at least at some stage in their history, that food allergy or intolerance underlies their urticaria. However, this can only rarely be substantiated. Parasite infestation represents another popular but hardly ever confirmed culprit. As long ago as 1972 a careful study of an Indian population with a high prevalence of gastrointestinal parasite infestation failed to demonstrate any correlation between parasite load and severity of urticaria.[51] Anxiety and depression undoubtedly account for flare ups but are not causative. Other alleged causes of chronic urticaria include viruses and bacteria, including *Helicobacter pylori*[26] and yeast infection. None of these have stood the test of time as recognized aetiological agents. Indeed, the author has been unable to implicate any of these aetiological factors in 25 years' experience running an urticaria clinic.

Foof allergy and intolerance

As discussed above, food allergy is a recognized cause of acute urticaria. Its role in chronic idiopathic urticaria is controversial. As long as ago as 1983 Mathews,[40a] in a review of urticaria and angio-oedema, asserted that, 'as a cause for chronic urticaria or angio-oedema food allergy can only rarely be implicated'. However, in a recent textbook on urticaria Henz describes food proteins, preservatives and colorants as a major cause of chronic urticaria.[27] The concept that preservatives and dye additives in foods and drugs is a significant cause of chronic urticaria was popularized in the 1970s and 1980s. Michaelsson and Juhlin[42] challenged 52 patients with chronic urticaria and angio-oedema, and 33 controls with a series of dyes and preservatives. Thirty-nine patients (but none of the controls) developed positive responses, mainly to azo dyes, benzoic acid and aspirin. These patients were subsequently said to have been successfully treated by appropriate dietary restrictions. A similar study by Douglas[13] in 1975 in

131 patients (no controls) gave positive responses in 35% of patients with chronic idiopathic urticaria. However, these studies were neither placebo-controlled nor blinded and the reproducibility of positive reactions was not investigated. More recently, Supramanian and Warner[55a] described 43 children with angio-oedema and urticaria said to have previously responded to an additive-free diet who were subsequently challenged on a double blind placebo-controlled basis. Of these, 24 reacted to one or more additives (tartrazine and sunset yellow were the main culprits) and only one to placebo. The 24 children with positive reactions were offered an appropriate diet and 21 had no relapse. This study was more convincing than earlier reports but the reproducibility of positive challenge tests was not investigated.

There are numerous publications reporting the results of questionnaires or case histories in patients with chronic urticaria and angio-oedema which purport to confirm the importance of food intolerance as an aetiological factor. Figures range from 1.4 per cent[11] to 57 per cent[48] of patients. The importance of placebo-controlled challenge in confirming a particular food item as a culprit is illustrated by the example of aspartame, an artificial sweetener. After an anecdotal report of aspartame-induced urticaria,[36] sales of aspartame plummeted. This was despite a subsequent study utilizing double blind placebo-controlled challenge testing in 61 patients who were allegedly sensitive to aspartame, none of whom reacted to aspartame challenge.[16] The author's experience of routine use of placebo-controlled single blind challenge testing for food additive intolerance indicates that no more than 5% of patients referred to this hospital urticaria clinic with a diagnosis of chronic idiopathic urticaria can be reproducibly shown to react to food additives.[9]

Patients with physical urticaria as the sole or predominant problem are not tested, by challenge since there is little or no evidence to suggest that food factors play any role. The author concurs with May[41] who advises that the only procedure capable of establishing a correct diagnosis of food allergy is the placebo-controlled double blind food challenge, to which this author would also add testing for reproducibility as a *sine qua non*. Conclusions derived from exclusion diets[58] are unsatisfactory. Diagnosis of food intolerance by challenge testing would be greatly facilitated if biochemical markers of exacerbation of urticaria (e.g. increased histamine or tryptase levels in the plasma) were available and authenticated.

Histamine-releasing factors and autoimmunity

That circulating immunoreactants may be involved in the pathogenesis in at least some patients with chronic idiopathic urticaria was first proposed by Rorsman.[52] He reported lowered peripheral blood basophil leukocyte counts in patients with chronic urticaria, the mean values in patients with non-physical urticarias being significantly lower than in those with physical urticarias. Rorsman proposed that, where basopenia was marked, 'antigen antibody reactions or histamine liberating substances bring about degranulation of basophils'. This has recently been confirmed by Grattan et al.[19] and Sabroe et al.[54] Previously Greaves et al.[21] observed that anti-IgE-evoked histamine release from basophils of chronic idiopathic urticaria sufferers was reduced compared to healthy individuals, although release evoked by compound 48/80 was normal, suggesting 'desensitization' of these cells in chronic urticaria, a finding subsequently independently confirmed.[34] The concept of basophil histamine releasability dependent on the degree of desensitization has been evoked to explain the remitting–relapsing course of chronic urticaria.[54]

A number of histamine-releasing factors have been studied. These include cytokines,[40] IgG–anti-IgE autoantibodies[25] and, most recently, IgG–anti-high affinity IgE receptor (anti-Fcε-RI) autoantibodies[29,47] subsequently confirmed independently by Fiebiger et al.[15] and by other groups. We first noted that over 60% of patients with chronic idiopathic urticaria possessed a wheal-producing serum factor as manifested by a positive autologous serum test.[17] This was tentatively proposed to be an anti-IgE autoantibody but subsequently turned out to be mainly attributable to anti-Fcε-RIα autoreactivity.[29,47] Of 163 patients with chronic idiopathic urticaria, 28% proved to have functional IgG–anti-Fcε-RIα autoantibodies and 5% anti-IgE autoantibodies. The corresponding figure for anti-Fcε-RIα autoantibodies in Fiebiger's study[14a] was 33%. Recent evidence[15] indicates that the IgG isotypes involved are predominantly IgG_1 and IgG_3. Functional anti-Fcε-RI autoantibodies have not been found in normal individuals, patients with physical urticarias, asthma, atopic dermatitis, psoriasis or autoimmune disorders, and are specific to chronic idiopathic urticaria. In our laboratory they are detected routinely by demonstrating release of histamine from basophil leukocytes of normal donors, which is blocked by preincubation with the human recombinant alpha subunit of Fcε-RI. Most but not all patients with a positive autologous serum skin test possess anti-Fcε-RIα or anti-IgE autoreactivity. A few of these patients have a factor which is mast cell-specific, i.e. it releases histamine from tissue mast cells but not from basophils, and is not an immunoglobulin and acts on mast cells independently of Fcε-RI. This factor is undergoing characterization.

That a subset of around 30–35% of patients with chronic urticaria have an autoimmune disease involving functional anti-Fcε-RIα (or less often anti-IgE) autoantibodies has prompted non-specific immunotherapy in severely affected patients who are unresponsive to conventional regimens. These have included cyclosporin,[3] intravenous immunoglobulin[49] and plasmapheresis.[18] The concept of chronic urticaria as an autoimmune disorder is not too surprising. It has long been recognized that there is a positive association between chronic idiopathic urticaria and autoimmune thyroid disease,[38] and the recent finding of an increase in certain HLA DR and DQ alleles in autoimmune patients is in accord with this view.[50]

However, it is evident that there is still a large proportion of patients with chronic idiopathic urticaria (more than 50%) who remain 'idiopathic' and in whom the cause is elusive. With more sensitive detection techniques it seems likely that at least some of these will prove to have autoimmune anti-Fcε-RIα urticaria,[15] but presumably other aetiological factors will emerge.

Diagnosis of chronic urticaria

This has been the subject of a recent review by the author,[20] to whom the reader is referred for a detailed discussion. Assuming that a careful history and clinical examination has been carried out (including a full drug history), the first step is to exclude physical urticarias by appropriate challenge testing (see above). This is because, if a physical urticaria is the patient's sole or principal problem, no further investigations are indicated. It is also necessary to exclude C'1 esterase deficiency in patients with angio-oedema. Although, strictly, urticaria is not a feature of angio-oedema caused by C1 inhibitor deficiency, patients' histories are not reliable in this regard, and the serum complement C'4 level should be undertaken as a screening test. If it is low then the

C'1 esterase inhibitor (functional and quantitative) should be measured. The next step is to exclude urticarial vasculitis in patients with an appropriate history and clinical picture (see below). Food intolerance is investigated by placebo-controlled challenge testing. A total of 34 identical numbered capsules are administered, half of which are placebos. The additives represented in the remaining capsules are listed in Table 44.1. (Details of the formulations of the capsules can be obtained on request from the Chief Pharmacist, St John's Institute of Dermatology, London SE1 7EH, UK.) Capsules are administered on a daily basis, and the patient maintains their regular diet and routine antihistamine treatment. A careful daily diary records any flare ups in relation to the capsule number ingested the same day. Any positive results must be confirmed by re-challenging to establish reproducibility.

If all the above prove unfruitful, then consideration should be given to the possibility that the patient falls into the group (comprising about 30% of the total) with autoimmune chronic urticaria due to function Fcε-RIα or occasionally anti-IgE autoantibodies. Unfortunately, this group has no distinguishing clinical or histological features. Recourse must therefore be made to autologous serum skin testing. Fifty μl of the patient's own serum, obtained during a period when the disease is active, is injected into the patient's own clinically normal forearm skin during a period of remission. If the resultant wheal diameter (read at 30min) is 1.5mm greater than the diameter of the control saline wheal, a positive response is recorded. Positively reacting sera are then tested for histamine-releasing properties against basophils of normal donors with and without preincubation with human recombinant Fcε-RIα. Patients with severe recalcitrant urticaria showing a positive response may be considered for immunotherapy (see above). An immunoassay for detection of anti-Fcε-RIα autoantibodies in serum has been developed,[15] but its sensitivity and specificity remains to be established.

It is acknowledged that having followed all these diagnostic procedures, the cause of chronic urticaria remains elusive in at least 50% of patients. These truly 'idiopathic' cases may in any case respond well to conservative measures, including H1-antihistamines. Their prognosis is for eventual remission in an average of 2–5 years.[11]

Management

The routine management of chronic urticaria is beyond the scope of this chapter and the reader is referred to a recent review.[20]

Food additive placebo-controlled oral challenge for chronic urticaria	
Tartrazine 10mg	Annatto 10mg
Sodium benzoate 500mg	Butyl-oxytoluene 50mg
4-OH benzoic acid 200mg	Butyl-oxyanisole 50mg
Yeast extract 600mg	Sorbic acid 600mg
Penicilin 0.5mg	Sodium nitrite 100mg
Aspirin 100mg*	Sodium nitrate 100mg
Newcoccine 10mg	Quinoline yellow 10mg
Canthaxanthine 100mg	Sodium glutamate 200mg
Sunset yellow 10mg	
* Only included if patient gives a negative history of reactivity to aspirin or other NSAIDs.	

Table 44.1 Food additive placebo-controlled oral challenge for chronic urticaria. Test capsules alternate with placebo (identical lactose capsules).

URTICARIAL VASCULITIS

Urticarial vasculitis is frequently overlooked by dermatologists and allergologists alike. It is important to make this diagnosis because its investigation and treatment differs in many important ways from that of other forms of chronic urticaria.

Pathology

A skin biopsy of a wheal is essential to establish the diagnosis of urticarial vasculitis. Features to be sought include venular endothelial swelling, leukocyte invasion of endothelium, nuclear dust caused by leukocytoclasis, red blood cell extravasation and fibrin deposition. Direct immunofluorescent examination of biopsy material does not usually help in distinguishing vasculitic from non-vasculitic pathology. The histological features have been reviewed by Russell Jones et al..[53]

Clinical features

These have been well reviewed by O'Donnell and Black[48a]. Urticarial vasculitis may occur at any age. Individual weals almost invariably last for more than 24 h, a feature not seen in other forms of chronic urticaria except for delayed pressure urticaria. Wheals, which are otherwise unremarkable in appearance, tend to fade, leaving staining of the skin due to haemosiderin. Itching is variable and lesions may be painful or tender. They may also cluster at sites of local pressure. Associated systemic features, including arthralgia, fever, malaise, eye and gastrointestinal involvement, occur in a minority of patients.

Aetiology

Urticarial vasculitis can be an important cutaneous manifestation and is sometimes a presenting feature of autoimmune connective tissue diseases, particularly systemic lupus[8] and Sjögrens syndrome.[1] Urticarial vasculitis can also occur in rheumatoid arthritis, cryoglobulinaemia and hepatitis B infection, and is generally believed to be caused by immune complex deposition or, rarely, to paraproteinaemia. A rare form of urticarial vasculitis, Schnitzler's syndrome, associates urticarial vasculitis and bone pain with IgM paraproteinaemia and, in some cases, with interleukin-1 autoantibodies.[7] Food intolerance is not a recognized cause of urticarial vasculitis.

Diagnosis

A skin biopsy is an essential step in the diagnosis, which should not be considered to be confirmed in the absence of supportive histology (see above). Endothelial damage, red blood cell extravasation and leukocytoclasis are major diagnostic criteria.

Other laboratory abnormalities occasionally found include a raised ESR, red cells and protein in the urine, and a lowered serum complement C'3 level. In addition, serological and immunopathological evidence of systemic lupus and Sjögren's syndrome should be sought and hepatitis B should be excluded. However, in most patients urticarial vasculitis remains confined to the skin.

Management

The prognosis is generally that of chronicity and the response to drug treatment is disappointing. Antihistamines are poorly effective and systemic steroids are only suppressive in unacceptably high dosage. Dapsone, colchicine and antimalarial drugs help a few patients. Immunosuppressive therapy (azathioprine or ciclosporin) have also proved disappointing. Plasmapheresis may help severely affected patients.

REFERENCES

1 Alexander EL, Provost TT. Cutaneous manifestations of primary Sjögren's syndrome: a reflection of vasculitis and association with anti-Ro (SSA) antibodies. *J Invest Dermatol* 1983; 80: 386–91.

2 Aoki T, Kojima M, Horiko T. Acute urticaria: history and natural course of 50 cases. *J Dermatol* 1994; 21: 73–7.

3 Barlow RJ, Black AK, Greaves MW. Treatment of severe chronic urticaria with cyclosporin. *Eur J Dermatol* 1993; 3: 273–5.

4 Barlow RJ, Warburton F, Watson K, Black AK, Greaves MW. Diagnosis and incidence of delayed pressure urticaria in patients with chronic urticaria. *J Am Acad Dermatol* 1993; 29: 954–8.

5 Barlow RJ, Ross EL, MacDonald DM, Black AK, Greaves MW. Adhesion molecule expression and the inflammatory cell infiltrate in delayed pressure urticaria. *Br J Dermatol* 1994; 131: 341–7.

6 Barlow RJ, Ross EL, MacDonald DM, Black AK, Greaves MW. Mast cells and T lymphocytes in chronic urticaria. *Clin Exp Allergy* 1995; 25: 317–22.

7 Berdy SS, Bloch K. Schnitzler's syndrome: a broader clinical spectrum. *J Allergy Clin Immunol* 1991; 87: 849–54.

8 Bisaccia E, Adamo V, Rozan SW. Urticaria vasculitis progressing to systemic lupus erythematosus. *Arch Dermatol* 1988;124: 1088–90.

9 Black AK, Greaves MW, Champion RH, Pye RJ. The urticarias 1990. *Br J Dermatol* 1991; 124: 100–8.

10 Black AK, Lawlor F, Greaves MW. Consensus meeting on the definition of physical urticarias and urticarial vasculitis. *Clin Exp Dermatol* 1996; 21:424–6.

11 Champion RH, Roberts SOB, Carpenter RG, Roger JH. Urticaria and angioedema: a review of 554 patients. *Br J Derm* 1969; 81: 588–97.

12 Commens CA, Greaves MW. Tests to establish the diagnosis in cholinergic urticaria. *Br J Dermatol* 1978; 98: 47–51.

13 Douglas HMG. Reactions to aspirin and food additives in patients with chronic urticaria including the physical urticarias. *Br J Dermatol* 1975; 93: 135–44.

14 Dover JS, Black AK, Milford Ward A, Greaves MW. Delayed pressure urticaria: clinical features, laboratory investigations and response to therapy of 44 patients. *J Am Acad Dermatol* 1988; 18: 1289–98.

14a Fiebiger E, Maurer DT, Holub H et al. Serum IgG autoantibodies directed against the alpha chain of FceR1: a selective marker and pathogenetic factor for a distinct subset of chronic urticaria patients. *J Clin Invest* 1995; 96: 2606–12.

15 Fiebiger E, Hammerschmid F, Stingl G, Maurer D. Anti FcεRIα autoantibodies in autoimmune-mediated disorders. Identification of a structure, function relationship. *J Clin Invest* 1998; 101: 243–5.

16 Garriga MM, Berkebile C, Metcalfe DD. A combined single blind double blind placebo controlled study to determine the reproducibility of hypersensitivity reactions to aspartame. *J Allergy Clin Immunol* 1991; 87: 821–7.

17 Grattan CEH, Francis DM, Hide M, Greaves MW. Detection of circulating histamine releasing auto antibodies with functional properties of anti-IgE in chronic urticaria. *Clin Exp Allergy* 1991; 21: 695–704.

18 Grattan CEH, Francis DM Slater NGP, Barlow RJ, Greaves MW. Plasmapheresis for severe unremitting chronic urticaria. *Lancet* 1992; 339: 1078–80.

19 Grattan CEH, Walpole D, Francis DM. *et al.* Flow cytometric analysis of basophil numbers in chronic urticaria: basopenia is related to histamine-releasing activity. *Clin Exp Allergy* 1997; 27: 1417–24.

20 Greaves MW. Current concepts: chronic urticaria. *New Engl J Med* 1995; 332: 1767–72.

21 Greaves MW, Plummer VM, McLaughlan P, Stanworth DR. Serum and cell bound IgE in chronic urticaria. *Clin Allergy* 1974; 4: 265–71.

22 Greaves MW, Shuster S. Responses of skin blood vessels to bradykinin histamine and 5-hydroxytryptamine. *J Physiol* 1967; 193: 255–67.

23 Greaves MW, Sondergaard JS. Urticaria pigmentosa and factitious urticaria. Direct evidence for release of histamine and other smooth muscle contracting activity in dermographic skin. *Arch Derm* 1970; 101: 418–26.

24 Greaves MW, Plummer VM, McLaughlan P, Stanworth DR. Serum and cell bound IgE in chronic urticaria. *Clin Allergy* 1974; 4: 265–71.

25 Gruber BL, Baeza MC, Marchese MJ, Agnello V, Kaplan AP. Prevalence and functional role of IgE auto antibodies in urticaria syndromes. *J Invest Dermatol* 1988; 90: 213–17.

26 Greaves MW. Chronic idiopathic urticaria (CIU)and *Helicobacter pylori* – not directly causative, but could there be a link? *Allergy & Clinical Immunology International* 2001; 13: 23–6.

27 Henz BM, Zuberbier T. Causes of urticaria. In: (Henz B, Zuberbier T, Grabbe J, Monroe E, eds)*Urticaria: clinical diagnostic and therapeutic aspects*, Springer–Verlag, Berlin–Heidelberg, 1998; p. 19.

28 Herxheimer A. The nervous pathway mediating cholinergic urticaria. *Clin Sci* 1956; 15: 194–205.

29 Hide M, Francis DM, Grattan CEH, Hakimi J, Kochan JP, Greaves MW. Autoantibodies against the high affinity IgE receptor as a cause of histamine release in chronic urticaria. *N Engl J Med* 1993; 328: 1599–604.

30 Hirschmann JV, Lawlor F, English SJC, Louback JB, Winkelmann RK, Greaves MW. Cholinergic urticaria. *Arch Dermatol* 1987; 123: 462–7.

31 Jorizzo JL. Cholinergic urticaria. *Arch Dermatol* 1987; 123: 455–7.

32 Kaplan AP, Horakova Z, Katz SI. Assessment of tissue fluid histamine levels in patients with chronic urticaria. *J Allergy Clin Immunol* 1978; 61: 350–4.

33 Kaplan AP, Natbony SF, Tawil AP, Fruchter L, Foster M. Exercise induced anaphylaxis as a manifestation of cholinergic urticaria. *J Allergy Clin Immunol* 1981; 65: 319–24.

34 Kern F, Lichtenstein LM. Defective histamine release in chronic urticaria. *J Clin Invest* 1976; 57: 1369–77.

35 Kidd JM, Cohen SH, Sosman AJ, Fink JN. Food dependent exercise-induced anaphylaxis. *J Allergy Clin Immunol* 1983; 71: 407–11.

36 Kulcycki A. Aspartame-induced urticaria. *Ann Int Med* 1986; 104: 207–10.

37 Lawrence CM, Jorizzo JL, Black AK, Coutts A, Greaves MW. Cholinergic urticaria with associated angioedema. *Br J Dermatol* 1981; 105: 543–50.

38 Leznoff A, Sussman GL. Syndrome of idiopathic chronic urticaria and angioedema with thyroid autoimmunity. A study of 90 patients. *J Allergy Clin Immunol* 1989; 84: 66–71.

39 Logan RA, O'Brien TJO, Greaves MW. The effect of psoralen photochemotherapy (PUVA) on symptomatic dermographism. *Clin Exp Dermatol* 1989; 14: 25–8.

40 MacDonald SM, Rafnar T, Langdon J, Lichtenstein LM. Molecular identification of an IgE-dependent histamine-releasing factor. *Science* 1995; 269: 688–90.

40a Mathews KP. Urticaria and angioedema. *J Allergy Clin Immunol* 1983; 72: 1–14.

41 May CD. Are confusion and controversy about food hypersensitivity really necessary? *J Allergy Clin Immunol* 1985; 75: 329–33.

42 Michaelsson G, Juhlin L. Urticaria induced by preservatives and dye additives in food and drugs. *Br J Dermatol* 1973; 88: 525–32.

43 Murphy GM, Black AK, Greaves MW. Persisting cholinergic erythema: a variant of cholinergic urticaria. *Br J Dermatol* 1983; 109: 343–8.

44 Murphy GM, Zollman PE, Greaves MW, Winkelmann RK. Symptomatic dermographism (factitious urticaria) – passive transfer experiments from human to monkey. *Br J Dermatol* 1987; 116: 801–4.

45 Murphy GM, Greaves MW, Zollman P, Stanworth D. Cholinergic urticaria. Passive transfer experiments from human to monkey. *Dermatologica* 1988; 177: 338–40.

46 Natbony SF, Phillips ME, Elias JM, Godfrey HP, Kaplan AP. Histologic studies of chronic idiopathic urticaria. *J Allergy Clin Immunol* 1983; 71: 177–83.

47 Niimi N, Francis DM, Kermani F *et al.* Dermal mast cell activation by auto antibodies against the high affinity IgE receptor in chronic urticaria. *J Invest Dermatol*, 1996; 106: 1001–6.

48 Nizami RM, Baboo MT. Office management of patients with urticaria: an analysis of 215 patients. *Ann Allergy* 1974; 33: 78–85.

48a O'Donnell BF, Black AK. Urticarial vasculitis. *Int Angiol* 1995; 14: 166–74.

49 O'Donnell BF, Barr RM, Black AK *et al.* Intravenous immunoglobulin in autoimmune chronic urticaria. *Br J Dermatol* 1998; 138: 101–6.

50 O'Donnell BF, O'Neill CM, Welsh KI, Barlow RJ, Black AK, Greaves MW. HLA associations in chronic urticaria. *Br J Dermatol* 1999 140: 853–8

51 Pasricha JS, Pasricha A, Prakash OM. Role of gastrointestinal parasites in urticaria. *Ann Allergy* 1972; 30: 348–51.

52 Rorsman H. Basophilic leucopenia in different forms of urticaria. *Acta Allergologica* 1962; 17: 168–84.

53 Russell Jones R, Bhogal B, Dash A, Schifferli J. Urticaria and vasculitis: a continuum of histological and pathological changes. *Br J Dermatol* 1983; 108: 695–703.

54 Sabroe RA, Francis DM, Barr RM, Black AK, Greaves MW. Anti-FcεRI auto-antibodies and basophil histamine releasability in chronic idiopathic urticaria. *J Allergy Clin Immunol* 1998; 102: 651–8.

55 Sheldon JM, Mathews KP, Lovell RG. The vexing urticaria problem. Present concepts of aetiology and management. *J Allergy* 1954; 25: 525–60.

55a Supramanian G, Warner JO. Artificial food additive intolerance in patients with angioedema and urticaria. *The Lancet* 1986; 2: 907–10.

56 Varjonen E, Vainio E, Kalimo K. Life-threatening recurrent anaphylaxis caused by allergy to gliadin and exercise. *Clin Exp Allergy* 1997; 27: 162–6.

57 Wong E, Eftekhari N, Greaves MW, Milford Ward A. Beneficial effects of danazol on symptoms and laboratory changes of cholinergic urticaria. *Br J Dermatol* 1987; 116: 553–6.

58 Zuberbier T, Chantramine-Hess S, Hartmann K, Czarnetzki BM. The role of food intolerance in chronic urticaria – a prospective study. *Acta Derm Venereol (Stockh)* 1995; 75: 484–7.

59 Zuberbier T, Ifflander J, Semmler C, Czanretski BM. Acute urticaria – clinical aspects and therapeutic responsiveness. *Acta Derm Venereol (Stockh)* 1996; 76: 295–7.

Chapter 45

Skin contact reactions to foods and spices

L. Kanerva

INTRODUCTION

Skin is the most frequently affected organ of systemic IgE-mediated allergy to foods.[15,98] However, contact with food may cause a localized 'contact' reaction, either at the site of skin contact or upon contact with the lips and oral mucosa (oral allergy syndrome[15]), or a more generalized skin reaction (systemic contact dermatitis). Skin contact reactions to foods and spices may occur both in the work place and at home. It is well known that chefs, caterers, farmers, and food handlers and preparers are occupationally exposed to foods and spices but the list of jobs in which exposure to these allergens may occur is extensive (Table 45.1). Spices are also used in cosmetics, perfumes and medicaments, and allergic contact dermatitis (ACD) may be caused by these products.[15] Contact dermatitis to vanilla was recognized more than a century ago[15] and, since then, numerous reports on skin reactions from foods and spices have been published.[15] Skin contact with foods and spices may result in irritant contact dermatitis (ICD), ACD, contact urticaria (CU), protein contact dermatitis (PCD), chemical photosensitivity (phototoxic and photoallergic reactions), and systemic ACD (Table 45.2). These reactions can result from contact with a natural food or spice, and food additives such as preservatives, flavourings, stabilizers, emulsifying agents, enzymes and antioxidants.

Often a combination of factors will contribute to skin contact reactions. An individual with hand dermatitis who works as a chef may have both ICD from wet work and frequent hand washing and ACD caused by garlic or onion, as well as a *Candida*[1] or protein contact paronychia.[88] The most common clinical picture of contact dermatitis to spices and foods is hand eczema. However, eczema and CU can also localize to the fingers and palms, with extension up the arms and involvement of the face and mouth.[17] Protection and good skin care helps to prevent some of the symptoms. Atopic individuals are genetically predisposed to hand dermatitis and have a greater incidence of ICD and type I allergic reactions.[17] Patch and prick testings are necessary to identify or rule out the possibility of causative allergens.

This chapter is based on several recent book chapters or reviews on contact skin reactions caused by foods and spices.[2–4,12,15,21,53,73,82] Much data in contact dermatitis are based on case reports and many of the original references can be found in the above articles.

Detailed job descriptions of several occupations in which there is exposure related to food and spices have been described (Table 45.1).[2,53] The present review does not deal with systemic IgE-mediated allergy to foods[98] as this is discussed elsewhere in this book.

IRRITANT CONTACT DERMATITIS

ICD is the most common skin reaction to foods.[12] Individuals working with foods are chronically involved in wet work, frequently washing their hands with soaps and detergents. Several foods are known irritants, e.g. garlic, onion, citrus fruits and potatoes. ICD of the hands, whether caused by foods or other agents,

Jobs recently described in which skin allergy from foods and spices may occur	
Agricultural fieldwork	Dairy workers and farmers
Aromatherapists	Detergent workers
Bakers	Farmers
Bartenders	Fishing industry
Beekeepers	Florists
Biotechnical industry workers	Food preparation workers and food handlers
Butchers and slaughterhouse workers	Gardeners
Candy and confectionery industry	Hairdressers
Cannery workers	Houseworkers
Catering workers	Masseurs
Cashew oil factory workers	Millworkers
Cheesemakers	Poultry processors
Chefs	Slaughterhouse workers (see butchers)
Child daycare workers	Sugar artists
Cigarette and cigar makers and tobacco workers	Tobacco industry (see cigarette makers)
Cosmetologists	Winemakers

Table 45.1 Jobs recently described[2,53] in which skin allergy from foods and spices may occur.

Reaction patterns to foods and spices, and skin test method for diagnosis			
Skin eruption	Skin test method	Other test method	Main causative agents/remarks
Irritant contact dermatitis	No specific test methods; prick testing and patch testing are needed to exclude allergy		LMWC, proteins, other agents
Allergic contact dermatitis	Patch testing		LMWC, exceptionally proteins
Contact urticaria	Prick testing	RAST	Proteins, exceptionally LMWC
Protein contact dermatitis	Prick testing. Allergic patch test reactions may be caused by LMWCs in (food) proteins	RAST	Proteins
Systemic contact dermatitis	Patch testing		LMWC, exceptionally proteins
Phototoxic contact dermatitis	Photopatch testing to exclude photoallergy		Furocoumarins in plants the most common causes
Photoallergic contact dermatitis	Photopatch testing		Photoallergy to foods and spices is rare

LMWC, Low molecular weight chemicals; RAST, radioallergosorbent test.

Table 45.2 Reaction patterns to foods and spices, and skin test method for diagnosis.

often starts in the web spaces as erythema and scaling. There is no objective test available for ICD. Clinically, an ACD cannot be eliminated without appropriate skin testing, i.e. patch and prick testing.

ALLERGIC CONTACT DERMATITIS

Studies have shown varying rates of sensitization to foods and spices,[17] ranging from 27 to 90%. Vegetables commonly causing ACD are given in Table 45.3.[12,82] Garlic and onion belong to the most common food allergens.[12,15] Clinically, the skin reaction to garlic is similar to that seen in handlers of tulip bulbs (tulip fingers), with involvement of the first, second and third fingers that hold the garlic as it is cut. The chief allergen in garlic is diallyl-disulphide. Other allergens include allylpropyl disulphide and allicine.[17,61,77] The reaction to onions is often seen in patients with ACD to garlic, but they are not believed to crossreact.[12,15,82] The most common spices to cause sensitization in the USA include cinnamon, cloves, nutmeg, vanilla and cayenne pepper.[12,15,82] The essential oils of the spices can irritate the skin but can also be sensitizers.[12,15,82] Gloves, soaps and cleaners used in the work place need to be remembered in the differential diagnosis.

A clue to ACD from food and spices can be obtained from patch testing with various series, including the standard series. An allergic patch test reaction to fragrances, balsam of Peru or colophony in the standard series may reflect ACD to a common

Vegetables causing allergic contact dermatitis (type IV allergy)	
Vegetable	**Allergen**
Artichoke	Sesquiterpene lactones
Asparagus	1,2,3-Trithiane-5-carboxylic acid
Carrot	Pinene, terpinol, limonene, cineole
Celery	Celery oil? (Lovell)
Chicory	Sesquiterpene lactones, lactucin
Chives	Diallyl disulphide (Lovell)
Endive	Sesquiterpene lactones
Garlic	Diallyl disulphide, allylpropyl disulphide, allicine
Horseradish	Allyl isothiocyanate
Leek	Diallyl disulphide (Lovell)
Lettuce	Sesquiterpene lactones, lactucin
Onion	Propanthiol-S-oxide?, tuliposide A?

Table 45.3 Vegetables causing allergic contact dermatitis (type IV allergy).[82]

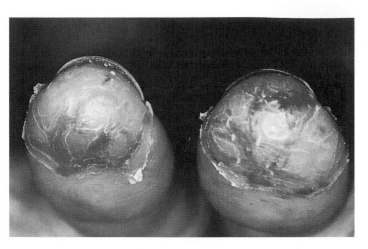

Fig. 45.1 Severe allergic fingertip dermatitis of a cold buffet manager. Patch testing showed her to be allergic to sesquiterpene/lactone mix and lettuce.

chemical in these patch test substances and foods and spices, respectively (Table 45.4). An allergic patch test reaction to, for example, preservatives when patch testing antimicrobials can be a sign of sensitization to a preservative used as a food additive (Table 45.2). Plants and their low molecular weight allergens,

especially sesquiterpene lactones, may be important in detecting allergy to foods and spices (Table 45.5). Sesquiterpene lactones in Compositae plants may reveal a chef's ACD to lettuce and other vegetables (Fig. 45.1). A so-called 'bakery series' containing allergens used in bakeries as well as those in other foods (antioxidants, preservatives, flavours, etc.) is commercially available from Chemotechnique Diagnostics (Malmö, Sweden) (Table 45.6) and can screen for allergy to foods and spices.

SYSTEMIC ALLERGIC CONTACT DERMATITIS

If a substance to which a person has developed cellular immunity (type IV allergy) because of contact with the skin is subsequently ingested or otherwise absorbed, a variety of cutaneous reactions

Patch test allergens/series that may reveal allergic contact dermatitis to foods and spices		
Series	**Chemical/agent**	**Remarks**
Standard series	Colophony, balsam of peru, fragrances	May contain same, or crossreacting allergens as foods and spices
Bakery series		Many additives, fragrances
Cosmetic series		Cosmetics and foods and spices may contain same additives (preservatives, antioxidants)
Fragrance series LMWC		Fragrances and foods and spices may contain the same, or crossreacting
Antimicrobials		May contain same antimicrobials as food additives
Plant allergens (pure chemicals or plant extracts)	Sesquiterpene lactones and other LMWC allergens	Same allergens as in foods and spices, also crossreacting allergens
Photopatch test series		Allergic reactions to photoallergens in foods and spices rare, usually photoirritant reactions
Textile colours		Same colours may be used in foods as in textiles

Table 45.4 Patch test allergens/series that may reveal allergic contact dermatitis to foods and spices. Low molecular weight chemicals (LMWC) may additionally be present in many food additives.

	Patch test substances with a series of allergenic plant chemicals		
	Contact allergen	**Source**	**Concentration (%)**
1	Primin	Allergen in primula (*Primula obconica*)	0.01
2	Tuliposide A	Allergen in tulips and alstroemerias (*Tulipa* sp.; *Alstroemeria* sp.; *Lilium* sp.)	0.1
3	Parthenolide	Allergen in feverfew (*Tanacetum parthenium*)	0.1
4	Alantolactone	Allergen in elecampane (*Inula helenium*)	0.1
5	Diallyl disulphide	Allergen in garlic (*Allium sativum*)	1
6	Allicin	Allergen in garlic (*Allium sativum*)	1
7	3-Methyl-2-butenyl-caffeate	Allergen in propolis (bee-glue)	0.1
8	Phenylethyl caffeate	Allergen in propolis (bee-glue)	0.1
9	Lichen acid mix*	Atranorin, usnic acid, evernic acid	0.3
10	Sesquiterpene/lactone mix*	Allergens in Compositae, frullania and bayleaf	0.1
11	Compositae mix	Allergens in Compositae (sesquiterpene lactones and other allergens)	6
12	2,6-dimethoxy-1,4-benzoquinone	Allergen of more than 50 different plant and wood species	10

Table 45.5 Patch test substances with a series of allergenic plant chemicals. The same (or crossreacting) chemicals may be present in foods and spices.

	The 'bakery' patch test series of Chemotechnique Diagnostics (Malmö, Sweden)		
	Allergen	**Patch test concentration (%)**	**Comment**
1	Vanillin	10	Flavouring agent in beverages, confectionery, foods, galenicals
2	Eugenol	2	Fragrance. Used in the production of vanillin
3	Isoeugenol	2	Fragrance, also in foods. Used in the production of vanillin
4	Sodium benzoate	5	Preservative, especially for food products (drinks, jellies, jams, pickles, syrups, etc.). Also common in cosmetic and pharmaceutical products
5	2,6-ditert-butyl-4-cresol (BHT)	2	Antioxidant
6	Menthol	2	In confectionery, perfumery, cigarettes, liqueurs
7	Cinnamic alcohol	2	Component in perfumed cosmetic products and deodorants. Cross reacts with balsam of Peru and propolis
8	Cinnamic aldehyde	1	Flavour in toothpaste, sweets, ice cream, soft drinks, chewing gums and cakes. Also present in balsam of Tolu and Peru, hyacinth plant, spices, cinnamon, Ceylon and cassia oil
9	2-tert-butyl-4-methoxyphenol (BHA)	2	Antioxidant
10	Anethole	5	Flavouring agent in food
11	Sorbic acid	2	Preservative in foods like cheese, syrup, etc.

continued

Table 45.6 The 'bakery' patch test series of Chemotechnique Diagnostics (Malmö, Sweden).

		The 'bakery' patch test series of Chemotechnique Diagnostics (Malmö, Sweden)	
	Allergen	**Patch test concentration (%)**	**Comment**
12	Benzoic acid	5	Preservative in foods, fats, fruit juices, etc. Also used for curing tobacco
13	Propionic acid	3	Food additive for the preservation against moulds in, e.g. cheese products. Also used in the production of fruit flavours and perfume bases
14	Octyl gallate	0.25	Antioxidant for use in cosmetic and pharmaceutical products and in food products such as margarine and peanut butter
15	Dipentene (limonene)	1	Peel of citrus fruits. Also used as solvent
16	Ammonium persulphate	2.5	Antioxidant, flour colour improver
17	Benzoyl peroxide	1	Oxidizer in flours, bleaching oils, etc.
18	Propyl gallate	1	Antioxidant for use in cosmetic and pharmaceutical products and in food products such as margarine and peanut butter
19	Dodecyl gallate	0.25	Antioxidant for use in cosmetic and pharmaceutical products and in food products such as margarine

Table 45.6 *continued.*

may occur. This is called systemic ACD.[23,72] The reaction can be a flare up of the previous site of involvement, resulting most commonly in hand dermatitis. Other presentations can include an exfoliative erythroderma, erythema multiforme, a widespread eruption favouring the buttocks and flexures known as the baboon syndrome, systemic symptoms such as nausea, vomiting and diarrhoea, cheilitis or perianal eczema.[23] Systemic ACD does not occur in all individuals sensitized to foods or spices.

CONTACT URTICARIA

Contact urticaria (CU) occurs immediately after contact with food and generally resolves within 24 h. Longlasting CU has also been reported.[48] CU can be immunological or non-immunological. Lipophilic allergens may penetrate the skin via the hair follicles.[98] Non-immunological CU may be caused by release of histamine and other substances that dilate blood vessels.[4] Allergic CU is an IgE-mediated reaction and is not detected by patch testing. The symptoms can be classified according to morphology and severity (Table 45.7).[3,4] The mildest form is the 'invisible' CU, when only subjective symptoms such as itching, tingling or burning without any objective change or just a mild erythema occur.[3,4] These reactions are often seen from fruits and vegetables. Wheal and flare at the contact area is the prototype of CU, while generalized urticaria after a local contact is less common.

Extracutaneous symptoms may also occur as part of a more severe reaction and may include rhinoconjunctivitis, asthmatic attack and orolaryngeal or gastrointestinal dysfunctions. Finally, anaphylaxis and death may occur as the most severe manifestation of CU. The term 'contact urticaria syndrome' is often used to describe the different stages of the symptoms (Table 45.7).[3,4]

CU is primarily attributed to fish and seafood, onions, fruits and vegetables.[3,4] The list of foods and spices that have caused CU is extensive (Table 45.8).[3,4] Prick (or in some cases, scratch) testing will help to diagnose such a reaction. Radioallergosorbent

	The contact urticaria syndrome: staging by symptomatology[3,4]
Cutaneous reactions only	
Stage 0	'Invisible', non-specific skin symptoms (itching, tingling, burning, etc.)
Stage 1	Localized urticaria Dermatitis (protein contact dermatitis)
Stage 2	Generalized urticaria
Cutaneous and extracutaneous reactions	
Stage 3	Rhinoconjunctivitis Orolaryngeal symptoms Bronchial asthma Gastrointestinal symptoms
Stage 4	Anaphylactic symptoms

Table 45.7 The contact urticaria syndrome: staging by symptomatology.[3,4]

(RAST) testing to certain foods may be of help and is more useful than basophil histamine release testing or passive transfer testing.[3,4] Many individuals with CU have a history of atopy.[17] Cooking of food often results in loss of the type I reaction because the antigens responsible may be heat-labile.[3,4]

In Finland, cooks, chefs and cold buffet managers are in the fourth position of any occupation with regard to frequency of occupational CU (this includes PCD).[51]

PROTEIN CONTACT DERMATITIS

In 1976 Hjorth and Roed-Petersen[41] reported on patients who developed itching within 30 min of contact with specific foods on involved or previously involved skin and who developed an

Foods and food additives causing contact urticaria			
Animal products	**Plant products**	Nuts	Rapeseed
Fish and seafood	Fruits	Almond	Rocket
Cod	Apple	Brazil	Rutabaga (Swede)
Crab	Apricot	Peanuts	Shallot
Herring	Apricot stone	Peanut butter	Soybean
Lobster	Banana	Seeds	Spinach
Oysters	Grapefruit	Sesame seeds	Stock (*Matthiola incana*)
Plaice	Kiwi	Sunflower seeds	Tomato
Shrimp	Lychee	Vegetables	Water cress
Frog	Lemon	Asparagus	Winged bean
Liver	Lemon peel	Beans	
Calf	Lime	Cabbage	*Flavourings and fragrances*
Chicken	Mango	Carrot	Balsam of Peru
Pig	Melon	Castor bean	Benzaldehyde
Meat	Orange	Cauliflower	Benzoic acid
Beef	Peach	Celery	Cassia (cinnamon) oil
Chicken	Pineapple flesh	Chives	Cinnamic acid
Lamb	Plum	Coffee been (green)	Cinnamic aldehyde
Pork	Strawberry	Coriander	Menthol
Sausage	Water melon	Cucumber	Vanillin
Turkey	Fungi	Dill	
Other animal products	Mushrooms	Endive	*Condiments and spices*
Cheese	Salami-casing moulds	Garlic	Cayenne pepper
Eggs	Grains	Green pepper	Caraway
Honey	Buckwheat	Leek	Cinnamon
Milk	Flour	Lettuce	Coriander
	Maize	Mustard	Curry
	Malt	Onion	Paprika (*Capsicum annuum*)
	Rice	Parsley and parsley root	Thyme
	Wheat	Parsnip	
	Wheat bran	Potato	

Table 45.8 Foods and food additives causing contact urticaria. For references see Amin et al.[4] and Ale and Maibach.[3]

eczematous reaction with erythema and vesiculation rather than the typical wheal and flare reaction seen in CU. They called the condition PCD. Foods most often involved are seafood, vegetables such as onion and meats such as pork.[3,4] A large number of agents have been reported to cause PCD (Table 45.9).[43,45] Clinically these patients have hand dermatitis after contact with food proteins, but the mechanism of action is poorly understood. It is not a type IV reaction because it can be elicited within minutes.[41] These individuals have a positive prick test excluding ICD as the cause, and the clinical picture is inconsistent with CU.[12] In some cases of PCD no *circulating* specific IgE can be detected in the serum despite strong positive skin prick test reactions.[52,98] IgE bound to Langerhans' cells may be involved in this type of contact dermatitis.[6,11,49,52] The reaction often seems to be a combination of type I allergy and irritation, the latter causing a defective skin barrier function.

FOODS

Onion family

Garlic and onion are members of the family *Alliaceae*. Allergens found in garlic include diallyl disulphide, allylpropyl sulphur and allicine.[15,61,77] Garlic sensitization typically manifests as a finger-

tip eczema of the first, second and third fingers of the non-dominant hand which holds the garlic for slicing. It can involve the palmar surface with desquamation and hyperkeratosis.[15] Garlic dermatitis is a major occupational problem in caterers. In a study in London, 28 of 34 individuals who were allergic to garlic were involved in the catering or food industry.[65] Patch testing for garlic or onion may be performed with a 10% aqueous extract of these vegetables or 50% in olive oil[15,17] if the pure allergens are not available.

Citrus fruits

Limonene is a terpene that is the most common allergen in citrus fruits. It is found in orange and lemon peel.[56] It is also found in dill, caraway oil, celery seed oil, nutmeg, perfumes, spearmint and lemon wood. Crossreactions can occur with turpentine and bergamot. Limonene is also used as a solvent.[55] D-Limonene-containing products were launched to replace the environmentally persistent chlorinated hydrocarbons and chlorofluorocarbons as solvents. The main allergens are oxidation products created when D-limonene is exposed to air, e.g. limonene oxide, L-carvone and limonene hydroperoxides.[55,56] Limonene has many other uses.[56] Individuals may have been sensitized via D-limonene-containing food products and then relapse from contact at work when limonene is used as solvent. Alternatively, sensitization may have been from solvents

Table 45.9 Proteins (sources) that have caused protein contact dermatitis. For references see Janssens *et al.*[43] and Kanerva.[45]

Proteins (sources) that have caused protein contact dermatitis			
Fruits and vegetables	**Animal proteins**	**Grains**	**Enzymes**
Almond	Amniotic fluid	Barley flour	Alpha amylase
Banana	Blood	Rye flour	Glucoamylase
Bean	Pig	Wheat flour	
Caraway	Cow	Oat flour	
Carrot	Lamb		
Castor bean	Amphibian serum		
Cauliflower	Cheese		
Celery	Cheddar		
Chicory	Cheese products		
Chrysanthemum	Emmenthal		
Cress	Egg yolk		
Cornstarch	Epithelium/dander		
Cucumber	Cow		
Curry	Pork		
Dill	Fish		
Eggplant	Cod		
Endive	Cuttlefish		
Fig	Herring		
Garlic	Lobster		
Hazel nut	Mackerel		
Horseradish	Perch		
Kiwi fruit	Plaice		
Lemon	Rainbow trout		
Lettuce	Salmon		
Mushroom	Squid		
Onion	Shellfish		
Paprika	Shrimps		
Parsley	Whitefish		
Parsnip	Gut: pig		
Peanuts	Liver		
Pineapple	Calf/ox		
Potato	Chicken		
Rubber latex	Lamb		
Tomato	Meat		
	Beef/cow		
	Pork		
	Chicken		
	Horse		
	Lamb		
	Mesenteric fat: pig		
	Milk		
	Cow		
	Milk products		
	Parasites		
	Anisakis		
	Placenta: calf		
	Saliva: cow		
	Skin		
	Chicken		
	Turkey		
	Worms		
	Nereis diversicolor		

and allergic reaction may then be seen to food products. A patch test preparation (dipentene) is available from suppliers of patch test allergens. Alternatively, patch testing can be performed with the peel itself.[15]

Vegetables

Vegetables reported to cause contact sensitization include chicory (*Cichorium intybus*), endive (*C. endiva*) and lettuce (*Lactuca sativa*). Lettuce can cause an ACD[76] and angio-oedema.[59] It contains the sensitizing sesquiterpene lactones lactucin and lactupicrin.[40] Fresh lettuce should be used for patch testing. Potatoes (*Solanum tuberosum*) typically cause an irritant dermatitis of the hands.[9] ACD[14] and urticarial eruptions[60] are rare. In the Compositae-like artichokes (*Cynara scolymus*), sensitivity is caused by the sesquiterpene lactone, cynaropicrina.[15]

Asparagus

Dermatitis from handling asparagus has been recognized for more than a century.[2] *Asparagus officinalis* L. is cultivated throughout Europe, Asia Minor, Africa and North America. White asparagus is produced by growing the plant under a fine silt of dirt, which protects it from sunlight and creates a tender white asparagus especially popular throughout Europe. When the stalks are peeled before cooking, the juice runs along the palm and volar wrist of the person holding the stem. It has long been suspected as containing one or more irritants,[2] and investigation has revealed a sulphur-containing growth inhibitor, 1,2,3-trithiane-5-carboxylic acid, which is thought to be the contact sensitizer.[39] Asparagus has also caused immunological CU.[84]

Umbelliferae

The Umbelliferae include carrots, parsnips, parsley, celery, dill and fennel. Carrots (*Daucus carota*) can produce contact cheilitis, ICD[79,96] and ACD,[32] as well as phototoxic reactions.[78] Allergens include pinene, terpineol, limonene and cineole.[12] Testing can be performed with, for example, a raw slice of carrot.[15] Crossreactivity to parsnip and celery has been reported.[58] Celery can cause an allergic or photocontact dermatitis. Crossreactions can be observed to essential oil of orange, lemon, bergamot, caraway and balsams.[29]

Mango

Mango is a member of the Anacardiaceae. These plants have a common sensitizer, urushiol or 3′,5′-pentadecylcatechol, and include mango, poison ivy, poison oak, cashew and gingko. Thus, patients with sensitivity to poison ivy can develop a reaction to mango peel or leaves.[35] Mango fruit peel is a common sensitizer and patients often develop a contact cheilitis from contact with the peel.[15] Ingestion can also cause an anaphylactic reaction.[67] Other fruits include pineapple, which contains bromelin that can cause an irritant reaction[80] and CU, and kiwi fruit that can cause a CU.[94]

SPICES

Spices are the aromatic parts of plants such as the seeds, fruits, roots, buds, flowers and barks. The boundary between spices, vegetables and aromatic plants is vague. For example, garlic, cayenne and paprika might be regarded as either vegetables or spices. The term herb is used for aromatic plants whose dried or fresh leaves or shoots are used. The flavouring constituents of spices are usually found in their ethereal oils, the main components of which are often known. Spices may cause delayed-type contact allergy, and/or immediate allergy.[50,72,74] Spice oils and their constituents are also used in perfumery. Spice oils contain substances which may both irritate and cause type IV allergy (Table 45.10). Spices also contain proteins which may cause immediate allergy.

Delayed allergy to spices

Clove, Jamaica pepper (allspice), garlic, cinnamon, nutmeg, paprika, vanilla and ginger are the most frequent causes of ACD.[41,72,73,90] Other causes of ACD are laurel (bay leaf),[33] cardamon,[68] turmeric[36] and mustard.[18] There is a correlation between allergies to perfumes and spices because of their identical or related substances. Therefore, on patch testing with the standard series, fragrance mix and balsam of Peru may detect contact allergy to, for example, clove, nutmeg, cinnamon and cayenne pepper.[90]

Some pure allergens of spice oils are available from patch test allergen suppliers (Table 45.10). Patch tests can also be performed with ethereal oils of spices. In patch tests, dry powders of spices are put in Finn Chamber® on a moistened filter paper.[73] Garlic, mustard and cayenne are too irritant to be tested as such (Table 45.10). At the Finnish Institute of Occupational Health, patch testing of both garlic and mustard is performed at 10% in water and at 25% in petrolatum. Patch tests with other native spices may also elicit irritant reactions[66,73] and dilution tests may be needed.

Cinnamon

Cinnamon is made from the bark of the cinnamon or cassia tree. Oil of cinnamon contains the allergens cinnamic aldehyde and eugenol (Table 45.10).[19,73] Cinnamon is a common flavour enhancer and is found in toothpaste,[62] chewing gum, tobacco, aperitifs and bitters, vermouth[25] and cola beverages. In addition, it is commonly used as an odour enhancer and is found in perfumes, aftershave lotions[23] and air deodorizers.[71] An ACD can occur in exposed individuals, particularly bakers,[63] candy makers and cooks. Sensitization to balsam of Peru can result in crosssensitivity to cinnamon.[15]

Cayenne pepper

Cayenne pepper, or *Capsicum frutescens*, from which the oleoresin of capsicum is derived, is a powerful irritant and is used in tear gas.[15] Ginger ale and liqueurs flavoured with capsicum can produce an ACD.[82]

Nutmeg

The nutmeg tree (*Myristica fragrans*) produces both nutmeg and mace, which are extensively used in flavouring foods. The fatty oils of nutmeg are found in soaps and perfumes and may be the cause of allergic dermatitis.[90]

Clove

The clove (*Syzygium aromaticum*) is the unexpanded flower bud of the tree. Oil of cloves is rich in essential oils, especially eugenol and vanillin. Eugenol is both a primary irritant and sensitizer and is also found in cinnamon oil and many toothpastes, perfumes, soaps and mouthwashes. Indians use cloves to flavor the betelnut. It is also used in dental preparations such as cement, impression pastes and surgical packings. It can cause stomatitis and allergic eczematous eruptions in dental personnel.[46] Crossreactions to balsam of Peru can be seen. Patch testing can be performed with a 10% solution in olive oil or a 5% solution in petrolatum. Oil of clove can be used as a 1–2% alcoholic solution.[29,73]

Vanilla

Vanilla is an extract made from the pod of the vanilla plant, *Vanilla planifolia*. Vanillin is a benzaldehyde which is the fragrant

Patch test materials for some spices

Native (powdered) spices*	Ethereal oils of spices†	Known allergens of spice oils‡
Basilica	Oil of basil 4%	Linalool (2–30%)
Bay (laurel) leaf	Oil of sweet bay 4%	Costunolide (0.055%), eugenol (1–5%), pinene (1–15%)
Caraway	Oil of caraway 4%	Dipentene (limonene) (1–2%), carvone (2%, 5%)
Cardamom	Oil of cardamom 4%	Dipentene (1–2%)
Capsicum frutescens**	–	–
Cayenne pepper (see Capsicum frutescens)	–	–
Cloves	Oil of clove 2%	Eugenol (1–5%), vanillin (10%)
Cassia (Chinese cinnamon), cinnamon of Ceylon	Oil of cassia 4%; oil of cinnamon, Ceylon 8%	Cinnamic aldehyde (cinnamal), (1–2%), eugenol (1–5%)
Cinnamon, see cassia		
Coriander	Oil of coriander 6%	Linalool (2–30%)
Garlic**	–	Diallyl disulphide (1–5%)
Ginger	Oil of ginger 4%	Phellandrene (5%), citral (2%)
Jamaica pepper (allspice, pimenta)	Oil of pimenta 8%	Eugenol (1–5%)
Laurel (see bay leaf)		
Mace. The nutmeg tree (Myristica fragrans) produces both nutmeg and mace. See nutmeg		
Marjoram	Oil of marjoram 6%	–
Mustard (seeds of white and black mustard)**	Allyl isothiocyanate	–
Nutmeg	Oil of nutmeg 8%	Eugenol (1–5%), dipentene (1–2%), geraniol (1–5%), pinene (1–15%)
Oregano	Oil of origanum 2%	–
Paprika (Capsicum annuum)**	–	–
Spearmint	Oil of spearmint 2%	Dipentene (1–2%), carvone (2%, 5%), pinene (1%, 12%, 15%)
Vanilla	–	Vanillin (10%)

*All may irritate when tested as such. In doubtful cases, 25% and 10% dilutions in petrolatum may be used.[73] **Not suitable to be tested as such. Dilutions (in petrolatum) may be used: cayenne[19] as 0.5%, paprika[73] as 25%, garlic and mustard[50] as 10%. †The presented concentrations do not irritate and are considered safe for patch testing.[19] ‡The test concentrations are given in parentheses. These concentrations are based on the reports of de Groot[19] and Niinimäki.[73]

Table 45.10 Patch test materials for some spices.[19,50,73]

constituent of vanilla. Clinically, contact dermatitis occurs in individuals who are exposed through cultivation, trade or industry. Symptoms can include oedema, erythema, rhinitis and asthma. Synthetic vanilla is a different compound, and individuals can be sensitized to the natural spice and not the synthetic compound, and vice versa. For patch testing, a 10% vanillin in petrolatum or a 10% alcoholic extract of vanilla in acetone can be used.[29]

Bay tree

The sweet bay or bay tree, *Laurus nobilis*, is native to the Mediterranean and Asia Minor. The usual allergen is laurenobiolide, which can crossreact with similar chemicals in the Compositae family and with magnolia.[15,54] Laurel oil is also used in the textile industry to improve the lustre of felt hats and can produce a hatband dermatitis. Laurel (or bay) leaves are used in cooking for their flavour and antioxidant properties, and are found in meat and fish preservation, pickled gherkins, condensed soups and spiced sauces. Extensive exposure and use have caused sensitization.[33,34] Patch testing may be performed with a 2% concentration in petrolatum or 4–5% concentration of essential oil in alcohol.[29,73]

Immediate allergy to spices

Paprika, mustard, coriander, caraway, cayenne, anis, dill, fennel, mustard, celery seed and parsley are the most common causes of type I skin allergy.[73,74]

Crossreactions between spices and other vegetables and fruits are common.[73,86,92,98–100] Positive type 1 skin reactions to spices and elevated spice-specific serum IgE values (RASTs) have been seen, especially in subjects with birch or mugwort pollen allergy.[73,74] The term 'celery–carrot–mugwort–spice syndrome' has been proposed[98–100] as these subjects also frequently react to fresh fruits and vegetables.

Prick tests can be performed with native spices as such. The selection of spices used in tests depends on the individual's exposure history. Prick tests are performed with native spices as follows: a small amount (2–5 mg) of powdered spice and a drop of saline are first mixed on the skin and then pricked into the skin. Reactions are read after 15 min. Reactions with a diameter of at least 3 mm larger than the negative control (saline) are regarded as positive.[73] In cases of fresh materials, prick–prick tests or scratch–chamber tests[73] can be used. The prick tests (size of the wheal) are easier to evaluate than the scratch tests. Determination of spice-specific IgE may also be used when evaluating the clinical significance of the reactions. RAST may be negative in prick test-positive cases.[75]

CHEMICAL PHOTOSENSITIVITY

Chemical photosensitivity describes skin diseases caused by the interaction of light and an exogenously acquired chemical. Both the chemical and the radiation are necessary. Exposure to the chemical can be either systemic or topical. The mechanism of the response can be irritant (toxic) or allergic. Chemical photosensitivity is classified into four clinical entities: photoirritant contact dermatitis (PICD), photoallergic contact dermatitis (PACD), photoallergy to a systemic agent and phototoxicity to a systemic agent.[3]

Furocoumarins

Phototoxic reactions have been described primarily after contact with foods containing furocoumarins (Table 45.11) such as celery, parsnip, parsley, figs and lime.[15] Furocoumarins are photosensitizing chemicals that occur naturally in the plant kingdom. They have also been synthesized and used as fragrance materials and therapeutic agents. The latter usage is dependent on the photosensitizing potential of these agents in photochemotherapy of skin disease. The most common agents used therapeutically are 8-methoxypsoralen (8-MOP) and 5-methoxypsoralen (5-MOP) and tripsoralen.[3]

Persian lime

The most frequent cause of phytophotodermatitis in the USA is the Persian lime, *Citrus aurantifolia*.[3] The active agent is 5-MOP. Limes contain large amounts of furocoumarins in the exocarp

Food and spice agents commonly inducing photoirritant contact dermatitis		
Furocoumarins		
Therapeutic		
8-methoxypsoralen		
4,5,8-trimethylpsoralen		
5-methoxypsoralen (Bergapten)		
Fragrance materials*		
Plants†		
Rutaceae	*Umbelliferae*	*Moraceae*
Lime	Carrots	Fig
Lemon	Cow parsley	
Bergamot	Wild chevril	*Cruciferae*
Burning bush	Fennel	Mustard
Bitter orange	Dill	
Gas plant	Parsnip	*Ranunculceae*
Common rue	Celery	Buttercup

* Berloque dermatitis; † phytophotodermatitis (not all-inclusive).

Table 45.11 Food and spice agents commonly inducing photoirritant contact dermatitis.[21]

(coloured part of the skin), and handling this and other citrus fruit may lead to phytophotodermatitis in, for example, bartenders. There can be a history of squeezing the juice for use in a drink followed by sun exposure. The eruption appears an average of 48 h later.

Umbelliferae

The Umbelliferae family includes parsnips and celery. The plant most often reported to induce phytophotodermatitis in the workplace is celery. Celery phototoxicity is caused by 5-MOP. It was initially believed that only celery infected with pink-rot fungus (*Sclerotinia sclerotiorum*) was capable of inducing this response. The infection induced increased production of furocoumarins in the celery and therefore led to the reaction.[7,57] Ordinary celery may also induce dermatitis. Reactions have been reported in cannery workers, grocery store cashiers, baggers, produce clerks and chefs.[3] There have been case reports of grocery workers developing a phytophotodermatitis from handling celery followed by intense sunbathing or tanning salon exposure.[15] Parsnips contain 5-MOP and 8-MOP. Wild parsnip is often found in open fields in the midwestern USA, where exposed persons can develop a linear vesiculobullous eruption which later develops hyperpigmentation.[12] Farmers and other outdoor workers are also at risk of developing phytophotodermatitis from exposure to the food products and other plants listed in Table 45.11. Many such reactions will present with linear lesions, as for poison ivy contact dermatitis.

Other plants

Plants other than those containing furocoumarins may also, in rare cases, cause phytophotodermatitis. For example, the condition has been reported in fieldworkers from *Cneoridium dumosum*, a native bush in the chaparral vegetation zone in California and Mexico.[89] Photodermatitis can also be caused by the juice of the rind of the Persian lime *Citrus aurantifolia*, which is widely grown in south Florida and Mexico.[37] Phototoxic reactions often leave areas of hyperpigmentation which are disfiguring and longlasting.

Photopatch testing

Photopatch testing is patch testing with the addition of radiation to induce formation of the photoantigen. Application of antigens and scoring criteria are the same as in conventional patch testing.[64]

Sunscreens, drugs and antibacterial drugs are the most common causes of PACD, but in some centres many plant allergens are also used for photopatch testing (Table 45.12).[3,97] A number of fragrance ingredients have been associated with PACD. The three most common include musk ambrette, 6-methylcoumarin and sandalwood oil. Both musk ambrette and 6-methylcoumarin are synthetic fragrances, and allergy to these is probably not related to spice allergy. Sandalwood oil is a 'woodsy' smelling fragrance ingredient. It is a rarely reported photosensitizer. The Scandinavian photopatch test series contains many plant allergens such as (+)-usnic acid, wood mix (pine, spruce, birch, teak), evernic acid, balsam of Peru and fragrance mix, but very little is known about the association of photoallergy to foods and spices and the above chemicals.[3,22,97]

When an individual develops PICD to a fragrance product it usually appears as a hyperpigmented macule at the site of application of perfume or cologne. This is the so-called 'berloque dermatitis'.[3]

Photopatch test allergens

Plants (13)
  Achillea millefolium
  Alantolactone
  Alpha-methylene-gammabutyrolactone
  Arnica montana
  Chamomilla romana
  Chrysanthemum cimerariafolium
  Diallyl disulphide
  Lichen acid mic
  Parthenolide
  Propolis
  Sesquiterpene lactone mix
  Tanacetum vulgare
  Taraxacum officinale

Sunscreens (8)

Fragrances (3)
  6-Methylcoumarin
  Musk ambrette
  Sandalwood oil

Drugs (4)
Antibacterials (8)
Miscellaneous (2)

Table 45.12 Photopatch test allergens.[21,22] Number of patch test allergens commonly used is given in parentheses.

FOOD ADDITIVES

A great number of food additives (Table 45.13), such as preservatives, antioxidants, emulsifying agents, stabilizers, bleaching agents to improve flour, insecticide sprays on fruits, colours and dyes, and synthetic flavouring agents may cause allergic or irritant skin eruptions.[82] Allergic reactions are rare.

Preservatives

Preservatives have antibacterial and antifungal properties and are found in many foods. The parabens[42] and sorbic acid are the most common causes of contact dermatitis from food preservatives. Parabens (methylparaben and propylparaben) can cause ACD, and can be found in ketchup, canned tomato goods, pickled goods, fruit juices, syrups, jams, milk preparations, soft drinks and packaged meat and fish.[82] Sorbic acid can be found in flour and salad dressings, and can produce both ACD and a CU.[16,27,83] Benzoates may also cause dermatitis.[42]

Antioxidants (Table 45.13)

Oxidation of fruits causes a brownish discolouration, whereas oxidation of fatty foods causes them to become rancid. Antioxidants are used to prevent this process. The most common antioxidants include butylated hydroxytoluene (BHT), butylated hydroxyanisole (BHA), nordihydroguaiaretic acid esters of gallic acid and tocopherols. BHA and BHT are used in oils and fats and can be found in many foods, including beverages, ice cream, candy, baked foods, gelatin, soup bases, potato flakes, glazed fruits, breakfast cereals, dry yeast, shortening and smoked dry sausage.[82] The incidence of ACD is low. Systemic symptoms such as asthma, headache and flushing[30] have been reported after oral administration of small amounts of these substances.

Other allergenic antioxidants

Other allergenic antioxidants include sodium bisulphite which is used as an additive to salads to prevent browning.[24] Sulphites used to maintain the appearance of freshness were challenged several years ago by the Food and Drug Administration (FDA), which proposed they not be allowed on 'fresh' potatoes intended to be sold or served unpackaged and unlabelled at retail food establishments or institutions such as hospitals and nursing homes.[2] These agents (usually sodium or potassium metabisulphite) are known to cause allergic-type reactions, including urticaria, itching, dizziness, nausea, diarrhoea, dyspnoea and, in rare instances, anaphylaxis and death. According to an FDA report,[31] 1 million people in the USA were estimated to be type 1 sulphite-sensitive, most of them asthmatic. Contact delayed-type hypersensitivity to sodium and potassium metabisulphite, although uncommon, has also been reported.[2,31,70,93,95]

There have been several reports of sensitization to gallate esters. Contact allergy to dodecyl (lauryl) gallate (found in margarine)[10] and octyl gallate have been reported in food workers.[20] Propyl gallate allergy to cosmetics and topical preparations has frequently been reported.[32] Tocopherols, or vitamin E, are natural antioxidants used in natural food preparations and in most vegetable oils. ACD has been reported from tocopherols[32] but not in food preparations.

Emulsifying agents[21]

Propylene glycol is a contact allergen which can be found in a wide variety of prepared foods, including salad dressings and

Table 45.13 Food additives.

Food additives	
Additive	**Comment**
Acacia (gum arabic)	Stabilizer
Agar agar	Stabilizer
Ammonium alginate	Stabilizer
Ammonium persulphate	Antioxidant, flour colour improver
Benzoic acid	Preservative
Benzoyl peroxide	Antioxidant, flour colour improver
Butylated hydroxyanisole (BHA), see 2-tert-butyl-4-methoxyphenol (BHA)	Antioxidant, prevents rancidity
Butylated hydroxytoluene (BHT), see 2,6-ditert-butyl-4-cresol (BHT)	Antioxidant, prevents rancidity
Calcium alginate	Stabilizer
Calcium disodium EDTA	Stabilizer, chelating agent
Calcium propionate	Antimould for bread
Carbo bean gum	Stabilizer
Chlorophyll	Colour for pastry
Cholic acid	Emulsifying agent
Chondrus extract	Stabilizer
Citric acid	Preservative
2,6-Ditert-butyl-4-cresol (BHT), see butylated hydroxytoluene	Antioxidant, prevents rancidity
Dodecyl gallate	Antioxidant
Dyes, certified	Colouring agents
Desoxycholic acid	Emulsifying agent
Discetyl tartaric acid esters of monoglycerides and diglycerides	Emulsifying agent
Enzymes	Flour additives
Flavouring agents and spices	Cause contact dermatitis
Ghatti gum	Stabilizer
Glycocholic acid	Emulsifying agent
Guaiac gum	Preservative
Guar gum	Stabilizer
Gum arabic (acacia)	Cream and cheese additive, stabilizer
Gum benzoin	Antioxidant
Karaya gum	Pastry filler, stabilizer
Lauryl gallate	Antioxidant
Lanolin	Chewing gum additive
Monoglycerides and diglycerides	Emulsifying agent
Monoglycerol citrate	Preservative
Nickel	May be added to hydrogenated fats
Nordihydroguaiaretic acids (NDGA)	Antioxidant
Octyl gallate	Antioxidant
Parabens	Preservative
Polysorbate	Preservative
Potassium alginate	Stabilizer
Potassium persulphate	Insecticide sprayed on fruits
Propionic acid	Preservative
Propylene glycol	Emulsifying agent
Propylene glycol alginate	Filler in many salad dressings
Propyl gallate	Antioxidant
Sodium alginate	Stabilizer
Sodium benzoate	Preservative
Sodium bisulphite	Antioxidant
Sodium silicon aluminate	Lump preventer in cake mix
Sorbic acid	Preservative
Sterculla (karaya) gum	Pastry filler, stabilizer
Taurocholic acid	Emulsifying agent
2-tert-butyl-4-methoxyphenol, see butylated hydroxyanisole (BHA)	Antioxidant, prevents rancidity
Tetramethylthiuram disulphide	Insecticide sprayed on bananas
Thiabendazol	Insecticide sprayed on citrus fruits
Tocopherols (see vitamin E)	Antioxidant
Tragacanth	Vegetable gum filler, stabilizer
Vitamin E (see tocopherols)	Antioxidant
Yeast	Flour additive

cake mixes, and which can cause systemic ACD. Fifteen of 38 patients with an allergic skin reaction to propylene glycol developed an exanthem 3–16 h after ingestion of 2–15 ml of propylene glycol.[38]

Stabilizers (Table 45.13)

There is a wide variety of waxes and gums used as stabilizers in foods. Some of these crossreact with balsam of Peru. Karaya, or sterculia gum, is a rare sensitizer that, as a component of meringue, has been reported to cause dermatitis in a baker.[32] In addition, it can be found in hair waving lotions, denture adhesive powders, furniture polishes and a cement for ileostomy appliances.[13]

Bleaching agents and food allergens in the baking industry

Bleaching agents used to whiten flour have caused ACD. Ammonium and potassium persulphate were previously used in Europe as a flour whitener, but have been banned in many countries after reports of sensitization. Ammonium persulphate is also used in hair bleaches to enhance the action of hydrogen peroxide.[28] In the USA, benzoyl peroxide is used in flour as a bleaching agent and has been reported to cause a contact dermatitis in a baker which was exacerbated after application of a benzoyl peroxide acne preparation.[26]

Synthetic flavouring substances

Synthetic flavouring substances (Table 45.14) contain many well known allergens and are putative causes of skin allergy from foods and spices.[82]

Synthetic flavouring substances
Acetaldehyde
Acetoin
Aconitic acid
Anethole
Benzaldehyde
N-Butyric acid
D- or L-Carvone
Cinnamaldehyde
Citral
Decanal
Diacetyl
Ethyl acetate
Ethyl butyrate
Ethyl vanillin
Eugenol
Geraniol
Geranyl acetate
Glycerol tributyrate
Limonene
Linalool
Linalyl acetate
1-Malic acid
Methyl anthranilate
3-Methyl-3-phenyl glycidic acid ethyl ester
Piperanol
Vanillin

Table 45.14 Synthetic flavouring substances.

Enzymes

Enzymes and other flour additives are being increasingly used in bakeries to improve the properties of the baked products and accelerate the baking process. Amylases are starch-cleaving enzymes used worldwide in the baking industry as flour additives (especially alpha amylase, obtained from *Aspergillus oryzae*).[47,69] Other enzymes, such as proteases, are additionally used in the USA and Canada, and cellulase is used in Finland. Lipo-oxygenases are also added to bleach flour.[47] Alpha amylase has long been known to produce skin and respiratory allergic symptoms.[3,47,81] Sandiford and coworkers[85] have shown that beta amylases are also allergenic. Many cases of occupational asthma, rhinitis[3,8,47,81,85,87,91] and dermatitis[69,87,91] caused by alpha amylase in bakers have been reported. These are immunological reactions and specific IgE antibodies have been found in the patients.[5] Baur *et al.*[5] studied 118 bakers, 35 of whom had bronchial asthma, rhinitis and/or conjunctivitis after contact with flour. Morren *et al.*[69] studied 32 bakers with hand dermatitis; seven had a positive immediate reaction to alpha amylase with the scratch chamber test and two also had a positive delayed reaction. Quirce *et al.*[81] reported five bakers sensitized to alpha amylase, four of whom were also sensitive to cellulase. In a Finnish study, 12 workers in four bakeries, three in one flour mill and four in a bread factory were skin prick-positive to both alpha amylase and cellulase.[91]

TREATMENT AND PREVENTION

Identification and avoidance of the causative allergen is critical. General principles to treat contact dermatitis should be used.[44] However, some studies have shown that, despite detection of the allergen and removal of the causative agent from the environment, not all patients will clear.[17] This may be caused by the multifactorial origins of many eruptions, which can include components of irritant and allergic reactions, endogenous eczema and unknown factors.

KEY FACTS

Skin and mucosal side effects from contact with foods and spices are characterized by several important features:

1. Irritant contact dermatitis (ICD) is the most common diagnosis in individuals exposed occupationally.
2. The diagnosis of ICD can only be made if extensive skin testing has been performed to exclude type I and type IV allergy.
3. The occupations most commonly affected from contact to foods and spices are chefs, caterers, farmers, food handlers and food preparers.
4. Allergic contact dermatitis (ACD) can only be diagnosed after patch testing.
5. ACD is mostly caused by low molecular weight chemicals (LMWC) present in foods and spices. Exceptionally, proteins in foods and spices can cause ACD.
6. The LMWCs may be endogenous components of foods and spices or may be added to improve the quality of foods and spices.
7. The clue to ACD from foods and spices may come from allergic patch test reactions to agents such as balsam of Peru, colophony, fragrances, etc. These agents may contain

the same chemicals as foods and spices, or the chemicals in foods and spices may crossreact with the above agents.

8. Patch testing with plant extracts and pure plant allergens may reveal food and spice allergy.

9. Contact urticaria (CU) occurs immediately after contact with food and generally resolves within 24 h. CU can be immunological or non-immunological. Allergic CU is an IgE-mediated reaction and is not detected by patch testing.

10. The symptoms of CU can be classified according to morphology and severity. The mildest form is the 'invisible' CU, when only subjective symptoms such as itching, tingling or burning without any objective change or just a mild erythema occur. Wheal and flare at the contact area is the prototype of CU, while generalized urticaria, rhinoconjunctivitis, asthmatic attack, anaphylaxis and orolaryngeal or gastrointestinal dysfunctions are less common.

11. In some cases protein food additives such as enzymes can be the cause of allergy.

12. Protein contact dermatitis (PCD) is clinically often identical to ACD but, on skin testing, only type I allergy is present.

13. Photodermatitis caused by foods and spices is in most cases caused by phototoxic reactions, but may also be photoallergic. The diagnosis of photoallergic reactions requires photopatch testing.

REFERENCES

1 Adams RM. Dermatitis in food service workers. *Allergy Proc* 1990; 11: 123–4.

2 Adams RM. *Occupational Skin Disease*, 3rd ed, WB Saunders Co, Philadelphia, 1999: 792 pp.

3 Ale SI, Maibach HI. Occupational contact urticaria. In: *Handbook of Occupational Dermatology*, (Kanerva L, Elsner P, Wahlberg JE, Maibach HI, eds), Springer-Verlag, Berlin, Heidelberg, New York, 2000; 200–16.

4 Amin S, Lahti A, Maibach HI. *Contact Urticaria Syndrome*. CRC Press LLC, Boca Raton, New York, 1997.

5 Baur X, Fruhmann G, Haug B, Rasche B, Reiher W, Weiss W. Role of *Aspergillus* amylase in baker's asthma. *Lancet* 1986; i, 43.

6 Bieber T. IgE-Rezeptoren auf Langerhans-Zellen. *Hautarzt* 1992; 43: 753–62.

7 Birmingham DJ, Key MM, Tubich GE, Perone VB. Phototoxic bullae among celery harvesters. *Arch Dermatol* 1961; 83: 73–87.

8 Blanco Carmona JG, Picon SJ, Sotillos MG. Occupational asthma in bakeries caused by sensitivity to α-amylase. *Allergy* 1991; 46: 274–6.

9 Bruce RS. Potato sensitivity, an occupational allergy in housewives. *Acta Allergol* 1986; 21: 507.

10 Brun R. Eczema de contact à un antioxidant de la margarine (gallate) et changement de metier. *Dermatologica* 1970; 40: 390–4.

11 Bruijnzeel-Koomen CAFM, van Wichen DF, Toonstra J. The presence of IgE molecules on epidermal Langerhans cells in patients with atopic dermatitis. *Arch Dermatol Res* 1986; 278: 199–205.

12 Camarasa JF. Foods. In: *Practical Contact Dermatitis, A Handbook for the Practitioner* (Guin J, ed.); McGraw-Hill, New York, NY, 1995: 519–37.

13 Camarasa JMB, Alomar A. Contact dermatitis from a karaya seal ring. *Contact Dermatitis* 1980; 6: 139–40.

14 Carmichael AJ, Foulds IS, Tan CY. Allergic contact dermatitis from potato flesh. *Contact Dermatitis* 1989; 20: 64–5.

15 Chan EF, Mowad C. Contact dermatitis to foods and spices. *Am J Contact Dermatitis* 1998; 9: 71–9.

16 Clemmensen O, Hjorth N. Perioral contact urticaria from sorbic acid and benzoic acid in salad dressings. *Contact Dermatitis* 1982; 8: 1–6.

17 Cronin E. Dermatitis of the hands in caterers. *Contact Dermatitis* 1987; 17: 265–9.

18 Dannaker CJ, White IR. Cutaneous allergy to mustard in salad maker. *Contact Dermatitis* 1987; 6: 212–4.

19 de Groot AC. *Patch Testing*. Elsevier, Amsterdam, 1994.

20 De Groot AC, Gerkens F. Occupational airborne contact dermatitis from octyl gallate. *Contact Dermatitis* 1990; 23: 184–205.

21 DeLeo V. Occupational phototoxicity and photoallergy. In: *Handbook of Occupational Dermatology*, (Kanerva L, Elsner P, Wahlberg JE, Maibach HI, eds), Springer–Verlag, Berlin, Heidelberg, New York, 2000; 314–24.

22 DeLeo V, Gonzalez E, Kim J, Lim H. Phototesting and photopatch testing: when to do it and when not to do it. *Am J Contact Dermatitis* 2000; 11: 57–61.

23 Dooms-Goossens A, Dubelloy R, Degreef H. Contact and systemic contact-type dermatitis to spices. *Dermatol Clin* 1990; 8: 89–93.

24 Epstein E. Sodium bisulfite. *Contact Dermatitis Newsletter* 1970; 7: 115–16.

25 Fisher AA. Contact dermatitis due to cinnamon and cinnamic aldehyde. *Cutis* 1975; 16: 383–8.

26 Fisher AA. Dermatitis of the hands from food additives. *Cutis* 1982; 30: 304–18.

27 Fisher AA. Hand dermatitis – a baker's dozen. *Cutis* 1982; 29: 214–21.

28 Fisher AA, Dooms-Goossens A. Persulphate hair bleach reactions. *Arch Dermatol* 1976; 112: 1407–9.

29 Fisher AA, Mitchell JC. Toxicodendron plants and spices. In: *Fisher's Contact Dermatitis*. (Rietschel RL, Fowler JF, eds), Williams & Wilkins, Baltimore, MD, 1995: 461–523.

30 Fisherman EW, Cohen G. Chemical intolerance to butylated-hydroxyanisole (BHA) and butylated-hydroxytoluene (BHT) and vascular response as an indicator and monitor of drug intolerance. *Ann Allergy* 1973; 31: 126–33.

31 Food and Drug Administration. Sulfiting agents on potatoes. *JAMA* 1988; 259: 794.

32 Foulds I, Sadhra S. Allergic contact dermatitis from carrots. *Contact Dermatitis* 1990; 23: 261.

33 Foussereau J, Benezra CL, Ourisson G. Contact dermatitis from laurel. I. Clinical aspects. *Trans St Johns Hosp Dermatol Soc* 1967; 53: 141–6.

34 Foussereau J, Muller JC, Benezra C. Contact allergy to *Frullania* and *Laurus nobilis:* Cross-sensitization and chemical structure of the allergens. *Contact Dermatitis* 1975; 1: 223–30.

35 Geroso AM, Elpern DJ. Some observations on mango and mohikana from Hawaii. *Contact Dermatitis* 1992; 26: 346–58.

36 Goh CL, Ng SK. Allergic contact dermatitis to *Curcuma longa* (turmeric). *Contact Dermatitis* 1987; 17: 186.

37 Guin JD. Foods. In: *Practical Contact Dermatitis*, McGraw-Hill Inc, New York, 1995.

38 Hannuksela M, Förström L. Reactions to peroral propylene glycol. *Contact Dermatitis* 1978; 4: 41–5.

39 Hausen BM, Wolf C. 1,2,3-Trithiane-5-carboxylic acid, a first contact allergen from *Asparagus officinalis (Liliaceae)*. *Am J Contact Dermatitis* 1996; 7: 41–6.

40 Hausen BM, Andersen KE, Helander I, Gensch KH. Lettuce allergy; sensitising potency of allergens. *Contact Dermatitis* 1986; 15: 246–9.

41 Hjorth N, Roed-Petersen J. Occupational protein contact dermatitis in food handlers. *Contact Dermatitis* 1976; 2: 28–42.

42 Jacobsen DW. Adverse reactions to benzoates and parabens. In: *Food Allergy, Adverse Reactions to Food and Food Additives* (Metcalfe DD, Sampson HA, eds), Blackwell Scientific, Boston, 1991; 276–87.

43 Janssens J, Morren M, Dooms-Goossens A, Degreef H. Protein contact dermatitis: myth or reality. *Br J Dermatol* 1995; 132: 1–6.

44 Kanerva L. Contact dermatitis. In: *European Handbook of Dermatological Treatments* (Katsambas A, Lotti T, eds), Springer–Verlag, Berlin, Heidelberg, New York, Tokyo 1999: 117–26.

45 Kanerva L. Occupational protein contact urticaria and paronychia from natural rubber latex. *J Eur Acad Derm Venereol* 2000; 14(6): 504–6.

46 Kanerva L, Estlander T. Dental nurse's occupational allergic contact dermatitis from eugenol used as a restorative dental material with poly-methylmethacrylate. *Contact Dermatitis* 1998; 38: 339–40.

47 Kanerva L, Vanhanen M. Industrial enzymes. In: *Handbook of Occupational Dermatology*, (Kanerva L, Elsner P, Wahlberg JE, Maibach HI, eds), Springer–Verlag, Berlin, Heidelberg, New York, 2000: 517–23.

48 Kanerva L, Estlander T, Jolanki R. Long-lasting contact urticaria from castor bean. *J Am Acad Dermatol* 1990; 23: 351–5.

49 Kanerva L, Estlander T, Jolanki R. Long-lasting contact urticaria. Type I and type IV allergy from castor bean and a hypothesis of systemic IgE-mediated allergic dermatitis. *Derm Clinics* 1990; 8: 181–8.

50 Kanerva L, Estlander T, Jolanki R. Occupational allergic contact dermatitis from spices. *Contact Dermatitis* 1996; 35: 157–62.

51 Kanerva L, Toikkanen J, Jolanki R, Estlander T. Statistical data on occupational contact urticaria. *Contact Dermatitis* 1996; 35: 229–33.

52 Kanerva L, Pajari-Backas M. IgE-mediated RAST-negative occupational protein contact dermatitis from taxonomically unrelated fish species. *Contact Dermatitis* 1999; 41: 295–6.

53 Kanerva L, Elsner P, Wahlberg JE, Maibach HI. *Handbook of Occupational Dermatology*, Springer–Verlag, Berlin, Heidelberg, New York, 2000: 1300 pp.

54 Kanerva L, Estlander T, Alanko K, Jolanki R. Patch test sensitization to Compositae mix, sesquiterpene–lactone mix, Compositae extracts, laurel leaf, Chlorophorin, Mansonone A and dimethoxydalbergione. *Am J Contact Dermatitis* 2001; 12(1): 18–24.

55 Karlberg A-T, Magnusson K, Nilsson U. Air oxidation of d-limonene (the citrus solvent) creates potent allergens. *Contact Dermatitis* 1992; 26: 332–40.

56 Karlberg A-T, Dooms-Goossens A. Contact allergy to oxidized d-limonene among dermatitis patients. *Contact Dermatitis* 1997; 36: 201–6.

57 Klaber R. Phytophotodermatitis. *Br J Dermatol* 1942; 54: 193–211.

58 Klauder JV, Kimmich JM. Sensitization dermatitis to carrots. *Arch Dermatol* 1956; 74: 149–58.

59 Krook G: Occupational dermatitis from *Latuca sativa* and *Chichorium* (endive): simultaneous occurrence of immediate and delayed allergy as a cause of contact dermatitis. *Contact Dermatitis* 1977; 3: 27–36.

60 Larkö O, Lindstedt G, Lundberg PA, Mobacken H. Biochemical and clinical studies in a case of contact urticaria to potato. *Contact Dermatitis* 1983; 9: 108–14.

61 Lembo G, Balato N, Patruno C, Auricchio L, Ayala F. Allergic contact dermatitis due to garlic (*Allium sativum*). *Contact Dermatitis* 1991; 25: 330–1.

62 Magnusson B, Wilkinson DS. Cinnamic aldehyde in toothpaste. *Contact Dermatitis* 1975; 1: 70–6.

63 Malten KE. Four bakers showing positive patch tests to a number of fragrance materials, which can also be used as flavors. *Acta Derm Venereol* 1979; Suppl. 59: 117–21.

64 Marks JG, DeLeo VA. *Contact and Occupational Dermatology*, Mosby–Yearbook Inc, Philadelphia PA, 1996.

65 McFadden JP, White IR, Rycroft RJ. Allergic contact dermatitis from garlic. *Contact Dermatitis* 1992; 27: 333–4.

66 Meding B. Skin symptoms among workers in a spice factory. *Contact Dermatitis* 1993; 29: 202–5.

67 Miell J, Papouchado M, Marshall AJ. Anaphylactic reaction after eating a mango. *BMJ* 1988; 297: 1639–40.

68 Mobacken H, Fregert S. Allergic contact dermatitis from cardamom. *Contact Dermatitis* 1975; 1: 175–6.

69 Morren MA, Janssen V, Dooms-Goossens A *et al*. Alfa-amylase, a flour additive: an important cause of protein contact dermatitis in bakers. *J Am Acad Dermatol* 1993; 29: 723–8.

70 Nater JP. Allergic contact dermatitis due to potassium metabisulfite in developers. *Dermatologica* 1968; 136: 477–8.

71 Nethercott JR, Pilger C, O'Blenis L, Roy AM. Contact dermatitis due to cinnamic aldehyde induced in a deodorant manufacturing process. *Contact Dermatitis* 1983; 9: 241–2.

72 Niinimäki A. Delayed-type allergy to spices. *Contact Dermatitis* 1984; 11: 34–40.

73 Niinimäki A. Spices. In: *Handbook of Occupational Dermatology*, (Kanerva L, Elsner P, Wahlberg JE, Maibach HI eds), Springer–Verlag, Berlin, Heidelberg, New York 2000; 767–70.

74 Niinimäki A, Hannuksela M. Immediate skin test reactions to spices. *Allergy* 1981; 36: 487–93.

75 Niinimäki A, Hannuksela M, Mäkinen-Kiljunen S. Skin prick tests and *in vitro* immunoassays with native spices and spice extracts. *Ann Allergy* 1995; 74: 280–6.

76 Oliwiecki S, Beck MH, Hausen BM. Compositae dermatitis aggravated by eating lettuce. *Contact Dermatitis* 1991; 24: 318–19.

77 Papageorgiou C, Corbet JP, Menezes-Brandao F, Pecegueiro M, Benezra C. Allergic contact dermatitis to garlic (*Allium sativum* L). Identification of the allergens: the role of mono-, di-, and trisulfides present in garlic. A comparative study in man and animal (guinea-pig). *Arch Dermatol Res* 1983; 275: 229–34.

78 Pathak MA. Phytophotodermatitis. *Clin Dermatol* 1986; 4: 102–21.

79 Peck SM, Spolyar LW, Mason HS. Dermatitis from carrots. *Arch Dermatol Syphil* 1944; 49: 266–9.

80 Polunin I. Pineapple dermatoses. *Br J Dermatol* 1951; 63: 441–55.

81 Quirce S, Cuevas M, Diez-Gomez M *et al*. Respiratory allergy to *Aspergillus*-derived enzymes in bakers' asthma. *J Allergy Clin Immunol* 1992; 90: 970–8.

82 Rietschel RL, Fowler JF. *Fisher's Contact Dermatitis*. Williams & Wilkins, Baltimore, MD, 1995.

83 Roed-Petersen J, Hjorth N. Contact dermatitis from antioxidants. Hidden sensitizers in topical medications and foods. *Br J Dermatol* 1976; 94: 233–41.

84 Sánchez MC, Hernández M, Morena V *et al*. Immunologic contact urticaria caused by asparagus. *Contact Dermatitis* 1997; 37: 181–2.

85 Sandiford CP, Tee RD, Taylor AJ. The role of cereal and fungal amylases in cereal flour hypersensitivity. *Clin Exp Allergy* 1994; 24: 549–57.

86 Stäger J, Wüthrich B, Johansson SGO. Spice allergy in celery-sensitive patients. *Allergy* 1991; 46: 475–8.

87 Tarvainen K, Kanerva L, Grenquist-Nordén B, Estlander T. Berufsallergien durch Cellulase, Xylanase und Alpha-Amylase (Occupational allergy from cellulase, xylanase and alpha-amylase). *Z Hautkr* 1991; 66: 964–7.

88 Tosti A, Guerra L, Morelli R, Bardazzi F, Fanti PA. Role of foods in the pathogenesis of chronic paronychia. *J Am Acad Dermatol* 1992; 27: 706–10.

89 Tunget CL, Turchen SG, Manoguerra AS, Clark RF, Pudoff DE. Sunlight and the plant: a toxic combination: severe phytophotodermatitis from *Cneoridium dumosum*. *Cutis* 1994; 54: 400–2.

90 van den Akker ThW, Roesyanto-Mahadi ID, van Toorenenbergen AW, van Joost Th. Contact allergy to spices. *Contact Dermatitis* 1990; 22: 267–72.

91 Vanhanen M, Tuomi T, Hokkanen H *et al*. Enzyme exposure and enzyme sensitization in the baking industry. *Occup Environ Med* 1996; 53: 670–6.

92 van Toorenenbergen AW, Huijskes-Heins MIE, Leijnse B, Dieges PH. Immunoblot analysis of IgE-binding antigens in spices. *Int Arch Allergy Appl Immunol* 1988; 86: 117–20.

93 Vena GA, Foti C, Angelini G. Sulfite contact allergy. *Contact Dermatitis* 1994; 31: 172–5.

94 Veraldi S, Schianchi-Veraldi R. Contact urticaria from kiwi fruit. *Contact Dermatitis* 1990; 22: 224.

95 Vestergaard L, Andersen KE. Allergic contact dermatitis from sodium metabisulfite in topical preparation. *Am J Contact Dermatitis* 1995; 6: 174–5.

96 Vickers HR. The carrot as a cause of dermatitis. *Br J Dermatol* 1941; 53: 52–7.

97 Wrangsjö K, Ros AM. Compositae allergy. *Semin Dermatol* 1996; 15: 87–94.

98 Wüthrich B. Food-induced cutaneous adverse reactions. *Allergy* 1998; 53 (Suppl. 46): 131–5.

99 Wüthrich B, Dietschi R. Das 'Sellerie-Karotten-Beifuss-Gewürz-Syndrom': Hauttest- und RAST-Ergebnisse. *Schweiz Med Wochenschr* 1985; 115: 358–64.

100 Wüthrich B, Hofer T. Nahrungsmittelallergie: das 'Sellerie-Beifuss-Gewurz-Syndrom'. Assoziation mit einer Mangofrucht-Allergie? *Dtsch Med Wochenschr* 1984; 109: 981–6.

Dermatitis herpetiformis

Jonathan Leonard and Lionel Fry

INTRODUCTION

Dermatitis herpetiformis (DH) is a specific disease entity. Although the clinical and histological features of the rash are not diagnostic, the demonstration by immunofluorescence of immunoglobulin (Ig)A deposits in the papillary dermis of un-involved skin leaves little doubt over the diagnosis. Patients with DH have an associated gluten-sensitive enteropathy, and over-whelming evidence has been presented during the past 30 years that gluten, a protein found in many cereals, is causally related to the development of both the rash and the enteropathy of DH in genetically predisposed individuals. Over 90% of patients with DH have the histocompatibility antigens HLA B8, DR3 and DQ2. The exact mechanisms by which gluten causes the lesions are not clear though there is evidence of disordered immunity. This chapter will present a background to the disease and review the evidence that gluten is responsible for the rash. It will also discuss the mechanisms that have been proposed to explain the patho-genesis of the rash.

BACKGROUND

Clinical features of dermatitis herpetiformis

DH is a rare disease. Precise estimates as to its prevalence are not possible, but it appears to be about 20% as common as coeliac disease – its aetiological counterpart. Gawkrodger et al.[43] esti-mated the incidence of DH in the Lothian region of Scotland as 11 per 100 000, but there is wide variation in different regions of the UK.

DH may present at any time from weaning to old age, but onset before the age of 10 years is rare. The usual age of onset is in early adult life with a peak in the mid-thirties. Men are affected about twice as often as women. The incidence of spontaneous remission is low,[33,43] between 5% and 15%. In the majority of patients the illness, once acquired, persists for life.

DH presents clinically as an itchy, blistering rash. The lesions consist of herpetiform clusters of vesicles on an urticarial back-ground. Because the lesions are so itchy, most patients with DH scratch the tops off the vesicles at an early stage. The predominant

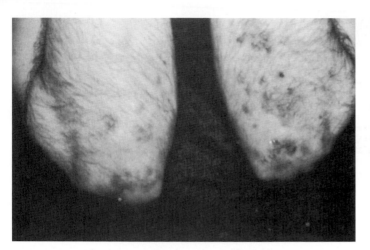

Fig. 46.1 Vesicles and excoriated papules distributed symmetrically over the extensor aspects of the elbows and forearms.

morphological feature, therefore, is of excoriated papules on an urticarial base (Fig. 46.1). The characteristic sites are the elbows, knees and buttocks, though the lesions may occur anywhere on the skin.

Histology of the lesions

The site of vesicle formation is subepidermal. There is an intense polymorphonuclear infiltrate in the mature lesion, with a variable amount of eosinophilia. Collections of polymorphs in the dermal papillae are the most characteristic feature. These are seen in an early lesion or adjacent to the main blister of a mature lesion and are termed papillary microabscesses (Fig. 46.2). They are not diagnostic of DH, however, and may be found in other subepidermal bullous dermatoses such as pemphigoid.[6]

Response to drug therapy

The response of the rash to therapy with sulphones (e.g. dapsone) and some sulfonamides (e.g. sulfapyridine and sulfamethoxypyridazine) is impressive. Itching subsides within 24 h of starting therapy and new lesions stop appearing after 48 h. Cessation of therapy leads to rapid recurrence of the rash. For many years the therapeutic response of the rash to these drugs was considered to be diagnostic for DH. Since the early 1970s, however, the demonstration of IgA deposits in the uninvolved skin has become the diagnostic criterion for DH.

Dapsone

Dapsone is of help in a variety of skin diseases that are characterized histologically by a polymorphonuclear infiltrate. Evidence has been presented that dapsone acts by inhibition of polymorph migration towards chemotactic agents released into the skin by complement activation.[58] Alternative explanations for its action include inhibition of polymorphonuclear myeloperoxidase activity, suppression of complement activity and suppression of the Arthus reaction.[86,110,114]

Side effects of dapsone

The use of dapsone is limited by its side effects. It is a powerful oxidizing agent. In therapeutic dosages of about 100 mg daily it causes a chemical haemolysis. This may be severe in some patients, especially those with glucose-6-phosphate dehydrogen-

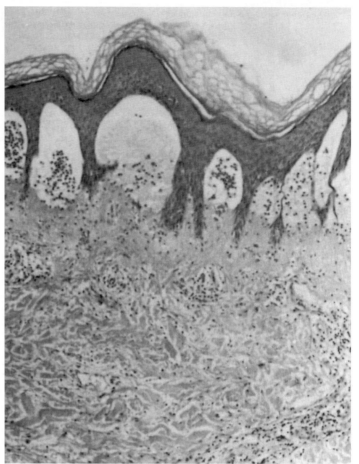

Fig. 46.2 Low power view of the histology of dermatitis herpetiformis showing papillary microabscesses adjacent to the main bulla.

ase deficiency. Elderly atherosclerotic patients tolerate poorly even moderate degrees of haemolysis. Dapsone also has idiosyncratic side effects such as headache and lethargy. The combined effect of all of these unwanted effects leads to withdrawal of dapsone therapy in about 25% of patients in whom it is prescribed.[33,74,83] Substitution with sulfonamides such as sulfapyridine or sulfamethoxypyridazine will usually bring about adequate therapeutic control without causing haemolysis, and many centres now prefer to use these drugs as a first line of therapy.

A significant problem arises when patients with DH are not able to tolerate sulfa drugs at all. There have been reports of successful suppression of the lesions using cyclosporin A and combinations of tetracyclines and nicotinamide.[111,134]

Effects of iodides on the rash

The deleterious effect of iodides on the rash of DH has been known for many years. Oral ingestion of iodides causes a generalized outbreak of the rash, while topical application leads to a local lesion that is histologically indistinguishable from a spontaneous one.[1,52,81] The mechanism by which iodides cause this reaction is not known. It is inhibited by sulfone therapy and cannot be elicited in patients whose rash is controlled by a gluten-free diet (GFD).

IMMUNOGLOBULIN DEPOSITION IN THE SKIN

Immunofluorescence techniques have given dermatologists an invaluable tool for distinguishing between the bullous dermatoses. The first report on immunoglobulins in the skin of patients with DH was by Cormane,[15] who found immunoglobulins in both the involved and uninvolved skin, though no mention was made of their class. In 1969, van der Meer[124] reported IgA deposits in the uninvolved skin in 10 of 12 patients with a previous diagnosis of DH. Van der Meer had shown that DH had an immunological basis and one that was distinct from other bullous dermatoses.

The presence of IgA in the dermal papillae of uninvolved skin in patients with DH is now the major laboratory criterion for diagnosing the disease.

Patterns of immunoglobulin A deposition

Chorzelski et al.[9] were the first to recognize the different sites of IgA deposition in the bullous diseases. They described two patterns of fluorescence, one in the dermal papillae (Fig. 46.3) and the other in a homogeneous line along the dermoepidermal junction (Fig. 46.4). Other groups of workers have confirmed these initial findings[65,71,102] and shown that the papillary pattern is more

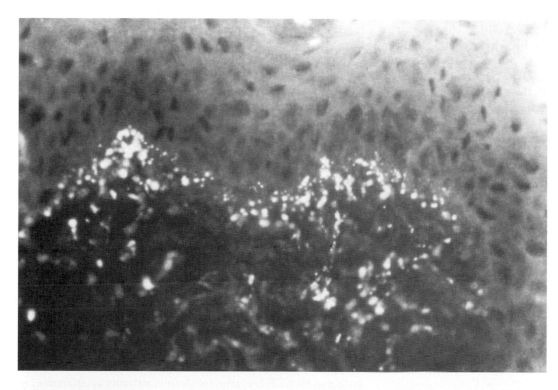

Fig. 46.3 Direct immunofluorescence of uninvolved skin showing the papillary pattern of deposition of IgA in dermatitis herpetiformis (courtesy G.P. Haffenden).

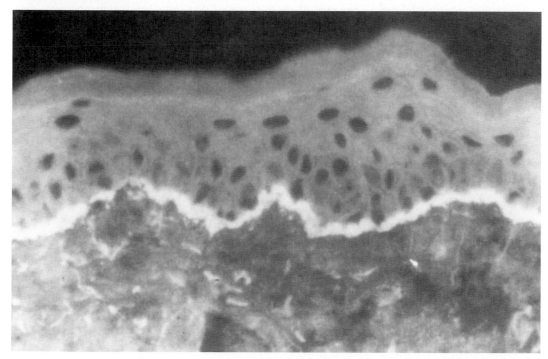

Fig. 46.4 Direct immunofluorescence of uninvolved skin showing the linear pattern of deposition of IgA in linear IgA bullous dermatosis (courtesy G.P. Haffenden).

common, occurring in 80–90% of patients with IgA deposits. The nosological classification of patients with the linear IgA pattern of deposition has caused much argument over recent years. The current view of most workers in the field is that the linear pattern represents a distinct disease entity from DH and it is now termed linear IgA disease.[13,73] The term DH should only refer to those with IgA deposited in the papillary dermis.

Site of attachment of immunoglobulin A in dermatitis herpetiformis

Early studies comparing the pattern of IgA fluorescence with that produced by silver stains suggested that IgA was bound to reticulin in the papillary dermis.[101] More recently, immunoelectron microscopy has shown that it is bound within clumps in the dermal papillae, closely associated either with anchoring fibrils[133] or with the microfibrillar component of elastic dermal microfibrillar bundles.[112] Haffenden and Ring[50] reported that the IgA was localized in large aggregates in the papillary dermis and in small deposits lying in the bundles of collagen fibres.

Diagnostic specificity of papillary immunoglobulin A deposits

IgA deposits in the uninvolved skin of patients with DH have diagnostic value,[10,29,65,77] although IgA has been reported in some patients with coeliac disease.[97] It is likely that these patients had latent DH.

In one study of the clinically normal skin of 22 patients with established coeliac disease, two were found to have immunoglobulins deposited in the skin, one patient having IgM and the other IgA in the papillary dermis.[108] It was apparent on further study of the second patient that she had had an itchy rash on the elbows and knees which had cleared on the GFD given for the coeliac disease. In another group of 16 patients[38] in whom IgA was not found in the skin, but who had a rash clinically consistent with DH (and which responded to dapsone), an alternative diagnosis could be made in 13.

Origin of immunoglobulin A

The association of DH with a gluten-sensitive enteropathy suggests that the IgA is of gut origin. This view was supported by Unsworth et al.,[122] who showed that the IgA in the skin of patients with DH contained J chain and was able to bind secretory component in vitro. The IgA was therefore predominantly dimeric and probably of mucosal origin. However, Hall and his colleagues,[54] using monoclonal antibodies against IgA1 and IgA2, found that all 22 patients tested had IgA1 whereas none had IgA2 and came to the opposite conclusion about the origin of the IgA deposits.

Efforts to elute the IgA from the skin and allow its characterization have been unsuccessful.[20–22,63] Although claims have been made of identification of IgA-like material, the extraction process has denatured the IgA in the eluate. Clearly these techniques need to be refined to allow isolation and characterization of the IgA.

Other classes of immunoglobulins in the skin of patients with dermatitis herpetiformis

By definition, all patients with DH have IgA deposition, but IgG and IgM are found in addition in about 10% of patients. Chorzelski et al.[9] found IgG in six of 19 patients, with IgM in five. Seah and Fry[102] found IgG in three of 78 biopsies and IgM in

eight. Of the nine patients who had IgG or IgM in addition to IgA, the pattern of immunofluorescence was the same in eight. In the single biopsy in which there was a difference, IgA was present in the homogeneous linear pattern and IgM in the papillary pattern. (This patient would now be classified as having linear IgA bullous dermatosis.)

There appears to be no correlation between the presence of immunoglobulins other than IgA and any clinical or prognostic factor in patients with DH. Repeat biopsies taken over a period of time from any given patient with DH consistently show papillary IgA, but the presence of other immunoglobulin classes is variable. It is possible that these other immunoglobulins represent secondary antibodies following damage to the basement membrane. Alternatively, they may simply represent the deposition of the immune complexes of different classes with different affinity for the various structures of the basement membrane zone.[28]

Complement in the skin

C3 has been found in the uninvolved skin of patients with DH by a number of workers.[31,51,60,94,124] However, IgA is not thought to be able to activate complement by the classical pathway, but aggregated IgA appears capable of activating complement by the alternative pathway.[45] A study of C3 and C1q deposition in relation to immunoglobulin deposition in both the involved and the uninvolved skin in 34 biopsies from 19 patients showed that IgA was present in all these biopsies, IgG in three and IgM in nine.[106] C3 was found in 16 (47%) of the specimens. The highest frequency was found in the subgroup of biopsies taken from an early lesion (eight of nine). However, C3 was also found in the uninvolved skin in three of nine patients whose rash was controlled by diet. C1q was present in only three of the 34 biopsies; in one, IgG was present and in two IgM was also present.

These results suggest that complement fixation in the skin of patients with DH occurs through the alternative rather than the classical pathway and can be attributed to IgA. This view was supported by the work of Provost and Tomasi,[92] who found properdin and Factor B (evidence of alternative pathway activation) in the skin of patients with DH. These studies demonstrate that complement is present in the skin of patients with DH and is likely to play some part in the pathogenesis of the skin lesion. After a GFD in DH,[31] C3 was found in the skin in 12 of 18 patients who were taking a normal diet and requiring dapsone to suppress the rash, but in only three of 19 patients whose rash was controlled by a strict GFD alone.

Immunogenetics of dermatitisis herpetiformis

The suggestion that genetic factors play a role in the pathogenesis of the disease was supported by the finding that DH, in common with coeliac disease,[24,113] is accompanied by a high incidence of certain histocompatibility antigens. Before precise diagnostic techniques became available for DH, reports showed that between 58 and 78% of patients have HLA B8.[44,66] When the presence of papillary IgA in uninvolved skin became the absolute diagnostic criterion for DH, the true incidence[95,105] of HLA B8 rose to over 80%. Pehamberger et al.[89] reported an increased incidence of the Class II histocompatibility antigen HLA DR3 in patients with DH. The incidence of this antigen was found to be in excess of 90%, a finding similar to that previously reported in coeliac disease.[67]

In 1983, Park et al.[88] reported that 93% of patients with DH had the Te24 antigen compared to 26% of normal controls. This antigen was later identified as the Class II antigen HLA DQ2. Sachs and coworkers,[99] in 1986, continued the strong association of DQ2 in patients with DH (DQ2 95% versus 41% in controls). Hall et al.[53] reported the antigenic frequency of a third group of expressed HLA Class II antigens located centromeric to HLA DR and DQ on the short arm of chromosome 6. These are termed HLA DP antigens, but no increased frequency was found when corrected for the linkage disequilibrium of the strong HLA DR3 and DQ2 associations in the disease. Although a strong association has been found between HLA B8, DR3 and DQ2 in both DH and coeliac disease, there are no clear discriminators between the two diseases. Reunala described four pairs of monozygotic twins using skin immunofluorescence to detect DH; two pairs were concordant for DH and the other two had one twin with DH and the other with coeliac disease.[96]

The HLA Class III locus codes for several complement components as well as tumour necrosis factor (TNFα) and is located next to the Class II region. A causative gene could well lie within this region. TNFα is a cytokine with a broad range of post-inflammatory modulating, immunomodulating and catabolic activities. Wilson et al.[130] examined the TNFα genotype in patients with DH and compared the associations with those of the Class II alleles. Although the gene for TNFα is strongly associated with DH this was found to be weaker than the association with Class II loci.

EVIDENCE THAT GLUTEN IS RESPONSIBLE FOR DERMATITIS HERPETIFORMIS

Evidence that gluten was implicated in the pathogenesis of DH was first seen in the late 1960s. Although some of the earlier descriptions of DH mentioned ill health, loss of weight and mental symptoms occurring in patients, these were attributed to the effects of chronic skin irritation which is a major feature of the disease. In 1966 and 1967 there were three reports of a high prevalence of structural changes of the jejunal mucosa in patients with DH.[26,82,126] The changes resembled those of idiopathic steatorrhoea. The finding of abnormalities in small intestinal structure and function, as well as haematological changes in 12 patients with DH, suggested that gluten was the cause of the disease.[32] In addition to the enteropathy, a high incidence of increased faecal fat excretion, reduced serum levels of folate and iron, and low serum IgM levels with evidence of splenic atrophy were also seen. The analogy was made with coeliac disease, where the enteropathy had been clearly shown to be caused by gluten.[98]

Specificity of gluten
Further conclusive evidence of the association between DH and coeliac disease was provided when it was shown that there was an improvement in the small intestinal mucosa, reduction in faecal fat excretion and restoration of normal serum levels of folate and iron with treatment by a GFD. On reintroduction of gluten into the diet, these changes were reversed, demonstrating the specificity of gluten in the pathogenesis of DH.[35,37]

Incidence of enteropathy
The incidence of enteropathy in patients with DH[26,32] was initially thought to be 70%. However, further studies have shown that a gluten-sensitive enteropathy occurs in all patients with DH but to varying degrees. Firstly, multiple biopsies of the small intestine

have shown the enteropathy to be patchy, so that if only one biopsy had been taken it would have been possible to have missed a morphologically abnormal area.[8] When eight biopsies were taken simultaneously from the upper small intestine, the incidence of morphological abnormality rose to 95%. Secondly, Weinstein[128] was able to induce structural changes in a previously normal looking small intestine by giving patients with DH an increased amount of gluten in the diet. This response to gluten loading does not generally occur in normal individuals, but there has been a recent report of its occurrence in relatives of patients with coeliac disease and in normal individuals with HLA B8.[19] Thirdly, it has been shown that, irrespective of the morphological change in the small intestine, a histological abnormality can be demonstrated in the majority of patients with DH.

Histological evidence
The most useful marker is the increased infiltration of the epithelium with lymphocytes, as this can be easily quantified. The intraepithelial lymphocyte count is expressed as the number of lymphocytes per 1000 epithelial cells.[36] There is also an increase in the number of lymphocytes in the lamina propria, but the cells here are more difficult to count reliably. The lymphocytes are presumably attracted to the mucosal surface as part of the immunological response to gluten. Although the number of lymphocytes infiltrating the epithelium is increased in patients with DH, the predominance of CD8+ T cells seen in the normal gut is maintained.[78]

It is possible that there is an increased permeability of the small intestine to large molecules in patients with DH who have a morphologically normal looking small intestine. This was supported by early studies describing techniques using probe molecules such as polyethylene glycol;[62] using a ^{51}Cr-labelled absorption test[5] may help to demonstrate a physiological abnormality in this group. However, Griffiths et al.,[49] in a study of sugar permeability in patients with DH, came to the conclusion that abnormal intestinal permeability is the result of gluten-induced damage to the mucosa rather than an inherent primary defect. It was therefore thought improbable that the rash is purely a manifestation of increased permeation of antigen.

Effect of a gluten-free diet on the rash
It has now been established beyond all reasonable doubt that the skin lesions in DH are associated with gluten sensitivity. Within 2 years of the initial report of structural changes in the small intestine in DH, the beneficial effect of a 6-month gluten-free period on the skin lesions of seven patients was described.[34,35] It was found that two patients were able to stop taking dapsone and another three showed a significant reduction in the dose required to suppress the rash. There was a correlation between the fall in dapsone requirements and the improvement in small intestinal structure, i.e. both skin and intestinal lesions improved on the GFD. The same group of workers showed that the skin lesions of patients who had taken a GFD for 1 year would reappear when gluten was reintroduced to the diet. The dapsone had to be reintroduced or increased in dosage to suppress the rash.

The intestinal abnormalities paralleled the dapsone requirements in that there was a deterioration in the structure and function of the small intestine on reintroduction of the gluten. It was suggested that the skin lesions, as well as the intestinal lesions, were related to gluten and that there was a direct relationship between the two.[35] The fall in dapsone requirement on treatment with a GFD could not simply be attributed to improved intestinal absorption of the drug since some patients were able to stop taking dapsone altogether, yet the rash relapsed on gluten challenge.

Failures on diet

A number of other reports[109,115,129] stated that the rash did not improve with a GFD and that the relationship between the skin and small intestine was indirect. However, it has to be stressed that the diet has to be strict to be successful and must be taken for many months before the rash can be controlled by diet alone.[37] It was evident from reports by Shuster et al.[109] and Weinstein et al.[129] that, in the reported cases of failure, the diet had not been taken for long enough to be effective (only one patient had taken the diet for over 9 months), or that it had not been strict enough (the enteropathy was still present in some patients on repeat biopsy while the patient was allegedly adhering to the diet). Support for the efficacy of a strict GFD in the treatment of DH has now come from many sources.[27,43,57,59,65,77,87,94]

Long-term follow up

The long-term follow up of patients with DH with and without treatment by a GFD has been reviewed.[33,39] A total of 78 patients were included in a study reported by Fry et al.,[33] of whom 42 opted for a GFD while 36 took a normal diet and controlled their rash with drugs alone. Thirty of the 42 patients (71%) taking a GFD were able to discontinue the drugs previously required to control the rash compared with five of the 36 patients (14%) taking a normal diet. The mean (range) time taken to reduce drug requirements for patients taking a GFD was 8 (4–30) months and for stopping the drugs 29 (6–108) months. The incidence of morphological abnormality of the small intestine decreased from 69% to 15%, and there was a significant reduction in the mean intraepithelial lymphocyte count in those patients controlled by diet alone. The improvement in skin and intestinal lesions was related to how strictly the diet was taken. Of the 42 patients who opted for a GFD, 23 were considered by the dietitian to be strictly adhering to the diet; 22 of these patients (96%) were able to stop drug therapy.

Gawkrodger et al.[43] found that 27 of 51 patients (53%) on a strict diet were able to stop taking dapsone, and in 12 others (24%) the drug requirements were reduced by at least half. The remaining 12 patients were not able to reduce their drug dosage, but four of these had been on the diet for less than 12 months. The mean (range) time for cessation of drug therapy in the 27 patients eventually controlled by a GFD alone was 25 (1–91) months, which is similar to the figure of Fry and his colleagues.[33]

Treatment of DH using GFD has been in use at St Mary's Hospital since 1967. Garioch reviewed the first 25 years' experience;[39] 78 patients had been on a strict diet and achieved complete control of the rash by diet alone. Of the 77 patients taking a normal diet, eight entered spontaneous remission, a rate of 10%. The advantages of a GFD in the management of patients with DH were summarized as: first, the need for medication is reduced or abolished; second, there is a resolution of the enteropathy; and, third, patients experience an improved sense of well being. Lewis et al.,[76] in a retrospective multicentre study of 487 patients with DH, showed that lymphoma developed in eight, the expected incidence being 0.21. All lymphomas occurred in patients in whom DH had been controlled without a GFD or in those who had been treated with a GFD for less than 5 years. These results suggested that a GFD has a protective effect against lymphoma in patients with DH, and gives further support for advising patients to adhere to a strict GFD for life.

Central role of gluten

The effects of reintroduction of gluten into the diet provide conclusive evidence for the central role of gluten in the pathogenesis of DH.[72] Twelve patients with DH whose rash had been controlled with a strict GFD alone for an average period of 7.6 years were challenged. The rash returned in 11 of the 12 patients after an average interval of 11.9 weeks from the start of the challenge. Biopsies of the small intestine performed before the challenge and again at reappearance of the rash showed a deterioration of the mucosa in seven of the 11 patients. The patient who failed to relapse on challenge probably represents the 10% of patients with DH who enter spontaneous remission.[33,43]

The question remains as to why all patients with DH do not respond to a GFD. The success rate of the diet depends on how strictly the diet is taken.[33] It should be noted that not all patients with coeliac disease respond to a strict GFD[55] and the same may be true for DH. Interesting data were presented in the early 1980s by van der Meer and his colleagues,[125] who treated patients that could not be managed with either dapsone or a GFD using an elemental diet composed of amino acids, sugars and carbohydrates. All the patients who could tolerate such an elemental diet responded within 2 weeks, with a sharp reduction in dapsone requirement. There has been a report that a milk-free diet in addition to a GFD may be necessary to control the rash in some patients with DH but this remains to be substantiated.[91] However, the most likely reason for failure of a GFD is non-adherence.

Other cereals implicated in a gluten-free diet

Avoidance of wheat, barley and oats has always been advocated in a GFD. Wheat, rye and barley are members of the grass tribe *Triticeae*; oats belong to a different tribe, *Aveneae*. The seed storage proteins of oats differ structurally from those of other species of grass. The toxic proteins of wheat (gliadin), rye (secalin) and barley (hordein) have amino acid sequences that are much richer in prolamine than those of oats (avenins). Also, avenin accounts for only 5–10% of the total proteins found in oats, whereas gliadin accounts for 40% of total protein in wheat.

Hardman et al.[56] reported the absence of toxicity of oats in patients with DH. They studied 10 patients with DH who had been treated with a GFD for an average of 15.8 years, with control of the rash and enteropathy. The patients added oats (average daily intake 62.5 g) to their diet and there was no adverse effect to the skin or gut. They stressed the importance of ensuring that the oats were not contaminated with other cereals, either from residue of crop rotation or during the milling process.

Effect of gluten on the intensity of immunoglobulin A fluorescence

Harrington and Read[57] reported a series of 10 patients with DH treated with a GFD. They found that two patients no longer required dapsone after 6 months on the diet and that IgA was no longer demonstrable in the skin biopsies once the rash had been controlled by diet alone. Others have not been able to demonstrate such a rapid disappearance of the IgA but have found that the intensity of the fluorescence was slowly reduced. It disappeared from the skin in only four of the 23 patients who had been on a strict GFD for a minimum of 7 years.[33] Similarly, Reunala and Salo found that only six of 42 patients on a strict GFD lost the IgA from their skin, and then only after a number of years.[93] Another interesting observation is that IgA can still be demonstrated in the skin of patients who have entered spontaneous remission.[72] Garioch *et al.*[39] reported loss of IgA from the skin of patients with DH in 10 of 41 (24%) taking a strict GFD for a mean (range) of 10 (3–16) years.

Gluten challenge of gluten-free diet-controlled patients

Twelve patients with DH (three of whom had lost their IgA staining), whose rash had been controlled with a strict GFD alone for a number of years, were challenged.[72] After 1 month, IgA deposits were demonstrated in the skin of all three patients who had previously lost their staining. Two of these patients relapsed clinically, although the other has still not relapsed 3 years after challenge commenced. In the other nine patients there was no detectable increase in the intensity of IgA fluorescence at the time of relapse of the rash compared to that before challenge.

MECHANISMS BY WHICH GLUTEN MAY CAUSE RASH

Serum immunoglobulins

Although some changes in the serum levels of immunoglobulins have been reported, they occur only in a minority of patients. A small proportion of patients have raised serum IgA levels.[32] Low serum IgM levels are present in one-third of patients with DH taking a normal diet;[25] this is possibly because of the lymphoreticular dysfunction and splenic atrophy that are known to occur in patients with DH.[90]

Evidence of a type I hypersensitivity reaction

Although an urticarial background to the vesicles is characteristic of DH, and although there is an increased incidence of atopy in patients with DH,[17] no evidence has been submitted that convincingly implicates a type I, IgE-mediated hypersensitivity mechanism in the pathogenesis of the rash. In our experience, neither H_1 nor H_2 antagonists have any influence on the rash. Oral disodium cromoglycate does not influence either the enteropathy or the dapsone requirements of patients with the condition.[30] Furthermore, the 28 months that it takes following gluten withdrawal for the rash to be controlled by diet alone,[33] is too long to readily support a type I hypersensitivity reaction as being responsible.

Circulating antibodies in dermatitis herpetiformis
Autoantibodies

A high incidence of tissue-reactive autoantibodies occurs in the serum of patients with DH.[17,84,103,127] Gastric parietal cell antibodies, thyroid antibodies and antinuclear antibodies are the most common. The incidence of circulating autoantibodies in DH is higher than that found in coeliac disease, which suggests that there may be a more widespread immunological disturbance in DH than in coeliac disease.[103]

Ljunghall *et al.*[79] found that autoantibodies were present in 29 of 43 patients with DH and that 12 of these had more than one

autoantibody. Antinuclear antibodies were the most commonly found in their series. Zone and Cunningham[135] found an increased prevalence of thyroid antibodies in patients with DH. Of 50 patients studied, two were hyperthyroid, five were hypothyroid, three had thyroid nodules requiring thyroidectomy, and five had symptomatic goitres. Microsomal thyroid antibodies were found in 38% of patients with DH compared to 12% of controls matched for age and sex, but not for HLA. The incidence of thyroglobulin antibodies was lower, occurring in 12%. Gawkrodger *et al.*[43] found gastric parietal or thyroid antibodies in 38% of 76 patients with DH; two cases of pernicious anaemia and three of thyroid disease were detected.

Bodvarsson and his colleagues[7] observed that there was a structural similarity between high molecular weight glutenin and elastin, a component of the dermis to which IgA seems to be attached. They postulated that DH may be an autoimmune disease caused by crossreactivity between dietary glutenin and dermal elastin.

Antireticulin antibodies

In 1971 an autoantibody was described in the serum of patients with DH which appeared to be directed against a component of connective tissue.[107] It could be demonstrated by indirect immunofluorescence on a composite block of rat tissues (Fig. 46.5). The staining was not abolished by pretreatment of the sections with collagenases but was absorbed by treatment of the serum with adult human spleen reticulin. The pattern of staining was similar to that obtained with silver[104] and it was concluded that the antibody was directed against reticulin.

Incidence of antireticulin antibodies

The incidence of the antireticulin antibody (ARA) in patients with DH[69,104] is approximately 20%, but it is higher, approximately 40%, in adults with coeliac disease.[2,69,104] The highest incidence of ARA is found in childhood coeliac disease[103,104,107] where it lies between 30% and 70%. It seems that the incidence of ARA is related to the severity of the gluten-sensitive enteropathy, which is most severe in childhood coeliac disease and least severe in DH. In addition, in patients with DH or coeliac disease, the incidence of ARA was related to the severity of the enteropathy on jejunal biopsy.[69] In patients in whom ARA is present in the serum, a GFD results in a gradual fall and eventual disappearance of the antibody.[80,104]

Significance of antireticulin antibodies

The true significance of ARA has yet to be determined. The recent observation by Unsworth *et al.*[117,123] that gliadin binds *in vitro* to reticulin is of interest (Fig. 46.6), particularly in view of the higher incidence of ARA in patients with a severe enteropathy. It is possible that in some way gluten damages the reticulin of patients with a gluten-sensitive enteropathy and renders it immunogenic, leading to the production of the antibody. Although the IgA in the skin of patients with DH is thought to be attached to reticulin, there is little evidence for implicating ARA in the pathogenesis of the rash. Firstly, the incidence of ARA is much higher in patients with coeliac disease and, secondly, the majority of reports show the class of ARA to be IgG rather than IgA. An exception was the report of Ljunghall and her colleagues,[79] who found that 12 of 15 patients with positive sera had ARA of IgA class.

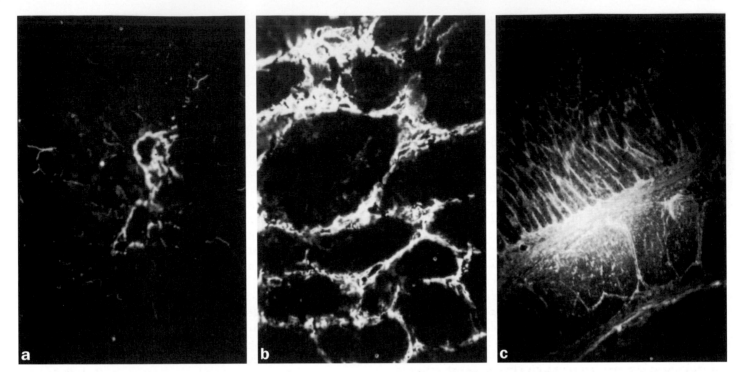

a b c

Fig. 46.5 Indirect immunofluorescence showing RI pattern of antireticulin antibody using a composite block of rat tissue as the substrate: (a) liver; (b) kidney; (c) stomach (courtesy D.J. Unsworth).

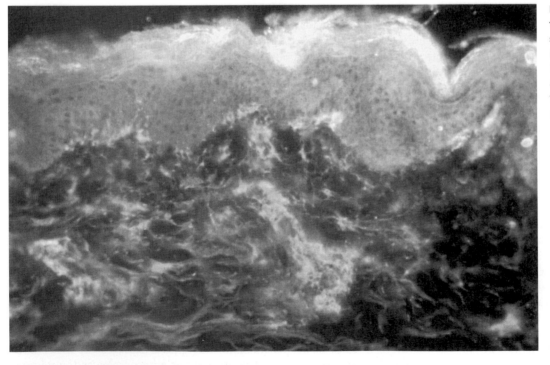

Fig. 46.6 Gliadin binding in vitro to reticulin of normal human skin. The cryostat section was incubated with gliadin prior to indirect immunofluorescence using a rabbit antigliadin antibody and fluorescinated antirabbit antiserum (courtesy D.J. Unsworth).

Antigliadin antibodies

The gluten-sensitive enteropathy associated with DH has given rise to speculation that antibodies against gluten may play a pathogenic role in the condition. Previous studies, however, have shown only 20% of patients with DH to have antigluten antibodies in the serum.[23,61,68,85] In contrast, a newly developed immunofluorescence technique[116,121] and a modification of the ELISA method have allowed the detection of antibodies to gliadin (the alcohol-soluble component of gluten) in the serum of 46% of adults with DH.[119]

The presence of antigliadin antibodies (AGA) correlates well with the severity of the gluten-sensitive enteropathy.

Using similar techniques on the sera of patients with coeliac disease, Unsworth et al.[118] found that all untreated children had AGA, and that the titre of antibody fell on treatment with a GFD. Patients with gluten-sensitive enteropathy, whether caused by coeliac disease or associated with DH, tended to have AGA of the IgG class with or without those of IgA class. Although IgG AGA were more common, Salvilahti et al.[100] have shown that

IgA AGA, when present, are a better indicator of gluten-sensitive enteropathy. The titres fell with time on a GFD, in keeping with the clinical improvement of the patients and the morphological improvement of the gut, whereas IgG AGA persisted for longer.

Diagnostic value of antigliadin antibodies

The value of AGA in screening tests for gluten-sensitive enteropathy associated with DH is limited by an unacceptably high incidence of false-positives (IgG class) and false-negatives (IgA class). IgG AGA are found in other skin and gut diseases that are unrelated to gluten sensitivity.[116] Their presence in these diseases has not yet been satisfactorily explained. IgA AGA are more specific,[116,121] but are not very sensitive as a screening test as not all patients with gluten-sensitive enteropathy proven by biopsy have them. Nevertheless, when present, the fall in the titre of IgA AGA is a useful guide to the response of the enteropathy to a GFD.

AGA have not fulfilled their initial promise. The observations that gliadin bound in vitro to reticulin[117,123] suggested that an immune complex consisting of gliadin and IgA AGA might be produced in the small intestine and circulate to the skin, where it could bind to dermal reticulin through the gliadin. However, the inability to demonstrate gliadin in the skin of patients with DH and the finding that there is a high incidence of AGA in patients with coeliac disease make this suggestion untenable. Similarly, the possibility that AGA crossreact with the reticulin in the papillary dermis of patients with DH but not those with coeliac disease seems unlikely.

Antiendomysial antibodies

In 1983, Chorzelski et al.[11] described an IgA class antibody to a component of smooth muscle. Silver staining showed the antigen to be the reticular component of the endomysium and the term IgA endomysial antibodies was introduced. The best substrate was found to be monkey oesophagus, although recently human umbilical cord has been shown to be as effective. The presence of IgA-EmA is related to the degree of gluten-sensitive enteropathy regardless of the presence of skin lesions.[14]

The overall frequency of positive results in patients with DH was 75 of 104 (72.1%) and in 10 of 10 cases of jejunal mucosal atrophy of grades III and IV. In addition, the levels of IgA-EmA paralleled the response to diet and changes to the antibody levels precede morphological changes of the gut mucosa.[12] The antibody appears to be specific to gluten-sensitive enteropathy since findings were negative in patients with other gut diseases, including inflammatory bowel disease and milk enteropathy.[4] IgA-EmA is the best serological screening test for gluten-sensitive enteropathy.[75]

IgA antibodies to endomysium are a particularly sensitive indicator of gluten-sensitive enteropathy, suggesting that the endomysium contains one or more target autoantigens that play a role in the pathogenesis of the disease. The identification of the endomysial autoantigen has remained elusive. Dieterich et al.[18] recently identified tissue transglutaminase as the unknown endomysial autoantigen. Gliadin is a preferred substrate for this antigen, giving rise to novel antigenic epitopes.

Circulating immune complexes

The regular finding of IgA and C3 in the skin of patients with DH has led to the suggestion that these individuals have circulating immune complexes that give rise to the cutaneous deposition of immune reactants in the skin. Cox and Friedman[16] injected autologous serum intradermally and induced lesions in 18–24 h in 24 of 30 patients with active DH but in none of the controls with bullous pemphigoid, linear IgA disease or inactive DH, suggesting that immune complexes may play a role. Circulating immune complexes have been reported in a variable proportion of patients with DH, ranging from 20 to 30% in the majority of studies.[65,131] Most of the assays used in these studies, however, were only able to detect IgG- and IgM-containing complexes. Zone et al.[136] described an immunofluorescence assay for the detection of immune complexes of IgA class and found them to be present in 30% of their patients.

Role of immune complexes

The role of circulating immune complexes in the pathogenesis of DH is uncertain. A major problem is the lack of satisfactory methods for the detection of IgA-containing immune complexes. The finding of Lane et al.[70] that patients with DH and coeliac disease have gluten in their sera and the knowledge that these groups of patients have AGA indicates that such complexes should exist. Also, the observation by Unsworth et al.[123] that gliadin could bind to reticulin in a lectin-like manner gave credence to a gliadin–IgA complex possibly arising from the gut being involved in the pathogenesis of DH. However, the inability to demonstrate gluten in the skin of patients with DH indicates that such complexes, if they do exist, may not be pathogenic. Zone and his colleagues[137] were able to induce immune complexes in patients with DH by feeding them gluten. Conversely, Yaney et al.[132] demonstrated that gluten challenge does not influence the levels of circulating immune complexes in patients with DH.

A further failing of the current methods for detecting immune complexes is that they do not allow for detailed analysis of the components of the complex. Unsworth et al.[120] applied sucrose density centrifugation techniques to enable both the demonstration and analysis of immune complexes in patients with DH and coeliac disease, but had disappointing results. Although there was evidence for complexes containing AGA, these were present in only 30% of patients and were of the IgG class.

The current situation in DH is that there is no good evidence to implicate the role of immune complexes in the pathogenesis of the disease. It is worthwhile remembering at this stage that the clinical observations argue against DH being an immune complex disorder. It takes an average of 28 months for the skin lesions to clear on a GFD and 3 months for relapse after a gluten challenge.

Evidence for a cell-mediated type IV hypersensitivity reaction

The poor solubility of gliadin in reagents other than alcohol makes the preparation of materials suitable for skin testing containing this antigen impracticable. Garioch et al.[41] gave intradermal injections of Frazer fraction III, the peptic digest of gluten which is known to be antigenic to both patients and controls. Both groups experienced a wheal and flare reaction within a few minutes of injecting the antigen and this persisted for up to 6 h. No skin reactions were present at 48 h in either group. There was no increase in T cells in the skin, suggesting that cells which are sensitive to gluten in patients with gluten-sensitive enteropathy are unable to migrate to the skin.[3,40,41]

Recent studies looking at expression of 11 T cell receptor Vβ families showed overrepresentation of Vβ2, Vβ5.2/5.3 and Vβ5.3 in the skin from 10 patients, suggesting that recognition of an antigen or superantigen is involved in the pathogenesis of DH skin lesions.[42]

The infiltration of polymorphonuclear cells into the upper dermis which characterizes the skin lesions of DH has never been satisfactorily explained. Graeber *et al.*[46,47] showed that lesional skin of patients with DH had increased expression of endothelial leukocyte adhesion molecules in the deep dermis, combined with a markedly increased staining for IL8 in the basal epidermal layer. Dendritic cells were also observed at the dermoepidermal junction of lesional skin and these stained for granulocyte-macrophage colony stimulating factor. These cytokines are all known to promote the activation and infiltration of polymorphonuclear cells suggesting that they may be relevant in the pathogenesis of DH.

CONCLUSIONS

There is overwhelming evidence that gluten is the cause of both the rash and enteropathy of patients with DH. The precise details of the pathogenic pathways have not yet been elucidated, but type 1 hypersensitivity mechanisms have not been shown to be responsible. They are undoubtedly complicated and multifactorial, involving genetic and environmental agents. There is good evidence for disordered immunity in these patients and the presence of IgA in the skin supports an immune basis for the disease.

REFERENCES

1 Alexander JO'D. *Dermatitis herpetiformis*. WB Saunders, London, 1979; 318–21.

2 Alp MH, Wright R. Autoantibodies to reticulin in patients with idiopathic steatorrhoea, coeliac disease and Crohn's disease and their relationship to immunoglobulins an dietary antibodies. *Lancet* 1971; 2(7726): 682–5.

3 Baker BS, Garioch JJ, Bokth S *et al.* Absence of gluten specific T lymphocytes in the skin of patients with dermatitis herpetiformis. *J Autoimmun* 1995; 8: 75–82.

4 Beutner EH, Chorzelski TP, Kumar V *et al.* Sensitivity and specificity of IgA class antiendomysial antibodies for dermatitis herpetiformis and findings relevant to their pathogenic significance. *J Am Acad Dermatol* 1986; 15: 467–73.

5 Bjarnasson I, Peters TJ, Veall N. A persistent defect in intestinal permeability in coeliac disease demonstrated by a Cr-labelled EDTA absorption test. *Lancet* 1983; i: 323–5.

6 Blenkinsopp WK, Fry L, Haffenden GP, Leonard JN. Histology of linear IgA disease, dermatitis herpetiformis and bullous pemphigoid. *Am J Dermatopathol* 1983; 5(6): 547–54.

7 Bodvarsson S, Jonsdottir I, Freydottir J *et al.* Dermatitis herpetiformis – an autoimmune disease due to cross reactivity between dietary glutenin and dermal elastin. *Scand J Immunol* 1993; 38: 546–50.

8 Brow JR, Parker F, Weinstein WE *et al.* The small intestinal mucosa in dermatitis herpetiformis. II. Relationship of the small intestinal lesion to gluten. *Gastroenterology* 1971; 60: 355–61.

9 Chorzelski TP, Beutner EH, Jablonska S *et al.* Immunofluorescence studies in the diagnosis of dermatitis herpetiformis and its differentiation from bullous pemphigoid. *J Invest Dermatol* 1971; 56: 373–80.

10 Chorzelski TP, Jablonska S. Diagnostic significance of the immunofluorescent pattern in dermatitis herpetiformis. *Int J Dermatol* 1975; 14: 429–34.

11 Chorzelski TP, Sulej J, Chorzewska H *et al.* IgA class antiendomysium antibodies in dermatitis herpetiformis and coeliac disease. *Ann NY Acad Sci* 1983; 420: 325–34.

12 Chorzelski TP, Beutner EH, Sulej J *et al.* IgA antiendomysium antibody – a new immunological marker of dermatitis herpetiformis and coeliac disease. *Br J Dermatol* 1984; 111: 395–402.

13 Chorzelski TP, Jablonska S, Beutner EH, Wilson BD. Linear IgA bullous dermatosis. In: *Immunopathology of the Skin*, 3rd edn, (Beutner EH, Chorzelski TP, Kumar V, eds), John Wiley & Sons, New York, 1987; 407–20.

14 Chorzelski TP, Jablonska S, Beutner EH *et al.* Antiendomysial antibodies in dermatitis herpetiformis and coeliac disease. In: *Immunopathology of the Skin*, 3rd edn, (Beutner EH, Chorzelski TP, Kumar V, eds), John Wiley & Sons, New York, 1987; 477–82.

15 Cormane RH. Immunofluorescent studies of the skin in lupus erythematosus and other diseases. *Pathol Eur* 1967; 2: 170–5.

16 Cox NH, Friedman PS. Induction of lesions of dermatitis herpetiformis by autologous serum. *Br J Dermatol* 1991; 124: 69–73.

17 Davies MG, Marks R, Nuki G. Dermatitis herpetiformis – a skin manifestation of a generalised disturbance in immunity. *QJ Med* 1978; 47: 221–48.

18 Dieterich W, Ehris T, Bauer M *et al.* Identification of tissue transglutaminase as the autoantigen of coeliac disease. *Nature Medicine* 1997; 3: 797–802.

19 Doherty M, Barry RE. Gluten induced mucosal changes in subjects without overt small bowel disease. *Lancet* 1981; i: 517–20.

20 Egelrud T, Back O. Dermatitis herpetiformis: preparation of papillary dermis and the effect of proteolytic enzymes on the IgA deposits. *J Invest Dermatol* 1984; 82: 501–5.

21 Egelrud T, Back O. Dermatitis herpetiformis: biochemical preparation of the granular deposits of IgA in papillary dermis. Characterisation of SDS-soluble IgA like material and potentially antigen binding IgA fragments released by pepsin. *J Invest Dermatol* 1985; 84: 239–45.

22 Egelrud T, Back O. Dermatitis herpetiformis; pH optimum for the release of potentially antigen-binding IgA fragments from papillary dermis of uninvolved skin by peptic digestion. *Arch Dermatol Res* 1985; 278: 44–8.

23 Eterman PK, Feltkamp TEW. Antibodies to gluten and reticulin in gastrointestinal disease. *Clin Exp Immunol* 1978; 31: 92–9.

24 Falchuk ZM, Strober W. HLA antigens and adult coeliac disease. *Lancet* 1972; ii: 1310.

25 Fraser NG, Dick HM, Crickson WB. Immunoglobulins in dermatitis herpetiformis and various other skin diseases. *Br J Dermatol* 1969; 71: 89–95.

26 Fraser NG, Murray D, Alexander JO'D. Structure and function of the small intestine in dermatitis herpetiformis. *Br J Dermatol* 1967; 76: 509–18.

27 Frodin T, Gotthard R, Hed J *et al.* Gluten free diet for dermatitis herpetiformis. The long term effect on cutaneous, immunological and jejunal manifestation. *Acta Derm Venereol (Stockh)* 1981; 51: 405–11.

28 Fry L. Dermatitis herpetiformis – basic findings. In: *Immunpathology of the Skin*, 2nd edn, (Beutner EH, Chorzelski TP, Bean SF, eds), John Wiley & Sons, New York, 1979: 283–301.

29 Fry L, Seah PP. Dermatitis herpetiformis. An evaluation of diagnostic criteria. *Br J Dermatol* 1974; 90: 137–46.

30 Fry L, Swain AF, Leonard J, McMinn RMH. Disodium cromoglycate in dermatitis herpetiformis. *Br J Dermatol* 1981; 105: 83–6.

31 Fry L, Haffenden GP, Wojnarowska F *et al.* IgA and C3 component of complement in the uninvolved skin in dermatitis herpetiformis and gluten withdrawal. *Br J Dermatol* 1978; 99: 31–7.

32 Fry L, Kier P, McMinn RMH *et al.* Small intestinal structure and function and haematological changes in dermatitis herpetiformis. *Lancet* 1967; ii: 729–33.

33 Fry L, Leonard JN, Swain AF *et al.* Long term follow up of dermatitis herpetiformis with and without dietary gluten withdrawal. *Br J Dermatol* 1982; 107: 631–41.

34 Fry L, McMinn RMH, Cowan JD et al. Effects of a gluten free diet on dermatological, intestinal and haematological manifestations of dermatitis herpetiformis. Lancet 1968; i: 557–61.

35 Fry L, McMinn RMH, Cowan JD et al. Gluten free diet and reintroduction of gluten in dermatitis herpetiformis. Arch Dermatol 1969; 100: 129–35.

36 Fry L, Seah PP, Harper PG et al. The small intestine in dermatitis herpetiformis. J Clin Pathol 1974; 27: 817–24.

37 Fry L, Seah PP, Riches DJ et al. Clearance of skin lesions in dermatitis herpetiformis after gluten withdrawal. Lancet 1973; i: 288–91.

38 Fry L, Walkden V, Wojnarowska F et al. A comparison of IgA positive and IgA negative dapsone responsive dermatoses. Br J Dermatol 1980; 102: 371–82.

39 Garioch JJ, Lewis HM, Sargent SA et al. 25 years' experience of a gluten free diet in the treatment of dermatitis herpetiformis. Br J Dermatol 1994; 131: 541–5.

40 Garioch JJ, Baker BS, Leonard JN, Fry L. T lymphocytes in lesional skin of patients with dermatitis herpetiformis. Br J Dermatol 1994; 131: 922–6.

41 Garioch JJ, Unsworth DJ, Baker BS et al. Failure of intradermal skin testing with gluten to produce delayed hypersensitivity reactions in patients with dermatitis herpetiformis. Br J Dermatol 1995; 132: 698–702.

42 Garioch JJ, Baker BS, Leonard JN, Fry L. T cell receptor Vβ expression is restricted in dermatitis herpetiformis skin. Acta Dermatol Vener (Stockh) 1997; 77: 184–6.

43 Gawkrodger DJ, Blackwell JN, Gilmour HM et al. Dermatitis herpetiformis: diagnosis, diet and demography. Gut 1984; 25: 151–7.

44 Gebherd RL, Katz SI, Marks JM et al. HLA antigen type and small intestinal disease in dermatitis herpetiformis. Lancet 1973; ii: 760–2.

45 Gotze O, Muller-Eberhard HJ. The C3 activator system – an alternative pathway of complement activation. J Exp Med 1971; (Suppl.) 134(3): 134–905.

46 Graeber M, Baker BS, Garioch JJ et al. The role of cytokines in the generation of the skin lesions in dermatitis herpetiformis. Br J Dermatol 1993; 129: 530–2.

47 Graeber M, Baker BS, Garioch JJ et al. A proposed mechanism for infiltration and localisation of polymorphonuclear cells in dermatitis herpetiformis. Br J Dermatol 1993; 129: 530–2.

48 Griffiths CEM, Barrison IG, Leonard JN et al. Preferential activation of CD4 lymphocytes in the lamina propria of gluten sensitive enteropathy. Clin Exp Immunol 1988; 72: 280–3.

49 Griffiths CEM, Menzies IS, Barrison IG et al. Intestinal permeability in dermatitis herpetiformis. J Invest Dermatol 1988; 91: 147–9.

50 Haffenden GP, Ring NP. Immuno-electron microscopy studies. In: Proceedings of the XVIth International Congress of Dermatology (Kukita A, Seiji M, eds). University of Tokyo Press, 1983: 408–11.

51 Haffenden GP, Wojnarowska F, Fry L. Comparison of immunoglobulin and complement deposition in multiple biopsies from the uninvolved skin in dermatitis herpetiformis. Br J Dermatol 1979; 101: 39–45.

52 Haffenden GP, Blenkinsopp WK, Ring NP et al. The potassium iodide patch test in dermatitis herpetiformis in relation to treatment with a gluten free diet and dapsone. Br J Dermatol 1980; 103: 313–17.

53 Hall RP, Sanders ME, Duquesnoy RJ. Alterations in HLA-DP and HLA-DQ frequency in patients with dermatitis herpetiformis. J Invest Dermatol 1989; 93: 501–5.

54 Hall RP. Dermatitis herpetiformis. J Invest Dermatol 1992; 99: 873–81.

55 Hamilton JD, Chambers RA, Wynn–Williams A. Role of gluten, prednisolone and azathioprine in non-respective coeliac disease. Lancet 1976; 1(7971):1213–16.

56 Hardman CM, Garioch JJ, Leonard JN et al. Absence of toxicity of oats in patients with dermatitis herpetiformis. N Engl J Med 1997; 337: 1884–7.

57 Harrington CI, Read NW. Dermatitis herpetiformis: effect of a gluten free diet on skin and jejunal structure and function. BMJ 1977; 1(6065): 872–5.

58 Harvath L, Yancey KB, Katz SI. Selective inhibition of neutrophil chemotaxis by sulfones. J Invest Dermatol 1983; 80: 321(Abstract).

59 Heading RC, Patterson WD, McClelland DBL et al. Clinical response of dermatitis herpetiformis skin lesions to a gluten free diet. Br J Dermatol 1976; 94: 509–14.

60 Holubar K, Doralt M, Eggerth G. Immunofluorescent patterns in dermatitis herpetiformis. Investigations on skin and intestinal mucosa. Br J Dermatol 1971; 85: 505–10.

61 Huff JC, Weston WL, Zirker DK. Wheat protein antibodies in dermatitis herpetiformis. J Invest Dermatol 1979; 73: 570–4.

62 Jackson PG, Lessoff MH, Baker RWR et al. Intestinal permeability in patients with eczema and food allergy. Lancet 1981; i: 1285–6.

63 Jones P, Kumar V, Beutner EH, Chorzelski TP. A simple method of elution of IgA deposits from the skin of patients with dermatitis herpetiformis. Arch Dermatol Res 1989; 281: 406–10.

64 Katz SL. Dermatitis herpetiformis – the skin and the gut. Ann Intern Med 1980; 93: 857–74.

65 Katz SL, Strober W. The pathogenesis of dermatitis herpetiformis. J Invest Dermatol 1978; 70: 63–75.

66 Katz SL, Falchuk ZM, Dahl MV et al. A genetic link between dermatitis herpetiformis and gluten sensitive enteropathy. J Clin Invest 1972; 51: 2977–80.

67 Keuning JJ, Pena AS, van Leuven A et al. HLA-Dw3 associated with coeliac disease. Lancet 1976; i: 506–7.

68 Kumar P, Ferguson A, Lancaster-Smith M et al. Food antibiotics in patients with dermatitis herpetiformis and adult coeliac disease – relationship to jejunal morphology. Scand J Gastroenterol 1976; 11: 5–10.

69 Lancaster-Smith M, Kumar PJ, Clark ML et al. Antireticulin antibodies in dermatitis herpetiformis and adult coeliac disease. Their relationship to a gluten free diet and jejunal morphology. Br J Dermatol 1975; 92: 37–42.

70 Lane AF, Huff JC, Weston WL. Detection of gluten in human sera by an enzyme linked immunoassay: comparison of dermatitis herpetiformis and coeliac disease patients with normal controls. J Invest Dermatol 1982; 79: 186–8.

71 Leonard JN, Haffenden GP, Ring NP et al. Linear IgA disease in adults. Br J Dermatol 1982; 107: 301–16.

72 Leonard JN, Haffenden GP, Tucker WFG et al. Gluten challenge in dermatitis herpetiformis. N Engl J Med 1983; 308: 816–19.

73 Leonard JN, Griffiths CEM, Powles AV et al. Experience with a gluten free diet in the treatment of linear IgA disease. Acta Dermatol Vener (Stockh) 1987; 67: 145–7.

74 Leonard JN, Fry L. Treatment and management of dermatitis herpetiformis. In: Clinics in Dermatology (Ahmed AR, Jablonska S, eds), 1992; 10: 403–8.

75 Lerner A, Kumar V, Lancer TC. Immunological diagnosis of childhood coeliac disease: comparison between antigliadin, antireticulin and antiendomysial antibodies. Clin Exp Immunol 1994; 95: 78–82.

76 Lewis HM, Reunala TL, Garioch JJ et al. Protective effect of a gluten free diet against development of a lymphoma in dermatitis herpetiformis. Br J Dermatol 1996; 135: 363–7.

77 Ljunghall K, Tjerlund U. Dermatitis herpetiformis – effect of gluten restricted and gluten free diet on dapsone requirement and on IgA and C3 deposits in uninvolved skin. Acta Dermatol Venereol (Stockh) 1983; 63: 129–36.

78 Ljunghall K, Loof L, Forsum U. T lymphocyte subsets in the duodenal epithelium in dermatitis herpetiformis. Acta Dermatol Venereol (Stockh) 1982; 62: 485–9.

79 Ljunghall K, Scheynius A, Forsum U. Circulating reticulin autoantibodies of IgA class in dermatitis herpetiformis. Br J Dermatol 1979; 100: 173–6.

80 Ljunghall K, Scheynius A, Jonsson I et al. Gluten free diet in patients with dermatitis herpetiformis. Effect on the occurrence of antibodies to reticulin and gluten. Arch Dermatol 1983: 119: 970–4.

81 Marks JM. Dogma and dermatitis herpetiformis. Clin Exp Dermatol 1977; 2: 189–207.

82 Marks JM, Shuster S, Watson AJ. Small bowel changes in dermatitis herpetiformis. Lancet 1966; ii: 1280–2.

83 McFadden JP, Leonard JN, Powles AV et al. Sulphamethoxypyridazine for dermatitis herpetiformis, linear IgA disease and cicatricial pemphigoid. Br J Dermatol 1989; 121: 759–62.

84 McFadden JP, Leonard JN, Powles AV, Fry L. Autoimmunity in dermatitis herpetiformis: effect of a gluten free diet. J Dermatol Treat 1991; 2: 87–90.

85 Menzell EJ, Pehamberger H, Holubar K. Demonstration of antibodies to wheat gliadin in dermatitis herpetiformis using ^{14}C-radioimmune assay. *Clin Immunol Immunopathol* 1978; 10: 193–201.

86 Millikan LE, Conway FR. Effect of drugs on Pillemer pathway – dapsone. *J Invest Dermatol* 1974; 62: 541(Abstract).

87 Marks R, Whittle MW. Results of treatment of dermatitis herpetiformis with a gluten free diet after one year. *BMJ* 1969; ii: 772–5.

88 Park MS, Terasaki PI, Razzaque Ahmed A. The 90% incidence of HLA antigen (Te24) in dermatitis herpetiformis. *Tissue Antigens* 1983; 22: 263–6.

89 Pehamberger H, Holubar K, Mayr WR. HLA-antigens in dermatitis herpetiformis. *Br J Dermatol* 1981; 104: 321–4.

90 Petit JE, Hoffbrand AV, Seah PP et al. Splenic atrophy in dermatitis herpetiformis. *BMJ* 1972; 28: 438–41.

91 Pock-Steen OC, Niorsson AM. Milk sensitivity in dermatitis herpetiformis. *Br J Dermatol* 1970; 83: 614–19.

92 Provost TT, Tomasi TB. Evidence for activation of complement via the alternate pathway in skin disease. II. Dermatitis herpetiformis. *Clin Immunol Immunopathol* 1974; 3: 178–86.

93 Reunala T, Salo OP. Effects of long term gluten free diet in dermatitis herpetiformis. In: *Proceedings of the XVIth International Congress of Dermatology* (Kukita A, Seiji M, eds), University of Tokyo Press, 1983: 411–13.

94 Reunala T, Blomquist K, Tarpilla S et al. Gluten free diet in dermatitis herpetiformis. *Br J Dermatol* 1977; 97: 473–80.

95 Reunala T, Salo OP, Tillikainen A et al. Histocompatibility antigens and dermatitis herpetiformis with special reference to jejunal abnormalities and acetylator phenotype. *Br J Dermatol* 1976; 94: 139–43.

96 Reunala T. Incidence of familial dermatitis herpetiformis. *Br J Dermatol* 1996; 134: 394–8.

97 Ross IN, Thompson RA, Montgommery RD et al. Immunoglobulin staining in the skin of patients with gastrointestinal disease. Specificity and significance of IgA deposition in dermatitis herpetiformis. In: *Perspectives in Coeliac Disease* (McNicholl B, McCarthy CF, Fottrell PF, eds), MTP Press, Lancaster, 1978: 217.

98 Rubin CE, Brandborg LL, Flick AL et al. Studies of coeliac sprue. 111. The effects of repeated wheat instillation into proximal jejunum of patients on a gluten free diet. *Gastroenterology* 1962; 43: 621–41.

99 Sachs JA, Awad J, Navarette C et al. Different HLA associated gene combinations code for susceptibility to coeliac disease and dermatitis herpetiformis. *Gut* 1986; 27: 512–15.

100 Salvilahti E, Vilander M, Perkkio M et al. IgA antigliadin antibodies – a marker of mucosal damage in childhood coeliac disease. *Lancet* 1983; i: 320–2.

101 Seah PP. *Immunological studies in dermatitis herpetiformis*. University of London, Doctoral thesis, 1975.

102 Seah PP, Fry L. Immunoglobulins in the skin in dermatitis herpetiformis and their relevance in diagnosis. *Br J Dermatol* 1975; i: 834–6.

103 Seah PP, Fry L, Hoffbrand AV et al. Tissue antibodies in dermatitis herpetiformis and adult coeliac disease. *Lancet* 1971; 1(7704): 834–6.

104 Seah PP, Fry L, Holborow EJ et al. Antireticulin antibody: incidence and diagnostic significance. *Gut* 1973; 14: 311–15.

105 Seah PP, Fry L, Kearney JW et al. A comparison of histocompatibility antigens in dermatitis herpetiformis and coeliac disease. *Br J Dermatol* 1976; 94: 131–8.

106 Seah PP, Fry L, Mazaheri MR et al. Alternate pathway complement fixation by IgA in the skin in dermatitis herpetiformis. *Lancet* 1973; ii: 175–7.

107 Seah PP, Fry L, Rossiter MA et al. Antireticulin antibodies in childhood coeliac disease. *Lancet* 1971; ii: 681–2.

108 Seah PP, Fry L, Stewart JS et al. Immunoglobulins in the skin in dermatitis herpetiformis and coeliac disease. *Lancet* 1972; i: 611–14.

109 Shuster S, Watson A, Marks JM. Coeliac syndrome in dermatitis herpetiformis. *Lancet* 1968; i: 1101–6.

110 Stendahl O, Molin L, Dahlgreen C et al. The inhibition of polymorphonuclear leucocyte cytoxicity in the treatment of dermatitis herpetiformis. *J Clin Invest* 1978; 62: 214–20.

111 Stenveld H, Starink TM, van Joost T, Stoof TJ. Efficacy of cyclosporin in two patients with dermatitis herpetiformis. *J Am Acad Dermatol* 1993; 28: 1014–15.

112 Stingl G, Honigsmann H, Holubar K et al. Ultra structural localisation of immunoglobulins in the skin of patients with dermatitis herpetiformis. *J Invest Dermatol* 1976; 67: 607–12.

113 Stokes PJ, Asquith P, Holmes GKT et al. Histocompatibility antigen associated with adult coeliac disease. *Lancet* 1972; ii: 162–4.

114 Thompson DM, Souhami RL. Suppression of the Arthus reaction in the guinea pig by dapsone. *Proc R Soc Med* 1975; 68: 273(Abstract).

115 Trier JS. Dermatitis herpetiformis and coeliac sprue. *Gastroenterology* 1971; 60: 468–9.

116 Unsworth DJ. *Humoral immunity in gluten sensitive enteropathy*. University of London, Doctoral thesis, 1982.

117 Unsworth DJ, Johnson GD, Haffenden GP et al. Binding of wheat gliadin in vitro to reticulin in normal and dermatitis herpetiformis skin. *J Invest Dermatol* 1981; 76: 88–93.

118 Unsworth DJ, Kieffer M, Holborow EJ et al. IgA antigliadin antibodies in coeliac disease. *Clin Exp Immunol* 1981; 46: 286–93.

119 Unsworth DJ, Kieffer M, Holborow EJ et al. IgA antigliadin antibodies in coeliac disease. *Clin Exp Immunol* 1981; 46: 286–93.

120 Unsworth DJ, McCarthy DA, Leonard JN et al. Circulating immune complexes containing IgG antigliadin antibody in dermatitis herpetiformis detected by sucrose density centrifugation and subsequent serological analysis. In: *Proceedings of the First Immunodermatology Symposium* (MacDonald DM, ed.), Cambridge University Press, Cambridge, 1984: 231–5.

121 Unsworth DJ, Manuel PD, Walker-Smith JA et al. A new immunofluorescent test for gluten sensitivity. *Arch Dis Child* 1981; 56: 864–71.

122 Unsworth DJ, Payne AW, Leonard JN et al. The IgA in dermatitis herpetiformis skin is dimeric. *Lancet* 1982; i: 478–9.

123 Unsworth DJ, Leonard JN, Hobday CM et al. Gliadins bind to reticulin in a lectin-like manner. *Arch Dermatol Res* 1987; 279: 232–5.

124 van der Meer JH. Granular deposits of immunoglobulins in the skin of patients with dermatitis herpetiformis – an immunofluorescent study. *Br J Dermatol* 1969; 81: 493–503.

125 van der Meer JH, Zeedjuk N, Poen H et al. Rapid improvement of dermatitis herpetiformis after elemental diet. *Arch Dermatol* 1981; 271: 455–9.

126 von Tongren JHM, van der Staak WJBM, Schilling PHM. Small bowel changes in dermatitis herpetiformis. *Dermatologica* 1967; 140: 231–4.

127 Weetman AP, Burrin JM, Mackay D et al. The presence of thyroid antibodies in dermatitis herpetiformis. *Br J Dermatol* 1988; 118: 377–83.

128 Weinstein WM. Latent coeliac sprue. *Gastroenterology* 1974; 66: 489–93.

129 Weinstein WM, Brow JR, Parker F et al. The small intestinal mucosa in dermatitis herpetiformis. II. Relationship of the small intestinal lesions to gluten. *Gastroenterology* 1971; 60: 362–9.

130 Wilson AG, Clay FE, Crane AM et al. Comparative genetic association of human leucocyte antigen Class II and tumour necrosis factor-alpha with dermatitis herpetiformis. *J Invest Dermatol* 1995; 104: 856–8.

131 Yancey KB, Lawley TJ. Circulating immune complexes: their immunocytochemistry, biology and detection in selected dermatologic and systemic disease. *J Am Acad Dermatol* 1984; 10: 711–32.

132 Yancey KB, Cason JC, Hall RP et al. Dietary gluten challenge does not influence the levels of circulating immune complexes in patients with dermatitis herpetiformis. *J Invest Dermatol* 1983; 80: 468–71.

133 Yaoita H, Katz SL. Immuno-electro microscopic localisation of IgA in the skin of patients with dermatitis herpetiformis. *J Invest Dermatol* 1976; 67: 502–6.

134 Zemstov A, Neldner KH. Successful treatment of dermatitis herpetiformis with tetracycline and nicotinamide in a patient unable to tolerate dapsone. *J Am Acad Dermatol* 1993; 28: 505–6.

135 Zone JJ, Cunningham MC. An increased prevalence of thyroid abnormalities in dermatitis herpetiformis patients. *J Invest Dermatol* 1983; 80: 363(Abstract).

136 Zone JJ, LaSalle BS, Provost TT. Circulating immune complexes of IgA type in dermatitis herpetiformis. *J Invest Dermatol* 1980; 75: 152–5.

137 Zone JJ, LaSalle BS, Provost TT. Induction of IgA circulating immune complexes after wheat feeding in dermatitis herpetiformis patients. *J Invest Dermatol* 1982; 78: 375–80.

Section D Central Nervous System

Chapter 47

Effects of food allergy on the central nervous system

Iris R. Bell

INTRODUCTION

This chapter will discuss the issues surrounding the effects of adverse food sensitivities, allergies and intolerances on the central nervous system (CNS). Foods, food additives and contaminants can affect central nervous system function in several different ways.[3,4,90,141] These include:

- pharmacological/toxicological effects – e.g. exorphins, xanthines, tyramine, histamine
- immunological processes – e.g. immune complexes
- endogenous mediators – e.g. peptides, other hormones, cytokines, prostaglandins
- metabolic changes – e.g. neurotransmitter precursors; enzyme defects
- neurophysiological effects – e.g. limbic and mesolimbic pathway sensitization
- psychobiological factors – e.g. classical conditioning, expectation/suggestion.

Notably, none of the above possible mechanisms derives directly from an IgE-mediated process. Consequently, although both patients and physicians may refer to CNS effects of foods as 'food allergy', the phenomena may be better termed 'food sensitivities' or 'food intolerances'.[141] It is likely that one or more of the above-listed mechanisms, rather than IgE, plays a primary role in the mediation of symptomatology. This chapter will focus on the neuropsychiatric symptoms that clinicians have reported in their patients[48,68,91] and indicate how certain mechanisms, many of which are discussed at length in other chapters of this volume, might play a role.

HISTORICAL BACKGROUND

Historically, a number of allergists reported anecdotal case observations of neurobehavioural disturbances that they attributed to food and sometimes pollen allergies.[48,68,91] These allergists included Duke,[52] Vaughan & Sullivan,[136] Shannon,[117] Rowe,[113] Randolph,[105,106] Davison[48] and Speer.[126] The most common symptoms of these allergic reactions, which may or may not have had reaginic mechanisms, included the 'tension-fatigue syndrome',[126] involving fatigue, weakness, nervousness and/or irritability. Randolph[108] went on to propose that a large proportion of patients with this type of food allergy also had multiple chemical intolerances or sensitivities (MCS), which, he suggested, could elicit the same polysymptomatic picture. Acute exposures to any of a wide range of foods or structurally unrelated chemicals could set off symptom flares, which would resolve upon avoidance of the inciting agent(s). Symptoms encompassed not only neurobehavioural, but also musculoskeletal, gastrointestinal and other bodily systems. Feingold[58] later popularized the controversial hypothesis that certain food dyes and related dietary constituents could trigger childhood hyperactivity. In terms of neurological conditions, clinical observers have most often reported that specific foods triggered epileptic seizures[1,43,46,49,50,139] or sleep disorders (hypersomnias or insomnias)[6,8–11,73,74,87,129] in individual patients. The lack of objective tests to confirm or disconfirm the diagnosis of food sensitivity/allergy/intolerance of this type has hindered progress in research on the problem.

This chapter will emphasize the possible role of food intolerances in the psychobiology of panic disorder, depression, somatization disorder and addiction, and sleep disorders. Other chapters in this volume address the literatures on migraine, epilepsy and childhood hyperactivity and food allergies/sensitivities/intolerances. Because of the evidence that food and chemical intolerances co-occur in the same individuals and result in similar symptoms,[15,18,20,23,40,51,92,119] the present discussion will address relevant studies on both types of environmental intolerance.

CONTROLLED STUDIES AND PSYCHIATRIC MORBIDITY

Some controlled studies attempted to address the food reaction component of this type of patient, with largely negative findings on laboratory challenge using either capsule challenges[101] or diluted antigen.[72] Despite many weaknesses in the latter studies and the existence of positive findings in studies with other designs,[44,54,77,115,144] mainstream allergists and allergy researchers have recently shown little interest in pursuing the possibility of neurobehavioural effects of foods. Some investigators[40,119,131] found elevated rates of psychiatric comorbidity in patients with multiple food and chemical intolerances and concluded that the psychopathology was a satisfactory explanation that could account for most cases. However, a substantial subset of these cases do not have any psychiatric history, yet they exhibit the same clinical presentation as do patients with psychopathology.[63,120] These data suggest that while psychological distress may contribute to the problem, it cannot be the sole explanation of the reported phenomena.[7,29,62]

Nonetheless, some of the psychiatric findings may provide valuable clues to understanding the pathophysiology of symptoms in some food- and chemical-sensitive patients. Controlled studies on patients with self-reported multiple chemical and food sensitivities have found elevated rates of either premorbid or comorbid psychiatric diagnoses, with depression most common, followed by anxiety disorders of various types, and finally somatization disorder.[24,62] The psychiatric diagnoses that best approximate the clinical picture of the tension-fatigue syndrome are also anxiety disorders such as panic disorder, depression and somatization disorder. Each type of psychiatric disorder has its own literature on phenomenology, epidemiology and psychobiology that raises possible directions for further research.

PANIC DISORDER

For example, among MCS patients with panic-spectrum symptoms, either intravenous lactate infusion[38] (an established panicogen in panic patients, relatives of panic patients and some non-panic patients) or awareness of an acute chemical laboratory exposure[82] will trigger panic symptoms. The effects of foods on panic are untested. Of note, however, the ambient air constituent carbon dioxide[67] and the peptide hormone cholecystokinin-4[42] are two other panicogenic agents in the biological psychiatry literature. Systematic studies indicate not only specificity of responsivity but also physiological hyperreactivity to these substances in panic patients.

Brainstem chemoreceptor specific hypersensitivity to carbon dioxide in panic disorder

Carbon dioxide is a marker for poor indoor air quality[146] at concentrations capable of inducing panic in susceptible patients.[67] Psychiatric researchers have evidence that patients with panic disorder show a specific hypersensitivity to carbon dioxide in

their respiratory system regulation that simple air hunger or voluntary hyperventilation do not fully mimic.[67,98,103] Thus, if a subset of food and chemical intolerant patients meet criteria for panic disorder and can exhibit lactate-induced panic attacks, it is likely that tests will also reveal the capacity of carbon dioxide at low levels to trigger panic attacks more reliably than do various sham procedures in a subset of food/chemical-intolerant patients as well. If so, then it is likely that such patients living or working in buildings with poor indoor air quality and mildly elevated carbon dioxide levels will experience increased CO_2-induced panic symptoms (shortness of breath, anxiety, autonomic disturbances, fatigue) in those settings.

Cholecystokinin in digestion, irritable bowel syndrome and panic disorder

Cholecystokinin (CCK) in particular may be relevant to panic symptoms in patients with food intolerances. Certain food constituents such as lipids and proteins activate digestive CCK release from the gut.[5] Various forms of this peptide act as neurotransmitters in the brain or as digestive hormones in the gut. We have found increased histories of physician-diagnosed irritable bowel syndrome as well as food sensitivities in MCS patients[20] and in community individuals with chemical intolerance[18,23] compared with normals. Other research has shown that patients with irritable bowel syndrome secrete elevated levels of gut CCK in response to a high-fat meal.[121] Thus, the food sensitivity literature may provide an important clue that could link abnormal CCK release in response to foods in some patients to both panic attacks and irritable bowel symptoms.

Apart from excessive CCK release, CCK peptide and/or receptor polymorphisms in the brain and gut may also contribute to vulnerability to conditions such as irritable bowel syndrome or panic disorder. This hypothesis is currently under study in panic disorder.[140] Finding individual differences in CCK receptor responsivity could eventually lead to related studies in food intolerant patients and expand our understanding of possible real-world triggers for the multisystem symptomatology of food- and chemical-sensitive patients.

Exogenous agents and classical conditioning

Thus, although specific causal attribution may or may not be correct in a given patient, chemicals and foods may trigger panic attacks via hyperreactive brainstem chemoreceptor and/or peptide receptor mediation. Testable hypotheses would be that carbon dioxide and foods could elicit panic attacks in a subset of MCS patients using neurophysiological mechanisms mobilized by (a) their direct, biological effects; (b) their indirect, conditioned effects; or (c) both modalities. Demonstration of one modality cannot logically exclude the presence of the other. In fact, conditioning implies the original involvement of direct, biological effects.[26]

That is, classical conditioning is a form of neurophysiological learning which occurs when a biologically active stimulus (unconditioned stimulus [UCS], such as a food) is paired with an initially inactive stimulus (conditioned stimulus [CS], such as a particular physical environment). After sufficient numbers of pairings, the CS takes on the capacity to elicit a response in the absence of the UCS. Researchers have begun to demonstrate that negatively, but not positively, valenced odours can act as CSs in triggering hyperventilation, a hallmark symptom of panic disorder.[134,135] Even so, a CS cannot mobilize these responses without an original UCS. Furthermore, the conditioning in the Van den Bergh et al.[134,135] studies did not generalize from negatively valenced to the positively valenced odours, making it less likely that conditioning could account for the global odour intolerance seen in many persons with severe chemical intolerance (CI). Finally, drugs that block excitatory amino acid neurotransmitters can block classical conditioning.[127] Thus, conditioning is a neurobiological process. The most important methodological question in this area would be determining the experimental parameters that best elicit the unconditioned response and which best elicit the conditioned response: this is not an either-or issue; rather, it is likely that both pathways could lead to the final common outcome of symptomatology in the same individual.

Olfactory-limbic involvement in food/chemical odour hyperreactivity: kindling as a special case of neural sensitization: application of animal models

The panic-disorder link also suggests that certain areas of the brain may contribute to symptoms in food- and chemical-sensitive persons. For instance, a recent animal study demonstrated that strong odours such as peppermint or the solvent toluene can kindle abnormal electrophysiological firing in specific brain structures within the limbic system.[79] That is, repeated olfactory exposures to these ambient substances induce a progressive and persistent lowering of the threshold for firing of neurons in the olfactory-limbic pathways, i.e. 'kindling' the brain.[79] Kindling is a special case of neural sensitization that involves the capacity of certain pathways in the brain to develop long-lasting changes in function, up to the point of tonic–clonic seizures, as a result of repeated, intermittent exposures to an electrical or chemical stimulus with initially no such effects.[112] Certain pesticides can facilitate or initiate kindling and subconvulsive kindling in animals.[66] It is currently unknown whether or not pesticide residues in foods can initiate the same type of dysfunction in vulnerable human populations.

Odours more benign than those of toluene or pesticides can activate abnormal slow-wave activity in the electrophysiology of the human brain. For instance, the odour of sweet orange elicits increased amounts of the electroencephalographic (EEG) delta (slow-wave) activity in panic-disorder patients who report symptoms of limbic dysfunction, i.e. depersonalization or derealization, but not in panic patients without limbic symptoms or in normals.[83] Other panic patients have evidence of subclinical seizure activity on continuous monitoring.[142] These data are potentially highly relevant, in view of Miller and Mitzel's[92] finding of an increased frequency of derealization symptoms in MCS patients, most of whom also report food sensitivities. Limbic structures such as the amygdala are part of the olfactory pathways of the brain and are markedly susceptible to kindling and related neural sensitization procedures.[13]

Kindling is an animal model for temporal lobe epilepsy, a neurological condition that involves discrete attacks of multiple behavioural, psychological, sensory and somatic symptoms.[89] The amygdala also modulates the activity of the dopaminergic mesolimbic pathway via excitatory amino acid neurotransmitter efferents.[75] The mesolimbic pathway, which is itself susceptible to sensitization,[4,123] plays a major role in responses to appetitive (and aversive) stimuli such as foods, alcohol and other drugs.[114] If limbic sensitization is a contributory factor in food and chemical intolerance, at least in those patients with panic-spectrum

symptoms, then the symptoms should overlap those of patients with limbic dysfunction, i.e. temporal lobe epilepsy, and should show other evidence of heightened sensitizability of their limbic and mesolimbic pathways.

Consistent with the limbic hypothesis,[13,24] our laboratory has replicated the finding in persons with self-reported food and chemical sensitivity in terms of increased scores on the 33-item McLean Limbic Symptom Checklist (MLSC).[19,31] The MLSC[130] is a scale assessing the frequency of symptoms usually seen in patients with temporal lobe epilepsy (TLE), the prototypical seizure disorder involving limbic nervous system foci. Moreover, women with TLE[69] and women with MCS[20] both report elevated rates of ovarian cysts. Herzog et al.[69] have pointed out that limbic dysfunction can disrupt hypothalamic regulation of reproductive hormone release and thereby induce a milieu at the ovaries conducive to cyst formation. We[34] have further shown sensitization (a progressive increase from one week to the next) of EEG delta activity to musk odour in community-based individuals with self-reported chemical intolerance, but not in normal controls. As indicated in the Locatelli et al. study,[83] delta activity in the waking EEG reflects, in part, temporal lobe disturbances. Overall, then, the data suggest that limbic dysfunction could underlie some of the neuropsychiatric features of individuals with food/chemical intolerances.

DEPRESSION

One of the simplistic hypotheses in the debate over food allergies and intolerances is that many of these patients have increased levels of depression, which then must account in full for their symptoms. Phenomenologically, depression and food/chemical intolerance do share many symptoms. These overlapping symptoms include low mood, anhedonia, weight changes, insomnia or hypersomnia, psychomotor agitation or retardation, fatigue, indecisiveness and difficulty concentrating. The time patterning of symptoms differs, however. Food-intolerant patients usually report episodic flares of mood changes at various times of day, related in a delayed fashion to meals, whereas a large proportion of depressives note their lowest mood each morning. Although depression is the most common past or current psychiatric diagnosis in persons with food intolerances,[62,63] the psychophysiological data on possible relationships between depression and food/chemical intolerance also do not support the equivalence of the two conditions.

Previous research has shown that depressed patients have a type of lateral asymmetry in the EEG alpha activity of their frontal regions.[2,47] That is, in depression, patients exhibit a greater amount of alpha activity on the left than on the right frontal side. The presumptive reason is the differential roles that the two sides play in regulation of affect. Greater right-sided activation (less alpha on the right) and/or lesser left-sided activation (more alpha on the left) is associated with more negative affect. While this observation has exceptions, it has generated a large body of research on the electrophysiology and neurobiology of emotion in normals as well as in persons with affective disorders. We compared women with chemical intolerances (43% with food tolerances and 57% with irritable bowel diagnoses) to a group of women with depression (but low scores for chemical intolerance) and a group of normals.[31] We found that the depressed group showed the frontal lateral asymmetry of EEG alpha activity

D

previously reported in depression, but that their pattern differed significantly from that of the women with CI. The women with CI had a different type of alpha lateralization pattern, with relatively similar amounts of EEG alpha on the right and left. Therefore, despite increased levels of subjective depression in the CI group, their brain waves diverge from those of the depressed group.

In the same subjects, we examined the levels and associations of serum neopterin.[32] Neopterin is a nonspecific endogenous marker of inflammation that both immunological and nonimmunological events can release. It is more stable in the bloodstream than are various other potential mediators of symptomatology. The groups with CI, depression and normals did not differ in neopterin levels. However, the groups did differ significantly in the nature of the correlations they showed between neopterin and several measures of somatization. Higher neopterin levels correlated strongly with higher degrees of somatization on the Symptom Checklist 90 (revised), the McLean Limbic Somatic Symptom Subscale and the Profile of Mood States Fatigue Subscale, only in the women with CI. In contrast, for the depressives, neopterin did not correlate at all with the SCL-90-R or McLean Somatic Subscale but did with the POMS Fatigue Subscale and, interestingly, with an index of CI. The data suggest that neopterin may indicate recent inflammatory events associated with somatic symptomatology in persons with CI, but not necessarily in those with depression.

Consequently, the mechanisms of somatic symptoms in CI and in depression may differ. Notably, Sugerman et al.[128] reported that patients with major depression, alcohol dependence or schizophrenia without evidence of allergic disease have elevated titres of allergen-specific immunoglobulin (Ig)E antibodies compared with normals: for the 10 depressives, 22% of 210 food tests were positive *versus* 6% of 231 food tests positive in the 11 normals. All of the depressives, whereas only 1/11 (9%) of the normals, showed egg as a positive food item for allergen-specific IgE titres. In a survey of 379 college students, we replicated and extended the finding of increased atopic allergy histories (71%) in persons with a lifetime history of a professional diagnosis of depression.[12] It is as yet unknown if the food or inhalant-specific IgE in the psychiatric patients plays any causative role in their symptoms. It is also unknown if persons with CI and those with depression would differ in their food-specific IgE titrers. However, previous research has demonstrated that elderly people with CI and their normal peers, both scoring low on a standardized measure of depression, do not differ in levels of milk-specific IgE and IgG antibodies.[22] Nevertheless, the polysomnographic sleep records,[22] plasma β-endorphin levels,[21] and cognitive test performances[25] of the two groups did differ. Therefore, neither depression nor food-specific antibodies are necessary for persons with CI to exhibit neurobehavioural disturbances.

SOMATOFORM DISORDERS AND ADDICTION

Randolph[105–107] was the first clinician to postulate that food allergies with behavioural and somatic manifestations might actually reflect a dynamic, addiction-like process. He observed that his patients often ate certain foods compulsively and excessively and that they underwent drug withdrawal-like syndromes during the early phases of food elimination programmes. He also noted that many alcoholics use foods containing sugar or caffeine in an addictive manner and claimed that sober alcoholics reported hangover-like conditions after acute food challenges with offending items. Randolph asserted that affected patients would temporarily relieve symptoms and feel better after ingesting the craved food, but that the passage of time after the meal would lead to an inevitable worsening of symptoms and escalating food cravings. He further claimed that the only way to determine if a craved or favourite food was responsible for recurrent chronic symptoms was to avoid it completely for a period of 4–5 days and then reintroduce it in a test meal. Under these challenge conditions, troublesome foods would reveal their capacity to induce intense adverse symptoms rather than symptom relief. Most investigators have ignored this aspect of his work, despite a growing research literature on the addictive nature of food use in conditions such as bulimia and other eating disorders[3] and on the neurobiology of addiction.[80]

In several studies,[19,33,35] we have shown increased ratings for carbohydrate and other food cravings in individuals with high levels of CI. Despite the cravings, such individuals also report increased rates of food intolerances and irritable bowel diagnoses. The latter could represent the 'withdrawal' side of a food addiction process. In a replicated finding, individuals of all ages who are high in CI rate themselves as ill more often than do normals if they miss or delay a meal[16,17] (see also Fig. 47.1). These observations take on further importance in considering other evidence that links food and chemical intolerances with alcohol and drug addiction research (Table 47.1).

For example, women far outnumber men among the subset of the population with MCS, food intolerances and/or CIs. Several studies suggest that MCS patients and community persons with food or chemical intolerances also have an increased prevalence of somatization disorder diagnoses[119] or elevated scores on standardized scales measuring multiple somatic symptoms, i.e. somatization.[20,23,32,40] Women with somatization disorder, like MCS patients, have increased lifetime histories of ovarian cysts and irritable bowel syndrome.[97]

Somatization disorder is a chronic, disabling psychiatric condition, primarily of women, involving multiple physical symptoms, beginning before age 30. Current diagnostic criteria include multiple pain complaints, gastrointestinal disturbances (including food intolerances), sexual dysfunction and pseudoneurological or conversion symptoms, all without medical explanation. Notably, adoption, twin and sibling studies show that alcoholism has heritable components.[60] However, careful studies have also shown that the adopted-away daughters of male alcoholics meet criteria for somatization disorder at increased rates, without a concomitant elevation in alcoholism.[41,45,70] One hypothesis that derives from these findings is that daughters of alcoholics inherit the psychobiology of addiction, including neural sensitizability, but that it manifests in food cravings and food and chemical intolerances rather than in alcohol or other drug cravings and addiction.[35,36]

To date, clinical and preclinical data support the above hypothesis. Among over 900 young adult college students, those with higher levels of CI ratings also report increased rates of drug problems in their families but not themselves.[19] We replicated and extended this finding in three other smaller samples.[31,35,37] When we ask specifically about parental substance abuse problems, alcoholism in the father is markedly increased among individuals meeting research criteria for MCS (46%) compared with normal controls (7%).[35] Black[39] recently reported a similar finding of family histories of alcoholism in long-term MCS patients. Thus,

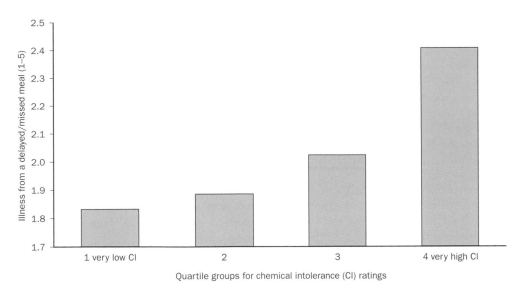

Fig. 47.1 Addictive-like phenomena in young adults with chemical intolerance: food 'withdrawal' symptoms. Highest illness from a delayed meal in the most chemically intolerant quartile (N_{tot} = 932). $F(3928)$ = 11.69; P = 0.0000.

Similarities between alcoholism and food/chemical intolerance	
Descriptive data	
Somatization disorder in female offspring of Cloninger's Type II male alcoholics	Somatization disorder and higher somatization scores in chemical intolerance (CI) Increased family/paternal histories of alcoholism in CI
Sweet cravings in alcoholics	Sweet/food cravings in CI
Biological data	
Increased EEG alpha in offspring of alcoholics	Increased EEG alpha in CI
Autonomic sensitization in offspring of alcoholics; EEG alpha sensitization to cocaine in animals	Autonomic and EEG sensitization (delta and alpha) in CI
Increased plasma β-endorphin after alcohol in persons at risk for alcoholism	Increased plasma β-endorphin after foods in CI

Table 47.1 Similarities between alcoholism and food/chemical intolerance.

the epidemiological associations that are predicted are consistent with a possible genetic link between alcohol/drug addiction and chemical/food intolerances.

If MCS patients and those with CI have inherited vulnerability to sensitization, then (a) they should exhibit physiological characteristics similar to those of alcoholics and/or their offspring and (b) they should demonstrate heightened sensitizability in the laboratory. Again, the data support the hypothesis. For example, sons of alcoholics and daughters of alcoholics with premenstrual syndrome both exhibit increased amounts of EEG alpha activity at rest and especially after alcohol ingestion.[55,56] We found that middle-aged women with CI have significantly higher amounts of EEG alpha activity at rest with eyes closed than do women with depression (but no CI) or normals.[31] Fernandez[61] observed that women with CI also have higher amounts of EEG alpha activity than do women with sexual abuse histories or normals.

Moreover, in both the Bell *et al.*[31] (at rest) and Fernandez *et al.*[61] (during chemical odorant exposures) studies, the groups with CI show sensitization (increases over sessions) in EEG alpha compared with decreases or stable levels in the normal controls.

Sons of alcoholics sensitize autonomic nervous system variables over repeated alcohol ingestion sessions in the laboratory.[96] Similarly, elderly individuals with CI[27] and middle-aged women with CI[37] show sensitization of diastolic blood pressure and/or heart rate over sessions in the laboratory involving, respectively, food ingestion or chemical exposures. In addition to the EEG and cardiovascular findings, researchers have demonstrated that individuals with genetic vulnerability to alcoholism have increased levels of β-endorphin after alcohol ingestion.[65] In parallel, elderly individuals with CI have, on average, significantly higher levels of plasma β-endorphin 90 min after food ingestion (milk or soy beverage) than do normals without CI.[21] In summary, as predicted, the data in human subjects suggest that the offspring of alcoholics and persons with CI share some key physiological traits.

Preclinical studies also support possible links between vulnerability to alcohol and drug addiction and chemical/food intolerances. One brain pathway which appears involved in most drug addictions is the dopaminergic mesolimbic system, from the ventral tegmental area (VTA) to the nucleus accumbens.[3,76,123] Afferents from other regions, including prefrontal cortex and

D

limbic amygdala, involving neurotransmitters such as dopamine, γ-aminobutyric acid and excitatory amino acids regulate mesolimbic function.[76] The mesolimbic system is susceptible to the process of neural sensitization. Sensitization is the progressive increase in host responsivity to a given stimulus over repeated, intermittent re-exposures;[3,4,123] it is proposed to underlie drug cravings.[111] However, the mesolimbic pathway also regulates hedonic responses to palatable foods such as sweets and fats, which induce increased mesolimbic dopamine release.[86]

Stress, stimulant drugs, alcohol, opiates, environmental chemicals, and certain endogenous mediators such as interleukin-2 or substance P agonists, can all initiate and elicit mesolimbic sensitization.[3,4,29,36,66,76,124,125,138] Increased spontaneous sucrose ingestion[118] and female gender[102] are among the individual difference factors that predict heightened vulnerability to sensitization. Repeated exposure to toluene[138] or formaldehyde[124,125] in animals causes cross-sensitization of locomotor responsivity to apomorphine or cocaine, respectively. Both of the latter drugs activate dopaminergic pathways.

Of possible relevance to the EEG alpha findings in human subjects above, repeated exposure to stimulant drugs in animals sensitize increases in EEG alpha, which results from progressive involvement of dopamine D2 receptors in the brain.[59] Animal studies indicate that solvents such as toluene exert effects on spatial memory via changes in dopamine D2 receptor function.[137] Interestingly, solvent-exposed workers, who have increased rates of chemical[94] and alcohol intolerance,[84] also show increased dopamine synthesis on positron emission tomography scans,[53] and increased EEG delta and alpha activity after work.[95] Taken together, the data indicate the possible involvement of mesolimbic dopaminergic D2 neurons in the clinical and neurophysiological alterations of persons with chemical and/or food intolerance.

NARCOLEPSY AND FOOD ADDICTION/INTOLERANCE

Clinical and preclinical data from research on narcolepsy may also relate to the hypothesized associations between food addiction/intolerance and mesolimbic dopamine. Narcolepsy is a neurological disorder, a disorder of rapid-eye-movement (REM) sleep, characterized by excessive daytime sleepiness with overpowering sleep attacks, disrupted nocturnal sleep, cataplexy (sudden waking muscle atonia elicited by strong emotion) and hypnagogic hallucinations. Polysomnography in narcoleptics reveals short sleep-onset latency and early onset REM sleep. We first reported in the mid-1970s[6,8–10] that narcoleptics endorse significantly more food cravings, especially for milk and sweets, as well as more food-induced gastrointestinal upsets (e.g. from alcohol, Mexican food, candy, onion, pork, sausage, popcorn, soda and chocolate)[6] than do normal controls. One patient anecdotally reports on over 20-year follow up the ability to avoid using medications for her cataplexy if she avoids eating specific foods to which she considers herself sensitive.

It is possible to induce attacks of cataplexy reliably in the canine model for narcolepsy by offering the animals food. The emotional excitement associated with eating triggers the cataplexy. Recently, Reid et al.[109] showed that local perfusion of the VTA with D2 and D3 dopamine agonist drugs leads to a marked increase in cataplexy in narcoleptic dogs. Local perfusion with a D2 dopamine blocking drug in the VTA slightly decreased the cataplexy. As a result, Reid et al.[109] suggested that food-induced cataplexy may partly reflect receptor dysfunction and/or neurochemical imbalances affecting specific dopaminergic neurons in the VTA. These animal data are consistent with the clinical findings on foods in narcoleptics described above and suggest dysfunction in the mesolimbic pathways of people and animals with narcolepsy.

FOOD AND/OR CHEMICAL INTOLERANCES: SELF-REPORT DATA

We have performed several large-scale surveys in young adult college students and in community-dwelling elderly individuals to delineate the characteristics of non-patients who report food and/or chemical intolerances.[15–19,23] For example, 23 (11%) of 211 University of Arizona college students (mean age 19, SD 3) enrolled in an introductory psychology course reported both physician diagnoses of asthma, hay fever or rhinitis, eczema, or hives and foods as triggers of these conditions in themselves. The food allergic group included more women than did the non-allergic group (food allergics 87% versus normals 64% women, Fisher's Exact Test $P=0.034$ two-tailed). From a short list of specific foods that might induce symptoms, these food-allergic young adults endorsed significantly more frequent illness on a 5-point Likert scale for milk, chocolate, corn, candy, coffee and alcohol, but not pizza, bread, grapes, food dyes or chlorinated water. Figure 47.2 illustrates that these food allergics scored significantly higher than did their healthy peers on the MLSC. These findings remained significant after controlling for the only psychological variable on which the groups differed, i.e. the Marlowe–Crowne Social Desirability Scale, a measure of denial of negative traits about oneself (food allergics: 3.7, SD 3.3 versus normals 5.0, SD 3.0, $F(1209)=4.0$, $P=0.047$). The groups did not differ significantly for overall psychological distress on the General Severity Index or the Positive Symptom Distress Index of the SCL-90-R, the Barsky Somatic Symptom Amplification Scale (a measure of subjective exaggeration of physical sensations) or the Social Reticence Scale (a measure of trait shyness).

Interestingly, the list of offending foods in this study overlaps those seen in patients with atypical food reactions that were unconfirmed on double-blind testing, such as milk and sugar.[99] However, unlike the atypical food allergics in the Parker et al.[100] sample, the young adults in the Bell et al. (unpublished data) study above did not differ significantly from their healthier peers in degree of psychological distress on the SCL-90-R. The offending items diverged only in part from those reported in MCS patients by Miller & Mitzel.[92] They found that chlorinated tap water and food dyes were among the most common offending ingestants for MCS patients, in contrast with the Bell et al. food allergics' problem items; but the Miller & Mitzel MCS patients also noted that milk, alcohol, chocolate, coffee, cola and corn were common offenders, similar to those foods found in the Bell et al. study above. The different findings may relate to methodological and recruitment differences between studies and highlight the problem of generalizing from one population to another in this complex field.

Nevertheless, the Limbic Checklist data, together with the EEG delta findings, reinforce the possibility that the limbic regions of the brain may have lower thresholds for activation, though not necessarily clinical seizure disorders, in community

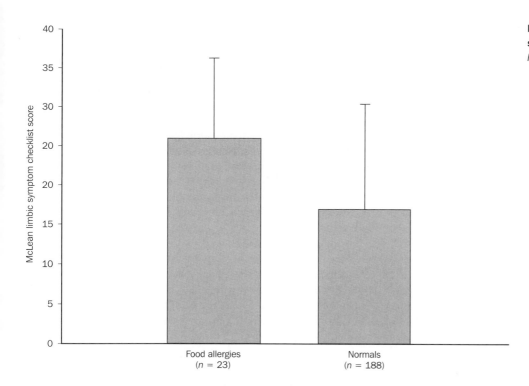

Fig. 47.2 **Higher limbic system checklist scores in food allergics than in normals.** $F(1206) = 7.5$; $P = 0.007$.

persons who report food allergies and/or chemical intolerances. The food allergies and chemical intolerances per se may or may not have a direct causative role in the limbic disturbances.[13,36] Limbic regions regulate affective tone, autonomic nervous system function, immune responsivity and endocrine hormone release.[7,13,19,29,36] Consequently, dysfunction in this part of the brain could lead to the multiple somatic disturbances and many of the symptoms that individuals with adverse food and chemical reactions report.

The food allergic sample above more likely captured a subset of persons with atopic allergies, as opposed to most other studies, which examine the traits of persons with food intolerances, with and without IgE-mediated allergies. In a more general sample of 24 community-recruited middle-aged individuals with food intolerances *versus* 15 healthy controls, Bell *et al.*[15] found that 50% also endorsed environmental chemical sensitivities, 38% drug sensitivities and 33% natural inhalant sensitivities. Symptoms for which the food-intolerant group had significantly higher ratings included depression, anxiety, difficulty concentrating, sluggishness/lethargy, difficulty making decisions, dopeyness/grogginess, ringing in the ears, fatigue, tension/nervousness, spaciness, irritability, clumsiness, abdominal bloating, confusion, excessive mucous production and earache. The food-intolerant group exhibited greater heart rate acceleration during performance of a mental arithmetic task than during isometric exercise, opposite to the pattern seen in the normals. These data are consistent with the early clinical descriptions of patients with the tension-fatigue syndrome. Complaints like 'dopeyness/grogginess', 'spaciness', and 'clumsiness' again imply CNS problems that may not meet criteria for a specific neurological diagnosis, but which suggest at least subclinical dysfunction different from the typical presenting complaints of patients with psychiatric disorders such as depression.

In other large-sample studies of non-clinical populations, we examined the traits of persons with self-reported intolerances to foods alone (FI), chemicals alone (CI), both classes of substance (FI/CI) or neither (NOILL). Among 490 college students, Bell *et al.*[16] divided the sample into those above and below median for the sums of frequency of illness ratings on 5-point Likert scales for three foods (wheat, dairy and eggs) and for five chemicals (pesticide, paint, new carpet, car exhaust and perfume). The four groups differed significantly for ratings of nervous system-related symptoms, including memory trouble (FI/CI>CI, NOILL), insomnia (FI/CI>NOILL), headaches (FI/CI, CI, FI>NOILL), difficulty concentrating (FI/CI, CI>NOILL), daytime grogginess (no posthoc differences) and ringing in the ears (FI/CI>NOILL). Again, the FI/CI group had significantly higher scores on measures of depression and anxiety than did the NOILL group; the FI/CI group also exceeded the CI-only group for level of depression. Similarly, Bell *et al.*[17] divided 263 community-living elderly individuals into a comparable set of four groups and again found that the FI/CI group significantly exceeded the NOILL group for insomnia ratings, but it was the CI-only who were higher than the NOILL for difficulty concentrating. Thus, these data suggest that it is the subset of younger and perhaps older adults reporting high levels of illness from both foods and chemicals who have the most significant neuropsychiatric picture.

FOOD AND/OR CHEMICAL INTOLERANCES: OBJECTIVE DATA

Cognitive tests

In view of questions raised by inconsistent results of actual food challenges in the laboratory, it is reasonable to ask whether or not food- and/or chemical-intolerant people have objective evidence of their neuropsychiatric symptomatology. Most studies have not found marked differences in baseline performance (without food or chemical challenges) between MCS patients and normals. A notable exception is the similar findings by Fiedler *et al.*[63] in MCS patients and by Bell *et al.*[30] in community middle-aged CI with lifestyle changes (60% of whom reported physician-diagnosed food sensitivity *versus* 8% of the normal controls) of increased rates of false alarms (to correct hits) on a standardized test of visual memory performance (Continuous Visual Memory Test, CVMT). Other research suggests that the CVMT may tap abilities that the frontal lobes regulate,[110] thereby raising the possibility of a specific type of frontal lobe dysfunction in certain persons with food and chemical intolerances.

In addition, however, community-recruited persons with CI who deny concomitant lifestyle changes do not exhibit the same difficulties with the CVMT. Rather, middle-aged persons with CI demonstrate a progressive worsening of divided attention test (DAT) performance with practice compared with both normals and those with CI and lifestyle changes.[30] Moreover, elderly with CI show slowed performance on the same test of visual divided attention, even at baseline, compared with normal elderly.[25] Given the literature on brain regions involved in divided attention,[64] the DAT findings raise the possibility that a different subset of persons with food and/or chemical sensitivities may have problems in the temporoparietal areas. The latter possibility is further reinforced by a replicated finding among elderly individuals with CI of more deficits in free recall verbal memory than in normal controls.[14,28]

The differences in ability to detect cognitive problems between studies may relate in part not only to lack of food or chemical challenges but also to age differences in the subject populations. The data suggest that older age may be a risk factor in those with CI for measurable deficits in both verbal memory and visual divided attention. At least in the elderly, those with subjective memory complaints and demonstrable memory problems do show a greater subsequent decline in memory test performance than do controls.[116] Moreover, we have found evidence of higher supine blood pressures upon awakening in elderly with CI[27] and elevated rates of antihypertensive medications in middle-aged persons with CI[34] compared with controls. Hypertension in mid- to later life is a predictive risk factor for subsequent development of geriatric dementias.[81,122] In particular, Alzheimer's disease, the most common late life dementia, typically affects temporoparietal function bilaterally.[93] No cross-sectional studies have as yet directly compared cognitive dysfunction in persons with FIs alone, CIs, both types, or neither complaint, in any age group; and no prospective studies have assessed FI and/or CI as risk factors for subsequent dementia. The preliminary findings in this area suggest such research would be useful.

Sleep studies

A common symptom among food- and/or chemical-intolerant persons is insomnia. In 17 children with a treatment-resistant degree of this problem (median age 13.5 months), Kahn et al.[74] found that sleep logs kept by parents showed significant improvements on a cow's milk-free diet over a period of 4–6 weeks. Parameters that improved included sleep-onset latency, number of arousals and total sleep time per 24 hours. A subsequent double-blind crossover challenge with diets containing *versus* not containing milk demonstrated re-emergence of insomnia from milk in all except one child. The children maintained the benefits of the exclusion diet through 24 months of age. Notably, family histories of atopy were positive in 10/17 families, but total serum IgE levels were elevated in only 1/12 children tested. Anti-β-lactoglobulin antibodies were abnormal in 9/14 children tested. A substantial proportion of the children had eczema, night-time wheezing, rhinitis or otitis, or recurrent diarrhoea or vomiting, on careful assessment. The elimination diet also reportedly led to reduced sweating at night and behavioural improvements during the day.

Kahn et al.[73] examined the polysomnographic sleep patterns of nine infants (including five of those studied above). They observed significant decreases in number of arousals and increases in total sleep time. Sleep stages were redistributed when sleep improved, with more of non-REM stages 2 and 3 and less non-REM stage 1. They did not find gastro-oesophageal reflux or sleep apnoea responsible for the milk-related sleep problems. Although they did not investigate specific mediators, they speculated that the poor sleep could result from excessive histamine release or reduced synthesis of serotonin, certain peptides or interleukin-1.

Another polysomnographic study was on healthy elderly individuals with histories of CI, but not milk or soy intolerance.[22] These individuals were placed on 3-week elimination diets in crossover design involving daily ingestion of customary/baseline diet, 24 ounces (680 g) of 1% fat milk or 24 ounces of a soy-based nondairy beverage. Diet plans were otherwise matched for nutrient intake, including wheat gluten. The group with high CI did not differ from the low CI group in terms of levels of IgE or IgG antibodies specific to milk. On the dairy diet, groups were also comparable in levels of plasma β-casomorphin (a milk-derived opioid peptide) measured 90 min after morning laboratory ingestion of 8 ounces (226 g) of milk. However, on sleep recordings (two successive laboratory nights at the end of each of the three diet conditions, with milk and soy counterbalanced in order), the high CI group had significantly more total sleep time on the soy-based diet compared with their own baseline or milk conditions, whereas the low CI group slept better on both milk and soy diets compared with their own baseline. During this study, it was stage REM sleep that was reduced in the high CI group. The high CI elderly individuals exhibited a trend towards a higher respiratory disturbance index on the milk than on the baseline or soy diets, compared with the low CI elderly individuals. The data indicate that infants and elderly individuals who reportedly sleep more poorly on milk-containing diets both show objective evidence of insomnia, but the nature of the sleep stage disruptions differs between age groups. Taken together, the objective observations are consistent with subjective sleep disturbances that persons with food and/or chemical intolerances report, but much research is needed to determine the physiological bases of the insomnia.

The findings again raise questions about possible humoral mediators of the food-related sleep disturbance: perhaps those released by non-immunological inflammatory responses as well as by immunological processes. The study of elderly individuals offers some additional possibilities. For example, the high CI elderly individuals had overall elevations of plasma β-endorphin, an endogenous opioid peptide, in the mornings, measured 90 min after ingestion of either milk or soy beverage.[21] The β-endorphin levels were also strikingly labile from session to session within diet types for the high CI, but not the low CI group. In addition to their own capacity to affect opioid receptors, endogenous opioids can induce non-immunological release of mast cell histamine.[88] Moreover, the high CI elderly individuals exhibited a trend towards ingesting more fat, especially saturated fat, than did their low CI peers.[21] In view of the research demonstrating that dietary fat mobilizes CCK release in the gut,[143] it is also possible that fluctuations in CCK levels contributed to the disturbed sleep. In cats, CCK induces earlier onset REM sleep;[57] a relative drop in CCK from the lack of fatty food intake during the night, i.e. food withdrawal, might then cause reductions in REM. Changes in cytokines are also plausible mechanisms for altered sleep in milk-intolerant individuals. These hypotheses are all testable with available research tools. Findings from this type of investigation may provide valuable new insights into the ways in which specific foods might affect CNS function in patients who report food and chemical intolerances.

CONCLUSIONS

The field of food allergy has engendered intense, dualistic debate. Proponents of direct biological effects insist that foods induce behavioural, psychiatric and neurological disturbances from nervous system dysfunction and often ignore possible psychological factors. Skeptics of these concepts emphasize evidence for concomitant psychological disturbances and infer exclusively psychogenic mediation.[71,132] Investigators appear to feel that they can put the question to rest by demonstrating one or the other category of mechanism. This type of limited thinking is in marked contrast with interdisciplinary advances in the fields of behavioural medicine, health psychology and even psychiatry. The schism between body and mind models for adverse food reactions overlooks the more integrative, interactive way of evaluating the problem. As illustrated above, finding psychiatric symptoms is not a final explanation in itself; rather, it suggests possible mechanisms by which the symptoms could occur.

In a seminal essay on a framework for modern psychiatry, for example, Kandel[78] describes five principles, which may also assist in taking a scientifically more balanced view of issues in food sensitivity:

1) all mental processes, even the most complex psychological processes, derive from operations of the brain; 2) genes and their protein products are important determinants of the pattern of interconnections between neurons in the brain and the details of their functioning; 3) altered genes do not, by themselves, explain all of the variance of a given major mental illness ... all of "nurture" is ultimately expressed as "nature;" 4) alterations in gene expression induced by learning give rise to changes in patterns of neuronal connections; 5) insofar as

psychotherapy or counseling is effective and produces long-term changes in behavior, it presumably does so through learning, by producing changes in gene expression that alter the strength of synaptic connections and structural changes that alter the anatomical pattern of interconnections between nerve cells of the brain.

As a corollary of Kandel's argument, a testable hypothesis is that foods are environmental stimuli from more than one point of view, e.g. both pharmacological and psychological, and thus impact brain function via biological final common pathways within the susceptible individual.[3] The pharmacological properties of foods potentially derive from their nutrient and drug constituents (e.g. xanthines), neurotransmitters or neuromodulatory peptides, neuroactive contaminants and/or the capacity to activate release of endogenous mediators by either immunological or non-immunological means.[3,90,141,143] The psychological properties of foods potentially derive from cultural influences, learned past experiences as in classical conditioning, beliefs and expectations, all of which the brain can translate into altered neurobiology, including modifying the release of endogenous mediators such as insulin or vasopressin, with profound somatic effects.[3]

In conclusion, the CNS effects of food allergies or intolerances require a great deal of additional study. Recent advances in the basic and clinical neurosciences should enable investigators to examine the various hypotheses that emerge from the current state of the art. At this point, we know more about the individuals who report food allergies than we do about the relationship of specific foods to specific symptoms. It is likely that both neural sensitization and classical conditioning processes, alone or together, could play a role in the clinical phenomenology of food and chemical intolerance in particular individuals. Genetic factors, especially family histories of alcoholism or drug abuse, may contribute to risk for this type of problem. The actual endogenous mediators that may generate symptoms at end organs could be diverse, ranging from β-endorphin to neopterin to histamine to numerous cytokines and related substances.[21,29,32,85,90] It is clear that the issues in this area are far more complicated than originally believed, beyond the question of whether or not IgE is a mediator of adverse nervous system reactions to foods.[104,133]

REFERENCES

1 Adamson WD, Sellers ED. Observations on the incidence of a hypersensitive state in 100 cases of epilepsy. *J Allergy* 1932; 4: 315–23.

2 Allen JJ, Iacono WG, Depue RR, Arbisi P. Regional EEG asymmetries in bipolar seasonal affective disorder before and after phototherapy. *Biol Psychiatry* 1993; 33: 642–6.

3 Antelman SM. Time-dependent sensitization as the cornerstone for a new approach to pharmacotherapy: drugs as foreign/stressful stimuli. *Drug Devel Res* 1988; 14: 1–30.

4 Antelman SM. Time-dependent sensitization in animals: a possible model of multiple chemical sensitivity in humans. *Toxicol Industr Health* 1994; 10: 335–42.

5 Backus RC, Rosenquist GL, Rogers QR, Calam J, Morris JG. Elevation of plasma cholecystokinin (CCK) immunoreactivity by fat, protein, and amino acids in the cat, a carnivore. *Regulatory Peptides* 1995; 57: 123–31.

6 Bell IR. Diet histories in narcolepsy. In: *Narcolepsy* (Guilleminault C, Dement WC, Passouant P, eds), Spectrum, New York, 1976: 221–7.

7 Bell IR. Neuropsychiatric aspects of sensitization to low level chemicals: a neural sensitization model. *Toxicol Industr Health* 1994; 10: 277–312.

8 Bell IR, Guilleminault C, Dement WC. Questionnaire survey of eating habits of narcoleptics versus normals. *Sleep Research* 1975; 4: 208.

9 Bell IR, Hawley CD, Guilleminault C, Dement WC. Diet and symptom histories in food allergics versus narcoleptics and normals. *Sleep Research* 1976; 5: 155.

10 Bell IR, Isaacs JG, Guilleminault C, Dement WC. Specific food and chemical sensitivities in narcolepsy. *Sleep Research* 1976; 5: 156.

11 Bell IR, Guilliminault C, Dement WC. Hypersomnia, multiple-system symptomatology, and selective IgA deficiency. *Biol Psychiatry* 1978; 13: 751–7.

12 Bell IR, Jasnoski ML, Kagan J, King DS. Depression and allergies: survey of a nonclinical population. *Psychother Psychosom* 1991; 55: 24–31.

13 Bell IR, Miller CM, Schwartz GE. An olfactory-limbic model of multiple chemical sensitivity syndrome: possible relationships to kindling and affective spectrum disorders. *Biological Psychiatry* 1992; 32: 218–42.

14 Bell IR, Amend D, Kaszniak AW, Schwartz GE. Memory deficits, sensory impairment, and depression in the elderly. *Lancet* 1993; 341: 62.

15 Bell IR, Markley EJ, King DS *et al*. Polysymptomatic syndromes and autonomic reactivity to nonfood stressors in individuals with self-reported adverse food reactions. *J Am College Nutrition* 1993; 12: 227–38.

16 Bell IR, Schwartz GE, Peterson JM, Amend D. Symptom and personality profiles of young adults from a college student population with self-reported illness from foods and chemicals. *J Am College Nutrition* 1993; 12: 693–702.

17 Bell IR, Schwartz GE, Peterson JM, Amend D, Stini WA. Possible time-dependent sensitization to xenobiotics: self-reported illness from chemical odors, foods, and opiate drugs in an older adult population. *Arch Environ Health* 1993; 48: 315–27.

18 Bell IR, Schwartz GE, Amend D, Peterson JM, Stini WA. Sensitization to early life stress and responses to chemical odors in older adults. *Biol Psychiatry* 1994; 35: 857–63.

19 Bell IR, Hardin E, Baldwin CM, Schwartz GE. Increased limbic system symptomatology and sensitizability of young adults with chemical and noise sensitivities. *Environ Res* 1995; 70: 84–97.

20 Bell IR, Peterson JM, Schwartz GE. Medical histories and psychological profiles of middle-aged women with and without self-reported illness from environmental chemicals. *J Clin Psychiatry* 1995; 56: 151–60.

21 Bell IR, Bootzin RR, Davis TP *et al*. Time-dependent sensitization of plasma beta-endorphin in community elderly with self-reported environmental chemical odor intolerance. *Biol Psychiatry* 1996; 40: 134–43.

22 Bell IR, Bootzin RR, Ritenbaugh C *et al*. A polysomnographic study of sleep disturbance in community elderly with self-reported environmental chemical odor intolerance. *Biol Psychiatry* 1996; 40: 123–33.

23 Bell IR, Miller CS, Schwartz GE, Peterson JM, Amend D. Neuropsychiatric and somatic characteristics of young adults with and without chemical odor intolerance and chemical sensitivity. *Arch Environ Health* 1996; 51: 9–21.

24 Bell IR, Schwartz GE, Baldwin CM, Hardin EE. Neural sensitization and physiological markers in multiple chemical sensitivity. *Reg Toxicol Pharmacol* 1996; 24:S39–S47.

25 Bell IR, Wyatt JK, Bootzin RR, Schwartz GE. Slowed reaction time performance on a divided attention task in elderly with environmental chemical odor intolerance. *Int J Neurosci* 1996; 84: 127–34.

26 Bell IR, Schwartz GE, Baldwin CM *et al*. Individual differences in neural sensitization and the role of context in illness from low level environmental chemical exposures. *Environ Health Perspectives* 1997; 105 (Suppl 2): 457–66.

27 Bell IR, Schwartz GE, Bootzin RR, Wyatt JK. Time-dependent sensitization of heart rate and blood pressure over multiple laboratory sessions in elderly individuals with chemical odor intolerance. *Arch Environ Health* 1997; 52: 6–17.

28 Bell IR, Walsh ME, Goss A, Gersmeyer J, Schwartz GE, Kanof P. Cognitive dysfunction and disability in geriatric veterans with self-reported intolerance to environmental chemicals. *J Chronic Fatigue Syndrome* 1997; 3: 15–42.

29 Bell IR, Baldwin CM, Schwartz GE. Illness from low levels of environmental chemicals: relevance to chronic fatigue syndrome and fibromyalgia. *Am J Med Suppl* 1998; 105(3A): 74S–82S.

30 Bell IR, Bootzin RR, Schwartz GE, Baldwin CM, Ballesteros F. Differing patterns of cognitive dysfunction and heart rate reactivity in chemically-intolerant individuals with and without lifestyle changes. *J Chronic Fatigue Syndrome* 1999; 5(2):3–25.

31 Bell IR, Schwartz GE, Hardin EE, Baldwin CM, Kline JP. Differential resting qEEG alpha patterns in women with environmental chemical intolerance, depressives, and normals. *Biol Psychiatry* 1998; 43(5): 376–88.

32 Bell IR, Patarca R, Baldwin CM, Klimas NG, Schwartz GE, Hardin EE. Serum neopterin and somatization in women with chemical intolerance, depressives, and normals. *Neuropsychobiology* 1998; 38: 13–18.

33 Bell IR, Baldwin CM, Stoltz E *et al*. Psychophysiological differences between fibromyalgia patients with and without environmental chemical intolerance. Presented at the Society of Behavioral Medicine, San Diego, CA, March 1999.

34 Bell IR, Szarek MJ, DiCenso DR, Baldwin CM, Schwartz GE, Bootzin RR: Patterns of waking EEG spectral power in chemically intolerant individuals during repeated chemical exposures. *Int J Neurosci* 1999; 97: 41–59.

35 Bell IR, Baldwin CM, Fernandez M, Schwartz GER. Paternal alcoholism in multiple chemical sensitivity: a genetic link with the biology of neural sensitization? Submitted for publication.

36 Bell IR, Baldwin CM, Fernandez M, Schwartz GER. Neural sensitization model for multiple chemical sensitivity: overview of theory and empirical evidence. *Toxicol Industr Health* 1999; 15: 295–304.

37 Bell IR, Baldwin CM, Russek LG, Schwartz GE, Hardin EE. Early life stress, negative paternal relationships, and current chemical odor intolerance in middle-aged women: support for a neural sensitization model. *J Women's Health* 1998; 7: 1135–47.

38 Binkley KE, Kutcher S. Panic response to sodium lactate infusion in patients with multiple chemical sensitivity syndrome. *J Allergy Clin Immunol* 1997; 99: 570–4.

39 Black DW. Nine year follow-up of persons diagnosed with multiple chemical sensitivity. Presentation at the 216th National Meeting of the American Chemical Society, 23–27 August ,1998.

40 Black DW, Rathe A, Goldstein RB. Environmental illness. A controlled study of 26 subjects with '20th century disease'. *JAMA* 1990; 264: 3166–70.

41 Bohman M, Cloninger CR, von Knorring AL, Sigvardsson S. An adoption study of somatoform disorders. III. Cross-fostering analysis and genetic relationship to alcoholism and criminality. *Arch Gen Psychiatry* 1984; 41(9): 872–8.

42 Bourin M, Baker GB, Bradwejn J. Neurobiology of panic disorder. *J Psychosom Res* 1998; 44: 163–80.

43 Campbell MB. Neurologic manifestations of allergic disease. *Ann Allergy* 1973; 31: 485–98.

44 Carter CM, Urbanowicz M, Hemsley R *et al*. Effects of a few food diet in attention deficit disorder. *Arch Dis Children* 1993; 69: 564–8.

45 Cloninger CR. Neurogenetic adaptive mechanisms in alcoholism. *Science* 1987; 236: 410–16.

46 Crayton JW. Epilepsy precipitated by food sensitivity: report of a case with double-blind placebo-controlled assessment. *Clin Electroencephalogr* 1981; 12: 192–8.

47 Davidson RJ, Schwartz GE, Saron C, Bennett J, Goleman DJ. Frontal versus parietal EEG asymmetry during positive and negative affect. *Psychophysiology* 1979; 16: 202–3.

48 Davison HM. Allergy of the nervous system. *Q Rev Allergy Immunol* 1952; 6: 157–88.

49 Dees SC, Lowenbach H. Allergic epilepsy. *Ann Allergy* 1951; 9: 446–58.

50 Dees SC. Neurologic allergy in childhood. *Pediatr Clin N Amer* 1954; 1: 1017–27.

51 Doty RL, Deems DA, Frye RE, Pelberg R, Shapiro A. Olfactory sensitivity, nasal resistance, and autonomic function in patients with multiple chemical sensitivities. *Arch Otolaryngol Head Neck Surg* 1988; 114: 1422–7.

52 Duke WW. Food allergy as a cause of illness. *JAMA* 1923; 81: 886–9.

53 Edling C, Hellman B, Arvidson B *et al*. Do organic solvents induce changes in the dopaminergic system? Positron emission tomography studies of occupationally exposed subjects. *Int Arch Occup Environ Health* 1997; 70: 180–6.

54 Egger J, Carter CM, Soothill JF, Wilson J. Oligoantigenic diet treatment of children with epilepsy and migraine. *J Pediatrics* 1989; 114: 51–8.

55 Ehlers CL, Schuckit MA: Evaluation of EEG alpha activity in sons of alcoholics. *Neuropsychopharmacology* 1991; 4: 199–205.

56 Ehlers C, Phillips E, Parry BL. Electrophysiological findings during the menstrual cycle in women with and without late luteal phase dysphoric disorder: relationship to risk for alcoholism? *Biol Psychiatry* 1996; 39: 720–3.

57 Fara JW, Rubinstein EH, Sonnenschein RR. Visceral and behavioral responses to intraduodenal fat. *Science* 1969; 166: 110–111.

58 Feingold BF. Behavioral disturbances linked to the ingestion of food additives. *Del Med J* 1977; 49: 89–94.

59 Ferger B, Stahl D, Kuschinsky K. Effects of cocaine on the EEG power spectrum of rats are significantly altered after its repeated administra-

tion: do they reflect sensitization phenomena? *Naunyn-Schmied Arch Pharmacol* 1996; 353: 545–51.

60 Ferguson RA, Goldberg DM. Genetic markers of alcohol abuse. *Clinica Chimica Acta* 1997; 257: 199–250.

61 Fernandez M, Bell IR, Schwartz GER. Sensitization during chemical exposure in women with and without idiopathic chemical sensitivity. *Toxicol Industr Health* 1999; 15: 305–12.

62 Fiedler N, Kipen H. Chemical sensitivity: the scientific literature. *Env Health Perspect* 1997; 105(suppl 2): 409–15.

63 Fiedler N, Kipen HM, DeLuca J, Kelly-McNeil K, Natelson B. A controlled comparison of multiple chemical sensitivities and chronic fatigue syndrome. *Psychosom Med* 1996; 58. 38–49.

64 Fink GR, Halligan PW, Marshall JC, Frith CD, Frackowiak RSJ, Dolan RJ. Where in the brain does visual attention select the forest and the trees? *Nature* 1996; 382: 626–8.

65 Gianoulakis C, De Waele JP, Thavundayil J. Implication of the endogenous opioid system in excessive ethanol consumption. *Alcohol* 1996; 13: 19–23.

66 Gilbert ME. Repeated exposure to lindane leads to behavioral sensitization and facilitates electrical kindling. *Neurotoxicol Teratol* 1995; 17: 131–41.

67 Gorman JM, Papp LA, Coplan JD *et al*. Anxiogenic effects of CO_2 and hyperventilation in patients with panic disorder. *Am J Psychiatry* 1994; 151: 547–53.

68 Hall K. Allergy of the nervous system. *Ann Allergy* 1976; 36: 49–64.

69 Herzog AG, Seibel MM, Schomer D, Vaitukaitis J, Geschwind N. Temporal lobe epilepsy: an extrahypothalamic pathogenesis for polycystic ovarian syndrome? *Neurology* 1984; 34: 1389–93.

70 Hill SY, Smith TR. Evidence for genetic mediation of alcoholism in women. *J Substance Abuse* 1991; 3: 159–74.

71 Howard LM, Wessely S. Psychiatry in the allergy clinic: the nature and management of patients with non-allergic symptoms. *Clin Exp Allergy* 1995; 25: 503–14.

72 Jewett DL, Fein G, Greenberg MH. A double-blind study of symptom provocation to determine food sensitivity. *N E J Med* 1990; 323: 429–33.

73 Kahn A, Francois G, Sottiaux M *et al*. Sleep characteristics in milk-intolerant infants. *Sleep* 1988; 11: 291–7.

74 Kahn A, Mozin MJ, Rebuffat E, Sottiaux M, Muller MF. Milk intolerance in children with persistent sleeplessness: a prospective double-blind crossover evaluation. *Pediatrics* 1989; 84: 595–603.

75 Kalivas PW, Alesdatter JE. Involvement of N-methyl-D-aspartate receptor stimulation in the ventral tegmental area and amygdala in behavioral sensitization to cocaine. *J Pharmacol Exp Ther* 1993; 267: 486–95.

76 Kalivas PW, Stewart J. Dopamine transmission in the initiation and expression of drug- and stress-induced sensitization of motor activity. *Brain Res Rev* 1991; 16: 223–44.

77 Kaplan BJ, McNicol J, Conte RA, Moghadam HK. Dietary replacement in preschool-aged hyperactive boys. *Pediatrics* 1989; 83: 7–17.

78 Kandel ER. A new intellectual framework for psychiatry. *Am J Psychiatry* 1998; 155: 457–69.

79 Kay LM. Support for the kindling hypothesis in multiple chemical sensitivity syndrome (MCSS) induction. *Society for Neuroscience* 1996; 22: 1825.

80 Korenman SG, Barchas JD (eds). *Biological Basis of Substance Abuse*. Oxford University Press, Oxford, NY: 1993.

81 Launer LJ, Masaki K, Petrovitch H, Foley D, Havlik RJ. The association between midlife blood pressure levels and late-life cognitive function. The Honolulu-Asia Aging Study. *JAMA* 1995; 274: 1846–51.

82 Leznoff A. Provocative challenges in patients with multiple chemical sensitivity. *J Allergy Clin Immunol* 1997; 99: 438–42.

83 Locatelli M, Bellodi L, Perna G, Scarone S. EEG power modifications in panic disorder during a temporolimbic activation task: relationships with temporal lobe clinical symptomatology. *J Neuropsychiatry Clin Neurosci* 1993; 5: 409–14.

84 Lundberg I, Michelsen H, Nise G *et al*. Neuropsychiatric function of housepainters with previous long-term heavy exposure to organic solvents. *Scand J Work Environ Health* 1995; 21(Suppl): 1–44.

85 Maier SF, Watkins LR. Cytokines for psychologists: implications of bidirectional immune-to-brain communication for understanding behavior, mood, and cognition. *Psychol Rev* 1998; 105: 83–107.

86 Martel P, Fantino M. Mesolimbic dopaminergic system activity as a function of food reward: a microdialysis study. *Pharmacol Biochem Behav* 1996; 53: 221–6.

87 May E. Attacks of unnatural somnolence of anaphylactic origin. *Bull Soc Med Hosp Paris* 1923; 47: 704.

88 Mediratta PK, Das N, Gupta VS, Sen P. Modulation of humoral immune responses by endogenous opioids. *J Allergy Clin Immunol* 1988; 81: 27–32.

89 Mesulam MM. *Principles of Behavioral Neurology*. F.A. Davis, Philadelphia, 1985: 289–326.

90 Metcalfe DD. Diagnostic procedures for immunologically-mediated food sensitivity. *Nutr Rev* 1984; 42: 92–7.

91 Miller K. Psychoneurological aspects of food allergy. In: *Stress, the Immune System, and Psychiatry* (Leonard BE, Miller K eds). John Wiley and Sons, Chichester, 1995: 185–206.

92 Miller CS, Mitzel HC. Chemical sensitivity attributed to pesticide exposure versus remodeling. *Arch Environ Health* 1995; 50: 119–29.

93 Miller BL, Chang L, Oropilla G, Mena I. Alzheimer's disease and frontal lobe dementias. In: *Textbook of Geriatric Neuropsychiatry* (Coffey CE, Cummings JL, eds). American Psychiatric Press, Washington, DC, 1994: 390–404.

94 Morrow LA, Ryan CM, Hodgson MJ, Robin N. Alterations in cognitive and psychological functioning after organic solvent exposure. *J Occup Med* 1990; 32: 444–50.

95 Muttray A, Lang J, Mayer-Popken O, Konietzko J. Acute changes in the EEG of workers exposed to mixtures of organic solvents. *Int J Occup Med Environ Health* 1995; 8: 131–7.

96 Newlin DB, Thomson JB. Chronic tolerance and sensitization to alcohol in sons of alcoholics. *Alc Clin Exp Res* 1991; 15: 399–405.

97 Orenstein H. Briquet's syndrome in association with depression and panic: a reconceptualization of Briquet's syndrome. *Am J Psychiatry* 1989; 146: 334–8.

98 Papp LA, Klein DF, Martinez J *et al*. Diagnostic and substance specificity of carbon-dioxide-induced panic. *Am J Psychiatry* 1993; 150: 250–7.

99 Parker SL, Leznoff A, Sussman GL, Tarlo SM, Krondl M. Characteristics of patients with food-related complaints. *J Allergy Clin Immunol* 1990; 86: 503–11.

100 Parker SL, Garner DM, Leznoff A, Sussman GL, Tarlo SM, Krondl M. Psychological characteristics of patients with reported adverse reactions to foods. *Int J Eating Disorders* 1991; 10: 433–9.

101 Pearson DJ, Rix KJ, Bentley SJ. Food allergy: how much in the mind? A clinical and psychiatric study of suspected food hypersensitivity. *Lancet* 1983; i: 1259–61.

102 Peris J, Decambre N, Coleman-Hardee ML, Simpkins JW. Estradiol enhances behavioral sensitization to cocaine and amphetamine-stimulated striatal [^{3}H] dopamine release. *Brain Res* 1991; 566. 255–64.

103 Perna G, Cocchi S, Bertani A, Arancio C, Bellodi L. Sensitivity to 35% CO_2 in healthy first-degree relatives of patients with panic disorder. *Am J Psychiatry* 1995; 152: 623–5.

104 Peveler R, Mayou R, Young E, Stoneham M. Psychiatric aspects of food-related physical symptoms: a community study. *J Psychosom Res* 1996; 41: 149–59.

105 Randolph TG. Fatigue and weakness of allergic origin (allergic toxemia); to be differentiated from 'nervous fatigue' or neurasthenia. *Ann Allergy* 1945; 3: 418–30.

106 Randolph TG. Allergy as a causative factor of fatigue, irritability, and behavior problems of children. *J Pediatrics* 1947; 31: 560–72.

107 Randolph TG. The descriptive features of food addiction. Addictive eating and drinking. *Q J Stud Alcohol* 1956; 17: 198–224.

108 Randolph TG. Specific adaptation. *Ann Allergy* 1978; 40: 333–45.

109 Reid MS, Tafti M, Nishino S, Sampathkumaran R, Siegel JM, Mignot E. Local administration of dopaminergic drugs into the ventral tegmental area modulates cataplexy in the narcoleptic canine. *Brain Res* 1996; 733: 83–100.

110 Retzlaff PD, Morris GL. Event-related potentials during the Continuous Visual Memory Test. *J Clin Psychol* 1996; 52: 43–7.

111 Robinson TE, Berridge KC. The neural basis of drug craving: an incentive-sensitization theory of addiction. *Brain Res Rev* 1993; 18: 247–91.

112 Rossi J. Sensitization induced by kindling and kindling-related phenomena as a model for multiple chemical sensitivity. *Toxicology* 1996; 111: 87–100.

113 Rowe AH. Allergic toxemia and migraine due to food allergy. *Calif West Med* 1930; 33: 785–92.

114 Salamone JD. The behavioral neurochemistry of motivation: methodological and conceptual issues in studies of the dynamic activity of nucleus accumbens dopamine. *J Neurosci Methods* 1996; 64: 137–49.

115 Schmidt MH, Mocks P, Lay B, Eisert HG *et al.* Does oligoantigenic diet influence hyperactive/conduct-disordered children – a controlled trial. *Eur Child Adol Psychiatry* 1997; 6: 88–95.

116 Schofield PW, Marder K, Dooneief G, Jacobs DM, Sano M, Stern Y. Association of subjective memory complaints with subsequent cognitive decline in community-dwelling elderly individuals with baseline cognitive impairment. *Am J Psychiatry* 1997; 154: 609–15.

117 Shannon WR. Neuropathic manifestations in infants and children as a result of anaphylactic reaction to foods contained in their dietary. *Am J Dis Children* 1922; 24: 89–94.

118 Sills TL, Vaccarino FJ. Individual differences in sugar intake predict the locomotor response to acute and repeated amphetamine administration. *Psychopharmacology* 1994; 116: 1–8.

119 Simon GE, Katon WJ, Sparks PJ. Allergic to life: psychological factors in environmental illness. *Am J Psychiatry* 1990; 147: 901–6.

120 Simon GE, Daniell W, Stockbridge H, Claypoole K, Rosenstock L. Immunologic, psychological, and neuropsychological factors in multiple chemical sensitivity. A controlled study. *Ann Internal Med* 1993; 19: 97–103.

121 Sjolund K, Ekman R, Lindgren S, Rehfeld JF. Disturbed motilin and cholecystokinin release in the irritable bowel syndrome. *Scand J Gastroenterol* 1996; 31: 1110–14.

122 Skoog I, Lernfeld B, Landahl S *et al.* A 15-year longitudinal study of blood pressure and dementia. *Lancet* 1996; 347: 1141–5.

123 Sorg BA, Hooks MS, Kalivas PW. Neuroanatomy and neurochemical mechanisms of time-dependent sensitization. *Toxicol Industr Health* 1994; 19: 369–86.

124 Sorg BA, Willis JR, Nowatka TC, Ulibarri C, See RE, Westberg HH. A proposed animal neurosensitization model for multiple chemical sensitivity in studies with formalin. *Toxicology* 1996; 111: 135–45.

125 Sorg BA, Willis JR, See RE, Hopkins B, Westberg HH. Repeated low-level formaldehyde exposure produces cross-sensitization to cocaine: possible relevance to chemical sensitivity in humans. *Neuropsychopharmacology* 1998; 18: 385–94.

126 Speer F. The allergic tension-fatigue syndrome in children. *Int Arch Allergy* 1958; 12: 207–14.

127 Stewart J, Druhan JP. Development of both conditioning and sensitization of the behavioral activating effects of amphetamine is blocked by the non-competitive NMDA receptor antagonist, MK-801. *Psychopharmacology* 1993; 110: 125–32.

128 Sugerman AA, Southern DL, Curran JH. A study of antibody levels in alcoholic, depressive, and schizophrenic patients. *Ann Allergy* 1982; 48: 166–71.

129 Suwa K, Toru M. A case of periodic somnolence whose sleep was induced by glucose. *Folia Psychiatr Neurol Jpn* 1969; 23: 253–62.

130 Teicher MH, Glod CA, Surrey J, Swett C. Early childhood abuse and limbic system ratings in adult psychiatric outpatients. *J Neuropsychiatry Clin Neurosci* 1993; 5: 301–6.

131 Terr AI. Multiple chemical sensitivities (editorial). *Ann Intern Med* 1993; 119: 163–4.

132 Terr AI. Psychoimmunology and the practice of allergy. *Clin Exp Allergy* 1995; 25: 483–4.

133 Ursin H. Sensitization, somatization, and subjective health complaints. *Int J Behav Med* 1997; 4: 105–16.

134 van den Bergh O, Kempynck PJ, van de Woestijne KP, Baeyens F, Eelen P. Respiratory learning and somatic complaints: a conditioning approach using CO_2-enriched air inhalation. *Behav Res Therapy* 1995; 33: 517–27.

135 van den Bergh O, Stegen K, Van de Woestijne KP. Learning to have psychosomatic complaints: conditioning of respiratory behavior and somatic complaints in psychosomatic patients. *Psychosom Med* 1997; 59: 13–23.

136 Vaughan WT, Sullivan CJ. On possibility of allergic factor in essential hypertension. *J Allergy* 1937; 8: 573.

137 von Euler G, Ogren SO, Li XM, Fuxe K, Gustafsson JA. Persistent effects of subchronic toluene exposure on spatial learning and memory, dopamine-mediated locomotor activity and dopamine D2 agonist binding in the rat. *Toxicology* 1993; 77: 223–32.

138 vonEuler G, Ogren S, Eneroth P, Fuxe K, Gustafsson J. Persistent effects of 80 ppm toluene on dopamine-regulated locomotor activity and prolactin secretion in the male rat. *Neurotoxicology* 1994; 15: 621–4.

139 Wallis RM, Nicol WD, Craig M. The importance of protein hypersensitivity in the diagnosis and treatment of a special group of epileptics. *Lancet* 1923; i: 741–3.

140 Wang Z, Valdes J, Noyes R, Zoega T, Crowe RR. Possible association of a cholecystokinin promotor polymorphism (CCK-36CT) with panic disorder. *Am J Med Genetics* 1998; 81: 228–34.

141 Warner JO. Food and behavior. *Clin Exp Allergy* 1995; 25(Suppl 1): 23–6.

142 Weilberg JB, Schacter S, Worth J *et al.* EEG abnormalities in patients with atypical panic attacks. *J Clin Psychiatry* 1995; 56: 358–62.

143 Wells AS, Read NW, Uvnas-Moberg K, Alster P. Influences of fat and carbohydrate on postprandial sleepiness, mood, and hormones. *Physiol Behav* 1997; 61: 679–86.

144 Weiss B, Williams JH, Margen S *et al.* Behavioral response to artificial food colors. *Science* 1980; 207: 1487–9.

145 Woods SC. The eating paradox: how we tolerate food. *Psychol Rev* 1991; 98: 488–505.

146 Yang Y, Sun C, Sun M. The effect of moderately increased CO_2 concentration on perception of coherent motion. *Aviation Space Environ Med* 1997; 68: 187–91.

Chapter

48

Psychological aspects of food intolerance

David S. King

INTRODUCTION

Food effects upon subjective states such as mood or cognitive functioning have long been anecdotally reported, but have also been a vexing source of controversy on several fronts in recent decades. Scientific issues at times may have been intertwined with the polarizing effects of professional differences in viewpoints, testing methods, and treatment modalities. Ideally, all such concerns should be resolved by properly controlled research, but such resolution has not been forthcoming because of inconsistent research findings, limited numbers of well-controlled studies, and the inherent difficulty of conducting double-blind experiments with food, particularly when assessing 'soft' symptoms such as subjective discomfort or dysphoria rather than skin wheals or wheezing. As such, the question of psychological effects of food intolerance (that is, food-mediated effects on brain functioning) falls at the interface of allergy and the behavioural sciences.

Clinical practice in medicine, as in clinical psychology, is not always guided by the results of controlled research. Clinical judgement must be exercised, especially when there is a lack of an adequate body of controlled research.

The dilemma of novel treatments

Similarly, a dilemma may emerge with the appearance of novel treatments with only anecdotal or clinical experience evidence for support. Does the clinician rely on the perhaps equally untested old clinical wisdom, or the new?

Therefore, in areas with little scientific foundation and in which practitioners hold widely divergent opinions, it is difficult to ascertain who is right and who is wrong, despite the conviction with which beliefs are espoused.

Hyperactivity caused by food intolerance?

In recent years, several major reviews have examined the evidence concerning the psychological effects of food intoler-

D

ance. In a position paper, Bruijnzeel-Koomen et al.[2] concluded both that 'there is no convincing evidence that hyperreactivity' [hyperactivity?] is caused by an adverse food reaction and that 'there is no convincing evidence of an IgE-mediated relationship between the intake of food and hyperreactivity, ... depression' and other listed symptoms, despite two significant clinical trials from the Hospital for Sick Children in Great Ormond Street. In contrast, another report concluded that '[t]he relationship between food and behaviour is a contentious issue and clearly there can be a link',[3] and called for additional careful research. A recent National Institutes of Health[8] consensus conference on the diagnosis and treatment of attention deficit hyperactivity disorder concluded that '[s]ome of the dietary elimination strategies showed intriguing results' and also called for more research.

The validity of testing methods for food intolerance

Major reviews have focused on food testing methods and their validity. The shaky scientific basis for controversial tests of food intolerance such as sublingual testing is often noted, as is appropriate. However, it is important that all testing techniques be judged by identical standards of validity. Terr[27] states that, in contrast to controversial techniques which he reviewed, 'the oral double-blind placebo-controlled food challenge test' is a 'reliable, well-standardized' technique that uses 'specified objective physical measurements or observations', although no references are provided. Pearson[25] stated that capsule challenge 'has been found to be reliable and reproducible' and cites five papers. Unfortunately, it is not clear that the papers support this conclusion, and problems with some of the studies have been discussed elsewhere.[17]

A tale of two studies

Consider the experiments of Jewett et al.[12] and Bernstein et al.,[1] both of which were published in prestigious journals. The two studies also bear a number of conceptual similarities: In both studies, patients with alleged food sensitivities were challenged under double-blind conditions (intradermal injection by Jewett et al.,[12] capsule challenge by Bernstein et al.[1]). In both studies placebo controls were employed and no statistically significant difference was found between the 'actives' and the placebos overall (in Bernstein et al.[1], responses occurred to 28% of the foods, and to 27% of the placebos). At this point, the studies diverge. In the case of the Jewett et al.[12] study, an accompanying editorial concluded, 'Thus, this diagnostic technique and neutralization procedure ... are in fact based on a placebo response'.[10] However, in the case of the Bernstein et al. study,[1] it was instead concluded that double-blind capsule challenge 'is an effective test of adult food sensitivity...'.

Diametrically opposed conclusions

Although differences between the experiments are present, it is clear that strikingly divergent conclusions were drawn from essentially identical results. If Jewett et al.[12] had applied the other study's logic to their findings, they would have concluded that intradermal testing was effective because positive responses did occur on food challenges. If Bernstein et al.[14] had applied the other study's logic to their results, they would have concluded that capsule challenges are based on a placebo response. In fact, neither sweeping conclusion is justified by a single study.

The problem of both positions and negative study findings

Negative findings can present difficulties in scientific inference. A myriad of mistakes, omissions, or even bad luck can produce negative findings which do not necessarily disprove the hypothesis in question. Conversely, positive findings must also be regarded with caution. The editorial[10], cited above also stated that

> [I]f the trial [Jewett et al.] had produced positive evidence that symptoms could be reproduced by the injection provocation technique, it would have obliged those of us in clinical science to accept the entity of multiple food (and environmental) sensitivity...

Oddly, King[15] did obtain positive evidence of sublingual testing producing cognitive and emotional symptoms above placebo levels, but was not cited by the author as 'obliging acceptance' with regard to food sensitivity. The more general problem of food test reliability and validity has been addressed in some detail.[17]

This chapter focuses on several issues that may have made the reaching of clear findings regarding the psychological aspects of food intolerance difficult. These include statistical power; perceptions and beliefs about food effects; and other methodological problems in research. My colleagues and I have conducted several studies that are summarized below.

METHODOLOGIC AND STATISTICAL ISSUES

Psychological symptoms

Because psychological states tend to vary naturally for a variety of reasons, attribution to food challenges may require statistical tests to rule out alternative explanations for reported changes. To establish the existence of a phenomenon such as cognitive or emotional changes caused by food in patients intolerant to a food, double-blind research is essential.

Science explicitly adopts the principle that if error is to occur, it is much better to err that no effect is present when this is incorrect than to falsely find that an effect is present when in truth it is not. Statistically speaking, with the conventional 0.05 probability level, this means that when no effect is present in nature, there is only a 5% chance that the null hypothesis will be falsely rejected. A correct decision (when there is not an effect in nature) is made 95 times out of 100; thus, the likelihood of error is relatively small under this assumption. Thus, all things being equal, 95% of experiments of food effects would be negative if no such effect truly exists. Perhaps contrary to intuition, a 50/50 split among well-controlled experiments or even a plurality of negative results does not indicate that no effect exists in nature. When no effect is present, chance would produce approximately only one significant finding for 20 identical studies.

Negative results do not cancel out positive findings

Two conclusions can be considered. One is that negative results do not cancel out positive findings in a boxscore tally approach. The best way to demonstrate this and to statistically evaluate divergent research findings is to use a meta-analysis. Excellent references on this subject are available.[22,26]

A second implication is that the difference between statistical significance and effect size must be remembered when evaluating a body of research. Statistical significance indicates nothing more than that the evidence is considered sufficient to reject the null hypothesis of no effect of foods or whatever the variable is under study. It is not directly related to the equally important question of the size and clinical relevance of the effect supported by the statistically significant finding.

With a large effect size, very few subjects would be required to obtain statistical significance. In contrast, a study of 10,000 allergy patients receiving drug Y and 10,000 allergy patients receiving placebo could well find a statistically significant effect, but be useless in clinical practice. The drug might have a real but trivial impact on allergy symptoms; although present, the improvement in symptoms might be so slight (e.g., one fewer sneeze per day) as to be not worth the trouble to take the medication.

Several key variables affect statistical power. These include the size of the effect present and the number of subjects studied. An excellent discussion of this problem as well as statistical power in general is found in Cohen.[5]

Is power generally good or poor in investigations of the psychological effects of foods? No single answer is possible, because the determination of statistical power is partially related to assumptions.

In the question of whether or not foods can have psychological effects in those intolerant of them, statistical power is a critical issue in evaluating experiments with negative outcomes, because the possibility of falsely failing to find an effect must be considered.

Statistical power and effect size

In Table 48.1, statistical power for various combinations of assumptions is provided from Cohen,[5] and Table 48.2 is derived from the same source. In the tables, d is a metric used by Cohen to indicate the effect size under investigation. Thus, $d = 0.2$ would indicate a small effect size; $d = 0.5$ is a medium effect size; and $d = 0.8$ indicates a large effect size in the behavioural sciences. As Cohen notes, a small effect size in the behavioural sciences would correspond to the difference in mean height between 15- and 16-year-old girls (about 0.5 inches). A medium effect size ($d = 0.5$) would be exemplified by the difference in mean IQ between semiskilled labourers and clerical workers (approximately 8 IQ points) or in mean height between 14- and 18-year-old girls (about 1 inch). Cohen states that, in general, medium effect sizes should be discernible to the naked eye. In addition, according to Cohen, a large effect size ($d = 0.8$) is

Statistical power for different effect sizes*			
n	d = 0.20	d = 0.50	d = 0.80
8	7	15	31
10	7	18	39
20	9	33	69
30	12	47	86
80	24	88	>99

* n = Number of each group; α= 0.05, two-tailed t test.

Table 48.1 Statistical power for different effect sizes.* (By permission of the author and publisher from Cohen J.[5]).

Statistical power for different effect sizes (repeated measures)*			
d	n	r = 0.4	r = 0.6	r = 0.8
0.20	8	8	9	14
	10	9	11	17
	20	13	17	31
	30	17	23	44
	80	38	52	85
0.50	8	23	30	54
	10	28	38	65
	20	52	68	98
	30	70	85	>99
	80	98	>99	>99
0.80	8	48	64	>73
	10	58	75	>84
	20	88	97	>99
	30	>99	>99	>99
	80	>99	>99	>99

* n = Number of paired scores, α = 0.05, two-tailed t test for paired observations. When n < 25, power may be overestimated. Linear interpolation was used.

Table 48.2 Statistical power for different effect sizes (repeated measures)*. (Derived by permission of the author and publisher from Cohen.[5])

'grossly perceptible' and could be illustrated by the difference in mean IQ between PhDs and college freshmen.

Let us assume that Dr Smith wishes to rigorously test the possibility that foods can cause psychological effects in those intolerant of certain foods. We will ignore the complexities of most aspects of the design and focus on her decision to use two groups, randomly assigned for a double-blind, placebo-controlled challenge experiment. A t test will be used to compare mean scores on her measure of psychological effects, whatever it may be, between the food and placebo groups. If foods have no effect in nature, we know that there is only a 5% chance that she will falsely observe a statistically significant difference between the two groups. But Dr Smith, being aware of statistical power and its relation to sample size, wonders how many patients should be included in her study to ensure a reasonable probability of being able to detect a real world effect in her experiment, assuming it exists. She consults Cohen,[5] and finds power analysis functions such as provided in Table 48.1. The table shows that if food effects are small ($d = 0.2$) in her study and if 8 or even 10 patients are included in each group, there is only a 7% chance that she will find a genuine effect. In other words, since there is a 93% probability of a mistake being made if an effect is 'real' and small, there would be no point in conducting the experiment.

D

The value of negative findings

Clearly, the negative findings likely to occur would be of virtually no value in publishing (they could have some limited use in a meta-analysis when combined with the findings of larger studies which would carry more weight in the analysis), and would convey a serious risk of being misinterpreted as proving that foods cannot cause psychological symptoms. As Table 48.1 illustrates, increasing the sample size per group to 30 only provides a 12% probability of correctly detecting a genuine effect; with a larger effect size (0.5), the probability is still 53% that a genuine effect will be missed. In the repeated measures case (each patient receives a placebo and a food), power can be enhanced, although the correlation between each patient's two scores must be included. Table 48.2 provides power characteristics under different assumptions of intercorrelation and sample size.

The difficulty of drawing potentially false conclusions from negative statistical findings was highlighted by Cohen:[5]

> Research reports in the literature are frequently flawed by conclusions that state or imply that the null hypothesis is true. For example, following the finding that the difference between two sample means is not statistically significant, instead of properly concluding from this failure to reject the null hypothesis that the data do not warrant the conclusion that the population means differ, the writer concludes, at least implicitly, that there is *no* difference. The latter conclusion is always strictly invalid, and is functionally invalid as well unless power is high.

PERCEPTIONS AND BELIEFS ABOUT PSYCHOLOGICAL AND BEHAVIOURAL EFFECTS OF FOODS

Self-reporting of symptoms

A crucial variable in selecting adults or children for participation in double-blind research on possible psychological and behavioural effects of foods is self-reporting of such effects (or, for children, reporting by a parent). Occasionally, physician reports of sensitivity or intolerance are used. In all cases, statistical power and the validity of conclusions may depend on how trustworthy this reporting is. Consider the following hypothetical scenario:

> An elderly patient tells her physician that she has trouble with her memory. He responds, 'OK, you have Alzheimer's disease' and prescribes Aricept (donepezil hydrochloride).

Clearly, such a simple-minded approach to diagnosis is unacceptable, since a multitude of factors may explain the patient's complaint other than Alzheimer's disease. Self-report of memory difficulty is not assumed to be *veridical* with regard to actual level of memory functioning. Some patients with memory complaints may have normal functioning, and other individuals may have a decline in memory without their awareness. Thus, in the case of self-reported memory functioning, as with self-reported food intolerance, objective reality may or may not correlate with subjective report.

With regard to research, consider the following scenario:

> To study Alzheimer's disease, a researcher advertises for elderly persons who have memory problems. He compares 10 such individuals to 10 others without such complaints on a standard memory test. No statistically significant difference is found

between the two groups. Many of the patients with memory complaints were found to be depressed. Psychological testing revealed others to have results compatible with a possible conversion disorder. The researcher concludes that Alzheimer's disease has no organic basis, and is probably psychogenic in origin.

The scenarios, of course, are ludicrous, and the errors of logic are obvious. Yet, similar scenarios and errors of logic can be found in clinical research on food intolerance, particularly with regard to psychological and behavioural effects. For example, patients are selected for inclusion in studies of the psychological effects of foods solely on the basis of their claim that they have such effects. No screening is performed; it is as if all patients are assumed to be alike and equally trustworthy and accurate in their self-report.

Is self-reporting of food intolerance accurate?

Are people accurate in their self-report of food effects upon themselves? A mail survey of college students at a large university in the northeastern United States showed widespread belief that food can affect behaviour and psychological states.[21] The survey examined students' general beliefs about food effects on cognition, affect, and behaviour as well as the effects of foods on themselves specifically. Results were provocative and bear upon the issue of using only self-report of food intolerance to select patients for controlled experiments.

The results showed that most students tended to endorse items that suggested that foods can have behavioural effects. For example, a large majority reported believing that sugar can cause or aggravate hyperactivity (89% strongly agree or agree). Similarly, students reported believing that food allergy or food sensitivity could cause or aggravate depression (74%), irritability (85%), fatigue (83%), anxiety/tension (73%), and difficulty in thinking clearly (71%). In contrast, a minority (44%) endorsed the belief that sleepiness or drowsiness can be caused by sugar consumption. Only 24% reported a belief that food dyes could cause or aggravate hyperactivity.

In regard to perceived personal effects of foods, responses to sugar were queried. The results of the statement 'Sugar affects how I feel,' are shown in Fig 48.1. Eighty percent of the respond-

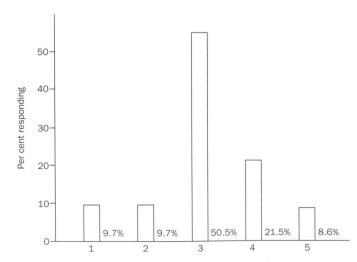

Fig. 48.1 Per cent responding to the statement: 'Sugar affects how I feel.' 1 = never; 3 = sometimes; 5 = always.

ents said that sugar intake affected them at some time or other. Of the sample, 37% indicated that a food other than sugar, caffeine, or alcohol affected them behaviourally. On an open-ended item with symptom checklists for foods listed by participants, most respondents who listed such a food provided only one. Some listed foods were difficult to categorize (e.g., Chinese food or 'fatty, sugary foods'), but responses included beef or other meats (8%), milk or dairy products (7%), starchy foods/grains/pasta (5%), fruits (5%), beans (3%), other vegetables (3%), MSG (3%), Nutrasweet (2%), shellfish/seafood (2%), nuts (2%), chocolate (1%) saccharine (1%), and turkey (1%).

Frequency of symptoms reported for sugar and other foods

Table 48.3 lists reported symptom frequencies for food effects in oneself, both for sugar and for the listed other food item, if any. Percentages refer to proportion of entire sample, not just those who reported a food symptom. The most frequently reported

effect of sugar was euphoric/high (39.4%), which evokes the popular stereotype of sugar acting as a stimulant. However, when symptoms were ranked by the size of their correlation with the student's reported frequency of response to sugar, a different pattern emerged. A symptom with high positive correlation indicated that frequent responders reported the symptom more than those claiming infrequent response to sugar. From data shown in Table 48.4, the symptom with the largest correlation with frequency of sugar response was fatigue ($r = 0.43$).

These correlations suggest that those individuals who reported more frequent reactions to sugar were more likely to attribute fatigue than euphoria to sugar consumption.

A breakdown of the proportion checking fatigue as a response to sugar by the reported frequency of their response to sugar confirmed that this was the case. A linear trend was apparent, with 88% of those who reported always being affected by sugar indicating that sugar caused them to feel fatigue, whereas only

Table 48.3 Frequency of symptoms reported for sugar and for other foods.

Frequency of symptoms reported for sugar and for other foods			
Sugar (n = 94)		**Other foods (n = 95)**	
Symptom	**Frequency (%)**	**Symptom**	**Frequency (%)**
Euphoric/high	39.4	Bloated stomach	15.8
Happy	36.2	Cramps	11.6
Headaches	36.2	Intestinal gas	11.6
Anxiety/tension	35.1	Fatigue	11.6
Fatigue	31.9	Headaches	9.5
Moody	28.7	Irritability	7.4
Irritability	26.6	Difficulty in thinking clearly	4.2
Difficulty in thinking clearly	22.3	Moody	4.2
Depression	18.1	Diarrhoea	4.2
Bloated stomach	18.1	Other	4.2
Cramps	12.8	Anxiety/tension	3.2
Intestinal gas	10.6	Calm	3.2
Diarrhoea	10.6	Constipation	3.2
Anger/aggression	8.5	Depression	3.2
Other	8.5	Nasal symptoms	3.2
Skin disorder	7.4	Skin disorder	3.2
Calm	7.4	Anger/aggression	2.1
Constipation	4.3	Happy	2.1
Asthma	2.1	Euphoric/high	1.1
Nasal symptoms	1.1	Asthma	0

Symptom correlation with sugar intake	
Fatigue $r = 0.43$	Moody $r = 0.36$
Depression $r = 0.34$	Happy $r = 0.32$
Anxious $r = 0.31$	Headache $r = 0.30$
Euphoric/high $r = 0.29$	

Table 48.4 Symptom correlation with sugar intake.

11% of respondents who marked '2' (between 'never' and 'sometimes') did so.

Dietary alterations and clinical response

When asked about dietary alterations, 68% of the sample reported that they had either eliminated or reduced consumption of a food. Because open-ended responses were permitted, more than one food could be listed by a respondent. Those reducing or eliminating foods listed sweets, candy or sugar (22%); meat (21%); fried or other fatty foods (21%); milk or other dairy products (8%); salt (4%); and alcohol (3%). Other responses listed specific foods, food additives, or unclassifiable items. Students reported that the following symptoms improved as a result of a dietary reduction or elimination: intestinal gas (24%), bloated stomach (23%), fatigue (23%), irritability (21%), anxiety or tension (19%), cramps (19%), and headache (18%).

Although a portion of these reported symptoms suggest recognized mechanisms such as lactose intolerance, others (e.g., fatigue, irritability, and anxiety or tension) are not generally recognized as being directly produced by food intolerance. Even if veridical, such symptoms could also reflect non-direct mechanisms. Double-blind research is essential to sort things out, but it remains of importance that relatively high rates of reported symptoms were found in the general student population.

These findings suggest two possibilities: either the students are correct, and a high rate of food intolerance (including food intolerance which results in psychological symptoms) exists in the general population; or self-reporting of food intolerance is unreliable and overreported to an unknown but substantial degree. Either possibility has important implications for research on this topic.

The relation of demographic characteristics to respondents' tendency to believe that foods can influence behaviour was explored by correlating these factors with a total score on the general food belief questionnaire. A significant relation was found between such belief and years of education (r (89) = −0.38, $P < 0.001$) such that the higher the level of education, the greater the tendency to report beliefs that foods affect behaviour. A linear trend in this belief was apparent across years of undergraduate education, and graduate students as a group scored significantly higher in such belief than undergraduates (t (89) = 3.42, $P = 0.001$). In contrast, belief in food effects was not significantly related to gender, parental social class, or race.

A skew distribution of results?

Given that the return rate was 41%, the likelihood that the results may have been biased must be considered. That is, individuals who tended to believe in a relation between food and behaviour may have been more likely to complete and return the survey, whereas skeptics discarded it (wastebasket bias). Under such conditions, the proportion of students found to endorse items concerning food–behaviour links would be distorted upward, and the findings could not be generalized to similar populations.

Even if the extreme case was assumed, and results were computed as if every nonrespondent had disagreed with the items on the general food questionnaire, instead of 89% of respondents reporting a belief that sugar can affect hyperactivity, the corresponding figure under the wastebasket hypothesis is 36% (95% confidence interval = 0.30 to 0.45). In contrast, between 6% and 14% of the respondents would endorse a relation between hyperactivity and food dyes or colourings.

Effect of age and education

In regard to personal symptoms, under these assumptions, 30–43% of the respondents believe that sugar has had an effect on how they have felt. These analyses suggest that assuming the most extreme possible bias does not alter the conclusion that substantial portions of the student population believe that diet influences behaviour in sensitive or allergic people and in themselves by producing psychological symptoms. This conservative analysis suggests that belief in personal reactions to foods appears to be pervasive in the student population and therefore cannot simply be ascribed to psychopathology. The finding that college freshmen are the most skeptical about food reactions, whereas graduate students express the strongest belief in them, is also difficult to reconcile with the view that such a belief reflects psychopathology. These data are comparable to other studies.[23] For example, McLoughlin & Nall[23] found no apparent difference between undergraduate and graduate students in rate of agreement about behavioural effects of foods, but graduate students tended to *disagree* less often than undergraduates that foods could have such effects in children.

The results suggest that reliance on self-report of behavioural response to a food or foods alone is a potentially weak strategy for research on this topic because, assuming that it is improbable that such a large proportion of the population has a response to sugar or other foods of this nature, nonresponders will be admitted to the study. In addition, physiological food intolerances cannot account for the education effect observed in this survey: either students become more aware of their actual food intolerances as they progress in their education, or social processes occur, leading to apparent misattributions of behavioural responses to foods in oneself. Another possibility not ruled out by the data is that sceptics drop out of school at a higher rate than students who believe in food reactions.

RESEARCH ON PSYCHOLOGICAL EFFECTS OF FOODS

In a study by King,[15] 30 adult patients received a total of 720 trials in a double-blind experiment that examined the cognitive and emotional effects of sublingual extracts on patients who reported such symptoms. Patients were not known by pretesting to be sensitive to the substances with which they were challenged, resulting in no response on 41% of the 'active' challenges. Also, sublingual provocative testing uses small doses. To the extent that an increasing dose–response curve applies to food intolerance reactions, the use of sublingual food challenges would tend (even in sensitive individuals) to produce a smaller effect size overall than normal meal-sized portions. Reliability and validity issues regarding sublingual provocative testing have been discussed elsewhere.[17]

The experiment included four conditions:

- a baseline condition to assess spontaneous symptoms;
- a screening condition to assess possible sensitivity to the placebo itself;
- a placebo condition;
- an 'allergen' or test substance condition.

Selected results are shown in Tables 48.5 and 48.6,[16] which show numbers of self-reported symptoms for double-blind trials

(trials considered suspicious for placebo awareness by any of several means were omitted in these analyses).

The primary findings

These were that even with quite conservative analyses, cognitive–emotional symptoms were significantly more frequent on 'active' trials than placebo trials, suggesting that the food and chemical extracts administered were causally responsible for producing such symptoms under double-blind conditions. That the analyses were quite conservative was made clear in Table 48.6. In this case, clearly somatic or physical symptoms reported on

Subject	Allergen	Placebo	Base rate	Screening
	Mean number of cognitive–emotional symptoms per trial (double-blind trials only)			
1	0.25	0.17	0.00	0.00
2	0.27	0.00	0.67	0.00
3	0.17	0.00	0.00	0.00
4	0.50	0.00	0.00	0.00
5	0.18	0.00	0.00	0.00
6	0.00	0.00	0.00	0.00
7	1.70	1.00	0.67	0.67
8	0.20	0.33	0.00	0.00
9	0.17	0.00	0.00	0.00
10	0.36	0.20	0.00	0.33
11	0.45	0.00	0.00	0.00
12	0.83	0.20	0.67	0.00
13	0.08	0.00	0.00	0.00
14	0.00	0.17	0.00	0.00
15	0.11	0.00	0.00	0.00
16	0.25	0.00	0.00	0.00
17	0.25	0.00	0.00	0.00
18	0.25	0.00	0.00	0.00
19	0.56	0.17	0.00	0.00
20	0.08	0.17	0.33	0.00
21	0.58	0.00	0.00	0.00

Allergen > placebo ($N = 20$, $x = 4$, $P = 0.006$).
Placebo = base rate.
Base rate = screening.

Table 48.5 Mean number of cognitive–emotional symptoms per trial (double-blind trials only). (Reproduced by permission of the editor and publisher from King.[16])

Subject	Allergen	Placebo	Base rate	Screening
	Mean number of somatic symptoms per trial (double-blind trials only)			
1	2.17	1.83	0.00	0.33
2	0.09	0.33	0.00	0.00
3	0.17	0.17	0.33	0.00
4	0.92	0.20	0.00	0.00
5	0.00	0.00	0.00	0.00
6	0.33	1.17	0.000	0.33
7	0.58	1.00	0.33	0.67
8	0.60	0.50	0.33	0.00
9	0.17	0.25	0.00	0.00
10	0.27	0.00	0.00	0.00
11	0.45	0.17	0.00	0.33
12	0.17	0.00	0.00	0.00
13	1.17	1.0	0.00	1.00
14	0.00	0.00	0.00	0.00
15	0.56	0.50	0.00	0.00
16	0.00	1.00	0.33	0.33
17	0.00	0.00	0.00	0.00
18	0.08	0.00	0.00	0.67
19	2.89	0.33	0.67	0.00
20	0.00	0.00	0.00	0.00
21	0.58	0.00	0.00	0.00

Allergen = placebo (NS, $P = 0.105$).
Placebo > base rate ($N = 13$, $x = 2$, $P = 0.011$).
Base rate = screening.

Table 48.6 Mean number of somatic symptoms per trial (double-blind trials only). (Reproduced by permission of the editor and publisher from King.[16])

'active' trials did not reach statistical significance compared with placebo trials. Placebo somatic symptoms were, however, in excess of baseline levels ($P < 0.02$). This pattern indicates, that patients were reporting physical symptoms in association with receiving placebos at a higher rate than in baseline periods, and did not report them at detectably higher levels on 'active' trials. This would further suggest that placebo awareness could not account for these results.

Interpretation of the negative somatic/physical response to sublingual testing

Although several interpretations could be offered for this negative result, it does suggest that sublingual testing of this type cannot distinguish between somatic symptoms provoked by a test substance and somatic symptoms due to placebo influences above baseline variability in the individual case. As shown in the study by King,[15] statistically significant differences overall did appear for cognitive–emotional symptoms and for 'mixed' symptoms. When only numbers of symptoms were considered, combined symptoms of all types did not differ from placebo levels, while placebo levels were significantly increased over baseline scores. Again, it is difficult to reconcile this finding with the argument that patients were not blind in an attempt to discount the findings for cognitive–emotional symptoms. The negative findings for somatic symptoms do not prove that such symptoms cannot be provoked by sublingual testing: they suggest that either the effect is nonexistent or that the effect size is too small to be detected with the experiment's level of statistical power. Statistical power was adequate for the larger effect size demonstrated by cognitive–emotional symptoms. In the somatic analysis, the effect size for the placebo was greater than the effect size for test substances (which could not be reliably distinguished from zero effect size).

One way to enhance statistical power is to increase the sensitivity of measures. Increased sensitivity in this case was attempted by examining the severity of symptom ratings as well as the number of symptoms reported. This analysis produced much the same pattern as for numbers of symptoms, except that, now, overall symptom scores did significantly differentiate between test substances and placebos. Somatic scores still did not differ significantly for test substances and placebos. It is likely that the increased statistical power of including severity ratings showed in the total symptom score grouping becoming significant.

Double-blind study of sublingual testing for food intolerance in children

To further explore the possible behavioural effects of foods upon selected individuals, a follow-up study was conducted.[19] (see also Ref.14.) To eliminate concerns about blinding, a method in which sublingual doses of test substances were disguised in a prune juice base was developed and pretested for adequacy of blinding.

This study included 15 children (14 male, 1 female; age range 6–12 years) who had no known food sensitivity or any serious medical condition. (Another child was recruited but failed to appear for the experiment and was therefore excluded from the study.) The 19 food extracts in 50% glycerol base (Hollister-Stier, 1:10 w/v) were selected because of the food's common occurrence in children's diets and are shown in Table 48.7.

Each child received 19 pairs of sublingual doses, and each pair represented one food. Dose pairs were administered in an individually randomized sequence by using a random number table

The 19 food extracts tested double blind in 15 children		
Beef	Fish	Potato
Chicken	Milk	Rice
Chocolate	Oats	Soybeans
Cola	Oranges	Sugar (beet and cane)
Corn	Peanut	Tomato
Egg	Pork	Wheat
Yeast (combined baker's and brewer's)		

Concentrated prune juice was used as diluent and placebo.

Table 48.7 The 19 food extracts tested double blind in 15 children.

and were of four possible types: food–food, food–placebo, placebo–food, and placebo–placebo. For each food, sets of four children were randomly assigned to receive the four pair types. Thus, each child received a random order of food pairs and a random type of pair for each food test.

Children were tested individually and were told that they would receive 'squirts of food' under the tongue. Some squirts would be just prune juice, while others would be prune juice mixed with another food. A written list of the 19 possible other foods was shown to each child and was read as needed to the one or two children who had difficulty reading. After receiving each dose, the child guessed whether it was prune juice or prune juice mixed with another food. All doses were expectorated after 15 seconds.

There was no significant correlation between dose order and accuracy, defined as correctly guessing the dose identity as prune juice or prune juice with an added food ($r = -0.02$).

More importantly, several analyses showed no evidence of discernible taste differences among the test doses as the median number of correct identifications of a food extract was 0. Further, a Pearson correlation between whether the child guessed the dose to be some food or just prune juice and the actual identity of the dose was nonsignificant ($r = 0.04$), nor could the children discern whether a pair of doses was the same or different ($r = 0.08$).

Overall, the blinding of the sublingual food doses with prune juice was successful in children.

Effect on behaviour of sublingual challenge with food

In the second phase of this project, 122 children were screened for behavioural response to a food under double-blind conditions. All were reported to have a behavioural reaction to a food, none had a serious medical illness, and none was taking daily prescribed medication.

Screening tests

On the basis of parental reports, up to five foods were selected for double-blind sublingual screening tests with placebo controls. In the screening procedure, each sublingual food dose was paired with placebo in random sequence. After each 10-min test period, the blinded experimenter globally rated both behavioural change and somatic symptom/sign change on 10-point scales based on observation and the self-report of the child. If a rating showed greater behavioural change on a food trial than in its paired placebo trial, the child was eligible to enter the experimental phase with that test food.

Experimental phase

The 24 children (17 male, 7 female) who participated in the experimental phase were 5.5–13 years old (median age, 8 years). On the Conners' Abbreviated Parent Questionnaire,[6] 8 of the 22 children for whom ratings were obtained scored 15 or higher, indicating that at least one-third of the sample were in the attention deficit/hyperactivity disorder range on this instrument.

The children were randomly assigned to receive a double-blind sequence of six sublingual doses, consisting of three identical doses of their test food and three doses of placebo. The foods used were beet or cane sugar, oranges, milk, peanuts, egg, beef, bakers' and brewers' yeast, tomato, cola, chocolate, wheat, and pork. The protocol for each trial is shown in Table 48.8.

Each trial lasted about 15 min. Ten-minute washout (play) periods followed each trial. A parent behind a one-way mirror made behavioural ratings after each trial, as did two blind judges, who later independently viewed videotapes of the trials after training. Judges rated global behavioural change (from before the dose), global somatic symptom/sign change, and guessed whether the dose was a test food or a placebo. Confidence in their guess was rated on a 10-point scale. Inter-rater reliability was $r = 0.56$ for behavioural change ratings and $r = 0.53$ for somatic change ratings. Interestingly, there was no relation between parental ratings (behavioural and somatic) and judges' ratings, either individually or averaged together. This might suggest a lack of validity for parent ratings overall in this study.

Results of sublingual challenge

Heart rate

After 1 min of sitting quietly before the first dose, heart rate did not differ for test foods and placebos. However, it was significantly higher on test food trials than on placebo trials for the 2-min postdose recording period, reflecting a mean increase of 1.6 beats/min ($P = 0.014$). Heart rate did not differ at the end of the trial.

Heart rate variability (standard deviation of six scores during the 1-min period) showed no difference for foods and placebos before the dose or at the end of the trial. At the 2-min postdose point, there was a significant interaction effect ($P = 0.034$), which was due to a slight suppression of heart rate variability on the second food dose as compared with the second placebo dose ($P = 0.055$).

Continuous performance test score

CPT performance was assessed for mean reaction time for correct responses, reaction time variability, misses, and false-positive responses. Test foods did not affect reaction time or misses. Variability in reaction time displayed a trend to be greater on test food trials. A significant statistical interaction effect emerged for false-positive responses ($P < 0.03$). This complex finding showed that significantly fewer false-positive responses occurred on third food doses than for third placebo doses overall ($P = 0.006$), with no effect on other dose pairs of foods and placebos.

Fingertapping test

This test produced a pattern similar to that obtained for the CPT false-positive findings: a significant interaction effect ($P < 0.05$) was produced by the children tapping significantly more after receiving the third food dose than after receiving the third placebo dose ($P = 0.036$).

Judges' ratings

These ratings showed quite small averaged behavioural change scores overall (M = 1.03, SD = 1.06) and for somatic symptom/sign change (M = 0.49, SD = 0.80) on a scale where 0 indicated no change and 1 indicated very slight change. The judges' averaged behavioural ratings produced a significant statistical interaction effect ($P = 0.032$). Further analyses found that delayed behavioural responses may have been occurring, as well as suggesting cumulative dose effects for the test foods.

Cumulative dose effects may also have been present for second-dose foods and second placebos, although simple delayed responses, as for first food trials, cannot be excluded. Thus, it was found that children who received their second test food dose immediately after the first food dose displayed a significant increase in behavioural ratings ($P = 0.044$) as compared with the other children. Further, the 12 children who received adjacent first and second food doses had significantly higher behavioural change ratings for the second food dose than for the second placebo dose ($P = 0.02$). The post-hoc nature of these rating findings renders them tentative but provocative (no pun intended). Behavioural and somatic change ratings were not highly related ($r = 0.16$), and somatic change scores were low, as noted. Somatic change scores were not significantly related to test food doses.

Effect size ranking for individual foods was also examined. Although unstable because of small sample sizes, the highest scores were obtained for pork, chocolate, and tomato. Interestingly, sucrose was administered to seven children, but its effect size was nearly zero.

Conclusion

Thus, this experiment provides evidence for limited cardiac and behavioural effects of sublingual food challenges under double-blind conditions, but the effects were subtle. Larger doses of foods might provoke more clinically relevant reactions. Also of concern was the suggestive evidence of possible delayed behavioural responses to a test food. Further, there was no evidence in this small sample of large, unmistakable, and even catastrophic responses to sublingual food doses that were not found on placebo trials. Instead, statistical tests were necessary to detect findings. In other words, effect sizes for dependent measures were not large and obvious.

Further study with food challenges

The small effects observed in the above experiment, albeit with small dosages of foods, suggested that it would be desirable to

Experimental trial protocol
1. Heart rate reading preceding sublingual dose of test food/placebo
2. Heart rate reading continuous performance test (CPT); 5 min fingertapping of nondominant hand. Final heart rate reading

Table 48.8 Experimental trial protocol.

blind larger, ideally meal-sized portions of common foods for potentially larger, more clinically relevant effects in susceptible individuals.

Blind oral challenge development was undertaken at the facilities of the Nutrition Department at the University of California, Berkeley.[20] Individualized test food–placebo pairs were produced, although overlap in base ingredients was common. Preparations tended to have a gelatinous (pudding) consistency after chilling.

We were not able to blind adequate doses of such foods as peanut, banana, fish (cod/haddock), and cheese by any edible combination of ingredients. Metcalfe[24] reported similar difficulties with peanut and other foods. A common problem with masking these foods and others, such as cocoa or baker's/brewer's yeast, was a single taste or odour component that was resistant to masking. Sometimes an entirely new ingredient would then be effective; for example, cumin was found to obscure a persistent distinctive aftertaste for chicken. Contrary to our initial expectations, sucrose was not easy to disguise in the dose we wished to provide (67 g). We abandoned efforts to develop a beverage base and, instead, placed the sucrose in a pudding base, with fructose in the placebo to achieve equivalent sweetness.

Development of satisfactory active-placebo pairs for pretest in a pudding format was obtained for 15 test foods. Common base ingredients in the formulations were agar, anise oil, apricot concentrate, rice flour, tapioca flour, and water.

Were placebo and test food distinguishable?

A double-blind test was conducted over 2 days, with seven foods tested the first day (apple, chicken, cocoa, corn, milk, potato, yeast), and eight on the second (beef, egg, grape, orange, soy, sucrose, tomato, wheat). Each participant received an individually randomized sequence of test servings on each test day. Servings were given in randomly assigned pairs of 30 g doses. Each pair consisted of either a food–food, placebo–placebo, food–placebo, or placebo–food sequence.

After eating both samples, the participants guessed whether or not the serving contained the specified test food and rated their confidence that their guess was correct on a 5-point scale (1 = not at all confident, 5 = extremely confident). They then rated the taste of the pudding on an 11-point scale (1 = extremely unpleasant, 6 = neither pleasant nor unpleasant, 11 = extremely pleasant). After 10 min, the same procedure was followed for the second dose of the pair. However, after the guess certainty measure and before the taste rating, participants were also asked to guess whether the two servings in the pair were the same or different, and to rate the certainty of this guess. This procedure was repeated for each test pair.

Results showed no evidence of an order effect with regard to participant accuracy, suggesting that neither palate fatigue nor practice effects were present. Neither sex nor age was related to guess accuracy.

There was no overall relation between guessed dose identity (specified food present or not) and actual identity. Nor was there any significant correlation between guessed identity of a pair (same or different) and actual identity overall. Confidence was not related to accuracy.

The data for apple (Table 48.9) were significant on the guessed dose identity measure, suggesting that apple was not adequately blinded, despite our single-blind taster screen.

Accuracy of guesses on pretest, by food				
	Guessed dose identity (N = 58)		Guessed pair identity (N = 29)	
Food	**r**	**P**	**r**	**P**
Apple	0.43	0.001	–0.18	0.36
Beef	0.07	0.61	0.25	0.21
Chicken	–0.06	0.64	–0.22	0.26
Cocoa	–0.08	0.55	–0.16	0.42
Corn	0.03	0.82	0.03	0.88
Egg	–0.14	0.29	–0.02	0.91
Grape	–0.04	0.79	0.18	0.36
Milk	–0.04	0.76	0.38	0.04
Orange	0.07	0.61	0.24	0.21
Potato	0.26	0.051	–0.10	0.60
Soy	0.10	0.47	0.24	0.21
Sugar	0.00	0.99	–0.45	0.014
Tomato	0.13	0.32	0.10	0.60
Wheat	0.03	0.80	0.17	0.37
Yeast	–0.14	0.29	–0.17	0.38

Table 48.9 Accuracy of guesses on pretest, by food.

Milk showed an apparently significant effect for the pair measure, but participants were completely unable to identify which test puddings contained milk and which did not (P = 0.76). If not spurious, it is unclear how one would interpret this pattern, and its practical significance would probably be minimal.

Potato was of borderline significance for the guessed dose identity measure, with no suggestion of consistency for the pair measure, and produced an overall non-significant result (r = 0.19).

Sugar (sucrose) was clearly non-significant on the guessed dose identity measure.

Oral challenge with whole food formulations

The advantage of the oral challenge formulations developed here is that a reasonably large portion of the test food is given through the normal route of ingestion in a demonstrably blinded fashion.

Table 48.10 provides the blinded portions of test foods in the servings, along with the estimated number of capsules required to duplicate the dose, which, in any case, would be unacceptably large with most of the foods tested.

It remains true that any method of blinded oral challenge under research conditions requires rigorous verification of the adequacy of blinding. This would appear to require a food-by-food approach if there is any reason to believe that the foods differ to a significant extent in how easily they may be detected. Ideally, then, a method

Food mixture descriptions and capsule equivalents

Test food	Approximate typical serving	Serving in pudding	Comment	Weight of total mix* (g)	Calories	Dry content of food (%)	Food dose eqivalent in capsules
Beef	85 g	47	lean, cooked London broil	310	825	25	24–59
Cocoa	5.5 g – ?[†]	11		335	390	100	22–55
Corn	82 g	80	skin removed	330	810	25	40–100
Egg	50 g[‡]	60 g		330	900	25	
Grape	20 grapes = 100 g	100 g	strained	360	840	19	?
Milk	244 g	120 g	whole	470	920	13	33–83
Orange	121 g	80 g	medium, peeled, strained	345	865	14	19–47
Potato	156 g	67 g	baked, skin removed	300	745	20	27–68
Soy	?	13 g	flour	355	800	92	25–63
Sugar	5–100 g	100 g	50% cane/50% beet	315	870	99.5	133–331
Tomato	135 g	80 g	raw, strained	340	810	6	10–24
Wheat	28 g–?[§]	37 g	50% whole, 50% white flour	450	1030	88	66–165
Yeast	?	2 g bakers', 1 g brewers'		375	950	?	?

* Weight of total mix may vary by ±10 g because of slightly different evaporative or pan losses. This variation may result in calorie differences of about 1–3%.
† 1 cup hot cocoa = 5.5 g cocoa powder.
‡ 1 egg = 50 g.
§ 1 slice bread = 28 g.

Table 48.10 Food mixture descriptions and capsule equivalents.

of oral challenge would include data documenting both the success of the blinding and the ability of the technique to provoke symptoms (above placebo levels) in those known to be sensitive to the food.

If positive research findings are obtained, but the success of the double-blind study was not checked, results may be vulnerable to a placebo or even baseline variability explanation. Negative results may render success of the blinding moot. However, the analogous problem emerges of the negative findings possibly being due to too low a dose of test food or because the preparation is in some way inadequate to provoke symptoms, even in those truly sensitive to the food.

Psychological and behavioural responses to food challenge

In a follow-up study to the development of adequately blinded test foods, described above, adults were recruited for a double-blind experiment to investigate the psychological and behavioural responses to foods.[18] Adults reporting a psychological or behavioural reaction to a food or foods were recruited by means of advertisements and physician referral. Those with no medical contraindication for participation were provided a hypoallergenic diet to follow for 5 days before and during the subsequent screening phase of the project.

Double-blind screening test

Participants received one test dose daily of a test food or placebo mixture. Three test foods were selected for each participant on the basis of their self-report and dietary records. The three test foods and placebo were assigned to a random sequence for each participant. Dependent measures were self-report of symptoms with rated severity, self-ratings on the profile of mood states (POMS), and heart rate. The first two measures were collected before and 2 hours after consumption of the blinded feeding, while heart rate was measured periodically throughout the session.

Participants who apparently had a behavioural response to one of the test foods were admitted to the concurrent inpatient hospital phase of the project. In the double-blind, crossover design, they consumed three consecutive meals of either the relevant test food or placebo on Tuesday of their week-long stay (admission was on Friday), and either placebo or test food on Thursday. Dependent measures included self-report of symptoms with rated severity, POMS ratings, reaction time on a CPT, free recall of word lists, and heart rate. Measures were collected before each feeding, at 1 and 2 hours after each feeding, and on the morning after the feedings.

Analysis of findings

To analyse symptom reports, two blinded judges independently sorted all symptoms into cognitive–emotional or other (somatic) categories. They further differentiated somatic symptoms into gastrointestinal and other somatic symptoms. The latter sort was performed because true food allergy can produce such symptoms, and also to check on possible irritant properties of the base ingredients. The screening phase was completed by 57 participants, 15 of whom finished the hospital phase. Although we were well aware of statistical power considerations, budgetary restrictions unfortunately prevented the acquisition of a larger sample for inpatient study.

Results were analysed for both phases as separate studies using MANOVA or univariate repeated-measures analysis of variance (with Huynh–Feldt adjusted degrees of freedom). In the hospital study, comparisons of test food and placebo-dependent measures produced no statistically significant differences. However, a statistically significant effect for day (first test day *versus* second test day) was found for symptom scores, POMS, and reaction time, such that scores were elevated generally on the first day. This finding suggests that participants were in a different psychological state for the initial hospital test day, perhaps because of factors such as anxiety, excitement, or heightened arousal. Whatever the nonspecific basis for this finding, it indicates that a 'first-day' effect produced demonstrably non-comparable psychological states for the 2 test days.

Gastrointestinal symptom scores

Despite the small sample size, another puzzling finding emerged. Gastrointestinal symptom scores showed a significant statistical interaction effect, indicating that scores differed for participants in the two test orders (i.e. active, placebo *versus* placebo, active) over the repeated measures, regardless of whether a test food or placebo had been consumed. This might suggest that, despite random assignment, participants in the two orders of testing differed in some way. Because the order of test food first, placebo second reported more gastrointestinal symptoms overall than the reverse order, it is possible that participants either tended to report more symptoms in general of this type, or perhaps they were in some cases intolerant of base ingredients. A parallel pattern also occurred for CPT reaction time. The group who received the test food first showed significantly slower reaction time after challenges than the group who received placebo first. Could they have been intolerant to a base ingredient?

Problems in selection of truly food-intolerant individuals

Statistical analysis of all 57 participants in the screening phase found no difference as a group overall for test foods and placebos for cognitive–emotional symptoms or the POMS. Multivariate analysis of variance did reveal a significant statistical interaction effect for heart rate ($P < 0.04$), but the effect was slight and uninterpretable. This result suggested a different pattern of heart rate increases and decreases over the test session's repeated measures for test foods and placebos, but this finding may be spurious. More relevant and problematic was the finding that the first test dose's scores were higher than those of the other day's doses, regardless of whether the dose was a test food or placebo.

This unexpected finding could have serious detrimental effects on the purpose of the screening trials. If nonresponders reported more cognitive–emotional symptoms on their first dose because

of psychological factors such as expectation or anxiety, a non-specific increase in symptom report on that dose could be mistakenly attributed to the first dose – especially if after breaking the blind, the dose was discovered to be a test food. Odds were good that this would occur, because three of the four doses were test foods. Such nonresponders could then be mistakenly admitted to the hospital phase as food-intolerant.

Future research using a similar design

Subsequent investigators may wish to discard first doses and lengthen the test procedure accordingly to minimize initial dose effects. Effects on statistical power, even with repeated measures, are obvious when nonresponders are included in a small sample.

As part of the inpatient phase, the 15 hospitalized participants and one pilot participant completed the Minnesota Multiphasic Personality Inventory (MMPI). Such data are of potential interest with regard to the type of individuals who believe themselves to be food-intolerant, and who would be willing and able to volunteer for an elaborate experiment requiring a week in the hospital. Visual inspection of the scored MMPIs revealed potentially interesting patterns, although admittedly post hoc in nature.

MMPI scores

In examining these scores, it was noticed that a striking proportion of the participants appeared to score in the abnormal range on the R scale. In contrast, scales commonly thought to reflect depression, somatoform disorders, and vulnerability to conversion disorders (scales 1, 2, and 3) were not as pronounced. Scale 1 (hypochondriasis) is designed to assess 'neurotic concern over bodily functioning'.[11] Scale 2 (depression) assesses depression, as the scale name implies. Scale 3 (hysteria) assesses specific somatic complaints as well as a tendency to present oneself as well adjusted. Histrionic personality dynamics may be tapped, and the high-scoring individual may be prone 'to develop conversion-type symptoms as a means to resolve conflict' and avoid responsibility.[11]

For the current sample, the median T score for scale 1 was 59 (2 in the abnormal range). For scale 2, the median score was 61.5 (4 abnormal), and for scale 3, the median score was 65 (6 abnormal). In contrast, for the R scale, the median score was 82.5, with 10 of the 16 participants scoring in the abnormal range. The post-hoc nature of this finding mandates caution in interpretation, but the implications of this result may be useful.

R scale in MMPI: atypical volunteers

The R scale has been described as a measure of repression or constriction.[4, 11] Men who score highly on the R scale were found to be 'submissive, unexcitable persons who readily made concessions rather than face unpleasantness of any sort, sidestepping troubles or disagreeable situations.'[7]

It is possible that an atypical type of person was drawn to volunteer for this study, one in which being submissive to directed regimens of diet and hospitalization was required. If such persons self-selected for admission to the study while truly food-intolerant individuals found the study requirements too burdensome, they would tend to be viewed as being reactive to the first screening dose presented to them because of the first-day effect discussed above. If their first dose was a food (75% would be), admission of a probable nonresponder to the hospital phase would follow. Apparent screening test food responses would then not be replicated in the inpatient phase, because they were not caused by a test food in the screening phase. The possibility of a first-trial effect was checked by King,[15] but no significant effect was found, perhaps because of two major procedural differences. First, the first few trials consisted of placebo screening doses and baseline periods, allowing for dissipation of novelty effects. Secondly, the patients in King's study[15] were actively involved with sublingual testing before beginning their research testing as part of the normal clinic operations. Receiving test doses and indicating symptoms were part of this procedure as well; thus, no novelty effect would necessarily be expected, because testing procedures were familiar.

CONCLUSIONS

Scientific investigation of the psychological and behavioural effects of food in intolerant individuals presents specific difficulties not found with other areas of study, such as drug effects on cardiac functioning. These difficulties include definition of the target population; selection of such individuals and matching them with the appropriate food to which they are intolerant; providing a sufficient dose of the test food; and properly designing the experiment to allow adequate statistical power despite placebo and baseline symptom variability.

Thus, the population studied in examining the effects of ragweed exposure on symptoms of rhinitis or other objective symptoms is indeed limited to those allergic to ragweed. It would not necessarily be valid to include individuals in such a study simply because they report that they are allergic to ragweed, particularly if such allergy has never been confirmed by skin testing. In the case of food intolerance, the population to be studied should be those truly intolerant of a food, and with some type of brain-related effect. The fact that no simple equivalent to a skin test for ragweed is available in this food-intolerant subject does not eliminate the equivalent logic in study design.

With the difficulties in conducting valid research in this area, how could the hypothesis that foods can produce behavioural effects be disproven? After all, if we assume that no such effect exists in nature, obviously one cannot successfully identify responders that do not exist. The answer is that well-designed experiments with sufficient statistical power can rule out the possibility of any nontrivial effect. Even better, meta-analyses conducted on a body of well-controlled, double-blind experiments can effectively establish that no behavioural effects of any consequence are present. For example, if statistical power was sufficient to detect a nontrivial effect with 95% probability, it would be reasonable to discard the hypothesis in question. However, if reliable effects of foods are found, such meta-analyses could also statistically examine dose–response curves, and identify variables that correlate with larger effect sizes for foods.

Given these and other constraints on the validity of research in this field, it is relevant that studies that have best attempted to meet these criteria have been successful in detecting behavioural effects (e.g., Egger et al.[9] and Kaplan et al.[13]) It is hoped that future research will consider the discussed factors in their design.

SUMMARY OF KEY POINTS

1. Effects of food on emotional state or cognition have long been anecdotally reported but are the subject of controversy among researchers.
2. Inconsistent research findings, too few well-controlled studies, and the inherent difficulty of conducting double-blind experiments with food have prevented resolution of the controversy about psychological effects of food intolerance.
3. Scientific investigation of the psychological and behavioural effects of foods presents special difficulty in defining the target population, selecting food-intolerant persons for study, matching persons to the foods they cannot tolerate, providing sufficient doses of test food, and designing the experiment to allow adequate statistical power.
4. For testing food intolerance, researchers should not rely completely on self-reported behavioural response to foods; instead, researchers should select for study persons who are intolerant to a food as shown by some type of objectively observable, brain-related effect.
5. Unlike the effects of alcohol on cognitive function – effects which presumably are universally detrimental – the putative effects of foods must be verified by determining the response of individual test subjects.
6. In studies of the psychological effects of foods, statistical power is critical for evaluating negative outcomes, because insufficient statistical power increases the likelihood that an actual effect will not be detected.
7. In a mailed questionnaire study of students at a large university in the northeastern United States, most respondents (especially graduate students) reported believing that foods produce psychological symptoms in sensitive or allergic people and in the students themselves.
8. Any method of blinded oral challenge to determine food effects requires rigorous verification of the adequacy of the blinding procedure and requires a food-by-food approach if the foods differ in their susceptibility to detection.

Acknowledgements

Portions of the author's research were supported by National Institutes of Mental Health grant MH38395. Sun-Diamond Growers of Pleasanton, California provided fig concentrate; Ritter International provided prune concentrate; and Gama Foods of Wapato, Washington supplied other fruit concentrates.

The Medical Editing Department of Kaiser Foundation Research Institute provided editorial assistance.

REFERENCES

1 Bernstein M, Day JH, Welsh A. Double-blind food challenge in the diagnosis of food sensitivity in the adult. *J Allergy Clin Immunol* 1982; 70: 205–10.

2 Bruijnzeel-Koomen C, Ortolani C, Aas K, Bindslev-Jensen C, Bjorksten B, Moneret-Vautrin D. Adverse reactions to food. European Academy of Allergology and Clinical Immunology Subcommittee. *Allergy* 1995; 50: 623–35.

3 BSACI Special Interest Group Report on Food Allergy and Intolerance. Conclusions and recommendations. *Clin Exp Allergy* 1995; 25 (Suppl 1): 43–4.

4 Caldwell AB. *MMPI Supplemental Scale Manual*. Caldwell Report, Los Angeles; 1988.

5 Cohen J. *Statistical Power Analysis for the Behavioral Sciences* (Rev. ed). Academic Press, New York, 1977.

6 Conners CK. *Food Additives and Hyperactive Children*. Plenum Press, New York, 1980.

7 Dahlstrom WG, Welsh GS, Dahlstrom LE. *An MMPI Handbook (Vol. 1)*. University of Minnesota Press, Minneapolis, 1972.

8 Diagnosis and treatment of attention deficit hyperactivity disorder. NIH Consensus Statement Online Nov 16–18, 1998.

9 Egger J, Carter CM, Graham PJ, Gumley D, Soothill JF. Controlled trial of oligoantigenic treatment in the hyperkinetic syndrome. *Lancet* 1985; 1: 540–5.

10 Ferguson, A. Food sensitivity or self-deception? [editorial] *N Engl J Med* 1990; 323: 476–8.

11 Greene RL. *The MMPI-2/MMPI: An interpretive manual*. Allyn and Bacon, Boston; 1991.

12 Jewett DL, Fein G, Greenberg MH. A double-blind study of symptom provocation to determine food sensitivity. *N Engl J Med* 1990; 323: 429–33.

13 Kaplan BJ, McNicol J, Conte RA, Moghadam HK. Dietary replacement in preschool-aged hyperactive boys. *Pediatrics* 1989; 83: 7–17.

14 King DS. Biologic and social factors in food sensitivities. *Toxicol Ind Health* 1992; 8: 137–44.

15 King DS. Can allergic exposure provoke psychological symptoms? A double-blind test. *Biol Psychiatry* 1981; 16: 3–19.

16 King DS. Food and chemical sensitivities can produce cognitive–emotional symptoms. In: *Nutrition & Behavior* (Miller SA, ed). Franklin Institute Press, Philadelphia, 1981; 119–30.

17 King DS. The reliability and validity of provocative food testing: a critical review. *Med Hypotheses* 1988; 25: 7–16.

18 King DS, Bell IR, Margen SM, Markley EJ. Double-blind food challenge effects upon hospitalized adults. Presented at the 1st annual meeting of the American Psychological Society, Alexandria, VA, June 1989.

19 King DS, Margen S, Ogar D, Durkin N. Double-blind food challenges affect selected children's behavior and heart rate. Presented at the 92nd annual meeting of the American Psychological Association, Toronto, Canada, August 1984.

20 King DS, Markley EJ, Bell IR *et al*. Development and testing of blind oral food challenges. Presented at the 94th Annual Convention of the American Psychological Association, Washington, DC, August 1986.

21 King DS, Wisocki P. A survey of student beliefs about the effects of food on behavior. Paper presented at the 99th annual convention of the American Psychological Association, San Francisco, August 17, 1991.

22 Light RJ, Pillemer DB. *Summing up: the science of reviewing research*. Harvard University Press, Cambridge, Massachusetts, 1984.

23 McLoughlin JA, Nall M. Teacher opinion of the role of food allergy on school behavior and achievement. *Ann Allergy* 1988; 61: 89–91.

24 Metcalfe DD. Food hypersensitivity. *J Allergy Clin Immunol* 1984; 73: 749–62.

25 Pearson DJ. Pseudo-food allergy. *Rheum Dis Clin North Am* 1991; 17: 343–9.

26 Rosenthal R. *Meta-Analytic Procedures for Social Research*. Sage, Beverly Hills, California, 1984.

27 Terr A. Unconventional theories and unproven methods in allergy. In: *Allergy: Principles and Practice*, 4th edn. (Middleton E, Reed CE, Ellis EF *et al.*, eds). Mosby, St. Louis, 1993; 1767–93.

Chapter
49

The psychologization of illness

Ellen M. Goudsmit

INTRODUCTION

Psychologization describes the emphasis on psychological factors where there is little or no evidence to justify it.[33] It is a process where relevant findings are ignored or downplayed in favour of data from incomplete examinations, flawed research or anecdotal reports. In a clinical context, differential diagnoses may be dismissed prematurely while psychological explanations are readily accepted.

Psychologization does not refer to situations where there is sound evidence that psychological factors play a significant role, or where all the arguments are discussed and the psychological explanations are deemed the most persuasive.

Psychologization is a serious issue because it leads to misdiagnosis, inappropriate treatment and unnecessary psychological distress.[76] Moreover, it undermines the general population's confidence in orthodox medicine and reduces their trust in its practitioners. Yet, despite the dangers, psychologization has received little attention in medical texts. In this article, I will discuss the main reasons underlying psychologization and examine whether it has influenced views about food allergies and intolerance.

PSYCHOLOGIZATION IN CLINICAL PRACTICE

Many cases of psychologization in clinical practice occur because doctors jump to conclusions without checking that their psychological explanations are correct. For instance, Treasure et al.[96] described how three women suffering from 'breathlessness and panic symptoms' were admitted to their Accident and Emergency Department. The initial diagnosis was hysterical hyperventilation, as a result of which two of the patients were referred to a psychia-

trist while the third was discharged with a prescription for diazepam. Within 3 days, however, the women returned and tests revealed that they were suffering from diabetes. According to Treasure et al.,[96] the assumption that the problem was psychological had led to

> the dangerous omission of physical examination, basic nursing observations, and urine analysis. In all these patients a simple test for glycosuria would have made the diagnosis obvious and the consequent and considerable risk to the patients could have been avoided.

Another typical example is that of a woman[13] who developed anxiety, fatigue and intermittent cramp-like abdominal pains after changing her job. Her GP diagnosed irritable bowel syndrome (IBS) precipitated by the stress at work, and advised a short period of sick leave. As the pain did not subside, she continued to consult her GP but neither he, nor the other doctors who saw her, questioned the diagnosis. A few months later, she noticed that the pain was associated with 'spasms visible through the abdominal wall', but the doctors who examined her at the local casualty department continued to blame IBS. When the patient consulted the author of the report, she found 'an easily palpable mass in the left iliac fossa' and an emergency operation confirmed cancer of the sigmoid colon. As in the case above, doctors had overlooked organic disease and wrongly attributed all the symptoms to a psychological cause.

PSYCHOLOGIZATION IN THE LITERATURE ON AETIOLOGY

Some of the most interesting examples of psychologization can be found in the theoretical discussions of disease. For instance,

D

Booth[9] offered a psychodynamic view of tonsillitis, arguing that many cases represented a love relationship with a bacteria in which the patient establishes

> libidinous contact on the earlier oral instead of the later genital level ... the object of the oral strivings is no longer another human being, but bacteria ... Such substitutions of bacteria for a human being makes biologic sense considering the fact that the basic object of the sex act is the copulation of the sex cells: primitive unicellular organisms like bacteria.

This is a typical case of psychologization, not only because of the poor quality of the supportive evidence but also because the author ignored all the relevant data to the contrary. For more recent examples of speculative and oversimplistic hypotheses, see Hay[36] and Millenson.[58]

Most cases of psychologization are not as extreme and indeed, may not be recognized except by colleagues who are familiar with the research. Perhaps the best examples of the more subtle forms of psychologization can be found in the British medical literature on myalgic encephalomyelitis (ME) and chronic fatigue syndrome (CFS*).

The 'reassessment' of ME

The problems began in 1970, with the publication of a paper on the epidemic which closed the Royal Free Hospital during the summer of 1955. 'Royal Free disease' resembled a viral infection and affected over 200 members of staff, the majority of whom were female. It was eventually reclassified as ME, but one of the consultants involved in their treatment noted later that he and his colleagues had considered the possibility of hysteria. However,

> the occurrence of fever in 89%, of lymphadenopathy in 79%, of ocular palsy in 43% and of facial palsy in 19% rendered it quite untenable.[73]

Fifteen years after the event, psychiatrists McEvedy and Beard were given access to some of the incomplete reports as well as the notes of those who were *not* thought to have had 'Royal Free disease'.[56] However, instead of restricting their conclusions to the sample studied, they dismissed the whole outbreak as a case of mass hysteria.

They based their view on three main arguments: first, they claimed that most of those affected had been young and socially segregated young females; secondly, they argued that the illness had not spread beyond the institutional population; and thirdly, they alleged that it had not affected a significant number of men. Notable omissions in their account included what might have triggered the anxiety among the older and more experienced health professionals involved, or what may have led to the lymphadenopathy or the morphological abnormalities seen in circulating lymphocytes.[19,57]

Arguments against the theory of mass hysteria

In fact, there are many arguments against the mass hysteria theory,[24,44,73] although these tend to be ignored by those writing

on the subject.[51,100] For example, the nurses were not socially segregated as suggested by McEvedy & Beard[29] and in terms of age, the illness was more common amongst those over 40 years old.[19] As for the predominance of females, this was true only in relation to the nonresident staff. The attack rates for resident men and women were 20 and 19 per 100, respectively.[19]

It has been pointed out that if the epidemic had resulted from anxiety in a segregated group of women, then one would have expected a higher proportion of cases in the Elizabeth Garrett Anderson Hospital and Maternity Home.[31] These institutions were part of the Royal Free Hospital group and were run for and staffed entirely by women. However, less than 7% of the patients came from these units – and only the Eastman Dental Hospital recorded fewer cases.[19]

Another argument against McEvedy & Beard's explanation is that some of the features of the outbreak were simply not typical of mass hysteria. According to Sirois,[85] most of these episodes last between 10 and 20 days, and primarily affect adolescent women. In contrast, the outbreak at the Royal Free Hospital lasted for 4 months (from 13 July 1955 until 24 November) and only a minority of those affected were younger than 20.[19]

Just a virus?

Finally, the literature on sporadic cases which clearly resembled those seen in the epidemic proved that the outbreak not only spread beyond the institutional population[42,72,81] but also beyond London.[73] Moreover, there was evidence of viral involvement, both in the Royal Free patients (Parish 1994, pers comm) and in people with an identical disorder examined later.[42] On the basis of these findings alone, the suggestion that all the cases at the Royal Free were the result of mass hysteria is unsustainable.

In the light of the available evidence, McEvedy & Beard's article should have been dismissed as deeply flawed and biased. Instead, it was widely accepted and became highly influential. For many years, their conclusions diverted the scientific community's attention away from the virological and neurological aspects of the disease and thus limited the research, and our understanding of ME. More importantly, their dualistic 'mind or body' approach provided the basis for the organic versus psychological debate, which has dominated the literature on the illness for the past two decades.[51,98,102]

THE CAUSES OF PSYCHOLOGIZATION

Stereotypical views of women

Although the literature shows that men are not immune, most of the reports relating to psychologization feature women. In older texts, female patients were often portrayed as suggestible, emotionally unbalanced, irrational, manipulative and unable to cope with even relatively minor 'stress'. For instance, authors writing about dysmenorrhoea claimed it was more common in 'highly strung', 'nervous' or 'neurotic' women, and speculated how a 'faulty outlook' might lead to 'an exaggeration of minor discomfort'.[52]

Premenstrual syndrome was also regarded as a mild and benign problem which women should be able to endure without medical intervention. As in the accounts of dysmenorrhoea, authors often implied a link with somatization, with suggestions that certain women were guilty of exaggerating their distress, perhaps to escape responsibility or effort.[62] Conversely, most of these articles did not consider the effect of recurring symptoms on the women's self-

---

*It is generally accepted that CFS is not a single entity, but that the term covers a number of disorders, all characterized by unexplained fatigue. The evidence supports the view that ME should be regarded as a subgroup of CFS. Many articles on these conditions feature highly selective discussions of the scientific data, with an emphasis on findings relating to psychiatric morbidity and a tendency to ignore or dismiss evidence of disease.[32]

confidence and self-esteem, or the possibility that this could explain the raised scores on psychometric tests.[30] Ignoring virtually all arguments to the contrary, many authors regarded emotional problems as the cause, rather than the result of ongoing ill health.[52]

The influence of gender and ethnic background: a clinical judgement

A more specific illustration of the influence of gender stereotypes was reported by Roberts.[78] She related the story of a brother and sister, both of whom suffered from migraines.[78] When the doctor was asked about his thoughts on the woman, he attributed her headaches to her social situation – tensions and problems caused by the fact that she was not married, did not have children, and that she was a 'career woman'. In contrast, he regarded her twin brother's migraines as having a genetic and biochemical basis and refused to consider a social explanation.

One reason why some doctors may be more inclined to psychologize the illnesses reported by women is the way in which many *express* their distress. Discussing her experiences as a physician, Gillespie[28] suggested that: 'men tend to speak from fact, women tend to speak from emotion'. Thus, women may refer to pain in terms of ruining their marriage and destroying their life. They relate the effects of their symptoms rather than their nature. According to Gillespie, this emphasis on the mental anguish can mislead some doctors into assuming a psychological aetiology.

A similar phenomenon has been documented in relation to ethnic groups. In one study, Zola[110] found that Italian Americans were given more psychiatric diagnoses than patients with an Anglo-Saxon or Irish background. Accounting for the findings, Zola noted that Italians had a tendency to report the effects of their symptoms and he suggested that their behaviour could have been interpreted as 'overacting'. As in the case of women, the way in which these patients described their symptoms might have influenced the clinicians to focus on one explanation and to dismiss another.

Medical training and gender stereotyping

Some of the stereotypical ideas about female patients may have originated during medical training. As one female student told Howell:[40] 'women's illnesses are assumed psychosomatic until proven otherwise'. Another observed that women are often

> portrayed as hysterical or as nagging mothers or as having trivial complaints. Men are almost never pointed to as having a psychological component to their illnesses – this is generally attributed to women.

Howell also reported that mothers were sometimes described as 'complaining', and that older women were deemed to be 'demanding and bitchy'.

The belief that psychological factors play a major role in the conditions reported by women may be one reason why they are often investigated less thoroughly than the same symptoms in men. For example, a small study by Armitage et al.[5] revealed that physicians ordered more extensive tests and procedures for men than for women with the same complaint. Discussing the findings, the authors suggested that the physicians

> might have been responding to current stereotypes that regard the male as typically stoic and the female as typically hypochondriacal.

Such a view is supported by Ayanian & Epstein,[6] who studied patients hospitalized for coronary heart disease and found that the women underwent fewer diagnostic and therapeutic procedures than the men. Likewise, Steingart et al. reported that women with cardiac disease were offered fewer procedures such as coronary bypass surgery than men, even though the women were more disabled and those procedures could have significantly lessened the symptoms.[88] The authors stated that the symptoms of chest pain in women were more likely to be attributed to noncardiac causes, but they did not speculate which. In a more recent study, Pope et al.[68] assessed patients with acute cardiac ischaemia who were mistakenly discharged from the emergency departments of 10 American hospitals. They found that discharge was more likely if the patient was a woman aged 55 years or younger, 'nonwhite', or if the principal symptom was shortness of breath. Although this study does not illustrate overt psychologization, it shows that in this age of evidence-based medicine, variables such as gender, age and race continue to influence some doctors' clinical judgement.

Despite the large number of reports detailing apparent 'sex-discrimination', the extent of gender bias in medicine is difficult to assess. For instance, several analogue studies found no significant differences in the percentage of men and women who were given a psychogenic diagnosis or psychotropic drugs.[55] However, it is probably fair to say that stereotypical attitudes still play a role in many cases of psychologization, though to varying degrees and alongside other variables such as ethnic background and age.

Lack of clarity relating to symptoms

Another important factor underlying many cases of psychologization is the difficulty in diagnosing certain conditions. For instance, Himmelhoch et al.[37] described eight patients with subacute encephalitis, of whom seven were initially diagnosed as having functional psychiatric disorders. They concluded that

> the bizarre behaviour induced physicians to ignore neurological findings, to overlook evidence of organic syndromes (such as intermittent lucidity and markedly abnormal electroencephalograms) and to make functional diagnoses.

Likewise, Randy Shilts[82] noted in his history of the AIDS epidemic that

> doctors frequently missed the damage to the central nervous system, writing off the often vague symptoms of dementia as related to stress or depression.

Similarly, the predominance of non-specific symptoms such as weakness and fatigue have been blamed for the failure to correctly diagnose cases of myasthenia gravis.[61]

Lack of evidence

The lack of clarity in relation to symptoms is not the only factor which can complicate the diagnostic process. There are now so many laboratory tests available that some doctors may interpret 'absence of evidence' as 'evidence of absence'.[35] Thus, if tests fail to identify a physical cause, some may reason that there is no physical cause to be identified and that the symptoms therefore have a non-organic, i.e. psychological cause. Consequently, patients may be told that 'there is nothing wrong' or that the illness 'is all in your head', two assessments which not only contradict actual experience but which also imply that the distress is not legitimate. Where this occurs, the physician's failure to define the illness as a 'disease state' is often an additional source of suffering which can undermine the patient's psychological health. As Stewart & Sullivan[90] observed, the emotional conflicts and tension caused by the 'misdiagnosis' of pathology can lead to 'a type of iatrogenic disease' characterized by symptoms such as 'feelings of frustration, worry and intermittent periods of depression'.

One person to have experienced this type of psychologization is the late Jacqueline Du Pré. In her biography of the cellist, Carol Easton[23] wrote:

> There is no specific test for multiple sclerosis. Its early symptoms – fatigue, loss of sensation, weakness and visual changes – are frequently misdiagnosed as psychoneurosis or an even more severe psychiatric disorder, such as hysteria, particularly in women. When doctors could find no organic cause for her complaints, they prescribed a year's rest, and referred her to a psychiatrist … When she consulted a doctor in Australia about her tenacious fatigue and occasional double vision in her right eye, he dismissed her symptoms as 'adolescent trauma' and suggested she take up a relaxing hobby.

According to the Multiple Sclerosis Society (pers comm), such an experience is not rare and after months or years of having been told their symptoms are psychological or psychosomatic, many patients actually feel relieved when they learn that they have MS. Robinson[79] confirmed this in his study, stating that

> the disclosure of the diagnosis gave back to many respondents their credibility and legitimised their strange behaviours which had previously been labelled as neurotic, hypochondria, malingering or drunk.

Further evidence that diagnostic uncertainty can influence attitudes towards patients comes from a study conducted among nurses.[92] They were asked to rate the degree of suffering, the need for pain relief and the personality of patients with severe pain. One of the vignettes they were given listed signs of objective pathology, the other did not. The results showed that the nurses attributed less intense pain when the patient in the vignette had no signs of pathology or when the condition was chronic. Moreover, ratings of the patient's personality were significantly more positive when pathology was present than when it was negative. According to the researchers, the nurses relied on the biomedical model of pain which suggests that this symptom is a physical response to tissue damage. The failure to find evidence of tissue injury led to a psychogenic labelling, as did chronicity, the suggestion being that after a time these patients should have adapted to their pain.

Cause or effect?

Some cases of psychologization may be due to the reversal of cause and effect. For instance, in their review of articles on severe dysmenorrhoea, Lennane & Lennane[52] found that doctors tended to view their patients' fear and dislike of menstruation as a cause of their pain, rather than as a result. Similarly, the frustration and irritability documented in women with mastalgia were for many years dismissed as an expression of psychoneurosis, rather than the effects of recurrent pain. In fact, when researchers studied these women, they were found to be 'no more neurotic' than people with varicose veins.[69] It is now generally accepted that most cases of mastalgia are related to a hormonal imbalance (Brush, pers comm).

The tendency to view psychological states and traits as a cause rather than the result of illness might also explain some of the psy-

chological explanations for Parkinson's disease,[20] premenstrual syndrome,[30] cancer,[47] multiple sclerosis[50,67] and the diabetes personality.[91]

Interpretation of research findings

When research reveals an apparent association between illness on the one hand and psychological symptoms, states and traits on the other, it is often difficult to determine the direction of the relationship. In addition to the possibility that the psychological variable caused the disease, there are a number of other explanations which should be considered.[63] They include:

a. *Coincidence*. The likelihood that both the illness and the psychological variable may have been caused by independent agents and that they are not related.
b. *The presence of an external agent*. A third variable, for instance, environmental pollution, might have caused both phenomena.
c. *The existence of an internal agent*. For example, heredity or an immunological or neurological dysfunction may have influenced both psychological and physical variables.
d. *The influence of a behavioural agent*. Certain behaviours may have induced emotional states and affected the person's health. For instance, eating a poor diet could result in depressed mood as well as disease.
e. *The presence of an intervening agent*. Here an event or state intervenes between the psychological and biological factors, causing them to correlate. For example, depression caused by bereavement may compromise immune function, which then increases one's predisposition to or exacerbates ill health.
f. *Disease causation*. A sixth possibility is that a disease caused a particular psychological reaction. Since it is often difficult to pinpoint the actual onset of a disease, it is possible that certain physiological changes preceded the psychological ones. Thus, depression may be the first symptom of pancreatic cancer, multiple sclerosis or Parkinson's disease.[80]

The interpretation of an apparent link between illness and psychological variables is further complicated by methodological problems, notably the use of different diagnostic criteria and measures. This has resulted in an astonishing range of prevalence figures for psychiatric morbidity in people with cancer, diabetes, multiple sclerosis and CFS.[32,59,60,109] Examples of psychologization include the citation of higher estimates in support of a 'psychosomatic' explanation, and not documenting, or unfairly dismissing, lower rates. In other cases, authors may deliberately overlook the flaws associated with a particular measure, leading them to exaggerate the significance of psychiatric illness associated with a disease.

Medical symptoms and psychiatric diagnosis

It is well known that estimates may be inflated as a result of confounding, i.e. the inclusion of symptoms of the medical condition as criteria for the diagnosis of psychiatric disorders.[3,22,74,94] The symptoms most often used for this purpose include fatigue, insomnia, loss of appetite, psychomotor retardation and difficulties with concentration.[14,15,18,26,48,87] Not surprisingly, omitting one or more of these from the list of criteria can have a significant effect on the estimates of psychopathology. For example, in their study on chronic fatigue, Katon *et al.* eliminated fatigue as a criterion of depression and found that this alone reduced the prevalence rate from 15.3% to 10.2%.[46]

The inclusion of disability-related items in self-rating scales can cause similar problems. For instance, Yeomans & Conway[109] reported that 33% of their patients with ME scored 11 or more on the depression subscale of the Hospital Anxiety and Depression (HAD) questionnaire. However, when they excluded the item 'I feel as if I am slowed down', no one exceeded the cut-off point for caseness.

The reliance on symptoms can also lead to false positives in relation to somatization disorder (SD). For instance, estimates of SD in patients with CFS have varied from 0% to 98%.[45] When one team of researchers excluded seven somatic items from the diagnostic criteria, this reduced the prevalence rate from 46% to 20%.[46] Reduced rates have also been noted by others, leading Johnson et al.[45] to conclude that the 'diagnosis of SD is of limited use in populations in which the aetiology of the illness has not been established'.

To assess whether the psychological disturbances reported by people with CFS represent a reaction to their illness or the presence of a primary psychiatric condition, researchers have compared this population with people suffering from multiple sclerosis,[49,65] rheumatoid arthritis,[46] cystic fibrosis,[99] spinal cord injuries[32] and muscle disorders.[101,106] Unfortunately, it is difficult to interpret most of these studies because they failed to match the samples with regard to the degree of impairment or the severity of symptoms. In relation to fatigue, the levels recorded by the comparison groups were often significantly lower than those of the patients with CFS. Where fatigue was not assessed, other illness-related variables showed that the controls had fewer symptoms and perceived their health to be better.[46]

Despite the various flaws, most reviewers have concluded that patients with CFS have higher rates of psychiatric disorders than other disabled groups. However, the failure to control for the degree of impairment means that their emphasis on psychopathology as a major factor in the perpetuation of CFS is probably not justified.[1,21,95]

Psychologization and the illusion of control

While psychologization can have serious and occasionally fatal consequences,[10,35,54] it also offers certain advantages.[53,93] For instance, Taylor[93] found that many women with breast cancer believed that stress management techniques and a positive attitude would prevent a recurrence. Although there is little research evidence which supports this view,[25,71] both she and Turnquist et al.[97] consider these 'illusions' to be adaptive, enabling more women to cope with the fear, vulnerability and helplessness associated with their illness.

The reverse is true when outsiders claim that patients create and are responsible for their symptoms.[36,56] A discussion of victim-blaming statements can be found in texts by Sontag[86] and Wilkinson & Kitzinger.[104] For instance, Sontag documents how cancer patients were once described as having a 'great tendency for self-pity' and as being 'empty of feeling and devoid of self'. In more general terms, it was alleged that the 'sick man himself creates his disease' and that 'illness is in part what the world has done to a victim, but in a larger part it is what the victim has done with his world, and with himself'.

In her response, Sontag concludes that

such preposterous and dangerous views manage to put the onus of the disease on the patient ... The view of cancer as a disease of the failure of expressiveness condemns the cancer patient; expresses pity but also conveys contempt.'

To that might be added that the emphasis on the spiritual flaws of the sick and disabled will make many patients feel guilty, thus further increasing their distress.

Blaming the victim

Outsiders might be tempted to play down the influence of factors such as viruses and pollution – over which mankind has relatively little control – to enhance their 'sense of mastery' over their lives.[93] By attributing them to personal flaws (which one doesn't share), one reduces one's own perceived risk of being struck down by a feared disease.

A variation on this theme is the suggestion by Lerner & Simmons[53] that 'blaming the victim' helps people to maintain their belief in a 'just world', where people get what they deserve and deserve what they get. According to this hypothesis, individuals can avoid adversity through their own activities; but this also implies that those struck by misfortune are deemed to have somehow merited their fate.

Surprisingly, such a view of illness is not restricted to a small group of 'New Age' philosophers or the odd clinical text.[36] Wortman & Dunkel-Schetter[108] wrote that health care professionals

often have ambivalent feelings towards their patients – patients they are supposedly trying to help. Past research has suggested that even a single encounter with a victim can be a powerfully distressing experience, and can result in blame and derogation of the victim.

Thus, the occasional comment which insinuates that the patient's character made them ill may be part of a coping strategy which allows practitioners to protect themselves from unpleasant emotions, even though it will almost certainly undermine the relationship with those in their care.

The role of politics

Finally, blaming the victim may result from strongly held political views.[104] For instance, some believe that health is a matter of personal responsibility and that people increase their risk of disease by engaging in behaviours such as smoking or eating an unhealthy diet. The politically motivated may exaggerate the influence of lifestyle factors or apply this reasoning to other conditions, to limit funds destined for research and restrict patients' eligibility for certain benefits. Thus, they will argue that if the cause of illness lies in people's character and behaviours, then fewer resources have to be spent evaluating the effects of environmental pollutants, pesticides and other external factors implicated in disease. Unless governments redirect the savings to educational projects concerned with prevention, or to support those already affected, blaming the victim is a useful way of freeing-up funds and diverting resources.

PSYCHOLOGIZATION OF FOOD ALLERGY AND INTOLERANCE

Examples of psychologization can also be found in the literature on food sensitivities. Most of these focus on the apparently high prevalence of psychiatric disorders in this population, with the implication that these are the main source of the patients' complaints.[39] However, as will be argued in the following section, such suggestions should be interpreted with care.

A major difficulty in assessing the actual role of psychological factors in food allergy and intolerance is that the majority of the studies have included patients with multiple chemical sensitivities and 'environmental illness'.[8,84] To complicate matters, some of the subjects were engaged in legal action for compensation at the time,[11] and many had supposed rather than proven allergies.[77] Indeed, few studies have restricted participation to patients with properly diagnosed food sensitivities and even fewer have assessed delayed reactions to food, presenting 24 hours or more after ingestion.

Another problem is the assessment of psychiatric morbidity and the use of measures which include the symptoms of food sensitivity as criteria of psychopathology. As noted above, such confounding can lead to diagnostic false positives[8,84] and give a misleading view of these patients' mental health.

This is certainly the case in relation to somatization disorder, where the criteria in DSM-IV (Diagnostic and Statistical Manual of Mental Disorders, 4th edn) require the presence of seven symptoms from a list which includes nausea, bloating and intolerance to several different foods, as well as headache and abdominal pain.[3] Accordingly, it is advisable to obtain additional evidence such as the presence of conflicts and other stressors at meal times or obvious signs of secondary gain, before attributing these symptoms to SD. If the aetiology is unclear, it may also be useful to engage the patient in an experiment, for instance, to compare the effects of standard treatments such as avoidance with the results of psychotropic medication.[89] A positive response to the latter does not prove that the reaction to food was mediated by emotional as opposed to immunological factors but it could give useful insights into the mechanisms underlying specific symptoms and clarify the role of contributory factors.

Some clinicians consider the documented rates of psychopathology to be reliable, arguing that symptoms such as depression are generally not triggered by food.[77] However, others remain unsure and have pointed to evidence linking diet with a number of psychological disturbances, including affective disorders and schizophrenia.[4,12,58,70]

Mood disorders and psychologization

As noted above, the finding of high rates of psychopathology does not prove that those disorders caused the patients' symptoms. Depression and anxiety may be due, at least in part, to factors such as uncertainty. In several studies, uncertainty relating to conditions such as myocardial infarction, multiple sclerosis and CFS was significantly correlated with psychological distress.[16,32,105] It is therefore possible that this variable also plays a role in people with food allergies and sensitivities. Similarly, any mood disturbances may be exacerbated and perpetuated as a result of continued psychologization by physicians and family.[75,90,107] These are just two of the factors which should be considered when assessing the psychological status of individuals with food sensitivities.[32] Focusing exclusively on the prevalence of affective disorders could lead to mistakes.

Other influences

In differentiating cause and effect, a prior history of psychiatric illness is often regarded as suggestive of a psychological vulnerability.[83] The problem here is obvious. Without corroboration

from accurate medical notes, much depends on the patient's memory and interpretation of the complaint.[84] Moreover, if one has to rely on the patient, it must be remembered that current psychological distress could increase the tendency to recall some symptoms and health events at the expense of others. Past symptoms were the result of conditions such as malabsorption and altered gut ecology, which also predisposed patients to develop sensitivities to food later in life.[41] Leaving these considerations aside, there is at present little evidence that people with proven food reactions are more likely to have a history of psychiatric morbidity or that they have a greater psychological vulnerability than people who do not experience reactions to foods.[66]

Finally, it has been suggested that blaming symptoms on allergies and environmental toxins may help people with psychiatric disorders to avoid the stigma of mental illness.[39,102] In a society where the general population and certain physicians still regard psychiatric disorders as less worthy of attention and respect than physical ones, it is understandable that some patients might choose to blame their unexplained symptoms on allergies rather than depression or anxiety. One can also postulate that these erroneous attributions may be reinforced by some self-help groups and articles in the popular press.[38] However, there is still no convincing evidence that most patients with food allergies are motivated by prejudiced views of mental illness. Moreover, until every patient is also assessed for conditions such as dysbiosis and tested for immune activation,[43] one cannot assume that their attributions are incorrect.

Clarification of the relationship between psychiatric illness and reactions to food

In summary, most of the claims that psychological factors are the source of food sensitivities seem to be based on methodologically flawed research and a biased interpretation of the findings. Moreover, the lack of studies on well-defined groups means that writers have tended to generalize from one population to another, which may not be justified. In this respect, it is worth noting the findings of Peveler *et al.*[66] They assessed patients from the community and found that individuals who attributed their symptoms to food sensitivity suffered less psychological impairment than those who attributed their complaints to stomach or bowel disorders and stress. The estimated rate of psychiatric illness was also relatively low, and they noted a strong relationship between the patients' attribution of symptoms to foods and the clinical judgement of food sensitivity. These findings show that the research relating to allergy clinic patients and people with alleged allergies or various environmental syndromes cannot be generalized to people with food intolerance from the general population. They also suggest that many patients' beliefs about food sensitivity are probably accurate and that the claims of widespread misattribution were premature.

SOLUTIONS

Perhaps the most important and effective remedy for psychologization in the clinic is for scientists to stop using psychological explanations as a convenient 'dustbin' for complex cases or troublesome patients. In this hi-tech age, where doctors depend more and more on the results from laboratory tests and objective clinical signs, a psychological diagnosis can explain the otherwise inexplicable. It is often plausible, difficult to disprove and can be altered to suit changing circumstances. To put it another way, a psychological explanation may be an attractive option for practitioners who lack financial resources and/or time. However, as many writers have pointed out,[34] it might serve healthcare professionals better to be 'agnostic' every now and then.

As for the examples in the literature, a more objective and critical approach by reviewers and editors should help to avoid most cases of bias. For instance, McEvedy & Beard's assessment of the outbreak at the Royal Free Hospital was largely based on information from selected case notes and a highly subjective evaluation of the evidence.[73] Their misrepresentation of the data constituted a clear case of psychologization, reflecting not only their own lack of respect for science but also the editors' failure to address the paper's many flaws.

The same lack of editorial interest in accuracy and balance has allowed more recent articles to exaggerate the role of psychiatric morbidity in CFS.[7,95,103] Here writers rarely consider alternative explanations for the associated mood disorders, such as the effect of uncertainty, the strain of the illness and the lack of social support.[32,102] This bias illustrates the editors' continued preference for simple, psychological explanations at a time when the actual evidence points to a heterogeneous population and a multifactorial aetiology.[2,17,27,64] In fact, the predilection for simplistic

theories and lack of interest in alternative views features in many cases of psychologization, not just those related to CFS.

People are entitled to their opinion and I am not suggesting that speculation has no place in scientific texts. However, unsubstantiated or poorly supported claims should be acknowledged as such and interpreted with care. In this age of evidence-based medicine, writers must consider all reasonable explanations, and take account of methodological flaws and valid criticisms.

It is my belief that articles with a strong bias towards one explanation *and* an unbalanced or unfair approach to the available data, do not belong in scientific publications unless marked as an opinion piece. Respect for plausible alternative views and the evaluation of all the relevant evidence are not luxuries to be indulged in should space permit. A broader editorial policy may produce more readable and provocative articles but it also leads to psychologization and, accordingly, to misunderstanding, inappropriate advice and to much needless distress. It deserves to be challenged.

ACKNOWLEDGEMENTS

I wish to thank all those who helped me with the preparation of the manuscript, especially Ms Mary Sullivan MSc, Mrs Sandra Howes and Mrs Doris Jones MSc.

REFERENCES

1 Abbey SE. Somatization, illness attribution and the sociocultural psychiatry of the chronic fatigue syndrome. In: *Chronic Fatigue Syndrome* (Bock GR, Whelan J eds). John Wiley and Sons, Chichester, 1993.

2 Ablashi DV, Eastman HB, Owen CB *et al.* Frequent HHV-6 reactivation in multiple sclerosis (MS) and chronic fatigue syndrome (CFS) patients. *J Clin Virol* 2000; 16: 179–91.

3 American Psychiatric Association. *Quick Reference to the Diagnostic Criteria from DSM-IV*. APA, Washington, 1994.

4 Anthony H, Birtwistle S, Eaton K, Maberly J. *Environmental Medicine in Clinical Practice*. BSAENM Publications, Southampton, 1997.

5 Armitage KJ, Schneiderman LJ, Bass RA. Response of physicians to medical complaints in men and women. *JAMA* 1979; 241: 2186–7.

6 Ayanian JZ, Epstein AM. Differences in the use of procedures between women and men hospitalized for coronary heart disease. *N Engl J Med* 1991; 325: 221–5.

7 Barsky AJ, Borus JF. Functional somatic syndromes. *Ann Int Med* 1999; 130: 910–21.

8 Black DW, Rath A, Goldstein RB. Environmental illness. A controlled study of 26 subjects with '20th century disease'. *JAMA* 1990; 264: 3166–70.

9 Booth G. Psychodynamics in Parkinsonism. *Psychosom Med* 1948; 10: 1–14.

10 Brahams D. Fatal case of undiagnosed diabetes. *Lancet* 1990; 335(8690): 652.

11 Brodsky CM. 'Allergic to everything': a medical subculture. *Psychosomatics* 1983; 24: 731–44.

12 Brostoff J, Gamlin L. *The Complete Guide to Food Allergy and Intolerance*. Bloomsbury, London, 1989.

13 Brozovic M. With women in mind. *Br Med J* 1989; 299: 689.

14 Bukberg J, Penman D, Holland JC. Depression in hospitalized cancer patients. *Psychosom Med* 1984; 46: 199–212.

15 Cavanaugh SA. Depression in the medically ill. In: *Handbook of Studies on General Hospital Psychiatry*. (Judd FK, Burrows GD and Lipsett DR eds). Elsevier, Amsterdam, 1991.

16 Christman NJ, McConnell EA, Pfeiffer C, Webster KK, Schmitt M, Ries J. Uncertainty, coping and stress following myocardial infarction:

transition from hospital to home. *Research in Nursing and Health* 1988; 11: 71–82.

17 Christodoulou C, DeLuca J, Johnson SK, Lange G, Natelson BH. Efforts to reduce heterogeneity in chronic fatigue syndrome. In: *Chronic Fatigue Syndrome* (Yehuda S and Mostofsky DI eds). Plenum Press, New York, 1997.

18 Clark DC, Cavanaugh S, Gibbons RD. The core symptoms of depression in medical and psychiatric patients. *J Nerv Ment Dis* 1983; 171: 705–13.

19 Crowley N, Nelson M, Stovin S. Epidemiological aspects of an outbreak of encephalomyelitis at the Royal Free Hospital in the summer of 1955. *J Hygiene (Cambridge)* 1957; 55: 102–22.

20 Dakof GA, Mendelsohn GA. Parkinson's disease: the psychological aspects of a chronic illness. *Psychol Bull* 1986; 99: 375–87.

21 David AS. Postviral fatigue syndrome and psychiatry. *Br Med Bull* 1991; 47: 966–88.

22 Dutton DG. Depression/somatization explanations for the chronic fatigue syndrome: a critical review. In: *The Clinical and Scientific Basis of Myalgic Encephalomyelitis/Chronic Fatigue Syndrome* (Hyde BM, Goldstein J, Levine P eds). The Nightingale Research Foundation, Ottawa; 1992.

23 Easton C. *Jacqueline Du Pré. A Biography*. Hodder & Stoughton, London, 1989.

24 Editorial. *Br Med J* 1978; 1: 1436–7.

25 Fox BH. Psychogenic factors in cancer, especially its incidence. In: *Topics in Health Psychology* (Maes S, Spielberger CD, Defares PB, Sarason ID, eds). John Wiley and Sons, Chichester, 1988.

26 Frank RG, Beck NC, Parker JC *et al.* Depression in rheumatoid arthritis. *J Rheumatol* 1988; 15: 920–5.

27 Friedberg F. A subgroup analysis of cognitive-behavioral treatment studies. *J Chronic Fatigue Syndrome* 1999; 5: 3–4, 149–59.

28 Gillespie L. *You Don't Have to Live with Cystitis*. Century, London, 1988.

29 Gosling PH. Epidemic malaise. *Br Med J* 1970; 1: 499–500.

30 Goudsmit EM. Psychological aspects of premenstrual symptoms. In: *Functional Disorders of the Menstrual Cycle* (Brush MG, Goudsmit EM, eds). John Wiley & Sons, Chichester, 1988.

31 Goudsmit EM. All in her mind! Stereotypic views and the psychologisation of women's illness. In: *Women and Health. Feminist Perspectives* (Wilkinson S, Kitzinger C, eds). Taylor and Francis, London, 1994.

32 Goudsmit EM. The psychological aspects and management of chronic fatigue syndrome. Doctoral thesis, Brunel University, 1996.

33 Goudsmit EM, Gadd R. All in the mind? The psychologisation of illness. *The Psychologist* 1991; 4: 449–53.

34 Guggenbuhl-Craig A, Micklem N. No answer to Job: reflections on the limitations of meaning in illness. In: *The Meaning of Illness* (Kidel M, Rowe-Leete S, eds). Routledge, London, 1988.

35 Hartnell L. Personal view. *Br Med J* 1987; 294: 1029.

36 Hay L. *You Can Heal Your Life*. Eden Grove, London, 1988.

37 Himmelhoch J, Pincus J, Tucker G, Detre T. Sub-acute encephalitis: behavioural and neurological aspects. *Br J Psychiatry* 1970; 116: 531–8.

38 Howard L, Wessely S. The psychology of multiple allergy. *Br Med J* 1993; 307: 747–8.

39 Howard LM, Wessely S. Psychiatry in the allergy clinic: the nature and management of patients with non-allergic symptoms. *Clin Exp Allergy* 1995; 25: 503–14.

40 Howell MC. What medical schools teach about women. *N Engl J Med* 1974; 291: 304–7.

41 Hunter JO. Food allergy – or enterometabolic disorder? *Lancet* 1991; 338: 495–6.

42 Innes SGB. Encephalomyelitis resembling benign myalgic encephalomyelitis. *Lancet* 1970; i: 969–71.

43 Jacobsen MB, Aukrust P, Muller F *et al*: Relation between food provocation and systemic immune activation in patients with food intolerance. *Lancet* 2000; 356: 400–1.

44 Jenkins R. Introduction. In: *Post-Viral Fatigue Syndrome* (Jenkins R, Mowbray J, eds). John Wiley & Sons, Chichester, 1991.

45 Johnson SK, DeLuca J, Natelson BH. Assessing somatization disorder in the chronic fatigue syndrome. *Psychosom Med* 1996; 58: 50–7.

46 Katon W, Buchwald DS, Simon GE, Russo JE, Mease PJ. Psychiatric illness in patients with chronic fatigue and those with rheumatoid arthritis. *J Gen Intern Med* 1991; 6: 277–85.

47 Kowal SJ. Emotions as a cause of cancer. *Psychoanal Rev* 1955; 42: 217–27.

48 Krupp LB, Alvarez LA, LaRocca NG, Scheinberg LC. Fatigue in multiple sclerosis. *Arch Neurol* 1988; 45: 435–7.

49 Krupp L, Sliwinski M, Masur DM, Friedberg F, Coyle PK. Cognitive functioning and depression in patients with chronic fatigue syndrome and multiple sclerosis. *Arch Neurol* 1994; 51: 705–10.

50 Langworthy OR. Relation of personality problems to onset and progress of multiple sclerosis. *Arch Neurol Psychiatry* 1984; 59: 13–28.

51 Leitch AG. The chronic fatigue syndrome reviewed. *Proc Roy Coll Physicians Edinb* 1994; 24: 480–508.

52 Lennane KJ, Lennane RJ. Alleged psychogenic disorders in women – a possible manifestation of sexual prejudice. *N Engl J Med* 1973; 288: 288–92.

53 Lerner MJ, Simmons CH. Observer's reaction to the 'innocent victim': compassion or rejection? *J Pers Soc Psychol* 1966; 2: 203–10.

54 Longden D. *Diana's Story*. Bantam Press, London, 1989.

55 Lopez SR. Patient variable biases in clinical judgement: conceptual overview, and methodological considerations. *Psychol Bull* 1989; 106: 184–203.

56 McEvedy CP, Beard AW. Royal Free epidemic of 1955: a reconsideration. *Br Med J* 1970; 1: 7–11.

57 Medical Staff of the Royal Free Hospital. An outbreak of encephalomyelitis in the Royal Free Hospital Group, London in 1955. *Br Med J* 1957; 2: 895–904.

58 Millenson JR. *Mind Matters. Psychological Medicine in Holistic Practice*. Eastland Press, Seattle, 1996.

59 Millon C, Salvato F, Blaney N *et al*. A psychological assessment of chronic fatigue syndrome/chronic Epstein–Barr virus patients. *Psychology and Health* 1989; 3: 131–41.

60 Minden SL, Orav J, Reich P. Depression in multiple sclerosis. *Gen Hosp Psychiatry* 1987; 9: 426–34.

61 Nicholson GA, Wilby J, Tennant C. Myasthenia gravis: the problem of a 'psychiatric' misdiagnosis. *Med J Aust* 1986; 144, 632–8.

62 Notman M. The psychiatrist's approach. In: *Premenstrual Tension. A Multidisciplinary Approach* (Debrovner CH, ed). Human Sciences Press, New York, 1982.

63 Panagis DM. Psychological factors and cancer outcome. In: *Psychological Aspects of Cancer* (Cohen J, Cullen JW, Martin LR, eds). Raven Press, New York, 1982.

64 Paul L, Wood L, Behan WMH, Maclaren WM. Demonstration of delayed recovery from fatiguing exercise in chronic fatigue syndrome. *Eur J Neurol* 1999; 6: 63–9.

65 Pepper CM, Krupp LB, Friedberg F, Doscher C, Coyle PK. A comparison of neuropsychiatric characteristics in chronic fatigue syndrome, multiple sclerosis and major depression. *J Neuropsychiatry Clin Neurosciences* 1993; 5: 200–5.

66 Peveler R, Mayou R, Young E, Stoneham M. Psychiatric aspects of food-related physical symptoms: a community study. *J Psychosom Res* 1996; 41: 149–59.

67 Philippopoulos GS, Wittkower ED, Cousineau A. The etiological significance of emotional factors in onset and exacerbations of multiple sclerosis. *Psychosom Med* 1958; 6: 459–74.

68 Pope JH, Aufderheide TP, Ruthazer R *et al*. Missed diagnoses of acute cardiac ischemia in the emergency department. *N Engl J Med* 2000; 342: 1163–70.

69 Preece PE, Mansel RE, Hughes LE. Mastalgia: psychoneurosis or organic disease? *Br Med J* 1978; 1: 29–30.

70 Radcliffe MJ, Ashurst P, Brostoff J. Unexplained illness: the mind versus the environment. *J R Soc Med* 1995; 88: 678–9.

71 Ramirez AJ, Craig TKJ, Watson JP, Fentiman IS, North WRS, Rubens RD. Stress and relapse of breast cancer. *Br Med J* 1989; 298: 291–3.

72 Ramsay AM. Encephalomyelitis in North London. An endemic infection simulating poliomyelitis and hysteria. *Lancet* 1957; 2: 1196–200.

73 Ramsay AM. *Myalgic Encephalomyelitis and Postviral Fatigue States*, 2nd edn. Gower Medical Publishing, London, 1988.

74 Ray C. Chronic fatigue syndrome and depression: conceptual and methodological ambiguities. *Psychol Med* 1991; 21: 1–9.

75 Rippere V. The mental state of dismissed patients – an enquiry into dismissal injury. II. Dismissal as unfinished business. *Newsletter of the Society for Environmental Therapies* 1991; 11: 72–9.

76 Rippere V. The mental state of dismissed patients – an enquiry into dismissal injury. V. Repercussions of psychogenic dismissal. *Newsletter of the Society for Environmental Therapies* 1992; 12: 138–48.

77 Rix KJB, Pearson DJ, Bentley SJ. A psychiatric study of patients with supposed food allergy. *Br J Psychiatry* 1984; 145: 121–6.

78 Roberts H. *The Patient Patients*. Pandora Press, London, 1985.

79 Robinson I. *Multiple Sclerosis*. Routledge, London, 1988.

80 Rodin GM, Craven J, Littlefield C (eds). *Depression in the Medically Ill. An Integrated Approach*. Brunner Mazel, New York, 1991.

81 Scott BD. Epidemic malaise. *Br Med J* 1970; 1: 170.

82 Shilts R. *And the Band Played On*. Penguin, London, 1988.

83 Simon GE, Katon WJ, Sparks PJ. Allergic to life: psychological factors in environmental illness. *Am J Psychiatry* 1990; 147: 901–6.

84 Simon GE, Daniell W, Stockbridge H, Claypoole K, Rosenstock L. Immunologic, psychological, and neuropsychological factors in multiple chemical sensitivity. A controlled study. *Ann Int Med* 1993; 119: 97–103.

85 Sirois F. Epidemic hysteria. In: *Hysteria* (Roy A, ed). John Wiley and Sons, Chichester, 1983.

86 Sontag S. *Illness as Metaphor*. Penguin, London, 1977.

87 Starkstein SE, Preziosi TJ, Forrester AW, Robinson RG. Specificity of affective and autonomic symptoms of depression in Parkinson's disease. *J Neurol Neurosurg Psychiatry* 1990; 53: 869–73.

88 Steingart R, Packer M, Hamm P *et al*. Sex differences in the management of coronary heart disease. *N Engl J Med* 1991; 325: 226–30.

89 Stewart DE, Raskin J. Psychiatric assessment of patients with '20th century disease' ('total allergy syndrome'). *Can Med Assoc J* 1985; 133: 1001–6.

90 Stewart DC, Sullivan TJ. Illness behavior and the sick role in chronic disease. *Soc Sci Med* 1982; 16: 1397–404.

91 Surwit RS, Scovern AW, Feinglos MN. The role of behavior in diabetes care. *Diabetes Care* 1982; 5: 337–42.

92 Taylor AG, Skelton JA, Butcher J. Duration of pain condition and physical pathology as determinants of nurses' assessments of patients in pain. *Nursing Res* 1984; 33: 4–8.

93 Taylor SE. Adjustment to threatening events. A theory of cognitive adaptation. *Am Psychol* 1983; 38: 1161–73.

94 Thase ME. Assessment of depression in patients with chronic fatigue syndrome. *Rev Infect Dis* 1991; 13 (Suppl 1): S114–118.

95 Thomas PK. The chronic fatigue syndrome: what do we know? *Br Med J* 1993; 306: 1557–8.

96 Treasure RAR, Fowler PBS, Millington HT, Wise PH. Misdiagnosis of diabetic ketoacidosis as hyperventilation syndrome. *Br Med J* 1987; 294: 630.

97 Turnquist DC, Harvey JH, Andersen BL. Attributions and adjustment to life-threatening illness. *Br J Clin Psychol* 1988; 27: 55–65.

98 Vollmer-Conna U, Lloyd A, Hickie I, Wakefield D. Chronic fatigue syndrome: an immunological perspective. *Aust NZ J Psychiatry* 1998; 32: 523–7.

99 Walford GA, McNelson W, McCluskey DR. Fatigue, depression, and social adjustment in chronic fatigue syndrome. *Arch Dis Child* 1993; 68: 384–8.

100 Wessely S. Mass hysteria: two syndromes? *Psychol Med* 1987; 17: 109–20.

101 Wessely S, Powell R. Fatigue syndromes: a comparison of chronic 'postviral' fatigue with neuromuscular and affective disorders. *J Neurol Neurosurg Psychiatry* 1989; 52: 940–8.

102 Wessely S, Hotopf M, Sharpe M (eds). *Chronic Fatigue and Its Syndromes*. Oxford University Press, Oxford, 1998.

103 Wessely S, Nimnuan C, Sharpe M. Functional somatic syndromes: one or many? *Lancet* 1999; 354: 936–9.

104 Wilkinson S, Kitzinger C. Towards a feminist approach to breast cancer. In: *Women and Health. Feminist Perspectives* (Wilkinson S, Kitzinger C, eds). Taylor and Francis, London, 1994.

105 Wineman NM. Adaptation to multiple sclerosis: the role of social support, functional disability, and perceived uncertainty. *Nursing Res* 1990; 39: 294–9.

106 Wood GC, Bentall RP, Gopfert M, Edwards RHT. A comparative psychiatric assessment of patients with chronic fatigue syndrome and muscle disease. *Psychol Med* 1991; 21. 619–28.

107 Woodward RV, Broom DH, Legge DG. Diagnosis in chronic illness: disabling or enabling – the case of chronic fatigue syndrome. *J R Soc Med* 1995; 88: 325–9.

108 Wortman CB, Dunkel-Schetter C. Interpersonal relationships and cancer: a theoretical analysis. *J Soc Issues* 1979; 35: 120–55.

109 Yeomans JDI, Conway SP. Biopsychosocial aspects of chronic fatigue syndrome (myalgic encephalomyelitis). *J Infect* 1991; 23: 263–9.

110 Zola IK. Problems of communications, diagnosis, and patient care: the interplay of patient, physician and clinic organisation. *J Med Educ* 1963; 38: 829–38.

Chapter 50

Food allergy and the central nervous system in childhood

Joseph Egger

INTRODUCTION

Food allergy as a cause of disorders of the central nervous system (CNS) has been much neglected because it is not easy to diagnose and because a connection between the gut and the brain is not obvious. Moreover, emotional factors often appear to trigger symptoms and so relatively greater importance has been given to them. Food-allergic symptoms of the CNS rarely occur soon after eating: they usually appear gradually, hours or days afterwards. Thus, especially with common foods, the relationship between ingestion and symptoms may not be obvious. Diagnosis is difficult because there are no laboratory tests to identify provoking foods. The management of food allergy is equally difficult; provoking foods have to be avoided, sometimes only temporarily, but often the offending foods are those the patient likes most.

MIGRAINE IN CHILDHOOD

Headaches in childhood have been relatively neglected and have frequently been interpreted as a symptom of nervous tension. The work of Bille[4] was highly significant in calling attention to migraine as a frequent disorder in childhood.

As a single event, headaches usually occur in the context of an intercurrent illness. Recurrent headaches are divided into vascular (usually migraine), psychogenic (to be distinguished from the Munchausen syndrome and Munchausen syndrome by proxy[46]) and organic (in which the headache is due to structural, metabolic or infectious disease). Often a new headache may be assigned to one of the three categories only with passage of time, pending re-examination for the development of possible neurological signs.

Diagnosis

Criteria for the diagnosis of migraine are outlined in Table 50.1. The problem of a generally acceptable clinical definition of migraine versus psychogenic headaches is almost insurmountable. Most studies have been content to identify migraine and to leave the issue of psychogenic headaches ambiguous.

Criteria for the diagnosis of migraine	
Essential criteria	**Necessary symptoms**
Recurrent headaches with symptom-free intervals, plus	three of the following: abdominal pain or nausea or vomiting unilateral throbbing relief after sleep aura (visual, sensory, motor) family history

Table 50.1 Criteria for the diagnosis of migraine.

The principal variables that form the basis of the symptomatic diagnosis of headache are occurrence (periodic versus continuous), the quality of painful discomfort and associated symptoms. The chief clinical characteristic of vascular headaches, in the majority of cases, is their periodic occurrence. In contrast the usual psychogenic headache is thought to be continuously present.

The quality of pain in vascular headaches varies from an aching sensation to sharp pain. Throbbing pain is more often reported by older children but rarely before puberty. In psychogenic headaches the more commonly used description is of sensations of frontal or occipital pressure or tightness.

Associated symptoms are important for the diagnosis of vascular headaches; during an episode of migraine, children are almost always pale and frequently mention photophobia and vertigo. Visual symptoms are not especially common in children, but abdominal symptoms are, and sometimes motor and sensory hemisyndromes occur. The symptoms thought to be associated with psychogenic headaches are those related to the psychiatric disorder and may consist of depression, irritability, apathy and outbursts of temper.

Association with underlying disease

Any headache in childhood may be symptomatic of underlying systemic, cranial or intracranial disease (Table 50.2), and it must

Causes of symptomatic headache	
Trauma	Congenital malformation and
Tumour	hydrocephalus
Arachnoid cyst	Paranasal sinusitis
Arteriovenous malformations	Epidural abscess
Berry aneurysm	Cerebral abscess
Acute subarachnoid haemorrhage	Meningitis
Connective tissue disease	Encephalitis
Hypertension and hypertensive	Phaeochromocytoma
encephalopathy	Hypoglycaemia
Childhood stroke (haemorrhagic,	Ornithine transcarbamylase
embolic, thrombotic)	deficiency

Table 50.2 Causes of symptomatic headache.

Epidemiology of headache in children 7–15 years of age	
Never had headaches	4%
Infrequent non-migrainous headaches	48%
Frequent non-migrainous headaches	7%
Migraine	4%

Table 50.4 Epidemiology of headache in children 7–15 years of age (n = 9059).

be remembered that brain tumours are more frequent in the first 6 years of life than at any time thereafter. History, clinical signs, CCT and other laboratory tests may be helpful in distinguishing migraine from symptomatic headaches.

More difficult is the separation of psychogenic headaches from migraine, as there are no tests available. In my experience, psychogenic headaches are overestimated and are uncommon under 12 or 13 years of age; probably many of the patients who are relegated to the psychogenic group have migraine and are likely to respond to similar treatments. However, juvenile migraine is often aggravated by psychological factors.

Classification
Different types of migraine are recognized (Table 50.3). They reflect the involvement of different parts of the brain and do not differ in response to treatment,[12] except alternating hemiplegic migraine, which is probably a different disorder.[37]

Epidemiology
Most epidemiological studies of headaches have been conducted on adult populations.[7,28] The incidence varies considerably and has been reported as 23% in women and 15% in men. In children, the classic study is that of Bille,[4] who analysed questionnaires given to

9059 schoolchildren between ages 7 and 15 in Uppsala, the results of which can be seen in Table 50.4. Four per cent had migraine, as defined by the criteria of Vahlquist,[44] i.e. paroxysmal headaches separated by free intervals and at least two of the following four: one-sided pain, nausea, visual aura and family heredity. Due to the restricted definition, Bille's data probably underestimate the frequency of vascular headaches in childhood. However, using the same criteria, Sillanpää[40] obtained similar results.

Pathogenesis
The cause of migraine is not known. Perhaps it is best regarded as a neurovascular syndrome with a generalized vasomotor instability and vulnerability to multiple extraneous factors. The apparent precipitating factors (Table 50.5) may be the final event leading to decompensation of the system.

A number of humoral factors (Table 50.6) have been incriminated as a cause of migraine. However, like platelet hyperaggregability,[25] changes occur mainly during migraine attacks and are therefore likely to be effects rather than the cause of the disease.

Genetic factors
There are a number of reports on the inheritance of childhood migraine;[2,10,35] the family incidence ranged from 72% to 89%. However, there are no series of comparable controls and it is my experience that almost everybody has relations with recurrent headaches. Controlled studies are urgently needed to establish whether there is really a genetic factor involved or not. In contrast, there is a high familial incidence in hemiplegic migraine.[5,20]

Food idiosyncrasy and food allergy also play a role in the causation of migraine; these will be discussed below.

Types of migraine
Common migraine[17]
Classical migraine[35]
Complex and complicated migraine syndromes
Hemiplegic migraine[9]
Basilar artery migraine[3]
Ophthalmoplegic migraine[16]
Migrainic vertigo[34]
Confusional migraine[18]
Migraine and syncope[27]
Migraine and epilepsy[39]
Migraine and stroke[6]
Migraine and fever[47]
Migraine and cerebrospinal fluid (CSF) pleocytosis[36]
Cluster headaches[24]
Alternating hemiplegic migraine[37]

Table 50.3 Types of migraine.

Precipitating factors
Emotional
Food
Trauma
Exertion
Upper respiratory tract infections
Hypoglycaemia
Lactose intolerance
Irregular sleep
Travel
Bright light
Hormonal

Table 50.5 Precipitating factors.

Humoral factors suspected to be involved in the pathogenesis of migraine
Serotonin
Histamine
Prostaglandins
Leukotrienes
Substance P
Peptide kinins
Catecholamines
Tyramine
Phenylethylamine

Table 50.6 Humoral factors suspected to be involved in the pathogenesis of migraine.

Abdominal migraine and the periodic syndrome

Wyllie and Schlesinger[47] created the concept of the periodic syndrome. Children with this condition usually present themselves with one or a combination of the following symptoms: cyclical vomiting, recurrent abdominal pains, recurrent headaches, dizzy spells, periodic attacks of fever and periodic limb and joint pains.

Recurrent central abdominal pains (abdominal migraine) occur in one of 10 children of school age.[1] Frequent associated symptoms are pallor, vomiting and headaches. Abdominal migraine has to be separated from recurring appendicitis, mesenteric enteritis, Meckel's diverticulum and school phobia. It is indistinguishable from the 'irritable bowel syndrome' which is largely provoked by foods[26]. Carbohydrate intolerance (enzyme deficiency) or protein intolerance (allergy) may be causatively involved, although often an infant may be both protein and carbohydrate intolerant.[48] It is perhaps not surprising that patients with the irritable bowel syndrome often have recurrent headaches (Hunter, pers comm).

The features of the periodic syndrome are reminiscent of juvenile migraine and, indeed, follow-up studies have shown that the incidence of later migraine and/or psychiatric disorders is considerably higher compared to control groups.[22]

THERAPY

The aim of therapy is to interrupt a step in the pathogenesis of migraine. The measures consist of reassurance, pharmacotherapy, behavioural modification, acupuncture and diet.

Reassurance

In double-blind studies of treatment of patients with migraine, 20–30%, and occasionally more, responded to administered placebo. Reassurance of the benign nature of the recurring syndrome may be all that is necessary, especially if the headaches are mild and infrequent. Reassurance should be combined with general advice about lifestyle, including avoidance of trigger factors (see Table 50.5).

Pharmacotherapy

If the headaches are severe but infrequent (<3 to 4 times per month) treatment may be focused on the individual attacks and aspirin is the first thing to try.[31] If the headaches are of sufficient frequency (>3 times per month) daily prophylactic pharmacotherapy may be the treatment of choice. Derivatives of ergot have a long history of successful use in the treatment of migraine,[17] but the risk of side effects such as retroperitoneal fibroplasia,[21] thrombophlebitis[8] and possibly stroke due to the additional vasoconstriction have to be considered. Propranolol, clonidine and pizotifen have all been reported to be effective, but double-blind, placebo-controlled studies showed that in children the effect was not superior to placebo.[14,19,41] A number of other drugs have been reported to be effective.[2]

Behavioural treatment

Behavioural modification techniques have become increasingly popular and useful for the management of migraine as well as psychogenic headaches. The development of relaxation skills and the recognition of environmental influences are the basic issues and the components of treatment involve training in meditative relaxation, electromyographic biofeedback and assessment of headache occurrence.[32]

Acupuncture

Acupuncture can remove headaches of organic origin, at least temporarily. Its usefulness was assessed by Loh et al.,[30] who undertook a trial of acupuncture versus medical treatment in 48 patients with severe migraine and other types of headaches. A larger proportion preferred acupuncture to medical treatment. A beneficial response to acupuncture was more likely when the patient had local tender muscular points. The technique of acupuncture is painful for the patient and time consuming for the doctor. Another disadvantage is that the majority of patients need to come back for more treatment at intervals of 2–6 months. However, it is a safe and cheap method and its use is undoubtedly justified in adults, but children do not accept it easily because it is painful.

DIET

Although the production and marketing of headache remedies involves a major proportion of the modern pharmaceutical industry, their value in childhood migraine is limited[10,14,19,41] and in many cases their safety is in question. Acupuncture is difficult to adopt in children and often works only as long as it is applied regularly.[30] Apart from behaviour modification programmes, whose effects have as yet to be established by controlled trials, dietary treatment is a logical approach in view of the evidence that food intolerance is responsible for much migraine. Publications concerning the relationship between migraine and dietary factors can be separated into two major groups: tyramine hypothesis, and food allergy hypothesis.

Tyramine hypothesis

Hannington[23] reported that foods containing tyramine, a vasoactive amine, may precipitate headaches, particularly in patients who are treated with monoamine oxidase inhibitors (see Table 50.6). Foods rich in tyramine include cheese, pickled herring, chicken livers, canned figs and the pods of broad beans. Other vasoactive amines too were suspected to cause migraine such as phenylethylamine, present in chocolate, and 5-hydroxytryptamine, present in bananas, pineapple and tomatoes. A defect in the conjugation of tyramine and phenylethylamine has been incriminated by some authors[38] and others proposed a deficiency of platelet phenolsulphotransferase.[29] However, these enzymes were found to be reduced only during migraine attacks and therefore seem to represent an effect rather than the cause of migraine. Moreover, double-blind administration of tyramine to patients who benefited from a low tyramine diet did not provoke migraine.[10]

Food allergy hypothesis

A role for food allergy in migraine has been postulated since the second half of the 19th century, and oral sodium cromoglycate was found to have a protective effect in some patients.[12,33] The value of an oligoantigenic diet was demonstrated by a double-blind, placebo-controlled crossover trial[12] where 93% of children with severe and frequent migraine (> once per week) were shown to benefit.

During the sequential reintroduction of food at weekly intervals, 90% of the responders relapsed with one or more foods (Tables 50.7, 50.8 and 50.9) and recovered again avoiding them. The interval between eating a provoking food and migraine varied between different patients and between different foods in the same patient (Table 50.10). Forty-six children in whom a provoking food was identified entered a double-blind placebo-controlled crossover trial of the provoking food and, highly significantly, more patients had headaches with active material ($P < 0.001$) than with placebo (Table 50.11).

The oligoantigenic approach

Patients with migraine are not usually aware of foods that provoke migraine. Moreover, causative foods are as a rule favourite ones. Unfortunately, skin prick tests and other laboratory tests are not helpful in identifying provoking foods[12] and at present the only method of sorting them out is an oligantigenic diet, followed by sequential reintroduction of foods.

Who should be treated by diet?

Oligoantigenic diets are very demanding and potentially dangerous from the point of view of malnutrition[43] and anaphylaxis when foods are reintroduced.[11] Therefore only patients with severe and frequent attacks of migraine should be considered for such treatment. The patients reported in our trial[12] were selected because they had migraine at least once a week. Oligoantigenic diets should not be attempted in patients with fewer headaches, because the diet would be worse than the disease and because it would not be possible to gauge the progress.

Patients with migraine attacks at least four times a month should be considered for prophylactic pharmacotherapy. However, such treatment does not lead to improvement or recovery in 90%. Rotation diets (diets in which major items are eliminated one or two at a time) are sometimes used in patients with fewer attacks of migraine but their effect has yet to be studied.

Diet and associated symptoms

Migraine often affects other organs apart from the brain, causing a number of symptoms (Table 50.12). Patients with and without such associated symptoms respond equally well to oligoantigenic diets[12] and usually the associated symptoms also resolve.

The incidence of gastrointestinal symptoms (nausea, abdominal pain, flatulence, vomiting and diarrhoea) is given as ranging from 70% to 100% in a compilation of eight reported series.[35]

Provoking foods in 88 patients treated by diet			
Food	Tested	Symptoms	%
Cow's milk	75	29	39
Chocolate	64	24	37
Benzoic acid	46	17	37
Eggs	71	26	36
Tartrazine	45	15	33
Wheat	71	22	31
Cheese	48	15	31
Citrus	72	22	30
Coffee	21	5	24
Fish	51	11	22
Maize	53	9	17
Grapes	23	4	17
Goat's milk	44	7	16
Tea	44	7	16
Pork	60	8	13
Beef	64	8	12
Beans	42	9	12
Malt	33	3	9
Lentils	21	2	9
Apples	74	6	8
Yeast	54	4	7
Pears	69	4	6
Apricots	48	3	6
Sugar	56	3	5
Potatoes	78	4	5
Peas	37	2	5
Banana	78	4	5
Carrots	76	3	4
Chicken	73	3	4
Peaches	51	2	4
Lamb	75	2	3
Rice	75	1	1
Brassica	76	1	1

Table 50.7 Provoking foods in 88 patients treated by diet.

When provoking foods are given, abdominal symptoms usually recur first (the allergic reaction may therefore occur in the gut, and the other manifestations may result from released mediators or from circulating antigen or antigen–antibody complexes).

Results of specific food challenge in those of the 76 patients who reacted to antigenically related material		
Food	Tested	Symptoms
Reacted to cow's milk		
Soya	16	11
Sheep's milk	2	0
Pregestamil	1	0
Reacted to cow's cheese		
Sheep's cheese	3	0
Reacted to wheat		
Rye	27	12
Oats	22	8

Table 50.8 Results of specific food challenge in those of the 76 patients who reacted to antigenically related material.

Number of provoking foods in individual patients	
Patients	Foods
8	0
17	1
14	2
16	3
8	4
2	5
2	6
2	8
2	10
2	11
2	12
1	13
1	14
1	16
1	22
1	24

Table 50.9 Number of provoking foods in individual patients.

Intervals between eating the provoking food and symptoms	
<1 day	63 times
2 days	56 times
3 days	51 times
4 days	14 times
5 days	8 times
6 days	1 times
>7 days	14 times

Table 50.10 Intervals between eating the provoking food and symptoms.

Double-blind placebo-controlled crossover trial: occurrence of headaches			
	AP	PA	Total
Neither food	2	6	8
Active food	14	12	26*
Placebo	0	2	2
Both foods	1	3	4
Total	17	23	40

* Difference between active and placebo; $P < 0.001$. Data from Egger et al.,[12] with permission.

Table 50.11 Double-blind placebo-controlled crossover trial: occurrence of headaches.

Associated symptoms and signs		
	Patients completing oligoantigenic diet ($n = 88$)	
	Before diet	On diet
Abdominal symptoms	61	8
Behaviour disorder	41	5
Aches in limbs	41	7
Rhinitis	34	15
Recurrent mouth ulcers	15	2
Epilepsy	14	2
Vaginal discharge	11	1
Enuresis	8	2
Asthma	7	3
Eczema	6	3

Table 50.12 Associated symptoms and signs.

Other symptoms

Periodic limb pain of considerable severity,[47] myalgia[42] and somnolence and lassitude alternating with irritability and restlessness are common complaints and enuresis nocturna,[13] epilepsy[39] and fevers without infection[47] occur more frequently in a migraine population than one would expect. Although asthma and eczema may improve on diet, the frequency of atopy is not increased in migraineurs.[12]

History of associated symptoms

A history of associated symptoms is not always given spontaneously by the patients, perhaps because they are mainly worried about the headaches, and only careful questioning will reveal the presence of other symptoms. Sometimes different symptoms are provoked by different foods in the same patient.

Diet and nonspecific triggers

Rarely the expression of migraine only occurs with specific precipitating factors. More commonly, most migraine episodes are apparently spontaneous, and only occasionally may an identified trigger be responsible for an attack (see Table 50.5). In either circumstance recognition of such factors is of value because some of them can be avoided. Recognized trigger factors, however, fail to provoke migraine in patients who are on appropriate diets (Table 50.13), which is important in migraine provoked by changes of climate or by other factors which cannot be avoided. On diet, only cigarette smoke, pollens, perfumes and other inhalants continue to trigger attacks of migraine which would suggest a causative role of inhaled antigens too.

SUMMARY

Migraine is a common and sometimes disabling disorder in childhood. A number of factors are known to provoke migraine, but the mechanisms are not understood. Foods and synthetic additives can provoke migraine; more than 90% of children with severe and frequent attacks of migraine recover or improve on oligoantigenic diets. Provoking foods can be identified by elimination followed by sequential reintroduction.

All types of migraine as well as the associated symptoms may respond to diet. Other recognized trigger factors lose importance once provoking foods are avoided. Future work has to concentrate on the development of useful *in vitro* tests, by which provoking foods can be identified.

Nonspecific provokers of migraine in 38 patients		
	Before diet	**On diet**
Exercise	13	1
Trauma	11	1
Emotional	10	0
Perfumes or cigarette smoke	10	9
Travel	9	0
Bright light	5	0
Heat	2	1
Noise	2	0

Data from Egger *et al.*,[12] with permission.

Table 50.13 Nonspecific provokers of migraine in 38 patients.

REFERENCES

1 Apley J, Naish N. Recurrent abdominal pains: a field survey of 1000 school children. *Arch Dis Child* 1958; 33: 165–70.
2 Barlow CF. *Headaches and migraine in childhood*. Blackwell Scientific Publications, Oxford: JB Lippincott, Philadelphia; 1984.
3 Bickerstaff ER. Basilar artery migraine. *Lancet* 1961; i: 15–17.
4 Bille B. Migraine in schoolchildren. *Acta Paediatr [Suppl]* 1962; 51: 136–51.
5 Blau JN, Whitty CWM. Familial hemiplegic migraine. *Lancet* 1965; iii: 1115–16.
6 Bousson MG, Baron JC, Chiras J. Ischaemic strokes and migraine. *Neuroradiology* 1985; 27: 583.
7 Bruyn GW. Epidemiology of migraine: a personal view. *Headache* 1983; 23: 127–33.
8 Carter ER. Bilateral thrombophlebitis after a single dose of ergotamine tartrate for migraine. *Br Med J* 1958; ii: 1453.
9 Clarke JM. On recurrent motor paralysis in migraine, with a report in which recurrent hemiplegia accompanied the attacks. *Br Med J* 1910; ii: 1534–8.
10 Congdon PJ, Forsythe WI. Migraine in childhood: a study of 300 children. *Dev Med Child Neurol* 1979; 21: 209–16.
11 David DJ. Anaphylactic shock during elimination diets for severe atopic eczema. *Arch Dis Child* 1984; 59: 983–6.
12 Egger J, Carter CM, Wilson J *et al*. Is migraine food allergy? A double-blind controlled trial of oligoantigenic diet treatment. *Lancet* 1983; ii: 865–9.
13 Filipowics A. Migraine in children with functional nocturnal enuresis – a long-term prospective study of 32 cases. *Cephalalgia [Suppl]* 1985; 5: 186.
14 Forsythe WI, Gilles D, Sills MA. Propranolol (inderal) in the treatment of childhood migraine. *Dev Med Child Neurol* 1984; 26: 737–41.
15 Friedman AP, Merrit HH. Treatment of headache. *J Am Med Assoc* 1957; 163: 1111.
16 Friedman AP, Harter DH, Merrit HH. Ophthalmoplegic migraine. *Arch Neurol* 1962; 7: 320–7.
17 Friedman AP, Finley KH, Graham JR *et al*. Classification of headache. *Arch Neurol* 1962; 6: 173–6.
18 Gascon G, Barlow CF. Juvenile migraine presenting as an acute confusional state. *Pediatrics* 1970; 45: 628–35.
19 Gillies D, Sills M, Forsythe J. Pizotifen (Sanomigran) in childhood migraine. A double-blind controlled trial. *Eur Neurol* 1986; 25: 32–5.
20 Glista GG, Mellinger JF, Rooke ED. Familial hemiplegic migraine. *Mayo Clin Proc* 1975; 50: 307–11.
21 Graham JR, Suby HI, LeCompte PR, Sadovsky NL. Fibrotic disorders associated with methysergide therapy for headache. *N Engl J Med* 1966; 274: 359–68.
22 Hammond J. The late sequelae of recurrent vomiting of childhood. *Dev Med Child Neurol* 1974; 16: 15–22.
23 Hannington E. Preliminary report on tyramine headache. *Br Med J* 1967; ii: 550–1.
24 Harris W. *The Facial Neuralgias*. Oxford Medical Publications, London, 1937.
25 Hilton BP, Cumings JM. 5-Hydroxytryptamine levels and platelet aggregation responses in subjects with acute migraine headache. *J Neurol Neurosurg Psychiatry* 1972; 35: 505–9.
26 Jones A, McLaughlan P, Shorthouse M *et al*. Food intolerance: a major factor in the pathogenesis of irritable bowel syndrome. *Lancet* 1982; ii: 1115–17.
27 Lance JW, Anthony M. Some clinical aspects of migraine. *Arch Neurol* 1966; 15: 356–61.
28 Leviton A. Epidemiology of headache. *Adv Neurol* 1978; 19: 341–51.
29 Littlewood J, Glover V, Sandler M. Platelet phenol-sulphotransferase deficiency in dietary migraine. *Lancet* 1982; ii: 983–6.
30 Loh L, Nathan PW, Schott GD, Zilkha KJ. Acupuncture versus medical treatment for migraine and muscle tension headaches. *J Neurol Neurosurg Psychiatry* 1984; 47: 333–7.
31 Majerus PW. Why aspirin? *Circulation* 1976; 54: 357–9.
32 Masek B, Russo DC, Varni JF. Behavioral approaches to the management of chronic pain in children. *Pediatr Clin North Am* 1984; 31: 1113–32.
33 Monro J, Carini C, Brostoff J. Migraine is a food-allergic disease. *Lancet* 1984; ii: 719–21.
34 Moretti G, Manzoni GC, Caffarra P, Parma M. Benign recurrent vertigo and its connection with migraine. *Headache* 1980; 20: 344–6.
35 Prensky AL. Migraine and migrainous variants in pediatric patients. *Pediatr Clin North Am* 1976; 23: 461–71.
36 Rossi LN, Vasella F, Bajc O *et al*. Benign migraine-like syndrome with CSF pleocytosis in children. *Dev Med Child Neurol* 1985; 27: 192–8.

37 Salmon MA, Wilson J. Drugs for alternating hemiplegic migraine. *Lancet* 1984; ii: 980.

38 Sandler MMBH, Hannington E. A phenyethylamine oxidizing defect in migraine. *Nature* 1974; 250: 335.

39 Seshia SS, Reggin JD, Stanwick RS. Migraine and complex seizures in children. *Epilepsia* 1985; 26: 232–6.

40 Sillanpää M. Changes in the prevalence of migraine and other headache during the first seven school years. *Headache* 1983; 23: 15–19.

41 Sills M, Congdon P, Forsythe WI. Clonidine and childhood migraine. A pilot and double-blind study. *Dev Med Child Neurol* 1982; 24: 837–41.

42 Simons DJE, Day E, Goodell H, Wolff HG. Experimental studies on headache: muscles of the scalp and neck as sources of pain. *Assoc Res Nerv Dis Proc* 1943; 23: 228–44.

43 Tripp JH, Francis DE, Knight JA, Harries JT. Infant feeding practice: a cause for concern. *Br Med J* 1979; ii: 707–9.

44 Vahlquist B. Migraine in children. *Int Arch Allergy* 1955; 7: 348–55.

45 Walker-Smith JA. Cows milk intolerance as a cause of post-enteritic diarrhoea. *J Pediatr Gastroenterol Nutr* 1982; 1: 163–75.

46 Warner JO, Hathaway MK. Allergic form of Meadow's syndrome (Münchhausen by proxy). *Arch Dis Child* 1984; 59: 151–6.

47 Wyllie WG, Schlesinger B. The periodic group of disorders in childhood. *Br J Child Dis* 1933; 30: 1–21.

D

Chapter

51

The hyperkinetic syndrome

Joseph Egger

INTRODUCTION

The first recorded description of a hyperactive child that we know about was in a poem written in 1844 by a German physician named Hoffmann. The poem includes the following lines:[28]

...But Fidgety Phil,
He won't sit still,
He wiggles and giggles,
And then, I declare,
Swings backwards and forwards,
And tilts up his chair,
Just as a rocking-horse –
'Philip! I am getting cross!'
See the naughty, restless child,
Growing still more rude and wild,
Till his chair falls over quite,
Philip screams with all his might...

This poem encapsulates in a colourful style the kind of child who is the subject of this chapter. The typical child with the hyperkinetic syndrome is generally brought to professional attention early in his elementary school years. However, careful questioning usually reveals symptoms present from early childhood. The clinical picture is that of overactivity, impulsivity, distractability and excitability.[8] Aggressive and antisocial behaviour, specific learning problems and emotional lability are often considered part of the syndrome.[40] However, careful clinical studies reveal that only a small but significant minority of hyperkinetic children present with antisocial behaviour when initially seen.[52,60] Since antisocial behaviour is seen more frequently in older hyperkinetic children, it may develop as a secondary reaction.

Comparison with conduct disorder

Hyperkinetic behaviour has to be distinguished from conduct disorder. This is a diagnostic category for children who are rebel-lious, defiant, cruel, bullying, aggressive, frequently fighting, disobedient and who also lie and steal. However, it is claimed that 75% of hyperkinetic children are antisocial and that about 40% of conduct-disordered children are hyperactive.[8,50]

Two-thirds of overactive children are reported by their parents to be underachieving at school and up to a half are rated as below average in school by their teachers.[51] Learning difficulties are evident not only in reading disability but also in spelling, language and conceptual areas and in mathematical skills. Attentional deficits are common in hyperkinetic children, consisting of distractability, poor concentration, short interest span and a flitting disorganized approach to task demands. These problems present particular difficulties in the classroom and contribute to the child's frequent learning delays.

Normal activity

We lack a standard of what is a normal level of activity on which to base comparisons. Activity measures such as actometers, wiggle chairs and stabilometric cushions have been largely unsuccessful since overactive and normal children do not differ greatly on such measures.[4]

The same applies for other cardinal symptoms; there are no measurements of impulsivity and attention. Because of the frequency of attention deficits in overactive children, many authors prefer the term attention deficit syndrome and distinguish attention deficits with and without overactivity. However, attention deficits do not as yet have any precise definition; the term is as broad as hyperactivity itself and equally heterogeneous, and not all overactive children have attention deficits.

Thus far, reliable and valid tests of overactivity are not possible. Moreover, the overactive child may behave quite reasonably in the clinician's room, especially at the first visit. For practical purposes, behaviour rating scales are used such as that of Conners,[13] and classification is by the criteria of the *Diagnostic and Statistical Manual*[1] (Table 51.1).

Conners' abbreviated rating scales				
Observation	**Degree of activity**			
	Not at all	**Just a little**	**Pretty much**	**Very much**
Restless or overactive				
Excitable, impulsive				
Disturbs other children				
Fails to finish things				
Short attention span				
Constantly fidgeting				
Inattentive, easily distracted				
Demands must be met immediately				
Easily frustrated				
Cries often and easily				
Mood changes quickly and drastically				
Temper outbursts				
Explosive and unpredictable behaviour				
Scoring:	0	1	2	3

Score > 15 Hyperactivity likely.

Table 51.1 Conners' abbreviated rating scales.

Prevalence

Prevalence estimations of the hyperkinetic syndrome range from 1.2% to 20%[6,30,31,61] of all school children. There are more boys with diagnosed overactivity than girls, with male to female ratios ranging from 4:1 to 6:1. However, the results of a recent study[5] suggest that girls with the syndrome may be underidentified because cognitive deficits have a more prominent role in girls, whereas behavioural disturbances are more often seen in boys.

Follow-up studies have shown that the difficulties first evident in early childhood all too often have sequelae that persist into adult life. Overactivity per se diminishes with age,[37,38,60] but psychotic and criminal behaviour often become major problems.[36]

AETIOLOGY

Many causes of overactivity have been proposed (Table 51.2). The simplistic equation of 'hyperactivity equals brain damage' has to be rejected, as there is no evidence for it. Moreover, overactivity does not seem to represent a single disease entity; 92 terms have been used to describe hyperactive children,[55] reflecting a number of diagnostically distinctive subgroups. Less than 5% of hyperactive children show any signs of neurological impairment[48] and the presence of soft neurological signs such as deficiencies in motor coordination, reflex asymmetries, mild visual, hearing or language impairment, general clumsiness, right–left discrimination difficulties, choreiform jerks and athetoid movements in some of the children with overactive behaviour do not justify the term 'minimal brain dysfunction' for all.

Suspected causes of overactivity
Inherited hyperkinetic syndrome
Adverse psychosocial situations
Brain damage
Brain dysfunction
Epilepsy
Anticonvulsants
Lead poisoning
Maternal smoking and alcohol intake during pregnancy
Atopy
Sensitivity to salicylates and synthetic food additives
Food allergy

Table 51.2 Suspected causes of overactivity.

Family studies

A number of studies suggest a genetic link. There is a 100% concordance rate for the hyperkinetic syndrome in monozygotic twins[33] and a 50% concordance rate in full siblings compared to 14% in half sibs[49] and there was no increased prevalence for psychiatric illness or the hyperkinetic syndrome in the non-biological relatives of adopted hyperkinetic children.[8] Few of the studies have been able to disentangle genetic from environmental influences such as family problems[12] or problems at school,[3] lead poisoning,[27] maternal smoking and alcohol intake.[2]

Effect of diet

Feingold reported that 70% of overactive children responded to a diet avoiding colourings, preservatives and salicylates,[24] but controlled studies did not show such an effect.[14,26,56,57,59,62]

Randolph[44] proposed that any food could cause the trouble, and this hypothesis was supported by a double-blind, placebo-controlled crossover trial.[20]

The latter part of this chapter presents detailed outlines of the principles and practice of dietary therapy for hyperactive children.

THERAPY

Hyperactivity is not just a chemical defect that needs the right pill to correct it. A number of treatments have been used, of which psychostimulant drugs, behavioural approaches and diet changes are the commonest.

Psychostimulant drugs

The major stimulant drugs are the amphetamines (e.g. amphetamine sulphate (Benzedrine); dexamphetamine sulphate (Dexedrine)) and methylphenidate (Ritalin). The beneficial effects are increased alertness and control of attentional processes and decreased socially inappropriate behaviour. Negative side effects include insomnia, appetite suppression, increased heart rate, abdominal pain, weight loss, growth suppression, headaches and personality and mood changes.[3] Moreover, while there is agreement that stimulant medication may have positive effects on some aspects of the behaviour in the short term, the picture is disappointing in the long term. Medicated children show no long-term benefits in either social or academic areas[11] and, although drug treatment may increase the time spent focusing on a task, it does not necessarily improve task performance.[25]

Behavioural approaches

A wide variety of target behaviours, settings and programmes have been used.[34] These aim at reduction of excess behaviours and of disruptive antisocial behaviour, together with increases in desirable behaviour such as improved on-task attention, more adaptive cognitive strategies and enhanced academic achievement.[17] These needs derive from the multifaceted nature of hyperactivity, which involves the difficulties children experience in dealing with their environment and the difficulties parents and teachers experience with the children's behaviour.[43]

While there is little agreement that behavioural methods can be effective in modifying problem behaviour in the short term, there is no evidence of a long-term effect. In addition, behavioural therapy requires a high degree of consistent, sustained and often dedicated effort on the part of teachers and parents[43] and sometimes parents have so many adjustment difficulties of their own that they would not make good candidates for a successful behavioural programme.[39]

Diet

Concern about the undesirable effects of drug treatment as well as the mounting evidence for the lack of long-term efficacy of both drug treatment and of behavioural methods has led to a focus on diets as treatment. Publications concerning the relationship between the hyperkinetic syndrome and food allergy can be broadly separated into two major groups: Feingold's hypothesis, and the food allergy hypothesis.

THE FEINGOLD HYPOTHESIS

In June 1973 a preliminary report was presented by Feingold in which it was proposed that hyperkinesis in childhood is associated with the ingestion of salicylates, of compounds which crossreact with salicylates and with common food additives such as artificial flavours and colours. Feingold noted that an adult patient with aspirin sensitivity showed remission of psychiatric disturbances when placed on a diet free of natural salicylates, food colours and artificial flavours. Because of the supposed crossreactivity of salicylates and dyes, Feingold treated hyperactive children with a diet free of so-called natural salicylates and all artificial colours and flavours and claimed success in 70% of them.[24]

Criticisms

A number of criticisms were immediately raised against his claims, and indeed his findings were impressionistic, anecdotal and lacking in objective evidence. Included among the criticisms were that the patients reported were not described by any standard methods, no controls were utilized, no objective measures of change were employed, the observer of change was not blind to the treatment being evaluated and alternative explanations based on commonly accepted placebo phenomena were not considered.

Double-blind trials

Subsequently a number of double-blind trials involving control diets and diets eliminating artificial colours, flavours and natural salicylates were conducted on children with well-defined hyperkinetic syndrome. Two groups of psychologists, Conners et al.[14] and Harley et al.,[26] each carried out a similar investigation in which they carefully studied hyperactive children for a baseline period of 1 month before the children were placed on special diets. The children had several types of psychological and other tests to determine their usual behaviour. They were then randomly and alternately placed on either the Feingold diet for 1 month or on a control diet which seemed equally difficult. After each diet, psychological tests and evaluations were repeated.

Results: Study 1

In Conners' study, both parents and teachers agreed that the Feingold diet reduced the children's activity compared to the baseline period. The teachers noted a few children who had highly significant reductions of symptoms on the Feingold diet but not on the control diet. The control diet ratings did not differ from the baseline period ratings for either parents or teachers.

It was concluded that there may be a small subgroup of hyperkinetic children who might benefit from the Feingold diet, although the final results were inconclusive, partly because the few hyperactive children who improved were generally the ones who received the Feingold diet after the placebo diet.

Results: Study 2

In another study of Feingold's hypothesis[62] 26 children were randomly assigned to treatment conditions whereby they were given active or placebo medications in combination with challenge biscuits with artificial food colours or control biscuits without the additives. The children were crossed over into each of the four treatment conditions, and double-blind assessments and behaviour checklists were completed by teachers and parents. Although stimulant medications were more effective than diet in reducing hyperactive behaviour, both parent and teacher ratings indicated that there was some reduction in symptoms in one-quarter of the children who received the Feingold diet.

Results: Study 3

Harley et al.[26] studied 36 school-age hyperactive boys and 10 hyperactive preschool boys under experimental and control diet conditions. Parental ratings revealed positive behaviour changes for the experimental diet, but teacher ratings, objective classroom and laboratory observational data, attention–concentration and psychological measures yielded no support for Feingold's hypothesis.

Results: Study 4

Swanson et al.[56] studied 40 children for 5 days on a diet free of artificial food dyes and other additives. Twenty of the children were hyperactive and the behaviour of the other 20 was normal. Oral challenges with large doses (100–150 mg) of synthetic food dyes or placebo were administered on days 4 and 5 of the experiment. The performance of the hyperactive children on paired associate learning tests on the day they received the colours was impaired relative to their performance after they received the placebo ($P < 0.01$). The performance of the non-hyperactive group was not affected by the challenge with the food dyes. The Conners' rating scale was also filled out twice daily, but no difference between the dye and placebo conditions was manifested on this measure of social behaviour.

Results: Study 5

Weiss et al.[59] challenged 22 children, maintained on a diet excluding certain foods, with a blend of seven artificial colours in a double-blind placebo-controlled crossover trial. Parents' observations provided the criteria of response. One child reacted mildly to the challenge and another one reacted dramatically. The doses of synthetic additives employed in this study were about 50 times lower than the maximum allowable daily intakes recommended by the Food and Drug Administration. The challenge was given once on each of 8 days randomly distributed among weeks 3 to 10 of the study period. It was concluded that Feingold's diet was effective in a small subgroup of hyperactive children.

Results: Study 6

In another study of Feingold's hypothesis,[57] 10 institutionalized children were maintained on an additive-free diet for 2 weeks, followed by 2 weeks in which two high, consecutive doses of artificial food colours were administered orally in a placebo-masked, double-blind experimental design. For the three psychometric measures examined (Porteus mazes, paired-associate learning test and actometer readings) the trend was in the direction hypothesized, i.e. group scores deteriorated under colour challenge. However, the results failed to reach statistical significance. The teachers' ratings changed in the opposite direction to that predicted. However, as with the psychometric tests, the behavioural rating measures did not reach statistical significance.

Conclusion

The results of the controlled studies of Feingold's hypothesis are all somewhat equivocal, but the broad conclusions were that his claims were probably exaggerated. The reason for the uncertainty was the lack of comparability between studies because of the heterogeneity of subject groups used, differences in dietary manipulations and additive substances given and the diversity of dependent variables employed. Overriding all these problems were inadequate research designs; Conners et al.[14] and Harley et al.[28] used a control diet whose effects on behaviour were not studied before. Williams et al.,[62] Harley et al.,[28] Swanson and Kinsbourne,[56] Weiss et al.[59] and Thorley[57] did not insert washout periods in between the test periods, which were probably disturbed by carry-over effects. Williams et al.,[62] Swanson and Kinsbourne[56] and Thorley[57] disguised the active and placebo ingredients in chocolate and sugar-containing materials, although it was known that these substances are likely to have adverse effects on behaviour. Swanson and Kinsbourne[56] and Weiss et al.[59] administered the challenges only for 1 or 2 days, thus not allowing the symptoms to develop. However, all studies showed that some hyperactive children or certain subgroups of them may benefit from an additive-free diet.

THE FOOD ALLERGY HYPOTHESIS

A role for food allergy in the hyperkinetic syndrome has been postulated since the early 20th century.[15,16,29,44,45,46,54] Because of the lack of scientific documentation, this hypothesis was rejected until the highly significant results of a double-blind, placebo-controlled crossover trial were published.[20] During a previous double-blind, controlled trial of the effect of diet on migraine, it was noted that any combination of foods could cause symptoms in children.[21] What was also of interest was that many responders had also been overactive and that their overactivity usually improved with food avoidance, in some instances with avoidance of foods other than those causing migraine. We therefore undertook a trial of diet in hyperkinetic children, and, in those who responded, provoking foods were identified by sequential reintroduction and tested in a double-blind crossover trial.

Double-blind trial
Clinical characteristics
Seventy-six children took part in the experiment. All were socially handicapped by their behaviour, and overactivity and inattention were prominent features. The children were selected for severe overactivity and may not be representative of hyperkinetic children in the general population. A surprisingly high proportion had associated symptoms such as headaches, abdominal pains and seizures and only 10 did not have any such symptoms. The study was criticized for the selection method, because headaches and recurrent abdominal pains are not usually recognized as part of the hyperkinetic syndrome. However, only a few patients and parents gave a history of associated symptoms because they were troubled more by the behaviour problems and only careful questioning revealed the presence of these other symptoms.

Results
Of all the children, 82% responded to an oligoantigenic diet. However, only 27% recovered completely (Table 51.3). Most of the associated symptoms also improved with diet (Table 51.4). During the subsequent reintroduction, the commonest substances that caused problems were tartrazine and benzoic acid but no child reacted to these alone. Forty-six other provocative foods were also identified (Table 51.5) and most patients reacted to several (Table 51.6). The interval between eating the provoking

Changes in severity of symptoms of hyperactivity with diet				
	Total	No improvement	Improved	Recovered
Mild	6	1 (17%)	0 (0%)	5 (83%)
Moderate	31	5 (16%)	16 (52%)	10 (32%)
Severe	39	8 (21%)	25 (64%)	6 (15%)

No improvement = grade unchanged; improved = 1 or 2 grades less severe; recovered = requires normal management only.

Table 51.3 Changes in severity of symptoms of hyperactivity with diet.

Clinical features of 76 children with the hyperkinetic syndrome		
Feature	Start of study	On diet
Number of subjects	76	76
Age (years, mean and range)	7.3 (2–15)	–
Sex (male/female)	60/16	–
Adverse psychosocial factors in the family	37	–
Overactivity		
Normal	0	21
Mild	6	28
Moderate	31	19
Severe	39	8
Mean Conners' score	24	12
Antisocial behaviour	32	13
Emotional difficulties	7	0
Severe mental retardation	6	
Specific developmental delay	10	
Headaches	48	9
Fits	14	1
Abdominal discomfort	54	8
Chronic rhinitis	33	9
Aches in limbs	33	6
Skin rashes (eczema, etc.)	28	9
Mouth ulcers	15	5
Atopy	30	–

Table 51.4 Clinical features of 76 children with the hyperkinetic syndrome.

food and reaction varied from a few minutes to more than 7 days, but was usually 2–3 days. There was no difference between synthetic additives and foods.

Reintroduction of provoking food

Altogether 28 patients completed the double-blind, placebo-controlled crossover trial of the effect of reintroduction of a provoking food. The parents kept daily Conners' scores and a paediatrician and a psychologist independently made an assessment of the children's behaviour for each arm of the double-blind trial. At the end of the second period parents also recorded preference based on difference of symptoms. The psychologist employed actometer readings, matching familiar figures tests and the Porteus maze test. Parents, the paediatrician and the psychologist assessed the period in which the placebo material was administered as being linked more often with better behaviour (Table 51.7). There was no significant order effect. However, Conners' scales scored by the parents showed a significant but expected treatment order interaction (Fig. 51.1).

Psychological tests

Except for the actometer readings, all the psychological tests showed a trend in favour of the placebo material. However, the differences between the active and placebo periods were not significant, possibly because they did not measure those skills most helped by dietary treatment or they were not sensitive enough to detect the deterioration induced by a brief challenge with a limited dose of the provoking food. The number of patients studied was also small.

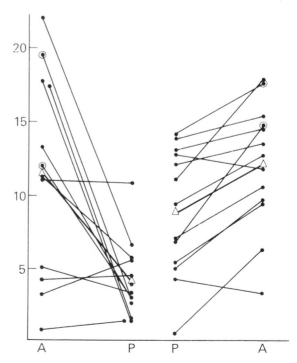

Fig. 51.1 Mean Conners' abbreviated scale scores (closed circle) while patients were on placebo (P) and active (A) material. Means of each group are shown by open triangles. Those values which include assigned maximum scores for a part of the period, after withdrawal of the material because of severity of the symptoms are encircled. (Reproduced with permission from the *Lancet.*[20])

Table 51.5 Reactions to foodstuffs.

Reactions to foodstuffs

Food	Number tested	Number reacted (%)	Food	Number tested	Number reacted
1 Foods universally tested			**2 Foods rarely tested and**		
Colourant and preservatives	34	27 (79)	positive‡		
Soya*	15	11 (73)	Plums	9	2
Cow's milk	55	35 (64)	Rabbit	6	3
Chocolate	34	20 (59)	Sago	5	2
Grapes	18	9 (50)	Duck	4	3
Wheat	53	28 (49)			
Oranges	49	22 (45)	**3 Foods tested only in**		
Cow's cheese	15	6 (40)	patients who reacted to		
Hen's eggs	50	20 (39)	antigenically related foods		
Peanuts	19	6 (32)	To cow's milk:		
Maize	38	11 (29)	Goat's milk	22	15
Fish	48	11 (23)	Ewe's milk	12	4
Oats	43	10 (23)	To wheat:		
Melons	29	6 (21)	Rye	29	15
Tomatoes	35	7 (20)			
Ham/bacon	20	4 (20)	**4 Foods to which there**		
Pineapple	31	6 (19)	was no reaction		
Sugar†	55	9 (16)	Cabbages	54	
Beef	49	8 (16)	Lettuces	53	
Beans	34	5 (15)	Cauliflowers	50	
Peas	33	5 (15)	Celery	49	
Malt	20	3 (15)	Goat's cheese	4	
Apples	53	7 (13)	Duck eggs	2	
Pork	38	5 (13)			
Pears	41	5 (12)			
Chicken	56	6 (11)			
Potatoes	54	6 (11)			
Tea	19	2 (10)			
Coffee	10	1 (10)			
Other nuts	11	1 (10)			
Cucumbers	32	3 (9)			
Bananas	52	4 (8)			
Carrots	55	4 (7)			
Peaches	41	3 (7)			
Lamb	55	3 (5)			
Turkey	22	1 (5)			
Rice	51	2 (4)			
Yeast	28	1 (4)			
Apricots	34	1 (3)			
Onions	49	1 (2)			

* Given only to those who reacted to cow's milk.

† Five reacted to both beet and cane sugar, three to cane sugar only and one to beet sugar only. The parents of several other patients thought that large quantities of sugar provoked symptoms, without definite confirmation.

‡ Tested in < 10 patients.

The oligoantigenic approach

Lack of diagnostic tests

Questioning of the patient and parents to identify possible provoking foods is worthwhile, but most children and parents do not give such a history, and its presence or absence is not a good predictor of response to diet. Skin prick tests and immunoglobulin E radio allergosorbent tests (IgE RASTS) to food antigens are also unhelpful in this respect.[21] Identification of food antigens can be achieved by oligoantigenic diets and subsequent sequential reintroduction of foods.[10]

This method was used to study the food allergy hypothesis of migraine and hyperkinetic behaviour (i.e. any food can cause the trouble). Each patient was first put on a very restricted oligoantigenic diet (few foods) for 4 weeks. If improvement occurred,

Number of foods causing symptoms in the patients	
Number of foods	Number of patients
1	5
2	4
3	4
4	8
5	4
6	9
7	3
8	4
9	3
10	3
11	2
12	2
18	1
21	1
27	1
30	2

Table 51.6 Number of foods causing symptoms in the patients.

this was followed by open sequential reintroduction of single foods. Response to a selected food was confirmed by double-blind food provocations where possible (Fig. 51.2).

The oligoantigenic diet
All foods are potential allergens and an oligoantigenic diet should contain as few foods as possible. A typical oligoantigenic diet contains one meat, one carbohydrate source, a few vegetables (brassicas) and one fruit (Table 51.8). Although the foods chosen may cause problems, they are less likely to do so than most others. Since adherence to such a strict and demanding diet is difficult, a modified oligoantigenic diet containing a greater variety of foods was developed, including some more foods which had seldom provoked symptoms in the early patients (Table 51.9). This diet can be altered to suit the individual. If medicines have to be given, preparations free of colours should be used.

Response to diet
If there is no improvement on the oligoantigenic diet it can be assumed that the patient is either intolerant to foods in the diet, or did not adhere to it or is not food intolerant. Unless adherence is suspect, an alternative diet with no foods in common with the first can be tried (see Table 51.8).

Children are treated at home, since hospitals are not usually capable of providing a wide variety of meals from only a few foods.

Symptoms may worsen for a few days when the diet is started and some patients show withdrawal-like reactions. Improvement normally occurs during the second week, but may be seen almost immediately or only after 3 weeks.

Double-blind trial of assessment of behaviour in hyperactive children											
	Overactivity									Any symptom		
	Paediatric neurologist			Parents			Psychologist			Parents		
	PA	AP	Both	PA	AP	Both	PA	AP	Both	PA	AP	Both
Behaviour better on:												
Neither	3	4	7	2	2	4	5	4	9	3	2	5
Placebo	12	8	20	13	10	23	7	6	13	12	11	23
Active	0	1	1	0	4	1	0	2	2	9	0	0
Total	15	13	28	15	13	28	12	12	24	15	13	28
P value												
PA versus AP	NS			NS			NS			NS		
A versus P	<0.001			<0.001			≏0.01			<0.001		
NS = not significant.												

Table 51.7 Double-blind trial of assessment of behaviour in hyperactive children.
(Reproduced with permission from the *Lancet*.)

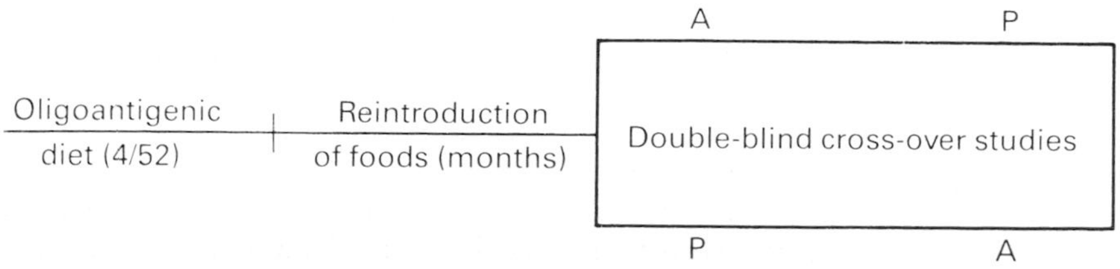

Oligoantigenic diet (4/52) — Reintroduction of foods (months)

A ——— P
Double-blind cross-over studies
P ——— A

Fig. 51.2 Method of the oligoantigenic approach to diagnosis of food-induced hyperactivity.

Ideal oligoantigenic diet (A) and alternative oligoantigenic diet (B)	
A	**B**
Turkey	Lamb
Cabbage, sprouts, cauliflower, broccoli	Carrots, parsnips
Potato, potato flour	Rice, rice flour
Banana	Pears
Soya oil, Tomor margarine	Sunflower oil
Water, salt	Water, salt
Calcium and vitamins	Calcium and vitamins

Table 51.8 Ideal oligoantigenic diet (A) and alternative oligoantigenic diet (B).

Modified oligoantigenic diet	
Meat	Include two meats, e.g. lamb and turkey. Also offal from these meats if liked
Carbohydrate	Rice, potatoes, arrowroot

Vegetables	Choose two of the following food families:
	    broccoli, cauliflower, cabbage, sprouts (brassicas)
	    carrots, parsnips, celery
	    cucumber, marrow, courgettes, melon
	    leeks, onions, asparagus

Fruit	Choose two of the following: apples, pears, bananas, peaches and apricots, pineapple

Fats	Milk-free margarine, e.g. Tomor–Van den Bergh
	    (typical analysis, palm and palm kernel oil with soya
	    or rape oils)
	Sunflower oil

Drinks	Pure fruit juice from included fruits, tap water, pure bottled water

Miscellaneous	Salt, pepper, pure herbs
	Plain potato crisps (preferably only one pack per day)
	Sugar and golden syrup and pure jam from included fruits
	Raising agents for baking
	A calcium (300 mg/day) and vitamin supplement is
	    advisable: calcium gluconate tablets (1 g) × 3 daily
	    or calcium lactate tablets (300 mg) × 6 daily.
	    Abidec (Parke Davis) 0.6 ml per day
	Avoid coloured toothpaste, medicines containing
	    artificial colour and preservative and discourage
	    chewing of chalks, etc.

Table 51.9 Modified oligoantigenic diet.

Open sequential reintroduction of foods

If recovery or definite improvement occurs during the period of oligoantigenic diet, foods are reintroduced one by one at weekly intervals with the new food being given daily in normal quantities. If no adverse reaction occurs with the new food, it is incorporated into the diet and the next food is introduced. If symptoms occur with a certain food, it is withdrawn and tested again at a later stage. After the child has recovered, another food is introduced. The order in which foods are introduced depends both on improving the nutritional adequacy and on the patients' preference (Table 51.10). If alarming reactions such as anaphylaxis, angiodema or status epilepticus are expected with the reintroduction of certain foods, the patient should be admitted to hospital for its reintroduction, which should begin with small quantities (e.g. 5 g).

Double-blind provocation

Diets have a powerful placebo effect, so double-blind provocations are a necessary step in most patients with suspected food allergy. This is also the only method to identify patients with the allergic Munchausen by proxy syndrome.[58]

Concealing a food in the necessary quantities presents problems. It is mixed with other foods to which the patient is known not to react and whose flavour, smell and appearance will conceal the food to be tested. The disguising material is given as a placebo. For example, if cow's milk was a provoking food and the child could drink soya, goat's milk or sheep's milk without problems, blind cow's milk preparations could be made by mixing it with one of these.[10] Each active and placebo material should be given daily for at least 1 week with a washout period of at least a week in between.

At present the oligoantigenic approach is the only method of identifying provoking foods. The provoking foods are not usually the ones the patient dislikes or the ones expected to be responsible, but are often frequently eaten or even craved. Therefore if only foods suspected by the patient are avoided, no response to diet will be seen, this being clearly shown by such an experiment.[42]

WHO SHOULD BE TREATED BY DIET?

Diets are socially disruptive, expensive and dangerous if not properly supervised, and are justified only in patients with severe disease. The patients selected for dietary treatment by Egger *et al.*[20] were handicapped by their behaviour problems and made life difficult for families and schools; patients less severely affected are not suitable for the dietary approach.

Associated symptoms

Children with severe hyperkinetic behaviour often suffer from a number of associated symptoms (see Table 51.4) although these are rarely the presenting ones.

Fatigue

Fatigue or the feeling that the child is 'rundown' is often a major complaint. The parents are concerned about his sluggishness, drowsiness and lack of interest in both schoolwork and play, although most of the time the child is restless, impulsive and highly irritable. This combination of behaviour pattern was seen in one-third of severely hyperkinetic children.[20]

Abdominal symptoms and headache

Recurrent abdominal pains and headaches are the most common associated symptoms. However, only a quarter of patients

Reintroduction of foods to diet of hyperactive children following oligoantigenic diet	
Chicken	Fresh or frozen chicken and chicken liver
Oats	Porridge oats, Scottish oatcakes, home-made flapjacks, etc., if sugar is already allowed
Beef	Fresh or frozen beef, any cut or offal
Wheat	Wholemeal or unbleached white flour for baking, spaghetti and pasta (egg-free), shredded wheat, puffed wheat
Yeast	Give homemade wholemeal bread, or buy wholemeal bread from a local baker or health food shop after checking there is no soya or preservative Wholemeal pitta bread
Cow's milk	Pasteurized cow's milk. If no symptoms arise, cream, pure plain yoghurt, pale uncoloured butter may be given
Cow's milk substitute	If cow's milk is not tolerated, substitutes can be tried one by one, diluted ewe's milk if available or goat's milk (boiled or pasteurized), or soya milk, e.g. Cow and Gate S Formula, or bovine casein hydrolysate, e.g. Nutramigen (Mead Johnson). Non-dairy or imitation cream, e.g. Sainsbury's 2 oz diluted to 1 pint (this contains some additives and is not a nutritional substitute for milk but it is a good vehicle for breakfast cereal, etc.)
Eggs	Use whole fresh eggs, e.g. 1 per day (a few who react will tolerate duck eggs)
Fish	Use fresh or frozen fish (not smoked, processed or battered, etc.) e.g. cod, herring. Try shellfish separately later
Orange	Pure natural unsweetened orange juice, oranges, satsumas, etc. If oranges are tolerated all citrus fruit probably is too
Tomatoes	Fresh tomatoes, additive-free canned and puréed tomatoes, and additive-free ketchup, e.g. Heinz
Pork	Fresh or frozen pork, any cuts or offal
Sugar	Use ordinary sugar (brown or white) on cereal, in puddings, drinks and in baking, etc. If sugar is not tolerated try cane and beet sugars separately. Tate and Lyle's sugar and syrup is of cane origin. Silver Spoon sugar and syrup is largely of beet origin but may contain some cane. If this is not tolerated, try glucose, fructose or glucose polymer
Chocolate	Try only if sugar is tolerated. If diet is milk-free, use milk-free chocolate, e.g. Terry's Bitter Chocolate and plain continental chocolate, e.g. Côte d'Or. If milk is taken, milk chocolate may be used. Cocoa powder may be used in cooking
Peas and beans	These include peas, runner beans, kidney beans, lentils. Also additive-free baked beans in tomato sauce if tomatoes are tolerated, e.g. Heinz
Rye	This is particularly worth trying if wheat is not tolerated e.g. Ryvita – the original rye crispbread, or Ryking (blue pack)
Malt	Rice Krispies if rice is tolerated, Weetabix and Shreddies if wheat is tolerated
Corn	Sweetcorn, homemade popcorn, cornflour, maize flour, corn oil, cornflakes if malt is tolerated
White flour	Use white flour in cooking and for homemade white bread. White pitta bread (white flour contains a bleaching agent)
Soya and propionate preservative	Supermarket white bread contains both of these. Its introduction tests for both, but a reaction necessitates distinguishing them
Tea	Add milk and sugar only if these are already in the diet
Coffee	
Colours and benzoic acid	Orange squash, e.g. Robinson's, usually contains tartrazine and benzoate preservative and can be tried if oranges and sugar are tolerated. Other items such as jelly, fruit gums, boiled fruit sweets, etc., contain colours but not benzoate preservative. Tartrazine and benzoic acid can also be tested using tartrazine or benzoic acid in capsules, e.g. 5 to 50 mg per day
Nitrites	These are preservatives in cooked or cured meats. Use ham and bacon if pork is tolerated, and corned beef if beef is tolerated
Sodium glutamate	Use stock cubes, e.g. Knorr cubes, or gravy mixes, e.g. Gravy Mate made by Bovril Ltd. provided their other ingredients are tolerated
Peanuts	Use plain or salted peanuts and peanut butter
Other nuts	These may be tried singly or mixed as preferred, e.g. almonds, walnuts, etc.

Other foods, e.g. fruits and vegetables, and manufactured foods such as ice cream, biscuits, etc., can be introduced weekly, taking into account avoidance of foods to which the patient is sensitive. If cereals or grains have to be avoided or restricted, buckwheat flour, wheatstarch, soya flour, grain (chickpea) flour and some of the special dietary products made for gluten-free and low protein diets may be tried but always check that the other ingredients are suitable for the individual.

Table 51.10 Reintroduction of foods to diet of hyperactive children following oligoantigenic diet.

mentioned them spontaneously, whereas careful questioning revealed their presence in more than half. Some had been investigated previously by gastroenterologists and/or neurologists.

Less frequently seen but not uncommon are aching limbs, excessive thirst, enuresis and fever.

Most of these symptoms are relieved on oligoantigenic diets and can be reproduced with provoking foods. Sometimes the foods causing associated symptoms differ from those which cause hyperkinetic behaviour. Of the 76 patients reported by Egger et al.,[20] 66 had associated symptoms relieved and reproduced on several occasions by avoiding and reintroducing certain foods and only 10 were hyperkinetic alone. Of the latter, nine responded to diet.

Hyperactivity combined with other symptoms has been reported by a number of authors[16,44,45,46,54] but was not mentioned by others.[5,14,26,56,57,59,62] No indication is given by the latter authors as to whether the children gave such a history or simply did not have the symptoms. It is my experience that only a minority of severely hyperactive children do not have associated symptoms if a careful history is taken.

The combination of symptoms often would suggest an underlying psychosomatic illness. Despite such an association, patients should not be excluded from a dietary experiment; it is possible that some so-called psychosomatic illnesses in fact are caused by food allergy, and polysymptomatic patients responded to diet as well as those with single symptoms.[20]

Family pressures

There is impressive evidence in support of 'family system' influences in the development of child behaviour problems, in particular the negative effects of marital discord, and continuous negative parent–child interactions have been incriminated.[12,41] Children in such unfavourable situations should not be regarded as unsuitable for dietary treatment, since the disturbances within the family might have arisen from food allergy in other family members, as food allergy is familial. Of the 72 families reported by Egger et al.[20] 35 had adverse psychosocial backgrounds. Although response to diet was less common in those families than in families not exposed to adverse psychosocial situations, such factors were present in more than 40% of the responders. Moreover, some family members with psychosocial problems, who underwent dietary treatment together with the children, reported relief of their symptoms. Others commented that the family life had improved simultaneously with the child's improvement.

PROGNOSIS

Some of our patients[20] ceased to react to provoking foods when they were tested again after about 1 year on the oligoantigenic diet. Others realized that their child was no longer intolerant to a particular food after mistakes had been made in the diet with no ill-effects. On the other hand, foods previously shown not to cause problems sometimes started to provoke symptoms, and this sometimes coincided with viral infections. The majority of children, however, continued to have problems when provoking foods were given.

Being on an acceptable diet did seem to make a remarkable difference to family life, and schoolwork improved in a number of children. Many of the patients, however, continued to have some behavioural problems and needed alternative management in addition to the diet.

Growing out of hyperactivity?

Early investigators thought that the hyperkinetic syndrome was a time-limited condition which disappeared as the child grew older.[22,32] It is now recognized that, although hyperactivity may diminish with age, antisocial behaviour, educational retardation, depression and psychosis are prevalent in grown-up hyperkinetic children.[35,36,60] It is too early to speculate whether dietary management will influence the prognosis of hyperkinetic children. However, there are reports suggesting that antisocial behaviour in young delinquents was often related to certain foods or food additives,[53] and that schizophrenics on a milk- and cereal-free diet were released from hospital twice as fast as those given the regular hospital diet.[18] More recently, Dohan et al.[19] tested this hypothesis by comparing the incidence of schizophrenia in a New Guinea population that consumes little or no grain or milk with one that consumes grain but no milk. They found that schizophrenia is infrequent in tribal populations where grains and milk are rare and more frequent in similar populations that do consume grains but no milk.

Prospective studies of the effect of dietary management into adulthood are urgently needed and the reports on dietary treatment of antisocial behaviour and psychiatric disorder in adults must be tested by double-blind, placebo-controlled trials.

SUMMARY

The hyperkinetic syndrome can be provoked by foods. There is no evidence as to which mechanism(s) is (are) involved, but the diversity of foods and the fact that children grow out of reactivity suggests allergy rather than idiosyncrasy. At present the only method of identifying provoking foods is an oligoantigenic diet followed by sequential reintroduction of foods. Food-allergic reactions may be immediate or slow (more than 7 days), therefore each food has to be tested for at least 1 week. Double-blind studies are essential, since diets have a powerful placebo effect. Only severe disease should be treated by diet and careful supervision by experienced doctors and dieticians is essential, because of the danger of malnutrition and the fact that diets are expensive and socially disruptive.

REFERENCES

1   American Psychiatric Association. *Diagnostic and Statistical Manual of Mental Disorders*. 3rd edn. American Psychiatric Association, Washington DC, 1980; 42–4.

2   Barkley RA. *Hyperactive Children: a Handbook for Diagnosis and Treatment*. Guilford Press, New York, 1981.

3   Barkley RA, Cunningham CE. Do stimulant drugs improve the academic performance of hyperkinetic children? A review of outcome studies. *Clin Pediatr* 1978; 17: 85–92.

4   Barkley RA, Ullman DG. A comparison of objective measures of activity and distractibility in hyperactive and nonhyperactive children. *J Abnorm Child Psychol* 1975; 3: 231–44.

5   Berry CA, Shaywitz SE, Shaywitz BA. Girls with attention deficit disorder: a silent minority? A report on behavioural and cognitive characteristics. *Pediatrics* 1985; 76: 801–9.

6   Bosco JJ, Robin SS. Hyperkinesis: prevalence and treatment. In: *Hyperactive Children: The social Ecology of Identification and Treatment* (Whalen C, Henker B, eds). Academic Press, New York, 1980: 173.

7   Cantwell D. A critical review of therapeutic modalities with hyperactive children. In: *The Hyperactive Child: Diagnosis, Management and Current Research* (Cantwell D, ed.). Spectrum Publications, New York, 1975.

8   Cantwell D. Genetic studies of hyperactive children: psychiatric illness in biologic and adopting parents. In: *Genetic Research in Psychiatry* (Fieve R, Rosenthal D, Brill H, eds). Johns Hopkins University Press, Baltimore, 1975.

9   Cantwell D. Hyperkinetic syndrome. In: *Child Psychiatry: Modern Approaches* (Rutter M, Hersov L, eds). Blackwell, Oxford, 1976; 524–55.

10 Carter CM, Egger J, Soothill JF. A dietary management of severe childhood migraine. *Hum Nutr Appl Nutr* 1985; 39A: 294–303.

11 Charles L, Schain R. A four-year follow-up study of the effects of methylphenidate on the behavior and academic achievement of hyperactive children. *J Abnorm Child Psychol* 1981; 9: 495–505.

12 Christensen A, Phillips S, Glasgow R, Johnson S. Parental characteristics and interactional dysfunction in families with child behavior problems: a preliminary investigation. *J Abnorm Child Psychol* 1983; 11: 153–66.

13 Conners CK. Rating scales for use in drug studies with children. *Psychopharmacol Bull [Special Issue – Pharmacotherapy with children]* 1973; 24–84.

14 Conners CK, Goyette CH, Southwick DA *et al*. Food additives and hyperkinesis: a controlled double-blind experiment. *Pediatrics* 1976; 58: 154–66.

15 Cooke RA. Studies in specific hypersensitiveness. On the phenomenon of hyposensitization (the clinically lessened sensitiveness of allergy). *J Immunol* 1922; 7: 219.

16 Crook WG, Harrison WW, Crawford SE, Emerson BS. Systemic manifestations due to allergy. *Pediatrics* 1961; 27: 790–9.

17 Cunningham CE, Barkley RA. The role of academic failure in hyperactive behavior. *J Learn Disabil* 1978; 11: 274–80.

18 Dohan FC, Grasberger FJ. Relapsed schizophrenics: earlier discharge from the hospital after cereal-free, milk-free diet. *Am J Psychiatry* 1973; 130: 685–8.

19 Dohan FC, Harper EH, Clark MH *et al*. Is schizophrenia rare if grain is rare? *Biol Psychiatry* 1984; 19: 385–99.

20 Egger J, Carter CM, Graham PJ *et al*. Controlled trial of oligoantigenic diet treatment in the hyperkinetic syndrome. *Lancet* 1985; i: 540–5.

21 Egger J, Carter CM, Wilson J *et al*. Is migraine food allergy? A double-blind controlled trial of oligoantigenic diet treatment. *Lancet* 1983; ii: 865–9.

22 Eisenberg L. The management of the hyperkinetic child. *Dev Med Child Neurol* 1966; 8: 593–8.

23 Feingold BP. *Introduction to Clinical Allergy*. Charles C Thomas, Springfield, Illinois, 1973.

24 Feingold BF. Hyperkinesis and learning disabilities linked to artificial food flavours and colors. *Am J Nurs* 1975; 75: 797–803.

25 Flintoff MM, Barron RW, Swanson JM *et al*. Methylphenidate increases selectivity of visual scanning in children referred for hyperactivity. *J Abnorm Child Psychol* 1982; 10: 145–63.

26 Harley JP, Ray RS, Tomasi L *et al*. Hyperkinesis and food additives: testing the Feingold hypothesis. *Pediatrics* 1978; 61: 818–28.

27 Harvey PG. Lead and children's health: recent research and future questions. *J Child Psychol Psychiatry* 1984; 25: 517–22.

28 Hoffmann H. *Der Struwelpeter: oder lustige Geschichten und drollige Bilder*. Insel Verlag, Leipzig, 1845.

29 Hoobler BR. Some early symptoms suggesting protein sensitization in infancy. *Am J Dis Child* 1916; 12: 129.

30 Huessy H. Study of the prevalence and therapy of the choreatiform syndrome or hyperkinesis in rural Vermont. *Acta Paedopsychiatr (Basel)* 1967; 34: 130–5.

31 Lambert NM, Sandoval J, Sassone D. Prevalence of hyperactivity in elementary school children as a function of social system definers. *Am J Orthopsychiatry* 1977; 48: 446.

32 Laufer M, Denhoff E. Hyperkinetic behavior syndrome in children. *J Pediatr* 1957; 50: 463–74.

33 Lopez R. Hyperactivity in twins. *Can Psychiatr Assoc J* 1965; 10: 421–6.

34 Mash EJ, Dalby JT. Behavioral interventions for hyperactivity. In: *Hyperactivity in Children: Etiology, Measurement and Treatment Implications* (Trites RL, ed.). University Park Press, Baltimore, 1978.

35 Mendelson W, Johnson N, Stewart M. Hyperactive children as teenagers: a follow-up study. *J Nerv Ment Dis* 1971; 153: 237–9.

36 Menkes MM, Rowe JS, Menkes JH. A twenty-five year follow-up study on the hyperkinetic child with minimal brain dysfunction. *Pediatrics* 1967; 39: 393–9.

37 Minde K, Weiss G, Mendelson N. A five-year follow-up study of 91 hyperactive school children. *J Am Acad Child Psychiatry* 1972; 11: 595–610.

38 Minde K, Weiss G, Lavigueuer H *et al*. The hyperactive child in elementary school: a 5 year, controlled follow-up. *Except Child* 1971; 38: 215–22.

39 O'Leary K, O'Leary S. *Classroom Management: The Successful Use of Behavior Modification*, 2nd edn. Pergamon, New York, 1977.

40 O'Malley J, Eisenberg L. The hyperkinetic syndrome. *Semin Psychiatry* 1973; 5: 5–17.

41 Patterson G, Jones R, Whittier J, Wright M. A behaviour modification technique for the hyperactive child. *Behav Res Ther* 1965; 2: 217–26.

42 Pearson DJ, Rix KJB, Benley SJ. Food allergy: how much in the mind? *Lancet* 1983; i: 1259–61.

43 Prior M, Griffin M. *Hyperactivity, Diagnosis and Management*. William Heinemann Medical Books, London, 1965.

44 Randolph TG. Allergy as a causative factor of fatigue, irritability, and behavior problems of children. *J Pediatr* 1947; 31: 560–72.

45 Rapp DJ. *Allergies and the Hyperactive Child*. Cornerstone Library, 1979.

46 Rowe AH. Allergic toxemia and fatigue. *Ann Allergy* 1950; 8: 72.

47 Rutter ML. Relationships between child and adult psychiatric disorders. *Acta Psychiatr Scand* 1972; 48: 3–21.

48 Rutter ML. Brain damage syndromes in childhood: concepts and findings. *J Child Psychol Psychiatry* 1977; 18: 1–21.

49 Safer DJ. A familial factor in minimal brain dysfunction. *Behav Genet* 1973; 3: 175–86.

50 Safer DJ, Allen RP. *Hyperactive Children: Diagnosis and Management*. University Park Press, Baltimore, Maryland, 1976.

51 Sanson AV. *Sub-Classification of Hyperactive Children*. La Trobe University, Victoria, Australia, 1984.

52 Satterfield JH, Hoppe CM, Schell AM: A prospective study of delinquency in 110 adolescent boys with attention deficit disorder and 88 normal adolescent boys. *Am J Psychiatry* 1982; 139: 795–8.

53 Schoenthaler SJ. Diet and delinquency: a multi-state replication. *Int J Biosoc Res* 1983; 5: 70–117.

54 Speer F. *Allergy of the Nervous System*. Charles C Thomas, Springfield, Illinois, 1970.

55 Sulzbacher SJ. The learning-disabled or hyperactive child: diagnosis and treatment. *J Am Med Assoc* 1976; 234: 939–41.

56 Swanson JM, Kinsbourne M. Food dyes impair performance of hyperactive children on a laboratory learning test. *Science* 1980; 207: 1485–7.

57 Thorley G. Pilot study to assess behavioural and cognitive effects of artificial food colours in a group of retarded children. *Dev Med Child Neurol* 1984; 26: 56–61.

58 Warner JO, Hathaway MJ. Allergic form of Meadow's syndrome (Munchausen by proxy). *Arch Dis Child* 1984; 59: 151–6.

59 Weiss B, Williams JH, Margen S *et al*. Behavioral response to artificial food colors. Science 1980; 207: 1487–9.

60 Weiss G, Minde K, Werry JS *et al*. Studies on the hyperactive child. VIII 5-year follow-up. *Arch Gen Psychiatry* 1971; 24: 409–14.

61 Wender PH. *Minimal Brain Dysfunction in Children*. Wiley-Interscience, New York, 1971.

62 Williams JJ, Cram DM, Tausig FT, Webster E. Relative effects of drugs and diet on hyperactive behaviors: an experimental study. *Pediatrics* 1978; 61: 811–17.

Chapter 52

The potential role of trace elements in child hyperkinetic disorders

Neil I. Ward

INTRODUCTION

Hyperkinetic disorders include:

- hyperkinesis or hyperactivity (HA)
- learning disability
- developmental balance
- perceptual handicap
- minimal brain dysfunction
- attention deficit disorder (ADD)
- attention deficit hyperactivity disorder (ADHD).

All of these disorders are complex health problems, characterized in part by excessive levels of motor activity, reduced attentiveness and concentration, distractibility, low frustration, hyperexcitability, poor impulse control and excessive restlessness.[9,38,58,136] In recent years ADHD has become the most widely researched of these disorders.

In diagnosing ADHD, children must have observable changes in three patterns of behaviour: they are (1) consistently inattentive, (2) hyperactive and (3) impulsive.[58] Signs of inattention include becoming easily distracted, failing to pay attention to details, losing or forgetting things, avoiding tasks that require sustained mental effort and rarely following instructions carefully and completely. Signs of impulsivity include feeling restless, excessive mobile activity, difficulty in waiting in line or for a turn, and providing spontaneous verbal responses without listening to all instructions.

Hyperactive children often show persistent symptoms of a short attention span coupled with low frustration levels. Other indicators include symptoms of excessive thirst, poor appetite, multi-allergic reactions and a tendency to develop asthma and/or eczema following exposure to a particular chemical, nutritional or environmental agent.[1,2,60]

The UK-based Hyperactive Children's Support Group (HACSG)[27,29] have reported that in infancy hyperactivity symptoms include:

- excessive crying, screaming, restlessness
- excessive dribbling and thirst
- head banging, cot rocking, fits and tantrums
- limited response to maternal cuddling and not easily pacified
- need of sleep.

The above features may appear in the early life of children with hyperkinetic disorders, especially before the age of 7, and they may result in behavioural changes that create real social interactive problems at home, school or within other social settings.[29] In some cases, especially ADHD children, the impact of some of these behavioural abnormalities results in disinhibition of future social relationships and a tendency to develop future antisocial attitudes.[39] Some parents have reported that neither praise nor punishment is effective in responding to the hyperkinetic child's behaviour. As a result many of these children become 'loners' and social outcasts, especially after continued dis-turbance at the playgroup, nursery/school, homes of friends and relatives.[29]

In older children hyperkinetic disorders may induce:[29]

- erratic disruptive behaviour
- aggressive activity towards others, especially children
- lack of concentration and may become withdrawn
- clumsiness, impulsive and accident prone
- self-abusive
- high pain threshold
- uncooperative, defiant and disobedient
- poor appetite and reduced hand and eye coordination
- continued excessive thirst and sleeping problems.

The aetiology of child hyperkinetic disorders is multifactorial, involving clinical, biological, nutritional and environmental determinants. An extensive list of research subjects are being evaluated, including genetic predisposition;[114] endocrine dysfunction;[50] enzyme deficiencies; immune dysfunction; neurodevelopmental disorders;[111,112,116,136] metabolism dysfunction; multiallergic reactivity[20,21,36,37,126] imbalances or deficiencies in nutritional requirements, especially essential trace elements, fatty acids and vitamins;[13,14,28,54–56,65,82,95,108,109] diet;[11,18,24,27,36,37,45,61,67,73,81,129,130,135] and environment.[49,80,124,125]

Nutrient deficiencies of essential trace elements and fatty acids may play an important role in hyperkinetic disorders. Several studies have reported low levels of zinc in hyperactive children, especially in relation to increased hyperactivity behavioural problems, asthma and eczema.[120,124] Lower levels of zinc have also been shown to be associated with decreased immunity and changes in gut permeability.[124] Other studies have confirmed decreased levels of other essential elements, including magnesium, iron, copper and calcium, in hyperactive children.[65] One study has indicated that decreased levels of fatty acids in ADHD children were correlated with low zinc status.[13,14] It has also been suggested that essential trace element, fatty acid and vitamin deficiencies are involved in immune dysfunction and behavioural variations through changes in food eating habits, decreased nutrient levels in foods and increased toxic heavy metal levels, especially lead and cadmium.[58,125,127]

Deficiencies of dihomogamma linolenic acid (DGLA), arachidonic acid (AA) and docosahexaenoic acid (DHA) were found in 44 children with ADHD compared with 45 age and sex-matched controls.[95] Many of these ADHD children suffered from polydypsia and polyuria (clinical signs of essential fatty acid deficiency). It has been proposed that a subset of ADHD children may have a problem in converting essential fatty acids (EFAs) to long-chained polyunsaturated fatty acid derivatives (LC-PUFAs).[95] Results of a randomized, double-blind trial in ADHD children with clinical signs of fatty acid deficiency showed that supplementation with a combination of DHA, eicosapentaenoic acid (EPA), AA and DGLA was successful in reducing ADHD symptoms.[95]

In addition, exposure to environmental toxins, especially lead, cadmium, mercury and aluminium may contribute to some of the behavioural features of hyperkinetic disorders.[49,80,124,125] Extensive research has also focused on chemical additives widely used in certain commercial foodstuffs and beverages. Tartrazine (E_{102}) is the colourant most widely studied in terms of food intolerance, behavioural changes and hyperactivity in children.[6,30,44,48,66,71,89,96–98,111,120,124,125]

During the last decade there has been an increasing awareness of an increase in numbers of children diagnosed with hyperkinetic disorders, especially ADHD. In 1998, the USA reported that approximately 4 million or 10% of all school-aged children had been diagnosed with either ADD or ADHD.[113] The Hyperactive Children's Support Group has recently reported an ever-increasing request from distraught and desperate parents for more help to deal with their hyperkinetic child's problems.[29] As a result, numerous investigators have been evaluating suitable remedial measures for such children. At present there is a vigorous debate over the methods of treatment being used, especially in relation to conventional orthodox medicine or complementary/nutritional alternatives.

Ritalin (methylphenidate) is increasingly being prescribed for both ADD and ADHD children.[99] It has similar pharmacological properties to amphetamine and various major side effects have been reported, including irritability, insomnia, depression, delayed growth, skin rash, mood swings, nausea and stomach pain, appetite and weight loss.[113] While Ritalin appears to be highly effective, it helps up to 70–90% of children with ADHD, there is a growing concern about the common side effects and possible, still yet unknown, long-term health effects on children.[19] As such, Ritalin is also a habit-forming drug and with a lack of understanding about its therapeutic mechanism of action in these disorders, the long-term effects on children are an area of serious concern for many medical researchers.

Complementary and nutritional alternatives are usually based on dietary management programmes in which food intolerances are identified and eliminated from the diet.[21,113] In addition, diet modification and/or supplementation with nutritional materials (EFAs, vitamins, trace elements, amino acid chelates, flavonoids) are becoming increasingly popular therapies for ADD and ADHD. Atopic children with ADHA have been shown to respond well to elimination diets.[24,36,37,101] The most common foods targeted for elimination are dairy products, sugar, wheat, eggs and chocolate and salicylate-rich foods such as apples, cherries, grapes, berries, tomatoes and oranges.[29] It should be stressed that not all hyperkinetic disorder children are sensitive to one or more of these foods, and in some cases it may be the addition of artificial chemicals to the food that is related to their behavioural effects.[58,124,125] In some cases it has been shown that the Feingold diet is an effective approach for improving the behavioural problems of ADD/ADHD children.[40,41,47,48] The Feingold diet eliminates artificial colourings, flavourings, artificial sweeteners (such as aspartame, saccharin, sucralose), several preservatives and foods containing salicylates. Some studies have also suggested that a combination of a sugar-restricted and high protein diet can have a positive effect on hyperkinesis.[113]

Nutrient supplementation has focused on the addition of:

1. ω-3 fatty acids – EPA and DHA, usually via the use of fish or linseed (flaxseed) oils
2. vitamin B complex, especially vitamin B_3 (niacinamide) and vitamin B_6 and vitamin C
3. zinc, chromium, copper, iron, magnesium and calcium, usually as single or multi-mineral supplements
4. amino acid chelates or other metabolites (for example, S-adenosylmethionine)
5. flavonoids (oligomeric proanthocyanidins).

Many of these nutrients act as metalloenzymes, neurotransmitter precursors and detoxifying agents (antioxidants).[90,91] Although the use of such supplements can provide a reduction in hyperkinetic activity in some children, there is an urgent need for more randomized, double-blind, placebo-controlled trials using either single and/or multinutrient preparations in relation to these disorders. In particular, the choice of treatment (including nutrient, chemical form, dose), duration and assessment of clinical benefits for the different types of child (or even adult) hyperkinetic disorder needs to be established before such complementary/nutritional alternatives will be recognized by some orthodox medical groups.

CHEMICAL FACTORS IN HYPERACTIVE CHILDREN

During October 1992 and June 2000, in association with the HACSG, the Allergy Support Group of Oxford (ASGO) and various other child health charities, a series of studies were undertaken to assess the chemical factors influencing children with hyperkinetic disorders. In nearly all cases the children in these studies were classified as hyperactive according to the symptoms outlined above.

Preliminary data (October 1992 to July 1995) showed that various synthetic colourings, flavourings and preservatives were linked to hyperkinetic behaviour in some of these children.[120,124] Due to the changing commercial environment of removing or modifying some of these chemicals in foods or beverages and household products, it was decided to extend the database up to the period of June 2000.

A questionnaire evaluation of 382 hyperactive (HA) and 148 control (C) children was undertaken by parents, social workers and dieticians between August 1995 and June 2000. The comprehensive questionnaire (prepared by the HACSG) contained questions on early life, early symptoms, symptoms in the older child, other health problems and what food or chemical substances affected the child's behaviour. The substances were subdivided into:

- synthetic colours/flavours
- preservatives
- antioxidants
- solvents
- petrol/diesel
- perfume
- detergents
- soaps
- sugar
- dairy products (milk, butter, cream)
- wheat and other grains
- monosodium glutamate
- artificial sweeteners
- chocolate
- salicylates.

The hyperactive group consisted of 76% male (86% Caucasian, 3% Black and 11% Asian; aged between 4 and 15 years) and 24% female (92% Caucasian and 8% Asian; aged 6 to 13 years). The main features of the HA children were 58% fair hair, 56% blue eyes and 82% very fair skin complexion. Comparison of the population statistics for this group (August 1995 to June 2000) with the previously reported group (October 1992 to July 1995)[124] show some slight changes in the subgroupings for the HA children. In particular, there is the addition of some non-Caucasian cases

(especially Asian children) and increased numbers of HA female cases (from 18% to 24%). The sex- and age-matched control group consisted of children with no predominance of hair or eye colour, skin complexion, all had typical body mass indexes (BMIs) for their age, and none were clinically diagnosed for a disorder for a period of 12 months prior to the study. None of the control children were on special diets or nutrient supplements.

The percentage of hyperactive (HA) and control (C) children reporting a positive response to foods or chemical substances in foods, beverages and the domestic environment are reported in Fig. 52.1 (study period: October 1992 to July 1995) and Fig. 52.2 (study period August 1995 to June 2000). In the initial study period (Fig. 52.1) more than 60% of the HA children reported a positive response (that is an increase in behavioural problems) in relation to synthetic colourings and flavourings, food and beverage preservatives, cow's milk and associated products, chemical detergents and perfume. In contrast, 12% of the control group also reported similar, but generally milder, responses to synthetic colourings/flavourings and chemical solvents. The second study group (Fig. 52.2) show some interesting differences. While the general pattern of substances for the two groups is the same, there are some important trend changes. In particular, the percentage number of HA children reporting positive responses to synthetic colourants/flavourings, preservatives or antioxidants, detergents/soaps, dairy products and salicylates have decreased, their responses for solvents, petrol/diesel, sugar, artificial sweeteners and chocolate have all increased.

Possible explanations for these trends include increased parental awareness of particular foodstuffs that HA children must avoid, changes in the types of chemical substances being used in foods, beverages and domestic products, and the continual changes in child dietary fads, especially in relation to sugar-based foodstuffs and beverages. A particular alarming trend is in the increased positive response to petrol/diesel, which may be related to the changes in the chemicals used in non-leaded petrol and/or exposure to new chemical pollutants arising from changes in the

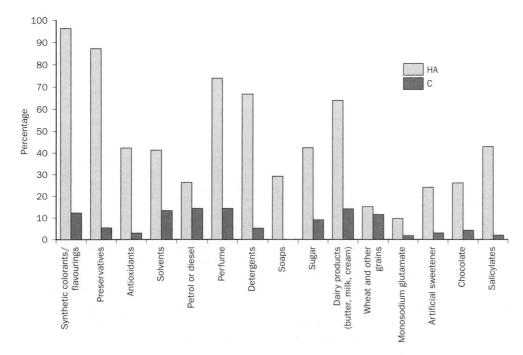

Fig. 52.1 Percentage of hyperactive (HA) and control (C) children reporting a positive response to foods or chemical substances in foods/beverages and the domestic environment: study period October 1992–July 1995.

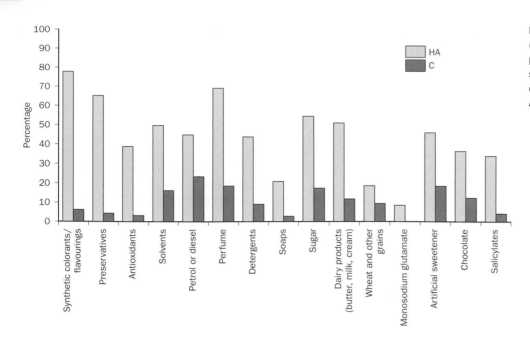

Fig. 52.2 Percentage of hyperactive (HA) and control (C) children reporting a positive response to foods or chemical substances in foods/beverages and the domestic environment: study period August 1995 to June 2000.

types of fuels being used and the steady increase in fuel consumption and traffic congestion. Similarly, the increased positive response to artificial sweeteners was shown by both the HA and C groups, which may in part be related to the types of chemicals now being used and the increased use of such substances in beverages.

An evaluation of the associated health problems of the two study groups of HA children showed that more than 60% or more had a persistent thirst problem and a continual problem with developing eczema, ear and/or chest infections (Table 52.1). Many of these cases also reported a history of taking numerous courses of antibiotics in early childhood.

During the period of completing the questionnaire the hyperactive and control children investigated in study period 2, namely August 1995 to June 2000, were also asked to have their behavioural activity evaluated by using an abbreviated questionnaire (prepared by the HACSG) of the Connors Scale Score.[30,125] In this questionnaire the parent, social worker or dietician records the responses from the child/parent in relation to the following observations:

- restless or overactive
- excitable, impulsive
- disturbs other children
- fails to finish things he/she starts – short attention span
- constantly fidgeting
- inattentive, easily distracted
- demands must be met immediately, easily frustrated
- cries often and easily
- mood changes quickly and drastically
- temper outbursts, explosive and unpredictable behaviour.

Each observation was graded according to the degree of activity: (1) not at all, (2) a little, (3) pretty much and (4) very much. The 10 observation rating scale was then calculated by assigning 1–3 for the various degrees of activity. A child showing a high level of hyperkinetic behavioural activity will score a grand total above 20. While it is acknowledged that this procedure is very subjective, a previous study using the Connors Scale Scores for assessing the

Percentage of hyperactive children (HA) diagnosed with particular health problems for the two study periods		
Health problem	**Oct 1992 to Jul 1995**	**Aug 1995 to Jun 2000**
Overactive	62	68
Dyslexic	6	12
Autistic	4	8
Epileptic	4	6
Asthma	44	58
Eczema	78	73
Ear infections	92	89
Chest infections	58	49
Excessive thirst	68	61
Catarrh	83	78
Excessive sweating	18	12
Allergies (food/chemicals)	78	82

Table 52.1 Percentage of hyperactive children (HA) diagnosed with particular health problems for the two study periods.

behavioural activity of hyperactive, excessive allergy, dyslexia and control children showed clear total score differences between the different groups.[125] Table 52.2 reports the Connors Scale Scores for the children evaluated in the second study period. There is a clear difference in the range of scores between the two groups of children. The values for the 382 hyperactive children is similar to those reported in another study using this assessment method, i.e. scores of 24–30.

	Hyperactive (HA)	Control (C)
Number	382	148
Scores	21–30	<12

Table 52.2 Connors Scale Scores for hyperactive (HA) and control (C) children: study period August 1995 to June 2000.

(Table heading within table) Connors Scale Scores for hyperactive (HA) and control (C) children: study period August 1995 to June 2000

TRACE ELEMENT LEVELS IN HYPERACTIVE AND CONTROL CHILDREN

To evaluate the trace element status of hyperactive (HA) and control (C) children, samples of scalp hair, mid-stream flow urine and blood serum were collected during the period of October 1992 and June 2000. Unfortunately, it is not always possible to collect all three samples from children, especially blood serum samples. In all cases written consent was obtained from the parents before sample collection. During the sampling period the total number of samples presented for analysis were: scalp hair – 1238 (HA) and 436 (C); mid-stream flow urine – 687 (HA) and 198 (C); and blood serum – 518 (HA) and 178 (C). Scalp hair samples were collected from the nape of the neck, at a point mid-position between the shoulders, and cut as close as possible to the skin surface. Approximately 0.2–0.5 g of hair material is necessary for analysis. All hair samples were washed using an acetone/distilled-deionized water ultrasonic procedure to remove surface contaminants (exogenous contributions). After washing the hair, samples were dried at 60°C for 6 hours and dry-ashed

at 450°C for 12 hours. The homogenized ash was digested in 6 md/l Aristar nitric acid. Blood serum and urine samples were collected at a standard time of 7:30–9:00 am following overnight fasting. This time procedure is used to minimize dietary contributions and diurnal variations. All body fluids (2–5 ml) were wet-ashed in Teflon digestion vessels using 12 mol/l Aristar nitric acid and 30% hydrogen peroxide (heated at 100°C for 12 hours).

All trace element measurements were undertaken using a Finnigan MAT SOLA inductively coupled plasma quadrupole mass spectrometer (ICP-QMS) located in the ICP-MS Facility, Department of Chemistry, University of Surrey (UniS). A series of five multielement standard solutions were prepared (over the analyte range of 0.1–1500 µg/l). Quality control checks were performed using various international certified reference materials to ensure high levels of accuracy and precision.[26,110] All reagent blanks, calibration standard solutions, certified reference material solutions and sample solutions were spiked with three internal standards (Be, In and Bi at 100 µg/l) to evaluate and correct, when necessary, any changes in instrument performance throughout the measurement period.

Tables 52.3–52.5 summarize the trace element concentrations for washed scalp hair, mid-stream flow urine and blood serum samples collected from the hyperactive (HA) and control (C) children.

In interpreting the data in Tables 52.3–52.5 it should be stressed that each media provides a different picture of the absorption, metabolism, utilization and excretion of the trace elements under investigation. Scalp hair represents the long-term trace element profile in response to the slow growth rate of ~1–2 cm per month.[110] Assessment of trace element status using this media must be treated with caution, as deficiencies or supplementation of some essential trace elements, especially zinc, can

Element (all µg/g or ppm)	Hyperactive (HA) n = 1238	Control (C) n = 436	Statistical level†
Aluminium	8.3 (1.8–22.3)	2.2 (0.8–6.9)	S** HA > C
Cadmium	1.8 (0.2–3.6)	0.3 (0.1–0.8)	S** HA > C
Calcium	384 (298–577)	548 (387–923)	S** HA < C
Chromium	0.38 (0.22–0.76)	0.72 (0.36–1.22)	S** HA < C
Copper	13.8 (8.6–25.4)	14.2 (9.7–24.3)	NS
Iron	18.9 (5.4–46.8)	26.8 (14.3–48.8)	S** HA < C
Lead	6.7 (2.1–11.8)	2.7 (1.1–5.4)	S** HA > C
Magnesium	38 (27–53)	47 (24–72)	S* HA < C
Manganese	0.92 (0.65–1.84)	0.94 (0.70–1.83)	NS
Selenium	0.38 (0.26–1.08)	0.78 (0.36–1.67)	S** HA < C
Zinc	94 (73–143)	141 (101–173)	S** HA < C

(Table heading within table) Trace element content of washed scalp hair samples for hyperactive (HA) and control (C) children: sampling period October 1992 to June 2000

Table 52.3 Trace element content of washed scalp hair samples for hyperactive (HA) and control (C) children: sampling period October 1992 to June 2000.

†Concentrations are reported as a mean (range), statistical two-tailed Student t-test: S** – very highly significant, $P < 0.001$; S* – $P < 0.01$; NS – not significant, $P > 0.10$.

D

Trace element content of mid-stream flow urine samples for hyperactive (HA) and control (C) children: sampling period October 1992 to June 2000			
Element (μg/ml[a] or μg/l[b])	**Hyperactive (HA)** $n = 687$	**Control (C)** $n = 198$	**Statistical level[†]**
Aluminium[b]	10.5 (3.5–32.6)	7.2 (1.8–22.8)	S** HA > C
Cadmium[b]	1.6 (0.6–4.2)	1.4 (0.7–3.0)	NS
Calcium[a]	98 (56–138)	102 (60–146)	NS
Chromium[b]	1.6 (0.7–2.8)	3.2 (0.6–6.3)	S* HA < C
Copper[b]	77 (32–98)	80 (35–109)	NS
Iron[b]	78 (43–156)	133 (67–178)	S** HA < C
Lead[b]	21 (10–37)	19 (9–34)	NS
Magnesium[a]	64 (55–83)	73 (61–92)	S** HA < C
Manganese[b]	15 (8–23)	18 (11–36)	S* HA < C
Selenium[b]	32 (12–56)	44 (18–78)	S** HA < C
Zinc[a]	0.18 (0.07–0.49)	0.68 (0.09–0.97)	S** HA < C

[†]Concentrations are reported as a mean (range), statistical two-tailed Student t-test: S** – very highly significant, $P < 0.001$; S* – $P < 0.01$; NS – not significant, $P > 0.10$.

Table 52.4 Trace element content of mid-stream flow urine samples for hyperactive (HA) and control (C) children: sampling period October 1992 to June 2000.

Trace element content of blood serum samples for hyperactive (HA) and control (C) children: sampling period October 1992 to June 2000			
Element (μg/ml[a] or μg/l[b])	**Hyperactive (HA)** $n = 518$	**Control (C)** $n = 178$	**Statistical level[†]**
Aluminium[b]	4.3 (0.8–9.3)	3.9 (0.7–7.9)	NS
Cadmium[b]	1.70 (0.45–2.30)	1.51 (0.34–1.98)	NS
Calcium[a]	87 (83–95)	92 (85–99)	NS
Chromium[b]	0.18 (0.08–0.34)	0.23 (0.13–0.27)	S* HA < C
Copper[a]	0.92 (0.88–1.02)	0.91 (0.86–1.03)	NS
Iron[a]	0.73 (0.59–0.93)	0.97 (0.77–1.19)	S** HA < C
Lead[b]	3.2 (0.7–7.3)	1.8 (0.8–3.4)	S* HA > C
Magnesium[a]	20 (17–24)	21 (18–25)	NS
Manganese[b]	0.44 (0.23–0.61)	0.47 (0.24–0.59)	NS
Selenium[b]	54.1 (39.6–78.3)	72.5 (51.7–80.3)	S** HA < C
Zinc[a]	0.62 (0.48–0.73)	0.92 (0.71–1.08)	S** HA < C

[†]Concentrations are reported as a mean (range), statistical two-tailed Student t-test: S** – very highly significant, $P < 0.001$; S* – $P < 0.01$; NS – not significant, $P > 0.10$.

Table 52.5 Trace element content of blood serum samples for hyperactive (HA) and control (C) children: sampling period October 1992 to June 2000.

be influenced by the change in the growth pattern and thereby the deposition of trace elements into the hair fibres.[110]

Urinary trace element analysis reflects the excretion performance of the kidneys in regulating the electrolyte and water metabolism of the body.[104,119] Such analysis may provide a direct method of assessing physiological changes within the body or any irregularities in the mode of absorption or excretion. This may be important in terms of children with hyperkinetic disorders, as suggestions have been made that such children have changes in gut permeability resulting in a more leaky gut than normal children.[124] In addition, previous reports that hyperactive children have lower zinc levels[14,100,115,120,124] may also affect gut permeability. Zinc deficiency has been linked to gastrointestinal changes in the enterocytes and damage to the microvilli.[46] Urinary toxic trace element levels are also very important, especially for cadmium, which has a tendency to accumulate in the kidneys.

Some questions have been raised about the use of mid-stream flow urine samples, especially as the trace element levels may be directly related to daily variations in dietary intake. However, for studies involving children, the use of 24-hour urine samples is impractical. Previous studies have been reported using mid-stream flow urine samples for assessing trace element status in hyperactive and control children.[124]

Blood serum is a good indicator of recent trace element changes in the body.[26,110] Some questions have been asked about the usefulness of blood serum analysis. Particular problems may be associated with the homeostatic regulation of essential trace elements in this body fluid. Such conditions can result in small trace element concentration variations in response to physiological conditions.[110,118] In addition, it is not always possible to collect blood serum samples from children. Some studies have used various blood fractions (serum, erythrocytes) and other blood components (haemoglobin, haematocrit, red and white blood count, total iron-binding capacity, globulin/albumin and ferritin) in assessing trace element (Mg, Zn, Fe, Al, Cd, Pb) changes in children with hyperkinetic disorders.[13,14,105,107,115,120,124]

In this study there are some significant trends in the trace element levels between hyperactive and control children. For all three media (scalp hair, urine and blood serum) the hyperactive children are significantly (Student t-test) lower (HA < C) in chromium, iron, selenium and zinc. Magnesium shows the same trends for scalp hair and urine. In contrast, hyperactive children show significantly higher levels (HA > C) of aluminium (scalp hair and urine), cadmium (scalp hair) and lead (scalp hair and blood serum) relative to the control group of children. At present it is difficult to suggest from these trends whether the data reflect any cause or effect in relation to hyperactivity. However, in comparing the trace element trends with other published studies in this area it may be possible to assess whether there is a consistency in trace element levels or patterns in children with hyperkinetic disorders.

ESSENTIAL TRACE ELEMENTS

Probably the most important essential trace element in relation to human behaviour is zinc. The relationship between this trace element and human brain function has been demonstrated through deficiency conditions in pregnancy causing impaired synthesis of brain DNA and histopathological abnormalities in the hippocampal brain region.[34]

Numerous studies have evaluated the zinc levels of hyperactive or ADHD children and all have reported lower zinc levels in these children.[13,14,100,115,120,124] One study has postulated that it is possible that the high prevalence of conduct disorder and aggressive behaviour in ADHD patients could be related to reduced melatonin and serotonin (5HT) associated with zinc deficiency.[100] Since melatonin production is regulated by zinc, it is possible that alterations in brain zinc metabolism may be involved in the dramatic reduction of melatonin production.[100] The involvement of reduced melatonin in ADHD patients and the role of the pineal gland has been reviewed by other authors.[100] Zinc is an important regulator of melatonin biosynthesis.[35] A dramatic increase in melatonin production in early childhood may also create an increased demand for zinc. Other studies have reported lower levels in HA or ADHD children that may be due to diminished nutritional zinc and poor or reduced zinc absorption and metabolism.[29,120,124,125] All of these postulations could result in a limited capacity of the pineal gland to synthesize melatonin. One study suggested that zinc supplementation might enhance the therapeutic efficacy of amphetamines in a subgroup of patients with ADHD.[5] It has been shown that amphetamines increase melatonin production.[8,53,69] It is therefore postulated that the effects of amphetamines on ADHD may be partially mediated through pineal melatonin and is directly linked to zinc status.[100]

Another study reported blood serum zinc levels of 60.6 ± 9.9 (range 46–82) µg/dl for 48 ADHD cases and 105.8 ± 13.2 (85–139) µg/dl for 45 control children.[14] This study also reported a significant correlation between decreased serum free fatty acid (FFA) concentrations and zinc levels in the ADHD group and postulated that FFA deficiency is secondary in ADHD. This latter hypothesis has been extensively challenged by various studies.[28,42,54–56,95,108,109,125]

Lower serum zinc levels were reported in 43 ADHD children (aged 6–16 years), although no significant correlation existed between serum zinc levels and dosages of methylphenidate (0–20 mg/day).[115] The authors reported that although the ADHD children were on a balanced diet many were selective eaters and did not sit at the table to consume their food. They also commented that a possible effect of stimulant-related appetite suppression should be considered with ADHD children taking methylphenidate.

Another possible biochemical link may exist between hyperadrenal condition and zinc deficiency.[51] Dysfunction of the adrenergic and the dopaminergic systems has indeed been implicated in ADHD.[62]

Three publications have used scalp hair to assess the zinc status of hyperactive children. In an uncontrolled study, hair samples from 31 of 46 hyperactive children showed zinc levels below the normal range.[28] Another study reported mean washed scalp hair levels of 65 and 128 mg/kg (dry weight) for 22 hyperactive and 18 control children prior to undertaking a dietary modification or nutrient supplementation programme.[125] Mean washed scalp hair zinc levels of 82 (range 66–138) µg/g for 486 hyperactive and 138 (98–155) µg/g for 172 control children were reported in a multi-element study assessing the chemical factors in child hyperactivity.[124] This study postulated that poor zinc (and iron) status in hyperactive children may be related to numerous factors, including poor dietary status, abnormal intestinal absorption or gut permeability and reduced utilization as a result of complexation or competitive interaction with other trace elements, such as copper, cadmium and lead.[124] The metal-induced interactions between low essential trace element levels (calcium, copper, iron, magnesium and zinc) and raised non-essential or toxic trace element levels (aluminium, lead, cadmium and mercury) in relation to human behaviour is an area that urgently needs researching.[125]

It has also been reported that low zinc levels have been associated with increased susceptibility to infection and impaired cell-mediated immunity.[63] This may be an important factor in child hyperactivity, as many of these children are reported to suffer from more frequent coughs, ear and chest infections and skin problems, such as eczema. One study reported that no correlation was found between zinc levels and measures of inattentiveness, hyperactivity and antisocial behaviour (using parent and teacher reports) in a general population of preadolescent children.[72]

Nutritional iron deficiency is associated with a reduction in brain non-haem iron, diminished density of D_2 dopamine receptors and lowered behavioural responses to the dopamine antagonists apomorphine and d-amphetamine.[7,134] Iron deficiency has been shown to impair learned motor behaviour and cognitive function.[133] Iron levels may also play an important role in hyperactivity, poor cognitive learning and attention deficit.[105]

Many children with hyperkinetic disorders, in particular hyperactivity and ADHD, have been reported to have lower iron levels in blood serum and scalp hair.[65,124] Statistically significant (Student t-test; $P<0.001$) lower iron levels have been published for hyperactive children relative to age and sex-matched controls for blood serum, urine and washed scalp hair.[124] Similar findings are reported in this study (see Tables 52.3–52.5). Several studies have shown that the administration of iron supplements to non-anaemic iron-deficient infants can improve their developmental scores[32,86] and cognitive development and attention behaviour.[32]

One study showed that ADHD children (aged 7–11 years) displayed normal serum iron, iron-binding capacity, ferritin and mean corpuscular volume levels.[105] Interestingly, this study reported that the administration of an oral iron supplement (ferrous calcium citrate) resulted in an increase in ferritin levels and an improvement in the parent Connors Rating Scale score. However, the authors noted that this finding should be viewed with some degree of caution as no placebo control group was included in the study.

Magnesium is the fourth cation in terms of abundance in the human body. Its high concentration in cells is similar to that of potassium. There are many similarities between these two elements in terms of metabolism, although magnesium is much harder to displace from the cell than potassium.[91] One of the main roles of magnesium is in oxidative phosphorylation. All enzymes that are known to be catalysed by adenosine triphosphate (ATP) show a requirement for magnesium. Both magnesium and ATP are involved in the synthesis of nucleic acids. Ribosomes (involved in the biosynthesis of protein) require magnesium ions in order to maintain their physical stability. Intestinal malabsorption is a common factor in magnesium deficiency.[84] Alcoholism is also recognized as a cause of magnesium deficiency.[42] Some of the symptoms reported for hypomagnesaemia in adults include sweating, apathy, depression and poor memory, mild to severe delirium (confusion, disorientation, hallucination), convulsions, muscular twitching and tremor.[84]

Interestingly, in this study the hyperactive group show a statistically significant (Student t-test, $P < 0.01$ – scalp hair, or <0.001 – urine) lower magnesium levels than the control group.

The lower magnesium levels in HA urine may be related to changes in dietary intake.[84]

In recent years the HACSG has reported that many of the trace element tests undertaken on hyperactive children have consistently shown lower chromium levels. This observation is supported by the results in this study in which all three media show statistically lower levels of this essential trace element in hyperactive children. Chromium has been shown to be associated with various enzyme systems and pathways, but its main role is in the form of the glucose tolerance factor (GTF).[74,75,77,78,85] It also participates in lipoprotein metabolism, gene expression and the maintaining of the structure of nucleic acids.[85] Chromium deficiency has been demonstrated in protein–calorie malnutrition and in patients receiving total parenteral nutrition (TPN) devoid of chromium supplements. There are few foodstuffs with appreciable amounts of chromium. Spices and yeast have the highest concentrations but these foodstuffs are not on the personal preference list of children. Refining processes are known to reduce the content of chromium in some foods, especially sugar.[103] Hyperkinetic disorder children tend to be selective eaters and in many cases the removal of sugar from their diet is beneficial in terms of reducing their behavioural problems. Therefore, the low chromium levels measured in this study may be a simple reflection of low dietary chromium intake. However, the link between chromium, impaired GTF and hypoglycaemic reactions[3,4,23] implies that in some hyperkinetic disorder children low chromium status may be linked with hypoglycaemic problems. Interestingly, some hyperactive children have shown reduced levels of overactivity following the removal of sugar from the diet and the oral supplementation of brewer's yeast.

Selenium is an essential trace element involved in the enzyme glutathione peroxidase (Se-GSHPx). This enzyme is involved in antioxidant systems of the cell and has the role of destroying potentially injurious hydrogen peroxide and lipid peroxides in the cell cytosol and probably in the plasma.[137] Including Se-GSHPx, more than 13 selenoproteins have been identified.[15,16] Glutathione peroxidase and phospholipid hydroperoxide glutathione peroxidase, both selenium-containing enzymes, represent a significant antioxidative defence mechanism. Selenium also has numerous effects on cellular and hormonal immune functions. Selenium deficiency affects a wide range of enzyme activities and metabolic processes, including changes in thyroid hormone metabolism,[10] and an increased incidence of different carcinoma disorders.[43,79,131]

The role of selenium in children is an area of limited research. At present the results in this study showing a statistically significant (Student t-test, $P < 0.001$) lower level of this important trace element in hyperactive children are difficult to explain. Human selenium status is closely linked to the amount and bioavailability of selenium in the diet. Various studies have shown that selenium levels in children are about 80% of adult levels in the first few years.[117] There is an increasing concern that selenium levels in foods, which correlate with levels in local soils, are decreasing.[93,94] The interesting results in this work confirm that there is an urgent need to undertake further research into the involvement of selenium in relation to the health of children.

NON-ESSENTIAL OR TOXIC TRACE ELEMENTS

There is also a significant effect of non-essential or toxic trace elements (lead, cadmium, aluminium and mercury) in relation to human behaviour. Low lead levels have been linked to hyperactivity and impulsivity in children, resulting in negative ratings by teachers with respect to classroom behaviour.[22] Lead has also been linked to juvenile delinquency and violent behaviour.[123] In many cases the effect of lead is due to it acting as an 'anti-nutrient', hindering the utilization of magnesium, zinc, vitamin B_1, etc. Minor elevations in blood lead and tooth lead have been associated with the impairment of psychological test performance and behavioural problems. The neurological effects of lead relate to acetylcholine, catecholamines, dopamine and γ-aminobutyric acid (GABA) transmitters.[34]

Low levels of cadmium have also been linked to childhood aggression. Cadmium has an adverse effect on brain metabolism.[34] Low doses of cadmium have been reported to have a depressive effect on the levels of norepinephrine, serotonin and acetylcholine. Only a limited number of studies have considered aluminium as a behavioural toxin.[83,87] Reports have shown an association between aluminium and antisocial behaviour and learning development.[83,121-123] Aluminium is ubiquitous in our environment. Individual human vulnerability not only depends upon dietary and environmental exposure but also on its chemistry with regard to biochemical processes, in particular its competition with other metal ions (Mg^{2+}, Ca^{2+}, Fe^{2+}/Fe^{3+} and Zn^{2+}). Some studies have reported that aluminium directly competes for the binding sites of biochemical receptors associated with the above metal ions.[17,131] It has been suggested that the possible suboptimal dietary intake of zinc and/or iron may explain the uptake of aluminium and the associated effects this trace element has on learning.[83,122]

In a previous evaluation of the trace element status of hyperactive children, aluminium, cadmium and lead were also shown to be elevated in the scalp hair and urine (but not blood serum) of the children.[124] In particular, the mean aluminium washed scalp hair levels for the hyperactive ($n = 486$) children were 9.4 (range 3.8–27.4) µg/g Al and for control ($n = 172$) children 2.4 (range 0.9–9.0) µg/g Al. The aluminium, cadmium and lead values reported in Table 52.3 are very similar to those in the previous study.[124]

The relationship between raised non-essential or toxic trace element levels in association with low essential trace element levels in some of the hyperactive children may be a marker for other future problems. As previously stated, there are several reports that behavioural abnormalities in ADHD children result in a tendency to develop future antisocial attitudes.[52] One study suggested that a person with untreated hyperactivity at an early age has a high possibility of developing schizophrenic symptoms before the age of 25.[52] Hyperactivity has also been identified as a primary cause of restlessness among the youth of today, leading them into such activities as truancy, vandalism, smoking, alcohol and drug abuse, violence, delinquency and crime.[52]

Throughout the 1980s and 1990s several studies suggested links between nutrition and criminal behaviour.[102] It was hypothesized that sugar can cause antisocial behaviour in juvenile offenders. Subsequent studies in 1982 linked low vitamin and mineral intakes as being a cause of antisocial behaviour in long-term young offenders. Blood tests showed that more than 33% of juveniles studied had low levels of one or more vitamins and minerals.[102] Following supplementation, there were 22% fewer assaults on staff and a 21% reduction in both violent and non-violent antisocial behaviour. A subsequent investigation reported

that the behaviour of incarcerated young offenders may, in part, be directly due to the exposure of neurotoxins such as lead, cadmium and mercury, or from nutritional deficiencies or malabsorption of essential nutrients in their diet. Trace element analysis of the three groups of young offenders – namely, 28 violent offenders, 15 who had committed armed robbery, and 25 who had committed burglary – showed clear evidence of raised lead, aluminium and cadmium, and decreased iron, chromium, calcium, selenium and zinc in blood serum or washed scalp hair.[123] The main statistical differences existed between controls and the young offenders who had committed violent acts against society.

HYPERACTIVITY AND A PREVIOUS HISTORY OF ANTIBIOTIC USAGE

In a previous study it was noted from the results of a questionnaire evaluation of 486 hyperactive children that many had reported a history of taking several courses of antibiotics in early childhood.[124] Inspection of the questionnaire study of August 1995 to June 2000 of 382 hyperactive and 148 control children showed that 178 hyperactive children (HA) reported having used three or more courses of antibiotics by 3 years of age. Interestingly, 42 of the control group (C) reported the same trend. Tables 52.6 and 52.7 report the washed scalp hair and blood serum values for some of the essential trace elements as a function of reported antibiotic usage in early childhood.

While the same essential trace element trends exist between hyperactive (HA) and control (C) children – namely, lower levels of Ca, Fe, Mg, Se and Zn (scalp hair); Fe, Se and Zn (blood serum) – there are some interesting differences shown in both groups in relation to a history of antibiotic usage. As with the previous study,[124] lower levels of zinc exist in those children who used

Mean trace element content of washed scalp hair samples for hyperactive (HA) and control (C) children reporting antibiotic usage in early childhood				
Element (all µg/g or ppm)	**Hyperactive (HA)**		**Control (C)**	
	AH ($n=178$)	**NAH ($n=104$)**	**AH ($n=42$)**	**NAH ($n=106$)**
Calcium	390	422	540	612
Chromium	0.33	0.37	0.69	0.76
Copper	12.8	13.8	13.2	12.9
Iron	22.8	21.9	33.8	29.8
Magnesium	38	36	54	51
Manganese	0.89	0.90	0.91	0.96
Selenium	0.36	0.42	0.83	0.98
Zinc	102	113	134	156

NAH, no antibiotic history (<3 years age); AH, three or more antibiotic courses (<3 years).

Table 52.6 Mean trace element content of washed scalp hair samples for hyperactive (HA) and control (C) children reporting antibiotic usage in early childhood: sampling period 1992 to June 2000.

Mean trace element content of blood serum samples for hyperactive (HA) and control (C) children reporting antibiotic usage in early childhood				
Element (all µg/g[a] or µg/l[b])	**Hyperactive (HA)**		**Control (C)**	
	AH ($n=56$)	**NAH** ($n=47$)	**AH** ($n=22$)	**NAH** ($n=38$)
Calcium[a]	89	90	91	91
Chromium[b]	0.17	0.25	0.19	0.24
Copper[a]	0.94	0.93	0.93	0.95
Iron[a]	0.75	0.78	0.93	0.98
Magnesium[a]	21	22	20	21
Manganese[b]	0.43	0.44	0.45	0.47
Selenium[b]	52.8	56.8	68.9	73.9
Zinc[a]	0.58	0.67	0.85	0.91

NAH, no antibiotic history (<3 years age); AH, three or more antibiotic courses (<3 years).

Table 52.7 Mean trace element content of blood serum samples for hyperactive (HA) and control (C) children reporting antibiotic usage in early childhood: sampling period October 1992 to June 2000.

antibiotics (three or more antibiotic courses before 3 years of age). In addition, a similar trend is observed for calcium (hair only), chromium and selenium.

It has been reported that alterations in trace element metabolism are typical of acute-phase response to a number of stressors, including inflammation and bacterial and viral infections. These changes are normally characterized by a redistribution of body zinc, iron and copper.[12,128] Similar observations have been made for calcium, magnesium, manganese, cobalt and chromium in response to acute stress and infectious diseases.[12]

Zinc is probably the most studied trace element in relation to immune function. It plays a key function in many enzymes that are crucial to cellular proliferation, especially the lymphoid system. Severe zinc deficiency is associated with alteration of various immune functions, such as T-helper, T-suppressor and T-killer function.[25,57] At present, the reasons for the above observations in hyperactive children are not clear, but zinc status may play an important role.

EFFECT OF AZO DYES ON HYPERACTIVE CHILDREN

Many food additives have been cited as inducing hyperactive behavioural problems in susceptible children. This subject has been extensively reviewed by others.[18,30,31,41,44,47,48,58,68,70,71,89,96–98,112,129]

A previous study reported the influence of a chemical substance, namely the food colourant tartrazine (E_{102}), on the zinc status of hyperactive children.[120] This double-blind placebo-controlled study showed that a negative relationship exists between the zinc levels of blood serum and saliva collected from hyperactive children given tartrazine. Urinary zinc excretion increased over a 24-hour period following the intake of tartrazine.

An assessment of associated physiological observations showed that only the hyperactive children given tartrazine had any changes in behaviour or emotional status. In fact, two children developed eczema and one asthma after a period of 30–45 min after taking the tartrazine drink.

The above study showed a possible direct relationship between a chemical and hyperactive behaviour in children. A follow-up study attempted to discover the possible mechanism of the effects of azo dyes on hyperactive children.[6] This work showed that tartrazine complexes with zinc in aqueous buffer and 50% ethanol solutions. However, it was not possible to show any *in vivo* relationship.

A subsequent assessment of the chemical factors in relation to child hyperactivity[124] used a questionnaire evaluation of 486 hyperactive children. This study showed that more than 60% of hyperactivity cases reported a positive behavioural response (that is increased problems) in relation to consuming synthetic colourings and flavourings. Some of these hyperactive children with a known behavioural response following the consumption of a beverage containing tartrazine (E_{102}), sunset yellow (E_{110}) or amaranth (E_{123}) showed significant reductions in blood serum zinc and increased urinary zinc output following the drinking of a beverage containing these chemicals. For the 23 children who consumed a tartrazine beverage, there were increased levels of overactivity, aggressive and/or violent activity, poor speech and coordination and the development of asthma and/or eczema. Most of these effects were severe or moderate changes. Although at present the mechanism behind these observations is not known, it is clear that two double-blind placebo-controlled studies have shown a strong link between chemicals and changes in child hyperactive behaviour, and that zinc is in some way involved in this chemical-induced activity. Many other studies have also suggested a link between tartrazine and food intolerance, resulting in behavioural changes in children.[31,70,96]

In the above study only zinc data has so far been evaluated. In 1999, a review of the study showed some other interesting trace element effects in relation to the consumption of food or beverage colourants. The following data relate to the group of hyperactive children with a known sensitivity to synthetic food colours who were given a dose of tartrazine ($n = 23$ children), sunset yellow ($n = 12$) or amaranth ($n = 12$). A sex- and age-matched control group ($n = 5$ children for each synthetic food colour group) was also studied. Figure 52.3 shows the zinc, iron, magnesium, copper and potassium levels in hyperactive (HA) and control (C) groups. Blood serum and urine samples were collected at 0, 30, 60, 90 and 120 min time periods (reported as a mean value for those cases providing a sample at that particular time interval) after the consumption of a drink (with a 50 mg dose of tartrazine, E_{102}).

Hyperactive children show a reduction in their blood serum zinc, iron, copper and potassium (but not magnesium) blood serum levels and an associated increase in urinary output over the 120-min period following the consumption of tartrazine. The maximum urinary output occurs after 60–90 min. Although no placebo HA or placebo C group were studied, previous work has shown that a non-tartrazine placebo beverage did not influence the zinc status (blood serum or urine) of either group of children.[120]

The effect of other synthetic food colours on the zinc levels of hyperactive and control children showed a difference between the types of synthetic beverage chemical consumed.[124] A review of the

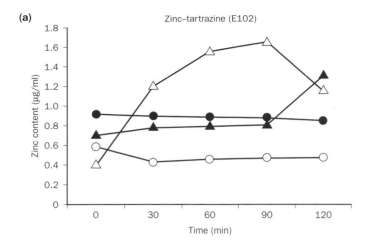

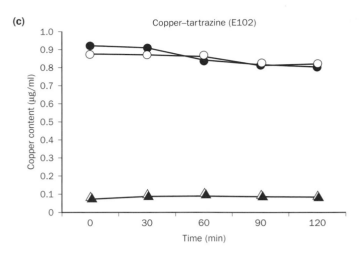

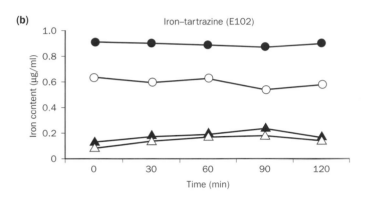

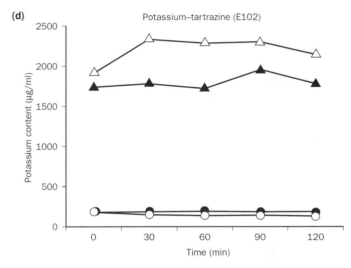

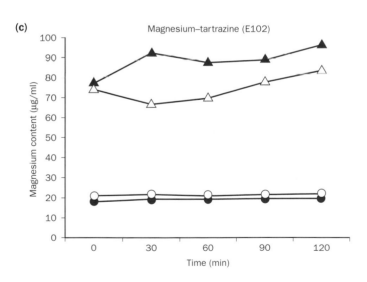

Fig. 52.3 Zinc (a), iron (b), magnesium (c), copper (d) and potassium (e) content (µg/ml) of blood serum and urine (tartrazine E$_{102}$).
○, Blood serum hyperactive (HA); ●, blood serum control (C); △, urine HA; ▲, urine C.

data for this study showed an interesting effect on another trace element. Figure 52.4 shows the magnesium levels in blood serum and urine samples for the two study groups after the consumption of a drink of sunset yellow (E$_{110}$) or amaranth (E$_{123}$).

In contrast to the small changes in magnesium content for blood serum and urine following the consumption of tartrazine and sunset yellow (Figs 52.3(c) and 52.4(a), respectively), amaranth (Fig. 52.4(b)) has a dramatic impact on magnesium levels in hyperactive children. Even after 120 min there is a continued decrease in magnesium blood serum levels and increased urinary

magnesium output. Interestingly, the magnesium levels of blood serum for the control group remain constant, with an associated steady release into the urine over the 120-min time period.

The fact that an ever-increasing number of studies have confirmed a link between the ingestion of synthetic food colours and hyperactivity raises the question about the possible mechanisms between azo dyes and biochemical systems. In the previous study, the reduction in blood serum zinc levels associated with an increase in urinary zinc excretion in hyperactive children given a dose of tartrazine may be related to the azo dye acting as a chelating agent that

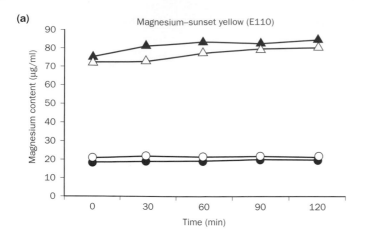

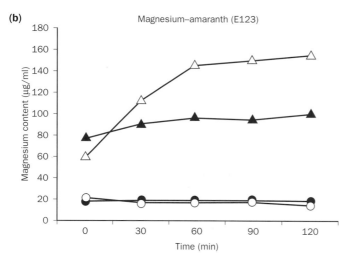

Fig. 52.4 Magnesium content (µg/ml) of blood serum and urine for (a) sunset yellow (E₁₁₀) and (b) amaranth (E₁₂₃). ○, Blood serum hyperactive (HA); ●, blood serum control (C); △, urine HA; ▲, urine C.

of azo dyes, such as sulphonated amines, may also appear in the urine or bile. One study showed that tartrazine was metabolized almost quantitatively to give sulphanilic acid, a reduction product, indicating that absorption before reduction by the gut flora is insignificant.[59] Therefore, if azo dyes are not readily absorbed, how do they 'interact' with these essential trace elements?

A possible suggestion is that the ingestion of strong chelating agents, such as tartrazine, may be able to shunt trace elements, such as zinc, away from its normal absorption route in the jejunum. One *in-vitro* study showed that mucosal zinc uptake from ethylenediaminetetracetic acid (EDTA)-containing media is greatly reduced, especially in the case of the intestines of zinc-depleted animals.[64] Therefore, hyperactive children who are low in zinc may be unable to absorb zinc (or other essential trace elements) in the presence of certain azo dyes or other chelating agents. In addition, since their digestive secretions, such as those from the pancreas, are high in endogenous zinc, further removal of this trace element from the body will occur.[64]

Another possible mechanism was reported in a study that showed that azo dyes inhibit trypsin activity by 50% following the addition of tartrazine and sunset yellow *in vitro*.[66] Similarly, the enzyme activity of amylase was reduced by 66% with tartrazine and 64% with erythrosine. If this effect could occur *in vivo*, low proteolytic enzyme activity would induce inadequate digestion. The direct consequences of this could be reduced nutrient availability, in particular the essential trace elements. This may also have an effect on the uptake of EFAs or increased antigenic loading of the gut.

Although, at present, the mode of action of these azo dyes and other chemical agents that induce behavioural changes in hyperkinetic children is not proven, a diet or environment free of these chemicals has been shown to improve the behaviour and well-being of many hyperkinetic disorder children.

ACKNOWLEDGEMENTS

The author would like to dedicate this chapter to Mrs Vicki Colquhoun and her daughter Mrs Sally Bunday of the UK-based Hyperactive Children's Support Group (HACSG) who through personal dedication and unlimited sacrifice have helped many families with hyperkinetic children obtain answers to their questions and thereby a better way of life. In addition, through their personal efforts they have also motivated many medical and scientific researchers to search for more answers, even when financial support is not forthcoming from recognized research-funding agencies.

binds any available blood zinc.[124] In this study it is apparent that the same metal ion chelation can occur with other trace elements.

It is not clear whether ingested azo dyes are readily absorbed by the stomach or small intestine. One study using rats found that only 2–4% of intake dye molecules manage to penetrate the mucosal barrier.[92] In the rat, amaranth was exclusively excreted in the bile, while tartrazine was almost exclusively excreted in the urine. For sunset yellow, 73% of the absorbed dye was excreted in the bile and 20% in the urine. Metabolities from the reduction

REFERENCES

1 American Psychiatric Association. *Diagnostic and Statistical Manual of Mental Disorders* 3rd edn. American Psychiatric Association, Washington, DC, 1987.

2 American Psychiatric Association. *Diagnostic and Statistical Manual of Mental Disorders*, 4th edn (DSM-IV). American Psychiatric Association, Washington, DC, 1994.

3 Anderson RA, Kozlovsky AS. Chromium intake, adsorption and excretion of subjects consuming self-selected diets. *Am J Clin Nutr* 1985; 41: 1177–82.

4 Anderson RA, Polansky MM, Bryden NA, Bhathena SJ, Canary J. Effects of supplemental chromium on patients with symptoms of reactive hypoglycemia. *Metabolism* 1987; 36: 351–6.

5 Arnold LE, Votolato NA, Kleykamp D, Baker GB, Bornstein RA. Does hair zinc predict amphetamine improvement of ADHD? *Int J Neurosci* 1990; 50: 103–7.

6 Ash J. *Investigations into the mechanisms of the effects of azo dyes on hyperactive children*. BSc (Hons) thesis, Department of Chemistry, University of Surrey, Guildford, 1994.

7 Ashkenazi R, Ben-Shachar D, Youdim MBH. Nutritional iron and dopamine binding sites in rat brain. *Pharmacol Biochem Behav* 1982; 17: 43–7.

8 Backstrom M, Wetterberg L. Increased N-acetylserotonin and melatonin formation induced by d-amphetamine in rat pineal gland organ culture via beta-adrenergic receptor mechanism. *Acta Physiol Scand* 1973; 87: 113–20.

9 Barkley RA. Attention-deficit hyperactivity disorder. *Sci Am* 1998; Sept: 66–71.

10 Beckett GJ, MacDougall DA, Nicol F, Arthur JR. Inhibition of type I and type II iodothyronine deiodinase activity in rat liver, kidney and brain produced by selenium deficiency. *Biochem J* 1989; 259: 887–94.

11 Behar D, Rapoport JL, Adams AJ. Sugar challenge testing with children considered behaviorally 'sugar reactive'. *Nutrition and Behavior* 1984; 1: 277–88.

12 Beisel WR. Trace elements in infectious processes. *Med Clin North Am* 1976; 60: 831–8.

13 Bekaroglu M, Deger O, Göktürk S. Investigation of zinc and copper levels in mentally-retarded children. *Turkish J Med Res* 1989; 7: 289–90.

14 Bekaroglu M, Aslan Y, Gedik Y *et al.* Relationships between serum fatty acids and zinc, and attention deficit hyperactivity disorder: a research note. *J Child Psychol Psychiatry* 1996; 37: 225–7.

15 Behne D, Hilmert H, Scheid S, Gessner H, Elger W. Evidence for specific selenium target tissues and new biologically important selenoproteins. *Biochim Biophys Acta* 1988; 966: 12–22.

16 Behne D, Scheid S, Kyriakopoulos A, Hilmert H. Subcellular distribution of selenoproteins in the liver of the rat. *Biochim Biophys Acta* 1990; 1033: 219–27.

17 Birchell JD, Chappell JS. Aluminium, chemical physiology, and Alzheimer's disease. *Lancet* 1988; I: 1008.

18 Boris M, Mandel FS. Foods and additives are common causes of attention deficit hyperactivity disorder in children. *Ann Allergy* 1994; 72: 462–8.

19 Brody JE. Diet change may avert need for Ritalin. *The New York Times*, Tuesday Nov. 2, New York, 1999.

20 Brostoff J. *The Complete Guide to Food Allergy and Intolerance*. Bloomsbury Press, London, 1992.

21 Brostoff J, Gamlin L. *Complete Guide to Food Allergies and Food Intolerance*. Bloomsbury Press, London, 1989.

22 Bryce-Smith D, Ward NI, Zaaijman J du T. Environmental influences on prenatal development. *Proc Int Conf Environ Pollut*, Thessaloniki, Greece, 21–25 Sept 1981.

23 Carter JP, Kattob A, Abd-El-Hodi, Davis JT, EL Cholmy A, Patwardhan VN. Chromium III in hypoglycemia and impaired glucose utilisation in Kwashiorkor. *Am J Clin Nutr* 1968; 21: 195–202.

24 Carter CM, Urbanowicz M, Hemsley R. Effects of a few foods diet in attention deficit disorder. *Arch Dis Childhood* 1993; 69: 564–8.

25 Chandra RK. Nutritional regulation of immunity and risk of infection in old age. *Immunology* 1989; 67: 1421–8.

26 Churchman DR. *The Analysis of Selenium in Human Blood Serum by Inductively Coupled Plasma Mass Spectrometry (ICP-MS)*. PhD thesis, Department of Chemistry, University of Surrey, Guildford, Surrey, UK, 1997; 1–382.

27 Colquhoun ID. AD/HD – a dietary/nutritional approach. *Therapeutic Care & Education* 1994; 3(2): 159–72.

28 Colquhoun I, Bunday S. A lack of essential fatty acids a possible cause of hyperactivity in children. *Medical Hypothesis* 1981; 7: 673–9.

29 Colquhoun I, Bunday S. *Attention Deficit Hyperactive Disorder – the Dietary/Nutritional Approach*. Hyperactive Children's Support Group, Chichester, UK, 1999; 1–32.

30 Connors CK, Goyette Charters, Southwick DA *et al.* Food additives and hyperkinesis: a controlled double-blind experiment. *Pediatrics* 1976; 58: 154–66.

31 David TJ. Reactions to dietary tartrazine. *Arch Dis Child* 1987; 62: 119–22.

32 Deinard AS, Murray MJ, Egeland B. Childhood iron deficiency and impaired attentional development or scholastic performance: Is the evidence sufficient to establish causality? *Pediatrics* 1976; 88: 162–3.

33 Deinard A, Gilbert A, Dodds M, Egeland B. Iron deficiency and behavioral deficits. *Pediatrics* 1981; 68: 828–33.

34 Dreosti JE, Smith RM. *Neurobiology of the Trace Elements, Vol 1. Trace Element Neurobiology and Deficiencies*. Humana Press, Clifton, NJ, 1983.

35 Ebadi M. Regulation of the synthesis of melatonin and its significance to neuroendocrinology. In: *The Pineal Gland* (Reiter RJ ed). Raven Press, New York, 1984: 1–37.

36 Egger J. Controlled trial of oligoantigenic treatment in the hyperkinetic syndrome. *Lancet* 1985; 1: 540–5.

37 Egger J, Stolla A, McEwen L. Controlled trial of hypersensitisation in children with food-induced hyperkinetic syndrome. *Lancet* 1992; 339: 1150–3.

38 Elia J, Ambrosini PJ, Rapoport JL. Treatment of attention-deficit-hyperactivity disorder. *N Engl J Med* 1999; 340: 780–8.

39 Eyestone LL, Howell RJ. An epidemiological study of attention-deficit hyperactivity disorder and major depression in a male prison population. *Bull Am Acad Psychiatry Law* 1994; 22: 181–93.

40 Feingold BF. *Why Your Child is Hyperactive*. Random House, New York, 1975.

41 Feingold BF. Hyperkinesis and learning disabilities linked to the ingestion of artificial food colors and flavors. *J Learn Disabil* 1976; 9: 19–27.

42 Flink EB, Flink PF, Shane SR, Jones JE, Steffes PE. Magnesium and free fatty acids in alcoholism. *Clin Res* 1973; 21: 884.

43 Goodwin WJ, Lane HW, Bradford K *et al.* Selenium and glutathione peroxidase levels in patients with epidermoid carcinoma of the oral cavity and oropharynx. *Cancer* 1983; 51: 110–15.

44 Goyette Charters, Conners CK, Petti TA. Effects of artificial colors on hyperkinetic children: a double-blind challenge study. *Pyscholopharmacol Bull* 1978; 14: 39–40.

45 Gross MD. Effect of sucrose on hyperkinetic children. *Pediatrics* 1984; 74: 876–8.

46 Halas ES. Behavioral changes accompanying zinc deficiency in animals. In *Neurobiology of the Trace Elements* (Dreosti I, Smith R eds), Humana Press, New Jersey, 1983: 213–43.

47 Harley JP, Ray RS, Tomasi L *et al.* Hyperkinesis and food additives: testing the Feingold hypothesis. *Pediatrics* 1978; 61: 818–28.

48 Harley JP, Matthews CG, Eichman PL. Synthetic food colours and hyperactivity in children: a double-blind challenge experiment. *Pediatrics* 1978; 62: 975–83.

49 Hartsough CS, Lambert NM. Medical factors in hyperactive and normal children. *Am J Orthopsychia* 1985; 55(2): 190–201.

50 Hauser P *et al.* ADD/HD in people with generalised resistance to thyroid hormone. *N Engl J Med* 1993; 328: 997–1001.

51 Hesse GW, Hesse KAF, Catalanotto FA. Behavioral characteristics of rats experiencing chronic zinc deficiency. *Physiol Behav* 1979; 22: 211–15.

52 Hippchen LJ. Ecologic-biochemical approaches to the treatment of delinquents and criminals. In: *Holistic Approaches to Offender Rehabilitation*. Charles C Thomas, Springfield, Illinois, 1982: 15.

53 Holtz RW, Deguchi TC, Axelrod J. Stimulation of serotonin N-acetyltransferase in pineal organ culture by drugs. *J Neurochem* 1974; 22: 205–9.

54 Horribin DF, Cunnane SC. Interactions between zinc, essential fatty acids and prostaglandins: Relevance to acrodermatitis enteropathica, total parenteral nutrition, the glucaconoma syndrome, diabetes, anorexia nervosa and sickle cell anaemia. *Medical Hypotheses* 1980; 6: 277–96.

55 Horribin DF, Bennett CN. New gene targets related to schizophrenia and other psychiatric disorders: enzymes, binding proteins and transport proteins involved in phospholipid and fatty acid metabolism. *Prostaglandins, Leukotrienes and Essential Fatty Acids* 1999; 60(3): 141–67.

56 Horribin DF, Bennett CN. Depression and bipolar disorder: relationships to impaired fatty acid and phospholipid metabolism and to diabetes, cardiovascular disease, immunological abnormalities, cancer, ageing and oeteoporosis. *Prostaglandins, Leukotrienes and Essential Fatty Acids* 1999; 60(3): 217–34.

57 Iwata T, Incefy GS, Tanaka T *et al.* Circulating thymic hormone levels in zinc deficiency. *Cell Immunol* 1979; 47: 100–8.

58 Jacobson MF, Schardt D. *Diet, ADHD & Behavior – A Quarter-Century Review*. Centre for Science in the Public Interest, Washington, DC, 1999.

59 Jones R, Ryan AJ, Wright SE. The metabolism and excretion of tartrazine in the rat, rabbit and man. *Fed Cosmet Toxicol* 1964; 2: 447.

60 Kaplan BJ, McNicol J, Conte R, Moghadam H. Physical signs and symptoms in pre-school age hyperactivity and normal children. *J Dev Behav Paediatr* 1987; 8: 305–9.

61 Kaplan BJ, McNicol J, Conte RA. Dietary replacement in preschool-ages hyperactive boys. *Pediatrics* 1989; 83: 7–17.

62 Kaplan HI, Sadock BJ, Grebb JA. Attention deficit disorders. In: *Synopsis of Psychiatry*, 7th edn, (Kaplan HI, Sadock BJ, Grebb JA eds). Williams and Wilkins, Baltimore, MD, 1994: 1063–8.

63 Keen C, Gershwin M. Zinc deficiency and immune function. *Ann Rev Nutr* 1990; 10: 415–31.

64 Kirchgessner M, Weigand E. Zinc absorption and excretion in nutrition. In: *Metal Ions in Biological Systems, Vol. 15, Zinc and its Role in Biology and Nutrition* (Sigel M ed). Marcel Dekker, New York, 1983.

65 Kozielec T, Starbrat E, Herhelin B. Deficiency of certain trace elements in children with hyperactivity. *Pol J Psychiatr* 1994; 28(3): 345–53.

66 Kroyer G. Artificial food colours as food additives. *Ernahrung Nutr* 1986; 10: 465–7.

67 Kruesi MJP, Rapoport JL, Cummings EM. Effects of sugar and aspartame on aggression and activity in children. *Am J Psychiatry* 1987; 144: 1487–90.

68 Levy F, Dunbrell S, Hobbes G *et al*. Hyperkinesis and diet: a double crossover trial with a tartrazine challenge. *Med J Austr* 1978; 1: 61–4.

69 Lynch HJ, Wang P, Wurtman RJ. Increase in rat pineal melatonin content following L-dopa administration. *Life Sci* 1973; 12: 145–51.

70 Mattes J, Gittleman-Klein RA. A crossover study of artificial colorings in a hyperkinetic child. *Am J Psychiatr* 1978; 135: 987–8.

71 Mattes J, Gittleman R. Effects of artificial colouring in children with hyperactive symptoms: a critical review and results of a controlled study. *Arch Gen Psychiatr* 1981; 38: 714–8.

72 McGee R, Williams S, Anderson J, McKenzie-Parnell JM, Silva PA. Hyperactivity and serum hair zinc levels in 11-year-old children from the general population. *Biol Psychiatry* 1990; 28: 165–8.

73 Menzies IC. Disturbed children: role of food and chemical sensitivities. *Nutrition & Health* 1984; 3: 39–54.

74 Mertz W. Biological role of chromium. *Fed Proc Fed Amer Soc Exp Biol* 1967; 26: 186–93.

75 Mertz W. Chromium occurrence and function in biological systems. *Physiol Rev* 1969; 49: 169–239.

76 Mertz W. Human requirements: basic and optimal. *Ann NY Acad Sci* 1971; 199: 191–9.

77 Mertz W. Biological function of chromium nicotinic acid-complexes. *Fed Proc Fed Amer Soc Exp Biol* 1974; 33: 659.

78 Mertz W, Roginski EE. Chromium metabolism: the glucose tolerance factor. In: *Newer Trace Elements in Nutrition* (Mertz W, Cornatzer WE eds). Dekker, New York, 1971.

79 Mikac-Devic M, Vukelic N, Kljaic K. Serum selenium level in patients with colorectal cancer. *Biol Trace Elem Res* 1992; 33: 87–94.

80 Milberger S *et al*. Further evidence of an association between maternal smoking during pregnancy and ADHD: findings from a high-risk sample of siblings. *J Clin Child Psychol* 1998; 27(3): 352–8.

81 Milich R, Pelham WE. Effects of sugar ingestion on the classroom and playgroup behavior of attention deficit disordered boys. *J Consulting Clin Psychol* 1986; 54: 714–8.

82 Mitchell E, Aman M, Turbott S. Clinical characteristics and serum essential fatty acid levels in hyperactive children. *Clin Paediatr* 1987; 26: 406–11.

83 Moon C, Marlow M. Hair-aluminium concentrations and children's classroom behaviour. *Biol Trace Elem Res* 1986; 11: 5–12.

84 Nielson JA, Thayson EH. Acute and chronic magnesium deficiency following extensive small gut resection. *Scand J Gastroenterol* 1971; 6: 663–6.

85 Okada S, Ohba H, Taniyama M. Alterations in ribonucleic acid synthesis by chromium (III). *J Inorg Biochem* 1981; 15: 223–31.

86 Oski FA, Honig AS, Helu B, Howanitz P. Effect of iron therapy on behavior performance in nonanemic, iron-deficient infants. *Pediatrics* 1983; 71: 877–80.

87 Petit TL. Aluminium neurobehavioural toxicology. In: *Neurobiology of the Trace Elements, Vol. 2, Neurotoxicology and Neuropharmacology* (Dreosti IE, Smith RM eds.) Humana Press, Clifton, New Jersey, 1983.

88 Pollit E, Leibel RL. Iron deficiency and behavior. *J Pediatr* 1976; 88: 372–81.

89 Pollock I, Warner JO. Effect of artificial food colours on childhood behaviour. *J Learn Disabil* 1990; 9: 19–27.

90 Prasad AS, Oberleas D. *Trace Elements in Human Health and Disease. Vol. I, Zinc and Copper*. Academic Press, New York, 1976.

91 Prasad AS, Oberleas D. *Trace Elements in Human Health and Disease. Vol. II, Essential and Toxic Elements*. Academic Press, New York, 1976.

92 Radomski JL, Mellinger TJ. The absorption, fate and excretion in rats of the water-soluble azo dyes FD & C Red no. 2, FD & C no. 4 and FD & C no. 6. *J Pharmacol Exptl Therapeutics* 1962; 136: 259–66.

93 Rayman MP. Dietary selenium: time to act. *Br Med J* 1997; 314: 387–8.

94 Rayman MP. The importance of selenium to human health. *Lancet* 2000; 356: 233–41.

95 Richardson AJ, Puri BK. The potential role of fatty acids in ADHD. *The Nutrition Practitioner* 2000; 2(2): 15–21.

96 Rose TL. The functional relationship between artificial food colors and hyperactivity. *J Appl Behav Anal* 1978; 11: 439–46.

97 Rowe KS Synthetic food colourings and 'hyperactivity': a double-blind crossover study. *Austr Paediatr J* 1988; 24: 143–7.

98 Rowe KS, Rowe KJ. Synthetic food coloring and behavior: a dose response effect in a double-blind placebo-controlled repeated-measures study. *J Pediatr* 1994; 125: 691–8.

99 Safer DF, Zito JM, Fine EM. Increased methylphenidate usage for attention deficit disorder in the 1990's. *Pediatrics* 1996; 98: 1084–8.

100 Sandyk R. Zinc deficiency in attention-deficit hyperactivity disorder [letter]. *Int J Neurosci* 1990; 52: 239–41.

101 Schmedt ME, Kruesi MJP, Elia J *et al*. Effect of dextroamphetamine and methylpenenidate on calcium and magnesium concentration in hyperactive boys. *Psychiatry Res* 1994; 54: 199–210.

102 Schoenthaler S, Amos S, Doras W, Rd MK, Muedeking G, Wakefield J. The effect of randomised vitamin–mineral supplementation on violent and non-violent antisocial behavior among incarcerated juveniles. *J Nutr Environ Med* 1997; 7: 343–52.

103 Schroeder HA. Losses of vitamin and trace minerals resulting from processing and preservation of foods. *Am J Clin Nutr* 1971; 24: 562–73.

104 Schroeder HA, Nason AP. Trace-element analysis in clinical chemistry. *Clin Chem* 1971; 17: 461–74.

105 Sever Y, Ashkenazi A, Tyano S, Weizman A. Iron treatment in children with attention deficit hyperactivity disorder. A preliminary report. *Neuropsychobiology* 1997; 35: 178–80.

106 Shafey H, van Dewetering C. Iron deficiency in two adolescents with conduct, dysthymic and movement disorder. *Can J Psychiatry* 1994; 39: 371–5.

107 Starobrat-Hermelin B, Kozielec T. The effects of magnesium physiological supplementation on hyperactivity with Attention Deficit Hyperactivity Disorder (ADHD). Positive response to magnesium oral loading test. *Magnesium Research* 1997; 10(2): 149–56.

108 Stevens LJ, Zentall SS, Deck JL *et al*. Essential fatty acid metabolism in boys with attention-deficit hyperactivity disorder. *Am J Clin Nutr* 1995; 62: 761–8.

109 Stevens LJ, Zentall SS, Abate ML, Kuczeek T, Burgess JR. Omega-3 fatty acids in boys with behavior, learning and health problems. *Physiol Behav* 1996; 59: 915–20.

110 Stovell AG. *Trace Elements and Human Fertility*. PhD thesis, Department of Chemistry, University of Surrey, Guildford, 1999; 1–333.

111 Swanson JM, Kinsbourne M. Food dyes impair performance of hyperactive children on a laboratory learning test. *Science* 1980; 207: 1485–6.

112 Swanson JM *et al*. Cognitive neuroscience of ADHD and hyperkinetic disorder. *Curr Opin Neurobiol* 1998; 8(2): 263–71.

113 Terrass S. Nutritional alternatives to Ritalin – a science-based approach. *The Nutrition Practitioner* 2000; 2(2): 24–7.

114 Thapar A *et al*. Genetic basis of attention deficit and hyperactivity. *Br J Psychiatry* 1999; 174: 105–11.

115 Toren P, Eldar S, Sela B-A *et al.* Zinc deficiency in attention-deficit hyperactivity disorder. *Biol Psychiatry* 1996; 40: 1308–10.

116 Uhlig T, Merkenschlager A, Brandmaier R. Topographic mapping of brain electrical activity in children with food-induced attention deficit hyperkinetic disorder. *Eur J Pediatr* 1997; 156: 557–61.

117 Ward KP, Arthur JR, Russell G, Aggett PJ. Blood selenium content and glutathione peroxidase activity in children with cystic fibrosis, coeliac disease, asthma and epilepsy. *Eur J Pediatr* 1984; 142: 21–4.

118 Ward NI, Bryce-Smith D, Minski MJ, Matthews WB. Multiple sclerosis: A multi-element survey. *Biol Trace Element Res* 1985; 7: 153–9.

119 Ward NI. Multi-element analysis of urine by neutron activation analysis: application to starvation and anorexia nervosa. *J Micronutr Anal* 1986; 2: 211–31.

120 Ward NI, Soulsbury K, Zettel VH, Colquhoun ID, Bunday S, Barnes B. The influence of the chemical additive tartrazine on the zinc status of hyperactive children – a double-blind placebo-controlled study. *J Nutr Med* 1990; 1: 51–7.

121 Ward NI. Multielement tissue status of sows exposed to aluminium in North Cornwall as a result of the Lowermoor Water Treatment Work incident. *Trace Elements in Man and Animals m-TEMA 7* (Momcilovic M ed). IMI, Zagreb, 1991: 23–1.

122 Ward NI, Ward AE. Element content of children's scalp hair and saliva in assessing reading development. *Trace Elements in Man and Animals m-TEMA 7* (Momcilovic M ed). IMI, Zagreb, 1991: 28–4.

123 Ward NI. Heavy metal status of incarcerated young offenders and control individuals. *Heavy Metals in the Environment.* CEP Consultants, Edinburgh, 1996: 227–80.

124 Ward NI. Assessment of chemical factors in relation to child hyperactivity. *J Nutr Environ Med* 1997; 7: 333–42.

125 Ward NI. Chemical substances and human behaviour. *The Nutrition Practitioner* 2000; 2(2): 43–5.

126 Warner JO. Behaviour and adverse food reactions in food allergy. In: *Adverse Reactions to Foods and Food Additives* (Metcalfe DD, Sampson HA, Simon RA eds), Blackwell Sciences, Oxford, 1997.

127 Watts M. The riddle of ADHD. *The Nutrition Practitioner* 2000; 2(2): 22–3.

128 Weinberg ED. Iron and susceptibility to infectious disease. *Science* 1974; 184: 952–8.

129 Weiss B. Food additives and environmental chemicals as sources of childhood behaviour disorders. *Am Acad Psychiatry* 1982; 21-2: 142–52.

130 Wender EH, Solanto MV. Effects of sugar on aggressive and inattentive behaviour in children with attention deficit disorder with hyperactivity and normal children. *Pediatrics* 1991; 88: 960–6.

131 Wenk GL, Stemmer KL. Suboptimal dietary zinc intake increases aluminium into the rat brain. *Brain Res* 1983; 288: 393–401.

132 Willett WC, Stampfer MJ. Selenium and cancer. Whether selenium protects against cancer is still unknown. *Br Med J* 1988; 297: 573–4.

133 Yehuda S, Youdim MBH, Mastofsky DI. Brain iron-deficiency causes reduced learning capacity in rats. *Pharmacol Biochem Behav* 1986; 25: 141–4.

134 Youdim MBH, Yehuda S. Iron deficiency induces several dopamine dependent circadian cycles: differential response to *d*-amphetamine and TRH. *Peptides* 1985; 6: 851–5.

135 Young E. Relationship of food to hyperactivity. In *MAAF Chief Scientist's Group Report of the Review of MAFF's Food Intolerance Research Programme*, Europa Gatwick Hotel, 22–23 October 1998; 39–40.

136 Zametkin AJ, Liotta W. The neurobiology of attention-deficit/hyperactivity disorder. *J Clin Psychiatry* 1998; 59(7): 17–23.

137 Zhang L, Maiorine M, Roveri A, Ursini F. Phospholipid hydroperoxide glutathione peroxidase: specific activity in tissues of rats of different age and comparison with other glutathione peroxidases. *Biochim Biophys Acta* 1989; 1006: 140–8.

Food addiction and criminal behaviour

Stephen J. Schoenthaler and Ian D. Bier

INTRODUCTION

Over the past two decades, many American juvenile correctional facilities have changed their institutional menus, replacing high sugar and fat manufactured foods with fresh fruits, vegetables and whole grain products.[10–12] In each of 13 institutional sites studied, the violent and non-violent antisocial behaviour fell significantly following these dietary changes. The four main findings[10,11,15] from these institutions may be summarized as follows:

1. a 48% reduction in antisocial behaviour was seen in a total of 7406 juveniles after implementation of similar diets
2. the incidence of assault, battery, fighting, suicide attempts, insubordination and hyperkinesis decreased more than 50%
3. all behavioural improvements were accounted for by changes in just 16–25% of the juveniles tested
4. the behaviour of juveniles who had been incarcerated for violent crimes improved, on average 55%, while those who had been confined for non-violent crimes improved, on average, 37%.

A year-long follow-up

In the longest trial conducted, behaviour improved gradually and linearly for 20 weeks and then levelled off at a rate 61% below baseline rates, where it remained stable for the next 32 weeks.[4,12] The gradual, linear nature of the improvements suggests that the primary cause of the improvements was the steady correction of undiagnosed marginal malnutrition. Placebo effects, although a possible explanation, do not produce the enduring improvements demonstrated.[4]

Nutrient intake and behaviour

These dietary replacement trials in 13 institutions were followed by five studies that compared nutrient intakes and behaviour in incarcerated adult and juvenile offenders.[12,13] Each study reported two associations between diet and behaviour. First, badly behaved incarcerated offenders were significantly more likely than well-behaved offenders to have a low dietary intake of vitamins and minerals. Each study used 70% of the US recommended daily allowances (RDAs) as the definition of 'low' dietary intake, the per cent of the RDA where the risk of malnutrition theoretically rises to 50% for each nutrient. Secondly, the offenders who were at risk of malnutrition due to intakes below 70% US RDA were significantly more likely to commit antisocial behaviour than offenders who were not deficient on any of 16 individual nutrients.

Does bad diet cause bad behaviour?

These five dietary studies suggested that bad diet causes bad behaviour, but they were not conclusive for two reasons: first, correlations do not prove causation; and secondly, the direction of effect is unclear. Perhaps bad offenders eat poor diets because they are bad offenders rather than the poor diet causing the bad behaviour. However, if malnutrition caused poor behaviour, and its correction caused the improvements in the dietary replacement studies, then a single daily multiple vitamin–mineral supplement ought to reduce infraction behaviour as well. This was simultaneously tested in two unpublished 3-month pilot studies on 40 offenders that used no control groups: official rule violations fell significantly – 37% in one study and 43% in the other – during supplementation. The pilot studies confirmed the need for a proper randomized placebo-controlled trial.

Vitamin and mineral supplements versus placebo

Three distinct randomized double-blind placebo-controlled trials followed on a total of 932 subjects between the ages 6 and 25 years. These trials were designed to overcome the methodological shortcomings of earlier dietary replacement designs[16–18] and pilot studies that lacked a control group. Each trial randomly assigned subjects to vitamin–mineral tablets or placebo tablets for 13–15 weeks. Each trial tested the hypothesis that additional micronutrients, such as those found in the fruits, vegetables and whole grains in the 13 dietary replacement studies, would cause behavioural improvements. The randomized controlled trials were conducted on schoolchildren aged 6–12 years old, confined teenage delinquents aged 12–17 years old and young adult felons aged 18–25 years old. Results in each group showed that the groups who ingested vitamin–mineral tablets produced about 40% less antisocial behaviour, with little differences across the three studies. In addition, these trials gathered pre- and post-test data on individual nutrient intakes from dietary analyses, blood vitamin and mineral concentrations, physical examinations, and even electroencephalograms (EEGs) on selected subjects. These data verified that micronutrient deficiencies resulted from the individual's 'addiction' to a narrow choice of foods that did not provide adequate vitamins and minerals, rather than an adverse effect of the high sugar and fat foods themselves.

This chapter reviews the above evidence on a relationship between diet and serious antisocial behaviour in (1) the two best dietary replacement studies; (2) the correlational studies on individual nutrients and behaviour; and (3) four randomized controlled trials, including one that measured brain functioning before and after nutritional intervention. This chapter also reviews the suspected micronutrient deficiencies and therapeutic concentrations that may have clinical utility.

THE DIETARY REPLACEMENT STUDIES ON DELINQUENTS

The first interrupted time-series design

All time-series designs record data on a dependent variable of interest before and after introduction of the independent variable in multiple time intervals rather than a single pre- and post-test. In this study, the dependent variable of interest was the official institutional rule violations before and after the diet change. However, a serious potential confounding factor may appear when studying institutional rule violation rates over sequential time intervals. Offenders are constantly being admitted and discharged from correctional facilities. A decline in rule violations may not be due to a new intervention, but due to the admission of better-behaved offenders. For example, the Bureau of Justice Statistics reports that prison rule violation rates differ based on age, gender, race and the type of crime that caused admission.[1]

The interrupted time-series design nicely eliminates such potential confounds by using what are called 'non-equivalent dependent variables'. The design records data on one or more additional variables that are not expected to change due to the intervention, but are known to affect the dependent variable. In this study, five additional variables were plotted, i.e. age, race, gender, type of crime that caused admission and any staff personnel changes. (The latter was deemed important because not only could the offenders be less trouble-prone, but also replace-

ment staff may not use the same standards when making the decision to record antisocial behaviour. This is called a change in instrumentation.)

Design of study

In short, this design involves a comparison of series of observations (O) over time on a dependent variable (a) that is expected to be affected by an intervention (X). It also involves a comparison series of observations (O) over time on at least one additional variable (b) that is not expected to be influenced by the same intervention.

> Although no research design guarantees correct inferences, the interrupted time-series design, with non-equivalent dependent variables is considered [to be] among the strongest of the non-experimental designs for drawing causal inferences … This design rules out the largest number of plausible alternative explanations for a hypothesized causal relationship.[21]

In spite of such strengths, such designs are almost unknown in medicine, with preference being given to the randomized placebo-controlled trial. This preference of one type of design over all others, regardless of the hypothesis being tested, is called methodological narcissism,[6] and may lead to the incorrect choice of a research design. For this study, the interrupted time-series design was the strongest design.

In this trial the effects of a diet change on behaviour were studied in a small Virginia juvenile correctional facility that housed children, aged 12–17 years old, who were awaiting trial. A month, rather than a year, was used as the unit of analysis, because monthly data are considered far superior for interpreting change and reducing history effects.[21] In other words, when the time intervals are short and a change occurs following treatment in a specific time interval, rival historical hypotheses are limited to changes that occurred in that short time interval. The management of the correctional institution avoided any personnel or policy changes close to the month the diet changed, to eliminate historical effects.

Confounding variables

In addition, the three most common psychological confounds[6] that creep into nutrition research – Hawthorne, Pygmalion and placebo effects – were controlled. Hawthorne effects are changes in behaviour because the subjects know that they are being studied. Pygmalion effects are an expectation of change in the observers who record the data. Placebo effects are an expectation of change in the subjects due to assumptions that the treatment will work.

The study was conducted after obtaining IRB approval, without the knowledge of the staff or inmates of the facility. The governor of the institution, although well respected by staff, had a reputation as 'a health food advocate'. This caused the staff to misinterpret the diet policy change as simply his desire to see the children eat more like him. In addition, data were not retrieved from the files, which were kept in another location until after the experimental period had ended. As a result, no staff member was aware that a study had even been conducted, which was established at a staff debriefing at the end of the study. This confirmed that the Hawthorne effect was not a confounding factor. Debriefing also verified that no staff member thought that the diet change might improve behaviour, and none had ever thought about the possibility before debriefing. This verified the absence of Pygmalion effects. Debriefing also confirmed that no staff remembered any of the 15 juveniles who experienced the change in the institutional fare vocalize a belief that the new diet could improve their behaviour. This strongly suggested, though did not confirm, the absence of placebo effects.

Thus, this study was the first to measure the effects of a diet change on behaviour controlling for the psychological confounds that normally occur. The variable of interest became the mean number of official disciplinary actions taken by the institution for 'rule violations' per juvenile during 13 four-week periods before the diet change and the same measure for the 13 four-week periods after the diet change.

Figure 53.1 depicts mean changes between the baseline and intervention year. After the diet policy change, the average rate

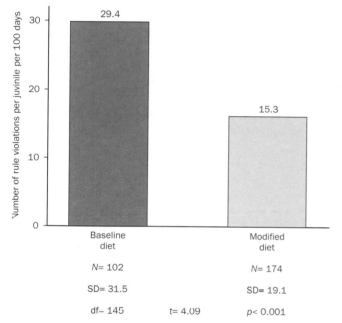

Fig. 53.1 Disciplinary actions taken for rule violations by group: 48% less violations when served a more nutritious diet.

of delinquency per juvenile was 48% lower among the 174 experimental youths than the 102 baseline youths ($P < 0.001$).

Number of juveniles in study

These data may give the false impression that fewer juveniles must have been confined in the facility during the baseline year. After former residents reach 18 years of age, their records are purged from the institutional archival files. Thus, the oldest boys from the baseline year were excluded. To control for this potential confound, the data were analysed with and without the oldest juveniles during the intervention period to measure the effect of this confound. The elimination of the older offenders would have increased the difference between the groups. Therefore, only the smaller 48% difference in behaviour was originally reported.

Does diet change reduce delinquency?

Although these data suggest that the diet change lowered delinquency, such a conclusion would be premature, since it is not possible to verify from this research design whether the behavioural improvements were due to the policy change or the result of a pre-existing downward trend. To answer this question an intervention analysis was completed.

Intervention analysis

The underlying principle of an intervention analysis is fairly simple. The trend before the policy went into effect is compared with the trend after the policy went into effect, and various intervention models are tried to see which best explains the trend seen. Three intervention models were considered. First, the possibility existed that, after intervention, the delinquency rate would drop sharply immediately and remain at a lower level for the remainder of the trial. Secondly, the policy change might have had a small initial impact that grew larger over time. Thirdly, the crime rate may have been reduced initially, but then returned to previous levels as time passed, similar to a placebo effect. The results are shown in Fig. 53.2. The trend during the baseline months was a slight increase in delinquency with the slope of

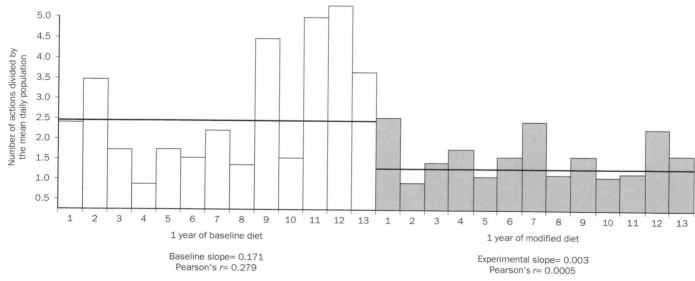

Fig. 53.2 Disciplinary actions taken for rule violations by group for 26 four-week intervals before and after dietary change: 46% less violations when served a more nutritious diet.

0.17 for the least squares regression line. During the intervention phase, the slope of the line decreased to 0.00. Three conclusions followed: delinquency was rising slightly during the baseline period; fell 45% from the baseline rate after the intervention; and remained at that level throughout the remaining 13 four-week periods.

Further confounding variables in the data set

Since the 102 juveniles during the pre-intervention period were not the same children as the 174 during the intervention period, one potential confound remained. It was possible that the two groups were not equal in proneness to delinquency due to a lack of random assignment. Accordingly, both groups were compared on confounding variables that are thought to influence official delinquency rates: age, race, gender and type of offence that caused their arrest. The data were re-examined by comparing pre- and post-rates on each of the potential confounds. In each contrast, the juveniles who received the diet containing more fruit, vegetables and whole grains produced lower delinquency rates than the juveniles who consumed a diet that was low in these foods, as illustrated in Figs 53.3–53.6. These figures show that the juveniles who received the revised diet had less anti-social behaviour regardless of the charges that brought them to the institution, their ages or their races. Two changes in staff that recorded the rule violations in the last 3 months of the study and the admission of females to the institution for 1 month also had negligible effects during the intervention time period.

Finally, a comparison was made on the types of rule violations that occurred within the institution before and after the diet changes. Figure 53.7 shows a marked decrease in all behaviour categories, including both violent and non-violent offences.[9]

What was most remarkable about the study is the fact that these children awaiting trial were only confined, on average, about 3 weeks. The short period of confinement effectively rules out any chance of the improvement being due to a placebo effect. In order for a placebo effect to be responsible for the lower rate of

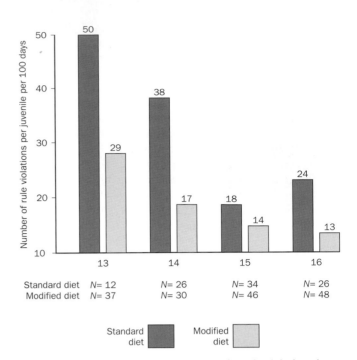

Fig. 53.4 Official disciplinary actions taken for rule violations by age of offender and type of diet.

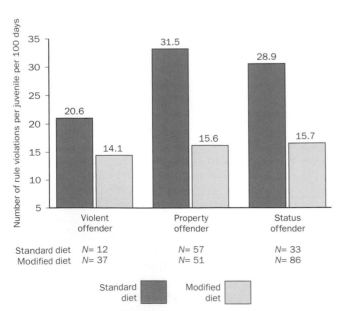

Fig. 53.3 Official disciplinary actions taken for rule violations by type of offender and type of diet.

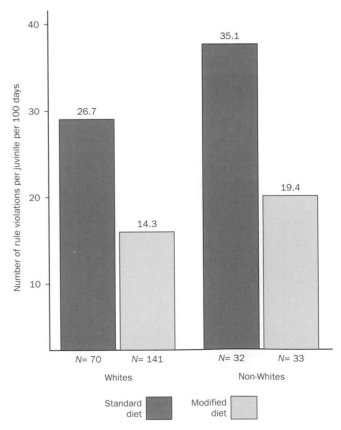

Fig. 53.5 Disciplinary actions taken for rule violations by race and type of diet.

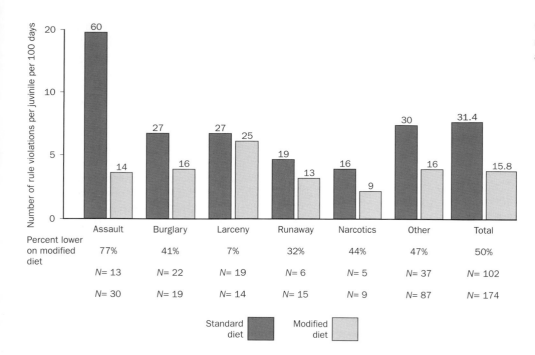

Fig. 53.6 Disciplinary actions taken for rule violations by formal charge at arrest and type of diet.

Percent lower on modified diet	Assault	Burglary	Larceny	Runaway	Narcotics	Other	Total
	77%	41%	7%	32%	44%	47%	50%
	N= 13	N= 22	N= 19	N= 6	N= 5	N= 37	N= 102
	N= 30	N= 19	N= 14	N= 15	N= 9	N= 87	N= 174

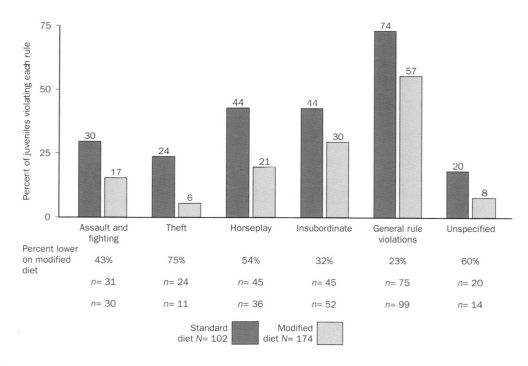

Fig. 53.7 Types of rule violations by type of diet. (*n* = the number of juveniles committing each offence. Each per cent was calculated by summing the number of juveniles who committed each type of offence and dividing by the appropriate population, either 102 or 174).

Percent lower on modified diet	Assault and fighting	Theft	Horseplay	Insubordinate	General rule violations	Unspecified
	43%	75%	54%	32%	23%	60%
	n= 31	n= 24	n= 45	n= 45	n= 75	n= 20
	n= 30	n= 11	n= 36	n= 52	n= 99	n= 14

rule violations over the next year, the following implausible scenario would have had to occur. At least one of the 15 juveniles who experienced the diet transition would have had to (1) believe in a diet and crime relationship; (2) convince other juveniles of that 'fact' without staff awareness; and (3) then successfully transmit that 'fact' to 13 succeeding populations of juveniles who were awaiting trial in that facility (since the population turned over 13 times over the next 12 months).

The primary weakness of the study lies in the absence of knowledge about the long-term effects of the diet change on a specific group of individuals. These effects were studied in the second time-series design trial.

The second interrupted time-series design

A group of 125 convicted delinquents who were incarcerated for long terms of confinement were compared for 1 year before and after a diet change similar to that used in the Virginia trial.[12,13] Again, the monthly rate of official rule violations served as the dependent variable and antisocial behavior fell, on average, 42% as shown in Fig. 53.8. Unfortunately, this chart does not illustrate the long-term effects. Figure 53.9 shows that the monthly baseline rates remained flat over a 52-week period prior to the initiation of the dietary change. After the diet change, rule violations fell gradually and linearly for 20 weeks, then levelled off and remained constant for the next 32 weeks at a new level 61% below the baseline

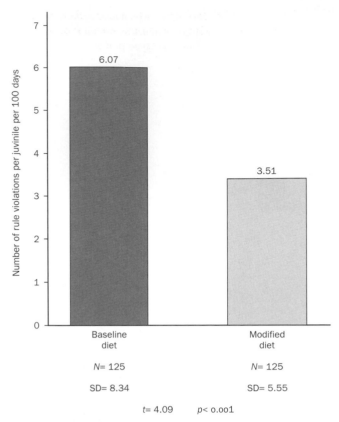

Fig. 53.8 Disciplinary actions taken for rule violations before and after dietary changes for 125 delinquents: 42% less violations when served a more nutritious diet.

to the first studies on the eating habits of confined juveniles and adults. The gradual nature of improvements strongly suggested that malnutrition was the cause, rather than reactive hypoglycaemia or a toxic effect of sugar, as was suspected previously.[8]

The two notable differences between the results found in the Tidewater Virginia study shown in Fig. 53.2 and The Alabama Youth Authority study in Fig. 53.9 are the magnitude and speed of behavioural improvements. Tidewater's 48% behavioural improvements occurred within a matter of days, while the Alabama institution took 18 weeks for the antisocial behaviour to reach its floor level, 61% lower. These differences were expected due to the different purposes of the two facilities and the different degrees of poor nutriture before intervention.

Tidewater is a pre-adjudication detention facility, while the Alabama site is a post-adjudication site. Detention facilities hold juveniles anywhere from a few days to a few weeks while they are awaiting their day in court. They usually arrive at the detention centre, shortly after being picked up by law enforcement, and suffer from both protein–calorie malnutrition as well as poor dietary habits. Detention facilities routinely report that youths who are released after 2–3 weeks in detention often have difficulty fitting into their clothes, due to weight gain. Accordingly, although both experimental diets were very similar, the children in the detention facility most likely had far worse baseline nutritional habits than children in the post-adjudication facility. This is because the youths in the post-adjudication facility had at least been receiving balanced meals from the institution for months before intervention. Accordingly, the post-adjudication offenders presumably entered the trial with superior nutrition when compared with the pre-adjudication youths, causing the initial improvements to be less dramatic.

On the other hand, the post-adjudicated youths had the benefit of the diet for months, not just weeks. It follows that longer exposure to intervention would produce greater effects over time and that is precisely what happened.

THE CORRELATIONAL STUDIES

This type of nutritional policy in juvenile correctional institutions became widespread across the United States in the 1980s. Every institution that was studied reported similar results, and no additional costs in the food budget were incurred. Yet, these

rate. This suggested that the diet was gradually correcting undiagnosed marginal malnutrition. Had the change in violations been due to the discontinuation of exposure to an unknown toxic property of sugar, behaviour would have improved rapidly. Because behaviour continued to improve gradually for 20 weeks before levelling off, correction of malnutrition is the most likely cause. Furthermore, since the same 125 juveniles were compared before and after intervention, there is no possibility that the change was due to differences in gender, race, type of committing offence, etc., such as was possible with the Virginia study. These results led

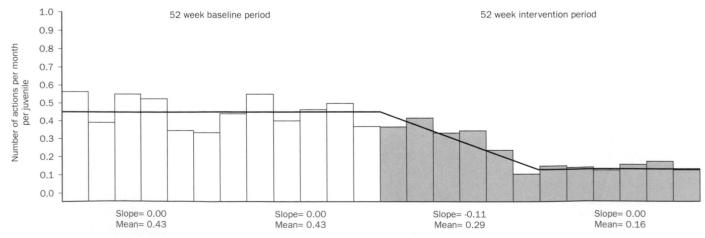

Fig. 53.9 Disciplinary actions taken for rule violations for 125 delinquents for 24 monthly intervals before and after dietary change: 61% less violations when served a more nutritious diet.

time-series designs left many questions unanswered. Confirmation that undiagnosed malnutrition was the underlying aetiology required further research. First, it would be necessary to examine the nutritional content of what correctional facilities served. Were they adequate or not on each nutrient for which a recommended daily allowance had been set? Secondly, there was a need to measure the nutrient-by-nutrient intakes of adult and juvenile offenders. Just because an institution serves nutritious foods does not mean the foods are being readily consumed. Thirdly, if the improvements in behaviour were due to bad diet, the juveniles and prisoners with the worst nutrient intakes should commit the majority of the rule violations.

Accordingly, the New York State Legislature commissioned a study to determine if incarcerated adult offenders who committed serious institutional rule violations consumed lower amounts of 16 micronutrients than incarcerated adult offenders who had not committed serious rule violations. Additionally, there were four other studies in Virginia, Florida, Oklahoma and California. Each study found that confined juveniles or adults who consumed fewer micronutrients were significantly more likely to commit institutional rule violations.[13] The New York results on 139 adult felons are illustrated in Table 53.1. It is important to note that the intake reported for zinc, magnesium, pyridoxine and folic acid were low, due to many foods not being assayed for these nutrients and reported in US government data at that time. Thus, offenders reported as having 0–4 deficiencies were likely to truly have had none, while offenders with 5 or more were likely to have had at least 1 deficiency.

It is important to note that the inmates who were involved in rule violations were more likely to be at risk of malnutrition on 16 of 16 evaluated nutrients, even though only 6 reached statistical significance in New York, as shown in Table 53.2.

One possible criticism of this work is that it was possible that the lower consumption rates of micronutrients reported were an artefact of the worst-behaved inmates consistently under-reporting consumption. In order to test this theory, atomic absorption spectrometry for minerals in hair and laboratory assays on blood vitamin concentrations were performed on subjects. The analyses confirmed that in both adult and youthful offenders, low concentrations of these nutrients are associated with higher rates of institutional rule violations,[7,17] as shown in Table 53.3. More specifically, offenders who commit serious rule violations have

Per cent of inmates below 70% of the recommended daily allowance (RDA) on selected nutrients by number of serious rule violations for 139 felons				
	Number of rule violations			
Nutrient	0	1–15	t	P
Vitamin A	2%	12%	4.05	0.012
Riboflavin	2%	12%	4.05	0.012
Vitamin B$_{12}$	2%	10%	2.89	0.023
Vitamin C	0%	4%	2.18	0.035
Vitamin D	6%	27%	9.26	0.001
Calcium	0%	5%	2.75	0.025

Table 53.2 Per cent of inmates below 70% of the recommended daily allowance (RDA) on selected nutrients by number of serious rule violations for 139 felons.

Blood nutrient deficiency rates for offenders who did or did not commit serious rule violations					
Adult offenders	Mean	Standard deviation	n	F	P
With no rule violations	0.18	0.44	100	11.76	0.0007
With rule violations	0.45	0.74	158		

Table 53.3 Blood nutrient deficiency rates for offenders who did or did not commit serious rule violations.

more than twice the number of low blood vitamin and blood mineral concentrations.

Laboratory assays of nutritional deficiencies

These present some problems. For some nutritional indicators, such as iron, the norms are well established and published in classical texts.[19] This, however, is not the case for most vitamins and minerals. Commercial laboratories offer norms, but they are not referenced to peer-reviewed articles and leading texts. Furthermore, even if they were, that does not mean that the norms for good health must be the same as those for good behaviour. They needed to be empirically tested.

Blood norms were subsequently established for behaviour and then validated in correctional institutions using the following procedure. Blood samples were taken from confined offenders who managed to officially stay out of all trouble while confined for no less than 6 months. Ranges were calculated on ten measures of vitamin status, eight measures of mineral status and five measures of iron status. Values within the range were defined as 'normal and adequate' for appropriate behaviour. Values below the range were defined as being 'at risk of deficiency' for appropriate behaviour. The data in Table 53.4 show textbook norms for five indices of possible iron deficiency: haemoglobin, haematocrit, mean corpuscular volume (MCV), mean corpuscular haemoglobin (MCH) and mean corpuscular haemoglobin concentration

Malnutrition and antisocial behaviour in a New York correctional institution for adults			
Number of official serious incidents	Number of nutrients below 70% of the US RDA*		Total
	0–4	5–9	
0	45 (41%)	3 (10%)	48
1–15	64 (39%)	27 (90%)	91
Total	109	30	139

$\chi^2 = 10.18441$; df = 1; P < 0.001.
*US RDA = United States recommended daily allowances.

Table 53.1 Malnutrition and antisocial behaviour in a New York correctional institution for adults.

Blood nutrient ranges on 34 adult offenders with no history of institutional rule violations					
Nutritional indices	Sample	Method	Unit	'Textbook' deficiency	Ranges found
Vitamins					
Vitamin A	S	Functional	IU/dl	65	80–199
Vitamin E	S	Functional	mg/dl	0.50	0.56–1.40
Thiamin	W	Micro	ng/ml	25	29–50
Thiamin	S	Functional	µg/dl	5.0	4.8–7.5
Riboflavin	W	Micro	ng/ml	250	220–500
Niacin	W	Micro	µg/ml	3.5	3.8–9.0
Pantothenic acid	W	Micro	ng/ml	200	160–270
Pyridoxine	S	Micro	ng/ml	30	20–42
Pyridoxine	S	Functional	ng/ml	20	27–85
Folates	S	Functional	ng/ml	1.4	2.2–38
Minerals					
Calcium	RBC	AAS	ppm	16	18–36
Magnesium	RBC	AAS	ppm	34	36–57
Copper	RBC	AAS	ppm	0.54	0.54–0.77
Iron	RBC	AAS	ppm	670	710–1100
Zinc	RBC	AAS	ppm	6.1	7.0–14.1
Selenium	RBC	AAS	ppm	0.14	0.16–0.31
Manganese	RBC	AAS	ppm	0.015	0.012–0.034
Chromium	RBC	AAS	ppm	0.023	0.027–0.120
Iron indices					
Haemoglobin	RBC	CBC	g/dl	14	14–17
Haematocrit	RBC	CBC	%	40	39–51
MCV	RBC	CBC	µm³	80	75–96
MCH	RBC	CBC	pg	27	26–33
MCHC	RBC	CBC	%	33	32–36

S = serum, W = whole blood, RBC = red blood cell, HPLC = high-pressure liquid chromatography, AAS = atomic absorption spectrophotometry, micro = microprotozoan. For the iron indices, CBC = complete blood count; MCV = mean corpuscular volume; MCH = mean corpuscular haemoglobin; and MCHC = mean corpuscular haemoglobin concentration. Textbook deficiencies come from Simko[19] for the CBC, while vitamin and mineral deficiencies come from commercial laboratories.

Table 53.4 Blood nutrient ranges on 34 adult offenders with no history of institutional rule violations.

(MCHC). Validation of the procedure used to establish the 23 indices of 'at risk of deficiency' was subsequently tested using the five iron status indices. More specifically, the mean difference was calculated between each previously validated index of anaemia and the low end of the range found in the well-behaved offenders. It was reasoned that if the lower end of the range found among this well-behaved population was an accurate and precise measure of nutrient deficiency for the 23 assessments, then the procedure should also generate five anaemia indices very close to the textbook reference norms. If the magnitude of the differences was very small, the results would suggest that the procedure used to establish 'at risk of deficiency' was valid and that reference norms for health and behaviour were identical.

'Normal' range of iron indices

The differences in magnitude between each iron index and the lower end of the range were negligible. 0 or 1 unit for four indices and 6% for the fifth. Each difference was within the split-sample coefficient of variation. This means that there is no evidence that the five empirically derived reference norms for iron differ at all from the five textbook norms. Accordingly, the reference norms for behaviour on the remaining 18 indices are likely to be valid as well.

These analyses suggest that the procedure for establishing deficiency was valid and that the norms for good health coincide with those for good behaviour, at least on iron. This procedure also created more confidence in the unpublished commercial laboratory norms for other vitamins and minerals, because their definitions of deficiency were close to the low end of the range for most nutrients. Obviously, further testing is warranted; however, there is now an empirical basis for the definitions of 'at risk of deficiency' in blood (Table 53.4).

Vitamin and mineral intake

From the dietary intake data, it was possible to determine which vitamin and mineral intakes were significantly different between the worst and best behaved. Furthermore, it was possible to measure how much of each nutrient per day would be needed to raise the intake of the worst-behaved offenders up to the mean of the well-behaved intakes. For example, the worst offenders tended to consume about 3000 international units (IU) of vitamin A each day, while the best-behaved offenders averaged about 8000 IU, a difference of about 5000 IU. Rather than create a supplement formula based on theoretical assumptions of how much of each vitamin and mineral is needed, it was possible to empirically construct a formula based on these differences for 13 vitamins and 9 minerals. The formula ended up being a very close approximation to 100% of the US RDAs. This formula was subsequently used in research.

These findings led to a pilot study in which confined California and Oklahoma juvenile delinquents were given a daily vitamin–mineral tablet to determine: (1) if a significant reduction in rule violations would follow and (2) if the improvements would be immediate (within 2 days) or be gradual. If successful, a randomized placebo-controlled trial would be warranted. The results are shown in Table 53.5 and Fig. 53.10. Figure 53.10 demonstrates that behaviour did improve significantly in both sites. Rule violations fell an average 40% when measured for a 6-week period and a 12-week period beginning after 3 days of intervention. Of interest is how quickly the violations fell in this study compared with the Tidewater Virginia study (see Fig. 53.2) and The Alabama Youth Authority study (see Fig. 53.9). In both of the previous studies diet was used as the intervention, while in these studies a vitamin–mineral supplement was used. It is probable that the concentrated vitamins and minerals in the supplements were able to raise nutrient levels quicker then diet alone.

Adverse reactions to supplements

However, a potential adverse reaction was uncovered, which is shown in Table 53.5. On the left side of the table, 22 juveniles ceased to be behavioural problems after intervention. In the middle, there are slight improvements or deteriorations in behaviour among 14 juveniles that may be attributed to chance. But, on the right side are two juveniles in both institutions who showed marked deterioration. It was hypothesized that since the tablet contained synthetic food colours and flavours, that these four juveniles may have suffered from a food intolerance[5] to these tablets. Accordingly, we only used hypoallergenic placebos and supplements in the subsequent randomized controlled trials and found no additional cases of marked deterioration in 464 juvenile or adult delinquents examined.

THE OKLAHOMA RANDOMIZED TRIAL

A further placebo-controlled double-blind study

A further randomized, double-blind trial was performed in an Oklahoma juvenile correctional facility. All 71 delinquents, aged 13–17 years old, who resided in the facility, volunteered to

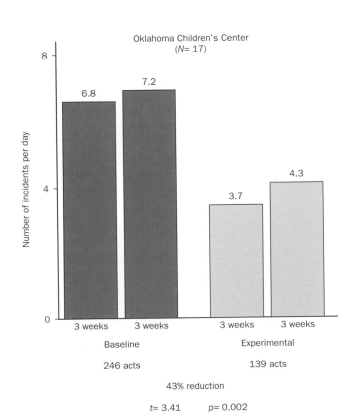

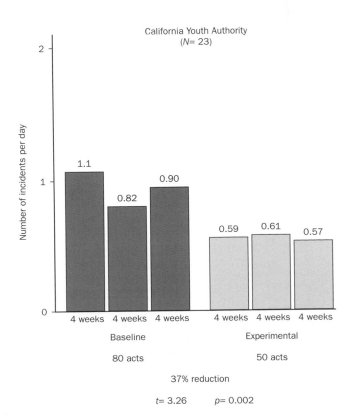

Fig. 53.10 Official disciplinary reports in two state juvenile correctional facilities that started to use vitamin–mineral supplements.

Rule violations per juvenile before and during supplementation in two correctional facilities

A Oklahoma Children's Center rule violations per person before and during supplementation (N = 17).

Eliminated		Some decrease		Some increase		Large increase	
(Case)	Pre – Post	(Case)	Pre – Post	(Case)	Pre – Post	(Case)	Pre – Post
(1)	27 – 0	(1)	7 – 2	(1)	10 – 11	(1)	13 – 27
(2)	24 – 0	(2)	9 – 3	(2)	15 – 19	(2)	4 – 12
(3)	11 – 0	(3)	25 – 10				
(4)	10 – 0	(4)	6 – 3				
(5)	8 – 0	(5)	26 – 15				
(6)	5 – 0	(6)	20 – 15				
		(7)	26 – 22				

43% reduction, $t = 3.41$, $P = 0.002$

B California Youth Authority rule violations per person before and during supplementation (N = 23).

Eliminated		Some decrease		Some increase		Large Increase	
(Case)	Pre – Post	(Case)	Pre – Post	(Case)	Pre – Post	(Case)	Pre – Post
(1)	7 – 0	(1)	4 – 1	(1)	5 – 6	(1)	7 – 12
(2)	7 – 0	(2)	6 – 5	(2)	4 – 6	(2)	7 – 18
(3)	6 – 0			(3)	0 – 2		
(4)	4 – 0						
(5)	3 – 0						
(6)	3 – 0						
(7)	2 – 0						
(8)	2 – 0						
(9)	2 – 0						
(10)	2 – 0						
(11)	2 – 0						
(12)	2 – 0						
(13)	2 – 0						
(14)	1 – 0						
(15)	1 – 0						
(16)	1 – 0						

37% reduction, $t = 3.26$, $P = 0.002$

participate and were rank-ordered on institutional violence rates based on a 3-month pre-intervention period. After exclusion of subjects who had not been institutionalized a minimum of 4 weeks (to ensure reliable violence rates), adjacent subjects on the violence rate scale were placed in pairs and randomly assigned to either the intervention or control group.[16]

The design included medical history, physical examinations for clinical signs and symptoms of malnutrition, blood and hair assays for nutritional status, a 7-day diet analysis and counselling by research staff on what types of dietary measures may be taken to correct any clinical signs and symptoms. At the end of the study, blood and hair were assayed again, and the 7-day dietary analysis was repeated. The post-intervention assays and diet analysis allowed the research team to determine which delinquents, if any, successfully changed their diets and which eliminated micronutrient deficiencies.

Sixty-two of the 71 delinquents were given either vitamin–mineral supplements or placebos for 13 weeks with minor attrition due to parole. During the experimental period, there were significantly less violent and non-violent rule infractions among the 32 juveniles who received supplements than the 30 who received placebos, as shown in Tables 53.6 and 53.7.

Only six offenders who received placebos showed significant improvements. There were no improvements or deterioration in the remaining 24 placebo subjects. Blood assays confirmed that all juveniles who produced the significant improvements in violence, regardless of group assignment, consistently had low concentrations of vitamins in their blood before supplementation began, and had corrected these deficiencies by the end of the study. Table 53.8 shows the change in violence among the six placebo responders and the ten best active responders as well as the specific pre- and post-nutritional deficiencies. Violence among these 16 fell from 110 to 11 acts during the intervention period, with 6 of these 11 violent acts occurring during the first week of intervention! It is also noteworthy that all of the six children in the placebo group that showed significant decreases in violent behaviour changed their diets after the initial counselling; thereby, their pre-intervention vitamin deficiencies were eliminated by the time of the post-test. None of the other children given placebos changed their diet. As expected, none of them had eliminated their vitamin deficiencies by the post-test, and no significant changes were seen in their rates of violent behaviour.

Speed of response to diet and supplements

A modest difference was observed in how long it took for improvement in antisocial behaviour to show in the children on placebo who had changed to a better diet *versus* those on the active supplement tablet. Antisocial behaviour had fallen as far as it would within the first week among those who received the supplement tablet. In contrast, the antisocial behaviour improved more slowly among the six children who had changed their diets. This was similar to the rate of change seen in the earlier interrupted time-series design dietary intervention studies. A number of possible explanations exist. Perhaps the children who changed their diets did so gradually during the study. Perhaps the dose levels in the tablets was greater than the average increase in nutrients these children who changed their diets received, so their malnutrition was corrected more slowly. However, a slight difference remains between how quickly proper diet or tablets reduce violence, with supplementation producing the quicker change. This remains a fertile area for future research.

Mean rule violation rates per subject for three measures of crime by group and condition*							
Type of serious rule infraction	Baseline		Experimental		Change		Net difference
	Active	Placebo	Active	Placebo	Active	Placebo	
Violent rule infractions	0.389	0.372	0.078	0.163	0.311	0.209	0.10
Non-violent rule infractions	3.05	2.57	0.515	1.03	2.54	1.27	1.27
Total rule infractions	3.44	2.94	0.587	1.31	2.85	1.63	1.22

*Means reflect the number of infractions divided by number of weeks confined for each resident. ANCOVA statistics and *P*-values are presented for these data in Table 53.7.

Table 53.6 Mean rule violation rates per subject for three measures of crime by group and condition.

Summary of analysis of variance and covariance for three indices of crime within a correctional setting using $\log_{10}$ transformations						
Indices	Differences in initial rates (between treatment groups)		Pre- post-period difference		Treatment period interaction	
	F	P	F	P	F	P
Violent rule infractions	0.0013	0.9710	0.986	0.325	4.236	0.044
Non-violent rule infractions	0.1608	0.6898	9.456	0.003	7.646	0.008
Total rule infractions	0.1537	0.6965	8.894	0.004	8.517	0.005

Table 53.7 Summary of analysis of variance and covariance for three indices of crime within a correctional setting using $\log_{10}$ transformations.

No.	Group	Changed diet	Violence		Vitamin C		Vitamin B₁		Niacin		Vitamin B₅		Vitamin B₆		Folates	
			Pre	Post	Pre	Post	Pre	Post	Pre	Post	Pre	Post	Pre	Post	Pre	Post
1	Placebo	Yes	23	1	–	–	–	–	–	–	–	–	25	–	–	–
2	Placebo	Yes	18	1	–	–	24	–	–	–	–	–	–	–	3.3	–
3	Placebo	Yes	9	0	–	–	–	–	–	–	128	–	–	–	3.4	–
4	Placebo	Yes	6	0	–	–	22	–	–	–	–	–	20	26	3.2	–
5	Placebo	Yes	8	2	0.50	–	–	–	–	–	–	–	14	–	3.3	–
6	Placebo	Yes	10	2	–	–	22	–	–	–	–	–	23	–	–	
7	Active	Yes	18	1	–	–	–	–	–	–	–	–	27	–	–	–
8	Active	Yes	9	0	–	–	24	–	–	–	–	–	–	–	–	–
9	Active	Yes	6	0	–	–	19	–	–	–	–	–	–	–	–	
10	Active	Yes	5	0	–	–	–	–	–	–	122	–	27	–	–	
11	Active	Yes	6	2	0.34	–	–	–	–	–	–	–	25	27	–	–
12	Active	Yes	3	0	–	–	–	–	2.8	–	–	–	25	–		
13	Active	No	4	2	–	–	–	–	2.8	–	–	–	25	–	3.0	
14	Active	No	2	0	–	–	25	–	–	–	–	–	–	–	3.4	
15	Active	No	2	0	–	–	–	–	–	–	–	–	28	–	–	
16	Active	No	2	0	–	–	–	–	–	–	–	–	18	–	–	
Totals			**131**	**11**	2	0	6	0	2	0	2	0	11	2	7	0
Below the range of 34 non-violent juveniles					<0.55 mg/dl		<26 ng/ml		<3.0 µg/m		<142 ng/m		<29 ng/ml		<3.6 ng/ml	

[–] = normal.

Table 53.8 Low pre- and post-test blood vitamin concentrations in 16 habitually violent offenders whose violence fell from 131 to 11 acts in 3 months.

Significance of blood vitamin deficiencies

Equally important, no child in the supplement group showed a significant reduction in violence post-test, unless they had pre-intervention blood vitamin deficiencies. The lack of change among offenders without low blood vitamin status confirms the multicausal nature of violence, with nutritional biochemistry being one of the primary causes, but not the only cause. These data suggest, rather convincingly, that the correction of low blood nutrient concentrations may be associated with a reduction in violent acts.

From the beginning with dietary replacement studies, the research had now shown an underlying biochemical change in nutrient status from dietary replacement that could very plausibly explain the change seen in behaviour. What was now necessary was to demonstrate how nutrient status could affect brain function.

BRAIN FUNCTION AND NUTRITIONAL STATUS

A study of 335 violent offenders compared those who were chronically violent, to those who only had one violent episode.[22] It showed that 57% of chronically violent subjects had an abnormal EEG, compared with only 11% in those with only one violent episode, which is the same as that seen in the general population. The authors concluded that the cause of habitual violence may be rooted in abnormal brain functioning. We reasoned that, if the mediating mechanism between violence and nutritional biochemistry is abnormal brain function, this should be readily testable within the Oklahoma placebo-controlled trial. Institutional staff were used to identify the 10 juvenile offenders whose violence was the most chronic, and whose violence could not be understood as a rational response to environmental situations. A review of medical files, to look for a history of head trauma or known neurological abnormalities was used to eliminate 4 of the 10. The remaining 6 underwent brain electrical activity mapping (BEAM) before and after the trial. Four of those received active tablets and 2 received placebos. All 6 had low pre-intervention blood vitamin concentrations and an abnormal EEG at baseline. Table 53.9 shows that the 2 offenders who received placebos did not show a significant change in brain abnormalities, as measured by BEAM, while all 4 of the offenders who received active tablets did.[14] More specifically, the 2 placebo subjects had a total of 8 abnormalities at baseline and 8 at the post-test, while the 4 subjects on active tablets had 14 at baseline and just 2 at the post-test. The differences were statistically significant ($\chi^2 = 9.125$, df = 1, $P < 0.01$).

Pre- and post-EEG abnormalities in standard deviation (SD) units for subjects given, supplements or placebos							
		Pre-intervention			**Post-intervention**		
		Eyes			**Eyes**		
Group and case	**Brain wave type**	**Open**	**Shut**	**Abnormal region**	**Open**	**Shut**	**Abnormal region**
Placebo	delta	normal	normal		normal	normal	
	theta	normal	normal		normal	normal	
Case 1	alpha	normal	normal		normal	normal	
	beta1	normal	normal		normal	normal	
	beta2	+4.71	+2.53	posterior	+3.12	+4.82	posterior
	beta3	normal	normal		normal	normal	
Placebo	delta	normal	normal		normal	normal	
	theta	normal	normal		normal	normal	
Case 2	alpha	normal	normal		normal	normal	
	beta1	−2.63	−2.30	occipital	−2.61	−2.69	occipital
	beta2	−2.12	−2.56	posterior	−2.86	−2.06	posterior
	beta3	−2.10	−2.05	occipital	−2.20	−2.21	occipital
Active	delta	normal	normal		normal	normal	
	theta	normal	normal		normal	normal	
Case 1	alpha	normal	normal		normal	normal	
	beta1	normal	normal		normal	normal	
	beta2	normal	−2.14	posterior	normal	normal	
	beta3	normal	normal		normal	normal	
Active	delta	normal	normal		normal	normal	
	theta	normal	normal		normal	normal	
Case 2	alpha	normal	normal		normal	normal	
	beta1	normal	normal		normal	normal	
	beta2	+3.21	normal	temporal	normal	normal	
	beta3	normal	normal		normal	normal	
Active	delta	+4.28	+2.52	posterior	normal	normal	
	theta	+3.79	normal	occipital	normal	normal	
Case 3	alpha	+4.32	normal	vertex	normal	normal	
	beta1	+2.15	normal	posterior	normal	normal	
	beta2	+3.23	normal	parietal	normal	normal	
	beta3	normal	normal		normal	normal	
Active	delta	+4.28	+2.52	posterior	normal	normal	
	theta	+3.79	normal	occipital	normal	normal	
Case 4	alpha	+4.32	normal	vertex	normal	normal	
	beta1	+2.05	−2.00	posterior	normal	normal	
	beta2	+2.27	−2.34	posterior	normal	−2.06	posterior
	beta3	−2.17	−2.20	temporal	normal	−2.53	posterior

Table 53.9 Pre- and post-EEG abnormalities in standard deviation (SD) units for subjects given supplements or placebos

Closer examination was done on the BEAM data for all subjects. For the 2 subjects on placebos who showed no change in the number of EEG abnormalities, the abnormalities were maintained in the same regions, the same direction (higher or lower amplitude) and under the same conditions (eyes open or closed). This shows that not only was there no change in the number of abnormalities, but that no change occurred in the brain functioning of the placebo subjects.

Conversely, the 4 experimental subjects showed improvements in multiple brain regions (posterior, occipital, parietal, temporal and vertex); in normalizing abnormalities in both directions (higher and lower amplitude); and under conditions where the eyes were closed or open. This suggests changes in multiple causal factors in brain functioning. For example, if the aetiology was as simple as improving metabolism alone, one would not expect supplementation to normalize the height of a brain wave whose amplitude was too high before treatment. These data confirm that in this small study the correction of low blood vitamin concentrations through supplementation can normalize anomalous brain functioning due to multiple abnormalities. This transition from nutrient status to brain functioning, which determines cognition, is a very small, but very important empirical step.

THE CALIFORNIA RANDOMIZED TRIAL

The Oklahoma study was replicated on 402 young adult, incarcerated, male felons who made up over 90% of the population of two California institutions.[17] The men were assigned to one of three groups and given either placebo or one of two strengths of supplements. The weaker supplement formula was based on 100% of the US RDA for 13 vitamins and 7 minerals (iron, copper, zinc, manganese, chromium, selenium and molybdenum). The stronger formula contained more ascorbic acid, thiamin, riboflavin, niacin, pantothenic acid, pyridoxine and cobalamin set at 300% of the US RDA. Both active tablets also contained about 20% of the US RDA of calcium and magnesium due to size limitations of using only two tablets. The main difference between the California and the Oklahoma studies was the absence of a 7-day dietary assessment and physical examination/nutritional education in California. Additionally, the experimental period lasted 15 weeks in the California trial instead of 13 weeks.

Another important difference was the decision by the California Legislature's Research Oversight Committee to attempt to eliminate any accidental researcher bias by having all crime data sent directly to the University of California, Berkeley, where it was analysed under blind conditions by a separate biostatistician. The concern was that the criminal justice department at California State University, Stanislaus, had done nearly all of the previous research on nutrition and crime. Thus, the biostatistician, the Stanislaus research staff and the institutional staff were blind as to treatment condition. An analysis of covariance on serious rule violations adjusted and weighted for days at risk was significant ($P = 0.025$). The biostatistician's main findings are shown in Table 53.10. It shows that behaviour in these institutions deteriorated in the placebo group and improved in both experimental groups, with the differences being significant between placebo and the 100% formula. The most provocative finding is the fact that the group who received the lower dose formula produced a larger decline in violence than the group who received the stronger formula, a finding that begs for further investigation. However, most important of all, the study serves as an independent replication on a slighter older group of felons that is very representative of adult criminals.

THE ARIZONA RANDOMIZED TRIAL

The previous randomized trials showed that institutional offenders, aged 13–17 years old, or 18–25 years old, produced about 40% less violence and other antisocial behaviour when given vitamin–mineral tablets compared with placebo controls. However, generalization could not be made to children aged less than 12 years old or to schoolchildren without criminal histories without a controlled trial of that population. The objective of this trial was to determine if schoolchildren, aged 6–12 years old, who were given low-dose vitamin–mineral tablets would produce significantly less violence and antisocial behaviour in school than classmates who were given placebos. This is especially important because of the potential benefit that could be derived from correcting behaviour in children. It has been demonstrated that children who commit such antisocial behaviour at a very young age in school have a greater chance of becoming incarcerated in the future.[23] To answer this question, a randomized controlled trial was completed in two elementary schools among 468 children aged 6–12 years old.[18] Randomization was done within each teacher's classes to eliminate any possible confound that the results might be due to teachers being the source of most rule violation reports. Daily vitamin–mineral supplementation lasted for 4 months at 100% of the adult US RDA. The primary dependent variable of interest became rule violations that resulted in formal disciplinary proceedings. The most typical types of offences, rank-ordered, were disorderly conduct, fighting, being defiant, endangering others, being disrespectful, uttering obscenities, verbal threats, theft, destruction of property, threatening, refusal to work, truancy and possession of a weapon. Between September and May, 80 of these schoolchildren were disciplined for the above offences and became the final study sample.

Results of nutritional supplementation

During intervention, the 40 children who received active tablets were disciplined, on average, a total of 1.00 times each, a 47% lower mean rate of antisocial behaviour than the 1.875 times total each for the 40 children who received placebos ($P = 0.038$). None of the examined potential covariates – school attended, teacher's class, grade, age, sex or student's IQ – were significant and thus did not modify the final statistical model. Table 53.11 shows the initial amount of each measured antisocial behaviour and the magnitude of change.

Mean rule violation rates by group and condition unadjusted and unweighted for days at risk						
Serious rule violations	**Baseline period**		**Experimental period**		**Change**	**Difference from placebo**
	$\bar{X}$	**SD**	$\bar{X}$	**SD**		
All groups ($n = 402$)	0.868	(1.57)	0.746	(1.25)	−12%	
Placebo ($n = 139$)	0.734	(0.98)	0.878	(1.34)	+20%	
100% US RDA ($n = 129$)	0.907	(1.36)	0.535	(0.88)	−41%	−61%
300% US RDA ($n = 134$)	0.970	(2.14)	0.813	(1.43)	−16%	−36%
*US RDA = United States recommended daily allowance.						

Table 53.10 Mean rule violation rates by group and condition unadjusted and unweighted for days at risk.

Table 53.12 clarifies what happened to produce such dramatic reductions in violent and non-violent antisocial behaviour among these 80 schoolchildren. The table shows that all differences in behaviour between the groups can be explained by chronic behavioural problems in 9 students who were disciplined from three to ten times during the intervention period. For example, one child was disciplined 10 times, one child 8 times, one child 6 times, two children 4 times and four children 3 times during the 4-month intervention period. In marked contrast, only one child who received active tablets was even disciplined 3 times. The rest appreciated the seriousness of their actions after going through the disciplinary procedures once or twice. This clearly shows that the school system had in place an effective disciplinary system with effective sanctions for bad behaviour and rewards for appropriate behaviour that worked fine with well-nourished children. However, the disciplinary procedures failed badly with the poorly nourished who, presumably, did not cognitively appreciate the seriousness of their actions and continued to disrupt the school. The study also suggests that the proportion of schoolchildren, aged 6–12 years old, who may be so malnourished as to not appreciate sanctions or rewards is only 9 of 234, or about 4%. However, this estimate may be low, since this assumes that the tablets were adequate for correcting all malnutrition regardless of intensity, a dubious assumption.

Number of rule violations per child during intervention by group		
Number of incidents per child	Placebo	Active
0	7 (18%)	10 (25%)
1	17 (43%)	21 (53%)
2	7 (18%)	8 (20%)
3	4 (10%)	1 (2.5%)
4	2 (5%)	0 (0%)
6	1 (2.5%)	0 (0%)
8	1 (2.5%)	0 (0%)
10	1 (2.5%)	0 (0%)

Note: Only 1 of 40 children receiving active tablets committed 3 or more offences while 9 of 40 children receiving placebo tablets committed 3 or more offences.

Table 53.12 Number of rule violations per child during intervention by group.

Mean difference in types of serious rule violations during intervention			
	Placebo (n = 40)	Active (n = 40)	Per cent fewer violations
Vandalism	0.100	0.000	–100%
Refusal to work/serve	0.125	0.000	–100%
Uttering obscenities	0.175	0.050	–71%
Disrespectful	0.125	0.075	–40%
Disorderly conduct	0.450	0.225	–50%
Assault/battery	0.400	0.350	–13%
Defiance	0.300	0.225	–25%
Endangerment	0.225	0.175	–22%
Other	0.475	0.275	–42%
Mean violations per person	2.375	1.375	–42%

Note: In May, the month after the trial ended, an additional 20 incidents in the placebo group and 15 incidents in the active group were committed and included in this table. They were not included in the analysis of covariance in Table 53.2, because they were beyond the intervention period. Their inclusion here raises the number of incidents to 95 and 55 in the placebo and active groups, respectively.

Table 53.11 Mean difference in types of serious rule violations during intervention.

A secondary hypothesis in the Arizona study concerned what effects, if any, would the supplementation produce on hyperkinesis using the Conner's Parent–Teacher Rating Scale. The 29 teachers were asked to fill out this scale on 4 consecutive weeks during the fall and 4 weeks during the spring for the children that they considered the most hyperactive in their class. Pre-intervention and intervention mean scores were then calculated. For children who reached a mean score of 15, Conner's minimum threshold for hyperactivity, analysis of covariance was performed. The children who swallowed active tablets produced lower hyperactivity scores than the children who swallowed placebos; however, the difference failed to reach statistical significance ($P = 0.08$). This was most probably due to a low statistical power, because of the small number of children participating in the hyperactivity portion of the trial. The data also showed a remarkable improvement in eight children on placebos. In each of these cases, another hyperactive child in the same class had markedly improved while taking active tablets. This suggests a social basis for hyperkinetic behaviour, in addition to a biological one. Replication is clearly warranted in this area.

There can be little doubt that a relationship exists between diet, crime and delinquency, but much more research is needed on the mechanism, which nutrients are causal, how low is too low on each nutrient (in intake and laboratory analysis) and how much is needed for correction. Still, we do know that government recommendations for a diet[20] containing 2–4 servings a day of fruit, 3–5 servings of vegetables and 6–11 servings of whole grain food nicely corrects much aberrant behaviour and is good for health as well.

REFERENCES

1   Anonymous. *Prison Rule Violators*. US Department of Justice, Office of Justice Programs, Bureau of Justice Statistics, Special Report, December 1989.

2   Conners CK. Rating scales for use in drug studies with children. *Psychopharmacol Bull* 1973; 9: 24–8.

3   Cook TD, Campbell DT. *Quasi-Experimentation: Design and Analysis Issues for Field Settings*. Houghton Mifflin, Boston, 1979.

4   Doraz WE. Diet and delinquency: the grounding of four leading theories in human physiology and sociology. In: *Nutrition and Brain Function* (Essman W, ed). Karger Press, Basel, Switzerland, 1987.

5   Egger J, Carter CM, Graham PJ *et al*. A controlled trial of oligoantigenic diet in the treatment of the hyperkinetic syndrome. *Lancet* 1985; 1: 940–5.

6   Hagen FE. *Research Methods in Criminal Justice and Criminology*. Allyn and Bacon, London, 1997.

7   Muedeking GD, Doraz WE, Schoenthaler SJ. Can hair trace mineral analysis predict violent behavior? An empirical test of the Walsh hypothesis. A paper presented at The Western Society of Criminology, 1 March 1986.

8   Schoenthaler SJ. Diet and crime: an empirical examination of the value of nutrition in the control and treatment of incarcerated juvenile offenders. *Inter J Biosocial Res* 1983; 4(1): 25–39.

9   Schoenthaler SJ, Doraz WE. Types of offenses which can be reduced in an institutional setting using nutritional intervention. A preliminary empirical evaluation. *Inter J Biosocial Res* 1983; 4(1): 25–39.

10 Schoenthaler SJ. Diet and delinquency: a multi-state replication. *Inter J Biosocial Res* 1983; 5(2): 70–8.

11 Schoenthaler SJ. Nutritional policies and institutional antisocial behavior. *Nutrition Today* 1985; 20(3): 16–25.

12 Schoenthaler SJ. Diet and delinquency: empirical testing of seven theories. *Inter J Biosocial Res* 1986; 7(2): 108–31.

13 Schoenthaler SJ. Malnutrition and maladaptive behavior. In: *Nutrition and Brain Function* (Essman W, ed). Karger Press, Basel, Switzerland, 1987.

14 Schoenthaler SJ, Amos SP, Doraz WE, Kelly M, Wakefield, J. Controlled trial of vitamin mineral supplementation on intelligence and brain function. *Personality and Individual Differences* 1991; 12(4): 343–50.

15 Schoenthaler SJ, Moody J, Pankow L. Applied nutrition and behavior. *J Appl Nutrition* 1991; 43: 31–9.

16 Schoenthaler SJ, Amos SP, Doraz WE, Kelly M, Wakefield J. The effect of nutritional counseling and vitamin-mineral supplementation on violent and non-violent antisocial behavior among incarcerated juveniles. *J Nutr Environ Med* 1997; 7(4): 343–52.

17 Schoenthaler SJ, Amos SP, Hudes M. A randomized trial of the effect of vitamin-mineral supplementation on serious institutional rule violations. (submitted for publication, 2000).

18 Schoenthaler SJ, Bier I. The effect of vitamin-mineral supplementation on juvenile delinquency among American schoolchildren: a randomized, double-blind placebo-controlled trial. *J Alter Compl Med* 2000; 6(1): 7–17.

19 Simko M, Cowell C, Gilbride J. *Nutrition Assessment*. Aspen, Publications, Rockville, Maryland, 1984.

20 Sizer F, Whitney E. *Nutrition Concepts and Controversies*. West Publishing, London, 1997.

21 Stolzenberg S, D'Alessio, Stewart J. 'Three strikes and your out': the impact of California's new mandatory sentencing law on serious crime rates. *Crime and Delinquency* 1997; 43(4): 457–69.

22 Williams D. Neural factors related to habitual aggression – consideration of differences between habitual aggression and others who have committed crimes of violence. *Brain* 1969; 92: 503–20.

23 Wolfgang M, Figlio R, Sellin T. *Delinquency in a Birth Cohort*. University of Chicago Press, Chicago, 1972.

INTRODUCTION

Historically and understandably, the whole subject of nutrition and dietary manipulation in the field of rheumatoid disease has been highly controversial. Many of the early reports of benefit from dietary changes were anecdotal and many of the early trials were poorly designed with results of doubtful credibility.

Diseases such as rheumatoid arthritis (RA) have fluctuating disease activity, which makes it all too easy to misinterpret improving fluctuations during dietary treatment as genuine improvements resulting from the changes in the diet. Moreover, since rheumatological diseases are frequently painful, there is a high potential placebo-response rate that may be increased by any form of treatment which involves frequent visits to a sympathetic physician, particularly if a complex, unusual form of treatment, such as dietary manipulation is involved. In such cases, placebo-response rates may reach over 40% – which makes well-designed and controlled research studies essential if results are to be believed.

Until the 1980s such well-designed studies were rare, and a highly unsatisfactory situation occurred – which has persisted to some degree even until the present day – in that patients, suffering from painful, chronic diseases of unknown cause and without a cure, have in desperation sought help from outside the conventional treatment offered to them. They have turned to practitioners of alternative medicine who have given advice which has ranged in value from useful to frankly ridiculous.

The result of this situation has been, and largely still remains, a stalemate, in which patients politely refrain from telling their doctors what alternative medical manoeuvres they are using while their doctors assume that any improvements in disease activity result only from the medication they have given to their patients and ignore any effects which may have resulted from dietary manipulation. Many doctors are also unaware that rates of compliance with conventional drug regimens for different illnesses tend to converge to only approximately 50%.[123]

Such a situation is obviously unacceptable: since much of the damage done to joints in diseases such as rheumatoid arthritis occurs in the first months or years of the disease,[147] effective drug treatment must not be delayed by ineffective dietary manipulation. Furthermore, patients need to be protected from the cost of expensive alternative treatment unless this is of proven benefit.

Unless orthodox researchers investigate unusual forms of therapy, our patients will have no scientific evidence on which to base their choice of treatment.

The role of nutrition in diseases such as arthritis has been understood more fully by the development of nutritional biochemistry, immunology and pharmacology, and the ever-increasing scientific data on free-radical disease, antioxidants, prostaglandins, flavonoids, etc., have lifted the subject of nutrition out of the realm of anecdotal uncertainty into the province of credible science.

Definitions

The study of nutrition in arthritis may be divided into two areas: *elimination therapy*, in which foods are removed from the diet, and *supplementation therapy*, in which substances are added to the diet.

Supplementation therapy

The best-studied supplements are fish oils, evening primrose oil (EPO), New Zealand green lipped mussel, vitamins and selenium. Garlic, honey, with or without cider vinegar, herbs, kelp, royal jelly and ginseng are also popular among patients but have little scientific evidence to support their use in arthritic disease.

In the context of this book, this chapter will only consider conditions in which foods and their constituent parts are believed to play a part in the development of arthritis and rheumatological disease, either by their presence or by their absence.

DIETARY ELIMINATION THERAPY

Fasting

Fasting can be considered to be an extreme form of elimination dieting.

Fasting, for short periods, although undoubtedly helpful to some patients with RA[60,84,133] is not to be recommended regularly since it may lead to malnutrition. However, used briefly and occasionally, it may give some predictable benefit.

Fasting, either as water only or with fruit and vegetable juices to supply up to 500 calories per day, may exert its beneficial effects by reducing inflammation, altering pain perception and immune function and may reduce gut permeability. It should only be undertaken with an ample fluid intake and never for more than an absolute maximum of 7 days.

Fasting is usually ineffective in osteoarthritis and should be avoided in patients with a tendency towards gout, since it causes a rise in lactic acid levels in the blood and this may provoke acute gouty arthritis.

Rheumatoid arthritis

A proportion of patients with rheumatoid arthritis improve and may remain well for long periods of time by removing certain foods from their diet. This response to diet is not universal in RA but occurs in a significant minority of patients (35–40% of RA patients on dietary therapy in our Rheumatology Unit).

The elimination diet programme is in three phases: first, an *elimination phase* in which the patient has only a small number of foods, albeit consumed liberally, and all other foods are excluded. The second phase, usually after 7 days, is the *reintroduction* of foods, one at a time, to determine which foods cause symptoms. The third phase, essential for scientific creditability,

is of *double-blind testing* to confirm that foods identified as culpable in the reintroduction phase are really culpable and not just subject to a placebo response or to other factors.

In 1980, Hicklin *et al.*[68] reported clinical improvement in 24 out of 72 RA patients on exclusion dieting and, in 1981, Parke & Hughes[111] described a patient with RA who responded well to restriction of dairy products by objective, clinical improvement (grip strength, Ritchie index, visual analogue pain score), by a fall in erythrocyte sedimentation rate (ESR) and by disappearance of circulating immune complexes, with reversal of these improvements on rechallenging with dairy produce. Williams[145] in 1981 described another patient with RA who showed clinical improvement and a significant fall in ESR on withdrawal of corn, and rapid deterioration on its blind reintroduction.

In 1983, however, Denman *et al.*[36] found no link between food and RA in 18 patients. This study, however, failed to eliminate wheat and other foods commonly incriminated in the production of symptoms and also used a diet programme from which 13 out of 18 patients defaulted early.

In 1983, Panush *et al.*[109] used a commercially popular diet (the Dong diet) in a 10-week, controlled, double-blind randomized trial in 26 RA patients. They obtained a good response in only a small percentage of patients but that subgroup responded excellently, suggesting that individualized dietary manipulation may be beneficial for certain RA patients as a subgroup response.

In 1986, we published results of a placebo-controlled study of 6 weeks of dietary manipulation therapy in 53 RA patients.[31] Significantly greater benefit occurred with diet than with placebo, with significant improvement in pain by day, by night and in 24 hours, duration of morning stiffness, number of painful joints, grip strength, time to walk 20 yards (18 m), ESR, haemoglobin, fibrinogen, platelet and C3 levels (Tables 54.1–54.4). Twenty-five per cent of patients in both treatment and control groups did not respond to dietary treatment, 40% showed some improvement, but about 35% responded well and were considered to be a subgroup of good responders.

Significant changes in diet group after first week, on elimination diet			
Parameter	**Baseline**	**Week 1**	**P**
Per cent with severe pain			
By day	44	4	<0.01
By night	40	4	<0.01
Pain in 24 hours	5.3 ± 2.5	2.9 ± 2.0	<0.001
Duration of morning stiffness (min)	60	10	<0.01
No. of painful joints	20.0 ± 9.4	15.6 ± 9.7	<0.005
Grip strength (mmHg)			
Right	142 ± 83	174 ± 84	<0.01
Left	142 ± 83	168 ± 84	<0.005
Fibrinogen (mg/dl)	371 ± 88	421 ± 119	<0.05

Table 54.1 Significant changes in diet group after first week, on elimination diet. (From Darlington et al., © The Lancet 1986; (i): 236–8.[31])

Significant changes in diet group after 6 weeks of dietary therapy

Parameter	Baseline	Week 6	P
Per cent with severe pain			
By day	44	14	<0.05
By night	40	0	<0.01
Pain in 24 hours	5.3 ± 2.5	1.9 ± 1.7	<0.001
No. of painful joints	20.0 ± 9.4	13.6 ± 10	<0.02
ESR (mm/h)	33.5 ± 18.6	28.1 ± 15.8	<0.02
Platelets (× 10⁹/l)	377 ± 104	341 ± 108	<0.05
C3 (IU/ml)	151 ± 34	130 ± 24	<0.001

C3 is a component of the complement pathway; ESR = erythrocyte sedimentation rate.

Table 54.2 Significant changes in diet group after 6 weeks of dietary therapy. (From Darlington et al., © The Lancet 1986; (i): 236–8.[31])

Significant changes in control group, in crossover stage of trial, after first week on elimination diet

	Baseline	Week 1	P
Per cent with severe pain			
By day	27	5	<0.01
By night	14	9	<0.02
Pain in 24 hours	4.1 ± 2.5	3.0 ± 2.6	<0.01
Duration of morning stiffness (min)	45	10	<0.01
No. of painful joints	25.1 ± 13.1	20.3 ± 12.3	<0.005
Time to walk 20 yards (18 m) (s)	14.3 ± 3.4	13.2 ± 2.7	<0.02
Haemoglobin (g/dl)	11.7 ± 3.0	13.1 ± 1.0	<0.001

Table 54.3 Significant changes in control group, in crossover stage of trial, after first week on elimination diet. (From Darlington et al., 1986 © The Lancet 1986; (i): 236–8.[31])

Significant changes in control group, in crossover stage of trial, after 6 weeks of dietary therapy

	Baseline	Week 1	P
Pain in 24 hours	4.1 ± 2.5	2.2 ± 2.0	<0.02
No. of painful joints	25.1 ± 13.1	18.4 ± 12.3	<0.005
Platelets (×10⁹/l)	389 ± 102	337 ± 112	<0.05
C3 (IU/ml)	149 ± 38	116 ± 17	<0.02

C3 is a component of the complement pathway.

Table 54.4 Significant changes in control group, in crossover stage of trial, after 6 weeks of dietary therapy. (From Darlington et al., 1986 © The Lancet 1986; (i): 236–8.31)

Energy deprivation is believed to affect immune response[48] and it was thought possible, therefore, that improvement on dietary treatment could be related to weight loss. In 1987, therefore, we investigated the mean weight loss of 4.78 kg occurring in 41 RA patients who underwent dietary therapy for 6 weeks.[29] Correlation coefficients were calculated between weight reduction and variables that improved significantly during the diet, but no significant correlations were found, suggesting that weight loss did not play a causal role in the improvement of RA patients during dietary elimination therapy.

In 1987 also, we investigated 59 patients with RA for evidence of a type 1 (immediate hypersensitivity) reaction which would suggest 'food allergy'.[29] A history of atopy was given by 45.8% of patients but 83% had normal total immunoglobulin E (IgE) levels (i.e. <300 IU/ml), with median total IgE levels before and after dietary therapy of 62.5 IU/ml and 62.0 IU/ml, respectively. Mean absolute eosinophil counts were normal (i.e. <440/mm³) before and after dietary therapy and there were no significant correlations to suggest a type 1, immediate hypersensitivity, reaction being involved in RA patients on dietary treatment.

In 1987, Wojtulewski described a group of 41 RA patients on a 4-week elimination diet. The 23 patients who improved were challenged with four different food groups, with positive reactions to challenge in 10 patients. Disodium cromoglycate did not protect.[146]

In 1987, we sought to identify foods to which patients with RA were most often intolerant.[28] Forty-eight RA patients underwent 6 weeks of dietary elimination therapy. Forty-one patients identified foods producing symptoms. Cereal foods were particularly troublesome, with corn and wheat each giving symptoms in more than 50% of symptomatic patients and, indeed, cereal foods comprised four of the top seven symptom-inducing foods (Table 54.5).

Foods most likely to cause intolerance in patients with rheumatoid arthritis

Food	Symptomatic patients affected by food (%)	Food	Symptomatic patients affected by food (%)
Corn	57	Malt	27
Wheat	54	Cheese	24
Bacon/pork	39	Grapefruit	24
Oranges	39	Tomato	22
Milk	37	Peanuts	20
Oats	37	Sugar (cane)	20
Rye	34	Butter	17
Eggs	32	Lamb	17
Beef	32	Lemons	17
Coffee	32	Soya	17

Table 54.5 Foods most likely to cause intolerance in patients with rheumatoid arthritis. (From Darlington & Ramsey © Br J Rheumatol 1993; 32: 507–14.[30])

It has been suggested that the offending element in wheat may be gluten, composed of glutenins and gliadins. O'Farrelly et al.[106] tested 93 RA patients for humoral sensitization to gliadin and compared their small intestinal biopsies with those from controls. Of 93 RA patients, 44 had raised levels of IgG to gliadin and, of these, 38 (86%) were also positive for IgA rheumatoid factor (RF). Patients with raised antibody levels had lower villous surface/volume ratio and lower intestinal lactose concentrations on jejunal biopsy than patients without antibodies or age-matched controls. The authors concluded that the gut may play a more important part in the immunopathogenesis of some cases of RA than of others, and that the former may be identified by raised levels of IgA RF and wheat protein IgG.

Blind challenge studies are needed to confirm symptoms obtained during unblind food challenge. In 1986, Panush et al.[110] described prospective, placebo-controlled blind challenges with milk in an RA patient, with exacerbation of arthritis on milk challenge (shown by deterioration in duration of morning stiffness and in numbers of tender and swollen joints).

Beri et al. (1988) in India, published an uncontrolled study with 71% of good responses[6] and, in 1989, we completed a prospective, blind, challenge study during which 15 RA patients undertook an exclusion diet followed by reintroduction of foods, after which three symptomatic foods were selected for each patient with which that patient was challenged. Results suggested that, although RA patients improved significantly on dietary manipulation, 3 weeks of food challenge rapidly produced deterioration.[32]

In 1990 Panush[108] reported food sensitivities, confirmed by double-blind challenges in three patients with palindromic arthritic symptoms sensitive to milk, shrimps and nitrate, respectively.

In 1991, Kjeldsen-Kragh et al.[78] reported good responses to dietary elimination therapy. Their patients were treated for 1 month on a health farm, where for 7–10 days they took only herbal teas and vegetable juices. This was followed by reintroduction of foods: any foods that provoked symptoms were excluded for 7 days, re-tested and, if they still caused symptoms, they were excluded permanently. Milk, eggs, gluten and citrus fruits continued to be avoided for $3\frac{1}{2}$ months, at which stage they were tested individually and reintroduced if they did not produce symptoms. Patients thus treated with diet improved significantly when compared with a placebo group. There was a subset of 'responders' (44% of the total), and 30.6% of the diet group were described as having a 'high improvement index'[112] – a percentage very similar to our 35% of 'good responders'.[31] Benefit was maintained for 1 year and most of Kjeldsen-Kragh's good responders showed improvement in laboratory as well as clinical variables.[80]

Certain Swedish trials reported similar fasts, followed either by a normal diet,[132] by a vegan diet[116,131] or by a lacto-vegetarian diet[137] with some benefit. Gamlin & Brostoff, in 1997, suggested that an elimination process may be required to give sustained benefit and that a vegetarian or vegan diet alone is insufficient.[52]

One study which reported a much smaller proportion of patients with symptoms provoked by food is that by Panush, in 1990, who estimated that only 5% of patients with RA were sensitive to food.[108] Gamlin & Brostoff[52] suggest that this may be an underestimate: they doubt whether patients can be sure that they have food sensitivities or can determine culpable foods without going through an elimination diet. They also query whether the food challenges undertaken by Panush contained sufficient quantities of food in the capsules given to the patients, since *food-intolerant* patients (in contrast to *food-allergic* patients) are believed to need a reasonable quantity of the food concerned to provoke a response.

In 1992, van de Laar & van der Korst described a double-blind, controlled trial of clinical effects of elimination of milk allergens and azo dyes in 94 RA patients[140] Only subjective improvements were seen on treating patients with two types of artificial, elementary food, but a subgroup of patients showed favourable responses, followed by marked disease exacerbation during rechallenge, and the authors felt that food intolerance may influence the activity of seropositive RA, at least in some patients. The same authors in a further paper,[141] also described six patients with seropositive RA who showed a marked improvement after 4 weeks of a hypoallergic, artificial diet, with placebo-controlled rechallenges showing intolerance for specific foodstuffs in four patients. Improving changes in biopsy material from synovial membrane and proximal small intestine in three RA patients treated with the hypoallergenic diet showed changes 'suggesting an underlying immuno-allergological mechanism'.

In 1995, Kavanagh et al. found a significant improvement in grip strength ($P = 0.008$) and Ritchie score ($P = 0.006$) in patients on an *elemental* diet when compared with a control group, i.e. an effective, albeit unpopular and unsustainable, alternative to an elimination diet.[77]

Our own experience (Darlington & Ramsey, unpublished work, 1998) has been that a subgroup of patients remain well – off all medication and controlled by diet alone – for follow-up periods of up to 12 years. Other patients relapsed, either spontaneously or on failing to comply with the diet.

As we described in 1993[30] there are certain practical problems associated with elimination diets:

- they are not universally effective
- they may cause nutritional difficulties
- they may cause social disruption
- they require considerable commitment from the patient
- they may be taken to extremes by patients if not correctly supervised.

Thus, they should only be undertaken under medical supervision.

Mechanisms affecting response to dietary manipulation
Improvement of patients on dietary therapy may be the result of a number of different mechanisms, acting singly or in combination.

Placebo response
It is important that the placebo response to dietary treatment should be investigated. In our experience, the placebo effect detected was insufficient to explain the significant improvement on treatment.[31] Furthermore, if benefit were due only to placebo, one would expect the benefit to fade after a few months on diet – which is not the case, as confirmed by the study by Kjeldsen-Kragh et al.,[78] which showed persistent benefit for a follow up of 1 year.

Suppression of a type 1 reaction
Sensitivities to foods in patients with RA are not acute, allergic (type 1) reactions. We have not shown abnormal IgE levels in patients with RA undergoing dietary therapy[29] and neither did Little et al.,[87] nor did they show positive skins tests to food extracts.

Weight loss

Since energy deprivation is believed to affect the immune response,[48] it is possible that weight loss during a diet could cause improvement; but many RA patients lose weight, without benefit during periods of disease activity. Furthermore, in studies of weight loss during dietary therapy, no correlation was shown between weight loss and variables that improved significantly.[29,78]

Reduced gastrointestinal permeability and bacterial antigens

In 1968, Olhagen & Mansson[107] reported that two-thirds of patients with RA have an abnormally abundant faecal flora of atypical *Clostridium perfringens*, and an increase in C. *perfringens* α-antitoxin titre. Controls do not. In 1978, Bennett[5] suggested that gut bacteria have a role in the development of RA.

Animal work

Pigs on a diet rich in fish developed abnormal gut flora, with increased numbers of atypical C. *perfringens* type A, and this was followed by arthritis, believed to result from an immunological reaction to the altered intestinal flora.[96]

When rabbits were fed cow's milk daily, they developed infiltrative synovial lesions, believed to result from stimulation by antigens absorbed from the gut.[24]

RA patients untreated by nonsteroidal anti-inflammatory drugs (NSAIDs) have normal gastrointestinal permeability, but patients on NSAIDs[7,99] and perhaps also on disease-modifying antirheumatic drugs (DMARDs)[3] show increased permeability. Such increased permeability may allow food or bacterial antigens to be absorbed in greater quantities than usual, overwhelming normal gut defences and, possibly, producing symptoms of RA. Dietary manipulation could, in theory, reduce gastrointestinal permeability, with reduced absorption of food and/or bacterial antigens.

In 1985, Ebringer et al.[38] proposed that both ankylosing spondylitis and RA are forms of reactive arthritis, to *Klebsiella* spp. and *Proteus* spp. respectively, probably mediated by cross-reactivity to human leucocyte antigens (HLA).

In 1988 Ebringer et al.[39] reported raised levels of antibodies against *Proteus mirabilis* – a bacterium found in the gut and urinary tract in patients with RA – and, in 1992 suggested a mechanism involving molecular mimicry between *Proteus* antigen and part of the HLA-DR1/DR4 molecule, which is associated with an increased risk of RA.[40]

The molecular mimicry hypothesis is not considered to have been proven, however, and a range of hypotheses have been suggested for association of HLA B27 with spondyloarthropathies.[104] Nonetheless, in 1995, Kjeldsen-Kragh et al.[81] investigated antibodies against P. *mirabilis* and against *Escherichia coli* in patients treated with diet. Patients on the vegetarian diet had a significant reduction in mean anti-*Proteus* titres compared with baseline values ($P < 0.05$). No significant change in titre was observed in patients taking an omnivorous diet. Good responders showed greater antibody reduction than non-responders or omnivores. Antibodies against E. *coli* were almost unchanged in all patient groups during the trial.

In view of the various types of bacteria suggested as playing a role in the pathogenesis of RA[38,95,96] it remains theoretically possible that different bacteria could be relevant to different subgroups of RA.

Seignalet proposed that RA is due in part to food, or bacterial peptide crossing the gut wall and proceeding towards the joints.[128]

In 1991 Hunter et al.[71] suggested that a disturbance of normal gut flora may occur, perhaps originating from a severe bout of diarrhoea or prolonged antibiotic therapy, which results in beneficial bacteria becoming less abundant and being replaced by more damaging organisms. The gut wall may become irritated by toxins released by the bacteria and become more permeable to undigested food molecules, which could pass through it and promote either an immunological reaction or, perhaps, act as exorphins. Alternatively, the more damaging bacteria may feed on particular foods and then produce toxins that produce symptoms. If abnormal bacterial toxins were produced, enzyme defects might also be relevant, and the lack of certain detoxification enzymes could exacerbate the effects of the disturbed gut flora.

Mechanisms for effects of dietary therapy on gut flora are at present hypothetical. The mechanism may be simple, with dietary manipulation removing from the diet certain nutrients needed by the relevant bacteria and reducing their pathogenicity. Alternatively, dietary toxins, e.g. lectins, may affect bacteria or the gut itself directly. Furthermore, when patients underwent dietary therapy with an individually adjusted vegetarian diet, their faecal bacterial fatty acids have been shown by Peltonen in 1994 to alter in ways which differed according to whether they responded well or not.[112]

In 1997, Peltonen et al.[113] investigated faecal microbial flora and disease activity in RA during a vegan diet and concluded that a vegan diet changes the faecal microbial flora and that these changes are associated with improvement in disease activity.

In 1998, Nenonen et al.[102] investigated effects of an uncooked vegan diet, rich in lactobacilli, in patients with RA and found that subjective symptoms of RA were reduced. They concluded that large amounts of living lactobacilli consumed daily may have positive effects on objective measures of RA.

Conclusion

There are still too few data definitely to confirm or refute the suggestion that dietary manipulation may have a beneficial effect on disease activity by affecting gut flora, but the hypothesis is interesting and further investigation is required.

Secretory IgA (SIgA) deficiency

Evidence exists that people with food intolerance may have less secretory IgA (SIgA) than healthy people,[13] but this is not thought to be sufficient alone to cause food intolerance, since many severely SIgA-deficient patients have no greater evidence of food intolerance than the general population.

Direct immunological response

There may be a direct immunological response to food. Most patients with food-sensitive RA do not have raised IgE levels,[29] although Parke & Hughes' milk - and cheese-sensitive patient was an exception.[111] IgG antibodies to relevant foods were described by Panush in two patients with food intolerance[108] and by Ratner in 1984[117] in a patient with juvenile RA, but the significance of such antibodies in many patients is arguable, since food antibodies may be present without being of pathogenic significance, and further work will be necessary to clarify their role. We investigated patients with RA who were undergoing a programme of elimination dieting followed by reintroduction of foods and we could not detect any pattern of elevated immunoglobulin or food antibody results (Darlington & Panush, unpublished work, 1989).

Application of elimination dieting to a range of arthritic diseases	
Disease	**Result**
Rheumatoid arthritis	Subgroup achieve benefit
Palindromic arthritis	Frequently helpful
Osteoarthritis	Any benefit is probably by weight reduction
Gout	Drugs are usually required to lower uric acid significantly but a low purine diet may assist
Enteropathic arthritis	Crohn's disease: dietary change may help but medical supervision essential Coeliac disease: gluten-free diets help bowel and joint symptoms Ulcerative colitis: no benefit from diet
Psoriatic arthritis	Variable responses reported
SLE (systemic lupus erythematosus)	Avoid alfalfa products which contain 6-canavanine, because these increase disease activity
Ankylosing spondylitis	Insufficient data to comment
Behçet's syndrome	Insufficient data to comment

Table 54.6 Application of elimination dieting to a range of arthritic diseases. (From *Diet and Arthritis* by LG Darlington & L Gamlin 1996, Vermilion Press, London.)[27]

In 1995, Kjeldsen-Kragh in a comprehensive review of his patients found only one food-sensitive patient with raised levels of antibody to the food which provoked symptoms.[79]

Other immunological changes which have been described include immediate and delayed reactivity of skin and mononuclear cells to the food in question[110] and impaired clearance of heat-damaged red cells, which may suggest an abnormally functioning reticuloendothelial system.[110] Little *et al.*, in 1983,[87] described release of 5-hydroxytryptamine, 5HT (serotonin), from platelets in response to food challenges. Kjeldsen-Kragh *et al.*, in 1995,[80] found that platelet counts and levels of calprotectin fell, as patients improved on dietary treatment, and were lower in responsive than in unresponsive patients.

Immune complexes are not raised in food-sensitive patients,[108] nor do they fall when patients respond to dietary therapy.[80]

Conclusion

Whatever the mechanism(s) of action, and although dietary elimination therapy only helps a proportion of patients, for those who do respond it can be a safe and useful way to control symptoms in a range of rheumatological diseases (Table 54.6).

LITERATURE ON NUTRITION AND ARTHRITIS

In an attempt to see what patients were reading about nutrition and arthritis, we investigated 21 books offering dietary advice for arthritic patients.[33] These books were unselected but readily available from book shops and health food shops. Seventeen books were strongly in favour of dietary therapy, three stated that diet was of no value in the control of arthritic symptoms and one was non-committal.

Dietary advice varied from book to book and was sometimes completely contradictory; it is hardly surprising, therefore, that patients are confused. However, patients will continue to read the literature available to them in such books and they need to be protected from conflicting and often inappropriate advice from such sources.

EPIDEMIOLOGICAL DATA ON NUTRITION AND ARTHRITIS

Rheumatoid arthritis has been described as being more prevalent in developed rather than in developing countries.[129] This could be explained on the basis of genetic factors, but the need for some environmental factor, such as diet, to trigger the genetic predisposition is enforced by the finding from 1995 by McDaniel *et al.*[93] that African-Americans with RA do not have the usually accepted genetic markers for RA.

EPIDEMIOLOGICAL DATA ON NUTRITIONAL MACRONUTRIENTS AND RHEUMATOID ARTHRITIS

Meat

Meat has been studied by several researchers as a possible dietary component contributing to the development of RA. In 1969, Epstein[43] considered that sodium nitrate in meat was associated with palindromic rheumatic symptoms. In 1986, Sköldstam reported improvement in 12 out of 20 Swedish patients with RA given a vegan diet for 3–4 months[131] and, in 1991, Kjeldsen-Kragh *et al.*[78] described a statistically significant improvement in RA symptoms in 34 patients on a vegetarian diet for 1 year, although some of the beneficial effect of this dietary manipulation could have resulted from the elimination diet and avoidance of other foods which caused symptoms.

In addition to the fact that meats are rich in purines and break down to form uric acid, which is associated with gout, Hergenrather *et al.* in 1981[67] stated that meats contain pesticides, hormones and other additives (the significance of which for arthritis is poorly understood): they also have a high saturated fat content, which may encourage inflammation.

In 1997, W.B. Grant (pers comm) used a multi-country approach to study the link between diet and rheumatoid arthritic. Data for female prevalence of RA from 15 countries prior to 1988 were compared statistically with macronutrients of national dietary supply for up to 4 years prior to the prevalence data. Meat fat had the highest statistical association, with the prevalence of RA $r^2 = 0.666$, $P = <0.001$. Time-series data of RA effects from six European countries from 1965 to 1977 were felt to confirm the meat fat finding. Grant hypothesized that meat fat changes the flora of the intestines, increases intestinal permeability and produces an inflammatory response. He also suggested that meat contains hormones and pesticides that may interfere with the body's immune system and lead to RA.

In view of these data from humans and the arthritogenic effects of a protein-rich diet in pigs,[5] the possible role of meat in the pathogenesis of arthritis requires further work to clarify the situation.

Dietary fat

The quantitative and qualitative effects of fat in the diet have been explored in some detail. In 1990, Jacobsson *et al.*[73] reported that patients with RA have low concentrations of the essential fatty acids linoleic acid and linolenic acid in the blood and high concentrations of total saturated fatty acids in both blood and adipose tissue.

The possible benefits from reducing saturated fat in the diet of patients with RA need further investigation, but such lower-fat diets have at least the appeal of potential cardiovascular protection.

Dietary fibre

It is possible that a tendency towards RA may be exacerbated by the highly processed, relatively low fruit and vegetable diet common to Western, established market economies. In 1995, Fine *et al.*[49] described how an increased intestinal flow rate leads to smaller pore size in the gut and, presumably, to a slower rate of absorption from the gut. This would agree with the description of high fruit and vegetable diets improving symptoms of RA,[78] since high fibre diets lead to higher flow rates through the gut.

Fish

The roles of fish and fish oil are considered later in this chapter.

Weight loss, i.e. elimination of calories

Historically, the most frequent advice given to patients with osteoarthritis (OA) has been that there is no evidence that dietary intervention will help in OA, but there are mechanisms which suggest that nutritional factors may influence its natural history.

It is known that obesity increases the risk of development of OA of the knees and possibly also of both hips and hands.[46] Since obese people do not necessarily carry increased load across their hands, the exact mechanism for the association between obesity and osteoarthritis remains unconfirmed, but data from the Framingham OA Study suggest that weight loss of approximately 5 kg will reduce the risk of developing OA of the knees during the subsequent 10 years by 50%.[47]

Lectins

Lectins are molecules of non-immune origin that bind to specific carbohydrate receptors with high affinity (in the same range as the affinities of antibodies and sometimes higher).[50]

Much food is full of lectins and, although lectins may be inactivated by cooking for a long time and at fairly high temperatures, this cannot safely be assumed. Raw and relatively unprocessed foods are now encouraged for health reasons, and health conscious people are now probably exposed to greater doses of dietary lectins than at any time for many decades.

Since some ingested lectins are profoundly damaging to the intestinal wall, it is not surprising that a systemic immune response to them is seen,[115] and the possible role of lectins in the pathogenesis of food intolerance in RA deserves careful attention.

Coeliac disease

One disease of the gastrointestinal tract that is associated with arthritis and responsive to elimination of a *specific* food is coeliac disease.

Coeliac disease is a condition in which there is an abnormal jejunal mucosa; it improves morphologically when the patient is treated with a gluten-free diet and relapses when gluten is reintroduced.

Gluten is a high-molecular-weight, heterogeneous compound that can be fractionated to produce α-, β-, and ω-gliadin peptides. α-Gliadin can injure the mucosa of the small intestine. The exact mechanism of how damage is produced is also uncertain, but there may be an immunogenetic mechanism, a lectin may be involved or a virus may play a role, in view of the amino acid sequence homology between gliadin and adenovirus 12.[53]

Toxic amines

A chronic, disabling osteoarthritic disease (Kashin–Beck disease) has been described in Eastern Siberia, and the cause found to be cereal grain contaminated with the fungus *Fusarium sporotrichiella*. The denatured grain proteins in the bread produce toxic amines that cause vasoconstriction, believed to interfere with joint nutrition.[103]

Nutrition and pH

The body is normally kept at a pH of approximately 7.4 by an effective buffering process. Contrary to the belief of patients, fruit and vegetables form *alkali* in the body, while cheese, meat, alcohol and cereal products produce *acid*.[11,118]

Roebuck (pers comm, 1998) described changes in urinary and salivary pH, correlating with each other and brought about by the long-term use of a diet low in acid-forming foods. Roebuck reported a reduction in rheumatological symptoms as pH rose in two patients over a prolonged period of time. Symptoms relapsed and pH fell when acid-forming foods were eaten.

Such data are of interest but need to be confirmed in a larger group of patients and with a control population. Such a study is under way in our Rheumatology Unit.

Gouty arthritis

Hyperuricaemia is exacerbated by a purine-rich diet and may provoke associated gouty arthritis. A reduction in dietary purines makes only a small impact on the uric acid level in the blood, and drugs will usually be required to avoid gouty arthritis in hyperuricaemic subjects.

Patients who are unable or unwilling to tolerate drug treatment can lower uric acid to some degree by avoiding foods rich in purines; these are listed in Table 54.7.

Foods rich in purines	
High purine levels	**Moderately high purine levels**
Liver, kidney and offal	Pulses
Meat extracts	Soya and gram flour
Pâté	
Sausages	
Fish roe, sardines, mackerel, herring	
Crab, shrimps	
Alcoholic drinks, especially beer	
Yeast extract and tablets	

Table 54.7 Foods rich in purines.

E

Candida species

Candida albicans is a yeast that is present normally in the human gut, and which feeds on simple carbohydrates such as glucose.[142]

It has been suggested that a low-sugar, low-alcohol diet may benefit patients with arthritis by an effect on *Candida* spp.

Candidiasis of the gut, mouth, vagina and skin is acknowledged but it is still debatable whether *Candida* can cause rheumatological symptoms, as suggested by Chaitow in 1985.[17]

SUPPLEMENTATION THERAPY

Hypothesis

It is possible that diets poor in certain nutrients may predispose to arthritic disease and that supplementation with the nutrients which are in poor supply could, therefore, reduce arthritic activity.

OXIDATIVE STRESS AND ANTIOXIDANTS

Reactive oxygen species (ROS), i.e. highly reactive atoms and molecules with unpaired electrons, are formed continuously in tissues by endogenous and exogenous mechanisms.[51] ROS can damage many macromolecules, including cell membranes, lipoproteins, proteins and deoxyribonucleic acid (DNA).[2]

There is evidence that intra-articular cells such as chondrocytes produce ROS[66] and that oxidative damage is important in arthritic processes.[65] Superoxide anions can affect adversely the structure and integrity of collagen *in vitro* and may cause depolymerization of hyaluronate in synovial fluid.[55,92]

Diseases such as rheumatoid arthritis, systemic lupus erythematosus (SLE) and psoriatic arthritis involve chronic inflammation of joint tissues, with oxidant-associated deterioration of joint structure.[20,35,130,136]

Intra-articular injection of agents which generate hydrogen peroxide (H_2O_2) causes severe joint damage in experimental animals[125] and there is much *in vitro* evidence suggesting that ROS can damage, or interfere with, joint components including hyaluronic acid,[57,92] glycoproteins,[25] collagens[34] and tissue and fluid proteinase inhibitors such as α-antiproteinase.[143]

There is also a considerable body of evidence that oxidative stress occurs within the inflamed joint *in vivo*[8,18,56,57,89,122] and that joints are probably damaged by ROS. Inflamed joints are infiltrated by activated neutrophils and rheumatoid pannus contains many macrophage-like cells. Both of these cell groups produce $O_2^{\cdot-}$ and H_2O_2[105,121] and perhaps also NO.[45] Neutrophils can also make HOCl. $O_2^{\cdot-}$ and H_2O_2 become converted into the highly reactive hydroxyl radical $OH^{\cdot}$ in the presence of free iron ions, and synovial fluid from RA patients often contains measurable quantities of iron[58] capable of catalysing oxidative damage *in vivo*.[59]

The question arises, therefore, whether diets poor in antioxidants may predispose to arthritic disease.

ANTIOXIDANTS

Many raw food materials contain natural antioxidants which affect oxidative processes in living cells. These include *enzymes* such as superoxide dismutase, glutathione peroxidase and glucose oxidase and catalase, which are usually inactivated during food processing, *non-enzyme antioxidants* such as carotenoids, especially astaxanthin (e.g. in fish), *tocopherols* (in oils) and other *phenolic compounds in plants*. Non-enzymic antioxidants such as β-carotene

and vitamins A and E can remain active after heating and, possibly, after food consumption. Vitamin C acts as a reducing substance which acts synergistically with other antioxidants and, indeed, two or more antioxidants can act synergistically together.

In the human body, antioxidant enzymes, such as superoxide dismutase, catalases and peroxidases, provide the major part of the intracellular defence while, in the extracellular space where there are few antioxidant enzymes, small-molecule antioxidants play an important defensive role.[12] These small-molecular antioxidants include α-tocopherol (vitamin E), β-carotene (a vitamin A precursor), other carotenoids and ascorbate (vitamin C), and their plasma concentrations are largely determined by dietary intake.

Micronutrient antioxidants may protect against tissue injury when intracellular enzymes are overwhelmed and, thus, protect against ROS-mediated damage which accumulates with age and causes chronic diseases.[61,74,120]

More work is required on tissue distributions and bioavailability of antioxidant molecules within joints, since lipophilic antioxidant molecules such as vitamin E or β-carotene may not have the same access to tissues as hydrophilic antioxidants such as vitamin C. It may be that different effects in disease processes may depend on lipophilia or hydrophilia of the antioxidant molecules concerned in different tissue areas.

Tocopherols and ascorbic acid

Tocopherols, of which α-tocopherol (vitamin E) is the most effective, protect cell membranes and other lipids by scavenging free radicals, such as lipid peroxyl radicals, much more quickly than these radicals can react with adjacent fatty acid side chains or with membrane proteins. Vitamin E is consumed but may be regenerated by reduced glutathione (GSH) and by ascorbic acid (vitamin C). Since ascorbic acid is a water-soluble vitamin which cannot enter the hydrophobic interior of membranes, this mechanism presupposes that the tocopherol radical can move close to the membrane surface for reduction by ascorbic acid outside the membrane.

Certain cells contain enzymes that can reduce dehydroascorbate back to ascorbate using either nicotinamide adenine dinucleotide (NADH) or GSH. Any dehydroascorbate that does not enter cells for regeneration may break down; hence, ascorbate tends to be lost irretrievably at sites of oxidative damage.

α-Tocopherol (vitamin E)

Benefit from vitamin E treatment has been suggested from rheumatological studies in humans.[37]

Vitamin E blocks arachidonic acid formation from phospholipids and inhibits lipoxygenase activity, although it has little effect on lipoxygenase. It is possible, therefore, that vitamin E has a mild anti-inflammatory effect, which could be beneficial in synovial inflammation.

Osteoarthritis and nutrition/antioxidants

Osteoarthritis can be regarded as a prototypical, age-related, degenerative disease and there is evidence that cells within joints produce ROS, and that oxidative damage is important.[65]

It is of interest that intra-articular *superoxide dismutase* (orgotein), a superoxide radical inhibitor, has been used for a long time to treat equine osteoarthropathy and has also been used, with benefit, in placebo-controlled clinical trials to treat human OA.[88,94]

Several small studies of OA in humans have suggested benefit from vitamin E treatment, such as the 6-week, randomized double-blind, placebo-controlled trial of 400 mg, α-tocopherol (vitamin E) in 50 patients with OA, among whom those treated with vitamin E experienced greater improvement in every efficacy measure.[9]

Ascorbic acid (vitamin C)

When McAlindon et al.[91] investigated, in 1996, the association of reported dietary intake of antioxidant micronutrients among participants followed up longitudinally in the Framingham Knee OA Cohort Study their data did not support the hypothesis that diets rich in antioxidant micronutrients reduced the risk of incident knee OA but they did suggest that antioxidants might protect people with established disease from disease progression.

Combined supplementation with vitamins C and E is more immunopotentiating than supplementation with either vitamin alone.[76]

Vitamins C and E also have non-antioxidant effects. Vitamin C has biochemical effects which may be of importance in OA. Vitamin C deficiency is associated with defective connective tissue, and ascorbate stimulates procollagen secretion.[114] Vitamin C is needed via the vitamin C-dependent enzyme lysyl hydroxylase for the post-translational hydroxylation of specific prolyl and lysyl residues in procollagen – actions necessary for the stabilization of the mature collagen fibril.[134] Vitamin C is also thought to be necessary for glycosaminoglycan synthesis.[127] Furthermore, Schwartz & Adamy[127] found a decreased level of arylsulphatase A and B in the presence of ascorbic acid and also that sulphated proteoglycan biosythesis, a presumed measure of repair, was increased significantly in chondrocyte cultures in the presence of ascorbic acid.

Selenium

Abnormalities in the metabolism of the essential trace element selenium (Se) have been described in patients with RA – selenium concentrations are relatively low in the serum of patients with RA when compared with healthy controls.[1] Selenium is an essential part of the enzyme glutathione peroxidase (SeGSHpx), at the active centre of which selenium catalyses reduction of hydroperoxides produced from oxidized species.[23]

In 1987, Tarp et al.[139] described long-term supplementation of RA patients and controls with selenium. Even after 26 weeks of treatment, patients with RA had granulocyte SeGSHpx activities still significantly lower than those of controls. The low granulocyte SeGSHpx activities of patients with RA, regardless of nutritional selenium status, may result in maintenance of inflammation from intracellular accumulation of reactive oxygen radicals. The unresponsiveness of granulocyte SeGSHpx to selenium treatment may explain the predominantly negative effects after treatment with selenium in RA.[138]

Data are conflicting: some clinical improvement has been reported for patients with RA treated by selenium[101] but other evidence suggests that any role of SeGSHpx in RA must be indirect since D-penicillamine is a specific inhibitor of SeGSHpx.[19]

Vitamin A

In 1988, Faimey et al.[44] reported a difference in vitamin A metabolism or intake between patients with RA and controls: serum retinol levels were lower in RA than in matched control sera ($P<0.01$) and in OA patients ($P<0.001$). Serum retinol-binding protein (RBP) values were lower in RA than in matched control sera ($P<0.001$), but in OA they were not different from normal ($P<0.3$). The mean serum osteocalcin was higher than normal in both RA and OA ($P<0.001$ and <0.005, respectively).

β-Carotene

If the diet of healthy volunteers is supplemented with a dietary achievable level of β-carotene, significant increases have been reported in the percentage of monocytes expressing the major histocompatibility complex (MHC) Class II molecule, HLADR, and the intercellular adhesion molecule 1 (ICAM1) and leukocyte function-associated antigen 3.[70] It is possible that β-carotene also quenches singlet oxygen, which may reduce the free radical burden and protect membrane lipids from peroxidation in arthritis and other diseases associated with oxidative stress.

It has been suggested that the French diet, rich in antioxidants in the form of fruit, vegetables and red wine, could be the reason for the 'French paradox', i.e. the fact that cardiovascular disease in France is a lesser problem than would be expected from the fat content of the average French diet.[119] The antioxidant-rich diet of the French could also be protective.

A study in Finland[64] in 1994 measured antioxidant levels in the blood of over 1400 people and then reviewed their health after 20 years. During that period 14 people developed rheumatoid arthritis. Elevated risks of RA were observed at low levels of α-tocopherol, β-carotene and selenium. A significant association was observed with a low antioxidant index (P for trend − 0.03, the relative risk of RA between the lowest tertile and the higher tertiles of its distribution being 8.3, 95% confidence interval 1.0–71.0). This was particularly interesting work since it measured antioxidant levels before the onset of disease and, hence, may well have measured a contributory factor in the pathogenesis of RA rather than simply measuring the effects of the disease, i.e. exhausted antioxidant supplies.

Systemic lupus erythematosus and antioxidants

In 1997, Mohan & Das[100] suggested that measurement of lipid peroxides, nitric oxide and antioxidants can be used as markers to predict progress in patients with SLE.

Conclusion

Much more work is required to clarify the role of antioxidants in arthritic disease and their possible therapeutic potential.

DIETS POOR IN BENEFICIAL POLYUNSATURATED FATTY ACIDS (PUFAs)

Fish oil in arthritis

The suggestion that a diet rich in fish oil may protect against arthritis has a long history. Conversely, a diet poor in fish and fish oil may fail to offer this protection.

For many years both patients and normal, healthy people have taken oils in an attempt to improve their health. In a recent review of our own patients with RA, as yet unpublished, two-thirds had tried fish oil and one-third had tried evening primrose oil (EPO).

There is a huge market for such oils, which have a traditional reputation for being good for health and protective against arthritis, but long-term safety has been assumed, which is unwise, and efficacy is uncertain in the small doses taken by many people.

E

The anti-inflammatory properties of fish oil and its therapeutic role in RA have been reviewed in 1991 by Cleland[21] and in 1993 by Darlington.[26] It is accepted that ingestion of long-chain n-3 fatty acids such as eicosapentaenoic acid (EPA) and docosahexaenoic acids (DHA) from fish oil is likely to have an anti-inflammatory effect, whereas saturated fatty acids tend to exacerbate inflammation.

Enthusiasm for fish oils is widespread among arthritic patients but doctors have been cautious.[41]

In 1959, Brusch & Johnson,[14] reported that arthritic patients on cod liver oil showed biochemical and clinical improvement, and, in 1987, Sperling et al.,[135] in an open study, showed a significant decrease in joint pain index and in patients' assessment of disease activity after 6 weeks of dietary supplementation with concentrated fish oil (20 g MAXEPA/day).

In 1985, Kremer et al.[82] in an open study, gave 10 g MAXEPA/day for 12 weeks to patients with RA, in combination with other dietary modifications, and reported modest improvement in morning stiffness and in the number of painful joints – improvements which deteriorated during follow up after cessation of treatment.

Kremer in 1987 then completed a well-controlled, crossover study[83] using 15 g MAXEPA/day *versus* 15 g olive oil and reported significantly fewer tender joints and improvement in time to onset of fatigue after 14 weeks of fish oil compared with olive oil treatment.

In 1988, Belch et al.[4] investigated the effect of EPO, alone and in combination with fish oil, on the requirements for NSAIDs in 49 patients with RA and claimed that EPO, both alone and when combined with fish oil, produced significant subjective improvement and allowed more than 70% of patients to reduce, or even to terminate NSAID therapy, although no significant objective changes in clinical or laboratory measurements were demonstrated.

Possible risks associated with long-term fish oil therapy

The concept that fish oil therapy, while of uncertain therapeutic benefit in the doses taken by most people, is at least completely safe is now less certainly correct.

In 1991, Meydani et al.[97] in a 3-month fish oil supplementation study (1.68 g EPA/day and 720 mg DHA/day) in 25 women found significant reductions in plasma triglycerides and a fall in plasma α-tocopherol, with an increase in lipid peroxide. Sanders & Hinds[124] found that the blood level of α-tocopherol (vitamin E) was decreased to below the normal range during supplementation with fish oil. These results of the Meydani et al.[97] and Sanders & Hinds[124] studies indicate that the vitamin E content of fish oil supplements may not be sufficient to provide adequate antioxidant protection, and that increased fish oil may require an increment in vitamin E intake – a fact not appreciated by many doctors and certainly not known by many patients who take fish oil. Such *increased oxidative stress induced by fish oil* appears to vary between species but certainly may be seen in primates other than man.[63]

In 1993, Meydani et al.[98] described a reduced delayed-type hypersensitivity (DTH) response in a measurement of cell-mediated immunity *in vivo* for several antigens, in subjects supplemented with 1.23 g EPA and DHA/day. When fish oil supplements of 1.27 g/day EPA and DHA were given for 24 weeks, they found a fall in the percentage of peripheral blood CD4+ cells and an increase in the percentage of CD8+ cells.

Fish oil reduces cytokine production, interleukins IL1α, IL1β, IL2, IL6 and tumour necrosis factor α (TNFα),[10,16,42,97,124] from human peripheral blood mononuclear cells *ex vivo*, in addition to a reduction in proinflammatory leukotrienes.[126]

In 1995, Hughes et al.[69] found that supplementation with n-3 PUFAs depressed immune reactivity by suppressing expression of monocyte surface molecules associated with their antigen-presenting function.

Effects of fish oil administration on lymphocyte functions *in vitro*, as judged by mitogen stimulation, have consistently shown reduced responses in human and non-human primate studies.[148]

In summary, the long-term consequences of alteration of the n-3/n-6 balance in favour of the n-3 is incompletely understood in man but it is possible that it could lead to detrimental immunological and haematological effects; so, if fish oil is to be taken, the lowest possible effective dose should be used, i.e. 500–750 mg EPA/day. More studies are required to investigate the *safety* of long-term supplementation with fish oil in man.

Furthermore, studies are needed to determine whether *low-dose* fish oil, as taken by patients without prescription, is *effective*, since many of the good results so far reported have been in studies using high-dose fish oil concentrates not available without prescription and fairly expensive to prescribe.

Other oils have been used to supplement the diet to give greater protection in arthritic disease. Their use is largely outside the remit of this chapter but benefit has been demonstrated from *evening primrose oil* (EPO) in RA,[4,62,75] *olive oil* in RA,[15,22] *borage seed oil* or *starflower oil* in RA[86] *blackcurrant seed oil* in RA[144] and, more controversially, *mussel oil* in RA and OA.[54,72,85]

SUMMARY

We accept the statement by McAlindon & Felson in 1997[90] that research into the effects of nutritional factors in arthritic disease may be made more difficult by many factors, such as the potential for confounding, problems with outcome definitions, absence of indicators of disease activity, imprecision and misclassification in measurement of dietary variables and many other factors.

We also believe, however, that nutritional immunology, biochemistry and pharmacology are research areas now recognized as fields of great scientific interest, too long under-researched.

The time has arrived for nutrition in arthritis to be researched fully, to ensure a dialogue between doctors and patients and to expose quackery and ill-founded hypotheses in rheumatology and, hence, to protect our patients.

Acknowledgements

The author gratefully acknowledges untiring help from Ms L. Gamlin, and from Mr Gordon Smith, Mrs Marion Morrison and Mrs Fiona Rees from the Sally Howell Library at Epsom General Hospital, and also the unfailing support of Mrs Alison Smith and Mrs Glenda Primarolo.

REFERENCES

1 Aeseth J, Munthe E, Førre Ø, Steinnes E. Trace elements in serum and urine of patients with rheumatoid arthritis. *Scand J Rheumatol* 1978; 7: 237–40.

2 Ames BN, Shigenaga MK, Hagen TM. Oxidants, antioxidants and the degenerative diseases of aging. *Proc Natl Acad Sci USA* 1993; 90: 7915–22.

3 Behrens R, Devereaux M, Hazleman B et al. Investigation of auranofin-induced diarrhoea. *Gut* 1986; 27: 59–65.

4 Belch JJF, Ansell D, Madhok R, O'Dowd A, Sturrock RD. Effects of altering dietary essential fatty acids on requirements for non-steroidal anti-inflammatory drugs in patients with rheumatoid arthritis: a double-blind placebo-controlled study. *Ann Rheum Dis* 1988; 47: 96–104.

5 Bennett JC. The infectious etiology of rheumatoid arthritis – new considerations. *Arthritis Rheum* 1978; 21: 531–8.

6 Beri D, Malaviya AN, Shandiya R, Singh RR. Effects of dietary restrictions on disease activity in rheumatoid arthritis. *Ann Rheum Dis* 1988; 47: 69–72.

7 Bjarnason I, Williams P, So A et al. Intestinal permeability and inflammation in rheumatoid arthritis. Effects of non-steroidal anti-inflammatory drugs. *Lancet* 1984; ii: 1171–4.

8 Blake DR, Hall ND, Treby DA, Halliwell B, Gutteridge JMC. Protection against superoxide and hydrogen peroxide in synovial fluid from rheumatoid patients. *Clin Sci* 1981; 61: 483–6.

9 Blankenhorn G. Clinical effectiveness of Spondyvit (vitamin E) in activated arthroses. A multicenter placebo-controlled, double-blind study. *Z Orthop* 1986; 124: 340–3.

10 Bonner SA, Rotondo D, Davidson J. Eicosapentaenoic acid supplementation modulates the immune responsiveness of human blood. Prostaglandins. *Leukot Essen Fatty Acids* 1997; 57(2): 462–71.

11 Breslau NA, Brinkley L, Hill KD, Pak CYC. Placebo controlled, blind study of dietary manipulation therapy in rheumatoid arthritis. *J Clin Endocrin & Metabol* 1998; 66(1): 140–6.

12 Briviba K, Seis H. Nonenzymatic antioxidant defense systems. In: *Natural Antioxidants in Human Health and Disease* (Frei B, ed.). Academic Press, San Diego, CA, 1994; 107–28.

13 Brostoff J, Gamlin L. *What Causes Food Intolerance? The Complete Guide to Food Allergy and Intolerance.* Bloomsbury, London; 1989; 76–7.

14 Brusch CA, Johnson ET. A new dietary regimen for arthritis. Value of cod liver oil on a fasting stomach. *J Nat Med Assoc* 1959; 51: 266–70.

15 Brzeski M, Madhok R, Capell HA. Evening primrose oil in patients with rheumatoid arthritis and side effects of non-steroidal anti-inflammatory drugs. *Br J Rheumatol* 1991; 30: 370–2.

16 Caughey GE, Mantzioris E, Gibson RA, Cleland LG, James MJ. The effect on human tumor necrosis factor- and interleukin-1 β production of diets enriched in n-3 fatty acids from vegetable oil or fish oil. *Am J Clin Nutr* 1996; 63: 116–22.

17 Chaitow L. *Candida albicans: Could Yeast be Your Problem?* Thorsons Publishers, Wellingborough, England, 1985: 86.

18 Chapman ML, Rubin BR, Gracy RW. Increased carbonyl content of proteins in synovial patients with rheumatoid arthritis. *J Rheumatol* 1989; 16: 15–18.

19 Chaudière J, Wilhelmsen EC, Tappel AL. Mechanism of selenium-glutathione peroxidase and its inhibition by mercapto carboxylic acids and other mercapatans. *J Biol Chem* 1984; 259: 1043–50.

20 Chidwick K, Winyard PG, Zhang Z, Farrell AJ, Blake DR. Inactivation of the elastase inhibitory activity of alpha 1 antitrypsin in fresh samples of synovial fluid from patients with rheumatoid arthritis. *Ann Rheum Dis* 1991; 50: 915–16.

21 Cleland LG. Diet and arthritis. *Current Therapeutics* Sept 1991; 51–6.

22 Cleland LG, French JK, Betts WH, Murphy GA, Elliott MJ. Clinical and biochemical effects of dietary fish oil supplements in rheumatoid arthritis. *J Rheumatol (Canada)* 1988; 15: 1471–5.

23 Comb GF Jr, Comb SB. In: *The Role of Selenium in Nutrition.* Academic Press, New York; 1986: 205–63.

24 Coombs RRA, Oldham G. Early rheumatoid joint lesions in rabbits drinking cow's milk. *Int Arch Allergy Appl Immunol* 1981; 64: 287–92.

25 Cooper B, Creeth JM, Donald ASR. Studies of the limited degradation of mucus glycoproteins – the mechanism of the peroxide reaction. *Biochem J* 1985; 228: 615–26.

26 Darlington LG. Fish oils: what is the current view on their benefits in various diseases? *Medical Dialogue* 1994; No. 429.

27 Darlington LG, Gamlin L. *Diet and Arthritis.* Vermilion, London, 1996; 79–251.

28 Darlington LG, Ramsey NW. Dietary manipulation therapy in rheumatoid arthritis. In: *Progress in Rheumatology III* (Machtey I, ed). Rheumatology Service, Golda Medical Center, Petah-Tiqva, Israel, 1987: 128–32.

29 Darlington LG, Ramsey NW. Weight loss, IgE levels and fish oils in rheumatoid arthritis. In: *Progress in Rheumatology III* (Machtey I, ed). Rheumatology Service, Golda Medical Centre; Petah-Tiqva, Israel, 1987: 137–40.

30 Darlington LG, Ramsey NW. Clinical review. Review of dietary therapy for rheumatoid arthritis. *Br J Rheumatol* 1993; 32: 507–14.

31 Darlington LG, Ramsey NW, Mansfield JR. Placebo-controlled, blind study of dietary manipulation therapy in rheumatoid arthritis. *Lancet* 1986; i: 236–8.

32 Darlington LG, Jump A, Ramsey NW, Spurgeon S, Street P. A prospective study of clinical and serological responses to single or double-blind food challenges in patients with rheumatoid arthritis subject to dietary manipulation. *Br J Rheumatol (Abstracts suppl)* 1989; 28: 116.

33 Darlington LG, Jump A, Ramsey NW. Literature on dietary treatment of rheumatoid arthritis available to the public. *The Practitioner* 1990; 234: 456–60.

34 Davies JMS, Horwitz DA, Davies KJA. Potential roles of hypochlorous acid and N-chloroamines in collagen breakdown by phagocyte cells in synovitis. *Free Radical Biol Med* 1993; 15: 637–43.

35 Davies JMS, Horwitz DM, Davies KJA. Inhibition of collagenase activity by N-chlorotaurine, a product of activated neutrophils. *Arthritis Rheum* 1994; 37: 424–7.

36 Denman AM, Mitchell B, Ansell BM. Joint complaints and food allergic disorders. *Ann Allergy* 1983; 51: 260–3.

37 Doumerg C. Etude clinique experimental de l'alpha-tocopheryle-quinone en rheumatologie et an reeducation. *Therapeutique* 1969; 43: 676–8.

38 Ebringer A Ptaszynska T, Corbett M et al. Antibodies to proteus in rheumatoid arthritis. *Lancet* 1985; ii: 305–7.

39 Ebringer A, Cox NL, Abuliadayel I et al. *Klebsiella* antibodies in ankylosing spondylitis and *Proteus* antibodies in rheumatoid arthritis. *Br J Rheumatol* 1988; 27(ii): 72–85.

40 Ebringer A, Cunningham P, Ahmadi K, Wrigglesworth J, Hosseini R, Wilson C. Sequence similarity between HLA-DR1 and DR4 subtypes associated with rheumatoid arthritis and proteus serratia membrane haemolysins. *Ann Rheum Dis* 1992; 52: 1245–6.

41 Editorial. Fish oils in rheumatoid arthritis. *Lancet* 1987; ii: 720–1.

42 Endres S, Meydani SN, Ghorbani R, Schindler R, Dinarello CA. Dietary supplementation with n-3 fatty acids suppresses interleukin-2 production and mononuclear cell proliferation. *J Leuk Biol* 1993; 54: 599–603.

43 Epstein S. Hypersensitivity to sodium nitrate. A major causative factor in case of palindromic rheumatism. *Ann Allergy* 1969; 27: 343–9.

44 Fairney A, Patel KV, Fish DE, Seifert MH. Vitamin A in osteo- and rheumatoid arthritis. *Br J Rheumatol* 1988; 27: 329–30.

45 Farrell AJ, Blake DR, Palmer RMJ, Moncada S. Increased concentrations of nitrite in synovial fluid and serum samples suggest increased nitric oxide synthesis in rheumatic diseases. *Ann Rheum Dis* 1992; 51: 1219–22.

46 Felson DT. Weight and osteoarthritis. *J Rheumatol Suppl* 1995; 43: 7–9.

47 Felson DT, Xhang Y, Anthony JM, Naimark A, Anderson JJ. Weight loss reduces the risk for symptomatic knee osteoarthritis in women. The Framingham Study. *Ann Intern Med* 1992; 116: 535–9.

48 Fernandes G, Yunis EJ, José DG, Good RA. Dietary influence on anti-nuclear antibodies and cell-mediated immunity in NZB mice. *Int Arch Allergy Appl Immunol* 1973; 44: 770–82.

49 Fine KD, Santa Ana CA, Porter JL, Fordtran JS. Effect of changing intestinal flow rate on a measurement of intestinal permeability. *Gastroenterology* 1995; 108: 983–9.

50 Freed DL. Lectins. *Br Med J* 1985; 290: 584–5.

51 Frei B. Reactive oxygen species and antioxidant vitamins: mechanisms of action. *Am J Med* 1994; 97 (suppl 3A): 5–13S: discussion 22S–28S.

52 Gamlin L, Brostoff H. Food sensitivity and rheumatoid arthritis. *Environ Toxicol Pharmacol* 1997; 4: 43–49.

53 Clark ML, Kumar PJ. Gastroenterology: In: *Clinical Medicine* (P. Kumar and M Clark, eds). Baillière Tindall, London, 1994: 208.

54 Gibson RG, Gibson SLM, Conway V, Chappell D. Perna canaliculus in the treatment of arthritis. *Practitioner* 1980; 224: 955–60.

55 Greenwald RA, Moy WW. Inhibition of collagen gelation by action of the superoxide radical. *Arthritis Rheum* 1979; 22: 251–9.

56 Grootveld M, Halliwell B. Aromatic hydroxylation as a potential measure of hydroxyl-radical formation *in vivo*. Identification of hydroxylated derivatives of salicylate in human body fluids. *Biochem J* 1986; 237: 449–504.

57 Grootveld M, Henderson EB, Farrell A, Blake DR, Parkes HG, Haycock P. Oxidative damage to hyaluronate and glucose in synovial fluid during exercise of the inflamed rheumatoid joint. Detection of abnormal low-molecular-mass metabolites by proton-n.m.r. spectroscopy. *Biochem J* 1991; 273: 459–67.

58 Gutteridge JMC. Bleomycin-detectable iron in knee-joint synovial fluid from arthritic patients and its relationship to the extra-cellular antioxidant activities of caeruloplasmin, transferrin and lactoferrin. *Biochem J* 1987; 245: 415–21.

59 Gutteridge JMC, Rowley DA, Halliwell B. Superoxide-dependent formation of hydroxyl radicals and lipid peroxidation in the presence of iron salts. Detection of 'catalytic' iron and anti-oxidant activity in extracellular fluids. *Biochem J* 1982; 206: 605–9.

60 Hafström I, Ringertz B, Gyllenhammar H *et al*. Effects of fasting on disease activity, neutrophil function, fatty acid composition, and leukotriene biosynthesis in patients with rheumatoid arthritis. *Arthritis Rheum* 1988; 3: 585–92.

61 Hankinson SE, Stampfer MJ, Seddon JM *et al*. Nutrient intake and cataract extraction in woman: a prospective study. *Br Med J* 1992; 305: 335–9.

62 Hansen TM, Lerche A, Kassio V, Lorenzen E, Søndergaard J. Treatment of rheumatoid arthritis with prostaglandin E precursors cis-linoleic acid and gamma-linolenic acid. *Scand J Rheumatol* 1983; 12: 85–8.

63 Harbige LS, Ghebremeskel K, Williams G, Summers P. N-3 and N-6 phosphoglyceride fatty acids in relation to *in vitro* erythrocyte haemolysis induced by hydrogen peroxide in captive common marmosets (*Callithrix jacchus*). *Comp Biochem Physiol* 1990; 97B: 167–70.

64 Heiövaara M, Knekt P, Aho K, Aaran R-K, Alfthan G, Aromaa A. Serum antioxidants and risk of rheumatoid arthritis. *Ann Rheum Dis* 1994; 53: 51–3.

65 Henrotin Y, Deby-Dupont G, Deby C, Franchimont P, Emerit I. Active oxygen species, articular inflammation and cartilage damage. *EXS* 1992; 62: 308–22.

66 Henrotin Y, Deby-Dupont G, Deby C, Debruiyn M, Lamy M, Franchimont P. Production of active oxygen species by isolated human chondrocytes. *Br J Rheumatol* 1993; 32: 562–7.

67 Hergenrather J, Hlady G, Wallace B, Savage E. Pollutants in breast milk of vegetarians. *New Engl J Med* 1981; 304: 792.

68 Hicklin JA, McEwan LM, Morgan JE. The effect of diet in rheumatoid arthritis. *Clin Allergy* 1980; 10: 463.

69 Hughes DA, Pinder AC, Piper Z, Lund EK. N-3 poly-unsaturated fatty acids (PUFA) modulate the expression of functionally associated molecules on human monocytes. *Biochem Soc Trans* 1995; 23: 303S.

70 Hughes DA, Wright AJ, Finglas PM *et al*. The effect of beta-carotene supplementation on the immune function of blood monocytes from healthy male non-smokers. *J Lab Clin Med* 1997; 129: 309–17.

71 Hunter JO. Food allergy – or entero metabolic disorder? *Lancet* 1991; 338: 495–6.

72 Huskisson EC, Scott J, Bryans R. Seatone is ineffective in rheumatoid arthritis. *Br Med J* 1981; 282: 1358–9.

73 Jacobsson L, Lindgärde F, Manthorpe R, Äkesson B. Correlation of fatty acid composition of adipose tissue lipids and serum phosphatidylcholine and serum concentrations of micronutrients with disease duration in rheumatoid arthritis. *Ann Rheum Dis* 1990; 49: 901–5.

74 Jacques PF, Chylack LT Jr. Epidemiological evidence of a role for the antioxidant vitamins and carotenoids in cataract prevention. *Am J Clin Nutr* 1991; 53: 352S–355S.

75 Jantti J, Nikkari T, Solakivi T, Vapaatalo H, Isomäki H. Evening primrose oil in rheumatoid arthritis: changes in serum lipids and fatty acids. *Ann Rheum Dis* 1989; 48: 124–7.

76 Jeng K-CG, Yang C-S, Sim W-Y, Tsai Y-S, Liao W-J, Kuo J-S. Supplementation with vitamins C and E enhances cytokine production by peripheral blood mononuclear cells in healthy adults. *Am J Clin Nutr* 1996; 64: 960–5.

77 Kavanagh R, Workman E, Nash P, Smith M, Hazleman BL, Hunter JO. The effect of elemental diet and subsequent food reintroduction on rheumatoid arthritis. *Br J Rheumatol* 1995; 34: 270–3.

78 Kjeldsen-Kragh J, Haugen M, Borchgrevink CF *et al*. Controlled trial of fasting and one-year vegetarian diet in rheumatoid arthritis. *Lancet* 1991; 338: 899–902.

79 Kjeldsen-Kragh J, Hvatum M, Haugen M, Førre Ø, Scott H. Antibodies against dietary antigens in rheumatoid arthritis patients treated with fasting and a one-year vegetarian diet. *Clin Exp Rheumatol* 1995; 13: 167–72.

80 Kjeldsen-Kragh J, Mellbye OJ, Haugen M *et al*. Changes in laboratory variables in rheumatoid arthritis patients during a trial of fasting and one-year vegetarian diet. *Scand J Rheumatol* 1995; 24: 85–93.

81 Kjeldsen-Kragh J, Rashid T, Dybwad A *et al*. Decrease in anti-*Proteus mirabilis* but not anti-*Escherichia coli* antibody levels in rheumatoid arthritis patients treated with fasting and a one-year vegetarian diet. *Ann Rheum Dis* 1995; 54: 221–4.

82 Kremer JM, Michalek AV, Lininger L *et al*. Effects of manipulation of dietary fatty acids on clinical manifestations of rheumatoid arthritis. *Lancet* 1985; i: 184–7.

83 Kremer J, Jubiz W, Michalek A *et al*. Fish oil fatty acid supplementation in active rheumatoid arthritis. *Ann Inter Med* 1987; 106: 497–503.

84 Kroker GP, Stroud RM, Marshall RT *et al*. Fasting and rheumatoid arthritis. A multi-centre study. *Clin Ecol* 1984; 2: 137–44.

85 Larkin JG, Capell HA, Sturrock RD. Seatone is rheumatoid arthritis: a six month placebo-controlled study. *Ann Rheum Dis* 1985; 44: 199–201.

86 Levanthal LJ, Boyce EG, Zurier RB. Treatment of rheumatoid arthritis with gammalinolenic acid. *Ann Intern Med* 1993; 119: 867–73.

87 Little CH, Stewart AG, Fennessy MR. Platelet serotonin release in rheumatoid arthritis: a study in food intolerant patients. *Lancet* 1983; ii: 297–9.

88 Lund-Olesen K, Menander-Huber KB. Intra-articular orgotein therapy in osteoarthritis of the knee. A double-blind, placebo-controlled trial. *Arzneimittelforschung* 1983; 33: 1199–203.

89 Lunec J, Blake DR, McCleary SJ, Brailsford S, Bacon PA. Self-perpetuating mechanisms of immunoglobulin G aggregation in rheumatoid inflammation. *J Clin Invest* 1985; 76: 2084–90.

90 McAlindon T, Felson DT. Nutrition risk factors for osteoarthritis. *Ann Rheum Dis* 1997; 56: 397–400.

91 McAlindon TE, Jacques P, Zhang Y *et al*. Do antioxidant micronutrients protect against the development and progression of knee osteoarthritis? *Arthritis Rheum* 1996; 39(4): 648–56.

92 McCord JM. Free radicals and inflammation: protection of synovial fluid by superoxide dismutase. *Science* 1974; 185: 529–31.

93 McDaniel DO, Alarcón GD, Pratt PW, Reveille JD. Most African-American patients with rheumatoid arthritis do not have the rheumatoid antigenic determinant (epitope). *Ann Intern Med* 1995; 123: 181–7.

94 McIlwain H, Silverfield JC, Cheatum DE *et al*. Intra-articular orgotein in osteoarthritis of the knee: a placebo-controlled efficacy, safety, and dosage comparison. *Am J Med* 1989; 87: 295–300.

95 Mansson I, Olhagen B. Intestinal *Clostridium perfringens* in rheumatoid arthritis and other connective tissue disorders. *Acta Rheum Scand* 1966; 12: 167–74.

96   Mansson I, Norberg R, Olhagen B, Björklund N-E. Arthritis in pigs induced by dietary factors. Microbiologic, clinical and histologic studies. *Clin Exp Immunol* 1971; 9: 677–93.

97   Meydani M, Natiello F, Goldin B *et al.* Effect of long-term fish oil supplementation on vitamin E status and lipid peroxidation in women. *J Nutr* 1991; 121: 484–91.

98   Meydani SN, Lichtenstein SH, Cornwall S *et al.* Immunologic effects of national cholesterol education panel step-2 diets with and without fish-derived n-fatty acid enrichment. *J Clin Invest* 1993; 92: 105–13.

99   Mielants H, de Vos M, Goemaere S *et al.* Intestinal mucosal permeability in inflammatory rheumatic diseases. II. Role of disease. *J Rheumatol* 1991; 18: 394–400.

100 Mohan IK, Das UN. Oxidant stress, anti-oxidants and essential fatty acids in systemic lupus erythematosus. *Prostaglandins, Leukotrienes and Essential Fatty Acids* 1997; 56(3): 193–8.

101 Munthe E, Aeseth J, Jellum E. Trace elements and rheumatoid arthritis (RA) – pathogenic and therapeutic aspects. *Acta Pharmacol Toxicol* 1986; 59 (suppl. 1): 365–73.

102 Nenonen MT, Helve TA, Rauma A-L, Hänninen OO. Uncooked, lactobacilli-rich, vegan food and rheumatoid arthritis. *Br J Rheumatol* 1998; 37: 274–81.

103 Nestérov AI. The clinical course of Kashin–Beck disease. *Arthritis Rheum* 1964; 7: 29–40.

104 Nuki G. Ankylosing spondylitis, HLAB27, and beyond. *Lancet* 1998; 351: 767–9.

105 Nurcombe HL, Bucknall RC, Edwards SW. Neutrophils isolated from the synovial fluid of patients with rheumatoid arthritis: priming and activation *in vivo. Ann Rheum Dis* 1991; 50: 147–53.

106 O'Farrelly C, Melcher D, Price R *et al.* Association between villous atrophy in rheumatoid arthritis and a rheumatoid factor and gliadin-specific IgG. *Lancet* 1988; ii: 819–22.

107 Olhagen B, Mansson I. Intestinal *Clostridium perfringens* in rheumatoid arthritis and other collagen diseases. *Acta Med Scand* 1968; 184: 395–402.

108 Panush RS. Food induced ('allergic') arthritis: clinical and serologic studies. *J Rheumatol* 1990; 17: 291–4.

109 Panush RS, Carter RL, Katz P, Kowsari B, Longley S, Finnie S. Diet therapy for rheumatoid arthritis. *Arthritis Rheum* 1983; 26: 462–71.

110 Panush RS, Stroud RM, Webster EM. Food induced (allergic) arthritis. Inflammatory arthritis exacerbated by milk. *Arthritis and Rheumatism* 1986; 29: 220–6.

111 Parke AC, Hughes GRV. Rheumatoid arthritis and food. A case study. *Br Med J* 1981; 282: 2027–9.

112 Peltonen R, Kjeldsen-Kragh J, Haugen M *et al.* Changes of faecal flora in rheumatoid arthritis during fasting and one-year vegetarian diet. *Br J Rheumatol* 1994; 33: 638–43.

113 Peltonen R, Nenonen M, Helve T, Hänninen O, Toivanen P, Eerola E. Faecal microbial flora and disease activity in rheumatoid arthritis during a vegan diet. *Br J Rheumatol* 1997; 36: 64–8.

114 Peterkofsky B. Ascorbate requirement for hydroxylation and secretion of procollagen: relationship to inhibition of collagen synthesis in scurvy. *Am J Clin Nutr* 1991; 54: 1135S–40S.

115 Pusztai A, Clarke EMW, Grant G, King TP. The toxicity of *Phaseolus vulgaris* lectins. Nitrogen balance and immunochemical studies. *J Sci Food Agric* 1981; 32: 1037–46.

116 Rasmussen GG, Svendsen H. Fasting and vegan diet in rheumatoid arthritis. *Scand J Rheumatol* 1984; Suppl. 53: 88.

117 Ratner D, Eshel E, Vigder K. Juvenile rheumatoid arthritis and milk allergy. *J R Soc Med* 1984; 78: 410–13.

118 Remer T, Manz FJ. Potential renal acid load of foods and its influence on urine pH. *J Am Diet Assoc* 1995; 95: 791–7.

119 Renaud S, De Lorgeril M. Wine, alcohol, platelets, and the French paradox for coronary heart disease. *Lancet* 1992; 339: 1523–6.

120 Rimm EB, Stampfer MJ, Ascherio A, Giovannucci EL, Colditz GA, Willett WC. Vitamin E supplementation and the risk of coronary heart disease in men. *N Engl J Med* 1993; 328: 1450–6.

121 Robinson J, Watson F, Bucknall RC, Edwards SW. Activation of neutrophil reactive-oxidant production by synovial fluid from patients with inflammatory joint disease. Soluble and insoluble immunoglobulin aggre-

gates activate different pathways in primed and unprimed cells. *Biochem J* 1992; 286: 345–51.

122 Rowley DA, Gutteridge JMC, Blake DR, Farr M, Halliwell B. Lipid peroxidation in rheumatoid arthritis: thiobarbituric acid – reactive material and catalytic iron salts in synovial fluid from rheumatoid patients. *Clin Sci* 1984; 66: 691–5.

123 Sackett DL, Snow JC. The magnitude of compliance and non-compliance. In: *Compliance in Health Care* (Haynes RB, Taylor WD, Sackett DL, eds). The Johns Hopkins University Press, Baltimore and London, 1979: 11–22.

124 Sanders TAB, Hinds A. The influence of a fish oil high in docosahexaenoic acid on plasma lipoprotein and vitamin E concentrations and haemostatic function in healthy male volunteers. *Br J Nutr* 1992; 68: 163–73.

125 Schalkwijk J, van den Berg WB, van de Putte LBA, Joosten LAB. An experimental model for hydrogen peroxide-induced tissue damage. Effects of a single inflammatory mediator on (peri-)articular tissues. *Arthritis Rheum* 1986; 29: 532–8.

126 Schmidt EB, Dyerberg J. N-3 fatty acids and leucocytes. *J Intern Med* 1989; 22: 151–8.

127 Schwartz ER, Adamy L. Effect of ascorbic acid on arylsulfatase activities and sulfated proteoglycan metabolism in chondrocyte cultures. *J Clin Invest* 1977; 60: 96–106.

128 Seignalet J. Les associations entre HLA et polyarthrite rhumatoide 11. – Une théorie sur la pathogenie de la polyarthrite rhumatoide. *Rev Int Rhumatoide* 1989; 19: 155–70.

129 Silman AJ, Hochberg MC. *Epidemiology of the Rheumatic Diseases.* Oxford University Press, Oxford, UK, 1993.

130 Situnayake RD, Thurnham DI, Kootathep S *et al.* Chain-breaking antioxidant status in rheumatoid arthritis: clinical and laboratory correlates. *Ann Rheum Dis* 1991; 50: 81–6.

131 Sköldstam L. Fasting and vegan diet in rheumatoid arthritis. *Scand J Rheumatol* 1986; 15: 219–23.

132 Sköldstam L, Magnusson K-E. Fasting, intestinal permeability, and rheumatoid arthritis. *Rheum Dis Clin N Am* 1991; 17: 363–71.

133 Sköldstam L, Larsson L, Lindström FD. Effects of fasting and lactovegetarian diet on rheumatoid arthritis. *Scand J Rheumatol* 1979; 8: 249–55.

134 Spanheimer RG, Bird TA, Peterkofsky B. Regulation of collagen synthesis and mRNA levels in articular cartilage of scorbutic guinea pigs. *Arch Biochem Biophys* 1986; 246: 33–41.

135 Sperling RA, Weinblatt M, Robin JL *et al.* Effects of dietary supplementation with marine fish oil on leucocyte lipid mediator generation and function in rheumatoid arthritis. *Arthritis Rheum* 1987; 30: 988–97.

136 Stevens CR, Benboubetra M, Harrison R, Sahinoglu T, Smith EC, Blake DR. Localisation of xanthine oxidase to synovial endothelium. *Ann Rheum Dis* 1991; 50: 760–2.

137 Sundqvist T, Lindström F, Magnusson K-E, Skoldstam L, Stjernstrom L, Tagesson C. Influence of fasting on intestinal permeability and disease activity in patients with rheumatoid arthritis. *Scan J Rheumatol* 1982; 11: 33–8.

138 Tarp U, Overvad K, Thorling EB, Grandal H, Hansen JC. Selenium treatment in rheumatoid arthritis. *Scand J Rheumatol* 1985; 14: 364–8.

139 Tarp U, Hansen JC, Overvad K, Thorling EB, Tarp BD, Grandal H. Glutathione peroxidase activity in patients with rheumatoid arthritis and in normal subjects. Effects of long-term selenium supplementation. *Arthritis Rheum* 1987; 30: 1162–6.

140 van de Laar MAF J, van der Korst JK. Food intolerance in rheumatoid arthritis. I. A double-blind, controlled trial of the clinical effects of elimination of milk allergens and azo dyes. *Ann Rheum Dis* 1992; 51: 298–302.

141 van de Laar MAFJ, Aalbers M, Bruins FG, van Dinther-Janssen ACHM, van der Korst JK, Meijer CJLM. Food intolerance in rheumatoid arthritis. II Clinical and histological aspects. *Ann Rheum Dis* 1992; 51: 303–6.

142 Vargas SL, Patrick CC, Ayers GD, Hughes WT. Modulating effect of dietary carbohydrate supplementation on *Candida albicans* colonization and invasion in a neutropenic mouse model. *Infect Immun* 1993; 61: 619–26.

143 Wasil M, Halliwell B, Moorhouse CP, Hutchison DCS, Baum H. Biologically significant scavenging of the myelo peroxidase-derived

oxidant hypochlorous acid by some anti-inflammatory drugs. *Biochem Pharmacol* 1987; 36: 3847–50.

144 Watson J, Byars ML, McGill P, Kelman AW. Cytokine and prostaglandin production by monocytes of volunteers and rheumatoid arthritis patients treated with dietary supplements of blackcurrant seed oil. *Br J Rheumatol* 1993; 32: 1055–8.

145 Williams R. Rheumatoid arthritis and food: a case study. *Br Med J* 1981; 283: 563.

146 Wojtulewski JA. Joints and connective tissue. In: *Food Allergy and Intolerance* (Brostoff J, Challacombe SJ, eds). Baillière Tindall, London, 1987; 723–35.

147 Wolfe F, Cathey MA. The assessment and prediction of functional disability in rheumatoid arthritis. *J Rheumatol* 1991; 18: 1298–1306.

148 Wu D, Meydani M, Hayek MG, Huth P, Nicolosi RJ. Immunologic effects of marine- and plant-derived n-3 polyunsaturated fatty acids in non-human primates. *Am J Clin Nutr* 1996; 63: 273–80.

Chapter 55

Ankylosing spondylitis and diet

A. Ebringer and C. Wilson

INTRODUCTION

The discovery that HLA B27 is linked to ankylosing spondylitis (AS) has provided a new approach to the study of the possible causation of this disease. It is the association between HLAs and arthritic complications occurring after enteric infections that has provided the vital clues to identification of the specific microbial agents involved in AS and related diseases. The majority of AS patients not only possess HLA B27, but during active phases of the disease have elevated levels of total serum immunoglobulin (IgA) suggesting that a microbe from the gastrointestinal tract is acting across the gut mucosa. Microbiological, immunological and biochemical studies have revealed an association between the Gram-negative microbe *Klebsiella pneumoniae* and AS. It has been suggested that *K. pneumoniae*, found in the bowel flora, might be the trigger factor for this disease and therefore reduction in the size of the bowel flora, especially *K. pneumoniae* microbes, by dietary manipulation could be of some benefit in the treatment of patients. This chapter will concentrate on the association between HLA B27, *K. pneumoniae* and AS, as well as the role of a 'low starch diet' in the management of the disease.

ANKYLOSING SPONDYLITIS

AS is a chronic inflammatory disorder affecting mainly the lumbar spine and sacroiliac joints. Onset of disease is often insidious with lower back pain and early morning stiffness. Inflammation can lead to fibrosis and ossification where bridging spurs of bone known as syndesmophytes form, especially at the edges of the intervertebral discs. This form of ossification is primarily seen at the sacroiliac joints and lumbar spine from where it ascends and, in extreme cases, can effectively solidify the vertebral column. The bony ankylosis may also affect the hips, leading to generalized restriction of movement. Although AS is a chronic disease, its activity fluctuates between periods of exacerbations and remissions. In the advanced stage, fusion of the spine occurs which often results in the formation of a characteristic stooped posture known as the 'Bechterew stoop'. In severe cases, the disease can progress to form the classic 'bamboo spine'. AS occurs approximately three times more frequently in men than in women, and the diagnosis is based on the patient satisfying the New York criteria. It is well established that HLA B27 is associated with AS in all racial groups examined,[10,35] but it must be noted that the majority of HLA B27 carriers are healthy individuals, free from any disease. However, there is a substantial proportion of healthy HLA B27 individuals who complain of frequent attacks of backache and early morning stiffness, which is usually relieved by exercise, but who do not go on to develop full blown classical AS. In a study of 200 healthy individuals belonging to the Anthony Nolan Bone Marrow Donor Panel, the frequency of backache was investigated. Backache was defined as being present if the individual had visited his or her family doctor. An individual who had backache, but had never visited a general practitioner with the complaint, was scored as negative for the complaint. The study was organized in such a way that 100 individuals positive for HLA B27 were compared to 100 individuals negative for HLA B27. It was found that 45 of 100 HLA B27-positive healthy individuals had consulted a doctor for backache, while only five of

100 HLA B27-negative healthy individuals had sought medical attention for their back problems. This difference was significant (χ^2 with Yates correction, 40.6; $P<0.001$).

Association of HLA B27 and ankylosing spondylitis

The association between HLA B27 and AS has altered our perception of rheumatology in that no viable model of the disease can be proposed which does not also provide some explanation for this immunogenetic observation. Two main theories have so far been proposed to explain the association: the receptor theory and the molecular mimicry theory.

Receptor theory

This theory states that both Class I and II MHC molecules act as a receptor cavity that binds pathogenic peptides (8–20 amino acids in length) and thereby cause disease.[7,8] However, to date no specific pathogenic peptides which occupy the HLA B27 cavity have been identified and, until such a peptide is found, no therapeutic test can be designed to determine whether withdrawal of antigens containing such peptides can modify the course of the disease. The lack of a special pathogenic peptide binding to HLA B27 is a serious weakness of the receptor theory.

Molecular mimicry theory

This theory is based on the idea that the HLA molecule shares molecular similarity with some antigens present in infectious organisms and, after exposure, disease occurs through reactive inflammation and immune mechanisms.[20]

Reactive arthritis is known to occur in HLA B27 individuals after infection with *Salmonella*, *Shigella*, *Yersinia*[3] and *Chlamydia*.[40] These observations provide a possible clue to any putative infectious agent that may be involved in AS. The agent could probably be related to those that are associated with reactive arthritis and be a member of the normal bowel flora.

Molecular mimicry between HLA B27 and *Klebsiella* molecules

The molecular mimicry theory[20] was first proposed by this group in 1976, when it was suggested that several Gram-negative microorganisms, including *K. pneumoniae*, carry antigens which crossreact with HLA B27. Studies showed that allogeneic human HLA B27 tissue typing antisera bind preferentially to *K. pneumoniae* antigens.[6,67] Subsequently, Van Bohemen *et al.*[65] reported that mouse monoclonal anti-HLA B27 sera showed increased binding for *Klebsiella*, *Shigella* and *Yersinia* antigens. In a later study, Kono and coworkers[37] carried out the reverse experiment, when they described an anti-*Yersinia* monoclonal antibody which reacted with 12 of 12 HLA B27 lymphoblastoid cell lines, but with only four of 31 which were HLA B27-negative. However, three of the four reactive HLA B27-negative cell lines carried HLA B7, an antigen that crossreacts with HLA B27. Further studies by Ogasawara *et al.*[50] reported that the anti-HLA B27 (M2) monoclonal antibody bound specifically to a 70 kDa component of *K. pneumoniae*, whereas no such reactivity was demonstrated with five other monoclonal antibodies. Molecular mimicry has also been demonstrated down to the level of amino acids.

Nitrogenase reductase

Schwimmbeck and colleagues[53] reported molecular mimicry between HLA B27 and *K. pneumoniae* nitrogenase reductase

enzyme, in that the sequence Gln Thr Asp Arg Glu Asp (QTDRED) is common to both molecules. Husby and coworkers,[33] using rat antisera raised against 16-mer synthetic peptides of *K. pneumoniae* nitrogenase reductase containing the QTDRED sequence, were able to detect by immunoperoxidase synovial biopsies obtained from HLA B27-positive AS patients but not B27-negative biopsies obtained from patients with rheumatoid arthritis. Furthermore, AS patients have elevated levels of antibodies to *K. pneumoniae* nitrogenase reductase, especially during active phases of disease.[2]

Pullulanase

Another molecule in *Klebsiella* microbes also has a sequence which crossreacts with a part of the HLA B27 molecule. Protein database analysis of published *K. pneumoniae* protein sequences has shown that molecular mimicry is present between *K. pneumoniae* secretion protein (pul D) of the inducible, starch-debranching enzyme pullulanase (DRDE) and HLA B27 (DRED)[29] (Fig. 55.1). Additionally, amino acid homology has been described between the extracellular starch-induced enzymes pullulanase (pul A) and types I, III and IV collagens.[29] If the molecular mimicry theory is to be considered as a valid model for the pathogenesis of AS, then a logical expectation is that both antigen (*K. pneumoniae*) and antibody against *K. pneumoniae* should be detectable in patients during active phases of the disease.

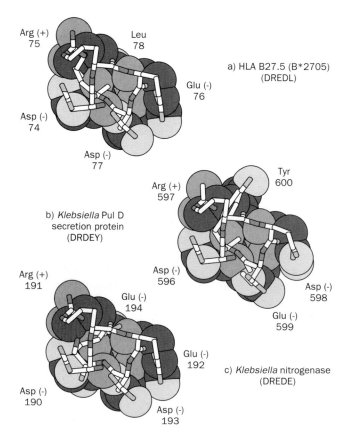

Fig. 55.1 Comparison of space-filling models. (a) HLA B27.5 (B*2705) (**DREDL**) predicted from known crystallographic structure; (b) *Klebsiella pneumoniae* pul D secretion protein (**DRDEY**); (c) *Klebsiella pneumoniae* nitrogenase enzyme (**DREDE**). (Reproduced with permission from Dr M. Fielder, PhD thesis (1995). Molecular modelling by Dr C. Ettelaie.)

Microbiological studies

Initial study involving 63 patients with AS showed that *K. pneumoniae* could be isolated more frequently during active phases of the disease.[28] In the second sequential study, involving 163 patients with AS, it was shown that a clinical relapse was preceded by the appearance of *K. pneumoniae* in faecal samples[27] and active inflammatory disease was associated with elevation in total serum IgA, suggesting that a microbial agent was acting across a mucosal surface such as the gut.[13] Other independent groups have also found an association between isolation of *Klebsiella* and active disease in these patients.[17,32,38] These studies, involving several centres, clearly lead to the suggestion that *K. pneumoniae* is somehow involved in producing pathological changes during active phases of the disease. It is clearly demonstrated that there is crossreactivity between HLA B27 and *K. pneumoniae* proteins. Together with the observation that this microbe is found in patients with AS during active phases of the disease, this crossreactivity is consistent with the predictions of the molecular mimicry theory. However, the molecular mimicry model makes a further prediction in that it is not sufficient only for the antigen (*K. pneumoniae*) to be present, but antibodies to that microbe and components must also be demonstrated. This is because the pathogenetic process involves antibodies produced against crossreactive antigens and, together with immunocompetent cells, this leads to autoimmune cellular and tissue damage.

Immunological studies

It has been well established that total serum IgA is elevated in patients with AS[66] and that it is usually associated with inflammatory phases of disease activity.[13,17,32,38,41,66] Elevation in total serum IgA indicates antigenic stimulation acting across a mucosal surface, such as the gastrointestinal tract. Plasma cells in the gut mucosa are the main source of serum IgA,[39] and therefore Gram-negative bowel flora could be responsible for this immunoglobulin elevation.[25] Elevations in immune responses to *K. pneumoniae* in patients with AS have been reported from several countries over the past 18 years (Table 55.1).

Immunoglobulin A levels

Early studies by Trull *et al.*[64] reported that the mean IgA anti-*Klebsiella pneumoniae* level was significantly higher in 43 patients with active AS as compared to 39 with inactive AS, 57 healthy control subjects, 35 patients with psoriatic arthritis, and 54 patients with rheumatoid arthritis (RA) (see also reference 12). However, there was no significant elevation of antibody levels against *Escherichia coli* and *Candida albicans* in any of the five groups examined (Fig. 55.2). In a second study an elevation in mean titre of anti-*Klebsiella* antibodies was reported in 24 patients with active AS, whereas no such elevation was found in 28 with inactive disease, 30 patients with RA and 41 healthy control subjects.[63] This observation was later confirmed by this group using several other immunological techniques.[1,22,55] Mäki-Ikola *et al.*,[42] in an extensive study from Finland, measured antibodies to *Salmonella*, *Yersinia*, *Campylobacter*, *Borrelia*, *Klebsiella*, *E. coli*, *Proteus* and *Chlamydia* in sera from 99 patients with AS and 100 healthy control subjects, showing increased levels of IgA and IgG antibodies against *Klebsiella*. Cellular as well as humoral responses are detected in patients with AS.[31] Others have shown elevated anti-*Klebsiella* antibodies not only in AS but also in Crohn's disease.[49]

Geographical distribution of antibodies against *Klebsiella* in patients with ankylosing spondylitis		
Country	Reference	Year
England	Trull et al.[64]	1983
	Trull et al.[63]	1984
USA	Schwimmbeck et al.[53]	1987
Finland	Mäki-Ikola et al.[42]	1991
Scotland	O'Mahony et al.[49]	1992
Canada	Thomson et al.[60]	1993
Germany	Sahly et al.[52]	1994
Spain	Collado et al.[12]	1994
Mexico	Garcia-Latorre et al.[31]	1995
Japan	Tani et al.[58]	1997
The Netherlands	Blankenberg-Sprenkels et al.[9]	1998

Table 55.1 Geographical distribution of antibodies against *Klebsiella* in patients with ankylosing spondylitis.

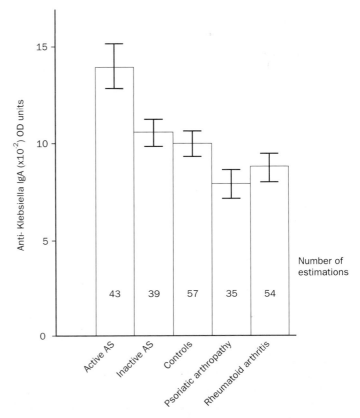

Fig. 55.2 Serum immunoglobulin A (IgA) antibody to *Klebsiella pneumoniae* (mean ± SE) measured in patients with active and inactive ankylosing spondylitis (AS) healthy controls and patients with psoriatic and rheumatoid arthritis. (Reproduced with permission from A. Ebringer.)

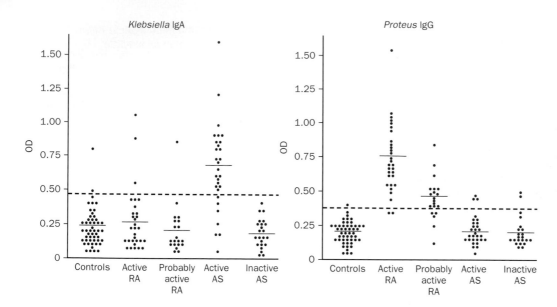

Klebsiella IgA

Proteus IgG

Fig. 55.3 IgA *Klebsiella* antibodies and IgG *Proteus* antibodies in patients with rheumatoid arthritis (RA) (active and probably active), patients with ankylosing spondylitis (AS) (active and inactive) compared to control subjects. The broken line represents 95% confidence limits of the distribution of the controls, the bars represent means. (Reproduced with permission from A. Ebringer.)

Lipopolysaccharide antibodies

Lipopolysaccharide (LPS) antibodies against *Klebsiella* and *Shigella* are elevated in patients with AS but not against LPS from *E. coli*, *Salmonella*, *Yersinia* and *Campylobacter*.[60] The antibodies are detected against a restricted number of *K. pneumoniae* capsular polysaccharides in patients with AS.[52]

Klebsiella *and* Proteus *antibodies*

Tani *et al.*[58] found elevated levels of antibodies to *K. pneumoniae* but not to *Proteus mirabilis* in 54 patients with AS, while elevated levels of antibodies to *P. mirabilis* were present in 50 patients with RA, each group thereby being a specificity control for the other disease (Fig. 55.3). Blankenberg-Sprenkels and colleagues[9] reported elevated levels of antibodies to *K. pneumoniae* in AS and acute anterior uveitis (AAU) patients compared to healthy control subjects. Apart from antibodies to whole *K. pneumoniae* being present in patients with AS, IgG antibody levels were also reported to be elevated against homologous synthetic peptides of HLA B27 (DRED), *K. pneumoniae* nitrogenase reductase (DRED)[53] and pullulanase (DRDE)[29] enzymes.

The presence of specific anti-*Klebsiella pneumoniae* antibodies in patients with AS and the observation that molecular mimicry between HLA B27 and *K. pneumoniae* has been defined down to the level of similarity of amino acids, found in both the suspect bacteria and the genetically susceptible individuals, clearly suggests that this microbe could be the environmental trigger factor in AS.

Molecular mimicry and pathology of ankylosing spondylitis

A conclusion from these extensive studies is that patients with AS have specific antibodies against *K. pneumoniae* and to no other bacteria. However, only a small proportion or a subset of the antimicrobial antibodies will also have antiself or autoimmune activity. The crossreacting antibodies which are produced in these patients in response to *K. pneumoniae* may well bind to HLA B27 because of molecular mimicry. The bacterial antigens, carrying the cross-reactive sequences, will be immunogenic, especially around the edges of the mimicking sequences, because it is at these sites that the immune system will not recognize that it is dealing with a self-antigen. Hence, there is no breakdown of tolerance, and the

production of anti-self bacterial antibodies or autoimmune activity is part of the normal immune response when encountering partially crossreacting antigens. When such crossreacting antibodies are present in small quantities, there is no complement activation and therefore neither cytotoxic events nor inflammation follow (Fig. 55.4). However, when such antibodies are present in high concentrations, the complement cascade is activated, with consequent stimulation of inflammation that may eventually result in localized tissue damage and fibrosis, especially in the enthesis around the lumbar spine, neck, sacroiliac joints, peripheral large joints and uvea.[19,34] The persistent infection would appear to act across the bowel mucosa of the gastrointestinal tract. Therapeutic intervention, aimed at removal of *K. pneumoniae* microbes and reduction of anti-*Klebsiella pneumoniae* antibodies, should lead to

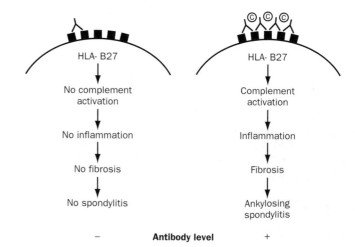

Fig. 55.4 Anti-*Klebsiella* antibody present at low concentration, binds to HLA B27 lymphocyte, but complement cascade is not activated, cells are not damaged and therefore no inflammation occurs. Conversely, anti-*Klebsiella* antibodies present at high concentrations bind to HLA B27 lymphocyte. Proximity of Fc parts of immunoglobulins leads to complement activation with cell death and inflammation therefore occurs. The result of inflammation is deposition of fibrous tissue, thereby limiting joint mobility and producing spinal ankylosis. (Reproduced with permission from A. Ebringer.)[26]

a reduction in inflammation and arrest the progression of the disease. The main source of substrates on which colonic microbes depend are the residual dietary nutrients entering the large bowel following incomplete digestion.

CARBOHYDRATES AND GROWTH OF *KLEBSIELLA PNEUMONIAE*

One of the major substrates available in the gut for microbial fermentation is monosaccharides and disaccharides, derived from complex carbohydrates.[5,47] Finegold and coworkers[30] carried out bacterial cultures on 47 subjects on a high carbohydrate/low protein diet and compared these to 45 subjects on a low carbohydrate/high protein diet. The mean number of *Klebsiella* microorganisms in the high carbohydrate group was 30 000 bacteria per gram of faeces compared to a value of 700 bacteria per gram of faeces in the low carbohydrate group. In a related study, equal amounts (5 g/l) of simple sugars and amino acids were compared for their ability to act as nutrients for the growth of *K. pneumoniae* in 24-h cultures and the number of bacteria obtained compared for the different substrates. The mean number of *K. pneumoniae* microbes was 10 times higher for three different sugars (glucose, sucrose and lactose) per gram of substrate compared to the value obtained after incubation with 11 different amino acids.[18] The source of these carbohydrates could be dietary starch. Nearly all normal subjects failed to absorb appreciable amounts (5–20%) of starch in wheat flour, commonly present in bread and pasta, as assessed by oral hydrogen excretion studies, following a test meal. This is because of the formation of insoluble complexes between some carbohydrate and protein components in wheat. Breath hydrogen concentrations were measured for 5 h after an overnight fast followed by a test meal containing equal amounts of either sucrose or bread/pasta. The sucrose meal produced no increase in oral hydrogen but significant amounts were detected at 4 and 5 h after a test meal with either bread or pasta (Fig. 55.5).[5] These observations suggest that *K. pneumoniae* microbes grow better on carbohydrate than on protein substrates. Therefore, an exclusion diet removing complex carbohydrates such as starch but not simple carbohydrates such as glucose and sucrose might inhibit the growth of *K. pneumoniae* and could also affect disease activity in patients with AS. Studies carried out on healthy individuals showed that serum IgA can be controlled by dietary intake of starch (Fig. 55.6). Since it is well established that serum IgA is elevated in AS, a similar approach might produce a drop in serum IgA as well as in IgA anti-*Klebsiella pneumoniae* antibodies which could lead to clinical improvements in AS patients.

LOW STARCH DIET AS TREATMENT

Ebringer and colleagues[18] reported a significant drop in the erythrocyte sedimentation rate (ESR) and total serum IgA in 36 patients with active AS on a low starch diet (Table 55.2) when studied over a period of 9 months. However, no such difference was observed in the same group of patients when examined retrospectively for the same period of time before they went on the low starch diet. Most patients in the study reported that the severity of their symptoms declined and in some cases completely disappeared. Many patients also noticed that their requirement for non-steroidal anti-inflammatory drugs (NSAIDs) also decreased.

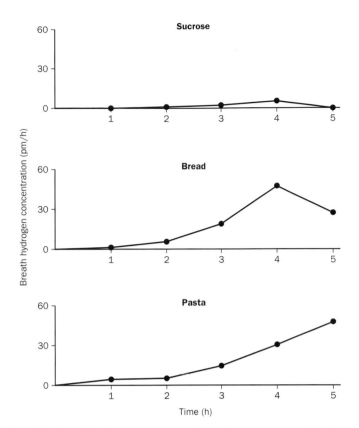

Fig. 55.5 Breath hydrogen concentrations after an overnight fast followed by a test meal containing equal amounts of either sucrose or bread/pasta. (Adapted from I.H. Anderson *et al.*[5], with permission.)

| Composition of a low starch diet for the treatment of patients with ankylosing spondylitis ||
Increase	**Reduce**
Red meat	Bread
White meat	Potatoes
Fish	Chips
Beans and peas	Rice
Nuts	Spaghetti
Vegetables and salads	Cereals
Milk	Cakes
Fruit	Biscuits
Data from Ebringer and Wilson[24], with permission.	

Table 55.2 Composition of a low starch diet for the treatment of patients with ankylosing spondylitis.

Over the past 18 years, the low starch diet has been used in the treatment of over 450 patients with AS attending the AS clinic at the Middlesex Hospital in London.[24] It normally takes some time, around 3–6 months for the effect of the diet to become obvious. The majority of these patients do not require any

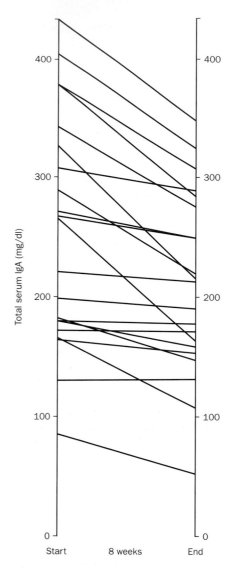

Fig. 55.6 Total serum IgA concentrations before and after an 8-week high protein, low starch diet in 21 healthy control subjects. (From Dr T.M.A. Ptaszynska, PhD thesis, 1985, with permission.)

medication and are treated by diet alone. Furthermore, some of the patients on the low starch diet required lower doses of sulfasalazine-EN to achieve the desired therapeutic effect, thereby avoiding some of the side effects of NSAIDs. A minority of patients find adherence difficult, it which case they have to be treated with high doses of NSAIDs.

Case study 1

Mrs B, aged 20 years and HLA B27-positive, was first seen at the AS Clinic in 1976. She had almost continuous, unremitting pains affecting large peripheral joints, the thoracic cage and the whole of the spinal column, eventually leading to complete ankylosis. During a 7-year period, her ESR was never below 20 mm/h and she acquired the radiological and clinical stigmata of advanced AS. She started on the low starch diet in 1983 and her clinical condition improved over the subsequent months. She was last seen in June 2001 when her ESR and haemoglobin were both normal. She takes an occasional NSAID for the mechanical pains produced by her rigid spine (Fig. 55.7).

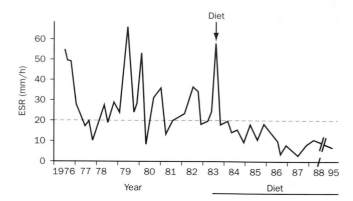

Fig. 55.7 Erythrocyte sedimentation rate (ESR, mm/h) in a patient from 1976 to 1995, showing the effect of diet. (From A. Ebringer and C. Wilson,[24] with permission.)

Case study 2

This was a 29-year-old HLA B27 woman, who had her first visit to the AS Clinic in 1993, at which time her ESR was 120 mm/h. She could not tolerate sulfasalazine because of skin reactions and was treated by diet alone. Her ESR steadily dropped to normal levels and she continues to be in clinical remission.

ASSOCIATION OF ANKYLOSING SPONDYLITIS WITH INFLAMMATORY BOWEL DISEASE

The association of AS with overt bowel disease is well established. There is an increased prevalence of inflammatory bowel disease (IBD) of up to 5% in families of patients with AS. Mielants and coworkers,[48] in a study of ileocolonoscopic findings in 232 patients with seronegative spondyloarthropathy, observed inflammatory gut lesions in 57% of patients with AS. Furthermore, in a follow up study 25% of those patients who had chronic inflammatory changes on initial biopsy had developed Crohn's disease.[14] Although the cause of Crohn's disease is unknown, a microbial link has long been suspected in the aetiology of the disease and antibodies to several microbes have been found. These include antibodies to *Saccharomyces cerevisiae* as well as *Candida albicans*,[46] *E. coli*[56] and *Mycobacterium paratuberculosis*.[59] Furthermore, an abnormal immune response to some species of anaerobic coccoid rods has been demonstrated in patients with Crohn's compared to healthy controls.[11]

Intestinal permeability

It has been suggested that abnormal intestinal permeability may be responsible for the non-specific immune response to various microbes observed in patients with Crohn's disease.[4] However, studies carried out by this group are not in agreement with those of others, in that a specific immune response to *K. pneumoniae* in Crohn's disease has been demonstrated. In a recent study, patients with AS and IBD have been shown to have elevated levels of antibodies to *K. pneumoniae*, but not to *Eubacterium*, *Bacteroides*, *Peptostreptococcus*, *E. coli* or *Proteus mirabilis*.[62] In a subsequent study, elevated levels of IgG, IgA and IgM antibodies were reported to whole *K. pneumoniae* and capsular extracts of many serotypes of the organism in patients with Crohn's, but not in those with ulcerative colitis, coeliac disease and normal controls.

Low starch diet

The above findings suggest a specific immune response to *K. pneumoniae* in both AS and Crohn's disease. It could be speculated that dietary manipulation using a low starch diet might modify the disease outcome in patients with Crohn's as it does in patients with AS. Interestingly, there have been many diet studies in patients with Crohn's disease, the results of which show a significantly increased consumption of refined carbohydrate[43] and sugars.[45]

Mayberry and coworkers[44] have suggested that the greater intake of sugar by patients with Crohn's may be of importance in the aetiology of the disease. The increased sugar consumption may be associated with a change in the bacterial flora of the intestine.[68] Clearly the role of *K. pneumoniae* in AS and Crohn's disease requires further study.

DIET AS THERAPY IN ANKYLOSING SPONDYLITIS AND RHEUMATOID ARTHRITIS

The concept of diet therapy has also been used in the treatment of RA. Early studies demonstrated that patients with active disease have elevated antibody levels to *Proteus mirabilis* and that there was crossreactivity between HLA DR4 and *P. mirabilis*.[23] Several independent groups have since confirmed these initial observations.[15,51,54] In 1992, Ebringer and colleagues[21] showed that there was molecular mimicry between the RA-associated motif Glu Gln Arg Arg Ala Ala (EQRRAA) (which is present in the HLA DR alleles linked to RA) and Glu Ser Arg Arg Ala Leu (ESRRAL) of *P. mirabilis* haemolysin. Wilson and coworkers[69] also showed molecular mimicry between *P. mirabilis* urease Ile Arg Arg Glu Thr (IRRET) and type XI collagen Leu Arg Arg Glu Ile (LRREI). In addition, patients with RA were found to have elevated antibody levels to the ESRRAL sequence, *P. mirabilis* haemolysin and urease proteins.[69] Moreover, other groups have reported elevated antibody levels to ESRRAL[16] and EQRRAA sequences[57] in patients with RA. Wilson and coworkers[70] also found a correlation between anti-*Proteus* antibody levels and the number of *P. mirabilis* colony-forming units isolated from urine specimens obtained from patients, with RA suggesting that they might be suffering from persistent subclinical upper urinary tract infection. Recent studies by Kjeldsen-Kragh and colleagues[36] have shown that these patients on a 1-year vegetarian diet had a decrease in anti-*Proteus* antibody levels while the levels of *E. coli* antibodies remain unchanged. It was suggested that a high fruit and vegetable intake will contain fructose which competes with both *P. mirabilis* and *E. coli* for adhesion molecules present on uroepithelial cells. A combination of high fluid intake containing fruit and vegetable extracts could be of therapeutic benefit in patients with RA in the same way as the low starch diet is in AS.

CONCLUSIONS

Molecular mimicry between HLA B27 and *Klebsiella pneumoniae* has been demonstrated down to the level of amino acids. Furthermore, *K. pneumoniae* can be isolated from patients with AS at a higher frequency than in healthy control subjects. In addition, patients with AS and Crohn's disease have elevated levels of antibodies against *K. pneumoniae*. These findings suggest that *K. pneumoniae* may be involved in the aetiopathogenesis of both diseases. Dietary manipulation using a low starch diet might modify the outcome of both diseases and a different dietary regime could benefit patients with RA.

REFERENCES

1 Abuljadayel I, Ebringer A, Cox NL. Antibodies to *Klebsiella* measured by immunofluorescence. *Clin Rheum* 1989; 8: 25.

2 Ahmadi K, Wilson C, Tiwana H *et al*. Antibodies to *Klebsiella pneumoniae* nitrogenase reductase in patients with ankylosing spondylitis. *Ann Rheum Dis* 1998; 57: 441.

3 Aho K, Ahvonen P, Lassus A *et al*. HLA-B27 in reactive arthritis. *Lancet* 1973; ii: 157.

4 Ainsworth M, Eriksen J, Rasmussen JW *et al*. Intestinal permeability of (^{51}Cr-EDTA) in patients with Crohn's disease and their healthy relatives. *Scand J Gastroenterol* 1989; 24: 993–8.

5 Anderson IH, Levine AS, Levitt MD. Incomplete absorption of carbohydrate in all-purpose wheat flour. *New Engl J Med* 1981; 304: 891–2.

6 Avakian H, Welsh J, Ebringer A *et al*. Ankylosing spondylitis, HLA-B27 and *Klebsiella*. II. Crossreactivity studies with human tissue typing sera. *Br J Exp Pathol* 1980; 61: 92–6.

7 Benjamin R, Parham P. Guilt by association: HLA-B27 and ankylosing spondylitis. *Immunol Today* 1990; 4: 137–42.

8 Bjorkman PJ, Saper MA, Samraou B *et al*. Structure of human class I histocompatibility antigen HLA-A2. *Nature* 1987; 329: 506–12.

9 Blankenberg-Sprenkels SHD, Fielder M, Feltkamp TEW *et al*. Antibodies to *Klebsiella pneumoniae* in Dutch patients with ankylosing spondylitis and acute anterior uveitis and to *Proteus mirabilis* in rheumatoid arthritis. *J Rheumatol* 1998; 25: 743–7.

10 Brewerton DA, Caffrey MFP, Hart FD *et al*. Ankylosing spondylitis and HLA-A27. *Lancet* 1973; i: 904–7.

11 Bull K, Matthews N, Rhodes J. Antibody response to anaerobic coccoid rods in Crohn's disease. *J Clin Pathol* 1986; 39: 1130–4.

12 Collado A, Gratacos J, Ebringer A *et al*. Serum IgA anti-*Klebsiella* antibodies in ankylosing spondylitis patients from Catalonia. *Scand J Rheumatol* 1994; 23: 119–23.

13 Cowling P, Ebringer R, Ebringer A. Association of inflammation with raised serum IgA in ankylosing spondylitis. *Ann Rheum Dis* 1980; 39: 545–9.

14 De Vos M, Mielants H, Cuvelier C *et al*. Long-term evolution of gut inflammation in patients with spondyloarthropathy. *Gastoenterology* 1996; 110: 1696–703.

15 Deighton CM, Gray J, Bint AJ *et al*. Specificity of the *Proteus* antibody response in rheumatoid arthritis. *Ann Rheum Dis* 1992; 51: 1206–7.

16 Dybwad A, Forre O, Sioud M. Increased serum and synovial fluid antibodies to immunoselected peptides in patients with rheumatoid arthritis. *Ann Rheum Dis* 1996; 55: 437–41.

17 Eastmond CJ, Wilshaw HE, Burgess SE *et al*. The frequency of faecal *Klebsiella aerogenes* in patients with ankylosing spondylitis and controls with respect to individual features of the disease. *Ann Rheum Dis* 1980; 39: 118–23.

18 Ebringer A, Baines M, Childerstone M *et al*. Etiopathogenesis of ankylosing spondylitis and the cross tolerance hypothesis. *Adv Inflam Res* 1985; 9: 101–28.

19 Ebringer A, Baines M, Ptaszynska T *et al*. Spondyloarthritis, uveitis, HLA-B27 and *Klebsiella*. *Immunol Rev* 1985; 86: 101–16.

20 Ebringer A, Cowling P, Ngwa Suh *et al*. Crossreactivity between *Klebsiella aerogenes* species and HLA-B27 lymphocyte antigens as an aetiological factor in ankylosing spondylitis. In: *HLA and Disease* (Dausset J, Svejgaard A, eds), INSERM, Paris, 1976; 58: 27.

21 Ebringer A, Cunningham P, Ahmadi K *et al*. Sequence similarity between HLA-DR1 and DR4 subtypes associated with rheumatoid arthritis and *Proteus/Serratia* membrane haemolysins. *Ann Rheum Dis* 1992; 51: 1245–6.

22 Ebringer A, Ghuloom M, Ptaszynska T *et al*. Role of micro-organisms in the aetiopathogenesis of HLA-B27 diseases. In *Spondyloarthropathies – Involvement of the Gut* (Veys E, Mielants H, eds), Elsevier, Excerpta Medica, Amsterdam, 1987; 235–47.

23 Ebringer A, Ptaszynska T, Corbett M *et al*. Antibodies to *Proteus* in rheumatoid arthritis. *Lancet* 1985; ii: 305–7.

24 Ebringer A, Wilson C. The use of low starch diet in the treatment of patients suffering from ankylosing spondylitis. *Clin Rheumatol* 1996; 15(Suppl. 1): 62–6.

25 Ebringer A. The relationship between *Klebsiella* infection and ankylosing spondylitis. In: *The Gut and Rheumatic Disease* (Rooney PJ, ed.), *Baillière's Clin Rheumatol* 1989; 3: 321–38.

26 Ebringer A. Ankylosing spondylitis is caused by *Klebsiella*. *Rheum Dis Clin N Am* 1992; 18: 105–31.

27 Ebringer R, Cawdell DR, Cowling P *et al*. Sequential studies in ankylosing spondylitis: association of *Klebsiella pneumoniae* with active disease. *Ann Rheum Dis* 1978; 37: 146–51.

28 Ebringer R, Cooke D, Cawdell DR *et al*. Ankylosing spondylitis: *Klebsiella* and HLA-B27. *Rheumatol and Rehab* 1977; 16: 190–6.

29 Fielder M, Pirt J, Tarpey I *et al*. Molecular mimicry and ankylosing spondylitis: possible role of a novel sequence in pullulanase of *Klebsiella pneumoniae*. *FEBS Letts* 1995; 369: 243–8.

30 Finegold SM, Sutter VL, Sugihara PT *et al*. Fecal microbial flora in Seventh Day Adventist populations and control subjects. *Am J Clin Nut* 1977; 30: 1781–92.

31 Garcia-Latorre EA, Dominguez-Lopez ML, Jimenez-Zamudio LA *et al*. Cellular immune response to different antigenic fractions to *Klebsiella pneumoniae* in ankylosing spondylitis. *Ninth International Congress Immunology*, San Francisco 1995, Abstract Vol. 165.

32 Hunter T, Harding GKM, Kaprove RE *et al*. Fecal carriage of various *Klebsiella* and *Enterobacter* species in patients with active ankylosing spondylitis. *Arthritis Rheum* 1981; 24: 106–8.

33 Husby G, Tsuchiya N, Schwimmbeck PL *et al*. Crossreactive epitope with *Klebsiella pneumoniae* nitrogenase in articular tissue of HLA-B27 positive patients with ankylosing spondylitis. *Arthritis Rheum* 1989; 32: 437–45.

34 Khan MA, Kushner I, Braun WE. Comparison of the clinical features of HLA-B27 positive and negative patients with ankylosing spondylitis. *Arthritis Rheum* 1977; 20: 909–12.

35 Khan MA. Genetics of HLA-B27. *Br J Rheumatol* 1988; 27(Suppl. 2): 6–11.

36 Kjeldsen-Kragh J, Rashid T, Dybwad A *et al*. Decrease in anti-*Proteus mirabilis* but not anti-*Escherichia coli* antibody levels in rheumatoid arthritis patients treated with fasting and a one year vegetarian diet. *Ann Rheum Dis* 1995; 54: 221–4.

37 Kono DH, Ogasawara M, Effros RB *et al*. Ye-1, a monoclonal antibody that crossreacts with HLA-B27 lymphoblastoid cell lines and an arthritis causing bacteria. *Clin Exp Immunol* 1985; 61: 503–8.

38 Kuberski TT, Morse HG, Rate RG *et al*. Increased recovery of *Klebsiella* from the gastrointestinal tract of Reiter's syndrome and ankylosing spondylitis patients. *Br J Rheumatol* 1983; 22(Suppl. 2): 85–90.

39 Lamm ME. Cellular aspects of immunoglobulin A. *Adv Immunol* 1976; 22: 223–90.

40 Lauhio A, Leirisalo-Repo M, Lahdevirta J *et al*. Double-blind, placebo-controlled study of three-month treatment with lymecycline in reactive arthritis, with special reference to *Chlamydia* arthritis. *Arthritis Rheum* 1991; 34: 6–14.

41 Mackiewicz A, Khan MA, Reynolds TL *et al*. Serum IgA and acute phase proteins in ankylosing spondylitis. *Ann Rheum Dis* 1989; 48: 99–103.

42 Mäki-Ikola O, Lehtinen K, Granfors K *et al*. Bacterial antibodies in ankylosing spondylitis. *Clin Exp Immunol* 1991; 84: 472–5.

43 Martini GA, Brandes JW. Increased consumption of refined carbohydrates in patients with Crohn's disease. *Klin Wschr Berlin* 1976; 54: 367–71.

44 Mayberry JF, Rhodes J, Hughes LE. Incidence of Crohn's disease in Cardiff between 1934 and 1977. *Gut* 1979; 20: 602–8.

45 Mayberry JF, Rhodes J, Newcombe RG. Breakfast and dietary aspects of Crohn's disease. *BMJ* 1978; ii: 1401.

46 McKenzie H, Main J, Pennington CR *et al*. Antibodies to selected strain of *Saccharomyces cerevisiae* (baker's and brewer's yeast) and *Candida albicans* in Crohn's disease. *Gut* 1990; 31: 536–8.

47 McNeil NI, Bingham S, Cole TJ *et al*. Diet and health of people with an ileostomy. 2. Ileostomy function and nutritional state. *Br J Nutr* 1982; 47: 407–15.

48 Mielants H, Veys EM, Cuveleir C *et al*. Ileocolonoscopic findings in seronegative spondyloarthropathies. *Br J Rheumatol* 1988; 27(Suppl. 2): 95–105.

49 O'Mahony S, Anderson N, Nuki G *et al*. Systemic and mucosal antibodies to *Klebsiella* in patients with ankylosing spondylitis and Crohn's disease. *Ann Rheum Dis* 1992; 51: 1296–300.

50 Ogasawara M, Kono DH, Yu DTY. Mimicry of human histocompatibility HLA-B27 antigen by *Klebsiella pneumoniae*. *Infect Immun* 1986; 51: 901–8.

51 Rogers P, Hassan J, Bresnihan B *et al*. Antibodies to *Proteus* in rheumatoid arthritis. *Br J Rheumatol* 1988; 27(Suppl. II): 90–4.

52 Sahly H, Podschum R, Sass R *et al*. Serum antibodies to *Klebsiella* capsular polysaccharides in ankylosing spondylitis. *Arthritis Rheum* 1994; 37: 754–9.

53 Schwimmbeck PL, Yu DTY, Oldstone MBA. Autoantibodies to HLA-B27 in the sera of HLA-B27 patients with ankylosing spondylitis and Reiter's syndrome: molecular mimicry with *Klebsiella pneumoniae* as potential mechanism of autoimmune disease. *J Exp Med* 1987; 166: 173–81.

54 Senior B, McBride P, Morley K *et al*. The detection of raised levels of IgM to *Proteus mirabilis* in sera from patients with rheumatoid arthritis. *J Med Microbiol* 1995; 43: 176–84.

55 Shodjai-Moradi F, Ebringer A, Abuljadayel I. IgA antibody response to *Klebsiella* in ankylosing spondylitis measured by immunoblotting. *Ann Rheum Dis* 1992; 51: 233–7.

56 Tabaqchali S, O'Donoghue DP, Bettelheim KA. *Escherichia coli* antibodies in patients with Crohn's disease. *Gut* 1978; 19: 108–13.

57 Takeuchi F, Kosuge E, Matsuta K *et al*. Antibody to a specific HLA-DRB1 sequence in Japanese patients with rheumatoid arthritis. *Arthritis Rheum* 1990; 33: 1867–8.

58 Tani Y, Tiwana H, Hukuda S *et al*. Antibodies to *Klebsiella*, *Proteus*, and HLA-B27 peptides in Japanese patients with ankylosing spondylitis and rheumatoid arthritis. *J Rheumatol* 1997; 24: 109–14.

59 Tanka K, Wilks M, Coates PJ *et al*. *Mycobacterium paratuberculosis* and Crohn's disease. *Gut* 1991; 32: 43–5.

60 Thomson GTD, Alfa M, Orr K *et al*. Humoral immune response to bacterial lipopolysaccharide in adult idiopathic spondyloarthropathies. *American College of Rheumatology: 57th Annual Meeting*, San Antonio, 1993. Abstract Vol: 5224, C218.

61 Tiwana H, Walmsley RS, Wilson C *et al*. Characterisation of the humoral immune response to *Klebsiella* species in inflammatory bowel disease and ankylosing spondylitis. *Br J Rheumatol* 1998; 37: 525–31.

62 Tiwana H, Wilson C, Walmsley RS *et al*. Antibody response to gut bacteria in ankylosing spondylitis. Rheumatoid arthritis, Crohn's disease and ulcerative colitis. *Rheumatol Int* 1997; 17: 11–16.

63 Trull AK, Ebringer A, Panayi GS *et al*. HLA-B27 and immune response to enterobacterial antigens in ankylosing spondylitis. *Clin Exp Immunol* 1984; 55: 74–80.

64 Trull AK, Ebringer R, Panayi GS *et al*. IgA antibodies to *Klebsiella pneumoniae* in ankylosing spondylitis. *Scand J Rheumatol* 1983; 12: 249–53.

65 Van Bohemen CHG, Grumet FC, Zamen HV. Identification of HLA-B27 M1 and M2 cross-reactive antigens in *Klebsiella*, *Shigella* and *Yersinia*. *Immunology* 1984; 52: 607–9.

66 Veys EM, Van Laere M. Serum IgG, IgM and IgA levels in ankylosing spondylitis. *Ann Rheum Dis* 1977; 32: 493–6.

67 Welsh J, Avakian H, Cowling P *et al*. HLA-B27 and *Klebsiella*. I. Crossreactivity studies with rabbit antisera. *Br J Exp Pathol* 1980; 61: 85–91.

68 Wensinck F. The faecal flora of patients with Crohn's disease. *Antonie van Leeuwenhoek* 1975; 41: 214–15.

69 Wilson C, Ebringer A, Ahmadi K *et al*. Shared amino acid sequences between major histocompatibility complex class II glycoproteins, type XI collagen and *Proteus mirabilis* in rheumatoid arthritis. *Ann Rheum Dis* 1995; 54: 216–20.

70 Wilson C, Thakore A, Isenberg D *et al*. Correlation between antibodies and isolation rates of *Proteus mirabilis* in rheumatoid arthritis. *Rheum Int* 1997; 16: 187–9.

Section F Other Organs

Chapter 56

Food sensitivity: the kidney and bladder

D. Sandberg

INTRODUCTION

Of the organ systems referred to in this book, the kidney has been most subjected to investigation of immunological mechanisms of disease. A majority of these studies have focused on reactions to microorganisms, self antigens, tumour antigens, drugs, etc. There has been only slight interest in a possible role of food components as sensitizing agents. In part this reflects the lack of adequate published data suggesting such a link. Some of the renal disorders in which immune mechanisms appear to play an important role are shown in Table 56.1.[2,14,30,31]

Perhaps the clearest published reports suggesting a relationship of food allergy to renal disease are those of Matsumura's group in Japan and our group's studies of food sensitivity in childhood nephrosis.[33,35,49,50] We have also studied a small number of children with the nephrotic syndrome associated with membranous glomerulonephropathy and anaphylactoid purpura nephritis. Williams recently reviewed the subject of allergy and the kidney and could find no other information implicating food allergy in renal disease except in nephrosis and anaphylactoid purpura nephritis.[61]

The lower urinary tract and bladder have also been investigated for a possible role of allergy, and specifically of food sensitivity as a cause of recurrent and chronic symptoms such as frequency, dysuria, enuresis, etc.[3–5,9,12,17,38,47,52,63] In addition, haematuria and interstitial and eosinophilic cystitis have characteristics suggesting a relationship to environmental sensitivities.[22,23] There is substantial clinical evidence, collected over many years, which suggests that in some individuals allergy, and specifically food sensitivity, may be a significant factor in the aetiology of these symptoms.

FOOD SENSITIVITY AND THE KIDNEY

There is general agreement among nephrologists that immunological mechanisms play a major role in many diseases involving the kidney. Post-streptococcal glomerulonephritis and serum sickness are prototypes of disease processes involving renal injury by humoral and/or cellular immune mechanisms. These disorders have been studied in great detail both in humans and in animal models. Extension of those studies has identified a number of other diffuse disease processes in which immunological mechanisms appear to be related to renal tissue injury.[2,14,31]

Through study of these various diseases, it has become evident that the entire range of pathophysiological immune mechanisms may be involved, including IgE-mediated processes. A considerable part of what is known about immune mechanisms in disease has been learned through study of those renal disorders in which hypersensitivity plays a role.

Minimal change disease nephrosis

Of those kidney disorders investigated, childhood nephrosis is the disease most clearly identified as having foods as precipitating factors. This association has been reported by Matsumura and coworkers in Japan, Laurent and coworkers and by our group.[26,27,33,35,49,50] Triggering of nephrotic relapses by inhaled allergens had previously been reported to occur in a minority of individuals with minimal change disease (MCD).[49,61] More recently

Renal disorders in which immune mechanisms play a role
Glomerulonephritis, various types
Goodpasture's syndrome
Systemic lupus erythematosus
Nephrotic syndrome
IgA nephropathy
Proteinuria

Table 56.1 Renal disorders in which immune mechanisms play a role.

this has been noted by others.[10,24,25,44] However, other investigators have questioned an aetiological relationship between allergy and the nephrotic syndrome, although accepting that childhood nephrosis occurs more frequently in atopic than in non-atopic individuals.[8,36]

Nephrotic syndrome

The nephrotic syndrome is the most frequent presentation of persistent glomerular disease in the paediatric age group.[18] It occurs more frequently in children than in adults.

Histopathology

The predominant histopathological lesion in children is MCD, although when the nephrotic syndrome presents in older children, the likelihood increases that it may be associated with another histological lesion. In biopsies from patients with minimal change type of childhood nephrosis, only very slight abnormalities can be recognized under light microscopy and immunofluorescence microscopy does not demonstrate immunoglobulin or complement deposition in the kidney (Fig. 56.1). There is also no evidence of an inflammatory response in the kidney. A report of deposition of IgE in the glomerulus has not been confirmed.[49] Approximately 10% of children with nephrotic syndrome have focal segmental glomerular sclerosis. If extensive, this change reflects a poorer prognosis. It is not clear that this is a distinct subset rather than the extreme of severity of the disease process.

Response to prednisone therapy

This is so consistent in MCD that induction of remission with prednisone provides sufficient support for the clinical diagnosis. Renal biopsy is not considered necessary in most children with MCD (Fig. 56.2). The decrease in weight associated with diuresis and the decrease in protein excretion after approximately 1–4 weeks of therapy are indicative of a good clinical response with induction of remission. Biopsy is reserved for patients who do not respond, older children or adults who may have other disease processes, and children whose course is complicated by frequent relapses and poor control with prednisone leading to consideration

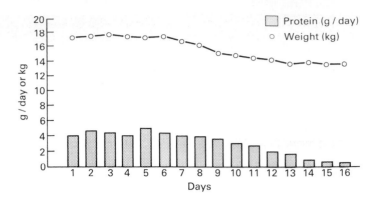

Fig. 56.2 Result of prednisone therapy for an initial episode of minimal change nephrotic syndrome.

of immunosuppressive therapy with ciclophosphamide or other cytotoxic drugs.

Inhalant allergy and minimal change disease

Many years ago association in an adult of MCD and pollen sensitivity was described by Hardwicke and coworkers.[19] In that patient immunotherapy appeared to induce prolonged remission. Subsequently other investigators reported coexistence of nephrosis with allergy.[10,49] More recently still, Laurent and coworkers have reported similar patients with nephrosis and relapse associated with inhaled allergens such as house dust, pollen and cat dander.[24,25] Reeves *et al.* have documented a seasonal pattern of nephrotic syndrome.[44] In Soothill's group, Thompson demonstrated an incidence of atopic disease in children with steroid-responsive nephrotic syndrome twice that of a group of age-matched controls.[54] Meadow and colleagues have noted a similar relationship with steroid-responsive nephrosis and atopy, although they did not find a relationship between atopic status and tendency to relapse.[36]

Further adding to the confusion, therapy with antihistamines, sodium cromoglycate or doxantrazole has been shown to be ineffective in preventing relapse.[10] Levinsky and coworkers demonstrated the presence of unusual circulating immune complex-like particles in patients with nephrosis.[28] Moorthy and colleagues[37] and Eyres and coworkers[13] have provided data suggesting involvement of the cellular immune system in MCD. Shaloub has proposed that minimal change nephrotic syndrome is caused by abnormal T cell function.[51] Further supporting evidence for a role for allergy or hypersensitivity in MCD includes reports that a variety of environmental substances, including drugs, insect stings, poison ivy etc., have triggered relapses.[49] In Soothill's group, Trompeter has also reported an association of short time to relapse after ciclophosphamide treatment with an increased frequency of HLA B12 in steroid-responsive nephrotic syndrome in children[55] (Table 56.2). An association with atopy was not shown. No significant differences were observed in incidence of atopic history, elevated serum total IgE concentration, positive prick tests for grass pollen or house dust mite or elevated serum IgE antibody to those two antigens. This is consistent with the view that a non-IgE-related mechanism for food sensitivity is involved in this disease process.[55] Florido *et al.* have reported a relationship of relapse to episodes of seasonal allergic respiratory symptoms.[15] Although substantial data have accumulated linking allergy to childhood nephrosis, it has not been clear whether the relation-

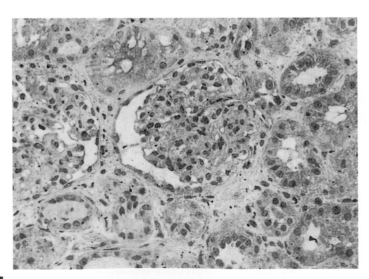

Fig. 56.1 Haematoxylin and eosin stain of a renal biopsy from a 3-year-old. WM, with minimal change nephrotic syndrome (×100). The essentially normal appearance of the glomeruli is evident.

Frequency of HLA B12 and relation with atopic features in children with steroid-responsive nephrotic syndrome						
	Group A		Group B		Combined		British blood donors
	+	−	+	−	+	−	+
HLA B12	54	46	44	56	50	50	24
Atopic history	37	3	15	32	29	16	
Total IgE > 150 U	48	13	17	32	34	24	

Values are percentages. Group A consisted of 71 children who were consecutive outpatients; group B comprised 72 of 81 children treated with ciclophosphamide. All were in remission and off treatment. Twenty-seven of group B were included previously in group A, while 45 were a new series not previously evaluated for HLA type and atopy.

Table 56.2 Frequency of HLA B12 and relation with atopic features in children with steroid-responsive nephrotic syndrome.[55]

ship is a direct one or whether the relationship is between allergy and the tendency to relapse.

Food sensitivity

Matsumura and his group reported in 1961 and again in 1971 results of clinical studies of a large number of children with nephrosis who were shown to have sensitivity to foods and in whom the use of limited diets was apparently helpful in achieving prolonged remission of their disease.[33,35] They also reported an association of food sensitivity with postural proteinuria (see below). In 1977, our group reported studies of six children with frequently relapsing steroid-dependent MCD in whom cow's milk sensitivity was associated with relapse.[50] We subsequently described further studies in the same children and investigation of an additional group of 13 children.[49] Richards and coworkers in 1977 described a girl who had nephrosis as well as a history of asthma, eczema and urticaria who appeared to have relapsed on ingestion of chicken eggs.[45] Lagrue and his colleagues[23a] have reported results of study of the human basophil degranulation test (HBDT) to investigate food sensitivity in 34 patients with MCD nephrosis. Five food allergens were used: wheat, milk, egg, beef and pork). Of the 34 patients, 64% had at least one positive test whereas a positive reaction was seen only once in a group of 19 blood donors ($P < 0.001$). Only nine showed one sensitization; eight reacted to two and three to three foods. All five foods were found to be reactive in multiple patients; this included five patients reactive to egg, six to milk and beef, and nine to wheat and pork. The HBDT was positive whether patients were in relapse or remission, whether on or off corticosteroid therapy, and whether serum IgE was elevated or not. There was little correlation between standard skin tests, radioallergosorbent tests (RAST) and HBDT.

Matsumura's group of patients with nephrosis is of importance to our understanding since they were not selected for a pattern of frequent relapse. In contrast, the children studied in Miami had had numerous relapses requiring frequent administration of prednisone or had been treated with an immunosuppressive agent such as cyclophosphamide.[49,50] Matsumura reported a high degree of successful control of the nephrosis in his patients using limited diets. Evidence of food sensitivity was obtained in those patients by individual oral food challenges.

Milk allergy and relapsing minimal change disease

The six children with frequently relapsing steroid-responsive MCD studied in Miami[50] were shown to be sensitive to cow's milk by intradermal titration skin testing and by *in vivo* alteration of plasma C3 complement using crossed immunoelectrophoresis. Oral challenge with cow's milk provoked relapse in five patients. Fig. 56.3 indicates one patient's response to challenge with cow's milk. The changes in protein excretion following milk ingestion were dramatic. Transient changes in serum IgG and IgM were also demonstrated. One girl did not relapse when prednisone was discontinued, although she had required intermittent, frequent prednisone therapy for several years because of relapse whenever prednisone was discontinued previously. Subsequently, 13 more children with steroid-dependent MCD were studied and reported in 1984,[48] as well as further studies of three of the original group. All 19 had had persistent disease; in nine treatment with cytotoxic drugs was undertaken because of inadequate control with prednisone or undesirable side effects of the latter drug. In 17 children, sensitivity to one or more foods was documented. Although these patients were not selected because of a history of allergic disease, seven had asthma, four eczema, one allergic rhinitis and one chronic urticaria. Thirteen of 19 children had positive intradermal skin tests to one or more foods. One child was unresponsive to prednisone; however, he responded well to diet restriction and food extract injections, with good control of his nephrosis. Although our initial report documented provocation of relapse with cow's milk, all but two patients who could not be adequately evaluated were found to be sensitive to multiple foods.

Study protocol

The study protocol consisted of discontinuance of prednisone while in remission, and admission to the Clinical Research Center when relapse occurred. Vivonex, a chemically defined formula feed, was provided as the sole diet and, following decrease in proteinuria, oral challenge with cow's milk was carried out. Urinary 24-h protein excretion, weight and fluid intake and output were monitored daily. Four patients developed increased proteinuria while on Vivonex. Protein excretion decreased in those patients when another limited diet or spring water was substituted for the Vivonex.[49,50] Eleven of the 19 patients were treated with food

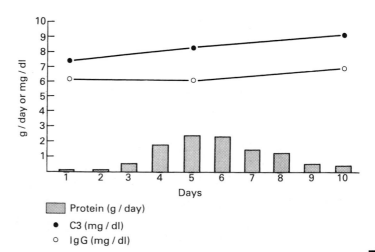

Fig. 56.3 Effect of milk ingestion on protein excretion in a child with minimal change nephrotic syndrome. The solid bars depict values for 24-hour protein excretion.

extracts either subcutaneously or sublingually, in addition to limited diets. In some instances, patients were also tested for inhaled allergens and, when appropriate, were given immunotherapy for those antigens to which they had positive reactions.

Long-term follow up: case histories

Long-term follow up of three of the original six patients has been possible (Table 56.3). One boy had no further relapses and no further need for prednisone. He was treated with a limited diet

and food extract injections twice weekly for several months; after that period, other foods were gradually added to his diet after skin testing. When skin tests were positive, he was treated subcutaneously or sublingually with the appropriate food extract, and later that food was included in his diet. Treatment was discontinued after 2 years without subsequent recurrence of the nephrotic syndrome and with maintenance of normal urine and plasma laboratory values.

The two other boys had a few brief relapses lasting a few days which were either associated with acute infections or lapses in their restricted diets. The last relapse noted was at age 16 years in one and at age 19 years in the other. All three individuals are now on normal diets. Table 56.4 shows results of the last laboratory values obtained on four of the six patients.

Long-term follow up was also available for six other patients with MCD. Two had no subsequent relapses; one had two relapses and then none thereafter, but did develop a chronic anaemia of uncertain aetiology. Table 56.5 shows the results of the most recent laboratory values in these six patients. One (THo) had early evidence of renal failure at that time, while values for the other five individuals were within normal limits. Two boys continued to have relapses, one in spite of careful diet and environmental control, and food and inhalant injection therapy.

In 1985, Howanietz and Lubec described a single female child who developed nephrotic syndrome at age 22 months.[21] She had

Studies of food sensitivity in nephrosis. Long-term follow-up of three children with minimal change disease			
Patients	Number of significant relapses	Prednisone therapy*	Other problems
EN	2	2	None
JR	1	1	None
TN	0	0	None

*Number of relapses since beginning management for food sensitivity which required prednisone therapy.

Table 56.3 Studies of food sensitivity in nephrosis. Long-term follow-up of three children with minimal change disease.

Studies of food sensitivity in nephrosis. Laboratory values with long-term follow up of four children with minimal change disease					
Patients	Protein excretion (mg/24 h)	Albumin TP/albumin (mg/dl)	Cholesterol (mg/dl)	IgG (mg/dl)	BUN/creatinine (mg/dl)
EN	80	7.2/4.8	—	950	14/0.9
JR	45	6.9/4.3	—	1150	16/1.1
TN	35	7.8/5.2	190	1260	14/1.1
JM*	40	7.2/4.9	205	920	11/0.8

*This patient did not relapse when prednisone was discontinued. BUN, blood urea nitrogen; TP, total protein.

Table 56.4 Studies of food sensitivity in nephrosis. Laboratory values with long-term follow up of four children with minimal change disease.

Studies of food sensitivity in nephrosis. Laboratory values with long-term follow up of six of 19 patients with MCD*					
Patients	Protein excretion (mg/24 h)	TP/albumin (mg/dl)	Cholesterol (mg/dl)	IgG (mg/dl)	BUN/creatinine (mg/dl)
VL	40	6.2/3.9	201	800	7/0.8
YB	65	7.3/4.2	165	940	9/0.8
TL	195	5.6/3.4	187	695	9/0.4
TW	60	6.2/3.8	230	580	13/0.8
THo†	1800	5.4/3.2	330	410	27/1.2
TH	35	6.8/4.5	181	1130	10/0.6

* These values were obtained from a recent follow up visit. † These values were representative of the status before dialysis and transplantation. TP, total protein; BUN, blood urea nitrogen.

Table 56.5 Studies of food sensitivity in nephrosis. Laboratory values with long-term follow up of six of 19 patients with MCD*.

a history of vomiting after ingestion of egg at age 6 months. Corticosteroid therapy produced prompt resolution of the nephrosis. She developed a relapse while on continued low dose corticosteroid therapy. Biopsy showed MCD. She was treated for 2 months with cyclophosphamide and was in remission. After eating a meal containing fish she became ill, with oedema of eyelids, vomiting and abdominal 'sensations' and had an appendectomy. Some years later she was evaluated in the author's institution outpatient department and found to have hypoproteinaemia with proteinuria ranging between 2 and 5 g/24 h. Serum total IgE levels on two occasions were 380 and 110 kU/l. There was no history of skin, intestinal or respiratory symptoms but she had an aversion to fish and pork. She was on corticosteroid therapy at the time. After fish and pork were excluded from her diet, she developed complete remission and corticosteroid therapy was discontinued. She remained in remission until the following year when she ate a schoolmate's lunch containing pork and bread. By the following day she had developed proteinuria (10 g/24 h) and her serum total IgE was 540 kU/l. Corticosteroid therapy was started, with remission within some days. Proteinuria had not recurred at the time of submission of the report.

Association of enteropathy with steroidnephrotic syndrome

In 1987, Genova and colleagues studied 12 children, aged 4–16 years, with steroid-resistant nephrotic syndrome with history suggestive of food intolerance (diarrhoea, atopic dermatitis or failure to thrive).[16] Duration of the nephrotic syndrome ranged from 9 months to 3.5 years. Corticosteroid and/or cyclophosphamide therapy had not induced complete remission. Histological findings were mesangioproliferative glomerulonephritis (nine patients) with progression to focal sclerosis in two of those individuals, and membranoproliferative glomerulonephritis in one patient. Two patients had elevated serum total IgE levels. Positive RAST to one or more food extracts were noted in six of the 12 children, and positive skin prick tests to one or more foods were found in four of the six children. While xylose absorption tests were within normal limits in all 12 patients, intestinal mucosal biopsies in 10 of 12 showed what was described as massive submucosal lymphocytic infiltration, sometimes epithelial, on light microscopic examination. They also described irregular villous shortening in six cases and in three of six reduced villus:crypt ratios. Immunofluorescence detected fibrinogen deposits in submucosa and in extravillous sites. Two children had positive faecal occult blood. These investigators interpreted these findings as evidence of inflammation resulting from a local immune response. The authors used an oligoantigenic exclusion diet in the 12 children, planned to ensure adequate nutrition and protein intake. In four patients, proteinuria decreased and the nephrotic syndrome improved within 1 month of dietary therapy. In two other children remission occurred later and became complete only after further exclusion of tomato and ham. After 4–6 months on diets, food challenge tests were begun with reintroduction of each food for 7 days before adding another food. In three patients there was immediate recurrence of proteinuria, especially with milk. Repeat jejunal biopsy in the six patients who responded showed improvement in pre-diet histopathology in five of the six children.

Laurent and coworkers have described six children with minimal change nephrotic syndrome in whom they documented a relationship to allergy and, more specifically, to sensitivity to foods, who responded to treatment of their allergic problems

with sustained remission.[27] The patient described in detail had a history of two episodes of asthmatic bronchitis. At the age of 25 months he had onset of typical moderately severe nephrotic syndrome which responded to corticosteroid therapy with complete remission in some days. The dose was very gradually reduced over 15 months. Subsequently, after 8 months without treatment, two relapses occurred at 6-month intervals, both episodes responding quickly to corticosteroid therapy. Thirteen months later, after 1 year without therapy, he developed a milder more chronic proteinuria with only mild signs of nephrotic syndrome. The proteinuria continued at about 2–3 g/24 h over the next 4 months. During that time he was not treated with corticosteroids. At the same time he had intermittent rhinitis and conjunctivitis. He was also noted to have a history of distaste for milk products for some years. He then had a medical evaluation which demonstrated positive skin tests for house dust, grass pollens, wheat, milk, eggs and potato. Serum total IgE concentration was 343 IU/l and RASTs were positive (class III) for grass pollens and wheat. Basophil histamine release tests (HBDT) were positive for house dust and mite extracts, grass pollens, cat and dog extracts, chicken, ovalbumin, pork, carrot and *Candida* extracts. He was then treated with ketotifen orally, nasal cromolyn sodium, as well as a diet excluding gluten, cow's milk, eggs, potato, chicken and carrot. Proteinuria disappeared after 4 days, and did not recur with reintroduction into the diet of gluten or cow's milk. Addition of potato was associated with some episodes of transitory proteinuria. Subsequently adding other excluded foods did not provoke proteinuria or relapse although transient proteinuria was observed after occasional meals eaten outside the home when there were lapses in his careful dietary controls. Throughout this period, consumption of eggs, potato and chicken were limited and cow's milk remained excluded from the diet. During the next year, he did not require further treatment with corticosteroids and remained free of symptoms and signs of relapse. The authors then evaluated 26 other patients with idiopathic nephrotic syndrome for a possible role of food sensitivity in their disorder. They found six patients, ranging in age from 4 months to 20 years, in whom complete remission occurred with treatment with limited diets. Foods identified as triggers included milk, wheat or gluten, eggs, chicken, pork and beef. Remission with corticosteroid therapy was observed for periods ranging from 1 to 5 years. They then evaluated 13 patients with idiopathic nephrotic syndrome, after failure of corticosteroid therapy, using an oligoantigenic diet comprising five or six foods for 10–15 days. Diets were selected based on testing as previously described. Eight of this group had a previous history of allergic problems: six had elevated serum total IgE concentration. Positive RASTs were found in five, with positive intradermal skin tests in another five patients. Positive histamine release tests were found in 11 of 13 patients. During the diet trials, proteinuria disappeared in five and was reduced by more than 50% in four patients . In eight of nine individuals, protein excretion returned to the previous abnormal range with reintroduction of their usual diet. In the ninth patient, remission of proteinuria continued with maintenance of a limited diet. The response to a limited diet was repeated during subsequent relapses. In another patient in whom the diet could not be repeated, administration of cromolyn sodium (300 mg before meals three times daily) for 10 days during three relapses produced reductions in proteinuria from 15 to 3–4 g/24 h with increase in proteinuria after discontinuation of treatment.

Diet in adult idiopathic nephrotic syndrome

In 1987, Laurent and colleagues also carried out similar studies in 13 adults with idiopathic nephrotic syndrome.[26] These individuals had not responded well to corticosteroid therapy. Characteristics of these patients were similar to those of the children described above. The authors identified food sensitivity by skin tests (five), RAST (five) and HBDT (11). They noted reduced proteinuria in all 13 individuals after a 10-day period eating an oligoantigenic diet (typically one each of a meat, 'carbohydrate', vegetable and fruit). Foods positive on tests were excluded. Response was considered as a decrease in protein excretion of more than 50% below initial levels of excretion. This occurred in nine of the 13 patients (complete remission was seen in five cases). Decrease in excretion was not seen until patients had been on the diets for 1 week. Median protein excretion at the start and end of study were 10 and 1 g/day, respectively. Of nine individuals in remission after the diet, eight relapsed soon after the diet was stopped. In three cases, restarting a limited diet resulted in remission. The authors concluded from this study that they would begin to use the diet for management of future adult patients with idiopathic nephrotic syndrome.

Gastrointestinal candidiasis

These patients are at risk from gastrointestinal colonization with *Candida albicans* as a result of chronic prednisone therapy as well as frequent antibiotic treatment, and are prone to hypersensitivity. It is possible that C. *albicans* could serve as an allergen to which such patients are chronically exposed. This could explain why some children with MCD develop a pattern of frequent relapses and why evaluation and treatment of food and inhaled allergen sensitivity does not explain persistent disease in some patients. Truss has suggested that the known capacity of C. *albicans* for altering the immune system can lead to multiple food sensitivities through interference with immunoregulation.[56-58]

Membranous glomerulonephropathy

A role for food sensitivity in membranous glomerulonephropathy (MG) and the nephritis associated with anaphylactoid purpura has been reported.[49] Close study of a small number of patients suggests that such a relationship exists; however, further confirmation is needed through study of more patients with these disorders.

Histopathology

MG is an uncommon cause of the nephrotic syndrome in children; it is somewhat more frequent in older children and adults. The histopathological lesion comprises minimal mesangial proliferation and hypertrophy of glomerular epithelial cells. The glomerular capillary walls are thickened by diffuse subepithelial deposits (Fig. 56.4). Immunofluorescence staining of these deposits usually indicates the presence of IgG and, less commonly, IgA and IgM; in addition, complement components are commonly present.[31]

Clinical features

This disorder is usually associated with a mild nephrotic syndrome, although occasionally the process will be severe and chronic and may progress to renal failure.[2,39] It has not been shown that therapy with corticosteroids or other immunosuppressive drugs alters the course of this disease process. Its variable clini-

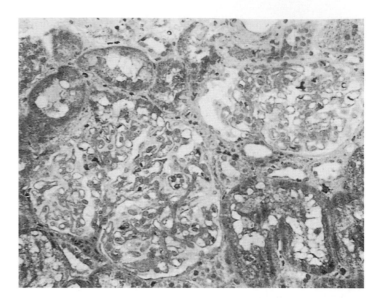

Fig. 56.4 Haematoxylin and eosin stain of a renal biopsy from a child with membranous glomerulonephropathy and the nephrotic syndrome (×100). The diffuse deposits along the glomerular capillary basement membrane are clearly visible.

cal expression makes it difficult to evaluate response to a specific therapy.

The immune deposits have been considered to be immune complexes. The subepithelial site of deposition suggests that these complexes are small. A variety of antigens have been demonstrated to be present in a few patients with concomitant diseases such as hepatitis B or malignancy.[49] In addition, MG has been associated with other infections such as syphilis and streptococcal disease, and with sickle cell disease and lupus erythematosus.

This renal lesion has also been related to reactions to some medications, i.e. troxidone (trimethadione, penicillamine, gold etc.). So far food or inhaled allergens have not been detected in immune deposits or circulating immune complexes from these patients.

Food allergens

In a study of three children, aged 13–15 years, with MG[49] and asthma (one had atopic dermatitis), all were demonstrated to be sensitive to multiple foods both by oral challenge and intradermal skin testing. They were also demonstrated to have acute *in vivo* alteration of plasma C3 following oral milk challenge. It was possible in all three to show increased protein excretion after ingestion of cow's milk as well as other foods. Figure 56.5 depicts changes in protein excretion and body weight after successive challenges with milk in one female patient.[49] It also shows the decrease in proteinuria and oedema indicated by decrease in body weight when she was taking only Vivonex.

Two of the children showed an excellent response to treatment using some diet limitation and food and inhalant extract injection therapy; with long-term follow up, both are free of demonstrable renal disease at this time although neither have allowed repeated renal biopsy. One of the two is still on weekly injections for inhaled allergens and a milk product-free diet. The third patient had more severe and chronic renal disease from the onset. She did not respond adequately to treatment, eventually developed renal failure and required renal transplantation. Table 56.6 shows lab-

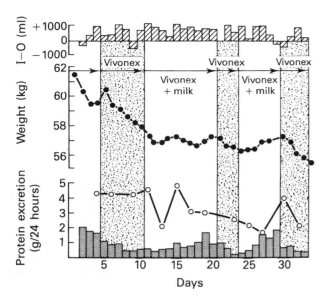

Fig. 56.5 Changes in weight, net water balance and protein excretion during dietary changes in a patient with the nephrotic syndrome associated with membranous glomerulopathy. I–O = 24-hour fluid intake minus urine output. g/24 hours = protein excretion during a 24-hour period. (From Sandberg et al.,[49] courtesy of Charles C. Thomas, Springfield, Illinois.)

oratory values obtained after long-term remission of the nephrotic syndrome in two patients and shows continued presence of the nephrotic syndrome in the third patient.

Anaphylactoid purpura nephritis

Anaphylactoid purpura involves the skin, gastrointestinal tract, joints and kidney. The incidence of renal involvement has been variously estimated at 22–70% (25% is a generally accepted figure). The nephropathy is an important component since prognosis of the disease is related to the severity of the renal lesion. In fact, the severity of skin, gastrointestinal and joint involvement has no apparent relationship to severity of the kidney disease. Renal manifestations include gross or microscopic haematuria, proteinuria and occasionally renal failure. Approximately 50% of patients develop the nephrotic syndrome, but it may also be a presenting manifestation.

Family history of allergy

There is a strong history of allergy in approximately 25% of patients, and recurrent bouts of acute nephrotic syndrome apparently related to food allergy have been described.[49] Other

reported associated factors include medications, immunizations, tuberculosis and insect stings. There is a tendency to relapse. Successive episodes may be accompanied by further renal involvement, and episodes of acute nephrotic syndrome may occur in the absence of other manifestations of anaphylactoid purpura.

Laboratory findings

There are no characteristic laboratory abnormalities in anaphylactoid purpura. Serum C3 concentrations are usually normal but decreased concentration of C4, C5 and C3PA have been reported, suggesting activation of the alternative pathway. Cryoglobulinaemia has been reported; these cryoglobulins contained predominantly IgA. An increased incidence of demonstrable circulating antibody to bovine proteins with simultaneous presence of circulating bovine globulin and casein antigen have also been noted. Immunohistological studies reveal predominantly mesangial deposits of IgA and, to a lesser extent, fibrinogen, complement, IgG and IgM. These suggest an immune complex pathogenesis. In general, this syndrome is a benign, self-limiting disorder; long-term prognosis is almost entirely related to renal involvement.

Histopathology

The predominant renal lesion observed is a focal and segmental proliferative glomerulonephritis. Other lesions described include minimal change, focal and segmental endocapillary glomerulonephritis, diffuse endocapillary proliferation and membranoproliferative glomerulonephritis. Treatment is considered to have no influence on the course of the renal disease.

Food sensitivity: case histories
Case I

We have reported food sensitivity in two patients with nephrotic syndrome related to anaphylactoid purpura nephritis.[49] Renal biopsy was obtained from both children, and showed severe nephritis in one and moderately severe nephritis in the other. In the latter patient, renal biopsy showed crescent formation in over 50% of glomeruli in the specimen (Fig. 56.6). The renal lesion, as indicated by this biopsy, was very severe with a high probability of subsequent development of renal failure. The patient was found to have widespread sensitivity to foods as well as to inhaled allergens and various chemical agents. He was maintained on rigid environmental control in the home and a meticulous limited diet with food and inhalant extract injections for approximately 4 years. The strict regimen was gradually relaxed and he is presently living a relatively normal

Studies of food sensitivity in nephrosis. Follow up of three patients with membranous glomerulonephropathy					
Patients	**Protein excretion (mg/24 h)**	**TP/albumin (mg/dl)**	**Cholesterol (mg/dl)**	**IgG (mg/dl)**	**BUN/creatinine (mg/dl)**
SS	40	7.4/5.3	175	1150	12/0.8
SL	50	6.8/3.9	195	1250	10/0.8
JW*	2410	5.3/2.9	340	520	45/3.7

* These values were representative of this patient's status shortly before institution of dialysis. TP, total protein; BUN, blood urea nitrogen.

Table 56.6 Studies of food sensitivity in nephrosis. Follow up of three patients with membranous glomerulonephropathy.

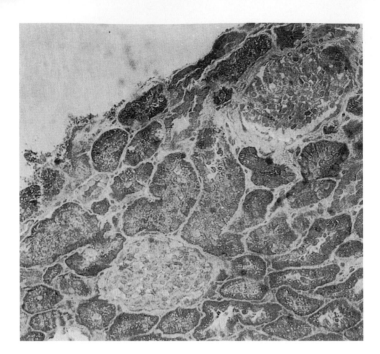

Fig. 56.6 Haematoxylin and eosin stain of a renal biopsy from a patient with severe anaphylactoid purpura nephritis and the nephrotic syndrome (×100). The glomeruli show severe injury with crescent formation.

life except for some dietary restrictions. Renal function studies have been normal except for a slightly increased 24-h urine protein excretion in the range of 300 mg/24 h. He and his parents have not consented to a second biopsy.

Case 2
The other child had a milder but chronic course with continued protein excretion in the range of 1–2 g/24 h and mild hypoproteinaemia and minimal oedema. During initial studies while taking only Vivonex, protein excretion decreased and serum IgG, C3, total protein and albumin concentrations increased towards normal. Oral challenge with cow's milk caused an increase in protein excretion to 2.4 g/24 h, which decreased after removal of milk from the diet. Urinary red blood cell excretion increased in both children after milk feeding, and decreased on Vivonex as the sole diet. Intradermal skin testing was positive to multiple food and inhaled allergens. Nephritis was undetectable after approximately 1 year and all therapy was discontinued.

Postural proteinuria
Matsumura and coworkers have reported very interesting clinical studies of food sensitivity associated with postural proteinuria.[32,34] They evaluated both orthostatic and lordotic proteinuria in 36 patients using standard clinical methods, including history, food diaries, elimination diets and challenge with individual foods.

Food challenge
The foods were tested by inclusion in the diet for 3 days in usual amounts or as a single meal with a food suspected to be the cause of postural proteinuria. They identified 72 foods as a cause of postural proteinuria in the 36 patients. Milk, egg and soya were identified 30, 20 and 17 times, respectively; pork, red beans and tuna were also found to precipitate postural proteinuria.

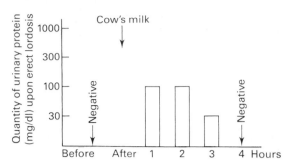

Fig. 56.7 Lordotic proteinuria resulting from administration of a single feeding of cow's milk. (From Matsumura[32] courtesy of Charles C. Thomas, Springfield, Illinois.)

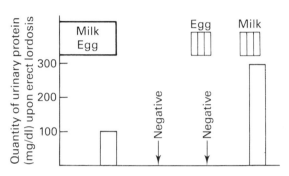

Fig. 56.8 Lordotic proteinuria resulting from successive 3-day periods of administration of egg and milk. (From Matsumura[32] courtesy of Charles C. Thomas, Springfield, Illinois.)

Frequently more than one food was identified for an individual, with one food in 14 patients, two in 12, three in six, and four in four individuals.

Other symptoms
Other associated symptoms were commonly observed, including headache, abdominal pain, fatigue and diarrhoea. Figure 56.7 shows lordotic proteinuria produced by a single feeding of cow's milk. Figure 56.8 illustrates results from 3-day challenges with milk and egg and also shows disappearance of lordotic proteinuria on a diet eliminating those foods. The sensitivity of this testing procedure allowed documentation of proteinuria after ingestion of minute amounts of an offending food.

FOOD SENSITIVITY AND THE LOWER URINARY TRACT

Recurrent cystitis and/or symptoms of dysuria, frequency, suprapubic pain or bleeding are common medical problems which have been reported by physicians and their patients for over 50 years to be triggered by environmental agents.[3–5,9,12,17,38,47,52,59,60,63] A large number of clinical observations suggest that food components may induce these problems. In many instances the urinary symptoms accompany other system involvement; however, it has also been pointed out that the urinary tract may be the sole target of an allergic reaction.

Enuresis

Enuresis, or involuntary emptying of the bladder beyond an age when bladder control should have been established, has been studied extensively and reasonable data have been obtained supporting a role for food sensitivity. In 1954, Powell and Powell reported a study of 82 women with lower urinary tract allergy.[41] They followed this paper with reports of continuing studies of allergy of the lower urinary tract.[40,42,43] These investigators could demonstrate that foods caused urinary tract symptoms in a majority of the women studied; the foods causing symptoms are shown in Table 56.7. Speer commented on his experience that milk was a common offender.[53] He also noted (as did the Powells) that black pepper was the most common triggering condiment. The authors did not provide evidence of the mechanism operating in these reactions. Specific mechanisms, in fact, have not been demonstrated in any of these studies, leaving room for doubt as to participation of immune factors in the process.

Pointers to an allergic cause

In evaluating possible allergic mechanisms of recurrent urinary tract infections, a positive history for other allergic problems in the patient and in the family may be helpful in supporting the need for further allergic study. Blood and urine eosinophilia and elevated serum total IgE concentrations may be helpful, but if not present do not rule out an allergic aetiology for the urinary tract symptoms.[20] The only valid confirming evidence is ability to provoke symptoms with specific challenges and ability to control symptoms with avoidance of incriminated substances such as foods or treatment with specific extracts in the absence of other environmental changes.

Food sensitivity

Breneman, Pastinszky, Gerrard and Crook, among others, have provided studies supporting a role for food sensitivity in evocation of lower urinary tract symptoms.[4,5,7,12,38] Bray, many years before, had noted that when children with asthma avoided food allergens to which they were sensitive, their enuresis sometimes disappeared.[3] Enuresis, of course, has other possible aetiological factors, as listed in Table 56.8. Cystoscopic findings included mucosal pallor and oedema, occasionally accompanied by bleeding. The urine may be clear or may contain red or white blood cells and, on occasion, eosinophils.

Food causing lower urinary tract symptoms in 82 women	
Food	Percentage affected
Citrus	60
Tomato	34
Condiments	20
Chocolate	15
Grape	15
Apple	9
Water melon	7

Table 56.7 Food causing lower urinary tract symptoms in 82 women.

Aetiology of enuresis
Allergy, including bladder spasm
Difficulty in arousal from deep sleep
Nocturnal diuresis after daytime water retention
Genetic factors
Psychological and emotional factors
Nocturnal epilepsy
Urinary tract infection
Increased urine volume secondary to diabetes mellitus or insipidus
Obstructive uropathy
Chronic renal failure with impaired concentrating ability

Table 56.8 Aetiology of enuresis.

Benign chronic haematuria

This condition is another disorder for which some reports have implicated food sensitivity in the aetiology.[23,45] That immune reactions can produce haematuria is recognized. In 1930, Coca described allergic haematuria in the absence of protein and red cell casts consistent with lower urinary tract origin.[6] Ammann and Rossi also reported investigation of allergic haematuria and have noted it to be related to sensitivity to foods.[1]

Eosinophilic infiltration

Eosinophilic infiltration of the bladder and lower urinary tract have been described associated with symptoms typical of cystitis. Horowitz reported a patient with chronic eosinophilic cystitis and asthma, and reviewed nine patients with the same disorder; two of these had coexistent asthma.[22] His patient progressed to renal failure in spite of treatment with corticosteroids. More recently, Sanchez-Palacios and coworkers,[48] and Yamada and colleagues[62] described patients with food-induced interstitial and eosinophilic cystitis. Littleton and colleagues have recently reviewed the literature pertaining to eosinophilic cystitis.[29] They found 39 cases reported and noted that a variety of antigens were implicated as aetiological factors, including medications, topical agents and foods. Parasites have also been identified as possible antigenic sources. This group emphasized the necessity for including other forms of cystitis in the differential diagnosis. An editorial in the *Lancet* discussed chronic interstitial cystitis but did not mention allergy or food sensitivity as a possible aetiological factor.[11]

The provoking agents of lower urinary tract symptoms include foods, although drugs and inhaled allergens such as moulds may play an important role in some individuals. The foods commonly implicated have been milk, wheat, corn, chicken, tomato, chocolate, cola drinks, citrus, egg, food colours, nuts and some condiments such as black pepper. Some instances of food-related bladder symptoms may be a result of non-specific irritation by spicy foods such as red pepper, etc. rather than an immunological mechanism.

CONCLUSION

In the intervening time since the first edition of this book was published, further studies have explored the multiple immunological processes involved in renal disorders. However, there has not been much progress in elucidation of a role for food hypersensitivity in either upper or lower urinary tract disorders. Such studies are still needed, but improvements in therapy of diseases such as the nephrotic syndrome have decreased interest in identifying environmental triggers, e.g. food elements, inhaled allergens, chemicals, etc. It is hoped that such investigation will be undertaken in the near future.

The availability of objective measures of renal function and the ability to monitor relatively easily renal and urinary tract function make this an excellent organ system for study of a potential role of environmental factors in these disorders. If the reported observations are confirmed and expanded, control of diet and other environmental factors *could* provide more specific and effective approaches to therapy.

KEY FACTS

1. A large proportion of renal disorders have an important immunological basis.
2. The nephrotic syndrome is associated with an allergic diathesis in a high percentage of patients.
3. In those patients with the nephrotic syndrome, food sensitivities may play an important role in provoking proteinuria.
4. Dietary management can play a key role in management of some patients with the nephrotic syndrome.
5. Postural proteinuria may also be triggered by food sensitivities.
6. Chronic haematuria may also be triggered by food sensitivities.
7. Food sensitivity may also play a role in some patients with lower urinary tract symptoms; this includes urinary frequency, dysuria, bleeding and enuresis.
8. In most instances allergic triggers of urinary tract disorders do not produce their effects via IgE antibody mechanisms.

REFERENCES

1 Ammann P, Rossi E. Allergic hematuria. *Arch Dis Child* 1966; 41: 539.
2 Barratt TM, Avner ED, Harmon W, eds. *Pediatric nephrology*, 4th edn, Lippincott, Williams and Wilkins, Baltimore, MD, 1999.
3 Bray GW. Enuresis of allergic origin. *Arch Dis Child* 1931; 6: 251.
4 Breneman JC. Allergic cystitis: the cause of nocturnal enuresis. *Gen Pract* 1959; 20: 85.
5 Breneman JC. Nocturnal enuresis: a treatment regimen for general use. *Ann Allergy* 1965; 23: 185–91.
6 Coca AF. Specific sensitiveness as a cause of symptoms in disease: essential hematuria and localized retinal edema as possible allergic symptoms. *Bull NZ Acad Med* 1930; 6: 593.
7 Crook WG. Genito-urinary allergy. In: *Allergy and Immunology in Childhood*, (Speer F, Dockhorn RJ, eds), Charles C Thomas, Springfield, 1974.
8 Dippell J, Wonne R. Atopie, HLA-System, und steroidsensibles nephrotisches Syndrome in Kindesalter. *Monatsschr Kinderheilkd* 1981; 129: 684–7.
9 Duke WW. Food allergy as a cause of irritable bladder. *J Urol* 1923; 10: 173.
10 Editorial. Atopy and steroid-responsive childhood nephrotic syndrome. *Lancet* 1981; i: 964–5.
11 Editorial. Chronic interstitial cystitis. *Lancet* 1985; ii: 134.
12 Esperanca M, Gerrard JW. Nocturnal enuresis. Comparison of the effect of imipramine and dietary restriction on bladder capacity. *Can Med Assoc J* 1969; 101: 721.
13 Eyres K, Mallick NP, Taylor G. Evidence for cell mediated immunity to renal antigens in minimal-change nephrotic syndrome. *Lancet* 1976; i: 1158–9.
14 Fish AJ, Michael AF, Good RA. Pathogenesis of glomerulonephritis. In: *Diseases of the Kidney*, 2nd edn, (Strauss MB, Welt LG, eds), Little, Boston, 1963.
15 Florido Diaz Pena JM, Beldie J, Estrada JL, Garcia Ara MC, Ojeda JA. Nephrotic syndrome and respiratory allergy in childhood. *J Investig Allergol Clin Immunol* 1992; 2: 136–40.
16 Genova R, Sanfilippo M, Rossi ME, Vierucci A. Food allergy in steroid-resistant nephrotic syndrome. *Lancet* 1987; i: 1315–16.
17 Gerrard JW. Nocturnal enuresis. In *Food Allergy: New Perspectives*, (Gerrard JW, ed.), Charles C Thomas, Springfield; 1980: 169.
18 Grupe WE. Primary nephrotic syndrome in childhood. In: *Advances in Pediatrics*, Year Book Medical Publishers, Chicago, 1979; 163.
19 Hardwicke J, Soothill JW, Squire JR *et al*. Nephrotic syndrome and pollen hypersensitivity. *Lancet* 1959; i: 500–2.

20 Horesh AJ. Allergy and recurrent urinary tract infections in childhood (Part II). *Ann Allergy* 1976; 36: 174.
21 Howanietz H, Lubec G. Idiopathic nephrotic syndrome, treated with steroids for five years, found to be allergic reaction to pork. *Lancet* 1985; ii: 450.
22 Horowitz J, Slavin S, Pfau A. Chronic renal failure due to eosinophilic cystitis. *Ann Allergy* 1972; 30: 502.
23 Kittredge WE, Johnson C. Allergic hematuria due to milk. *New Orleans Med Surg J* 1948–9; 101: 419.
23a Lagrue G, Heslan JM, Belghiti D *et al*. Basophil sensitization for food allergens in idiopathic nephrotic syndrome. *Nephron* 1986; 42: 123–7.
24 Lagrue G, Laurent J. Role de l'allergie dans la nephrose lipoidique. *Nouv Presse Med* 1982; 11: 1465–6.
25 Laurent J, Lagrue G, Belghiti D *et al*. Is house dust allergen a possible causal factor for relapses in lipoid nephrosis? *Allergy* 1984; 39: 231.
26 Laurent J, Rostoker G, Robeva R, Bruneau C, Lagrue G. Is adult nephrotic syndrome food allergy?: Value of oligoantigenic diets. *Nephron* 1987; 47: 7–11.
27 Laurent J, Wierzbicki N, Rostoker G, Lang P, Lagrue G. Idiopathic nephrotic syndrome and food hypersensitivity. Value of an exclusion diet. *Arch Fr Pediatr* 1988; 45: 815–19.
28 Levinsky RJ, Malleson PN, Barratt TM *et al*. Circulating immune complexes in steroid-responsive nephrotic syndrome. *N Engl J Med* 1978; 298: 126.
29 Littleton RH, Rarab RN, Cerny JC. Eosinophilic cystitis: an uncommon form of cystitis. *J Urol* 1982; 127: 132–3.
30 McIntosh RM, Ozawa T. Immunologically mediated cell injury. In: *Pediatric Nephrology: Epidemiology, Evaluation and Therapy*, vol. 2, (Strauss J, ed.), Symposia Specialists, Miami, 1976; 161.
31 McIntosh RM, Griswold WR, Chernack W *et al*. The glomerulonephropathies-etiopathogenesis. In: *Pediatric nephrology: current concepts in diagnosis and management*, vol. 1. (Strauss J, ed), Miami: Symposia Specialists, 1974; 89.
32 Matsumura T. Postural proteinuria. In: *Clinical ecology*. (Dickey L, ed.) Springfield: Charles C Thomas, 1976; 233.
33 Matsumura T, Kuroume T. The role of allergy in the pathogenesis of the nephrotic syndrome. *Jpn J Pediatr* 1961; 14: 921.
34 Matsumura T, Kuroume T, Fukushima I. Significance of food allergy in the etiology of orthostatic albuminuria. *J Asthma Res* 1966; 3: 325.
35 Matsumura T, Kurome T, Matsui A *et al*. Therapy of the nephrotic syndrome by eradication of foci and elimination diets. *Proc 13th Int Cong Pediatr* 1971; 41.

36 Meadow SR, Sarsfield JK. Steroid-responsive nephrotic syndrome and allergy: clinical studies. *Arch Dis Child* 1981; 56: 509–16.

37 Moorthy AV, Zimmerman SW, Burkholder PM. Inhibition of lymphocyte blastogenesis by plasma of patients with minimal change nephrotic syndrome. *Lancet* 1976; i: 1160.

38 Pastinszky I. The allergic diseases of the male genitourinary tract with special reference to allergic urethritis. *Urol Int* 1959; 9: 258–305.

39 Pollak VE, Pirani CL, Clyne DH. The natural history of membranous glomerulo-nephropathy. In: *Glomerulonephritis*, (Kincaid Smith P, Mathew TH, Becker EL, eds.), Part 1. New York: Wiley, 1973; 429.

40 Powell NB. Allergies of the genitourinary tract. *Ann Allergy* 1961; 19: 1019–20.

41 Powell NB, Powell BB. Vesical allergy in females. *South Med J* 1954; 47: 841.

42 Powell NB, Boggs PB, McGovern JP. Allergy of the lower urinary tract. *Ann Allergy* 1970; 28: 252–5.

43 Powell NB, Powell BB, Thomas OC *et al.* Allergy of the lower urinary tract. *J Urol* 1972; 107: 631–4.

44 Reeves WG, Cameron JS, Johansson SGO *et al.* Seasonal nephrotic syndrome. *Clin Allergy* 1975; 5: 121–37.

45 Richards W, Olson D, Church JA. Improvement of idiopathic nephrotic syndrome following allergy therapy. *Ann Allergy* 1977; 39: 332–3.

46 Rowe AH, Rowe AH Jr. Diagnosis and control of the causes of hematological allergy. In: *Food allergy: its manifestations and control and the elimination diets.* Springfield: Charles C Thomas, 1972; 430.

47 Rowe AH, Rowe AH Jr. Urogenital allergy-bladder allergy. In: *Food allergy: its manifestations and the elimination diets.* Springfield: Charles C Thomas, 1972; 409.

48 Sanchez-Palacios A, Quintero-de-Juana A, Martinez-Sagarra J *et al.* Eosinophilic food-induced cystitis. *Allergol Immunopathol* 1984; 12: 463–9.

49 Sandberg DH, McLeod TF, Strauss J. Renal disease related to hypersensitivity to foods. In: *Food allergy: new perspectives.* (Gerrard JW, ed.), Springfield: Charles C Thomas, 1980; 144.

50 Sandberg DH, McIntosh RM, Bernstein CW *et al.* Severe steroid-responsive nephrosis associated with hypersensitivity. *Lancet* 1977; i: 388.

51 Shalhoub RJ. Pathogenesis of lipoid nephrosis: a disorder of T-cell function. *Lancet* 1974; ii: 556–60.

52 Siegel S, Rawitt L, Sokoloff B *et al.* Relationship of allergy, enuresis and urinary tract infections in children 4 to 7 years of age. *Pediatrics* 1976; 57: 526.

53 Speer F. *Food Allergy*, 2nd edn. J Wright, Boston, 1983: 34.

54 Thompson PD, Stokes CR, Barratt TM *et al.* HLA antigens and atopic features in steroid-responsive nephrotic syndrome of childhood. *Lancet* 1976; ii: 765–8.

55 Trompeter RS, Barratt TM, Kay R *et al.* HLA, atopy, and cyclophosphamide in steroid-responsive childhood nephrotic syndrome. *Kidney Int* 1980; 17: 113–17.

56 Truss CO. Tissue injury induced by *Candida albicans*: mental and neurologic manifestations. *J Orthomol Psychiatry* 1978; 7: 17–37.

57 Truss CO. Restoration of immunologic competence to *Candida albicans*. *J Orthomol Psychiatry* 1980; 9: 287–301.

58 Truss CO. The rule of *Candida albicans* in human illness. *J Orthomol Psychiatry* 1981; 10: 225–38.

59 Unger DL, Kubik F, Unger L. Urinary tract allergy. *J Am Med Assoc* 1959; 70: 1380.

60 Walter CK. Allergy as the cause of genitourinary symptoms: clinical considerations. *Ann Allergy* 1958; 16: 158.

61 Williams DG. Allergy and the kidney. In: *Allergy: Immunological and Clinical Aspects*, (Lessof MH, ed.), Wiley, New York, 1984: 373.

62 Yamada T, Taguchi H, Nisimura H *et al.* Allergic study of interstitial cystitis. I. A case of interstitial cystitis caused by squid and shrimp hypersensitivity. *Arerugi* 1984; 33: 264–8.

63 Zaleski A, Shokeir MHK, Gerrard JW. Enuresis: familial incidence and relationship to allergic disorders. *Can Med Assoc J* 1972; 106: 30.

F

Chapter 57

Cardiovascular disease in response to foods and chemicals

William J. Rea and Gerald H. Ross

INTRODUCTION

Environmental insults have long been known to influence man's health. Even in his book, *Air, Water, and Places*, Hippocrates emphasized environmental effects on the health of his patients.[46] Early environmental records indicate that excess heat and cold influence bodily functions, with extreme exposure resulting in vascular spasm, hypoxia, gangrene of the extremities and death.

Treatment and prevention of cardiovascular disease must not only encompass the understanding of many factors including biological (pollen, bacteria, virus, fungus and parasites) but also chemical factors (organic and inorganic) and physical forces (weather, cyclic phenomena, sound and electromagnetic effects) in addition to genetics. The cardiovascular system has complex physiology that must be kept in efficient homeostasis by avoidance of as many triggering agents as possible and maintenance of optimum nutrition of the vessels in order to deliver optimum amounts of oxygen to the end organ to ensure the body's optimum function. The causes of cardiovascular disease are almost always multifactoral and are not always easy to eliminate.

AGENTS AFFECTING THE CARDIOVASCULAR SYSTEM

The cardiovascular system can be affected by a variety of agents including chemical agents, water, food, outdoor and indoor air pollution and electrical phenomena.

Chemical agents

While chemical incitants may trigger a maladaptation response in virtually any of the smooth muscle systems, those of the cardiovascular system appear to be the most susceptible[41] and critical to maintain homeostatic function. Recent literature and our vast experience at the Environmental Health Center in Dallas (EHC-Dallas) with over 20 000 environmentally triggered cardiovascular cases have verified previous findings regarding the harmful effects of a variety of chemicals on the cardiovascular system as shown in Table 57.1. Some of the most common of these chemicals are insecticides, chlorinated and non-chlorinated solvents, formaldehyde, phenols, carbon monoxide, nitrous oxide, sulphur dioxide, heavy metals (lead, cadmium, mercury) and amines.[83] If a pollutant overload occurs, for acute survival, the toxic substance will be parked in the fatty tissue or fat layers of cells or in the connective tissue matrix. Once in place, this toxic substance can be mobilized under the stress response, thus creating a new internal toxic exposure. There are now 60 000 man-made chemicals in our environment. When they enter the body, they must be utilized, compartmentalized or eliminated in order to maintain optimum vascular function. These substances will be contained in air, food, and water, each being discussed separately.

Water

Water usually contains minerals, toxic metals, organic chemicals, particulate matter (mould, sand, leaves) and radiation.[82] Chemically contaminated water is a major component of the

Chemical agents affecting the cardiovascular system				Table 57.1 Chemical agents affecting the cardiovascular system.
Chemical	**Reference**	**Chemical**	**Reference**	
Fluorocarbons	Harkavy 1963 Taylor and Hern 1970	Formaldehyde	Rea and Mitchell 1982	
Phenol	Nour-Eldon 1970	Chlorine	Finn 1979	
Petroleum alcohol and its products	Yervick 1975	Cigarette smoke	Fisher 1981	
Glycerine	Fregers 1980	Chlorophenothane	Rea and Mitchell 1982	
Toluene	Rea and Mitchell 1982	Turpentine	Rea and Mitchell 1982	
Hydralazine	Suhonen 1980	Chlorinated hydrocarons	Balaz 1981	

total environmental load. Most public water systems are loaded with organic and inorganic chemicals, which may increase the body burden of some chemicals several-fold (Fig. 57.1). These include trihalomethanes,[122] pesticides,[12,71,77,88] formaldehyde,[66] solvents,[66] oils,[123] heavy metals (lead, mercury, cadmium),[66] tetra-chloroethylene, trichloroethylene, phthalates, methyl-tert-butyl gas additive, and other metals such as copper,[66] zinc and manganese. Public drinking water has been described by Laseter *et al.*[55] and others[97] as containing most of the contents of an organic chemical laboratory. An example of how water contaminants can influence the cardiovascular system is illustrated in the following case.

Case report. A 35-year-old male physician developed pericarditis along with multiple other symptoms of fatigue, fibromyalgia and endocrine dysfunction. His drinking water was contaminated by a dry-cleaning company's spill in his village, which eventually contaminated the drinking and bathing water. The community was told that not enough tetra-chlorethylene, which was in the low parts per million, was in the drinking water to cause problems. He eventually became incapacitated. Blood levels showed only tetrachloroethylene. He was placed in an environmentally controlled environment and cleared his symptoms. Double-blind, inhaled challenge with the ambient doses of tetrachloroethylene triggered his tachycardia and chest pain. He was rehabilitated and able to practice medicine again using a programme of massive avoidance of pollutants in air, food, and water, injection therapy and nutritional supplementation.

When water is ingested, all of its components must be metabolized, catabolized or excreted. In developed nations, the prevalence of many chronic diseases, particularly cardiovascular diseases, can be associated with various water characteristics related to hardness. Those involved include coronary heart disease, hypertension and stroke. The protective agents found in hard water are calcium, magnesium, vanadium, zinc, lithium, chromium and manganese.[66] Recent studies report fewer heart attacks, less coronary disease and lower mortality rates in patients with existing cardiovascular disease in areas where there is hard water.[30]

Suspected harmful agents include sodium, and the metals cadmium, lead, aluminium, bismuth, copper and zinc, which tend to be found in higher concentrations in soft water as a result of its relative corrosiveness. Copper and zinc can also aid blood vessel health. Nitrates in water pose immediate threats to children under 3 months of age. Excessive levels have been known to react with haemoglobin in the blood to produce methaemoglobinaemia. Though barium occurs naturally in the environment, it can enter water supplies through industrial waste discharges. Barium can bring about an increase in blood pressure and even death.[26] Patients susceptible to water contaminants may exhibit multiple sensitivities and be especially sensitive to airborne chemicals.[77]

Food

There are at least three aspects of food to consider in evaluating a patient's cardiovascular health: food sensitivity, food additives (natural and man-made toxins) and the nutritive quality.

Involvement of the cardiovascular system in food sensitivities, which has been reported by a number of researchers, was first shown by Hare in 1905.[40] He recognized tachycardia and bradycardia in patients following ingestion of some foods. Since then, a variety of cardiovascular disease states have been reported to be related to food, including increased heart rates, angina pectoris, arrhythmias, myocardial infarction, extrasystoles and atrial and ventricular fibrillation.[41] Other researchers have reported phlebitis and vasculitis that were triggered by foods.[78,87,107] Of the 20 000 cardiovascular patients treated at the EHC-Dallas, 80% have specific food sensitivities as part of the triggering agents for their vessel dysfunction.

The widespread contamination of food supplies is witnessed by the increasing use of pesticides, herbicides and nitrogen fertilizers in growing food and the presence of food additives, preservatives and dyes in the manufacturing and processing of commercially available food products. Urticarial reactions, vascular abnormalities and immunological changes as a function of exposure to a number of chemicals and food additives have been reported by a number of authors.[7,8,39,49,58,64,79,85,122] At the EHC-Dallas, we have treated over 5000 patients with cardiovascular disease who can eat less chemically contaminated organic food without symptoms. However, when they eat the same foods with additives and preservatives, the symptoms of their cardiovascular disease exacerbates.

Natural toxins such as cardiac glycosides in food can trigger cardiovascular responses. Many other natural toxins such as trypt-

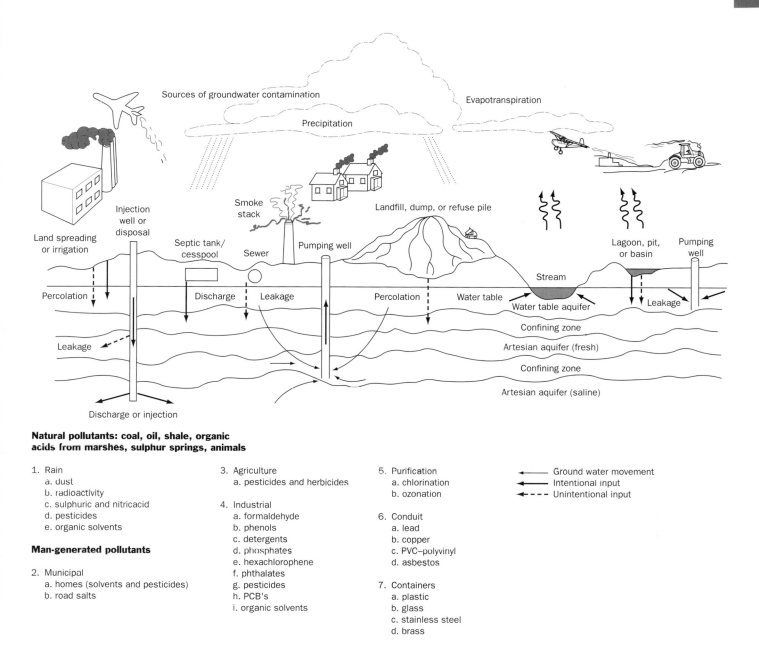

Natural pollutants: coal, oil, shale, organic acids from marshes, sulphur springs, animals

1. Rain
   a. dust
   b. radioactivity
   c. sulphuric and nitricacid
   d. pesticides
   e. organic solvents

Man-generated pollutants

2. Municipal
   a. homes (solvents and pesticides)
   b. road salts

3. Agriculture
   a. pesticides and herbicides

4. Industrial
   a. formaldehyde
   b. phenols
   c. detergents
   d. phosphates
   e. hexachlorophene
   f. phthalates
   g. pesticides
   h. PCB's
   i. organic solvents

5. Purification
   a. chlorination
   b. ozonation

6. Conduit
   a. lead
   b. copper
   c. PVC–polyvinyl
   d. asbestos

7. Containers
   a. plastic
   b. glass
   c. stainless steel
   d. brass

← Ground water movement
← Intentional input
←--- Unintentional input

Fig 57.1 Water cycle of contamination that affects the chemically sensitive individual adversely. (Adapted from Concern, Inc., December 1986. *Drinking Water: a Community Action Guide*. Washington, DC, p. 2.)

amine in bananas and cheese can trigger high blood pressure. There are now many natural toxins in food that can affect the cardiovascular system.

Intake of high fat plus sugar in combination with additive-rich food will damage blood vessels, yielding plaque deposition with resultant arteriosclerosis or non-specific vasculitis. Many discussions appear in the literature on this subject and it will not be further discussed here.

Selenium deficiency causes cardiomyopathy,[117] popularly called Keshan's disease in China.

Air pollution

Air pollution, either indoors or outdoors, is able to trigger cardiovascular disease. The total load of the toxic pollutants can initiate, propagate and cause occlusion in environmentally triggered cardiovascular disease.

Outdoor air pollution

The physical factors of the weather include not only heat and cold but also humidity, barometric pressure, electromagnetic and electric fields, seasons and weather cycles. It has been estimated that 25–30% of the population are sensitive to weather changes.[45] Some authors have suggested that triggering of cardiovascular disease, including myocardial infarction, may be related to the weather.[22,45]

Outdoor air pollution has long been thought to enhance disease processes. Prior to the 19th century, air pollution as we know it was virtually unknown as was arteriosclerotic cardiovascular disease. The term 'smog' was first used in England to denote a combination of smoke and natural fog, which may produce ill-effects.[36] The term is now used in all industrialized countries, but often denotes air pollution of vastly different compositions. For example, Los Angeles smog is largely composed of petrochemicals and their byproducts,[36] while in China it is composed mainly of coal effluent. Both types can adversely affect the cardiovascular system. According to the Environmental Protection Agency (EPA) studies,[36] there has been no 'fresh' air in the United States in 20 years.

Contaminants involved in air pollution include inorganic chemicals (sulphur dioxide, carbon monoxide, nitrogen oxides, ozone, lead, etc.), organic chemicals (petroleum-derived hydrocarbons, etc.), particulates (pollen, moulds, dust, car and factory emissions), and electromagnetic and electric emissions.[22]

London smog

A combination of weather inversions occurred in London during a 4-day period in December 1952. The London-type smog of particulates, sulphur oxides and fog caused approximately 4000 deaths in the following week. Between 80% and 90% of the deaths were due to respiratory and cardiovascular disease, which were mainly of a chronic nature. A majority of deaths occurred in people over the age of 65 years.[118] A similar incident occurred in Donora, Pennsylvania, a highly industrialized valley, during a 6-day period in October 1984. Out of a population of 44 000, 42% became ill and 18 deaths resulted.[60] This highlights the clinical effect of outdoor air pollution. Pesticides, hydralizines and other sulphur amino acids can cause dissecting aneurysms. Organochlorines can cause Behçet's disease (Ishikawa, pers comm) including vascular aneurysms.[5]

Indoor air pollution

Historically, contaminated indoor air began with the soot on the ceilings of prehistoric caves that resulted from open fires. Home air was very bad for health during the times of the great plagues and tuberculosis outbreaks. Changes in cleanliness in the home resulted in the virtual elimination of many diseases such as tuberculosis. More recently, the use of rapidly disintegrating synthetic materials, fossil fuels, formaldehyde and pesticides, coupled with the sealing of buildings in an attempt to conserve fuel by prevention of heat or cold loss, has led to a new type of indoor pollution, which, although not as visible, appears to be more damaging to the blood vessels.

Typically, people spend more than 90% of their time indoors. Some contaminants have been found to be in higher concentrations indoors than outdoors, such as aeroallergens, microorganisms, asbestos fibres, formaldehyde, pesticides, nitrogen dioxide, carbon monoxide, radon decay products, tobacco smoke and electromagnetic fields. All of these have now been implicated in some type of cardiovascular diseases, including vasculitis with or without spasm, arteriosclerosis and collagen vascular diseases.

Electrical phenomena

There seems little doubt that electromagnetic fields (EMF) can have clinical effects on the cardiovascular system and that EMF may contribute to the overall environmental load. This, in turn, may make patients more susceptible to chemicals in foods and, thus, to vascular dysfunction.

Electromagnetic fields

Some natural areas of the earth, e.g. over water veins and geological faults, have higher levels of EMF than others. There are increased areas found radiating from the poles and widening over the equator[6] and now from the proliferation of mobile phones.

High-frequency emitters in the United States consist of the whole of the EMF spectrum, including the AM radio band (0.535–1.604 MHz) and FM and TV band (54–806 MHz). Low-frequency electromagnetic exposures emanate from the electrical power systems (60 Hz in the United States, 50 Hz in Europe and Russia). Common sources of indoor electromagnetic fields include hair dryers (10–25 G), electric shavers (5–10 G) and televisions (1–5 G).[6] However, environmental exposures are very small compared with the 10^{-1} V/m across a live cell membrane.[6]

Clinical effects of electromagnetic fields

Electromagnetic fields can trigger any system in the body, because the body functions on electricity. However, specific alterations can occur directly on the blood vessel or indirectly on the autonomic nervous system or the endocrine system.

Animals and humans exposed to EMF may exhibit significant changes in electrocardiograms,[11] sinus arrhythmia[11] and brachycardia[29,76] (Fig. 57.2). Alterations in heart function such as falling arterial pressure[76] and increased heart rate[6] have been noted in humans. Both short- and long-term hypotensive effects have been reported,[61] along with decreases in efficient cardiac output.[29] Autonomic nervous system dysfunction was reported in individuals who were continuously exposed to higher levels of EMF, whereas very low-frequency exposures were found to cause neurovascular instability in some individuals.[96] At the EHC-Dallas, we have been seen this phenomenon repeatedly in patients with cardiovascular disease as measured by the pupillography and heart rate variability. Many anaesthetics and other toxics have been shown to trigger the cardiovascular system. The chlorinated insecticides and solvents are high on the list of substances whose effects are enhanced by EMF.

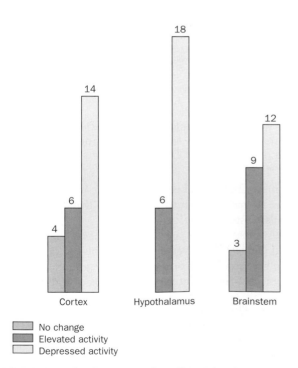

Fig 57.2 Relation of EEG response from the cortex, hypothalamus and brainstem due to exposure at 3 GHz. The numbers indicate rabbits with a given response. (*Source:* Becker RO, Marino AA: *Electromagnetism and Life.* State University of New York Press, Albany, 1982.)

Haematological effects

Changes in the cellular composition of blood of a variety of laboratory animals exposed to EMF have been shown. Changes in the number of red and white blood cells have been noted and the changes were found to be dependent on time and the magnitude of the EMF. A variety of other changes in haematological parameters in response to EMF have been reported and are discussed elsewhere,[38,52,54,60,96] including changes in iron metabolism, fibrinolytic activity and coagulation.[54]

Charged electrical conditions

Negative ions have been shown to affect the carbon dioxide combining power of plasma and to increase blood pH.[120,121] Stimulation of heart rate and cortical α-rhythm[27,95] with decreases in α-frequency has been seen in humans exposed to air ions of either polarity. Increases in blood pressure and 17-ketosteroids under positive ionization have been noted, accompanied by cholesterol decreases. Tchijevsky[106] and Vasiliev[112] proposed, as a mechanism, the penetration of charged particles through the alveolar wall into the blood vessels where the charges are transferred to blood cells and colloids.

MECHANISMS OF ENVIRONMENTALLY INDUCED VASCULAR DAMAGE

The entry of pollutants into the body depends on the integrity of the skin and oily layer or mucosa at the site of entry, as well as on the amount of IgM, IgA and IgG, the quantity of vitamins A, E and C and the quantity and quality of the antipollutant enzymes superoxide dismutase, glutathione peroxidase and catalase.

Environmental pollutants have many ways of triggering vascular responses while disturbing the immune and biological detoxification systems, but whatever mechanisms are involved the effects of pollutants once they have entered the body can be seen on the vessel walls, in the clotting equilibrium/dysequilibrium mechanism and the intravascular cellular contents.

The mechanism of vascular damage is now quite clear, with toxic chemicals triggering the vascular wall directly, the surrounding connective tissue myogenic matrix and the autonomic nervous system, resulting in vascular inflammation and/or triggering of the clotting mechanism. The end result of pollutant triggering is either vasodilation or vasospasm, with the latter being the most common. Vasospasm can then result in hypoxia which, if chronic, will trigger a whole host of physiological and pathological responses, including the non-specific mesenchyme reaction,[43] which can set in process the dyshomeostatic physiology resulting in either vasculitis or arteriosclerosis.[114]

Pollutant effects on vessel walls

As the pollutants enter the body, they may create free radicals.[65] These may be O−, OH+, lipid peroxide or others, and may damage mitochondrial and cellular membranes of the vascular tree, causing inflammation, vessel leakage and loss of energy.

These aforementioned substances can affect the vasomotor tone. Vasomotor tone is a complex interaction involving connective tissue content, with its matrix response around blood vessels as well as the endothelial wall. The vasomotor tone of vascular smooth muscles is due to neuromyogenic mechanisms, metabolic action, autoregulatory forces, extravascular compressive forces and possibly others mechanisms we do not understand.

Metabolically, there are many vascular relaxant factors that are necessary for normal vascular function. These factors include nitric oxide,[111] carbon dioxide, prostacycline (eicosanoid), adenosine,[111] lack of free radicals, lactic acid, citrate, acetate, histamine (certain levels), serotonin (certain levels), lack of glucose, sodium, potassium, magnesium and bradykinin. Balance of these factors will help the vessels deliver appropriate oxygen to the end-organ tissue.[113]

According to Zeek,[125] vessel wall damage may be mild, with leak of fluid, but as it progresses, the leaks get larger, allowing red blood cells to migrate. This will cause petechiae, spontaneous bruises or purpura. With severe damage to the wall, clotting may occur after severe inflammation has been induced, giving distal peripheral tissue damage from hypoxia.

Attempts at healing may occur in various ways, leading to granulomatous or fibrous scar formation. Triggering agents may be infectious (bacteria, virus, fungi, parasitic), chemical (sulphur dioxide, phenol, hydrocarbon),[80,123] nutritional,[80] or traumatic (physical environmental agents, as discussed above).

Any toxic chemical can trigger inflammation which, if severe enough, will then cause the coagulation mechanism to be triggered. Countless medical and surgical procedures have been associated with chemically triggered inflammation and clotting reactions. Nickel sensitivity has been reported secondary to the use of skin clips, and in a patient with a nickel steel heart valve who developed valve thrombosis. All synthetic heart valves and artificial hearts and lungs are known to be able to trigger the clotting mechanism as well as the inflammatory response. This is why chronic anticoagulation is used in the patients. For example, cardiopulmonary bypass immediately triggers the inflammatory responses the minute the synthetic cannula is inserted. If heparin is not used prior to insertion, clotting occurs. If the bypass apparatus is not terminated after a moderate period of time (2 hours), more inflammation occurs generally and the individual becomes very ill and may have difficulty surviving. Haemolysis has been associated not only with the cardiopulmonary bypass syndrome but also with necrotizing dermatitis, and this can occur after exposure to the epoxy resin in needles and polyvinylchloride tubing as well as from long-term exposure to synthetic surfaces such as artificial pumps. People with more advanced vascular damage who receive another environmental pollutant exposure that is enough to cause a vascular reaction may develop severe adverse clinical responses. These subjects may develop vascular spasm that results in hypoxia, which will then trigger arrythmia (if the heart is involved), or develop an acute coronary occlusion, cerebral vascular accident or hypertension and heart failure.

Pollutant effects on cells

Pollutant effects on the intravascular cells may result in oxidant damage to the red cells, leukocytes, the plasma and the platelets. This damage occurs in the form of free radicals, causing free radical damage with degeneration of the elements, which results in more generalized homeostatic destruction of both the immune and non-immune system.

Chemicals such as dichlorodiphenyltrichloroethane (DDT) suppress the mast cells so thoroughly that angioedema and/or anaphylaxis is less likely to occur.[33,34] However, the resultant damage can lead to chronic vascular disease if the pollutant load is not removed.

F

Other toxic substances, such as the heavy metal cadmium[4] and the organic fungicide hexachlorobenzene, can suppress the mononuclear phagocyte system, resulting in recurrent infections. Ozone can cause lipid plastic parathyroiditis with leukocytic infiltration and capillary proliferation.[102] Some substances such as phenol have an affinity for the cardiovascular system,[67] which results in endothelial as well as vaso-vasorum damage. Yevick[123] demonstrated cardiovascular changes in sea animals exposed to oil spills that appear to be similar to those seen in humans exposed to petroleum products. Chloracne perivasculitis lesions have been produced in monkeys fed a pesticide, Arochlor 1248 (polychlorinated biphenyl).[91] Chloro and fluorocarbons can cause arrhythmias.[3] Red blood cells can be damaged by pollutant-induced free radicals that cause lack of end-organ O_2 supply, resulting in chronic hypoxia with metabolic and tissue changes.

Ground regulation system

The mechanisms of vascular damage from foods and chemicals are broad. After *incitants* enter the body, damage may start at the endothelial level but also may occur at the connective tissue matrix and extracellular fluid, which contains part of the ground regulation system (GRS).[44,74] The GRS regulates local, regional and generalized homeostasis. The matrix around the vessel also contains and is the receptor for the environment.[44] The GRS consists of the connective tissue matrix and extracellular fluid, the fibrocyte and the macrophage, the end autonomic nerve, the end capillary and the basement membrane of the capillary to the basement membrane of the end organ (Fig. 57.3).[74] Vascular damage can be local, with excess food or chemical, or can occur from autonomic nerve imbalance due to noxious incitant stimuli. Finally, direct injury can occur to the vascular wall (Fig. 57.4) matrix, resulting in vasculitis. Toxic chemicals can damage nitric oxide production, resulting in vascular spasm, hypoxia and, finally, tissue changes, again resulting in occlusive fibrotic lesions, either non-arteriosclerotic or arteriosclerotic.

Non-immune triggering of the vessel wall may also occur via many mediators. Complement may be triggered directly via the alternative pathway by moulds, foods or toxic chemicals.[85] Mediators such as kinins and prostaglandins may also be directly triggered. Interestingly, in addition to allergic responses, pollens have been shown to have toxic substances that will trigger haemolysis and other responses.[31]

Endocrine effects in the vascular system (Fig. 57.5)

Oestrogen has long been known to have a mildly suppressive effect on the cardiovascular system. The late onset of arteriosclerosis in females with the onset of menopause is commonly observed. A study by Couch and Wortman[17] supports this observation in that they found a significantly greater number of occurrences of migraine in pathologically anovulatory females (polycystic ovary, galactorrhea, amenorrhea) compared with pregnant women or women taking the contraceptive pill. They suggested that this might also be due to hypothalamic abnormalities. Excess oestrogen has been shown to have an adverse effect on vessel walls, giving rise to venous inflammation, which results in thrombophlebitis and pulmonary emboli.[17] It has been shown that progesterone therapy decreases the risks of coronary artery heart disease in post-menopausal women.[50] Also, when oestrogen was combined with vitamin E, cardiovascular risks decreased function. Vitamin E plus oestrogen improved vascular endothelium-depen-

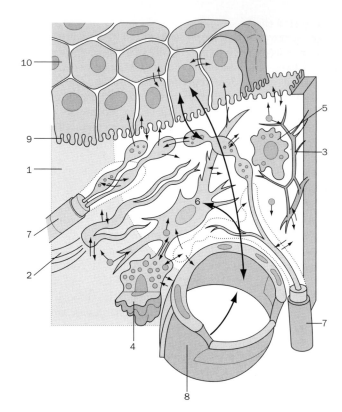

Fig 57.3 Reciprocal relationships (arrows) between capillaries (8), ground substance (matrix), proteoglycans and structural glycoproteins (1), collagen (2), elastin (3), connective tissue cells (mast cell (4), defence cell (5)), fibrocyte (6), terminal autonomic axons (7) and organic parenchymal cells (10). Basement membrane (9). The fibrocyte (6) is the regulatory centre of the ground substance. Only this type of cell is able to synthesize extracellular components. The *amin* mediators and filters of information are the proteoglycans, structural glycoproteins and the cell-surface sugar film (glycocalyx: dotted line on all the cells, collagen and elastin). (*Source* Heine, H: 1996: pers comm, 1996 with permission.)

dent vasodilator responsiveness, consistent with increased nitric oxide in post-menopausal women, despite divergent effects on atherogenic effects on lipoproteins. Oestrogen reduces the levels of atherogenic proteins, markers of inflammation and fibrinolysis inhibition, which are potentially important in the pathogenesis of atherosclerosis.

Testosterone has been shown to have an ameliorating effect on vessel walls.[20,57,73,116] Other effects of androgen supplementation are decrease in cholesterol and retarded arteriosclerosis in men.[20] Webb *et al.*[116] found physiological concentrations induce coronary dilatation and increase coronary blood flow in men with coronary artery disease.

Neurogenic vascular responses to external stimuli

When noxious stimuli that affect the nervous system are first detected there is a retrograde impulse to the dorsal nerve root ganglia through the afferent fibres of peripheral nerves (slow C or rapid delta A), or the gastrointestinal plexus. The sensory neurotransmitter, substance P, will cause immediate vasodilatation and increased permeability of the microcirculation in the area of the nerve and activate the non-IgE-mediated release of histamine via the mast cells. In addition, the release of leukotactic factors and leukotrienes is stimulated. Somatostatin is released in other cells

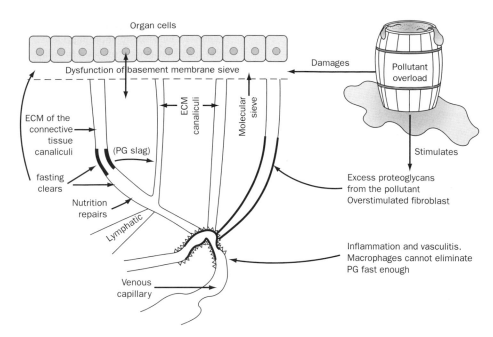

Fig 57.4 The basement membrane and the extracellular matrix (ECM) canaliculi of the connective tissue going to the blood vessels and lymphatics must be kept flowing properly or the vasculitis of the chemically sensitive individual occurs. The ground regulation system plays a key role in healing, with a return to homeostasis when it is unloaded. PG = proteoglycans.

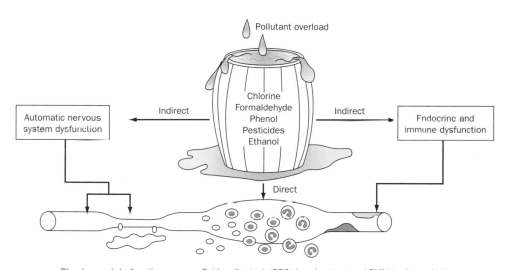

Fig 57.5 Mechanisms of pollutant injury to the blood vessels. A = arteriole; V = venule; ——, nerve conduction or release of cellular mediator; ——, stimulation or increase inhibition.

of the dorsal root, but can also be released from the central nervous system and the pancreas. The relationship between somatostatin and substance P is complicated and both have effects on other cell interactions. Autonomic dysfunction is seen in all forms of environmentally triggered vasculitis, sinus arrhythmias and reflex sympathetic dystrophy[78]. (Figure 57.6; Table 57.2). These can be measured objectively by pupillography and heart rate variability tests.

Immune-mediated vascular function

The intrinsic mechanisms by which blood vessels are damaged can be mediated either via the immune system or via the non-immune biological detoxification system. The immune hypersensitivity responses in the vessel wall can be any of four types and frequently can be a combination of types.

Type I hypersensitivity is mediated through the IgE mechanisms on the vessel wall. The classic examples are angioedema, urticaria and anaphylaxis due to sensitivity to pollen, dust, mould or food.[107]

Type II cytotoxic damage may occur with direct injury to the cell and thus the vessel wall. A clinical example of this is seen with exposures to mercury,[35] although this might also be directly toxic rather than antibody-mediated.

Type III immune complex syndromes (IgG plus complement) include lupus vasculitis. Numerous chemicals, including procaineamide[93] and chlorothiazide,[93] are known to trigger the autoantibody reactions of lupus. Other chemicals such as vinyl chloride[56] will produce microaneurysms in vessels of the fingers of exposed workers.

Type IV cell-mediated immunity occurs with sensitization and stimulation of T lymphocytes. Numerous chemicals such as phenol, pesticides, organohalides and some metals will also alter immune responses, possibly triggering lymphokines and causing a Type IV reaction.[119] Clinical examples are polyarteritis nodosa, hypersensitivity angitis, Henoch–Schönlein purpura and Wegener's granulomatosis.[78] Implant syndromes from silicone, Teflon, other plastics, and metals can cause Raynaud's syndrome and scleroderma[9,10,15,16,21,24,25,28,32,42,48,59, 62,90,92,94,98,100,101,103,108,109,115,124]

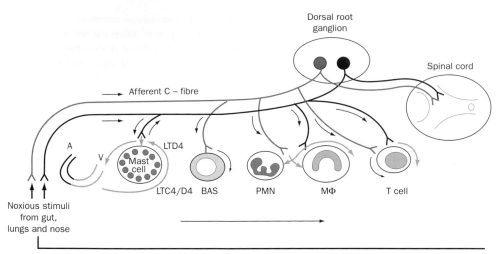

Fig 57.6 Modulation of immunological responses by sensory neuropeptides after pollutant stimuli as seen in some chemically sensitive individuals.

Overall results of pupillography in 720 patients *versus* normal controls					
	Total	Male	Female	Ages	Abnormal
Patient group	720*	231	489	4–89	69%
Comparison group	181	90	91	5–84	

* Each measurement was performed three times.
Source: Sujisawa I, Suyama H, Namba T. 1989–1991. EHC-Dallas.

Table 57.2a Overall results of pupillography in 720 patients *versus* normal controls.

Light reflex analysis by pupillography: double-blind inhaled challenge after 4 days deadaptation in the ECU (50 patients)*			
Toxic chemical (No. of patients)	Ambient dose (ppm)	Response	Pupil
Pesticide (20)	<0.0034	Cholinergic nerve increase	A1 decrease CR increase VD decrease
Toluene (6)	<3.0	Sympathetic nerve decrease	CR increase T5 increase
Phenol (22)	<0.0024	Sympathetic nerve increase Cholinergic nerve decrease	CR decrease
Chlorine (13)	<0.33	Non-specific change	CR decrease

Notes: Increase or decrease ($P<0.05$); increase–excited; decrease–inhibited; A1=pupil area; T5=dilation time; CR=contraction ratio; VD=velocity of dilation.
* Some patients reacted to more than one chemical.
Source: Homma K. 1993. EHC-Dallas.

Table 57.2b Light reflex analysis by pupillography: double-blind inhaled challenge after 4 days deadaptation in the ECU (50 patients)*

Diagnosis of vascular dysfunction

A variety of laboratory tests can be performed, with the most relevant ones being indicated by clinical experience. Angiograms and magnetic resonance angiographs should be carried out to rule out fixed lesions as required. Frequently, spasm will be seen if the larger vessels are involved. If skin lesions are present, biopsies may show either necrotizing vasculitis with polymorphonuclear leukocyte infiltration or non-necrotizing lesions with eosinophils and/or the most common with lymphocytes around or in the vessel wall. However, only active lesions are likely to be positive when biopsy of the petechiae and bruises is done. Blood levels for T and B cells, cell cycles, blastogenic index and phagocytic indexes may also be used to evaluate the immune status. Direct measurement of blood solvents (i.e. hexanes, benzenes, chlorinated hydrocarbons, insecticides) are now available. Also, antipollutant enzymes such as superoxide dismutase, glutathione peroxide and catalase can be measured in the blood of those who have compromised heart or blood vessels. Heart rate variability and pupillography will measure the electrical and neurovascular responses. These technologies have been efficacious in viewing new parameters for the prevention of fixed-named vascular disease.

Challenge tests

Challenge tests should be done to define triggering agents. These may be done via oral, inhaled or intradermal routes. Care should be taken to do challenge tests under steady-state environmental conditions to reduce variability. The patient should avoid a substance for 4 days to decrease the total body load, placing the patient in the state of deadaptation before challenges. Also, provocation intradermal challenges can be used for accurate diagnosis of biological, inhalant, food, and chemical sensitization.

Environmental control unit

The use of an environmental control unit (ECU) with its reduction of pollutants in air, food and water, in order to put the patient in the de-adapted state with the total load reduced, can lead to the most precise diagnosis and treatment for the environmental aspects of cardiovascular diseases. It is particularly useful for the severely compromised patient. Since these units are not commonly available, controlled areas in hospitals and offices may have to be used as a less satisfactory substitute. An improvement on reduction of the total load, with deterioration on subsequent challenge, is the key to diagnosing triggering agents of cardiovascular disease (Fig. 57.7).

Clinical manifestations of vascular injury

Vascular injury gives rise to a variety of clinical manifestations depending on the types of vessels involved (vein, capillary, large or small artery) and the intensity and duration of the insult. Injury can result in acute life and limb catastrophies (myocardial infarction, strokes, gangrene of the limbs) or – in the vast majority of people – chronic hypoxia states that cause chronic fatigue, fibromyalgia and cerebral dysfunction. Several specific clinical entities are now discussed.

Hypersensitivity vasculitis

The hypersensitivity vasculitides are a group of disorders characterized by small-vessel inflammation. Manifestations are often mild and self-limited. Although any organ can be involved, the most common is the skin: lesions are found on the buttocks, ankles

and legs, and the causes for some of these have now been found. Theorell et al.[107] showed occurrences of purpura and other signs of vasculitis after challenge with moulds, cedar and some foods. We have also observed such vascular lesions after challenge with phenol, formaldehyde, petroleum, alcohol, insecticide (2,4-DNP or organophosphate), chlorine and beef. Hypersensitivity vasculitis is a diverse group of disorders that includes serum sickness reactions, Henoch–Schönlein purpura (Fig. 57.8), essential mixed cryoglobulinaemia and the connective tissue diseases, particularly rheumatoid and lupus vasculitis and scleroderma.[47]

Foreign serum proteins can cause serum sickness reactions, and similar reactions may occur after the use of penicillin,[104] sulphonamide,[89] streptomycin,[14] thiouracils[14] and hydencompounds.[14] We have seen a case of Henoch–Schönlein purpura triggered by pollen, dust, moulds, foods and chemicals (Fig. 57.8).

Periarteritis nodosa

Periarteritis nodosa (PAN) generally follows a prodromal fever with arthralgia and malaise; it may manifest itself as acute gastrointestinal distress, myocardial infarction, neuritis, muscle pain, or gangrene of the extremities. PAN generally presents in the muscular arteries, involves all three layers of the arterial walls and adjacent veins and is usually segmental.

Biopsy of skin, subcutaneous nodules or smooth muscle reveals acute healing vasculitis without giant cells. The infiltrative process involves polymorphonuclear leukocytes, eosinophils and oedema followed by fibrinoid necrosis. The areas of fibrinoid necrosis are subsequently replaced by fibroblasts, and scar tissue forms.

Systemic lupus erythematosus

Apparently, many foreign substances can trigger a systemic lupus erythematosus (SLE)-like syndrome with vasculitis. Chemical

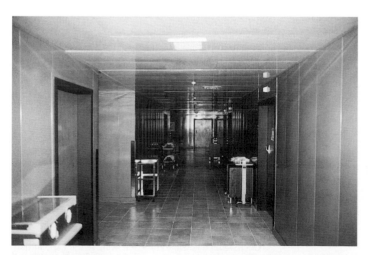

Fig 57.7 Porcelain environmental control unit (ECU) – Northeast Community Hospital.

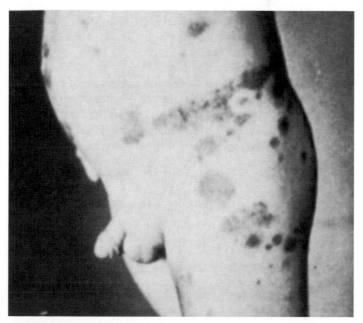

Fig 57.8 Henoch–Schönlein purpura (anaphylactoid purpura) in a 14-year-old boy, with associated urticarial erythematous lesions with purpura, painful articular swelling and microscopic haematuria.
(*Source:* Olsen T. Peripheral vascular disease, necrotizing vasculitis and vascular-related diseases. In: *Dermatology* (Moschella SL, Hurley HJ, eds) Vol. 1, 2nd edn. WB Saunders, Philadelphia, 1985.)

triggering of lupus has been well-established in the literature.[110] The following case report is an example of a patient whose symptoms were environmentally induced.

Case study. A 36-year-old, white female had developed recurrent bouts of vomiting at the age of 5. These gave way to migraine at the age of 11, which persisted. At the age of 16, she developed a polyarthritis, and a diagnosis of systemic lupus erythematosus (SLE) was made. Her disease progressed over the next several years, with further involvement of the gastrointestinal, genitourinary, respiratory and vascular systems. Spontaneous bruising and petechiae occurred, together with peripheral oedema. She was eventually placed on cortisone and cytotoxic drugs. Antinuclear antibodies and LE preparations were positive on numerous occasions. She was placed in the ECU, and all medications were discontinued. The stiffness and swelling of her joints gradually disappeared. Her sedimentation rate fell from 63 to 15 mm. This was the lowest it had been for many years. The circumference of her fingers diminished by 1.5–2 cm while fasting, reflecting the massive decrease of oedema. She was able to open and close her hands for the first time in many years. Challenges with 20 out of 30 different foods precipitated a return of her symptoms. The inhalation of chemicals such as perfume, phenol and natural gas also triggered symptoms. She has done well without medications on an avoidance programme for several years.

Wegener's granulomatosis

PAN is closely related to Wegener's granulomatosis, which is characterized by necrotizing granulomas in the respiratory tract and vasculitis of the medium-size arteries, veins, arterioles and venules. The onset may be acute or chronic. Though pathologically well-defined, the aetiology of the disease is still obscure. Recent studies indicate that looking for incitants is worthwhile. A case followed for years at the EHC-Dallas illustrates the environmental triggering resulting in severe vasculitis that results in devastating symptoms.

Case study. A 48-year-old nurse was first seen at the EHC-Dallas at the age of 33 years. She complained of leg, arm and back lesions that started as bruises, became ulcers, and then eventually healed, or if they remained raw, became inflamed. As a result of the inflammation, she was frequently unable to walk. All treatments were refractory to medication, and the course was unrelenting. The patient had severe vascular spasm that resulted in excruciating pain and eventually resulted in occlusion of her superior and inferior vena cava, femoral and subclavian veins. The patient was severely malnourished, having difficulty with food intake due to the vasculitis in the intestine. She proved to have sensitivity to multiple foods and chemicals. Her past history was significant in that she was born with a gastroschisis and had to be operated on at birth. Her intestinal tract had never functioned properly in her life. Multiple biopsies of the vascular lesions showed leukocytoclastic vasculitis followed by lymphocytic vasculitis. Eventually a diagnosis of Wegener's granulomatosis was suggested, but it was never proven. This patient had multiple surgery for clotting in the inflamed vessels, many due to insertion of plastic catheters and others due to severe vascular spasm. At one time, she had early renal failure, which reversed when environmental control was tightened. She is on a rigid avoidance programme, avoiding the biological inhalants, foods and chemicals that trigger her vasculitis. She built an environmentally controlled house and has taken injection therapy for her biological inhalant, food and chemical sensitivities. Nutritional therapy is also part of her treatment programme. This patient has maintained reasonable health over the last 15 years, and is still a viable human being.

Diseases such as rheumatoid arthritis exhibit a variety of vascular manifestations and biopsy evidence of vasculitis. Although the aetiology of this disease is generally not known, evidence of immune changes in patients with rheumatoid arthritis following food and chemical challenges has been found. Two controlled series have been reported, defining triggering agents in rheumatoid arthritis,[53,68] and a recent report has clearly shown the efficacy of diet in rheumatoid arthritis.[18]

Eosinophilic vasculitis

Eosinophilic vasculitis has now been reported in some disease processes, i.e. eosinophilic granulomas and Goodpasture's syndrome. Lymphocytic vascular inflammation has been seen in some infectious diseases[68] and other syndromes[53] and by many chemical triggering agents.[78]

Small-vessel vasculitis

The most common vascular entity that occurs is inflammation of the end arterial, capillary and venous vessels. The inflammation can occur in any organ system but often is generalized, resulting in homeostatic dysfunction.

Rea *et al.*[87] described a group of patients with multisystem involvement distinguished by a wide variety of symptoms. All evidenced frequent peripheral vasospasm, spontaneous cutaneous bruising or petechiae and peripheral oedema (Table 57.3). Often, adult-onset acne vasculitis was part of the syndrome.

Small vessel vasculitis			
Patient:	36-year-old, white female		
Symptoms:	Vomiting, migraine, bruising, petechiae, peripheral oedema		
		Patient	Control
Laboratory:	Sedimentation rate	48	10 ± 10 mm/h
	Total complement CH_{50}	181%	100 ± 20%
	C-reactive protein	Positive	Negative
	Total eosinophil count	325	125 ± 75% m³
	Antinuclear antibody	+	–
	LE test	+	–
Triggering agents:	Moulds	Dust	20 foods
Discharge status:	Improving: clear of symptoms without medication on discharge		
Follow-up:	Long-term follow-up (5 years): doing well without medications		
	Occasional mild symptoms following acute exposures		

Table 57.3 Small vessel vasculitis.

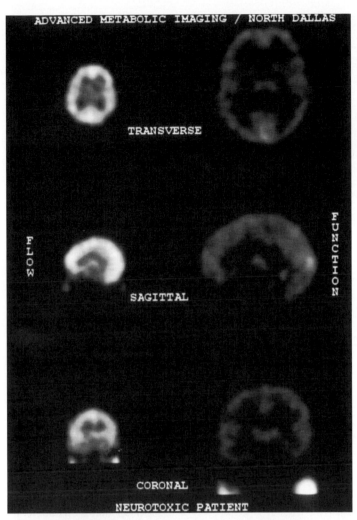

Fig 57.9 SPECT brain scan showing discrepancy between flow and function patterns in a neurotoxic chemically sensitive patient. (*Source* Simon T, Hickey D. *Metabolic Imaging*, 1993. pers comm)

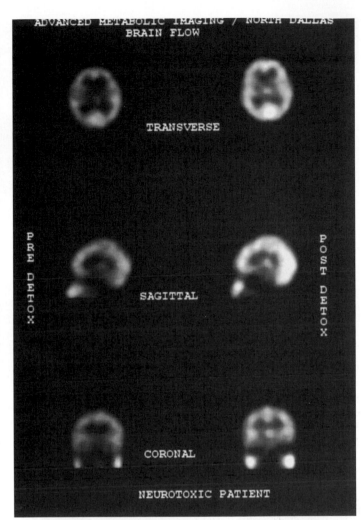

Fig 57.10 Triple camera SPECT brain scan of cerebral blood flow before and after detoxification. (*Source*. Simon T, Hickey D. *Metabolic Imaging*, 1993. pers comm)

Following challenge, most patients produced a sequential progression of symptoms of colour change of the hands, feet, nose and skin, followed by pulse alteration, periorbital and peripheral oedema, petechiae or spontaneous bruising. Biopsies showed perivascular lymphocytic infiltrates. We have now diagnosed and treated several thousand of these patients at the EHC-Dallas. One of the most common syndromes seen with small-vessel vasculitis is characterized by short-term memory loss, imbalance with stressed positive tandom Romberg and inability to stand on the toes with the eyes closed, vertigo and inability to concentrate with chronic fatigue. Triple camera brain scans (CT, SPECT) show decreased flow and function and clearing after total environmental treatment (Figs 57.9 and 57.10).

Large-vessel vasculitis

Large-vessel involvement associated with sensitivities has also been reported.[23,37] Rea detailed the case of a 65-year-old female who exhibited large-vessel involvement. She was found to be sensitive to 10 foods and three synthetic chemicals. All appeared to trigger spasm of her femoral arteries (Fig. 57.11).[86]

Large-vessel vasculitis may ultimately have more devastating results than other vascular disorders since the blood supply to

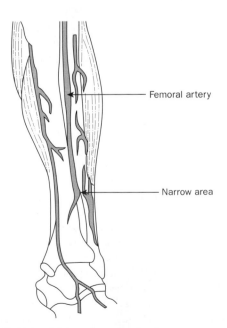

Fig 57.11 Angiogram of femoral artery showing spasm associated with sensitivities after a corn challenge.

Transient hemiplegia				
Patient	Side	Number of occurrences	Triggering agents	Long-term without neurological damage (years)
1	R	6	Foods Multiple chemicals	5
2	R	20	Moulds Foods Multiple chemicals	3
3	L	3	Foods	10
4	L	2	Chemicals	15
5	R	5	Moulds Foods Multiple chemicals	8

Source: EHC-Dallas. 1991.

Table 57.4 Transient hemiplegia.

major organs is affected. Organ ischaemia or necrosis may result in severe disability or even death. The author has now seen five patients with spastic carotid phenomena resulting in transient cerebrovascular accidents (Table 57.4). A 35-year-old surgeon had transient hemiplegia with vascular spasm due to pesticide (Fig. 57.12).

Vasculitis: Raynaud's disease

Raynaud's disease refers to any localized peripheral digital vascular spasm or collapse of unknown aetiology. It may lead to gangrene.[86]

Triggering agents can be identified and culprits include both foods and chemicals. One patient's symptoms could be reproduced by challenge with multiple foods and five inhaled chem-

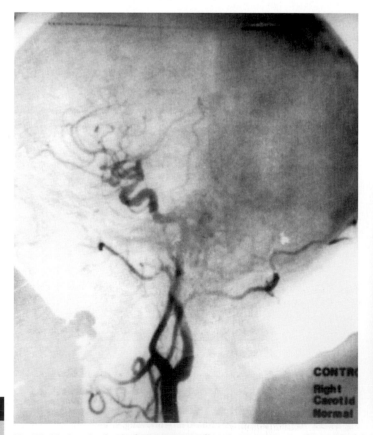
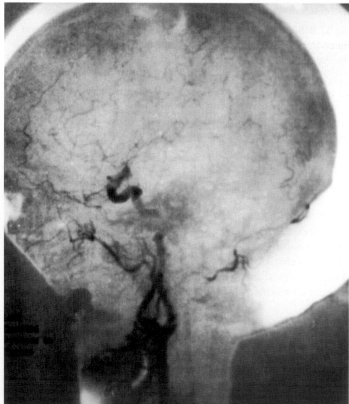

Fig 57.12 Cerebral arteriograms revealing decreased carotid and left intracerebral flow due to arterial spasm.

icals. Follow-up over an 8-year period showed total clearing of the problem with exacerbations occurring only when massive exposures occurred.

The extreme of environmentally triggered vasculitis is illustrated in the following case report of a 4-year-old child.

Case study. The child was well until her neighbours had their lawn treated with insecticide (Fig. 57.13). The child played on the lawn. She developed a sudden pain in her feet and her left leg turned red. This rapidly progressed to severe spasm, followed by severe hypoxia. She was treated with intravenous steroids, anticoagulants and antibiotics. The vascular surgeon felt that she was going to need a hip dysarticulation due to the severe gangrene. She was evacuated by air from her home in Florida to Dallas, where she was placed in the environmental wing of the hospital. She was tested and fasted, placed on 15 g of intravenous vitamin C, daily around the clock, and 6 L/min of oxygen. Within 48 hours, her spasm was relieved and we were able to salvage all gangrenous tissue except for the end of two toes (Fig. 57.14). The patient was treated with a rotary diet, biological inhalant and food injections, organic food and spring water bottled in glass. She did well for 18 months until the same neighbour sprayed the lawn again. The pesticide drift caused the left leg to become red again, but the whole syndrome was aborted by vitamin C, 15 g intravenously, oxygen, 4 L/min, and fasting. The child has remained well for the last 6 years.

We have evaluated over 300 patients with essential hypertension who were triggered by multiple foods and chemicals. Figure 57.15 shows a series of 53 patients who had their BP significantly lowered without medication by removing the incitants.

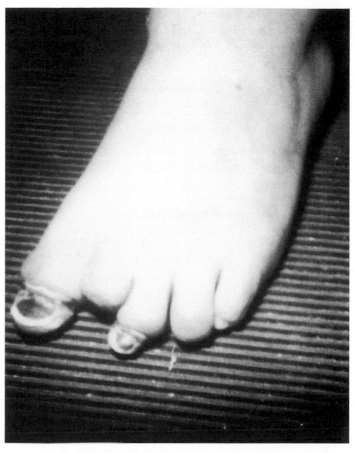

Fig 57.14 Four-year-old white female. After ECU treatment, minimal loss of toes; foot and leg intact.

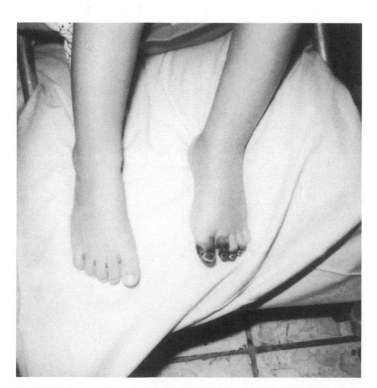

Fig 57.13 Four-year-old white female. After exposure to lawn pesticides, gangrene of the foot developed.

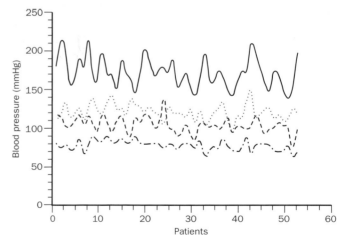

Fig 57.15 Comparison of blood pressure in 53 hypertensive patients before and after environmental treatment. ——, Before, systolic blood pressure; – – –, before, diastolic blood pressure; ······, after, systolic blood pressure; —·—·— after, diastolic blood pressure. (*Source*: EHC-Dallas, 1990.)

Recurrent phlebitis

Conner[41] noted two patients whose phlebitis was triggered by fish and citrus fruits. Others have identified numerous triggering agents including foods, chemicals and inhalants. It has become apparent that, in many patients, phlebitis is only part of a more generalized and severe vasculitis.[86] A study of 10 patients (Table 57.5) treated in an environmental control unit (ECU) shows that symptoms can generally be reproduced following the relevant challenge and that treatment is effective both in the short term and the long term. The treated group showed a remarkable improvement in walking distance and exercise on a stationary bicycle (Table 57.6). These

Thrombophlebitis: associated signs and symptoms and results of challenge studies in 10 patients in an environmental control unit		
Associated signs and symptoms reproduced	**Offending agents**	**Phlebitis reproduced**
1 Diarrhoea Pulse increase (30 beats/min) Nasal congestion Bigeminy Multifocal premature ventricular contractions	Beef, chicken, cigarette smoke, shrimp, pork, gas heat, ingested chemicals	Pork Shrimp Inhaled chemicals
2 Vomiting Pulse increase	Wheat, rice, inhaled chemicals	No
3 Wheezing Rhinorrhoea Red nose Nasal stuffiness Tender muscles Cystitis	Corn, cane sugar, eggs, inhaled chemicals	Corn Eggs Inhaled chemicals
4 Peripheral pulse from 4 to 1+ Tachypnoea Shortness of breath Cyanosis Belching	Beef, potatoes, corn, ingested chemicals	Beef Corn Inhaled chemicals
5 Oedema (generalized) Tender muscles Colitis Dizziness	Pork, pork fumes, ingested chemicals, inhaled chemicals	
6 Syncope Wheezing Muscle tenderness Hives Paroxysmal atrial tachycardia	Legumes, seafood, cane sugar, wheat, chicken, cigarette smoke, inhaled chemicals	Cigarette smoke Ingested chemicals Inhaled chemicals Seafood
7 Gastrointestinal bloat Belching Premature ventricular contractions Ventricular tachycardia	Beef, chicken, lettuce, ingested chemicals, inhaled chemicals	Wheat Potatoes
8 Decrease in pulse, left arm only Left neck and arm tenderness Tender over arm veins	Turkey, chicken, peas, beef, cigarette smoke, inhaled chemicals	No
9 Dyspnoea Wheezing Eyes watering Hoarseness Pulse increase (50 beats/min)	Coffee, peanut butter, cane sugar, chemicals	Apple Corn, wheat Inhaled chemicals
10 Cystitis Diarrhoea Skin rash Itching Dyspnoea Pulse increase	Corn, wheat, beef, eggs, inhaled chemicals	Chicken Beef Inhaled chemicals

Table 57.5 Thrombophlebitis: associated signs and symptoms and results of challenge studies in 10 patients in an environmental control unit.

Results of thrombophlebitis treated in an environmental control unit (ECU)						
	Phlebitis		Exercise			
			Before treatment		After treatment	
	Cleared	Reproduced	Times walking around a 10 ft × 10 ft room	Exercycle miles at 150 kpm resistance	Times walking around a 10 ft × 10 ft room	Exercycle miles 150 kpm resistance
ECU	10	8	0.5	0	36.6	2.85
Control	0	10 (continued)	2.1	0	3.1	0

Table 57.6 Results of thrombophlebitis treated in an environmental control unit (ECU).

results have both clinical and important financial implications, since all 10 of the treated patients were able to return to work whereas only one out of the 10 patients with triggering agents not defined was able to do so.

We at the EHC-Dallas have now seen several hundred intractable cases of chronic thrombophlebitis that can be diagnosed and treated by environmental techniques.

Cardiac arrhythmias

Food and chemical inhalation and ingestion can cause cardiac arrhythmias or coronary spasm.[99,105] The causal role of coffee and cigarettes in the triggering of atrial arrhythmias is well known. Pollutants can also harm the heart.[85]

Details of 12 patients and their cardiovascular response to chemical exposure are shown in Table 57.7.

Reaction to double-blind exposure to fumes of chemicals (1 to 15-min exposure ambient dose) for 12 patients in an environmental control unit									
Patient	Saline control (three challenges)	Petroleum alcohol (<0.5 ppm)	Phenol (<0.002 ppm)	Chlorine (<0.33 ppm)	Pesticides (mixture) (<0.134 ppm)	Pine-scented floor wash	Formaldehyde (<0.2 ppm)	Arrhythmia spectrum	
1	–	+	+	+	+	+	+	Sinus tachycardia (above 130 beats/min)	10
2	–	+	+	+	+	+	+	Sinus bradycardia (below 45 beats/min)	10
3	–	–	+	+	+	–	–	Sinus arrhythmia	11
4	–	–	+	+	+	+	+	Atrial fibrillation (PAT)	4
5	–	+	+	+	+	–	–	Coronary sinus rhythm	12
6	–	+	+	+	+	–	–	1° AV block	8
7	–	+	+	–	+	+	+	PVC	8
8	–	+	+	+	+	+	+	Ventricular tachycardia	2
9	–	+	+	+	–	–	–		
10	–	+	+	+	+	+	+		
11	2–,1+	–	–	–	–	–	–		
12	–	–	–	–	–	–	–		

1° AV, first-degree atrioventricular; PAT, paroxysmal atrial tachycardia; PVC, premature ventricular contraction.
Source: Rea WJ. Environmentally triggered cardiac disease. Ann Allerg 1978; 40(4):243–51, with permission.

Table 57.7 Reaction to double-blind exposure to fumes of chemicals (1 to 15-min exposure ambient dose) for 12 patients in an environmental control unit.

Case study. An undertaker whose bedroom was located above the embalming room of his mortuary had a myocardial infarct at the age of 35 and a quadruple bypass operation at the age of 37. This did not clear his recurrent chest pain and ventricular arrhythmias, and he was refractory to medication (Fig. 57.16). In addition, this patient had recurrent sinusitis, bronchitis and gastrointestinal upsets. After 5 days in the ECU, he became symptom-free, being in sinus rhythm and not taking any medication. Following the ambient dose bronchial challenge with formaldehyde (<0.2 ppm), the patient sequentially developed rhinorrhoea, sinus pain, coughing chest pain and ventricular ectopic beats. He continued to run his business in an office distant to the mortuary.

Case study. A 45-year-old, white male had a 6-month history of uncontrollable bradycardia–tachycardia syndrome with associated irritable bowel syndrome (57.17). Following challenge with phenol, he developed bradycardia and then sinus arrest (Fig. 57.18). On another occasion he responded to a natural gas exposure with a tachycardia of over 200 beats/min for over 1 hour. The patient constructed an environmentally controlled office and home. He has worked without medication or severe exacerbations for the last 20 years, living a healthy life.

At least 20 000 patients with some type of cardiovascular dysfunction have been seen at the EHC-Dallas over the last 25 years. They can be diagnosed and treated by environmental techniques discussed in this chapter.

Arteriosclerosis

Certainly, von Ardenne[114] and Hauss[43] have shown that a vascular change can occur due to pathological processes that result in vasospasm; this results in capillary endothelial swelling, with a shunting of oxygen past certain areas of the target tissue, causing more local tissue hypoxia distal to the stimulation, and producing a high peripheral venous oxygen (PvO_2). High composite PvO_2 is found in the antecubital vein. This shunting of oxygen is detrimental to local tissue metabolism, and results in appropriate function with poor detoxification as seen in the chemically sensitive patient. Hauss[43] has further shown that toxic exposures through inhalation and ingestion of substances such as lead, mercury and organic hydrocarbons disturb the microcirculation, and result in local tissue hypoxia, which triggers the non-specific

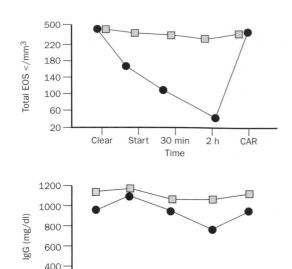

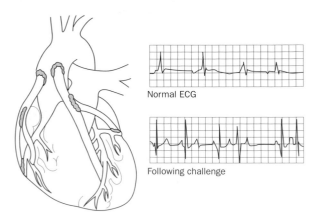

Fig 57.16 Electrocardiograms before and after challenge with formaldehyde in a 37-year-old undertaker.

Fig 57.17 A 37-year-old white male, double-blind challenge (formaldehyde inhaled, <0.2 ppm) after 4 days deadaptation with total load decreased in the ECU. Reproduced symptoms included recurrent PVCs, chest pain, fatigue, sinusitis, bronchitis, gastrointestinal upset and vasculitis. ■, Saline control; ●, formaldehyde challenge. (*Source:* EHC-Dallas, 1978.)

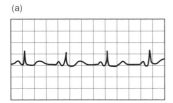

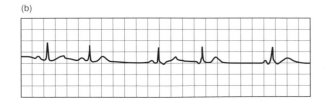

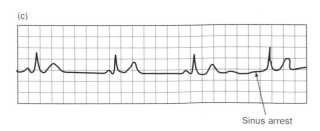

Fig 57.18 Electrocardiograms: (a) prechallenge; (b) 30 seconds after chemical challenge with spa spring water, showing sinus arrhythmia; and (c) sinus bradycardia and sinus arrest 5 min after challenge with phenol. (45-year-old white male after 4 days of deadaptation in the ECU.)

mesenchyme reaction, stimulating fibroblasts to produce PGs/GAGs (prostaglandins/glycosaminoglycans) in an attempt to reassert homeostatic control.

Non-specific mesenchyme reaction (NSMR)

This appears to be instigated early in arteriosclerosis or connective tissue and vascular inflammation as well as fibrosis.[43,114] This NSMR reaction may also be involved in the emergence of alteration of homeostasis, resulting in abnormal lung function parameters following exposure to pollutant or other noxious stimuli and after physical exertion. In the NSMR, many cells become activated, including endothelial cells of the vascular intima, fibroblasts, fibrocytes, smooth muscle cells of the vascular media, etc. This mesenchymal reaction supersedes that of all other cell reactions in the organism. It is clearly a dyshomeostatic reaction. The stimulation of the mesenchyme in the aortic wall is followed by incorporation of lipids into the macrophages, causing more dyshomeostasis and eventually resulting in arteriosclerosis. This lipid incorporation into the mesenchyme of the vessel walls and the quantity and extent of lipid deposits depends on the strength and duration of the pollutant stimuli.

The steps of atherogenesis

First, there is an injury to the vascular intima and connective matrix by trauma, bacteria, virus or toxic substance. Often, the injury is multifactorial and, if the total pollutant load remains high, the process will be unrelenting. Because of the injury and increased total body pollutant load, there is a failure of homeostasis to contain local injury. Activation of the monocyte macrophage system by oxidized low-density lipoproteins occurs. There is an expression of monocyte chemotactic activating factors, such as leukocyte CXCR 2 and homologue. Then a migration of these factors occurs, resulting in neointima formation, which is dependent on plasmin generated from plasminogen from the extracellular matrix. The matrix metal proteases are liberated from the matrix, which causes proteolysis in the lipid deposition area, with fragmentation of the internal elastic lamina and more accumulation of lipids. This accumulation causes triggering of the vascular smooth muscle cells, which proliferate, resulting in coronary stenosis that is very stable. However, unstable coronary lesions lead to myocardial infarction. This situation occurs when the plasminogen activates an inhibitor (PAI-a) found in vessel walls (especially in Type II diabetes). In the case of the acute coronary syndrome, the plaques are more lipid-laden and acellular. There are not many smooth muscle cells involved, because they are inhibited by the release of PAI 1. Thus, the intima is covered by a thin fibrous cap prone to rupture. The activated macrophages then precipitate the plaque rupture. Rupture of the intramural plaque results in haemorrhage and thrombosis. More luminal compression occurs, resulting in obstruction and the acute coronary syndrome.

Pollutant load

If the total body pollutant load is decreased, the structural changes in the vessel wall usually regress after the sclerogenous noxae have been removed; thus, homeostasis can be restored. However, if the sclerogenous irritation or oxygen deficiency lasts for a long time (reduced clearance capacity due to energy deficiency), the non-decomposable metabolic waste products (collagen, fibre bundle, calcification, etc.) accumulate in the way shown on electromicrographs. The structural damage to the vessel wall caused

by the breakdown products no longer recedes (irreversible stage). At this stage, the increase in diffusion time (oxygen, nutrients, etc.) in both the peripheral and the central vessel wall begins to alter the metabolism. For example, the diffusion time through the length of a capillary may decrease from 80 to 30 times, thus altering metabolism. Oxygen therapy plus strict fasting and then dietary alteration under environmentally controlled conditions will often reverse this arteriosclerotic process up to a certain point. This point is where structural vessel wall changes (i.e. aneurysm, total occlusion) occur which make the process irreversible.

A similar structural change in response reaction in the fine capillaries causes the vessel wall to change in diabetes. In diabetes, there is a basement membrane thickening due to protein deposits, which results in the development of microangiopathies. This process of the NSMR narrows the vessel wall lumen, directly hampering local tissue oxygen supply and resulting in a vicous downward dyshomeostatic cycle by the positive feedback characteristic. A similar process can also occur in the membranes of the myelin sheath, leading to the neuropathies in diabetics. According to von Ardenne,[114] this pathogenic basement membrane thickening can be broken down by multi-step step oxygen therapy. However, again, it appears that if structural changes result in fibrotic scars, the nerves and basement membranes are irreversibly damaged. This type of therapy then will not work.

The chemically sensitive and chronically diseased patient appears to have severe problems with oxygenation at the tissue level.[84] When studying the microcirculation in the chemically sensitive, there appears to be a higher demand for oxygen at the end-tissue level, thus altering the capillary sphincter mechanism function over that seen in the normal individual. Capillary sphincter response appears altered, with blood shunting in different areas of the end-organ tissue; this results in more dyshomeostasis and hypoxia, with a vicious downward cycle by the positive feedback homeostatic characteristic. It is not uncommon to see antecubital vein PO_2 as high as 40–50 mmHg in the chemically sensitive and the chronically diseased patients compared with normal control values of 22 ± 5 mmHg.[84,114] This inability to extract sufficient oxygen results in inefficient metabolic breakdown of toxins (at the end-capillary level) by the oxygen-driven cytochrome detoxification systems, which leads to inadequate detoxification by oxidation, acetylation, acylation (peptide conjugation) sulphonation, methylation and glucuronide processes. Also, decreased tissue oxygen will lead to more tissue deterioration, which causes a straining of the homeostatic repair mechanism and eventually triggers the NSMR.

TREATMENT

Treatment of environmentally triggered cardiovascular disease involves massive avoidance of pollutants in air, food and water; injection therapy for biological inhalants; foods, some chemicals, neurotransmitters, intestinal peptides, as well as oral and intravenous nutrition; heat depuration (sauna) with physical therapy including exercise and massage; immune modulators; oxygen therapy; and, in some cases, surgery to remove inflamed organs or synthetic implants that are disrupting homeostasis.

Acute reactions

Acute angioedema reactions triggered by a sudden exposure can best be treated by avoidance or removal of the offending

Treatment of acute reactions
Laxative
Oxygen 40–100% for 2 hours
Sodium bicarbonate, 50 mEq intravenously
Vitamin C 7.5–15 g intravenous, oral to gastrointestinal tolerance (oral 2 tsp)

Table 57.8 Treatment of acute reactions.

substance(s) immediately. This can be done by placing the individual in a less-polluted office, room at home, or hospital. If the toxic agent is ingested, treatment should be given as outlined in Table 57.8, using a laxative such as milk of magnesia (magnesium oxides) or Epsom salts (magnesium sulphate). Less-polluted water and organic food should be used along with 15 g of intravenous vitamin C, $MgSO_4$ or $MgCl_2$ 20–40 mEq, 2 mL of multiple minerals including chromium, zinc, manganese, selenium and copper, plus 2 mL of vitamin B complex with glutathione 600 mg plus 2 g of taurine given daily until symptoms clear. Oxygen is administered at 2–4 L/min. If the neutralization dose of the specific antigen that triggered the reaction is available, administration is useful. If it is not available, the neutralization dose of histamine or serotonin should be given. Trisalts consisting of sodium, potassium and calcium bicarbonate 3:2:1, using one teaspoonful in a glass of water every hour until the reaction stops, should be taken. If heart failure is a problem, the sodium should be omitted. Repeat the whole cycle of removal of the incitant, alkalinization, oxygen and neutralization injection until the reaction has ceased. Rapid institution of these procedures within the first 1–2 hours after exposure will usually stop an acute reaction and allow the patient to return to his basal state. This regime may be effective up to 24 hours after an acute exposure.

Chronic inflammatory vascular disease

The treatment of chronic, recurrent inflammatory vascular disease (whether it be phlebitis, arthritis, arteriosclerosis or vasculitis) again involves avoidance of as many triggering agents as possible, thus reducing the total incitant load. This can be done by drinking less-polluted water (spring, distilled, ceramic, charcoal-filtered), and eating less-contaminated food (fewer additives, preservatives, pesticides, etc.). If a patient has a food sensitivity (usually non-IgE-mediated), avoidance of those foods is necessary. Rotary diets, where the patient does not eat the same food more often than 4–5 days, helps decrease the total body load. Injection therapy for treatment of the food and biological inhalant sensitivity is usually needed. Maintenance of vessel integrity and dilatation to eliminate vasospasm by oxygenation is necessary for the wall of the blood vessels. Immune modulation, such as transfer factor or autogenous lymphocytic factor, can be used to enhance immune response. Occasionally, surgery is needed to remove inflamed, infected organs or artificial implants. Long-term treatment is usually necessary with day-in and day-out lowering of the total noxious incitant load; replacement of nutrition and oxygen are essential for reversal and maintenance of vessel wall integrity.

Avoidance modalities

Systematic avoidance for the treatment of chronic or inflammatory vascular disease can now be used in place of, or in addition to, medication therapy. The two should go hand-in-hand, but avoidance with removal of triggering agents should be emphasized, since it is the most powerful tool available to the clinician. If the pollutants are avoided successfully most of the time, medications are not necessary. Avoidance has been the cornerstone of treatment of infectious disease and applies as well to other non-infectious inflammatory diseases such as vasculitis and arteriosclerosis.

Avoidance of pollutants in indoor air will reduce the entry of potential triggering agents into the body. This includes constructing a less-polluted home environment. For severely affected patients, an oasis should be created in the bedroom by removing all possible pollutants, including pesticides, fossil fuels, carpets, toxic mattresses, formaldehyde-saturated plywood, particle board, etc., synthetic and dry-cleaned clothes and curtains. Some severely ill patients may have to change jobs or areas of work. Complete cessation of smoking in the home is mandatory.

Injection therapy

For patients with the hypersensitive state of vasculitis, injection therapy for biological inhalants, food and some chemicals such as metals and intestinal peptides are necessary for stopping the vasculitis. Injection therapy is usually performed daily to every 4 days and is one of the most powerful tools for decreasing vascular spasm. The neutralizing dose of histamine and serotonin has been extremely efficacious in aiding our vascular patients at the EHC-Dallas.

Injections of the neutralizing doses of intestinal peptides are usually given every 4 days, but sometimes, for a brief period, daily or every other day doses are necessary. Injection neutralization for intestinal peptides of various substances, such as vaso-active intestinal peptides, gastrin and choleocystokinin, can be used and will often aid in stopping vascular deregulation. If the proper neutralizing injections can be found, they can be administered daily to every 4 days.

Nutritional replacement and supplementation

Correction of nutritional deficiencies is important when trying to correct vascular damage. Often this is simple, but many times it is complex, depending upon the severity of the vascular damage. We now discuss these in detail.

Vitamin C

Vitamin C can be depleted with chemical exposures particularly to substances like benzene,[1, 51] carbon monoxide,[13] ethanol, smoking,[2] nitrous compounds,[119] vinyl chloride,[119] heavy metals[119] and pesticides.[55] Amorphous ground substance of the vessel wall is somewhat dependent on vitamin C, which lies in the basement membrane. Vitamin C supplements can be used not only to strengthen the blood vessel wall but also as a free-radical scavenger and antioxidant.[70] Usually an oral dose of 1–10 g per day of powdered vitamin C has been used in patients with vascular dysfunction. One must be careful of the source, since many individuals become intolerant of the food of origin, such as corn, sago palm, potato and carrot.

Vitamin A

β-Carotene (precursor of vitamin A) is used as a potent antioxidant and has been shown to positively affect free-radical activity as well as keeping the gap junctions tight to preserve vascular wall integrity. From 5000 to 25 000 units daily have been used in our centre without side effects. The patients with vascular acne-like lesions sometimes will respond to vitamin A-*cis*-retinoic acid. Care has to be taken to avoid multiple potential side effects.[72] Careful monitoring of vitamin A compounds should be carried out to avoid liver damage. Vitamin A has been shown to blunt the effects of radiation, probably through its free-radical scavenger effect.[75] It should not be taken for a long period of time without attempting to find the triggering agents.

Vitamin D
Vitamin D is needed to help regulate calcium metabolism. People who live in northern climates have more difficulty generating vitamin D, due to less exposure time to the sun. It has been shown that persons living where oxidant pollutant levels are high may have a concomitant decrease in vitamin D accumulations by as much as 15% over a 25-year period. Pasteurization also eliminates vitamin D. Supplementation must be carefully monitored to avoid toxicity. The safest therapy is exposure to sunlight.[72]

Vitamin E
Vitamin E, which is necessary for vascular wall integrity, is an effective antipollutant. From 400 to 1400 units have been used in some vascular patients.[19]

Bioflavanoids
Bioflavanoids are also needed to strengthen the vascular wall. Two capsules daily are needed.

Vitamin B complex
Vitamin B complex (50–100 mg), B_{12} (1000 IU) and folic acid (400 μg) may be used as a protective in reducing homocysteine, which has been implicated in myocardial infarctions.

Calcium
Calcium is clearly one mineral that is necessary for membrane stability and, thus, vascular wall tone. It is also a cofactor in many metabolic steps. The calcium level has been found to be inversely proportional to radiostrontium; thus it would be of use in protecting a patient against this pollutant. One to three grams of calcium have been given daily to patients with vascular disease without problems. Many forms have been used due to the patient's sensitivity. These are calcium plus magnesium, calcium chloride, calcium gluconate plus calcium carbonate. The complications of excess calcium ingestion are well known.

Magnesium
Magnesium is a membrane stabilizer and vasodilator. It is anti-vasospastic. It is complexed with ATP and ADP, and therefore is a mandatory cofactor for all kinases and other enzymes with nucleotides as a substrate or product cytosol. Occasionally, intravenous challenge is necessary to correct a total body deficiency. Magnesium is an integral factor for vascular membrane function: up to 1500 mg may be used. One can push to bowel tolerance. A combination of calcium and magnesium in a 2–3:1 ratio may be necessary.[72]

Zinc
Zinc is needed for wound healing and immune regulation. Zinc supplements are capable of reducing lipid peroxidation; conse-quently, zinc loading has been found to stabilize cell membranes. It has reduced the damage induced by carbon tetrachloride in animals. Zinc also catalyses many other metabolic reactions in the body and is essential in the antipollutant enzyme superoxide dismutase. Up to 45 mg of elemental zinc has been used in patients with vascular disease without problems.[72]

Selenium
Selenium has immune-stimulating properties. It enhances the capacity of phytohaemagglutinin (PHA) to increase blastogenic transformation of lymphocytes.[63,69] Up to 300 μg of selenium have been given safely. It is necessary for many direct biochemical detoxification reactions[69] and also for the maintenance of the antipollutant enzyme glutathione peroxidase, which is needed to stop pollutants at the point of entry. Care should be taken to avoid overdose, since severe toxic symptoms of weakness and muscle pain may occur.

Chromium
Chromium, 200 μg/day, is an antiglucose factor and may be used for patients who have glucose elevations that alter blood vessels, such as in diabetes mellitus.

Copper
In most cases of deficiency 2 mg of copper is used. Excess copper can cause angiogenesis, which in certain areas can be harmful.

Glutathione
Glutathione, 600 mg to 2 g, is a powerful sulphur-containing antioxidant that helps neutralize free radicals generated by toxins. In particular, glutathione binds heavy metals such as mercury, lead and cadmium.

Taurine
To stabilize cardiac membranes 1–2 g/day is needed. Taurine is another sulphur-containing antioxidant that is a membrane stabilizer in heart muscle.

Coenzyme Q-10
This substance has been used at the EHC-Dallas to stabilize patients with early heart failure, myocardial infarctions and arrhythmias. Intravenous coenzyme Q-10, 300 mg is used over a 4-hour period along with 40 mEq of $MgSO_4$ and oxygen administration and oxygen therapy at 6 L/min. Table 57.9 shows the cessation of acute myocardial infarction in four cases with subsequent 6 months follow-up without sequelae. Chronic oral administration is 150–300 mg daily.

Arginine
Arginine is a precursor to nitric oxide, which is a potent natural vasodilator in the body; 2 g daily are used in some patients with spastic vascular phenomena.

Medications
Prednisone (10 mg four times daily) may be given and will usually diminish reactivity in some patients as a result of its anti-inflammatory and immunosuppressive properties. Just as often, prednisone will aggravate the problem, making the patient much worse. The complications of long-term use of prednisone are well known and will not be discussed here.

Acute myocardial infarction aborted by intravenous coenzyme Q-10, 300 mg, plus 40 mEq MgSO$_4$ over a 4-hour period and 12 hours of oxygen							
Age (years)	Race/sex	ECG injury current	Significant enzyme elevation	Crushing chest pain (2+ hour duration)	Exercise tolerance (6 months)	Post-treatment follow-up without symptoms*	
56	White/male	+	+	+	Walk 1.6 miles at one time	6 months	
79	White/male	+	+	+	Walk 1 mile at one time	9 months	
60	White/female	+	+	+	Walk unlimited	1 year	
64	White/male	+	+	+	Walk 3 miles at one time	6 months	

* All patients were placed on an oral regimen of coenzyme Q-10, 300 mg/day; 1000 mg of magnesium citrate/day; 800 U of vitamin E/day; 2 g of taurine/day; folic acid 400 µg/day; vitamin B$_{12}$ 1000 U/day.

Table 57.9 Acute myocardial infarction aborted by intravenous coenzyme Q-10, 300 mg, plus 40 mEq MgSO$_4$ over a 4-hour period and 12 hours of oxygen.

Cytotoxic agents (Plaquenil and methotrexate) have been used in some patients with leukocytoclastic vasculitis. Cyclophosphamide has been used but may not induce a significant long-term remission since the patient is well into fixed end-stage disease at this point.

Over all, drug treatment is not recommended for the long-term prevention and treatment of cardiovascular disease without removal of the incitants and replacement of the nutrients. Digitalis is the time-honoured treatment for heart failure. Vasodilators can also be used temporarily. Standard medical therapy for end-stage disease will not be discussed, due to common knowledge in medicine.

Heat depuration/physical therapy (exercise and massage)

These modalities, utilizing environmentally controlled saunas, exercise and massage, have been used in over 2000 patients. Initially, blood toxins increase (Table 57.10) and then decrease after 1–3 weeks, and the patients improve their symptoms. These modalities have been exceptionally good for hypertensive and Raynaud's patients.

Oxygen administered at 2–4 L/min for 10–40 min relieves vascular spasm and helps stabilize an individual after a reaction.

Immunomodulators

Immunomodulators such as transfer factor have been used by a few groups. We have a small group of patients who appeared to respond to biweekly injections of transfer factor. However, no patient was totally cleared of his vascular malady. T cell autogenous lymphocytic factor is an immune modulator developed at the EHC-Dallas. This substance has been used in over 600 chemically sensitive patients with 88% responding ($P < 0.001$) with less chemical sensitivity, more resistance to exposure plus immune and vascular enhancements.

Oxygen therapy

Oxygen therapy is directed at preventing the triggering of vascular spasm and hypoxia, which results in end-organ triggering of the NSMR. Once this process is set in motion, tissue changes may occur in the vascular wall, causing arteriosclerosis or vascular wall inflammation that results in occlusive fibrous vessels.

Von Ardenne[114] has shown that 2 hours of oxygen at 6 L/min for 18 days will relieve the spasm of the microcirculation and venous endothelium swelling, causing an increase in tissue oxygen absorption with the resulting decrease in venous PO$_2$. We have used this technique in over 500 patients with vascular spasm extensively using an especially designed oxygen delivery apparatus. This type of oxygen therapy is efficacious in a subset of chemically sensitive patients with vasculitis.

Surgery

Removal of chronically inflamed organs such as the gall bladder, uterus, colon (partially), small bowel (partially) or other affected organs or occlusive vessels will decrease the total body load and thus vascular inflammation.

Removal of any synthetic prostheses such as breast and abdominal wall implants and vascular and orthopaedic grafts will also decrease the total body load and allow for a decrease in vascular inflammation.

Exercise

Exercise as a treatment for cardiovascular disease is a double-edged sword. When used early in the preventive and treatment cycle, it may well blunt reactions and exclude incitants from harming the vessel wall. When it is used later in the disease process, the vasculitis and arteriosclerotic patient responds just as in exercise-induced asthma. We have seen many patients attempting to exercise in a late stage of vascular disease only to be incapacitated with muscular aches, dizziness and weakness. It is well known that marathon runners who ignore their cardiac signs and symptoms can die suddenly. Clearly, exercise in moderation appears to help strengthen the cardiac muscle in other patients.

CONCLUSION

The prospect for the future is very bright when one studies the physiology and preventive aspect of cardiovascular disease. A concept and method have now been established for the scientific definition of chemical- and food-triggering agents for inflammatory cardiovascular diseases, including spastic vascular pheno-

Chemical	Marked			Efficacious			Ineffective			Total effective rate +	++
	No.	%+	++	No.	%+	++	No.	%	++		
n-Pentane	1	7.1	20	3	21.4	50	10	71.4	30	29.6	70
2,2-Dimethylbutane	4	36.4	75	0	0	23	7	63.6	2	36.4	98
Cyclopentane	3	60.0	70	1	20.0	22	1	20.0	8	80[a]	92
2-Methylpentane	0	0	60	4	28.6	31.6	10	71.4	8.4	28.6	91.6
3-Methylpentane	1	7.1	73.2	4	28.6	15.8	9	64.3	20	35.7	89
n-Hexane	1	7.1	90	5	35.7	7.0	8	57.1	3	42.9[a]	97
n-Heptane	–	–	xxx	–	–	100	–	–	0	–	100
Benzene		55.6	85		10	12	12	44.4	13	55.6	87
Toluene		7.1	88	88	42	42.9	10	50.0	2	50	98
Ethylbenzene		66.7	75		0	21.8		33.3	3.2	66.7	96.8
Xylene		42.9	100	42	14.2	20		42.9	20	57.1	80
Styrene		100	100		0	0		0	0	100	100
Trimethylbenzene		0*	83[b]		0	16		*	1	*	99[a]
Chloroform		50	50[b]		25	40		25	10	75[a]	90
Dichloromethane		30.8	60		15.4	30		53.8	10	46.2	90
1,1,1-Trichloroethane		13.3	25		33.3	50		53.3	25	48.6	75
Trichloroethylene		66.7	73		0	20		33.3	7	66.7	93
Dichlorobenzene		7	50[b]		0	40		*	10	*	90
Tetrachloroethylene		23.1	40		23.1	40		53.8	20	46.2	80

Notes:
* Blood levels below detection limit before and after.
xxx Ten patients
a Most easily cleared.
b 10 patients only.
Source: EHC-Dallas, 1993.

Table 57.10 Effective clearance number and rate for volatile allphatic panel in whole blood of first 14+ patients++ and last 100 patients out of 1000.

mena such as migraines and other vascular headaches, angina due to coronary spasm, Raynaud's disease, etc., many autoimmune vasculitides, i.e. lupus, rheumatoid and other early collagen vasculitis, in addition to small- and large-vessel vasculitis with Henoch–Schönlein purpura, etc., cardiac arrhythmias, non-traumatic phlebitis and arteriosclerosis. There are now many articles in the scientific literature supporting the view that cardiovascular diseases can be caused by reactions to food and environmental irritants. We have been increasingly confident in defining and eliminating the triggering agents, augmenting nutrition and clearing and managing the various aspects of cardiovascular dysfunction.

REFERENCES

1 Askari EM, Gabliks J. DDT and immunological responses. I. Altered histamine levels and anaphylactic shock in guinea pigs. *Arch Environ Health* 1979; 26(6): 309–19.

2 Astaldi G, Karanoic D, Vettori PP *et al.* Phytohemagglutinin (PHA) stimulation of peripheral-blood lymphocytes and stem cell. *Biol 1st Seroten Milanesi* 1974; 53: 599.

3 Balaz T. *Cardiac Toxicology.* Vols I and II. CRC Press, Boca Raton, Florida, 1981.

4 Barnes DW, Munson AE. Cadmium-induced suppression of cellular immunity in mice. *Toxicol Appl Pharmacol* 1978; 45(1): 350.

5 Bartlett SJ, McCarthy III SW, Palmer AS, Flynn WR, Beryman JJ, Yao JS. Multiple aneurysms in Behcet's disease. *Arch Surg* 1988; 123: 1004–8.

6 Becker RO, Marino AA. *Electromagnetism and Life.* State University of New York Press, Albany, 1982.

7 Bell, I, Kind D. Psychological and physiological research relevant to clinical ecology: an overview of the recent literature. *Clin Ecology* 1982: 1(1).

8 Bjorkner BH. Sensitization capacity of acrylated prepolymers in ultraviolet curing inks tested in the guinea pig. *Acta Derm Venereol (Stockh)* 1981; 61(1): 7–10.

9 Black CM, Welsh KI. Occupationally and environmentally induced scleroderma-like illness: etiology, pathogenesis, diagnosis, and treatment. *IM* 1988; 9(6): 136–54.

10 Black CM, Pereira S, McWhirter A, Welsh K, Caurent R. Genetic susceptibility to scleroderma-like syndrome in symptomatic and asymptomatic workers exposed to vinyl chloride. *J Rheum* 1986; 13: 1059–62.

11 Blanchi D, Cedrini L, Ceria F *et al.* Exposure of mammals to strong 50-Hz electric fields. *Arch Fisiol* 1980; 70: 33.

12 Bunter RG, Carrol JH, Randolph JC. Water in the urban environment: Real Estate Lakes. US Dept of Interior/Geological Survey, 11–19.49. *Pest Monit J* 1980; 14(3): 102–7.

13 Calabrese EJ. *Pollutants and High Risk Groups: the Increased Human Susceptibility to Environmental and Occupational Pollutants.* John Wiley and Sons, New York, 1978.

14 Cluff LE. Serum sickness and related disorders. In: *Harrison's Principles of Internal Medicine* (Wintrobe MM, Thorn GW, Adams RD *et al.* eds.), McGraw-Hill, New York, 1970: 374–6.

15 Cohen IS, Mosher MB, O'Keefe EJ, Klaus SN, De Conti RC. Cutaneous toxicity of bleomycin therapy. *Arch Dermatol* 1973; 107(4): 553–5.

16 Cordier JM, Fievez MJ, Sevrin A. Acro-osteolysis and exposure to vinyl chloride. *Cah Med Travail* 1966; 4: 14–19.

17 Couch, JR, Wortman J. Anovulatory states as a factor in occurrence of migraine. Paper presented at The Migraine Trust, Fifth International Symposium, Sept., 1984.

18 Darlington LG, Ramsey NW, Mansfield JR. Placebo-controlled, blind study of dietary manipulation therapy in rheumatoid arthritis. *Lancet* 1986; i: 236–8.

19 Davis A. *Let's Get Well.* Harcourt Brace, New York, 1965; 41–2.

20 Debled G. *L'Andropause: Cause, Consequences and Remedies.* Malione, Paris, 1989.

21 Delena MA, Guzzon S, Monfardini S, Bonadonna G. Clinical radiologic and histopathologic studies on pulmonary toxicity induced by treatment with bleomycin (NSC-125066). *Cancer Chemother Rep* 1972; 56: 343–56.

22 De Pasquale NP, Burch GE. The seasonal incidence of myocardial infarction in New Orleans. *Am J Med Sci* 1961; 242: 468–78.

23 Dickey JW Jr. Drifting hematomas. *Surg Gynecol Obset* 1979; 148: 209.

24 Dinman BD, Cook WA, Whitehouse WM, Magnuson HJ, Mich AA, Ditcheck T. Occupational acroosteolysis: I. An epidemiological study. *Arch Environ Health* 1971; 22: 61–73.

25 Dodson VN, Dinman BD, Whitehouse WM, Nasr ANM, Magnuson HJ. Occupational acroosteolysis. III. A clinical study. *Arch Environ Health* 1971; 22: 83.

26 EPA. *What Everyone Should Know about Their Drinking Water.* Environmental Protection Agency, 1987.

27 Erban L. A study of biochemical and hematological changes under the application of ionized air. *Int J Bioclimatol Biometeorol* 1958; 3(vi).

28 Finch WR, Buckingham RB, Rednan GP, Prince RK, Winkelstein A. Scleroderma induced by bleomycin. In: *Systemic Sclerosis (Scleroderma)* (CM Black, AR Myers, eds), Gower Medical, New York, 1985; 114–21.

29 Fischer G, Waibel R, Richter T. Influence of line-frequency of electric fields on the heart rate of rats. *Zentralbl Bakteriol Mikrobiol Hyg [B]* 1976; 162: 374.

30 Fourth International Symposium on Magnesium, and American College of Nutrition 26th Annual Meeting. 1985; 4(3): 303–404.

31 Freed DJL, Buckley CH, Tsiviori Y *et al.* Non-allergenic haemolysis in grass pollens and housedust mites. *Allergy* 1983; 38: 477–86.

32 Fries JF, Lindgren JA, Bull JM. Scleroderma-like lesions and the carcinoid syndrome. *Arch Intern Med* 1973; 131: 550–3.

33 Gabliks J, Askari EM, Yolen N. DDT and immunological responses. I. Serum antibodies and anaphylactic shock in guinea pigs. *Arch Environ Health* 1975; 26(6): 305–8.

34 Gabliks J, Al-Tubaidy T, Askari E. DDT and immunological responses. III. Reduced anaphylaxis and mast cell population in rats fed DDT. *Arch Environ Health* 1975; 30(2): 81–4.

35 Gaworski CL, Sharma RP. The effects of heavy metals on (3H) thymidine uptake in lymphocytes. *Toxicol Appl Pharmacol* 1978; 46(2): 305–13.

36 Gilpin A. *Air Pollution*, 2nd edn. University of Queensland Press, St. Lucia, Queensland, 1978.

37 Grant EC. Oral contraceptives, smoking, migraine and food allergy. *Lancet* 1968; ii: 581–9.

38 Groza P, Nicolescu E, Laz'ar D *et al.* The influence of magnetic fields on some humoral parameters and on resistance to hyperthermia in rats. *Physiologie* 1982; 19(1): 15–24.

39 Hannington E. Diet and migraine. *J Hum Nutr* 1978; 34: 175–80.

40 Hare F. *The Food Factor in Disease.* Longmans, London, 1905, Chapter 10.

41 Harkavy J. *Vascular Allergy and Its Systemic Manifestations.* Butterworths, Washington, 1963.

42 Harris DK, Adams WGF. Acro-osteolysis occurring in men engaged in the polymerization of vinyl chloride. *Brit Med J* 1956; 3: 712–14.

43 Hauss WH. Rolle der mesenchymzelen in der pathogenese der arteriosklerose. *Doc Angiol* 1970; 2: 11.

44 Heine H (ed.). *Matrix and Matrix Regulation. Basis for a Holistic Theory in Medicine* (Pischinger A, Engl trans N Maclean.), Editions Haug International, Brussels, 1991.

45 Heyter HE, Teng HC, Barris WB. The increased frequency of acute myocardial infarction during summer months in warm climates. *Am Heart J* 1953; 45: 741.

46 Hippocrates. *On the Theory and Practice of Medicine.* Citadel Press, 1964.

47 Katz P. Hypersensitivity vasculitis. *AFP* 1982; 26(1): 171–5.

48 Keifer O. Über die nebenwirkungen der bleomycintherapie auf der haut. *Dermatologica* 1973; 146: 229–43.

49 Kleibel K, Rackova M. Cutaneous allergic reactions to dithiocarbonates. *Contact Dermatitis* 1980; 6(5): 348–9.

50 Koh KK, Blum KA, Hathaway I *et al.* Vascular effects of estrogen and vitamin E therapies in postmenopausal women. *Circulation* 1999; 100(18): 1851–7.

51 Kollwe LD. Altered immune response by environmental contaminants. *International Symposium on Pathobiology of Environmental Pollutants: Animal Models and Wildlife as Monitors*, CPI (59), Reg No. A7722, 1977.

52 Korobetson MA, Malenuik Bu. Glucocorticoids and the blood anticoagulation system under the effect of SHF-range electromagnetic waves. *Kosm Biol Aviakosm Med* 1978; 1213: 60–3.

53 Kroker GF, Stroud RM, Marshall R *et al.* Fasting and rheumatoid arthritis: a multi-center study. *Clin Ecology* 1984; 2(3): 137–44.

54 Kuksinsky VYe. Coagulative properties of blood and tissue of the cardiovascular system following exposure to an electromagnetic field. *JPRS* 1978; 71595: 1.

55 Laseter JL, DeLeon IR, Rea WJ, Butler JR. Chlorinated hydrocarbon pesticides in environmentally sensitive patients. *Arch Clin Ecol* 1983; 2(1).

56 Lelbach WK, Marsteller HJ. Vinyl chloride associated disease. *Ergeb Inn Med Kinderheilkd* 1981; 47: 1–100.

57 Levine SA, Likoff WB. The therapeutic value of testosterone propionate in angina pectoris. *N Engl J Med* 1943; 229: 770–2.

58 Lindemayer H, Schmidt J. Intolerance to acetylsalicyclic acid and food additives in patients sufering from recurrent urticaria. *Wien Klin Wochenschr* 1979; 91(24): 817–22.

59 Luna MA, Bedrossian Wm, Lichtiger B, Salem PA. Interstitial pneumonitis associated with bleomycin therapy. *Am J Clin Path* 1972; 58: 501–10.

60 Marino AA, Berger TJ, Mitchell JT *et al*. Electric field effects in selected biologic systems. *Ann NY Acad Sci* 1974; 238: 436.

61 Markov VV. The effects of continuous and intermittent microwave radiation on weight and atrial pressure of animals in chronic experiments. *JPRS* 1973; 63321: 95.

62 Markowitz SS, McDonald J, Fethiere W, Kerzner MS. Occupational acroosteolysis. *Arch Dermatol* 1972; 106: 219.

63 Martin J, Spallholz J. *Proceedings of the Symposium on Selenium–Tellurium in the Environment*, Industrial Health Foundation, Pittsburg, 1976; 204–25.

64 Monroe EW, Schulz CI, Maize JC, Jordan RE. Vasculitis in chronic urticaria: an immunopathologic study. *J Invest Dermatol* 1981; 76(2): 103–7.

65 Mustafa MG, Tierney DF. Biochemical and metabolic changes in the lung with oxygen, ozone, and nitrogen dioxide toxicity. *Am Rev Respir Dis* 1978; 118: 1061–90.

66 National Research Council. Water hardness and health. In: *Drinking Water and Health*. National Academy of Sciences, New York, 1977; 439–47.

67 Nour-Elden R. Uptake of phenol by vascular and brain tissue. *Microvasc Res* 1970; 2: 224.

68 Parish WR. Studies on vasculitis, immunoglobulins β1C, C-reactive proteins and bacterial antigens in cutaneous vasculitis lesions. *Clin Allergy* 1971; 1: 97–110.

69 Passwaters, RA. *Selenium as Food and Medicine*. Keats Publishing, New Canaan, Connecticut, 1980; 88–95.

70 Pauling L. *Vitamin C, Common Cold, and Flu*. WH Freeman, San Francisco, 1976: 191–3.

71 *Pest Toxic Chem News* 1984; 12(32).

72 Pfeiffer CC. *Mental and Elemental Nutrients*. Keats Publishing, New Canaan, Connecticut, 1975.

73 Phillips GB, Pinkernell BH, Jing TY. The association of hypotestosteronemia with coronary artery disease in men. *Arterioscler Thromb* 1994; 14: 701–6.

74 Pischinger, A. *Matrix and Matrix Regulation: Basis for a Holistic Theory in Medicine* (Heine H. ed., Eng trans N Maclean). Editions Haug International, Brussels, 1975.

75 Primer on allergy and immunologic disease. *J Am Med Assoc* 1982; 248: 20.

76 Prokhvatilo YeV. Reduction of functional capacities of the heart following exposure to an electromagnetic field of industrial frequency. *JPRS* 1977; 70101: 76.

77 Randolph TG. *Human Ecology and Susceptibility to the Chemical Environment*. Charles C Thomas, Springfield, Illinois, 1962.

78 Rea WJ. Environmentally triggered small vessel vasculitis. *Ann Allergy* 1977; 38: 245–52.

79 Rea WJ. Recurrent environmentally triggered thrombophlebitis. *Ann Allergy* 1981; 47: 338–44.

80 Rea WJ. Elimination of oral food challenge reaction by injection of food extracts: a double-blind evaluation. *Arch Otolaryngol* 1984; 110: 248–52.

81 Rea WJ. *Chemical Sensitivity*, Vol. 1. Lewis, Boca Raton, Florida, 1992.

82 Rea WJ. *Chemical Sensitivity*, Vol. 2. Lewis, Boca Raton, Florida, 1994.

83 Rea WJ. *Chemical Sensitivity*, Vol. 3. Lewis, Boca Raton, Florida, 1996.

84 Rea WJ. *Chemical Sensitivity*, Vol. 4. Lewis, Boca Raton, Florida, 1997.

85 Rea WJ, Suits CW. Cardiovascular disease triggered by foods and chemicals. In: *Food Allergy: New Perspectives*. (Gerrard JW, ed.). Charles C Thomas, Springfield, Illinois, 1980.

86 Rea WJ, Bell IR, Smiley RE. Large vessel vasculitis. In: *Allergy: Immunology and Medical Treatment*, (Johnson F, Spence JT, eds). Symposia Specialist, Chicago, 1975.

87 Rea WJ, Smiley RE, Edgar RE *et al*. Recurrent environmentally triggered thrombophlebitis: a five-year follow-up. *Ann Allergy* 1981; 47: 338–44.

88 Reag WJ, Butler JR, Laseter JL, DeLeon IR. Pesticides and brain function changes in a controlled environment. *Arch Clin Ecol* 1984; 2(3): 145–50.

89 Read H, Holt S, Housley E *et al*. Raynaud's phenomenon induced by sulphasalzine. *Postgrad Med* 1980; 56: 106–7.

90 Reinl W. Sklerodermie dureh Trichloroethylene-Einwirkung? *Bull Hy* 1957; 32: 678.

91 Rier SE, Martin CD, Bowman RE, Dmowski WP, Becker JL. Endometriosis in rhesus monkeys (*Macaca mulatto*) following chronic exposure to 2,3,7,8-tetrachlorodibenzo-*p*-dioxin. *Fundamen Appl Toxicol* 1993; 21: 433–41.

92 Rodnan GP, Benedek TG, Medsger TA, Cammarata RJ. The association of progressive systemic sclerosis (scleroderma) with Coal Miners' pneumoconiosis and other forms of silicosis. *Ann Intern Med* 1967; 66: 323–34.

93 Romaquera C, Grimalt F. Sensitization to benzoyl peroxide, retinoic acid and carbon tetrachloride. *Contact Dermatitis* 1980; 6(6): 422.

94 Saihan EM, Burton JL, Heaton KW. A new syndrome with pigmentation, scleroderma, gynaecomastia. Raynaud's phenomenon and peripheral neuropathy. *Brit J Dermatol* 1978; 99: 437–40.

95 Silverman D, Kornblueh IH. Effect of artificial ionization of the air on the electro-encephalogram. *Am J Phys Med* 1957; 36: 352–8.

96 Smith CW. Electromagnetic phenomena. In: *Living Biomedical Systems, Frontiers of Engineering and Computing. Health Care* Sept. 15–16, 1984.

97 Spalding RF, Junk GA, Richard JJ. Water: pesticides in ground water beneath irrigated farmland in Nebraska. *Pestic Monit J* 1980; 1(2): 70–3.

98 Sparrow GP. A connective tissue disorder similar to vinyl chloride disease in a patient exposed to perchlorethylene. *Clin Exp Dermatol* 1977; 2(1): 17–22.

99 Spizer FE, Wegerman DH, Ramires A. Palpitation rate associated with fluorocarbon exposure in a hospital setting. *N Engl J Med* 1975; 272: 624.

100 Stachów A, Joblonska S, Kencka DL. Tryptophan metabolism in scleroderma and eosinophilic fascitis. In: *Systemic Sclerosis (Scleroderma)* (CM Black and AR Myers, eds). Gower Medical, New York, 1985: 130–4.

101 Sternberg EM, Van Woert MH, Young SN *et al*. Development of a scleroderma-like illness during therapy with L-5-hydroxytryptophan and carbidopa. *N Engl J Med* 1980; 303: 782–7.

102 Stokingert HE. Ozone toxicology. A review of research and industrial experience. 1954–1964. *Arch Environ Health* 1965; 10.

103 Suciu I, Drejman I, Valaczkai C. Investigation of the disease caused by vinyl chloride. *Med Int* 1963; 15: 967–78.

104 Svedhem A, Alestis K, Jertborn M. Phlebitis induced by parenteral treatment with fluxoxacillin and doxacillin: a double-blind study. *Antimicrob Agents Chemother* 1980; 18: 349–52.

105 Taylor GS, Hern WS. Cardiac arrhythmias due to aerosol propellants. *J Am Med Assoc* 1970; 219: 8.

106 Tchijevsky AL. Die Wege des Eindringens von Luftionene in den organismus und die physiologische wirkung von luftionen. *Acta Med Scand* 1934; 83: 219–72.

107 Theorell H, Blombock M, Kockum C. Demonstration of reactivity to airborne and food antigen in cutaneous vasculitis by variation in fibrino peptide and others, blood coagulation, fibrinolysis, and complement parameters. *Thrombo Haemo Sts (Stattz)* 1976; 36: 593.

108 Tomlinson IW, Jayson MIV. Systemic sclerosis after therapy with appetite suppressants. *J Rheumatol* 1984; 11(2): 254.

109 Tribukh SL, Tikhomirova NP, Levina SV, Kozlov LA. Conditions of work and measures of industrial hygiene in the production of, and manufacture from, vinyl chloride plastics. *Gig Sanit* 10: 38–44, cited in WK Lelbackh and HJ Marsteller, 1981; Vinyl chloride associated disease. *Adv Int Med Pediatr* 47: 1–110.

110 Tumulty PA. Systemic lupus erythematosus. In: *Harrison's Principles of Internal Medicine* (Wintrobe MM, Thorn GW, Adams RD *et al.*, eds). McGraw-Hill, New York, 1970; 1962–7.

111 Vane JR, Anggard EE, Botting RM. Regulatory functions of the vascular endothelium. *N Engl J Med* 1990; 323: 27–36.

112 Vasiliev LL. *Theory and Practice of Aeroionotherapy*. University of Leningrad Press, Leningrad, 1951.

113 Verries ED, Boyle EM Jr. Endothelial cell injury in cardiovascular surgery: an overview. *Ann Thoracic Surg* 1997; 64(4 Suppl): 52–8.

114 Von Ardenne M. Oxygen multistep therapy. Physical and technical foundations (trans. P Kirby and W. Krüger). George Thieme Verlag, Stuttgart, 1990; 148.

115 Walder BK. Do solvents cause scleroderma? *Int J Dermatol* 1983; 22: 157–8.

116 Webb CM, McNeill JG, Hayward CS, de Zeigler D, Collins P. Effects of testosterone on coronary vasomotor regulation in men with coronary heart disease. *Circulation* 1999; 100(16): 1690–6.

117 Werbach MR. *Foundations of Nutritional Medicine: A Sourcebook of Clinical Research*, Third Line Press, Tarzana, California, 1997: 11.

118 Whehner AP. Electro-aerosols, air ions, and physical medicine. *Am J Phys Med* 1969; 48(3): 19–49.

119 Winslow SG. The effects of environmental chemicals on the immune system; a selected bibliography with abstracts. Toxicology Information Response Center, Oak Ridge National Laboratory, Oak Ridge, Tennessee, 1981: 1–36.

120 Worden JL. The effect of unipolar ionized air on the relative weights of selected organs of the golden hamster. *Sci Stud* 1953; 15: 71–82.

121 Worden JL. The effect of air ion concentrations and polarity on the CO_2 capacity of mammalian blood plasma. *Fed Proc* 1954; 13: 557.

122 Wuthrich B, Fabio L. Acetylsalicylic acid and food intolerance in urticaria, bronchial asthma, and rhinopathy. *Schweiz Med Wochenschr* 1981; 1(39): 1445–50.

123 Yevick P. Oil pollutants in marine life. *Eighth Advanced Seminar, Society of Clinical Ecology*. Dallas, Texas, 1975: Instatape, Tape II.

124 Zarafonetis CJD, Lorber SH, Hanson SM. Association of functioning carcinoid syndrome and scleroderma. *Am J Med Sci* 1958; 236: 1–14.

125 Zeek PM. Periarteritis nodosa and other forms of necrotizing angitis. *N Engl J Med* 1953; 248: 764.

INTRODUCTION

Untoward reactions to foods were recognized in ancient times by Hippocrates (460–370 BCE),[40] and some 600 years later by Galen (131–210 CE).[30] Although Magendie, in 1839, found that repeated injections of egg albumin in rabbits were lethal,[52] food-induced diseases were not systematically investigated until the 20th century when life-threatening or even fatal reactions to certain foods were observed.[43,65,77,80] Because of similarities between those acute, alarming symptoms in humans and systemic anaphylaxis induced in animal models[63,67], it was assumed that the clinical disorders were immunological in nature. Indeed, the putative antibodies for immediate-type hypersensitivity reactions in humans were discovered in the 1920s by injecting serum from a fish-sensitive subject intradermally into an individual who was allergic to grass pollen but not food, reinjecting the test site with an extract of fish tissue and noting the subsequent immediate local weal and erythema[69] – the classical Prausnitz–Küstner reaction.

During the next three decades, increasing numbers of cases of allergic reactions to foods were described and the spectrum of clinical abnormalities in these cases was broadened to include reactions that were often slower in onset and involved the gastro-intestinal tract, skin or respiratory system.[6,21] In these reports, however, a cause and effect relationship between the exposure to the food and the production of the clinical abnormalities was often not established. The diagnoses were usually based on the clinical history and improvement after elimination of the suspected allergen from the diet. The reactions were not verified by subsequent purposeful oral challenge with the food, and appropriate immunological methods to investigate the problem had not been developed.

DESIGN OF CLINICAL INVESTIGATIONS FOR FOOD ALLERGY

Because of the paucity of objective information, many leaders in academic medicine in the mid 20th century felt that very little, if any, credence could be given to the concept of food allergy, and they cautioned that non-allergic mechanisms were responsible for most food-related disorders. In concert with those concerns, one of the present authors (A.S.G.) considered at that time whether postulates modified from those sequentially developed by Bassi,[9] Henle[38] and Koch[48] for investigating infectious diseases would be useful in designing investigations of food hypersensitivities (Table 58.1). We recommended that controlled test feedings with the suspected allergens to reproduce the symptoms would be the 'gold standard' for deciding whether the patient was allergic to a food.

Cow's milk allergen challenge

The lack of purified food allergens for oral challenges, however, precluded investigations until the 1960s when sufficient quantities of

Criteria for identifying the causal role of food allergens in disease

1. Symptoms disappear after the suspected allergen has been eliminated.
2. The allergen is isolated in a pure form for experimental use.
3. The administration of the allergen by the natural route produces reactions in experimental subjects that are similar to the original symptoms.
4. The allergen in its natural or modified form reacts with sensitized B or T cells or antibodies from the patient.
5. Immunological responses generated by the allergen reacting with the immune system of the recipient are responsible for the pathogenesis of the untoward reactions.

Criteria modelled by A.S.G. after Koch's postulates for the identification of the causal role of infectious agents in disease.

Table 58.1 Criteria for identifying the causal role of food allergens in disease.

isolated cow's milk proteins were made available for such a study.[33] In that study, a large group of children (mainly infants who were never breast fed) who were suspected of being sensitive to cow's milk were first taken off cow's milk in the diet to ascertain if their symptoms disappeared. If this occurred, then the child was challenged orally, first with a standard preparation of skimmed, lactose-free cow's milk, and then, if reactive, with purified preparations of bovine casein, β-lactoglobulin, α-lactalbumin or serum albumin. The results established a number of points that served as guidelines for future studies (Table 58.2). Perhaps the most important was that oral challenges usually reproduced the types of reactions that had been historically attributed to cow's milk.

Immunological basis of reactions

This was investigated by direct skin testing[34] and serological methods[76] with the antigens employed in the oral challenge experiments. Few clues to an immunological basis for the reactions were found, except that those patients who developed anaphylactic reactions during food challenges displayed very strongly positive immediate reactions at skin test sites with the same cow's proteins to which they reacted after oral challenge.

Double blind challenges with food

Over a decade later a double blind design was employed in oral challenge tests by May and Bock and their colleagues for the investigation of food hypersensitivity to minimize observer bias.[14,56,57] Although purified food proteins were not employed and the initial investigations were limited to a highly selected group of older children with severe asthma, it was demonstrated that food hypersensitivities could be detected by provoking the reactions by oral challenge. The coupling of dietary elimination with oral challenge has remained the cornerstone of experimental studies and practical clinical diagnosis of food hypersensitivities. This has recently been reaffirmed.[81]

DIAGNOSIS OF FOOD ALLERGY

Since non-immunological causes of adverse food reactions are common and may mimic food hypersensitivities,[3,4] it is important to consider those disorders in a given case. These include the following.

1. Food contaminants such as pathogenic microorganisms or their toxins.[27]
2. Food additives such as tartrazines.
3. Enzymatic defects (e.g. galactosaemia[47]), which block the metabolism of a nutrient.
4. Acquired insults to the intestinal tract owing to enteric microbial pathogens (rotavirus, salmonellosis, shigellosis) that interfere with the digestion or absorption of food (e.g. disaccharidase deficiencies[45]).

In addition, other common infections and different pathological processes that produce respiratory, gastrointestinal or skin abnormalities must be considered in the differential diagnosis.[3,4]

The principal foods responsible for allergic reactions may be age-dependent and may be contingent upon ethnic and cultural factors. Food allergens in infants are usually limited to the major types of foreign proteins in the diet (Table 58.3).

Elimination of suspected food allergen

If the history suggests that a food is the responsible allergen, it is eliminated from the diet and the patient is observed to determine whether the symptoms disappear. The test period of elimination depends upon the type of food-induced disorder. In more

Important findings from dietary elimination and oral challenge with cow's milk protein allergens

1. Past symptoms suggestive of food allergy are provoked by the oral administration of purified preparations of cow's milk proteins.
2. Most patients are sensitive to two or more milk proteins.
3. Onset, duration and type of reactions elicited by oral challenge are highly reproducible in individual patients.
4. Oral challenge reactions vary in their onset, duration, intensity and organ system involvement.
5. Multiple symptoms involving one or more organ systems are commonly found.
6. An inverse relationship is found between the dose of the allergen necessary to provoke a reaction and the rapidity with which the reaction develops and its severity.
7. Reactions to oral challenge with cow's milk proteins occur principally in infants not breast fed and usually do not persist in school age children.

Table 58.2 Important findings from dietary elimination and oral challenge with cow's milk protein allergens.

Principal foods responsible for allergic reactions[18]

Infants	Older children
Cow's milk	Peanuts
Cereal	Nuts
Eggs	Fish
Peanuts	Shellfish
Soya	

Table 58.3 Principal foods responsible for allergic reactions.[18]

Factors involved in eliminating a suspected food allergen
Age of patient
Compliance
Parents
Type of food

Table 58.4 Factors involved in eliminating a suspected food allergen.

common types of sensitivities, the symptoms disappear within several days after the offending food is removed from the diet, whereas in more complex types of food hypersensitivities (such as cow's milk-induced pulmonary haemosiderosis) the pathology resolves more slowly.

The degree of difficulty in eliminating a suspected food allergen depends upon a number of factors, shown in Table 58.4. In general, the diet of young infants is easily controlled. If cow's milk is the suspected allergen, the diet can be restricted to a soya milk or casein or whey hydrolysate formulations. Hydrolysate preparations may be preferable because of their low antigenicity and because some patients who are allergic to cow's milk also react to soy proteins.[68] If other foods are suspected, then the infant's diet can be restricted to cow's milk for the test period. The elimination of basic foods such as cow's milk is much more difficult in older children, because their occurrence is widespread in food products. Elimination of such foods, even for a test period, therefore requires careful planning and often the aid of a dietitian.

Oral food challenge with suspected food allergen

Although oral challenge with the suspected food allergen is necessary for diagnosis, there are certain pitfalls and shortcomings in the procedure (Table 58.5). For example, patients who present with urticaria should be particularly monitored for anaphylaxis during the challenge.[33]

Disadvantages and pitfalls of oral food challenges
1. In the face of a compelling history of severe reactions such as anaphylaxis, oral challenge with the suspected food allergen is usually precluded because of excessive morbidity.
2. Even in the absence of a history of anaphylaxis, such a reaction may occur during oral challenges. Affected individuals with a history of urticaria have a high risk for severe reactions.
3. If the challenge is conducted with a mixture of foods, a positive reaction may occur but the identity of the offending agent will remain uncertain.
4. An oral dose of allergen that often produces symptoms may not be sufficient to provoke a reaction in certain allergic patients.
5. The reaction may be missed because of a delay of several hours to a few days in the onset of some reactions.
6. Positive challenges may be because of intercurrent diseases such as an infection rather than an effect of the ingested food.
7. In the open challenge method, bias by the observer or the subject may be confounding.
8. The double blind challenge method is the gold standard for diagnosis, but the purified allergens and placebo preparations needed for the procedure are not available in most clinical care settings.

Table 58.5 Disadvantages and pitfalls of oral food challenges.

Objective findings after food challenges
Urticaria
Angio-oedema
Vomiting
Diarrhoea
Wheezing
Blood or eosinophils in stool mucus[68]
Inflammatory changes in intestinal tissues[28,78]
Altered lung function

Table 58.6 Objective findings after food challenges.

To minimize the severity of reactions and potential bias of observers, oral challenges should be conducted by a physician in a medical facility, and the diagnostic criteria limited to objective findings as shown in Table 58.6. Furthermore, the period of observation should be extended for at least 6 h because of the possibility of a late onset anaphylactic reaction.[75]

Preparation for oral challenge

Preparations for oral challenge are as follows.

1. The decision is made as to whether it is safe to conduct the challenge and what safeguards should be employed to minimize a serious reaction. This can to some extent be predicted by the history of the severity and duration of the clinical symptoms and the time of onset of the reaction after ingestion of the suspected allergen, and also by the type of allergen (such as peanut or other nuts) that is likely to provoke severe reactions.

2. An interim history is obtained to document that the patient has become asymptomatic during the dietary elimination of the suspected allergen and has not been exposed to any agent (for example, drugs) which would mimic or suppress a reaction.

3. A thorough physical examination is then performed to confirm that the patient is asymptomatic.

4. If the history suggests that the reaction might be serious, an intravenous line should be established to administer fluids, electrolytes and antiallergic medications and the oral dose of the allergen should be reduced considerably. Aqueous adrenaline (epinephrine), parenteral corticosteroids, antihistamines and equipment for respiratory resuscitation should be immediately available. It is essential that the personnel who are conducting the challenge have the expertise to detect and properly treat serious allergic reactions. Challenges performed on patients with suspected anaphylaxis should be conducted in the clinical setting, such as in an intensive care unit, where a team of physicians and nurses are available to monitor and rapidly treat serious reactions.

In cases of systemic anaphylaxis where the history concerning the offending food allergen is compelling, it is prudent to forego the challenge.

Single food challenge

The oral challenge is performed with a single food (preferably a purified component) in a dose which is judged to incite a reaction. Double blind challenges with or without the suspected allergen hidden in an elemental diet or in capsules[7,10,13,14,56,57,81] are preferable for research purposes, but the procedure is impractical for standard clinical use.

The start of the challenge is timed. The patient is monitored intensively during the first hour after the challenge to detect and treat early signs of anaphylaxis. The time of appearance and the intensity of abnormal findings should be carefully recorded to document the outcome of the challenge. An example of such a documentation is included in Table 58.7. Recently, a two-stage double blind oral challenge method was reported to detect a late onset type of food-induced reaction that could not be detected by the single oral challenge method.[7] Delayed onset reactions were supposedly IgE-mediated. If so, then it is likely that the reactions involved the recruitment and activation of eosinophils and other types of inflammatory leukocytes and the participation of proinflammatory cytokines. It was not clear from the report whether the effects of the double challenge method could be duplicated by simply increasing the dose of the allergen given in a single challenge.

Exercise-induced anaphylaxis

In cases of anaphylaxis that are suspected to be because of an interaction between food allergy and exercise,[50,72] the oral challenge must be conducted shortly before a suitable degree of measured exercise on a treadmill, stationary bicycle, or another appropriate device. Such challenges are therefore usually performed in a clinical cardiology or pulmonology facility.

Labial food challenge

A non-blinded study of labial food challenges has recently been reported.[70] The sensitivity of the method as compared to single blinded oral challenges was 77%. Most patients reacted either to egg white or peanuts. Since the patients were selected in part because of positive immediate reacting skin tests and/or positive radioallergosorbent tests (RAST) with the food antigens in question, the method is not necessarily applicable to patients who display non-IgE-mediated, slower onset reactions.

Colonic food challenge with suspected food allergen

Caecal food allergen challenges for the diagnosis of gastrointestinal food allergies in adults have recently been explored.[11] Mucosal weal and flare reactions were observed endoscopically within 20 min of the provocation in 54 of 70 patients with suspected food allergy. The method was not validated by the oral challenge method, and it was unclear whether gastrointestinal problems decreased after the food to which the patients responded was eliminated from the diet.

Laboratory tests for suspected food allergy

Because of the cumbersome nature and possible danger of the oral challenge method and the potential for self-deception, many efforts have been made to discover the immunological basis of food sensitivities and thereby develop appropriate laboratory procedures to diagnose these disorders. As discussed elsewhere in this book, some food reactions, particularly sudden severe ones, appear to be mediated by IgE antibodies, whereas other types of adverse reactions, particularly those with a delayed onset after oral challenge, are presumably because of other immunological mechanisms. In 1978, a close correlation was demonstrated between the presence of IgE antibodies to cod and allergic reactions after

Example of one oral challenge										

Patient's name: B.P.
Patient ID number: 24001-X
Sex: Male
Age: 4 months
Suspected food allergen:
Symptoms before allergen elimination:
Period of dietary elimination:
Effects of dietary elimination:
Prechallenge physical examination:
Type and time of challenge:

Date of birth: 6/2/84
Date of challenge: 10/8/84
Observer: G.P.

Cow's milk
Vomiting, diarrhoea and weight loss
Two weeks
Disappearance of symptoms. Weight gain of 400 g in 2 weeks.
No abnormalities
100 ml of skimmed cow's milk given by mouth at 10.00 a.m.

Time	General	Pulse rate	Respiration rate	BP	Skin	Respiratory system	Gastrointestinal system	Other	Treatment
9.30 a.m.	Active	100	24	84/62	N	N	N	–	–
10.00 a.m.	Challenge	104	26	82/62	N	N	N	–	–
10.05 a.m.	N	102	24	82/60	N	N	N	–	–
10.10 a.m.	Crying	116	30	86/64	N	N	Vomiting	–	–
10.15 a.m.	Crying	112	30	88/62	N	N	Vomiting	–	–
10.30 a.m.	N	104	26	80/64	N	N	N	–	–
11.00 a.m.	N	104	26	80/64	N	N	N	–	–
1.40 p.m.	Crying	112	30	88/64	N	N	Diarrhoea	–	–
2.00 p.m.	Fussing	108	28	86/62	N	N	Diarrhoea	–	–
3.00 p.m.	N	108	26	80/60	N	N	Diarrhoea	–	–
4.00 p.m.		120	28	84/60	N	N	N	–	–

Specific remarks: Stool mucus obtained at 3.00 p.m. containing many eosinophils.
BP = arterial blood pressure, N = normal.

Table 58.7 Example of one oral challenge.

feedings with that antigen.[1] Currently employed *in vivo* and *in vitro* techniques for detection of IgE antibodies to food allergens, however, do not appear to be generally useful in predicting clinical reactions to the foods, especially those involving the gastrointestinal tract or those that have a delayed onset after oral challenge.

Skin testing and radioallergosorbent tests

Skin testing and RAST have limited reliability because of the paucity of purified food allergens and poor correlation between the results of immunological tests and those of oral challenge.[8,10,34,73,81] In fact, both types of tests tend to overestimate greatly the population of patients who will react clinically to specific foods, although strongly positive skin tests to certain foods may be useful in diagnosis of allergic reactions that have a very rapid onset,[33,74,75] such as urticaria, bronchospasm, laryngospasm, or systemic anaphylaxis. A recent innovation in radioallergosorbent methods has improved the binding of antibodies to immobilized allergens. This method has been found to be more useful in the detection of allergies to certain food such as hen egg, but was poorly predictive for allergies to other foods such as soy and wheat.[74] Although continued advances in the methods for detecting IgE-mediated reactions to food may occur in the near future, one should remain circumspect about the predictive value of skin or serological tests for IgE antibodies to foods in the diagnosis of food allergy.

Pollen/food allergen crossreactivity

One very interesting exception, however, has been the discovery that some allergens in birch pollen crossreact immunologically with certain allergens in fruits such as apples and vegetables such as carrots.[23] In such circumstances, immediate reacting skin tests may be an important diagnostic tool.

Other immunological tests

The measurement of serum or secretory antibodies of other immunoglobulin classes produced in response to food antigens,[58] the detection of blood lymphocytes sensitized to these allergens,[41] investigations of oral tolerance,[46] complement activation[55] and other abnormalities of the immunological functions of the gastrointestinal tract are promising, but are as yet not clinically applicable. It should also be stressed that the clinical usefulness of such laboratory diagnostic methods will require validation by careful oral challenge experiments in selected patients with the food allergens in question.[2]

DISORDERS ASSOCIATED WITH FOOD ALLERGENS

Based upon the use of dietary elimination and oral challenge studies and the exclusion of other disorders, certain clinical manifestations have been suspected to be caused by immunological reactions to food proteins.

Gastrointestinal reactions

Gastrointestinal disorders are the most common reactions to food allergy. The manifestations include perioral erythema, fissuring of the mouth, palatal itching, abdominal pain, colic, diarrhoea, gastrointestinal blood loss, protein-losing enteropathy, carbohydrate and/or fat malabsorption[51,78,84] and possibly ulcerative colitis.[82] The most common problems are as follows.

Vomiting

Vomiting is one of the most common symptoms in food allergy and usually occurs within 10 to 30 min of ingestion of the allergens. The emesis usually consists of gastric secretions and ingested food, and ranges from mild spitting to projectile vomiting.

Abdominal pain – colic

In children who are old enough to describe their symptoms, abdominal pain owing to food allergy varies from dull to severe. The pain is usually located in the upper abdomen or the periumbilical region. Even when the pain is severe, abdominal tenderness is usually absent.

Infant colic

A great deal of controversy persists regarding the role of food allergy in the production of colic in infants. Although there are convincing reports of colic induced by ingested foods, it is unclear for the following reasons whether food allergens commonly cause colic. In some studies, objective criteria for the diagnosis of colic by history or oral challenge were not stated. In fact, the degree of irritability or crying that constitutes pathological colic is difficult to define.[15] In addition, it was not clarified in some investigations whether the subjects in studies were selected at random from cases of colic in the community or whether the cases were chosen because of a strong suspicion of food allergy. Furthermore, certain studies suggest that crying is a natural behaviour in most infants during the first 2–3 months of life.[15]

Diarrhoea

Diarrhoea is probably the most common clinical manifestation of food allergy. The degree of diarrhoea ranges from loose to explosive watery stools. In cow's milk and soy protein-induced enterocolitis[51,68], stool mucus obtained after oral challenge often contains eosinophils, and proctoscopy reveals an erythematous, friable, ulcerated mucosa.

Gastrointestinal bleeding

Gastrointestinal blood loss often occurs in infants who are allergic to cow's milk.[33,86,87] This may occur in the presence or absence of diarrhoea and the bleeding may be gross or more often occult. Those infants who experience blood loss in the absence of diarrhoea are usually deficient in iron and the degree of loss appears to be directly proportional to the amount of ingested cow's milk.[86,87] The bleeding ceases within several days of the elimination of cow's milk, and the disorder disappears in most infants by 2 years of age.

Allergic gastroenteropathy

Some cases of protein-losing enteropathy because of cow's milk have been reported.[84] Affected infants present with oedema due to hypoproteinaemia. Fat malabsorption, gastrointestinal blood loss, iron-deficiency anaemia or eosinophilia are found in some individuals.

Fat malabsorption

Directly after World War II, Dicke and his colleagues[22] in the Netherlands recognized a large number of infants and preschool age children who displayed steatorrhoea and growth failure caused by wheat and related cereals. The responsible component in the cereal proved to be gluten. Although the number of reported cases decreased as the amount of gluten in the diet of infants declined, gluten intolerance, also known as coeliac disease, continues to be one of the principal causes of fat malabsorption. In this condition the villi of the small intestine are flattened and an increased number of inflammatory cells are often found in the lamina propria.[65,78] The steatorrhoea and intestinal pathology usually resolve a few weeks after eliminating gluten from the diet. A very similar, if not identical, syndrome may be provoked by cow's milk[28,51] and a number of other foods.[83]

Ulcerative colitis

A few decades ago it was reported that cow's milk might play a role in the pathogenesis of ulcerative colitis.[82] To our knowledge, no other cases caused by ingested foods have been reported.

Respiratory diseases
Asthma and rhinitis

A wide variety of respiratory symptoms, including rhinitis, cough and asthma.[13,14,33,37,44,56,57] have been documented to be triggered by food allergens, especially as part of immediate systemic reactions. However, in a highly atopic population of patients with atopic dermatitis with asthma and/or allergic rhinitis where food allergy was suspected, only a small number of patients developed lower airway obstruction during food challenges.[44] Furthermore, it is unclear whether food allergens are often responsible for chronic, recurrent respiratory disorders. For example, the majority of asthma attacks in young infants are associated with viral respiratory infections, especially respiratory syncytial virus and rhinovirus.[85] Nevertheless, food allergens should be considered in the pathogenesis of allergic respiratory disease, particularly in infants who present also with dermal and/or gastrointestinal symptoms.

Otitis media and food allergy

There is considerable controversy regarding the possible association of otitis media with food allergy. One report suggested that such an association is likely,[12] but a subsequent well controlled study did not confirm the impression,[29] and investigations of unselected cases of acute otitis media indicate that infections are the most common cause.[42]

Cow's milk-induced pulmonary haemosiderosis

In the early 1960s Douglas Heiner and his colleagues discovered a novel type of cow's milk hypersensitivity in young infants.[36,37] The disorder is characterized by pulmonary haemosiderosis, gastrointestinal blood loss, iron-deficiency anaemia, failure to thrive, eosinophilia and high serum titres of precipitating antibodies to cow's milk proteins. The manifestations of the sensitivity disappeared within several weeks of elimination of cow's milk from the diet, and the abnormalities reappeared when cow's milk was reintroduced into the diet. Although this syndrome is less common than gastrointestinal reactions to cow's milk, it is perhaps the best documented type of cow's milk sensitization because of the close relationship between the exposure to cow's milk, the elevation of serum IgG antibodies to the allergens and the clinical abnormalities.

Skin diseases

Two types of dermal reactions, urticaria and atopic dermatitis, have been found to be provoked by food allergens, but the number of cases that can be attributed to food allergens is controversial. In surveys of chronic recurrent urticaria,[54] a cause was found in only 10–15% of cases. In the absence of other symptoms, a search for food allergens may be fruitless unless there is a temporal relationship between food ingestion and the onset of urticaria or if the reactions occur in young infants. The role of yeasts in urticaria is controversial, and will require further investigation

The role of food allergens in the pathogenesis of atopic dermatitis remains puzzling. Some investigators have presented reasonable evidence that certain cases of this chronic dermatitis are provoked by food allergens, but it is unclear whether these patients are representative of most cases of atopic dermatitis or whether they were selected for study because of a strong suspicion of food allergy. For example, in one study the median age of affected cases supposedly due to food allergy was 11 years,[73] whereas atopic dermatitis usually begins in the first year of life and remits by the age of 5 years.[71] It is therefore difficult to decide whether food allergens are aetiological agents in a subpopulation of patients with atopic dermatitis or whether the dermatological manifestations of these cases are only similar to atopic dermatitis.

To confirm the role of foods in a population of children with atopic eczema, Atherton et al.[5] showed quite clearly in a double blind placebo-controlled study that foods were important allergens in this skin disease.

Further studies with larger groups of children confirmed the value of diet in children with severe atopic eczema.[66]

Systemic anaphylaxis

The manifestations of anaphylaxis because of food allergens are identical to those reported in anaphylaxis caused by other agents. They include urticaria, angio-oedema, laryngeal oedema, bronchospasm, diarrhoea, convulsions and shock. Anaphylactic reactions are not as common as other disorders induced by food allergens. In most cases the diagnosis is evident because of the rapid onset of the reaction after food ingestion. It is difficult, however, to identify the responsible allergen in some patients because of the complexity of the mixture of food ingested or because of hidden food additives. Some adults and older children present with anaphylaxis caused by an interaction between physical exercise and the ingestion of a particular food allergen.[50,72] The nature of this interaction in the pathogenesis of the reaction is unknown.

Central nervous system abnormalities

Seizures, anxiety, lethargy, headaches and other central nervous symptoms have been reported to be caused by food allergens. There is little objective evidence for the occurrence of these abnormalities in food allergies. However, there is good evidence for a role of food allergens in the production of chronic behavioural disturbances such as ADHD from two excellent dietary studies from Great Ormond Street Children's Hospital in London.[19,24] Immunotherapy can also be useful in these children.[26]

It is of interest that an elimination diet can also be of benefit in childhood epilepsy but only if there is an associated migraine.[25]

The role of food allergens in the production of headaches is controversial, since the finding is subjective and few double blind trials with suspected food antigens have been performed in affected subjects. The problem is further compounded by the occurrence of vasoactive amines in many foods (tyramine in cheese, phenylethylamine in chocolate) which may trigger vascular headaches. Thus, such reactions associated with foods may not only be due to specific immunological events.

Uncertain associations

Although many other symptoms or disorders, such as sudden infant death syndrome, thrombocytopenia, enuresis, vasculitis syndromes, cardiac arrhythmias and disorders of the musculoskeletal system, have been attributed to food allergens, there is little scientific evidence to support these claims.[3,4]

CONCLUSIONS

Food sensitivities are most likely to occur in young infants who are not breast fed.[20] The principal food allergens are cow's milk, cereals, eggs, soya protein, shellfish, peanuts and tree nuts. The most frequent symptoms produced by food allergens are gastrointestinal reactions. In addition, respiratory symptoms, dermatoses, anaphylaxis and certain specific disorders, such as fat malabsorption and pulmonary haemosiderosis, are attributable in some cases to food allergens.

The diagnosis of food hypersensitivity is dependent upon the amelioration of symptoms after elimination of the suspected food antigen, and the development of similar clinical reactions after oral challenge with the food antigen. The oral challenge method should be conducted under careful medical supervision to recognize and quickly abort serious reactions and to obtain objective information about the presence or absence of reactions. Double blind challenges are the gold standard for research but are impractical in many clinical settings. Other diagnostic procedures, though of considerable research interest, have not always proved to be reliable in the diagnosis of food sensitivities.

The immunological/inflammatory mechanisms responsible for many types of allergic reactions to foods remain uncertain. Consequently, there are shortcomings either with the specificity or sensitivity of laboratory methods in the diagnosis of food allergy in many patients. The situation should change, however, given rapid advances in information concerning macromolecular absorption, oral tolerance, the TCR repertoire, Th1 and Th2 cytokines, the molecular pathways of hypersensitivities and mucosal immunology, and our understanding of the complex way in which the gastrointestinal tract deals immunologically with food antigens. In addition, researchers should investigate the genetic aspects of food allergy, particularly in families where two or more members display the same food hypersensitivities. This is particularly pertinent in this era of molecular genetics, where responsible genes may be mapped or identified before their protein products are discovered. If a more rational understanding of the genesis of hypersensitivities to foods is forthcoming in the near future, then it should be possible to develop more appropriate immunological methods for the diagnosis of food allergies.

A new question concerning food allergy has also emerged with the creation of genetically modified (GM) foods. The potential allergenicity of these new foods will require careful prospective assessment, since some may contain antigenic determinants that crossreact with those found in natural food allergens. The genetic expression of a Brazil nut allergen in soya beans is a warning of the potential danger of GM foods.[62] A further warning has been expressed concerning the regulation of GM crops and the concept of 'substantial equivalence'.[60] Further, some genetically engineered foods may display new antigenic determinants that are prone to provoke allergic reactions in susceptible humans.[59]

Finally, more attention should be paid to preventing untoward food reactions in infants and young children by encouraging breast feeding. In that regard, there is increasing evidence that human milk contains not only anti-infectious factors but also a host of anti-inflammatory[32] and immunomodulating agents.[31] In addition, there may be prolonged tolerogenic effects of human milk, as evidenced by the long-term decrease in alloreactivity to maternal transplant antigens in children who have been breast fed.[16,17] However, it should also be recognized that breastfeeding may transmit foreign food antigens and may be responsible for the induction of allergic reactions in the recipient infant.[35] Thus, research will be required to discover the determinants of the protection against food allergy by breastfeeding in most infants and the induction of allergic reactions by breastfeeding in some infants.

REFERENCES

1   Aas K. The diagnosis of hypersensitivity to ingested foods: reliability of skin prick testing and the radioallergosorbent test with different materials. *Clin Allergy* 1978; 8: 39–50.

2   American Academy of Allergy. Position statements controversial techniques. *J Allergy Clin Immunol* 1978; 67: 333–8.

3   American Academy of Allergy and Immunology Committee on Adverse Reactions to Foods and National Institute of Allergy and Infectious Diseases. *DHEW Publication No. (NIH)* 1984; 4-2442: 43–102.

4   American Academy of Allergy and Immunology Committee on Adverse Reactions to Foods and National Institute of Allergy and Infectious Diseases. *DHEW Publication No. (NIH)* 1984; 4-2442: 103–24.

5   Atherton DF, Sewell M, Soothill JF, Wells RS, Chilrens CE. A double blind controlled crossover trial of an antigen-avoidance diet in atopic eczema. *Lancet* 1978; i: 401–3.

6   Bachman KD, Dees SC. Milk allergy. II. Observations on incidence and symptoms of allergy in allergic children. *Pediatrics* 1957; 20: 400–7.

7   Baehler P, Chad Z, Gurbindo C, Bonin AP, Bouthillier L, Seidman EG. Distinct patterns of cow's milk allergy in infancy defined by prolonged, two-stage double-blind, placebo-controlled food challenges. *Clin Exp Allergy* 1996; 26: 254–61.

8   Bahna SL. *RAST or Skin Test versus Oral Challenge in Food Sensitivity.* Presented at the 5th International Food Allergy Symposium. American College of Allergists, Atlanta, 1984.

9   Bassi A. Del mal del segno calcinaccio o moscardino malattia cheaffigge i bachi da seta a sul modo di liberame le bigattaje anche le piu infestate, 2 vols, Lodi, Orcesi, 1837: 1835–6.

10 Bergtsson U, Nilsson-Balknas U, Hanson LÅ, Ahlstedt S. Double blind, placebo controlled food reactions do not correlate to IgE allergy in the diagnosis of staple food related gastrointestinal symptoms. *Gut* 1996; 39: 130–5.

11 Bischoff SC, Mayer J, Wedemeyer J *et al.* Colonoscopic allergen provocation (COLAP): a new diagnostic approach for gastrointestinal food allergy. *Gut* 1997; 40: 745–53.

12 Bluestone CD. Eustachian tube function and allergy in otitis media. *Pediatrics* 1978; 61: 753–60.

13 Bock SA, Atkins FM. Patterns of food hypersensitivity during sixteen years of double-blind, placebo-controlled food challenges. *J Pediatr* 1990; 117: 561–7.

14 Bock SA, Lee W-Y, Remigio LK, May CD. Studies of hypersensitivity reactions to foods in infants and children. *J Allergy Clin Immunol* 1978; 62: 327–34.

15 Brazelton TB. Crying in infancy. *Pediatrics* 1974; 29: 579–88.

16 Campbell DA Jr, Lorber MI, Sweeton JC, Turcotte JG, Beer AE. Maternal donor-related transplants: influence of breast feeding on reactivity to the allograft. *Transplant Proc* 1983; 15: 906–9.

17 Campbell DA Jr, Lorber MI, Sweeton JC, Turcotte JG, Niederhuber JE, Beer AE. Breast feeding and maternal-donor renal allografts. *Transplantation* 1984; 37: 340–4.

18 Canadian Paediatric Society, Allergy Section. Fatal anaphylactic reactions to foods in children. *Can Med Assoc J* 1994; 150: 337–9.

19 Carter CM, Urbanowicz M, Helsley R *et al*. Effects of a few food diets in attention deficit disorder. *Arch Dis Child* 1993; 69: 564–8.

20 Chheda S, Keeney SE, Goldman AS. Immunology of human milk and host immunity. In: *Fetal and Neonatal Physiology*, 2nd edn, (Polin RA, Fox WW, eds). WB Saunders, Philadelphia PA, 1998; 2022–32.

21 Clein NW. Cow's milk allergy in infants and children. *Int Arch Allergy Appl Immunol* 1958; 13: 245–56.

22 Dicke WK, Wiejers HA, van de Kamer JH. Coeliac disease. II. The presence in wheat of a factor having a deleterious effect in cases of coeliac disease. *Acta Paediatr Scand* 1953; 42: 34–42.

23 Ebner C, Hirschwehr R, Bauer L *et al*. Identification of allergens in fruits and vegetables: IgE cross-reactivities with the important birch pollen allergens Bet v 1 and Bet v 2 (*Birch profilin*). *J Allergy Clin Immunol* 1995; 95: 962–9.

24 Egger J, Carter CM, Graham PJ, Gumley D, Soothill JF. Controlled trial of oligoantigenic treatment in the hyperkinetic syndrome. *Lancet* 1985; i: 540–5.

25 Egger J, Carter CM, Soothill JF, Wilson J. Oligoantigenic diet treatment of children with epilepsy and migraine. *J Pediatr* 1989; 114: 51–8.

26 Egger J, Stolla A, McEwen LM. Controlled trial of hyposensitisation in children with food-induced hyperkinetic syndrome. *Lancet* 1992; 339: 1150–3.

27 Finberg L. Toxic substances in the food supply in infants and children. *Pediatr Ann* 1979; 8: 706–9.

28 Fontaine IL, Navarro J. Small intestinal biopsy in cow's milk protein allergy in infancy. *Arch Dis Child* 1975; 50: 357–62.

29 Friedman RA, Doyle WJ, Casselbrent MC, Bluestone C, Fireman P. Immunologic-mediated Eustachian tube obstruction: a double-blind crossover study. *J Allergy Clin Immunol* 1983; 71: 442–7.

30 Galen. *De Sanitate Tuenda (Hygiene)*. RM Green, translator. Charles C. Thomas, Springfield IL, 1951: 210.

31 Goldman AS, Garofalo R, Chheda S. Spectrum of immunomodulating agents in human milk. *Int J Pediatr Hematol/Oncol* 1997; 4: 491–7.

32 Goldman AS, Thorpe LW, Goldblum RM, Hanson LÅ. Antiinflammatory properties of human milk. *Acta Paediatr Scand* 1986; 75: 689–95.

33 Goldman AS, Anderson DW Jr, Sellers WA, Saperstein S, Kniker WT, Halpern S. Milk allergy. I. Oral challenge with milk and isolated milk proteins in allergic children. *Pediatrics* 1963; 32: 425–43.

34 Goldman AS, Sellers WA, Halpern SR, Anderson DW, Furlow TE, Johnson CH. Milk allergy. II. Skin testing of allergic and normal children with purified milk proteins. *Pediatrics* 1963; 32: 572–9.

35 Goldman AS. Editorial. Association of atopic diseases with breast-feeding, food allergens, fatty acids and evolution. *J Pediatr* 1999; 134: 5–7.

36 Heiner DC, Sears JW. Chronic respiratory disease associated with multiple circulating precipitins to cow's milk. *Am J Dis Child* 1960; 100: 500–2.

37 Heiner DC, Sears JW, Kniker WT. Multiple precipitins to cow's milk in chronic respiratory disease. A syndrome including poor growth, gastrointestinal symptoms, evidence of allergy, iron deficiency anemia and pulmonary hemosiderosis. *Am J Dis Child* 1962; 103: 634–54.

38 Henle FGJ. *Von den Miasmen und contagien*. Pathologische Untersuchungen, Berlin, 1840; 1–82.

39 Hide DW. Food allergy in children. *Clin Exp Allergy* 1994; 24: 1–2.

40 Hippocrates: The Hippocratic Collection. *Encyclopedia Britannica* 1983; 8: 942–3.

41 Hoffman KM, Ho DG, Sampson HA. Evaluation of the usefulness of lymphocyte proliferation assays in the diagnosis of allergy to cow's milk. *J Allergy Clin Immunol* 1997; 99: 360–6.

42 Howie V, Pollard RB, Kpeyn K *et al*. Presence of interferon during bacterial otitis media. *J Infect Dis* 1982; 145: 811–14.

43 Hutinel V. Intolerance pour le lait et anaphylaxie chez les nourrissons. *Clinique (Paris)* 1908; 3: 227–31.

44 James JM, Bernhisel-Broadbent J, Sampson H. Respiratory reactions provoked by double-blind food challenges in children. *Am J Resp Crit Care Med* 1994; 149: 59–64.

45 Johnson JD, Kretchmer N, Simoons FJ. Lactose malabsorption: its biology and history. *Adv Pediatr* 1974; 21: 197–237.

46 Kagnoff MF. Induction and paralysis: a conceptual framework from which to examine the intestinal immune system. *Gastroenterology* 1974; 66: 1240–56.

47 Kailckav HM, Kinoshita JH, Donnell GN. Galactosemia, biochemistry, genetics, pathophysiology, and developmental aspects. In: *Biology of Brain Dysfunction*, vol 2, (Gaull GE, ed.), Plenum Press, New York, 1973; 31.

48 Koch R. *Untersuchungen über die aetiologie der Wundinfectionkrankheiten*; F.C.W. Vögel, Leipzig, 1878.

49 Kollmann TR, Pettoello-Mantovani M, Katopodis NF *et al*. Inhibition of acute in vivo human immunodeficiency virus infection by human interleukin 10 treatment of SCID mice implanted with human fetal thymus and liver. *Proc Natl Acad Sciences (USA)* 1996; 93: 3126–31.

50 Kidd IM III, Cohan SH, Sosman AJ, Fink JN. Food dependent exercise induced anaphylaxis. *J Allergy Clin Immunol* 1975; 71: 407–11.

51 Kuitunen P, Visakorpi JK, Savilahti E, Pelkonen P. Malabsorption syndrome with cow's milk intolerance. *Arch Dis Child* 1975; 50: 351–6.

52 Magendie F. *Lectures on the Blood*, Harrington, Barrington, Haswell, Philadelphia, 1839; 244–9.

53 Majamaa H, Mettinen A, Laine S, Isolauri E. Intestinal inflammation in children with atopic dermatitis: faecal eosinophil cationic protein and tumor necrosis factor-alpha as non-invasive indicators of food allergy. *Clin Exp Allergy* 1996; 26: 181–7.

54 Mathews KP. Management of urticaria and angioedema. *J Allergy Clin Immunol* 1980; 66: 347–57.

55 Mathews TS, Soothill JF. Complement activation after milk feeding in children with cow's milk allergy. *Lancet* 1970; ii: 893–5.

56 May CD. Objective clinical and laboratory studies of immediate-hypersensitivity reactions to food in asthmatic children. *J Allergy Clin Immunol* 1976; 58: 500–15.

57 May CD, Bock SD. A modern clinical approach to food hypersensitivity. *Allergy* 1978; 33: 166–88.

58 McDonald PJ, Goldblum RM, Van Sickle GJ, Powell GK. Food protein-induced enterocolitis: altered antibody response to ingested antigen. *Pediatr Res* 1984; 18: 751–5.

59 Metcalfe DD, Astwood JD, Townsend R, Sampson HA, Taylor SL, Fuchs RL. Assessment of the allergenic potential of foods derived from genetically engineered crop plants. *Critical Reviews Food Science Nutrition* 36 (suppl.): S165–86.

60 Millstone E, Brunner E, Mayer S. Beyond substantial equivalence. *Nature* 1999; 401: 525–6.

61 Noma T, Yoshizama I, Kou K *et al*. Correlation of interleukin-2 (IL-2) responsiveness by eggwhite-stimulated lymphocytes with hen egg oral provocation test in atopic children. *Jap J Allergology* 1966; 45: 660–71.

62 Nordlee JA, Taylor SL, Townsend JA, Thomas LA, Bush RK. Identification of a Brazil-nut allergen in transgenic soybeans. *N Engl J Med* 1996; 334: 688–92.

63 Otto R. Zur Frage der Serum-Ueberempfindlichkeit. *München Med Wochenschr* 1907; 54: 1665–70.

64 Park EA. A case of hypersensitivity to cow's milk. *Am J Dis Child* 1920; 19: 46–54.

65 Paulley JW. Observations on aetiology of idiopathic steatorrhea: jejunal and lymph-node biopsies. *BMJ* 1954; ii: 1318–21.

66 Pike MG, Carter CM, Boulton P, Turner MW, Soothill JF, Atherton DJ. Few food diets in the treatment of atopic eczema. *Arch Dis Child* 1989; 64: 1691–8.

67 Portier P, Richet C. De l'action anaphylactique des certaines venins. *C R Soc Biol (Paris)* 1902; 54: 170–2.

68 Powell GK. Milk and soy induced enterocolitis of infancy. Clinical features and standardization of challenge. *J Pediatr* 1978; 93: 553–60.

69 Prausnitz C, Küstner H. Studien fiber die Ueberempfindlichkeit. *Zentralbl Bakteriol Orig* 1921; 86: 160–9.

70 Rance F, Dytau G. Labial food challenge in children with food allergy. *Pediatr Allergy Immunol* 1997; 8: 41–4.

71 Rasmussen JE, Provost TT. Atopic dermatitis. In: *Allergy, Principles and Practice 2*, (Middleton E, Jr, Reed CE, Ellis EF, eds), Mosby, St Louis, 1983; 1297–312.

72 Romano A, Di Fonso M, Giuffreda F *et al*. Diagnostic work-up for food dependent, exercise-induced anaphylaxis. *Allergy* 1995; 50: 817–24.

73 Sampson HA. Role of immediate food hypersensitivity in the pathogenesis of atopic dermatitis. *J Allergy Clin Immunol* 1983; 71: 473–80.

74 Sampson HA, Ho DG. Relationship between food-specific IgE concentrations and the risk of positive food challenges in children and adolescents. *J Allergy Clin Immunol* 1997; 100: 444–51.

75 Sampson HA, Mendelson L, Rosen JP. Fatal and near fatal food anaphylaxis reactions in children and adolescents. *N Engl J Med* 1992; 327: 380–4.

76 Saperstein S, Anderson DW, Goldman AS, Kniker WT. Milk allergy. III. Immunological studies with sera from allergic and normal children. *Pediatrics* 1963; 32: 580–7.

77 Schlossman A. Ueber die Giftwirkung des artfremden Eiweisses in der Milch auf den Organismus des Sauglings. *Arch Kinderheilkd* 1905; 41: 99–103.

78 Shiner M, Ballard J, Brook CG, Herman S. Intestinal biopsy in the diagnosis of cow's milk protein intolerance without acute symptoms. *Lancet* 1975; ii: 1060–3.

79 Sutas Y, Hurme M, Isolauri E. Oral cow's milk challenge abolishes antigen-specific interferon-gamma production in the peripheral blood of children with atopic dermatitis and cow's milk allergy. *Clin Exp Allergy* 1997; 27: 277–83.

80 Talbot FB. Idiosyncrasy to cow's milk: its relationship to anaphylaxis. *Boston Med Surg J* 1916; 175: 409–10.

81 Terho EO, Savolainen J. Diagnosis of food hypersensitivity. *Eur J Clin Nutr* 1996; 50: 1–5.

82 Truelove SC. Ulcerative colitis provoked by milk. *BMJ* 1961; i: 154–65.

83 Vitoria JC, Camarero C, Sojo A, Ruiz A, Rodriguez-Soriano J. Enteropathy related to fish, rice and chicken. *Arch Dis Child* 1982; 57: 44–8.

84 Waldmann TA, Wochner RD, Laster L, Gordon RS Jr. Allergic gastroenteropathy. A cause of excessive gastrointestinal protein loss. *N Engl J Med* 1967; 276: 762–9.

85 Welliver RC. Viral infections and obstructive airway disease in early life. *Pediatr Clin North Am* 1983; 30: 819–28.

86 Wilson JF, Heiner DC, Lahey ME. Studies on iron gastrointestinal dysfunction in infants with iron deficiency anemia: a preliminary report. *J Pediatr* 1962; 60: 787–800.

87 Wilson JF, Lahey ME, Heiner DC. Studies on iron metabolism. V. Further observations on cow's milk-induced gastrointestinal bleeding in infants with iron-deficiency anemia. *J Pediatr* 1974; 84: 335–44.

INTRODUCTION

Whatever laboratory or clinical techniques may be deployed to assist in the diagnosis of food allergy or intolerance, at some stage it is necessary to attempt to demonstrate a cause and effect relationship between food ingestion and the occurrence of symptoms.

When immunoglobulin (Ig) E-mediated immediate food allergy reactions are involved, the relationship of the typical symptoms of anaphylaxis or oral allergy to the specific ingestant is often clear from the history. When this history is strongly supported by correlating evidence from either skin prick test or a test of circulating IgE antibody such as radioallergosorbent test (RAST), then there is little need for evidence from ingestion challenge. However, in practice difficulties do commonly occur.

The presence of small quantities of the offending food as an unexpected or unlabelled ingredient can cause confusion. Reactions to food additives may be unsuspected and labelling of commercially prepared foods may be unhelpful. Also, the fact that in approximately 20% of cases, a cause for anaphylaxis cannot be identified despite comprehensive investigation[34] suggests that within this group are patients who react to an unidentifiable dietary trigger.

When non-immediate food intolerance reactions are involved, the history is generally unhelpful and the situation far more confusing. It has been suggested that divergent views are held in this area more than in any other in medicine. Researchers have used non-standardized methods of dietary elimination and blinded challenge techniques to investigate the presence of non-immediate food reactions in a variety of clinical presentations (Table 59.1). In doing so, food intolerances totally unsuspected by the patient have often been demonstrated.

The converse situation arises when studies of suspected food-allergic patients use the standardized technique known as the double blind placebo-controlled food challenge (DBPCFC).[7] In this test the suspected food or food additive is usually administered concealed in a capsule or capsules. A variation of the technique uses a strongly flavoured or textured edible vehicle to achieve the necessary blinding of the test substance (e.g. soup or ice cream). Observations from the clinical history are frequently unconfirmed by this technique. A study of 688 children by double blind food challenge was inconsistent with the clinical history in 60% of children challenged.[6] Proponents of DBPCFC assert that a history of adverse reaction to food is more often inaccurate than it is accurate,[19] and that patients in whom adverse reaction to food is confirmed react demonstrably to fewer foods than they suspect.[5]

Whatever technique is employed, it is clearly critical that the test should be devised to minimize both false-negative and false-positive outcome. It has been suggested that the DBPCFC test should be regarded as the 'gold standard' for the diagnosis of adverse reactions to foods.[5] However, before accepting this claim it is important to consider its possible limitations and, in particular, the likelihood of false-negative response.

Examples of conditions in which there is some evidence that food (and food additive) intolerance reactions cause symptom provocation usually in the absence of evidence of immune response	
Respiratory	Asthma
	Rhinitis
	Secretory otitis media
Gastrointestinal (infancy and childhood)	Cow's milk-sensitive enteropathy
	Other food-sensitive enteropathies
	Infantile colitis
	Colic
	Crohn's disease
	Oro-facial granulomatosis
	Occult intestinal haemorrhage
	Failure to thrive
	Pyloric stenosis
	Recurrent abdominal pain
	Constipation
Gastrointestinal (children and adults)	Coeliac disease
	Crohn's disease
	Irritable bowel syndrome
	Aphthous ulceration
	Oropharyngeal pruritus
	Vomiting
Skin	Atopic eczema
	Urticaria
	Purpura and vasculitis
	Dermatitis herpetiformis
Central nervous system	Headache and migraine
	Hyperactivity
	Epilepsy when coexistent with migraine in children
	Hypersomnia
	Anxiety
	Somatoform disorders
Cardiovascular	Large vessel vasculitis
	Small vessel vasculitis
	Arrhythmias
Musculoskeletal	Arthralgia
	Arthritis
	Myalgia
	Palindromic rheumatism
	Henoch–Schönlein syndrome
Renal tract	Enuresis
	Nephrotic syndrome
	Non-bacterial cystitis

Table 59.1 Examples of conditions in which there is some evidence that food (and food additive) intolerance reactions cause symptom provocation usually in the absence of evidence of immune response.

THE GOLD STANDARD

Three important criteria measure the accuracy of any test. The precise method of application of elimination and challenge will affect the performance under each heading.

1. *Reproducibility*. The ability to produce the same result on different occasions. This will be poor if the circumstances of the food challenge vary between tests (e.g. amount, processing, cooking, time since last ingestion, presence or absence of the symptom(s), factors affecting digestion and absorption).
2. *Specificity*. The absence of false-positive results. This will be poor in the presence of significant risk of placebo effect.
3. *Sensitivity*. The absence of false-negative results. This will be poor if the circumstances of the food challenge vary between the test challenge and the real life challenge. For example, the amount, processing, cooking, time since last ingestion, presence or absence of the symptom(s), and factors affecting digestion or absorption may all affect sensitivity.

The design of the DBPCFC test is intended to maximize reproducibility and specificity. It is likely to perform well in the particular situation of immediate food allergy if account is taken of the risk of anaphylaxis. However, in the particular situation of non-immediate food intolerance, where an elimination and challenge test is vital for diagnosis, the DBPCFC test is likely to show poor sensitivity for a number of reasons.

1. *Quantity*. It is not easy to determine the dose needed to elicit a response.[6] The amount required may be much larger than suspected.[16] Such quantities may be difficult or impossible to blind and the investigator may have to resort to dehydrated forms, thus risking denaturing the antigen.
2. *Form of administration*. The specificity of reaction to the food, whether cooked or uncooked, has been studied both when the sensitivity is only to the raw form[14] and when the sensitivity is only to the cooked form.[23] The use of dehydrated foods adds another untested variable.
3. *Concomitant exposure*. It is clearly possible that a reaction could be dependent upon the concurrent ingestion of two or more allergens. Although unproven in the food allergy context, validation in the context of contact sensitivity suggests that this possibility should not be discounted.[17]
4. *Total load concept*. This concept asserts that maximal symptom control from allergen avoidance follows comprehensive environmental (ingestant, inhalant and contact) allergen avoidance. Similarly, to achieve the most robust challenge test response requires the prior establishment of such comprehensive symptom control. In its simplest form, it explains why single allergen avoidance and challenge may fail to influence symptoms. For example, an adult with asthma related to multiple food intolerances may not improve with the removal of one of the implicated foods. Similarly, challenge testing with this single food may not perceptibly provoke the asthma.
5. *Problems of blinding*. It may be difficult or impossible to conceal the amount, texture and flavour of the dose required to elicit a response. The masking of taste and/or smell introduces an artefact. As the mechanisms of response are largely unknown, it would be unwise to assume that any influence of taste or smell operates only in a psychosomatic manner. Doty and associates have shown that subolfactory threshold levels of common odours can increase by two to three times the nasal resistance of chemically sensitive individuals when compared to controls.[11]
6. *Placebo activity*. It is difficult to ensure inactivity within the placebo. The choice of another food – one that is not under

suspicion (e.g. strongly flavoured soup or ice cream) – presupposes that suspicion is an accurate determinant of food intolerance. Placebos widely used in a pharmaceutical context can be inappropriate in testing for food allergy (e.g. lactose). Attention has been drawn to the possibility that food-derived sugars (such as dextrose), despite purification, may still convey the reaction-inducing capacity of the parent food (corn in the case of dextrose).[26]

7. *Use of capsules.* Reactions to food occurring within the mouth may be missed.[6] Remote reactions may depend on the oral route for their precipitation.[31] In bypassing the oral component of the digestive process, delay of qualitative modification of that process may occur. This may influence any reaction. The gelatin from which capsules are usually made is often of beef or pork origin and therefore reaction to the gelatin cannot be discounted. Provocation of headache by gelatin capsules has now been confirmed by double-blind challenge.[28a]

8. *Use of nasogastric tube.* The same difficulties resulting from bypassing the mouth (see above) may result.

9. *Inactive phase latency.* It may be necessary for a disease to be in an active phase for a food challenge response to occur.[20] This may or may not be a function of the total load concept (see above). For example, some patients may have their hay fever exacerbated by foods which apparently cause no problems outside the hay fever season.[13]

10. *Masking and unmasking.* These concepts (discussed more fully below) are poorly defined scientifically, but observational studies suggest that an understanding may be vital for the success of studies in this area. Put simply, the juxtaposition of successive challenges with the same or differing allergens may induce a state of partial 'immunity' to subsequent challenge during a latent period which may last for several days.

11. *Partial tolerance.* It appears that in some cases, a period of remission of symptoms through the avoidance of a demonstrably symptom-provoking food results in the eventual tolerance of an isolated ingestion of that food. In other cases, repeated reintroduction challenge with that food over a number of hours or even days seems necessary to induce symptom recurrence even at the commencement of that period of remission. In this situation food intolerance may exist but be impossible to prove by single ingestion challenge. This difficulty seems to occur with cereal grains in particular.

From an examination of the above it should be clear that an adequate ingestion test of intolerance of a food is virtually impossible to achieve. The investigator is faced with a stark choice, to use the double blind placebo-controlled method with the risk of false-negative outcome described above, or to use elimination and open challenge and encounter the risk of false-positive and psychological reactions.

At the present time no laboratory test of food intolerance demonstrates adequate reproducibility or correlation with clinical outcome. Therefore, whilst clinical dietary elimination and challenge must remain the gold standard for the diagnosis of food intolerance, no particular method fulfils all the necessary criteria to establish it as ideal.

The double blind placebo-controlled food challenge

It is important to stress that, in spite of the drawbacks, double blind placebo-controlled methods have been successfully used under clinical trial conditions to confirm the role of food intolerance in a wide range of conditions (e.g. asthma,[21] irritable bowel syndrome[2]). In undertaking such studies a remarkably wide range of symptoms has been triggered (e.g. enuresis in children being investigated for migraine[12]). An examination of these studies shows that careful adaptation of the double blind method can minimize the drawbacks. Clearly, the method needs to remain at the cornerstone of the research investigation of non-IgE-mediated food intolerance until something better replaces it. Meanwhile, every attempt should be taken to ensure that the test is applied under conditions that will maximize its sensitivity.

The routine use of such techniques in patient management carries the risk of underperformance. Each case will need to be considered on its merits, and the use of carefully designed blinding techniques limited to certain cases.

FOOD ADDICTION AND MASKING

Food addiction

The term *addiction* is usually applied to the mostly conscious compulsive phenomena seen with habit-forming drugs, both inhaled and ingested. The occurrence of withdrawal symptoms is its most constant characteristic feature. Alcohol addiction and caffeine addiction represent dietary examples of this. However, an examination of the circumstances that determine food intolerance shows that hidden addictions often distinguish this mode of symptom presentation. Food cravings, at times intense, may occur to a regularly consumed food or foods to which the individual is sensitive. Withdrawal symptoms triggered by the omission of that food could occur. In such cases, the facts may be clear from an examination of the dietary history.

In other cases, the affected individual is unaware that this is happening. The fact that the next 'fix' is being subconsciously timed in order to forestall withdrawal manifestations may not be apparent even if the dietary history is scrutinized in close detail. In this case, it may be the accidental or deliberate avoidance of the food that initiates a symptom response. This situation is seen in caffeine addiction, where symptoms of lethargy, irritability and cognitive impairment may occur in response to prolonged avoidance. In another common example, a migraine sufferer with undiagnosed milk intolerance may typically experience migraine after a morning lie-in, unaware that the migraine has been triggered by omitting their morning cereal with milk.

The term *tolerance* is used to describe the diminishing of intensity of symptoms that may occur over time. Typically, a food that originally caused symptoms is later temporarily tolerated without apparent problem. In some cases, this appears to occur spontaneously. In some cases, tolerance may be deliberately induced by a period of weeks or months of avoidance followed by a gradual return to regular, but occasional, ingestion of the previously troublesome food. The maintenance of temporary tolerance appears to be dependent on the actual rate of frequency of exposure. This is the principle that underlies the 4-day rotation diet.

Loss of tolerance may subsequently occur, temporarily or permanently, typically after an increase in the frequency of use of this particular food or following a major physiological or emotional stress.

In practice, both tolerance and addiction can be seen as manifestations of a state in which a precise cause and effect relationship between the eating of a food and the precipitation of symptoms becomes distorted. The response to a specific food challenge in a particular subject may vary from nil to maximal, depending upon how recently that subject was regularly exposed to that or to a closely related food. If insufficient time has elapsed since the ingestion of that food (or if the food is still being ingested in small amounts inadvertently), the challenge test may produce a false-negative response. Conversely, if too much time has elapsed since regular exposure (as may happen in a prolonged sequential food challenge protocol), then the heightening of symptom response may wane.

Masking

This state of insusceptibility to specific challenge is termed *masking*. This concept appears to be without scientific equivalent; none the less, it is useful. The patient who is 'masked' through the regular ingestion of a food or foods capable of triggering symptom responses may cause the investigator considerable confusion in diagnosis. The investigator's ability to understand this concept and manipulate the circumstances to achieve challenge testing in the unmasked state is critical to successful outcome.

Ashford and Miller, in discussing the subject of chemical (including food chemical) sensitivity generally, have proposed a set of postulates after the fashion of the postulates proposed by Koch for verification of microbial causation.[4]

Ashford and Miller's postulates

1. When a subject simultaneously avoids all chemical, food and drug incitants, remission of symptoms occurs (unmasking).
2. A specific constellation of symptoms occurs with the re-introduction of a particular incitant.
3. Symptoms resolve when the incitant is again avoided.
4. With re-exposure to the same incitant, the same constellation of symptoms reoccurs, provided that the challenge is conducted within an appropriate window of time. Clinical observations suggest that an ideal window is 4–7 days after the last exposure to the test incitant.

This 4–7-day interval is based on the observation that a period of heightened (in terms of both speed of onset and severity) or hyperacute responsiveness follows the phase of withdrawal.

In an examination of the effects of passage of time and frequency of exposure on the height and nature of the food intolerance symptom response, Rinkel proposed a cyclic concept.[28] A graphical representation based on Rinkel's original 1944 exposition is given in Fig. 59.1. It remains a valid and useful account of the clinical phenomena encountered in the investigation of food intolerance.

Comprehensive environmental control

It has been suggested that food intolerance most commonly presents as part of a wider multiple chemical sensitivity problem.[25] This phenomenon, distinct from classical toxicity, has been much debated and is ill understood at the present time.[4] It raises the possibility that amongst sufferers a continuum of reactivity to inhaled and ingested chemical substances may exist. The masked state in such sufferers may be maintained by inhalation of chemical incitants as much as by their ingestion.

In addition, the common coexistence of classical IgE-mediated allergy in such sufferers reinforces yet further the need for a comprehensive environmental approach. To achieve this degree of

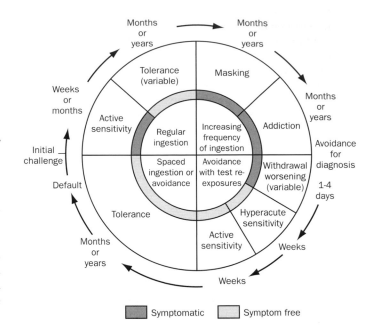

Fig. 59.1 The cyclic concept of food intolerance. The upper part of the figure represents the natural history before diagnosis starting with an initial challenge in infancy. The lower part the sequence which follows test avoidance and challenge for specific diagnosis.

comprehensive control would require a purpose-built hospital-based clinical research facility. Although few units of this type exist at present, Environmental Control Units are being established, particularly in the USA, and at least one has a University affiliation.

IMPORTANCE OF A FULL MEDICAL HISTORY

A full and carefully taken medical history is extremely important to place in context the condition or symptoms under investigation. The presence of undiagnosed organic disease must be eliminated if suspected. Occult neoplastic, connective tissue disease or infection may be difficult to suspect from the history, and a minimal screening process should be considered in all cases where the patient is generally unwell.

As well as taking a full personal and family history, it is helpful to ask about factors that may have been associated with the onset of the condition. Certain conditions tend to be associated with the precipitation of food intolerance. Amongst these are viral illnesses, broad-spectrum antibiotic therapy (particularly when prolonged or recurrent) and major life stresses.

Excluding unsuitable subjects

History-taking should also be used to establish the suitability of the subject for this type of investigation. Psychologically disturbed subjects present a particularly difficult challenge. On the one hand, establishing the presence of genuine food intolerance reactions may dramatically improve the quality of life and substantially reduce the need for subsequent medical treatment (see case history, below). On the other, cases may be encountered in which the attempt to reduce symptoms of environmental causation produces exacerbation and complication of symptoms of mental or psychosomatic illness.

The iatrogenic exacerbation of an eating disorder or a phobic illness is a very real risk. The obsessional pursuit of an allergic explanation for every bodily sensation encountered can become a way of life for certain psychologically vulnerable individuals. The investigator must be aware that 'suggestion can produce virtually any subjective symptom, as well as many measurable organic changes'.[22]

Cases may be encountered in which this type of obsessional behaviour pattern has already become established. In such cases, it is important to take a broad view. The history may suggest that there are unresolved emotional conflicts, and it may be important to seek a psychiatric opinion before proceeding. Often the dietary factor cannot be ignored (there may be a risk of nutritional inadequacy) and it may be necessary to 'meet half way' over the dietary elimination issue. Compromises in the elimination strategy with due regard to the possibility of genuine food intolerances and the search for a socially and nutritionally acceptable outcome should be the goal.

In the case of children, the psychological vulnerability of their parent(s) must be considered. The field of food intolerance appears to offer special scope for the exaggeration or fabrication of children's symptoms by their parent(s) and a form of Munchausen syndrome (by proxy) has been described.[30]

Other unsuitable cases may be encountered in which it may prove impossible to undertake a food intolerance investigation. This may be because of the lack of adequate motivation, inconsistency between the dietary precision needed and the patient's lifestyle or because of inadequate intellect.

Special situations

No patient who has had an actual or potentially severe reaction to food such as anaphylaxis or laryngeal or tongue oedema should be allowed to undertake a challenge exposure with that food except under close supervision. Neither should such patients undertake unsupervised challenge testing of related foods (such as another legume in the case of a person sensitive to soya) where any doubt exists as to the possibility of sensitivity to that food.

Even when patients with a history of anaphylaxis are excluded, anaphylaxis can still occur after oral challenge.[15] For this reason, subjects who suffer IgE-mediated disease should be considered capable of developing anaphylaxis, even if this has not previously occurred. The type, severity and duration of symptoms, and the speed of onset after any suspected allergen exposure can all be used to predict the risk of challenge exposure.

There is an additional risk in undertaking elimination and challenge testing of brittle asthmatics. Typically, the brittle asthmatic may have no idea that a regularly consumed food may be exacerbating their asthma.[4a] A hyperacute response may be anticipated if such a food is scrupulously avoided and then challenged after a 5–14-day interval (see Masking, above).

Patients suffering from poor nutrition should have their nutrient intake improved before starting on an elimination diet. The use of a hypoallergenic elemental food formula in place of the standard elimination diet might be considered both in the malnourished and in those with certain inflammatory disease (e.g. Crohn's disease, rheumatoid arthritis).

A small number of patients are sensitive to and disabled by a wide range of environmental exposures (e.g. inhaled fumes, aeroallergens). In many cases, accurate identification of food symptom responses is impossible, as these cannot be teased out from all the other reactions that are taking place. In such patients admission to an Environmental Control Unit for full allergy investigation involving an initial period of fasting may be preferable.

USE OF THE DIET DIARY

An examination of the pattern of food ingestion and the pattern of symptom response provides a valuable initial dietary assessment and can help the physician decide what form of exclusion regime it would be most helpful to employ.

A frequently used device is the diet diary. The patient records the nature and time of consumption of all foods, beverages, snacks and medications, together with a timed record of activity and symptoms. It may be necessary to instruct the patient in the evaluation of symptoms, as often they tend to disregard lower levels of symptoms as a symptom-free state. Those with complex allergic problems should in addition record such activities as exposure to dust, moulds, feathers, animals and chemical fumes. Women should note also the possible correlation of symptoms with the menstrual cycle.

Although immediate cause and effect relationships between food and symptoms are likely to have already been spotted by the patient, they should nevertheless be sought at this stage. Diets high in chemical additives or nutritionally unsound should be earmarked for correction before the start of an exclusion regime. Marked improvement often occurs with simple dietary advice about wholefood nutritional principles, making the complex process of food allergy diagnosis unnecessary.

The possible presence of reaction to food additives should be borne in mind at this stage.

Pattern of symptoms

An addictive food ingestion pattern may be apparent from the food diary. More subtle single food responses can become known if it is remembered that symptoms from a single ingestion may occur later the same day or during the night or following day. In some cases, symptoms from a single ingestion may occur on two or three consecutive nights with relative freedom from symptoms during the intervening daytime hours.

Certain other diurnal patterns of symptom occurrence can suggest a masked food allergy without necessarily implicating a specific food. Such diurnal patterns may be made up of exacerbations and quiescent periods of the symptom constellation characteristic to that subject (e.g. headache, lethargy, muscular pain, nasal congestion, etc.). This is a characteristic pattern of response to masked staple food intolerance, e.g. wheat, milk, corn, egg, potato, etc. With a low grade response, the only clear exacerbation of such symptoms may be during the first hour or two after rising.

With a higher degree of sensitivity, an increase in both the frequency and intensity of exacerbations may be seen. Typically, such episodes occur 1–2 h after rising and then ebb and flow throughout the day at 3–5-h intervals. In some cases a further exacerbation of symptoms will awaken the sufferer from sleep at 2.00 to 4.00 am.

The effect of alcohol

One other factor in symptom provocation is worth noting, as it is quite helpful in diagnosis. This is the apparent ability of alcohol to act as a catalyst to the food intolerance response. For example, a hidden sensitivity to potato might show up as an immediate exacerbation after a meal containing potato and alcohol.

There is also the possibility that the alcoholic beverage that is derived from a particular food may be capable of producing a reaction in an individual sensitized to that food.[27] For example, a rhinitis sufferer might notice that a particular alcoholic beverage produces sneezing and rhinorrhoea. Closer study might reveal such a sufferer to be sensitive to corn and suffer no reaction on consuming a non-grain-derived alcoholic beverage (e.g. Jamaica rum). A similar relationship between the food and its botanical source has also been proposed for sugars.[26]

Incomplete avoidance

The diet diary may show that a specific food, already suspected as being troublesome in that patient, is being inadequately avoided. Such is the ubiquity in the modern diet of many of our staple foods, that the individual's own attempts to avoid that which is known to cause symptoms is usually ineffective. The child who avoids milk but eats yoghurt and the adult who avoids fish but eats ice cream (which usually contains fish oils), may be preventing full symptom remission because of inadequate compliance.

Lastly, the diet diary may show patients who are poorly motivated, or use only ready-made meals with no access to facilities for their own food preparation. Such patients are unlikely to do well with a test elimination regime.

METHODS OF DIETARY ELIMINATION

Whether the elimination planned is a selective elimination of one to three foods, a basic elimination diet or an elemental diet, the method of implementation of the dietary procedure is the same in each case.

The involvement of a dietician is a particular advantage at this stage. As well as being well versed in the practical aspects, both social and nutritional, of diet change, the dietician will have access to comprehensive information about the distribution of foods, both obvious and hidden, within the modern diet. The need for objectivity and an understanding of the placebo response

will have been covered within the dietician's training, and due regard for nutritional adequacy is less likely to be a problem if the dietician is involved from the outset.

The patient (or the parents in the case of a child) will be responsible for the recording of symptoms, so it is desirable that a baseline period of self-observation precedes the test diet. This should be conducted on the patient's normal diet. Investigator and patient should decide together what symptoms should be the subject of daily scores.

Care should be taken to ensure that the patient does not exclude the recording of certain symptoms simply because they do not think that the particular symptom does not apply to food intolerance. For example, a patient being studied for migraine may have unexplained bladder irritability and may not realize that the same food or foods could be triggering both types of response. Any self-measurable parameter of disease activity (e.g. peak flow rate, grip strength) can be added to the symptom chart (Fig. 59.2).

Hidden ingredients

If the food to be eliminated is not widely used as an ingredient by the food industry (e.g. coffee), its elimination is reasonably straightforward.

Unfortunately, an increasing number of foods are now used in this way and their elimination is no simple matter. As stated above, the help of a dietician experienced in this work is invaluable.

Milk: casein, caseinate, lactose and whey are all milk derivatives. Most 'non-dairy' milk and cream substitutes contain one of these derivatives. Powdered artificial sweeteners contain lactose, as do many medications. For the following foods it should be assumed that milk is present unless one has specific evidence to the contrary: bread, margarine, ice cream (even when labelled 'non-milk fat'), sausages, hamburgers, plain chocolate, sherbet and other sweets.

Egg: vitellin, ovovitellin, livetin, ovomucin, ovomucoid and albumin are all egg derivatives. They are found both labelled and

Date	Specific symptoms				Notes	Weight (kg)
	Migraine	Oedema	Lethargy	Joint Pain		
30.5.96	1-3	3	2	3		85.9
31.5.96	1-3	3	2	3		
1.6.96	0-2	3	2	3		85.9
2.6.96	0-1	3	2	3		85.9
3.6.96	2-3	2	2	3		85.9
4.6.96	3-5	2	2	3-5	Took 1 Imigran	85.0
5.6.96	2-3	2	2	4		84.1
6.6.96	1-2	1	1-2	3		83.6
7.6.96	1-0	1	1	3		83.2
8.6.96	2	1	1	1		82.7
9.6.96	3-0	0	0	1	Took 1 Imigran	82.3
10.6.96	0	1	0	0		82.7
11.6.96	0	1	0	0		81.8
12.6.96	0	1	0	0		81.8
13.6.96	0	0.5	0	0		81.4
14.6.96	0	1	0	0		80.5

(Left margin: Normal Diet (30.5.96–3.6.96); Test Diet (4.6.96–14.6.96))

Fig. 59.2 Actual elimination symptom chart of a severe migraine and daily headache and oedema sufferer who subsequently became free from migraine (apart from elimination diet transgressions) with the avoidance of all grains and potato. 0, none; 1, very mild; 2, mild; 3, moderate; 4, severe; 5, very severe.

unlabelled in baking powder, cakes, cake mixes, croissants, glazed bread and rolls, pastry, meringue, sauces, salad dressings, icing, sweets, sausages and luncheon meats. Egg is used in the production of wines, some instant coffee and root beer.

Wheat: this category includes wheat grain, germ, starch and 'food starch', flour, bran and farina. Wheat starch may be classified as gluten-free if its purity is within the *Codex alimentarius* definition. However, this may be a quite unsuitable standard for the wheat-allergic patient. Major wheat-containing foods are easily identifiable. Hidden sources include baking powder, sausages, vinegar and alcoholic beverages. Rye and barley frequently cross-react with wheat and, for practical purposes, should be classified together. Even 'pure' rye flour contains up to 10% wheat as the seed is commonly contaminated. Malt is derived from barley, sometimes from wheat or corn as well, and is present in many non-wheat breakfast cereals.

From the above it can be seen that a number of foods commonly contain all three of these frequently encountered food allergens.

For this reason, the author frequently uses a diet eliminating all three, giving the patient a list of foods to be avoided together with recipes for biscuits, cakes and crackers made from rice, soya, sago, chickpea and potato flours. Books containing recipes for such patients are available.[32]

Other foods commonly found as allergens and widespread as hidden ingredients include corn, soya, yeast, fish, pork and beef. Corn is probably the most difficult to avoid. As oil, starch, syrup or sugar (e.g. glucose, fructose, dextrose), it is present in virtually all factory processed foods. It is also very widely distributed in alcoholic beverages. A fuller account of hidden natural ingredients has been prepared by Miller.[18]

Quite clearly, even the avoidance of a single food can be quite difficult. It follows that, if the patient is to avoid more than one or two foods, a more structured approach is needed.

Medications

Drugs often contain excipient materials that may be troublesome. Capsules may be made from gelatin of beef or pork origin and tablets may contain food starches and sugars. Drugs in any form may contain preservatives or colourings (particularly azo dyes). The continuation of any of these during the period of dietary elimination may interfere with the specificity of the test. All non-essential drugs should be considered and, if possible, stopped. In the case of drugs that may produce withdrawal effects, this should be done well in advance.

Essential drugs (e.g. thyroxine, insulin) will need to be continued. In other situations, disease-modifying drugs (e.g. cortico-steroids in Crohn's disease or asthma) can be continued and consideration given to discontinuing them if a good response to dietary control is established.

In some cases, it may be possible to substitute for one particular preparation of a drug another that is less likely to contain a troublesome excipient. For example, a simple aqueous suspension of a medication may be prepared in place of a tablet known to contain, for example, potato starch. Soluble tablets do not contain insoluble food starches, and a white soluble tablet, if available, may be the better choice to replace a drug that cannot be stopped.

In some cases, there may be an advantage in switching to a closely related drug to avoid a particular excipient.

Standard elimination diets

Basic elimination diets are based on the inescapable fact that giving the patient one list of foods to be avoided (containing, for example, milk) is difficult. Adding together numerous lists for various avoidances (for example, food additives, milk, egg, wheat, corn and soya) would make adherence complex and compliance virtually impossible to achieve. Diets that tell the patient what to eat rather than what not to eat are simpler to apply.

Numerous basic regimes have been used. Those employed most frequently by the author are shown (Tables 59.2–59.4).

With all these standard regimes, the two biggest difficulties for most patients are a substitute for tea or coffee and a substitute for bread. There are no truly satisfactory grain-free bread substitutes, although reasonable tea and coffee substitutes are available (e.g. Rooibosch tea and dandelion coffee).

It must be stressed that these diets are for short-term diagnostic use only, especially if used in young children. Generally the more liberal the regime (e.g. the wheat milk and egg free diet or the Stone Age diet) the longer it can be successfully and safely applied. In the case of symptoms that are infrequent (e.g. headaches that only occur once a fortnight), an elimination diet may have to be continued for longer to be convincing.

The elemental diet

Alternative techniques include the use of proprietary 'elemental' diets (e.g. Elemental EO28, Scientific Hospital Supplies). These have been employed where it has been thought that the number of involved allergens may be large and in particular when prolonged avoidance is thought necessary to secure a remission. They have been used in the investigation of eczema in children,[29] rheumatoid arthritis[9] and following 7–10-day intravenous nutrition in the investigation of inflammatory bowel disease.[1]

However, neither of these forms of alternative nutrition can be claimed to be free of antigenic activity. Both contain sugar derivatives of corn which have been shown to perpetuate chronic effects attributable to corn when administered both orally and intravenously.[26]

Such extreme measures can be advocated only for the most complex of problems. In most cases, the simple elimination diets described above and administered with careful preparation and attention to detail will produce good results.

Prerequisites for successful elimination diet

Laxative: in the absence of a history of regular normal bowel habit, the patient should take a dose of Epsom salts or milk of magnesia on the first morning to obtain a satisfactory bowel evacuation.

Fluid intake: a large quantity of fluid should be drunk. Bottled spring water is to be preferred, allowing for the testing of tap water as a challenge test.

Absolute adherence: the degree of avoidance necessary to induce remission is likely to vary. However, it should be assumed that adherence needs to be total. For example, spurious reactions have been traced to licking a food-soiled finger in the preparation of food for others. Another example of the role of minute quantities would be an urticarial reaction after exposure to the odour of a food being cooked.[10] The problem of hidden food ingredients has been referred to above.

Fresh foods: foods used in exclusion diets should be fresh if possible, but frozen or dried if not. However, the latter two heighten the risk of hidden ingredients of both natural and synthetic

Wheat, milk and egg-free diet

	Foods not allowed			Foods allowed
	Wheat (including rye and barley)	**Milk**	**Egg**	
Bakery goods	Bread, rolls, scones, fruit loaf, biscuits, cake	Some biscuits, cakes, breads	Some breads and rolls (especially glazed), most cakes and biscuits, croissants	Special breads and bread mixes which are wheat, milk and egg-free, gluten-free breads are usually wheat, egg and milk-free (ask pharmacist), plain rice cakes, oat cakes, papadums
Pasta and soups	Spaghetti, pasta, noodles, soups thickened with flour barley or noodles	Some pasta sauces, creamed soups	Some pastas, egg noodles, noodles in some soups, macaroni	Rice noodles, pure buckwheat pasta (e.g. buckwheat spaghetti), clear soups without noodles
Flour	Wheat rye or barley flour, malt cake and pastry mixes	Some cake and pastry mixes	Some cake and pastry mixes	Cornflour, arrowroot, rice flour, potato flour, soya flour, gram flour, cornmeal
Cereals	Most, including bran, wheatgerm, most muesli, some porridge oats contain added wheat (especially 'own label' brands)	Prepared porridge, milk added to cereals		Cornflakes, rice cereals (eg Rice Krispies), wheat-free porridge oats, wheat-free muesli, (use cereals with fruit juice or milk substitute)
Puddings and sweets	Custard, white sauce pies and pastries, sponge and suet puddings, sweets and pudding mixes, pancakes and batters, waffles, mincemeat, fruit crumbles, Liquorice 'Allsorts', many sweets and candies, sherbet, ice cream cones and wafers	Custard, custard powder, white sauce, pies and pastries, sponge and suet puddings, ice cream, milk chocolate, most *plain* chocolate, sweets with chocolate	Pancakes, batters, commercially prepared pudding mixes, egg custard, soufflés, waffles, meringue, pavlovas, doughnuts, marshmallows, some ice creams, 'dolly mixture', Opal Fruits	All fresh, frozen, canned or dried fruits, special recipe cakes, sweets and pastries, wheat-free batters made with alternative flours (e.g. buckwheat), boiled sweets
Vegetables and salads	Avoid sauces, breadcrumbs or gravies used in preparation	Avoid sauces or butter, some gravies and salad dressings	Scrambled and hard boiled egg added to salads, salad dressings	All fresh frozen or tinned vegetables, all salad foods
Meat and meat products, fish and fish products	Sausages, salami, flour used in thickening, gravies and sauces, breadcrumb or batter coatings, hamburgers, pies, pasties, pizza, stuffing, fish cakes, fishfingers	Cooking in butter, white sauce, milk or cheese, sausages, mortadella, Spam, polony, gravies	Pre-crumbed foods (e.g. fish), hamburgers and sausages, fartar sauce, meat loaf, Béarnaise and Hollandaise sauce	All fresh fish, meat, most precooked meats if free from binders or stuffing, batters made from alternative flours, alternatives to breadcrumbs (e.g. crushed cornflakes)
Beverages	Ovaltine, Bengers, Horlicks, malted or barley-containing drinks, root beer (whisky, beer and lagers can contain wheat or barley derivatives)	Chocolate drinks, Ovaltine, Horlicks, some tea and coffee whiteners	Ovaltine, some instant coffees (some wines are cleared with egg white)	Tea, coffee, plain cocoa, fruit cordials, soft drinks, mineral water
Milk products	Commercial milk drinks, custard made with custard powder, white sauce, cheese sauce, ice cream with biscuit pieces or sauces	Milk, cheese, butter, most margarine, ice cream, milk powder, yoghurt, buttermilk	Some ice creams	Milk substitutes, tofu, apple puree (substitute for egg in cooking), vegetable puree (substitute for milk or egg in savory recipes), milk (and whey)-free margarine
Packet and tinned foods (check labels)	Wheat starch, wheat flour, gluten, wheat gluten, starch, food starch, wheat germ, bran, farina	Milk solids, skim milk, whey, milk proteins, non-fat milk, casein, caseinate, lactose	Vitellin, ovovitellin, livetin, ovomucin, ovomucoid, albumin	Check all purchased and packaged foods are free from items listed
Miscellaneous	Baking powder, malt vinegar, some soya sauce, communion wafers, some pepper powder		Some baking powder	Wheat and egg-free baking powder, wine or cider vinegar, wheat-free soya sauce

Table 59.2 Wheat, milk and egg-free diet.

The Stone Age diet	
Fresh or frozen meat	Any kind, including offal
Fresh or frozen fish	Any kind
Fresh or frozen poultry	Any kind
Fresh vegetables	Any kind except potato, tomato and soya (Yam or sweet potato can be substituted for potato)
Fresh fruit	Any kind except citrus fruits (orange, lemon, grapefruit, lime, satsuma, etc.)
Grain	Rice, rice cakes, rice noodles
Grain substitute	Buckwheat, Quinoa
Drinks	Spring water, additive-free juices of allowed fruits, herb and fruit teas (i.e. mint, rosehip, Rooibosch, Ruby Red)
Seasoning	Sea salt, fresh pepper and herbs
Oils	Olive oil, sunflower oil, safflower oil (avoid unidentified vegetable oil)

Table 59.3 The Stone Age diet. The diet is free from the more commonly non-tolerated foods. It excludes most cereal grains and sugars, milk and milk products, egg, chicken, citrus fruits, sugars, potato, soya, tomato, additives and a number of other possible hidden food allergens. The diet should be changed under certain circumstances (e.g. if allergy to fruits is suspected).

'Few foods' diet		
Cod	Swede	Courgette
Trout	Sweet potato	Cooked carrot
Mackerel	Quinoa	Safflower oil
Pear	Beansprouts	Sea salt
Avocado pear	Marrow	Olive oil

Table 59.4 'Few foods' diet. These foods appear to be amongst the least likely to produce non-immediate hypersensitivity (food intolerance).

origin. Ideally, chemically less contaminated food of organic origin should be used to eliminate the possibility of reactions occurring to pesticide or herbicide residues.

Pharmaceutical preparations: toothpaste, drugs and medicines (including the contraceptive pill) contain food substances and their discontinuation should be considered to avoid false-negative challenge tests because of incomplete unmasking. Teeth can be brushed with a little sodium bicarbonate and water.

Withdrawal effects

Elimination diets should not cause withdrawal symptoms in patients not suffering food intolerance. However, many (though not all) of those who eventually benefit will experience withdrawal symptoms. Early effects may appear in the afternoon or evening of the first day. Irrespective of the presenting complaint, headache is common, frequently migrainous in type.

Other common manifestations include nausea, diarrhoea, aching limbs, weakness, malaise, depression and agitation, thus allowing a direct comparison to be made between the withdrawal effects of foods, alcohol, drugs and tobacco. If not warned that such effects may occur, patients may discontinue the test, suspecting a coincident flu-like illness (but without the fever).

Although it can be criticized on the grounds of suggestion, patients should be warned about the possibility of exacerbation of symptoms on staple food elimination. Food cravings can occur and may be severe. If they occur, careful note should be made of the craved-for food or foods in this situation, as it is likely that they may be those responsible for the original symptoms.

Later manifestations of the withdrawal effect may include extreme muscle ache; the worst affected individuals may need to spend the second and third days of the test at rest. On the second, third and fourth days, fatigue, physical weakness and tachycardia with minimal exertion sometimes occurs, leading the sufferer and others to ascribe the symptom state to hunger; a break in the dietary regime may then follow. These symptoms are temporary and perseverance results in their rapid amelioration. If drugs are needed for symptom control, they should be chosen to try to avoid those with excipient food starches and dyes (see above).

Length of the elimination period

If withdrawal symptoms do occur, the elimination diet should continue until this is over and there have been 2–3 days of freedom from symptoms.

In the absence of withdrawal symptoms, adequately sustained symptom clearance should be the guide. It may appear that it would be inconclusive to follow an elimination diet to investigate a symptom which occurs very infrequently, *particularly when the patient is completely well between attacks*. However, one must bear in mind the possibility that a state of partial masking by a food consumed as frequently or more frequently than once a day may be determining this infrequent symptom occurrence. In this situation it is quite possible that there will be frequent, and perhaps daily, concomitant symptoms which are not as fully masked by regular ingestion but involving the same food(s). With luck, an investigation using the clearing and recurrence of the frequent symptoms as the endpoint may identify the food responsible for the infrequent symptom. What may happen is that the infrequent symptom (say, a classical migraine attack) is precipitated as a withdrawal response by the elimination regime, thus strengthening the observation.

No hard and fast rule can be laid down as to the necessary duration of an elimination diet in the investigation of frequently occurring symptoms, but in general 5–10 days are needed. Young patients seem to clear in a shorter time. Symptoms in some conditions where there is pronounced inflammation (such as arthritis, eczema, non-bacterial cystitis, Crohn's disease, cow's milk-induced pulmonary haemosiderosis and some cases of asthma) may take as long as 4–6 weeks to clear.

SEQUENTIAL FOOD INGESTION CHALLENGE

If food intolerance is suspected as the cause of a patient's symptoms, and there has been a positive outcome to the elimination diet, the assumption should be that there are a number of foods involved. The period of elimination should have converted the patient's food intolerance to the unmasked state and a hyperacute stage of reactivity should exist to those potentially reactive foods that have been scrupulously eliminated.

Failure to establish an unmasked state to the food under test can result in either marked attenuation or complete absence of symptoms on challenge.

Failure to establish this unmasked state can result from the incomplete avoidance of the food under test, the food being still consumed inadvertently. The period of elimination should not be too short (leading to incomplete withdrawal) or too long (leading to tolerance to single ingestion challenge). The latter situation is in danger of occurring when many sequential food challenges are to be undertaken, and particularly if a prolonged challenge (several days to a week) is to be undertaken for each food reintroduced.

It has been suggested that food intolerance must be tested by prolonged challenges of several days per food.[33] Whilst this may be feasible if only a few foods have been eliminated, it is cumbersome to apply if many foods are to be tested.

It is possible that in some clinical situations (e.g. eczema, arthritis) food intolerance reactions will require a number of days of challenge to trigger the precise symptom constellation under test. However, in such situations it is likely that there will be earlier manifestations of related, but different, symptoms. For example, a patient suffering from joint pain and stiffness relieved by cow's milk avoidance might not develop joint pain and stiffness until the second or third day after challenge. However, headache may have occurred within 2 h and diarrhoea within 6 h of challenge.

In practice, if care has been taken to establish the unmasked state, most food intolerance reactions have commenced (though may not be concluded) by 8 h. Anthony and Maberly[3] studied 1263 food challenges in 30 subjects suspected of having multiple food intolerances. Reactions occurred in 671 of 1263 challenges (53%). When time to onset of symptoms was studied, there was a tendency for this measurement to cluster by subject. The subjects appeared to divide into four groups. In group I (two of 30, 7%) most reactions to a range of food challenges had commenced by 20 min, and virtually all by 40 min. In group II (six of 30, 20%) most reactions had commenced by 40 min, and virtually all by 60 min. In group III (10 of 30, 33%) most reactions had commenced by between 40 and 60 min and virtually all by 4 h. In group IV (12 of 30, 40%) most reactions had commenced by between 1 and 4 h, and virtually all by 8 h.

Although very few reactions commenced after 8 h, this was a group studied in an Environmental Control Unit, and therefore likely to have been well prepared and closely studied.

The pulse test

Certain measurements may usefully be made in addition to the recording of symptoms. Where any simply measured parameter of disease activity exists in a particular condition (e.g. peak flow rates in asthma, grip strength measurements in arthritis), this should be measured at intervals after the test ingestion.

Another useful addition to subjective symptom assessment is measurement of pulse rate. This can be satisfactorily carried out by the patient when conducting the test at home, and it forms the basis of the pulse test originally described by Coca.[8]

Pulse change (a rise or fall of ≥ 10 beats/min) is not an invariable accompaniment of a food intolerance reaction.[3] However, it occurs in about half of all symptom-producing tests (Table 59.5) and there is a statistically significant correlation between pulse change and symptom production.[24] An examination of the data in Table 59.5 shows that a pulse rate change (usually a rise, but sometimes a fall) appears to precede the onset of other symptoms in some cases. This can be seen in the case of grains in particular, which tend in general to produce delayed symptom reactions.

The author has found the measurement of pulse rate change to be a useful addition to food challenge testing. The pulse should be taken after a brief period of rest immediately before food ingestion challenge and 20, 40 and 60 (and, in the case of grains, 90 and 120) min after ingestion. Generally, one food challenge test per day can be undertaken, ideally in the morning. If there is no response to the first ingestion, the same food may be eaten up to twice more on the same day. If no reaction is apparent by the next morning, the next test can proceed, the tolerated food being reintroduced back into the diet. In an individual case, examination of the results of early testing may allow an increase in the rate of testing to two foods per day.

Some investigators modify this regime in the case of the cereal grains, undertaking two or three test challenges on the day of the test, and leaving the next day free of testing in case of a delayed symptom response (Table 59.6).

In spite of the evidence suggesting that most food reactions commence within an 8-h period, there may still be occasions when an investigator decides to test a number of foods over a number of days of challenge test for each. This may happen when successful symptom clearance occurs with an elimination diet, but sequential food testing fails to identify the incitant.

In this case, an alternative regime would be to test foods by reintroducing them in groups rather than singly (e.g. grains, pulses, poultry, cabbage family, etc.). In this way, tests can be completed in a shorter period, without the risk of inducing tolerance inherent in a longer testing period.

Whilst symptom provocation is, quite clearly, the most reliable indicator of a positive response, in practice the pulse provides a useful crosscheck and may help avoid a false-negative test response. It must be stressed, however, that a pulse change is neither pathognomonic of food allergy nor a universal accompaniment of a reproducible symptom response.

Variations in the testing regime

For a number of reasons there is general agreement that neither the elimination diet nor the period of challenge testing should continue for too long. Ideally, foods should be tested in the hyperacute response phase that appears to start from about day 5 of elimination and lasts for about 1–3 weeks. If it seems likely that more than 4 weeks of food challenge may be needed, consideration should be given to introducing as a block challenge over a 3- or 4-day period those foods still untested at that time. This assumes that the most likely suspects have already been tested and that one or more have been identified as incitants of reaction.

This manoeuvre acts as a possible short cut if no new symptoms arise. If the block challenge does trigger a fresh reaction, the diet immediately before the block challenge can be resumed for a few days until any symptom has fully settled, and sequential challenge recommended. Any temporary tolerance that the period of prolonged avoidance may have produced is likely to

The total number (and percentage) of a series of 1256 oral challenges with different foods							
	No. of tests	No. (%) causing		Proportion of symptom reactions starting		Proportion of pulse reactions starting	
		Symptoms	Pulse changes	Early	Late	Early	Late
Meat	139	77(55)	42(30)	0.19	0.56	0.43	0.42
Fish	129	70(54)	27(21)	0.23	0.48	0.48	0.34
Dairy	113	68(60)	39(35)	0.31	0.32	0.49	0.23
Grains	127	85(67)	65(51)	0.20	0.53	0.68	0.16
Nuts	40	24(60)	13(33)	0.38	0.33	0.69	0
Seeds	51	24(47)	16(31)	0.33	0.37	0.44	0.32
Fruit	279	127(46)	67(24)	0.24	0.41	0.54	0.21
Vegetables	280	142(51)	59(21)	0.21	0.42	0.47	0.29
Drinks	67	37(55)	26(39)	0.38	0.27	0.50	0.16
Yeast	31	17(55)	5(16)	0.24	0.35	0.20	0.80
Total	1256	671(53)	359(28)	0.25	0.43	0.52	0.25

Data from Anthony HM, Maberly DJ. Time of onset of symptoms after food challenge. *J Nutr Med* 1991; 2: 121–30, with permission.

Table 59.5 The total number (and percentage) of a series of 1256 oral challenges with different foods which provoked symptoms (grade ≥ 3) and pulse changes (≥ 10 beats/min), and the proportions of these responses noted early (within 20 min) or late (after 1 h).

have been superseded by a restoration of the phase of hyperacute sensitivity.

CASE HISTORY

Patricia, a 40-year-old housewife, presented with a 30-year history of multiple health problems. In the preceding 5 years, she had been a frequent hospital inpatient and outpatient and a very frequent attender at the doctor's surgery. She had consumed a variety of different medications. During her worst year, 2 years previously, she had spent 30 days in hospital, made 20 outpatient attendances, saw her GP 28 times, and was taking as many as 11 different medications concurrently.

She had suffered severe migraine since the age of 12, urinary difficulties since her teens with subsequent non-bacterial cystitis and severe episodes of renal pain. Assuming a microangiopathy, her nephrologist had been treating her with warfarin for the previous 2 years. She had a history of depression, having made two suicide attempts in the previous 5 years. She had had two full courses of electroconvulsive therapy. As a child she had tonsillitis and since childhood had had perennial rhinitis. She was known to be sensitive to the house dust mite.

She was initially started on a simple egg and milk-free diet and suffered severe withdrawal effects, resulting in the worst migraine she had ever known. This fortuitously provided the opportunity to fast her for several days and she became free from symptoms and felt better than she could ever remember. The results of her challenge tests are given in Table 59.6. Since the establishment of a compatible diet, she has led a happy healthy family life. Her medical requirements over the next 5 years were met by four

visits to the surgery. She required no regular prescribed medications. Details of her medical needs over the past 10 years are summarized in Fig. 59.3.

CONCLUSIONS

The presence of immediate food allergy can usually be established by careful examination of the history supported by *in vitro*

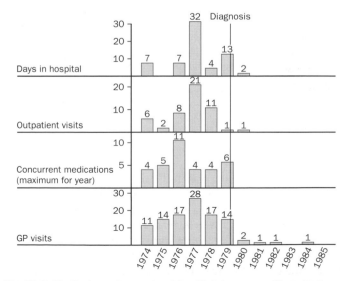

Fig. 59.3 Medical requirements of food intolerance sufferer before and after the diagnosis of food intolerance.

Individual sequential food ingestion challenge and concomitant changes in pulse rate								
Pulse rate								
	Time after ingestion (min)							
	Before ingestion	**20**	**40**	**60**	**80**	**100**	**120**	**Symptoms in the next 4 h**
Turkey	92	92	92	92	92			None
Potato	92	92	92	92	92			None
Cow's milk	90	90	98	**104**	**120**			Sneezing, chest tight, runny nose, pain in temples
Plaice	92	92	92	92	90			None
Soya	88	88	88	88	88			None
Pork	88	96	**100**	96	88			None
Tomato	80	80	**88**	88	88			Slight headache
Rice	92	92	92	94	94			None
Butter	84	84	**104**	**96**	**96**			Headache, agitated
Onion	82	82	**82**	82	82			None
Wheat 1	94	94	96	94	94	90	82	None
Wheat 2	82	84	**96**	84	80	80	80	None
Wheat 3	80	80	**80**	80	84	–	–	16 h very depressed, 22 h severe migraine
Banana	78	78	78	76	78			None
Egg	88	88	**100**	**116**	**120**			Frontal headache, nausea, renal pain
Mushroom	92	92	88	92	92			None
Corn 1	86	88	96	**100**	88	90	84	Nausea and fatigue, 12 h
Corn 2	–	–	–	–	–	–	–	–
Corn 3	–	–	–	–	–	–	–	–

Bold type indicates a significant rise in pulse rate.

Table 59.6 Individual sequential food ingestion challenge and concomitant changes in pulse rate.

(RAST) or skin prick test. Subsequent dietary elimination may be used to confirm that the food or foods have been comprehensively identified by establishing that full remission has occurred with their avoidance. Where doubt exists and confirmatory testing is indicated, careful supervised challenge can be undertaken.

There is no satisfactory *in vitro* test for food intolerance. Despite the failure of elimination diets to satisfy the necessary criteria for an ideal diagnostic test completely, they remain essential for the diagnosis of dietary intolerance. Properly performed, they provide information about the patient's intolerances that cannot be obtained in any other way.

While DBPCFC testing may be valid in the context of immediate food allergy, its use in this situation is rarely justifiable.

While DBPCFC tests have become an important part of the research approach to food intolerance, their routine use would be cumbersome, likely to lead to underdiagnosis, and cannot be recommended in most cases. However, considering the importance of the psychological factor, a circumspect approach is needed and there may be a place for the use of blinded tests in certain cases. When used, great care is required to ensure that the method of food avoidance and challenge takes into account the empirical phenomena of masking addiction and tolerance.

The ubiquitous distribution in the average diet of many of our staple foods must be borne in mind.

The risks of elimination diets must be remembered. Improperly applied, there are risks of producing handicapping psychological and social effects and exacerbating underlying psychological illness. The concomitant risk of nutritional inadequacy adds an extra dimension to these risks. Such risks are particularly likely to occur when treating psychologically vulnerable individuals. The importance of patient selection when undertaking this type of investigation must be emphasized. In the case of children, the psychological vulnerability of the parent(s) must be remembered.

All these techniques are subject to certain limitations, particularly to human error. This means that, for some of our patients, the diagnosis of food allergy with currently available techniques remains impossible. This human factor must not be overlooked. The technique requires time and patience on the part of the investigator, and dedication and care, together with appropriate objectivity, on the part of the patient. Accurate diagnosis is only possible when the patient's cooperation is enlisted from the outset, and when careful training of the patient in the method of diagnosis is a planned part of the diagnostic regimen.

REFERENCES

1 Alun-Jones VA, Hunter JO. Crohn's disease: maintenance of remission by diet. *Lancet* 1985; ii: 177.

2 Alun Jones V, Shorthouse M, McLaughlan P *et al.* Food intolerance, a major factor in the pathogenesis of the irritable bowel syndrome. *Lancet* 1982; ii: 1117–20.

3 Anthony HM, Maberly DJ. Time of onset of symptoms after food challenge. *J Nutr Med* 1991; 2: 121–30.

4 Ashford NA, Miller CS. *Chemical Exposures: low levels and high stakes.* Van Nostrand Reinhold, New York, 1998.

4a Baker JC, Tunnicliffe WS, Duncanson RC, Ayres JG. Double blind palcebo controlled food challenge in severe asthma. *Resp Crit Care Med* 1997; 155: A 894.

5 Bock SA. In vivo diagnosis: skin testing and oral challenge procedures. In: *Food Allergy: Adverse reactions to foods and food additives*, 2nd ed, (Metcalfe DD, Sampson HA, Simon RA, eds) Blackwell Science, Cambridge, Mass, 1997: 151–66.

6 Bock SA, Atkins FM. Patterns of food hypersensitivity during 16 years of double-blind placebo-controlled food challenges. *J Pediatr* 1990; 117: 561–7.

7 Bock SA, Sampson HA, Atkins FM *et al.* Double-blind, placebo-controlled food challenge (DBPCFC) as an office procedure: a manual. *J Allergy Clin Immunol* 1988; 82: 986–97.

8 Coca AF. *Familial Non-reaginic Food Allergy*, Charles C Thomas, Springfield, Illinois, 1942.

9 Denman AM, Mitchell EB, Ansell BM. Dietary exclusion in patients with rheumatoid arthritis. In: *The Second Fisons Food Allergy Workshop*, Medicine Publishing Foundation, Oxford, 1983: 84–5.

10 Derbes VJ, Krafchuk JD. *Arch Dermatol* 1957; 76: 103–4.

11 Doty R. Olfactory sensitivity, nasal resistance and autonomic function in patients with multiple chemical sensitivities. *Arch Otolaryngol Head Neck Surg* 1988; 114: 1422–7.

12 Egger J, Carter CH, Soothill JF *et al.* Effect of diet treatment on enuresis in children with migraine or hyperactive behaviour. *Clin Pediatr* 1992; 31: 302–7.

13 Eriksson NE. Food sensitivity reported by patients with asthma and hay fever. *Allergy* 1978; 33: 189.

14 Fries JH, Glazer I. Studies on the antigenicity of banana, raw and dehydrated. *J Allergy* 1950; 21: 169–75.

15 Goldman AS, Anderson DW Jr, Sellers WA *et al.* Milk allergy I. Oral challenge with milk and isolated milk proteins in allergic children. *Pediatrics* 1963; 32: 425–43.

16 Hill DJ, Hosking CS. Some limitations of double-blind placebo controlled food challenges in young children. *J Allergy Clin Immunol* 1991; 87: 136–7.

17 McLelland J, Schuster S. Contact dermatitis with negative patch tests: the additive effect of allergens in combination. *Br J Dermatol* 1990; 122: 623–30.

18 Miller JB. Hidden food ingredients, chemical food additives and incomplete food labels. *Ann Allergy* 1978; 41: 93–8.

19 Moffett AM, Swash M, Scott DF. Effect of chocolate in migraine: a double blind study. *J Neurol Neurosurg Psychiat* 1974; 37: 445–8.

20 Moore-Robinson M, Warin RP. Effect of salicylates in urticaria. *BMJ* 1967; 4: 262–4.

21 Onorato J, Merland N, Terral C *et al.* Placebo-controlled double-blind food challenge in asthma. *J Allergy Clin Immunol* 1986; 78: 1139–46.

22 Pearson DJ, Rix KJB. Psychological effects of food allergy. In: *Food Allergy and Intolerance*, (Brostoff J, Challacombe SJ, eds), Baillière Tindall, London; 1987: 688–708.

23 Prausnitz C, Kustner H. Studien uber die Ueberempfindlichkeit. *Centralblatt Bakteriol Parasitol* 1921; 86: 160–9.

24 Radcliffe MJ. Diagnostic use of dietary regimes. In: *Food Allergy and Intolerance* (Brostoff J, Challacombe SJ, eds), Baillière Tindall, London, 1987; 806–35.

25 Randolph TG. *Human ecology and susceptibility to the chemical environment.* Charles C Thomas, Springfield, Illinois, 1962.

26 Randolph TG. The role of specific sugars. In: *Clinical Ecology* (Dickey LD, ed.), Charles C Thomas, Springfield, 1976; 310–20.

27 Randolph TG. The role of specific alcoholic beverages. In: *Clinical Ecology* (Dickey LD, ed.), Charles C Thomas, Springfield, 1976; 321–33.

28 Rinkel HJ. Food allergy. I. The role of food allergy in internal medicine. II. The technique and clinical application of individual food tests. *Ann Allergy* 1944; 2: 504.

28a Strong FC. Why do some dietary migraine patients claim they get headaches from placebos? *Clin Exp Allergy* 2000; 30: 739–43.

29 Warner JO, Hathaway MJ. Dietary treatment of eczema due to food intolerance. In: *The Second Fisons Food Allergy Workshop*, Medicine Publishing Foundation, Oxford; 1983: 105–8.

30 Warner JO, Hathaway MJ. Allergic form of Meadow's syndrome (Munchausen by proxy). *Arch Dis Child* 1984; 59: 151–6.

31 Wilson CMW. Food sensitivities, taste changes, aphthous ulcers and atopic symptoms in allergic disease. *Ann Allergy* 1980; 44: 302–7.

32 Workman E, Hunter JO, Alun Jones V. *The Allergy Diet – how to overcome your food intolerance*, Martin Dunitz, London, 1984.

33 Wraith DG. Asthma. In: *Food Allergy and Intolerance* (Brostoff J, Challacombe SJ, eds), Baillière Tindall, London, 1987; 486–97.

34 Yocum MW, Khan DA. Assessment of patients who have experienced anaphylaxis: a 3-year survey. *Mayo Clin Proc* 1994; 69: 16–23.

INTRODUCTION

In this text, I will be using the term *food allergy* to mean the result of an abnormal immunological response after the ingestion of a food.[4] Immunological responses in food allergy can fall into any one of the four types of Gell and Coombs classification (Table 60.1).

There are suggested modifications to this classification which tend to vary in their terminology. The important point is to recognize that foods may express the immunological problem in a variety of ways. A single or multiple end-organ response may occur with food ingestion. This expression of food allergy must be in the physician's differential diagnosis when the patient is seen, especially for those diseases not normally associated with allergies. A few of these diseases, which may also be less-recognized expressions of food allergy, include irritable bowel syndrome,[1] Crohn's disease,[2] atopic eczema,[8] migraine headaches[29] nephrosis[43] and rheumatoid arthritis.[15]

The food allergy should be suspected and questioned to a greater degree than is frequently done, emphasizing that the history is very important in the potentially allergic patient. Sufficient time must be spent with the patient to get a complete history. A physician may see a patient who is somewhat emotionally disturbed and the physician is apt to dismiss many of the symptoms presented as not being associated with allergy. However, allergy may be expressed with the end-organ being

some part or multiple parts of the brain and/or other areas of the nervous system. Once the physician has a suspicion of food allergy, then some further procedure must be done to prove or disprove the existence of food allergy.

SCRATCH TESTS

The oldest form of skin testing dates back to the application of pollen to abraded skin by Charles Blackley in 1873.[9] Scratch tests are superficial epidermal abrasions approximately 2 mm long, to which an antigen is applied. This test was thought to be simple and quick, but has not been shown to be sufficiently sensitive or specific because of the variation in performing the tests. The disadvantages of scratch testing are the significant incidents of false positive reactions, the fact that the test is somewhat more painful than prick–puncture tests and it is not as reproducible as the prick-puncture and intradermal tests.[3,18] Consequently, because of the reproducibility issue, the Allergy Panel of the AMA Council of Scientific Affairs recommended that scratch testing not be performed.[3]

PRICK–PUNCTURE TESTS

Prick tests were first described by Lewis & Grant in 1926.[22] In the 1970s, Pepys[34] promulgated and popularized the prick test. He advised using a 25-gauge hypodermic syringe needle, which was pricked through the antigen, into the skin at a 45° angle to an approximately 1 mm depth, while tenting the skin to allow more antigen to enter. This procedure is subject to significant variability due to the difficulty of precisely reproducing the depth, penetration and the amount of skin lifting. In all of the prick tests, the antigen used is the concentrate, and each test uses a single antigen. The problem with any prick test is the inability to know with certainty what volume of the antigen enters the skin. Pepys has stated that using his modified prick test procedure permits 0.003 ml of the antigen to be absorbed (FJ Waickman pers comm, 1986).

Classifications of hypersensitivity reactions
Type I: mast cell mediated
Type II: antibody mediated
Type III: immune complex
Type IV: cell mediated

Table 60.1 Classifications of hypersensitivity reactions.

Modifications of prick testing

These came into being when Morrow Brown[12] introduced the vertical prick–puncture method using a single-point device measuring 1.25 ml in length. A guard prevented penetration of the needle beyond a predetermined depth. No skin lifting was used and, in using this instrument, there supposedly was less antigen delivered into the skin compared with the Pepys modified prick test. It did produce more reproducible skin testing and was very quick and easy to use. Recently, the Morrow Brown multi-well tray was introduced. This permits the concentrated antigen to be put into the wells, and the needles placed into the well and then transferred directly to the skin test. As a result, time is not needed to put the antigen directly onto the skin and then puncture through the antigen. This also conserves antigen. The advantage of the Morrow Brown needle is the consistency of the penetration of the skin, and consistency from one patient to another. However, this has a disadvantage in so far as some people have thicker corneum, some have thinner and others have very dry skin, which can affect the degree of accuracy of the test. Demoly et al.[16] demonstrated the variability of skin-prick tests using different methods – namely, the 25-gauge needle, the Pharmacia lancet, Stallerpointe, Pricker, Wyeth bifurcated needle, Allerprick, Morrow Brown precision needle and Stallerkit – all done by the same person. A recent device employing a different methodology is the Duotip-test. This device is removed from a previously filled dipwell tray, then pressed against the skin to make an indentation and twisted 360° (prick and scarification).

The Multi-Test has been available for 15 years and, recently, the Multi-Test II with dipwell tray became available. This consists of a plastic device containing eight heads, four on each side. Each head has nine prongs that are similar to the old-time device which was used for giving smallpox vaccinations. This device is very quickly and easily applied and it is possible to do 24 prick–puncture tests within a matter of 30 seconds. This becomes a cost effective way of answering allergy problems. There is a special review of this particular device published by Kniker in 1993.[20] In addition to the ease of administration of the antigens with the Multi-Test II, there is an economic advantage. If performed correctly, 500 tests can be done from a single 5 ml of concentrated extract. Another device used to deliver a quick application of tests is the Quick-Test (Quanti-Test System by Panatrex, Placentia, California). This device has elastic arms and is designed for adaption to uneven skin test sites; it is similar to the Multi-Test II, but has six prongs, whereas the Multi-Test II has nine prongs.

Numerous articles have been written attempting to compare one device with another. Demoly et al.[16] and Nelson et al.[31] demonstrated that there is considerable variability among the various devices. Variability may also occur due to the technique of the physician or technician doing the test. Those devices that do not scarify are more comfortable for the patient and reproducibility seems to be more consistent.

Precautions before skin testing

Before any skin testing is performed, there are certain precautions that should be followed for the patient's safety and for accuracy in testing. This is a modification of precautions as outlined in Allergy, Principles and Practice.[25]

1. No testing should be done without a physician being immediately available to treat a patient should a systemic reaction occur.

2. Emergency equipment with all necessary medicines, intubation equipment, etc., should be readily available and 1:1000 epinephrine should be immediately available in a syringe, such as an EpiPen.

3. The allergenic extracts used should be standardized and/or potent antigens and free of extraneous antigenic factors.

4. Test concentrations to be used must be appropriate for the degree of sensitivity of the patient as determined from the history.

5. A positive (histamine) and negative control solution should be included.

6. Before any skin tests are done, the skin must be surveyed to identify any defects, such as scars, so that the test is performed on reasonably normal skin.

7. Before the test, it should be determined whether a patient has dermographism, so that the test is done very precisely.

8. It must be determined ahead of time whether the patient is on any drugs, either prescription or over-the-counter (OTC) medicines that would interfere with accuracy of the skin tests, namely H_1- or H_2-blocking agents as well as certain tricyclic antidepressants.[18] Note: The author would disagree with the report in the previous reference for the item doxepin (Sinequan). One molecule of doxepin will block 3100 H_1 sites.[39] This is the most potent antihistaminic drug that I have encountered. It has been my experience that the minimum time that doxepin must be omitted is 40 days (unpublished case studies). This is based on a small group of patients who were on doxepin because of psychiatric problems. The histamine control may be positive before the 40 days, but it will not reach its full potential of size unless the drug is omitted for 40 days. This is required to prevent false negative tests.

9. An accurate record of the reactions and the timing must be kept, and each reaction must be accurately measured.

10. A health evaluation of the patient and an evaluation of their symptoms must be completed before any tests are done and close observation carried out during the test period for any symptoms that may arise that were not present prior to the testing being initiated. If anaphylactic symptoms occur, these should be treated immediately.

11. Regardless of the type of testing done, each prick–puncture device or needle should be used only once and then discarded, to prevent mixing of antigens as well as to prevent the introduction of infectious organisms.

Editors' note: While this is obviously the ideal technique to adopt, a survey of practitioners in both the UK and USA has suggested that a single lancet and wipe method appears to be used extensively in clinical practice. Brydon,[13] a specialist allergy nurse practitioner, reports a long personal experience of skin testing using this method without evidence of carry-over and has conducted experiments with histamine skin testing concluding that carry-over could not be induced in this way.[13]

Irrespective of which technique the clinical practitioner adopts, it is essential for clinical trial work that the lancet is used for each antigen. This method also avoids the potential for blood-borne pathogen exposure.

Common errors in prick–puncture testing

1. When doing prick or prick–puncture testing, with multiple antigens needing to be tested, there is a tendency to put the tests too close together, particularly in small children. Each of these tests should be 2 cm or more apart.[16,32] This is prevented when one uses a device such as the Multi-Test II, which has the heads

separated by $2\frac{1}{2}$ cm lengthwise and $1\frac{1}{2}$ cm sideways. The Quintest is another multi-type test (Bayer Corporation). It has one series of five heads that are separated by 3 cm. These devices prevent the physician or technician from getting the antigens too close together and prevents the overlap of reactions, which makes the reading of the response difficult.

2. Insufficient or excess penetration of the skin may occur when one is using an intradermal needle for the modified Pepys testing, whereas devices such as the Morrow Brown needle, Multi-Test II, Quick Test and Quintest have a specific depth, making the response more consistent and easier to evaluate from one antigen to another at that particular test setting.

3. It is important that no matter which device is used, the skin must be sufficiently penetrated for an adequate amount of antigen to be delivered, but at the same time, it should not be penetrated excessively deep, inducing bleeding which may lead to a false positive result.

Although prick–puncture tests appear to be safe, systemic reactions have been observed and reported.[33,45]

PRICK–PRICK TESTS

Prick–prick skin testing is done using fresh foods. One first pricks through the fresh food and then pricks the skin of the patient. Rance et al.[37] reported their results using skin-prick tests involving commercial extracts, fresh foods, food challenges and specific IgE. The skin-prick tests were positive 40% of the time with commercial extracts and 81% of the time using fresh foods. The overall concordance between a positive prick test and a positive challenge test was 58.8% with commercial extracts and 91.7% when fresh foods were used. When a history is positive, and a commercial food antigen prick test is negative, then a prick–prick test using fresh food should be considered. This is particularly true when one is considering doing a skin test for fruits, vegetables, or a food antigen where the commercial antigen is not available.

PATCH TESTS

Patch testing, as described by the American Academy of Dermatology, is indispensable in proving the cause of allergic contact dermatitis. It has been shown that patch testing may be helpful where a history of food allergy exists, but the prick test is negative. In this case, a patch test for a specific food might be of help in order to make a specific diagnosis. Majamaa et al.[23] tested 143 infants under 2 years of age by elimination and challenge because of suspected cow's milk allergy. The oral challenge tests had been performed in 1996. Of the 143 children who were challenged, 72 (50%) had a positive oral challenge. Of the 72 children, 26% showed elevated specific immunoglobulin E (IgE) to cow's milk by radioallergosorbent (RAST) testing, 14% had a positive skin-prick test and 44% had a positive patch test to cow's milk. It is interesting to note, that most of the positive patch test patients had a negative prick test for cow's milk. In another study, Majamaa et al.[24] studied a group of 39 infants under 2 years of age suffering from atopic eczema or gastrointestinal symptoms. Each child was tested for wheat by either a double-blind, placebo-controlled or open challenge. In addition, wheat-specific IgE RAST tests, skin-prick tests and patch tests for wheat were performed. Of the 39 wheat challenges, 22 (56%) were positive, 20% showed elevated IgE to wheat, 23% had a positive skin-prick

test and 86% had a positive patch test to wheat. In circumstances like this, the patch test would indicate some immunological response, but the physician must be certain that the immunological expression is meaningful from an active allergy standpoint today as opposed to this being an indication that a potential future allergy expression may result. This must be remembered for all types of testing.

Regardless of the type of prick or prick–puncture device used, the grading of the skin test is of importance. The tests should be read at the peak of their reaction. Histamine will give a peak at approximately 8–10 min, whereas antigens will peak between 10 and 20 min. Many physicians will use the wheal measurement as the determining factor, and this should be measured in millimetres. Many people also measure the erythema, but erythema is relative, as there may be a positive wheal and no erythema in some people, particularly dark skinned or deeply tanned individuals, as the erythema may not be visible, or there may be a skin test that shows erythema only and no whealing, as in a very fair-skinned person. It has been my observation that measuring the wheal size is the most consistent item in showing a positive and accurate response.[6,36]

The incidence of food allergy, as depicted in the literature, varies a great deal. Golbert[17] stated: 'Food allergy is uncommon. Its incidence among children is estimated at 0.3 percent.' The reference that he gives, however, refers to a study by Collins-Williams[14] in which he reviewed 3000 patients, omitting all patients who were seen because of allergy, suspected or proven. Of the remainder, he studied these to see how many milk allergies were missed. The number was 9 or 0.3% of the 3000 patients. A prospective study of 480 newborns, followed through their third birthday, showed 28% had food allergy.[10] In a recent survey from the United Kingdom, food intolerance was reported in approximately 20% of 7500 households, although blind food challenge undertaken in the same population was only able to confirm a prevalence of 1.4–1.8%.[46] Many of the references discuss milk allergy only, or multiple food allergies in the atopic individual or in a person with asthma. As a consequence, one must look on these numbers as being relative, since food allergy is certainly going to be more prevalent in children, in the patient with atopic dermatitis and with other diseases where allergy may be the causative factor. Therefore, when attempting to compare the incidence of food allergy, one must know what the cohort of patients are, be certain to evaluate the numbers with similar diseases and make sure the comparison is either with a single food test or a multitude of foods tested.

The largest series reporting systemic reactions to allergy skin tests is by Valyasevi et al.[45] They report an incidence of six patients having systemic reactions following skin testing in 497 656 skin tests performed on 18 311 patients. Skin puncture tests were performed on 16 505 patients, while skin puncture and intradermal skins tests were performed on 1806 patients. There was an overall rate of 33 systemic reactions per 100 000 skin tests. The largest number of reactions was with latex skin testing. The conclusions from this study would indicate that the systemic reaction rate to skin tests was very low, the systemic reactions were mild and all the patients fully recovered within 1 hour.

INTRADERMAL TESTS

Testing for food may also be done intradermally. If the initial prick test or prick–prick test is negative and the history is positive for a particular food, a single intradermal test may be performed. This is preferably done by using a dilution of 1:1000 or 1:5000 and making a very superficial intradermal 4 mm wheal which, relatively, will deliver 0.01 ml. This should be read in the same manner as the previous outline for prick testing. Murphree & Kniker[30] reported that a Multi-Test would be equivalent to an intradermal skin test of an aqueous dilution of 1:1000. Therefore, if the previous prick types of testing are negative, a 1:1000 dilution intradermally should be safe. If this is negative and the history is still considered positive, and one wishes to have some concrete evidence, then a 1:500 dilution of the aqueous food antigen may be used. Most of the time, such intradermal testing is not needed if the patient is properly tested by one of the prick–puncture techniques. Nevertheless, skin testing for food allergy may be unrewarding, as the food testing response may not be of an immunological nature, thereby giving a negative test.

There are errors occurring when intradermal tests are done, some of which are more common than others. The main problems occur as follows:

1. The skin tests are too close together and, as a result, false positives may occur. These tests should be 2 cm from each other.
2. Occasionally, a lymphatic vessel is injected and a 'splash' reaction seems to occur. This test is false, and the test should be redone at a different site.
3. When doing intradermal testing, one must know ahead of time, whether you are interested in obtaining a 4 mm wheal, which means an injection of 0.01 ml, or a 7 mm wheal, which is an injection of 0.05 ml. A greater amount of antigen injected than this amount will give a false-positive test.
4. If the skin test is too deep, and especially if it is subcutaneous, it will give a false-negative test. If intracutaneous bleeding is encountered during a test, the test should be crossed off and a more superficial, accurate skin test performed.
5. If an excessive number of tests are done using a strong concentration, then a systemic reaction may occur. If this occurs, then recognize which skin test is the most positive, and this is most likely the antigen causing the systemic reaction. This is not necessarily so, but it does occur in the majority of cases. This is a modification of the common errors in intradermal testing as set forth in *Allergies Principles and Practice*.[27]

PROVOCATION–NEUTRALIZATION TESTS

In 1959, an accidental occurrence on the part of Dr Carlton Lee when treating a patient began the sequence of events to introduce the test that was initially termed provocation/neutralization for food allergy. The history of this occurrence and the development of the test is presented in the 1999 American Academy of Environmental Medicine (AAEM) Instructional Course Part II Syllabus.[5]

Lee first documented his initial observations in 1961.[21] Rinkel, in Kansas City, Missouri, began to perfect the test and the initial formal presentation of this test was given in Vichy, France, 29 June 1963 at the First International Congress on Food and Digestive Allergy.[42] Miller further defined the procedure, as outlined in his book *Food Allergy, Provocative Testing and Injection Therapy*.[28] The dilutions used in this test comprise a series of 1:5

dilutions from the concentrate. These are referred to as dilution #1 (No. 1), dilution #2 (No. 2), etc. As with any other test in the medical arena, there have been refinements and corrections made over a period of time. Many articles for and against this procedure have occurred, many of which are used to denounce the test – most of these are items of information based on articles early in the evaluation of the test. This is not the place for a rebuttal, for or against these articles. A summary of some of these early articles was reported in 1983 by Podell.[35]

A review of the literature is confusing, because people doing the testing and reporting used different terms and different procedures; consequently, the results are not comparable. Today's definition for the provocative–neutralization test is a dose (0.05 ml) of a specific antigen given intradermally and superficially. If the result of that skin test does (1) not increase in diameter, (2) there is no blanching, (3) no hardness, (4) it is not raised, (5) it is not discoid and (6) does not produce any signs or symptoms, the test is negative. The first five items are the criteria that one uses to evaluate the skin wheal. In assessing signs and symptoms, it is very important to observe the patient and to ask non-leading questions. The study by King *et al.*[19] outlines how the intradermal provocation–neutralization test should be performed. They emphasize that 0.05 ml of the No. 1 (#1) dilution should be injected first. This should produce a 7 mm wheal initially immediately following injection. If this test is positive, it should grow in mean diameter during a 10-min observation period with a wheal that is blanched, hard, raised and discoid. If it is negative, it should not grow at all. Once a positive wheal is recognized, and/or symptoms occur, it is customary to inject 0.05 ml of the #2 dilution, proceeding if need be with injection of progressively weaker dilutions until the neutralizing dose is found. Typically, this dose (a) is the strongest dose to produce no whealing response and (b) relieves any symptoms, which may have been provoked by the preceeding stronger test dilutions.

Obviously, concerns have been raised in the past for doing such a test on people who give a history of severe reactions to a particular food. In this case, giving 0.01 ml of dilution #4 is generally regarded as safe. This should give initially a 4 mm wheal, and if this test does not increase in size, or does not increase to more than a 7 mm wheal in 10 min, then it is suggested that 0.05 ml of the #2 dilution can be given safely. However, if 0.01 ml of the #4 dilution is given, and this increases to a 9 mm wheal and symptoms occur, then progressively weaker dilutions and given until the first strongest negative wheal is reached and neutralization of signs and symptoms occurs.

Through the 30+ years that this test has been used, terms to describe the test have been confusing. The terms 'endpoint' and 'titration' should be restricted to their use in the serial dilution end point titration that is used for inhalant skin testing, as principally described by Rinkel,[40,41] or to the serial end point titration (SET), which is used by the American Academy of Otolaryngic Allergy. Using terms that imply two different tests has led to confusion and hopefully, this is controlled in the future. That is why in using the provocation–neutralization test, one should use the terms 'progressive, weaker dilutions' to reach a neutralizing dose or if one is going stronger, a progression of stronger doses to reach a provocative dose.

A study comparing double-blind food challenges and provocation–neutralization was reported by King *et al.*[19] Each patient was tested for five foods by oral challenge food test (OCFT) and intracutaneous provocation–neutralization food test (IPFT).

Sandberg *et al.*[44] explain their studies in relation to nephrosis and food allergy. They cited the response that they had with patients being treated with the neutralizing dose and correcting the nephrotic syndrome, as manifested in their cohort of patients.

A further discussion explaining provocation–neutralization is in the text *Environmental Medicine in Clinical Practice*.[7] These authors have used this test successfully. They also point out, as does Miller, that this test may be used for other antigens, not just foods.

One of the objections to the provocation–neutralization test has been an inadequate immunological explanation for this test. The exact mechanisms involved are not understood, although tentative hypotheses have been put forward. It is clearly an active phenomenon, since it is inhibited by indomethacin.[11] For those who are interested, a more detailed explanation has been outlined by Rea.[38]

DISCUSSION

Food allergy has been recognized from the days of Hippocrates. It is a problem that can arise in any physician's practice. As discussed above, the incidence of food allergy can vary from one author to another, and how one interprets the diagnosis, depending upon what test was used. It is imperative when discussing this subject, that each physician defines the parameters from which he or she speaks, and what food(s) tests and how they are interpreted.

Since food allergy is seen statistically more often in children than in adults, it should be a well recognized item in paediatric practice. As presented, under specified conditions, skin-prick tests, prick–prick tests and/or provocation–neutralization testing for foods can be appropriate as well as blinded or open food challenges. It is imperative that physician's opinions be changed to accept the fact that different end-organ responses may occur, and more than one end-organ response may occur with food challenges. These responses must not be looked on as emotional factors unless equal psychological or psychiatric types of testing are done to prove that the patient has emotional problems.

This is one advantage of the provocation–neutralization test. There is the aspect of observing the wheal response, as well as the signs and symptoms produced and neutralized. This should be done as a single-blinded test always, and the patient informed at the end of the testing session, what items are positive or negative. This has been a good approach to elucidating emotional factors, as a placebo skin test can be done any time to prove or disprove associated emotional factors.

SUMMARY

Skin testing has been described in a variety of ways. The use of the answers from these tests can be treatment for the positive foods.

Acknowledgement

Appreciation to my son Michael J. Waickman, MD, for his review and constructive criticism of this manuscript. Thanks also to Mary Beth Frohnapfel, RN, who is responsible for the typing of the manuscript.

REFERENCES

1 Alun Jones V, Shorthouse M, McLaughlan P, Workman E, Hunter JO. Food intolerance: a major factor in the pathogenesis of irritable bowel syndrome. *Lancet* 1982; Nov 20: 1115–17.

2 Alun Jones V, Workman E, Freeman AH, Dickinson RJ, Wilson AJ, Hunter JO. Crohn's disease: maintenance of remission by diet. *Lancet* 1985; Jul 27: 177–80.

3 AMA Council on Scientific Affairs, Panel on Allergy. *In vivo* diagnostic testing and immunotherapy for allergy. *JAMA* 1987; 258: 1363–7.

4 American Academy of Allergy and Immunology/NIAID. *Adverse Reactions to Foods* (Anderson JA, Sohn DD, eds). NIH Publication 1984; 84-2442: 1–6.

5 American Academy of Environmental Medicine. *Instructional Course Part II Syllabus*. 7701 East Kellogg, Suite 625, Wichita KS 67207-1705, USA, 1999.

6 Anon JB. Introduction to *in vivo* allergy testing. *Otolaryngol Head Neck Surg* 1993; 109: 593–600.

7 Anthony H, Birtwistle S, Eaton K, Maberly J. *Environmental Medicine in Clinical Practice*. BSAENM Publications, Totton, Southampton, 1997.

8 Atherton DJ, Soothhill JF, Sewell M, Wells RS. A double-blind controlled crossover trial of an antigen-avoidance diet in atopic eczema. *Lancet* 1978; Feb 25: 401–3.

9 Blackley CH. *Experimental Researches on the Causes and Nature of Catarrhus Aestivus*. Balliere, Tindall & Cox, London, 1873.

10 Bock SA. Prospective appraisal of complaints of adverse reactions to foods in children during the first 3 years of life. *Pediatrics* 1987; 79: 683–8.

11 Boris M, Schiff M, Weindorf S. Injection of low-dose antigen attenuates the response to subsequent broncho-provocative challenge. *Otolaryngol Head Neck Surg* 1988; 98: 539–45.

12 Brown HM, Su S, Thantrey N. Prick testing for allergens standardized by using a precision needle. *Clinical Allergy* 1981; 11: 95–8.

13 Brydon MJ. *Skin Prick Testing in Clinical Practice*. NADAAS, Norwich, 2000: 21.

14 Collins-Williams C. The incidence of mild allergy in pediatric practice. *J Pediat* 1956; 48: 39.

15 Darlington LG, Ramsey NW, Mansfield JR. Placebo-controlled, blind study of dietary manipulation therapy in rheumatoid arthritis. *Lancet* 1986; Feb 1: 236–8.

16 Demoly P, Bosquet J, Manderscheid JC et al. Precision of skin prick and puncture tests with nine methods. *J All Clin Immunol* 1991; 88: 758–62.

17 Golbert TM (ed.). Food allergy and immunologic diseases of the gastrointestinal tract. In: *Allergic Diseases* (Patterson R ed.). J.B. Lippincott Company, Philadelphia, 1972: p 355.

18 Hansel FK. *Allergy and Immunity in Otolaryngology*. MN American Academy of Ophthalmology and Otolaryngology, Rochester, 1975.

19 King WP, Rubin WA, Fadal RG et al. Provocation-neutralization: a two-part study. Part I. The intracutaneous provocative food test: a multi-center comparison study. *Otolaryngol Head Neck Surg* 1988; 99: 263–71.

20 Kniker, WT. Multi-Test skin testing in allergy: a review of published findings. *Ann Allergy* 1993; 71: 485–90.

21 Lee CH. Food desensitization. *Buchanan County Missouri Medical Bulletin* 1961; 25: 9.

22 Lewis T, Grant RT. Vascular reactions of the skin to injury. *Heart* 1926; 13: 219–25.

23 Majamaa H, Moisio P, Holm K, Kautiainen H, Turjanmaa K. Cow's milk allergy: diagnostic accuracy of skin prick and patch tests and specific IgE. *Allergy* 1999; 54(4): 346–51.

24 Majamaa H, Moisio P, Holm K, Turjanmaa K. Wheat allergy: diagnostic accuracy of skin prick and patch tests and specific IgE. *Allergy* 1999; 54(8): 851–6.

25 Middleton E, Reed CE, Ellis EF, Adkinson F, Yunginger JW, Busse WW. *Allergy Principles and Practice*, Vol. I. Mosby, St. Louis. 1998: 431.

26 Middleton E, Reed CE, Ellis EF, Adkinson F, Yunginger JW, Busse WW. *Allergy Principles and Practice*, Vol. I. Mosby, St. Louis. 1998: 434.

27 Middleton E, Reed CE, Ellis EF, Adkinson F, Yunginger JW, Busse WW. *Allergy Principles and Practice*, Vol. I. Mosby, St. Louis. 1998: 432.

28 Miller J. *Food Allergy, Provocative Testing and Injection Therapy*. Charles C. Thomas; Springfield, Illinois, 1972.

29 Monro J, Carini C, Brostoff J, Zilkha. Food allergy in migraine. *Lancet* 1980; Jul 5: 1–4.

30 Murphree JT, Kniker WT. Correlation of immediate skin test responses to antigens introduced by multi-test and intracutaneous routes. *Ann All* 1979; 43: 279–85.

31 Nelson HS, Lahr J, Buchmeier A, McCormack D. Clinical aspects of allergic disease: evaluation of devices for skin prick testing. *J Allergy Clin Immunol* 1988; 101: 153–6.

32 Nelson HS, Knoetzer J, Bucher B. Effect of distance between sites and region of the body on results of skin prick tests. *J Allergy Clin Immunol* 1996; 97: 596–601.

33 Novembre E, Bernardini G *et al*. Skin-prick-test-induced anaphylaxis. *Allergy* 1995; 50: 511–13.

34 Pepys J. Skin testing [suppl]. *Br J Hosp Med* 1975; 10: 1.

35 Podell RN. Intracutaneous and sublingual provocation & neutralization. *Clin Ecol* 1983; II(1): 13–20.

36 Poulsen LK, Bindslev-Jensen C, Rihoux JP. Quantitative determination of skin reactivity by two semiautomatic devices for skin prick test area

measurements. *Agents Actions* (special conference issue) 1994; 41: C134–5.

37 Rance F, Juchet A, Bremont F, Dutau G. Correlations between skin prick tests using commercial extracts and fresh foods, specific IgE, and food challenges. *Allergy* 1997; 52(10): 1031–5.

38 Rea WJ. *Chemical Sensitivity*, Vol. IV. Lewis Publishers, CRC Press, Boca Raton, Florida, 1997: 2481–503.

39 Richelson E. Tricyclic antidepressants and histamine H_1 receptors. *Mayo Clinic Proc* 1979; 54: 669–74.

40 Rinkel HJ. Inhalant allergy, part I: the whealing response of the skin to serial dilution testing. *Ann Allergy* 1949; 7: 625.

41 Rinkel HJ. The management of clinical allergy. part II. Etiologic factors and skin titration. *Archives Otolaryngol* 1963; 77: 42.

42 Rinkel HJ, Lee CH, Brown DW, Willoughby JW, Williams JM. The diagnosis of food allergy. *Arch Otolaryngol* 1964; 79: 71–9.

43 Sandberg DH, McIntosh RM, Bernstein CW, Carr R, Strauss J. Severe steroid-responsive nephrosis associated with hypersensitivity. *Lancet* 1977; 1: 388.

44 Sandberg DH, McLeod TF, Strauss J. Food hypersensitivity and the nephrotic syndrome of anaphylactoid purpura. *Pediatr Res* 1980 (abstract).

45 Valyasevi MA, Maddox DE, Li JTC. Systemic reactions to allergy skin tests. *Ann Allergy Asthma Immunol* 1999; 83: 132–6.

46 Young E, Stoneham MD, Petruckevitch A *et al*. A population study of food intolerance. *Lancet* 1994; 343: 1127–30.

Chapter 61

Laboratory diagnosis of food intolerance

D. L. J. Freed and F. J. Waickman

BASIC PRINCIPLES

The need for laboratory tests

In our combined 80 physician-years as allergists we have not yet discovered how to make an accurate diagnosis of food allergies or intolerances. The body has only a limited repertoire of disease states, and although some are often caused by food reactions, none is always so. If the patient gets better as a result of our ministrations we may be tempted to think that we must have got the diagnosis right, but this is not necessarily so (see below).

If all food intolerance syndromes were typical and occurred within a few minutes of ingestion every time the food were taken, there would be no need for laboratory tests and little need for allergists. Unfortunately, the onset of some food intolerance syndromes is delayed for several hours or days (perhaps longer) after taking the food. This statement can be made with confidence because of the efforts of numerous physicians (and patients) who over the years have taken the time and trouble to embark upon challenge programmes, sometimes double-blind.[100,177]

It can also be stated confidently that even when true food intolerance exists, food challenges will not necessarily cause symptoms every time. Some food reactions require the simultaneous presence of another stress factor, such as exertion,[148,175] histamine[122,282] or aspirin.[54] One needs to be exceptionally lucky to uncover such synergistic factors, so we do not know how often they are important. It follows that food challenges must give an unknown number of false-negative results. False-negatives also occur when the dose is not large enough or not repeated often enough[101] or when the challenge is delivered direct to the stomach via tube or capsules in an individual whose main route of antigen uptake is buccal.[173,201] After a period of avoidance, a patient may not respond again to a damaging food for several doses,[123,168] or indeed ever again[203] and it must also be remembered that reactivity can fluctuate with season,

with menstrual cycle or with intercurrent infections.[109] It follows, therefore, that it is never completely possible to disprove food intolerance, even in those cases when the patient is convinced that her symptoms (or her children's symptoms) are caused by foods and the doctor is convinced that they are not.[213,277] Failure to respond to 'oligoallergenic diets' or fasting does not disprove food intolerance either, since the illness may take a long time to remit and either starvation supervenes or the patient loses patience. In published series, the proportion of apparently food-sensitive patients who are confirmed by double-blind challenge tends to be rather low,[34,43,109,203,213] which suggests either that patients and clinicians are easily fooled or that the false-negative rate of this procedure is uncomfortably high.

Double-blind challenges (Table 61.1)

It is sometimes forgotten that the opposite proviso also applies: namely, that double-blind challenges cannot formally *prove* the existence of food intolerance.[214] At best they can make the null

Difficulties with double-blind challenges
Theoretical
Positive challenges do not prove intolerance
Negative challenges do not disprove intolerance
Practical
Expense of time, effort, money
Organization
Patient compliance
Choice of truly inert placebo
Danger of hypochondria

Table 61.1 Difficulties with double-blind challenges.

hypothesis implausible, as in the cases reported by Finn and Cohen,[100] who correctly distinguished active challenge from water each time in a series of 10 double-blind challenges. The probability of correctly guessing the answer in any individual double-blind challenge is 50%, i.e. $P = 0.5$. The probability of correctly guessing two in a row is $P = 0.5 \times 0.5 = 0.25$ and so on. To get below the conventional 5% probability level therefore requires five consecutive correct identifications, in a randomized series, as $P = (0.5)^5 = 0.031$, and clinicians who frequently subject their patients to the rigours of such challenge series should be aware that one in every 32 patients who 'pass' that test will have done so by chance. If the clinician recognizes that false-positive and false-negative challenges can occur, and permits one mistake in a series of six challenges,[213] the probability of passing that test by chance is $P = 0.11$ (binomial theorem), i.e. one in every nine patients.[214]

Added to these fundamental weaknesses of the double-blind challenge approach are the practical difficulties of expense, laboriousness, patient compliance, the choice of a placebo that is truly inert (patients are sometimes allergic to the gelatin of the challenge capsules[257]) and the danger that simply initiating a challenge programme will switch on a hypochondriacal response in patients predisposed to neuroticism.[277] In the case of children who must be challenged without understanding or giving consent the question of real suffering cannot be evaded. We personally do not therefore routinely subject our patients to double-blind challenges, taking the view that the risks of unnecessary elimination diets are lower than the risks of prolonged drug treatment. The only absolute indication for double-blind challenges is in order to convince sceptical doctors, though there are relative indications (Table 61.2).

We have given some emphasis to the question of double-blind challenge procedures, as these are the best clinical diagnostic tool for confirming food reactions (though unreliable for disproving them, as noted). Even the most skillfully elicited case history is unreliable[215] and skin tests are only a general guide to systemic sensitivity, and even then only in Type I (immunoglobulin (Ig)E-associated) hypersensitivity. A reliable laboratory test for food intolerance would be immensely valuable.

The validation of laboratory tests

The requirement is simply stated: laboratory tests should be positive in all patients who have a food sensitivity and negative in all people who do not. But if we cannot be certain of making the

Patients in whom *in-vitro* tests are indicated
1. Patients with an increased risk of adverse reactions from skin testing (a) individuals with near fatal reactions from minimal contact with allergens (b) individuals with limited reserves of pulmonary or cardiac function
2. Patients with suspected allergic disease who do not have normal skin (a) individuals with ichthyosis or other congenital or acquired skin disorders which make skin testing impossible (b) individuals with severe and extensive burns (c) individuals post transplantation, especially if graft-versus-host is present (d) severe eczema that does not respond to initial management
3. Patients who cannot cooperate with skin testing (a) mentally challenged adults or children
4. Patients receiving drugs which interfere with or increase the risk of skin testing (a) skin testing may be a better alternative if the drug can be temporarily discontinued or switched (b) drugs which can interfere with skin tests are antihistamines and tricyclic antidepressants (c) drugs which may increase the risk of skin tests are beta-blockers, including eye drops
5. Patients with suspected allergic reactions to low molecular weight molecules (a) occupational exposure to chemicals (b) drugs which may undergo extensive metabolism before becoming bound to a carrier protein (c) molecules which may be very unstable unless bound to a carrier protein
6. Investigations of fatal reactions which may have been caused by allergens
7. Determining which component of an allergen mixture caused a reaction
8. Individuals with HIV infections (a) relative risks of transmitting infection to health care workers (b) will the skin respond normally?
9. Young children (a) relative pain of skin testing *versus* drawing blood sample (b) sensitivity of skin tests *versus* in vitro tests in young children
10. Individuals needing evaluation for unusual allergens where skin test reagents may not be available

Table 61.2 Patients in whom *in-vitro* tests are indicated.

correct clinical diagnosis we have no yardstick against which to measure the reliability of our tests. We can only try to get as close as possible to accuracy.

Definitive clinical diagnosis can be approached most closely and relatively easily in Type I allergies in which response to challenge is usually swift and convincing and occurs every time. As the control group we need, *not* apparently food-sensitive patients with negative challenges (since the challenge results may have been false) but rather a group of healthy or sick volunteers, matched for age, sex, social class, smoking and dietary habits, who have no history or family history of allergies or food reactions, who are also challenged and emerge without reactions. Of course it is very difficult to assemble two comparable groups of this kind, but at least it is theoretically feasible and examples will be alluded to below. The percentage of genuinely intolerant individuals who show a positive test is referred to as the sensitivity; the percentage of non-intolerant people who show the corresponding negative test is termed the specificity, and the ideal test scores 100% in both. More realistically, comparison of true-positive, true-negative, false-positive and false-negative rates allows us to calculate the χ^2, which tells us how closely overall the test approximates to clinical reality (Table 61.3).

Statistically acceptable studies

Statistically acceptable double-blind challenge studies in delayed-onset non-IgE-associated food intolerances are rather rare; a flavour of the daunting difficulties involved can be obtained by a close perusal of the methods sections of the papers by Egger *et al.*[83] on childhood migraine and Alun Jones *et al.*[138] on irritable bowel syndrome. In a disease that may not be provoked unless challenges last for 1 week or more one cannot reasonably expect a series of five challenges to be administered to each patient. The reader who calculates the probabilities as outlined above on these two papers will conclude that food intolerance is virtually proven in a substantial proportion of these patients – but one cannot say *which* patients. As we do not know which patients to allot to which block in our contingency table, it would be impossible to work out the accuracy of laboratory tests by the χ^2 method; as it happens, however, the only test tried in these studies was RAST (radioallergosorbent test), whose 'true-positive' rate was so low that we do not need to look any further. Since it is so immensely

difficult to establish the necessary clinical yardstick in diseases of this type, it is not yet possible to assess the reliability in such cases of most of the tests alluded to in this chapter. It is of course quite illogical to argue that since a particular test is reasonably accurate in Type I allergies its positivity in a non-IgE condition proves the condition to be allergic – or (more dangerously) that its negativity disproves food intolerance[142] (see below).

A more popular approach to the validation of tests is to prescribe a diet based on the test results and see whether the patient feels better. If a good proportion of patients improve, at least in the short term, the test is considered valid, but this is not true. This kind of evidence – the evidence of success – actually tells us little about the accuracy of the test, for at least three good reasons:

1. Those patients who do badly tend either not to return to the doctor to report, or else give a falsely favourable report in order to please him.
2. Placebo-sensitive or attention-seeking patients may improve, at least for a while, after any dietary change (exclusion diets are stressful and expensive and cause radical realignments in family tensions).
3. There is always coincidence; a proportion of patients who improve on elimination dieting would have improved anyway.

It should also be acknowledged that exclusion diets of the kind that forbid additives and convenience foods usually force the patient to eat a more healthful diet, so that a marginal unsuspected nutrient deficiency that might have been causing immunological imbalance[53,103,114] is inadvertently corrected. The evidence of success is therefore not to be trusted when it comes to validating tests.

However, let us not throw out the baby with the bathwater of academic niceties. True, elimination diets have their dangers, especially if needlessly strict. All the same, success is success, and the primary purpose of doctors is not only to make accurate diagnoses but also to improve the health of ill people. Accurate diagnosis is only a means to that end, and not the only means. For some of the tests reviewed here, accuracy calculations are non-existent, but the tests still enable a good number of ill people to get better, and that is arguably the more important datum as long as it is honestly acknowledged. We will term this percentage the 'utility value' of the test.

Experienced allergists know what proportion of their patients will get better by the intelligent application of informed guesswork. For practical purposes, the clinician need only use tests that perform better than this.

Reproducibility and specificity

As well as the accuracy of a test, we need to consider its reproducibility when replicates of the same specimen are tested on the same, and on separate, occasions by the same and by different laboratories and staff, and when different specimens from the same patient are tested. The ideal test has a reproducibility of 100%, but it may come as a distressing surprise to some clinicians to realize that most clinical laboratories consider an error rate of around 10% rather good.

When ordering an *in vitro* study, a clinically competent physician, adequately trained in allergy should be aware of the potential errors in an *in vitro* test. That physician should be able to interpret the test results accurately, understand what the units mean, and know where a potential error may occur. The laboratory used should also be reviewed. Is the laboratory properly licensed? Are

Example of the χ^2 approach to validation of a test, applied to RAST (radioallergosorbent test) diagnosis of allergic rhinitis			
	Test result positive	**Test result negative**	**Totals**
Clinically sensitive	19 (true-positives)	14 (false-negatives)	33
Clinically not sensitive	2 (false-positives)	48 (true-negatives)	50
Totals	21	62	83

χ^2 = 27.4 $P<0.00025$.
This statistic tells us how probable it is that the test results and the clinical diagnoses are non-correlated. The lower the P value, the better the test's accuracy. Only P values below 0.05 (preferably below 0.01) need be of interest. (Data taken from Freed *et al.*[106])

Table 61.3 Example of the χ^2 approach to validation of a test, applied to RAST (radioallergosorbent test) diagnosis of allergic rhinitis.

high quality reagents used? Are potent or standardized antigens used? Are there positive and negative controls used on each run and/or for each antigen? Are the results in true quantitative terms and is the reference curve calibrated against an international standard, preferably the World Health Organization (WHO) standard for IgE? Is the laboratory monitored by a programme, such as that of the College of American Pathologists? If these points are known, then it is reasonable to place confidence in that laboratory.

THE VALUE OF A LABORATORY TEST IN THE DIAGNOSIS OF FOOD ALLERGY

We do not intend to cover the use of laboratory tests in initially deciding that an allergy diagnosis is appropriate, since that is properly done by taking a careful history. To base the initial diagnosis of allergy on a high total IgE level, for example, will yield many false results. The use of initial screening tests for this purpose is also an invitation to the doctor to stop thinking. Hamburger[121] notes that 'no serum IgE level, no matter how low, precludes a diagnosis of atopic allergy', and the same certainly goes for non-atopic allergy.

AlaTOP is a fluid-phase multi-antigen automated *in vitro* test that has a high degree of sensitivity and is comparable to prick skin testing for inhalants. It does not indicate which specific antigen in the test is positive, but it is a screening test to identify any food antigens that may be causing IgE-mediated disease. Although more informative than a total IgE level, it suffers from most of the same deficiencies. The only established value for screening for total IgE is in infancy, since a high cord-blood IgE level predicts the development of later atopy and should make exclusive breast-milk feeding mandatory.[51] The IUIS/WHO working group report on laboratory tests[133] states that a total IgE estimation is never essential except for the diagnosis of the hyperimmunoglobulin-aemia E – recurrent infection syndrome (Buckley's syndrome) – in which the information does not determine treatment.

We shall assume that the doctor has already formed the view that an allergy or intolerance may be the cause of the patient's illness and is now seeking guidance on the identification of the damaging ingestant. This is the rational way to use laboratory tests. Although history, skin tests, challenge studies and laboratory tests are each individually unreliable to some degree, if most or all of them point in the same direction the physician is justified in feeling some confidence in that identification.

General unsolved problems: Which allergen preparation?
Before considering each laboratory test in detail it will be advisable to contemplate the uncertain foundations upon which our edifice is built: that is, the unsolved problems that apply to all tests (Table 61.4).

To cook or not to cook?
Prausnitz and Küstner[219] noted that whereas Küstner was exquisitely sensitive to cooked fish he could consume large doses of raw fish without problem. The reverse of this situation is rather more common.[170,193] In spite of these known facts, extracts of uncooked foods are usually used in tests. The question breeds subquestions. How hot and how long? Dry heat, hot water or steam? With or without salt or spices? This subject is obviously in need of investigation but has not been properly approached because of the awesome size of the task.

General unsolved problems in laboratory food allergy diagnosis
Raw or cooked allergens?
Whole foodstuffs or digests?
Complex mixtures of antigens in each foodstuff
Antigenic crossreactivity
Labelling and chemical handling problems
Lectins
Stability of allergens
Limitations of the antibody titre
Non-immunological food intolerance
Interpretation of 'false-positive' results

Table 61.4 General unsolved problems in laboratory food allergy diagnosis.

Should digests be used?
Peptic/tryptic digestion of proteins leads to the destruction of some antigens[259] and the creation of new ones.[117] The former process is probably more common than the latter,[242] although failure to detect allergenic activity in digests is fraught with dangers of artefacts. Foods change their antigenic clothing continuously in the journey from plate to portal vein but undigested foods are almost universally used in tests. This problem, likewise, has not been properly approached, except for the case of gliadin in coeliac disease, in which digests retain toxicity[75] and lectin activity.[155]

Which part of the foodstuff should be looked at?
All foods are complex mixtures, and any or all of the components might be clinically relevant. The mixture may vary from batch to batch and from season to season. If saline extracts are used, the test ignores all materials in the insoluble residue, which are usually the majority.

Cow's milk, for example, contains over 20 separate antigenic proteins.[20] The principal whey antigens are α-lactalbumin, β-lactoglobulin, casein and bovine serum albumin (BSA); different patients have antibodies to one, several or all of these proteins. The fat globule membrane has its own separate antigens[71] besides adsorbing casein and other proteins from the milk plasma (Shakib, pers comm). To save effort, many investigators use whole pasteurized milk as test reagent, yet this approach is also risky, since the various antigens may mask each other in the test.[116,135] With the modern drive for the exclusive use of 'major allergens' in testing, patients allergic to minor allergens are increasingly in danger of being misdiagnosed and mistreated.[120] With the exception of cow's milk, egg and wheat, most foods used in tests are not yet chemically fractionated, although there are claims that the use of highly purified individual proteins in RAST increases the test's accuracy for codfish[3,69] which is unusual in that it contains just one major allergen[55]. Turner *et al.*[262] wryly observe that 'the choice of allergen for screening purposes is never clear-cut and some compromise is necessary'. In view of the complex mixtures of allergens in most foods, there is some relevance in finding out which are significant in each individual patient. There are several immunoelectrophoretic methods for separating food antigens (cross-electrophoresis and immunoblotting), developing with patient's serum and labelled anti-IgE.[160] The techniques are expensive and have not found a place in routine clinical practice though arguably they should.

Antigenic crossreactivity

Now that highly sensitive methods for antibody detection are used (radioisotope and enzyme techniques), antigenic crossreactions are frequently found. It is no surprise to find that wheat and rye share several antigenic determinants,[39,91] since these grasses are closely related botanically, and with more sensitive methods some crossreactivity is also demonstrated with (in decreasing order) barley, oats[89,259] and even to some extent rice and maize[42]. Similarly, there is considerable crossreactivity between goat's and cow's milk[20,170] and, indeed, between different species of mite.[92] Unexpected crossreactions between totally different botanical families also occur. In Scandinavia, where a short but vicious birch pollen season causes considerable allergy, high degrees of sensitization to birch pollen (assessed by RAST and skin prick tests) are strongly correlated with food intolerance, particularly to apple;[79,87,88] this clinical cross-sensitivity is reflected in the RAST[38] (see below). The profilins – a family of proteins involved in transmembrane cell signalling – are widely distributed in the plant kingdom and cause crossreactions between numerous pollens and plant foods (e.g. olive pollen, soya, peanut, sunflower seed).[241] Similarly, latex allergy predisposes to fruit allergy (e.g. banana, kiwi and avocado).[158] These instances of crossreactivity – and the many others no doubt yet undiscovered – cause an unknown number of false positive test results.

Solid-phase support and labelling problems

Most radioimmunoassays and enzyme methods require that the food extract either be chemically coupled on to a solid surface (paper, plastic, Sepharose, etc.) or labelled. These procedures affect antigenicity to a variable degree and are responsible for an unknown number of false-negatives. Some proteins in the mixture always bind better than others to the solid phase which can interfere with their expression once bound.

Lectins

These are carbohydrate-binding proteins of variable chemical nature, prominent in edible seeds such as grains and beans, and to a lesser extent in other plant, and some animal, tissues. Their binding affinities are in the same range as those of antibodies and often higher. Human immunoglobulin molecules have carbohydrate side chains as well as antigen-binding sites, and when an antibody binds to a foodstuff this could be because of antigen–antibody binding, lectin–carbohydrate binding or both.[251] Extracts of pea, for example, bind all IgE molecules so that any individual with a detectable serum IgE will also have an apparent positive RAST for pea.[1] The same is probably true for other legumes and, to a lesser extent, grains, and this will inevitably reduce the 'signal-to-noise' ratio. Peanut lectin, exceptionally, is a poor allergen in RAST and does not bind IgE nonspecifically.[26] Lectins could be removed from most foodstuffs, albeit laboriously, but the lectin molecules might be attached to relevant allergens. A better scheme would be to neutralize the lectin activity with simple sugar inhibitors (if they were known), leaving the antigenicity of the lectin unaltered. The complexities of this situation are enormous and, in the 18 years since the first edition of this book, have hardly begun to be explored.

Confusingly, there is a suggestion that allergen-bound IgE of food-allergic patients may be more susceptible to lectin competition than the IgE of patients allergic only to pollens.[167] Food lectins are particularly confusing in tests of lymphocyte activation (see below), since many lectins are polyclonal mitogens. The same is true for skin tests.

Stability and reliability of allergen extracts

Most water-based extracts deteriorate on storage, some (e.g. apple) within minutes,[79] unless preservatives are used, and sometimes even then.[10,287] The extent of this deterioration is usually unknown.[199] Although solid-phase allergens are generally very stable, some can apparently desorb from the matrix on storage.[145]

The limitations of a titre

The titre of an antibody is a function both of its concentration and its average binding avidity. Since the latter can vary by up to two orders of magnitude for IgE[273] and by more than that for other immunoglobin classes, the concentration and function of antibodies can vary widely between different sera having the same titre. This has important biological consequences – for example, the sensitivity of histamine release from basophils[189] – which we are only just beginning to explore. The term 'antibody level' is a convenient shorthand whose limitations should be understood.

Non-immunological food toxicity

Foods contain an impressive array of potential poisons, including alkaloids, lectins, anti-enzymes, antivitamins, hormone mimics, toxic amino acids, mycotoxins, saponins, goitrogens and many other categories,[61,221] some of which are resistant to cooking and digestion. May[177] notes that 'the prevalence of toxic reactions … is unknown and while the possibilities are legion, cases proven by blind challenge are uncommon'. This observation – a classic illustration of rigid thinking – is hardly surprising, as food toxins whose effects are rapid are well known in folklore, which is why acorns and deadly nightshade berries – full of nourishment though they are – are not generally eaten. The toxins that exist in foodstuffs are by definition those whose effects are gradual and insidious. If their effects become apparent within a week or two they might be detected by the kind of long-term challenges discussed in relation to migraine,[83] though some toxins take months or years to build up and are undetectable except by epidemiology, e.g. chickpea lathyrism[248] and carcinogens.[255] Some people are inevitably more sensitive to those poisons than others. No immunological tests can detect this kind of intolerance.

The significance of false-positive results

When a test result is positive for a food but the patient can consume the food without obvious harm, we usually conclude that the test result is wrong. But it could also mean

- that a previous allergy has waned while the immune function remains still abnormal,[60]
- that the patient has a subclinical degree of sensitization which could become clinical in the near future[176] or
- that there is a silent pathological mechanism in progress which might manifest itself in years ahead in an apparently non-allergic guise, such as heart attacks[71] or rheumatoid arthritis.[62]

TESTS FOR FOOD INTOLERANCE

Antibodies against foodstuffs

Precipitating antibodies against cow's milk proteins were observed at the turn of 20th century by Moro[192] in the blood of a baby suffering from cow's milk-induced marasmus. Food antibodies have been sought in serum since the 1920s for the diagnosis of food intolerance but it is now abundantly clear that the presence of these antibodies is a normal phenomenon.[60,261]

Antibodies to cow's milk and/or its constituents are occasionally found in cord blood and are usual by the age of 1–3 months, although initial feeding at the breast (or on protein hydrolysates) reduces the titres and delays their appearance.[81,116,153,237] Although food antibodies are normal, titres and prevalence are raised in selective IgA deficiency[27,49,237] (even though most of these patients can tolerate cow's milk), and in coeliac disease, inflammatory bowel disease and acute infectious gastroenteritis as well as in proven symptomatic food intolerance.[261] Most workers agree that *very* high titres are significant or at least suspicious. Overt food intolerance in infancy commonly remits spontaneously, after which the antibody titre may gradually fall; the same is observed after successful treatment of coeliac disease and inflammatory bowel disease.[60,146,236,237] Raised cow's milk antibody titres are associated with challenge-proven food intolerance (not necessarily milk intolerance[182]), chronic recurrent pulmonary diseases, iron deficiency anaemia in children, Wiskott–Aldrich syndrome, systemic lupus erythematosus (SLE) and conditions predisposing to aspiration, such as familial dysautonomia and Down's syndrome.[27,159]

Coeliac disease

This condition is a paradigm for food intolerances that are associated with immunological sensitization but not necessarily caused by it. Of all food intolerances it has the firmest clinical diagnostic criteria, which makes it the ideal condition against which to judge laboratory tests. Coeliac patients have high titres of antibodies (though not usually IgE) against not only gliadin but also most of the various wheat proteins as well as the proteins of rye, barley and oats.[59,149] This could be related to increased permeability of the gut in coeliac disease.[35,204,212,218] The ability to become orally sensitized to wheat proteins is a species characteristic; normal rabbits have as much antibody as coeliac humans, whereas guinea pigs can only be immunized parenterally to produce such antibodies.[63] This supports an alternative explanation, which is that the coeliac intestinal mucosa is more heavily bound by gluten lectins,[156] which then become the target for secondary immunological attack.

This explanation is further supported by the curious 'antireticulin' antibodies (Fig. 61.1) of many coeliac sera which bind to the intercellular matrix of mammalian tissues. Wheat lectin binds directly to connective tissue fibres in mammalian tissues, and when the 'reticulin' antibody test is done using sections of tissue that have been pretreated with wheat protein, the test becomes highly specific, excluding the diagnosis of coeliac disease when negative.[265] When antibodies of different classes are examined, antigliadin antibodies of the IgA class are found to be highly specific, falling on a gluten-free diet and rising after challenge.[239,264] A combination of these two tests with anti-endomysial antibodies offers a very firm diagnosis, and in recent years these serological tests have become increasingly used for preliminary diagnosis (especially of atypical presentations) and prevalence surveys, and have sometimes supplanted the traditional duodenal biopsy.[118,119]

Assay methods

The classical immunological techniques (precipitation, passive haemagglutination, complement fixation, passive cutaneous anaphylaxis (PCA) in guinea pigs) have all been employed with no one technique showing consistent superiority over the others, although Saperstein *et al.*[236] reported that the PCA technique discriminated far better than the others between milk-intolerant

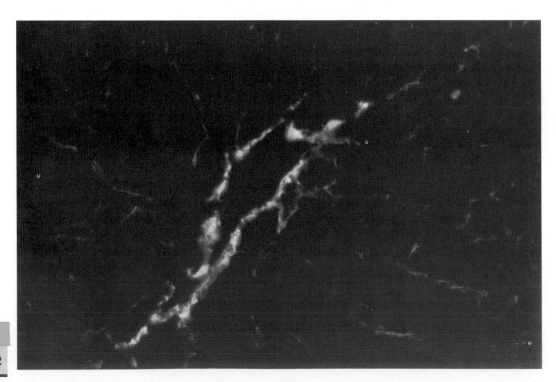

Fig. 61.1 Immunofluorescent demonstration of antireticulin antibodies.

and tolerant children. Since this technique requires the killing of several animals each time, it has never been popular.

Direct binding tests

Direct binding tests of this kind also include radioimmunoassays, enzyme-linked immunosorbent assays (ELISA) in their various forms, the fluorescent immunosorbent test[50] and the indirect fluorescent antibody test.[89] This last technique has the advantage that the whole foodstuff – a thin cross-section of a grain or bean, for example – is used as substrate, so worries about incomplete extraction are eliminated (Fig. 61.2a–d). The section can also be

cooked if desired. This is incubated with the patient's serum and, after washing, bound antibodies are 'developed' with fluorescent-labelled antihuman immunoglobulin serum (Fig. 61.3). With this method one may see which portion of the foodstuff is binding the antibody; for wheat, antibodies to gluten are easily distinguished from antibodies to other components of the grain. It is more sensitive to small changes in antibody titre than other solid-phase techniques.[139] Of course, the test cannot be applied to such foodstuffs as milk and egg.

Radioactive and other direct binding techniques can be used to distinguish antibodies of different immunoglobulin classes but,

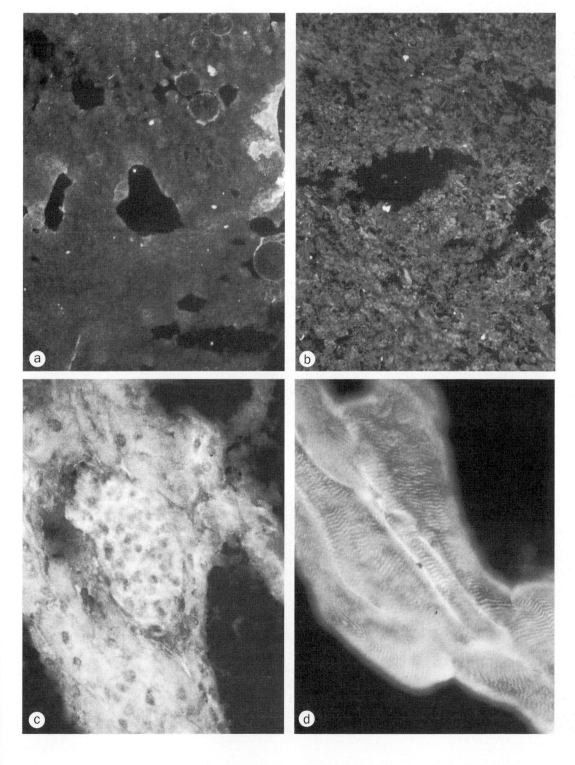

Fig. 61.2 Immunofluorescent demonstration of antibodies against (a) yeast, (b) peanut, (c) lamb's kidney, and (d) chicken.

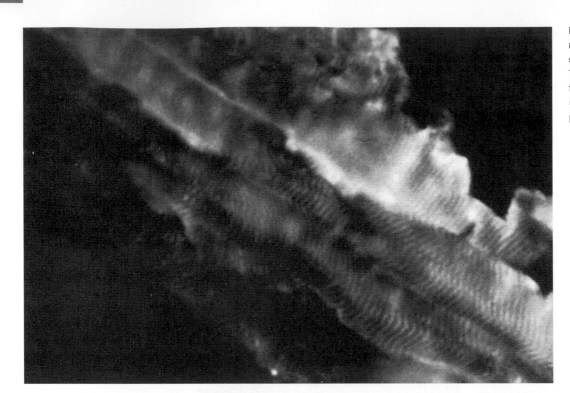

Fig. 61.3 Section of beef muscle showing fluorescent staining of anti-beef antibody. This is not autoantibody, although the appearances are identical (×400 approx). (Reproduced with permission from Freed *et al.*[104])

apart from the case of coeliac disease, there seems to be little diagnostic advantage in separately measuring the non-IgE classes of antibody (except for one isolated report of clinically relevant IgD antibodies).[110] Direct-binding techniques are far more sensitive than the classical methods but, because of this very sensitivity, false-positive rates are high and antigenic crossreactivity is a serious problem (see above).

Antibodies in faeces and other secretions

Coproantibody studies have not been followed with enthusiasm, not only because of the nature of the specimens but also because of the enormous difficulties involved. Unlike blood, whose composition is kept steady by many homeostatic mechanisms, faeces and other secretions vary greatly in concentration and composition, so that it is difficult to assign meaningful units to antibodies found therein.[105,174] In addition, most secretions contain protease enzymes, so protease inhibitors must be incorporated into the assay to prevent the destruction or desorption of the antigen. The choice of antiprotease is difficult as it must be effective and, at the same time, must not itself interfere with either antigen or antibody.[125,274]

IgA and IgG antibodies against cow's milk, wheat and pollen appear in faeces, tears and colostrum and appear to be a normal physiological phenomenon, while corresponding serum antibodies are frequently absent.[24,72,140,152] IgE antibodies are found in jejunal aspirate and faeces (albeit in semi-digested form) but appear to have no diagnostic value.[25,154] The levels of IgE and IgD antibodies to cow's milk and soya protein in duodenal fluid appear to be under the control of pancreozymin and secretin, raising the possibility that these antibodies play a role in normal digestion.[107]

IgE antibodies against foodstuffs – RAST (Fig. 61.4)

The radioallergosorbent test was first described by Wide *et al.*[281] in 1967, and because it had the glamour of immunology and an aura of scientific precision it became in a very short time the accepted standard allergy test. So accepted and standard, in fact, that some doctors came to regard RAST-negative patients as, by definition, not allergic – a fallacy that caused a giant step backwards in allergology, from which it has still not entirely recovered.[6]

In this test, solid-phase-immobilized allergen is incubated with the patient's serum and, after washing, the solid phase (cellulose, paper, etc.) is 'developed' with radiolabelled anti-IgE (Fig. 61.4). The label bound by the solid phase is a function of the antibody titre.[4–6,76,133,187] The isotope label can be replaced by an enzyme or fluorescent label with little difference in results.[205] In 1967, Wide *et al.*[281] in Sweden, developed the first *in vitro* assay for the measurement of specific serum IgE. This was developed 1 year after the discovery of IgE, a new class of immunoglobulin, by Johansson in Sweden[137] and Ishizaka in the United States.[132]

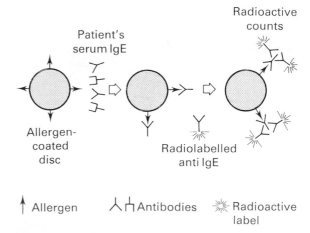

Fig. 61.4 Radioallergosorbent test (RAST). The allergen is made insoluble on a paper disc and the patient's serum containing immunoglobulin E (IgE) is then placed on the disc, allowing the IgE to bind to the allergen. Radiolabelled anti-IgE is added; the radioactive counts obtained reflect the amount of allergen-specific IgE in the serum.

RAST was first developed for commercial use by Pharmacia, Uppsala, Sweden.[85,113] They developed a scoring system that was somewhat illogical, but it was used for a period of time until the Modified RAST Test (MRT) was introduced in 1979 by Nalebuff and Fadal.[196–198] They proceeded to make several procedural and interpretive changes, which increased the sensitivity of the RAST without significantly decreasing the specificity. As time went on, a variety of other IgE-specific *in vitro* tests were developed. Table 61.5 lists the *in vitro* tests that are available for use today.

The various *in vitro* tests use different units in reporting the results. At the present time, it is not possible to make a direct comparison of one type of test to another in relation to accuracy, unless the same units are being measured.

In doing an *in vitro* test, there are certain factors that will influence specific IgE antibody levels. The technical factors include

1. the cutoff point separating positive and negative results
2. intra- and inter-assay variation
3. nature of solid- or liquid-phase support
4. quality of antigen coupled to the solid or liquid phase
5. incubation times
6. material used for the standard curve
7. nonspecific binding of IgE
8. interference by immunoglobulin G (IgG) antibodies
9. quality of labelled anti-human IgE
10. error(s) in reagent preparation, pipetting, and sequential reagent handling.

There are also non-technical factors such as

1. age
2. season
3. immunotherapy.

The major advantages of an *in vitro* test are fairly specific, namely

1. patient convenience
2. no patient risk
3. not influenced by concomitant drug intake
4. stable reagents
5. test of choice in select groups, namely
   (a) infants
   (b) patients with severe dermographism
   (c) patients with widespread dermatitis
6. an evaluation for patients who give a history of anaphylaxis to a specific food.

In the intervening years, the solid phase has gone from a paper disc to a micro titre plate using a fluorescent enzyme reagent. The latter was principally used in the Pharmacia CAP System (CAP). In the late 1980s, the AlaSTAT was introduced by Diagnostic Products Corporation (DPC) (Los Angeles, CA). This assay used a liquid instead of a solid phase, which permitted the assay to be more automated than the *in vitro* tests up to that time.

Automated systems offer repeatability both in terms of precision and accuracy. Consequently, more tests can be performed in a single assay, reducing turn around time and costs. Today, the Pharmacia CAP and the DPC systems are almost fully automated, requiring minimal hands-on time per run. These systems provide a computerized printout and same day reporting to the physician. They also have lower maintenance requirements, again, increasing cost-effectiveness.

Even though an automated procedure removes the chance of human error such as in pipetting, machines are subject to mechanical failure. Tubing may leak, mechanisms can break down and variations in measurements may occur. For accuracy's sake, positive and negative controls for each run should be performed and the laboratory supervisor should review each report as it is printed. Because of cost-cutting concerns, these procedures are not always carried out.

In an attempt to improve accuracy for an *in vitro* test, Ali developed the Third Heir Avidin Biotin Enzyme System Test [THABEST].[7] This is a semi-automated procedure with an absolute positive and negative control for each antigen on each run. Using this information the computer makes a correction for coefficient variables between the tested antigen and the standard curve. The CAP, DPC and THABEST tests are comparable and very useful in determining accurate levels of specific IgE in food allergy. This, in turn, is useful in providing evidence for a correct clinical diagnosis.

Difficulties with RAST and other IgE tests

1. The IgE molecules detected in the blood are in truth only in transit to the mast cells and basophils or the overspill therefrom. That is, they comprise the antibodies that are *not* being used in any real-life allergic reaction. RAST tells us nothing about those. Indeed, the serum IgE antibodies may actually block the action of their tissue-bound counterparts.

2. The solid phase has a nonspecific trapping effect, so that sera having a having a high level of total IgE may give spurious positive

In vitro tests currently in use	
Test name	**Units of measurement**
BioWhittaker FAST PLUS	IU/ml
DPC – Extended AlaSTAT	IU/ml
DPC – Extended Microplate	
DPC – Standard AlaSTAT	
DPC – Standard Microplate	
Hycor HY-TEC EIA	IU/ml
Hycor (Ventrex) Modified RAST	
MAST Immunosystems	LU (LUM)
MAST Immunosystems	mV (CLA)
Pharmacia & Upjohn CAP	% Ref-ASM
Pharmacia & Upjohn CAP	kU$_A$/L
Pharmacia & Upjohn UniCAP 100	% Ref-ASM
Pharmacia & Upjohn UniCAP 100	kU$_A$/L
Quidel Allergen Screen	Positive/negative only
THABEST – IgE	SIE units

Table 61.5 *In vitro* tests currently in use.

RAST results.[136] This can be avoided by diluting sera that have total IgE levels greater than 1000 units/ml. Total IgE levels (and the RAST antibodies that constitute them) are artifactually raised by extraneous influences, such as cigarette smoking,[22,278,288] which is in contrast to the immunosuppressive effect of smoking on other immunoglobulin classes.[11] Malnutrition,[223] acute infections[130] and, particularly, infectious mononucleosis,[21] and recent ingestion of the relevant food[115] can also elevate IgE levels, which may also vary seasonally.[253]

3. RAST results are artifactually low in the presence of IgG or IgD antibodies against the same antigen.[6,45,57,202,217] This may pose a special problem when patients are being desensitized. This can be overcome to some extent by further diluting the specimen[57,202] by using extra allergen[217] or by pretreating the specimen with staphylococcal protein A (although this may present further problems as some IgE is also removed by this procedure).[217]

4. Because of the expense of the labelled second antibody it is often used at suboptimal doses, leading to underestimation at high levels of IgE antibody;[171] the opposite, too high a dose, would run the risk of falsely high results when the true RAST level is low. This can be overcome by repeating the estimation on further diluted sera, or by eluting the bound IgE antibodies from the solid-phase allergen and measuring them immunochemically. However, there is little to be gained from accurately quantifying very high RAST levels.

5. There is a suggestion that IgE molecules are not all equally efficient at binding to basophils and inducing histamine release.[16,189] It is likely that histamine-release assays (see below) are more relevant, as they assess bound antibody and the 'releasability' of the cells.

6. Because of chemical limitations, RAST can only be used to study allergens containing amino acids, although polysaccharide antigens can sometimes be immobilized by adsorption on to plastic instead.[136]

7. Because of variable IgE avidities and the inherent problems of standardizing multicomponent allergens, RAST can never be more than semiquantitative.[184] Results obtained by the Phadebas RAST system cannot be meaningfully compared with those of other RAST or equivalent systems,[133] nor can RAST grades with regard to one allergen be compared with those for other allergens.[133]

8. The problem of crossreaction artefacts has been alluded to above and is particularly troublesome in RAST.[1,29,38,158]

9. Problems with the anti-IgE specificity have arisen in the past[33] and still cause some controversy[136] but these are less of a problem with more recent anti-IgE antibodies.[77,216] 'Home-made' anti-IgE sera are dangerous unless raised by experts.

10. Many atopic sera contain autoantibodies against IgE (a type of rheumatoid factor though not linked with rheumatoid disease),[131] which can interfere with the binding of the second antibody.

11. RAST gives no indication of the avidity of the IgE antibodies (see above), although it could be adapted to do so.[189,273]

12. RAST is far more expensive than skin testing when a wide range of allergens is to be investigated. It is also susceptible to commercial abuse.

13. There are notable inter- and intra-laboratory errors.[90,127]

Conclusions

With these provisos in mind, the IUIS/WHO working group on laboratory tests concluded in 1981[133] that RAST is 'not essential in any clinical situation' and 'no alternative to careful history taking and skin tests'. The working group disputed the contention[210] that RAST can be used as a screening test for allergy. These comments are still valid 20 years later. But these difficulties are not the only side of the coin, and some advantages of RAST are listed on the previous page.

Clinical accuracy of RAST

Early enthusiasm for the usefulness of RAST[284] has given way to a more realistic assessment (Table 61.6). In 'immediate', Type I syndromes, most workers now agree on an overall accuracy of about 75%, which means that one-quarter of patients will be wrongly assigned. This overall figure conceals the fact that some foods perform considerably better than others. RAST is most reliable in egg white and codfish allergies for which single major allergens are responsible. Cow's milk and cereal RAST are less accurate, while at the other end of the scale the RAST results for beans are virtually random,[2,3,69,111] perhaps because of the lectin problem noted above. IgE antibody levels are usually well correlated with antibodies of other classes,[180,260] so there is unlikely to be any profit from measuring RAST and antibodies of other classes simultaneously.

In 'slow' reactions, as exemplified by the migraine and irritable bowel studies cited above, early enthusiasm for RAST[284] has largely evaporated.[83,138,187] A novel use for RAST in migraine was reported by Monro et al. in 1980.[191] Although results were generally low (approaching perilously close to background error), when they were arranged relative to each other in a RAST profile those foods that stood out above the others were well correlated with clinical migraine triggers and enabled clinically efficacious diets to be prescribed in 23 of 26 patients. Other workers failed to confirm this claim,[183] but seem to have missed the point that conventional cutoff points were inappropriate. Therefore, the initial results still stand unrefuted, in stark contradiction to the consensus view and seem to have withered of inanition.

Reported accuracy, false-positive and false-negative rates of food RAST in selected papers			
Reference and year of publication	Accurate (%)	False-positives (%)	False-negatives (%)
249 (1979)	92	6	2
36 (1983) (if delayed reactions are classed as positive)	66	9	26
36 (1983) (if delayed reactions are classed as negative)	74	9	17
2 (1978)	78	20	2
144 (1983) egg	19	–	28
144 (1983) wheat	6	38	21
144 (1983) cow's milk	10	–	47

Table 61.6 Reported accuracy, false-positive and false-negative rates of food RAST in selected papers.

Cellular studies

Lymphocyte activation

Committed lymphocytes are involved in various capacities in all immunological responses and should be detectable by blastoid transformation in the presence of the relevant antigen (Fig. 61.5). Food antigens are problematic though, because of their lectin content (see above). Frew et al.[108] reported that a proportion of healthy people show lymphocyte transformation in response to wheat gliadin, or its chemical subunits. There are some day-to-day fluctuations. Also, the lymphocytes of atopic people are likely to be somewhat different in their intrinsic responsiveness to those of normals.[19,94,256] Any work involving living cells is technically more demanding than antibody work and therefore expensive and slow by comparison. Experience is in general rather limited for this reason.

The results of different groups have been in conflict. On the credit side, Baudon et al.[28] found positive lymphocyte transformation in response to β-lactoglobulin, although not α-lactalbumin or casein, in a majority of milk-sensitive children, and Shibasaki et al.[245] found the same with rice protein in sensitive patients; the IgE-binding determinants of rice protein were quite distinct from the lymphocyte-stimulating moiety. Endre and Osvath[86] found lymphocyte transformation to β-lactoglobulin or bovine serum albumin in 15 of 17 milk-allergic patients and in only one of eight control subjects.

In contrast, May and Alberto[178] were unable to distinguish patients from normals when testing milk- and egg-sensitive cells against the relevant antigens. These workers recorded false-positive rates of 87% and 64% for the two foods. On the other hand, Scheinmann et al.[240] reported a false-negative rate of 62% and a false-positive rate of only 10% in cow's milk intolerance. To some extent these differences are reflections of the very many variables between laboratories in performing this test. Although there is nothing wrong with the immunological credentials of this test, it has only been used by isolated enthusiasts for allergy diagnosis.

Gliadin adheres to the B lymphocytes of coeliac patients more than to normal lymphocytes,[272] presumably because of the differences in lectin receptors. It is therefore not surprising that coeliac lymphocytes transform in response to gliadin and, provided a precise gluten subfraction is used, their stimulation is far greater than that of normal lymphocytes, with very little overlap.[247] Ironically, the one condition in which the test could be of value is the one where it is not needed.

Lymphokine production

Of the various lymphokines produced by activated lymphocytes, only the leukocyte migration inhibition factor (LIF) has been much investigated for diagnosis of food intolerance. Peripheral blood leukocytes from atopic patients are somewhat different from those of normals in their intrinsic responsiveness to adrenaline and methacholine[220,224] so their responsiveness to lymphokines might also be different; the LIF test in such patients is therefore susceptible to at least two separate variables.

Ashkenazi et al.[14] applied a variation of the LIF test to cow's milk allergy using β-lactoglobulin as stimulant (Fig. 61.6), reporting virtually no overlap between challenge-proven milk-intolerant patients and controls (including patients with acute gastroenteritis, whose milk *antibody* levels were presumably raised or rising). Five out of 18 children who had become tolerant of milk after previously being sensitive were also positive. Three of these children in whom a previous LIF test had been done during the active illness now had lower results than when they were ill. A similar good discrimination was observed when using gliadin for coeliac disease, provided a defined subfraction of gliadin was used.[13] Once again, after healing of the disease on a gluten-free diet, 50% of the hitherto positive LIFs became negative after (in some cases) a transient rise.[15] Reversion to normal of the test thus appears to follow within months, on resolution of the illness – unlike antibody levels.

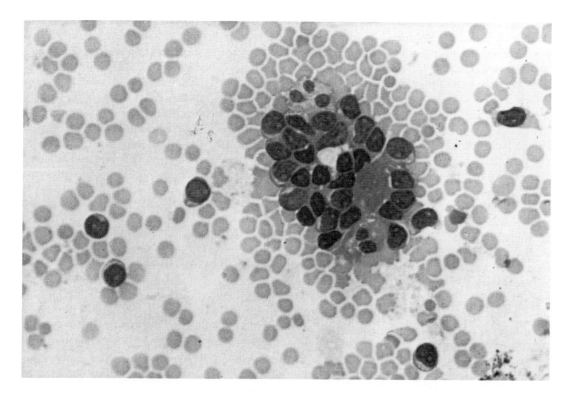

Fig. 61.5 Blastoid transformation of lymphocytes; small lymphocytes and many lymphoblasts can be seen.

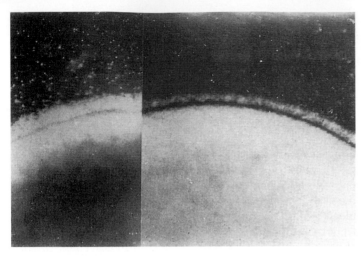

Fig. 61.6 Demonstration of positive LIF test. Left, control; right, 40% inhibition by 10 µg/ml β-lactoglobulin. (Reproduced by courtesy of Dr A. Ashkenazi.)

Considerable manual skill and experience is required of the technician who performs these tests (in common with most technologies involving living cells), but results are reproducible once this level is attained. Gettinby *et al.*[112] criticized Ashkenazi's technique on methodological grounds and Minor *et al.*[188] obtained poor discrimination when using the test in milk allergy and corn allergy. As with most tests involving living cells, this test remains a minority enthusiasm.

Food Allergy Cellular Test (FACT) – leucotriene release from buffy-coat cells

De Weck and colleagues developed an assay for leucotrienes C4, D4 and E4 using ELISA (enzyme-linked immunosorbent assay)[73] and this has been applied by Abrahams (personal communication) for food sensitivity diagnosis. Buffy-coat cells are first stimulated with interleukins IL3 and IL5, then incubated with food extracts, after which the leucotrienes in the supernatant are assayed. No accuracy calculations have been made by the laboratory marketing the test (Individual Wellbeing, London) but utility values for various conditions of 70–90% are reported. Clearly this will need to be tested by unbiased outside observers before the test's place can be decided.

Mediator release from basophils

Histamine release from peripheral blood leukocytes or basophils in response to antigen is a function of the final common pathway of Type I and Type III hypersensitivity. Although there is some correlation between serum and cell-bound IgE, the relationship is far from linear;[8] the two types of IgE may not be quite the same with respect to histamine-releasing efficiency.[16] The 'releasability' of atopic mast cells and basophils is also probably different from that of normal cells[99] and thus a functional measurement of cell-bound IgE is theoretically more likely to be clinically accurate than a RAST – the *in vitro* equivalent of a skin-test.[233] Histamine release can either be measured chemically or indirectly by observing degranulation of basophils. Both methods can be automated and give results consistent with each other.[74,181,270]

However, there are theoretical grounds for concern. The basophils of food-allergic children have high spontaneous histamine release, which can appear after positive food challenge and

last for months.[179] If the test is done in the presence of plasma, normal and atopic plasma will have different effects.[179,186] Histamine release is elevated in the presence of factors from activated platelets[157] and nonsteroidal anti-inflammatory drugs (NSAIDs),[283] and the binding of IgE to basophils is also influenced by interferon.[246] All of these effects are likely to modulate the response of the cells to antigen.

Nevertheless, Soifer and Hirsch[249] applied the test to 17 'selected patients with distinct and reliable clinical (food intolerant) syndromes' and 31 normal controls, reporting an accuracy of 69%. These authors did not find any fundamental difference in releasability between the two groups. Benveniste[32] popularized a semiautomated version of the test in France (TDBH: test de degranulation des basophiles humaines) and reported that true-positive results may be obtained in cases of drug reactions that do not usually show up with other methods. The TDBH should have been further evaluated but Benveniste became unpopular in the scientific community after an involvement with homeopathy and we have not seen the test mentioned since. McLaughlan and Coombs[169] reported histamine release in response to cow's milk proteins in 25% of normal infants and to a marked degree in 10%; they interpreted this not as a false-positive rate, but as evidence of silent and potentially harmful allergy. Degranulation tests remain a minority enthusiasm.

Non-immunological tests: cytotoxic test and its daughters

Vaughan[271] and then Rinkel[225] reported in the 1930s that open ingestion of a damaging foodstuff was followed within 60 min by a drop of total white cell count (the 'leukopenic index'). Squier and Lee[252] followed this up by demonstrating the same phenomenon *in vitro* using the whole blood of ragweed-sensitive hay fever sufferers. This did not occur with the blood of successfully treated patients. Two years later a paper appeared that purported to refute this observation[103] but it has been independently rediscovered since then,[129,230] and there seems to be no doubt that the phenomenon exists. In the 1950s and 1960s Black[40] and later the Bryans[48] popularized the test for the diagnosis of both inhalant and ingestant allergies, claiming utility values of up to 95%. This test has been taken up by a number of commercial laboratories but is generally ill-regarded by conventional allergists who consider it to be 'controversial',[9] 'untested',[46] 'not proven'[166] and (to be honest, if unkind) totally unbelievable. On the other hand, a 1981 paper from Finland reported that the test was in routine use at the Ear, Nose and Throat Hospital of Helsinki.[231]

The criteria of test positivity are slowing and rounding of polymorphs, with (in very strong reactions) apparent disintegration of polymorphs and degenerative changes in platelets and erythrocytes. Results are usually graded from 0 to 3.

Theoretical considerations

The test is performed in autologous plasma: this is essential for some but not all reactions.[126] It is often forgotten (by all but first-year physiology students) that the pH of blood is largely maintained by the buffering action of carbonic acid and bicarbonate ions; when whole citrated blood or serum is left to stand, the pH rises due to outgassing of carbon dioxide (Fig. 61.7), thus providing a culture medium in which the cells are already considerably stressed, to a variable and unknown degree. Although plasma is of fairly uniform composition, variations in its lipoprotein and mineral levels occur, and have a strong influence on lymphocyte

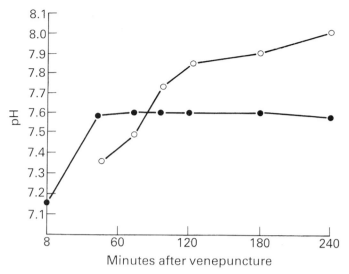

Fig. 61.7 Changes in pH of whole citrated blood (○) and serum (●) with time. The specimens were allowed to stand at room temperature in sealed screw-top tubes. (Demonstration performed by Ms K. Collison.)

Cytotoxic test result in patients with grass pollen or house dust mite allergy			
	Positive	**Negative**	**Totals**
Clinically sensitive	20	19	39
Clinically not sensitive	19	36	55
Totals	39	55	94

The χ^2 of this analysis was 1.99, which means that although these results do indeed point in the right direction (60% accurate), this could easily have been due to chance.

Table 61.7 Cytotoxic test result in patients with grass pollen or house dust mite allergy.

function.[102,114,254] To the buffy-coat cell suspension in autologous plasma is added an unspecified concentration of food extract or chemical, usually with some distilled water to counteract its 'dryness'. The resulting medium has an unknown pH, osmolarity and microbial content, and its composition must vary between laboratories and within laboratories, and between different foods and chemicals. This is clearly a test devised and performed by enthusiastic amateurs, which may partly explain the prejudice against it.

Reproducibility

In common with the RAST, it is reasonable to bear in mind that a difference between adjacent grades could be discounted as the distinction is hard to make for borderline results. Several workers have noted that about 20–30% of results vary from day to day over two or more grades,[31,56,161,231] which agrees with the variability reported to me in a joint study by the York Medical and Nutritional Laboratory, UK. In our study, about 2% of specimen replicates, whether taken from the same blood sample or from the same patient on different days, varied across three grades at least once (i.e. were said to be both grade 0 ['not allergic'] and grade 3 ['severely allergic']). Although this error rate may horrify the clinician reader, it is not much worse than that of some conventional laboratory tests of cellular immunology.[112]

Accuracy

Although the initial observations[40,252] implied that the test might be valuable for inhalant allergy, most enthusiasts now consider that the cytotoxic test should be reserved for use in 'masked food allergy', i.e. that kind of food intolerance that is associated with craving or addiction to the food in question and only becomes apparent after prolonged avoidance. A cynic might observe that thus limiting the claims restricts the test to those very cases in which its validation is most difficult, if not impossible. That this circumspection is wise is clear from a small collaborative study with the York Medical and Nutritional Laboratory on grass pollen and house dust mite allergy which yielded the results in Table 61.7.

Being controversial, the test has provoked some workers into making unfair criticisms without having become adept in its use.[56,161] Nevertheless, some well-conducted trials have been done[32,161] and report false-positive rates of up to 70%, noting that in several patients a strict adherence to the indicated diet would inevitably lead to malnutrition.[31] Clearly, the results need to be interpreted with great caution.[285]

Utility value

In spite of the above discussion it would be unfair to deny that many patients do become better, or well, when they embark on the diets indicated by the cytotoxic test.[44,263,266] It is entirely possible that were the test done in a defined, stable and sterile culture medium, with and without added serum, using food extracts of defined composition and concentration and using replicate estimations, a clinically accurate test might emerge having good utility value.[128,129] Following this dream, the cytotoxic test has in recent years sired the following daughters.

Antigen Leukocyte Cellular Antibody Test (ALCAT)

The ALCAT (AMTL Corporation, Hollywood, FL) is a whole blood assay intended for the determination of the effects of multi-pathogenic mechanisms involved in food sensitivities. It is an *in vitro* test that utilizes whole blood. This has the theoretical advantage that whole blood contains all of the circulating factors and chemical mediators, as well as the leukocytes and other cellular elements that may be involved in adverse food reactions. Reactions of aliquots of blood with individual food extracts are carried out under carefully controlled conditions and compared with control aliquots identically treated but not exposed to the food extracts. After separation of the white cell fraction, each aliquot is then analysed using a specially modified cell sizer and counter capable of separating the white cells into hundreds of subsets based on cell size. The analyser measures cell number, mean cell size and size distribution curves. Using computerized analysis, changes in cell number and size and distribution curves are measured quantitatively and per cent change calculated and printed numerically and graphically. Positive reactions are indicated by a change in cell size (increase or decrease) and/or absolute loss of cells. The primary reactive leukocyte fraction is the subset containing granulocytes and monocytes. The method requires minimal participation by technicians, and computerized measurement and calculations eliminate any error that might have otherwise been introduced by observer bias.

The ALCAT is strictly a screening test to be used when a patient gives a contradictory food history. If there is a possibility of multiple food reactions, it may be used to separate those foods that may be absolutely positive, potentially positive or negative. This test will not and should not be read as an absolute test but can be used to put a patient on a reasonable elimination diet and/or use the positive results for further challenge testing in order to prove that those foods reported as positive *are* truly positive. This test may help patients with suspected food sensitivities in whom the possibility of reactions to more than one food exists and in whom the likelihood of pathogenic mechanisms other than IgE exist. The term ALCAT is euphonious although possibly not accurate. We have not seen any attempt at accuracy calculations but excellent utility values are reported for ALCAT by independent observers, exceeding the results that most allergists would claim for the application of informed guesswork.[97,98,141,250] Interestingly, Fell[96] has shown that ALCAT responds to purified food toxins in the absence of immunological involvement (see above), even in healthy people. At the time of writing ALCAT appears to hold some promise.

NuTron

In this variant, whole blood aliquots are incubated in microtitre plates with food extracts. The red cells are then lysed and the remaining white cells evaluated for their electrical properties (radiofrequency and DC). A significant shift from control values is held to signify clinically relevant food intolerance. No accuracy calculations are presented by the laboratory but excellent utility values are claimed. We have seen no independent data from unbiased observers and are unable to hold an opinion until these have been provided.

Intestinal permeability and the detection of dietary antigens in the blood

The human intestine appears to undergo 'closure' *in utero* at around 34 weeks of gestation,[30,228,280] so that except for premature infants (especially during an episode of bloody stools[279]) only trace amounts of protein survive intact the translation from intestine to systemic blood.[207] Nevertheless, such small doses are often capable of evoking antibody formation and ingestion of food is normally followed by the appearance of circulating immune complexes, which presumably constitute a physiological pathway for clearance of these antigens.[47,207] Food-allergic patients appear to form more of these complexes,[207] which are larger,[47] often contain IgE and/or Clq[46,207] and are more slowly cleared[235] than normal complexes. Abnormal postprandial immune complexes are also associated with selective IgA deficiency[66,67] and some cases of glomerulonephritis.[52,269] Although these statements have been challenged,[84] this is largely because of the wide array of available immune-complex assays, most of which give results somewhat at variance with each other,[229] so that the assay to be used has to be selected intelligently.

Postprandial immune complexes

The abnormal postprandial immune complexes of food allergy seem to be a reflection of an increased gut permeability,[134] although this is controversial.[80] Food-allergy patients whose symptoms are limited to the gastrointestinal tract have been reported to have *lower* intestinal permeability than normals,[95] presumably because the antigens are trapped within local gut immune complexes[162,227] and do not proceed further. Gut permeability is nonspecifically enhanced by alcohol,[36,276] trauma[147,200] and inflammation, whether induced by toxins[200] or intestinal anaphylaxis.[41] Thus, the causal antigen may be prevented by local immune complexes from passing into the circulation at the same time as the uptake of 'bystander' antigens is encouraged. The presence of free dietary antigens in the circulation is not therefore diagnostic of allergy to that food[206] and if antibodies are also present these will mask the antigen.[70,206]

Several workers have attempted to split postprandial immune complexes in order to find out which antigens are involved. There are several methods of doing this,[12,17,67,208] and clinically relevant antigens have been detected.[67,208,209] It is too early to say if such complex splitting will prove to have diagnostic value.

DISCUSSION

As seen from Table 61.2, there are obvious reasons for doing testing *in vitro*. Granted, testing *in vitro* is more specific for inhalant allergies than for foods, however, when properly done, food-specific IgE tests *in vitro* are, in general, equally as sensitive as PSTs and provide similar information.[234]

In vitro tests can be most helpful where an anaphylactic reaction has occurred and there is more than one possible food involved. The *in vitro* tests can also be helpful when the patient's history is very complex and the patient is reluctant to accept allergy as a diagnosis. At times, a laboratory printout showing a positive result that a patient can *read* may mean more to that person than skin testing and/or the physician's clinical observations. *in vitro* tests may be helpful at times from a medicolegal standpoint, especially to confirm a possible anaphylactic reaction as the cause of death, if blood can be drawn early post mortem and *in vitro* tests done on the serum obtained.

Immunoassays for IgE antibodies have proven very helpful in shedding light on the problems of reactions from immunizations. In the cases of measles, mumps, and rubella (MMR) vaccine[143,144] as well as diphtheria and tetanus toxoids and acellular pertussis vaccine (DTaP),[195] gelatin proved to be the sensitizing antigen, rather than egg. Sakaguchi et al.[232] also reported another case of anaphylaxis from gelatin when recombinant erythropoietin (epoetin) was given intravenously. Some of the patients who reacted to the MMR vaccine also had hives when eating gelatin. This emphasizes the value of an accurate allergy history, especially in children. However, any physician should be alert to the possibility of collagen sensitivity wherever the exposure is possible.[194]

There are occupational exposures that may cause IgE-mediated reactions manifested by asthma. An example of this is the case report of a textile industry worker who was sensitive to cellulase, and had specific IgE antibodies to cellulase.[150]

In vitro tests are most helpful when the physician is seeing an emotionally disturbed patient who has an associated diagnosis of allergy but is on drugs which cannot be stopped and severely interfere with the accuracy of any skin tests. The *in vitro* tests are not altered by any H_1 or H_2 blocking agents. Also, these tests are helpful when a patients is on a β-blocker drug and there is concern for anaphylaxis occurring with some other type of test.

In the United States, there is no latex antigen approved by the Food and Drug Administration (FDA) to use for PST at this time. For this antigen, DPC and CAP latex *in vitro* tests are FDA approved. In view of the increasing incidence of latex sensitivity among medical personnel,[151] this is an important test to place in the differential diagnosis.

Caution must be taken not to overuse *in vitro* tests when simple prick tests can be used. The prick test can be just as correct if properly done as the *in vitro* test with less cost and minimal inconvenience. In the United States, health maintenance organizations (HMO) preferred provider organizations (PPO) and other health insurance providers frequently prohibit the use of *in vitro* tests because of costs. If these tests are necessary, the physician may have to obtain pre-approval from the insurance provider in order to have them done.

CONCLUSIONS

1. *In vitro* tests indeed have their place in medicine. There are times when they are necessary and there are times when they are used excessively. When used appropriately, they can be very helpful in making a correct diagnosis and helping to institute proper therapy.

2. Immunological reactivity against foods is a normal physiological phenomenon. Anti-food antibodies in the blood, although not universal, are common and do not correlate with clinical illnesses.

3. No laboratory test can prove food intolerance; at best it can add meaningful weight to a clinical suspicion and a starting point for dietary elimination experiments.

4. No laboratory test, if negative, can disprove food intolerance. Its use for this purpose is an abuse of the trust of patients and public.

5. The accuracy of a test is not the same as its utility value for the real-life task of improving patients' health.

6. RAST and histamine release are fairly (up to 75%) reliable in 'immediate' Type I allergies but unhelpful in slow (possibly non-IgE) types of intolerance.

7. RAST accuracy varies from food to food, being good for codfish and egg white, intermediate for milk and cereals and poor for soya and other beans.

8. Certain food antibody measurements (see text) have become quite accurate for diagnosis of coeliac disease.

9. Tests of lymphocyte activation and mediator release have their enthusiasts but have not become generally available for the clinic.

10. The 'cytotoxic test' and its daughters offer a possible way forward for management of patients with 'toxic' (non-immunological) food intolerances, although, as with antibody tests, they are not to be relied on, but interpreted with caution.

11. The case history, skin tests, challenges and laboratory tests are all individually unreliable to some extent, but can serve to strengthen the provisional diagnosis. The allergist should not fool either himself or the patient that he can make a definitive diagnosis; there will always be cases in which food intolerance can be neither proved nor disproved.

12. Although accurate diagnosis is usually held to be the bedrock of effective medicine, the allergist is forced to proceed on the basis of probabilities. However, this does not prevent us from converting many ill people into well people.

REFERENCES

1   Aalberse RC, Koshte V, Clemens JGJ. Immunoglobulin E antibodies that crossreact with vegetable foods, pollen and Hymenoptera venom. *J Allergy Clin Immunol* 1981; 68: 356–64.

2   Aas K. The diagnosis of hypersensitivity to ingested foods. Reliability of skin prick testing and the radioallergosorbent technique with different materials. *Clin Allergy* 1978; 8: 39–50.

3   Aas K, Lundkvist V. The radioallergosorbent test with a purified allergen from codfish. *Clin Allergy* 1973; 3: 255–63.

4   Adkinson NF. The radioallergosorbent technique: uses and abuses. *J Allergy Clin Immunol* 1980; 65: 1–4.

5   Adkinson NF. The radioallergosorbent test. *J Allergy Clin Immunol* 1980; 66: 174–5.

6   Adkinson NF. The radioallergosorbent test in 1981 – limitations and refinements. *J Allergy Clin Immunol* 1981; 67: 87–9.

7   Ali M. In vitro immunoassay techniques in clinical allergy. *J Clin Ecol* 1985; 3: 68–78.

8   Allen KR, Osmond S, Alston WC. A method for the simultaneous determination of serum and cell bound IgE. *Clin Allergy* 1977; 7: 273–7.

9   American Academy of Allergy. Position statements – controversial techniques. *J Allergy Clin Immunol* 1981; 67: 333–8.

10 Anderson MC, Baer H. Antigenic and allergenic changes during storage of a pollen extract. *J Allergy Clin Immunol* 1982; 69: 3–10.

11 Anderson P, Pedersen OF, Bach B, Bonde GJ. Serum antibodies and immunoglobulins in smokers and non-smokers. *Clin Exp Immunol* 1982; 47: 467–73.

12 Anonymous. On acupuncture. *Edinburgh Med Surg J* 1827; 27: 190–200.

13 Ashkenazi A, Levin S, Idar D *et al*. Immunological assay for the diagnosis of coeliac disease: interaction between purified gluten fractions. *Pediatr Res* 1980; 14: 776–8.

14 Ashkenazi A, Levin S, Idar D *et al*. In vitro cell-mediated immunologic assay for cow's milk allergy. *J Pediatrics* 1980; 66: 399–402.

15 Ashkenazi A, Levin S, Idar D *et al*. Effect of gluten-free diet on an immunological assay for coeliac disease. *Lancet* 1981; I: 914–16.

16 Assem ESK, Attallah NA. Increased release of histamine by anti IgE from leucocytes of asthmatic patients and possible heterogeneity of IgE. *Clin Allergy* 1981; 11: 367–74.

17 Baatrup G, Petersen I, Svehag S-E, Brandslund I. A standardized method for quantitating the complement-mediated immune complex solubilizing capacity of human serum. *J Immunol Meth* 1983; 59: 369–80.

18 Bamdad S, Goodwin BFJ, Hill JE. IgE antibodies to food allergens detected by ELISA, RAST and monkey PCA. *Clin Allergy* 1983; 13: 89–97.

19 Badger A, Young J, Poste G. Inhibition of PHA induced proliferation of human peripheral blood lymphocytes by histamine and histamine H1 and H2 agonists. *Clin Exp Immunol* 1983; 70: 205–6.

20 Bahna SL, Heiner DC. Cow's milk allergy: pathogenesis, manifestations, diagnosis and management. *Adv Pediatr* 1978; 25: 1–37.

21 Bahna SL, Heiner DC, Horwitz CA. Sequential changes of the five immunoglobulin classes and other responses in infectious mononucleosis. *Int Arch Allergy Appl Immunol* 1984; 74: 1–8.

22 Bahna SL, Heiner DC, Myhre BA. Immunoglobulin E pattern in cigarette smokers. *Allergy* 1983; 38: 57–64.

23 Baldo BA. Standardization of allergens: examinations of existing procedures and the likely impact of new techniques on the quality control of extracts. *Allergy* 1983; 38: 535–46.

24 Ballow M, Mendelson L, Donshik P *et al*. Pollen specific IgG antibodies in the tears of patients with allergic-like conjunctivitis. *J Allergy Clin Immunol* 1984; 73: 376–80.

25 Barnetson R St C, Merrett TG, Ferguson A. Studies on hyperimmunoglobulinaemia E in atopic diseases with particular reference to food allergens. *Clin Exp Immunol* 1981; 46: 54–60.

26 Barnett D, Baldo BA, Howden MEH. Multiplicity of allergens in peanuts. *J Allergy Clin Immunol* 1983; 72: 61–8.

27 Barnett DJ, Bertani L, Wara DW, Amman AJ. Milk precipitins in selective IgA deficiency. *Ann Allergy* 1979; 42: 73–6.

28 Baudon JJ, Fontaine J-L, Mougenot JF et al. L'intolerance digestive aux proteins du lait de vache chez le nourisson et l'enfant. *Arch Fr Pediatr* 1975; 32: 787–802.

29 Baux X. Studies on the specificity of human IgE – antibodies to the plant proteases papain and bromelain. *Clin Allergy* 1979; 9: 451–7.

30 Beach RC, Menzies IS, Clayden GS, Scopes JW. Gastrointestinal permeability changes in the preterm neonate. *Arch Dis Child* 1982; 57: 141–5.

31 Benson TE, Arkins JA. Cytotoxic testing for food allergy: evaluation of reproducibility and correlation. *J Allergy Clin Immunol* 1976; 58: 471–6.

32 Benviniste J. The human basophil degranulation test as an in vitro method for the diagnosis of allergies. *Clin Allergy* 1981; 11: 1–11.

33 Bernier GM, McIntyre OR. Contaminating antibodies in anti IgE antisera. *J Immunol Meth* 1976; 13: 81–5.

34 Bernstein M, Day JH, Welsh A. Double-blind food challenge in the diagnosis of food sensitivity in the adult. *J Allergy Clin Immunol* 1982; 70: 205–10.

35 Bjarnason I, Peters TJ, Veall N. A persistent defect in intestinal permeability in coeliac disease demonstrated by a ^{51}Cr-labelled EDTA absorption test. *Lancet* 1983; i: 323–5.

36 Bjarnason I, Ward K, Peters TJ. The leaky gut of alcoholism: possible route of entry for toxic compounds. *Lancet* 1984; i: 179–82.

37 Björksten B, Ahlstedt S, Björksten F et al. Immunoglobulin E and immunoglobulin G^4 antibodies to cow's milk in children with cow's milk allergy. *Allergy* 1983; 38: 119–24.

38 Björksten F, Halmepuro L, Hannuksela M, Lahti A. Extraction and properties of apple allergens. *Allergy* 1980; 35: 671–7.

39 Björksten F, Backman A, Järvinen KAJ et al. Immunoglobulin E specific to wheat and rye flour proteins. *Clin Allergy* 1977; 7: 473–83.

40 Black AP. A new diagnostic method in allergic disease. *Pediatrics* 1956; 17: 715–23.

41 Bloch KJ, Walker WA. Effect of locally induced intestinal anaphylaxis on the uptake of a bystander antigen. *J Allergy Clin Immunol* 1981; 67: 312–16.

42 Block G, Tse KS, Kijek K et al. Baker's asthma: studies of the cross-antigenicity between different cereal grains. *Clin Allergy* 1984; 14: 177–85.

43 Bock SA, Lee W-Y, Remigio LK, May CD. Studies of hypersensitivity reactions to foods in infants and children. *J Allergy Clin Immunol* 1978; 62: 327–34.

44 Boyles JH. The validity of using the cytotoxic food test in clinical allergy. *Ear Nose Throat J* 1977; 56: 168–73.

45 Bringel H, Vela C, Ureha V et al. IgD antibodies in vitro blocking activity of IgE mediated reactions. *Clin Allergy* 1982; 12: 37–46.

46 Brostoff J, Johns P, Stanworth DR. Complexed IgE in atopy. *Lancet* 1977; ii: 741–2.

47 Brostoff J, Carini C, Wraith DG et al. Immune complexes in atopy. In: *The Mast Cell* (Pepys J, Edwards AM, eds). Pitman, London, 1979; 380–93.

48 Bryan WTK, Bryan MP. Cytotoxic reactions in the diagnosis of food allergy. *Laryngoscope* 1969; 79: 1453–72.

49 Buckley RH, Dees SC. Correlation of milk precipitins with IgA deficiency. *New Engl J Med* 1969; 281: 465–9.

50 Burgin-Wolff A, Signer E, Friess HM et al. The diagnostic significance of antibodies to various cow's milk proteins (fluorescent immunosorbent test). *Eur J Pediatr* 1980; 133: 17–24.

51 Businco L, Marchetti F, Pellegrini G, Perlini R. Predictive value of cord blood IgE levels in 'at-risk' newborn babies and influence of type of feeding. *Clin Allergy* 1983; 13: 502–8.

52 Cairns SA, London A, Mallick NP. Circulating immune complexes following food delayed clearance in idiopathic glomerulonephritis. *J Clin Lab Immunol* 1981; 6: 121–6.

53 Calder PC. Dietary nucleic acids and Th1/Th2 balance: a clue to cow's milk allergy? *Clin Exp Allergy* 2000; 30: 908–11.

54 Cant AJ, Gibson P, Dancy M. Food hypersensitivity made life-threatening by ingestion of aspirin. *Br Med J* 1984; 228: 755–6.

55 Catsimpoolas N (ed). *Immunological Aspects of Foods*. Avi Publishing, Westport, Connecticut, 1977.

56 Chambers VV, Hudson BH, Glaser J. A study of the reactions of human polymorphonuclear leukocytes to various antigens. *J Allergy* 1958; 29: 93–102.

57 Cheung N-KV, Blessing-Moore J, Reid MJ et al. Reduction of interference by specific IgG with a modified microtiter solid-phase radioimmunoassay to measure honeybee venom IgE. *J Allergy Clin Immunol* 1983; 71: 283–93.

58 Chua YY, Bremner K, Llobet JL. Diagnosis of food allergy by the radioallergosorbent technique. *J Allergy Clin Immunol* 1976; 58: 477–82.

59 Ciclitira PJ, Ellis HJ, Evans DJ. A solid-phase radioimmunoassay for measurement of circulating antibody titres to wheat gliadin and its subfractions in patients with adult coeliac disease. *J Immunol Meth* 1983; 62: 231–9.

60 Collins-Williams C, Salama Y. A laboratory study on the diagnosis of milk allergy. *Int Arch Allergy* 1965; 27: 110–28.

61 Conning DM, Landsdown ABG (eds). *Toxic Hazards in Food*. Croom Helm, London, 1983.

62 Coombs RRA, Oldham G. Early rheumatoid-like joint lesions in rabbits drinking cow's milk. *Int Arch Allergy Appl Immunol* 1981; 64: 287–92.

63 Coombs RRA, Kieffer M, Fraser DR, Frazier PJ. Naturally occurring antibodies to wheat gliadin fractions and to other cereal antigens in rabbits, rats, guineapigs on normal laboratory diets. *Int Arch Allergy Appl Immunol* 1983; 70: 200–4.

64 Cuevas M, Moneo I, Urena V et al. Reverse enzyme immunoassay for the determination of Lolium perenne IgE antibodies. *Int Arch Allergy Appl Immunol* 1983; 72: 184–7.

65 Cukor P, Woehler ME, Persiani C, Fermin A. Iodinated versus fluorescent labelling in the RAST for the determination of serum IgE levels. *J Immunol Meth* 1976; 12: 183–92.

66 Cunningham-Rundles C, Brandeis WE, Good RA. Bovine antigens and the formation of circulating immune complexes in selective IgA deficiency. *J Clin Invest* 1979; 64: 272–9.

67 Cunningham-Rundles C, Brandeis WE, Safai B et al. Selective IgA deficiency and circulating immune complexes containing bovine proteins in a child with chronic graft vs. host disease. *Am J Med* 1979; 67: 883–9.

68 Dannaeus A, Inganäs M. A follow-up study of children with food allergy. Clinical course in relation to serum IgE and IgG antibody levels to milk, egg and fish. *Clin Allergy* 1981; 11: 553–9.

69 Dannaeus A, Johansson SGO, Foucard T, Ohman S. Clinical and immunological aspects of food allergy in childhood. I. Estimation of IgG, IgA and IgE antibodies to food antigens in children – food allergy and atopic dermatitis. *Acta Paediatr Scand* 1977; 66: 31–7.

70 Dannaeus A, Inganäs M, Johansson SGO, Foucard T. Intestinal uptake of ovalbumin in malabsorption and food allergy in relation to serum IgG antibody and orally administered sodium cromoglycate. *Clin Allergy* 1979; 9: 263–70.

71 Davies DF. Immunology of human atheroma. In: *Health Hazards of Milk* (Freed DLJ, eds), Ballière Tindall, Eastbourne, 1984; 202–13.

72 Davis SD, Bierman CW, Pierson WE et al. Clinical non-specificity of milk copro-antibodies in diarrhoeal stools. *New Engl J Med* 1970; 282: 612–13.

73 de Weck AL, Furukawa K, Dahindedn C, Maly FE. A new cellular assay for the diagnosis of allergy. In *Progress in Allergy and Clinical Immunology* (Myiamoto T, ed). 14th ICACI, Kyoto, 1992.

74 Diamant B, Patkar S. Histamine release from washed whole blood. A method suitable for routine diagnosis of Type I allergy. *Int Arch Allergy Appl Immunol* 1982; 67: 13–17.

75 Dissanayake AS. Coelic disease. In: *Topics in Gastroenterology*, Vol. I, (Truelove SC, Jewell DP, eds). Blackwell, Oxford, 1973; 167–83.

76 Dockhorn RJ. Using the RAST and PRIST with an overview of clinical significance. *Ann Allergy* 1982; 49: 1–8.

77 D'Onofrio I. Clinical accuracy of updated versions of Phadebas RAST. In: *Recent Developments in RAST and Other Solid-Phase Immunoassay Systems* (Kemeny DM, Lessof MF, eds). Excerpta Medica, Amsterdam; 1983; 86–92.

78 Donovan K, Torres-Pinedo R. Effects of d-galactose on the fluid loss in soy bean protein intolerance. *Pediatr Res* (abstract) 1978; 12: 433.

79 Dreborg S, Foucard T. Allergy to apple, carrot and potato in children with birch pollen allergy. *Allergy* 1983; 38: 167–72.

80 DuMont GCL, Beach RC, Menzies IS. Gastrointestinal permeability in food-allergic eczematous children. *Clin Allergy* 1984; 14: 55–9.

81 Eastham EJ, Lichauco T, Grady MI, Walker WA. Antigenicity of infant formulas: role of immature intestine on protein permeability. *J Pediatr* 1978; 93: 561–4.

82 Editorial. Food allergy and intolerance. *Lancet* 1980; ii: 1344–5.

83 Egger J, Carter CM, Wilson J *et al*. Is migraine food allergy? *Lancet* 1983; ii: 865–8.

84 Elkon KB, Lanham JG, Dash AC, Hughes GRV. The effect of a protein meal on a three fluid-phase assay for circulating immune complexes. *Clin Exp Immunol* 1981; 45: 279–82.

85 Emanuel IA. In vitro testing for allergy diagnosis: comparison of methods in common use. *Otolaryng Clin N Am* 1998; 31(1): 27–33.

86 Endre L, Osvath P. Antigen-induced lymphoblast transformations in the diagnosis of cow's milk allergic diseases in infancy and early childhood. *Acta Allergologica* 1975; 30: 34–42.

87 Eriksson NE, Formgren H, Svenonius E. Food hypersensitivity in patients with pollen allergy. *Allergy* 1982; 37: 437–43.

88 Eriksson NE, Wihl J-A, Arrendal H. Birch pollen-related food hypersensitivity: influence of total and specific IgE levels. *Allergy* 1983; 38: 353–7.

89 Eterman KP, Hekkens WThJM, Pena AS *et al*. Wheat grains, a substrate for the determination of gluten antibodies in serum of gluten-sensitive patients. *J Immunol Meth* 1977; 14: 85–92.

90 Evans R (Committee on in vitro tests, American Acad Allergy). Variability in the measurement of specific immunoglobulin E antibody by the RAST technique. *J Allergy Clin Immunol* 1982; 69: 245–52.

91 Ewart JAD. Immunochemistry of wheat proteins. In: *Immunological Aspects of Foods*. Avi Publishing, Westport, Connecticut, 1977; 87–116.

92 Falk ES, Dale S, Bolle R, Haneberg B. Antigens common to scabies and housedust mites. *Allergy* 1981; 36: 233–8.

93 Fällstrom S-P, Ahlstedt S, Hanson LA. Specific antibodies in infants with gastrointestinal intolerance to cow's milk protein. *Int Arch Allergy Appl Immunol* 1978; 56: 97–105.

94 Fällström S-P, Lindholm L, Ahlstedt S. Cow's milk protein intolerance in children is connected with impaired lymphoblastic responses to mitogens. *Int Arch Allergy Appl Immunol* 1983; 70: 205–6.

95 Fälth-Magnusson K, Kjellman N-IM, Magnusson K-E, Sundqvist T. Intestinal permeability in healthy and allergic children before and after sodium cromoglycate treatment assessed with different sized polyethylene glycols (PEG 300 and PEG 1000). *Clin Allergy* 1984; 14: 227–86.

96 Fell PJ. *Pilot study into the effect of naturally occurring pharmacoactive agents on the ALCAT test*. American Otolaryngic Allergy Association, Sept 1991, AMTL Corp, One Oakwood Blvd, Suite 130, Hollywood, FLA 33020.

97 Fell PJ, Brostoff J, Soulsby S: *ALCAT – a new cellular test for food sensitivity*. American in-vitro Allergy & Immunology Society, August 1990. AMTL Corporation, One Oakwood Blvd, Suite 130, Hollywood, FLA 33020.

98 Fell PJ, Soulsby S, Brostoff J. Cellular responses to food in irritable bowel syndrome – an investigation of the ALCAT test. *J Nutr Med* 1991; 2: 143–9.

99 Findlay SR, Lichtenstein LM. Basophil 'releasability' in patients with asthma. *Annu Rev Respir Dis* 1980; 122: 53–9.

100 Finn R, Cohen HN. Food allergy: fact or fiction? *Lancet* 1978; i: 426–8.

101 Ford RPK, Hill DJ, Hosking CS. Cow's milk hypersensitivity: immediate and delayed onset clinical patterns. *Arch Dis Child* 1983; 58: 856–62.

102 Fraker PJ. Zinc deficiency: a common immunodeficiency state. *Surv Immunol Res* 1983; 2: 155–63.

103 Franklin W, Lowell FC. Failure of ragweed pollen extract to destroy white cells from ragweed-sensitive patients. *J Allergy* 1949; 20: 375–7.

104 Freed DLJ. Laboratory diagnosis of food intolerance. *Clin Immunol Allergy* 1982; 2: 181–203.

105 Freed DLJ, Sinclair T, Topper R *et al*. IgA levels in rhinitic nasal secretions during short-term therapy with sodium cromoglycate, beclomethasone and anti-histamine. In: *The Mast Cell* (Pepys J, Edwards AM, eds). Pitman, London, 1979; 795–804.

106 Freed DLJ, Wilson P, Downing NPD, Musgrove D. The cytotoxic test in immediate-type respiratory allergies. *Int J Biosoc Res* (in press).

107 Freier S, Lebenthal E, Frier M *et al*. IgE and IgD antibodies to cow's milk and soy protein in duodenal fluid: effects of pancreozymin and secretin. *Immunology* 1983; 49: 69–75.

108 Frew AJ, Bright S, Shewry PR, Minro A. Proliferative response to lymphocytes of normal individuals to wheat protein (gliadins). *Int Arch Allergy Appl Immunol* 1980; 62: 162–7.

109 Fries JF. Food allergy: current concerns (editorial). *Ann Allergy* 1981; 46: 260–3.

110 Galant S, Nussbaum E, Wittner R *et al*. Increased IgD milk antibody responses in a patient with Down's syndrome, pulmonary hemosiderosis and cor pulmonale. *Ann Allergy* 1983; 1: 446–9.

111 Gavani UD, Hyde JS, Moore BS. Hypersensitivity to milk and egg white, skin tests, RAST results and clinical intolerance. *Ann Allergy* 1983; 51: 446–9.

112 Gettinby G, Connolly PJ, Anderson JM. Immunological assays for coeliac disease. *Lancet* 1981; i: 1156.

113 Gleich GJ, Yunginger JW. The radioallergosorbent test: its present place and likely future in the practice of allergy. *Adv Asthma Allergy* 1975; 2(2).

114 Good RA. Nutrition and immunity. *J Clin Immunol* 1981; 1: 3–11.

115 Goodwin BJF. IgE antibody levels to ingested soya protein determined in a normal adult population. *Clin Allergy* 1982; 12: 55–62.

116 Gunthur M, Aschaffenburg R, Matthews RH *et al*. The level of antibodies to the proteins of cow's milk in the serum of normal human infants. *Immunology* 1960; 3: 296–306.

117 Haddad ZH, Kaira V, Verma S. IgE antibodies to peptic and peptic tryptic digests of lactoglobulin: significance in food hypersensitivity. *Ann Allergy* 1979; 42: 368–71.

118 Hadjivassiliou M, Grunewald RA, Chattopadhyay AK *et al*. Clinical, radiological, neurophysiological and neuropathological characteristics of gluten ataxia. *Lancet* 1998; 352: 1582–5.

119 Hadjivassiliou M, Grunewald RA, Davies-Jones GAB. Gluten sensitivity: a many-headed hydra. *Br Med J* 1999; 318: 1710–11.

120 Hales BJ, Shen H-D, Thomas WR. Cytokine responses to Der p1 and Der p7; housedust mite allergens with different IgE-binding patterns. *Clin Exp Allergy* 2000; 30: 934–43.

121 Hamburger RN. The immunogenetics of IgE provides predictive value for the development of allergy. *Ann Allergy* 1982; 49: 9–11.

122 Haraparsad D, Wilson N, Dixon C, Silverman M. Oral tartrazine challenge in childhood asthma: effect on bronchial reactivity. *Clin Allergy* 1984; 14: 81–5.

123 Hill DJ, Davidson GP, Barnes GL. The spectrum of cow's milk allergy in childhood. Clinical, gastroenterological and immunological studies. *Acta Paediatr Scand* 1979; 68: 847–52.

124 Hoffken K, Bosse F, Steih V, Schmidt CG. Dissociation and isolation of antigen and antibody from immune complexes. *J Immunol Meth* 1982; 53: 51–9.

125 Hofmann A, LaBrooy J, Davidson GP, Shearman DJC. Measurement of specific antibodies in human intestinal aspirate: effect of the protease inhibitor phenylmethylsulphonyl fluoride. *J Immunol Meth* 1983; 64: 199–204.

126 Holopainen E, Palva T, Stenberg P *et al*. Cytotoxic leukocyte reaction. *Acta Otolaryngeal* 1980; 89: 222–6.

127 Homburger HA, Jacob GL. Analytic accuracy of specific immunoglobulin E antibody results determined by a blind proficiency survey. *J Allergy Clin Immunol* 1982; 70: 474–80.

128 Hopkins JM, Gorecka D. Tough cells and old age. *Lancet* 1983; ii: 1170–3.

129 Hopkins JM, Tomlinson VS, Jenkins RM. Variation in response to cytotoxicity of cigarette smoke. *Br Med J* 1981; 283: 1209–11.

130 Hsieh KH. Interferon-induced suppression of an in vitro IgE biosynthesis in asthmatic children. *Ann Allergy* 1982; 48: 302–4.

131 Inganäs M, Johansson SGO, Bennich H. Anti-IgE antibodies in human serum: occurrence and specificity. *Int Arch Allergy Appl Immunol* 1981; 65: 51–61.

132 Ishizaka K, Ishizaka T. Identification of gamma E-antibodies as a carrier of reaginic activity. *J Immunol* 1967; 99: 1187.

133 IUIS/WHO working group report. Use and abuse of laboratory tests in clinical immunology: critical considerations of eight widely used diagnostic procedures. *Clin Exp Immunol* 1981; 46: 662–74.

134 Jackson PG, Lessof MH, Baker RWR *et al.* Intestinal permeability in patients with eczema and food allergy. *Lancet* 1981; i: 1285–6.

135 Johansson SGO, Bennich HH. The clinical impact of the discovery of IgE. *Ann Allergy* 1982; 48: 325–30.

136 Johansson SG, Björksten F. Standardization of in vitro methods of atopic allergy. *Allergy* 1980; 35: 177–80.

137 Johansson SGO, Bennich H, Wide L. A new class of immunoglobulin in human serum. *Immunology* 1968; 14: 265.

138 Jones VA, McLaunglan P, Shorthouse M *et al.* Food intolerance: a major factor in the pathogenesis of irritable bowel syndrome. *Lancet* 1982; ii: 115–17.

139 Jonsson J, Schilling W. Some characteristics of immunofluorescence tests for antibodies against gluten using wheat grain sections or gliadin coated sepharose beads. *Acta Pathol Microbiol Immunol Scand* 1981; 89: 253–62.

140 Jonsson J, Schilling W, Forsberg M. Colostral IgA binding to wheat gluten and gliadin. *Clin Exp Immunol* 1982; 50: 203–8.

141 Kaats GR, Pullin D, Parker LK. *The short term efficacy of the ALCAT test.* The Bariatrician, Spring 1996; 18–23.

142 Kaplan GW, Wallace WW, Orgel HA, Miller JR. Serum IgE and incidence of allergy in group of neurotic children. *Orology* 1977; 10: 428–30.

143 Kelso JM. The gelatin story (editorial). *J Allergy Clin Immunol* 1999; 103: 200–2.

144 Kelso JM, Jones RT, Yuninger JW. Anaphylaxis to measles, mumps and rubella vaccine mediated by IgE to gelatin. *J Allergy Clin Immunol* 1993; 91: 867–72.

145 Kemeny DM, Mackenzie-Mills M, Lessof MH. Allergen-cellulose interactions in RAST: specificity and stability with purified bee venom proteins. In: *Recent Developments in RAST and Other Solid-Phase Immunoassay Systems* (Kemeny DM, Lessof MH, eds). Excerpta Medica, Amsterdam, 1983; 3–13.

146 Kenrick KG, Walker-Smith JA. Immunoglobulins and dietary protein antibodies in childhood coeliac disease. *Gut* 1970; 11: 635–40.

147 Kessel D, Cuthbert AW. Sidedness of the reaction to lactoglobulin in sensitized colonic epithelia. *Int Arch Allergy Appl Immunol* 1984; 74: 113–19.

148 Kidd JM, Cohen SH, Sosman AJ, Fink JN. Food dependent exercise-induced anaphylaxis. *J Allergy Clin Immunol* 1983; 50: 651–60.

149 Kieffer M, Frazier PJ, Daniels NWR, Coombs RRA. Wheat gliadin fractions and other cereal antigens reactive with antibodies in the sera of coeliac patients. *Clin Exp Immunol* 1982; 50: 651–60.

150 Kim HY, Nahm DH, Park HS, Choi DC. Occupational asthma and IgE sensitization to cellulase in a textile industry worker. *Ann Allergy Asthma Immunol* 1999; 82: 174–8.

151 Kim KT, Wellmeyer EK, Miller KV. Minimum prevalence of latex hypersensitivity in health care workers. *Allergy and Asthma Proc* 1999; 20(6): 387–91.

152 Kletter B, Freier S, Davies AM, Gery I. The significance of copro-antibodies in cow's milk proteins. *Acta Paediatr Scand* 1971; 60: 173–80.

153 Kletter B, Gery I, Freier S, Davies AM. Immune responses of normal infants to cow's milk. II. Decreased immune reactions to initially breast-fed infants. *Int Arch Allergy Appl Immunol* 1971; 40: 667–74.

154 Kolmannskog S, Haneberg B, Marhang G, Bolle R. Immunoglobulin E in extracts of faeces from children. *Int Arch Allergy Appl Immunol* 1984; 74: 50–4.

155 Kottgen E, Kluge F, Volk B, Gerok W. The lectin properties of gluten as the basis of the pathomechanism of gluten sensitive enteropathy. *Klin Wochenschr* 1983; 61: 111–12.

156 Köttgen E, Volk B, Kluge F, Gerok W. Gluten, a lectin with oligomannosyl specificity and the causative agent of gluten sensitive enteropathy. *Biochem Biophys Res Commun* 1982; 109: 168–73.

157 Krauer KA, Kagey-Sobotka A, Adkinson NF Jr, Lichtenstein LM. Platelet augmentation of IgE-dependent histamine release from human basophils and mast cells. *Int Arch Allergy Appl Immunol* 1984; 74: 29–35.

158 Lahti A, Bjorksten F, Hannuksela M. Allergy to birch pollen and apple and cross reactivity of the allergens studied with the RAST. *Allergy* 1980; 35: 297–300.

159 Lee SK, Kniker WT, Cook CD, Heiner DC. Cow's milk-induced pulmonary disease in children. *Adv Pediatr* 1978; 25: 39–57.

160 Lehman CW. The leukocyte food allergy test: a study of its reliability and reproducibility. Effect of diet and sublingual food drops on this test. *Ann Allergy* 1980; 45: 150–8.

161 Lieberman P, Crawford L, Bjelland J *et al.* Controlled study of the cytotoxic test. *J Am Med Assoc* 1975; 231: 728–30.

162 Lim PL, Rowley D. The effect of antibody on the intestinal absorption of macromolecules and on intestinal permeability in adult mice. *Int Arch Allergy Appl Immunol* 1982; 68: 41–6.

163 Lis H, Sharon H. The biochemistry of plant lectins (phytohemagglutinins). *Annu Rev Biochem* 1973; 42: 541–74.

164 Littlewood JM. RAST measurements in childhood. In: *The Second Fisons Food Allergy Workshop.* Medicine Publishing Foundation, Oxford, 1983; 49–51.

165 Lowell FC. Some untested diagnostic and therapeutic procedures in clinical allergy. *J Allergy Clin Immunol* 1975; 56: 168–9.

166 Lowell FC, Heiner DC. Food allergy: cytotoxic diagnosis technique not proven. *J Am Med Assoc* 1972; 220–1624.

167 Lowenstein H, Eriksson NE. Hypersensitivity to foods among birch pollen-allergic patients. Immunochemical inhibition studies for evaluation of possible mechanisms. *Allergy* 1981; 46: 44–6.

168 McGovern JJ. Re: sublingual provocative food testing (letter). *Ann Allergy* 1981; 46: 44–6.

169 McLaughlan P, Coombs RRA. Latent anaphylactic sensitivity of infants to cow's milk proteins: histamine release from blood basophils. *Clin Allergy* 1983; 13: 1–9.

170 McLaughlan P, Anderson KJ, Widdowson EM, Coombs RRA. Effect of heat on the anaphylactic-sensitising capacity of cow's milk, goat's milk and various infant formulae fed to guineapigs. *Arch Dis Child* 1981; 56: 165–71.

171 Magnusson CGM, Masson PL. Particle-counting immunoassay after immunoglobulin E antibodies after their elution from allergosorbents by pepsin: an alternative to the radioallergosorbent test. *J Allergy Clin Immunol* 1982; 70: 326–36.

172 Malm L, Wihl JA, Lamm CJ, Lindqvist N. Reduction of metacholine-induced nasal secretion by treatment with a new topical steroid in perennial non-allergic rhinitis. *Allergy* 1981; 36: 209–14.

173 Mathews JB, Fivaz BH, Sewell HF. Serum and salivary antibody responses and the development of oral tolerance after oral and intragastric antigen administration. *Int Arch Allergy Appl Immunol* 1981; 65: 107–13.

174 Matthews KP. Calculation of secretory antibodies and immunoglobulins. *J Allergy Clin Immunol* 1981; 68: 46–50.

175 Maulitz RM, Pratt DS, Schocket AL. Exercise-induced anaphylactic reaction to shellfish. *J Allergy Clin Immunol* 1979; 63: 433–4.

176 May CD. Food allergy: lessons from the past. *J Allergy Clin Immunol* 1982; 69: 255–9.

177 May CD. Food sensitivity. *Proc N Engl Soc Allergy* 2: 198–203.

178 May CD, Alberto R. In vitro responses of leukocytes to food proteins in allergic and normal children: lymphocyte stimulation and histamine release. *Clin Allergy* 1972; 2: 335–44.

179 May CD, Remigio L. Observations on high spontaneous release of histamine from leucocytes in vitro. *Clin Allergy* 1982; 12: 229–41.

180 May CD, Remigo L, Bock SA. Usefulness of measurement of antibodies in serum in diagnosis of sensitivity to cow's milk and soy proteins in early childhood. *Allergy* 1980; 35: 301–10.

181 May CD, Lyman M, Alberto R, Cheng J. Procedures for immunochemical study of histamine release from leucocytes with small volume of blood. *J Allergy* 1970; 46: 12–20.

182 May CD, Remigio L, Feldman J *et al.* A study of serum antibodies to isolated milk proteins and ovalbumin in infants and children. *Clin Allergy* 1977; 7: 583–95.

183 Merrett J, Peatfield RC, Rose FC, Merrett TG. Food related antibodies in headache patients. *J Neurol Neurosurg Psychiatry* 1983; 46: 738–42.

184 Merrett TG, Merrett J. The RAST principle and the use of mixed-allergen RAST as a screening test of IgE-mediated allergies. *Methods Enzymol* 1980; 70(A): 376–87.

185 Metzger WJ, Butler JE, Swanson P *et al.* Amplification of the enzyme-linked immunosorbent assay for measuring allergen-specific IgE and IgG antibody. *Clin Allergy* 1981; 11: 523–31.

186 Miadonna A, Tedeschi A, Zanussi C. Plasma of normal, but not atopic, persons reducing basophil degranulation induced by anti-IgE. *Clin Allergy* 1984; 14: 29–35.

187 Minford AMB, Macdonald A, Littlewood JM. Food intolerance and food allergy in children: a review of 68 cases. *Arch Dis Child* 1982; 57: 742–7.

188 Minor JD, Tolber SG, Frick OL. Leukocyte inhibition factor in delayed-onset food allergy. *J Allergy Clin Immunol* 1980; 66: 314–21.

189 Mita H, Yasueda H, Akiyama K. Affinity of IgE antibody to antigen influences allergen-induced histamine release. *Clin Exp Allergy* 2000; 30: 1582–9.

190 Moneret-Vautrin DA, Gerard H, Grilliat JP. Allergie alimentaire de type immediat: evaluation critique du RAST et du teste degranulation des basophiles. *Nouv Press Med* 1979; 8: 3176.

191 Monro J, Brostoff J, Carini C, Zilkha K. Food allergy in migraine. Study of dietary exclusion and RAST. *Lancet* 1980; ii: 3176.

192 Moro E. Kühmilchpräzipitin im Blute eines 4 1/2 Monate alten Atrophikers. *Munch Med Wochenschr* 1906; 53: 214.

193 Morrow Brown H. Milk allergy and intolerance: clinical aspects. In: *Health Hazards of Milk* (Freed DLJ, ed). Baillière Tindall, Eastbourne; 1984; 92–113.

194 Mullins RJ, Richards C, Walker T. Allergic reactions to oral, surgical and topical bovine collagen. Anaphylactic risk for surgeons. *Austral NZ J Ophthalmol* 1996; 24(3): 257–60.

195 Nakayama T, Aizawa C, Kuno-Sakai H. A clinical analysis of gelatin allergy and determination of its causal relationship to the previous administration of gelatin-containing acellular pertussis vaccine combined with diphtheria and tetanus toxoids. *J Allergy Clin Immunol* 1999; 103: 321–5.

196 Nalebuff DJ. An enthusiastic view of the use of RAST in clinical allergy. *Immunology Allergy Pract* 1981; 3: 18.

197 Nalebuff DJ, Fadal RG. The modified RAST assay: an aid in the diagnosis and management of allergic disorders. *Continuing Education for Family Physicians* 1979; 10: 64.

198 Nalebuff DJ, Fadal RG, Ali M. The study of IgE in the diagnosis of allergic disorders in an otolaryngology practice. *Otolaryngol Head Neck Surg* 1979; 87: 351.

199 Nelson HS. Effect of preservatives and conditions of storage on the potency of allergy extracts. *J Allergy Clin Immunol* 1981; 67: 64–9.

200 Nicklin S, Miller K. Local and systemic immune responses to intestinally presented antigen. *Int Arch Allergy Appl Immunol* 1983; 72: 87–90.

201 Niinimaki A, Hannuksela M. Immediate skin test reactions to spices. *Allergy* 1981; 36: 487–93.

202 Oggell JD, Dockhorn RJ. Staphylococcal protein A and enhancement of disc RAST sensitivity. *Ann Allergy* 1983; 50: 178–81.

203 Ogle KA, Bullock JD. Children with allergic rhinitis and/or bronchial asthma treated with elimination diet: a five year follow-up. *Ann Allergy* 1980; 44: 273–8.

204 O'Mahony CP, Stevens FM, Bourke M *et al.* ^{51}Cr-EDTA test for coeliac disease. *Lancet* 1984; i: 1355.

205 Ormonroyd P, Robertshaw D. A comparison of the Phadebas^R and Phadezym^R IgE paper immunosorbent test kits. *Clin Allergy* 1983; 13: 51–5.

206 Paganelli R, Levinsky RJ. Solid phase radioimmunoassay for detection of circulating food protein antigens in human serum. *J Immunol Meth* 1980; 37: 333–41.

207 Paganelli R, Atherton DJ, Levinsky RJ. Differences between normal and milk allergic subjects in their immune responses after milk ingestion. *Arch Dis Child* 1983; 58: 201–6.

208 Paganelli R, Levinsky RJ, Atherton DJ. Detection of specific antigen within circulating immune complexes. Validation of the assay and its application to food antigen/antibody complexes found in healthy and food-allergic subjects. *Clin Exp Immunol* 1981; 46: 44–53.

209 Paganelli R, Levinsky RJ, Brostoff J, Wraith DG. Immune complexes containing food proteins in normal and atopic subjects after oral challenge and effect of sodium cromoglycate on antigen absorption. *Lancet* 1979; i: 1270–1.

210 Pantin CFA, Merrett TG. The microcomputer as an aid to allergy investigation. *Ann Allergy* 1982; 49: 12–15.

211 Papageorgiou N, Lee TH, Nagakura T *et al.* Neutrophil chemotactic activity in milk-induced asthma. *J Allergy Clin Immunol* 1983; 72: 75–82.

212 Pearson ADJ, Eastham ET, Laker MF *et al.* Intestinal permeability in children with Crohn's disease and coeliac disease. *Br Med J* 1982; 285: 20–1.

213 Pearson DJ, Rix KJB, Bentley SJ. Food allergy: how much in the mind? *Lancet* 1983; i: 1259–61.

214 Pearson DJ, Bentley SJ, Rix KJB, Roberts C. Food hypersensitivity and irritable bowel syndrome. *Lancet* 1983; ii: 746–7.

215 Pecoud A, Bonstein HS, Frei PC. Value of the case history in the diagnosis of allergic state and the detection of allergens. *Clin Allergy* 1983; 13: 141–7.

216 Pecoud A, Ochsner M, Arrendal H, Frei PC. Improvement of the radioallergosorbent test (RAST) sensitivity by using an antibody specific for the determinant D2. *Clin Allergy* 1982; 12: 75–81.

217 Peelmutter L, Bergeron M, Mandy F. Assessment of the effect of IgG antibodies to ragweed and rye grass on the IgE antibody disc RAST. *Ann Allergy* 1983; 50: 393–7.

218 Pitcher-Wilmott RW, Booth I, Harries J, Levinsky PJ. Intestinal absorption of food antigens in coeliac disease. *Arch Dis Child* 1982; 57: 462–6.

219 Prausnitz C, Küstner H. Studies on supersensitivity. *Centralbl f Bakteriol 1 Abt Orig* 1921; 86: 160–9.

220 Radermecker M, Maldague M-P. Depression of neutrophil chemotaxis in atopic individuals: an H_2 histamine receptor response. *Int Arch Allergy Appl Immunol* 1981; 65: 144–52.

221 Rechcigl M (ed). CRC *Handbook of Naturally Occurring Food Toxicants.* CRC Press, Florida, Boca Raton, 1983.

222 Reid MJ, Cheung N-KV, Lewiston NJ: Microtiter solid-phase radioimmunoassay for specific immunoglobulin E. *J Allergy Clin Immunol* 1981; 67: 263–71.

223 Reyes MA, Saravia NG, Watson RR, McMurray DN. Effect of moderate malnutrition on immediate hypersensitivity and immunoglobulin E levels in asthmatic children. *J Allergy Clin Immunol* 1982; 70: 94–100.

224 Ring J, Mathison DA, O'Connor R. In vitro cyclic nucleotide responsiveness in leukocytes and platelets in patients suffering from atopic dermatitis. *Int Arch Allergy Appl Immunol* 1981; 65: 1–7.

225 Rinkel HJ. The leukopenic index in allergic diseases. *J Allergy* 1936; 7: 356.

226 Rinkel HJ, Randolph TG, Zeller M. *Food Allergy.* Charles C. Thomas, Springfield, Illinois, 1951.

227 Roberts SA, Reinhardt MC, Paganelli R, Levinsky J: Specific antigen exclusion and non-specific facilitation of antigen entry across the gut in rats allergic to food proteins. *Clin Exp Immunol* 1981; 45: 131–6.

228 Robertson DM, Paganelli R, Dinwiddie R, Levinsky RJ. Milk antigen absorption in the preterm and term neonate. *Arch Dis Child* 1982; 56: 33–42.

229 Rote NS, Caudle MR. Detection of circulating immune complexes with a Raji cell enzyme immunoassay. *J Immunol Meth* 1983; 56: 33–42.

230 Rubin JL, Griffiths RW, Hill HR. Allergen-induced depression of eutrophil chemotaxis in allergic individuals. *J Allergy Clin Immunol* 1978; 62: 301–8.

231 Ruokonen J, Holopainen E, Palva T, Backman A. Secretory otitis media and allergy with special reference to the cytotoxic leucocyte test. *Allergy* 1981; 36: 59–68.

232 Sakaguchi M, Kaneda G, Inouye S. A case of anaphylaxis to gelatin included in erythropoietin products. *J Allergy Clin Immunol* 1999; 103: 349–50.

233 Sampson H. In vitro diagnosis and mediator assays for food allergies. *Allergy Proc* 1993; 14: 259–61.

234 Sampson HA, Burks AW. Mechanism of food allergy. *Annu Rev Nutr* 1996; 16: 161–77.

235 Sanco J, Egido J, Rivera F, Harnando L. Immune complexes in IgA nephropathy: presence of antibodies in IgA nephropathy: presence of antibodies against diet antigens and delayed clearance of specific polymeric IgA immune complexes. *Clin Exp Immunol* 1983; 54: 194–202.

236 Saperstein S, Anderson DW Jr, Goldman AS, Kniker WT. Milk allergy. III. Immunological studies with sera from allergic and normal children. *Pediatrics* 1963; 32: 580–7.

237 Savilahti E. Cow's milk allergy. *Allergy* 1981; 36: 73–88.

238 Savilahti E, Pelkonen P, Visakorpi JK. IgA deficiency in children. A clinical study with special reference to intestinal findings. *Arch Dis Child* 1971; 46: 665–70.

239 Savilahti E, Viander M, Perkkiö M *et al*. IgA anti-gliadin antibodies: a marker of mucosal damage in childhood coeliac disease. *Lancet* 1983; i: 320–2.

240 Scheinmann P, Gendrel D, Charles J, Paupe J. Value of lymphoblast transformation test on cow's milk protein intestinal intolerance. *Clin Allergy* 1976; 6: 515–21.

241 Schenner S, Wangorsch A, Haustein D, Vieths S. Cloning of the major allergen Api g4 profilin from celery (*Apium graveolens*) and its cross-reactivity with birch pollen profilin Bet v2. *Clin Exp Allergy* 2000; 30: 962–71.

242 Schwartz HR, Nerurkar LS, Spies JR *et al*. Milk hypersensitivity: RAST studies using new antigen-generated by pepsin hydrolysis of beta-lactoglobulin. *Ann Allergy* 1980; 45: 242–5.

243 Scott ML, Thornley MJ, Coombs RRA. Comparison of red-cell linked anti IgE and ^{125}I-labelled anti IgE in a solid-phase system for the measurement of IgE specific for castor bean allergen. *Int Arch Allergy Appl Immunol* 1981; 64: 230–5.

244 Sepulveda R, Longbottom JL, Pepys J. Enzyme-linked immunosorbent assay (ELISA) for IgG and IgE antibodies to protein and polysaccharide antigens of *Aspergillus fumigatus*. *Clin Allergy* 1979; 9: 359–71.

245 Shibasaki M, Suzuki S, Nemoto H, Kuroume T. Allergenicity and lympho-stimulating property of rice protein. *J Allergy Clin Immunol* 1979; 64: 259–65.

246 Shurkovich S, Shurkovich B, Bellanti JA, Banergee DK. Interferon increases IgE binding to basophils. *Ann Allergy* 1983; 50: 505–8.

247 Sikora K, Anand BS, Truelove SC, Ciclitira PJ. Stimulation of lymphocytes from patients with coeliac disease by a subfraction of gluten. *Lancet* 1976; ii: 389–91.

248 Silverstone GA. Possible sources of food toxicants: plants, some foods of animal origin, microorganisms, food additives. In: *Diet-Related Diseases: The Modern Epidemic* (Seely S, Freed DLJ, Silverstone GA, Rippere V, eds). Croom Helm, London, (in press).

249 Soifer MM, Hirsch SR. The direct basophil degranulation test and the intracutaneous test: a comparison using food extracts. *J Allergy Clin Immunol* 1975; 56: 127–32.

250 Solomon BA. The ALCAT test – a guide and barometer in the therapy of environmental and food sensitivities. *Environ Med* 1992; 9: 54–9.

251 Spengler GA, Weber R-M. Interactions of PHA and human normal serum proteins. Lectins. *Biol Biochem Clin Biochem*, Vol. I, 1981; 231–40.

252 Squier TL, Lee HJ: Lysis in vitro of sensitized leukocytes by ragweed antigen. *J Allergy* 1947; 18: 156–63.

253 Stempel DA, Davis VL, Morissey LJ, Helms RW. Seasonal variations of serum IgE levels in normal children. *Ann Allergy* 1981; 47: 14–16.

254 Stenback EI. The influence of human plasma lipoproteins and fatty acids in immunological reactions. *Allergy* 1984; 39: 1–11.

255 Stoddart RW. The generation of cancer: irritation, promotion, progression and the multiple influences of the environment. *Nutr Health* 1983; 2: 153–62.

256 Strannegard O, Strannegard IL. In vitro differences between the lymphocytes of normal subjects and atopics. *Clin Allergy* 1979; 9: 637–43.

257 Strong FC III. Why do some dietary migraine patients claim they get headaches from placebos? *Clin Exp Allergy* 2000; 30: 739–43.

258 Subba Rao PV, McCartney-Francis NL, Metcalfe DD. An avidin-biotin micro ELISA for rapid measurement of total and allergen-specific human IgE. *J Immunol Meth* 1983; 57: 71–85.

259 Sutton R, Hill DJ, Baldo BA, Wrigley CW. Immunoglobulin E antibodies to ingested cereal flour components: studies with sera from subjects with asthma and eczema. *Clin Allergy* 1982; 12: 63–74.

260 Taylor B, Fergusson DM, Mahoney GN *et al*. Specific IgA and IgE in childhood asthma, eczema and food allergy. *Clin Allergy* 1982; 12: 499–505.

261 Truelove SC, Jewell DP. The intestine in allergic diseases. In: *Clinical Aspects of Immunology* (Gell PGH, Coombs RRA, Lachman PJ, eds). Blackwell, Oxford, 1975; 1441–65.

262 Turner MW, Paganelli R, Levinsky RJ, Williams A. Antigen-binding radioimmunoassays for human IgG antibodies to bovine-lactoglobulin. *J Immunol Meth* 1983; 56: 175–83.

263 Ulett GA, Perry SG. Cytotoxic testing and leucocyte increase as an index to food sensitivity. *Ann Allergy* 1974; 33: 23–32.

264 Unsworth DJ, Kieffer M, Holborow EK *et al*. IgA anti-gliadin antibodies in coeliac disease. *Clin Exp Immunol* 1981; 46: 286–93.

265 Unsworth DJ, Manuel PD, Walker-Smith JA *et al*. A new immunofluorescent blood test for gluten sensitivity. *Arch Dis Child* 1981; 46(2): 864–8.

266 Updegraff TR. Food allergy and cytotoxic tests. *Ear Nose Throat J* 1977; 56: 450–9.

267 Valverde E, Vich JM, Garcia-Calderon JV, Garcia-Calderon PA. In vitro response of lymphocytes in patients with allergic tension-fatigue syndrome. *Ann Allergy* 1980; 45: 185–8.

268 Valverde E, Vich JM, Garcia-Calderon JV, Garcia-Calderon PA. In vitro stimulation of lymphocytes in patients with chronic urticaria induced by additives and food. *Clin Allergy* 1980; 10: 691–8.

269 Van der Woude FJ, Hoedemaeker PhJ, Van der Giessen M *et al*. Do food antigens play a role in the pathogenesis of some cases of human glomerulonephritis? *Clin Exp Immunol* 1983; 51: 587–94.

270 van Toorenenbergen AW, Kramps JA, van der Burgh JF, Dijkman JH. Use of automatic counting of basophil leukocytes: correlation of basophil degranulation with histamine release. *J Immunol Meth* 1982; 49: 209–13.

271 Vaughn. Food allergens III: the leucopenic index preliminary report. *J Allergy* 1934; 5: 601.

272 Verkasalo MA. Adherence of gliadin fractions to lymphocytes in coeliac disease. *Lancet* 1982; i: 389–91.

273 Vervloet D, Bongrand P, Charpin J. Absolute determination of IgE antibodies to grass pollen allergens. *Allergy* 1978; 33: 203–10.

274 Viscidi R, Laughton BE, Hanvanich M *et al*. Improved enzyme immunoassays for the detection of antigens in fecal specimens. Investigation and correction of interfering factors. *J Immunol Meth* 1984; 67: 129–43.

275 Wahn U, Herold U, Danielsen K, Lowenstein H. Allergoprints in horse allergic children. *Allergy* 1982; 37: 335–43.

276 Walzer M. Allergy of the abdominal organs. *J Lab Clin Med* 1941; 26: 1867.

277 Warner JO, Hathaway MJ. Allergic form of Meadow's syndrome (Munchausen by proxy). *Arch Dis Child* 1984; 59: 151–6.

278 Warren CPW, Holford-Strevens V, Wong C, Manfreda J. The relationship between smoking and total immunoglobulin E levels. *J Allergy Clin Immunol* 1982; 69: 370–5.

279 Weaver LT, Laker MF, Nelson R. Enhanced intestinal permeability in preterm babies with bloody stools. *Arch Dis Child* 1984; 59: 280–1.

280 Weaver LT, Laker MF, Nelson R. Intestinal permeability in the newborn. *Arch Dis Child* 1984; 59: 236–41.

281 Wide L, Bennich H, Johansson SGO. Diagnosis of allergy by an in vitro test for allergen antibodies. *Lancet* 1967; ii: 1105–7.

282 Wilson N, Vickers H, Taylor G, Silverman M. Objective test for food sensitivity in asthmatic children: increased bronchial reactivity after cola drinks. *Br Med J* 1982; 284: 1226–8.

283 Wojnar RJ, Hearn T, Starkweather MS. Augmentation of allergic histamine release from human leucocytes by NSAI – analgesic agent. *J Allergy Clin Immunol* 1980; 66: 37–45.

284 Wraith DG, Merrett J, Roth A *et al*. Recognition of food-allergic patients and their allergens by the RAST technique and clinical investigation. *Clin Allergy* 1979; 9: 25–36.

285 York Alternative Medical Practice. *Physician's Cytotoxic Handbook: Explanatory Literature*.

286 Zeiss CR, Grammer LC, Levitz D. Comparison of the RAST and a quantitative solid-phase RIA for the detection of ragweed-specific immunoglobulin E antibody in patients undergoing immunotherapy. *J Allergy Clin Immunol* 1981; 67: 105–10.

287 Zetterström O, Ohman S, Nilson G, Dreborg S. Stability of freeze-dried and reconstituted Timothy pollen allergen extract and hymenoptera venoms reconstituted in saline with and without albumin. *Allergy* 1982; 37: 25.

288 Zetterström O, Osterman K, Machado L, Johansson SGO. Another smoking hazard: raised serum IgE concentration and increased risk of occupational allergy. *Br Med J* 1981; 283: 1215–17.

Diagnosis of gastrointestinal food-allergic diseases in childhood

A. D. Phillips and J. A. Walker-Smith

INTRODUCTION

Various approaches have been addressed to the problem of diagnosis of gastrointestinal food allergic disease. As described in Chapter 42, the types of adverse reaction can be broadly divided into quick and slow onset following food ingestion. The quick-onset reactions are relatively easy to recognize, whereas the slow-onset reactions are difficult to diagnose; hence the search for reliable and practical objective diagnostic tests. So far the gastrointestinal tests which have been employed in the diagnosis of the slow-onset reactions have been based either on proximal small intestinal biopsy, colonic biopsy or on tests of gut function (Table 62.1).

Gastrointestinal tests employed in the diagnosis of gastrointestinal food-allergic disease
Upper endoscopy
Small intestinal biopsy
Light microscopy
Morphometry
Electron microscopy
Mucosal immunoglobulins
Disaccharidase estimation
Intestinal permeability
Breath hydrogen test
Colonoscopy
Colonic biopsy

Table 62.1 Gastrointestinal tests employed in the diagnosis of gastrointestinal food-allergic disease.

Cow's milk and cow's milk-based formulae are the major offenders in the first years of life. When soy formulas are used to treat cow's milk allergy, sensitization to soy may occur. Proteins in eggs, nuts, fish and cereals have all been described as eliciting immunoglobulin E (IgE)-mediated gastrointestinal food allergy, often accompanied with skin symptoms, but they can also cause small intestinal mucosal damage on occasion.

CLINICAL CRITERIA FOR DIAGNOSIS

An absolute and essential first criterion for the diagnosis of gastrointestinal food allergy must be a response to a food elimination diet. This response will include clinical and laboratory observations.[70]

A second criterion for diagnosis is a positive food challenge, but this is not always essential for routine clinical practice. Food challenge is not required when the characteristic clinicopathological diagnostic features are present at initial diagnosis. These include chronic diarrhoea with failure to thrive, in association with the biopsy findings of partial, often patchy, villous atrophy, accompanied by a thin mucosa and a moderate rise in intraepithelial lymphocyte count.[43,64] The need for challenge in children with gastrointestinal food allergy will depend upon the individual clinical syndrome. ESPGAN has made recommendations for diagnostic criteria.[59]

Clinical diagnosis
Response to an elimination diet

In each category a response to an elimination diet is essential. In children with multiple food allergies, however, this may be incomplete. Typically, there should be relief of all symptoms, gain in weight and normal growth.

Response to a food challenge

The diagnosis can only be definitely established in each category at present by a food challenge. In the past when there was scepticism about the existence of gastrointestinal food allergy, strict diagnostic criteria, such as the Goldman criteria[17] using three challenges under clinical control, were demanded. This is no longer necessary or practical in the 1990s for routine diagnosis, especially in small infants when there may be a risk of acute anaphylaxis.

In older children with multiple food allergy, placebo-controlled food challenges may be necessary, but these should not be done in infancy.

Diagnosis of quick-onset allergy

There is usually a clear history of symptoms in association with food ingestion. There is relief of symptoms on withdrawal of the offending food and rapid return on challenge. Symptoms include acute vomiting, facial urticaria, lip swelling and sometimes wheezing and acute diarrhoea.

Laboratory diagnosis

In early infancy and especially in breast-fed babies who develop acute cow's milk allergy, the presence of a specific elevation of IgE antibodies to cow's milk and a specifically positive radioallergosorbent test (RAST) or skin-prick test to cow's milk may be diagnostically valuable. The usefulness of skin-prick and patch testing for the diagnosis of cow's milk allergy was studied in 193 Finnish children aged between 2 and 36 months, who then underwent either double-blind placebo controlled or open cow's milk challenge. Prick tests were positive in 67% of infants with quick-onset reactions to cow's milk when patch tests were largely negative. Patch tests were positive in 87% of infants who had delayed eczematous reactions to cow's milk, while skin-prick tests were often negative. Small intestinal mucosal changes were not studied.[24] A positive skin-prick test for egg in children with egg allergy is diagnostically useful. Its persistence usually means continuing intolerance to egg, although antigen-specific IgE antibodies may persist when the child has lost all evidence of clinical sensitivity.[14]

In older children such investigations may reveal the presence of several positive skin-prick tests and RAST tests not only to foods but also to inhaled antigens and so indicate an atopic tendency rather than specific food allergy.

Diagnosis of food allergy associated with gastrointestinal pathology

Initial diagnosis concerns investigation of infants with chronic diarrhoea, usually with failure to thrive. Sometimes infants with failure to thrive, and older children with gastrointestinal symptoms including rectal bleeding, have been investigated either by a small bowel biopsy or colonoscopy with multiple biopsies. The pathological features revealed by these biopsies demonstrate pathology that has the features of gastrointestinal food allergy.

This chapter primarily concentrates therefore on the diagnosis of gastrointestinal milk hypersensitivity, since the majority of studies have dealt with this food. Other foods will be mentioned as appropriate.

UPPER ENDOSCOPY

Some children with a history of gastro-oesophageal reflux and/or abdominal pain have been implicated as having cow's milk allergy.[5,15] The diagnosis has been based on the presence of oesophagitis, positive β-lactoglobulin serum antibody and a clinical response to cow's milk elimination. The use of the β-lactoglobulin antibody ELISA (enzyme-linked immunosorbent assay) has also been used in children with small intestinal evidence of cow's milk allergy, i.e. cow's milk-sensitive enteropathy.

SMALL INTESTINAL BIOPSY

Light microscopy

The diagnostic role of small intestinal biopsy for cow's milk-sensitive enteropathy has evolved with time. The first observation made with this technique was that cow's milk protein could produce severe small intestinal mucosal damage in young infants who were failing to thrive. This relationship between cow's milk protein and mucosal damage was recognized by means of serial biopsies taken before and after milk provocation[33,67] and led to the recognition of cow's milk-sensitive enteropathy as a definite diagnostic entity.[71] It has been suggested that evidence of small intestinal mucosal damage should be included in the criteria for the routine diagnosis of all cases of gastrointestinal cow's milk allergy in infancy,[26] but this is not generally practicable. However it is essential in children with failure to thrive. Also, biopsies have established that histological damage following cow's milk ingestion does not always lead to the development of clinical symptoms[58,61] and, conversely, not all children with gastrointestinal symptoms that are clearly produced by cow's milk ingestion have recognizable small intestinal mucosal damage.[16,22]

Food-induced small intestinal mucosal damage

There are conflicting reports on the incidence and degree of small intestinal mucosal damage following cow's milk challenge, ranging from 0 to 100% of patients studied (Table 62.2). Some variables which may explain these differences are as follows:

1. Time and the type of allergic reaction induced in the gut are important. Time is needed for histological damage to occur after cow's milk ingestion in those with a slow-onset reaction and the degree of damage may depend upon the amount of time elapsed following milk ingestion. Mucosal changes have been seen within the first 24 hours,[60,61] and after several weeks[58] of continuing milk ingestion. More often they occur within 24–48 hours.[68] With quick-onset reactions usually only small amounts of milk can be taken because either it is rapidly vomited, or serious reactions preclude further drinking. This gives little opportunity for mucosal damage to occur. However, from experimental studies in animals it appears that minimal histological changes would be seen.[10] Thus, normal mucosa may be present with quick-onset reactions. However, both type I and IV reactions may coincide.

2. The degree of mucosal damage may relate to the amount of milk ingested. In the first reports of cow's milk-induced mucosal damage,[35] infants had had prolonged exposure to milk and showed severe mucosal damage. Later studies,[22] with biopsies performed at the onset of symptoms when relatively little milk had been

Light microscopy mucosal changes in gastrointestinal milk allergy				
Authors	**Symptomatic patients**		**Biopsy timing***	**Number (%) of abnormal biopsies**
	Number	**Age range**		
Kuitunen et al.[32]	6	2–4 months	Varied	6 (100%)
Walker-Smith et al.[71]	5	0–3 months	24 hours	5 (100%)
Iyngkaran et al.[27]	7‡	0–3 months	24 hours	7 (100%)
Kuitunen et al.[35]	48	0–9 months	When symptomatic	47 (98%)
Fontaine & Navarro[11]	31	3–7 months	Varied	30 (97%)
Silver & Douglas[62]	3	2–4 months	NS†	2 (66%)
Shiner et al.[60,61]	6	5–8 months	6–23 hours	4§ (66%)
Freier et al.[16]	6	0–3 months	NS	2 (33%)
Hill et al.[22]	9	7–17 months	At onset of symptoms	3 (33%)
Lubos et al.[39]	18	3 months to 8 years	NS	0 (0%)

* Time elapsed from cow's milk ingestion to small bowel biopsy.
† NS = not stated.
‡ Four other children had moderate changes but no symptoms.
§ Two of these children were asymptomatic.

Table 62.2 Light microscopy mucosal changes in gastrointestinal milk allergy.

given, reported both a lower incidence and a decreased severity of mucosal damage.

3. Age and nutritional status are likely to influence the degree of small bowel mucosal damage. With increasing age, an increased tolerance to milk is seen, and mucosal damage may be more limited. This may explain the lack of mucosal damage in the older group of patients studied by Lubos et al.[39] In children with a poor nutritional status, as in some of the earlier studies, mucosal damage may be modified by the associated depression of the immune and inflammatory response.

4. Coincidental gastrointestinal infection and parasitic infestation (mostly giardiasis) must be carefully excluded. In fact, cow's milk-sensitive enteropathy and post-enteritis enteropathy may overlap and may be difficult to distinguish between.

5. Technical details of the biopsy – the numbers of samples taken, the orientation and interpretation of the section – and application of quantitative techniques must be also taken into consideration when evaluating the literature on this subject.

6. The selection of the patients in the above studies was varied. In some studies only those patients who had less severe small intestinal mucosal damage were studied.

Small intestinal biopsy on its own is not a specific test for gastrointestinal food allergy, but it plays a useful diagnostic role in detecting gastrointestinal food allergy, especially in infants less than 1 year old. Its main value has been to establish unequivocally, by means of serial biopsies with dietary challenge, that a number of foods – namely, soya,[1] chicken meat, ground rice, fish[66] and eggs[25] – may all temporarily damage the small intestinal mucosa, thus introducing the concept of food-sensitive enteropathy. However, it is clear that a normal small intestinal mucosa may be found in some children with clinical gastrointestinal food allergy.

Morphometry

In addition to histological evaluation of the small intestinal mucosa by light microscopy, accurate measurements of tissue dimensions and cell numbers can be made, providing a quantitative, objective assessment of small bowel appearance. This technique of quantitative morphometry has been applied to the mucosa of children with cow's milk-sensitive enteropathy.[31,54,63] When on a milk-containing diet the mucosa is thinner than in normal controls, with crypt depth lengthening, shortening of the villi and reduction of epithelial cell height (Table 62.3).[43] The numbers of intraepithelial lymphocytes are increased in the untreated disease. When treated with a cow's milk-free diet, their numbers diminish to below normal levels, and on challenge rise to within the normal range.[55]

This mucosal lesion is mild in comparison to that seen in coeliac disease.

Morphometric changes in the intestinal mucosa in milk-sensitive enteropathy
Thin mucosa
Crypt lengthening
Villus shortening
Epithelial cell height reduced
Intraepithelial lymphocytes increased

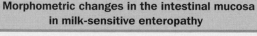

Fig. 62.3 Morphometric changes in the intestinal mucosa in milk-sensitive enteropathy.

Electron microscopy

This technique gives greatly improved resolution, allowing study of cellular detail, but no specific abnormalities have been detected. Shortened microvilli and increased lysosomal bodies are seen in the epithelium and increased collagen deposition may be apparent in the basement membrane.[33,60]

Electron microscopy can be particularly useful in excluding acute viral infection, which can be misinterpreted as an acute reaction to milk. Rapid stool virology using negative-staining electron microscopy is of more practical value than ultrastructure of a biopsy specimen and may indeed postpone a small intestinal biopsy in the situation where a child develops a nosocomial infection.

Mucosal immunoglobulins

Immunoglobulins can be demonstrated in the gastrointestinal mucosa by immunofluorescence and immunoperoxidase-staining techniques (see Chapter 8), but there is conflicting evidence over the classes of antibodies that are involved in the immune response in children with gastrointestinal cow's milk allergy (Table 62.4).

Shiner et al.[60,61] presented evidence that an IgE-mediated reaction occurs within the first 24 hours of milk challenge, followed by mast cell degranulation. No changes were found in the numbers of IgA plasma cells, but IgM and IgE plasma cells were increased.

An increase in IgE-producing plasma cells was also demonstrated in children with colic related to cow's milk ingestion,[19] although no diarrhoea was present.

Increases of IgA-producing plasma cells have been found by others,[29,58,70] as well as some elevation of IgM-producing plasma cells. Small bowel biopsies in these studies were performed after a longer (several days) exposure to milk and the increased mucosal IgA levels were reflected by increased IgA levels in serum and faeces. This increase in IgA plasma cells is likely to be a morphological response of the small intestine to damage and not a primary abnormality.[46]

Disaccharidase estimation

Disaccharidases are the enzymes, situated on the brush border of the small intestine, hydrolyse disaccharides into their component monosaccharides. The disaccharidase activity of the mucosa is usually depressed when there is mucosal damage. Lactase activity appears to be the most vulnerable of the disaccharidase activities.

Adverse gastrointestinal reactions to cow's milk protein may result in damage to the small bowel mucosa, which in turn may cause secondary lactase depression. The degree of lactase depression in children with milk-sensitive enteropathy varies from 0 to 100% and this appears to be closely related to the extent of mucosal damage (Table 62.5). Poley et al.[57] found mucosal abnormalities and lactase depression in all their patients, while Lubos et al.[39] found none.

Although, generally, the degree of lactase depression seems to correspond to the amount of intestinal mucosal damage, Harrison & Walker-Smith[21] found that in individual patients the levels of lactase did not necessarily closely correlate with mucosal morphology.

Lactose intolerance may play an important part in the symptoms of children with cow's milk protein intolerance. It has been clearly demonstrated that, although cow's milk protein alone can cause adverse gastrointestinal symptoms in milk-allergic infants, these symptoms of diarrhoea, abdominal pain and irritability can be potentiated by the addition of lactose.[37] Harrison et al.[20] found both lactase depression and a degree of lactose malabsorption in the majority of their milk-hypersensitive children after milk challenge. McNeish[40] has suggested that lactose malabsorption may be common in milk allergy, but that frank clinical lactose intolerance was probably uncommon.

Challenge tests *in vitro*

The technology is available to keep small intestinal biopsy tissue growing in tissue culture medium for several days or weeks.[29] It is therefore theoretically possible to challenge the small bowel

Immunoglobulin mucosal changes in gastrointestinal cow's milk allergy							
Authors	Number	Patient age	Biopsy timing*	Immunoglobulin-producing plasma cells[†]			
				IgG	IgA	IgM	IgE
Shiner et al.[60,61]	4	5–8 months	6–23 hours	+	–	++	++
Kilby et al.[30]	2	2–4 months	4–6 days	ND[‡]	ND	ND	++
Harris et al.[19]	7	2–6 months	NS[§]	–	–	–	++
Savilahti[58]	8	2–8 months	2–24 days	–	+++	+	–
Jos[29]	7	NS	NS	–	++	+/–	ND
Maffei et al.[42]	10	2–20 months	NS	ND	++	–	ND
Stern et al.[63]	10	9 months, mean	NS	++	++	++	++

* Time elapsed from cow's milk challenge to small bowel biopsy.
† Increase in numbers of immunoglobulin-producing plasma cells: – = no change, +/– = variable, + = slight, ++ = moderate, +++ = marked.
‡ ND = not done.
§ NS = not stated.

Fig. 62.4 Immunoglobulin mucosal changes in gastrointestinal cow's milk allergy.

Lactase levels in gastrointestinal cow's milk allergy					
Authors	Number	Patient's age	Abnormal biopsies	Reduced lactase	Reduced sucrase
Lubos et al.[39]	18	3 months to 8 years	0 (0%)	0 (0%)	NS*
Hill et al.[22]	8	8–16 months	3 (30%)	2 (25%)	NS
Iyngkaran et al.[26]	18	1–12 months	18 (100%)	17 (94%)	17 (94%)
Poley et al.[57]	7	1–11 months	7 (100%)	7 (100%)	7 (100%)
* NS = not stated.					

Table 62.5 Lactase levels in gastrointestinal cow's milk allergy.

mucosa *in vitro* with suspected foods and observe any subsequent tissue damage. This type of procedure has been applied in coeliac disease.[29] However, great caution is needed when extrapolating these results to the clinical condition *in vivo*. This technique can still only be viewed as a research tool.

GUT FUNCTION TESTS

Other methods have been used to try and measure the effects of food upon the function of the small intestinal mucosa. In principle, the integrity of the small bowel can be assessed by its ability to absorb various substances and the tests used to determine changes in permeability will be discussed.

Intestinal permeability
The differential absorption of two or more inert sugars appears to be a useful test of intestinal permeability and, indirectly, a reflection of mucosal integrity. A major advantage of this technique is that by expressing the urinary excretion of the sugars as a ratio, the effects of the many variables influencing the individual sugar probes can be overcome. These variables include the adequacy of ingesting the oral load, gastric emptying time, intestinal transit time, the dilution of the marker by intestinal secretions, renal clearance and the completeness of the urine collection. The disadvantages are the difficulty in collecting any urine in small children with diarrhoea and the complexity of the assay. Sugar permeability of a combination of lactulose and mannitol or lactulose and rhamnose are most often used in practice.

Lactulose and rhamnose
After an overnight fast of at least 6 hours, an isotonic load containing 3.5 g lactulose and 0.5 g rhamnose in 50 ml is given by mouth. All urine passed in the subsequent 5 hours is collected, the volume recorded and an aliquot, preserved with Merthiolate (thimerosal), is kept at –20°C until analysis. Stored in this way, it remains stable for many months. Urinary concentrations of each sugar are measured by quantitative thin-layer chromotography. Results are expressed as a ratio of the percentages of the oral sugar loads excreted in the 5-hour urine collection.[13] The lactulose : rhamnose ratio is normally less than 0.08.

In general, abnormal intestinal permeability is associated with mucosal damage of the small intestine and this investigation can be used as a screen for mucosal damage. Occasionally, abnormal permeability can occur in the presence of a normal mucosa.[51]

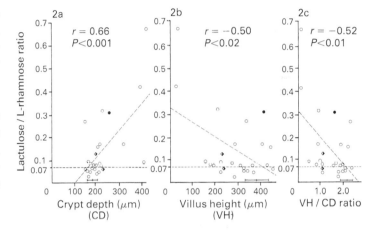

Fig. 62.1 Relationship between intestinal permeability and proximal small bowel morphology.

In a study using lactulose and mannitol, Sullivan et al.[61] found that although in general there is a correlation between morphology and permeability, there was not a direct quantitative correction between small intestinal mucosal damage, assessed by morphometry, and lactulose–mannitol absorption. Normally, the urinary lactulose : mannitol ratio should be less than 0.008.

Also using lactulose and mannitol, Andre et al.[2] have shown that in patients with food allergy there is a decrease in mannitol recovery and an increase in lactulose recovery after ingestion of the offending food allergen, thereby indicating the value of this test in the challenge situation. Oral sodium cromoglycate, administered before a food provocation test in patients with gastrointestinal food allergy, protected against the development of abnormal intestinal permeability.

Permeability of the small intestinal mucosa to lactulose and rhamnose has been shown to be altered in young children with iron deficiency.[3] There is a lower urinary recovery of rhamnose, which passes across the epithelium via the transcellular route, but normal recovery of lactulose, which passes through a paracellular route. Permeability returns to normal when a normal iron status is achieved. Thus, iron status must be taken into account when interpreting results of permeability studies.

These tests of differential sugar absorption therefore appear to have potential in the investigation and diagnosis of small intestinal mucosal abnormality in childhood because they are non-invasive and should give an objective measurement of significant changes in the integrity of the intestinal mucosa; their precise role in diagnosis still awaits clarification. They cannot by themselves replace small intestinal biopsy, although in centres where this test is available and biopsy is not, sugar permeability provides a useful screen and may be a useful test for diagnosis of food allergy with small intestinal mucosal change.

The other techniques available to measure intestinal permeability have serious drawbacks. The ^{51}Cr-labelled EDTA (ethylenediaminetetraacetic acid) method[4] uses only one probe molecule and this loses the advantage of the differential absorption technique. It is dependent upon a radioisotope, and thus is not suitable for regular or repeated use in children. It also requires an accurate 24-hour urine collection, which is not practicable for routine use with children. The other method is based on the differential absorption of polyethylene glycol (PEG) fractions[6] which also requires a 24-hour urine collection. In addition, the smaller fractions of PEG are lipid soluble, and thus its absorption is not only a function of its permeability.[49]

COLONIC BIOPSY

Those infants and children who have chronic bloody diarrhoea require colonoscopy with multiple colonic mucosal biopsies. The colonoscopic features of cow's milk-sensitive colitis are erythema, friability of the mucosa and sometimes ulceration. This appearance is not specific and it needs to be distinguished from inflammatory bowel disease.[7]

Multiple mucosal biopsies taken at the time of colonoscopy characteristically show an eosinophilic infiltration of the mucosa,[27] although Gryboski[18] describes changes not unlike ulcerative colitis. Cow's milk, soya protein and probably other foods can produce such a colitis.

DIAGNOSTIC APPROACH TO GASTROINTESTINAL FOOD ALLERGY

We have discussed the techniques that are presently available to assess the gastrointestinal status of a patient in relation to gastrointestinal food-allergic disease. Many of these tests may be impracticable for routine use, may not be reliable or may not yet have been sufficiently validated to be worthwhile. We therefore present our approach to the child presenting with possible gastrointestinal food-allergic disease.[70]

Quick-onset reactions
Children with quick-onset reactions to foods are usually not a diagnostic problem, as the symptoms are usually florid and closely associated with the ingestion of a particular food. The children are usually atopic and investigations show an elevated total IgE. Also the response to skin-prick test and RAST are positive. The approach to these children is discussed in Chapter 42.

Slow-onset reactions
Food-sensitive enteropathy
This diagnosis should be suspected in a child with chronic diarrhoea and poor weight gain. Food-allergic disease is only one of a number of causes for such a clinical picture, many of which can be identified by small intestinal biopsy (see Table 62.6). A scheme for approaching this problem is given in Fig. 62.2. This is most important when a child is under 2 years of age.

Conditions causing chronic diarrhoea and poor growth which may be distinguished from food-sensitive enteropathy by small intestinal biopsy
Coeliac disease
Giardiasis
Sucrase–isomaltase deficiency
Lactase deficiency
A β-lipoproteinaemia
Lymphangiectasia
Hypogammaglobulinaemia
Cystic fibrosis
Autoimmune enteropathy
Microvillous atrophy

Table 62.6 Conditions causing chronic diarrhoea and poor growth which may be distinguished from food-sensitive enteropathy by small intestinal biopsy.

Small intestinal biopsy is most helpful when performed at the presentation of the illness when the child is still on the original diet. If the child has an enteropathy, i.e. a light microscopic abnormality, then the major diagnostic decision is between coeliac disease and food-sensitive enteropathy, although other conditions must be considered (Table 62.7). It is therefore of paramount importance to determine whether or not the child has been taking gluten in the diet.

Flat mucosa, on gluten
If gluten has been taken and the biopsy appears uniformly damaged, and there is a high intraepithelial lymphocyte count, then coeliac disease is the most likely diagnosis and a gluten-free diet should be implemented. However, if there is no response to this diet, then the elimination of other foods should be considered, as a small number of children with coeliac disease may subsequently develop sensitivities to other food proteins.[11] Where there is a positive clinical response to a gluten-free diet, it is necessary to perform serial biopsies while off and on gluten to confirm the diagnosis.[47]

Transient gluten intolerance
There are now clear criteria for the scientific diagnosis of 'transient gluten intolerance'. These are, first, the need to provide

Conditions in which an enteropathy is found
Coeliac disease
Food-sensitive enteropathy
Giardiasis
Gastroenteritis and post-enteritis enteropathy
Tropical sprue
Acquired hypogammaglobulinaemia
Microvillous atropy
Autoimmune enteropathy

Table 62.7 Conditions in which an enteropathy is found.

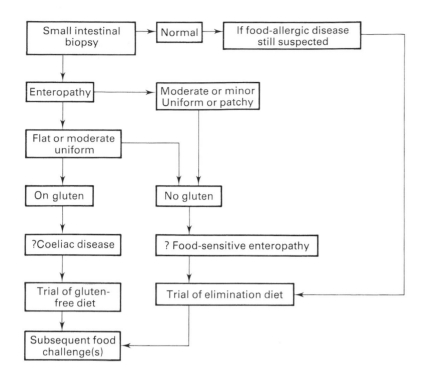

Fig. 62.2 Diagnostic approach to the investigation of possible food-sensitive enteropathy.

evidence that gluten toxicity was in fact present and that the apparent response to gluten restriction was not fortuitous.[41] In practice this is very difficult to do. Second, is the need to show the presence of a normal small intestinal mucosa 2 years or more after the return to a normal gluten-containing diet. A retrospective diagnosis of transient gluten intolerance can be made when a child with features of an abnormal mucosa previously has responded to a gluten-free diet but after 2 years on a normal diet has a normal mucosa. However, reports of the delayed relapse of coeliac disease after more than 2 years on a gluten-containing diet make the final diagnosis of transient gluten intolerance very difficult.[55]

Mucosal damage, no gluten

If there is an enteropathy that is not uniformly flat, then this is more likely to be caused by food sensitivity, but similar appearances occur in post-enteritis enteropathy. This type of mucosal damage is characteristically patchy.[44] Most children presenting in this way are in their first 6 months of life and not taking gluten. A trial elimination diet, usually avoiding cow's milk, is then indicated. If there is a positive clinical response, then it is best to proceed on the elimination diet until the age of 18 months, when milk can usually be safely reintroduced into the diet.

Mucosal damage with gluten

Finding a patchy thin enteropathy in a child taking gluten is unlikely to be coeliac disease. Such findings are typical of food-sensitive or post-enteritis enteropathy.

Normal mucosa

If there is no enteropathy, this does not necessarily exclude the possibility of food-allergic disease. If other conditions have been excluded and food is still suspected as causing the symptoms, then the only practical approach is an empirical trial of an elimination diet. Again, milk is the most commonly implicated food, but other foods may be incriminated by a carefully taken dietary history. Indeed, this is more typical of multiple food allergy. If there is a clinical response to such an elimination diet, then food provocation is needed to confirm the diagnosis.

Response to elimination diet

Once a child is seen with the clinical and biopsy features of cow's milk-sensitive enteropathy, a milk protein-free diet should be commenced. This should be a protein hydrolysate. A soy formula is not recommended as children may become intolerant to soy, developing a soy-sensitive enteropathy in at least 15% of cases.[53] There should be a rapid symptomatic response to cow's milk-free diet, i.e. relief of diarrhoea and gain in weight, with histological evidence (at some point) of morphological improvement of the small intestinal mucosa on the elimination diet.

The ESPGAN Working Group on diagnostic criteria for food allergy with predominantly intestinal symptoms[59] has recommended that morphological studies of the gastrointestinal tract are indicated in two clinical situations:

- infants with chronic diarrhoea and failure to thrive in which food-sensitive intestinal enteropathy is possible
- infants with rectal bleeding in which food allergy is suspected.

In the former situation, small intestinal biopsy is indicated and in the latter, colonoscopy with biopsy. Such a biopsy has a diagnostic role for food-sensitive or food-allergic colitis.[68]

Food-sensitive colitis

Children with chronic bloody diarrhoea require colonoscopy with multiple colonic mucosal biopsies; such clinical features suggest chronic inflammatory bowel disease, but can occur in food-sensitive colitis.

Diagnosis of cow's milk colitis

These infants typically have bloody diarrhoea or rectal bleeding[9] but are well nourished and not failing to thrive. There may be an association with atopic disease.[28] It occurs in early infancy in bottle-fed infants and in breast-fed infants whose mother is drinking cow's milk.

Infection with *Campylobacter* and *Shigella* must be excluded. The definitive diagnostic investigation is endoscopy and biopsy. The major differential diagnosis is chronic inflammatory bowel disease (usually ulcerative colitis). Characteristically, there is a dense infiltration of eosinophils in an otherwise normal mucosa, although non-specific inflammatory changes have also been described.

The second step in diagnosis is to demonstrate a complete relief of symptoms on an elimination diet (which should include the mother if the child is breast-fed, when breast-feeding can be continued), i.e. cessation of rectal bleeding. With recognition of this syndrome, an early diagnostic milk challenge is not essential routinely.

Some clinicians will elect to do a follow-up endoscopy and biopsy, others will not. Usually an early cow's milk challenge is best avoided and delayed until the age of 9–12 months. Follow-up is essential to exclude chronic inflammatory bowel disease.

Multiple food allergy

This is the most difficult and sometimes controversial area for diagnosis. It is in this group, which usually occurs in older children, that 'blinded' food challenges are necessary. The small intestinal mucosa is typically normal. There is often an atopic background. Response to food elimination may be partial. Some children have been reported to respond to disodium cromoglycate.[65] However, an appropriately blinded, placebo-controlled trial has not yet established its role in these patients.

Food challenge

There are many problems encountered when attempting to provoke symptoms and small intestinal mucosal changes with foods. These problems need to be carefully appraised to achieve a balanced and practical approach to food challenges. Again, milk allergic reactions have been the ones most commonly investigated and to which this discussion will be primarily related.

An objective approach to the diagnosis of milk allergy by milk provocation was first made by Goldman *et al.*[17] whose diagnostic rules have become known as Goldman's criteria. They are as follows:

(a) symptoms should subside following milk elimination
(b) symptoms should occur within 48 hours following a trial feeding of milk
(c) three such challenges should be positive and similar with respect to onset, duration and clinical features
(d) symptoms should subside following each challenge reaction.

These criteria have subsequently been adopted for the diagnosis of hypersensitivity to other foods. This approach to the diagnosis of cow's milk hypersensitivity was an important milestone in the history of the study of food intolerance. Although these criteria led to the collection of more objective evidence, and seemed to eliminate both coincidental illness with milk challenge and fortuitous recovery with milk elimination, these criteria had many serious drawbacks:

1. Some children are so sensitive to some food proteins that it may be considered unsafe to give repeated food challenges, which would impose unnecessary morbidity to the child and distress to the parents.
2. The time of onset of symptoms may be greater than 48 hours.[35]
3. Symptoms may change with successive challenges, depending upon circumstances such as the rate of food administration and the age of the child.[16]
4. The child may have outgrown the hypersensitivity to milk by the time of the second or third challenge, and thus the diagnosis of food hypersensitivity may be incorrectly excluded.
5. Conditioned reflexes to the challenge food might have been developed, and thus adverse reactions may be predominantly psychological manifestations.[38] Double-blind studies showing this effect have been on older children and adults[45,46] and not on infants.
6. The adverse reaction may be due to other factors and not related to the food protein at all; e.g. lactose or sucrose intolerance.
7. Subclinical reaction may be missed if the assessment is purely clinical.[35]

Although Goldman himself recognized many of these faults, much use has nevertheless been made of these criteria to recognize the existence of cow's milk protein intolerance, but they are no longer used in routine clinical practice. Improved criteria for the diagnosis of food allergy must therefore take these problems into consideration and may need to incorporate variations to suit the circumstances of individual adverse clinical reactions.

An early cow's milk challenge is not diagnostically essential in a child with chronic diarrhoea and failure to thrive who has both the typical small intestinal enteropathy and a rapid clinical response to an elimination diet. An early (i.e. less than 1 year) challenge carries the risk of anaphylaxis.[9] Thus, in practice, the timing of milk challenge is best delayed to the age of 1 year or more. By then, in fact, most children with cow's milk-sensitive enteropathy will have recovered and the cow's milk challenge merely decides the safety of cow's milk reintroduction. In view of the risk, albeit small, of acute anaphylaxis, food challenges should ideally be done in hospital. For children with previous enteropathy, it is best to precede challenge with a small bowel biopsy to demonstrate healing or at least improvement in morphology.

Generally we favour the use of open challenges. In our experience we have found that the rate of positive double-blind, placebo-controlled challenge has been the same as the rate of positive open challenges in children under 5 years of age. This suggests that psychological conditioning is not an important factor in the persistence of symptoms in the early years of life and most children that we see can tolerate milk by 3 or 4 years of age. In addition, children with food-sensitive enteropathies often require large amounts of milk over several days to provoke symptoms and it becomes logistically very difficult to give these volumes under double-blind conditions.

We would advocate double-blind, placebo-controlled challenge in older children with persisting symptoms, especially in those who report unusual symptoms. Adults who report bizarre symptoms have been found to be uniformly unresponsive to food provocation under double-blind conditions.[52]

Age at challenge

The age at which the initial food provocation challenge should be done is debatable. By performing challenges in the first 6 months of life there is more likelihood of observing a positive reaction as the child has had little time to develop tolerance to the food. But such a reaction is likely to be more severe in this age group than in older children, with the risk of life-threatening reaction occurring.[9] It is our practice, in children with a convincing history of a food allergy who have clinically responded to an elimination diet, to wait until they are at least 12 months old before formally challenging them. The drawback of this approach is that the diagnosis cannot be confirmed in children who have outgrown their food allergy by the time of their food provocation, and one then merely establishes the safety of reintroducing milk. One then has to revert to the less satisfactory diagnosis of milk elimination responsive enteropathy.[23]

We recommend that the initial food challenges should be commenced under careful supervision because of both the occasional occurrence of severe reactions and the need for careful observation. There may be a considerable time delay until the development of symptoms, so it is often impossible to definitely state whether or not the food provoked the symptoms observed. For example, intercurrent gut infection may cause diarrhoea. Hence the need for some reliable objective test that indicates if an adverse response has occurred.

SUMMARY

The diagnosis of gastrointestinal food-allergic disease remains a predominantly clinical one, i.e. the response to food elimination and subsequent challenge, and so the various laboratory and clinical tests put forward for its diagnosis must still be evaluated and compared with the clinical response. It is important to ensure that symptoms associated with food provocation are not due to coincidental illness or psychological conditioning. The diagnosis of quick-onset food allergy is fairly straightforward but slow-onset syndromes, especially multiple food allergy, remain a problem.

For diagnosis of food-sensitive enteropathy small intestinal biopsy seems to be the most useful investigation test, but it is not pathognomonic. It helps exclude other gastrointestinal conditions. Mucosal damage due to food allergy might be detected with more sensitivity by tests of gut function, but no such test for routine use has been found to be particularly helpful. Tests of gut function require further study: at present, sugar permeability is most valuable. When the pathogenesis of temporary food-sensitive enteropathies of infancy are better understood, then diagnostic tests may become more specific and sensitive. Until that time, clinical history, small intestinal biopsy and food elimination with food challenge remain the cornerstones of diagnosis.

For diagnosis of cow's milk colitis, endoscopic biopsy with response to cow's milk elimination is required.

For the present, observation of the structure of the mucosa of the gastrointestinal tract remains centre stage. However, the hope must remain that less invasive tests will soon replace these investigations.

REFERENCES

1. Ament ME, Rubin CE. Soy protein – another cause of the flat intestinal lesion. *Gastroenterology* 1972; 62: 227–34.
2. Andre C, Andre F, Colin L, Cavagna S. Measurement of intestinal permeability to mannitol and lactulose as a means of diagnosing food allergy and evaluating therapeutic effectiveness of disodium cromoglycate. *Ann Aller* 1987; 59: 127–30.
3. Berant M, Khourie M, Menzies IS. Effect of iron deficiency on small intestinal permeability in infants and young children. *J Ped Gastr Nutr* 1992; 14: 17–20.
4. Bjarnason I, Peters TJ, Veall N. A persistent defect in intestinal permeability in coeliac disease demonstrated by a ^{51}Cr-labelled EDTA absorption test. *Lancet* 1983; i: 323–5.
5. Cavataio F, Iacono G, Montalto G *et al.* Gastro-oesophageal reflux associated with cow's milk allergy in infants: which diagnostic examinations are useful? *Am J Gastroenterol* 1996; 91(6): 1215–20.
6. Chadwick VS, Phillips SF, Hofmann AF. Measurements of intestinal permeability using low molecular weight polyethylene glycols (PEG 400). *Gastroenterology* 1977; 73: 247–51.
7. Chong SKF, Bartram C, Campbell CA *et al.* Chronic inflammatory bowel disease in childhood. *Br Med J* 1982; 284: 101–4.
8. Cobden I, Rothwell J, Axon ATR. Intestinal permeability and screening test for coeliac disease. *Gut* 1980; 21: 512–18.
9. De Peyer E, Walker-Smith JA. Cow's milk intolerance presenting as necrotizing enterotozing enterocolitis. *Helv Paediatr Act* 1977; 32: 509.
10. Ferguson A. Pathogenesis and mechanisms in the gastrointestinal tract. In: *Proceedings of the First Fisons Food Allergy Workshop*. Medicine Publishing Foundation, Oxford, 1980: 28–38.
11. Fontaine JL, Navarro J. Small intestinal biopsy in cow's milk protein allergy in infancy. *Arch Dis Child* 1975; 50: 357–63.
12. Ford RPK, Barnes GL, Hill DL. Gastrointestinal milk hypersensitivity: the diagnostic value of gut function tests. *Aust J Paediat* 1986.
13. Ford RPK, Menzies IS, Phillips AD *et al.* Intestinal sugar permeability: relationship to diarrhoeal disease and small bowel morphology. *J Pediatr Gastroenterol Nutr* 1985; 4: 568–75.
14. Ford RPK, Taylor B. Natural history of egg hypersensitivity in childhood. *Arch Dis Child* 1982; 57: 649–52.
15. Forget P, Arends JW. Cow's milk protein allergy and gastro-oesophageal reflux. *Eur J Pediatr* 1985; 144: 298–300.
16. Freier S, Kletter N, Gery I *et al.* Intolerance to milk protein. *J Pediatr* 1969; 75: 623–31.
17. Goldman AS, Anderson DW, Sellers WA *et al.* Milk allergy. 1. Oral challenge with milk and isolated milk protein in allergic children. *Paediatrics* 1963; 31: 425–43.
18. Gryboski JD. Gastrointestinal milk allergy in infants. *Pediatrics* 1967; 40: 354–62.
19. Harris M, Petts V, Renny P. Cow's milk allergy as a cause of infantile colic: immunofluorescent studies on jejunal mucosa. *Aust Paediatr J* 1977; 13: 276–81.
20. Harrison M, Kibly A, Walker-Smith JA *et al.* Cow's milk protein intolerance: a possible association with gastroenteritis, lactose intolerance, and IgA deficiency. *Br Med J* 1976; i: 1501–4.
21. Harrison M, Walker-Smith JA. Re-investigation of lactose intolerant children: lack of correlation between continuing lactose intolerance and small intestinal morphology, disaccharidase activity and lactose tolerance tests. *Gut* 1977; 18: 48–52.

22 Hill DJ, Davidson GP, Cameron DJS, Barnes GL. The spectrum of cow's milk allergy in childhood: clinical, gastroenterological and immunological studies. *Acta Paediatr Scand* 1979; 68: 847–52.

23 Hutchins P, Walker-Smith JA. End-organ effects. The gastrointestinal system. *Clin Immunol Allergy* 1982; 2: 34–77.

24 Isolauri E, Turjanmaa K. Combined skin prick and patch testing enhances identification of food allergy in infants with atopic dermatitis. *J Allergy Clin Immunol* 1996; 97: 9–15.

25 Iyngkaran N, Abidain Z, Meng LL, Yadav M. Egg protein-induced villous atrophy. *J Pediatr Gastroenterol Nutr* 1982; 1: 29–35.

26 Iyngkaran N, Davis K, Robinson MJ et al. Cow's milk protein-sensitive enteropathy: an important contributing cause of secondary sugar intolerance in young infants with acute infective enteritis. *Arch Dis Child* 1979; 54: 39–43.

27 Iyngkaran N, Robinson MJ, Prathap K et al. Cow's milk protein sensitive enteropathy: combined clinical and histological criteria for diagnosis. *Arch Dis Child* 1978; 53: 20.

28 Jenkins HR, Milla PJ, Pincott TR et al. Food allergy: the major cause of infantile colitis. *Pediatr Arch Dis Child* 1984; 59: 326–9.

29 Jos J. Immunohistochemical study of the intestinal mucosa in children (Abstract). *Acta Paediatr Scand* 1970; 59: 447.

30 Kilby A, Walker-Smith JA, Wood CBS: Small intestinal mucosa in cow's milk intolerance. *Lancet* 1975; i: 351.

31 Kuitunen P, Kosnai I, Savilahti E. Morphometric study of the jejunal mucosa in various childhood enteropathies and special references to intraepithelial lymphocytes. *J Pediatr Gastroenterol Nutr* 1982; 1: 525–31.

32 Kuitunen P, Visakorpi JK, Hallman N. Histopathology of duodenal mucosa in malabsorption syndrome induced by cow's milk. *Ann Paediatr* 1965; 205: 54–63.

33 Kuitunen P, Rapola J, Savilahti E, Visakorpi JK. Light and electron microscopic changes in the small intestinal mucosa in patients with cow's milk induced malabsorption syndrome. *Acta Paediatr Scand* 1972; 61: 237.

34 Kuitunen P, Rapola J, Savilahti E, Visakorpi JK. Responses of jejunal mucosa to cow's milk in the malabsorption symptoms with cow's milk intolerance. A light- and electron-microscopic study. *Acta Paediatr Scand* 1973; 62: 585–95.

35 Kuitunen P, Visakorpi JK, Savilahti E, Pelkunen P. Malabsorption syndrome with cow's milk intolerance, clinical findings and course in 54 cases. *Arch Dis Child* 1975; 50: 351–6.

36 Levitt MD. Production and excretion of hydrogen gas in man. *N Engl J Med* 1969; 281: 122–7.

37 Liu HY, Tsao MU, Moore B, Giday Z. Bovine milk protein induced intestinal malabsorption of lactose and fat in infants. *Gastroenterology* 1968; 54: 27–34.

38 Loveless MH. Milk allergy: a survey of its incidence: experiments with masked ingestion test. *J Allergy* 1950; 21: 489–99.

39 Lubos MC, Gerrard JW, Buchan DJ. Disaccharidase activities in milk-sensitive and celiac patients. *J Pediatr* 1967; 70: 325–31.

40 McNeish AS. The role of lactose in cow's milk intolerance (Abstract). *Acta Paediatr Scand* 1974; 63: 651.

41 McNeish AS, Rolles CJ, Arthur LJH. Criteria for diagnosing temporary gluten intolerance. *Arch Dis Child* 1976; 51: 275–8.

42 Maffei HV, Kingston D, Hill ID, Shiner B. Histopathologic changes and the immune response within the jejunal mucosa in infants and children. *Paediatr Res* 1979; 13: 733–6.

43 Maluenda C, Phillips AD, Briddon A, Walker-Smith JA. Quantitative analysis of small intestinal mucosa in cow's milk sensitive enteropathy. *J Pediatr Gastroenterol Nutr* 1984; 3: 349–56.

44 Manuel PD, Walker-Smith JA, France NE. Patchy enteropathy in childhood. *Gut* 1979; 20: 211–15.

45 Maslansky L, Wein G. Chocolate allergy: a double blind study. *Conn Med* 1971; 35: 5–9.

46 May CD. Objective clinical and laboratory study of immediate hypersensitivity reaction to foods in asthmatic children. *J Allergy Clin Immunol* 1976; 58: 500–15.

47 Meeuwisse G. Diagnostic criteria in coeliac disease. *Acta Paediatr Scand* 1970; 59: 461–3.

48 Menzies IS. Absorption of intact oligosaccharides in health and disease. *Biochem Soc Trans* 1974; 2: 1042–7.

49 Menzies IS. Transmucosal passage of inert molecules in health and disease. *Falk Symposium* 1984.

50 Menzies IS, Laker MF, Pounder R et al. Abnormal intestinal permeability to sugars in villous atrophy. *Lancet* 1979; ii: 1107–9.

51 Pearson ADJ, Eastham EJ, Laker MF, Craft AW, Nelson RH. Intestinal permeability in children with Crohn's disease and coeliac disease. *Br Med J* 1982; 285: 20–1.

52 Pearson DJ, Rix KJB, Bently SJ. Food allergy: how much in the mind. *Lancet* 1983; 1: 1259–61.

53 Perkkio M, Savilahti E, Kuitunen P. Morphometric and immunohistochemical study of jejunal biopsies from children with intestinal soy allergy. *Eur J Pediatrics* 1981; 137: 63–9.

54 Phillips AD, Rice SJ, France NE, Walker-Smith JA. Small intestinal lymphocyte levels in cow's milk protein intolerance. *Gut* 1979; 20: 509–12.

55 Polanco I, Larraui J. Does transient gluten intolerance exist? In: *Coeliac Disease: 100 Years* (Kumar PJ, Walker-Smith JA, eds). University Printing Service, Leeds, 1989: 236–31.

56 Poley JR, Klein AW. Scanning electron microscopy of soy protein-induced damage of small bowel mucosa in infants. *J Pediatr Gastroenterol Nutr* 1983; 2: 271–8.

57 Poley JR, Bhatia M, Welsh JD. Disaccharidase deficiency in infants with cow's milk protein intolerance: response to treatment. *Digestion* 1978; 17: 97–107.

58 Savilahti E. Immunochemical study of the malabsorption syndrome with cow's milk intolerance. *Gut* 1973; 14: 491–501.

59 Savilahti E, Heyman M, MacDonald TT et al. Diagnostic criteria for food allergy with predominantly intestinal symptoms. *J Paediatr Gastroenterol Nutr* 1992; 14: 108–12.

60 Shiner M, Ballard J, Smith ME. The small-intestinal mucosa in cow's milk allergy. *Lancet* 1975; i: 136–40.

61 Shiner M, Ballard J, Brook CGD, Herman S: Intestinal biopsy in the diagnosis of cow's milk protein in tolerance without acute symptoms. *Lancet* 1975; ii: 1060–3.

62 Silver H, Douglas DM. Milk intolerance in infancy. *Arch Dis Child* 1968; 43: 17–22.

63 Stern M, Dietrich R, Muller J. Small intestinal mucosal in coeliac disease and cow's milk protein intolerance. Morphometric and immunofluorescent studies. *Eur J Pediatr* 1982; 139: 101–15.

64 Sullivan PB, Lunn PG, Northrop Clews C et al. Persistent diarrhoea and malnutrition – the impact of treatment on small bowel structure and permeability. *J Ped Gastr Nutr* 1992; 14: 208–10.

65 Syme J. Investigation and treatment of multiple intestinal food allergy in childhood. In: *The Mast Cell: Its Role in Health and Disease* (Pepy SJ, Edwards AH, eds). Pitman Medical, Tunbridge Wells, 1979: 438–42.

66 Vitoria JC, Camarero C, Sojo A et al. Enteropathy related to fish, rice and chicken. *Arch Dis Child* 1982; 57: 44–8.

67 Walker-Smith JA. Cow's milk protein intolerance. Transient food intolerance of infancy. *Arch Dis Child* 1975; 50: 347–50.

68 Walker-Smith JA. Fibre-optic techniques for investigation of gastrointestinal diseases in children. *Paed Allergy Immunol* 1993; 4 (Suppl 3): 40–3.

69 Walker-Smith JA. Food sensitive enteropathy: overview and update. *Acta Paediatricia Japonica* 1994; 36: 545–50.

70 Walker-Smith JA. Diagnostic criteria for gastrointestinal food allergy in childhood. *Clin Exp Allergy* 1995; 25 (Suppl 1): 20–3.

71 Walker-Smith JA, Harrison M, Kilby A et al. Cow's milk sensitive enteropathy. *Arch Dis Child* 1978; 53: 375–80.

INTRODUCTION

The diagnosis of food-allergic disease affecting the gut presents problems. The symptoms produced by food reactions are commonly diarrhoea, abdominal pain, wind and bloating, and these are seen in many other conditions affecting the gut. There are misconceptions over definitions of food intolerance and food allergy, and no simple tests exist to identify those patients who may be suffering from these conditions, or to identify the foods concerned.

The diagnosis of food intolerance is, therefore, partly one of exclusion. A comprehensive history and a careful physical examination, including sigmoidoscopy, are essential. Dietary history is usually disappointingly misleading, as most food intolerances involve staple foods such as wheat and dairy products. As these are often eaten daily, it is unusual for patients to make the link between eating such foods and chronic symptoms. A number of investigations, including full blood count sedimentation rate, serum albumin, liver and thyroid function tests, urea and electrolytes, acute phase proteins, gliadin and endomysial antibodies, stool cultures and, in those over 40, a barium enema, may be necessary to exclude chronic infection, inflammatory bowel or coeliac disease, and colonic neoplasia.

Psychological disorders also cause problems because, like food intolerance, these may produce abdominal symptoms with no sign of organic pathology. Clinical depression is usually fairly easily recognized. Anxiety, which is often associated with air swallowing, is more common and may lead to considerable difficulties because it often coexists with food intolerance, especially in patients who have suffered unexplained gut symptoms for many years with no accurate diagnosis being made. Air swallowing leads to flatulence, bloating and pain, but is rarely associated with chronic diarrhoea. Symptoms of chronic hyperventilation such as breathlessness, chest pain, palpitations, sweating, paraesthesiae, faintness, dizziness and chronic fatigue may also be present and, if not volunteered by the patient, must be specifically sought.

Considerable confusion is now arising over the relationship between food intolerance and the irritable bowel syndrome (IBS). Although the name has been hallowed by long usage, IBS is not a distinct entity but merely a collection of disorders which are characterized by abdominal symptoms but no obvious organic pathology. G.W. Thompson[32] forecast in 1985: 'the IBS is organic; that is, all sufferers will eventually be found to have measurable, unique pathophysiologic defects'.[1] When that happy day arrives, the term IBS will no longer be used, and each patient will receive a more precise diagnosis. Until then, it is sufficient to appreciate that food intolerance represents an important proportion of the conditions which together make up IBS. Food intolerance is always present in coeliac disease[4] and in the great majority of cases of Crohn's disease,[15] but these conditions are fully discussed in Chapters 40 and 41, respectively.

ADVERSE FOOD REACTIONS

Adverse food reactions may be divided into three groups: food poisoning, food intolerance and food aversion.[31] Further subdivisions are indicated in Fig. 63.1. Food poisoning occurs after the ingestion of pathogenic microorganisms or toxic chemicals. Examples include *Campylobacter* gastroenteritis or scombrotoxicosis from eating mackerel which has been inadequately frozen. Food poisoning is usually a single episode, and will not be considered further here. Food aversion refers to psychological reactions to or avoidance of foods, and is also outwith the discussion of true food intolerance.

Food allergy is commonly misinterpreted as an adverse reaction to food but most food reactions are not true allergic reactions.[18,33] A food allergy by definition constitutes an immune-mediated reaction to the food.[14] Food intolerance on the other hand is a much wider concept embracing adverse reactions whatever their mechanisms may be, and includes food allergy amongst others. Food intolerance refers to a reproducible unpleasant non-physiological reaction to a specific food or ingredient.[31]

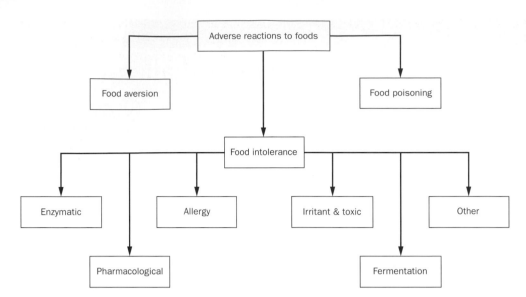

Fig. 63.1 Classification of adverse food reactions.

In food intolerance a number of mechanisms may be responsible for the reactions observed. These include pharmacological or toxic effects of chemicals in foods, enzyme deficiencies in the patient, and the effects of fermentation of malabsorbed food residues in the colon. Toxic or irritant effects include those commonly noted after excess ingestion of substances such as alcohol or spices and the cause is usually readily apparent. Chemicals in food which may have a pharmacological effect include caffeine and vasoactive amines such as tyramine and histamine, found in chocolate, cheese, bananas and citrus fruits. These may produce gastrointestinal effects such as oesophageal reflux and diarrhoea, or systemic symptoms, including headaches and palpitations. The commonest enzyme deficiency encountered in clinical practice is hypolactasia, which may lead to diarrhoea, bloating and pain after ingestion of lactose. Monoamine oxidase inhibitors, used in the treatment of depression, reduce the hepatic breakdown of vasoactive amines and may cause hypertension and headache if the patient does not follow a diet which is low in these chemicals.[17]

DIAGNOSIS OF TRUE FOOD ALLERGY

Adverse allergic immunologically mediated reactions may cause a variety of symptoms. Acute attacks of vomiting, diarrhoea and abdominal pain may be accompanied by systemic symptoms such as skin rashes and even anaphylaxis. Those reactions which occur within minutes of eating the food are termed immediate reactions; examples are reactions to shellfish and peanuts. True allergy is mediated by immunoglobulin (Ig) E and the concentration of IgE in the plasma may be raised. As specific IgE molecules to the foods concerned circulate in the plasma it is possible to diagnose true food allergens allergy by objective tests.[27]

The longest established and most widely used test for true allergy is the skin prick test, in which a small amount of allergen is placed on the skin and a prick made through it. A positive weal forms after a few minutes and may be compared with the effect of the weal produced by the histamine control. Common allergens used include house dust mite, grass pollen, dog, cat and horse dander, as well as some food allergens such as egg, fish, nuts, cows' milk and wheat.

The radioallergosorbent test (RAST) also relies on circulating IgE. In this test the patient's serum is exposed directly to an allergen onto which the patient's antibodies may be absorbed. These antibodies may subsequently be quantified by the addition of ^{125}I-specific anti-IgE and measuring the amount of ^{125}I absorbed.

Both the skin prick test and the RAST may give false-positive results which may be misleading and the range of food allergens available is restricted. Both therefore have limitations on their value for the diagnosis of food allergy.[31]

A number of other tests available only from private laboratories have been promoted for the diagnosis of allergy. These include hair analysis for trace elements, the 'cytotoxic test' in which the patient's white cells are incubated with food allergens and cell damage recorded, the provocation of symptoms by sublingual application of food allergens and the 'Vega' test, in which changes in potential difference are sought when the patient is in contact with various food stuffs. None of these tests has been shown to be reliable when tested double blind and all may lead to patients following diets which prove nutritionally inadequate.[30]

As IgE-based tests for allergy may give false-positive results[27] it is important to use them as a simple guide and to confirm the food allergy by asking the patient to follow a diet from which the foods concerned have been excluded, to see if the symptoms clear. If it is considered necessary and desirable, double blind confirmatory challenge tests may be undertaken, although these may sometimes be dangerous, especially if the patient suffers from anaphylactic reactions. The use of double blind placebo-controlled food challenges (DBPCFC) is discussed later.

DIAGNOSIS OF FOOD INTOLERANCE

The symptoms of food intolerance are very similar to those of true food allergy, although anaphylactic reactions do not occur. Those affecting the gut include abdominal pain, diarrhoea or constipation, wind and bloating (Table 63.1). There may also be systemic symptoms, characteristically headache, fluid retention, skin rashes, arthralgia and chronic fatigue. In young women, the symptoms often become worse in the week preceding the menses.

As food intolerance may arise in several different ways, there is no objective test available to screen for the condition or to

Symptoms suffered by 122 patients subsequently identifying food intolerances	
Symptom	%
Abdominal pain	73
Diarrhoea	60
Tiredness	42
Headaches	38
Constipation	22.5
Abdominal distension	21.5
Fluid retention	20
Related conditions Migraine	11
Atopy	10

Table 63.1 Symptoms suffered by 122 patients subsequently identifying food intolerances.[12]

identify the foods concerned. The only accurate way to make the diagnosis is to alleviate symptoms on a limited diet, and then to confirm that harmful effects follow when foods are reintroduced prospectively.

Hypolactasia may be identified by observing changes in the breath excretion of hydrogen after the ingestion of 50 g lactose. The resting breath hydrogen is normally less than 20 ppm, and a rise of 20 ppm or more after lactose administration implies hypolactasia or bacterial overgrowth in the small bowel. Unfortunately, this test is of limited value in clinical practice as some patients with demonstrable hypolactasia do not develop symptoms on challenge, whereas others with normal concentrations of jejunal lactase may be intolerant of other components of milk, such as protein or fat. Thus in a study conducted in Cambridge of 120 consecutive patients with suspected food intolerance, of which only two were not Caucasian, 33 (27.5%) had positive lactose hydrogen breath tests. Of these, 23 followed a lactose-free diet but only nine responded. Nine of the 14 who failed to respond went on to try exclusion diets and five then responded (56%). As those patients intolerant of lactose respond well to exclusion diets, it appears that the simplest way to investigate these subjects is by the exclusion diet alone.[22]

DIETARY DIAGNOSIS OF FOOD INTOLERANCE

The basic principle of the dietary diagnosis of food intolerance is for the patient to follow a limited diet to allow his symptoms to clear. This may take anything from 4 to 14 days. When the patient has become free of symptoms, foods are reintroduced singly to see which provoke a return of symptoms, and any which do so are subsequently excluded. Finally, further food challenges are performed, either open or blind, to confirm that suspected reactions are genuine and not coincidental, and the resulting diet is assessed for nutritional adequacy.

A number of diets are available to serve as a starting point for testing. In general, the more restricted the diet, the more likely

it is to prove successful in identifying food intolerance, but patient compliance is always inversely related to the difficulty of the diet, and these diets should always be followed under the supervision of a state registered dietician. The main diets in current use are the elimination and exclusion diets.

The elimination diet
The elimination diet was one of the earliest dietary regimes introduced to investigate food intolerance. It involves the consumption of one fruit, usually pear, one meat (usually chicken or lamb) and water for up to 7 days. Sometimes rice is allowed as well. This diet places considerable burdens on the patient, particularly as during the first 2 or 3 days the symptoms, especially headache, may be greatly exacerbated. Nevertheless, it may be highly effective. Hunter et al.[12] found that 144 (79%) of 182 patients who completed the diet improved after 1 week. The foods used for the first phase of the diet in this study are shown in Table 63.2. Of the 182 patients using this diet, 122 (67%) succeeded in detecting food intolerances. In 16 (9%) symptoms returned after reintroduction of food, but accurate identification of the foods concerned was not possible, and six (3%) improved but identified no particular foods as causing symptoms. The elimination diet has the disadvantages, however, that it is nutritionally inadequate, and that when the patient has reached remission a formidable list of foods to be tested lies ahead. For this reason it has largely been superseded by the exclusion diet.

The exclusion diet
Exclusion diets may be defined as diets in which a number of foodstuffs which are believed likely to be responsible for food intolerances are forbidden. The grounds for such food exclusion may vary from the scientific to the whimsical. The 'Stone Age' diet excludes all foods believed to have been introduced into the human food chain as a result of agriculture. The 'Candida diet'

Foods used during first 7 days of elimination diet	
Food	Number (%) eating food
Lamb	136 (75)
Turkey	2 (1)
Fish	18 (10)
Chicken	5 (3)
Beef	4 (2)
Pears	151 (83)
Pineapple	1 (0.5)
Banana	3 (2)
Apples	10 (5.5)
Rice	97 (53)
Water alone	17 (9)

Table 63.2 Foods used during first 7 days of elimination diet ($n = 182$).

excludes those which it is claimed promote the growth of the yeast. An exclusion diet in widespread use today is the Addenbrooke's exclusion diet, which was developed from the elimination diet used for patients with IBS.[21]

The elimination diet showed that the majority of people were upset by similar foods. It was therefore decided to construct a diet which excluded all those foods upsetting more than 20% of those who successfully completed the elimination diet (Table 63.3).

Wines were also excluded because of their yeast content, and tap water even though it produced symptoms in only 10% of patients. This was because it was drunk frequently, especially by those denied tea and coffee.

Food intolerance reported by patients in initial study			
Food	**Patients affected (%)**	**Food**	**Patients affected (%)**
Cereals		Vegetables	
wheat	60	onions	22
corn	44	potatoes	20
oats	34	cabbage	19
rye	30	sprouts	18
barley	24	peas	17
rice	15	carrots	15
		lettuce	15
Dairy products		leeks	15
milk	44	broccoli	14
cheese	39	soya beans	13
eggs	26	spinach	13
butter	25	mushrooms	12
yoghurt	24	parsnips	12
		tomatoes	11
Fish		cauliflower	11
white fish	10	celery	11
shellfish	10	green beans	10
smoked fish	7	cucumber	10
		turnip/swede	10
Meat		marrow	8
beef	16	beetroot	8
pork	14	peppers	6
chicken	13		
lamb	11	Miscellaneous	
turkey	8	coffee	33
		tea	25
Fruit		nuts	22
citrus	24	chocolate	22
rhubarb	12	preservatives	20
apple	12	yeast	20
banana	11	sugar cane	13
pineapple	8	sugar beet	12
pear	8	alcohol	12
strawberries	8	saccharin	9
grapes	7	honey	2
melon	5		
avocado pear	5		
raspberries	4		

Table 63.3 Food intolerance reported by patients in initial study (n = 122).

Subsequently, the exclusion diet was further modified in the light of changes in the frequency of food intolerances discovered as the diet was used (Table 63.4). This meant that sheep and goat's milk, and beef were also excluded.[21]

MANAGEMENT OF PATIENTS WHO FAIL TO IMPROVE ON THE EXCLUSION DIET

Although the exclusion diet is simpler than the elimination diet, and more popular with patients, it has the disadvantage that the allowance of a wider range of foods may mean that those patients who have unusual food intolerances fail to respond. This difficulty may be overcome by careful study of the food diary. In those patients who fail to improve on the basic exclusion after 2 weeks or those whose symptoms fluctuate in the second week, foods eaten in the 24 h before a good day are compared with those eaten in the 24 h before a bad day. Those foods preceding a bad day which score highly in the food frequency table (Table 63.3) are then excluded. In this way, unusual food intolerances may be detected. Parker et al. found that 22% of their patients had unusual intolerances (Table 63.5).[21]

The exclusion diet may fail for reasons other than unusual food intolerances. Figure 63.2, modified from Parker et al.,[21] suggests a possible route for the management of this problem. Patients who do not comply with the diet should be encouraged to return to normal eating. In those patients who fail to respond, having faithfully followed the diet the diagnosis must be reconsidered. Patients with multiple food intolerances may also fail to improve on the exclusion diet and, because of the possibility of nutritional problems if their diets are further restricted, this group is also best encouraged to return to normal eating and to be managed in other ways.

Hawthorne et al. performed a similar study of 38 patients with IBS using a diet which excluded all milk products, wheat, corn, yeast, rye, spices, tomato, alcohol, peas, banana, coffee and tea.[10] Food reintroduction began for those who were asymptomatic after 2 weeks, each food being tested over a period of 2 days. Likewise, Nanda et al. used a similar exclusion diet, but allowed products derived from sheep or goat's milk.[20] The results of these studies have confirmed that 47–50% of patients showed improvement on the basic exclusion diet. In Nanda's study, 42% were able to identify food intolerances compared with 63% in that of Parker. Wheat was shown to be the most important food intolerance, with dairy products following.

THE PRACTICAL APPROACH TO AN EXCLUSION DIET

Before the diet is started, a detailed dietary history is taken to ascertain the patient's current eating pattern and any known food intolerances are noted. Alternatives are suggested for any current medications known to contain wheat or lactose.

It is important that the practicalities of the diet are discussed with the patient so that they understand what is involved. The diet is a lengthy process which requires self-discipline and motivation and which may take 2–3 months to complete. It is not possible to eat the same as family and friends, and holidays and eating out cause problems, as the diet must not be broken during the first 2 weeks. A simple guide has been published which many patients find helpful.[13]

Main components of modified exclusion diet	
Foods to avoid	**Foods allowed**
Beef	All other meats and poultry
Fish in batter or breadcrumbs	White and fatty fish tinned in brine or oils, e.g. sunflower, soya, olive
Potatoes, onions, sweetcorn, tinned vegetables in sauce	All other vegetables fresh or frozen or tinned
Citrus fruits	All other fruits fresh or tinned
Wheat, rye, oats, barley, corn	Rice, arrowroot, tapioca, sago, millet, buckwheat, soya flour
Dairy products, sheep and goat's milk, eggs	Soya milk, milk-free margarine
Tea, coffee, alcohol, citrus fruit juices and squashes, tap water	Herbal teas, other fruit juices, blackcurrant squash, mineral water
Yeast, gravy mixes, marmalade, salad cream and dressings, blended oils, corn oils	Salt, herbs, spices, honey, syrup, sugar, gravy browning (caramel and salt only)
Vinegar, nuts, chocolate	Dried fruit and seeds, carob

Table 63.4 Main components of modified exclusion diet.

Unusual food intolerances identified during the modified exclusion diet			
Pork	5	Liver	1
Gammon/bacon	3	Lamb	1
Dried fruit	3	Turkey	1
Ham	2	Prawns	1
Tinned fish in soya oil	2	Apples	1
Smoked fish	2	Apple juice	1
Bananas	2	Grapes	1
Peas	2	Grape juice	1
Cauliflower	2	All fruit	1
Cabbage	2	Lettuce	1
Peppers	2	Parsnips	1
Broccoli	1	Cucumber	1
Sugar	1	Spices	1
Fried rice	1	Rice	1
		High fibre food	1

Table 63.5 Unusual food intolerances identified during the modified exclusion diet.

If the patient is not fully compliant with the diet (even at one meal), all previous efforts will have been wasted and he will have to begin again. It is necessary to be organized and to plan foods in advance. The diet is also more expensive than a normal diet and many alternatives such as millet, buckwheat and gram flour may only be found in health food shops.

The patient should be warned that symptoms may become worse in the first few days on the diet. This may in part be due to caffeine withdrawal, especially if large amounts of tea or coffee were consumed previously. If analgesics are required, soluble paracetamol or soluble aspirin should be used, as many other preparations may contain corn or wheat starch. Many lose weight in the first week of the diet because of diuresis and the effects

of adapting to unusual foods. A sample meal plan is shown in Table 63.6.

It is essential that the patient maintains an accurate food diary, including the time and nature of all symptoms experienced, the menses and bowel habit. Any dietary indiscretions may be spotted and unusual food intolerances identified.

However, should the patient improve it is likely that the symptoms are because of a food intolerance and hence can be controlled by diet. The process of food reintroduction then begins; this may take 6–8 weeks to complete, depending on the number of food reactions.

Food reintroductions

A single food is tested over a period of 2 days. This is because immediate reactions are unusual and a response may not be noted

Sample menu	
Breakfast	Rice cereal, soya milk and sugar
	Rice cakes, milk-free margarine and jam
	Apple juice, herbal tea
Lunch	Meat/fish/chicken
	Rice or rice cakes
	Vegetables/salad
	Fruit/soya yoghurt
Supper	Meat/fish/chicken
	Rice/rice pasta/sweet potato
	Vegetables/salad
	Fruit salad/soya ice cream/sorbet
	Milk pudding made with soya milk

Table 63.6 Sample menu.

A

until the second or third day. The food being tested should be eaten in moderate amounts at least twice on each day. The order of food reintroductions is shown in Table 63.7. The food and symptom diary is continued throughout this period.

If a food produces a reaction it should be avoided for several weeks, but retested at the end of the reintroduction process to confirm that the first reaction was not coincidental. After each reaction, no further foods should be tested until the patient is again asymptomatic. Sodium bicarbonate, 5–10 g in 300 ml water, may be taken to help relieve any adverse side effects.

If, after 2 days, the patient remains free of symptoms it can be assumed that the food being tested is safe to eat and the patient may subsequently include this food in the diet as desired. Wheat is tested towards the end as it has been shown to provoke reactions in many patients. It is also tested over a longer period (7

Number of patients with nutritional deficiency (as defined by DHSS Recommended Intakes of Nutrients for the UK)	
No. of patients	**Nutrient**
18	Ca
7	Fe
3	Vitamin A
3	Vitamin D
2	Vitamin C
1	Protein

Table 63.8 Number of patients with nutritional deficiency (as defined by DHSS Recommended Intakes of Nutrients for the UK).

Order of reintroduction of foods on the modified exclusion diet	
Tap water	
Potatoes	
Milk	1 pint a day
Yeast	3 brewer's yeast tables or 2 tsp fresh yeast
Tea	
Rye	Rye crispbread or rye bread (if yeast OK)
Beef	
Butter	
Onions	
Eggs	
Oats	
Coffee	
Chocolate	Plain chocolate or cocoa
Citrus fruits	
Corn	
Cheese	
White wine	
Yoghurt	
Wheat	As bread if yeast OK or wheat breakfast cereals or pasta
Nuts	
Barley	Barley flakes
Vinegar	

Table 63.7 Order of reintroduction of foods on the modified exclusion diet.

days) as it often produces symptoms slowly and insidiously. It is therefore an advantage to have previously reintroduced many other foods and thus to have built up a more varied safe diet before trying wheat. Patients who complete the food testing process without detecting any reactions are usually intolerant of wheat and should test it again over a longer period.

After the process has been completed and suspect foods retested, the diet should be assessed by a qualified dietitian to ensure that it is nutritionally adequate, especially in those with multiple food intolerances and those who are upset by staple foods. In a study by Hunter et al.[12] the diets of 122 patients who had previously diagnosed food intolerances were reviewed. It was found that 28% had nutritionally inadequate diets, the details of which are shown in Table 63.8. Calcium deficiencies are common because of the high incidence of intolerance to diary products. Foods provoking symptoms should be retested after 3–6 months to confirm genuine intolerances. Patients should then remain on their limited diets as long as is necessary. Many find that food intolerances slowly improve, and we therefore recommend that they retest annually to ensure that foods still provoke symptoms.

DOUBLE BLIND PLACEBO-CONTROLLED FOOD CHALLENGE

The gold standard for the diagnosis of food intolerance remains the DBPCFC. However, it is difficult to design and perform reliable challenges and therefore, except for research purposes and to identify cases of pseudoallergy, they are not often used in routine practice.

The difficulties of food challenge are well exemplified by coeliac disease. Here, both symptoms and an objective change in the jejunal mucosa are known to be caused by a food protein, gluten. However, no uniform protocol has been agreed for the gluten challenge in coeliac disease and review of the literature reveals wide variation in the form and amount of gluten administered, and the length of time of the study (Table 63.9). When such difficulties are encountered in establishing a standard challenge technique in a disease which has been known for over 40 years to be caused by intolerance of a single protein, it is not surprising that such difficulties exist over DBPCFC in food intolerance where no objective changes are apparent. Similar difficulties have been encountered with challenge in lactose intolerance.[22]

Challenges used in coeliac disease				
Daily amount (g)	**Material**	**Site**	**Duration**	**References**
7.5	α-Gliadin	Jejunum	6 h	11
10	Gluten	Oral	6 weeks	3
10–20	Gluten	Oral	7 days	16
20	Gluten	Oral	Days or weeks	24
20	Gluten	Oral	3 months	25
20	Gluten	Duodenum	1 dose	28
25–40	Gluten	Oral	1 dose	16
30	Gluten	Duodenum	1 dose	5
30	Gluten	Oral	Daily	23
30	Gluten	Oral	7 days	2
40	Gluten	Oral	2 months	7
40	Gluten	Oral	6 weeks	6
60	Gluten	Oral	6 daily	19
3	Gluten flour	Oral	Daily	29
150	Wheat	Proximal ileum	9–11 days	26
25	Bread	Oral	Daily	9

Table 63.9 Challenges used in coeliac disease.

True food allergies may be satisfactorily confirmed by tests in which allergens are concealed in opaque plastic capsules. This technique is rarely adequate in food intolerance where the amounts of the food concerned may be too large to be easily contained in small capsules. There may also be difficulties in deciding for how long the challenge should continue. As many cases of food intolerance may be caused by colonic malfermentation, the physical state of the food, e.g. roast or mashed potato, may affect the amount reaching the colon and available to provoke symptoms.

We find it is better to give the liquidized food by nasogastric tube or to disguise it in a flavoured soup, rather than use capsules. Alun Jones et al. performed double blind food challenges in six patients who were free of symptoms on limited diets.[1] The patients were admitted to hospital for 4 days and breakfast was given as a double blind challenge via nasogastric tube. Two test and two control food were given over 4 days.

In a study by Farah et al. DBPCFCs were performed to confirm intolerances.[8] In this study food was administered in three opaque capsules, three times daily, 1 h before meals. This was carried out for 1 week, during which time the patients remained on the exclusion diet. Each patient was tested with the food which had earlier been identified as provoking symptoms, and the order of placebo and active capsule administration was

randomized. All symptoms were recorded and rated on a scale of 0–4 according to severity.

Twenty-three per cent of food intolerances were correctly identified using the capsules compared to four of six (67%) in Alun Jones et al.'s nasogastric tube study.

Although the use of DBPCFC may be necessary to screen out patients whose food allergies are not genuine, it is clear that challenges incorrectly performed may confuse rather than clarify the issue.

CONCLUSIONS

The diagnosis of food-allergic disease affecting the gastrointestinal tract is challenging. The main symptoms are common to many conditions and no specific or simple test to diagnose and distinguish between food intolerance and food allergy exists. The diagnosis of food intolerance is largely one of exclusion. The elimination diet has largely been superseded by the exclusion diet where foods presumed to be causing symptoms are forbidden. Foods commonly causing intolerance include cereals (wheat, corn and oats), dairy products (milk and cheese), citrus fruits and coffee. Foods provoking symptoms should be retested after a few months to confirm genuine intolerances. Annual retesting is recommended to determine whether foods can be reintroduced.

REFERENCES

1 Alun Jones V, Shorthouse M, McLaughlan P *et al*. Food intolerance: a major factor in the pathogenesis of irritable bowel syndrome. *Lancet* 1982; Nov 20: 1115–17.

2 Bayliss CE, Houston AP, Alun Jones V, Hishon S, Hunter JO. Microbiological studies on food intolerance. *Proc Nutr Soc* 1984; 43: 16a.

3 Congdon P, Mason MK, Smith S, Crollick A, Steel A, Littlewood J. Small bowel mucosa in asymptomatic children with coeliac disease. *Am J Dis Child* 1981; 135: 118–21.

4 Dicke WK, Weijers HA, van de Kamer JH. The presence in wheat of a factor having a deleterious effect in the case of coeliac disease. *Acta Paed* 1953; 34: 34–42.

5 Doe WF, Henry K, Holt L, Booth CC. An immunological study of adult coeliac disease. *Gut* 1972; 13: 324–5.

6 Doherty M, Barry RE. Gluten induced mucosal changes in subjects without overt small bowel disease. *Lancet* 1981; i: 517–20.

7 Egan-Mitchell B, Fottrell PF, McNicholl B. Prolonged gluten tolerance in treated coeliac disease. In: *Perspective in Coeliac Disease* (McNicholl B, Fottrell PF, McCarthy CF, eds), MTP Press, Lancaster, 1978.

8 Farah DA, Calder I, Benson L *et al*. Specific food intolerance: its place as a cause of gastrointestinal symptoms. *Gut* 1985; 26: 164–8.

9 Hamilton JR, McNeill LK. Childhood coeliac disease: response of treated patients to a small uniform daily dose of wheat gluten. *J Paediat* 1972; 81: 885–93.

10 Hawthorne B, Lambert S, Scott D *et al*. Food intolerance and the irritable bowel syndrome. *J Human Nutr Dietetics* 1991; 3: 19–23.

11 Hekkens WTJM, Haex AJC, Willinghagen RGJ. Some aspects of gliadin fractionation and testing by a histochemical method. In: *Coeliac Disease* (Both CC, Dowling RH, eds),Churchill Livingstone, Edinburgh, 1970.

12 Hunter JO, Workman EM, Alun Jones V. Chapter 12. In: *Topics in Gastroenterology* (Jewell DP, Gibson PR, eds), Blackwell Scientific Publications, London, 1985.

13 Hunter JO, Workman EM, Woolner JT. *The New Allergy Diet*, Vermilion, London, 2000.

14 Kaplan AP (ed.). *Allergy*. Churchill-Livingstone, New York, 1985.

15 King TS, Woolner JT, Hunter JO. Dietary management of Crohn's disease. *Alim Pharmacol Therapeut* 1997; 11: 17–31.

16 Lancaster Smith M, Kumar PJ, Dawson AM. The cellular infiltrate of the jejunum in adult coeliac disease and dermatitis herpetiformis following the reintroduction of dietary gluten. *Gut* 1975; 16: 683–8.

17 Lessof MH. *Food Intolerance*. Food Safety Series 2. Chapman and Hall, London, 1992.

18 McCarthy EP, Frick OL. Food sensitivity: keys to diagnosis. *J Paediat* 1983; 102: 645–52.

19 McDonald GB, Earnest DL, Admirand WH. Hyperoxaluria correlates with fat malabsorption. *Gut* 1977; 18: 561–6.

20 Nanda R, James R, Smith H *et al*. Food intolerance and the irritable bowel syndrome. *Gut* 1989; 30: 1099–104.

21 Parker TJ, Naylor SJ, Riordan AM *et al*. Management of patients with food intolerance in irritable bowel syndrome: the development and use of an exclusion diet. *J Human Nutr Dietetics* 1995; 8: 159–66.

22 Parker TJ, Wodner JT, Prevost AT *et al*. Irritable bowel syndrome: is the search for lactose intolerance justified? *Eur J Gastroenterol Hepatol* 2001; 13: 219–25.

23 Pollock DJ, Nagle RE, Jeejeebhoy KN, Coghill NF. The effect on jejunal mucosa of withdrawing and adding dietary gluten in cases of idiopathic steatorrhoea. *Gut* 1970; 11: 567–75.

24 Rolles CJ, Anderson CM. The usefulness of a modified d-xylose absorption test in the preliminary diagnosis of coeliac disease and its later confirmation. *Clin Gastroenterol* 1973; 3: 127–44.

25 Rolles CJ, McNeish AS. Standardised approach to gluten challenge in diagnosing childhood coeliac disease. *BMJ* 1976; i: 1309–11.

26 Rubin CE, Brandborg LL, Flick AL, Phelps P, Parmentlier C, Van Niel S. Studies of coeliac sprue. III. The effect of repeated wheat instillation into the proximal ileum of patients on a gluten free diet. *Gastroenterology* 1962; 43: 621–41.

27 Rusznak C, Davies R. Diagnosis of allergy. *BMJ* 1998; 316: 686–9.

28 Schmerling DH, Shiner M. The response of the intestinal mucosa to the intraduodenal instillation of gluten in patients with coeliac disease. In: *Coeliac Disease* (Booth CC, Dowling RH, eds), Churchill Livingstone, Edinburgh, 1970.

29 Schwartz MK, Sleisenger MH, Pert JH, Roberts KE, Randall HT, Almy TP. The effect of a gluten free diet on fat, nitrogen and mineral metabolism in patients with sprue. *Gastroenterology* 1957; 32: 232–46.

30 Sethi TJ, Kemeny DM, Tobin S *et al*. How reliable are commercial allergy tests? *Lancet* 1987; i: 92–4.

31 Thomas B (ed.). *Manual of Dietetic Practice*, 2nd edn, Chapter 4.31, *Food allergy and food intolerance*. Blackwell Scientific, London, 1994.

32 Thompson WG. The irritable bowel. One disease or several, or none? In: *Irritable Bowel Syndrome*, Vol. 1, (Read NW, ed.), Grune and Stratton, London, 1994.

33 Zwetchkenbaum JF, Burakoff R. Food allergy and the irritable bowel syndrome. *Am J Gastroenterol* 1988; 83(9): 901–4.

Chapter 64

Non-immunological adverse reactions to food

Gisèle Kanny and D. Anne Moneret-Vautrin

INTRODUCTION

False food allergies (FFA) or non-immunological adverse reactions to food are defined by the ability of certain food substances to induce clinical reactions mimicking allergy, without IgE-dependent specific release of chemical mediators. The first definition attributed FFA to a non-immunological mechanism involving histamine.[28] The field of FFA has since widened. Certain foods can induce FFA involving other mechanisms which are not exclusively histamine-based; other mediators such as biogenic amines, leukotrienes, prostaglandins and neuromediators could be implicated.

While food-allergic reactions are induced by a specific immunological mechanism involving antibodies or T lymphocytes, FFA are due to pharmacologic effects of various substances contained in foods.[25]

PHYSIOPATHOLOGY OF NON-IMMUNOLOGICAL REACTIONS TO FOOD

Non-immunological reactions to food can be categorized into three groups (Table 64.1).

Intolerance to biogenic amines

Biogenic amines are lightweight molecular substances derived from an amino acid by decarboxylation. Thus, histamine is derived

Types of non-immune reactions to food
Intolerance to biogenic amines
Non-immunological release of chemical mediators from intestinal mast cells and skin mast cells
Miscellaneous mechanisms

Table 64.1 Types of non-immune reactions to food.

from histidine and tyramine from tyrosine. They are naturally present in human food, particularly in fermented products such as cheese and wine, and in certain fish and meats. In the latter, they indicate poor preservation. The excessive consumption of starchy foods can provoke the proliferation of fermenting flora responsible for decarboxylation of amino acids into biogenic amines.

Histamine
Biogenic amines can induce toxic reactions.[34] Histamine present in excessive quantities in some foods is usually held responsible for these toxic reactions. Fish in particular can be rich in histamine if the commercial distribution system does not deliver perfectly

fresh fish. Histamine is not destroyed at high temperatures (210°C) and, for this reason, it may not be denatured by cooking.[5]

Neutralization of histamine

Physiologically, there are effective systems of neutralization and catabolism of histamin and biogenic amines in the digestive tract (Table 64.2). While a healthy subject tolerates 200–500 mg of histamine via the digestive route, intravenous administration of 7 μg can induce adverse effects.[33] The human protective systems against ingested histamine comprise the following:

- Digestive mucoproteins which can fix and inactivate some histamine.
- Intestinal microorganisms.
- The mechanical barrier represented by the intestinal epithelium; this is mainly enterocytes linked by tight junctions which effectively close intercellular spaces.
- Enzymes catabolizing histamine which are represented by diamine oxidase and histamine methyltransferase. Diamine oxidase is mainly located in enterocytes, whereas histamine methyltransferase is more widespread.[16]

Tyramine

Tyramine is a powerful adrenergic substance, capable of stimulating the release of other mediators (noradrenaline and histamine) and is catabolized by monoamine oxidase to become an inactive metabolite. Monoamine oxidase also catabolizes phenylethylamine, which is an agonist of alpha receptors.

Other biogenic amines, such as cadaverine and putrescine, present in the same foods could favour histamine reactions by competing with histamine catabolism, both in its linking to intestinal mucoproteins and in its enzymatic destruction by diamine oxidase, monoamine oxidase and histamine methyltransferase.[2]

Tyramine poisoning has been described in patients treated by monoamine oxidase inhibitors after the ingestion of cheese because of the block of normal enzyme destruction of this amine.

Neutralization of tyramine

Various substances can inhibit the activity of the enzymes involved in amine destruction. Diamine oxidase can be inhibited by food toxins such as gyromitrin, and certain additives such as sodium nitrite, metabolites of alcohol and numerous drugs.[9,36,38,39,42,45] Other drugs, e.g. antimalarial (quinacrine, chloroquine, amodiaquine), vecuronium and chlorhexidine, can inhibit the activity of histamine methyltransferase.[8,10]

Protective mechanisms against histamine in the human gastrointestinal tract
Mucoproteins can fix and inactivate histamine
Intestinal microorganisms
Mechanical barrier of intestinal epithelium
Enzymes catabolizing histamine, diamine oxidase and histamine methyltransferase

Table 64.2 Protective mechanisms against histamine in the human gastrointestinal tract.

Subjects presenting with FFA are characterized by an abnormal sensitivity to biogenic amines at a level well tolerated by healthy subjects. The role of ingested histamine has been demonstrated in adults.[33] Intraduodenal instillation of 200 mg of histamine bichloride (DHC, digestive histamine challenge) is well tolerated by controls, while in patients presenting intolerance to histamine this dose induces the appearance of clinical signs (pruritus, urticaria, headache) in 64% of cases. An increase of plasma histamine is noted in parallel in 72% of cases.[18] The passage of histamine through the digestive epithelium is demonstrated: ingested histamine induces interstitial oedema and capillary lesions of duodenal mucosa in these subjects.[20] An enzymatic deficiency, mainly in diamine oxidase, is postulated.[24]

Non-immunological release of chemical mediators from intestinal mast cells

Mast cells and basophils can be activated in a non-specific way by morphine and codeine. Certain foods, such as basic peptides and peptones, can induce non-specific histamine release of mast cells. The role of lectins which bridge carbohydrate chains of immunoglobulin (Ig) E Fc fragments has been suggested.[14] Fungal contaminants and bacterial endotoxins could activate C3 into anaphylatoxins and induce histamine release.[7] Other chemical mediators, such as leukotrienes and prostaglandins, are also involved.

Thus, ingestion of certain foods can provoke pseudoallergic reactions by non-specific histamine release. Strawberries are certainly the fruit most often held responsible. Chocolate, egg white and, in particular, ovomucoid are histamine releasers, as are crustaceans, fish and tomatoes. Certain exotic fruits, such as pineapple and papaya, contain proteases (bromelain and papain) which are histamine releasers, and various vegetables (peas, soya, green beans, lentils, beans, peanuts, cereals and nuts) contain lectins.

False food allergic reactions by non-specific histamine release are often observed in atopic young children and could provoke an exacerbation of atopic dermatitis the more so as skin mast cells are prone to release histamine easily.

Reactions owing to other mechanisms

The third group of FFA are related to various mechanisms which are often poorly understood.

Interference with metabolic routes of arachidonic acid

The inhibition of cyclo-oxygenase induces an increase of leukotriene synthesis by lipo-oxygenase. Certain substances such as sulphites, benzoic acid or azo dyes might act in this way by interfering with the metabolism of arachidonic acid.

Interference with the autonomic nervous system

Foods or, more often, food additives, can interfere with receptors in the autonomic nervous system, sometimes peripheral (adrenergic and cholinergic receptors) and sometimes in the central nervous system.

The 'Chinese restaurant' syndrome is related to the interference of glutamate with the synthesis of neuromediators. Sodium glutamate could interfere with glutaminergic neurons as well as γ-aminobutyric acid (GABA)ergic inhibitory neurons, as glutamic acid is the precursor of GABA. Glutamic acid and sodium are also precursors of acetylcholine synthesis.[11] High quantities of glutamate (>8 g) could favour excessive synthesis of acetylcholine. Caffeine (an additive of Coca Cola) and theine, have well known adrenergic properties.

Sulphites release sulphur dioxide in an acid medium and can stimulate bronchial epithelial receptors of irritation. This can induce a vagal reflex and provoke immediate bronchoconstriction in certain asthmatics.[26]

Abnormalities of enzymatic activities

The phenomenon of enzymatic inhibition probably plays an increasing part in the physiopathology of adverse reactions to food. It has been postulated that some antioxidants, such as sodium nitrite, vanilline, BHT and BHA are inhibitors of diamine oxidase.[12] These substances can interfere with histamine metabolism.

Certain additives can exert excessive pharmacological action in the presence of a pre-existing enzymatic deficiency. Thus, a deficiency in hepatic and pulmonary sulphite oxidase was demonstrated in certain cases of intolerance to sulphites.[43] This would result in abnormally high level of plasma and tissue sulphites, inducing inflammatory reactions by the increased production of oxidant free radicals from the membrane arachidonic acid.

A biological role of monoamine oxidase deficiency has been suspected in patients treated with inhibitors of this enzyme. These patients developed symptoms after the ingestion of certain foods, such as cheese. Deficiency of this enzyme induces the increase of circulating amines such as tyramine and phenylethylamine. A role of a deficiency of platelet monoamine oxidase has been suggested in patients with migraine.[37]

Factors enhancing pseudo-allergic reactions to food

A functional alteration of the digestive mucosa is probably an important factor. Indeed, the presence of factors which make mucosa more fragile at the onset of FFA is frequently observed, e.g. drug irritation from aspirin, non-steroidal anti-inflammatory drugs or spices, digestive fungal infestation or imbalance of the intestinal flora following antibiotherapy. The injection of 500 mg of aspirin induces an increase in intestinal permeability in 50% of subjects with chronic urticaria.[30] Certain substances such as alcohol, because of their effect on the digestive mucosa and their vasodilatory ability, are likely to enhance the passage of substances responsible for FFA.[23]

Abnormalities of histamine release are frequently found. A magnesium-deprived diet promotes hyperactivity to histamine.

CLINICAL ASPECTS OF FALSE FOOD ALLERGY

By definition, FFA mimics the symptoms of food allergy, but symptomatology is usually less severe. The clinical aspects are varied. A study carried out on 230 patients showed chronic urticaria or recurrent Quincke oedema in 75% of cases, digestive symptoms in 40%, vasomotor headaches in 16.8%, rhinitis in 10.8%, asthma in 5.6% and anaphylactoid shock in 1.7%.[29]

Histaminic shock

This is rare and milder, and appears later than anaphylactic shock, 2–3 h after meals. The subject experiences a hot flush with generalized erythema, nausea, vomiting or diarrhoea. A moderate and transitory drop in blood pressure is sometimes observed. Histaminic shock responds well in general to simple treatment (corticosteroids, antihistamines). Its relative mildness differentiates it from anaphylactic shock due to food allergy. It is, in general, related to the ingestion of foods particularly rich in histamine, such as tuna.[3,44]

Urticaria

Urticaria is the most frequent clinical symptom of FFA. The intraduodenal instillation of histamine (120 mg) induces hives in 64% of patients with chronic urticaria. An abnormal increase of plasma histamine was noted in 72% of cases.[18] A functional deficiency of diamine oxidase has been suggested.[24]

Histamine release reactions often occur in young children in the form of acute urticaria or exacerbation of atopic dermatitis. They are dose-dependent, e.g. urticaria may appear after eating a lot of strawberries, but not after the intake of a single fruit.

Digestive symptoms

Digestive symptoms are frequent and consist of either slowing of digestion, meteorism, epigastric or abdominal pain, or intermittent diarrhoea.

The frequency of abdominal pain in young children can lead to diagnosis of 'histaminic intestine' which could correspond either to a weakening of mast cells or to a greater reactivity of the smooth muscular tunic. It is very difficult to evaluate the part played by FFA in these digestive symptoms, which can be linked to irritable bowel syndrome, considered as an idiopathic abnormality of peristalsis and muscle tone.

Headaches

The triggering of migraine attacks owing to certain foods is frequently reported by patients. The mechanisms which underlie this phenomenon are unknown. It must, however, be noted that the foods most often blamed are rich in biogenic amines or histamine releasers, e.g. wine, chocolate, eggs, cooked meats and cheese.[22]

Histamine can induce a particular headache, the cluster headache. It occurs in the triggering of migraine.[21] Common headaches, lasting more than 1 h, are classically observed after intraduodenal instillation of histamine.

Hannington[13] has shown that it is possible to induce migraines by ingestion of 100 mg of tyramine, which corresponds to the quantity present in approximately 100 g of cheese. They are characterized by postprandial headaches, sometimes accompanied by pain in the right hypochondriac region, nausea and vomiting. Symptoms occur within 12 h of ingestion. The ingestion of 3 mg of phenylethylamine induced the appearance of migraine in 16 of the 38 migraine patients studied by Sandler and Youdim.[37] Sodium glutamate can also induce migraine, probably because of direct arterial vasospasm[41]. Tyramine is an agonist of glutamate. The association of tyramine and sodium glutamate increases the frequency and intensity of migraines.

Rhinitis and asthma

Respiratory symptoms are rare. Sulphites can induce bronchospasm in asthmatic subjects and nasal hyperreactivity syndrome in patients with nasal polyposis. Symptoms usually appear within 5 min of ingestion.

Worsening of atopic dermatitis

Eczematous skin is particularly rich in mast cells. The ingestion of histamine-releasing foods can induce a marked release of histamine in the skin, exacerbating pre-existing lesions and inducing pruritus and scratching which will accentuate lesions. Histamine-releasing foods have a stronger tendency to induce urticaria, oedema and erythema in subjects with atopic dermatitis.[1] This possibility must be considered, along with the classic implication of IgE-mediated food allergy particularly observed in atopic dermatitis of children.

The hyperactive child syndrome

This syndrome has benefited from much media attention, despite the lack of clinical and scientific studies reinforcing the hypothesis of a relationship between these emotional disorders and an additive intolerance. Several studies based on avoidance and reintroduction diets do not suggest the influence of additives on the children's behaviour, although sparse double blind[4] and crossover studies[40] are suggestive of such an association.

Other symptoms

Numerous neurovegetative (in particular neurosensory) symptoms are attributed to food by patients. Food neuroses may be confirmed after medical analysis and check-up. These symptoms must therefore be considered as a differential diagnosis which has a tendency to increase in frequency with media attention of food allergy and FFA.

DIAGNOSIS OF FALSE FOOD ALLERGY

The main diagnostic elements are summarized is Table 64.3.

1. Elimination of an immunological mechanism.
2. Proof of food category imbalance. Foods responsible for FFA are often consumed in excessive quantities in a diet which is frequently imbalanced.
3. Demonstration of abnormalities in the metabolism of histamine. Studies concerning abnormalities of the metabolism of certain substances, of which the best known are biogenic amines, are still rare and not easily applicable in common medical practice.

Category dietary analysis

Diagnosis begins by a careful dietary analysis of food eaten by the patient over 1 week. The patient notes all intake, including food, liquids or drugs, as well as quantities absorbed over 1 week. Analysis of labels of commercialized complex foods is an essential step to assess the consumption of additives.

Following this, the analytical study of this dietary diary estimates the weekly intake of histamine-rich food, histamine-releasing substances, tyramine, starchy foods, additives, etc.

Excessive consumption of these categories gives weight to the diagnosis of FFA. However, only a rough estimation is obtained, since reference values of usual intake by healthy subjects lack.

Elimination of immunological mechanisms

Establishing the diagnosis of FFA begins with the invalidation of a food allergy hypothesis. Skin prick tests with native food cur-

rently consumed by the patient must be extensive and eventually completed by challenge tests. Negative reactions are expected. The negative predictive value of these negative prick tests is excellent and food allergy can be discorded. Batch-tests have been lately recommended.

Detection of intestinal disorders

A parasite or yeast intestinal infestation may enhance FFA and has to be detected. The intestinal permeability is not altered.

Oral challenge tests

Skin tests allow elimination of an immediate hypersensitivity mechanism, but do not offer a positive argument in favour of the diagnosis of FFA. Only double blind challenge tests can prove the link between amines or additives on the one hand and the FFA symptoms on the other. Oral challenge tests can be very informative concerning FFA. They are carried out under strict medical control in a hospital environment with clinical follow up (skin, respiratory, ears, nose and throat, cardiovascular), along with blood pressure and pulse measurement. Assessment of the respiratory condition is currently made by measuring the peak expiratory flow, less commonly by forced expiratory volume in 1 second (FEV_1).

Challenge tests are carried out on quantities of blamed food substances normally eaten. These include certain biogenic amines (histamine, tyramine, phenylethylamine), aspirin and certain additives (sulphites, benzoic acid, tartrazine, sodium nitrite, etc.). Intraduodenal instillation of histamine at a dose normally well tolerated can reproduce the symptoms described by the patients: urticaria, headaches, functional digestive disorders, and more.[30] The use of enterosoluble capsules could constitute an interesting alternative in children by introducing histamine in a more acceptable way.[47] Aspirin has been considered as a pharmacological marker of intolerance to some additives and is often included in the battery of challenge tests.[32]

According to our experience of oral provocation tests with biogenic amine-rich or -poor cheese, challenge tests with histamine-rich and -poor foods could be valuable. Such tests need the cooperation of agro-alimentary industries[6,15,19,35,46].

Restriction diet

The restriction diet which must be envisaged is restricted in biogenic amines, without additives and, in addition, hypoallergenic. It commonly constitutes an alternative for diagnosis of FFA. It can be a necessary prerequisite in the case of severe symptomatology preventing the practice of challenge tests.[27] Its average length is 3–4 weeks.[17] During chronic urticaria, the percentage of improvement varies between 62 and 92% according to the authors. Tests of dietary reintroduction are not commonly used in FFA. In general, foods do not act exclusively by their own quality but by excessive consumption of a category of disparate foods containing the same compound (histamine, histamine releasers). In addition, excessive consumption acts in conjunction with an imbalanced diet and numerous enhancing factors.

TREATMENT

Rebalancing the diet

The marked reduction in consumption of the blamed foods should lead to the disappearance or the marked reduction in these dis-

Key elements in the diagnosis of false food allergy
Elimination of an immunological mechanism
Proof of food category imbalance
Demonstration of abnormalities in the metabolism of histamine

Table 64.3 Key elements in the diagnosis of false food allergy.

orders.[31,48] The correction of eating habits is a priority. Restoring a regular rhythm for meals is indispensable, which presupposes a similar rhythm regarding sleep and lifestyle. All non-specific causes of irritation of digestive mucosa should be suppressed (spices, alcohol, non-steroidal anti-inflammatory drugs, yeast or parasite intestinal infestation).

Antihistamines

Antihistamines constitute the symptomatic treatment, particularly in chronic urticaria. This type of treatment has only an adjuvant role, with the only long-term therapy being the establishment of a considered balanced diet.

Disodium cromoglycate is said to protect mast cells from degranulation. It has a variable effect in FFA in response to a histamine-releasing mechanism. The average prescription dose is 300 mg three times a day, taken approximately 45 min before meals.

CONCLUSIONS

The overall clinical picture of FFA mimics that of food allergy but can be distinguished by the absence of involvement of specific immunological mechanisms. FFA are characterized by the multiplicity of mechanisms which control them. In the absence of positive diagnostic tests, FFA must necessarily be a secondary diagnosis, the priority being the research and elimination of real food allergies, whose diagnosis can henceforth be currently established. Nutritional analysis, with the analysis of eating habits, food balance, research into excessive consumption of certain food categories, is therefore of extreme importance. It is advisable to eliminate borderline pathologies, and various forms of food neuroses. These facts underline the importance of nutritional consultation. The best result of treatment of FFA is complete recovery after the reintroduction of a balanced diet which is without additives, poor in histamine and in histamine-releasing foods, and after the correction of all exacerbating factors.

REFERENCES

1 Benton EC, Barnetson RC. Skin reactions to foods in patients with atopic dermatitis. *Acta Derm Venereol* 1985; 4: 129–32.

2 Bjeldanes LF, Schutz DE, Morris MM. On the etiology of scombroid poisoning: cadaverine potentiation of histamine toxicity in the guinea-pig. *Food Cosmet Toxicol* 1978; 16: 157–9

3 Boutin JP, Puyhardy JM, Chianea D et al. Les intoxications alimentaires histaminiques. *Santé Publique* 1998; 10: 29–37.

4 Carter CM, Urbanowicz M, Wemsley R et al. Effects of few food diets in attention deficit disorder. *Arch Div Childhood* 1993; 69: 564–8.

5 Chauchaix D, Pailler FM. L'histamine dans les denrées alimentaires. *Méd Armée* 1980; 8: 455–62.

6 Cliffort MN, Walker R, Ijomah P, Wright J, Murray CK, Hardy R. Is there a role for amines other than histamine in the aetiology of scombrotoxicosis? *Food Addit Contam* 1993; 8: 641–51.

7 De Weck AL. Pathophysiologic mechanisms of allergic and pseudo-allergic reactions to foods, food additives and drugs. *Ann Allergy* 1984; 53: 583–6.

8 Cohn VH. Inhibition of histamine metabolism by antimalarial drugs. *Biochem Pharmacol* 1965; 14: 1686.

9 Finazzi-Agro A, Floris G, Fadda MB, Crifo C. Inhibition of diamine oxidase by antihistaminic agents and related drugs. *Agents Actions* 1979; 9(3): 244–7.

10 Futo J, Kupferberg JP, Moss J. Inhibition of histamine N-methyltransferase (HMT) in vitro by neuromuscular relaxants. *Biochem Pharmacol* 1990; 39: 415–20.

11 Ghadimi H, Kumar S. Studies on monosodium glutamate ingestion: biochemical M-explanations of Chinese restaurant syndrome. *Biochem Med* 1971; 5: 447–56.

12 Goodman DL, McDonnel JT, Nelson HS, Vaughan TR, Weber RW. Chronic urticaria exacerbated by the antioxidant food preservatives, butylated hydroxyanisole (BHA) and butylated hydroxytoluene (BHT). *J Allergy Clin Immunol* 1990; 86: 570–5.

13 Hanington E. Preliminary report on tyramine headache. *BMJ* 1967; ii: 550–1.

14 Helm P, Froese A. Binding of the receptors for IgE by various lectins. *Int Arch Allergy Appl Immunol* 1981; 65: 81–4.

15 Hermann K, Hertenberg B, Ring J. Measurement and characterization of histamine and methylhistamine in human urine under histamine-rich and histamine-poor diets. *Int Arch Allergy Immunol* 1993; 101: 13–19.

16 Hesterberg R, Slattler J, Lorenz W et al. Distribution and metabolism of histamine. *Agents Actions* 1984; 14: 325–34.

17 Juhlin L. Additives and chronic urticaria. *Ann Allergy* 1987; 59: 119–23.

18 Kanny G, Moneret-Vautrin DA, Schohn H, Feldman L, Mallie JP, Gueant JL. Abnormalities in histamine pharmacodynamics in chronic urticaria. *Clin Exp Allergy* 1993; 23: 1015–20.

19 Kanny G, Bauza T, Frémont S et al. Wine histamine content does not influence the tolerance of wine in normal subjects. *J Allergy Clin Immunol* 1996; 97: 336.

20 Kanny G, Grignon G, Dauca M, Guedenet JC, Moneret-Vautrin DA. Ultrastructural changes in the duodenal mucosa induced by ingested histamine in patients with chronic urticaria. *Allergy* 1996; 51: 935–9

21 Krabbe AA, Olesen J. Headache provocation by continuous intravenous infusion of histamine. *Pain* 1980; 8: 253–9.

22 Larmande P, Ligeard P, Maillot F, Belin C. Le déclenchement alimentaire des crises de migraine. *Med Nut* 1993; 29(6): 263–7.

23 Lavo B, Jean F, Colombel F, Knutsson L, Hallgren R. Acute exposure of small intestine to ethanol induces mucosal leakage and prostaglandin E2 synthesis. *Gastroenterology* 1992; 102: 468–73.

24 Lessof MH, Gant V, Hinuma K, Murphy GM, Dowling RH. Recurrent urticaria and reduced diamine oxidase activity. *Clin Exp Allergy* 1990; 20: 373–6.

25 Malone G, Shea SM, Leventhal M. Histamine in foods: its possible role in non-allergic adverse reaction to ingestants. *N Engl Reg Allergy Proc* 1986; 7: 241–5.

26 Maria Y, Vaillant P, Delorme N, Moneret-Vautrin DA. Les accidents graves liés aux métabisulfites. *Rev Med Int* 1989; 10: 36–40.

27 Michaelsson G, Juhlin L. Urticaria induced by preservatives and dye additives in food and drugs. *Br J Dermatol* 1973; 88: 525–38.

28 Moneret-Vautrin DA. Approche diagnostique actuelle des accidents histaminiques d'origine alimentaire. *Med Hyg* 1975; 33: 1124–7.

29 Moneret-Vautrin DA. False food allergies. In: *Clinical Reactions to Food* (Lessof MH, ed.), Wiley, London, 1983: 135–53.

30 Moneret-Vautrin DA. Biogenic amines. In: *Food Allergy and Food Intolerance* (Somogyi JC, Müller HR, Ockhuisen T, eds), *Bibl Nutr Dieta*, Basel, 1991: 61–71. (Karger, ed. vol. 48.)

31 Moneret-Vautrin DA, Kanny G. Rational principles of diets in food allergy. *Adv Allergy Immunol* 1993; 2: 1–9.

32 Moneret-Vautrin D, Kanny G. Food and drug additives: hypersensitivity and intolerance. In: *Human Toxicology* (Descites J, ed.), Elsever Science, 1996: 259–80.

33 Mordelet-Dambrine M, Parrot JL. Action de l'histamine introduite par voie buccale ou formée dans le tube digestif. *Méd Nutr* 1970; 6: 59–73.

34 Morrow JD, Margolies GR, Rowland J, Roberts LJ. Evidence that histamine is the causative toxin of scombroid-fish poisoning. *N Engl J Med* 1991; 324: 716–20.

35 Oosting E, Keyzer JJ, Wilthers BG. Correlation between urinary levels of histamine metabolites in 24-hour urine samples of man: influence of histamine-rich food. *Agents Actions* 1989; 27: 205–7.

36 Saint-Blanquat G. Aspects toxicologiques et nutritionnels des nitrates et nitrites. *Ann Nutr Aliment* 1980; 34: 827–64.

37 Sandler M, Youdim MBH. A phenylethylamine oxidising defect in migraine. *Nature* 1974; 250: 335–7.

38 Sattler J, Hesterberg R, Lorenz W, Schmidt U, Crombach M, Stahlknecht CD. Inhibition of human and canine diamine oxidase by drugs used in an intensive care unit: relevance for clinical side effects? *Agents Actions* 1985; 16: 91–4.

39 Sattler J, Lorenz W, Kubo K, Schmal A, Sauer S, Luben L. Food induced histaminosis under diamine oxidase (DAO) blockade in pigs: further evidence of the key role of elevated plasma histamine levels as demonstrated by successful prophylaxis with antihistamines. *Agents Actions* 1989; 27: 212–14.

40 Schulte-Korne G, Deimel W, Gutenbrunner C *et al*. Effect of an oligo-antigen diet on the behavior of hyperkinetic children. *Z Kinder Jugenpsychiatr* 1996; 24: 176–83.

41 Scopp AL. MSG and hydrolyzed vegetable protein induced headache: review and case studies. *Headache* 1991; 31: 107–10.

42 Sessa A, Desiderio A, Perin A. Effect of acute ethanol administration on diamine oxidase activity in the upper gastrointestinal tract of rat. *Alcohol Clin Exp Res* 1984; 8: 185–90.

43 Simon R. Sulfite sensitivity. *Ann Allergy* 1983; 56: 281–91.

44 Taylor SL, Stratton JE, Nordlee JA. Histamine poisoning (scombroid fish poisoning): an allergy-like intoxication. *Clin Toxicol* 1989; 27: 225–40.

45 Uragoda CG. Histamine poisoning in tuberculous patients after ingestion of tuna fish. *Am Rev Respir Dis* 1980; 121: 157–9.

46 Van Gelderen CEM, Savelkoul TJF, Van Ginkel LA, Van Dokkum W. The effects of histamine administered in fish samples to healthy volunteers. *Clin Toxicol* 1992; 30: 585–96.

47 Vind S, Sondergaard I, Kaergaard Poulsen L, Gerner Svendsen U, Weeke B. Comparison of methods for intestinal histamine application: histamine in enterosoluble capsules or via a duodeno-jejunal tube. *Allergy* 1991; 46: 191–5.

48 Wantke F, Gotz M, Jarisch R. Histamine-free diet: treatment of choice for histamine-induced food intolerance and supporting treatment for chronic headaches. *Clin Exp Allergy* 1993; 23: 982–5.

INTRODUCTION

Dysfunctional breathing (DB) is a loss of breathing control. Hyperventilation (HV) is respiration above metabolic requirements. This leads to a reduction of the partial pressure of arterial carbon dioxide (P_aCO_2) (hypocapnia), respiratory alkalosis, vasoconstriction, central and peripheral hypoxia, reduced ionized calcium and destabilization of nerve and muscle membranes. We believe that symptomatic HV is usually based on chronic DB and will use the latter term. This is fully discussed later in the chapter. DB is a significant complication of three important allergic syndromes.

1. Chronic hypocapnia and loss of respiratory centre responsiveness to CO_2 are physiological consequences of asthma. Changes in the rate of breathing are a major cause of attacks of asthma.

2. The triad of psychological, irritable bowel, migraine syndrome, entitled PIMS (Fig. 65.1 and Table 65.1),[104] which is related to non-atopic allergy/intolerance, is complicated by symptoms of DB in approximately 70% of patients. A common complaint is: 'When I am careful with my diet I do not need to do my breathing exercises but when I eat the wrong thing I can't do them'. Ingestion of food allergen leads to an exacerbation of hyperventilation, delayed by between 10 min and 6 hours.

3. Fume sensitivity, often called 'multiple chemical sensitivity', usually triggers hyperventilation within 2–3 min.

In these conditions the symptoms generated by DB (Table 65.2) are often more dramatic and of more concern to the patient than those caused by straightforward allergy (see Table 65.1). Sufferers believe that symptoms due to DB are directly caused by allergy,

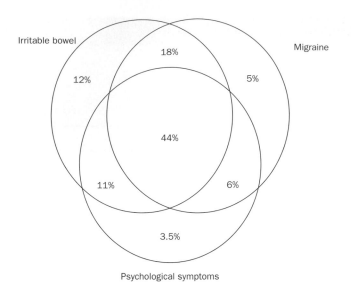

Irritable bowel

Migraine

12%

18%

5%

44%

11%

6%

3.5%

Psychological symptoms

Fig. 65.1 The psychological, irritable bowel, migraine syndrome (PIMS). Venn diagram showing overlap between complaints of mental problems (brain fag, confusion, memory lapses) irritable bowel and migraine in a consecutive series of adult patients attending an allergy clinic. The total cluster contains 113 patients with 50 (44%) having all three complaints. Atopic allergy in the airways identified a second separate group of migraineurs. Migraine not associated with atopy or other features of PIMS is unusual (5% in the diagram).

Symptoms associated with the psychological, irritable bowel, migraine syndrome (PIMS)
Psychological dysfunction: 'Brain fag': thinking process is 'slug-like' and coherent thinking takes a considerable effort, difficulties with concentration and memory, sensation of unreality   Addiction: usually to particular foods, e.g. bread or chocolate   Panic, depression
Irritable bowel syndrome: Diarrhoea/constipation   Abdominal bloating   Colic: intestinal or biliary
Migraine syndrome: Migraine: classical or common   Face ache: migraine equivalent in mask area   Headache: food-induced
Commonly associated problems with PIMS: Dysfunctional breathing (DB)   Hypomagnesaemia   Non-specific joint pains (hands/wrists often affected)   Fluid retention (variable weight and facial appearance)
Less frequently associated problems: • Urinary tract symptoms/vaginitis   • True fibromyalgia (diffuse pain centred on paraspinal muscles. Not aching due to hypomagnesaemia or DB)

Table 65.1 Symptoms associated with the psychological, irritable bowel, migraine syndrome (PIMS)

Symptoms of dysfunctional breathing (DB)
1. Mental: confusion, tension/lethargy, mood change, catastrophic misattribution, hallucinations (auditory and visual)   2. Eyes: blurred vision, photophobia   3. Ears: vertigo, dislike of loud noise   4. Muscles: 'draining' strength on exercise, chronic fatigue   5. Sensory: numbness, tingling, changes of awareness (may be asymmetrical   6. Heart: 'Palpitations', true arrhythmia, 'mitral valve prolapse' (reversible cardiac murmur), pseudoangina   7. Circulaton: pallor, cold extremities, easy flushing   8. Chest: Air hunger, pseudo-asthma   9. Throat: strained, dry, globus, voice problems   10. Bowels/bladder ugency

Table 65.2 Symptoms of dysfunctional breathing (DB). Observed symptoms of hyperventilation in allergy sufferers who tend to attribute these symptoms to allergies rather than dysfunctional breathing.

unless taught otherwise. This belief is reinforced by 'alternative' books on allergy and information from self-help groups which list the symptoms of hyperventilation as typical symptoms of allergy, 'Candida' or chronic fatigue syndrome. The 16-item Nijmegen questionnaire[146] (discussed below in 'Clinical management') is often used to screen patients for chronic symptomatic hyperventilation. However, the McEwen Hyperventilation Questionnaire (69 items, Appendix 1) allows for more comprehensive screening of DB and is more suitable for use in the preliminary stages of the investigation of patients who present with complex allergy problems.

Hyperventilation in an allergy clinic

A 3-min forced hyperventilation test (see below) has been used as a routine part of the examination of patients presenting with PIMS (see Table 65.1) or fume sensitivity. Symptoms supposed to be due to allergy are often reproduced during this test, confirming the relevance of hypocapnia. The demonstration of the true cause of symptoms is vital to the patient, since it also points to a direct form of therapy. At the start of this work patients were questioned using a checklist of symptoms of hyperventilation devised by Lum (Dr Claude Lum, pers comm, 1983). As experience increased, this was replaced by a wider checklist of complaints which appeared to be associated with DB in allergy patients. Table 65.3 shows the results of this checklist in 100 consecutive patients referred for the management of allergy but who were unable to complete the 3-min forced hyperventilation test and reproduced symptoms which they recognized. Using this information the McEwen hyperventilation questionnaire and scoring system (Appendix 1) was introduced in 1989. The use of physiotherapy for hyperventilation has been of significant benefit for these patients.

Physiological abnormalities in hyperventilation

The aetiology of hypocapnia in asthma is well understood and will be discussed later. Several publications have indicated other probable physiological links between allergic disease and hyperventilation.

1. Schmidt-Traub & Bamler[31] observed that 70% of panic disorder patients (total $n = 79$) displayed IgE-mediated type I

Symptoms reported by 100 consecutive patients referred for management of allergy

Mental symptoms

1. Concentration difficulty	83	
2. Floating sensation	75	
3. Memory lapses	74	
4. Confusion	60	
5. Sudden anger	60	
6. Tense	59	
7. Anxious	56	
8. Panic attacks	51	
9. Sudden tears	45	
10. Agoraphobia	42	
11. Fear of insanity	23	
12. Stupor (semiconscious episodes)	8	
13. Hallucinations	7	
14. Delusions	3	
15. Convulsions	2	

Sleep

16. Feels 'beaten up' in the morning	73
17. Vivid dreams	54
18. Wakes with symptoms at night	40

Ears

19. Vertigo	71
20. Dislike of noise	65
21. Tinnitus	38
22. Sounds distant	26

Eyes

23. Blurred vision	73
24. Dislikes bright lights	57
25. Altered perspective	17
26. Diplopia	12

Nervous system

27. Tingling	54
(a) Hands/feet	35
(b) Arms/legs	31
(c) Lips	10
(d) Face	9
(e) Tongue	4
28. Numbness	42
29. 'Thick head'/headaches	33
30. Migraine attacks	31

Autonomic nerves and circulation

31. Spontaneous sweating	41
32. Cold hands/feet	34
33. Poor circulation	21
34. Exaggerated reflexes	2
35. Incoordination	1

Respiratory system

36. Tight chest	49
37. (Frequent) yawning	45
38. Breathless	41
39. Can't get a satisfactory breath	30
40. (Frequent) sighing	30
41. Stop breathing	30
42. Dry throat	23
43. Irritable cough	21
44. Off key (singing)	20
45. Loss of singing voice	19
46. Asthma now	11
47. Asthma remitted	1

Heart

48. Palpitations	61
49. Dull pre-cordial ache	39
50. Angina-like pain	18
51. Pseudo coronary	3

Muscles

52. Constant weakness/fatigue	85
53. Draining strength	74
54. Muscle ache overall	35
(a) Limbs	50
(b) Neck	18
(c) Jaw	12
(d) Chest	9
55. Cramp	27
56. Twitch	25
57. Tremor	24
58. Exercise improves symptoms	21
59. Asymmetric weakness	4

Throat

60. Husky	43
61. Globus	37
62. Dysphagia	19
63. Submandibular swellings*	19
64. Restricted throat	2

Gastrointestinal

65. Excessive belching	38
66. Upper abdominal distress	26
67. Bowel movement urgent	7
68. Bowel movement uncontrolled	5
69. Bladder, uncontrolled	5
70. Bladder, urgent	5

*Sausage-shaped 'swellings' are hyoid muscles in spasm which come and go with other symptoms.

Table 65.3 Symptoms reported by 100 consecutive patients referred for management of allergy. Patients were unable to complete 3 min of forced hyperventilation and reproduced some recognized symptoms during the hyperventilation provocation test. The table shows the per cent of patients reporting a particular symptom. (For questionnaire as a diagnostic tool for hyperventilation in allergy patients, see McEwen Hyperventilation Questionnaire, Appendix 1).

allergic reactions in comparison to only 29% of normal controls (total $n = 66$).

2. Hypocapnia reduces the stability of mast cells (and magnesium has a stabilizing effect).[31]

3. In man, forced overbreathing significantly increases histamine levels in arterial and venous blood.[81]

4. Intracellular magnesium depletion is usual in asthma, irritable bowel and fume sensitivity. Fehlinger & Seidel[43] suggested that hyperventilation was primarily a manifestation of magnesium imbalance.

5. After 45 min of voluntary hyperventilation, the proportion of T suppressor cells was higher in patients with chronic DB compared with healthy controls ($P < 0.031$, Mann–Whitney U test).[111] At baseline the blood T lymphocyte helper/suppressor ratio ($T_H:T_S$) was slightly (although not significantly) higher in DB patients. Throughout the forced hyperventilation test the $T_H:T_S$ ratio was lower in the DB group compared with controls. The difference reached greatest significance after 30 min. This was chiefly due to a reduction in T suppressor cells in the control group compared with the DB patients, which reached greatest significance after 45 min (Fig. 65.2). Mooney et al.[111] propose that such a depressed $T_H:T_S$ ratio could be an indicator that patients with chronic DB become immunologically incompetent provided periods of acute HV are sufficiently frequent.

6. Irritable bowel, food intolerance and disturbed bowel flora are important features of PIMS, a syndrome related to non-atopic allergy described below. It seems likely that inappropriate secretion of gut hormone by the jejunum is responsible for many features of this syndrome. A possible link to DB is the demonstration that injection of the neuropeptide cholecystokinin provokes panic in up to 100% of patients with panic disorders (for a review, see van Megen et al.[147]).

7. The link between fume sensitivity and DB is probably more direct. Bell et al.[14] postulated a facilitated pathway from olfactory lobes to the amygdalae. Stimulation of the amygdalae can provoke panic.

Misattribution of symptoms of DB to allergy is harmful. Besides allergic disease, there are many other correctable causes of DB. The medical profession in general is underinformed on this subject. The practice of clinical allergy requires a holistic approach, with expertise in the environment, nutrition and psychology as well as in optimal conventional management of a variety of clinical problems. Skill in diagnosing and treating DB fits well with these interests. Most importantly, DB easily becomes a learned and self-perpetuating habit. When it complicates allergic disease, its recognition, education of the patient and retraining of the breathing may be essential for a full recovery (see 'Habituation' below).

Patients suffering from PIMS or fume sensitivity are the objects of strong medical disagreement. Other sections of this book put the case for hypersensitivity to environmental agents. This aetiology is dismissed by a large section of the medical profession, which asserts that these patients merely suffer from expressions of somatization, anxiety and panic. If the role of allergy/intolerance is ignored, true cure must be replaced by palliative drugs and treatment aimed at acceptance of symptoms. A false diagnosis of allergy leads to inappropriate restriction of lifestyle and diet, but a false diagnosis of psychosomatic illness is even more damaging. Hypersensitivity syndromes and panic are both associated with DB. Apart from the need to improve the management of hypersensitivity syndromes complicated by DB, allergists cannot defend their position without a working knowledge of DB and panic (Fig. 65.3).

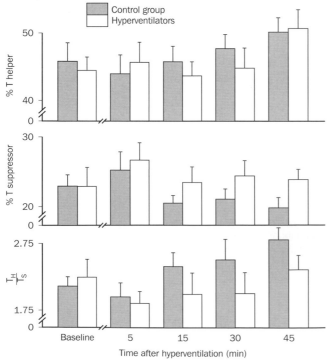

Fig. 65.2 Proportions of T helper and T suppressor lymphocytes before and after hyperventilation in healthy control subjects and in patients with hyperventilation. The TH:Ts ratio was more depressed in hyperventilation patients than in controls throughout the test period. This suggests that in recurring hyperventilation immunological functions may be compromised among hyperventilators. (Reprinted by permission of Elsevier Science from Moonay et al.[111] © 1986 by the Society of Biological Psychiatry.)

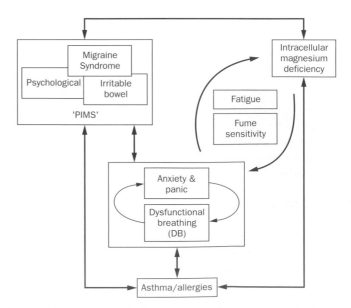

Fig. 65.3 Unrecognized dysfunctional breathing may complicate diagnosis and treatment of complex allergy problems and may be present in up to 70% of PIMS sufferers. Dysfunctional breathing is easy to recognize and responds well to therapy.

The psycho–physiological hypothesis of dysfunctional breathing

At the time of writing, patients suffering from DB may be treated by psychiatrists holding the view that hyperventilation is nearly always an expression of anxiety state and panic disorder. The hyperventilation syndrome[3,77] has chiefly interested physiologists, chest physicians and psychiatrists. Is the aetiology purely psychological? Kerr et al.[77] and Lum[98] emphasized that their patients had no organic disease. Bass & Gardner[7] recognized the importance of anxiety and panic but accepted that psychiatric morbidity could not always be confirmed. Later, Gardner & Bass[51] listed anxiety/panic alongside 11 physical causes of chronic hypocapnia, especially subclinical asthma (allergy was omitted). No distinction was made between hyperventilation driven by physical or psychological mechanisms. Wessely et al.[150] recognized the clustering of syndromes reported by McEwen,[104] which include hyperventilation, but interpreted them as a group of functional somatic syndromes. This has led further to the concept of a psychosomatic 'illness superhighway'.[101]

Chronic hypocapnia or normocapnia?

Some authors believe that patients suffering from chronic hyperventilation syndrome are by definition continously hypocapnic,[87] whereas others find that patients are often but not always hypocapnic.[46,53] Wilkinson et al.[153] for example, found that only 5% of patients subsequently diagnosed with chronic hyperventilation had a $P_{et}CO_2$ (end-tidal partial pressure of carbon dioxide) level of 30 mmHg (4 kPa) or less when first tested. In a paper read to the Society of Psychosomatic Medicine in 1985 Folgering reported that in his clinic the figure was 14%. In 1999 Folgering proposed strict diagnostic criteria which would be fulfilled by few patients:

1. patients should have a low arterial P_{CO_2}
2. somatic disease should be excluded
3. patients should present with current or previous hypocapnic complaints.

These proposals would restrict the definition of chronic hyperventilation to a purely psychiatric aetiology and require that hypocapnia be continuous. It may be true that transcutaneous monitoring of $P_{tc}CO_2$ (transcutaneous partial pressure of carbon dioxide) is less satisfactory than measurement of arterial blood gases, but measurement of end-tidal P_{CO_2} is valid and noninvasive. Folgering's definition excludes patients who are normocapnic at pre-test but who are plunged into dramatic and prolonged hypocapnia after overbreathing.[53] Folgering also ignores the many cases of symptomatic chronic hyperventilation driven by somatic complaints, such as subclinical asthma, which are discussed later in this chapter.

Dysfunctional breathing or hyperventilation?

These arguments arise from attempts to fit observation to preconceptions. The true nature of what has been known as the 'chronic hyperventilation syndrome' is revealed by observation of the pattern of breathing. Hyperpnoea is often imperceptible. By day, at rest, phases of normal breathing or subtle overbreathing last 3–5 min. The pattern may be disturbed by sighing and yawning. These phases alternate with intervals of apnoea which usually last between 20 and 40 seconds. The apnoeic intervals are easy to recognize. This irregular breathing pattern is evidence of disturbance of the respiratory control system. There is CO_2 chemore-

ceptor insensitivity.[45] The respiratory centre fails to respond to variations in the P_aCO_2 and does not reset carbon dioxide levels to normal.[45,51] The breathing is 'free-wheeling'. This is a homeostatic disturbance. Contrary to a widespread belief, hyperventilation can therefore be chronic as well as intermittent. A more accurate description is therefore *dysfunctional breathing* (DB). It is likely that lack of a correct understanding and imprecise diagnostic criteria (leading to poorly screened patient samples) has produced inconclusive research outcomes. This may be one of the main reasons why the hyperventilation syndrome has met with increasing criticism.[65,68,71]

Nocturnal dysfunctional breathing

The truth of the above description is particularly illustrated during sleep. DB continues but everything slows down. Hyperpnoea is replaced by appropriate respiration. The intervals of apnoea may increase to the point where the sufferer experiences symptoms of central sleep apnoea. The P_{CO_2} rises and settles to a near-normal level during the first few hours of sleep.[51] As discussed below, the rise in P_{CO_2} appears to play a role in the aetiology of nocturnal panics. The most common symptom arising from nocturnal DB is generalized muscle ache on waking. Feeling 'beaten up' is reported by over 70% of DB patients (Table 65.3) (McEwen, unpublished work).

PHYSIOLOGY OF DYSFUNCTIONAL BREATHING

Physiology of CO₂ metabolism

During a single passage through the lungs only 20% of the CO_2 dissolved in the blood should be lost to the expired air. The remaining 80% is retained in the blood as it leaves the lungs. Excess CO_2 is easily lost by increased breathing effort and the quantity retained is regulated by the respiratory centre's control of breathing. By washing out CO_2, hyperventilation reduces blood carbonic acid. The pH of arterial blood rises within 5–20 seconds. A few minutes after termination of hyperventilation the partial pressure of CO_2 and the pH return to normal.[18,20,85] The inverse relationship between rise in pH and hypocapnia is illustrated in Fig. 65.4. When the pH rises, ionized calcium falls. The electrical stability of nerve and muscle membranes depends on ionized

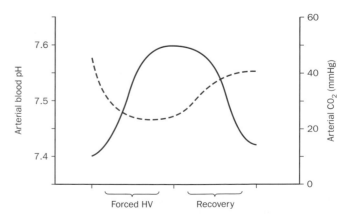

Fig. 65.4 Respiratory alkalosis induced by hypocapnia during voluntary hyperventilation (30 breaths/min) in healthy volunteers.
———, Arterial blood pH; – – – – –, arterial Co_2. (Adapted from Gorman et al. 1988).

calcium. The most immediate symptoms provoked by hyperventilation result from destabilization of peripheral autonomic and sensory nerves, leading to enhanced conduction, in particular along demyelinated nerve fibres.[128] As the alkalosis is sustained, anoxia becomes important and symptoms which develop more slowly have a complex aetiology.

Renal compensation

The kidneys compensate for the respiratory alkalosis by excreting bicarbonate. If overbreathing is sustained, the alkali reserve becomes significantly depleted. When prolonged overbreathing stops, the alkali reserve recovers more slowly than the P_{CO_2}. The blood contains other buffers and its pH is only partly dependent on dissolved CO_2/bicarbonate. This is much less true of the cerebrospinal fluid (CSF). Depletion of the CSF bicarbonate makes the central nervous system (CNS) vulnerable to the effect of short-term swings of dissolved CO_2. Lambertsen[83] emphasized the very slow equilibration of the CSF bicarbonate. The persistent low CSF alkali reserve and the resulting excess susceptibility to short-term hypocapnia form the physiological background to the 3-min forced hyperventilation test. Patients who have been sufficiently hypocapnic to develop symptoms at some time during the preceeding 24–48 h cannot forcibly hyperventilate for 3 min. Excessive symptoms force them to stop prematurely, sometimes after less than 30 seconds.

Paradoxically, overbreathing produces tissue anoxia. There are two reasons. First, the increased pH of capillary blood leads to a leftward shift of the oxyhaemoglobin dissociation curve (Bohr effect). The arterial blood is fully oxygenated but oxygen release is greatly reduced. The second reason for tissue anoxia is vasoconstriction.

The coronary blood flow may be reduced by 40%[30] and the cerebral blood flow is similarly reduced.[127] A 1 mmHg drop of P_aCO_2 causes a reduction of 2% in cerebral blood flow.[126] Even muscle is affected by these changes: lactate production during muscular exercise is increased by inappropriate overbreathing.[36]

Hypoxia

A sequel of chronic moderate cerebral hypoxia is a partial switch to anaerobic metabolism. During hyperventilation lactic acid accumulates in the brain.[135] Lambertsen[83] showed that acid and base transfer across the blood–brain barrier is very slow, and lactic acid has a prolonged half-life in the brain which is not adapted for anaerobic metabolism. Through this mechanism a single relatively short episode of hyperventilation (1 h) may generate mental symptoms which persist for 2–3 days. Intravenous infusion of lactic acid causes panic in normal subjects.[59]

Behavioural breathlessness[73] or air hunger is commonly reported by DB sufferers and it is often possible to reproduce air hunger by forced overbreathing. Although the aetiology of air hunger is unproven, it seems likely that this is another consequence of the failure of haemoglobin to part with its oxygen if the pH is too high. The carotid bodies sense lack of oxygen and drive the breathing inappropriately. Persistent overbreathing at the end of forced hyperventilation is an important diagnostic sign of DB. It seems likely that previous hyperventilation reduces the threshold of the response to signals from the carotid bodies, since air hunger is not generated by forced overbreathing in normal subjects.

The cause of symptoms

Most symptoms of hypocapnia are associated with increased neuronal excitability linked directly to the increased pH or to anoxia. The total blood calcium is unchanged but the pH shift leads to reduction of the proportion which is ionized. There is a consequent increase in the excitability of all cell membranes. This is most obvious in the peripheral nerves (for a review see Macefield & Burke[100]). Small unmyelinated autonomic fibres are the first to be affected.[128] The first signs of paraesthesiae occur usually at CO_2 levels of 29 mmHg or less.[124] The reduction of ionized calcium eventually leads to tetany[100] (Fig. 65.5).

The importance of this classical mechanism for increased neuronal excitability and tetany has been challenged by others who failed to measure an appropriate reduction in ionized calcium

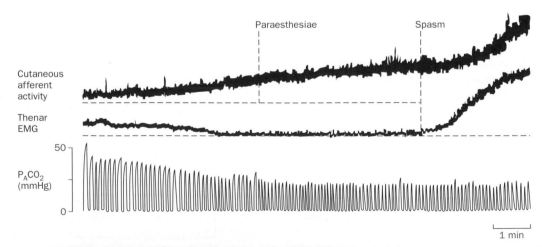

Fig. 65.5 Integrated neural activity recorded within a fascicle innervating digit IV (upper trace), integrated electromyogram (EMG) activity recorded with surface electrodes over the thenar muscles (middle trace) and alveolar P_ACO_2 (lower trace) during voluntary hyperventilation. The arrow in the middle trace indicates voluntary relaxation of the hand, on request. Background neural activity increased progressively as P_ACO_2 declined, reflecting the spontaneous discharge of cutaneous axons. Involuntary EMG leading to a tetanic spasm of the hand developed 8 min after neural activity began to increase. Paraesthesiae were reported first in the face, 4 min before tetany developed in the hand. Integrator time constants were 200 ms. (Reprinted from Macefield G & Burke D,[100] with permission.)

and suggest that increased neuronal excitability is associated with hypophosphataemia (for a review see Gardner[50]). The chief difficulty with this research is that outside forced hyperventilation experiments, most sufferers from DB are normocapnic most of the time. This has already been discussed above. Lum (pers comm, 1984) has also emphasized that CO_2 dissolves directly into excitable membranes. The strength of this stabilization is demonstrated by the importance of CO_2 narcosis at increased atmospheric pressure.

Central nervous disturbances such as vertigo, loss of consciousness, blurred vision, headache, ataxia, tremor and tinnitus have all been ascribed to reduction of cerebral blood flow and hypoxia.[122] Cold extremities and pseudoangina are caused by hypocapnic vasoconstriction. Blau et al.[16] have reported that the CNS symptoms of hyperventilation are often left-sided and frequently falsely diagnosed as epilepsy, ischaemia or demyelination. Hypocapnia may also give rise to contraction of hyoid muscles which are felt as sausage-shaped swellings below the jaw and are reported as 'glands'. A disc jockey complained that these 'glands' came up and the left side of his face became numb when he reached over his control panel to change a record. Two deep breaths reproduced the symptoms.

Role of magnesium
Magnesium deficiency

Fehlinger & Seidel[43] drew attention to the role of hypomagnesaemia in hyperventilation but this subject has attracted little attention despite the fact that intracellular magnesium is nearly always depleted in DB patients. This is a vicious circle. First, the kidneys attempt to correct the elevated blood pH by excreting bicarbonate. Hydrogen ions are conserved, but in the urine the bicarbonate anion must be accompanied by a cation. The metal cations available are sodium, potassium and magnesium. Sodium excretion is increased only transiently before it is limited by other homeostatic mechanisms. Potassium and magnesium can replace sodium, and their excretion will be increased. Dietary potassium is easily absorbed, and the urinary loss does not normally lead to hypokalaemia. On the other hand, dietary intake of magnesium is likely to be low in Western societies.[106] Magnesium is lost during cooking and refining of food,[132] and absorption from the gut is limited. When excretion is increased, magnesium deficiency is probable.

Homeostasis of extracellular magnesium is essential to the heart, and in chronic hypomagnesaemia the serum magnesium is always normal. This is maintained at the expense of the intracellular pool. Red cell magnesium is the most useful measure commonly available. There are patients in whom the red cell value is normal, but the myothermogram (MTG) reveals severe intracellular hypomagnesaemia within the muscles (see 'Muscle function' below). In a specialist laboratory the magnesium status can be confirmed by MTG or sweat mineral analysis. Galland[47] confirms that magnesium deficiency may predispose to hyperventilation. He also recognizes that severe magnesium depletion may lead to loss of hearing, migraine and transient ischaemic attacks. Egger et al.[37] demonstrated that an oral supplement of magnesium orotate could successfully treat the runaway hyperventilation and apnoeic convulsions which characterize Rett syndrome.

Magnesium and pH levels: a vicious circle

Like potassium, magnesium is chiefly an intracellular positively charged cation which reduces the negative charge across cell membranes. When the intracellular magnesium is depleted, this negative charge tends to increase. Hydrogen ions are the chief cation available as a substitute, so magnesium deficiency leads to intracellular acidosis. The cells of the respiratory centre respond to decreased intracellular pH by stimulating breathing, and the vicious circle is complete. Recognizing and treating magnesium deficiency is important.

Muscle function

Besides directly helping to regulate breathing dysfunction, correction of hypomagnesaemia is important in the treatment of physical fatigue. Cox et al.[29] demonstrated that chronic fatigue patients had significantly lower red cell magnesium than controls and that intravenous magnesium sulphate reduced fatigue, muscle pain and other symptoms. Muscle lengthening is an energy-consuming process which replaces calcium with magnesium on the myosin threads. Intracellular magnesium deficiency leads to greater heat production during muscular relaxation and repeated spikes of heat production while the muscle remains relaxed. This can be measured by the MTG. Fig. 65.6A is a tracing (courtesy of Dr. John Howard) from a thermocouple over the biceps of a patient suffering from PIMS, intracellular hypomagnesaemia, DB and chronic fatigue. The subject was asked to bend the elbow and straighten it again three times. The recording was made during a fourth repeat (Fig. 65.6B). Figure 65.6C shows the change after oral repletion of magnesium. In the author's experience, intracellular hypomagnesaemia within skeletal muscle demonstrated by MTG is not reliably reflected even by red cell or sweat magnesium.

Bicarbonate

Bicarbonate excretion leads to a reduced alkali reserve. A blood bicarbonate near or below the lower limit of the normal range is common in DB patients. This is often misinterpreted as evidence for metabolic acidosis although the real cause is respiratory alkalosis. Nevertheless, there is some truth in this assumption because, as we have seen, secondary magnesium deficiency leads to an intracellular acidosis. Fortunately this condition is usually treated with supplements of potassium and magnesium, loosely described as 'alkali', which help to break the vicious circle described above.

pH and magnesium levels

Diagnosis of DB depends on previous depletion of the alkali reserve. Although the 3-min forced hyperventilation provocation test has certain limitations as a diagnostic tool, particularly in dealing with panic patients,[69] it can nevertheless provide the clinician dealing with DB with useful information. Controlled overbreathing produces symptoms much more quickly if the bicarbonate reserves are low, particularly within the CNS (see above). A forced hyperventilation test will be negative if a patient who hyperventilates intermittently has not done so in the previous 24–48 h and there has been time for the alkali reserve to recover. The forced hyperventilation test should be continued until the patient is forced to stop. This gives the best chance of observing the prolonged involuntary overbreathing following the test, which is strong evidence of DB. The mechanism of this persistent air hunger has been discussed above.

Asthma

The threshold doses of histamine or methacholine aerosols required to provoke bronchospasm are greatly reduced in asthmatics. It is

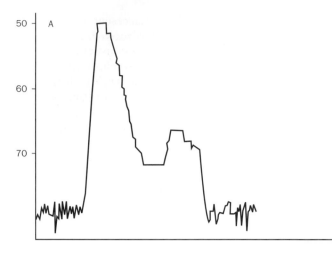

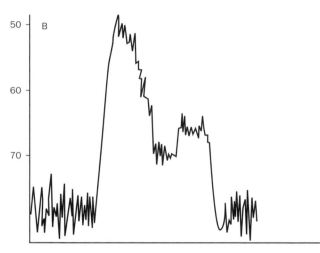

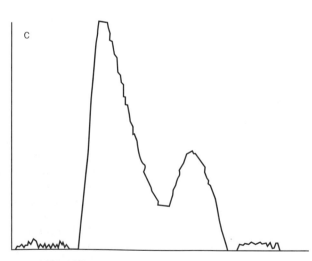

Fig. 65.6 Myothermograms. Heat produced by the biceps muscle recorded from a surface thermocouple. The elbow is flexed. The heat of contraction decays to a new plateau as the biceps remains shortened. Extending the muscle generates metabolic heat of relaxation and a return to the original baseline. (**A**) During hypomagnesaemia – the muscle has been resting; baseline, magnesium deficient. (**B**) During hypomagnesaemia. The elbow has been flexed three times isotonically. Note the spikes of heat production required during relaxation and the increased heat of relaxation. After slight isotonic exercise, magnesium deficient. (**C**) Same patient. Same conditions as (**B**). Hypomagnesaemia has been corrected. Same exercise, effective magnesium supplement for a month. (Courtesy Dr. John Howard.)

now recognized that depletion of magnesium is partly responsible for bronchial hyperreactivity in asthma.[19,35] Again it is the intracellular magnesium which is depleted. The red cell magnesium is likely to be low but the serum magnesium will be normal. Magnesium has bronchodilating properties, but there have been conflicting reports (for a review see Hill[66]). Some physicians now use intravenous (IV) magnesium sulphate as part of their emergency treatment of status asthmaticus.[86,140] The relationship of asthma to DB is further discussed below.

Fatigue

Fatigue is a common complaint in chronic hyperventilators, reported by 53–93% of patients.[27] Forced hyperventilation provokes a sensation of muscular weakness. Panic or agoraphobia associated with hyperventilation leads to sudden draining of strength. Folgering & Snik[46] studied fatigue in patients with hyperventilation syndrome. Electromyogram (EMG) analysis of fatigability failed to find a correlation between fatigue and P_{CO_2}, nor was EMG fatigability influenced by lactate in contracting muscles. Objective measurement of endurance time revealed that muscular strength was lost *more slowly* in hyperventilators. These authors concluded that hyperventilation-induced physical fatigue is a central sensation. Bazelmans *et al.*[10] compared patients with chronic fatigue syndrome with or without hyperventilation and found no differences with regard to fatigue, depression, number of complaints or activity level. Saisch *et al.*[129] also found only a weak association with hyperventilation in 31 patients with chronic fatigue syndrome. Naifeh[114] has suggested that hypocapnic bronchoconstriction may contribute to fatigue, since increased airway resistance increases the work of breathing. This may be true of hyperventilation associated with subclinical asthma but the majority of sufferers from chronic fatigue and DB do not have significant airway obstruction.

Many names such as effort syndrome, neurasthenia and chronic fatigue syndrome have been applied to hyperventilation-related fatigue,[88,116,117] but these names have often been used in such a way that fatigue from any unrecognized cause may be included. The term chronic fatigue syndrome is correctly used in a purely descriptive sense, not as a diagnosis in its own right. There is little doubt of the existence of a persistent fatigue syndrome which appears to be post-viral, but the experience of Pearson (pers comm, 1996) (described below) illustrates that the diagnosis of myalgic encephalomyelitis (ME) has been widely misused.

Intracellular hypomagnesaemia within skeletal muscle has been discussed above. This is usual in patients suffering from DB. The MTG shows that magnesium deficiency directly affects the energy requirements of the contractile process. A failure to study the MTG in parallel with the EMG may account for some of the present confusion concerning chronic fatigue, particularly as it relates to DB which is usually accompanied by hypomagnesaemia.

CAUSES AND SUSTAINING FACTORS OF DYSFUNCTIONAL BREATHING (Table 65.4)

Habituation

Following a prolonged episode of hypocapnia, hyperventilation may become habitual. An acute stressful stimulus such as a mugging or bereavement[28] or even a stressful concert performance[151] can trigger an initial period of hypocapnia, which may

Causes and sustaining factors of DB
Learned pattern of breathing (habituation), stress and phobias
Allergy and asthma
Psychological, irritable bowel, migraine syndrome (PIMS)
Fume sensitivity ('multiple chemical sensitivity')
Infection, fever, myalgic encephalomyelitis (ME), chronic fatigue syndrome (CFS)
Pain
Magnesium deficiency
Premenstrual syndrome (PMS)
Hypoglycaemia
Respiratory diseases
Middle ear diseases
Alcohol addiction/withdrawal

Table 65.4 Causes and sustaining factors of DB. Single and multiple aetiological factors of hyperventilation observed in one of the authors' (L.M.M.) clinical practice.

subsequently develop into DB or be maintained by, for example, persistent psychological stress or chronic pain. Due to selective referral, the experience of Lum (a chest physician) and L.M.M. (an allergist) inevitably differs from that of psychiatrists. Lum (pers comm, 1984) holds the view that hyperventilation need be nothing more than a learned and self-perpetuating pattern of breathing. This was illustrated by a patient who complained only of lifelong fatigue. He was happy and well adjusted but had suffered painful repair of a war wound 40 years previously. He lost his fatigue after one session of breathing instruction. The physiology of this habituation has been well illustrated in an experiment by Saltzman et al.[130] During a brief episode of forced hyperventilation the P_aCO_2 quickly drops from 40 mmHg to 20 mmHg. Once established, this hypocapnia is easily maintained by occasional deep breaths equivalent to a deep sigh or yawn. The role of conditioning of ventilatory responses has been extensively studied.[11,33,48,109] These investigators agree that emotions, cognitions and breathing behaviour are closely interconnected and respiratory responses can be conditioned (for a review see Ley[93]). Respiratory changes may trigger certain emotions and vice versa.

Preliminary confirmatory evidence for conditioning of hyperventilation was recently presented.[94,144] It lends support to Ley's dyspnoea/suffocation fear theory[91] which identified hypocapnic symptoms as the unconditioned stimulus for secondary panic attacks.

The psychiatric debate: cognitive versus biological models of panic

Hyperventilation may occur without panic and, similarly, panic may occur without hypocapnia (for a review see Bass et al.[9]). In the first author's series of 100 consecutive allergy patients who reproduced their symptoms in a 3-min forced hyperventilation test, only 51 had experienced panic attacks. Nevertheless, patients suffering from allergy/intolerance and DB often come under the control of psychiatrists holding the view that hyperventilation is mainly an expression of anxiety state and panic disorder. Liebowitz et al.[96] suggested that about half of all patients with panic disorders are chronic hyperventilators. Gorman[58] and Papp

and coworkers[120] found that panic disorder is associated with a significant reduction of $P_{et}CO_2$ and blood bicarbonate. The question whether (cognitive) panic precedes hyperventilation or vice versa continues to be disputed.[23,24,38,89,91,102] The cognitive model of panic[23] maintains that hypocapnic symptoms are secondary to anxiety and are epiphenomena of panics. Emphasis is put on catastrophic misattribution of bodily symptoms. For example, palpitations are misinterpreted as an impending heart attack. Such misinterpretations are common in patients with panic. According to a survey of a British general practice population (total of 3000, aged 18–65), 7.5% of registered patients had experienced a panic attack within the previous 8 weeks.[139] This agrees with other studies which show that at least occasional panic attacks are reported by about 10% of the adult population (for a review see Margraf & Ehlers[103]). Doctors are generally unaware that many of their patients regularly experience bizarre hypocapnic symptoms but feel unable to disclose their real concerns unless directly questioned.

The cognitive model of panic has been challenged[92] since it fails to explain the aetiology of nocturnal panics[63,108] which break into dreamless, non-rapid eye movement (REM) sleep.[90] Chronic hyperventilators may also experience relaxation-induced panic[5] and panic associated with a significant *increase* in PCO_2.[53,79] Klein[79] has suggested that panic is triggered by a physiological misfiring of the false suffocation alarm monitor, but Gardner[50] doubts this. These observations favour the concept of a failure of breathing control (DB) put forward in this chapter.

Allergies

Asthma

Asthmatics suffer from symptoms of chronic variable hypocapnia which are often misattributed to anoxia even by members of the medical profession. In asthma the carbon dioxide in the blood does not control the respiratory centre. If bronchospasm is suddenly totally relieved, alveolar ventilation and thus hypocapnia may increase. Bronchodilator drugs sometimes cause unpleasant symptoms through this mechanism. Bronchospasm and blood flow changes are not uniform throughout asthmatic lungs: some patches of lung are well aerated and some are not; some patches are well perfused and some are not. There is ventilation/perfusion mismatch and blood passes through areas of lung which are not aerated.[105] Blood which perfuses patches of good aeration becomes fully saturated with oxygen, but the mixed blood reaching the left side of the heart remains partly desaturated. This cannot be corrected by extra ventilatory effort; the carotid bodies respond by driving the breathing and hypocapnia results. This applies to all degrees of asthma except terminal respiratory failure. Unrecognized mild asthma may present as troublesome symptoms of chronic hyperventilation,[21,34,123] which can be relieved by steroid aerosol therapy.[52] Hypocapnia is an important cause of nonspecific bronchial hyperreactivity in asthma. Increases in the rate of breathing lead to increased bronchospasm. Herxheimer[64] described how hyperventilation triggers asthma attacks in susceptible individuals. Immediately before the onset of asthma attacks the P_aCO_2 may be as low as 21 mmHg (2.8 kPa).[105] Although the ventilation/perfusion mismatch model is undisputed, Gardner[49] has suggested that vagal receptor stimulation in the lungs, stimulation of chemoreceptors by hypoxia and the mechanical effect of hyperinflation may all contribute to inappropriate respiratory drive. The destabilizing effect of hypocapnia on mast cells[31] and the increased blood histamine after forced hyperventilation[81] have been referred to earlier in this chapter. It is a common clinical experience that a purely psychogenic attack of bronchospasm triggered by overbreathing requires the same treatment as asthma triggered by allergy. The teaching of relaxation and abdominal breathing to asthmatics can be helpful,[149] in particular where asthma is accompanied by panic, but research findings to date are mixed.[84]

More recently the Russian *Buteyko* breathing technique[136] has attracted publicity. It teaches asthma patients to counteract hyperventilation by prolonged breath holding (up to 2 min). Mouth breathing at night (which favours hypocapnia by reducing the respiratory dead-space) is prevented by wearing adhesive tape over the mouth when sleeping. A prospective blind controlled study of 39 asthmatics (age 12–70) with substantial medication use failed to show any change in airway calibre or changes in $P_{et}CO_2$ after 3 months. Nevertheless, use of inhaled steroid was reduced by 49% in the actively treated group.[17] At present the *Buteyko* method remains controversial[15,148] and further controlled research is needed to evaluate its efficacy.

Psychological, irritable bowel, migraine syndrome (PIMS)

McEwen & Birtwistle recognized that patients referred to allergy clinics for management of psychological difficulty ('brain fag'), irritable bowel or migraine often suffered from all three complaints. In McEwen's clinic the overlap was 44% (see Fig. 65.1). This led McEwen[104] to propose the psychological, irritable bowel, migraine syndrome (PIMS) (Table 65.4). This paper reported that PIMS (Table 65.1) is frequently associated with hyperventilation, giving rise to additional symptoms which may be more dramatic than the true symptoms of allergy. Further experience suggests that DB may be associated with PIMS in up to 70% of cases. The symptoms of DB are frequently assumed to be typical of allergy.

'Brain fag' is a difficulty in thought and concentration which resembles somnolence. The sufferer can think clearly and coherently but only with effort. In contrast, hyperventilation gives rise to racing, unfocused thoughts, and variable difficulty with memory. Sufferers from PIMS commonly experience both problems at different times.

Although PIMS is easy to identify, therapists and sufferers frequently define this disorder purely in terms of the hypersensitivities which are believed to be involved, such as 'multiple chemical sensitivity', 'total allergy syndrome' or 'Candida'. The hypomagnesaemia and DB associated with PIMS lead to muscle aching and physical fatigue. This may result in the diagnosis of chronic fatigue syndrome, ME or chronic fatigue immune deficiency syndrome (CFIDS). The term 'fibromyalgia' is now also being applied to the same syndrome. True idiopathic fibromyalgia is sometimes associated with PIMS, but the term is now being used when this is not the case. Pearson (pers comm, 1996) researched groups of 50 patients referred by general practitioners, first for 'total allergy syndrome', second for 'Candida' and third for 'myalgic encephalopathy'. The interval between each of the investigations was 5 years. Half of the patients referred for the second and third studies had presented previously with a different diagnosis (Pearson, pers comm, 1996). Wessely *et al.*[150] also recognized many names for one cluster of symptoms, but believed somatization to be the chief mechanism. The role of non-atopic hypersensitivity, chiefly to foods, as a cause of mental dysfunction,

irritable bowel and migraine is dealt with elsewhere in this book. Clinical experience suggests that in patients suffering from PIMS, dysfunctional breathing may be driven directly by intolerance and disturbed gut flora. The link to breathing may be through inappropriate secretion of cholecystokinin, which can provoke panic when injected (for a review see Ref.147). Patients trained to recognize their DB report that food intolerance can force them to hyperventilate: 'If I stay on my diet I do not need to do my breathing exercises. If I break my diet I cannot do them.'

Fume sensitivity

This problem, characterized by the rapid onset of multiple symptoms after smelling an odour, typically a perfume, is popularly but inaccurately called 'multiple chemical sensitivity' (MCS). Millqvist & Löwhagen[110] studied patients who reported stuffy nose, phlegm, dyspnoea, cough, hoarseness, pressure over the chest, fatigue, dizziness and headache after exposure to solvents, petrol fumes, perfumes, cigarette smoke, flower scents, physical exertion or cold air. Double-blind inhalation tests were performed while the subjects wore nose clips and were unable to smell the test materials. Symptoms were reproduced by perfume but not by placebo. The fatigue, dizziness and headache reported by these subjects suggest that contact with specific fumes was provoking hyperventilation. The effect of exercise and cold air also point to this mechanism. These authors showed that the response to methacholine inhalation was normal and there was no bronchospasm. They suggested a trigeminal nerve reflex was responsible for the condition.

The most common response to fumes appears to be triggered by smell and gives rise to a symptom pattern which scores highly in the McEwen questionnaire. Patients who have recently suffered a fume response usually reproduce recognized symptoms during a 3-min forced hyperventilation test and are unable to complete it, suggesting that they respond to the stimulus of specific odours by hyperventilation. (It should be remembered that if a subject has successfully avoided their fume stimulus for a few days this test may be negative.) This group has been studied by Bell and her collaborators.[12,13] Bell *et al.*[14] suggested that the pathway from olfactory lobes to amygdalae, which is important to flight animals, has become facilitated, leading to immediate panic on exposure to a harmful fume.

Although some individuals appear sensitive to the full range of stimuli reported by Millqvist & Löwhagen's patients,[110] many react only to one or two fumes, a pattern which suggests an allergic mechanism. This impression is supported by the result of the audit of enzyme-potentiated desensitization (EPD) by the American EPD Society in 1999. The report shows that 2944 patients with MCS have been treated with three or more doses of EPD. Of these, 64% report that their condition has been improved by more than 50%. Although the basis of MCS may be specific hypersensitivity, conditioning easily leads to phobic avoidance. Cognitive behavioural therapy is also useful.[61,138]

Other causes of Dysfunctional Breathing (DB)
Chronic fatigue

Pyrexia is known to stimulate the respiratory centre and may lead to hypocapnia.[49,99] Patients with chronic fatigue syndrome apparently started by a virus infection frequently suffer from DB, and it is possible that some ongoing infection is responsible for the persistent illness. The MTG would be essential to confirm whether or not hypomagnesaemia was not a cause of supposedly viral fatigue. Cox and collaborators[29] have shown that the red cell magnesium was reduced in a group of chronic fatigue patients and that intramuscular replacement of magnesium sulphate produced improvement.

Pain

Acute pain induces hyperventilation, which is known to have analgesic properties.[26,55] Ventilatory responses to pain may become conditioned,[44] and chronic pain may train a sufferer to continuously hyperventilate. Abdominal injuries/surgery also interfere with relaxed abdominal breathing and may teach a patient to breathe only with the chest, which favours hyperventilation. The patient cited in the section on habituation is an example.

Magnesium deficiency

The role of magnesium deficiency as a drive for DB and the value of magnesium supplements has been explained above.

Premenstrual syndrome

Progesterone is a strong respiratory stimulant.[57,78] The $P_a CO_2$ may drop by as much as 8 mmHg (1.07 kPa) premenstrually,[32] and hypocapnia can exacerbate premenstrual irritability and headaches.[50,99] The effect of progesterone on breathing control requires further investigation but may partly explain an increased biological vulnerability among women to panic disorder, hyperventilation disorder and 'functional syndromes' or why women are four times more frequently affected by PIMS than men.

Hypoglycaemia

Hypocapnic and hypoglycaemic symptoms can be indistinguishable[137] and the potential for misdiagnosis of hypoglycaemia in diabetics can have life-threatening consequences.[50] The cumulative effects of hypocapnic cerebral hypoxia (reducing blood flow to the brain by up to 40%) and low blood glucose levels can produce frightening symptoms for patients with DB. With blood glucose values between 70 and 75 mg% (still normal fasting blood sugar levels) only 3 min of overbreathing produced dramatic disturbances of the electroencephalogram (EEG) and cortical functions were significantly impaired.[40] Patients with DB need to be advised on how to maintain blood sugar levels above 100 mg% and to avoid fasting for longer than 6 h.

Respiratory diseases

Many disorders of the lungs and airways are associated with hypocapnia such as chronic bronchitis[97] or pneumonia.[76] Hill et al.[66a] recognized that the orifices of dry upper lobe bronchiectatic airways may resonate as air flows past them and fremitus may be palpated in the chest wall. Affected patients suffer symptoms of DB apparently stimulated by vibration. A number of McEwen's patients developed DB after an episode of viral pneumonia or staphylococcal pneumonia. The patients believed that they suffered from allergy or ME and their disability, entirely due to DB, had persisted for many years. It is possible that this is another example of a reflex sympathetic dystrophy which persists once it has been established.

Middle ear disease

Vertigo may stimulate hyperventilation. The hyperventilation reinforces the vertigo, leading to crippling chronic symptoms.

Fortunately this association is rare. A patient escaped the allergens provoking her vertigo in England by living in Tenerife, where she remains free of symptoms.

Alcohol addiction/withdrawal

Alcohol increases urinary loss of magnesium.[133] Alcoholism leads to a wide variety of acid–base and electrolyte abnormalities. The most common is hypomagnesaemia, occurring in 30% of 127 chronic alcoholics.[39] During alcohol withdrawal this may be associated with respiratory alkalosis.[39] The pathophysiology of magnesium during alcohol withdrawal is not completely understood[125] and the usefulness of routine administration of magnesium has been questioned.[41] Nevertheless, magnesium therapy appears to be beneficial during alcohol withdrawal and is generally recommended.[133] Unless magnesium is replaced in patients undergoing alcohol withdrawal, successful treatment of DB may be hampered.

CLINICAL DIAGNOSIS OF DYSFUNCTIONAL BREATHING (Table 65.5)

Symptom checklist – questionnaire

The 16-item Nijmegen questionnaire[146] (see Appendix 2), validated by van Dixhoorn,[145] has been widely used for the assessment of the hyperventilation syndrome in psychiatric settings. It correlates closely with the DSM IV diagnostic criteria for panic attacks.[4] McEwen first studied DB in his patients from 1983 using a questionnaire based on Lum's advice. From this experience he constructed a second-generation questionnaire and used it to collate the symptoms of 100 consecutive patients referred for general allergy (not panic disorder) who were unable to complete a 3-min forced hyperventilation test and reproduced recognized symptoms during this test (Table 65.3). From this information and further experience a third-generation questionnaire, the McEwen hyperventilation questionnaire, was constructed and introduced in 1989. This included a loaded scoring system intended to increase selectivity for DB (Appendix 1).

Diagnosis and treatment of DB: investigative sequence
Diagnosis
1. *History taking* with the additional help of the McEwen *hyperventilation questionnaire*, identification/exclusion of organic disorders
2. Observation of *respiratory pattern* (respiratory frequency, abdominal/upper chest breathing, sighing, yawning, apnoea, breathy speech)
3. Testing the effects of *respiratory coordination* (switching from upper chest to abdominal breathing)
4. Testing the effects of *controlled overbreathing* (3-min hyperventilation provocation test)
5. Testing the effects of *exercise* (treadmill, bicycle ergometer)
Treatment
1. *Cognitive re-education* and reassurance following hyperventilation *desensitization* (exposure therapy)
2. *Breathing retraining* and relaxation
3. *Magnesium* replacement therapy
4. *Medication* (tricyclic antidepressants, if appropriate)
5. *Treatment of other causes* of hyperventilation (e.g. asthma, allergy)

Table 65.5 Diagnosis and treatment of DB: investigative sequence.

This pathway of development, studying polysymptomatic patients who believed they were allergic and were selected only by their response to a forced hyperventilation test, appears to have led to an instrument adapted to recognize DB in a wider spectrum of patients, especially those in whom the breathing abnormality is related to physical disease rather than anxiety or panic. Although 51% of the subjects in the second study reported panic attacks, this was never a first complaint.

Preliminary data from a small study with 13 healthy college students[95] show significant positive correlation coefficients between the McEwen hyperventilation questionnaire and the Nijmegen questionnaire (Pearson's $r = 0.61$, df = 11, $P < 0.01$). However, whereas the latter showed a strong correlation with the Beck Anxiety Inventory ($r = 0.78$, df = 11, $P < 0.01$) the correlation with the McEwen hyperventilation questionnaire was weak and nonsignificant ($r = 0.31$, n/s). This suggests that the McEwen hyperventilation questionnaire complements the Nijmegen questionnaire and is more useful for the assessment of patients with DB related to allergy and other physical conditions rather than anxiety disorders.

So far the McEwen hyperventilation questionnaire has been used for the assessment of about 1000 patients presenting with polysymptomatic allergies and has proved to be a valuable additional diagnostic tool. The questionnaire has high sensitivity at the expense of selectivity and will recognize related breathing disturbances. For example, a high score in the sleep section may point to sleep apnoea (any cause) or nocturnal hypocapnia (Table 65.6). If properly understood this is an advantage. The general usefulness of this questionnaire is illustrated by a racing driver who had suffered severe injuries on several occasions. He did not complain of anxiety or panic but scored highly in the McEwen questionnaire. Curiously his symptoms disappeared in a race, possibly due to the semi-prone driving position and the physical exercise imposed by G-forces. Nevertheless, the result of the questionnaire suggested it was unsafe to continue.

A conclusion to be drawn from this work is that there are significant differences between the most commonly studied subjects who suffer from hyperventilation driven by anxiety/panic and a possibly larger group in whom dysfunctional breathing has other causes. This appears to be an area which deserves continued research.

The McEwen hyperventilation questionnaire is not to be filled in by the patients themselves. Patients are often reticent about symptoms of DB which they perceive to be bizarre: they fear the assumption that their illness is psychiatric. A second problem arises in patients who self-diagnose their symptoms. The pattern of symptoms which is presented has been tailored to fit a preconcieved cause. For example, patients may present this cluster of symptoms as evidence that the body is pervaded by (self-diagnosed) 'Candida'. Ascribing a symptom to a particular cause may result in denial. Specific questioning then elicits the response: 'Yes, but only when I eat certain food' or 'When I have Candida'. For these reasons a professional must go through the questionnaire with each patient, a point on which Lum has been insistent.

Clinical observation

The true breathing pattern can only be watched while the subject remains naive or is distracted at the first interview. A female assistant is best to act as observer, since the physician should make eye contact and prolonged study of the bosom without explanation

Three minutes after the end of forced overbreathing (duration 3 min), end-tidal CO_2 should have recovered to at least 67% of baseline (pre-test) levels. A slower recovery is suggestive of DB	
100% CO_2 (mmHg)	67% CO_2 (mmHg)
45	30.15
44	29.48
43	28.81
42	28.14
41	27.47
40	26.80
39	26.13
38	26.46
37	24.79
36	24.12
35	23.45
34	22.78
33	22.11
32	21.44
31	20.77
30	20.10
29	19.43
28	18.76
27	18.09
26	17.42
25	16.75

Table 65.6 Three minutes after the end of forced overbreathing (duration 3 min), end-tidal CO_2 should have recovered to at least 67% of baseline (pre-test) levels. A slower recovery is suggestive of DB.

will unnerve a female patient. The observer is unlikely to detect excessive breathing in DB sufferers, but apnoeic intervals are relatively easy to recognize. It is also usually easy to observe that movement of the upper chest predominates rather than normal diaphragmatic/abdominal breathing. This is easier to observe if the patient is asked to stand on some pretext. 'Chest heaving' is another sign: the subject appears to prefer to keep the chest in the inflated position; this seems more common in women, and hence the description.[67,141] Tobin et al.[143] measured rib cage movements in hyperventilators and were unable to confirm this respiratory pattern, but the necessary apparatus would alter the breathing pattern and naivety is unlikely. Excessive yawning/sighing is another characteristic which may triple the tidal volume:[79] this can be part of the continuing overbreathing after an episode of hyperventilation; for example, a patient who was embarrassed every Sunday by uncontrollable yawning in church after singing the first hymn. A further sign is 'breathy' speech: the subject exhales excessively as each word is spoken and has to stop to reinflate the chest at inappropriate points within sentences. Speaking more than a few sentences may provoke symptoms which stop further conversation.

Testing respiratory coordination

Most patients presenting with symptoms of DB breathe almost exclusively with the rib cage. They cannot switch to abdominal breathing until trained to do so. Nevertheless, abdominal breathing taught without dealing with rhythm and depth and without relaxation training will not cure DB. Trained singers and yoga enthusiasts with excellent breathing coordination can nonetheless be suffering from severe symptoms of DB (see yoga below).

Forced hyperventilation test

The subject sits and is asked to breathe fast and deeply for 3 min. A deep breath every 2 seconds is ideal. Breathing through the mouth cuts down dead space in the airway. The physician should listen to the chest to ensure good air entry and should coach the patient to maintain effort. This test gives three end points:

1. Patients who have suffered from DB in the previous few days will be unable to continue forced hyperventilation for the full 3 min. If the test can be completed, a diagnosis of DB is unlikely.
2. During the test, patients should reproduce some of symptoms they recognize, although their full pattern is unlikely. Immediately after the test, the physician should have a list of the patient's previously recorded symptoms and quickly enquire which have been reproduced. (The patient may be unable to recall later due to mental confusion at the end of the test.)
3. When told the test is over, normal subjects promptly stop breathing, often for 10–20 seconds. DB sufferers rarely show this apnoea, and some will continue to overbreathe.

When present, this sign is strongly in favour of a diagnosis of DB but it is not invariable. Persistent overbreathing is most likely in patients who complain of breathlessness (41% of patients in Table 65.3). It is also more likely if patients are coached to hyperventilate until it is impossible to continue rather than stopping when mild discomfort develops. Finally, if overbreathing persists it may be necessary to stop continuing symptoms by rebreathing into a paper bag.

Susceptibility to forced hyperventilation

This example illustrates an important point. The forced hyperventilation test identifies patients who quickly develop intolerable symptoms at a degree of hypocapnia which is tolerated for 3 min by individuals who have not suffered from DB within the previous few days. For example, a patient who suffered symptoms of DB associated with premenstrual tension could tolerate the test during the first 2 weeks of her cycle but not towards the end. In contrast, patients who only intermittently hyperventilate and whose alkali reserve has had time to recover in between hyperventilation episodes (see 'pH and magnesium levels') may need to overbreathe for longer than 3 min before symptoms develop.

Paced hyperventilation test

The patient breathes through a capnograph (see below) in time with a metronome. This is computer-controlled to bring down the expired PCO_2 through 20–30 min according to a predetermined slope. This test may reproduce a patient's usual symptoms more accurately (including hallucinations) and is useful in an academic setting.

The deep breathing technique

Lum (pers comm, 1984) has preferred a more subtle approach to provocation testing. He keeps the patient standing and examines the chest with his stethoscope, encouraging the patient to take repeated deep breaths. Lum finds that DB sufferers reproduce their symptoms within 4 min but warns that the physician must be ready to catch the patient as they stagger or fall. He considers that this technique is less hazardous and can be used on selected patients when working alone.

Exercise test

During exercise the respiratory centre responds to stimuli from moving joints by accelerating the breathing ahead of changes in the blood CO_2. These reflexes become exaggerated in DB, so that in moderate exercise the breathing effort may exceed the requirement to blow off extra CO_2 and hypocapnia develops. This is the mechanism of the sudden draining of strength reported by many DB sufferers during activities like shopping, but it is an unreliable sign. Treadmill exercises such as those described by Goff & Gaensler[56] (4.8 km/h, incline 8%) are recommended to elicit symptoms in patients with hyperventilation disorders. The treadmill test alone is not appropriate for diagnosis, but a positive result (e.g. inappropriate breathlessness, sudden draining or exaggerated hypocapnia, i.e. <30 mmHg during or immediately after exercise) provides the clinician with an additional indicator of respiratory disturbance. Nevertheless, if draining on exercise is a major complaint, it may pay to watch the patient while they undertake the activity which causes the problem. One woman believed she should adopt a military posture while walking in the street. She inflated her chest to do so. Another, an actress, tried to adopt a 'model' shape on stage, withdrawing her abdomen and tilting her hips backward. The posture made her struggle to breathe with her chest.

Value of capnograph

If a capnograph is available, monitoring of the expired PCO_2 shows that the patient has achieved an adequate degree of hypocapnia. For an introductory text to the use of a capnograph, see O'Flaherty.[118] The rate of recovery of PCO_2 after the test can also be monitored. A slow recovery to pre-test levels has been considered to be an important diagnostic sign of chronic hyperventilation in a big study with 100 chronic hyperventilators and 100 healthy controls.[62] Figure 65.7 shows the slower return of PCO_2 in patients to pre-test levels compared with healthy controls. We recommend that during the 3-min provocation test PCO_2 baseline levels should be reduced by 50% with approx 30 breaths/min. If a capnograph is available, the following protocol is useful. DB is suspected if:

(a) patients are unable to hyperventilate for 3 min because symptoms become intolerable and/or
(b) if patients reproduce and recognize a substantial number of symptoms from the McEwen hyperventilation questionnaire reported to the physician and/or

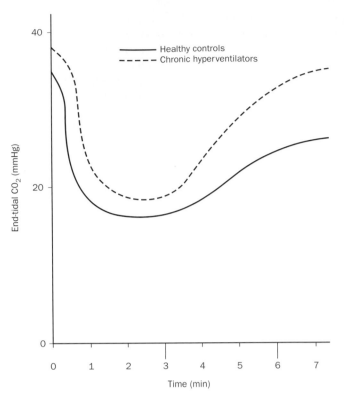

Fig. 65.7 Recovery of exhaled CO₂ after an episode of voluntary overbreathing. In patients with chronic dysfunctional breathing, recovery to pre-test levels is usually slower than in healthy individuals. – – – – –, Healthy controls; ————, chronic hyperventilators.

(c) if the recovery of P_{CO_2} to pre-test baseline levels is less than 67% 3 min after the end of the provocation (Table 65.6).

However, Hardonk's criteria (recovery of P_{CO_2} to at least 67% of pre-test levels within 3 min) have not been confirmed by others.[53,152] The comments above concerning persistent overbreathing may explain this discrepancy.

The use of a capnograph is not essential and is easily misunderstood. All subjects with normal lungs who cooperate can easily produce the necessary degree of hypocapnia during 3 min of forced hyperventilation. A positive test result is the patient's assertion that this produces intolerable symptoms. The tolerance to symptoms is subjective and the slow recovery of the P_{CO_2} is a reflection of continued overbreathing, which is easily observed and can be contrived. A well-informed journalist who wished to discredit a specialist in hyperventilation was able to mislead him even though a capnograph was used.

Precautions

Forced hyperventilation tests should be performed by a physician in an adequate clinical setting. An assistant should be in the room. L.M.M. considers an allergist's office equipped to deal with expected emergencies is adequate for this kind of work. In sickle cell disease, forced overbreathing may cause permanent neurological damage.[2] Hypocapnia causes coronary artery constriction and is dangerous if the vessels are diseased.[115,154] On the other hand, pseudoangina results from hyperventilation-induced constriction of normal coronary vessels. When angiography is negative, diagnosis and appropriate treatment may require provocation by forced hyperventilation, which is best undertaken

by a cardiologist. Controlled overbreathing triggers precordial pain in between 39%[6] and 50%[42] of patients with functional heart disease (the latter study included also 26% of patients with organic heart disease). In the former study, chest pain could be triggered in five patients simply by breath holding.[21] It is assumed that in addition to physiological factors, musculoskeletal and psychogenic factors are involved in the aetiology of chest pain.[8] In asthma there is no place for forced hyperventilation testing: hypocapnia is always present as a result of the mechanism of asthma. Forced hyperventilation will trigger an attack[64] which may be difficult to control. Nevertheless, when unrecognized subclinical asthma is the cause of DB, forced hyperventilation is unlikely to cause difficulty.

MANAGEMENT OF HYPERVENTILATION
(Table 65.7)

Diagnosis
Look for other causes of hyperventilation, listed in Table 65.4, and treat appropriately.

Reassurance and desensitization
Although panic is experienced by only 50% of PIMS sufferers who hyperventilate, episodes of hyperventilation are associated with alarming symptoms and often a sense of doom. Among patients referred to psychiatrists for panic, misattribution of symptoms to impending catastrophe is usual. When allergy is believed to be involved, misattribution leads to escalating fear of diet and environment as well as fear of death. It is essential to convince the patient that dysventilation is the direct cause of symptoms and that these can be controlled. As part of this cognitive-behavioural approach, patients undergo a 3-min hyperventilation provocation test which triggers symptoms of panic. The patients recognize the link between bodily symptoms, hyperventilation and catastrophic misattribution and learn how to deal with and control the symptoms by:

(a) rebreathing from a paperbag
(b) monitoring catastrophic thinking and replacing it with realistic appraisal.

Breathing retraining and relaxation
Physiotherapy
Diana Innocenti, teaching a combination of relaxation and breathing techniques at the Papworth Hospital in Cambridge, was the

Hyperventilation questionnaire: syndromes giving a positive score
1. Hyperventilation syndrome: 'yes' to 'draining', 'stop breathing' or 'better after exercise' make this certain
2. Sleep apnoea, any cause: a high score in the sleep section makes this obvious
3. Pickwick syndrome
4. Magnesium deficiency without hyperventilation (a maximum score of 30)
5. Limbic facilitation: fume reflex, benzodiazepine addiction

Table 65.7 Hyperventilation questionnaire: syndromes giving a positive score.

first to show that it is possible to cure DB.[74] Breathing retraining should be accompanied by relaxation training,[25,72] which in itself benefits patients suffering from anxiety and panic.[119] In a sample of 50 habitual overbreathers (37 with pseudoangina, 13 patients with organic heart disease), physiotherapeutic breathing retraining completely stopped recurrent symptoms in over 75% of patients who remained asymptomatic at follow ups of between 11 and 68 months.[42] Allergy patients generally learn slow relaxed diaphragmatic breathing fairly quickly, sometimes at the first lesson, but regular sessions of practise must follow, preferably 20 min twice per day. Pacing of the breathing by counting or other methods may help at the start of training but ultimately interferes with relaxation. The mechanism by which breathing retraining corrects DB remains unclear.[54] We postulate that time spent on breathing exercises is an opportunity to replace the CNS alkali reserve, thereby reducing susceptibility to symptoms of hypocapnia.

Grossman et al.[60] and Peper & Tibbets[121] developed the use of electronic biofeedback instruments to assist the patient to learn breathing technique. This refinement reduces the need for intervention by a skilled therapist and some patients may feel the benefit of being their own master. Others need the reassurance of the human touch and often benefit from relaxation tapes of their therapist's voice.

Yoga breathing exercises

Other forms of breathing exercises, such as yoga breathing, have been successfully used in bronchial asthma,[75,112,113] obsessive compulsive disorders[134] and chronic hyperventilation (for a review see Chandra[22]) Calming (trophotropic) breathing exercises induce relaxed wakefulness (i.e. EEG alpha states)[142] as well as mild respiratory acidosis,[82] and are thus beneficial for chronic hyperventilators (for a review see Chandra[22]). In contrast, excitatory (ergotropic) breathing (such as 'bhastrika' or 'bellows breathing') originated as a form of controlled hyperventilation intended to elicit transcendental experience. Excitatory breathing is strongly contraindicated for patients with DB.[22] Chandra warns about the dangers of referring patients to yoga instructors who lack the necessary medical expertise. Not surprisingly therefore experience with yoga therapy is often disappointing. Lum (pers comm, 1984) found that yoga did not help hyperventilators. McEwen referred 12 patients affected by DB to a therapeutic yoga centre: only one improved, the others became worse. At a different centre, a patient lost awareness of the left side of her body after practising hatha yoga under inappropriate supervision.

Magnesium supplementation

Replacing magnesium is usually necessary. In the absence of a more sophisticated measure of intracellular magnesium the red cell value may be used as a guide, but clinical response is more important. L.M.M. uses the MTG as a guide to muscle magnesium and has found that the red cell value may be in the normal range when there is significant hypomagnesaemia. A short-term response may be obtained from injections of magnesium sulphate. A suitable adult dose is 2 ml containing 10 mg/ml of magnesium sulphate by intramuscular injection on alternate days for six injections. Allergy patients, particularly those with irritable bowel, need long-term oral supplementation with preparations such as magnesium orotate, picolinate or chloride/fumarate, which are well absorbed. The dose should be adjusted for the individual. The range is 200–600 mg of magnesium daily. The RDA for magnesium is 300–350 mg. Many oral supplements of magnesium are based on insoluble magnesium oxide or carbonate. Only the fraction dissolved by stomach acid can be absorbed.

Antidepressants

Serotonin (5-hydroxytryptamine, 5HT) is involved in respiratory regulation. Antidepressant drugs such as imipramine interrupt breathing in children with Ondine's curse.[107] In contrast, doxapram (0.5 mg/kg), for example, triggers hyperventilation and panics in panic disorder patients even more strongly than 5% carbon dioxide or lactate challenges.[1] The respiratory centre is 5HT-ergic and tricyclic antidepressant drugs are 'among the most effective drugs for panic disorder'.[80] Patients who complain of waking with the sensation that they have been in a fight may benefit from protryptilene, 5–10 mg at night, which acts as a respiratory stimulant. If this drug is too activating and interferes with sleep, it may be accompanied by 10 mg of imipramine, a similar drug, but with sedative properties. It should not be assumed that symptoms relieved by an antidepressant drug are necessarily due to depression.

SUMMARY

Allergic disease may often be complicated by dysfunctional breathing (DB). DB is commonly underdiagnosed by the medical profession and hypocapnic symptoms may often be wrongly attributed to allergies. Addressing the underlying causes and sustaining factors of DB is vital for a positive therapeutic outcome. Initial patient assessment for DB includes the application of the McEwen hyperventilation questionnaire, respiratory challenges and the observation of breathing pattern. Diagnosis can be further confirmed by measuring end-tidal CO_2 by capnometry if available. The main aspects of the integrative treatment include cognitive behavioural training, breathing retraining, magnesium supplementation and medication (such as antidepressants) if appropriate. Full recovery of patients with allergic disorders may be hampered unless DB is adequately diagnosed and treated.

REFERENCES

1 Abelson JL, Nesse RM, Weg JG, Curtis GC. Respiratory psychophysiology and anxiety: cognitive intervention in the doxapram model of panic. *Psychosom Med* 1996; 58: 302–13.

2 Allen I, Imbus C. Neurologic impairment induced by hyperventilation in children with sickle cell anemia. *Pediatrics* 1976; 58: 124–6.

3 Ames F. The hyperventilation syndrome. *The Journal of Mental Science (The British Journal of Psychiatry)* 1955; 101 (424): 466–525.

4 APA. *Diagnostic and Statistical Manual of Mental Disorders IV (DSMIV).* American Psychiatric Association, Washington, DC, 1994.

5 Barlow DH. *Anxiety and Its Disorders: the Nature and Treatment of Anxiety and Panic.* Guilford Press, New York, 1988.

6 Bass C, Chambers JB, Gardner WN. Hyperventilation provocation in patients with chest pain and a negative treadmill exercise test. *J Psychosom Res* 1990; 35: 83–9.

7 Bass C, Gardner WN. Respiratory and psychiatric abnormalities in chronic symptomatic hyperventilation. *Br Med J (Clin Res Ed)* 1985; 290: 1387–90.

8 Bass C, Gardner WN, Jackson G. Psychiatric and respiratory aspects of functional cardiovascular syndromes. In: *Psychological and Behavioral Approaches to Breathing Disorders* (Timmons BH, Ley R, eds.). Plenum Press, New York, 1994.

9 Bass C, Kartsounis L, Lelliott P. Hyperventilation and its relationship to anxiety and panic. *Integr Psychiatry* 1987; 5: 274–91.

10 Bazelmans E, Bleijenberg G, Vercoulen JH, van der Meer JW, Folgering H. The chronic fatigue syndrome and hyperventilation [published erratum appears in *J Psychosom Res* 1998 Mar–Apr; 44(3–4): 517]. *J Psychosom Res* 1997; 43: 371–7.

11 Bekhterev VM. *General Principles of Reflexology* (E. Murphy, W. Murphy, Trans.). International Publishers, New York, (original work published 1917), 1932.

12 Bell IR, Baldwin CM, Schwartz GE. Illness from low levels of environmental chemicals: relevance to chronic fatigue syndrome and fibromyalgia. *Am J Med* 1998; 105: 74S–82S.

13 Bell IR, Peterson JM, Schwartz GE. Medical histories and psychological profiles of middle-aged women with and without self-reported illness from environmental chemicals. *J Clin Psychiatry* 1995; 56: 151–60.

14 Bell IR, Schwartz GE, Baldwin CM *et al*. Individual differences in neural sensitisation and the role of context in illness from low-level environmental chemical exposures. *Environ Health Perspect* 1997; 105: 151–60.

15 Berlowitz D, Denehy L, Johns DP, Bish RM, Walters EH. The Buteyko asthma breathing technique [letter]. *Med J Aust* 1995; 162: 53.

16 Blau JN, Wiles CM, Solomon FS. Unilateral somatic symptoms due to hyperventilation. *Br Med J (Clin Res Ed)* 1983; 286: 1108.

17 Bowler SD, Green A, Mitchell CA. Buteyko breathing techniques in asthma: a blinded randomised controlled trial. *Med J Aust* 1998; 169: 575–8.

18 Brassfield CR, Behrmann VG. A correlation of the pH of arterial blood and urine as affected by changes in pulmonary ventilation. *Am J Physiol* 1941; 132: 272–80.

19 Britton J, Pavord I, Richards K *et al*. Dietary magnesium, lung function, wheezing, and airway hyperreactivity in a random adult population sample. *Lancet* 1994; 344: 357–62.

20 Brown EB J. Physiological effects of hyperventilation. *Physiol Rev* 1953; 33: 445–70.

21 Chambers JB, Kiff PJ, Gardner WN, Jackson G, Bass C. Value of measuring end tidal partial pressure of carbon dioxide as an adjunct to treadmill exercise testing. *Br Med J (Clin Res Ed)* 1988; 296: 1281–5.

22 Chandra FA. Respiratory practices in yoga. In: *Psychological and Behavioral Approaches to Breathing Disorders* (Timmons BH, Ley R, eds). Plenum Press, New York, 1994; 221–32.

23 Clark DM. A cognitive approach to panic. *Behav Res Ther* 1986; 24: 461–70.

24 Clark DM. Cognitive mediation of panic attacks induced by biological challenge tests. *Adv Behav Res Ther* 1993; 15: 75–84.

25 Cluff RA. Chronic hyperventilation and its treatment by physiotherapy; discussion paper. *J Roy Soc Med* 1984; 77: 855–62.

26 Clutton-Brock J. The cerebral effects of overventilation. *Br J Anaesthesia* 1957; 29: 111–13.

27 Compernolle T, Hoogduin K, Joele L. Diagnosis and treatment of the hyperventilation syndrome. *Psychosomatics* 1979; 19: 612–25.

28 Conway A. Breathing and feeling. In: *Behavioral and Psychological Approaches to Breathing Disorders* (Timmons BH, Ley R, ed). Plenum Press, New York, 1994.

29 Cox IM, Campbell MS, Dowson D. Red blood cell magnesium and chronic fatigue syndrome. *Lancet* 1991; 337: 757–60.

30 Crea F, Davies G, Chierchia S *et al*. Different susceptibility to myocardial ischemia provoked by hyperventilation and cold pressor test in exertional and variant angina pectoris. *Am J Cardiol* 1985; 56: 18–22.

31 Cyrek-Vrowska S, Obrzut D, Hofman J. The relation between magnesium, blood histamine level and eosinophilia in the acute stage of allergic reactions in human. *Arch Immunol Ther Exp* 1978; 26: 709–14.

32 Damas-Mora J, Davies L, Taylor W. Menstrual respiratory changes and symptoms. *Br J Psychiatry* 1980; 136: 492–7.

33 Dekker E, Pelser HE, Groen J. Conditioning as a cause of asthma attacks. *J Psychosom Res* 1957; 2: 97–108.

34 Dent R, Yates D, Higgenbottom T. Does the hyperventilation syndrome exist? *Thorax* 1983; 38: 223.

35 Dominguez LJ, Barbagallo M, Di Lorenzo G *et al*. Bronchial reactivity and intracellular magnesium: a possible mechanism for the bronchodilating effects of magnesium in asthma. *Clin Sci (Colch)* 1998; 95: 137–42.

36 Edwards RHT, Clode M. The effect of hyperventilation on the lactacidaemia of muscular exercise. *Clin Sci* 1970; 38:269–76.

37 Egger J, Hofacker N, Schiel W, Holthausen H. Magnesium for hyperventilation in Rett's syndrome [letter]. *Lancet* 1992; 340: 621–2.

38 Ehlers A, Margraf J. The psychophysiological model of panic. In: *Anxiety Disorders* (Emmelkamp PM, Everaerd W, Kraaymaat F, vanSon M, eds). Swets, Amsterdam, 1989.

39 Elisaf M, Merkouropoulos M, Tsianos EV, Siamopoulos KC. Pathogenetic mechanisms of hypomagnesemia in alcoholic patients. *J Trace Elem Med Biol* 1995; 9: 210–14.

40 Engel GL, Ferris EG, Logan M. Hyperventilation: analysis of clinical symptomatology. *Ann Intern Med* 1947; 27: 683–704.

41 Erstad BL, Cotugno CL. Management of alcohol withdrawal. *Am J Health Syst Pharm* 1995; 52: 697–709.

42 Evans DW, Lum LC. Hyperventilation: an important cause of pseudoangina. *Lancet* 1977; 1: 155–7.

43 Fehlinger R, Seidel K. The hyperventilation syndrome: a neurosis or a manifestation of magnesium imbalance? *Magnesium* 1985; 4: 129–36.

44 Finesinger J, Mazick SG. Effect of a painful stimulus and its recall upon respiration in psychoneurotic patients. *Psychosom Med* 1940; 2: 333.

45 Folgering H, Colla P. Some anomalies in the control of P_ACO_2 in patients with a hyperventilation syndrome. *Bull Eur Physiopathol Respir* 1978; 14: 503–12.

46 Folgering H, Snik A. Hyperventilation syndrome and muscle fatigue. *J Psychosom Res* 1988; 32: 165–71.

47 Galland L. Magnesium, stress and neuropsychiatric disorders. *Magnes Trace Elem* 1991; 10: 287–301.

48 Gallego J, Perruchet P. Classical conditioning of ventilatory responses in humans. *J Appl Physiol* 1991; 70: 676–82.

49 Gardner WN. Diagnosis and organic causes of symptomatic hyperventilation. In: *Psychological and Behavioral Approaches to Breathing Disorders* (Timmons BH, Ley R, eds). Plenum Press, New York, 1994; 99–112.

50 Gardner WN. The pathophysiology of hyperventilation disorders. *Chest* 1996; 109: 516–34.

51 Gardner WN, Bass C. Hyperventilation clinical practice. *Br J Hosp Med* 1989; 41: 73–81.

52 Gardner WN, Bass C, Moxham J. Recurrent hyperventilation tetany due to mild asthma. *Respir Med* 1992; 86: 349–51.

53 Gardner WN, Meah MS, Bass C. Controlled study of respiratory responses during prolonged measurement in patients with chronic hyperventilation. *Lancet* 1986; 2: 826–30.

54 Garssen B, deRuiter C, vanDyck R. Breathing retraining: a rational placebo? *Clin Psychol Rev* 1992; 12: 141–53.

55 Glynn CJ, Lloyd JW, Folkhard S. Ventilatory response to intractable pain. *Pain* 1981; 11: 201–11.

56 Goff AM, Gaensler EA. Hyperventilation syndrome. *Respiration* 1969; 26: 359–68.

57 Goodland RL, Reynolds AB, McCoord AB, Pommerenke WT. Respiratory and electrolyte effects induced by estrogen and progesterone. *Fertil Steril* 1953; 4: 300–16.

58 Gorman JM, Cohen BS, Liebowitz MR *et al*. Blood gas changes and hypophosphatemia in lactate-induced panic. *Arch Gen Psychiatry* 1986; 43: 1067–71.

59 Griez E, Schruers K. Experimental pathophysiology of panic. *J Psychosom Res* 1998; 45: 493–503.

60 Grossman P, de Swart JC, Defares PB. A controlled study of a breathing therapy for treatment of hyperventilation syndrome. *J Psychosom Res* 1985; 29: 49–58.

61 Guglielmi RS, Cox DJ, Spyker DA. Behavioral treatment of phobic avoidance in multiple chemical sensitivity. *J Behav Ther & Exp Psychiat* 1994; 25: 197–209.

62 Hardonk HJ, Beumer HM. Hyperventilation syndrome. In: *Handbook of Neurology* (Vinken PJ, Bruyn GW, eds). North Holland Biomedical Press, Amsterdam, 1979; Vol. 38.

63 Hauri PJ, Friedman M, Ravaris CL. Sleep in patients with spontaneous panic attacks. *Sleep* 1989; 12: 323–37.

64 Herxheimer H. Hyperventilation asthma. *Lancet* 1946; 350: 83–7.

65 Hibbert G, Pilsbury D. Hyperventilation: is it a cause of panic attacks? *Br J Psychiatry* 1989; 155: 805–9.

66 Hill J. Magnesium and airway reactivity. *Clin Sci* 1998; 95: 111–12.

66a Hills LS, Thompson Z, Adam WJ. Is the hyperventilation syndrome simply a manifestation of occult bronchiectasis? *Thorax* 1987; 42(a): 737.

67 Holloway E. The role of the physiotherapist in the treatment of hypeventilation. In: *Psychological and Behavioral Approaches to Breathing Disorders* (Timmons BH, Ley R, eds). Plenum Press, New York, 1994; 157–75.

68 Hornsveld H, Garssen B. Hyperventilation syndrome: an elegant but scientifically untenable concept. *Neth J Med* 1997; 50: 13–20.

69 Hornsveld H, Garssen B, Dop MF, van SP. Symptom reporting during voluntary hyperventilation and mental load: implications for diagnosing hyperventilation syndrome. *J Psychosom Res* 1990; 34: 687–97.

70 Hornsveld H, Garseen B, van SP. Voluntary hyperventilation: the influence of duration and depth on the development of symptoms. *Biol Psychol* 1995; 40: 299–312.

71 Hornsveld HK, Garssen B, Dop MJ, van Spiegel PI, de Haes JC. Double-blind placebo-controlled study of the hyperventilation provocation test and the validity of the hyperventilation syndrome. *Lancet* 1996; 348: 154–8.

72 Hough A. *Physiotherapy in Respiratory Care: A Problem-Solving Approach*. Chapman and Hall, London, 1991.

73 Howell JB. Behavioural breathlessness. *Thorax* 1990; 45: 287–92.

74 Innocenti DM. Chronic hyperventilation syndrome. In: *Cash's Textbook of Chest, Heart and Vascular Disorders for Physiotherapists* (Downey PA, ed). Faber & Faber, London, 1987.

75 Jain SC, Talukdar B. Evaluation of yoga therapy programme for patients of bronchial asthma. *Singapore Med J* 1993; 34: 306–8.

76 Kassabian J, Miller KD, Lavietes MH. Respiratory center output and ventilatory timing in patients with acute airway (asthma) and alveolar (pneumonia) disease. *Chest* 1982; 81: 536–43.

77 Kerr WJ, Gliebe PA, Dalton JW. Physical phenomena associated with anxiety states; the hyperventilation syndrome. *Cal West Med* 1937; 48: 12–16.

78 Kimura HF, Hayashi A, Yoshida A, Watanabe S, Hashizume I, Honda Y. Augmentation of CO_2 drives by chlormadinone acetate, a synthetic progesterone. *J Appl Physiol* 1984; 56: 1627–32.

79 Klein DF. False suffocation alarms, spontaneous panics, and related conditions. An integrative hypothesis. *Arch Gen Psychiatry* 1993; 50: 306–17.

80 Klein DF. Panic disorder and agoraphobia: hypothesis hothouse. *J Clin Psychiatry* 1996; 57: 21–7.

81 Kontos HA, Richardson A, Jarrell R, Hassan ZU, Patterson JLJ. Mechanisms of action of hypocapnic alkalosis on limb blood vessels in man and dog. *Am J Physiol* 1972; 223: 1296–307.

82 Kuvalayananda S. Oxygen absorption and carbon dioxide elimination in prananyama. *Yoga Mimamsa* 1933; 4: 267–89.

83 Lambertsen CJ. Carbon dioxide and respiration in acid–base homeostasis. *Anaesthesiol* 1960; 21: 642–51.

84 Lehrer PM. Emotionally triggered asthma: a review of research literature and some hypotheses for self-regulation therapies. *Appl Psychophysiol Biofeedback* 1998; 23: 13–41.

85 Lepper EH, Martland M. Variations in the pH and bicarbonate of the plasma and of the alveolar CO_2 during forced breathing. *Biochem J* 1927; 21: 823–30.

86 Levy BD, Kitch B, Fanta CH. Medical and ventilatory management of status asthmaticus. *Intensive Care Med* 1998; 24: 105–17.

87 Lewis BI. Chronic hyperventilation syndrome. *J Am Med Assoc* 1954; 155: 1204–8.

88 Lewis T, Cotton TF, Barcroft J, Milroy TR, Dufton D, Parsons TR. Breathlessness in soldiers suffering from irritable heart. *Br Med J* 1916; 2: 517–19.

89 Ley R: Blood, breath and fears. a hyperventilation theory of panic attacks and agoraphobia. *Clin Psychol Rev* 1985; 5: 271–85.

90 Ley R. Panic attacks during sleep: a hyperventilation-probability model. *J Behavior Therapy Experimental Psychiatry* 1988; 19: 181–92.

91 Ley R. Dyspneic-fear and catastrophic cognitions in hyperventilatory panic attacks. *Behav Res Ther* 1989; 27: 549–54.

92 Ley R. Breathing and the psychology of emotion, cognition, and behavior. In: *Psychological and Behavioral Approaches to Breathing Disorders* (Timmons BH, Ley R, eds). Plenum Press, New York, 1994: 81–95.

93 Ley R. The modification of breathing behavior. Pavlovian and operant control in emotion and cognition. *Behav Modif* 1999; 23: 441–79.

94 Ley R, Ley J, Bassett C. Pavlovian conditioning of hyperventilation. *Psychophysiology* 1996; 33 (Suppl.): 55.

95 Ley R, Schleifer L. Abstracts of papers presented at the Fourth Annual Meeting of the International Society for the Advancement of Respiratory Psychophysiology (ISARP), North Falmouth, Massachusetts, USA, 13–15 October, 1997. *Biol Psychol* 1998; 48: 79–98.

96 Liebowitz MR, Gorman JM, Fyer AJ *et al*. Lactate provocation of panic attacks. II. Biochemical and physiological findings. *Arch Gen Psychiatry* 1985; 42: 709–19.

97 Loveridge B, West P, Kryger MH. Alteration in breathing pattern with progression of chronic obstructive pulmonary disease. *Am Rev Respir Dis* 1986; 134: 930–4.

98 Lum LC. The syndrome of habitual chronic hyperventilation. In: *Modern Trends in Psychosomatic Medicine* (Hill OW, ed). Butterworths, London, 1976; Vol. 3.

99 Lum LC. Hyperventilation syndrome; physiological considerations in clinical management. In: *Psychological and Behavioral Approaches to Breathing Disorders* (Timmons BH, Ley R, eds). Plenum Press, New York, 1994: 113–23.

100 Macefield G, Burke D. Paraesthesiae and tetany induced by voluntary hyperventilation. Increased excitability of human cutaneous and motor axons. *Brain* 1991;114: 527–40.

101 Madhill PV. Functional somatic syndromes (letter). *Lancet* 1999; 354: 2080.

102 Margraf J. Hyperventilation and panic disorder: a psychophysiological connection. *Adv Behav Res Ther* 1993; 15: 49–75.

103 Margraf J, Ehlers A. Recent research on panic disorder; review of Marburg studies. *German J Psychol* 1991; 15: 302–19.

104 McEwen LM. PIMS (psychological, irritable bowel, migraine syndrome). *J Soc Envir Ther* 1984; 4: 213.

105 McFadden ER, Lyons HA. Arterial blood gas tension in asthma. *N Engl J Med* 1968; 278: 1027–32.

106 McLean RM. Magnesium and its therapeutic uses: a review. *Am J Med* 1994; 96: 63–76.

107 Mellins RB, Balfour HH, Turino GM *et al*. Failure of automatic control of ventilation (Ondine's Curse). *Medicine* 1970; 49: 487–504.

108 Mellman TA, Uhde TW. Electroencephalographic sleep in panic disorder. A focus on sleep-related panic attacks. *Arch Gen Psychiatry* 1989; 46: 178–84.

109 Miller DJ, Kotses H. Classical conditioning of total respiratory resistance in humans. *Psychosom Med* 1995; 57: 148–53.

110 Millqvist E, Löwhagen O. Placebo-controlled challenges with perfume in patients with asthma-like symptoms. *Allergy* 1996; 51: 434–9.

111 Mooney NA, Cooke ED, Bowcock SA, Hunt SA, Timmons BH. Hyperventilation is associated with a redistribution of peripheral blood lymphocytes. *Biol Psychiatry* 1986; 21: 1324–6.

112 Nagarathna R, Nagendra HR. Yoga for bronchial asthma: a controlled study. *Br Med J (Clin Res Ed)* 1985; 291: 1077–9.

113 Nagendra HR, Nagarathna R. An integrated approach of yoga therapy for bronchial asthma: a 3–54-month prospective study. *J Asthma* 1986; 23: 123–37.

114 Naifeh KH. Basic anatomy and physiology of the respiratory system and the autonomic nervous system. In: *Psychological and Behavioral Approaches to Breathing Disorders* (Timmons BH, Ley R, eds). Plenum Press, New York, 1994.

115 Neill WA, Hattenhauer M. Impairment of myocardial O_2 supply due to hyperventilation. *Circulation* 1975:52(5) 854–6.

116 Nixon PG. Effort syndrome: hyperventilation and reduction of anaerobic threshold. *Biofeedback Self Regul* 1994; 19: 155–69.

117 Nixon PG. An appraisal of Thomas Lewis's effort syndrome. *Q J Med* 1995; 88: 741–7.

118 O'Flaherty D (ed). Capnography. *Principles and Practice Series* (Hahn CE, Adams AP, ed). BMJ Publishing Group, London, 1994. .

119 Öst LG. Applied relaxation: description of a coping technique and a review of controlled studies. *Behav Res Ther* 1987; 25: 397–409.

120 Papp LA, Martinez JM, Klein DF *et al*. Arterial blood gas changes in panic disorder and lactate-induced panic. *Psychiatry Res* 1989; 28: 171–80.

121 Peper E, Tibbets V. Fifteen months follow-up with asthmatics utilizing EMG/incentive inspirometer feedback. *Biofeedback and Self-Regulation* 1992; 17: 143–51.

122 Perkins GD, Joseph R. Neurological manifestations of the hyperventilation syndrome. *J Roy Soc Med* 1986; 79: 448–50.

123 Prior JG, Cochrane GM. Home-monitoring of peak expiratory flow rate using mini-Wright peak flow meter in diagnosis of asthma. *J Roy Soc Med* 1980; 73: 731–3.

124 Rafferty GF, Saisch SG, Gardner WN. Relation of hypocapnic symptoms to rate of fall of end-tidal PCO_2 in normal subjects. *Respir Med* 1992; 86: 335–40.

125 Ragland G. Electrolyte abnormalities in the alcoholic patient. *Emerg Med Clin North Am* 1990; 8: 761–73.

126 Raichle ME, Plum F. Hyperventilation and cerebral blood flow. *Stroke* 1972; 3: 566–75.

127 Raichle ME, Posner JB, Plum F. Cerebral blood flow during and after hyperventilation. *Arch Neurol* 1970; 23: 394–403.

128 Rogart RB, Ritchie JM. Pathophysiology of conduction in demyelinated nerve fibers. In: *Myelin* (Morell P, ed). Plenum Press, New York, 1977: 353–82.

129 Saisch SG, Deale A, Gardner WN, Wessely S. Hyperventilation and chronic fatigue syndrome. *Q J Med* 1994; 87: 63–7.

130 Saltzman HA, Heyman A, Sieker HO. Correlation of clinical and physiologic manifestations of sustained hyperventilation. *N Engl J Med* 1963; 268: 1431–6.

131 Schmidt-Traub S, Bamler KJ. The psychoimmunological association of panic disorder and allergic reaction. *Br J Clin Psychol* 1997; 36: 51–62.

132 Schroeder HA, Nason AP, Tipton IH. Essential metals in man. Magnesium. *J Chronic Dis* 1969; 21: 815–41.

133 Shane SR, Flink EB. Magnesium deficiency in alcohol addiction and withdrawal. *Magnes Trace Elem* 1991; 10: 263–8.

134 Shannahoff-Khalsa DS, Beckett LR. Clinical case report: efficacy of yogic techniques in the treatment of obsessive compulsive disorders. *Int J Neurosci* 1996; 85: 1–17.

135 Siesjo BK, Kjallquist A. A new theory for the regulation of the extracellular pH in the brain. *Scand J Clin Lab Invest* 1969; 24: 1–9.

136 Stalmatski A. Freedom from asthma. Kyle Cathie Ltd, London, 1997.

137 Steel JM, Masterton G, Patrick AW, McGuire R. Hyperventilation or hypoglycaemia? *Diabet Med* 1989; 6: 820–1.

138 Stenn P, Binkley K. Successful outcome in a patient with chemical sensitivity. Treatment with psychological desensitization and selective serotonin reuptake inhibitor. *Psychosomatics* 1998; 39: 547–50.

139 Stirton RF, Brandon S. Preliminary report of a community survey of panic attacks and panic disorder. *J Roy Soc Med* 1988; 81: 392–3.

140 Swain R, Kaplan-Machlis B. Magnesium for the next millennium. *South Med J* 1999; 92: 1040–7.

141 Timmons BH. Breathing-related issues in therapy. In: *Psychological and Behavioral Approaches to Breathing Disorders* (Timmons BH, Ley R, eds). Plenum Press, New York, 1994.

142 Timmons BH, Salamy J, Kamiya J, Girton D. Abdominal-thoracic respiratory movements and levels of arousal. *Psychonom Sci* 1972; 27: 173–5.

143 Tobin MJ, Chadha TS, Jenouri G, Birch SJ, Gazeroglu HB, Sackner MA. Breathing patterns. 2. Diseased subjects. *Chest* 1983; 84: 286–94.

144 Van den Bergh O, Stegen K, Van de Woestijne KP. Learning to have psychosomatic complaints: conditioning of respiratory behavior and somatic complaints in psychosomatic patients. *Psychosom Med* 1997; 59: 13–23.

145 van Dixhoorn J, Duivenvoorden HJ. Efficacy of Nijmegen Questionnaire in recognition of the hyperventilation syndrome. *J Psychosom Res* 1985; 29: 199–206.

146 van Doorn P, Folgering H, Colla P. Control of the end-tidal PCO_2 in the hyperventilation syndrome: effects of biofeedback and breathing instructions compared. *Bull Eur Physiopathol Respir* 1982; 18: 829–36.

147 van Megen HJGM, Westenberg HGM, den Boer JA, Kahn RS. Cholecystokinin in anxiety. *Eur Neuropsychopharmacol* 1996; 6: 263–80.

148 Weiner JM, Burdon JG. Severe allergen-induced asthma despite the use of Buteyko breathing technique [letter]. *Med J Aust* 1999; 171: 109.

149 Weiss JH. Breathing control. In: *Handbook of Phobia Therapy* (Lindemann C, ed). J. Aronson, New York, 1989: 299–326.

150 Wessely S, Nimnuan C, Sharpe M. Functional somatic syndromes: one or many? *Lancet* 1999; 354: 936–9.

151 Widmer S, Conway A, Cohen S, Davies P. Hyperventilation: a correlate and predictor of debilitating performance anxiety in musicians. *Medical Problems of Performing Artists* 1997; 12: 97–106.

152 Wientjes C, Grossman P, Defares P. Psychosomatic symptoms, anxiety and hyperventilation in normal subjects. *Bulletin Europeen Physiopathologie Respiratoire* 1984; 20: 90–1.

153 Wilkinson JB, King J, Nixon PGF. Hyperventilation and neurasthenia [letter]. *Br Med J* 1989; 298: 1577.

154 Yasue H, Nagao M, Omote S, Takizawa A, Miwa K, Tanaka S. Coronary arterial spasm and Prinzmetal's variant form of angina induced by hyperventilation and Tris-buffer infusion. *Circulation* 1978; 58: 56–62.

APPENDIX I

The McEwen Hyperventilation Questionnaire helps to determine the extent of dysfunctional breathing in patients with complex allergies.
It is used in the initial stages of patient assesment.

McEwen Hyperventilation Questionnaire

Scoring Instructions

In each box score full value even if only one symptom applies to patient. Do not increase the score if patient suffers from more than one of the symptoms in a box.

Sheet 1

Score	Value	Mental symptoms
	1	Sensation of floating/"spaced out"/unreal/"distant".
	1	Difficulty with memory.
	2	Difficulty with concentration.
	1	Mental confusion/"racing thoughts".
	1	Tension.
	1	Anxiety.
	3	Attacks of panic.
	2	Have to avoid/Fear of: Crowds, shops, queues, stuffy places, artificial lights, lifts, trains, underground trains, other.
	2	Feel physically ill / tight chested / collapse in these circumstances.
	1	Temporary delusion.
	1	See things which are not there (hallucination).
	1	Quick temper / sudden aggression / "short fuse". Quick/easy tears.
	1	Attacks of coma/stupor.
	1	Convulsions.

Score	Value	Sleep
	2	Vivid / frightening dreams.
	1	Waking in morning feeling "drugged"/with vertigo (dizzy). Waking in morning with headache. Waking in morning with muscles fatigued / aching / lethargy.
	1	Waking in the night choking / breathless. Waking in the night with panic. Waking repeatedly soon after going to sleep.

Score	Value	Eyes
	2	Blurred vision which varies with other symptoms.
	1	Double vision when other symptoms bad.
	1	Distortion of perspective: "The room tilts away."
	½	Dislike of bright lights.
	1	Some lights cause physical symptoms.
		TOTAL Sheet 1

Sheet 2

Ears

	2	Vertigo (dizziness) which varies. Worse with other symptoms / in certain places / with exercise.
	1	Tinnitus (Ringing/Buzzing in ears) which varies from hour to hour.
	1	Sounds sometimes seem distant. Sounds sometimes seem louder than they should be.
	½	Great dislike of loud noises.

Nervous System

	1	Incoordination / drops things / bumps things / clumsy.
	1	Headache/"Tension headache"/"Thick head"/"Hangover-like" for large part of many days. Headache during "attacks" / Caused by exercise.
	—	Migraine attacks.
	2	Numbness/"Deadness"/Tingling in extremities, limbs, lips, face, tongue. Touching certain objects gives tingling or unpleasant sensation. "Feels electric". (Not electric shock on making contact with an object.)
	1	Unpleasant sensations: In skin / Just below surface of skin. Cold/burning/aching/"creeping". Commonly in thighs/buttocks/feet. May be other parts of body. (These sensations may be fairly constant. May not vary with other symptoms. Are often one-sided.)

Autonomic Nerves

	1	Emotional sweating/sweaty armpits/sweaty palms.
	1	Easy flushing/blushing.
	½	Often very pale.
	1	Cold hands/feet (when rest of body is warm). Raynaud's disease.

Respiratory System

	2	Unreasonable breathlessness/Air hunger/Feeling of restricted chest.
	½	"I do exercises to improve my breathing."
	2	"I do not breathe enough/breathe deeply enough."
	3	"Sometimes I stop breathing/have to remember to breathe."
	1	Frequent sighs/yawns.
	1	Deep inhalation of aerosol drugs (for "asthma") / cigarette smoke provokes other symptoms on this chart.
	1	Singing voice: off-key / lost ability / become husky.
	1	Loud singing/speaking provokes symptoms on this chart.
	1	Speaking voice goes husky / feels strained.
	1	Throat dry / "rough" / sore.
	1	Asthma attacks now. Used to have asthma.
		TOTAL Sheet 2

Sheet 3

Heart

1	Attacks of fast/slow heartbeat. Attacks of irregular heartbeat, fast or slow.
1	Blood pressure changes easily: too high or too low.
2	Dull central chest pains/aching. Attacks of angina/coronary pain, but medical investigations negative.
1	Vaso-vagal fainting attacks are profound/frequent.

Muscles

1	* Constant weakness/fatigue: Whole body or limbs.
2	Exercise stopped by sudden unreasonable exhaustion.
3	Sudden loss of strength: "Draining" in other situations:- (Emotion/agoraphobia/other circumstances which provoke symptoms.)
3	Hard exercise improves symptoms/weakness. Swimming improves symptoms/weakness.
1	* Muscles feel stiff or "in spasm": Hand/Forearm/Shoulder/Leg.
1	* Muscles ache: Overall ("beaten up". "Been in a fight".) Chest (often a single area) Limb Neck (May cause headache) Jaw muscles (May cause headache)
1	Muscle tremor/Muscle twitching.
1	Tightness around eyes/mouth.

* May be symmetrical, one-sided or single limb.

Throat

2	Globus: Sensation of pressure or lump in throat at root of neck.
1	Sensation of restricted throat, normal on examination. Difficulty in swallowing.
1	Small aching sausage-shaped swellings in neck above voice box. (Increased tension in hyoid muscles usually described as "glands", but varies with other symptoms.)

Gastrointestinal

1	Excessive belching. Air swallowing.
1	Central discomfort / tension / sinking feeling / distress just below the tip of breast-bone.
½	Distended stomach.
1	During attacks of other symptoms: Urgent/uncontrolled bowel movement.
	TOTAL Sheet 3

Sheet 4

Urinary Tract

	1
	1

Frequent need to pass urine. Discomfort at neck of bladder. Aching bladder.

Severe urge to pass urine / incontinence <u>during attacks of other symptoms</u>.

Sex

	1
	1

Premature ejaculation.

Sex provokes prolonged exhaustion.

Sex improves all symptoms for a few hours.

TOTAL   Sheet 4

TOTALS

Sheet 1

Sheet 2

Sheet 3

Sheet 4

GRAND TOTAL

<u>Interpretation</u>

Grand total

> 15 or less   **Unlikely to overbreathe**
> 16 – 20   **Symptoms may be caused by DB**
> 21 or more   **Symptoms suggestive of DB**
> 25 or more   **Symptoms highly suggestive of DB**

APPENDIX 2

Nijmegen questionnaire (van Doorn et al.[146]). Patients with suspected 'hyperventilation syndrome' undergo a hyperventilation provocation test. A total score of 24/64 is considered positive. (For diagnosis of hyperventilation, i.e. dysfunctional breathing (DB) in allergy patients, see the McEwen hyperventilation questionnaire in Appendix 1).

Nijmegen questionnaire					
	Never	**Rare**	**Sometimes**	**Often**	**Very often**
Chest pain	0	1	2	3	4
Feeling tense	0	1	2	3	4
Blurred vision	0	1	2	3	4
Dizzy spells	0	1	2	3	4
Feeling confused	0	1	2	3	4
Faster or deeper breathing	0	1	2	3	4
Shortness of breath	0	1	2	3	4
Tight feelings in chest	0	1	2	3	4
Bloated feelings in stomach	0	1	2	3	4
Tingling fingers	0	1	2	3	4
Unable to breathe deeply	0	1	2	3	4
Stiff fingers or arms	0	1	2	3	4
Tight feelings around mouth	0	1	2	3	4
Cold hands or feet	0	1	2	3	4
Heart racing (palpitations)	0	1	2	3	4
Feelings of anxiety	0	1	2	3	4

INTRODUCTION

Diet has now been shown to influence symptoms in a number of conditions. With the rising incidence of atopic disease[36] and public awareness of food intolerance due to freely available information, there is an associated increasing demand for provision of appropriate assessment, information and dietary support to enable a positive outcome.

With the current lack of adequate and reliable tests for food intolerance, dietary investigation is the basis for both the assessment of the contribution of food intolerance to the condition and, where proven, for the management of subsequent dietary treatment and the maintenance of symptom relief. To be successful, clinicians need to be aware of an array of pitfalls encountered during the dietary process, including the everyday practical problems and the social and psychological problems encountered, which affect not only the dieter but also other family members.

The precise method of dietary management depends on the stage of investigation or treatment process. If the provoking food is clearly known – e.g. as in severe peanut allergy – advice is tailored to the individual for practical management to avoid that food totally. If the provoking foods are uncertain or unknown, a trial elimination diet may be used.

Several of the points discussed under one stage of the dietary investigation may apply to other phases of the dietary process.

PERCEPTION OF FOOD INTOLERANCE

Beliefs in the general population about food and food allergy may have serious consequences when diets are self-imposed, particu-

larly in children, and may result in failure to thrive. In a national survey of primary school children in the United Kingdom,[51] 4% of pupils were perceived as ever having had food intolerance with consequent food avoidance, of which half had never had any medical advice. Within this study group, those with perceived food intolerance were significantly shorter than other children, and this was associated with the number of foods avoided;[49] However, it is unclear whether this was due solely to food avoidance or whether it was associated with other factors such as family dynamics or the disease process itself. Conditions such as asthma and eczema are often associated with shortness.[39]

The perceived prevalence of food allergy among parents of pre-school children in Dublin was 12.5%, the most commonly reported symptom being hyperactivity.[38] This may reflect the age group studied and media attention given to this condition. One UK population study found the perceived incidence of food intolerance to be 20.4%, with an actual prevalence of 1.4% when controlled challenges to eight selected foods were performed.[61] However, there are methodological problems with this study, which probably underestimates the true incidence.[3] Studies of perceived prevalence of food intolerance have consistently produced greater incidence figures than studies using controlled challenges to confirm reported reactions. There are several reasons why this discrepancy may occur, including the population selection procedures, reaction type and method of challenges used.

However, the high incidence rate of public belief in food intolerance raises the issue of the importance of being open minded to the patients' concerns over the possibility of such a diagnosis, and the appropriateness of a dietary approach needs to be discussed. If there is an inadequate response by the medical profession, there is a danger of patients seeking inappropriate advice and following self-imposed diets[17] with possible adverse consequences.

ELIMINATION DIETS

Detailed information on the use of various elimination diets as a diagnostic tool is detailed in Chapter 59, and in other publications.[11] In summary, when the possibility of another organic cause of disease has been excluded, a trial elimination diet may be used for a specified length of time, which is dependent on the symptom type and frequency and on the degree of restricted diet. If the diet results in significant symptom relief, foods are reintroduced in an open manner to determine which of them provoke symptoms. When this phase is concluded, where eliminations are found beneficial and are to be maintained, advice is required to enable the patient to continue with a diet that is acceptable nutritionally, socially and practically.

The dietary process, therefore, involves the following stages:

1. assessment and selection of suitable patients
2. implementation of the appropriate elimination diet
3. reintroduction phase
4. maintenance diet.

For each individual stage, there are a number of factors which need to be considered throughout the process.

Assessment and selection of suitable patients

When deciding whether to use this diagnostic method for determining which potential sensitizers are capable of acting upon the individual, it should be considered whether the symptoms are severe enough to warrant this approach, particularly in children. In one study of 73 children seen in a dermatology outpatient clinic,[53] 71% had excluded one or more foods from their diet although most had only mild flexural dermatitis.[60]

In an ideal scenario patients should be well motivated, keen to take responsibility for their own health, intelligent and with sufficient resources in terms of time and finances. This combination of characteristics is, of course, not usual and in practice it is sometimes those judged to be unable to carry out the diet adequately but who wish to 'give it a go' who have a highly successful outcome.

Problem groups
Failure to thrive
There is always the concern that a change of diet may not be accepted, with consequent further weight loss; however, institution of the appropriate diet may enable catch-up weight gain. In children with atopic dermatitis and food hypersensitivity, reversal of subclinical malabsorption has been demonstrated when food allergens were removed from the diet.[24]

Cases of failure to thrive as a result of parental withholding of foods due to alleged food allergy have been recorded[27] in addition to erroneous diagnosis of food allergy due to deliberate parental misreporting[50] and has been described as an allergic form of Meadows syndrome or Munchausen by proxy.[59]

Conflict
There is a need to be aware of any existing conflict between parents and the child, which may escalate if dietary restrictions are imposed. There may be poor rapport between parents and child and an inability to control or discipline the child generally, which poses behavioural and management problems. This issue may need addressing in addition to any dietary management. Creation of conflict not already present is also an area of concern. Not adhering to the diet may be used as a way of rebelling, particularly in adolescents.

Equally, the suggestion of a dietary trial may create conflict between parents, if one or other is strongly in favour of the dietary trial against the wishes of their partner, with resulting distress for the child if inappropriately managed.

Parents may undergo a range of emotions if they feel that they have to institute a restricted diet on their child. They may feel guilt in that they may have passed on an inherited condition now requiring a treatment that they see as being cruel but necessary. However, most parents want to do whatever they can in the best interests of their child.

Reluctance to change
Although medical history may indicate that a dietary trial is appropriate, some patients will be reluctant to either accept that food may be a contributing factor or will be unwilling to make any dietary changes. Some patients take time to accept the idea and may need a period to consider the factors involved; however, those patients who reject the idea, should not be made to feel guilty if they do not feel able to manage such change.

Underweight
Adults who are underweight, with a body mass index (BMI) of under 19, may need to increase their weight before a trial elimination diet. However, this will depend on the possible cause and their weight and diet history, which needs to be established. They may be underweight due to the condition and, once on the correct diet, appetite increases, malabsorption is reduced and weight improves.

Conception and pregnancy
The primary concerns are nutritional adequacy and that no harm occurs to the fetus. Dietary trials in pregnancy are controversial and will depend on the extent of the symptoms: frequently, symptoms improve during pregnancy due to hormonal changes and any food challenges may give a different response during pregnancy than would normally occur.

Prior or current disease
Depending on the disease, nutritional status may be poor and need correcting prior to a dietary trial. Current nutritional status is an important determinant of the immune response[14] and may influence the result of any dietary investigation.

Elimination trials may be used in Crohn's disease, where malnutrition is frequently observed as a complication in those with active disease but has now also been shown in those in clinical remission.[26] Increased energy requirements have been demonstrated in children with atopic dermatitis, with increase in rate of scratching during sleep.[37]

Sports people
Both recreational and competitive athletes require a high carbohydrate diet to maintain performance. This is not such a concern at a recreational level as long as appropriate dietary advice is given; however, in the case of competitive athletes, an elimination diet may have serious consequences on their performance. The

timing of such an investigation will be critical in relation to their competitive programme.

Depression

Depending on mood state, not only is there the problem of sufficient motivation to change diet but there is also the very real possibility of precipitating a crisis, particularly when foods are reintroduced.

Highly fatigued

In cases of severe fatigue, help may be needed with the practical aspects, including the extra shopping and cooking.

Eating disorders

There is an increasing incidence of eating disorders in younger children, therefore focusing on diet may not be appropriate in some cases. Careful enquiry as to parental eating habits and attitude to diets may be needed, as this may influence the development of feeding disturbances in their children.[56]

A patient currently suffering from an eating disorder should not be put on a restricted diet. A range of symptoms – e.g. bloating, constipation and stomach pain – may occur in cases of food intolerance, but can be attributable to the eating disorder due to a smaller stomach, increased gut transit time and perception of abdominal size. If there is any doubt about such a diagnosis, there are a number of questionnaires available for assessment and further referral is advisable.

If the patient is not adequately recovered, having to focus on diet may precipitate the reappearance of the disorder. In cases considered to be sufficiently recovered, regular monitoring is essential; a reliable friend or family member is needed to assist in detecting the development of any problems.

However, the opposite scenario may occur where patients – particularly young women, with weight loss and symptoms of food intolerance such as abdominal bloating resulting in 'feeling fat' – may be wrongly labelled as having an eating disorder.

Learning disabilities

In this client group there are many issues around client consent in the administration of a restricted diet. Any such proposed changes need to be discussed fully with the client as appropriate, together with their carer or advocate and professions involved in the local teams for people with a learning disability. Depending on the degree of learning disability, there may be a practical problem instituting any change in diet and in the adequacy of monitoring change if symptoms cannot be well communicated.

Social situation

Social psychological stresses experienced can affect susceptibility to inflammatory disease and influence its course.[57] It may therefore not be advisable to conduct any trial elimination diets while the stressful situation continues, particularly where the dietary process is likely to increase the stress experienced: not only may the response to diet be altered but it is also unlikely that the patient could cope with the diet.

Financial situation

In the United Kingdom there is no longer any Department of Health provision for special diets. The possible increased cost of a new diet may be prohibitive for some. However, on careful enquiry of current food purchasing practices, it may be possible to help reduce the resulting dietary expense.

Already restricted diet

The diet may already be highly restricted for a variety of reasons: e.g. for religious reasons; through following a vegetarian or vegan diet; by being a fussy eater, with several foods disliked; or by following an elimination diet because of perceived or actual food intolerances. If such patients are not prepared to widen their diet with alternatives and, on reintroduction, find numerous additional foods cause symptoms, they may be left on an overly restricted diet.

Cooking capability

Because elimination diets avoid pre-prepared foods and ready-to-eat meals, a dislike of, or poor ability to cook poses a significant problem, and cooking skills may need to be learnt.

Diet and social history

Information concerning the patient's daily pattern and circumstances enables adequate assessment as to how to adapt and manage the elimination diet for the individual with respect to energy requirements, meal pattern, snack and recipe requirements. This can be adequately carried out verbally, as shown in a study[33] of children suffering a range of symptoms from irritability and poor appetite to loose stools and failure to gain weight. Employing a careful verbal diet and fluid history identified that the problems were caused by an excessive intake of fruit cordials, which provided over 30% of the children's energy intake. However, ideally, a written diary is most informative, and the process may not only assist the patient to identify problem areas but may also reveal that simple dietary measures are needed first.

A diet diary (Fig. 66.1) is an investigative tool that gives useful information on meal pattern, food type and frequency, use of convenience foods, fluids (type and amount) and whether eating away from home is common. Ideally it should cover at least 5 days, including a weekend. If patients are unable to complete this form, it may show lack of commitment to carry out any dietary investigation. To procure an honest response, it should be stressed that this investigation is not being undertaken to criticize the patient's diet.

Enquiry should be made into any previous diets tried and their outcome, with details of the method of identification of any suspected food intolerances. This needs careful clarification, as there are often influencing preconceived ideas resulting from articles read or 'alternative' tests that have been carried out without objective substantiation of any perceived intolerance.

It should be established which foods are disliked or avoided and for what reason. Nationality and religion influence food type, frequency and possible major allergens. For example, in Japan, allergy to soya and buckwheat is more common.

Information on activity level at work and during recreation helps to assess energy and dietary requirements. Details may be needed on other activities, including hobbies, where possible contact or inhalant allergens may be encountered which may influence symptoms.

Lack of adequate cooking and food-storage facilities may be a limiting factor in proceeding with a diet (e.g. a single electric ring in a bedsit) and will require practical management advice.

Name: **Day/Date:**

Time	Food or Drink	Description (e.g. Quantity, brand name, etc.)	Comments

Fig. 66.1 Diet diary.

Motivation

A great deal of self-discipline is required to follow a diet and it is important to recruit a positive attitude from the patient. The degree of motivation needs to be assessed and may depend on the severity of the condition. Where the disease process results in reduced scholastic achievement and self-esteem, bad self-image with poor peer relationships, or absenteeism and loss of employment, a diet trial would seem reasonable. However, it may be important to ask the question 'which is worse – the diet or the symptoms?'

There is the need to stress that the initial elimination diet, which restricts a number of possibly troublesome foods, is an investigative procedure for a defined and mutually agreed timescale and is not a diet for life. It is of course necessary at the outset to discuss what degree of symptom relief is expected and the level of dietary restriction that is possible and acceptable to the patient. It is important that patients understand there may not be total resolution of symptoms, otherwise some patients become obsessive to achieve complete symptom relief.

The actual diet used may be a compromise between the optimum diet, as assessed, and the diet the patient feels they can manage. Patients will have different priorities regarding diet versus other life events; however, once they have started the process their views may alter and they may become willing to undergo further change if needed.

Implementation of diet

Good dietary management is critical, as the overall process takes much time on the part of the patient, doctor and dietitian.

The choice of diet and degree of restriction will depend on age, medical and diet history and should be tailored to the individual's

ability and dietary preferences. With the changing patterns of food availability, both seasonal and increasing food importation, resulting in a possible change in the pattern of food intolerances, the choice of diet is becoming more complex.

Choice of milk substitute

Current feeding guidelines[23] recommend that infants up to 1 year of age should receive breast milk or infant formula. For infants and children with suspected cow's milk intolerance, where milk normally provides the majority of nutrition, an appropriate substitute formula should be used. The selection of formula will depend on a number of factors, including symptomatology, palatability and cost. Goat's and sheep's milk are unsuitable substitutes due to crossreactivity, microbiological uncertainty and inappropriate nutritional composition. For infants under 2 years of age, ordinary shop-bought carton soya milk may not be nutritionally adequate and a soya formula specifically prepared for infant feeding should be used where appropriate. Other options, where necessary, are the protein hydrolysates or amino acid based formulas. There are various protein hydrolysates available, including partially hydroysed and extensively hydrolysed formulas, which may be based on whey, casein, soya and pork. The use of these has been reviewed by Macdonald[46] and Carter.[11,12] One of the problems in the use of these formulas is their poor palatability and acceptability (particularly in those over a few months of age) and, therefore the nutritional adequacy of the diet.

Dietary assessment of a controlled trial of a few foods diet in children in atopic dermatitis compared nutritional intake in those using either a whey- or casein-based milk substitute (Table 66.1).[44] The median daily volume of casein hydrolysate taken was 10.5 ml/day compared with 267 ml/day in the whey group. There was a significant reduction in protein and calcium intake in both

Median intake during normal and few foods diet and change in nutrient intake		
Nutrient median intake (range)	**Whey hydrolysate**	**Casein hydrolysate**
Energy		
Normal	84 (20–170)	88 (28–156)
Few foods	82 (30–140)	87 (33–123)
Median change	–6.8	–12.8
Protein		
Normal	299 (128–632)	305 (162–530)
Few foods	245 (94–555)	226 (74–419)
Median change	–58	–61
Iron		
Normal	154 (95–426)	190 (113–300)
Few foods	227 (24–568)	208 (70–316)
Median change	+59	+19
Calcium		
Normal	242 (66–700)	210 (37–558)
Few foods	134 (23.5–583)	52 (12–232)
Median change	–116	–144

Table 66.1 Median intake during normal and few foods diet and change in nutrient intake. Median values and range expressed as % of dietary reference values; EAR for energy and protein; LRNI for nutrients.[44]

groups compared with normal diet and in energy intake in the casein hydrolysate group.

Diet sheets

Whichever diet is selected, information needs to be provided on which foods to avoid and, importantly, which foods patients *can* have. It is important to be positive about available alternatives. Information on how to interpret food labels is required, and the various supermarkets and manufacturers will provide their own 'free from' lists. Other information needs to include sources of unusual foods, recipes and general cooking tips, meal ideas and suitable cookbooks. It is helpful to discuss proposed dietary changes with the person who does the cooking.

Where relevant, advice on the prescribability of suitable products as approved by the Advisory Committee on Borderline Substances for the listed condition should be given as in the case of replacement formulas in cow's milk protein intolerance. However, multiple food intolerance is not a listed condition.

Symptom and behaviour chart

Use of a symptom (Fig. 66.2) or behaviour chart (Fig. 66.3) to monitor change and to document any loss of dietary compliance is essential, although many patients forget to bring it to their consultation!

Reactivity can fluctuate, depending on the condition, the season, and concurrent exposure to additional environmental allergens. Other factors that influence the degree of reactivity to foods include alcohol, exercise, aspirin intake, and the stage in the menstrual cycle. Recording of associated factors is crucial to prevent misinterpretation of a successful or unsuccessful outcome.

When assessing any change, the patient may report alteration in symptoms not previously considered relevant and they need to be warned that this can occur. However, it is also important to discourage obsessive listing of symptoms and continuing to focus on reactions for longer than is absolutely necessary.

Medications

Suitability of any medications and their contents needs to be investigated together with giving advice on any reduction programme.

Problem areas

Support and time

The amount of support needed will vary. This depends on the confidence of the patients or their carers, their degree of understanding, the severity of the disease and other associated medical problems. The patients' ability to attend appointments may be constrained by availability of time or money. Regular follow up by telephone may be needed.

Timing of diet

As there is the possibility of a withdrawal reaction lasting a few days, the start of the diet may need to be carefully planned. The timing of the investigation will be influenced by a number of social and business events:

- holidays/business travel
- birthdays/anniversaries
- social events/weddings.

Name: _____

Instructions

Record any symptoms you experience in the far left box of each table. Then each day give each symptom a score as follows:

0 = no problems	**1 = mild**	**2 = moderate**
3 = severe	**4 = very severe**	

In the brackets next to the week number record whether it is a control week (i.e. you have not started the diet), an elimination week (i.e. you have eliminated food from your diet as instructed) or a test week (i.e. you are testing different foods to see if you react).

Use the following codes: C = control, E = elimination, T = test.

If it is a test week, please record the food you are testing in the box at the bottom as shown.

SYMPTOM WEEK 1 ( )	M	T	W	TH	F	S	SU
Food being tested if applicable.							

SYMPTOM WEEK 2 ( )	M	T	W	TH	F	S	SU
Food being tested if applicable.							

Fig. 66.2 Symptom diary.

Babies/children

A number of factors may arise, which may influence the outcome: teething, coincidental infection and food cravings with loss of compliance may all cause difficulty. Compliance in children of school age may cause a particular problem. It may be necessary to liaise with the school and, usually, advice on suitable packed lunches is needed. For some it may be best to start the diet in the school holidays. There may be problems with foodstuffs that are contained in non-food items such as Playdoh®, and the eating of crayons, paints, etc.

It is important the reason for the diet is explained to the child and is that it is not seen as a punishment.

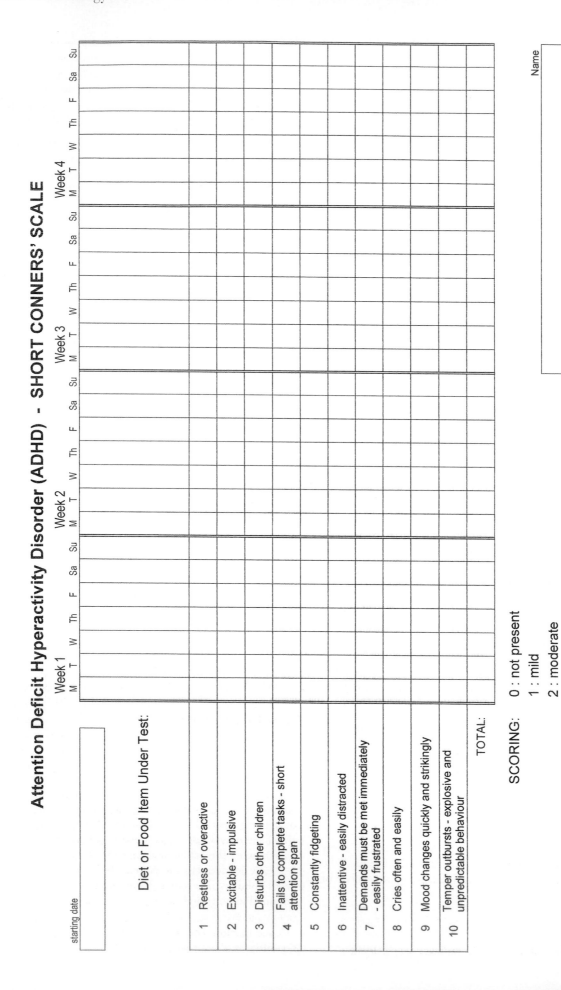

Fig. 66.3 Attention deficit hyperactivity disorder (ADHD) – Short Conners' Scale.

Multiple carers

Where there are several carers involved, it is important that a full explanation of what is being undertaken together with detailed dietary information is disseminated accurately to everyone involved.

Eating out

It is essential to be prepared for situations that may arise, such as business lunches and when away from home. Eating out is often difficult or even impossible during the restricted phase.

Family situation

Depending on the diet it may be supportive and easier for the whole family to follow the diet.

Treats

Foods are often used as treats and may be offered by a relative or friend as a temptation if there is insufficient understanding of what is being undertaken.

Drug treatment

Infection may be acquired during the diet requiring drug treatment. The medication used may contain a food or food additive that is being avoided.

All of these factors and others (Table 66.2) have the potential to result in a failure of the trial diet to improve symptoms. Several trials, particularly in the case of few foods diets, report a high withdrawal rate,[43] indicating the difficulty of adhering to such a strict diet. This also indicates the problem with results of such trials where adherence to diet is difficult to check.

Reintroduction phase
General considerations

If the diet results in symptom relief, confirmation of provoking foods is required. Foods should be reintroduced singly in as pure a form as possible. If symptoms do not reappear after the specified period, the foods can then be included back in the diet. The procedure for challenge will vary, depending on age, risk of severe reaction, disease and number of foods to test. Challenge protocols are available for cow's milk allergy (CMA) in infants.[35] David[15] has cited occasional anaphylactic reactions to food introductions in children with atopic dermatitis who have been on an elimination diet but have not previously reacted to that food. There is a period of heightened sensitivity in the immediate period post diet and patients need to be warned of this. Other

considerations are reviewed in Chapter 59 by Radcliffe. The symptom chart must be continued throughout the challenge process.

Choice of foods to reintroduce

The reintroduction schedule should include the following considerations:

- making the diet more palatable
- socially easier
- nutritionally complete
- based on patient preference and history
- food form – if the food usually consumed reacts, then advice on methods of food processing or cooking which may alter allergenicity needs to be given for further challenges, e.g. evaporated milk, eggs cooked in cakes rather than soft boiled.

Timescale

Advice on the number of days to challenge with each food will vary, depending on patient history, symptoms being investigated and food type under challenge, as some foods take longer to react, e.g. the grains.

Problems encountered

- When symptoms clear, some patients are so relieved that they become reluctant to test foods and may need to be encouraged to conduct food challenges.
- Where the diet appears to resolve symptoms that do not reappear on challenge, there may be other reasons for a successful outcome, including spontaneous remission, coincidence or placebo effect. It is also useful to check that no other treatment has been commenced at the same time!
- Timing of reintroductions may be problematic where reactions are severe enough to require time off school or work.
- It is important that other non-dietary factors that may provoke symptoms are recorded to avoid misattributing a reaction to a food, e.g. inhalant triggers in asthma.
- Where the reaction to challenge is uncertain, the foods should always be retested at a later date to avoid unnecessary dietary restrictions.
- Where there is a concurrent infection at this stage, the level of reactivity may change and challenge results become unreliable.
- If many challenge results are not clear cut, this can result in continued multiple avoidances and a nutritionally inadequate diet. The process must not become prolonged and the patient may need to be encouraged to abandon the procedure.
- There is always the risk that once a diet has been instigated the patient is lost to follow up and pursues an inappropriate dietary restriction.

How long do foods need to be excluded?

Once it has been established which foods cause a reaction, depending on the symptoms and severity of reaction, the extent and duration to which foods need to be avoided will vary. It is important that this is discussed with the patients or carers. In the case of life-threatening allergic reactions, avoidance needs to be 100% and may need to be lifelong.[8] However children often grow out of their intolerances and foods should be retested at 6–12-month intervals.

Confirmation of reaction by the double-blind, placebo-controlled food challenge (DBPCFC) is more usually used as a

Reasons for failure of the diet to improve symptoms
1. Diet allowed has not excluded culprit food/foods
2. Diet has not been followed for long enough
3. Intercurrent illnesses and medications
4. Incorrect reporting of symptoms by patient/carer
5. Diet has no influence on symptoms
6. Abnormal gut flora (see Chapter XX by K.E. Eaton)
7. Inability to follow diet through lack of understanding
8. Diet not followed strictly, as practically and socially unacceptable

Table 66.2 Reasons for failure of the diet to improve symptoms.

research tool and the problems encountered in its use have been reviewed, particularly with respect to slow-onset food intolerance.[13] However, the method may be useful in cases of suspected food aversion and a standardized tool has been developed for use in brittle asthma.[4]

In a study[54] of children with atopic dermatitis whose allergic reactions had been confirmed initially by DBPCFC, rechallenge in the same manner 1–2 years later showed that approximately one-third of the symptomatic food allergies had resolved. However, the likelihood of developing clinical tolerance varied depending on which food the child was reactive to. Development of tolerance to soy was common in contrast to peanut, which was rare. One report, however, does suggest that peanut allergy may resolve in a small proportion of pre-school children and may be more likely in those without other food intolerances.[34] It should be noted that challenges were not conducted in cases that had had a life-threatening reaction.

The prognosis of cow's milk protein allergy or intolerance (CMPA/CMPI) in infants is good, with a remission rate of 85–90% at 3 years of age.[31] However, this will vary, with a later age of presentation being associated with a greater duration of intolerance and reduced probability of growing out of it.

However, as tolerance may develop over time, patients often need encouraging to determine the quantity of a food that may no longer provoke symptoms. If one or two slices of bread every so often can be managed, this will make the situation more manageable when those unavoidable occasions arise. However, some patients become very rigid in their avoidances and will refuse to retest foods later, preferring to avoid them for life when this may be unnecessary.

Maintenance diet
Nutritional adequacy

The nutritional adequacy of the resulting diet will depend on the type and number of foods that have to be avoided in addition to which foods the patient self-selects. If the only food to be avoided is unlikely to make a significant difference to the nutritional intake, simple history taking and management advice will be all that is needed. However, if significant nutrient contributors to the diet are avoided, it is advisable to carry out a full dietary assessment, particularly in certain groups, e.g. children, vegetarians, vegans, and in cases of multiple intolerances.

Diet analysis

To do this analysis, the patient or carer needs to keep a detailed diet and fluid diary for 7 days. Ideally, the food should be weighed, but this is rarely practical and may unduly influence intake. Description in terms of household measures can, with experience and the aid of available information,[47] be interpreted into weights. The data can then be analysed to provide daily average intakes of most nutrients. There are a number of computer programs available to assist that use the UK food tables of McCance and Widdowson.[30] These tables are regularly updated by production of a series of supplements based on one or more food groups, providing more detailed nutritional information. Experience is required in their use, as there are a number of errors that can be made when using these databases, particularly within software analysis.[58]

A good working knowledge of the database and the way in which the results can be interpreted validly is required to translate analyses into appropriate practical advice. Problems include unavailability of data for some of the more unusual foods for one, more or all nutrients. There are also differences between various brands of products, particularly where they are supplemented to different levels, as in the case of calcium supplementation of various soya products. This information needs to be conveyed to the patient when a brand change is likely to make a significant difference to nutrient intake. The whole process is very time consuming for both the patient and the dietitian.

The result of analysis can be used to assess the likely adequacy of an individual's diet by comparing intakes of individual nutrients with appropriate recommended nutrient intakes, dietary reference values (DRVs)[22] for sex and age, as a guideline (see below). Where there are likely shortfalls, information on good suitable dietary sources should be given. Where these cannot be included in the diet to provide adequate intake, appropriate supplementation should be advised, bearing in mind possible additives and excipients that might be potential allergens. There are ranges of hypoallergenic formulas available, but few are prescribable. There are reports of reactions to pure mineral salts, although the mechanism is unknown.[19]

However, there are several points that need to be considered when using these data. This is an assessment of nutritional *intake*, which is the basic starting point to achieve a reasonable nutritional status, but tells us nothing about absorption, which may be abnormal in food-intolerant patients. The DRVs are recommendations for normal healthy populations and 'are not necessarily appropriate for those with different needs arising from disease, such as infections, disorders of the gastro-intestinal tract …' and are intended as recommendations for groups, not individuals. However, they can be used as a basis to compare the individual intake with the reference nutrient intake (RNI) for the nutrients concerned. The RNI level should be adequate for 97.5% of *healthy* individuals within a population group.

In addition, the assessment is only as good as the information provided and is a snapshot in time. Dietary intake will change over the year for a variety of reasons, with new foods being introduced and others dropped. If one food source is providing a very significant intake of a particular nutrient and dietary preferences change without adequate substitution, nutritional deficiencies could occur. Requirements also change with age, as for example with calcium, as shown in Table 66.3. This is particularly pertinent to children, who should be followed up on a regular basis to assess whether they are following an adequate growth pattern using centile charts[25] with reassessment of dietary intake.

Nutritional considerations

Dairy products, together with wheat, are among the more commonly implicated groups of foods causing symptoms. Milk and milk products provide about 56% of the calcium, 27% of riboflavin and are one of the few sources of iodine in the British diet. In a study of 7–8-year-old Scottish school children, milk contributed 10% of energy, 30% vitamin A, 36% vitamin B_{12}, 42% calcium and 33% riboflavin.[52] As dairy products are a major contributor to nutrients in the British diet, if these are excluded it is essential that suitable food sources of these nutrients are substituted. However, remaining food sources with significant amounts of the nutrient may be disliked or foods not common to the national diet. This can be demonstrated in the case of calcium, where there are only a few food sources with high calcium concentrations. If these are not regularly included in the diet, it may be dif-

Recommended nutrient intakes for calcium (mg/day)	
Age	RNI
0–12 months	525
1–3 years	350
4–6 years	450
7–10 years	550
11–18 years female	800
11–18 years male	1000
19–50 years	700
50+ years	700
Pregnancy	No increment
Lactation	+550
Data from Department of Health.[22]	

Table 66.3 Recommended nutrient intakes for calcium (mg/day).

Calcium content of a selection of foods	
Food group	Calcium content (mg/100 g)
Dairy products and soya substitutes	
Cow's milk	120
Baby milks	49–63
Soya milk – unsupplemented	13
Soya milk – supplemented	42–140
Yogurt – cow's	200
Soya yogurt – unsupplemented	<20
Soya yogurt – supplemented	100
Cheese – cheddar	720
Soya cheese	<20
Ice cream – cow's	130
Soya ice cream	13
Cereal products	
Bread – white	110
Bread – wholemeal	54
Cereals – bran flakes	50
Cereals – porridge made with water	7
Grains – pasta cooked	6
Grains – rice boiled	4
Fish, meat, eggs	
Sardines – tinned with bones	540
Tuna – tinned	8
Lamb, beef, pork	8
Eggs	57
Nuts/seeds	
Sesame seeds	670
Cashew nuts	32
Vegetables	
Curly kale – boiled	150
Broccoli – boiled	40
Baked beans	53
Swede	26
Fruits	
Figs – dried	250
Dates	45
Oranges – no skin	47
Bananas – no skin	6
Note: Actual calcium intake will depend on the portion size.	
Data from the Composition of Foods.[30]	
Crown copyright material is reproduced with the permission of the Controller of Her Majesty's Stationary Office.	

Table 66.4 Calcium content of a selection of foods.

ficult to eat sufficient of the remaining sources to provide requirements (Table 66.4).

Although there is an increasing amount of nutritional information available to the public, this still needs interpreting into practical information. There are many misconceptions about the nutritional content of foods, particularly regarding the adequacy of milk substitutes for infants. A case of soy milk-induced rickets has been reported where unsupplemented carton soya milk was used for a cow's milk-free diet from age 8 months on advice from a general practitioner.[2] It is also not widely appreciated that substitute formulas contain only half as much calcium as cow's milk (Table 66.4). The author has also come across the parental use of home prepared 'nut milks' for infants that are not nutritionally adequate.

It is important to stress that variety in the diet is important not only to establish a good nutritional intake but also to help prevent recruiting new intolerances. Reviewing the diet at this stage can also provide an opportunity to improve the diet of the whole family, as they often become more nutritionally aware, with an interest in diet and health.

Nutritional inadequacy

Although appropriate advice on a suitable maintenance diet is given at the start, dietary preferences may change and nutritional requirements will change with age.

Infants and children

In children avoiding cow's milk, it cannot be assumed that the prescription of a substitute formula ensures an adequate nutritional intake.[21,33,48] This will depend on the amount of formula actually taken and the age of the child. Older children are less likely to achieve necessary calcium intakes, as requirements increase with age, particularly in adolescence when calcium requirements are greatest to achieve peak bone mass.[29]

In a series of 23 children on an established avoidance diet for atopic eczema, 7 being the median number of foods avoided, 56% had a calcium intake of less than 75% of the RDA, with one developing rickets due to stopping their substitute formula.[19]

Ongoing dietetic supervision is essential in this age group with CMPA/CMPI when other intolerances may develop, particularly to egg, soy, peanuts, citrus, fish and cereals,[32] and care is needed that further diets are not instigated by parents without appropriate advice.

Multiple intolerances

Those patients with multiple intolerances will need much greater and continued input. Alternative dietary strategies may need to be considered, based on the individual's range of tolerated foods, including rotation diets or highly varied diets that reduce the dose of each food taken. Their strict interpretation should only be considered in extreme cases, as they are socially and practically difficult.

In a survey of 12 adults with multiple symptomatology due to proven food intolerance, dietary assessment revealed significantly lower intakes of energy, magnesium, calcium and riboflavin compared with controls.[9] However, of the nutrients studied, only calcium intake appears to be deficient, being just above the lower reference nutrient intake (LRNI).

Vegetarian and vegan diets

Vegetarianism is becoming more popular. Depending on the foods selected, the nutrients which are more likely to be inadequate are those that provide energy, vitamins D, B_{12}, B_2, iron, zinc, calcium and iodine. If they are intolerant to several foods, patients may need to be encouraged to start eating meat and fish in order to achieve a nutritionally adequate diet.

Inappropriate restrictions

Unnecessary self-imposed diets without dietary advice can lead to severe nutritional consequences, including osteoporosis and megaloblastic anaemia[5] and hypothyroidism with failure to thrive.[40]

Practicality

Although the diet may have had proven beneficial effects, the practical problems involved in maintaining the diet may be seen to be so great that it is abandoned; this may depend on degree of restriction, severity of disease and the age of the patient. In a review of 40 children with severe eczema associated with proven food intolerance, 21% under 3 years of age and 46% over 3 years of age gave up the diet with relapse of eczema.[28] In this group of highly motivated parents, it was felt the diet was worse than the disease. It is easier to maintain a diet in younger children before attending school where access to food is less controlled and other influences are introduced. However, in some cases, it can be the parents who cannot stick to the diet for the child due to guilt in having to restrict foods associated with pleasure, love and reward or indeed foods that they would miss themselves.

All the respondents (40%) to a survey of those adults with proven brittle asthma associated with food intolerance felt the diet was preferable to their symptoms.[4]

Everyday management considerations
Time

Special diets usually involve more time in all areas of food provision, including shopping, cooking, freezing and washing up.

Specialist food items are gradually becoming more widely available but may require additional shopping trips or need to be ordered from specialist mail order companies, both of which involve additional costs. The continual checking of labels while shopping can be highly time consuming. However, in one survey on the effect of diet on the family, although the time taken to check labels for food content was one of the most significant changes to shopping, in most cases it was found to be absorbed into shopping routines fairly easily. The additional shopping required was not seen as particularly time consuming, but this may reflect differing notions of time and timescale attached to different roles within households.[55]

Where there are several different diets in the household, one member may go without particular items. Having to cook two different types of pasta at one meal requires more cooker space, pans, fuel and provides more washing up. The diet may therefore become overly restrictive in order to simplify meal provision, particularly in families where there may be children with different combinations of dietary avoidances.

Although variety in the diet is very important and may help to prevent recruitment of further intolerances, many patients cannot be bothered and end up on an unnecessarily limited range of foods. It is helpful for patients to plan for themselves, with guidance, a week's menus and then to organize their shopping rather than cooking on an ad hoc basis.

Cooking

An increasing number of people rely on processed and prepacked meals; therefore, cooking skills may need to be acquired not only in terms of basic cooking methods but also of the different techniques required to use alternative products. Baking with wheat-free flours can require considerable skill and a range of recipes; cooking hints and tips on how to adapt usual family recipes need to be provided. Information on suitable alternatives to provide a particular physical function rather than nutritional value also needs to be considered, e.g. alternative products to use as a binding agent where egg has to be excluded.

Various items of kitchen equipment can make a considerable difference, enabling production of palatable, quick and easy replacement foods, e.g. a waffle maker provides a useful bread substitute.

Cost

Many alternative products on a weight-for-weight basis are 2–3 times more expensive than the usual product. In spite of the increasing range of products available, the prohibitive cost prevents patients attaining an adequately varied diet in some cases and may result in them abandoning the diet. Limited ranges of products are now being stocked by some supermarkets, resulting in a lower unit cost than an equivalent purchase from a health food shop. However, some alternative products are only available in smaller packet sizes than the equivalent 'normal' product, which again increases the unit cost.

The only published study calculating the cost of such special diets is based on figures in 1986.[45] The minimal costs were calculated for a normal diet, wheat-free, gluten-free, milk-free and a few foods elimination diet. Costs were quoted for intakes required to meet the RDA levels for a 4-year-old boy, an 8-year-old boy, a 15–17-year-old boy and a moderately active man. Costs to the patient were reduced where prescribable products could be used, as in milk-free children's diets and gluten-free diets for coeliac disease. In the case of elimination and wheat-free diets, all costs were increased, ranging from 37 to 109% additional expense. This does not include increased travel costs to purchase special items or additional fuel costs when having to cook different meals in the household.

Dietetic support is important for advice on the use of alternative foods and recipe adaptation to provide an acceptable healthy diet without having to resort to the purchase of these expensive substitutes.

Travelling and holidays

A suitable quick snack is often not available when away from home, which makes unplanned excursions a potential problem. When on holiday abroad, supplies of sufficient suitable foods may need to be taken and a knowledge of the language may be needed to read food labels and explain requirements to restaurants. Many patients feel that they have to limit their holidays to the self-catering option.

Eating out

The restaurant type and suitable menu choices may be restricted. However, it is important that patients are encouraged not to let the diet rule their life. Many establishments are able to provide suitable meals, particularly if given warning and information on what patients *can* have rather than just the restrictions. In addition, some patients may find benefit from the use of oral sodium cromoglycate on such occasions. However, eating out does present the greatest threat to those with anaphylactic reactions, as the statistics on peanut allergy fatality show.

Other problem areas

Social

Food plays a central role in nearly all social occasions, and giving food is often an expression of love. Having to avoid certain foods can therefore present significant problems socially and may limit the capacity for a normal life. Some patients choose not to accept social invitations rather than have to appear awkward and socially unacceptable when refusing foods and drink provided, or find that they receive fewer invitations. Some patients feel miserable watching other people eat and may therefore be tempted to eat foods they know will make them ill, leading to guilt at causing their own problem. Some patients find it embarrassing at social occasions when attention is drawn to their diet, resulting in cross-examination about their symptoms.[10] In restaurants quizzing waiters to ensure the food is suitable can cause offence to other diners.

Practical and emotional support can be crucial to maintaining the diet, and unhelpful pressure and scepticism from family and friends, maintaining that 'a little won't hurt', can add to the stress involved.

Within the household both the condition and the diet may impact on the whole family and alter family dynamics.[1] Other family members may feel the need to hide specific foods, eating them away from the 'diet' family member. The overall stress of the diet may significantly increase family conflict, with detrimental outcome.

Dietary obsession

Dietary avoidances may escalate unnecessarily either where treatment has been unhelpful or there is only partial improvement and 'more must be better'. Persistence with the idea of causative food allergy may lead to extending the dietary exclusion process.[17] In addition, some patients may impose on themselves some other form of dietary manipulation which they have read about, increasing their dietary restrictions without any further symptom improvement.

Where a true sensitivity to a particular food has been demonstrated, further food exclusions may be implemented either by a parent, resulting in an unsafe diet and failure to thrive,[50] or the patient may develop food phobia. The response of patients may depend on the severity of their reaction, psychological state and remaining fear of further reactions. Fear of the known problem food may extend to a range of other foods and result in a highly restricted diet. Even where a food has been eaten without any reaction, a further trial of the food may be refused in fear of a reaction. This fear of symptoms may result in hyperventilation and its associated manifestations when confronted with a food or even when mentally planning a meal, resulting in perceived symptom reinforcement.

Food is a part of everyday life and, as a result, the diet and symptoms may become a major preoccupation; the disease continues to rule, with the patient becoming increasingly aware of any physical changes. This may then develop into misattributing symptom changes to other foods, with further self-imposed dietary restriction.

Parents will naturally be concerned that their child should not feel different from their peers but can become overprotective and restrictive with excessive concern when their children are eating out, particularly at parties.

Initially, the patient may be grateful to have found that food provokes their symptoms, which enables their control. However, this initial elation may be dashed at the realization that something as simple as food, which most people are able to take for granted, can make them ill. Patients may lose all enjoyment in eating and find the whole process stressful. Without adequate support, they may view themselves as an allergy '*sufferer*' rather than as someone who reacts to foods. It can therefore be helpful for some patients to have contact with the various allergy support groups.

Labelling

With the ever-increasing range and availability of manufactured foods, the art of label reading becomes increasingly important for those avoiding certain food ingredients or food additives. Information needs to be provided on all the terminology used to describe individual food items and their components. For example, when avoiding cow's milk the ingredients casein and whey need to be avoided also. Patients on milk-free diets who have not been given dietetic advice commonly make this mistake and continue to use sunflower or other margarines containing whey. Although additives must be listed in the ingredients, the avoidance of particular food additives can be confusing to the consumer as manufacturers switch from using the additive number to the use of the chemical name. Lists of both should be made available.

Many food companies and supermarkets will provide 'free from' product lists, but these become out of date very quickly and need to be updated regularly.

Hidden ingredients

Although ingredients are listed on a product label appearing in descending order of weight, there may be hidden ingredients due to the current labelling regulations. If a compound ingredient constitutes less than 25% of the finished product, the component ingredients do not have to be listed except in the case of additives. For example, if a vegetable margarine is used in a biscuit recipe and comprises less than 25% of the contents of the biscuit, the components of the margarine (which may include whey), do not have to be listed. However, in the case of bread and bread flour, if the only additives used are the ones stipulated in the Bread and Flour Regulations (1984) which includes soya protein, they do not need to be listed on the label. There are current draft proposals to amend the EC labelling legislation to declare certain ingredients and food-stuffs that are now scientifically recognized as causing hyper-sensitivity, in order to assist consumers who have allergies or intolerances (Table 66.5).

The labelling used may be inadequate to provide sufficient information regarding suitability of the product as in the case of flavours covered by the single term flavouring(s) without refer-ence to their source. In addition, the terminology used can be misleading to consumers without adequate knowledge. Common mistakes include the assumption that all 'vegetarian' and 'soya' cheeses are dairy-free. Additional poor marketing of a product can mislead as to its suitability for certain diets. When first available in the UK market, Spelt – an old variety of wheat containing gluten – caused considerable confusion amongst those on wheat- and gluten-free diets. In addition, some foods may appear in unexpected roles, e.g. peanuts ground, reshaped and reflavoured to imitate other nuts.[42]

Mistakes can easily be made when products are reformulated without adequate change in the label format for recognition. The increasing production of brand extensions can cause a false sense of security. The original suitable branded chocolate bar may be used to produce other products such as an ice cream or mousse that will have different ingredients. In addition, one branded product may be produced using different technologies in differ-ent countries, with different contents, resulting in a different allergy status.

Currently, the problem of possible cross-contamination in product manufacture, particularly of nuts, is resulting in a large number of basic products bearing the warning 'may contain', which is reducing the possible range of products available to the consumer.

FUTURE DEVELOPMENTS

Transgenic foods

With the current trend for production of new plant varieties using recombinant DNA technologies, there may be the potential for the breeding and production of less allergenic varieties.[41] However, a major issue is the transfer of known allergenic proteins into new foods, as has happened with the transfer of a gene from the brazil nut to soybeans, with the resulting expression of a major allergen of the brazil nut. A further major concern is the transfer of unknown protein allergens into new foods, which may not be evident until the consumer is exposed to them. Although it is stated that there is no evidence that recombinant proteins will be any more allergenic than traditional proteins, this is an unknown quantity with the potential to be beneficial or prob-lematic to the food-intolerant patient.

CONCLUSION

This chapter covers what is currently a controversial area of dietet-ics but it is important that for patients with possible food intoler-ance an open-minded approach is required, with adequate monitoring of a trial diet and appropriate follow up. It is important to encourage the abandonment of inappropriate dietary restrictions.

Whichever physiological mechanism is involved in the reaction to a specific food or food form, the ultimate outcome for the patient is avoidance of that food in order to prevent symptom provocation. It may be that patients choose not to avoid the incriminated food or foods, but that is then their choice. If patients have the knowledge as to which foods (or their quantity) have the potential to upset them, they can then make their own decisions as to whether they choose to avoid the item. For many patients, this can be highly reassuring and reduces the stress of suspecting some other more sinister diagnosis.

Although this chapter has drawn particular attention to the problems involved in the dietary management of food intoler-ance, this form of treatment can be very positive for some patients, particularly for those patients who prefer to avoid med-ications and are keen to help themselves. It can lead to increased physical well being and social harmony, particularly in cases of attention deficit hyperactivity disorder.[6] However, for some patients, the stress of dieting may be too much and they must not be made to feel guilty if this is not an option for them. Ultimately, the dietary process must do no harm.

European Commission 1998 – proposed list of foodstuffs and ingredients which must be declared in the list of ingredients in the European Union
Cereals containing gluten and products of these
Crustaceans and products of these
Eggs and egg products
Fish and fish products
Peanuts and products of these
Soya beans and products of these
Milk and milk products (lactose included)
Tree nuts and nut products
Sesame seeds
Sulphite at concentrations of at least 10 mg/kg

Table 66.5 European Commission 1998 – proposed list of foodstuffs and ingredients which must be declared in the list of ingredients in the European Union.

REFERENCES

1 Aas K. Societal implications of food allergy: coping with atopic disease in children and adolescents. *Annals Allergy* 1987; 59: 194–9.

2 Ahmad T, Watson S, Eastham EJ. Soy milk induced rickets: case report. *J Nutr Med* 1990; 1(3): 227–9.

3 Anthony HM, Birtwhistle S, Brostoff J, Eaton K *et al*. Letter – food intolerance. *Lancet* 1994; 344: 136–7.

4 Baker JC, Tunnicliffe WS, Duncanson RC, Ayres JG. The development of a standardised method for double blind placebo controlled food chal-lenge in patients with brittle asthma and perceived food intolerance. In press.

5 Barratt JA, Summers GD. Scurvy, osteoporosis and megaloblastic anaemia due to alleged food intolerance. *Br J Rheum* 1996; 35(7): 701–2.

6 Bennett CPW, McEwen LM, McEwen HC, Rose EL. The Shipley project: treating food allergy to prevent criminal behaviour in community settings. *J Nutr Env Med* 1998; 8: 77–83.

7 Bernhisel-Broadbent J, Sampson HA. Cross-allergenicity in the legume botanical family in children with food hypersensitivity. *J Allergy Clin Immunol* 1989; 83: 435–40.

8 Bock SA, Atkins FM. The natural history of peanut allergy. *J Allergy Clin Immunol* 1989; 83: 900–4.

9 Brown M *et al*. Food allergy in polysymptomatic patients. *The Practitioner* 1981; 225: 1651–4.

10 Bunnin A. *The Career of the Food Allergy Sufferer*. Allergy Research and Education, London, 1989.

11 Carter C. The immune system – food allergy and intolerance. In: *Clinical Paediatric Dietetics* (Shaw V, Lawson M, eds). Blackwell Science, Oxford, 1994; 152–62.

12 Carter C. Dietary treatment of food allergy and intolerance. *Clin Exp All* 1995; 25 (Suppl 1): 34–42.

13 Carter C. Double-blind food challenges in children: a dietitian's perspective. *Current Medical Literature – Allergy* 1995; 3: 95–9.

14 Chandra RK. Nutrition and the immune system. *Am J Clin Nutr* 1997; 66: 460–3.

15 David TJ. Anaphylactic shock during elimination diets for severe atopic eczema. *Arch Dis Child* 1984; 59: 983–6.

16 David TJ. The overworked or fraudulent diagnosis of food allergy and food intolerance in children. *J Roy Soc Med* 1985; 78 (Suppl 5): 21–30.

17 David TJ. Unhelpful recent developments in the diagnosis and treatment of allergy and food intolerance in children. In: *Food Intolerance* (Dobbing J, ed). Baillière Tindall, London, 1987: 185–214.

18 David TJ. Hazards of challenge tests in atopic dermatitis. *Allergy* 1989; 44(Suppl 9): 101–7.

19 David TJ, Waddington E, Stanton RHJ. Nutritional hazards of elimination diets in children with atopic eczema. *Arch Dis Child* 1984; 59: 323–5.

20 Devlin J, David TJ. Intolerance to oral and intravenous calcium supplements in atopic eczema. *J Roy Soc Med* 1990; 83: 497–8.

21 Devlin J, Stanton RH, David TJ. Calcium intake and cows' milk free diets. *Arch Dis Child* 1989; 64: 1183–93.

22 Department of Health. *Rep Hlth Soc Subj 41: Dietary Reference Values for Food Energy and Nutrients for the United Kingdom*. HMSO, London, 1991.

23 Department of Health. *Rep Hlth Soc Subj 45: Weaning and the Weaning Diet*. HMSO, London, 1994.

24 Flick J, Sampson HA, Perman J. Intestinal permeability to carbohydrates in children with atopic dermatitis and food hypersensitivity. *Pediatr Res* 1988; 23: 303A.

25 Freeman JV, Cole TJ, Chinn S, Jones PRM, White EM, Preece MA. Cross sectional stature and weight reference curves for the UK, 1990. *Arch Dis Child* 1995; 73: 17–24.

26 Geerling BJ, Badart-Smook A, Stockbrugger RW, Brummer RM. Comprehensive nutritional status in patients with long-standing Crohn's disease currently in remission. *Am J Clin Nutr* 1998; 67: 919–26.

27 Gray J, Bentovim A. Illness induction syndrome: Paper 1 – A series of 41 children from 37 families identified at the Great Ormond Street Hospital for Children NHS Trust. *Child Abuse and Neglect* 1996; 20: 655–73.

28 Hathaway MJ, Warner JO. Compliance problems in the dietary management of eczema. *Arch Dis Child* 1983; 58: 463–4.

29 Henderson RC, Hayes PRL. Bone mineralization in children and adolescents with a milk allergy. *Bone and Mineral* 1994; 27: 1–12.

30 Holland B, Welch AA, Unwin ID, Buss DH, Paul AA, Southgate DAT. *McCance and Widdowson's The Composition of Foods*, 5th edn. Royal Society of Chemistry and Ministry of Agriculture, Fisheries and Food, Cambridge, 1991.

31 Host A, Halken S. A prospective study of cow milk allergy in Danish infants during the first three years of life. Clinical course in relation to clinical and immunological type of hypersensitivity reaction. *Allergy* 1990; 45: 587–96.

32 Host A. Cow's milk protein allergy and intolerance in infancy. Some clinical, epidemiological and immunological aspects. *Paediatr Allergy Immunol* 1994; 5(Suppl 5): 5–36.

33 Hourihane JO'B, Rolles CJ. Morbidity from excessive intake of high energy fluids: the 'squash drinking syndrome'. *Arch Dis Child* 1995; 72: 141–3.

34 Hourihane JO'B, Stephen AR, Warner JO. Resolution of peanut allergy: case-control study. *Br Med J* 1998; 316: 1271–5.

35 Isolauri E, Hill DJ. Guide for paediatricians on the diagnosis and treatment of severe cow milk allergy and multiple food protein intolerance in infancy. SHS International Ltd., Liverpool, 1997.

36 Jarvis D, Burney P. ABC of allergies – the epidemiology of allergic disease. *Br Med J* 1998; 316: 607–10.

37 Jenney MEM, Childs C, Mabin D, Beswick MV, David TJ. Oxygen consumption during sleep in atopic dermatitis. *Arch Dis Child* 1995; 72: 144–6.

38 Kilgallen I, Gibney MJ. Parental perception of food allergy or intolerance in children under 4 years of age. *J Hum Nutr Dietet* 1996; 9: 473–8.

39 Kristmundsdottir F, David TJ. Growth impairment in children with atopic eczema. *J Roy Soc Med* 1987; 80: 9–12.

40 Labib M, Gama R, Wright J, Marks V, Robins D. Dietary maladvice as a cause of hypothyroidism and short stature. *Br Med J* 1989; 298: 232–3.

41 Lehrer SB, Horner WE, Reese G. Why are some proteins allergenic? Implications for biotechnology. *Crit Rev Food Sci Technol* 1996; 36: 553–64.

42 Loza C, Brostoff J. Peanut allergy. *Clin and Exp Allergy* 1995; 25: 493–502.

43 Mabin DC, Sykes AE, David TJ. Controlled trial of a few foods diet in severe atopic dermatitis. *Arch Dis Child* 1995; 73: 202–7.

44 Mabin DC, Sykes AE, David TJ. Nutritional content of few foods diet in atopic dermatitis. *Arch Dis Child* 1995; 73: 208–10.

45 Macdonald A, Forsythe WI. The cost of nutrition and diet therapy for low-income families. *Hum Nutr Appl Nutr* 1986; 40A: 87–96.

46 MacDonald A. Which formula in cow's milk protein intolerance? The dietitian's dilemma. *Eur J Clin Nutr* 1995; 49(Suppl 1): 56–63.

47 Ministry of Agriculture Fisheries and Food. *Food Portion Sizes*. HMSO, London, 1993.

48 Paganus A, Juntunen-Backman K, Savilahti E. Follow-up of nutritional status and dietary survey in children with cow's milk allergy. *Acta Paediatr* 1992; 81: 518–21.

49 Price CE, Rona RJ, Chinn S. Height of primary school children and parents' perceptions of food intolerance. *Br Med J* 1988; 296: 1696–9.

50 Roesler TA, Barry PC, Bock SA. Factitious food allergy and failure to thrive. *Arch Pediatr Adolesc Med* 1994; 148: 1150–5.

51 Rona RJ, Chinn S. Parents' perceptions of food intolerance in primary school children. *Br Med J* 1987; 294: 863–6.

52 Ruxton CHS, Kirk TR, Belton NR. The contribution of specific dietary patterns to energy and nutrient intakes in 7–8 year old Scottish school children. 1. Milk drinking. *J Hum Nutr Diet* 1996; 9: 5–14.

53 Sampson HA. Food sensitivity and the pathogenesis of atopic dermatitis. *J Roy Soc Med* 1997; 90 (Suppl 30): S2–8.

54 Sampson HA, Scanlon SM. Natural history of food hypersensitivity in children with atopic dermatitis. *J Pediatr* 1989; 115: 23–7.

55 Spencer H, Gregory S, Hamilton M, Walker A. *The effect on the family of one member's change in diet*. Report to the Economic and Social Research Council, 1996. Unpublished.

56 Stein AS, Stein J, Walters EA, Fairburn CG. Eating habits and attitudes among mothers of children with feeding disorders. *Br Med J* 1995; 310: 228.

57 Sternberg EM, Gold PW. The mind–body interaction in disease. *Scientific American* 1997; Sept: 8–15.

58 Thomas B (ed) *Manual of Dietetic Practice*, 2nd edn. Blackwell Scientific Publications, Oxford, 1994: 18–21.

59 Warner JO, Hathaway MJ. Allergic form of Meadows syndrome (Munchausen by proxy). *Arch Dis Child* 1984; 59: 151–6.

60 Webber SA, Graham-Brown RAC, Hutchinson PE, Burns DA. Dietary manipulation in childhood atopic dermatitis. *Br J Dermatol* 1989; 121: 91–8.

61 Young E, Stoneham MD, Petruckevitch A *et al*. A population study of food intolerance. *Lancet* 1994; 343: 1127–9.

INTRODUCTION

The use of drugs in the treatment or prevention of adverse reactions to foods or other constituents of the diet is of interest for two reasons. First, the failure to identify an avoidable causal agent may require the consideration of drug therapy to prevent or relieve symptoms known or suspected to be food-related. Second, knowledge of the mode of action of drugs effective in this condition may provide clues to the pathogenetic mechanisms of food-induced clinical reactions.

THE ROLE OF DRUG TREATMENT IN FOOD ALLERGY

Symptoms may require and respond to treatment with appropriate drugs, irrespective of the cause. Urticaria in patients where there is a clearcut dietary trigger may respond just as well or as badly to treatment with antihistamines as that due to other causes. Such symptomatic treatment may be clinically effective but tells us little about the mechanisms of the reaction, except that histamine may be among the mediators involved. It is not proposed therefore to examine the whole range of drugs which may on occasion be indicated for the relief of food-related clinical syndromes. Such a survey would have to cover a wide area of the field of clinical therapeutics including, for example, eczema, urticaria/angioedema, asthma, rhinitis, migraine, arthritis and gastrointestinal upsets, both acute and chronic. This review will be confined to the more restricted topic of drug treatment which may have a particular experimental or specific therapeutic role in adverse reactions to foods. Most of the work in this area has, understandably, been directed to the more obviously food-related reactions, particularly those which reproducibly follow provocation testing. Since the mode of action of some of the drugs concerned is still a matter for debate, it is important not to draw too sweeping conclusions from such studies. The fact that sodium cromoglycate (SCG) inhibits mediator release from allergen-challenged mast cells does not prove, for example, that all conditions responding to this drug involve mediator release from mast cells. Other actions of SCG may be relevant to its effects, both in asthma and in food allergy.

Apart from SCG, the other drug for which claims have been made that it interferes in some more or less specific way with the genesis of food-allergic or pseudoallergic reactions is aspirin and, with it, the other non-steroidal anti-inflammatory drugs.

SODIUM CROMOGLYCATE

A number of studies have shown that acute adverse reactions to foods can be prevented or ameliorated by oral pretreatment with SCG. As in asthma, the efficacy of this compound seems to be most readily demonstrable in symptom-free patients subjected to provocation testing. The picture is much less clear when clinical improvement is sought in longer term studies of conditions thought to be food-related. This is understandable, since such trials usually include patients in whom a dietary factor may be only one among several significant precipitating factors, or in whom an initially allergen-induced condition has produced a long-standing non-specific hyperreactivity. Such conditions may be difficult to reverse without the use of more potent drugs. Recommendations as to the dose and mode of administration of SCG have been reviewed.[19]

The beneficial effect of SCG in milk intolerance was first proposed on the basis of an open study in four infants.[23] A single case of fish- or fruit-induced urticaria reproducibly blocked by SCG but not by placebo in a double blind study, was subsequently reported.[29] In a placebo-controlled crossover study, 20 children with multiple food allergies manifest as eczema, urticaria, asthma or gastrointestinal symptoms, were treated with a dose of 100 mg four times daily. Of the 16 assessed, 10 showed greater improvement on SCG than on placebo, with four showing no difference and only two preferring placebo.[16] Another study on 16 patients which included both children and adults showed a similar level of positive response.[33]

Asthma

In six patients with asthma exacerbated by IgE-mediated food allergy, supported in four cases by a history of attacks precipitated by specific foods and in the other two by improvement on an elimination diet, provocation tests were performed. Pretreatment with inhaled SCG for 24 h before the challenge was completely ineffective in preventing the response to the food concerned (soya protein, wheat or egg). In contrast, SCG administered orally at a higher dose over a similar period was effective in blocking the 25–40% fall in peak expiratory flow rate observed in all six patients after placebo. Neither route of administration was effective in preventing similar degrees of bronchoconstriction after aspirin challenge in six known aspirin-sensitive asthmatics. It was calculated that the amount of SCG absorbed was similar by both dosing routes, and it was therefore concluded that the site of action was the gastrointestinal tract.[13] This study confirmed and extended earlier work from the same authors,[12,14] but similar work by others failed to show the same effect.[26] Subsequent observations appear to support the concept that limitation of allergen absorption might account for the protective effect of SCG.[7,15,17,36] The failure to prevent aspirin-induced asthma may reflect the ready absorption of this drug from the normal gastrointestinal tract, or some basic difference in the nature or site of the triggering mechanism. This is of interest in view of the association of food intolerance with aspirin sensitivity in some patients with urticaria.[1]

Another study involved a well characterized group of patients in whom symptoms could be reliably induced by a specific food, in this case fish. Twenty patients who developed asthma within an hour of ingesting fish and with positive skin tests to fish extract were given 100 g of cod after 3 days of double blind treatment with oral placebo, SCG (400 mg four times daily) or ketotifen (1 mg twice daily). Protection was complete in eight, and partial in another eight on SCG treatment. Three of the four patients showing no protection were among the four with the highest total IgE levels.[21]

Gastrointestinal allergy

Several studies on food allergy with mainly gastrointestinal manifestations have been published, but these have generally been poorly controlled and have involved few patients. However, in one placebo-controlled study, 14 children aged 2–15 years with a history of diarrhoea within 48 h of ingesting various foods, were treated with SCG, 50–70 mg four times daily, for 2 days before oral challenge with cow's milk, soya-based milk substitute or beef. In 11 of 13 trials, SCG was effective in preventing or ameliorating the expected symptoms, whereas placebo was only effective in three of nine trials.[30] Such trials have difficulty in finding suitable subjects, since history of a severe adverse reaction to a food often leads to a prolonged period of avoidance, during which the intolerance may well be lost spontaneously. The current degree of sensitivity always needs to be established by unprotected studies.

Another problem is that an adverse reaction may be followed by a period of specific or non-specific non-responsiveness.

Eczema

The role of food allergy in eczema, particularly in childhood, has led to the investigation of SCG as a prophylactic or therapeutic agent in this condition. As in the case of urticaria, early reports were of single cases which showed impressive improvement.[39] SCG has been tried topically, with mixed results,[25,43] but more frequently by the oral route. Here too results have been most clearly shown when a food factor has been identified and eliminated, and the patient then challenged against a background of low eczema activity (see Chapter 35).

Children

In an open trial of 35 children in whom foods had been established as contributing significantly to their eczema, a period of combined SCG treatment and dietary avoidance was followed by improvement in 66%. Some, but not all, of these suffered a relapse on subsequently reintroducing the avoided foods.[31]

The addition of oral SCG to the treatment programme of 22 children already on a strict exclusion diet produced no additional improvement.[27] This lends support to the view that the activity of this compound is related to the food allergy component of the eczema, which is of variable importance in different groups, probably playing a role in only a minority of adults with the condition. This is paralleled in some ways by a single blind investigation of SCG in urticaria and angioedema, in which a higher proportion of those with an atopic background (five of seven) showed improvement than in the non-atopic group (one of nine).[32]

Another group of 26 young children with eczema treated by food avoidance together with SCG and placebo in a crossover design, followed in each phase by reintroduction of the avoided foods, appeared to demonstrate a strong carry-over effect in the half who received SCG before placebo.[10] If confirmed, this finding has interesting implications, including the possibility that food administration in an allergic patient protected by SCG might induce a state of tolerance. A further, open study of 13 children under 5 years of age, whose chronic eczema had improved on an elimination diet, demonstrated that, in about two-thirds, SCG was effective in preventing relapse upon return to a normal diet. Discontinuation of SCG in these patients was subsequently followed within 2 months by relapse.[11]

The most carefully controlled study in this group was a double blind (for both food and drug), crossover placebo-controlled study of 10 children with egg-induced eczema, proven by previous food challenge.[9] No evidence of reduction in the egg-induced exacerbations was seen in any subject after 30–40 mg/kg/day of SCG for 1 week. Some of the patients experienced not only eczema, or other rashes, but also rhinitis and abdominal symptoms. Criteria studied in relation to food response included amount of egg needed to initiate a response, time to onset of subjective symptoms or of objective signs, and duration of symptoms or signs.

In spite of many anecdotal cases and published case reports over two decades documenting impressive protective activity of oral SCG against food-induced acute allergic reactions, this treatment remains unproven in the properly controlled clinical trial context.

Adults

In adult eczema patients some studies have claimed marginal improvement but this has not generally been sufficiently encouraging to promote the widespread use of SCG in this group, reflecting perhaps the smaller role of food allergy in this age range. Even in children, however, some apparently well designed studies have failed to show benefit.[3]

Criteria of clinical improvement

Few studies in eczema have included measurements of any objective criteria which might relate to clinical improvement. These include claims that total IgE levels in the plasma can be reduced by this treatment, this effect only being observed in patients whose skin improved on SCG. Changes in IgE do not generally accompany remissions and exacerbations of eczema, so this observation is at least a step in the direction of finding an objective index of the drug's efficacy. However, only about 15–20% of patients with eczema show any benefit from SCG, and the IgE changes are not sufficiently clearcut to allow this to be a screening procedure to select suitable patients without submitting large numbers to a prolonged therapeutic trial. For example, in one large trial, only 40 of 196 patients showed a rise in IgE, and of these 19 nevertheless reported improvement. Of the 55 patients whose IgE fell, 38 showed clinical improvement, but 17 did not.[20]

In another study, an open phase of 8 months' oral SCG treatment (200 mg rising to 1200 mg daily) was followed by a 4-month double-blind phase in which the optimum dose for each patient was tested against placebo. Only three of 18 patients showed marked clinical improvement in the open phase, with a further seven showing lesser benefit and eight none. The incidence of food allergy was similar in all three groups (three of three, four of seven and five of eight, respectively in the good, moderate and non-responders). IgE measurements in these subjects showed 20% falls in 14 of the 18, but the subsequent double blind phase of the investigation failed to show any benefit from treatment.[6]

Urticaria

In patients with urticaria who have evidence of food or additives (preservatives or colourings) as triggering agents, protection by SCG against provocation has been demonstrated. In patients with chronic urticaria exacerbated by aspirin or tartrazine, the percentage increase in skin bleeding time was taken as an objective index of adverse reactions, with most of these patients showing a rise of 100% or more on provocation. (The 99% confidence limits for normal subjects were 52% for aspirin and 25% for tartrazine.) The provoking agent used was aspirin in 14 patients (50mg) or tartrazine in six (5 mg). The dose of SCG was 800 mg 15 min before provocation, and the study was placebo-controlled and double-blind. After SCG only six of the 14 aspirin-sensitive patients who had previously reacted gave a change over 52%, the corresponding figure for tartrazine being four of six (67%).[35]

This study, while having the merit of using an objective index of response, did not relate this to the severity of the clinical reaction, nor was it established whether bleeding time could be affected in normal subjects by oral SCG treatment. The site of action both for aspirin and SCG was proposed to be the gastric mucosa, though it seems more likely that aspirin's effect on platelets might be responsible for the effect observed on bleeding time.

Double blind study

The same group also reported an 8-week double-blind crossover study of 24 adults with food- and additive-induced adverse reactions, confirmed by at least two positive provocation tests after a strict exclusion diet. Increased bleeding time was again taken as an objective index of adverse reactions to foods, as well as to drugs or food additives. Symptom scores, which included skin, respiratory tract and gastrointestinal symptoms, were used to assess the patients' responses. These showed that in the fourth week of treatment there was significant advantage to the actively treated group, this being particularly noticeable in those who had received placebo in the first phase of the crossover. This group also showed clear patient and doctor preference for SCG but, because of the small numbers involved, this reached statistical significance only in the case of the doctors' preference, all nine patients assessed being judged better on active treatment and the corresponding figures for patient preference[2] being 10 of 13. One significant feature of this study is the small magnitude of the effect observed. This amounted to an improvement in symptom scores of less than 30%, which, while it may be statistically significant, may not be clinically significant. This is disappointing in view of the careful selection of cases for this trial. Bleeding times, which had been shown to change in an earlier study, do not appear to have been measured in the treatment phase of this investigation.

When SCG was tested in patients with positive provocation tests to food additives or drugs, it conferred no benefit in a placebo-controlled study of 15 adults.[40] Neither was benefit seen in 27 chronic urticaria patients in whom an exclusion diet had failed to elicit improvement.[18] This was in spite of the fact that the same authors were able to show clear SCG protection from multiple food-induced symptoms in two patients. The conclusion that it is specifically food-related urticaria which responds to SCG is supported by a study of 22 patients with chronic urticaria who had failed to respond to antihistamines. All had exacerbations induced by tartrazine and/or sodium benzoate. These patients showed a similar level of response (approximately 70%) to both dietary management and to SCG 200 mg before meals.[4]

Multiple food-associated symptoms

In a number of studies, patients with a variety of symptoms ascribed to specific food allergy or intolerance have been grouped together, and here again SCG treatment seems most effective when given to patients rendered symptom-free by an avoidance diet and subsequently challenged. In 14 patients, mostly adults, with a variety of allergic symptoms, within 24 h of food challenge, 64% of 30 food challenges produced reactions after placebo, with only 8% being positive in 32 treated with SCG. Nine of the 11 patients protected against formal challenge were subsequently able to eat a full diet while on SCG without relapse.[5] In another similar study, 24 of 32 patients were protected to some extent by SCG, although there was an unusually high incidence of adverse reactions to the drug, including some of the very symptoms attributed in other cases to the food intolerance, namely urticaria, headache and gastrointestinal disturbance.[24,41] Other similar studies have been mentioned elsewhere in this review[33] and include one study in which no effect was observed from SCG treatment.[26] The largest group investigated was 66 patients with a variety of symptoms ascribed to single or multiple food sensitivities. Many had asthma, along with other complaints. The treatment was combined in some of the patients with partial or total dietary avoidance. Of the 21 patients reporting total suppression of symptoms, 11 were also practising dietary avoidance. The study included a placebo phase, but was not blinded. Fifteen patients reported exacerbations and 25 partial remission. Doses ranged from 300 to 2000 mg daily. The group studied was so diverse that the only conclusion to be drawn was, as in some other studies, that there might be a subgroup who benefited from SCG, but that without dietary control the effect of the drug was only marginal.[42]

Studies employing objective methods of assessment

The unsatisfactory reliance on subjective factors in many of these studies, which makes their interpretation particularly difficult when the patients have a variety of different clinical syndromes attributed to their food intolerance, makes those few studies in which objective criteria are used of particular interest. Many of these, however, have the disadvantage already mentioned that the objective criteria are not related clearly to the subjective or clinical assessment, nor is it always clear how, if at all, they are relevant to the mechanisms of adverse reactions to foods or to the mode of action of the drugs.

Polyethylene glycol

One study in which SCG has shown such effects on objective criteria involved measurement of intestinal permeability. This was assessed in normal and allergic children by polyethylene glycol (PEG) urinary excretion in the 6 h following oral dosing with a mixture of two PEG fractions of molecular weight 400 and 1000. The dose of SCG used was 100 mg four times daily for 1 week and 200 mg 15 min before the PEG test. The allergic children with gastrointestinal manifestations showed less uptake of 'small' PEG than normal, whereas those with other allergies had greater than normal uptake. SCG reduced PEG recovery in all three groups, but variation within groups was large. The relative excretion of the different size probe molecules was used to calculate a 'filter constant' for the intestinal barrier, and by this criterion SCG treatment clearly reduced the absorption of the smallest fractions in most (10 of 11) of the allergic, and in several of the normal group. Analysis of a calculated index related to apparent pore size of the intestinal barrier showed a change in the allergy group described as 'normalization'; that is, it was consistent with reduction in pore size in those with gastrointestinal allergy, and with a rise in the group with other allergies.[22]

Immune complexes

Immune complexes containing food proteins were detected in the serum of healthy individuals after ingesting milk, and at higher levels in two food-allergic patients (after egg). A biphasic peak was seen, and this was abolished by two prechallenge doses of SCG 500 mg, which also prevented the clinical manifestations, namely bronchospasm and itch, seen after unprotected challenge.[36] This study might have been easier to interpret if the normal subjects had received the same food challenge as the patients, and if the effects of SCG had also been investigated in them.

Neutrophil chemotactic activity

Another study in three adult subjects with milk-induced asthma showed rises in blood neutrophil chemotactic activity corresponding in time to immediate airway obstruction. A fourth subject, who developed an isolated late reaction, showed no such rise. Both neutrophil chemotactic activity rise and immediate asthmatic reaction were inhibited by the prior oral administration of SCG or of beclomethasone dipropionate.[37]

ASPIRIN AND OTHER NON-STEROIDAL ANTI-INFLAMMATORY DRUGS

There has been much less investigation of the role of these cyclo-oxygenase inhibitors in the prophylaxis of adverse food reactions. Acute gastrointestinal and other 'allergic' reactions to foods which had previously provoked symptoms have been shown to be blocked by these drugs. This observation was made by a patient who discovered that an anti-inflammatory drug which she was taking for arthritis enabled her to eat without ill effects shellfish, which in previous and subsequent unprotected challenge caused severe vomiting and diarrhoea. Measurement of the levels of prostaglandins (PG) E_2 and $F_{2\alpha}$ in venous blood plasma and in the stool showed high levels coinciding with the onset of the clinical reaction. The peaks were shortlasting, but measurement of a stable metabolite of $PGF_{2\alpha}$ suggested that a prostaglandin-mediated process was responsible for this type of adverse food reaction, and that inhibiting the production of cyclo-oxygenase products could therefore explain the protective effect observed with the aspirin-like drugs.[8] Support for this hypothesis is found in the observation that gastrointestinal disturbances, including vomiting, colic and watery diarrhoea, are among the side effects most frequently observed during experimental or therapeutic intravenous administration of PGE_2 or $PGF_{2\alpha}$.

A study of patients with urticaria who mentioned aspirin among the factors precipitating their attacks disclosed that these patients very often had specific foods which could also cause symptoms. The induction of tolerance to aspirin by careful administration of increasing doses, and its maintenance by daily dosing, showed that this was accompanied by tolerance to the foods concerned. This incidental finding requires confirmation by placebo-controlled provocation studies. In these patients, too, there was evidence of an underlying biochemical abnormality to the arachidonate pathway, since there were consistently higher than normal levels[2] of $PGF_{2\alpha}$ and histamine in blood samples taken before challenge. Paradoxically, these mediator levels fell to normal during the drug-induced reactions and the subsequent tolerant phase. Further study of this group of patients may enable their biochemical lesion to be more exactly defined, but it will not necessarily cast much light on the mechanisms of other, non-aspirin-related, types of urticaria and asthma.

TREATMENT OF ACUTE LOCAL AND GENERALIZED ALLERGIC REACTIONS TO FOOD

Minor food reactions in sensitive individuals which are local in nature, such as contact urticaria or the oral allergy syndrome (fresh fruit-induced lip or tongue tingling, intraoral angioedema and perioral urticaria, usually seen in patients allergic to silver birch pollen), are usually transient and may not require medication. If they do, a single dose of a non-sedating antihistamine, such as loratadine (adult dose 10 mg) is usually effective either as treatment or prophylaxis. A more rapid onset of action, at the price of some sedation, may be obtained with oral chlorpheniramine. The choice of antihistamine in such cases, as in minor generalized reactions (flush, urticaria, itch, rhinitis or conjunctivitis), may be influenced by the patient's occupation. Drivers or machinery operators may not be able to take a sedative antihistamine and continue at work. Pregnant women should avoid unnecessary medication, but few currently available antihistamines are specifically contraindicated in pregnancy.

Food allergens in such forms as peanut dust in aeroplanes or prawn allergen aerosol in food factories can precipitate asthma exacerbations. These may require treatment with bronchodilator drugs such as beta-agonists, by metered dose aerosol, dry powder inhaler or nebulizer. Such reactions usually occur in known asthmatics, who should normally have such treatments available. In food allergen-induced asthma, whether by the inhaled or oral route, it is important for the patient to understand the importance of (a) always being prepared, especially if eating out, to treat an asthma exacerbation with their reliever medication, and (b) of keeping their asthma optimally treated, preferably with the aid of a written management plan, by adjusting the preventor medication dose according to symptoms, reliever use and peak flow measurements. Agreed and revised guidelines for asthma management along these principles have been widely published, for example in the *British National Formulary*, and are of particular relevance to the safety of this group of patients.

More severe systemic reactions, including anaphylaxis, may involve hypotensive episodes with loss of consciousness (anaphylactic shock), upper airway obstruction or laryngeal oedema. Such episodes are life-threatening emergencies and are, in practice, often treated with suboptimal regimens. Faintness, visual disturbance or dizziness can all be signs of a drop in blood pressure, the most effective first aid treatment for which is for the patient to adopt, or be put into, the lying position, with the head on a level with the heart. Sitting up in a car, or being propped up by helpers, can be dangerous in this situation by producing cerebral hypoperfusion. The most effective treatment for severe systemic allergic reactions, including anaphylactic shock, is undoubtedly epinephrine. This drug has multiple actions, including inhibition of mast cell mediator release, raising peripheral vascular resistance and cardiac output, reducing microvascular permeability to macromolecules and bronchodilatation, all of which can be beneficial in this situation.

There have been recent concerns that lack of familiarity with the use of epinephrine in this context, was leading in many cases to dangerous failures in first line medical care, either by delaying or omitting treatment, or by giving it by an inappropriately dangerous route, such as a bolus iv injection. These concerns have led to the recent publication of consensus guidelines by a project team of the Resuscitation Council (UK).[38] This committee included representatives from all the relevant disciplines, including accident and emergency staff, primary care doctors, allergists and paramedics. The appropriate nature of these recommendations has been confirmed in a recent *BMJ* editorial.[28] In summary,

the use of oxygen (if available), followed if stridor, wheeze, respiratory distress or clinical signs of shock are present, by 0.5 ml im epinephrine 1:1000 (500 µg) repeated after 5 min if no clinical improvement is observed, is recommended. This is followed by 10–20 mg chlorpheniramine im or by slow iv injection. In asthmatics, and all with severe or recurrent reactions, 100–500 mg of hydrocortisone should be given im or by slow iv injection. Rapid infusion of 1–2 l of intravenous fluid, preferably crystalloid, is recommended if clinical manifestations of shock do not respond promptly to drug treatment.

CONCLUSIONS

The place of drug therapy in food allergy is difficult to assess. The natural history of food-related allergic disease makes it difficult to obtain suitable patient populations for study. Food allergy or intolerance may cause a wide variety of symptoms, and these may vary greatly in one individual on different exposures, as in those with food-associated, exercise-induced anaphylaxis, to quote an extreme example. There is sometimes a lack of objective findings to support a patient's symptomatic response. When objective changes have been shown, their relevance has not always been apparent, and many studies lack critical controls to validate the tests applied. The interval between the last reported spontaneous reaction and a provocation, or between successive provocations, may profoundly affect the response. Allergen avoidance may reduce, or in other cases greatly increase, sensitivity to subsequent challenge. Food factors may be only one among several triggers in urticaria and other conditions. Few studies have involved more than a few patients, and it is often difficult to extrapolate from the formal challenge to the environmental exposure situation, or from one category of adverse reaction to another.

The efficacy of SCG is most readily demonstrated in subjects who have clearcut symptoms precipitated acutely by the ingestion of specific foods, including those in whom there is evidence of an IgE-mediated mechanism. Attempts to treat or to elucidate the mechanisms of other less well defined adverse food reactions with SCG have not generally been impressive. Aspirin appears to have a specific role, related to its ability to inhibit the cyclo-oxygenase pathway, in those adverse food reactions which are manifest mainly as gastrointestinal upsets. The relationship between aspirin-induced urticaria or asthma, food intolerance and induced aspirin or food intolerance, suggests a central role for cyclo-oxygenase products as mediators or modulators in this group of conditions. It is questionable whether the findings from such clearcut clinical syndromes as IgE-mediated food allergy or the urticaria induced by aspirin or foods, have much relevance to other forms of food intolerance. Until immunological or pharmacological clues to the mechanisms of such reactions are found, treatment must remain largely empirical and symptomatic.

REFERENCES

1 Asad SI, Youlten LJF, Lessof MH. Specific desensitisation in 'aspirin sensitive' urticaria; plasma prostaglandin levels and clinical manifestations. *Clin Allergy* 1983; 13: 459–66.

2 Asad SI, Murdoch R, Youlten LJF, Lessof MH. Plasma levels of histamine and prostaglandin in aspirin sensitive patients. *Ann Allergy* 1987; 59: 219–22.

3 Atherton DJ, Soothill JF, Elindgo J. A controlled trial of sodium cromoglycate in atopic eczema. *Br J Dermatol* 1982; 106: 681–5.

4 August PJ. Successful treatment of urticaria due to food additives with sodium cromoglycate and an exclusion diet. In: *The Mast Cell: Its Role in Health and Disease* (Pepys J, Edwards AM, eds), Pitman Medical, Bath, 1979; 584–90.

5 Basomba A, Campos A, Villalmanzo IG, Pelaez A. The effect of sodium cromoglycate in patients with food allergy. *Acta Allergol* (Suppl.) 1977; 13: 95–101.

6 Benton EC, Barnetson RSC, Merrett TG, Ferguson A. Long term studies of oral sodium cromoglycate in atopic eczema. In: *The Second Fisons Food Allergy Workshop*, Medicine Publishing Foundation, Oxford, 1983; 123–7.

7 Brostoff J, Carini C, Wraith DG, Johns P. Production of IgE complexes by allergen challenge in atopic patients and the effect of sodium cromoglycate. *Lancet* 1979; i: 1268–70.

8 Buisseret PD, Youlten LJF, Heinzelmann DI, Lessof MH. Prostaglandin-synthesis inhibitors in the prophylaxis of food intolerance. *Lancet* 1978; i: 906–8.

9 Burks AW, Sampson HA. Double blind placebo-controlled trial of oral cromolyn in children with atopic dermatitis and documented food hypersensitivity. *J Allergy Clin Immunol* 1988; 81: 417–23.

10 Buscino L, Bernincori N, Buscino E *et al*. Double blind crossover study with an oral solution of sodium cromoglycate in children with atopic dermatitis due to food allergy. In: *The Second Fisons Food Allergy Workshop*, Medicine Publishing Foundation, Oxford, 1983; 111–15.

11 Cavagni G. Atopic dermatitis due to food allergens. *Practitioner* 1981; 225: 1657–60.

12 Dahl R. Disodium cromoglycate and food allergy. The effect of oral and inhaled disodium cromoglycate in a food allergic patient. *Allergy* 1978; 33: 192–4.

13 Dahl R. Oral and inhaled sodium cromoglycate in challenge tests with food allergens or acetylsalicylic acid. *Allergy* 1981; 36: 161–5.

14 Dahl R, Zetterstrom O. The effect of orally administered sodium cromoglycate on allergic reactions caused by food allergens. *Clin Allergy* 1978; 8: 419–22.

15 Dannaeus A, Johansson SGO. Prevention of antigen absorption in food allergic patients with oral sodium cromoglycate. In: *The Mast Cell: Its Role in Health and Disease* (Pepys J, Edwards AM, eds), Pitman Medical, Bath, 1979; 447–9.

16 Dannaeus A, Foucard T, Johansson SGO. The effect of orally administered sodium cromoglycate in asthma and urticaria due to foods. *Clin Allergy* 1978; 8: 423–7.

17 Dannaeus A, Inganas M, Johansson SGO, Foucard T. Intestinal uptake of ovalbumin in malabsorption and food allergy in relation to serum IgG antibody and orally administered sodium cromoglycate. *Clin Allergy* 1979; 9: 263–70.

18 Denman AM, Platts-Mills T, Brereton PJ *et al*. Urticaria and dietary hypersensitivity. In: *Antigen Absorption by the Gut* (Hummings WA, ed.). University Park Press, Baltimore, 1978; 167–81.

19 Edwards AM. Drug management. In: *The First Food Allergy Workshop*. Medical Education Services, Oxford, 1980; 95–101.

20 Edwards AM. Report on a multi centre study to examine the effects of oral sodium cromoglycate on serum IgE levels in atopic dermatitis. In: *The Second Fisons Food Allergy Workshop*. Medicine Publishing Foundation, Oxford, 1983; 128–31.

21 Ellul-Micallef R. Effect of oral sodium cromoglycate and ketotifen in fish-induced bronchial asthma. *Thorax* 1983; 38(7): 527–30.

22 Faith-Magnusson K, Kjellman NIM, Magnusson KE, Sundqvist T. Intestinal permeability in healthy and allergic children before and after sodium cromoglycate treatment assessed with different-sized polyethylene glycols (PEG 400 and PEG 1000). *Clin Allergy* 1984; 14: 277–86.

23 Freier S, Berger H. Disodium cromoglycate in gastrointestinal protein intolerance. *Lancet* 1973; i: 913–15.

24 Gerrard JW. Oral cromoglycate: its value in treatment of adverse reactions to foods. *Ann Allergy* 1979; 42: 135–9.

25 Haider SA. Treatment of atopic eczema in children: clinical trial of 10% sodium cromoglycate ointment. *BMJ* 1977; i: 1570–2.

26 Harries MG, O'Brien IM, Burge PS, Pepys J. Effects of orally administered sodium cromoglycate in asthma and urticaria due to foods. *Clin Allergy* 1978; 8: 423–7.

27 Harris JM, Graham P, Hall-Smith SP, Price ML. The use of sodium cromoglycate and exclusion diets in childhood atopic eczema. In: *The Second Fisons Food Allergy Workshop*. Medicine Publishing Foundation, Oxford; 1983; 111–15.

28 Hughes G, Fitzharris P. Managing acute anaphylaxis. *BMJ* 1999; 319: 1–2.

29 Kingsley PJ. Oral sodium cromoglycate in gastro intestinal allergy. *Lancet* 1974; ii: 1011.

30 Kocoshis S, Gryboski JD. Use of cromolyn in combined gastrointestinal allergy. *JAMA* 1979; 242: 1169–73.

31 Molkhou P, Waguet JC. Food allergy and atopic dermatitis in children: treatment with oral sodium cromoglycate. *Ann Allergy* 1981; 47: 173–5.

32 Moneret-Vautrin DA, Claudot N. Allergie alimentaire de type I et pseudo-allergies alimentaires chez l'adulte. Effets du cromoglycate de sodium sur les manifestations cliniques. *Nouv Presse Med* 1980; 9: 2549–52.

33 Nizami RM, Lewin PK, Baboo MT. Oral cromolyn therapy in patients with food allergy: a preliminary report. *Ann Allergy* 1977; 39: 102–5.

34 Ortolani C, Pastorello E, Zanussi C. Prophylaxis of adverse reactions to foods. A double blind study of oral sodium cromoglycate for the prophylaxis of adverse reactions to foods and additives. *Ann Allergy* 1983; 50(2): 105–9.

35 Ortolani C, Cornelli U, Bellani M *et al*. Sodium cromoglycate and provocation tests in chronic urticaria. *Ann Allergy* 1982; 48: 50–2.

36 Paganelli R, Levinsky RJ, Brostoff J, Wraith DG. Immune complexes containing food proteins in normal and atopic subjects after oral challenge and effect of sodium cromoglycate on antigen absorption. *Lancet* 1979; i: 1270–2.

37 Papageorgiou N, Lee TH, Nagakura I *et al*. Neutrophil chemotactic activity in milk-induced asthma. *J Aller Clin Immunol* 1983; 72(1): 75–82.

38 Project Team of the Resuscitation Council (UK). The emergency medical treatment of anaphylactic reactions. *J Accident Emerg Med* 1999; 16: 243–7.

39 Shaw RF. Cromolyn therapy in chronic infantile eczema. *Arch Dermatol* 1975; 111: 1537.

40 Thormann J, Laurberg G, Zachariae H. Oral sodium cromoglycate in chronic urticaria. *Allergy* 1980; 35: 139–41.

41 Vaz GA, Tan LKT, Gerrard JW. Oral cromoglycate in treatment of adverse reactions to foods. *Lancet* 1978; i: 1066–8.

42 Wraith DG, Young GVW, Lee TH. The management of food allergy with diet and Nalcrom. In: *The Mast Cell: Its Role in Health and Disease* (Pepys J, Edwards AM, eds), Pitman Medical, Bath, 1979; 443–6.

43 Zachariae H, Afzelius H, Laurberg G. Topically applied sodium cromoglycate in atopic dermatitis. In: *The Mast Cell: Its Role in Health and Disease* (Pepys J, Edwards AM, eds), Bath: Pitman Medical, 1979; 568–9.

INTRODUCTION

Most food allergies, explicit or hidden, can be investigated and managed at home, but patients with multiple symptoms may get quicker relief from admission to a dedicated unit; for a few, admission may be necessary to get a good result. In this book adverse reactions to foods have been generally considered in isolation although this is not the situation in practice. Most patients with hidden food allergies also react to aeroallergens, or to chemicals in the environment, foods or medications, or to both. In the 1960s Dr Theron Randolph in Chicago realized that investigations of hidden food allergy in some polysymptomatic patients were failing because of contamination of the home and hospital environments.[18–20] This led him to establish the first environmentally controlled inpatient unit.[19,20] As he anticipated, in this relatively 'clean' environment he was able to identify the factors causing ill health in a wider range of patients with chronic illness.

The atmosphere in buildings is contaminated by pollution penetrating from outside and that generated inside. The latter predominates in most buildings, arising from the outgassing of volatile chemicals from building materials, synthetic fittings, wood treatments, toiletries, cleaning agents, DIY, newspapers, etc., as well as the products of combustion and accumulated allergens from house dust mites, moulds, etc. Sufficient reduction of pollution for *clinical* purposes can often be achieved in private houses by relatively simple means,[3] but much stricter controls are needed to reduce it to the level required for *diagnostic* and *research* purposes. These measures include filtering incoming air and water, the use of natural non-outgassing materials in construction, fittings

and furniture and strict running controls. Units which apply all the necessary precautions are known as comprehensive environmentally controlled units (ECUs).

In the early days, Randolph used separate rooms in a hospital, which gave some protection from the cigarette smoke, perfumes and cleaning agents in use in other rooms. In 1975 he started a separate Ecology Unit as a section of a Chicago hospital, in which far greater environmental control was possible. Over the next few years as he improved the adaptation of the building and introduced appropriate controls in the running of the unit, fewer patients failed to improve.[21] The use of large and effective air purifiers proved to be a major advance. When he discovered that the floor of his unit had been sprayed with chemical pesticide by a previous user, he had the floorboards removed and the floor tiled with ceramic tiles, and results improved further. Rea's units in Dallas drew on Randolph's experience; he adapted part of the hospital buildings by installing glazed ceramic tiled floors and covering walls with porcelainized-steel to form a barrier, and used effective air filters.[24] The Airedale Allergy Centre (AAC), the first purpose-built unit in the world, opened in 1985, drawing on all this experience. It is the only inpatient comprehensive ECU operating in the UK.

At the time of writing there are ECUs in the UK, Australia and China, but the unit in Dallas, Texas has unfortunately closed. In this chapter we shall describe the precautions employed to keep ECUs free of pollutants, the regimes used and some evidence about their efficacy and cost-effectiveness. Much of the data quoted will relate to the AAC, with which the authors are closely associated.

The role of the ECU

The AAC sees its role as fourfold:

- to investigate patients with multiple symptoms or intractable medical problems to establish whether adverse reactions to foods or environmental factors contribute to the aetiology
- to complete the investigation of patients in whom outpatient investigation has been only partly successful
- to investigate patients with uncontrolled, life-threatening allergic reactions under close supervision
- to initiate treatment with a view to making it possible for patients to remain well (or at least substantially better) and able to tolerate a nutritionally adequate diet and a socially manageable lifestyle when they leave the protected atmosphere of the ECU.

Treatment includes education about how to reduce exposure to aeroallergens and chemicals at home, the initiation of specific prophylaxis, planning an appropriate dietary regime and nutritional supplementation.

The first objective can usually be achieved within a week. The aim is to protect patients from all sources of exposure – external and internal – to allow rapid unmasking of hidden allergies. The regime therefore starts with a therapeutic fast, usually for 5 days. During a fast in the clean conditions of an ECU, environmentally provoked symptoms improve (after an initial worsening) and may resolve completely. If any patient shows no evidence of improvement within 10 days, an environmental aetiology can usually be ruled out, although in some chemically sensitive patients the process may not be complete for 2–3 weeks. Admission to an ECU can be a valuable exercise in patients with multiple sensitivities and those with intractable medical problems. At present there is no other way of eliminating the possibility that such conditions are provoked by environmental factors. A period in an ECU either opens up a constructive method of management or rules it out: each can be equally important, although in our experience the former is the usual outcome in patients who are able to cooperate.

A clean atmosphere is of vital importance in the investigation of such cases.[3,18–21,24] Many of the patients whose symptoms clear on admission to an ECU have previously been admitted to hospital, sometimes requiring repeated acute admissions. Many felt worse in the hospital environment even though their acute condition was controlled with medication. Sometimes the contribution of food intolerance has been suspected previously and even tested by subjecting them to a therapeutic fast in hospital, without any improvement to support the contention. The same patients have been shown to be highly food intolerant when tested in an ECU.[13] Other cases have given false negative responses to tests for chemical sensitivity when attending for testing from a polluted home environment but unequivocal positive results have been obtained after some days in an ECU.

CONSTRUCTION AND MANAGEMENT

The building

In addition to profiting from earlier experience, the AAC has the advantages of being a self-contained detached building, purpose-built in a relatively unpolluted location. It was difficult to isolate ECUs that were conversions of old buildings and Rea found it necessary to coat the walls and floor with impermeable material.[24]

In a new building the materials used in construction could be controlled and it was therefore not considered necessary to line all the walls with stainless steel, as in Dallas, or to tile the floor of the lounge. Results have been satisfactory,[14] but it is, of course, impossible to establish without doubt the necessity of any individual item of the precautions taken during construction.

The principles were to avoid using any material from which chemicals would outgas, to make sure that particles and pollutant chemicals were removed from incoming air and water and to arrange that the ventilation rate was high enough to keep the relative humidity too low to support the multiplication of house dust mites and moulds.[3] Mattresses in the unit are virtually house dust mite-free even after use for 12 years.

Natural materials

The AAC was constructed of natural materials – stone, African walnut (to avoid softwoods needing paint or varnish, and woods such as teak and pine which outgas terpene-like materials), glass, steel, copper, aluminium and ceramics, and using mortar, concrete and plaster with no accelerators or retardants. It is a small unit, built in a village in an unpolluted part of West Yorkshire close to the Yorkshire Dales. The original building was planned for a maximum of 12 inpatients but with land for extension. The inpatient area consists of a 25 ft (7.62 m) lounge area with picture windows down the long wall, open plan to a corridor with a nurses' office, testing room (with separately ventilated exposure booth), three bedrooms for two patients each (often housing one patient) and two single rooms; a toilet wing leads off this, beyond which there are two additional double rooms, one usually in use as a television room. The entrance hall, kitchen, utility room and staff changing rooms are isolated from the patient area by double doors. There is a small outpatient department off the entrance hall, not within the controlled area.

Hardwood doors, door and window frames and floors were permanently sealed with polyurethane varnish and allowed to mature before use. The floor of the lounge is hardwood, the rest is of ceramic tiles. Except where tiles were required, walls were plastered with plain plaster mix and decorated with simple emulsion. Electrical wiring was standard; switches have hard plastic buttons, since all-metal light switches were not permitted. All pipes are copper and were polished initially with wire wool and have remained bright and smooth.

Air filtration

The standards of air filtration for ECUs must be very high. Minimal penetration of unfiltered outdoor air into the AAC is ensured by sound construction with fixed, airtight windows, a system of double doors and positive pressure ventilation. Each entry has double doors far enough apart so that a single person cannot open them simultaneously; the outer doors open outward. There is forced air ventilation giving two–three air changes an hour overall with no recirculation, fine filtration to remove particles and high-quality filtration by activated carbon units to remove chemical contamination; filters and ducts are checked regularly. The sequence of filters starts with a fibre filter, then a closely packed carbon filter, then a second fibre filter and finally a high efficiency particle air filter (HEPA) excluding particles down to a diameter of 0.5 μm. Incoming air is warmed by going through a heat exchanger, but heating is from a separate circulating water-filled radiator system fuelled by a distant boiler, giving a temperature of 70°F (21°C). A single master air inlet serves inlets in the bedrooms, office, testing room and large lounge, with extracts in the passages, bathrooms and toilets; there is an extra air inlet in the corridor of the toilet wing. Air is exhausted from the main corridor through a heat exchanger to a main exhaust vent carefully situated away from the inlet vent. Continuous extraction direct to the outside from each toilet and bathroom gives a higher rate of air change in the toilet wing. Humidity is very low in winter, and low to normal in summer, varying between 5 and 35% RH, insufficient to support the growth of house dust mites or moulds: additional precautions are taken against mould growth in the bathrooms by swabbing regularly with borax.

The ventilation system contrasts with that of the Dallas ECU where external pollution was so high that the decision was taken to recirculate all the air, relying on continuous filtration, and refreshing with filtered air from outside only when pollution was lowest.[24] Rea monitored indoor air quality, and the detected levels of chemical pollutants were generally substantially lower than in the main hospital or outside; however, some chemical pollutants were present at higher concentrations, mostly those detected in the bloodstream of patients on admission or released by electric motors.[24] The AAC does not usually require to filter *indoor* air, although this has occasionally been necessary in a bedroom of a patient highly polluted on admission until the excretion of detectable amounts of chemicals (usually perfumes) is over.

As far as possible the furnishings of the AAC are of metal, hardwood and cotton. No carpets are used or soft plastics or synthetic fabrics. Curtains and covers are made from unbleached cotton dyed with vegetable dyes, and bedding and upholstery are cotton. Patients are allowed to bring in some articles made of hard plastics, but only if the experienced noses of the staff can detect no smell at all. A television is provided but it is housed in an isolated room which can be avoided by any patients who do not tolerate it.

Management

Strict operational controls keep pollution originating within the building to a minimum. Both patients and staff use perfume-free toiletries and staff change into dedicated footwear and cotton clothes before going on duty; patients wear clothes of natural vegetable fibres or silk and visitors put on gowns and shoe covers. Visitors smelling of perfumes, cleaning agents, cigarettes, etc., are not admitted, and nothing with any odour can be taken in. Every attempt is made to keep the standards at the AAC as high as possible, so that pollution is kept to an absolute minimum. This requires fairly spartan surroundings with no carpets or upholstery, and rigorous restrictions such as the banning of newspapers. These high standards are essential if definite conclusions about the environmental aetiology of intractable symptoms are to be reached.

All water is filtered to reduce chemical contamination, and drinking and cooking water is also subject to purification by reverse osmosis.

The cleaning materials used are limited to washing soda and borax for general cleaning, hypoallergenic non-biological non-scented detergent for washing clothes and bedlinen, or for very sensitive patients sodium bicarbonate only. Vegetable-based non-perfumed detergent is used for windows, washing-up and in the dishwasher.

In the kitchen area, which is separated from the rest of the unit by double doors and separate air extraction, cleaning policy is dictated by the hygiene inspectors: they insist on the use of disinfectants. Until recently among the products they were prepared to approve the one with the least smell was Dettox. They have recently approved the use of Germacert, an odourless product with proven effectiveness against a wide range of bacteria.

The Local Health Authority also require each institution to have a defined policy about methods to be used if there is spillage of body fluids – blood, urine or faeces. The AAC has therefore been required to stock 0.5% phenol for this purpose, but has not so far had to use it. At present Germacert is not deemed suitable, since there are no data about its virocidal activity.

Staffing

The nurses are led by an experienced nurse-manager. Trained nurses are on duty throughout the 24 hours; they are conventionally trained and fully qualified nurses who have been given additional training in environmental medical techniques at the AAC. In addition, there is an outpatient manager, a nutritionist, cooks and cleaners, all given extra training, and a visiting psychologist. All staff are non-smokers. The total staffing depends on the numbers of patients for which the AAC is currently licenced: for six beds about 11 full-time equivalents are employed, well above the statutory requirements.

The Medical Director of the AAC lives on site and other doctors visit as necessary.

TREATMENT PROTOCOL

Admission to the AAC is normally for a period of 3 weeks plus or minus 2–3 days. The initial admission period must be continuous; if it has to be broken for any reason the patient has to start again, entailing a longer total period of admission. After a 5-day fast to clear hidden or 'masked' food reactions, the factors which had been provoking the symptoms can be identified from tests for sensitivity to aeroallergens, and serial challenges with foods and extracts of chemical pollutants. Patients stay inside all the time until testing for aeroallergens and chemicals is complete and they are protected by specific prophylaxis (see Chapter 70). Occasional patients subsequently need to be readmitted for further testing or for adjustments to their vaccines; this may only take a few days and does not usually involve a repeat of the fast.

On admission a very full history is taken, the patient is examined and some investigations arranged. There are very few acute admissions and chronic illness has usually been investigated before admission, in particular to rule out malignancy. Routine investigations include standard haematology and biochemistry, total immunoglobulin E (IgE) levels and prick tests, and estimations of some aspects of nutritional status (serum trace elements, red cell magnesium, functional activity of vitamin B_1, B_2 and B_6 and others as indicated). In our experience, as in the USA,[28] these patients are commonly deficient in several micronutrients, particularly B vitamins, magnesium, zinc and essential fatty acids. Many other investigations were undertaken in the ECU in Dallas, including estimations of body burden of pesticides, organic solvents and other chemicals, and metabolic, immunological and other assessments, but reliable results depend on a high level of expertise and add greatly to the expense. Rea *et al.* reported that body burdens of chemicals fell significantly over the period of admission, although the raw data were not given.[24,26] Results of other investigations varied and no single test was helpful for all patients, but Rea claims that the phagocytosis index is a useful general monitor of progress.[24]

Physical examination is usually uninformative, merely confirming, for instance, the expected signs of involvement of the bowel, bronchi, skin and/or joints. However, some peripheral observations are of interest. Patients usually seem to have either very active reflexes or weak reflexes which may be impossible to elicit; reflexes have often reverted to normal if retested before discharge. In some cases muscle tone may also be unusually high (accompanied by pain in the muscles and/or joints) or low, and pupils may be large. There may be clinical evidence of nutritional deficiencies, particularly of B vitamins, or of bruising to which poor absorption of vitamin K seems to contribute. Some of the patients are suffering pain or disability obvious even to the casual observer and more evident when they are examined, although there is often minimal evidence of physical or X-ray changes to account for the disability.

INVESTIGATION AND MANAGEMENT

The therapeutic fast

On admission, adult patients fast for 5 days, but a shorter fast usually suffices for children. Previous medication is withdrawn, or reduced as far as possible and reconsidered daily. Many medications contain food products and continuing to take them during the fast may interfere with subsequent testing. Most of the drugs used before admission are no longer required by the end of the fast because symptoms have resolved. Intravenous infusions of zinc, magnesium and B and C vitamins with small amounts of other important trace elements (selenium, chromium, manganese, molybdenum and copper) are administered to most patients, guided by the results of investigations: in our experience, this speeds up recovery.

Patients are encouraged to rest on their beds during the fast, but most dress and move about to a limited extent. Curiously, after the first day, although patients tend to feel weak, few are plagued by hunger and a lot of patients are not bothered by it at all. If the patient is well enough, testing and neutralization titration for aeroallergens are carried out during this period (see Chapter 70): in view of the insensitivity of prick tests, relevant aeroallergens are tested intradermally even if the prick test is negative.

During this withdrawal period, pulse rate, temperature, blood pressure, fluid balance and body weight are monitored. Patients are observed day and night by experienced staff and record their symptoms regularly, mainly by subjective scoring; most patients prove to be surprisingly consistent in their scoring of symptoms. Asthmatics measure their peak expiratory flow rate (PEF) regularly, four times a day. PEF may fall temporarily during withdrawal, even without changes in medication.[13]

Most patients who will subsequently benefit suffer withdrawal symptoms, feeling unwell during the first part of the fast, often markedly so: the word 'lousy' is often used to describe it. They often have 'flu' symptoms, aching limbs, restless legs, irritability, poor concentration, nausea and headache (sometimes very severe), and need to be warned before admission. Plain paracetamol powder or milk of magnesia are given for mild symptoms, but diamorphine and/or Buccastem or prochlorperazine may be used

for severe symptoms since withdrawal is short-lived, the severe phase rarely lasting more than 2–3 days. However, withdrawal symptoms may be biphasic. If so, the initial phase seems to be due to the withdrawal of foods and aeroallergens and the secondary phase to withdrawal of chemicals.

During the fast most patients drink 2–3 litres of water a day but are in negative fluid balance, many losing as much as $3\frac{1}{2}$ kg of fluid in 5 days over and above the weight loss expected on the fast (calculated taking account of activity, sex, height and age):[2] occasional patients lose much more. This represents the resolution of chronic water retention.

Resting pulse rate often falls by 10 beats/min or more over the withdrawal period, but may rise temporarily before dropping to a steady baseline. Blood pressure often falls; if it falls to below normal this is usually transient, commonly recovering before the end of the fast. If it was raised before admission, the drop usually indicates that foods and/or environmental agents will be found to provoke hypertensive reactions.

Resolution of presenting symptoms

Presenting symptoms that were due to foods or aeroallergens usually resolve by the fifth or sixth day and patients often feel better than they have for years. Complete resolution is usual for symptoms of headache (including all forms of migraine), irritable bowel syndromes (which may include symptoms previously attributed to hiatus hernia or peptic ulceration) and emotional/cognitive, motor, sensory and general symptoms that show variations in severity. There is usually a marked improvement in asthma symptoms (wheeze, shortness of breath, cough and phlegm[13]) even though medication has been reduced or withdrawn, many patients becoming symptom-free. However, the more severe asthmatics may need to continue taking some preventive medication during admission and for a few months after discharge, while the reduction in triggering (and in the medication needed) allows inflammation to settle and hormone production to stabilize. Bladder symptoms, eczema, some of the arthritides and rhinitis due to foods respond more slowly, although there are usually signs that disease activity is reducing, for instance less itch. Some cases of ulcerative colitis have responded well.

Other changes are also noted. After the initial fall, PEF usually rises, even in patients whose asthma medication has been reduced or stopped. Figure 68.1 shows the PEF traces for two patients throughout admission; the morning PEF is represented by the solid line, the grey area shows the range of values over the day; with the foods provoking the most marked fall in PEF indicated. The initial drop in PEF was partly due to withdrawing medication (as shown); after that, the PEF rose steadily in each patient, with no medication. These traces illustrate our observation that the low morning PEF, often accepted as a characteristic of asthma, does not occur regularly in clean conditions; when it occurs it marks a reaction to food challenge the previous evening.[13]

Challenge phase

Controlled challenges with foods and synthetic and pollutant chemicals are possible in the setting of an ECU without the confounding effects of other exposures. After the end of withdrawal, there is a period of maximum sensitivity to challenge which varies in different individuals but usually lasts about 3–4 weeks. Challenges with extracts of chemicals are performed single blind using dilutions too weak to be identified (excepting cigarette

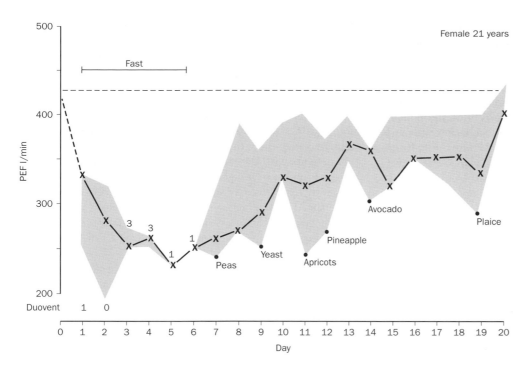

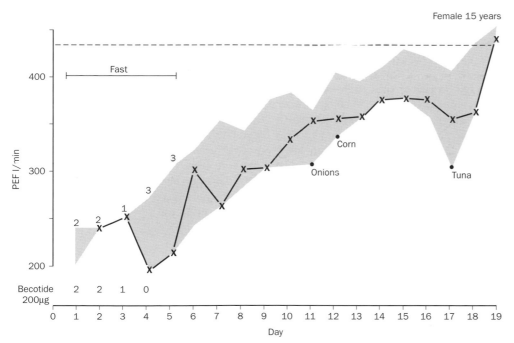

Fig. 68.1 Peak expiratory flow rate (PEF) measurements throughout ECU admission in two young women (top, 21 years old; bottom 15 years old) with asthma and eczema. Solid line, morning PEF; grey area, daily range. (Reproduced from Maberly & Anthony[13] with permission.)

smoke extract, sometimes recognized), but food challenges are by open consumption of the food.

Food challenge

The amount of food required to provoke reactions may be greater than that which it is possible to conceal,[4] and a negative result achieved by enclosing food in capsules cannot rule out a reaction initiated in the mouth or oesophagus.[7] The use of disguise in double-blind studies assumes that the disguising foods are safe: in our experience there is no food that can be considered safe until it has been tested and, during comprehensive testing, disguise could therefore only be applied secondarily to confirm a few individual reactions.

Is double-blind challenge needed?

Double-blind challenge may be needed to establish that a symptom can be provoked by a food, but in the clinical treatment situation, where the aim is to prepare protection for the patient on discharge, it is more important to make sure that an adequate challenge of each food is given, to avoid false negative results. In practice, patients are both surprised and dismayed at the foods to which they react, many of which are favourite foods eaten frequently;[12] patients are, nevertheless, relieved when provocation of their symptoms provides an explanation and a way of preventing the symptoms in future.

As long as symptoms have cleared sufficiently for exacerbations to be clearly recognizable, patients test their home water on the fifth day; unfiltered home water provokes symptoms in about one-third of the patients. Patients begin serial food challenges on the sixth day, taking a single food three times a day about 5 hours apart for the rest of their stay. The patient is asked to lie on the bed during challenges. He takes a resting pulse before the challenge and again 20, 40 and 60 min afterwards, and records the time of development of any symptoms, informing the nursing staff. Asthmatics take PEF readings at the same intervals and other readings (such as blood pressure) are taken by the staff. All patients record body weight morning and night, and usually before each meal. They grade the severity of symptoms from each reaction on a scale of 0–10 with the help of the doctor or charge nurse. Changes in pulse (rate and regularity[23]), blood pressure, weight, appearance and behaviour (when relevant) are taken into consideration as well as reported symptoms when interpreting the results of each challenge.

Testing individual foods

The foods tested are the foods the patient normally eats or wishes to eat. Details are decided with dietetic help to ensure that the patient builds up a satisfactory range of foods to form the basis of a nutritionally adequate 4-day rotation diet on discharge. The general plan is that a fruit is tested in the morning, a vegetable at lunchtime and a protein in the evening, because reactions to proteins are more likely to be delayed.[1] The exception is that the main grains (wheat and corn) are tested at lunchtime and repeated in the evening, if negative, since more than one meal of grains may be required before symptoms are provoked.

In most cases the patient is asked to eat a full portion of the single food, but patients with a history of severe immediate reactions eat a small amount first, proceeding to a larger quantity if no immediate reaction occurs. In patients with anaphylaxis, neutralization titrations may be performed *before* oral challenge (starting at the weakest end of the concentration range) so that the provisional neutralization endpoint can be administered before the meal as a precaution, and adjustments made subsequently if required.

Response to challenge

In most patients the results of challenge are clear cut. Some foods cause symptoms and may give objective changes in weight, pulse, blood pressure and/or appearance; other foods cause none of these changes. In our experience changes in pulse and weight correlate significantly with symptoms but occur in fewer patients;[1] however, the correlation between these reactions is incomplete – patients with a pulse response may not show a weight change. Asthmatics may show these changes as well as a fall in PEF but some patients with the most marked bronchospasm showed no changes in pulse or weight.[1] Clearly the profile of mediators released by reactions may vary.

The speed with which symptoms develop also varies widely. We have looked at the interval between the start of the meal and the first recorded symptom graded 3 or above (out of 10) for each challenge in a series of 1274 food challenges in 32 patients in the AAC:[1] the first symptom recorded was not necessarily the most severe. Most reactions were noticed between 1 h and 4 h from the beginning of the meal, although some started within minutes and others not for over 24 h. When the times of onset after each of approximately 40 food challenges were plotted cumulatively for each patient, the patients fell into four groups, for which the median cumulative onsets are shown in Fig. 68.2. In Group I nearly all the reactions had started by 20 min but in Group IV the patients showed fewer reactions and very few of those had started within the first 40 min; Groups II and III had intermediate patterns. There was some clustering of presenting symptom in the different groups; in particular, Group IV included most of the cases with angio-oedema or water retention as a main symptom.[1] The figure also shows a comparable plot for the first record of a pulse change of 10 beats/min or more: the patients are grouped in the same way, based on the pattern of onset of their *symptoms*. The cumulative onset patterns for symptoms and pulse changes are very similar, but there were only about half as many pulse changes as symptoms. This correlation of symptoms with the objective measurement of pulse rate indicates that the differences in timing have a biological basis.

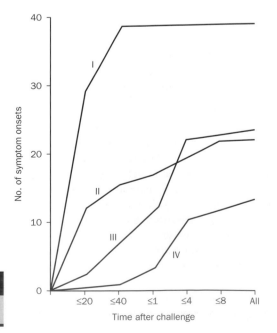

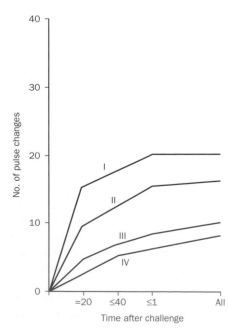

Fig. 68.2 Different patterns of reaction after food challenge. Cumulative reactions by time after challenge (from <20 min to >8 hours) following approximately 40 food challenges per patient in 32 patients, expressed as the median for patients grouped by symptom onset pattern. Left, symptoms; right, pulse changes. (Reproduced from Anthony & Maberly[1] with permission.)

The range of symptoms provoked

The range of symptoms provoked by challenge is very wide, often including all the symptoms the patients reported on presentation and sometimes others that they have had for years and attributed to something quite different. For instance, pain from an old injury may resolve during the fast and then recur to the patient's surprise with one or more food challenges. On the other hand, some severe symptoms may be relieved during the fast but not be provoked by challenge with any food, leading patients to worry that their symptoms may recur when they are discharged, since the cause of the most feared symptom has not been found. This is usually unfounded provided that neutralization prophylaxis has been employed for all the foods causing signs and/or symptoms, even if mild. The severe symptom may have been provoked previously by a combination of factors – more than one food or a combination of a food and another environmental, physical or emotional factor – as in food-dependent exercise-induced asthma or anaphylaxis.[8]

Some of the symptoms provoked can be quite bizarre. We have seen many patients who fall asleep after some foods or even in the middle of eating them and others who suffer from a form of collapse which does not seem to be anaphylaxis, epilepsy or a vasovagal attack. Other patients report hot areas on certain parts of the body, or one leg hot and the other cold, confirmed on examination. Brain fag, irritability and even marked aggression or panic attacks are not uncommon. Some patients suffer from a temporary failure of coordination, which may have a limited distribution. Muscle spasm or muscle weakness may also occur, sometimes very marked. Many of these reactions could easily have been interpreted as hysterical if the provocation by food challenge and the relief at the neutralization endpoint had not been witnessed.

The number of foods provoking symptoms on challenge varies from none (which is rare in patients admitted) to almost all of the 45 or so tested. There seems to be a positive correlation between the severity and duration of the illness and the number of foods to which the patient reacts. Most of the food reactions are confirmed by the relief of symptoms at the neutralization treatment dose.

Food intake

We have examined the food intake of patients on this regime. The content of all the nutrients was adequate with the exception of calcium. Moreover, when the intake was compared with the diet most of the patients were eating before admission the single food diet included a much wider range of foods and was better balanced nutritionally, as well as being free of additives and very low in contaminants.

The American ECUs tested only organic foods. When the AAC opened, these were very difficult to obtain in the UK and expensive, and this was not an option. Good-quality foods were therefore tested – organic for those items that were readily available, such as the grains and pulses – but patients were advised to eat organic food when possible on discharge. In general this has worked well, but a number of patients have subsequently found that they tolerate organic foods but have variable reactions to foods from standard sources; in one patient this has been tested double blind. We do not know which chemicals are responsible for such reactions but suspect it is mainly the pesticides.

Neutralization

Effect of neutralization on symptoms and signs after food challenge

Titration of the endpoint (treatment dose) by the neutralization technique (see Chapter 70) is normally undertaken for each food that causes symptoms. Unless symptoms are so severe as to be potentially life-threatening (for instance severe bronchospasm in patients with no reserve), this is the primary method used to relieve the symptoms provoked by challenge, and other treatments are only used if this fails or is only partly successful. In severe asthmatics a nebulizer is kept ready but patients rarely want it after they have experienced the effectiveness of the neutralization technique in relieving bronchospasm.

Neutralization after oral challenge

When the neutralization technique is used after oral challenge with a food, as in an ECU, there are two endpoints to consider – the first negative skin wheal and the dilution which relieves symptoms. These are usually the same. However, occasionally, a patient does not wheal but still gets relief from symptoms at a consistent dilution, suggesting that failure in the skin-whealing mechanism may be a temporary physiological anomaly, due perhaps to nutritional or enzyme deficiencies. In a few other patients the symptoms are not relieved at the dilution that gives the first negative wheal, but at a higher dilution, usually, but not always, the next fivefold dilution (more dilute). During titration, the skin reactions and the changes in pulse rate, symptoms and appropriate signs are all noted but the dilution which relieves symptoms is regarded as the endpoint if there is any discrepancy. Patients may need a further dose of the treatment dilution if symptoms are prolonged, or reactions biphasic, as demonstrated in asthma by Pelikan & Pelikan-Filipek.[17]

Symptom provocation by oral challenge and relief by the neutralization endpoint is most easily demonstrated by effects on lung function in asthmatics. The relief of symptoms varies from a mild or rather slow relief that requires more than one injection of the endpoint before it can confidently be regarded as effective, to a relief of bronchospasm so marked that PEF rises by as much as 170 l/min within a few minutes. The range of changes in a consecutive series of 19 asthmatic patients is shown in Table 68.1 (some primarily admitted for other symptoms), and charts for two patients in Fig. 68.3. The figure shows *all* the PEF readings in the early days of food challenge, days 6–9 and 7–10, respectively:[12] PEF was normally taken morning and night, before and three times after each food challenge, and during neutralization, but the intervals are shown in a standardized fashion. You will notice that PEF remained unchanged after challenge with a number of foods (for instance, pineapple and milk, lower trace) but dropped after others, although this was sometimes delayed (for instance after sole, lower trace). PEF usually recovered with neutralization (open arrows and open circles) with no need for bronchodilators, but no extract of buckwheat was available at that time (upper trace) and after the buckwheat challenge the PEF was still low the next morning and required bronchodilator therapy (black arrowhead). These long-lasting or recurrent episodes of bronchospasm after food challenge are in keeping with the findings of Wraith[29] and Pelikan & Pelikan-Filipek.[17] After cashews (top trace) there was severe wheeze and the PEF was not measured. The wheeze responded well to neutralization but peak flow was again low next morning, did not respond to

Table 68.1 Maximal peak expiratory flow rate (PEF) drop on challenge and rise on recovery during neutralization for each of 19 asthmatics

	Number of patients	
Maximum PEF change	Fall on challenge	Rise on EP titration
Over 130 l/min	4	2
100–130 l/min	7	3
70–100 l/min	3	4
30–70 l/min	3	3
Not assessable*	2	7
Total	19	19

*In two patients because of poor compliance: PEF recovery not monitored in five patients.

Table 68.1 Maximal peak expiratory flow rate (PEF) drop on challenge and rise on recovery during neutralization for each of 19 asthmatics. (Reproduced from Maberly & Anthony[12] with permission.)

salbutamol, but improved with a further dose of the cashew therapy dose, and after a further dose of salbutamol had recovered sufficiently to allow the next food, carrot, to be tested. Carrot caused a minor fall in PEF that was reversed by the carrot

endpoint alone. The AAC now carries a large range of food extracts, and inpatients do not normally test foods for which extracts are not available.

Which symptoms are relieved by neutralization?

The only symptoms that are relieved by the treatment dose are those provoked by that food or a closely related food which cross-reacts. This provides a useful method of confirming which food was responsible, particularly in patients with late reactions. The standard practice when patients develop symptoms is to titrate with the extract of the most recently eaten food. If this gives no relief, the treatment doses of earlier foods are repeated, or an earlier food which seemed 'safe' titrated. On occasions the latter has been omitted. One patient with severe asthma had no sign of reaction to cabbage but a severe reaction after the next meal – potato – which was not relieved by titration with potato extract and required repeated use of the nebulizer until next morning.[12] A week later cabbage was used as a 'safe' food and provoked exactly the same pattern of late reaction, which was relieved by titration with cabbage extract. The apparent reaction to potato must have been a late reaction to cabbage, so it is not surprising that it did not respond to titration with potato extract!

Testing three foods a day is feasible in outpatients only if patients react to few foods and have short-lived reactions. In the severely affected patients admitted to the AAC this schedule of testing could not be maintained without neutralization to curtail reactions. Even then, for patients who react to a large number of foods the challenge schedule is physically demanding and they

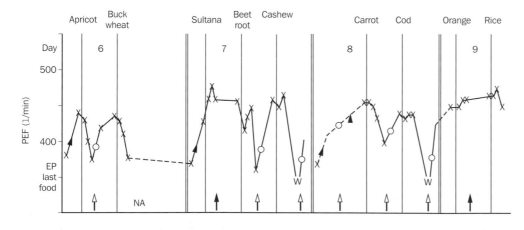

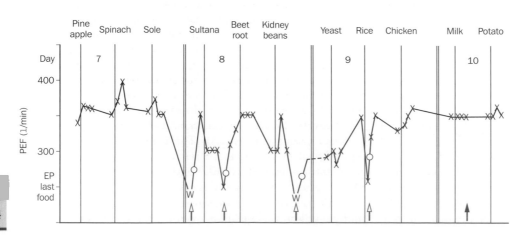

Fig. 68.3 Stylized plots of peak expiratory flow rate (PEF) measurements on four consecutive days at the beginning of food challenge in two patients admitted with moderately severe asthma, showing PEF falls after some challenges and recovery with neutralization when available. Day 6 was the first day of food challenge (shown by single vertical lines); double lines indicate nights. For each challenge PEFs before and 20, 40 and 60 min after the start of the meal are shown, with the PEF at the end of the neutralization titration if monitored; W indicates wheeze. Black arrowheads show use of salbutamol inhaler, no other medication taken. Open circles indicate recovery from bronchospasm following neutralization. Along the bottom, neutralization undertaken for other symptoms is indicated by black arrows; for bronchospasm by open arrows. NA, neutralization not performed because food extract not available. (Reproduced from Maberly & Anthony[12] with permission.)

sometimes become 'overloaded' after a number of tests, not clearing properly between reactions until after a rest from testing. A single safe food meal (or a food preceded by the specific treatment dose for that food) may be enough to allow them to recover but some need a full day of 'safe' foods or fasting.

Hormone testing

Some patients with premenstrual tension or period pains seem to be reacting to their hormones, and have been reported to improve with neutralization to oestrogen and progesterone.[15] Neutralization titrations with these hormones are used in some patients with these symptoms, and symptoms are often prevented by a prophylactic vaccine, usually included in one of the other vaccines.

Chemical testing

With most patients it is possible to start testing chemicals about day 14. Patients fast at breakfast or have a safe food before chemical testing so that the testing is less likely to be confused by reactions to foods. There are several ways in which chemical testing may be performed; in the AAC the routine is to use the sublingual route, although booth challenge or intradermal testing are used occasionally. Different dilutions of chemicals and chemical mixtures are given sublingually: in sensitive patients symptoms are provoked at one dilution and subsequently relieved by another dilution, the treatment dose. Most of the dilutions used are too weak to be identified by taste. They are applied single blind, starting with saline and including a number of saline placebos. If patients give negative results on sublingual testing with chemicals when the history suggests sensitivity, tests may be repeated by exposing them to the fumes in a special booth (as at the ECU at Dallas[27]), again using concentrations most of which are too low for identification. Whichever method has been used to provoke symptoms, titration of the relieving dilution is normally carried out sublingually. Some asthmatics develop bronchospasm with some chemicals but not others and chemical testing has been shown to cause effects on PEF similar to those illustrated above after foods, with recovery of PEF at the neutralization endpoint.[12]

A range of about 40 chemicals and chemical mixtures are used for testing at the AAC at the present time, some routinely, others when indicated. We do not test for pesticides, or routinely for food additives other than monosodium glutamate. This is not because they do not cause trouble. In the case of the additives it is partly because the large numbers used in food production would make such testing excessively time consuming and expensive but also because patients recover their tolerance more quickly if they are able to reduce chemical exposures substantially: for those for whom it is feasible, avoiding food additives is therefore part of the management. Testing with pesticides, and prophylactic use of vaccines containing them, would add to the load of these substances in the body even if they prevented symptoms: these substances were synthesized to interfere with body enzymes and it is probable that no dose is safe.

EVIDENCE OF THE EFFECTIVENESS OF ECUs

There have been no double-blind randomized controlled trials (DBRCT) comparing ECU treatment with either orthodox management or outpatient environmental management. This is for two main reasons. First, the 'blind' aspect of DBRCT methodology cannot be applied to managements which depend on the

patients' cooperation in altering their lifestyle. But crucially, the ECUs have all been private ventures and referral to them has usually required persistence on the part of the patient, and the availability of some source of funding (often NHS in the AAC): imposing randomization at this point would therefore be unacceptable, especially if one arm was to treatments the patient had already tried. A randomized trial would be possible if the randomization was applied *before referral*, and observer bias could be overcome by careful planning, with independent confirmation of changes in condition.

Patients admitted to an ECU have usually been ill for years (a median of >10 years[14]), and although the severity of symptoms will have been variable, the general trend has usually been downward. It is therefore valid to compare the condition on follow up of *groups* of these patients with pre-treatment condition, provided that the timescales are long enough (months/years). There can be less confidence in a comparison of this sort where one or two patients are concerned, except in the case of patients who improve in an ECU and maintain that improvement at home, even though they had previously failed to show improvement under consultants from several different specialties. Two patients with severe and disabling back pain of, respectively, 8 and 20 years' duration are an example. Both had had many previous referrals to physicians, neurologists, rheumatologists, psychiatrists and others, but had continued to deteriorate and were referred to the AAC as a last resort.[11] Both arrived in wheelchairs and were disabled by continuous severe pain but severity varied – on some days they were bed bound. On the standard regime of the AAC both were entirely pain free and moving normally within 10 days except when reacting to challenge with foods or chemicals – reactive pain was relieved and subsequently prevented by neutralization prophylaxis; both were well on discharge and had kept well and active when followed up, the last time over 5 years later.

Clinical audit of treatment

All the patients treated at the AAC have been subject to audit,[14] in three cohorts. The follow-up questionnaire, sent 6 months to $2\frac{1}{2}$ years later, asked the degree of life disruption caused by symptoms before admission and at follow up, whether the patients considered they were worse, the same or better (with degrees), and the frequency (0 to $++$) and severity ($+$ to $+++$) of each of 63 symptoms on admission and at follow up. Many of the patients had answered exactly similar questions about life disruption and symptoms at the time of admission and there was good correlation between these and the answers given retrospectively. Figure 68.4 is a pie chart showing marked reduction of life disruption at follow up. Figure 68.5 shows the range of symptoms on presentation and the decrease in the score of frequency/severity at follow up (combined scores for frequency and severity minus one, range 0–4), based on the 71 patients (81% of those mailed) who gave full symptom data in reply to the questionnaires sent out in 1990. The overall decreases in symptom score were highly significant for all the commoner symptoms, and for some of the less common symptoms such as palpitations and phlegm.

The published report compared the results attained by the AAC with those of the more severely affected patients (those requiring enzyme-potentiated densensitization (EPD)) of a Cambridge colleague (Dr S. Birtwistle). Results were very similar in the two series,[14] but she sent out her follow-up questionnaires

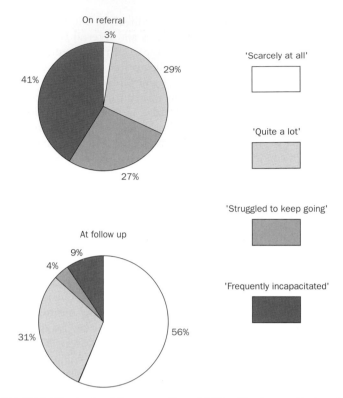

On referral

'Scarcely at all'

'Quite a lot'

'Struggled to keep going'

At follow up

'Frequently incapacitated'

Fig. 68.4 Pie charts of the proportion of AAC patients reporting each of the four degrees of life disruption on presentation and at follow up. (Reproduced from Maberly *et al.*[14] with permission.)

3–9 years after referral because the benefits of EPD in food reactions are much slower. In contrast, most of the improvement in AAC patients occurs during admission, i.e. within 3 weeks, but was investigated months later to assess long-term benefits.

Extensive analyses of the AAC data (which also involved independent replies to some questions from relatives) established both the validity and the reliability of the follow-up questionnaire.[14] Most patients reported multiple symptoms: at presentation the *median* number of symptoms in the worst category (F/S = 4) was 5 per patient and fell to 1 by follow up (*P* < 0.0001). This accurately reflects the multiplicity of symptoms in patients admitted to the AAC, greater than that for referred patients generally, since only the more severely affected (about one-fifth) are admitted, some as tertiary referrals from other environmental physicians.

Results in patients with asthma

Results during and after admission in a consecutive series of 19 asthmatic patients treated in the AAC have been reported.[13] All reacted to inhalant allergens. Ten reacted with bronchospasm after chemical challenge and all but one after food challenge. They were protected on discharge by neutralization vaccines, and on follow up all but two of those who replied to the questionnaire suffered less life disruption, with significant improvement in both the frequency and severity of chest and other symptoms, although taking less medication (*P* < 0.001).

Figure 68.6 shows the inpatient costs for a case of severe brittle asthma, a woman of 22 years with asthma from early childhood. For the last 3 years she had had repeated emergency admissions to hospital, often to intensive care, complicated by cardiac and respiratory arrests and fractured ribs, and had spent months living in the grounds of a hospital. She was unable to work or have any

social life. She was referred to the AAC and was well for 3 months after her first admission in 1990. Having been admitted on charity funds, she did not return when she deteriorated after a severe viral infection and had repeated conventional hospital admissions until she eventually came into the AAC for retitration of her specific prophylaxis in 1991. She then remained well except for one brief emergency admission with a chest infection. For the next 3 years she was able to work, living alone, cycling, swimming and having a full social life with minimal medication, until sudden death from anaphylaxis to an antibiotic. Only inpatient costs are shown in the figure: the cost of drugs, loss of earnings, continuous sickness benefit, repeated GP and hospital consultations and the estimated compensatory cost of the stress, severe suffering and lifestyle restriction of the earlier years should be added to arrive at the total costs for that period.

When 43 patients with rheumatoid arthritis were treated in ECUs,[10] there were significant improvements in functional activity and in objective assessments after a 6-day therapeutic fast; 40 patients no longer needed medication.

Rea[22] has reported results in a series of 10 patients with vasculitis. He also examined the cost benefit of investigation in an ECU for 10 patients with chronic intractable phlebitis,[25] comparing the outcome with that of 10 patients managed conventionally, during a 5-year follow-up period. The patients treated conventionally had a total of 41 episodes requiring hospital admission and ≥ 60 other episodes at a cost of $200 000: this contrasted with a total of two transient episodes costing $200 during the same period in the ECU group. The latter could walk without pain; control patients remained incapacitated.

EDUCATION AND RESEARCH

Interested health professionals are welcome to visit the AAC by arrangement, provided that they fulfil the strict odour criteria. ECUs provide what is probably the best introduction to the clinical practice of environmental medicine, since it is possible to observe the clearing of long-term symptoms within a period of days followed by the provocation of symptoms by some but not by other challenges. The AAC could be a valuable postgraduate training facility, but its potential is, at present, underexploited. Some medical students and nutrition or nursing students have been accepted for elective periods, including a medical student from Germany and one from Japan.

As a profession we should not accept serious medical conditions as *idiopathic* or *intrinsic* or *of unknown aetiology* without making every attempt to exclude the possibility that the condition is caused or exacerbated by reactions to foods or environmental factors, particularly for conditions which have increased in prevalence or severity over the last 50 years, as have virtually all the conditions which respond to environmental management. We should also be wary of accepting *psychological factors* as an aetiological explanation, since psychological symptoms are commonly provoked by challenge with foods and environmental factors in sensitive patients (Fig. 68.5 and King[9] and Anthony *et al.*[3]), and stress has well-documented effects on the immune system.

ECUs offer an unrivalled diagnostic facility for patients who can, and will, cooperate. They should be fully exploited. A successful investigation explains the aetiology of the problem and empowers patients to control their symptoms and understand those they choose not to prevent. At present the facility cannot

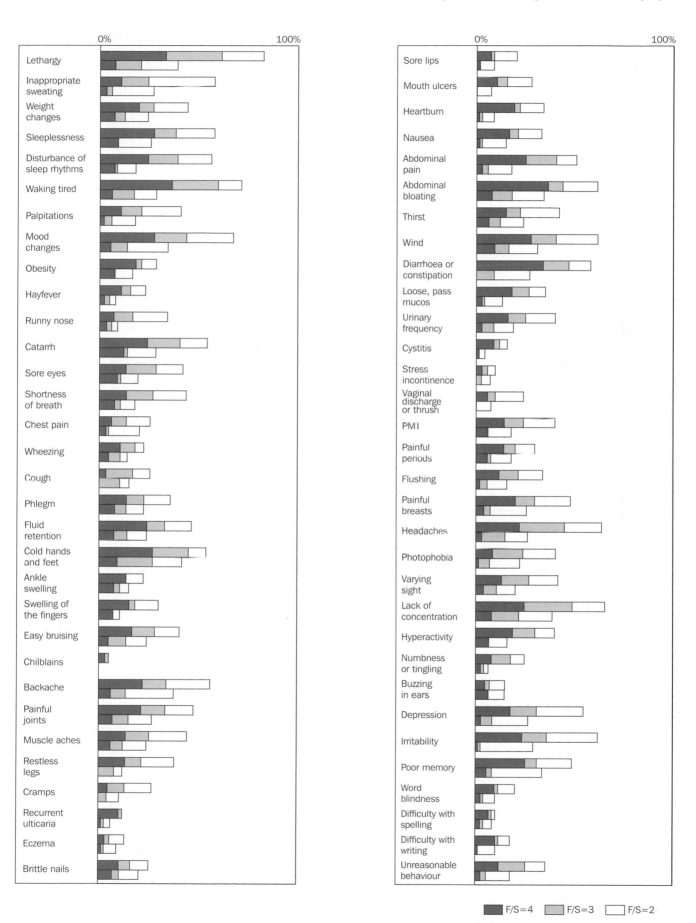

Fig. 68.5 Proportion of AAC patients reporting each symptom on presentation (upper bars) and at follow up (lower bars). (Reproduced from Maberly *et al.*[14] with permission.)

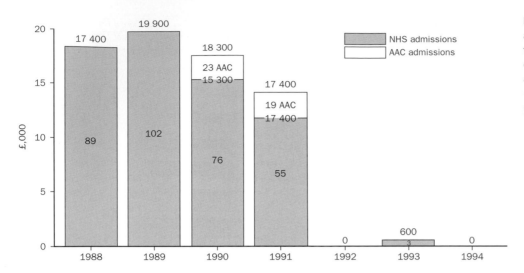

be extended to patients with severe psychiatric and behaviour problems because the AAC is not equipped to control transient severe and destructive exacerbations provoked by challenge. A physically and environmentally safe environment is needed to help to elucidate the aetiology of severe behaviour problems.

ECUs also make an essential contribution to research. The three main workshop reports[5,6,16] at a recent New Jersey symposium all deemed that valid research investigations of chemical sensitivity in humans required that the patients be admitted to an ECU.

Note

Since this chapter was written, the Airedale Allergy Centre has unfortunately been forced to close because the arrangements for funding of extra-contractual referrals in the National Health Service were changed. The incoming funding bodies were not confident about the funds at their disposal and refused (or delayed) approvals of funding for patients who had been referred, making it impossible to maintain the labour-intensive unit. Prior to that most patients had received NHS funding.

REFERENCES

1 Anthony HM, Maberly DJ. Time of onset of symptoms after food challenge. *J Nutr Med* 1991; 2: 121–30.

2 Anthony HM, Maberly DJ. Weight changes in chronically ill patients with evidence of multiple intolerance to foods, chemicals and inhalants. *J Nutr Med* 1991; 2: 131–41.

3 Anthony H, Birtwistle S, Eaton K, Maberly J. *Environmental Medicine in Clinical Practice.* BSAENM Publications, 1997; IBSN 0 9523397 2 2.

4 Atkins FM, Steinberg SS, Metcalfe DD. Evaluation of immediate adverse reactions to food in adult patients. 2. A detailed analysis of reaction patterns during challenge. *J Allergy Clin Immunol* 1985; 75: 356–63.

5 Bascom R, Meggs WJ, Frampton M *et al.* Working Group Report. Neurogenic inflammation: with additional discussion of central and perceptual integration of non-neurogenic inflammation. *Environmental Health Perspectives* 1997; 105(Suppl 2): 531–8.

6 Bell IR, Rossi J, Gilbert ME *et al.* Working Group Report. Testing the neural sensitisation and kindling hypothesis for illness from low levels of environmental chemicals. *Environmental Health Perspectives* 1997; 105(Suppl 2): 539–48.

7 Kaplan MS. The importance of appropriate challenges in diagnosing food sensitivity. *Clin Exp Allergy* 1994; 24: 291–3.

8 Katsunuma T, Iikura Y, Akasawa A *et al.* Wheat-dependent exercise-induced anaphylaxis: inhibition by sodium bicarbonate. *Ann Allergy* 1992; 68: 184–8.

9 King DS. Can allergic exposure provoke psychological symptoms? *Biological Psychiatry* 1981; 16: 3–17.

10 Kroker G, Stroud RM, Marshall R *et al.* Fasting and rheumatoid arthritis: a multicentre study. *Clin Ecol* 1984; 2: 137–44.

11 Maberly DJ, Anthony HM. A reversible back pain syndrome: report of two cases. *J Nutr Med* 1991; 2: 83–7.

12 Maberly DJ, Anthony HM. Asthma management in a 'clean' environment: 1. The effect of challenge with foods and chemicals on the peak flow rate. *J Nutr Med* 1992; 3; 215–30.

13 Maberly DJ, Anthony HM. Asthma management in a 'clean' environment: 2. Progress and outcome in a cohort of patients. *J Nutr Med* 1992; 3: 231–48.

14 Maberly DJ, Anthony HM, Birtwistle S. Polysymptomatic patients: a two-centre outcome audit study. *J Nutr Environ Med* 1996; 6: 7–32.

15 Mabray CR, Burditt ML, Martin TL *et al.* Treatment of common gynecologic–endocrinologic symptoms by allergy management procedures. *Obstet Gynecol* 1982; 59: 560–4.

16 Miller C, Ashford N, Doty R *et al.* Working Group Report. Empirical approaches for the investigation of toxicant-induced lack of tolerance. *Environmental Health Perspectives* 1997; 105(Suppl 2): 515–20.

17 Pelikan Z, Pelikan-Filipek M. Bronchial response to food ingestion challenge. *Ann Allergy* 1987; 58: 164–72.

18 Randolph T. *Human Ecology and Susceptibility to the Chemical Environment.* Charles C Thomas, Springfield, Ill, 1962.

19 Randolph TG. The Ecologic Unit. *Hospital Management* 1964; 97 March: 45–9; April: 46–8.

20 Randolph TG. Ecologic orientation in medicine; comprehensive environmental control in diagnosis and therapy. *Ann Allergy* 1965; 23: 7–22.

21 Randolph TG. *Environmental Medicine – Beginnings and Biographies of Clinical Ecology.* Clinical Ecology Publ., Colorado, 1987.

22 Rea WJ. Environmentally-triggered small vessel vasculitis. *Ann Allergy* 1977; 38: 245–51.

23 Rea WJ. Environmentally-triggered cardiac disease. *Ann Allergy* 1978; 40: 243–51.

24 Rea WJ. Chemical Sensitivity. Volume 4. Tools of Diagnosis and Methods of Treatment. Lewis Publishers, Boca Raton, 1997.

25 Rea WJ, Peters DW, Smiley RE *et al.* Recurrent environmentally-triggered thrombophlebitis: a five year follow-up. *Ann Allergy* 1981; 47: 338–44.

26 Rea WJ, Butler JR, Laseter JL *et al.* Pesticides and brain-function changes in a controlled environment. *Clin Ecol* 1984; 2: 145–50.

27 Rea WJ, Ross GH, Johnson AR *et al.* Confirmation of chemical sensitivity by means of double blind inhalant challenge of toxic volatile chemicals. *Clin Ecol* 1989; 6: 113–18.

28 Ross GH, Rea WJ, Johnson AR *et al.* Evidence for vitamin deficiencies in environmentally-sensitive patients. *Clin Ecol* 1989; 6: 60–6.

29 Wraith DG. Asthma and rhinitis. *Clin Immunol Allergy* 1982; 39: 349.

INTRODUCTION

Enzyme-potentiated desensitization (EPD) is a method of immunotherapy which offers several advantages. It is inherently safer than alternatives, few doses are needed, multiple allergies can be treated simultaneously and EPD is effective in different types of allergy including atopic, non-atopic and delayed-type hypersensitivity (DTH). EPD is based on a natural mechanism of immunostimulation by the enzyme β-glucuronidase (β-GL). Antigen-specific tolerance is achieved by using a precise low-dose formulation. Double-blind placebo-controlled (DBPC) trials have shown that EPD protects against immunoglobulin E (IgE)-mediated seasonal pollenosis, asthma due to house dust mite allergy and against non-atopic food hypersensitivity in children causing migraine or hyperactivity. The only side effects recorded were mild headaches, noticed in one trial.

An audit of all doses of EPD administered in the United States has been conducted by the American EPD Society. The 1998 data confirm safety and better than 70% efficacy in over 4500 patients who received three or more doses.

THE CLINICAL METHOD

EPD treatment consists of intradermal injections of 0.05 ml containing β-GL, cyclohexane-1,3 diol and allergens in precise low doses. Trials have shown that a single preseasonal injection is sufficient to provide protection from seasonal pollenosis although two injections are preferred in the first season. It is usually sufficient to give a single annual injection for 4–5 years to produce a long-term effect. For other conditions, more injections of EPD may be required. These are administered at intervals of not less than 8 weeks. The strength of the doses remains the same. When remission has been secured, the interval between injections is increased. Treatment is completed with two–three annual boosting doses. The average polysymptomatic non-atopic patient with multiple sensitivities completes treatment in less than 20 injections, although the best response may not develop until 8–10 doses have been given.

DEVELOPMENT OF THE EPD FORMULATION

During 1959, S. Popper attempted to dissolve nasal polyps using a commercially available preparation of mammalian hyaluronidase, which he injected into the inferior turbinates. This was not effective, but Popper noticed that some patients stopped excessive sneezing. He went on to give intranasal injections of hyaluronidase to patients while they were suffering from hay fever and found that a single injection sometimes cured the condition for 2 years. Popper's method remained dependent on the presence of allergen in the nose at the time of treatment.

Percutaneous allergen

McEwen[38] developed a technique for delivering hyaluronidase and allergen extracts through scarified skin which made it possible to control the dose of allergen accurately and to use non-inhalant allergens. Popper recognized batch variation in the immunological effect of the hyaluronidase he used but failed to identify the reason. McEwen showed that this was due to variable contamination of hyaluronidase with β-GL.[37]

Empirical use

From 1966, EPD was developed empirically. It became a useful clinical method long before advances in immunology provided the background necessary to begin to understand the mechanism. We now know of a variety of cytokines and adhesion molecules. Some are proposed as therapeutic agents but none except β-GL were first recognized because they produced a useful clinical effect even when impure.

Murine anaphylaxis
Sensitization with horse serum

During the early work the immunological effect of β-GL was not consistent from batch to batch and this led to a series of animal experiments, initially in guinea pigs and rats.[37] These models of immunotherapy were cumbersome. Murine pinnal anaphylaxis[17] proved a better investigative tool. Mice presensitized to horse serum were desensitized with a single very small dose of horse serum plus β-GL. One week later the effect of treatment was assessed by prick testing the ears with horse serum and measuring extravasation of intravenous pontamine sky blue dye.

Role of sugar contaminants

Using this technique it was found that the immunological effect of β-GL was controlled by the presence of sugar contaminants.[34] This action of the enzyme can be switched from hyposensitization to hypersensitization by changing the dose of glucose or other sugar, giving a characteristic W-shaped dose–response curve.[39] Two doses of sugar cause β-GL to stimulate hyposensitization. An intervening dose stimulates hypersensitization. A structure–function study revealed that control of the immune response to the enzyme depends on the presence of a simple chemical structure. Any substance bearing two hydroxyls separated by three carbons will reproduce the W-shaped dose–response of a sugar.[33,39] The most simple structure with the required activity is 1,3-propane diol. The substance which produces the characteristic W-shaped signature at the lowest concentrations is 1,3-cyclohexane diol.

Testing formulations for efficacy

It was possible to optimize the EPD formulation of allergen, enzyme and diol by testing variations 'blind' on groups of hay fever sufferers in winter. Intranasal grass pollen challenge 3 weeks after treatment revealed the effect of changing doses of the components in the formulation. The clinical relevance of the results

in mice was confirmed. The W-shaped dose–response curve for 1,3-cyclohexane diol is displaced 10-fold in man.[39] Further work with the same clinical protocol optimized the doses of protamine, used as a stabilizer of the enzyme,[40] and chondroitin sulphate, which prevents adsorption of the highly dilute allergens on to containers.

A UNIQUE OPPORTUNITY

This work was made possible in the early 1970s by the existence of the Hay Fever Clinic of the Wright–Fleming Institute, where up to 120 preselected patients were seen on winter afternoons for confirmation of their diagnosis and recommendation of treatment. Volunteers for the EPD trials were recruited and treated on the same day. They required a single visit for testing with intranasal grass pollen 3 weeks later. In March they each received a single preseasonal dose of EPD using a formulation known to be effective. Follow up in the autumn revealed that subjects who had been hypersensitized or hyposensitized in the previous winter were equally protected during the summer. Over 500 subjects took part in this work between 1970 and 1974.

It would now be difficult to construct similar clinical dose–response curves for a new complex therapeutic formulation. If a cytokine has important clinical activity only at a single, precise and ultra-low dose or requires clinical titration of an activator, the administrative, ethical and commercial pressures of present-day medicine will ensure that this remains undiscovered.

THE IMMUNOLOGICAL ROLE OF β-GLUCURONIDASE

β-GL appears to deliver a specific signal to the immune system. It is an active enzyme only at low pH. At neutral pH the enzyme functions as an adhesion molecule for T lymphocytes, causing adhesion to the extracellular matrix (ECM) and to keratinocytes.[20,27] This adhesion is reduced as the pH is lowered. The enzyme binds to the ECM and to keratinocytes in a saturable manner, suggesting that specific binding sites are involved.

Biology of β-glucuronidase

Large quantities of β-GL are normally present in the body. The enzyme is concerned with turnover of glycosaminoglycans (GAGs) such as dermatan and keratan sulphates and hyaluronic acid of the ECM. β-GL is also present in the lysosomes of polymorphs and macrophages, acting as enzyme in the acid milieu of digestive vacuoles. These cells extrude lysosomes when activated, so that a large quantity of β-GL enters the extracellular space during inflammation.

Other saccharolytic enzymes

These enzymes are also liberated by inflammation and free sugars are released from the polysaccharide ECM. These will give direction to the immunological effect of the enzyme, usually to increase immunity. Besides the β-GL reaching lymphocytes from elsewhere, naive CD4+ T lymphocytes synthesize β-GL *de novo* upon activation, while memory T cells store the enzyme and release it within minutes of activation.[20,27] The resting blood level of β-GL is 15–90 Fishman units/ml (Sigma test kit). This value is increased by inflammation or allergy: for comparison, an injection of EPD delivers 40 Fu.

Antigen presentation and 1,3-diol

Although our present knowledge goes some way to explain why β-GL might alter the appreciation of antigen by lymphocytes, we still do not know why a 1,3-diol should be able to determine the result of interaction between enzyme, antigen and receptor cell. The β-GL molecule is believed to exist as a homotetramer bearing four exposed enzyme clefts. Highly purified β-GL loses enzyme activity and specificity, gaining β-galacturonidase activity. β-GL activity and specificity is restored by propylene glycol (1,2-propane diol),[19,48] suggesting that association with a 1,2-diol brings about a configurational change at the enzymic sites. It seems that a different configuration, favoured by association with a 1,3-diol or a sugar, is important for immunological activity. A specific cell receptor may be involved.

LEUKOCYTE MIGRATION INHIBITION

The changes observed in these experiments were not antigen-specific, but they suggest that the mechanism by which β-GL provokes clinical hyposensitization may be by altering the behaviour of antigen-presenting cells (APCs) rather than lymphocytes. This would be consistent with the result of leukocyte migration inhibition experiments. The buffy coat leukocytes from patients with hay fever were studied and showed that cell migration was inhibited by low concentrations of grass pollen extract.[5] The experiment was repeated using leukocytes from cow's milk-sensitive patients suffering from eczema and found migration inhibition by highly dilute milk. When the patients had been desensitized by EPD, cow's milk no longer inhibited migration (J. Brostoff, pers comm).

In this experiment the migrating cells are chiefly monocytes and the milk antigen stimulates T lymphocytes to release macrophage inhibitory factor (MIF). The lymphocytes can respond to the milk antigen only when it is presented to them by APCs, which are chiefly macrophages, so this experiment illustrates two-way talk between APCs and lymphocytes. It now seems possible that EPD-induced tolerance may prevent the first part of this conversation.

TYPE 4 HYPERSENSITIVITY

EPD was discovered through its effect on clinical IgE-mediated type 1 allergy but the method has also proved to be effective for non-atopic allergy. The mechanism of this form of allergy (e.g. intrinsic asthma) is not yet understood but it may also depend on Th2 type CD4[+] T lymphocytes.[26,50]

The mechanism of conventional injection immunotherapy (SIT) is now better understood. A number of groups have shown that clinical desensitization is accompanied by a switch of allergen-sensitive T lymphocytes from the Th2 cytokine profile to Th1, which is characteristic of type 4 hypersensitivity (tuberculin type). If this interpretation is correct, SIT replaces type 1 hypersensitivity with type 4.[41] Allergists using EPD have gained the clinical impression that EPD may be used to downregulate type 4 contact hypersensitivities. If this is true it means that EPD and conventional immunotherapy produce different kinds of clinical tolerance.

Experimental contact dermatitis

An experimental model of type 4 contact allergy consists of sensitizing mice by painting their skin with 2,4-dinitrofluorobenzene (DNFB).[44] Three days later one ear is painted with DNFB and its thickness over the next 2 days is compared with the unpainted control ear. McEwen[36] studied mice which were allowed to recover completely after this procedure before being treated by EPD. They were injected with a small dose of the clinical formulation of β-GL plus 1,3-cyclohexane diol and an ultra-low dose of DNFB. Three weeks after this treatment, the mice were again challenged as before. Compared with control mice treated with a saline injection, the response of the EPD-treated group was reduced by approximately 50%. This is evidence that this form of immunotherapy can downregulate a pre-existing type 4 contact allergy.

CHANGES IN BLOOD CYTOKINES

Ippoliti *et al.*[28] have investigated the effect of EPD on blood cytokines. This group measured blood interleukins IL6 and IL10 in children who suffered from seasonal asthma due to grass pollen. The controls were normal children and the laboratory worked 'blind'. The experiment was conducted in early spring at the appropriate time for a therapeutic preseasonal dose of EPD. At this time the asthmatic children were not exposed to their allergen and were symptom-free. Nevertheless, compared with the controls, the pre-treatment blood levels of both cytokines were significantly raised and increased still further 24 h after the EPD injection. After 15 days the blood level of IL6 had fallen to the level in controls, but the elevation of IL10 persisted (Table 69.1).

Although IL10 is reported to favour differentiation of Th2 CD4[+] T lymphocytes, which might increase allergy, this cytokine has been shown to induce hapten-specific immune tolerance *in vivo*,[16] and to induce long-term antigen-specific CD4[+] T-cell anergy.[23] A possible mechanism is IL10-induced inhibition of B7 expression which has been demonstrated in human monocytes.[49] This provides a costimulus required for antigen presentation. When B7 is blocked, presentation leads to lymphocyte anergy.[21,45] The primary allogeneic T cell response to human epidermal Langerhans' cells is also inhibited by IL10.[25]

Cytokines and immunotherapy

In cultures of peripheral blood mononuclear cells (PBMCs) from patients desensitized to bee venom by SIT, Bellinghausen *et al.*[3]

Plasma IL6 and IL10 (ng/ml) in grass pollen-sensitive asthmatic and normal children before treatment, 24 h after EPD and 15 days later			
	Patients (n = 17)	**Controls (n = 17)**	**P**
IL6			
Baseline	17.08 ± 8.09	5.84 ± 2.15	< 0.002
24 hours	20.54 ± 12.37	6.89 ± 4.20	< 0.005
15 days	10.64 ± 6.29	9.10 ± 4.27	NS
IL10			
Baseline	112.46 ± 18.51	64.39 ± 10.15	< 0.005
24 hours	146.54 ± 26.31	53.65 ± 12.73	< 0.005
15 days	143.04 ± 12.57	66.87 ± 18.54	< 0.005

Table 69.1 Plasma IL6 and IL10 (ng/ml) in grass pollen-sensitive asthmatic and normal children before treatment, 24 h after EPD and 15 days later (from Ippoliti et al[28]).

have identified cells, previously thought to be anergic, which release IL10 in response to allergen. These authors suggest that the Th2 to Th1 shift alone cannot explain the clinical effect of SIT but the added contribution of IL10 secreting cells may be sufficient.

In their *in vitro* model, neutralization of IL10 restored proliferative responses to bee venom. IL10-producing regulatory CD4+ T cell clones designated Tr1 have also been shown to prevent colitis.[24]

EPD and IL10

EPD is the only form of immunotherapy which has been reported to increase circulating IL10. This will also reduce hypersensitivity responses in additional ways which are not antigen-specific. IL10 downregulates synthesis of many other cytokines and inhibits allergic inflammation,[25] 1,5-lipoxygenase[9] and prostaglandin H synthetase.[42]

The downregulation of IL6 may also be important. This is a proinflammatory cytokine and the raised pretreatment blood level in Ippoliti's subjects may have increased allergic responses in a nonspecific way.[28] This is another mechanism by which EPD may produce clinical improvement which is not antigen-specific.

The source of both the IL6 and IL10 induced by EPD is uproven. Keratinocytes may elaborate both,[10,47] but it seems unlikely that the small area of skin which is directly in contact with an EPD injection could be the only source of the IL10 measured in Ippoliti's experiments. The reduction in the IL6 blood level at 15 days must be due to an action of EPD at a distance from the injection.

THE RESPONSE TO INJECTION

The experiments described above show clearly that β-GL is immunologically active but do not explain the mechanism by which a single intradermal injection of EPD can affect the immune status of the whole body. The initial effect must be local, because the injected dose of β-GL will be submerged by the tissue level of the enzyme within a short distance of the site of injection. The blood glucose will also change the immunological effect of the enzyme. It seems likely that APCs in a small area of dermis are quickly programmed for antigen-specific tolerance and pass on this information after migration.

THE ROLE OF ANTIGEN

In vitro work has so far failed to demonstrate that β-GL can modify immunological responses in an antigen-specific way. Nevertheless, clinical experience shows that EPD changes sensitivity only to specific antigens which are included in the injection. In some cases this is not entirely true. First, crossreactivity between related allergens is more obvious when treating with EPD than during skin prick testing. Secondly, a large environmental exposure to allergen at the time of EPD may behave as part of the treatment (e.g. airborne grass pollen or a food).

Dose of antigen

The dose of antigen determines the outcome of an injection of EPD. A high dose (equivalent to allergen exposure which would provoke symptoms) may result in hypersensitization. Lower doses are necessary to achieve desensitization. For the treatment of rhinitis and asthma, the dose of inhalant allergen in an intradermal injection of EPD is similar to the dose delivered to the dermis by a diagnostic skin prick test. This is at least 10-fold less than a conventional diagnostic intradermal test. The dose of food allergens for EPD is 100-fold less than the dose of inhalants. In the treatment of atopic or non-atopic food allergy another ultra-low dose range may be used. This second optimum is 1 million-fold less than the first. Intermediate doses are ineffective. If repeated doses of EPD are required, the dose of allergen is unchanged.

EPD is not related to other 'low-dose' forms of immunotherapy. In the absence of β-GL the doses of allergen have no therapeutic effect. In their DBPC trial of EPD for Parietaria pollenosis, Astarita *et al.*[2] incorporated two control groups: the first group was treated with plain buffered saline, while the second group received the dose of allergen without β-GL. In the pollen season these control groups experienced almost identical symptoms.

Response to intradermal EPD

As might be expected, intradermal injections of allergen in doses equivalent to prick tests provoke wheal-and-flare skin responses. Astarita's group reported that their control injections of allergen without β-GL provoked intense itching and this group of controls could not be double blind. Injections of the full EPD formulation may elicit even larger wheal-and-flare responses, but there is no discomfort. Patients are unaware unless they see their response. This is not yet understood. The absence of discomfort and the single dose of EPD required for pollenosis have made it possible to arrange clinical trials in which treatment remains double blind in spite of the large skin responses.

Allergen doses in the ultra-low range do not usually produce significant skin responses. In his trials of EPD in childhood hyperactivity and migraine, Egger *et al.*[14,15] found that covering the injection site with sticking plaster was sufficient to obscure any differences between active and placebo injections.

SAFETY OF EPD

The low doses of allergen required for EPD mean that this treatment is exceptionally safe. The risk entailed in treating inhalant allergies is similar to skin prick testing. EPD can be used to treat allergies which would be unsafe to desensitize by other means. The observation that two narrow dose levels of antigen can be incorporated in EPD to produce hyposensitization while other doses may lead to hypersensitization emphasizes another safety aspect. EPD is essentially a method of immunostimulation. The increased responsiveness of T lymphocyte cultures to fresh APCs after incubation with β-GL also demonstrates this point.

The 1998 figures from the American database show that the clinical condition with the best response to EPD is repeated ear infection.[22] Of 245 patients with a history of repeated ear infections, 89% considered that this symptom was more than 50% improved. This confirms the clinical impression that EPD generally increases resistance to infection.

Increasing knowledge of immunological mechanisms has revealed a variety of signalling molecules and their T cell receptors in pathways which lead to allergy. Drugs or antibodies which disrupt one or more of these signals are presently considered to be potential therapeutic agents.[29] The problem with this approach is the lack of evidence that the pathways concerned have no protective function. The safety of any attempt to downregulate or divert the immune system in a way which is not antigen-specific must be proven over the human lifespan. EPD already has a long track record of safety. The first doses of an EPD formulation were given in 1966 and, by December 1970, 540 patients had been treated.

Patient selection

Although increased general immunity is desirable, it is theoretically possible for EPD to stimulate autoimmunity or unwanted hypersensitivity to unrecognized allergens which are significant for the patient. Experience shows that these risks are avoided by appropriate patient selection and management. EPD formulations have been used clinically since 1966, and approximately 300 000 doses have been given. The incidence of possible late side effects is low, and no consistent pattern has emerged, suggesting that most of the reported 'events' have been unconnected with EPD. A very small number of patients have been given injections of adrenaline (epinephrine) following doses of EPD. These patients did not suffer from IgE-mediated allergy and it seems doubtful that the reactions for which adrenaline was given were classical anaphylaxis.

The exception is a physician involved in the early development of EPD who had frequently inhaled unpurified β-GL powder over a number of years. He is sensitized to the purified product and developed a true IgE-mediated reaction after injection of EPD. This promptly responded to treatment.

MULTIPLE ALLERGENS

Since EPD appears to reinforce tolerance to agents which should not cause an immune response and does not elicit other immune responses to allergen such as increased blocking antibody, (Starr & Weinstock[46] and pers comm) it should not be harmful to include allergens to which a particular patient is not sensitive. In addition, allergens in the environment can contribute to the treatment in an uncontrolled way. It may be better to ensure that EPD contains optimal desensitizing doses of these allergens to override the environment. A third consideration is that a significant proportion of allergy sufferers who have not received immunotherapy start to react to new allergens as time passes. With this background it was decided to include mixed allergens in EPD injections, starting in 1970.

Increased sensitivity following EPD?

There has been no evidence of increased recruitment of new sensitivities among patients who have received mixed allergens. EPD was discontinued at St. Mary's Hospital in 1979. Approximately 600 patients with multiple allergies were booked for further treatment. EPD again became available 2 years later and, over time, approximately 300 of these patients relapsed and returned for further treatment. Since these patients had been diagnosed and started EPD before the treatment was withdrawn, the average time between diagnosis of the allergies and return for further doses of EPD was at least 5 years. Only 12 of the 300 patients reported that they had become sensitive to a new allergen. This extremely low incidence favours the hypothesis that administering mixed allergens in previous EPD treatments had protected against development of new allergies.

The 1998 WHO Position Paper on allergen-specific immunotherapy (SIT) lists 84 published DBPC trials of SIT which studied 27 different forms of vaccine.[4] Two successful trials used vaccine containing more than one allergen (cat and dog). All other trials studied vaccines containing extracts from a single source or mixtures of related allergens (grass pollens). SIT uses an escalating ladder of allergen doses and depends for success on a high final dose. Mixed allergens dilute one another, so that the final dose of each is reduced. Stability may also be reduced. In contrast, all the published DBPC trials of EPD for inhalant allergies (grass, Parietaria and olive pollens and house dust mite) were conducted with the same polyvalent mixed antigen which also contained dander and mould extracts. The totals of 117 actively treated subjects and 114 controls in these trials of a single immunotherapy product are equalled only by the 103 actively treated subjects included in trials of standardized alum-precipitated house dust mite vaccine listed in the WHO report. Similarly, in the published trials of EPD for food-sensitive migraine and attention deficit disorder (ADD), the same mixed food antigen was given to all subjects.

Single and multiple allergens

Experience with conventional immunotherapy has led to the belief that any form of polyvalent immunotherapy for allergy is bad practise. EPD has been considered unscientific for this reason. This criticism arises from a lack of understanding. The mechanism of EPD is not related to those of other methods of immunotherapy. The protocols for its correct use have been established since the 1970s and proven by DBPC trials and a large clinical audit.

Immunotherapy of ADHD

The efficacy of mixed antigens in EPD means that it is theoretically possible to desensitize 'blind', without extensive diagnostic tests to determine which allergens are important for the individual patient. In principle, this is not a satisfying approach but it may be necessary if patient compliance is a problem. This was demonstrated by Kaschnitz (pers comm). He used computer programs to assess a group of ADHD children who were subsequently given a 3-week diagnostic oligoantigenic diet to identify individuals in whom the ADD appeared to be due to dietary intolerances. After the diagnostic diet, all children returned to a full diet and their previous behaviour. No attempt was made to identify each child's specific allergies. A group of these children were given three doses of EPD at 2-month intervals. At the time of each treatment their diets were controlled for 1 week only. A second group was treated with methylphenidate (Ritalin) and a third group received psychotherapy. At the final assessment, children treated with EPD and the group using phenindamine performed equally well and significantly better than the children treated by psychotherapy.

CLINICAL STUDIES OF EPD

Five DBPC clinical trials of EPD for pollinosis have been published.[1,2,11,18,30] All studied the effect of single preseasonal injections of EPD or placebo. A sixth DBPC trial[6] observed the result of two doses of EPD or placebo in children suffering from asthma due to house dust mite sensitivity. All these trials showed that the active treatment gave statistically significant protection (Table 69.2).

A seventh DBPC trial[7] was a 2-year study of EPD (single-blind in the second year) in children suffering from rhinitis or asthma who were sensitized to pollens and/or dust mite. Greatest

Table 69.2 Trials of EPD for inhalant allergy.

					Trials of EPD for inhalant allergy		
Authors	**Allergens**	**DBPC**	**A**	**P**	**Symptoms (P)**	**Symptom-free days (P)**	**Use of drugs (P)**
Fell & Brostoff[18]	Grass	Yes	22	22	NS†	NS‡	<0.02
Di Stanislao et al.[11]	Grass	Yes	20	20	NS	< 0.005	<0.05
Longo et al.[30]	Grass	Yes	9	7	<0.001	<0.001	NS
Astarita et al.[2]	Parietaria Grass	Yes	10	10*	<0.001	—	—
Angelini et al.[1]	Parietaria Olive	Yes	11	10	0.001	<0.001	<0.001
Businco et al.[6]	Dust mite	Yes	10	10	<0.05	<0.01	<0.01
Caramia et al.[7]	Grass Dust mite	Yes	8 27	8 27	<0.001 <0.001	—	<0.001 <0.001

DBPC, double-blind placebo-controlled; A, active treatment, P, placebo. Total subjects: All DBPC studies of inhalant allergy: A, 117; P, 114.
* Excludes second control group treated with allergen alone who were not 'blind'.
† Unlimited intranasal steroid aerosol. All subjects titrated themselves to 'comfort'.
‡ Only 14-day observation period at peak of pollen season.

improvement was seen in the second year. These authors comment that if two injections of EPD were given each year for an appropriate period of time, asthma totally disappeared in all patients.

Fell & Brostoff[18] were interested in the cost-effectiveness of EPD. To demonstrate this, they gave a preseasonal injection of EPD or placebo and measured drug consumption during a 2-week period at the peak of the grass pollen season. Since intranasal steroid aerosol is highly effective and was allowed ad lib, the trial subjects took sufficient drug to achieve comfort and, not surprisingly, symptoms were similar in both groups. There were significant large differences in the consumption of steroid aerosol and antihistamines between the two groups. The authors concluded that EPD reduced drug consumption in the pollenosis season sufficiently to be cost-effective.

Di Stanislao et al.[11] allowed antihistamines ad lib, and the symptom scores of treated and control subjects were not significantly different. These authors studied their subjects for 12 weeks and found major differences in the number of days free of symptoms and drug consumption, except during the week of maximum pollen count. This is consistent with the hypothesis that EPD increases the threshold dose of allergen necessary to provoke symptoms but has less effect on the severity of symptoms once this threshold has been exceeded.

IgE CHANGES FOLLOWING EPD

Astarita et al.[2] studied EPD in patients sensitive to Parietaria pollen. The single preseasonal injection of EPD gave significant protection during the 3 months of high pollination. Compared with the baseline value in February, by June the Parietaria-specific IgE antibody had increased by 25.4% in the control group, ($P = 0.0002$). In the actively treated subjects the increase was 6%. By October this antibody was still 17.2% above the February value in the control group, but in the treated patients the

Parietaria-specific IgE had fallen to 6% below its spring value. Compared with the June value, this fall was significant ($P = 0.003$). EPD had downregulated the stimulation of specific IgE production which results from allergen exposure. Nevertheless, skin prick test responses remained unchanged in both groups of subjects.

These authors also studied CD3[+], CD4[+] and CD8[+] T lymphocytes in peripheral blood. In February the CD8[+] cell percentages of actively treated and placebo groups were 23.3% and 25.2%, respectively. By October the percentage of CD8[+] cells had risen to 28.3% in the treated group ($P = 0.033$) and fallen slightly to 23.8% in the placebo group. There were no significant changes in the CD3[+] or CD4[+] cells.

Astarita et al.[2] were the only authors to report any side effects of EPD during these trials. Mild headaches which started 24–48 h after the injection of active EPD and lasted about 2 days were experienced by 20% of subjects.

CONJUNCTIVAL TESTS

Businco et al.[6] studied the effect of EPD on children suffering from perennial asthma due to atopic sensitivity to *D. pteronyssinus*. Two injections of EPD or placebo with an interval of 8 weeks were given in November and January. Diary cards showed that during the follow-up period the number of days with asthma was reduced by 61% in the EPD-treated children *versus* the control group ($P < 0.01$). The number of days on which drugs were used for asthma was reduced by 71% ($P < 0.01$). The EPD injections in this trial produced no side effects apart from the initial skin responses.

Businco et al.[46] also studied the threshold concentration of *D. pteronyssinus* extract in the conjunctival test before and after EPD. In April the threshold concentration was 10-fold higher than before treatment in 7 out of 10 actively treated children *versus* 2 out of 10 in the control group ($P = 0.0349$).

NON-ATOPIC FOOD SENSITIVITY

At an early stage in our understanding of how to manage EPD for inflammatory bowel disease, McEwen conducted a single-blind controlled trial of EPD for ulcerative colitis which suggested that the treatment reduced the severity of the disease.[35] Lou has shown that attention deficit disorder with hyperactivity (ADHD) in children involves transient changes in the frontal cortex which closely resemble changes in a parietal lobe during an attack of migraine.[31,32] The two conditions often occur together and may have a similar mechanism. Trials have shown that the majority of children suffering from either of these conditions will improve while using a restricted oligoantigenic diagnostic diet. When excluded foods are reintroduced it is found that symptoms are provoked by specific foods and that different individuals are sensitive to different foods. This has been confirmed by double-blind dietary testing of harmful foods *versus* placebos.[8,12,13]

The mechanism by which specific foods can provoke migraine or alter behaviour has been unclear. Metabolic intolerance or a response to pharmacological agents in food has been proposed. An immunological response to food antigens is a third possibility.

The mechanism would be a form of non-atopic allergy, since IgE is not involved. Egger proposed that if children suffering from migraine or ADHD caused by diet responded to EPD, this would be strong evidence in favour of the non-atopic allergy hypothesis. Children with migraine or ADHD were selected for Egger's trials if they had a proven sensitivity either to foods which are essential for health or to an unacceptable number of foods. They were instructed to avoid foods which caused symptoms while three doses of EPD containing mixed food antigens were administered at 8–12 week intervals. Reintroduction of previously harmful foods began 3 weeks after the third injection. A single new food was introduced each week. In a DBPC trial in children suffering from ADHD,[14] 16 children were assessed following active EPD. All proved to be tolerant *versus* only 4 out of 18 in the placebo-treated group ($P < 0.001$). There were no side effects.

Using the same protocol, Egger's team conducted a parallel trial of EPD in children suffering from food sensitivity expressed as migraine.[15] Among 18 children receiving the active desensitization, 16 became tolerant. Of 15 placebo-treated children, 6 became tolerant ($P < 0.01$). Again, there were no side effects of EPD. These trials favour the hypothesis that non-atopic food allergy is a cause of childhood ADHD and migraine and that EPD is effective treatment.

AUDIT *VERSUS* FORMAL TRIALS

Formal controlled trials are not necessarily a good guide to the performance of a therapeutic modality in a normal clinical setting. A formal trial is designed to use a treatment in the most effective way. The subjects are selected because they are likely to comply with the protocol and according to narrow clinical criteria to give the best chance of response. As an example, all published trials of conventional immunotherapy have dealt with vaccines containing a single allergen and subjects in whom tolerance to this allergen would be easy to recognize.

This must be compared with the normal clinical practice of the majority of conventional allergists. Immunotherapy vaccines containing multiple allergens are widely prescribed to treat clinical sensitivities which have been diagnosed only by skin testing. Moreover, patients are not usually refused treatment if they do not appear likely to comply with instructions. Audit is essential to assess the impact of any form of therapy in the disadvantaged setting of a routine clinic but, until now, no form of allergy therapy has been studied in this way.

AUDIT OF EPD

In the United States the use of EPD has been controlled by Institutional Review Board (IRB) approval, which is enforced and inspected by the Food and Drugs Administration (FDA). It has been illegal to administer EPD unless a report signed by the patient is returned to an independent database set up by the American EPD Society. This has provided a unique opportunity for 'total audit' of EPD in the United States. More than 60 physicians have contributed. The settings for this work range from university hospitals to private clinics.

At the time of writing, the database figures for 1998 are provisional.[22] A total of 4636 patients who have received three or more doses of EPD have been assessed. Reasons for earlier dropout are recorded. The report forms filled by patients instructed that 'good' meant greater than 50% improvement in symptoms. Among patients treated for seasonal rhinitis or asthma, over 75% scored the result of their treatment as 'good' or better. For perennial rhinitis or asthma, the figure was over 70%. There are records of 434 patients treated for IgE-mediated immediate-type food allergies. Of these, over 70% considered the result 'good' or better and only 11% found the treatment unhelpful.

'Multiple chemical sensitivity' (MCS) is a term used to describe an important group of patients who react to inhaled aromatic fumes, formaldehyde, tobacco smoke, motor exhaust, etc. These sensitivities are untreatable by conventional immunotherapy but may respond to EPD if a suitable representative antigen mixture is used. The American EPD Society audit contains records of 2533 patients suffering from MCS of whom 65% consider themselves more than 50% improved by EPD, while 14% consider the treatment a failure.

Overall, for all indications, 9% of patients considered that the treatment has failed following their most recent dose of EPD. These preliminary figures do not discriminate between patients who have completed treatment and others who have received only three injections of EPD and will require further doses.

Audit of such a large number of treatments permits a useful estimate of safety. No patient required emergency treatment after a dose of EPD. This is particularly significant for the large number of patients suffering from IgE-mediated food allergy.

'EVIDENCE-BASED MEDICINE'

This term has become the watchword of those who wish to improve the standard of medicine and also of those responsible for conserving health finance. The results of the DBPC trials of EPD, supported by the data from clinical audit, are sufficient to propose that EPD is evidence-based medicine. No other method of immunotherapy has been subjected to similar scrutiny when used outside a strict academic setting.

REFERENCES

1 Angelini G, Curatoli G, D'Argento V, Vena GA. Pollinosi: una nuova metodica di immunoterapia. *Med J Surg Med* 1993; 4: 237–92.

2 Astarita C, Scala G, Sproviero S, Franzese A. A double-blind placebo-controlled trial of enzyme potentiated desensitisation in the treatment of pollenosis. *J Invest Allergol Clin Immunol* 1996; 6(4): 248–55.

3 Bellinghausen I, Metz G, Enk AH *et al*. Insect venom immunotherapy induces interleukin-10 production and a Th2 to Th1 shift, and changes surface marker expression in venom-allergic subjects. *Eur J Immunol* 1997; 27: 1131–9.

4 Bousquet J, Lockey RF, Malling HJ (eds). WHO Position Paper. Allergen immunotherapy: therapeutic vaccines for allergic diseases. *Allergy* 1998; 53 (44 Suppl): 1–42.

5 Brostoff J. Migration inhibition studies in human disease. *Proc Roy Soc Med* 1970; 63: 905–6.

6 Businco L, Cantani A, Monteleone MA, Ragno V, Lucenti P. Enzyme potentiated desensitisation in children with asthma and mite allergy: a double-blind study. *J Invest Allergol Clin Immunol* 1996; 6(4): 270–6.

7 Caramia G, Franceschini F, Cimarelli ZA, Ciucchi MS, Gagliardini R, Ruffini E. The efficacy of EPD, a new immunotherapy, in the treatment of allergic diseases in children. *Allergie et Immunologie* 1996; 28(9): 308–10.

8 Carter CM, Urbanowicz M, Hemsley R *et al*. Effects of a few food diet in attention deficit disorder. *Arch Dis Childhood* 1993; 69: 564–8.

9 Deleuran B, Iversen J, Kristensen M *et al*. Interleukins and 1,5-lipoxygenase activity in rheumatoid arthritis: *In vitro* anti-inflammatory effects by interleukin-4 and interleukin-10 but not by interleukin-1 receptor antagonist protein. *Br J Rheumatol* 1994; 33: 520–5.

10 Derocq JM. Interleukin-13 stimulates interleukin-6 production by human keratinocytes: similarity with interleukin-4. *FEBS Letter* 1994; 343: 32–6.

11 Di Stanislao C, Di Berardino L, Bianchi I, Bologna G. A double-blind, placebo-controlled study of preventive immunotherapy with EPD in the treatment of seasonal allergic disease. *Allergie et Immunologie* 1997; 30(2): 39–42.

12 Egger J, Carter CM, Wilson J, Turner MW, Soothill JF. Is migraine food allergy? *Lancet* 1983; 2: 865–9.

13 Egger J, Carter CM, Graham PJ, Gumley D, Soothill JF. Controlled trial of oligoantigenic treatment in the hyperkinetic syndrome. *Lancet* 1985; 1: 540–5.

14 Egger J, Stolla A, McEwen LM. Controlled trial of hyposensitisation in children with food-induced hyperkinetic syndrome. *Lancet* 1992; 339: 1150–3.

15 Egger J, Stolla A, McEwen LM. Hyposensibilisierung bei nahrungsmittelinduzierter migraine. In: *Aktuelle Neuropadiatrie* (Lischka A, Bernett G, eds). Ciba-Geigy Verlag, Wehr, 1992: 287–91.

16 Enk AH, Saloga J, Becker D, Madzadah M, Knop J. Introduction of hapten-specific tolerance by interleukin-10 *in vivo*. *J Exper Med* 1994; 179: 1517–27.

17 Feinberg JG. Pinnal anaphylaxis. An additional anaphylactic site. *Nature, Lond*. 1961; 191: 721.

18 Fell P, Brostoff J. A single-dose desensitisation for summer hay fever. Results of a double-blind study. *Eur J Clin Pharmacol* 1990; 38: 77–9.

19 Fishman WH, Green S. Enzymic catalysis of glucuronyl transfer. *J Biol Chem* 1957; 225: 435–52.

20 Gilat D, Hershkovitz R, Goldkorn I *et al*. Molecular behaviour adapts to context: heparanase functions as an extracellular matrix-degrading enzyme or as a T-cell adhesion molecule depending on local pH. *J Exper Med* 1995; 181: 1929–34.

21 Gimmi CD, Freeman GJ, Gribbe JG, Gray G, Nadler LM. Human T-cell clonal anergy is induced by antigen presentation in the absence of B7 costimulation. *Proc Nat Acad Sci* 1993; 90: 6586–90.

22 Great Lakes College of Clinical Medicine. Investigational Review Board Project Report, WA Shrader, chief investigator. 1998.

23 Groux H, de Bigler M, de Vries JE, Roncarolo MG. Interleukin 10 induces a long-term antigen-specific anergic state in human CD4+ T-cells. *J Exper Med* 1996; 184: 19–29.

24 Groux H, O'Garra A, Bigler M *et al*. A CD4+ T-cell subset inhibits antigen-specific T-cell responses and prevents colitis. *Nature* 1997; 389: 737.

25 Grunig G, Corry DB, Leach MW *et al*. Interleukin-10 is a natural suppressor of cytokine production and inflammation in a murine model of allergic bronchopulmonary aspergillosis. *J Exper Med* 1997; 185: 1089–99.

26 Haselden M, Larche M, Barata T, Robinson DS, Kay B. Asthma provoked by T-cell epitopes: a novel method of studying IgE-independent isolated late asthmatic reactions. *British Society for Allergy and Clinical Immunology*; Annual meeting: Abstract 11, 1997.

27 Hershkovitz R, Marikovsky M, Gilat D, Lider O. Keratinocyte-associated chemokines and enzymatically quiescent heparanase induce the binding of resting CD4+ T-cells. *J Invest Dermatol* 1996; 106(2): 243–8.

28 Ippoliti F, Ragno V, Del Nero A, McEwen LM, McEwen HC, Businco L. Effect of preseasonal enzyme potentiated desensitisation (EPD) on plasma IL-6 and IL-10 of grass pollen-sensitive asthmatic children. *Allergie et Immunologie* 1997; 29(5): 120, 123–5.

29 Le Gros G, Erb K, Harris N, Holloway J, McCoy K, Ronchese F. Immunoregulatory networks in asthma. *Clin Exper Allergy* 1998; 28: 92–6.

30 Longo G, Poli F, Bertoli G. Efficacia clinica di un nuovo trattamento iposensibilizzante, EPD (Enzime potentiated desensitisation) nella terapia della pollinosi. *Riforma Med* 1992; 107: 171–6.

31 Lou HC, Hendriksen L, Bruhn P. Focal cerebral hypoperfusion in children with dysphasia and/or attention deficit disorder. *Arch Neurol* 1984; 41: 825–9.

32 Lou HC, Henriksen L, Bruhn P, Børner H, Neilsen JB. Striatal dysfunction in attention deficit and hyperkinetic disorder. *Arch Neurol* 1989; 46: 48–52.

33 McEwen LM. Effects of sugars and diols on enzyme potentiated hyposensitisation. *J Physiol* 1972; 230: 65–66P.

34 McEwen LM. Enzyme potentiated hyposensitisation II. Effects of glucose, glucosamine, N-acetylamino-sugars and gelatin on the ability of β-glucuronidase to block the anamnestic response to antigen in mice. *Ann Allergy* 1973; 31: 79–83.

35 McEwen LM. A double-blind controlled trial of enzyme potentiated hyposensitisation for the treatment of ulcerative colitis. *Clin Ecology* 1987; 5: 47–51.

36 McEwen SM. MSc thesis, London University, 1998.

37 McEwen LM, Starr MS. Enzyme potentiated hyposensitisation 1. The effect of pre-treatment with β-glucuronidase, hyaluronidase and antigen on anaphylactic sensitivity of guinea pigs, rats and mice. *Int Arch Allergy* 1972; 42: 152–8.

38 McEwen LM, Ganderton MA, Wilson CWM, Black JHD. Hyaluronidase in the treatment of allergy. *Brit Med J* 1967; 2: 507–8.

39 McEwen LM, Nicholson M, Kitchen I, White S. Enzyme potentiated hyposensitisation III, Control by sugars and diols of the immunological effect of β-glucuronidase in mice and patients with hay fever. *Ann Allergy* 1973; 31: 543–50.

40 McEwen LM, Nicholson M, Kitchen I, O'Gorman J, White S. Enzyme potentiated hyposensitisation IV, Effect of protamine on the immunological behaviour of β-glucuronidase in mice and patients with hay fever. *Ann Allergy* 1975; 34: 290–5.

41 Mavroleon G. Restoration of cytokine imbalance by immunotherapy. *Clin Exp Allergy* 1998; 28: 917–20.

42 Niiro H, Otsuka T, Kuga S *et al*. Interleukin-10 inhibits prostaglandin E2 production by lipopolysaccharide-stimulated monocytes. *Int Immunol* 1994; 6: 661–4.

43 Peuget-Navarro J, Moulon C, Caux C, Dalbiez-Gauthier C, Banchereau J, Schmitt D. Interleukin-10 inhibits the primary allogeneic T-cell response to human epidermal Langerhans cells. *Eur J Immunol* 1994; 24: 884–91.

44 Phenuphak P, Moorhead JW, Claman HN. Tolerance and contact sensitivity to DNFB. 1. *In vivo* detection by ear swelling and correlation with *in vitro* cell stimulation. *J Immunol* 1974; 112(1): 115–23.

45 Robinson DS. T-cell costimulation: a potential therapeutic target in asthma. *Clin Exp Allergy* 1998; 28: 788–90.

46 Starr MS, Weinstock M. Studies in pollen allergy 3. *Int Arch Allergy Appl Immunol* 1970; 38: 514–21.

47 Ullriche SE. Mechanism involved in the systemic suppression of antigen presenting cell function by U.V. irradiation: keratinocyte-derived interleukin-10 modulates antigen-presenting cell function of splenic adherent cells. *J Immunol* 1994; 152: 3410–16.

48 Wakabayashi M, Fishman WH. The comparative ability of β-glucuronidase preparations (liver, *Eschericha coil*, *Helix pomatia* and *Patella vulgata*) to hydrolyse certain steroid glucosiduronic acids. *J Biol Chem* 1961; 236: 996.

49 Willems F, Marchant A, Delville JP *et al*. Interleukin-10 inhibits B7 and intercellular adhesion molecule-1 expression on human monocytes. *Eur J Immunol* 1994; 24: 1007–9.

50 Ying S, Humber M, Barkans J *et al*. Expression of IL-4 and IL-5 mRNA and protein product by CD4+ and CD8+ T-cells, eosinophils and mast cells in bronchial biopsies obtained from atopic and non-atopic (intrinsic) asthmatics. *J Immunol* 1997; 158: 3539–44.

INTRODUCTION

In general, food hypersensitivity is a transient phenomenon in early childhood, but in many atopic subjects immediate-type food allergy often is the first evidence of a genetic predisposition towards the development of atopic disease, predicting later-appearing allergic manifestations in the respiratory tract.[15,29] In such atopic children, food allergens (egg, nuts, peanuts and milk) dominate as sensitizing agents during the first 2–3 years of life. Differences in disappearance rate depend on the allergen and on individual factors in the person subject to the allergy. Young children with food allergy seem to have a more than twofold higher chance of outgrowing their food allergy than school children.[7,22] The likelihood of outgrowing a food allergy also depends on the allergen involved. Thus, most children with cow's milk allergy tolerate at least small amounts of cow's milk before 3 years of age. Egg allergy usually subsides before 7 years of age, while allergy to fish, soy and nuts tends to remain for a considerably longer time.[17,22,62]

When contemplating allergy preventive measures, the mostly good prognosis of the food allergy should be remembered, both as it relates to cost-effectiveness and when critically assessing the outcome of various preventive measures. As food allergy is often but the first step in the 'atopic march' and infants with an IgE-mediated food allergy run a high risk of developing respiratory allergies such as asthma and rhinoconjunctivitis later during child-

hood, a holistic approach to allergy prevention in infants and young children is important. In this chapter, I discuss pre- and postnatal sensitization to food allergens, predictive markers of possible use for the identification of at-risk infants, the possible protective role of breast feeding as well as the outcome of previous studies on primary and secondary prevention, mainly as they relate to food allergy. Finally, some possible future directions for general allergy prevention are indicated.

PRENATAL SENSITIZATION

During fetal life there is a close immunological interaction between the mother and her offspring, through the placenta. Relatively little is known about the exchange of immunological information however or the significance of this interaction. Recent studies indicate that this may occur already during fetal life as T cells of neonates may respond to food and inhalant allergens.[39,53,65] It is not known how this is related to maternal immunity or whether these immune responses are a normal part of the maturation of immunity.

Verified food sensitization resulting in immunoglobulin E (IgE) antibody formation *in utero* is uncommon.[9,36,47] On the other hand, several prospective studies have demonstrated that elevated IgE levels in cord blood are associated with an increased risk for allergic disease, indicating the possibility that factors encountered in fetal life could influence the likelihood for allergy (summarized in

Kjellman).[36] The possibility that maternal immunity may be an important environmental factor influencing the risk for allergic manifestations in her child is further strengthened by reports that drugs administered to women during pregnancy may have some immune regulatory activities. Observations include progesterone and the β-adrenergic receptor-blocking agent, metoprolol.[5]

Maternal diet during pregnancy

These observations have raised the question whether maternal food intake during pregnancy could affect the incidence of allergy in the offspring. In one randomized study of high allergy risk pregnancies, all products containing cow's milk and egg were avoided during the last trimester of pregnancy, but not after birth. The avoidance diet did not influence the development of IgE antibodies to foods in the children, nor the incidence or prevalence of food allergy and atopic disease up to 5 years of age.[18–20,40]

In another study high amounts of milk and egg were given during the last trimester based on the hypothesis that this would induce tolerance. This resulted in increased maternal serum IgG antibodies to milk and egg, but there was no effect on the development of allergy/atopic disease during early childhood.[40,41] Consequently, maternal dietary manipulation during pregnancy is not warranted. Such practice may even be harmful, as nutrition may be suboptimal unless the maternal diet is carefully monitored, preferably by a dietician.[18]

It has been argued that allergen avoidance should be instituted earlier in pregnancy as fetal T cell responses may appear before 20 weeks of gestation. These immune responses are however just as likely to be beneficial as potentially harmful and should not be taken as reason for instituting dietary manipulation during pregnancy. The conclusion of those well-designed and controlled studies in which a manipulation of the maternal diet during pregnancy was assessed is that a hypoallergenic diet is not warranted, particularly since it may impede an optimal nutrition during pregnancy.

POSTNATAL SENSITIZATION

The season of birth seems to be important not only for sensitization to inhalant allergens like pollens, house dust mites and pets, but also for foods. Thus, in a Dutch study the highest risk for egg and cow's milk sensitization was found in babies born during November and January.[1] Similar observations have recently been reported from Sweden.[48] Reasons for a seasonal effect on sensitization to foods are not known.

Supplementary feeds

Neonates appear to be particularly prone to food sensitization. As a consequence, even occasional cow's milk formula feeds should be avoided at the maternity ward. If supplementary feeding of babies is at all necessary, then only glucose water or an extensively hydrolysed, truly hypoallergenic formula should be given as substitute until the breast milk amounts are sufficient. On the other hand, in one study cow's milk formula given repeatedly and in large amounts in the maternity ward before breast milk was available was associated with a reduced risk for allergic disease in infants with a family history of allergy.[42] A follow-up investigation, when the children were 4–6 years of age, however, revealed no significant remaining effect.[43] Therefore, in the absence of supporting evidence from a randomized and blindly evaluated study,

intentional early introduction of highly allergenic foods must be regarded as experimental and should be avoided.

Enteromammary circulation

It has been established that food antigens eaten by the mother are present in human milk. As a consequence, food sensitization may occur via antigen present in breast milk.[13,24,33] This could explain why many infants manifest allergic symptoms when a certain food is given for the first time.

Early weaning and atopy

Introduction of cow's milk or solid foods into the diet of infants before 4–6 months of age has been shown to significantly increase the risk for atopic dermatitis and milk sensitization.[23] In another study, late introduction of all allergenic foods, in addition to breast feeding for 6 months or more, delayed the onset of food allergy and atopic eczema.[57] These findings were supported by a study reporting that the intake of four or more solid foods before 4 months of age significantly increased early developing atopic dermatitis and gave a nearly threefold increase in the occurrence of chronic and recurrent atopic dermatitis up to the age of 10 years.[21] In a well-designed Finnish study, however, it was reported that children with introduction of fish and citrus fruit after 12 months of age, had almost the same frequency of food allergy at 3 years of age as control children who started eating such food items between 3 and 6 months of age.[59]

Identification of at-risk individuals

Preventive programmes could either be generally recommended or be directed towards certain risk populations who would conceivably benefit from the measures. For economic and ethical reasons the latter procedure would be preferable. As propensity for atopic disease appears to be associated with various immunological abnormalities in early infancy, the allergy predictive capacity of several immunological tests have been assessed (Table 70.1). Although they generally show an association with subsequent atopic manifestations, the tests are too nonspecific, costly and/or complicated for clinical use (summarized in Kjellman *et al.*[38]). Thus, there are currently no predictive markers that would be useful for screening in the general population. A

Markers of atopic disease of possible use for the identification of at-risk infants who will develop allergic disease			
Marker	**Sensitivity**	**Specificity**	**Diagnostic accuracy**
SIgE	Low	High	Poor
IgE antibodies to	Low	High	Poor
Family history	High	Low	Poor
Phosphodiesterase	Low	Low	Poor
Eosinophils	Low	Low	Poor
Cytokines	?	?	?
SIgE, secretory immunoglobulin E.			

Table 70.1 Markers of atopic disease of possible use for the identification of at-risk infants who will develop allergic disease.

carefully obtained family history of allergy among the members of the immediate family, and the determination of secretory IgE (SIgE) levels in cord blood and early infancy, are the most commonly recommended procedures to identify allergy risk babies. None of these procedures are useful for general screening, however, due to poor sensitivity. In a large prospective study comprising 1700 newborn infants who were followed up to 11 years of age, less than 30% of those that developed allergic disease during the follow-up period, could have been identified.[15]

BREAST FEEDING

Breast feeding has many advantages over formula feeding, including providing an optimal nutrition for the baby, low cost and nearness between the baby and the mother. Furthermore, breast milk contains components from the mother's humoral and cellular immune defence and protects the baby against infections in the respiratory and gastrointestinal tracts.[16,32,55] Undoubtedly, it is the best infant food, at least for the first 6 months of life.

Human milk has also been recommended for the prevention of food allergy and other atopic disease, especially in infants with a high genetic propensity for development of allergy and atopic disease.[4] Already in 1936 infants fed cow's milk were reported to have a seven times higher incidence of atopic eczema than breast-fed infants.[26] Such large differences have not been confirmed since and several more recent studies have failed to demonstrate a clear benefit from exclusive breast feeding. This may depend on the present use of less allergenic heat-treated milk-based formula instead of natural cow's milk. It is also possible that unknown environmental factors have such a strong impact on the development of allergy as to obscure a modest protective effect of breast feeding.

Breast feeding, otitis media and asthma

Saarinen reported a reduced incidence of atopic symptoms and otitis media in infants fed breast milk for at least 6 months with no supplementary food before 6 months of age, as compared to a control group following routine feeding recommendations.[57] A very recent prospective study with a follow-up period up to 17 years by the same author indicated that the protective effects of breast feeding are particularly obvious for respiratory manifestations.[58] This study did not, however, control for a number of potentially confounding variables. For example, it is known that breast feeding for more than a few weeks is, in many Western industrialized societies, associated with a high level of education, less maternal smoking, postponed introduction of foreign foods and several other socioeconomic conditions. There is still no general agreement regarding an allergy preventive effect of breast feeding, as in many studies a protective effect was not confirmed.[3,4]

Breast feeding and allergy prevention

There are several possible explanations for the outcome of the various studies in which the protective effects of breast feeding were studied. It is thus possible that breast feeding is protective only in infants with a genetic propensity to allergy rather than in the general population. It is also conceivable that the effects on allergy are indirect: e.g. by protecting against infection, the incidence of allergy would be reduced. As a protection against allergy was demonstrated more clearly in earlier studies, it is possible that

Suggested design of studies intended to study the efficacy of primary and secondary prevention of food allergy
Prospective design
Adequate sample size (statistician and/or epidemiologist should be consulted in advance). Low numbers result in poor statistical power and handling of data, making conclusions and recommendations invalid
Study populations should be clearly defined whether they are selected from the general population or comprise genetically susceptible infants
Randomization, since self-selection infers bias
Several arms included, testing components of intervention
Feasible and reasonably simple programmes should be employed to avoid high drop-out rate or hidden non-compliance and to be useful in clinical routine if successful
Definitions of disease and allergy should be stated in advance and be identical in multi-centre trials. Well-defined inclusion and exclusion criteria
Good measurements of exposure
Objective parameters should be employed to measure outcome. All known and possible confounders should be included. Accuracy of tests and questionnaires should be evaluated
Truly blinded evaluation and not merely a double-blind design
Careful supervision of compliance to programme
Drop-outs should be accounted for
Follow-up period long enough to allow disease to develop

Table 70.2 Suggested design of studies intended to study the efficacy of primary and secondary prevention of food allergy.

unknown environmental triggers of allergy of more recent origin exert a strong influence and thus would obscure a modest protective effect of breast feeding. Furthermore, very few studies have fulfilled the criteria of a well-designed study to assess the role of breast feeding in allergy prevention (Table 70.2).

A reduced incidence of respiratory infections in breast-fed infants may also possibly be associated with less wheezing later in life. It seems reasonable to conclude from all these studies that if there is an allergy preventive effect of breast feeding it is marginal.

Protective effect of breast feeding against asthma and food allergy

How can this be explained? Low allergenicity is a less-likely explanation, since it is well established in experimental studies that extremely low amounts of antigens in the picogram range are sensitizing, often even more so than higher doses.[2,34] As discussed in a previous section, it is also well established that human milk contains various antigens from foods eaten by the mother and that sensitization to food is common in young infants, also during the period of exclusive breast feeding.[13,24,33]

Secretory IgA

Factors present in human milk that influence the immune system of the infant, including SIgA production and cellular immunity may be important for the enhancement of active immunity and tolerance in the neonate.[16,54,55] Human milk also contains low levels of IgE antibodies, metachromatically staining cells and eosinophils.[64] The possible role of these components is unknown.

Protection from allergy by maternal antibodies

The composition of the breast milk varies not only over time but also among mothers, and there are large individual variations in the composition of human milk from an immunological point of view. It has been suggested that the maternal antibody levels against, for example, cow's milk proteins would offer some protection against cow's milk allergy in the babies.[44] However, this was not confirmed in a larger, well-conducted study.[18,20,40] Recently, a prospective study of children who were followed from birth up to 8 years of age lended support to the suggestion that high levels of antibodies against foods may have a protective role against food allergy.[35]

Breast milk lipids

The composition of lipids in breast milk has also been suggested to affect any possible protective effects of breast milk against allergy. It has for many years been suggested, although never conclusively confirmed, that atopic disease, particularly eczema, is associated with a disturbed metabolism of the essential fatty acids linoleic (LA) and α-linolenic (LnA) acid and their long-chain metabolites of the n-6 and n-3 series.[10,66]

Differences in fatty acid composition (PUFA)

It has also been observed in some but not all studies that the fatty acid composition of breast milk differs in nursing mothers of healthy babies and infants with atopic dermatitis. We have recently confirmed such differences and that the composition of milk from atopic and non-atopic mothers differs.[67] Thus, the normal decrease in long-chain polyunsaturated fatty acids (PUFA) and concomitant increase in LA and LnA occurred more rapidly in atopic mothers, and the relationships between the levels of individual fatty acids differ in milk from atopic and non-atopic mothers. Furthermore, differences in the composition of the milk appeared to be related to the development of atopic dermatitis in the infants, independent of maternal allergy.

Maternal diet: allergens in breast milk

Allergens present in breast milk are regarded as important sensitizing agents. A maternal elimination diet during the first 3 months of lactation (complete avoidance of all cow's milk, egg and fish) reduced the occurrence of early food sensitization and food allergic symptoms.[28] Atopic eczema was significantly less common up to 6 months of age. When eczema developed it was significantly less severe in the infants of mothers on elimination diet compared with the control group. Only highly devoted mothers were included and the conclusion was that mothers who want to make special efforts to delay the onset of allergy could be recommended a strict elimination diet during lactation, provided they are supported and their dietary intake is surveyed by a dietician. A follow up, at 4 years, revealed a lower cumulative prevalence and period prevalence of atopic dermatitis in the diet group compared with the control group, but there was no effect on respiratory allergy.[63] The results are interesting but need to be confirmed in a truly randomized and blindly evaluated study.

In conclusion, the role of breast feeding for the protection against food allergy and other allergies is controversial. The results of previous studies showing a low incidence of food allergy in breast-fed infants are mostly not substantiated in more recent studies. It is possible that unknown environmental factors that have caused the large increase in the prevalence of allergy over the past 30–40 years overcome a modest protective effect of breast feeding that could previously be discerned.

FORMULA FOODS

Infant formulas for allergy protection

Highly hydrolysed casein preparations like Nutramigen, Pregestimil and Alimentum only rarely elicit anaphylactic reactions in milk-allergic subjects.[6,60] They have also been employed in the prevention of allergy in babies with a family history of allergy. A highly hydrolysed whey product (Profylac) has also passed the tests and can be recommended for preventive purposes, as the efficacy appears to be similar to that of Nutramigen.[27] All these extensively hydrolysed infant formulas appear to be associated with a reduced occurrence of atopic eczema in infancy but they seem to have no effect on the prevalence of asthma.[8,11,46]

Extensively hydrolysed casein preparations fulfilling the criteria for hypoallergenicity (Table 70.3) are currently recommended not only for children with proven cow's milk hypersensitivity but also sometimes as a possible means for the prevention of cow's milk allergy in high allergy risk infants when there is need for a substitute for breast milk.[8,11,14]

In contrast, claims that partial hydrolysates would be useful in allergy prevention have not been substantiated in carefully designed studies, meeting at least most of the criteria outlined in Table 70.2.

Maternal dietary avoidance and reduction of atopic eczema

The effect of maternal avoidance of highly allergenic foods (cow's milk, egg and peanuts) during late pregnancy and throughout lactation, combined with late introduction of milk, egg, fish, citrus fruits and peanuts into the infant's diet, was studied in a randomized study in 288 allergy-risk families.[68,69] A highly hydrolysed casein formula (Nutramigen) was given when needed as substitute for breast milk. The control group had an unrestricted diet. A threefold reduction in food-associated atopic dermatitis, hives and/or gastrointestinal disease was seen in the first 12 months in the prophylaxis group and the cumulative prevalence of food allergy was reduced by a factor of three at 12 and 24 months of age. The effects were only temporary as no differences were seen at 4 and 7 years with regard to current food allergy, atopic

Requirements for a 'hypoallergenic formula'
1. Nutritionally adequate and safe
2. Providing a feeling of satisfaction to the baby
3. Acceptable regarding taste and smell
4. Acceptable regarding price and availability
5. Hypoallergenic and virtually non-immunogenic, as confirmed by the following tests:
a. Immunization tests in animals
b. Crossed radioimmunoelectrophoresis, immunoblot technique or more sensitive assay with serum samples from subjects allergic to the raw material
c. Skin prick tests or histamine release from cells in children allergic to the raw material of the formula
d. Oral provocation tests in children allergic to the raw material

Table 70.3 Requirements for a 'hypoallergenic formula'.

dermatitis, allergic rhinitis, asthma, lung function and food or aeroallergen sensitization. Many practical problems were encountered during the study period and the conclusion was that the effects of food restrictions were limited to the first year of life and to dermatitis.

Hydrolysed milk formulas

Due to high costs and poor taste of highly hydrolysed milk-based products, less-hydrolysed products based on various cow's milk proteins have been launched. Although the allergenicity of the products is reduced compared with regular cow's milk formulas, they still contain 1000 times more of the major allergen β-lactoglobulin than the extensively hydrolysed products,[11] and severe reactions have been noted in children who were fed a partially hydrolysed whey protein formula.[8,50,56] The product contains low but considerable amounts of β-lactoglobulin. Since we know from animal experiments that low doses of allergen may be particularly sensitizing while high doses tend to induce tolerance,[2,34] these hydrolysates cannot be recommended for preventive purposes. New products should be subject to proper evaluation in randomized, blindly evaluated and controlled studies performed by independent scientists, focusing on high allergy-risk infants. They should be compared with those of the best available hypoallergenic formula and with a normal cow's milk formula as 'placebo'.

Extensive hydrolysis and allergy prevention

In a recent study the allergy-preventive capacity of an extensively and partially hydrolysed formula given after weaning were compared in 155 infants with a family history of allergy. No cow's milk was given during the first 9 months of life and no egg and fish up to 12 months of age. The extensively hydrolysed formula was associated with less eczema and other allergy up to 18 months of age than either the partial hydrolysate or a regular infant formula, thus confirming that formulas intended for allergy prevention need to be extensively hydrolysed in order to possess a low allergenicity.[51]

Soy formulas

Soy formula has been recommended for many years as a possible low allergenic alternative to cow's milk formula based on animal experiments indicating that sensitization is less often induced by soy than by cow's milk.[52] Soy sensitization is frequently seen in cow's milk hypersensitive subjects, however, although many of them tolerate soy, as judged from provocation tests.[25] In one study, no allergy preventive effect was seen when soy formula was given as compared with cow's milk formula at weaning in babies of two atopic parents.[37] Thus, the possible allergy preventive effect of soy formulas remains an open question. Since soy allergy tends to be more prolonged than cow's milk allergy, and it seems to be more difficult for soy allergic subjects to avoid soy completely than it is for cow's milk allergic subjects to avoid milk, soy formula is currently not recommended for preventive purposes in high-risk babies.[8]

Dietary and environmental measures in allergy prevention

Hide *et al.* assessed the effects of a complex protocol including dietary and environmental measures in a randomized study including 120 high allergy risk babies.[30] The intervention group received a hydrolysed soy formula, in addition to breast milk from mothers strictly avoiding egg, cow's milk, wheat and nuts. The babies avoided cow's milk up to 9 months of age, and they got wheat

from 10 months and egg from 11 months of age. The intervention group also slept on polyvinyl-covered mattresses and an acaricide was applied to carpets and upholstered furniture to reduce dust mite exposure. The control group had standard feeding recommendations and no environmental measures were suggested. At 12 months of age, the intervention group had less allergic problems, e.g. eczema and asthma, compared with the control group. At 2 years of age, the children in the intervention group still had a lower prevalence of allergy, and positive skin prick tests (SPT) were less common than in the control group. This was true not only for SPT to house dust mites but also for other allergens. There was a non-significant trend towards lower prevalence of food intolerance, eczema and asthma in the intervention group at 2 years of age. At 4 years, albeit the prevalence of sensitization was still lower in the intervention group, the presence of respiratory allergic manifestations were similar in the two groups. Even if a modest allergy preventive effect were to be confirmed in other studies, the feasibility and cost-effectiveness of this protocol is doubtful in the general population.

PREVENTIVE MEASURES

General recommendations

Allergy preventive measures have so far almost exclusively been recommended and tested in babies with a high risk for allergy, i.e. babies with a bilateral family history of allergy or a unilateral family history combined with a high serum IgE concentration in cord blood. As discussed above, a valid family history is not easily obtained, and neonatal IgE determination and other tests are not ideal for allergy risk screening due to low sensitivity.[36]

Maternal smoking

The effect of passive exposure to tobacco smoke is a well-established risk factor for respiratory allergies. Furthermore, maternal smoking during pregnancy is a major health problem. It is associated with numerous risks for the fetus, including growth retardation, perinatal complications and childhood allergy. Hence, a non-smoking environment for all children should be encouraged. Although there are no studies of the possible impact of environmental tobacco smoke exposure on food allergy, food allergic children run a high risk for subsequently developing manifestations of respiratory allergy and should therefore be subject to preventive measures.

Promotion of breast feeding

Breast feeding should be promoted. The WHO recommendation of breast feeding for at least 6 months, if feasible, may possible be advantageous also in the context of allergy prevention. Breast milk is from an immunological point of view characterized by its anti-inflammatory properties. SIgA antibodies do not activate complement and do prevent microorganisms from adhering to the mucosa. The cytokine profile is mainly of low inflammatory activity, e.g. with high levels of interleukin 10 (IL10) and tumour necrosis factor α (TNFα) and low levels of interferon γ (IFNγ).

To effectively promote breast feeding, the entire family, including the father, should be involved and motivated. In a maternity ward meeting the criteria for a 'baby friendly hospital' only glucose water should be given to a healthy infant if extra fluid is at all required. Formula should only be given on prescription from the attending paediatrician. If formula is deemed to be necessary, then a truly hypoallergenic formula should be used until it has been decided whether the mother is going to breast feed her baby or not.

Education of medical personnel, teachers, social welfare personnel and others regarding allergy and atopic disease should be improved to make life easier for subjects with allergic problems and, hopefully, to reduce the risk for development of allergy and atopic disease in the population.

Prevention in genetically susceptible infants

High allergy risk families (Table 70.4) should have access to information on available preventive measures (Table 70.5). Preventive measures should be put in perspective, however, and the families must be aware of the limited effects of dietary manipulations. This delay may make it well worth doing the efforts, however.

Mothers-to-be should avoid foods they do not tolerate but there is no evidence that eliminating certain allergenic foods would reduce the risk for allergy in their babies.

After birth, breast feeding should be encouraged and a safe alternative – i.e. a truly hypoallergenic formula – could be recommended. Partially hydrolysed infant formulas, although often aggressively marketed, should not be considered for allergy prevention.

Breast feeding should be recommended for the first 6 months, if possible without introducing any additional food. Introduction of egg, fish, citrus fruits, nuts and peanuts should be avoided for the first 12 months of life. New food items should be introduced one at a time with at least weekly intervals. By this procedure any sensitivity is more easily recognized.

Indications for considering special allergy preventive measures
1. Verified allergy/atopic disease in both parents or one parent and a sibling
2. Elevated cord blood IgE, i.e. >0.5 kU/l
3. Sensitization to any allergen during infancy
4. Motivated family

Table 70.4 Indications for considering special allergy preventive measures.

Recommendations for families of infants with a high risk for allergy and atopic disease
During pregnancy
• No smoking
• Promote breast feeding; instructions and information to both parents
After birth
• No smoking
• No cow's milk formula feeds in maternity wards, not even occasionally at night. Promote breast feeding for at least 4–6 months. Instructions and information to both parents
• Avoid other foods before 4 months of age
• Highly allergenic foods (egg, fish, nuts, peanuts) introduced only after 1 year of age

Table 70.5 Recommendations for families of infants with a high risk for allergy and atopic disease. Dietary restrictions should always be supported by a dietician.

Risks associated with allergy preventive measures
1. Malnutrition due to difficulty to include all necessary nutrients in many foods
2. High costs for the family and society
3. Anxiety in the family and overprotection of the child
4. Disturbed family interaction due to interference with daily life
5. Social isolation of the family as meals may be outside the home
6. Disappointment when symptoms develop despite the preventive measures
7. Poor compliance (e.g. intermittent cow's milk formula intake) is probably worse than regular intake

Table 70.6 Risks associated with allergy preventive measures.

No elimination diet to the mother should be recommended unless the family is highly motivated. The dietary intake of mother and child must be supervised and family members supported through the whole period of preventive measures. Otherwise, there is a risk for negative effects on the well-being and economy of the family (Table 70.6).

POSSIBLE FUTURE DIRECTIONS

Research should focus on immune mechanisms, the importance of adjuvant factors for sensitization and development of tolerance. Well-conducted randomized and blindly evaluated trials in large enough numbers of high allergy risk infants should compare the various allergy programmes, including the effect of complete avoidance of allergenic foods and adjuvants for sensitization in comparison with early continuous exposure to high doses of food allergens to settle the best way to prevent the development of allergy and atopic disease.

The possible role of the intestinal microbial flora for the maturation of the immune system in infants and for the development of tolerance against foods has very recently received attention. It is known that the microbial flora drives immunity.[31] Probiotic strains of lactobacilli are of particular interest in this respect. It has been shown that intestinal microbial flora differ in infants in Sweden with a high incidence of atopic disease and Estonia with a low incidence.[61] In the latter infants lactobacilli and eubacteria were more commonly encountered and the counts were higher than in the Swedish infants. In contrast, *Clostridium difficile* was demonstrated in one-third of the Swedish infants but not in the Estonian babies. Similar differences exist between allergic and non-allergic children at 2 years. Very recently, a Finnish placebo-controlled study demonstrated that the administration of a *Lactobacillus* strain reduced the clinical symptoms in infants with atopic dermatitis.[45] A prospective study to assess the possible role of lactobacilli in the primary prevention of food allergy in infants is currently being carried out.

Concluding remarks

Food allergy in infancy and early childhood is often the first manifestation of atopic disease. Thus, although the prognosis with regard to the food allergy is usually good, other allergic diseases in the respiratory tract are common some years later. There are currently very few simple and well-documented allergy preventive measures. One of them is strict avoidance of exposure to tobacco smoke. Other reasonable measures include promotion of exclusive breast feeding, preferably for 6 months. Only hypoallergic infant formulas may be considered for primary prevention, while various partially hydrolysed preparations and soy formulas are not recommended for this purpose.

REFERENCES

1 Aalberse RC, Nieuwenhuys EJ, Hey M, Stapel SO. 'Horoscope effect' not only for seasonal but also for non-seasonal allergens. *Clin Exp Allergy* 1992; 22: 1003–6.

2 Ahlstedt S, Björkstén B. Specific antibody responses in rats and mice after daily immunization without adjuvant. *Int Arch Allergy Appl Immunol* 1983; 71: 293–9.

3 Björkstén B. Does breast feeding prevent the development of allergy? *Immunol Today* 1983; 4: 215–17.

4 Björkstén B, Kjellman N-IM. Does breast-feeding prevent food allergy? *Allergy Proc* 1991; 12: 233–7.

5 Björkstén B, Finnström O, Wichman K. Intrauterine exposure to the beta-adrenergic receptor-blocking agent metoprolol and allergy. *Int Arch Allergy Appl Immunol* 1988; 87: 59–62.

6 Bock SA. Probable allergic reaction to casein hydrolysate. *J Allergy Clin Immunol* 1989; 84: 272.

7 Bock SS. The natural history of food sensitivity. *J Allergy Clin Immunol* 1982; 69: 173–7.

8 Bruijnzeel-Koomen C, Ortolani C, Aas K *et al*. Position paper: adverse reactions to food. *Allergy* 1995; 50: 623–35.

9 Businco L, Marchetti F, Pellegrini G, Perlini R. Predictive value of cord blood IgE levels in 'at risk' newborn babies and influence of type of feeding. *Clin Allergy* 1983; 13: 503–8.

10 Businco L, Ioppi M, Morse NL, Nisini R, Wright S. Breast milk from atopic mothers of children with newly developed atopic eczema has low levels of long chain polyunsaturated fatty acids. *J Allergy Clin Immunol* 1993; 91: 1134–9.

11 Businco L, Dreborg S, Einersson R, *et al*. ESPACI Position Paper: hydrolysed cow's milk formulae. Allergenicity and use for treatment and prevention. *Pediatr Allergy Immunol* 1993; 4: 101–11.

12 Businco L, Lucenti P, Arcese G, Ziruolo G, Cantani A. Immunogenicity of so-called hypoallergenic formula in at-risk babies: two case reports. *Clin Exp Allergy* 1994; 24: 42–5.

13 Cavagni G, Paganelli R, Caffarelli C *et al*. Passage of food antigens into circulation of breast-fed infants with atopic dermatitis. *Ann Allergy* 1988; 61: 361–5.

14 Committee on Nutrition of the American Academy of Pediatrics. Hypoallergenic formulas. *Pediatrics* 1989; 83: 1068–9.

15 Croner S, Kjellman N-IM. Development of atopic disease in relation to family history and cord blood IgE levels. Eleven-year follow-up in 1654 children. *Pediatr Allergy Immunol* 1990; 1: 14–20.

16 Duchén K, Björkstén B. Sensitization via the breast milk. In: *Immunology of Milk and the Neonate* (Mestecky, J ed). New York, Plenum Press, 1991: 427–36.

17 Esteban MM, Pascual C, Madero R, Diaz Pena JM, Ojeda JA. Natural history of immediate food allergy in children. In: *Proceedings of the First Latin Food Allergy Workshop* (Busino L, Ruggieri F, eds). Fisons SpA, Rome, 1985: 27–30.

18 Fälth-Magnusson K, Kjellman N-IM. Development of atopic disease in babies whose mothers were on exclusion diet during pregnancy – a randomized study. *J Allergy Clin Immunol* 1987; 80: 968–75.

19 Fälth-Magnusson K, Kjellman N-IM. Allergy prevention by maternal elimination diet during late pregnancy – a 5-year follow-up of a randomized study. *J Allergy Clin Immunol* 1992; 89: 709–13.

20 Fälth-Magnusson K, Kjellman N-IM, Magnusson K. Antibodies IgG, IgA and IgM to food antigens during the first 18 months of life in relation to feeding and atopic disease. *J Allergy Clin Immunol* 1988; 81: 868–75.

21 Fergusson D, Horwood L, Shannon F. Early solid feeding and recurrent childhood eczema, a 10-year longitudinal study. *Pediatrics* 1990; 86: 541–6.

22 Ford PK, Taylor B. Natural history of egg hypersensitivity. *Arch Dis Child* 1982; 57: 649–52.

23 Forsyth J, Ogston S, Clark A, Florey C, Howie P. Relation between early introduction of solid food to infants and their weight and illnesses during the first two years of life. *Br Med J* 1993; 306: 1572–6.

24 Gerrard J. Allergy in breast fed babies to ingredients in breast milk. *Ann Allergy* 1979; 42: 69–71.

25 Giampietro P, Ragno V, Daniele S, Cantani A, Ferrara M, Businco L. Soy hypersensitivity in children with food allergy. *Ann Allergy* 1992; 69: 143–6.

26 Grulee C, Sanford H. The influence of breast and artificial feeding on infantile eczema. *J Pediatr* 1936; 9: 223–5.

27 Halken S, Høst A, Hansen L, Østerballe O. Preventive effect of feeding high-risk infants a casein hydrolysate formula or an ultrafiltrated whey hydrolysate formula. A prospective, randomized, comparative clinical study. *Pediatr Allergy Immunol* 1993; 4: 173–81.

28 Hattevig G, Kjellman B, Sigurs N, Björkstén B, Kjellman N-IM. Effect of maternal avoidance of eggs, cow's milk and fish during lactation upon allergic manifestations in infants. *Clin Exp Allergy* 1989; 19: 27–32.

29 Hattevig G, Kjellman B, Björkstén B. Appearance of IgE antibodies to ingested and inhaled allergens during first 12 years of life in atopic and non-atopic children. *Pediatr Allergy Immunol* 1993; 4: 182–6.

30 Hide DW, Matthews S, Matthews L *et al*. Effect of allergen avoidance in infancy on allergic manifestations at age two years. *J Allergy Clin Immunol* 1994; 93: 842–6.

31 Holt PG. Environmental factors and primary T-cell sensitisation to inhalant allergens in infancy: reappraisal of the role of infections and air pollution. *Pediatr Allergy Immunol* 1995; 6: 1–10.

32 Howie PW. Protective effect of breast feeding against infection. *Brit Med J* 1990; 300: 11–16.

33 Jakobsson I, Lindberg T, Benediktsson B, Hansson B. Dietary bovine betalactoglobulin is transferred to human milk. *Acta Paediatr Scand* 1985; 74: 342–5.

34 Jarrett E, Hall E. The development of IgE-suppressive immuno-competence in young animals: influence of exposure to antigen in the presence and absence of maternal immunity. *Immunology* 1984; 53: 365–73.

35 Jenmalm MG, Björkstén B. Development of the immune system in atopic children. *Ped Allergy Immunol* 1998; 9 (suppl 11): 5–12.

36 Kjellman N-IM. IgE in neonates is not suitable for general allergy risk screening. *Pediatric Allergy Immunol* 1994; 5: 1–4.

37 Kjellman N-IM, Johansson S. Soy versus cow's milk in infants with a biparental history of atopic disease: development of atopic disease and immunoglobulins from birth to 4 years of age. *Clin Allergy* 1979; 9: 347–58.

38 Kjellman N-IM, Croner S, Fälth Magnusson K, Oderam H, Björkstén B. Prediction of allergy in infancy. *Allergy Proc* 1991; 12: 245–9.

39 Kondo N, Kobayashi Y, Shinoda S *et al*. Cord blood lymphocyte responses to food antigens for the prediction of allergic disorders. *Arch Dis Child* 1992; 67: 1003–7.

40 Lilja G, Dannaeus A, Fälth-Magnusson K *et al*. Immune response of the atopic woman and foetus; effects of high- and low-dose food allergen intake during late pregnancy. *Clin Allergy* 1988; 18: 131–42.

41 Lilja G, Dannaeus A, Foucard T, Graff-Lonnevig V, Johansson S, Öman H. Effects of maternal diet during late pregnancy and lactation on the development of atopic diseases in infants up to eighteen months of age – *in vivo* results. *Clin Exp Allergy* 1989; 19: 473–9.

42 Lindfors A, Enocksson E. Development of atopic disease after early administration of cow milk formula. *Allergy* 1988; 43: 11–16.

43 Lindfors A, Danielsson L, Enocksson E, Johansson S, Westin S. Allergic symptoms up to 4–6 years of age in children given cow milk neonatally. A prospective study. *Allergy* 1992; 47: 207–11.

44 Machtinger S, Moss R. Cow's milk allergy in breast-fed infants: the role of allergen and maternal secretory IgA antibody. *J Allergy Clin Immunol* 1986; 77: 341–7.

45 Majamaa H, Isolauri E. Probiotics: a novel approach in the management of food allergy. *J Allergy Clin Immunol* 1997; 99: 179–85.

46 Mallet E, Henocq A. Long-term prevention of allergic diseases by using protein hydrolysate formula in at-risk infants. *J Pediatr* 1992; 121: S95–S100.

47 Michel FB, Bousquet J, Greiller P, Robinet-Levy M, Coulomb Y. Comparison of cord blood immunoglobulin E concentrations and maternal allergy for the prediction of atopic disease in infancy. *J Allergy Clin Immunol* 1980; 65: 422–30.

48 Nilsson L, Björkstén B, Hattevig G, Kjellman B, Sigurs N, Kjellman N-IM. Season of birth as predictor of atopic manifestations. *Arch Disease Child* 1997; 76: 341–4.

49 Oldaeus G, Björkstén B, Einarsson R, Kjellman N-IM. Antigenicity and allergenicity of cow milk hydrolysates intended for infant feeding. *Pediatr Allergy Immunol* 1991; 4: 156–64.

50 Oldaeus G, Bradley CK, Björkstén B, Kjellman N-IM. Allergenicity screening of 'hypoallergenic' milk-based formulas. *J Allergy Clin Immunol* 1992; 90: 133–5.

51 Oldaeus G, Anjou K, Björkstén B, Moran JR, Kjellman N-IM. Extensively and partially hydrolysed infant formulas for allergy prophylaxis. *Arch Dis Child* 1997; 77: 4–10.

52 Piacentini G, Benedetti M, Spezia E, Boner A, Bellanti J. Anaphylactic sensitizing power of selected infant formulas. *Ann Allergy* 1991; 67: 400–2.

53 Piccini M-P, Mecacci F, Sampognaro S *et al.* Aeroallergen sensitization can occur during fetal life. *Int Arch Allergy Appl Immunol* 1993; 102: 301–3.

54 Pittard W, Bill K. Immunoregulation by breast milk cells. *Cell Immunol* 1979; 42: 437–41.

55 Prentice A. Breast feeding increases concentrations of IgA in infants' urine. *Arch Dis Child* 1987; 62: 792–5.

56 Ragno V, Giampietro P, Bruno G, Businco L. Allergenicity of milk protein hydrolysate formulae in children with cow's milk allergy. *Eur J Pediatr* 1993; 152: 760–2.

57 Saarinen UM. Prophylaxis for atopic disease: role of infant feeding. *Clin Rev Allergy* 1984; 2: 151–67.

58 Saarinen UL. Breastfeeding as prophylaxis against atopic disease: prospective follow-up study until 17 years old. *Lancet* 1995; 346: 1065–9.

59 Saarinen U, Kajosaari M. Does dietary elimination in infancy prevent or only postpone a food allergy? *Lancet* 1980; i: 166–7.

60 Saylor JD, Bahna SL. Anaphylaxis to casein hydrolysate formula. *J Pediatr* 1991; 118: 71–4.

61 Sepp E, Julge K, Vasar M, Naaber P, Björkstén B, Mikelsaar M. Intestinal microflora of Estonian and Swedish infants. *Acta Paediatr* 1997; 86: 956–61.

62 Sigurs N, Hildebrand H, Hultquist C *et al.* Sensitization in childhood atopic disease identified by Phadebas RAST, serum IgE and Phadiatop. *Pediatr Allergy Immunol* 1990; 1: 74–8.

63 Sigurs N, Hattevig G, Kjellman B. Maternal avoidance of eggs, cow's milk and fish during lactation: Effect on allergic manifestations, skin-prick tests and specific IgE antibodies in children at age 4 years. *Pediatrics* 1992; 89: 735–9.

64 Vassella C, Hjälle L, Björkstén B. Basophils and eosinophils in human milk in relation to maternal allergy. *Pediatr Allergy Immunol* 1992; 3: 184–9.

65 Warner J, Miles E, Jones A, Warner J. Is deficiency of interferon gamma production by allergen triggered cord blood cells a predictor of atopic eczema? *Clin Exper Allergy* 1994; 24: 423–30.

66 Wright S. Essential fatty acids and atopic dermatitis. *Pediatr Allergy Immunol* 1991; 2(suppl 1): 23–30.

67 Yu G, Duchén K, Björkstén B. Fatty acid composition in colostrum and mature milk from non-atopic and atopic mothers during the first 6 months of lactation. *Acta Paeditr* 1998; 87: 729–36.

68 Zeiger R, Heller S. The development and prediction of atopy in high risk children: follow-up at age seven years in a prospective randomized study of combined maternal and infant food allergen avoidance. *J Allergy Clin Immunol* 1995; 95: 1179–90.

69 Zeiger RS, Heller S, Mellon MH, Halsey JF, Hamburger RN, Sampson HA. Genetic and environmental factors affecting the development of atopy through age 4 in children of atopic parents: a prospective randomized study of food allergen avoidance. *Pediatr Allergy Immunol* 1992; 3: 110–27.

Index

The suffix 'f' refers to figures.
The suffix 't' refers to tables.